THE 5 MINUTE CLINICAL CONSULT

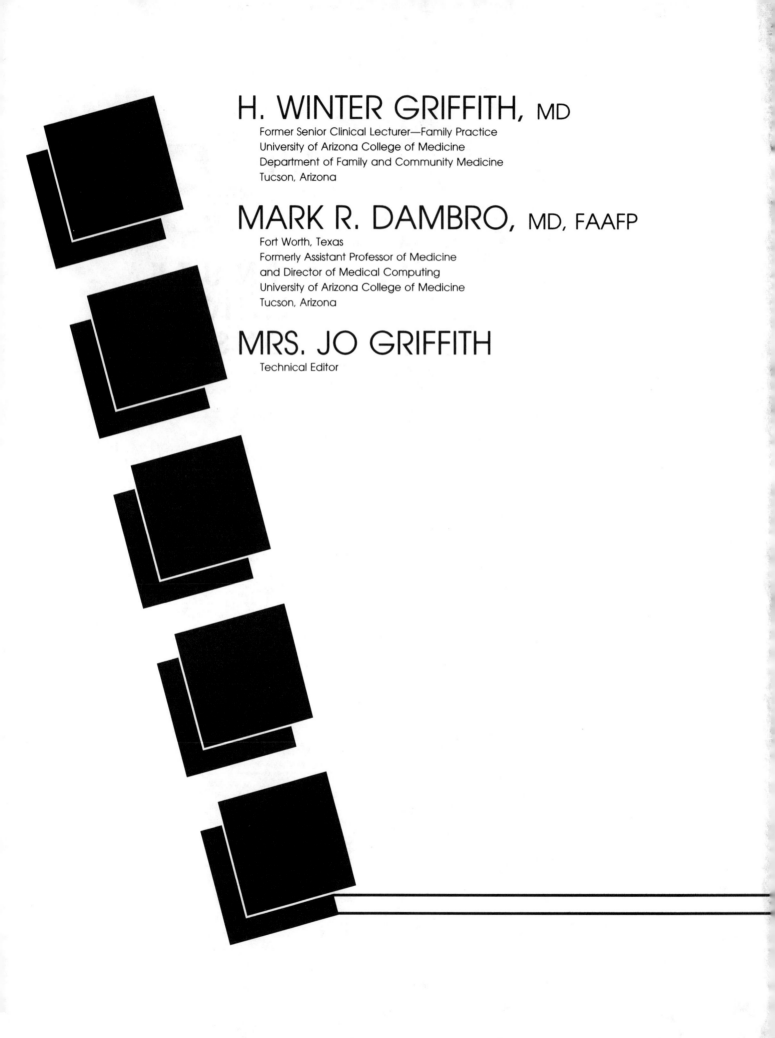

H. WINTER GRIFFITH, MD

Former Senior Clinical Lecturer—Family Practice
University of Arizona College of Medicine
Department of Family and Community Medicine
Tucson, Arizona

MARK R. DAMBRO, MD, FAAFP

Fort Worth, Texas
Formerly Assistant Professor of Medicine
and Director of Medical Computing
University of Arizona College of Medicine
Tucson, Arizona

MRS. JO GRIFFITH

Technical Editor

THE 5 MINUTE CLINICAL CONSULT

Lea & Febiger

PHILADELPHIA • BALTIMORE • HONG KONG
LONDON • MUNICH • SYDNEY • TOKYO

A WAVERLY COMPANY
1994

Lea & Febiger
Box 3024
200 Chester Field Parkway
Malvern, Pennsylvania 19355-9725
U.S.A.
(610) 251-2230

Executive Editor—Carroll C. Cann
Development Editor—Susan Hunsberger
Production Manager—Michael DeNardo

ISBN 0-8121-1753-0

NOTE: Although the author(s) and the publisher have taken reasonable steps to ensure the accuracy of the drug information included in this text before publication, drug information may change without notice and readers are advised to consult the manufacturer's packaging inserts before prescribing medications.

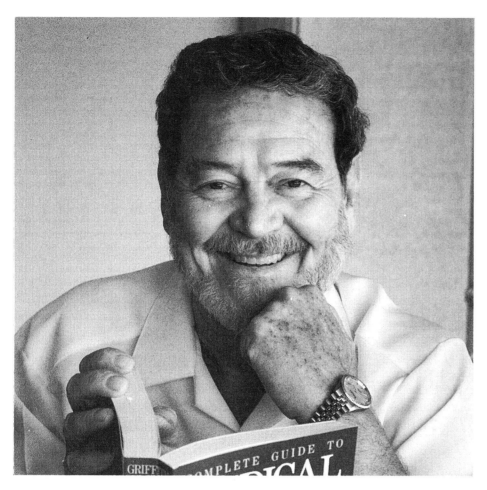

It was with a great deal of sorrow in my heart when, in the spring of 1993, I made my last visit to Winter Griffith. I had known this extraordinary man for many years and we had shared much. As a role model and teacher, he shared with me his creativity, enthusiasm and energy.

Winter viewed projects with an unsurpassed zeal that lead him to be a prolific author and ultimately lead us both to **THE 5 MINUTE CLINICAL CONSULT.** His outline concept in medical writing began years ago and he applied it over and over, refining it with each new publication. As an innovative thinker he believed, as I do, that medical information is often best organized in this now familiar style.

Perhaps you also knew Winter through one of his many projects. Or perhaps you knew him as a physician or as a friend. Perhaps as your golfing partner or your choir partner. Perhaps as your husband or father. Perhaps only as a familiar author on a book spine somewhere. Wherever you knew Winter, you knew that he did not worry about failure. Winter approached projects, indeed his whole life, with unparalleled optimism; he never concerned himself with how a project would be completed, only whether it was a worthwhile project. ``Good projects get done,'' he'd say. ``Just begin at the beginning; do not dwell on why not, but rather on how.''

Winter would advise us to spend our time accomplishing our goals and praising others rather than criticizing or worrying about failure. He would wish us a fine day, filled with a balance of creativity, spirituality, and love, and to make each day an example of your best.

I wish each of you your best, and may you be as fortunate as I to have known H. Winter Griffith.

MRD

DEDICATION

PREFACE

THE 5 MINUTE CLINICAL CONSULT–1994 represents Lea & Febiger's second annual edition of a quick medical reference for current medical diagnosis and treatment. These are the features:

SCOPE
1,000 topics arranged alphabetically and cross-indexed to synonyms of each. Approximately 550 **expanded** topics in a full format that contains enough detail to confirm the diagnosis and treat the problem. Approximately 450 **short** topics in a brief format, with data supplied in the public domain by the National Library of Medicine.

CONTRIBUTING AUTHORS
Over 300 experienced clinicians writing on medical and surgical problems within their areas of interest and expertise.

CONSULTANTS
Over 42 authorities in fields of general and specialty practice. Review was for accuracy, currency, appropriateness, completeness, and safety. All medication entries and dosages were verified by a Doctor of Pharmacy and rechecked by the contributing authors prior to publication.

UPDATES
Annual. Assures inclusion of the most recent norms of practice and consensus of the majority of experts.

FORMAT
For the 550 major topics, a consistent, two-page, graphic, chart-like format, similar to the skeleton format displayed below. The six major divisions and 35 information blocks cover the major aspects of each disorder and are repeated for each topic.

BASICS	DIAGNOSIS	TREATMENT	MEDICATION	FOLLOW-UP	MISCELLANEOUS
• Description	• Differential	• General measures	• Drug(s) of choice	• Monitoring	• Age-related factors
• Genetics	• Laboratory	• Activity	• Contraindications	• Prevention	• Pregnancy
• Prevalence	• Special tests	• Diet	• Precautions	• Complications	• Synonyms
• Age	• Pathology	• Patient education	• Interactions	• Prognosis	• ICD-9-CM
• Signs and symptoms	• Imaging		• Alternate drugs		• See also
• Causes	• Diagnostics				• Other notes
• Risk factors					• References

Preface

A glance at the format of this book will alert the reader to the fact that *THE 5 MINUTE CLINICAL CONSULT* aptly lends itself to the realm of electronic media. All the data, for both the expanded and short topics, will be available on CD-ROM for use by developers and end-users this year.

We wish to make this work continuously responsive to the needs of its users and invite you to express your wishes regarding chapters you would like to appear in future editions. Send comments and suggestions to:

Mark R. Dambro, MD
1650 W. Rosedale, Suite 307
Fort Worth, TX 76104

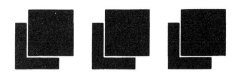

CONTRIBUTING AUTHORS

STONEY A. ABERCROMBIE, MD
Self Memorial Hospital
Greenwood, SC

ABDULRAZAK ABYAD, MD, MPH
Assistant Professor
Department of Family Medicine
American University of Beirut
New York, NY

RODNEY D. ADAM, MD
Assistant Professor of Medicine and Microbiology/Immunology
University of Arizona College of Medicine
Tucson, AZ

ALAN ADELMAN, MD, MS
Department of Family and Community Medicine
Milton S. Hershey Medical Center
Hershey, PA

RICHARD W. ALLINSON, MD
Clinical Assistant Professor
Department of Ophthalmology
University of Arizona College of Medicine
Tucson, AZ

PATRICIA ANDERSON, MD
Mt. Auburn Associates
Cincinnati, OH

DEIRDRE ANDRES, MD CCFP
Department of Family Medicine
University of Saskatchewan
Saskatchewan, Saskatoon
Canada

WATSON C. ARNOLD, MD
Director Pediatric Nephrology
Cook–Fort Worth Children's Medical Center
Fort Worth, TX

JEHAD Y. ASFOURA, MD
Assistant Professor, Clinical Internal Medicine
Northeastern Ohio Universities College of Medicine
Canton, OH

ROBERT L. ATMAR, MD
Department of Medicine
Baylor College of Medicine
Houston, TX

EDITH P. BAILEY, MD
Private Practice
Catalina Pediatrics
Tucson, AZ

TIMOTHY BAKER, MD
Family Practice Residency Program
St. Joseph's Hospital
Phoenix, AZ

COLIN R. BAMFORD, MD
Department of Neurology
University of Arizona College of Medicine
Tucson, AZ

MUSTAFA BARUDI, MD
Assistant Professor of Pediatrics
Northeastern Ohio Universities College of Medicine
TOD Children's Hospital
Youngstown, OH

ROBERT P. BAUGHMAN, MD
Associate Professor of Medicine
Pulmonary/Critical Care Division
University of Cincinnati Medical Center
Cincinnati, OH

KAY A. BAUMAN, MD, MPH
Associate Professor
Department of Family Practice and Community Health
University of Hawaii School of Medicine
Honolulu, HI

KARIL BELLAH, MD
Cardiology
Lawrence, KS

JAMES B. BENJAMIN, MD
Associate Professor of Surgery
University of Arizona College of Medicine
Tucson, AZ

PAUL J. BENKE, MD, PhD
University of Miami School of Medicine
Miami, FL

GEORGE R. BERGUS, MD
Assistant Professor
Department of Family Practice
University of Iowa
Iowa City, IA

WILLIAM H. BILLICA, MD
Assistant Director
Family Practice Residency Program
Good Samaritan Medical Center
Phoenix, AZ

RICHARD B. BIRRER, MD
Emergency Department
Catholic Medical Center
Jamaica, NY

TIMOTHY L. BLACK, MD, FACS, FAAP
Medical Director of Trauma
Cook–Fort Worth Children's Medical Center
Fort Worth, TX

Contributing Authors

BRUCE BLOCK, MD
Family Practice Residency Program
Shadyside Hospital
Pittsburgh, PA

MICHAEL BOESPFLUG, MD
Private Practice
Eugene, OR

JESS G. BOND, MD, MPH
Assistant Professor of Internal Medicine
Northeastern Ohio Universities College of Medicine
Akron, OH

MARJORIE A. BOWMAN, MD, MPA
Department of Family and Community Medicine
Bowman Gray School of Medicine
Winston-Salem, NC

JOHN T. BOYER, MD
Professor, Department of Medicine
University of Arizona College of Medicine
Tucson, AZ

GEORGE R. BRADBURY, MD
Section of Orthopedic Surgery
University of Arizona College of Medicine
Tucson, AZ

MARYLYN E. BROMAN, MD
Associate Professor of Clinical Pediatrics
Director of Adolescent Medicine
University of Miami School of Medicine
Miami, FL

DAVID E. BURTNER, MD
Department of Family and Community Medicine
Mercer University School of Medicine
Macon, GA

ABRAHAM R. (RUDY) BYRD, MD
Private Practice
Tucson, AZ

JOANNA M. CAIN, MD
Associate Professor
Department of Obstetrics and Gynecology
University of Washington Medical Center
Seattle, WA

CYNTHIA GAIL CARMICHAEL, MD
Clinical Assistant Professor
Department of Family Medicine and Community Health
University of Miami School of Medicine
Miami, FL

KEVIN CARMICHAEL, MD
Department of Family and Community Medicine
University of Arizona College of Medicine
Tucson, AZ

JOHN Z. CARTER, MD
Private Practice
Family Practice/Geriatrics
Northwest Hospital Medical Plaza
Tucson, AZ

L. PHILIP CARTER, MD
Professor
Department of Surgery
University of Arizona College of Medicine
Tucson, AZ

ROY R. CASIANO, MD
Assistant Professor
Department of Otolaryngology
University of Miami School of Medicine
Miami, FL

JASON CHAO, MD, MS
Assistant Professor
Department of Family Medicine
Case Western Reserve University
Cleveland, OH

HAROLD CHEVLEN, MD, FAAFP
Private Practice
Youngstown, OH

ANTHONY W. CHOW, MD, FRCPC, FACP
Professor of Medicine
Head, Division of Infectious Diseases
The University of British Columbia
Vancouver, British Columbia, Canada

THOMAS W. CLARK, MD
Department of Surgery
Akron General Medical Center
Northeastern Ohio Universities College of Medicine
Akron, OH

WILLIAM W. CLEVELAND, MD
Professor of Pediatrics
Director, Division of Endocrinology
University of Miami
Miami, FL

RICHARD D. CLOVER, MD
Department of Family Medicine
University of Texas Medical Branch
Galveston, TX

RICHARD W. COHEN, MD
Georgia Orthopaedics and Sports Medicine
Marietta, GA

RUSSELL G. COHEN, MD
University of Arizona College of Medicine
Tucson, AZ

JOHN J. COLEMAN, III, MD
Professor of Surgery
Director, Plastic Surgery
Indiana University Medical Center
Indianapolis, IN

MICHAEL G. CONNOLLY, MD
Private Practice
Birmingham, AL

JACK G. COPELAND, MD
Professor, Department of Surgery
Section of Cardiovascular and Thoracic Surgery
University of Arizona College of Medicine
Tucson, AZ

ANTHONY J. COSTA, MD
Residency Program Director
Barberton Citizens Hospital
Barberton, OH

CYNTHIA COTE, MD
Faculty
Department of Family Practice
Valley Medical Center
Renton, WA

ALAN J. CROPP, MD, FCCP
Associate Professor of Internal Medicine
Northeastern Ohio Universities College of Medicine
Youngstown, OH

PAUL T. CULLEN, MD
Director, Family Practice Residency Program
The Washington Hospital
Washington, PA

J.P.W. CUNNINGTON, MD, FRCP
Associate Professor of Medicine
McMaster University
Hamilton, Ontario
Canada

M. BEATRIZ CURRIER, MD
Department of Psychiatry
University of Miami School of Medicine
Miami, FL

ROBERT B. DAIGNEAULT, MD, FAAP
Assistant Clinical Professor
University of California, San Diego
San Diego, CA

JAMES E. DALEN, MD
Vice Provost for Health Sciences
Dean, College of Medicine
University of Arizona College of Medicine
Tucson, AZ

MARK R. DAMBRO, MD, FAAFP
Private Practice
Fort Worth, TX

NANCY N. DAMBRO, MD
Cook–Fort Worth Children's Medical Center
Fort Worth, TX

JERYL DANSKY, MD
Private Practice
Tucson, AZ

MARC DARR, MD
Family Practice Residency Program
St. Joseph's Hospital
Phoenix, AZ

JANICE E. DAUGHERTY, MD
Department of Family Medicine
East Carolina University School of Medicine
Greenville, NC

MEG DAVIDSON, MD
ACL Hospital
San Fidel, NM

KHALEEL DEEB, MD
Department of Family Practice
University Hospital of Cleveland
Cleveland, OH

LISA M. DERANEK, MD
Private Practice
Seven Hills, OH

EMIL S. DICKSTEIN, MD
Associate Professor of Medicine
Northeastern Ohio Universities College of Medicine
Youngstown, OH

J. HARLAN DIX, MD, FACP
Clinical Associate Professor
Northeastern Ohio Universities College of Medicine
Killbuck, OH

MICHEL J. DODARD, MD
Assistant Professor
Clinical Family Medicine and Community Health
Jackson Memorial Hospital
Miami, FL

ROBERT DOLIN, MD
Department of Medicine
Kaiser Permanente
Anaheim, CA

PATRICK J. DUEY, MD
Family Medicine Center
Phoenix Baptist Hospital
Phoenix, AZ

S. SHEVAUN DUIKER, MD
Assistant Professor
Department of Family Practice
University of Texas Health Science Center
Houston, TX

BURRIS DUNCAN, MD
Professor
Department of Pediatrics
University of Arizona College of Medicine
Tucson, AZ

M. PATRICE EIFF, MD
Assistant Professor
Family Medicine
Oregon Health Sciences University
Portland, OR

DONALD F. EIPPER, MD
Associate Professor Internal Medicine
Northeastern Ohio Universities College of Medicine
Akron General Medical Center
Akron, OH

STEVEN EISENSTEIN, MD
Private Practice
The Family Doctors of Northbrook
Northbrook, IL

NANCY ELDER, MD, MSPH
Assistant Professor
Oregon Health Sciences University
Portland, OR

GREG ELDERS, MD
Private Practice
Mountain Home, AR

CECILIA ELLIS, DO
Chief Resident
Akron City Hospital
Akron, OH

KURT ELWARD, MD, MPH
Clinical Assistant Professor, Department of Family Medicine
University of Virginia
Fellow, Thomas Jefferson Health Policy Institute
Charlottesville, VA

GARY A. ERBSTOESSER, DO
Family Medicine Center
Phoenix Baptist Hospital
Phoenix, AZ

MICHAEL J. ESSIG, MD
Chairman, Department of Family Practice
Medical Director, Mercy Family Health Center
Mercy Hospital of Pittsburgh
Pittsburgh, PA

Contributing Authors

ROBERT G. FANTE, MD, CAPT, MC, USAF
Clinical Instructor
Department of Ophthalmology
University of Nebraska
Omaha, NE

NANCY P. FAWCETT, MD
Department of Pediatrics
University of Miami
Miami, FL

ANDREW H. FENTON, MD
Department of Surgery
Akron General Medical Center
Northeastern Ohio Universities College of Medicine
Akron, OH

MICHAEL FERREBEE, MD
Fellow, Pediatric Critical Care
Division of Critical Care
Le Bonheur Children's Medical Center
Memphis, TN

SCOTT A. FIELDS, MD
Assistant Professor
Family Medicine
Oregon Health Sciences University
Portland, OR

DOUGLAS P. FINE, MD
University of Oklahoma Health Sciences Center
Veterans Administration Medical Center
Oklahoma City, OK

STANLEY FINEMAN, MD
Clinical Assistant Professor
Department of Pediatrics
Emory University School of Medicine
Marietta, GA

DANIEL B. FISHBEIN, MD
Coordinator, Scientific Studies
International Branch
Centers for Disease Control
Atlanta, GA

ROSMARY FLEMING, RN, BSN
Pulmonary Rehabilitation Association
Pulmonary Medicine Consultants
Youngstown, OH

JOSEPH A. FLORENCE, MD
Director, East Kentucky Family Practice Residency Program
University of Kentucky
Hazard, KY

GRANT C. FOWLER, MD
Assistant Professor
Department of Family Practice
Director, Hermann/LBJ Family Practice Program
Houston, TX

DAVID J. FRAMM, MD
Private Practice
Charlotte, NC

WESLEY FURSTE, MD, FACS
Clinical Professor, Emeritus
Department of Surgery
Ohio State University
Columbus, OH

GREGORY G. GAAR, MD
Medical Toxicology Consultants
Harborside Medical Tower
Tampa, FL

ERIC P. GALL, MD
Professor of Medicine
Chief, Rheumatology/Allergy and Immunology
University of Arizona College of Medicine
Tucson, AZ

JAMES M. GALLOWAY, MD, FACP
Clinical Assistant Professor, Division of Cardiology
Department of Medicine
University of Arizona College of Medicine
Tucson, AZ

GALE GARDNER, MD, FACS
Clinical Professor
Department of Otolaryngology
University of Tennessee, Memphis
Memphis, TN

WILLIAM G. GARDNER, MD
Chairman, Department of Medicine
Akron General Medical Center
Akron, OH

KENT R. GEBHARDT, DO
Clinical Assistant Professor of Family Medicine
College of Osteopathic Medicine of the Pacific
Tacoma, WA

JOHN P. GEYMAN, MD
Professor Emeritus of Family Medicine
University of Washington
Seattle, WA

JEFF RAY GIBSON, Jr., MD
Department of Anesthesiology
Scott and White Clinic
Temple, TX

BRUCE C. GILLILAND, MD
Professor of Medicine and Laboratory Medicine
School of Medicine
University of Washington
Seattle, WA

MARK GOLDBERG, MD
Section of Cardiology, Department of Medicine
University of Arizona College of Medicine
Tucson, AZ

PAUL R. GORDON, MD
Family and Community Medicine
University of Arizona College of Medicine
Tucson, AZ

R. SCOTT GORMAN, MD
Clinical Associate Professor of Medicine
University of Arizona College of Medicine
Tucson, AZ

CARMELO GRAFFAGNINO, MD, FRCP
Department of Neurology
Duke University Medical Center
Durham, NC

JULIE GRAVES-MOY, MD
Clinical Assistant Professor of Family Medicine
Department of Family Medicine
Baylor College of Medicine
Houston, TX

DAVID S. GRAY, MD
Community Hospital
Family Practice Residency
Santa Rosa, CA

J. THOMAS GRAYSTON, MD
Professor, Department of Epidemiology
University of Washington School of Public Health and Community
   Medicine
Seattle, WA

RONALD A. GREENFIELD, MD
Associate Professor
University of Oklahoma Health Sciences Center
Veterans Administration Medical Center
Oklahoma City, OK

DAVID A. GRIESEMER, MD
Section of Child Neurology
Departments of Pediatrics and Neurology
University of Arizona College of Medicine
Tucson, AZ

FRANKLIN W. GRIFF, MD
Associate Professor
Northeastern Ohio Universities College of Medicine
Canton, OH

H. WINTER GRIFFITH, MD
(Deceased)
Senior Clinical Lecturer–Family Practice
University of Arizona College of Medicine
Tucson, AZ

SHARON GRUNDFEST-BRONIATOWSKI, MD, FACS
Department General Surgery
Cleveland Clinic
Cleveland, OH

VLADIMIR C. HACHINSKI, MD, DSC, FRCP
Department of Clinical Neurological Sciences
The University of Western Ontario
London, Ontario, Canada

SAMI K.W. HADEED, MD
Pulmonary Medicine
Cook–Fort Worth Children's Medical Center
Fort Worth, TX

KAREN HALL, MD
Family Practice Residency Program
University of Florida
Gainesville, FL

LARRY W. HALVERSON, MD
Director, Cox Family Practice Residency Program
Cox Medical Centers
Springfield, MO

KAREN A. HARDY, MD
Chief, Pediatric Pulmonary and Cystic Fibrosis Center
California Pacific Medical Center
San Francisco, CA

CLYDE L. HARRIS, MD
Private Practice
Franklin, NC

IRWIN E. HARRIS, MD
Orthopedic Oncology
Pediatric Orthopedics
University of Arizona College of Medicine
Tucson, AZ

WILLIAM S. HAUBRICH, MD, FACP
Senior Consultant Emeritus
Scripps Clinic and Research Foundation
Clinical Professor of Medicine University of California, San Diego
La Jolla, CA

FERN R. HAUCK, MD, MS
Assistant Professor
Department of Preventive Medicine and Epidemiology
Loyola University Medical Center
Maywood, IL

CATHRYN HEATH, MD
Department of Family Medicine
Syracuse, NY

DARELL E. HEISELMAN, DO
Professor and Chief, Critical Care Medicine
Northeastern Ohio College of Medicine
Akron General Medical Center
Akron, OH

SCOTT T. HENDERSON, MD
Assistant Professor of Family Practice
Family Practice Residency Program, Cheyenne
University of Wyoming
Cheyenne, WY

ERIC HENLEY, MD, MPH
Albuquerque PHS Hospital
Albuquerque, NM

KEVIN M. HEPLER, MD, MBA
Associate Residency Program Director
Family Practice Residency Program
Good Samaritan/Penn State
Lebanon, PA

BARTON L. HODES, MD
Professor
Department of Ophthalmology
University of Arizona College of Medicine
Tucson, AZ

MICHAEL P. HOPKINS, MD
Professor
Department of Obstetrics and Gynecology
Northeastern Ohio Universities College of Medicine
Akron, OH

MARK HORATTAS, MD
Assistant Professor
Department of Surgery
Northeastern Ohio Universities College of Medicine
Akron, OH

LAURENE L. HOWELL, MD
Department of Otolaryngology
Oregon Health Sciences University
Portland, OR

THOMAS E. HURD, MD
Chairman
Department of Anesthesia
Kennestone Hospital
Marietta, GA

FRANK L. IBER, MD
Department of Gastroenterology
Edward Hines, Jr. Hospital
Hines, IL

STEPHEN J. JACKSON, MD
(Deceased)
Assistant Director
Division of Education
American Academy of Family Physicians
Kansas City, MO

CHARLES N. JACOBS, MD
Nephrologist
Waterville, ME

Contributing Authors

PHILIP E. JAFFE, MD
Assistant Clinical Professor of Medicine
University of Arizona College of Medicine
Director, GI Endoscopy Lab, VA Medical Center
Tucson, AZ

STEVEN L. JAFFE, MD
Associate Professor of Psychiatry
Director, Adolescent Programs
Emory University
Brawner Hospital
Atlanta, GA

PAUL J. JASTER, MD
Associate Director, Assistant Professor
Smoky Hill Family Practice Residency Program
Salina, KS

E.R. JEANS, MD, BSC
Fellow, Infectious Diseases and Microbiology
Chedoke-McMaster Hospitals
Hamilton, Ontario, Canada

ERIC L. JENISON, MD
Associate Professor
Obstetrics and Gynecology
Northeastern Ohio Universities College of Medicine
Akron, OH

CHARLES JENNINGS, MD
Lima Urology, Inc.
Lima, OH

PAUL JOHNSON, MD
Emergency Department
St. Luke's Hospital
Phoenix, AZ

FURNIE W. JOHNSTON, MD
Private Practice
Dothan, AL

SMITH L. JOHNSTON, III, MD, MSC
Project Physician, Medical Operations Space Station
Freedom NASA, Johnson Space Center
KRUG Life Sciences
Houston, TX

K. SHASHI KANT, MD
Professor of Medicine
Division of Nephrology and Hypertension
University of Cincinnati Medical Center
Cincinnati, OH

PAUL E. KAPLAN, MD
Bert C. Wiley Professor and Chairman
Physical Medicine and Rehabilitation
Ohio State University
Columbus, OH

WAYNE J. KATON, MD
Professor of Psychiatry
Department of Psychiatry, School of Medicine
University of Washington Medical School
Seattle, WA

RICK KELLERMAN, MD
Director
Smoky Hill Family Practice Residency Program
Salina, KS

MARY KELLIHER, MD
New England Medical Center Hospitals
Boston, MA

ROBERT M. KERSHNER, MD, FACS
Associate Professor
University of Utah Medical Center in Salt Lake
Chief, Section of Ophthalmology, Northwest Hospital
Tucson, AZ

MYRA K. KERSTITCH, MD
Department of Family Practice
University of Arizona College of Medicine
Tucson, AZ

GEORGE E. KIKANO, MD
Assistant Professor, Department of Family Medicine
University Hospitals of Cleveland
Case Western Reserve University
Cleveland, OH

MICHELLE D. KIMMEL, MD
Cushing Medical Associates
Cushing, OK

SCOTT A. KINCAID, MD
Assistant Clinical Professor of Family Medicine
Medical College of Virginia
Radford, VA

MITCHELL S. KING, MD
Assistant Director
Family Practice Residency
Bon Secours Hospital
Grosse Pointe, MI

JEFFERY T. KIRCHNER, DO
Clinical Instructor
Family and Community Medicine
Lancaster General Hospital
Lancaster, PA

EVAN W. KLIGMAN, MD
Chairman
Department of Family and Community Medicine
University of Arizona College of Medicine
Tucson, AZ

MARY E. KLINK, MD
Physicians Plus Medical Group
Medical Director, Sleep Disorders Program
Meriter Hospital
Madison, WI

AUBREY L. KNIGHT, MD
Assistant Director of Family Practice Education
Roanoke Memorial Hospitals
Roanoke, VA

STEVEN R. KNOPER, MD
Research Assistant Professor
Respiratory Sciences Center
University of Arizona College of Medicine
Tucson, AZ

ELLEN LACKERMANN, MD
Family Practice Department
Swedish Hospital Medical Center
Seattle, WA

ALVIN LANGER, MD
Professor of Obstetrics and Gynecology
Associate Dean for Clinical Education
Northeastern Ohio Universities College of Medicine
Canton, OH

RICHARD A. LARSON, MD
Associate Professor of Medicine
Director, Acute Leukemia Program
The University of Chicago Medical Center
Chicago, IL

MARC LeDUC, MD
Private Practice
Port Clinton, OH

MARK C. LEESON, MD, FACS
Associate Professor
Northeastern Ohio Universities College of Medicine
Akron, OH

GARY LEVINE, MD
Director of Southwest Georgia
Family Practice Residency Program
Phoebe Putney Memorial Hospital
Albany, GA

DANIEL O. LEVINSON, MD
Department of Psychiatry
University of Arizona College of Medicine
Tucson, AZ

RICHARD P. LEVY, MD
Professor of Internal Medicine
Northeastern Ohio Universities College of Medicine
Akron, OH

JAMES H. LEWIS, MD, FACP
Associate Professor of Medicine
Division of Gastroenterology
Georgetown University Medical Center
Washington, DC

THOMAS LEWIS, DDS
Private Practice
Bayside, CA

ELMER S. LIGHTNER, MD
Professor of Pediatrics
Department of Pediatrics
University of Arizona College of Medicine
Tucson, AZ

CAROL B. LINDSLEY, MD
Professor of Pediatrics
Director, Pediatric Rheumatology
University of Kansas Medical School
Kansas City, KS

JOHN M. LITTLE, MD
Director, Family Practice Residency Program
Clinical Associate Professor
Carolinas Medical Center
University of North Carolina
Charlotte, NC

DOROTHY LOWDER, RN
Holmes County Hospice
Millersburg, OH

ELYSE E. LOWER, MD
Associate Professor of Medicine
Hematology/Oncology Division
University of Cincinnati Medical Center
Cincinnati, OH

D.W. MACPHERSON, MD, MSC (CTM), FRCPC
Director, Parasitology Regional Laboratory
Assistant Professor
McMaster University
Hamilton, Ontario, Canada

KATHY E. MAGLIATO, MD
Department of Surgery
Akron General Medical Center
Akron, OH

BARBARA A. MAJERONI, MD
Director of Predoctoral Education
Department of Family Medicine
State University of New York at Buffalo
Buffalo, NY

SYLVIA A. MAMBY, MD
Assistant Professor of Medicine
Division of Cardiology
Mayo Clinic, Scottsdale
Scottsdale, AZ

RICHARD M. MANDEL, MD
Assistant Clinical Professor
Internal Medicine
University of Arizona College of Medicine
Tucson, AZ

COLIN D. MARCHANT, MD
Associate Professor of Pediatrics
Pediatric Infectious Disease Division
New England Medical Center Hospitals
Tufts University School of Medicine
Boston, MA

ROBERT A. MARLOW, MD
Associate Dean/Program Director
Family Practice Residency Program at Cheyenne
University of Wyoming
Cheyenne, WY

BRADLEY R. MARTIN, MD
Akron City Hospital
Akron, OH

L.E. (BRUNO) MASTERS, MD
Private Practice
Atlantic Beach, FL

SUSANA MAY, MD, MPH
Assistant Clinical Professor
Family Medicine
University of Tennessee
Memphis, TN

PATRICK J. McCARVILLE, MD
Private Practice
Valley, NE

ELIZABETH McCORD, MD
Instructor, Family Medicine
University of Illinois, College of Medicine
Rockford, IL

K. PATRICIA McGANN, MD, MSPH
Assistant Professor
Department of Family and Community Medicine
Bowman Gray School of Medicine
Wake Forest University
Winston-Salem, NC

DON McHARD, MD
Residency Director
Department of Family Practice
St. Joseph's Hospital
Phoenix, AZ

SEAN O. McMENOMEY, MD
Department of Otolaryngology
Oregon Health Sciences University
Portland, OR

STEVEN MEIS, MD
Assistant Professor
Department of Family Medicine
University of Iowa
Iowa City, IA

Contributing Authors

LEO C. MERCER, MD
Assistant Professor
Texas Tech University Health Sciences Center
El Paso, TX

DAVID C. METRIKIN, MD
Department of Ophthalmology
Southwestern Medical Center at Dallas
Dallas, TX

GARY M. MILLER, MD
Marietta Neurological Associates
Marietta, GA

JAMES P. MILLER, MD
Pediatric Surgical Associates of Fort Worth
Fort Worth, TX

JOSEPH I. MILLER, MD
Professor of Cardiothoracic Surgery
Department of Surgery
The Emory University Clinic
Atlantic, GA

SANDRA MILLER, MD
Family Practice Center
Good Samaritan Regional Medical Center
Phoenix, AZ

JEFFREY F. MINTEER, MD
Associate Director
Family Practice Residency Program
The Washington Hospital
Washington, PA

CHARLES D. MITCHELL, MD
Division of Immunology and Infectious Diseases
Department of Pediatrics
University of Miami School of Medicine
Miami, FL

REZA MOATTARI, MD
Associate Professor of Medicine
Northeastern Ohio Universities College of Medicine
Chief, Endocrinology, Akron General Hospital
Akron, OH

SUSAN LOUISA MONTAUK, MD
Associate Professor of Clinical Family Medicine
Department of Family Medicine
University of Cincinnati College of Medicine
Cincinnati, OH

T. GLENDON MOODY, MD
Clinical Lecturer
Department of Ophthalmology
University of Arizona College of Medicine
Mesa, AZ

DONALD W. MOORMAN, MD
Department of Surgery Education
Iowa Methodist Medical Center
DesMoines, IA

WILLIAM J. MORAN, DMD, MD, FACS
Otolaryngology–Head and Neck Surgery
University of Chicago Hospitals
Chicago, IL

VENITA MORELL, MD
Assistant Professor
Department of Family and Community Medicine
Bowman Gray School of Medicine
Winston-Salem, NC

KEVIN H. MOSSER, MD
Department of Family Medicine
York Hospital
York, PA

BRIAN MURRAY, MD
Medical Director
Student Health Services
University of California at San Diego
La Jolla, CA

WILLIAM MUTH, MD
Assistant Professor of Medicine and Microbiology/Immunology
University of Arizona College of Medicine
Tucson, AZ

JOSEPH MYERS, MD
Akron General Hospital
Akron, OH

ARI J. NAMON, MD
Otolaryngology–Head and Neck Surgery
University of Chicago Hospitals
Chicago, IL

JAMES A. NARD, MD
Department of Pediatrics
TOD Children's Hospital
Youngstown, OH

DIANE NEDDENRIEP, MD
Private Practice
Tucson, AZ

DONALD A.F. NELSON, MD
Family Health Center
Cedar Rapids Medical Education Program
Cedar Rapids, IA

JAMES C. NIEDERMAN, MD
Clinical Professor of Medicine and Epidemiology
Yale University School of Medicine
New Haven, CT

PETER T. NIEH, MD
Senior Staff
Department of Urology
Lahey Clinic Foundation
Burlington, MA

ROBERT NOECKER, MD
Department of Ophthalmology
University of Arizona College of Medicine
Tucson, AZ

RANDALL OATES, MD
Private Practice
Springdale, AR

MICHAEL A. ODDI, MD
Department of Surgery
Akron General Medical Center
Akron, OH

LINDA R. OLAFSON, MD
Clinical Instructor, Family Medicine
University of California, San Diego
San Diego, CA

EDWIN J. OLSEN, MD
Department of Psychiatry
University of Miami School of Medicine
Miami Beach, FL

SCOTT OWEN, MD
Department of Family Medicine
State University of New York at Buffalo
Buffalo, NY

BENITA PADILLA, MD
Department of Nephrology
University of Cincinnati Medical Center
Cincinnati, OH

TEJAL PARIKH, MD
Department of Family and Community Medicine
University of Arizona College of Medicine
Tucson, AZ

JOSE R. PARKER, MD
Family Medicine Center
Phoenix Baptist Hospital
Phoenix, AZ

EDWARD PAUL, MD
Program Director
Department of Family Medicine
Phoenix Baptist Hospital
Phoenix, AZ

GREG PENNOCK, MD
Department of Cardiology
University of Arizona College of Medicine
Tucson, AZ

JOHN E. PERCHALSKI, MD, FAAFP
Associate Professor
Department of Community Health and Family Medicine
University of Florida College of Medicine
Gainesville, FL

JOHN R. PERSON, MD
Fallon Medical Center
Worcester, MA

CLAUDIA A. PETERS, MD
Associate Professor
Hotel Dieu Family Medicine Center
Queen's University
Kingston, Ontario
Canada

DANA W. PETERSON, MD
Internal and Family Medicine Associates
Albuquerque, NM

DELANA PHILLIPS, MD
Assistant Professor
Department of Family Practice
University of California, Davis
Sacramento, CA

GREGORY A. POLAND, MD
Assistant Professor
Department of Internal Medicine
The Mayo Clinic
Rochester, MN

DAVID A. POPE, MD
Private Practice
Janesville, MN

WILLIAM A. PRIMACK, MD
Associate Professor of Pediatrics
University of Massachusetts Medical Center
Auburn, MA

LEE P. RALPH, MD
Department of Family Medicine
University of California, San Diego Medical Group
San Diego, CA

RAGHU RAM, MD
Family Practice Residency Program
Shadyside Hospital
Pittsburgh, PA

KATHRYN REILLY, MD, MPH
Family Practice Residency Program
University of Oklahoma
Oklahoma City, OK

J. RANDALL RICHARD, MD
Assistant Professor of Clinical Family Medicine
Northeastern Ohio Universities College of Medicine
Associate Residency Director
Barberton Citizens Hospital
Barberton, OH

CHARLES W. RICKETSON, MD, FRCP(C)
Greater Victoria Hospital Society
Victoria, British Columbia, Canada

MICHEL E. RIVLIN, MD
Department of Obstetrics and Gynecology
University of Mississippi Medical Center
Jackson, MS

TIMOTHY ROBINSON, DO
Emergency Department
Catholic Medical Center
Jamaica, NY

VANCE D. RODGERS, MD
Director, Inflammatory Bowel Disease Center
Scripps Clinic and Research Foundation
La Jolla, CA

DUANE C. ROE, MD
Associate Professor of Medicine
Northeastern Universities College of Medicine
Akron, OH

R. CURTIS ROGERS, MD
Greenwood Genetic Center
Greenville, SC

BRUCE M. ROTHSCHILD, MD
Director, Arthritis Center of Northeast Ohio
Professor
Northeastern Ohio Universities College of Medicine
Youngstown, OH

LAURIE ROWAN, DO
Akron General Hospital
Akron, OH

JAMES H. RUDICK, MD, FACP
Assistant Professor of Internal Medicine
Northeastern Ohio Universities College of Medicine
Canton, OH

BARRY S. RUSSMAN, MD
Professor
Pediatrics and Neurology
University of Connecticut Medical School
Newington, CT

GREGORY W. RUTECKI, MD
Associate Professor of Medicine
Northeastern Ohio Universities College of Medicine
Timken Mercy Medical Center
Canton, OH

ANDRÉS M. SALAZAR, MD
Professor of Neurology
Director, Defense and Veterans Head Injury Program
Uniformed Services University of the Health Sciences
Bethesda, MD

Contributing Authors

EDWARD C. SALTZSTEIN, MD
Professor and Regional Chairman, Surgery
Texas Tech University Health Sciences Center
El Paso, TX

RICHARD E. SAMPLINER, MD
Professor of Medicine
Chief of Gastroenterology Section
University of Arizona College of Medicine
Tucson, AZ

DOUGLAS H. SANDBERG, MD
Professor of Pediatrics
Division of Gastroenterology
University of Miami Children's Hospital Center
Miami, FL

ARTHUR SANDERS, MD
Professor, Section of Emergency Medicine
Department of Surgery
University of Arizona College of Medicine
Tucson, AZ

WILLIAM D. SAWYER, MD
China Medical Board of New York
New York, NY

DANIEL T. SCHELBLE, MD, FACEP
Chairman, Department of Emergency Medicine
Akron General Medical Center
Akron, OH

ROBERT M. SCHULTZ, MD
Private Practice
Pediatric Endocrinology
Atlanta, GA

WAYNE H. SCHWESINGER, MD
Department of Surgery
The University of Texas Health Science Center at San Antonio
San Antonio, TX

NAN SCOTT, PhD
Associate Professor
University of Oklahoma Health Sciences Center
Veterans Administration Medical Center
Oklahoma City, OK

ROBERT H. SCOTT, MD
Faculty
Family Practice Residency
Swedish Medical Center
Seattle, WA

DAVID P. SEALY, MD
Director, Research and Sports Medicine
Assistant Professor and Associate Director
Self Memorial Hospital Family Medicine Residency
Greenwood, SC

MARK E. SEXTON, MD
Associate Director
St. Joseph's Family Practice Residency Program and Center
Phoenix, AZ

WILLIAM V. SHARP, MD
Professor of Surgery
Northeastern Ohio Universities College of Medicine
Akron, OH

ALBERT T. SHIU, MD, FACOG
Assistant Professor
Department of Obstetrics and Gynecology
Northeastern Ohio Universities College of Medicine
Canton, OH

GARY J. SILKO, MD
Assistant Director
Family Practice Residency Program
The Washington Hospital
Washington, PA

RICHARD J. SIMENSEN, PhD
Associate Professor
Family Medicine
Self Memorial Hospital
Greenwood, SC

MARK S. SISKIND, MD
Internal Medicine
University of Arizona College of Medicine
Tucson, AZ

ARTHUR R. SLAUGHTER, MD
Associate Director, Family Practice Education
Carilion Health System
Roanoke Family Practice Residency Program
Roanoke, VA

ROBERT J. SLIMAN, MD
Assistant Professor
Department of Internal Medicine
Northeastern Ohio Universities College of Medicine
Canton, OH

W. PAUL SLOMIANY, MD
Assistant Director
Family Practice Residency Program
Washington Hospital
Washington, PA

H. GRATIN SMITH, MD, FAAP
Director of Pediatric Education
Family Practice Residency Program
Self Memorial Hospital
Greenwood, SC

JAY W. SMITH, MD
Vice Dean
University of Arizona College of Medicine
Tucson, AZ

STAN G. SMITH, MA, MB, FCFP(C)
Chairman, Department of Family Practice
University of Saskatchewan
Saskatchewan, Saskatoon, Canada

NANCY SNAPP, MD, MPH
Family Practice Faculty
Swedish Family Practice Residency
Swedish Hospital Medical Center
Seattle, WA

VERA Y. SOONG, MD
Assistant Professor
Department of Dermatology
The University of Alabama at Birmingham
Birmingham, AL

NICHOLAS J. SPIRTOS, DO
Associate Professor
Director, Northeastern Ohio Fertility Center
Northeastern Ohio Universities College of Medicine
Akron City Hospital
Akron, OH

JEFFREY A. STEARNS, MD
Assistant Professor
Family Medicine
University of Illinois College of Medicine
Rockford, IL

G. GAYLE STEPHENS, MD
Professor Emeritus
Department of Family and Community Medicine
University of Alabama at Birmingham
Birmingham, AL

THOMAS R. STRIGLE, MD
Department of Surgery
Northeastern Ohio Universities College of Medicine
Akron, OH

GREGG W. SUITS, MD
Department of Otolaryngology/Head and Neck Surgery
Oregon Health Sciences University
Portland, OR

JACK L. SUMMERS, MD
Professor, Urology
Northeastern Ohio Universities College of Medicine
Chairman, Urology, Summa Health Systems
Akron, OH

GEOFFREY R. SWAIN, MD
Assistant Professor
Department of Family Medicine
Medical College of Wisconsin
Milwaukee, WI

JAMES S. TAN, MD, FACP
Professor of Medicine
Chairman, Infectious Disease Section
Northeastern Ohio Universities College of Medicine
Akron, OH

ROBERT TARASZEWSKI, MD
Pulmonary Disease and Internal Medicine
Akron General Medical Center
Akron, OH

DAVID H. THOM, MD, PhD
Assistant Professor, Department of Medicine
Division of Family and Community Medicine
Stanford University School of Medicine
Palo Alto, CA

MARK D. THOMAS, MD
Private Practice
Sebastopol, CA

SUMNER E. THOMPSON, MD, MPH
Professor of Medicine
Director, AIDS Program
Emory University School of Medicine
Atlanta, GA

WILLIAM L. TOFFLER, MD
Associate Professor
Department of Family Medicine
Oregon Health Sciences University
Portland, OR

MOSHE S. TOREM, MD
Professor and Chairman
Department of Psychiatry
Northeastern Ohio Universities College of Medicine
Akron General Medical Center
Akron, OH

SHELDON M. TRAEGER, MD
Head, Intensive Care Service
Department of Internal Medicine
Summa Hospital System
Northeastern Ohio Universities College of Medicine
Akron, OH

FRANCISCO G. VALENCIA, MD
Section of Orthopedic Surgery
University of Arizona College of Medicine
Tucson, AZ

MICHAEL M. VAN NESS, MD
Gastroenterology Consultant
Canton, OH

BRUCE VANDERHOFF, MD
Staff
Akron City Hospital
Akron, OH

DINA K. VARON, DDS, MS
Adjunct Assistant Professor of Pediatrics
University of Miami College of Medicine
Miami, FL

ARUN K. VERMA, MD
Department of Gastroenterology
Edward Hines, Jr. Hospital
Hines, IL

RICHARD VIKEN, MD
Chairman
Department of Family Practice
The University of Texas Health Center at Tyler
Tyler, TX

CHRIS VINCENT, MD
Faculty
Family Practice Residency
Swedish Medical Center
Seattle, WA

KIMBERLE VORE, MD
Clinical Instructor
Washington Hospital
Washington, PA

ANTHONY F. VUTURO, MD, MPH
Professor, Family and Community Medicine
Associate Dean for Health Affairs
University of Arizona College of Medicine
Tucson, AZ

STANLEY WALLACH, MD
Endocrine Division and Metabolic Bone Disease Center
Hospital for Joint Disease
New York, NY

ANNE D. WALLING, MD
Vice-Chairman
Department of Family and Community Medicine
The University of Kansas Medical Center
Wichita, KS

BRIDGET T. WALSH, DO
Department of Rheumatology
University of Arizona College of Medicine
Tucson, AZ

ALBERTA L. WARNER, MD
Clinical Assistant Professor
Department of Medicine
University of Arizona College of Medicine
Tucson, AZ

CHATRCHAI WATANAKUNAKORN, MD
Professor of Internal Medicine
Northeastern Ohio Universities College of Medicine
St. Elizabeth Hospital Medical Center
Youngstown, OH

Contributing Authors

JOHN R. WATERSON, MD, PhD
Associate Professor of Pediatrics
Northeastern Ohio Universities College of Medicine
Akron, OH

KURT J. WEGNER, MD
Professor of Pediatrics
Neonatologist, Geneticist and Pediatric Consultant
Northeastern Ohio Universities College of Medicine
TOD Children's Hospital
Youngstown, OH

MARTIN E. WEINAND, MD
Assistant Professor of Surgery
Section of Neurosurgery
University of Arizona College of Medicine
Tucson, AZ

BARRY D. WEISS, MD
Professor
Family and Community Medicine
University of Arizona College of Medicine
Tucson, AZ

JEFFREY R. WELKO, MD
Director, Hyperbaric Oxygen Unit
Akron General Medical Center
Akron, OH

ROBERT L. WESTON, MD
Associate Physician
University of California, San Diego
La Jolla, CA

BERNHARD L. WIEDERMANN, MD
Associate Professor of Pediatrics
George Washington University
Director, Pediatric Residency Training Program
Children's National Medical Center
Washington, DC

FRED WILLIAMS, MD
University of Arizona College of Medicine
Tucson, AZ

GARY B. WILLIAMS, MD
Associate Professor of Surgery
Northeastern Ohio Universities College of Medicine
Akron, OH

WM. CAMERON WILLIAMS, MD, MSPH
Assistant Professor
Department of Family and Community Medicine
Bowman Gray School of Medicine at Wake Forest University
Winston-Salem, NC

FREMONT P. WIRTH, MD, FACS
Neurological Institute of Savannah
Savannah, GA

CHRISTOPHER M. WISE, MD
Associate Professor Medicine
Division of Rheumatology, Allergy, and Immunology
Medical College of Virginia
Richmond, VA

JEFFREY D. WOLFREY, MD
Assistant Director
Family Practice Residency Program
Good Samaritan Hospital
Phoenix, AZ

MARK ERIC WORSHTIL, MD
Assistant Director
Family Practice Residency Program
Washington Hospital
Washington, PA

FRANCES WU, MD
Assistant Director
Somerset Family Practice Associates
Somerville, NJ

T.C. YANG, MD, FRCPC
Department of Pathology
Regional Parasitology Laboratory
St. Joseph's Hospital
Hamilton, Ontario, Canada

ALAYNE YATES, MD
Department of Psychiatry
University of Arizona College of Medicine
Tucson, AZ

WILLIAM F. YOUNG, Jr., MD
Associate Professor of Medicine
Division of Hypertension, Endocrinology and Metabolism
Mayo Clinic and Foundation
Rochester, MN

RICHARD KENT ZIMMERMAN, MD, MPH
Assistant Professor
Department of Clinical Epidemiology and Family Medicine
University of Pittsburgh
Pittsburgh, PA

CHARLES I. ZUCKER, MD
Assistant Director
Family Medicine Center
Phoenix Baptist Hospital
Phoenix, AZ

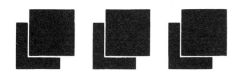

CONTENTS

EXPANDED TOPICS

Contents

Contents

Contents

Contents

Contents

SHORT TOPICS

Contents

Contents

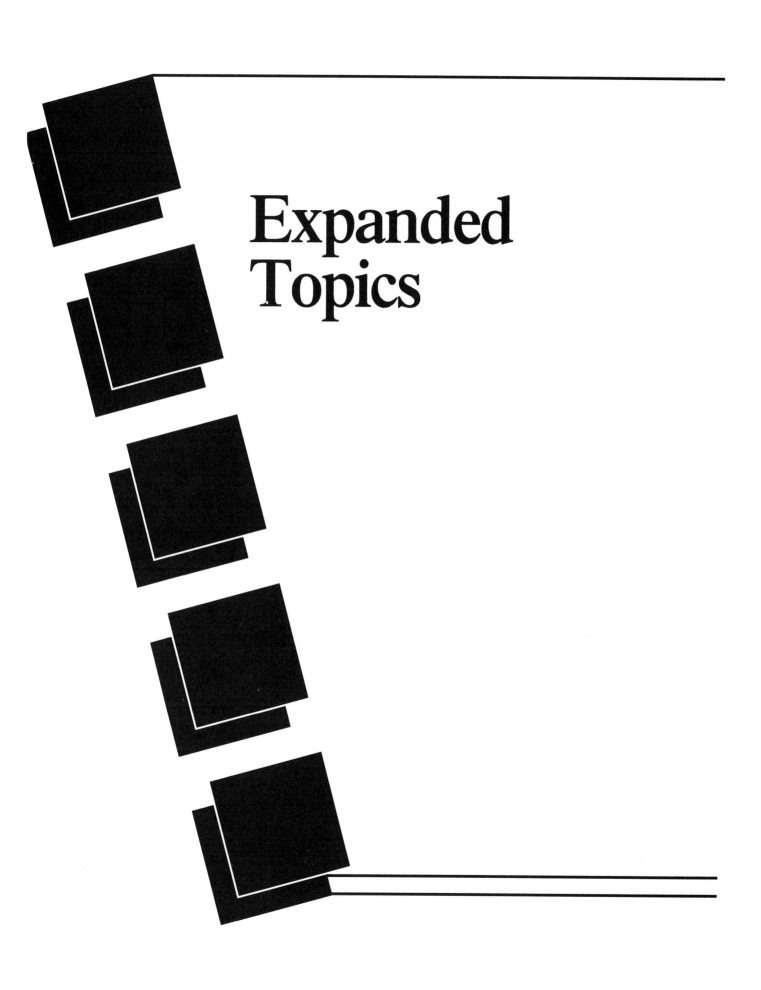

Expanded
Topics

Abortion, spontaneous

BASICS

DESCRIPTION Abortion is the separation of products of conception from the uterus prior to the potential for fetal survival outside the uterus. Gestationally, the point at which potential fetal viability exists has been the subject of much legal and scientific debate and definitions vary with locale and/or medical center; however, a "potentially viable" fetus is generally considered to weigh at least 500 grams and/or have a gestational age of greater than 20 weeks.
• Spontaneous abortion - refers to expulsion of all (complete abortion) or part (incomplete abortion) of the products of conception from the uterus prior to the 20th completed week of gestation. Incomplete abortion tends to occur more often after the 10th gestational week, when the placenta and the fetus tend to be expelled separately. The placenta, either in whole or in part, can be retained and leads to continuing vaginal bleeding (sometimes profuse). Abortion is "threatened" when vaginal bleeding occurs early in pregnancy, with or without uterine contractions, but without dilatation of the cervix, rupture of the membranes, or expulsion of products of conception. Cervical dilation, rupture of membranes or expulsion of products in the presence of vaginal bleeding portends "inevitable abortion."
• Must differentiate between threatened and inevitable abortion since management differs.
• Induced abortion - refers to the evacuation of uterine contents/products of conception by either medical or surgical methodology
• Missed abortion - occurs with the retention of embryonic or fetal parts for eight weeks or more following embryonic or fetal demise
• Infected abortion - infection involving the products of conception and the maternal reproductive organs
• Septic abortion - dissemination of bacteria (and/or their toxins) into the maternal circulatory and organ system
• Habitual spontaneous abortion - three or more consecutive spontaneous abortions. Although repeated spontaneous abortions are often "chance" occurrences, many investigators recommend karyotyping of the parents and maternal evaluation for abnormalities (such as incompetent cervix) in cases of habitual abortion.
System(s) affected: Reproductive
Genetics: Fetal (and to a much lesser extent maternal) chromosomal abnormalities greatly increase the incidence of spontaneous abortion
Incidence/Prevalence in USA:
• Estimated that 45-60% of all fertilized ova are spontaneously aborted. Most spontaneous abortions are clinically unrecognized because the fertilized/implanted ovum is expelled at or near the first missed period (i.e., prior to the traditional "hallmark" of potential pregnancy - amenorrhea).
• Approximately 10-15% of all recognized pregnancies (and 30% of all first pregnancies) end in clinically apparent spontaneous abortion

Predominant age:
• Young (≤ 15 years) and over 35 years of age
• Incidence of induced abortion tends to decrease with age
Predominant sex: Female only

SIGNS AND SYMPTOMS

In a previously diagnosed intrauterine pregnancy
◊ Vaginal bleeding (pink or brownish discharge)
◊ Uterine cramping
◊ Cervical dilation
◊ Ruptured membranes
◊ Passage of non-viable products of conception
◊ Fever
◊ Shock
◊ Soft, sub-involuted uterus

CAUSES
• The cause of most spontaneous abortions is unknown
• Defective germ plasm
• Improper implantation of fertilized ovum
• Abnormality of maternal reproductive organs
• Endocrine dysfunction
• Infectious systemic disease
• Poisons (including drugs)
• Placental insufficiency abnormality
• Defective spermatozoa
• Trauma
• Therapeutic or criminal intervention

RISK FACTORS
• Fetal chromosomal abnormalities (100-fold increase in spontaneous abortion)
• Uterine abnormalities
• Maternal alcohol/drug ingestion
• Increasing maternal age
• Deteriorating health status (i.e., diabetes/thyroid disease)
• Infections with certain viruses or bacteria

DIAGNOSIS

DIFFERENTIAL DIAGNOSIS
• Ectopic pregnancy - a potentially life-threatening complication, difficult to distinguish from threatened abortion. Ultrasound can quickly distinguish ectopic vs. intrauterine pregnancy. Culdocentesis may demonstrate free peritoneal blood.
• Cervical polyps, neoplasias, and/or inflammatory conditions can cause vaginal bleeding. This bleeding is not usually associated with pain/cramping and is readily apparent on speculum exam.
• Hydatidiform mole pregnancy usually ends in abortion prior to the 20th week of pregnancy. Bloody discharge prior to abortion is common. An intrauterine grape-like appearing mass on the ultrasound is diagnostic. HCG is often positive.
• Membranous dysmenorrhea - characterized by bleeding, cramps and passage of endometrial casts can mimic spontaneous abortion. Human chorionic gonadotropin (HCG) is negative.

LABORATORY
• Cultures - for group B Streptococcus, gonorrhea and chlamydia
• Decreased hemoglobin
• Decreased hematocrit
Human chorionic gonadotropin (HCG) - presumptive detection of pregnancy
◊ HCG (or its beta-subunit BHCG) can be assayed in urine and plasma, qualitatively and quantitatively
◊ Tests for the early detection of pregnancy detect HCG in concentrated urine within two weeks of ovulation
◊ Plasma assays of BHCG can provide presumptive evidence of pregnancy at implantation - one week after ovulation and one week prior to the first missed period
Human chorionic gonadotropin (HCG) - assessment of fetal viability
◊ HCG concentration in maternal plasma rises rapidly from the second through the ninth gestational week. If plasma HCG is stable or declining, fetal viability and/or normal pregnancy is doubtful
Drugs that may alter lab results:
• Plasma HCG - heparin anticoagulants or ethylenediaminotetraacetate acid (EDTA)
• Urine HCG - phenothiazines
Disorders that may alter lab results: Urine HCG - gross proteinuria, hematuria, elevated ESR

PATHOLOGICAL FINDINGS Conceptual fragments

SPECIAL TESTS N/A

IMAGING
• Ultrasound examination for fetal viability and to rule out ectopic pregnancy
• Ultrasound imaging can be sensitive enough to confirm an intrauterine pregnancy in the fourth or fifth gestational week

DIAGNOSTIC PROCEDURES
• Two positive signs of early pregnancy are identification of fetal heart sounds (usually accomplished by Doppler instrumentation at/or after the ninth week of gestation) and identification of fetal parts/gestational sac by ultrasound
• Presumptive signs of pregnancy - increasing uterine size with corresponding increase in abdominal size, softening of the cervix, amenorrhea, breast soreness/swelling, presence of HCG in urine or blood
• Sterile speculum exam to determine the source of bleeding. Obtain cultures for group B Streptococcus, gonorrhea and chlamydia. Obtain catheterized urine for urinalysis and culture.
• A bimanual exam to assess uterine size and consistency/dilation of the cervix
• Careful assessment for adnexal mass/tenderness
• Consider a diagnosis of spontaneous abortion in a woman, of childbearing age, presenting with abnormal vaginal bleeding

TREATMENT

APPROPRIATE HEALTH CARE
Outpatient or inpatient, depending on severity of symptoms

GENERAL MEASURES
• Explore all cases of first trimester vaginal bleeding
• Serial quantitative BHCG determination
• Threatened abortion: bed rest (usually at home) and insert nothing per vagina. If bleeding is more severe (i.e., more than a heavy period), hospitalization and close observation are advisable.
• Inevitable or incomplete abortion: Dilatation and curettage (D&C) (usually suction)
• Type and screen for possible transfusion requirements
• When completeness of an abortion is in doubt, a D&C for retained products should be performed

ACTIVITY
If appropriate, bed rest until resolution

DIET
No special diet

PATIENT EDUCATION
American College of Obstetricians & Gynecologists, 409 12th St., SW, Washington, DC 20024-2188, (800)762-ACOG

 MEDICATIONS

DRUG(S) OF CHOICE
• Bleeding following uncomplicated D&C/spontaneous abortion can usually be controlled by oxytocin (Pitocin) 3-10 units IM, or methylergonovine (Methergine) 0.2 mg IM
• Analgesics if needed
• Rh negative mother - give Rho D immune globulin
Contraindications: None
Precautions: Do not give methylergonovine IV. Refer to manufacturer's literature.
Significant possible interactions: Refer to manufacturer's literature

ALTERNATIVE DRUGS
N/A

 FOLLOWUP

PATIENT MONITORING
• Identification of products of conception within material expelled from the uterus confirms spontaneous abortion
• If abortion is complete, observe the patient for a period of time to check for further bleeding

PREVENTION/AVOIDANCE
• Any vaginal bleeding in a woman with a presumed or proven intrauterine pregnancy is abnormal and should be considered a "threatened" abortion until proven otherwise. In reality, vaginal bleeding during early pregnancy is fairly common and often the source of bleeding eludes diagnosis.
• In the event of habitual abortion, the abortus should be sent for karyotyping. Other causes of habitual abortion need to be explored with the couple to determine the best therapy techniques.
• Special care and attention for the patient who has a subsequent pregnancy
• Surgical reinforcement of cervix for habitual abortion

POSSIBLE COMPLICATIONS
• Complications of D&C include uterine perforation, infection and bleeding
• Repetitive abortion
• Depression and feelings of guilt (patient may need counseling help)

EXPECTED COURSE AND PROGNOSIS
• In cases of threatened abortion where bleeding ceases and parameters of pregnancy continue normal progression, maternal prognosis is excellent
• Following D&C for incomplete or inevitable abortion and following complete abortion, prognosis is excellent
• Habitual abortion - prognosis for successful pregnancy decreased

 MISCELLANEOUS

ASSOCIATED CONDITIONS
• Hypothyroidism
• Diabetes mellitus

AGE-RELATED FACTORS
Pediatric: N/A
Geriatric: N/A
Others: N/A

PREGNANCY
This problem confined to pregnancy

SYNONYMS
• Miscarriage
• Habitual abortion
• Recurrent abortion

ICD-9-CM
634.9

SEE ALSO
N/A

OTHER NOTES
N/A

ABBREVIATIONS
N/A

REFERENCES
• Cunningham, F.G., MacDonald, P.C. & Gant, N.F. (eds.): Williams Obstetrics. 18th Ed. Norwalk CT, Appleton and Lange, 1989
• Wilcox, A.J., et al.: Incidence of early loss of pregnancy. New Engl J Med, 1988; 319: 189-94
• Miller, J.F., et al.: Fetal loss after implantation: a prospective study. Lancet 1980; 2: 554-6
• Edmonds, D.K., et al.: Early embryonic mortality in women. Fert Sterility. 1982; 38: 447-53

Author K. Gebhardt, D.O. & C. Cote, M.D.

Abruptio placentae

 BASICS

DESCRIPTION Premature separation of otherwise normally implanted placenta. Sher's grade 1- minimal or no bleeding; detected as retroplacental clot after delivery of viable fetus. Sher's grade 2- viable fetus with bleeding and tender irritable uterus. Sher's grade 3- type A with dead fetus and no coagulopathy; type B with dead fetus and coagulopathy (about 30% of grade 3's).
System(s) affected: Reproductive, Cardiovascular
Genetics: N/A
Incidence/Prevalence in USA:
- 1% of all deliveries
- 15% if one prior episode
- 20% if ≥ 2 prior episodes
Predominant age: All childbearing ages
Predominant sex: Female only

SIGNS AND SYMPTOMS
- Third trimester vaginal bleeding greater than one pad or tampon per hour
- Back pain, abdominal pain
- Uterine contractions, tenderness and/or hypertonia
- Blood loss may be concealed; clinical signs of shock may exceed estimated blood loss
- Since blood volumes increase in pregnancy, volume lost may exceed 30% before signs of shock or hypovolemia. Vital signs may be preserved even with significant loss.
- Narrowed pulse pressure, increased diastolic pressure, positive tilt test, orthostatic changes, or tachycardia may be soft signs of volume depletion
- Difficulty hearing fetal heart tones or palpating fetus through a tender, tense, irritable uterus with bloody amniotic fluid
- Often constant pain with or without contractions
- In complete abruption, may find non-tender uterus

CAUSES
- Trauma of variable amounts; especially blunt abdominal trauma with anterior placental location in which external signs of trauma may be incongruent with fetal injury
- Sudden decompression of over-distended uterus as in hydramnios or twin gestation
- Cocaine use and abuse

RISK FACTORS
- Maternal smoking especially > 1 pack/day
- Multiparity
- Alcohol abuse
- Short umbilical cord
- Hypertension: pregnancy-induced and chronic
- Prior abruption
- Increased risk if hypertensive and parity >3
- Preterm rupture of membranes, especially if bleeding occurs during observation interval - 5%
- Vaginal bleeding before spontaneous rupture of membranes - 25%

 DIAGNOSIS

DIFFERENTIAL DIAGNOSIS Uterine rupture, placenta previa, vasa previa, marked bloody show, cervical and vaginal causes (e.g., chlamydia or gonorrhea with bloody, friable cervix), masses, other painful conditions (e.g., appendicitis, pyelonephritis), and labor.

LABORATORY
- Blood type, Rh, Coombs
- CBC with platelet count
- Prothrombin time (PT) , partial thromboplastin time (PTT), fibrinogen levels
- Cross match at least three units
Drugs that may alter lab results:
- Those affecting clotting parameters
- RhoD immune globulin less than 12 weeks prior may affect antibody test
Disorders that may alter lab results:
- Fibrinogen levels climb to 350-550 mg/dl in third trimester and must fall to 100-150 mg/dl before PTT will rise
- Fibrin split or degradation products are elevated in pregnancy so not very helpful in assessing disseminated intravascular coagulation (DIC)

PATHOLOGICAL FINDINGS
- Normocytic normochromic anemia with acute bleeding
- Elevated PT, PTT, fibrinogen levels below 100-150 mg/dl, platelets 20,000-50,000 if DIC active
- Positive Kleihauer-Betke reaction if fetal-maternal transfusion has occurred
- Positive antibody if RhoD isosensitization has occurred

SPECIAL TESTS
- Kleihauer-Betke for fetal-maternal transfusion
- Bedside clot test with red top tube of maternal blood with poor or non-clotting blood after 7-10 minutes indicating coagulopathy
- Apt test for fetal blood origin: mix vaginal blood with small amount tap water to cause hemolysis, centrifuge several minutes, mix pink hemoglobin containing supernatant with 1 cc 1% sodium hydroxide (NaOH) for each 5 cc supernatant, reading color in two minutes with fetal Hgb staying pink and adult turning yellow-brown
- Wright stain vaginal blood, observe for nucleated RBC's - usually of fetal origin
- Lecithin/sphingomyelin (L/S) ratio if delay of delivery is an option and length of pregnancy is preterm

IMAGING Although ultrasound may show sonolucent retroplacental clot, rounded placenta margin or thickened placenta, it is often not definitive - especially with posterior placement or mild abruption

DIAGNOSTIC PROCEDURES External uterine monitoring often shows elevated baseline pressure and frequent low amplitude contractions

 TREATMENT

APPROPRIATE HEALTH CARE
Hospitalize until stable

GENERAL MEASURES
- Remember a good history and physical with past medical history, allergies, prior ultrasounds this gestation, and time of last meal
- In general, severe abruption best managed by delivery of fetus
- Sher's grade 1- usual labor protocol
- Sher's grade 2- varies with situation urgency
- Sher's grade 3- vaginal delivery preferable if mother stable
- In trauma monitor inpatient at least 4 hours for evidence of fetal insult, abruption, fetal-maternal transfusion
- Early aggressive restoration of maternal physiology to protect fetus and maternal organs from hypoperfusion/DIC
- Stabilize vitals, keep Hct >30, urine output >30 cc/hr
- Bedrest with external fetal and labor monitoring, if fetus is viable
- Large bore 16-18 gauge IV crystalloid infusion, central line placement only after coagulation status has been assessed
- Attend to the basic ABC's with arterial blood gases (ABG) if acidosis suspected
- Follow hemoglobin/hematocrit (H/H) and coagulation status every 1-2 hours
- Place intrauterine pressure catheter (IUC) since fetal risk climbs with elevated pressure
- Role of amniotomy to prevent amniotic fluid embolism is debatable but will speed delivery
- Positioning on left side may enhance venous return and cardiac output up to 30%
- Oxygen for all patients since oxygen consumption up 20% in pregnancy and fetus especially hypoxia sensitive
- If trauma without compromise after observation or small abruption and preterm may observe outpatient encouraging reduction of risk factors
- May need c/s after maternal stabilization if fetus viable and situation urgent

ACTIVITY Bedrest until status defined

DIET NPO until status defined and cesarean section possibility ruled out

PATIENT EDUCATION In preterm mild abruption not necessitating delivery, teach about risks and causes

MEDICATIONS

DRUG(S) OF CHOICE
- Oxygen
- Saline or Ringer's lactate
- Whole blood and packed RBC's to keep hematocrit > 30
- May use Pitocin augmentation to speed delivery
- Tocolytics like terbutaline or ritodrine may be used in mild non-compromising preterm abruption
- RhoD immune globulin for RhoD negative mother if undelivered or indicated after delivery
- 300 mcg RhoD immune globulin/15 cc fetal blood transfused, if Kleihauer-Betke test returns positive
- Fresh frozen plasma and platelet transfusions for coagulopathy with cryoprecipitate and fibrinogen given if indicated

Contraindications: Tocolytics should be withheld in preterm labor until abruption ruled out and fetal status defined

Precautions:
- Suffusion of blood into myometrium with weakening may increase risk of uterine rupture with Pitocin augmentation
- Cryoprecipitate and fibrinogen may represent greater transfusion infection transmission risk

Significant possible interactions: Refer to manufacturer's profile of each drug

ALTERNATIVE DRUGS N/A

 ## FOLLOWUP

PATIENT MONITORING
- If not delivered, monitor for intrauterine growth retardation (IUGR)
- See regularly and assess for preterm labor

PREVENTION/AVOIDANCE Eliminate risk factors when possible

POSSIBLE COMPLICATIONS
- Infection transfusion risks: Hepatitis, cytomegalovirus infection, HIV and others
- Sensitization from blood product transfusion

EXPECTED COURSE AND PROGNOSIS
- 0.5% to 1% fetal mortality and 30-50% perinatal mortality
- With trauma and abruption 1% maternal and 30-70% fetal mortality
- Labor typically more rapid but hypotonus from blood suffusion may occur

 ## MISCELLANEOUS

ASSOCIATED CONDITIONS
- Preeclampsia and other forms of hypertension in pregnancy
- Hypertension from collagen diseases such as lupus erythematosus
- Postpartum hemorrhage
- Maternal and fetal organ damage from hypoperfusion

AGE-RELATED FACTORS
Pediatric: N/A
Geriatric: N/A
Others: Multiparity, advanced maternal age - more at risk

PREGNANCY This problem limited to pregnancy

SYNONYMS
- Placental abruption
- Premature separation of the placenta
- Couvelaire placenta

ICD-9-CM
641.2 Premature separation of placenta

SEE ALSO Placenta previa

OTHER NOTES
- Increased pregnancy pelvic flow may enhance blood loss
- Amniotic fluid embolism is rare but may present with DIC and severe respiratory distress
- Increased risk of fetal-maternal transfusion with trauma of anterior placenta

ABBREVIATIONS N/A

REFERENCES
- Scott, C.J., et al.: Emergencies in pregnancy. Patient Care. Aug 15,1991:132-150
- Lowe, T.W. et al.: Placental abruption. Clinical OB Gyn. Vol. 33, No 3, Sept. 1990

Author M. Sexton, M.D.

Acne rosacea

 BASICS

DESCRIPTION Chronic skin eruption with flushing and dilation of small blood vessels in the face, especially nose and cheeks
System(s) affected: Skin/Exocrine
Genetics: People of Northern European and Celtic background commonly afflicted
Incidence/Prevalence in USA: Common
Predominant age: 30-50
Predominant sex: Female > Male

SIGNS AND SYMPTOMS
• Skin flush - prominent at onset
• Redness - lower half of nose, sometimes whole nose, forehead, cheeks, chin
• Conjunctivae red - (sometimes)
• Erythema, dusky - (in advanced cases)
• Blood vessels in involved area collapse under pressure
• Acne lesions form papules, pustules, and nodules; comedones are rare
• Telangiectasia
• Rhinophyma (sometimes) more common in males

CAUSES
No proven cause. Possibilities include:
◊ Thyroid and gonadal disturbance
◊ Alcohol, coffee, tea, spiced food overindulgence (unproven)
◊ Demodex follicular parasite (suspected)
◊ Exposure to cold, heat, hot drinks
◊ Emotional stress
◊ Dysfunction of the gastrointestinal tract

RISK FACTORS   Listed with Causes

 DIAGNOSIS

DIFFERENTIAL DIAGNOSIS
• Drug eruptions (iodides and bromides)
• Granulomas of the skin
• Cutaneous lupus erythematosus
• Carcinoid syndrome
• Deep fungal infection
• Acne vulgaris
• Seborrheic dermatitis

LABORATORY   N/A
Drugs that may alter lab results: N/A
Disorders that may alter lab results: N/A

PATHOLOGICAL FINDINGS
• Inflammation around hypertrophied sebaceous glands, producing papules, pustules and cysts
• Absence of comedones and blocked ducts
• Vascular dilatation and dermal lymphocytic infiltrate

SPECIAL TESTS   N/A

IMAGING   N/A

DIAGNOSTIC PROCEDURES   N/A

 TREATMENT

APPROPRIATE HEALTH CARE
Outpatient

GENERAL MEASURES
• Reassurance
• Treat psychological stress if present
• Avoid oil based cosmetics. Others are acceptable and may help women tolerate the symptoms.
• Surgical treatment of rhinophyma
• Electrodessication of permanently dilated blood vessels

ACTIVITY   No restrictions. Support physical fitness.

DIET   Avoid any food or drink that causes facial flushing, e.g., hot drinks, spiced food, alcohol

PATIENT EDUCATION
• American Academy of Dermatology (708) 330-0230

MEDICATIONS

DRUG(S) OF CHOICE
• Low dose oral tetracycline 500-1000 mg/day
• Sulfur-containing local applications (Liquimat, Fostril, Rezamid, Sulfacet-R)
• Topical steroids should not be used as they may aggravate rosacea
• Topical metronidazole 0.75% gel - apply each morning and at bedtime to clean skin
• Topical erythromycin
• Topical clindamycin

Contraindications: Refer to manufacturer's literature

Precautions: Take tetracycline on empty stomach. Don't take with iron, antacids or milk.

Significant possible interactions: Refer to manufacturer's literature

ALTERNATIVE DRUGS
For severe cases, isotretinoin orally for 4 months. Extreme caution must be utilized as it is teratogenic. Pregnancy must be avoided while on the medication.

FOLLOWUP

PATIENT MONITORING
Occasional and as needed. Close followup for women using isotretinoin.

PREVENTION/AVOIDANCE
No preventive measure known

POSSIBLE COMPLICATIONS
• Rhinophyma (dilated follicles and thickened bulbous skin on nose), especially in men
• Conjunctivitis
• Blepharitis
• Keratitis

EXPECTED COURSE AND PROGNOSIS
• Slowly progressive
• Subsides spontaneously (sometimes)

MISCELLANEOUS

ASSOCIATED CONDITIONS
• Seborrheic dermatitis of scalp and eyelids
• Keratitis with photophobia, lacrimation, visual disturbance
• Corneal lesions
• Blepharitis
• Uveitis

AGE-RELATED FACTORS
Pediatric: Unlikely in this age group
Geriatric: Uncommon after age 60
Others: N/A

PREGNANCY
Use of oral isotretinoin contraindicated

SYNONYMS
Rosacea

ICD-9-CM
695.3 rosacea

SEE ALSO
N/A

OTHER NOTES
N/A

ABBREVIATIONS
N/A

REFERENCES
• Fitzpatrick, T.B. et al. (eds.): Dermatology In General Medicine. 3rd Ed. New York, McGraw-Hill, 1987
• Habif, T.: Clinical Dermatology. 2nd Ed. St. Louis, C.V. Mosby, 1990

Author J. Little, M.D.

Acne vulgaris

 BASICS

DESCRIPTION Acne is an androgenically stimulated, inflammatory disorder of the sebaceous glands, resulting in comedones, papules, inflammatory pustules and, occasionally, scarring
System(s) affected: Skin/Exocrine
Genetics: N/A
Incidence/Prevalence in USA: Virtually 100% of adolescents are affected to some degree. 15% will seek medical advice.
Predominant age: Early to late puberty, although some cases will persist into the third and fourth decade
Predominant sex: Male = Female (males tend to be more severely affected)

SIGNS AND SYMPTOMS
- Closed comedones (whiteheads)
- Open comedones (blackheads)
- Nodules or papules
- Pustules, with or without redness and edema ("cysts")
- Scars
- The lesions occur over the forehead, cheeks and nose, and may extend over the central chest and back

CAUSES Androgens stimulate the rate of keratin turnover in the sebaceous gland. The keratin plug, visible as a comedone, causes an accumulation of sebum in the gland. The presence of Propionibacterium acnes stimulates an inflammatory response to the sebum, which results in papule and pustule formation.

RISK FACTORS
- Adolescence
- Male sex
- Androgenic steroids, e.g., steroid abuse, some birth control pills
- Oily cosmetics, including cleansing creams, moisturizers, oil-based foundations
- Rubbing or occluding the skin surface, as may occur with sports equipment (helmets and shoulder pads), holding the telephone or hands against the skin
- Drugs - iodides or bromides, lithium, phenytoins
- Systemic corticosteroids
- Virilization disorders
- Hot, humid climate

 DIAGNOSIS

DIFFERENTIAL DIAGNOSIS
- Occupational exposure to tars, oils, grease
- Folliculitis
- Acne rosacea
- Steroid acne
- Perioral acne

LABORATORY N/A
Drugs that may alter lab results: N/A
Disorders that may alter lab results: N/A

PATHOLOGICAL FINDINGS
- Oiliness, thickening of the skin
- Hypertrophy of the sebaceous glands
- Perifolliculitis
- Scarring

SPECIAL TESTS Testosterone and its metabolites can be measured in those very rare cases when acne arises de novo in the previously unaffected adult

IMAGING N/A

DIAGNOSTIC PROCEDURES History and physical exam

 TREATMENT

APPROPRIATE HEALTH CARE
Outpatient

GENERAL MEASURES
- Comedone extraction - using a comedone extractor, after incising the thin layer of epithelium directly over the comedone
- Intralesional injection - of large cystic lesions with 0.5-1.0 mL of triamcinolone (Kenalog 20)
- Cleansing - gentle cleansing with a mild soap once or twice a day will control surface oiliness. More frequent washing will further irritate the skin and increase sebum production.
- Oil-free sun blocks - although UV light results in some improvement in untreated acne, it will react adversely with the medications used to treat acne. Long-term UV exposure causes permanent skin damage.
- Stress management - may be helpful for those whose acne flares under stress

ACTIVITY Full activity. Physical conditioning important.

DIET
- Counsel regarding good nutrition
- No special diet has been shown to diminish acne. Chocolate and fatty foods do not aggravate acne.

PATIENT EDUCATION
- It is important for the patient to know that there is no cure for acne, that treatment only controls the lesions
- Any treatment measure takes a minimum of 4 weeks to show results
- The topical agents can cause redness and drying of the skin and most people need encouragement to persist with these useful agents
- For patient education materials favorably reviewed on this topic: American Academy of Dermatology, 930 N. Meacham Rd., P.O. Box 4014, Schaumburg, IL 60168-4014, (708)330-0230

MEDICATIONS

DRUG(S) OF CHOICE
• Topical medications, best for comedones and mild inflammatory acne
• Benzyl peroxide starting at 5%, applied to dry skin at bedtime.
• Retinoic acid starting with .025% cream, applied to dry skin at bedtime. Gel is available and is more drying; better for chest and back. Retinoic acid often causes an initial flare of lesions as it increases the turnover of previously formed keratin plugs.
• Topical erythromycin applied to cystic lesions, or
• Clindamycin, 2% solution in water, often helps cystic acne lesions
• Tetracycline 250 mg qid for 7-10 days, then tapering to the lowest effective dose
• Erythromycin 250 mg qid for 7-10 days, then tapering to the lowest effective dose
• Oral contraceptives, especially those with a very low androgenic activity
• Isotretinoin (Accutane), although associated with serious, dose-related side effects, can help patients who have severe pustular acne in spite of all the previous measures. Dosage is 0.5-1.0 mg/kg/day, in two doses, given for 12-16 weeks. A second course can be given after an 8-week interval. Common side effects include very dry skin, mucous membranes and cheilitis in effective doses, and lipid and liver function abnormalities.

Contraindications:
• Allergy
• Severe hepatic dysfunction - all oral agents

Precautions:
• Refer to manufacturer's literature
• Isotretinoin: causes severe fetal malformations; effective contraception should be ensured one month prior to and one month following isotretinoin therapy.

Significant possible interactions:
• Tetracycline
  ◊ Dairy products, antacids: decreased absorption of tetracycline due to chelation by calcium and magnesium cations
• Erythromycin
  ◊ terfenidine (Seldane): ECG abnormalities

ALTERNATIVE DRUGS   See previous discussion

FOLLOWUP

PATIENT MONITORING
• Monthly visits until adequate response is obtained
• Pre-treatment and monthly serum lipids, liver function tests, and pregnancy tests for patients on isotretinoin

PREVENTION/AVOIDANCE   N/A

POSSIBLE COMPLICATIONS
• Acne conglobata - a severe confluent inflammatory acne with systemic symptoms
• Facial scarring
• Psychological scarring

EXPECTED COURSE AND PROGNOSIS   Gradual improvement over time

MISCELLANEOUS

ASSOCIATED CONDITIONS
• See risk factors
• Androgen-secreting tumors

AGE-RELATED FACTORS
Pediatric: Mild, self-limited acne can occur in the neonate
Geriatric: N/A
Others: N/A

PREGNANCY
• May result in a flare, or remission, of acne
• Isotretinoin: causes severe fetal malformations; effective contraception should be ensured one month prior to and one month following isotretinoin therapy.
• Erythromycin can be used during pregnancy, but would prefer topical agents whenever possible.

SYNONYMS   N/A

ICD-9-CM
706.1 Other acne

SEE ALSO   Acne rosacea

OTHER NOTES
• Acne is usually much more significant to the patient than it appears to the doctor
• Mother Nature cures acne in time; we only control it
• Acne is often an "entry ticket;" frequently the adolescent also wants advice about life-style, contraception, physiology, etc.

ABBREVIATIONS   N/A

REFERENCES
• Fitzpatrick, T.B. et al.: Color atlas and synopsis of clinical dermatology. New York, McGraw-Hill, 1983
• Fitzpatrick, T.B. et al. (eds.): Dermatology In General Medicine. 3rd Ed. New York, McGraw-Hill, 1987
• Pochi, P.E. & Quan, M.: Acne Vulgaris. Amer Fam Phys Monograph, Spring, 1992

Author   D. Andres, M.D.

Addison's disease

 BASICS

DESCRIPTION Adrenal hypofunction resulting from primary disease of the adrenal gland. The inadequate secretion of glucocorticoids and mineralocorticoids is caused by partial or complete destruction of the adrenal glands. An autoimmune process is the most common cause (80% of the cases) followed by tuberculosis. AIDS is becoming a more frequent cause.
• Addisonian (adrenal) crisis - acute complication of adrenal insufficiency (circulatory collapse, dehydration, nausea, vomiting, hypoglycemia)

System(s) affected: Endocrine/Metabolic
Genetics: Autoimmune adrenal insufficiency shows some hereditary disposition. Autosomal recessive pattern has been suggested.
Incidence/Prevalence: Approximately 4:100,000
Predominant age: All ages
Predominant sex: Females > Males

SIGNS AND SYMPTOMS
• Weakness
• Fatigue
• Weight loss
• Orthostatic hypotension
• Increased pigmentation (tanning, freckles, vitiligo, blue-black discolorations of areolas and mucous membranes)
• Anorexia
• Vomiting
• Diarrhea
• Decreased cold tolerance
• Dizziness
• Blood pressure low

CAUSES
• Autoimmune adrenal insufficiency
• Idiopathic atrophy of the adrenal cortex
• Tuberculosis
• Fungal disease (histoplasmosis, blastomycosis, coccidioidomycosis)
• Sarcoidosis
• Adrenal hemorrhage
• Hemochromatosis
• Bilateral adrenalectomy
• Neoplasm
• Amyloidosis
• Inflammatory necrosis
• AIDS
• Adrenoleukodystrophy

RISK FACTORS
• Family history of autoimmune adrenal insufficiency. About 40% of patients have a first- or second-degree relative with one of the associated disorders.
• Taking steroids for prolonged periods; then, experiencing severe infection, trauma or surgical procedures

 DIAGNOSIS

DIFFERENTIAL DIAGNOSIS
• Varying myopathies
• Other causes of hypoglycemia
• Syndrome of inappropriate antidiuretic hormone
• Salt-losing nephritis
• Bronchogenic carcinoma
• Heavy metal ingestion
• Hemochromatosis
• Anorexia nervosa
• Sprue syndrome
• Hyperparathyroidism

LABORATORY
• Low serum sodium (< 130 meq/L)
• High serum potassium (> 5 meq/L)
• Elevated BUN
• Depressed cortisol level, high renin level (radioimmunoassay)
• Elevated ACTH level
• Urea nitrogen elevated
• Moderate neutropenia (about 5000/µL)
Drugs that may alter lab results: Digitalis
Disorders that may alter lab results: Diabetes mellitus

PATHOLOGICAL FINDINGS Atrophic adrenals

SPECIAL TESTS
• Cosyntropin 0.25mg IV: measure pre-injection and postinjection cortisol level. Patients with Addison's disease have low or normal values that do not rise.

IMAGING
• Abdominal CT scan:
  ◊ small adrenal glands (idiopathic atrophy or long-standing TB)
  ◊ enlarged adrenal glands (early TB or potentially treatable disease)
• Abdominal x-ray: may show adrenal calcifications
• Chest x-ray: may show adrenal calcification, heart size decreased

DIAGNOSTIC PROCEDURES A work-up to determine the cause of Addison's disease

 TREATMENT

APPROPRIATE HEALTH CARE
• Outpatient
• Inpatient during adrenal crisis

GENERAL MEASURES
• Treatment for adrenal insufficiency is with glucocorticoid and mineralocorticoid replacement
• Appropriate treatment for underlying cause (e.g., tuberculosis)

ACTIVITY As tolerated

DIET Arrange for a diet that maintains sodium and potassium balances

PATIENT EDUCATION
• For patient education materials favorably reviewed on this topic, contact: National Addison's Disease Foundation, 505 Northern Blvd., Suite 200, Great Neck, NY 11021, (516)487-4992
• Patient should wear or carry medical identification with information about the disease and the need for hydrocortisone or other replacement therapy
• Instruct patient in self-administering of parenteral hydrocortisone for emergency situations (e.g., traveling in remote areas away from medical help)

MEDICATIONS

DRUG(S) OF CHOICE
For chronic adrenal insufficiency:
◊ Hydrocortisone 10 mg orally each morning and 5 mg each afternoon (dosage is variable - may require 20-30 mg of hydrocortisone per day in adults [children's dosage is less]),PLUS,
◊ Fludrocortisone 0.1-0.2 mg orally once/day
Therapy of stress
◊ During acute illness, or following minor trauma - double the steroid dosage until well
◊ For surgery - adjust dosage preoperative and postoperative as needed
Adrenal crisis
◊ Precipitated by infection, trauma, surgery, salt loss: profound asthenia, peripheral vascular collapse, renal shutdown, severe abdominal pains, subnormal temperature
◊ Treat immediately with hydrocortisone 100 mg IV over 30 seconds
◊ Follow with 1 L 5% dextrose in normal saline over 2 hours. Repeat to total dosage of 300 mg of hydrocortisone in 24 hours.
◊ Identify and correct any precipitating factor
Contraindications: Refer to manufacturer's literature
Precautions:
• Patients with hepatic disease may need a reduced dose
• Elderly should have a slightly reduced dose
• Refer to manufacturer's literature for other precautions
Significant possible interactions: Refer to manufacturer's literature

ALTERNATIVE DRUGS
Prednisone 5 mg in AM and 2.5 mg at hs

FOLLOWUP

PATIENT MONITORING
• Verify adequacy of therapy - normal blood pressure, serum electrolytes normal, normal plasma renin, improvement of appetite and strength, increase in heart size to normal, normal blood glucose fasting level
• Lifelong medical supervision for signs of continued adequate therapy and avoidance of overdose

PREVENTION/AVOIDANCE
• No preventive measures known for Addison's disease
Prevention of complications
◊ Anticipate adrenal crisis and treat before symptoms begin
◊ If nausea and vomiting preclude oral therapy, patient should seek medical help to start parenteral therapy
◊ Elective surgical procedures require adjustment in steroid dose
◊ Prevent exposure to infections

POSSIBLE COMPLICATIONS
• Hyperpyrexia
• Psychotic reactions
• Complications from underlying disease
• Over- or under-steroid treatment
• Hyperkalemic paralysis (rare)
• Addisonian crisis

EXPECTED COURSE AND PROGNOSIS
• Good outlook with appropriate treatment. With adequate replacement therapy, life expectancy approximates normal
• Active tuberculosis or fungal disease responds to specific chemotherapy

MISCELLANEOUS

ASSOCIATED CONDITIONS
• Diabetes mellitus
• Thyrotoxicosis
• Thyroiditis
• Hypoparathyroidism
• Pernicious anemia
• Ovarian failure
• Hypercalcemia
• Chronic moniliasis
• Schmidt's syndrome (multiple endocrine deficiency syndrome)
• Adrenoleukodystrophy

AGE-RELATED FACTORS
Pediatric:
• Hydrocortisone and fludrocortisone doses are lower than adults
• More difficult to diagnose
• Occurs in siblings
Geriatric: Acute adrenal crisis more likely
Others: N/A

PREGNANCY N/A

SYNONYMS
• Adrenocortical insufficiency
• Waterhouse-Friederickson syndrome (adrenal crisis)

ICD-9-CM 255.4

SEE ALSO N/A

OTHER NOTES N/A

ABBREVIATIONS N/A

REFERENCES
• Felig, P., Baxter, J.D., Broadus, A.E., et al. (eds.): Endocrinology and Metabolism. 2nd Ed. New York, McGraw-Hill, 1987
• Hershman, J.M.: Endocrine Pathophysiology: A Patient-Oriented Approach. 3rd Ed. Philadelphia, Lea & Febiger, 1988

Author E. Lightner, M.D.

Adenovirus infections

 BASICS

DESCRIPTION Usually a self-limited febrile illnesses characterized by inflammation of conjunctivae and the respiratory tract. Adenovirus infections occur in epidemic and endemic situations.

Common types
◊ Acute febrile respiratory illness (AFRI) affecting primarily children
◊ Acute respiratory disease (ARD) affecting adults, particularly military recruits
◊ Viral pneumonia affecting children and adults
◊ Acute pharyngoconjunctival fever (APC) affecting children, particularly after summer swimming
◊ Acute follicular conjunctivitis affecting all ages
◊ Epidemic keratoconjunctivitis (EKC) affecting adults
◊ Intestinal infections leading to enteritis, mesenteric adenitis and intussusception

System(s) affected: Pulmonary, Gastrointestinal, Renal/Urologic, Nervous, Hemic/Lymphatic/Immunologic, Musculoskeletal, Cardiovascular

Genetics: N/A

Incidence/Prevalence in USA: Very common infection, estimated at 2-5% of all respiratory infections. More common in infants and children.

Predominant age: All ages

Predominant sex: Male = Female

SIGNS AND SYMPTOMS
• Depends on type (see "Differential diagnosis")
In common with most respiratory forms:
• Headache
• Malaise
• Sore throat
• Cough
• Fever (moderate to high)
• Vomiting
• Diarrhea
• Mucosa exhibits patches of white exudate

CAUSES
• Adenovirus (DNA viruses 60-90 nm in size with 42 known serotypes)
• Different serotypes have different epidemiologies
Most common known pathogens are:
◊ Types 1, 2, 3, 5, 7 cause respiratory illness
◊ Type 3 causes pharyngoconjunctival fever
◊ Types 4, 7, 21 cause acute respiratory disease in military camps
◊ Several other types may cause epidemic keratoconjunctivitis

RISK FACTORS
• Large number of people gathered in a small area (military recruits, college students at the beginning of the school year, daycare centers, community swimming pools, etc.)
• Immunocompromised at risk for severe disease

 DIAGNOSIS

DIFFERENTIAL DIAGNOSIS
• Early diagnosis depends on clinical evaluation
The following are the primary characteristics of the major adenovirus infections.

Acute febrile respiratory illness:
◊ Nonspecific cold-like symptoms, similar to other viral respiratory illnesses (fever, pharyngitis, tracheitis, bronchitis, pneumonitis)
◊ Mostly in children
◊ Incubation period 2 to 5 days
◊ May be pertussis-like syndrome rarely

Acute respiratory disease:
◊ Malaise, fever, chills, headache, pharyngitis, hoarseness and dry cough
◊ Occurs mostly in military recruits
◊ Fever lasts 2 to 4 days
◊ Illness subsides in 10 to 14 days

Viral pneumonia
◊ Sudden onset of high fever, rapid infection of upper and lower respiratory tracts, skin rash, diarrhea
◊ Occurs in children aged a few days up to 3 years
◊ Common; severe illness occurs in subset

Acute pharyngoconjunctival fever
◊ Spiking fever lasting several days, headache, pharyngitis, conjunctivitis, rhinitis, cervical adenitis
◊ Conjunctivitis is usually unilateral
◊ Subsides in about 1 week

Epidemic keratoconjunctivitis
◊ Usually unilateral onset of ocular redness and edema, preorbital edema, preorbital swelling, local discomfort suggestive of foreign body
◊ Lasts 3 or 4 weeks

LABORATORY
• Viral cultures from respiratory, ocular or fecal sources can establish diagnosis
• Antigen detection in stool for enteric serotypes is available
• Serologic procedures such as complement fixation with a four fold rise in serum antibody titer identifies recent adenoviral infection

Drugs that may alter lab results: N/A
Disorders that may alter lab results: N/A

PATHOLOGICAL FINDINGS
• Varies with each virus, severe pneumonia may be reflected by extensive intranuclear inclusions
• Bronchiolitis obliterans may occur

SPECIAL TESTS Cultures and serologic studies if appropriate

IMAGING X-ray: bronchopneumonia in severe respiratory infections

DIAGNOSTIC PROCEDURES
• Biopsy (lung or other) may be needed in severe or unusual cases

 TREATMENT

APPROPRIATE HEALTH CARE Ambulatory except for severely ill infants or those with epidemic keratoconjunctivitis or infants with severe pneumonia

GENERAL MEASURES Treatment is supportive and symptomatic. Infections are usually benign and of short duration.

ACTIVITY Rest during febrile phases

DIET No special diet

PATIENT EDUCATION Avoid aspirin in children. Give instructions for nasal spray, cough preparations, frequent hand washing.

MEDICATIONS

DRUG(S) OF CHOICE
• Acetaminophen, 10-15 mg/kg/dose, for analgesia (avoid aspirin)
• Topical corticosteroids for conjunctivitis (after consulting an ophthalmologist)
• Cough suppressants and/or expectorants
Contraindications: Refer to manufacturer's literature
Precautions: Refer to manufacturer's literature
Significant possible interactions: Refer to manufacturer's literature

ALTERNATIVE DRUGS   N/A

FOLLOWUP

PATIENT MONITORING   For severe infantile pneumonia and conjunctivitis: daily physical exam until well

PREVENTION/AVOIDANCE
• Live types 4 and 7 adenovirus vaccine orally in enteric coated capsule reduces incidence of acute respiratory disease in recruits
• Frequent hand washing among office personnel and family members

POSSIBLE COMPLICATIONS
• Few if any recognizable long-term problems

EXPECTED COURSE AND PROGNOSIS
• Self-limited, usually without sequelae
• Severe illness and death in very young and in immunocompromised hosts

MISCELLANEOUS

ASSOCIATED CONDITIONS
• Hemorrhagic cystitis (can be caused by adenovirus)
• Viral enteritis
• Intussusception and mesenteric adenitis

AGE-RELATED FACTORS
Pediatric: Viral pneumonia in infants may be fatal
Geriatric: Complications more likely
Others: N/A

PREGNANCY   No special precautions

SYNONYMS   N/A

ICD-9-CM   079.0

SEE ALSO
• Conjunctivitis
• Intussesception
• Pneumonia, viral

OTHER NOTES   Conjunctivitis sometimes called "pink eye".

ABBREVIATIONS   N/A

REFERENCES
• Mandell, G.L. (ed.): Principles and Practice of Infectious Diseases. 3rd Ed. New York, Churchill Livingstone, 1990
• Fields, B.N. & Knipe, D.M. (eds.): Virology. 2nd Ed. New York, Raven Press, 1989

Author   BL Wiedermann, MD

Alcoholism (part 1)

BASICS

DESCRIPTION Alcoholism is an illness characterized by significant impairment that is directly associated with persistent and excessive use of alcohol. Impairment may involve physiological, psychological or social dysfunction.
System(s) affected: Nervous, Gastrointestinal
Genetics: Twin and adoption studies strongly support a genetic influence
Incidence/Prevalence in USA:
• 10% of men; 3.5% of women
• 7% of all drinkers have 3 or more symptoms of dependence
• Lifetime prevalence for adults of 11.5-15.7%
Predominant age:
• All ages
• Highest prevalence of drinking problems is in the 18-29 age group. Subgroups of some age categories have higher prevalence rates.
Predominant sex: Males > Female (slightly)

SIGNS AND SYMPTOMS
Behavioral
• Psychological and social dysfunction (early or late finding)
• Marital problems, divorce or separation
• Anxiety, depression, insomnia
• Social isolation or frequent moves to new areas
• Child or spouse abuse
• Alcohol related arrests or legal problems (less likely in women)
• Preoccupation with recreational drinking
• Repeated attempts to stop or reduce drinking
• Loss of interest in non-drinking activities
• Employment problems (tardiness, absenteeism, decreased productivity, interpersonal problems at work, frequent job changes)
• Blackouts (not remembering what happened during drinking spells)
• Complaints by family members or friends about alcohol related behavior

Physical
• Gastrointestinal - anorexia, nausea, vomiting, abdominal pain, stigmata of chronic liver disease, peptic ulcer disease, pancreatitis, gastrointestinal malignancies
• Cardiovascular - modest hypertension (e.g., 140/95 mm Hg), arrhythmias or palpitations (supraventricular), cardiomyopathy
• Respiratory - aspiration pneumonia, bronchitis and chronic pulmonary disease from associated cigarette smoking
• Genitourinary - impotence, menstrual irregularities, testicular atrophy
• Endocrine/metabolic - hypercholesterolemia, hypertriglyceridemia, cushingoid appearance, gynecomastia
• Dermatologic - signs of accidents and trauma, burns (esp. cigarette burns), bruises in various stages of healing, poor hygiene
• Musculoskeletal - old fractures and fractures in various stages of healing, myopathy
• Neurologic - cognitive deficits (e.g., mild impairment of recent memory), peripheral neuropathy, Wernicke-Korsakoff syndrome
• HEENT - plethoric facies, parotid hypertrophy, poor oral hygiene, head and neck malignancies

CAUSES
• Alcoholism is a complex disease with a multifactorial etiology including biological, psychological and sociocultural factors
• Possible biologic markers - brain neuro transmitters, cell membrane receptors, enzyme systems (monoamine oxidase and adenylate cyclase)
• No evidence for a characteristic personality predisposition

RISK FACTORS
• Anyone who drinks alcohol
• Use of other psychoactive drugs, including nicotine
• Family history of alcohol abuse
• Young single male
• Heavy drinking - defined as, five or more drinks in one sitting, getting drunk at least once per week
• Peer group pressure
• Family or sociocultural background promoting intoxication or accepting it as a norm
• Increased accessibility of alcohol
• Adolescents (alcohol and drug use by peers or parents, delinquency, sociopathy in the parents, poor self-esteem, social nonconformity, and stressful life changes)

DIAGNOSIS

DIFFERENTIAL DIAGNOSIS
• Wide variety of medical and psychiatric disorders
• Depression
• Anxiety states
• Bipolar or manic-depressive disease
• Essential hypertension
• Peptic ulcer disease
• Viral gastroenteritis
• Ischemic heart disease
• Cholelithiasis or viral hepatitis
• Diabetes
• Pancreatitis or cholelithiasis
• Hyperlipidemia
• Solar skin damage
• Breast tumor
• Primary endocrine disorder
• Primary seizure disorder

LABORATORY
• Three laboratory findings diagnostic of alcoholism, others are only suggestive, and when present, indicate advanced alcoholism
Blood alcohol concentration:
  ◊ > 0.1 mg percent during any office visit
  ◊ > 0.15 mg percent without obvious signs of intoxication
  ◊ > 0.30 mg percent at any time
Suggestive - if increased:
  ◊ Gamma-glutamyl transferase (GGT)
  ◊ Alanine aminotransferase (ALT)
  ◊ Aspartate aminotransferase (AST)
  ◊ Alkaline phosphatase
  ◊ Lactate dehydrogenase (LDH)
  ◊ Bilirubin (total)
  ◊ Amylase
  ◊ Uric acid
  ◊ Triglycerides
  ◊ Cholesterol (total and high density lipoprotein fraction)
  ◊ Mean corpuscular volume
  ◊ Prothrombin time
Suggestive - if decreased:
  ◊ Calcium
  ◊ Phosphorus
  ◊ Magnesium
  ◊ Blood urea nitrogen
  ◊ White blood cell count
  ◊ Platelet count
  ◊ Hematocrit
  ◊ Protein deficiency
  ◊ Coagulopathy
Drugs that may alter lab results: See manufacturer's profile for each drug patient takes
Disorders that may alter lab results: Liver, heart, and kidney diseases

PATHOLOGICAL FINDINGS
• Liver - inflammation or fatty infiltration (alcoholic hepatitis), periportal fibrosis (alcoholic cirrhosis - occurs in only 20% of alcoholics)
• Gastric mucosa - inflammation, ulceration
• Pancreas - inflammation, liquefaction necrosis
• Intestine - flattening of villi, loss of enzymes
• Heart - interstitial fibrosis and myofibril atrophy (identical to other dilated cardiomyopathies)
• Immune system - depression of granulocyte production, lymphocyte proliferation response, and cell-mediated immunity
• Endocrine organs - elevated plasma cortisol levels, testicular atrophy, suppression of reproductive hormones in women
• Brain - cortical atrophy, enlarged ventricles

SPECIAL TESTS
Psychological tests:
◊ Michigan Alcohol Screening Test (MAST): 25 item questionnaire, score > 5 indicates alcoholism, sensitivity 90%, specificity 74%
◊ Short MAST (SMAST): shortened version of the MAST, 13 questions, score > 3 indicates alcoholism, sensitivity 70%, specificity similar to MAST
◊ CAGE: 4 questions, lower sensitivity and specificity, easily administered during a clinical interview, score > 2 suggests alcoholism
Biologic tests:
◊ Mitochondrial AST-to-total AST ratio (still investigational, limited availability, sensitivity 85-100%, specificity 81%)
◊ Acetate (still investigational, limited availability, sensitivity 65%, specificity 92%)

IMAGING
• X-ray - multiple old rib fractures on chest x-ray suggests alcoholism
• CT scan, MRI of brain - cortical atrophy, structural lesions in the thalamic nucleus and basal forebrain

DIAGNOSTIC PROCEDURES Liver biopsy - for diagnosis of alcoholic hepatitis or cirrhosis

 TREATMENT

APPROPRIATE HEALTH CARE
Inpatient or outpatient depending on:
◊ Severity of alcoholism
◊ Risk of major alcohol withdrawal (delirium tremens)
◊ Patient's health
◊ Social situation
◊ In some cases, detoxification is done as an inpatient, with the remainder of treatment done as an outpatient
Indications for inpatient alcohol detoxification:
◊ Symptoms or complications of major withdrawal, history of delirium tremens
◊ Failure to complete prior outpatient detoxification
◊ Associated medical problem requiring hospitalization
◊ Significant psychiatric symptoms
◊ Depressive symptoms, particularly suicidal ideation
◊ Lack of physician or other care provider during withdrawal
◊ Lack of clear commitment to complete abstinence from alcohol
◊ Inadequate social support network (family/friends)

GENERAL MEASURES
• Supportive, non-judgmental attitude from the physician is critical in helping the patient to recognize their problems with alcohol and accept help
• Physicians not skilled in managing alcohol withdrawal, particularly when complicated by other drug use, may want to consult an addiction specialist

ACTIVITY Fully active as tolerated

DIET
• Well balanced diet (malnutrition from poor eating habits is common)
• Alcohol interferes with the metabolism of most vitamins
• Patients with alcoholic hepatitis or ketoacidosis may have specific vitamin deficiencies, particularly thiamine
• Other deficiencies include magnesium, phosphate and zinc

PATIENT EDUCATION
• Help the patient to understand that he is not to blame for having the disease of alcoholism, but that he is responsible for what he does or does not do about it
• Information, literature and emotional support (crisis hot line) available from local Alcoholics Anonymous group (number in phone book)

Alcoholism (part 2)

 MEDICATIONS

 FOLLOWUP

DRUG(S) OF CHOICE

For detoxification and management of alcohol withdrawal syndrome:

(dosage varies depending on the patient's tolerance to alcohol)

◊ Chlordiazepoxide (Librium)

◊ Diazepam (Valium)

◊ Lorazepam (Ativan) - for patients with severe liver disease

◊ Phenobarbital - used less often because of risk of respiratory depression

Detoxification adjunct:

Used, as adjuncts to (not in place of) benzodiazepines, in doses adequate to control withdrawal symptoms, suppress seizures and delirium tremens.

◊ Beta blockers (propranolol, atenolol) - for persistent sinus tachycardia when other withdrawal signs are controlled

◊ Clonidine - relieves symptoms of autonomic hyperactivity (tremor, tachycardia, hypertension)

To promote sobriety:

◊ Disulfiram - inhibits enzyme aldehyde dehydrogenase, causing build-up of blood acetaldehyde and a toxic reaction. Contraindicated if patient still in denial about alcoholism, and seeking a "quick fix", or if there is a serious medical condition or poor health status

Supplemental to all:

◊ Thiamine

Contraindications:

• Patients who continue to drink while taking detox medications

• See manufacturer's profile of each drug

Precautions:

• Use caution in patients with severe liver disease, organic pain, organic brain syndromes

• Monitor for nystagmus, ataxia, excessive somnolence, slurred speech, other signs of intoxication

• See manufacturer's profile of each drug

Significant Possible Interactions:

• Alcohol and benzodiazepines have additive effects

• Other sedative hypnotics

• See manufacturer's profile of each drug

ALTERNATIVE DRUGS N/A

PATIENT MONITORING

• During detoxification - daily visits, if in-patient, frequent monitoring of vital signs

• Soon after patient completes treatment program - more frequent visits, e.g. weekly

• As patient more established in recovery - less frequent visits

PREVENTION/AVOIDANCE

• Preventive counseling of patients with a family history of alcoholism or other risk factors

• Anticipatory guidance for patients at increased risk due to life changes

• Public health and education measures, e.g., raising drinking age and liquor taxes, non-alcohol youth activities, restrict alcohol advertisements to youth, teaching servers to monitor customers for intoxication and encourage less alcohol consumption

POSSIBLE COMPLICATIONS

• Relapse of drinking

• Wernicke-Korsakoff syndrome

• Alcoholic neuropathy

• Alcoholic dementia

• Increased susceptibility to infection

• Aseptic necrosis of the hip

• Malignancies - especially of gastrointestinal tract

• Cirrhosis (women develop it sooner than men)

EXPECTED COURSE AND PROGNOSIS

• Chronic relapsing disease

• Untreated, alcoholism is progressive and fatal

MISCELLANEOUS

ASSOCIATED CONDITIONS
• Nicotine addiction
• Depression, bipolar disorder and antisocial personality disorder
• Women - have associated reproductive tract disorders, history of sexual abuse or incest. Often a concurrent prescription drug abuse or dependence.

AGE-RELATED FACTORS
Pediatric:
• Substance abuse including alcohol has a profoundly negative impact on normal maturation and development, attainment of social, educational and occupational skills
• Signs and symptoms more often include depression, suicide thought or attempts, family disruption, disorderly behavior, violence or destruction of property, poor school or work performance, sexual promiscuity, social immaturity, lack of hobbies or interests, isolation, moodiness
• Usually multiple drug use
Geriatric:
• Alcoholism often missed, yet elderly receive highest proportion of alcohol related diagnoses when hospitalized
• More hidden due to social unacceptability
• Physicians less likely to suspect due to inaccurate stereotyping
• Self-reports of alcohol consumption inaccurate due to: Memory problems, difficulties in "mental averaging", high levels of denial
• Elderly more sensitive to the effects of alcohol
• Screening and assessment tools standarized on younger populations are often inappropriate
• Signs and symptoms may be different (often attributed to chronic medical problems, or dementia)
• Alcoholism beginning late in life may be related to life stresses
Others: N/A

PREGNANCY
• Alcohol is a teratogen - both morphological and behavioral
• Greatest teratogenic effect occurs during the early weeks of fetal development (woman may not know she is pregnant)
• Fetal alcohol syndrome (craniofacial abnormalities, mental retardation, major organ system malformations) occurs in infants born to women drinking heavily during pregnancy
• Fetal alcohol effects (more subtle morphologic abnormalities and cognitive-behavioral dysfunction)
• Many recommend women abstain when planning conception and throughout pregnancy

SYNONYMS
• Alcohol dependence
• Alcohol abuse
• Dipsomania
• Problem drinking

ICD-9-CM
303 Alcohol dependence syndrome
303.90 Other and unspecified alcohol dependence; unspecified drinking behavior

SEE ALSO N/A

OTHER NOTES N/A

ABBREVIATIONS N/A

REFERENCES
• Barnes, H., Aronson, M., Delbanco, T. (eds.): Alcoholism: A guide for the Primary Care Physician. (Frontiers of primary care). New York, Springer-Verlag, 1987
• Clark, W.: Alcoholism: Blocks to Diagnosis and Treatment. Am J Med. 71:275-286, 1981
• Johnson, B., Clark, W.: Alcoholism: a challenging physician-patient encounter. J Gen Internal Med. Vol 4 (Sept/Oct):445-452, 1989
• Hays, T., Spickard, A.: Alcoholism: early diagnosis and intervention. J Gen Internal Med. Vol 2 (Nov/Dec): 420-427, 1987
• Wallace, J.: The new disease model of alcoholism. West J Med. 152:502-505, 1990
• National Institute on Alcohol Abuse and Alcoholism. Seventh Special Report to the US Congress on Alcohol and Health. DHHS: Rockville, MD, 1990

Author M. Kerstitch, M.D.

Aldosteronism, primary

 BASICS

DESCRIPTION The clinical syndrome of hypertension, hypokalemia, low plasma renin activity, and increased aldosterone secretion
• Unilateral aldosterone-producing adenoma (APA) - most common form (60%) and cured with unilateral adrenalectomy
• Idiopathic hyperaldosteronism (IHA) due to bilateral zona glomerulosa hyperplasia - second most common form (34%); not cured with surgery. Chronic medical therapy is treatment of choice.
System(s) affected: Endocrine/Metabolic
Genetics: Unknown
Incidence/Prevalence in USA:
• 0.5 to 2% of the hypertensive population
Predominant age: Usually diagnosed third to sixth decades
Predominant sex: APA more common in women

SIGNS AND SYMPTOMS
• Usually asymptomatic
• Marked hypokalemia may be associated with muscle weakness and cramping, headaches, palpitations, polydipsia, polyuria, or nocturia
• Mild to severe hypertension
• Funduscopy - benign or grade 1-2
• Edema (rare)
• Hypokalemia
• Metabolic alkalosis
• Relative "hypernatremia"
• Impaired glucose tolerance
• Increased incidence of renal cysts

CAUSES
• Unilateral aldosterone-producing adrenal adenoma (APA)
• Idiopathic hyperaldosteronism (IHA)
• Aldosterone-producing adrenocortical carcinoma
• Other rare subtypes

RISK FACTORS   N/A

 DIAGNOSIS

DIFFERENTIAL DIAGNOSIS
• Diuretic use
• Renovascular hypertension
• Pheochromocytoma
• Renin-secreting tumor
• Malignant hypertension
• Congenital adrenal hyperplasia
• Deoxycorticosterone-producing tumor
• Exogenous mineralocorticoid
• High dose glucocorticoid therapy
• Apparent mineralocorticoid excess syndrome (congenital or acquired due to licorice ingestion)

LABORATORY
• Hypokalemia with inappropriate kaliuresis
• Unsuppressible urine or plasma aldosterone levels
• Low ambulatory plasma renin activity
• Normal glucocorticoid excretion
Drugs that may alter lab results: The list of drugs and hormones capable of affecting the renin-angiotensin-aldosterone axis is extensive; examples include - spironolactone, estrogens, diuretics, ACE-inhibitors, vasodilators, calcium channel antagonists, and adrenergic inhibitors
Disorders that may alter lab results: Malignant hypertension

PATHOLOGICAL FINDINGS Unilateral aldosterone-producing adrenal adenoma (APA), bilateral idiopathic adrenal hyperplasia (IHA), aldosterone-producing adrenocortical carcinoma

SPECIAL TESTS
• Posture study
• Spironolactone treatment trial
• Adrenal venous sampling

IMAGING Adrenal computerized tomography (CT preferred over MRI). Use 3 mm cuts.

DIAGNOSTIC PROCEDURES Adrenal venous sampling

 TREATMENT

APPROPRIATE HEALTH CARE
• Unilateral APA - unilateral adrenalectomy
• Bilateral IHA - chronic medical therapy

GENERAL MEASURES
• Unilateral APA - correct hypokalemia preoperatively with spironolactone
• Bilateral IHA - low sodium diet, regular isotonic exercise, maintenance of ideal body weight, tobacco avoidance, potassium-sparing agent, anti-hypertensive agent (e.g., calcium channel antagonist, ACE-inhibitor, low-dose thiazide diuretic)

ACTICITY   No limitations

DIET   Low sodium

PATIENT EDUCATION   N/A

MEDICATIONS

DRUG(S) OF CHOICE
• Potassium-sparing agent - spironolactone (Aldactone) or amiloride (Midamor)
• Anti-hypertensive agent - calcium channel antagonist, ACE-inhibitor, or low-dose thiazide diuretic
Contraindications: Potassium-sparing agent and ACE-inhibitors in renal failure, hyperkalemia, and pregnancy
Precautions: Monitor serum potassium closely after any adjustment in potassium replacement or potassium-sparing agent
Significant possible interactions: Lithium and diuretics, non-steroidal anti-inflammatory agents with diuretics and ACE-inhibitors

ALTERNATIVE DRUGS
Peripheral alpha-1 antagonists (e.g., terazosin (Hytrin), doxazosin (Cardura) or guanadrel (Hylorel) may be used to control hypertension during the diagnostic evaluation for primary aldosteronism.

FOLLOWUP

PATIENT MONITORING
• Blood pressure checks
• Serum potassium check
• 24-hour urine aldosterone following surgery

PREVENTION/AVOIDANCE N/A

POSSIBLE COMPLICATIONS
Cardiac arrhythmia associated with severe hypokalemia

EXPECTED COURSE AND PROGNOSIS
Surgical removal of an APA results in cure of hypertension in approximately 70% of cases. Hypertension does not resolve immediately post operatively, but rather over 1 to 4 months.

MISCELLANEOUS

ASSOCIATED CONDITIONS
Cystic renal disease

AGE-RELATED FACTORS
Pediatric: Bilateral adrenal idiopathic hyperplasia is the most common form in children
Geriatric: N/A
Others: N/A

PREGNANCY
Treat hypertension with agents proven to be safe during pregnancy; avoid spironolactone and ACE-inhibitors

SYNONYMS
• Conn's syndrome
• Hyperaldosteronism

ICD-9-CM
255.1 hyperaldosteronism

SEE ALSO
• Hypertension
• Hypokalemia

OTHER NOTES
All patients with hypertension and spontaneous hypokalemia should be screened

ABBREVIATIONS
APA = aldosterone-producing adenoma
IHA = idiopathic hyperaldosteronism

REFERENCES
• Young, W.F., Jr., Hogan, M.J., Klee, G.G., Grant, C.S., Van Heerden, J.A.: Hyperaldosteronism: Diagnosis and Treatment. Mayo Clinic Proc. 65:96, 1990
• Weinberger, M.H., et al.: Primary aldosteronism in diagnosis, localization and treatment. Ann Intern Med. 90:386, 1979

Author W. F. Young, Jr., M.D.

Alopecia

BASICS

DESCRIPTION Absence of the hair from skin areas where it normally is present
• Telogen effluvium - diffuse hair loss that results in decreased hair density but does not progress to complete baldness
• Anagen effluvium - diffuse shedding of hairs, including growing hairs, that may progress to complete baldness
• Cicatricial alopecia - also known as scarring alopecia and characterized by slick, smooth scalp without any evidence of follicular openings of hair
• Androgenic alopecia - hair loss occurring in either sex, caused by stimulation of the hair roots by male hormones
• Alopecia areata - patchy, non-scarring hair loss
• Traction alopecia - patchy, initially non-scarring hair loss
• Tinea capitis - patches of hair broken off close to the scalp, with or without associated inflammation, caused by fungus infection
System(s) affected: Skin/Exocrine
Genetics: In Caucasians, androgenic alopecia follows a dominant trait with incomplete penetrance. The hereditary incidence is notable not only in men but also in women with a strong family history of baldness.
Incidence/Prevalence in USA: 50% of Caucasian males by 50 years of age have noticeable male-pattern baldness. 37% of postmenopausal females show some evidence of hair loss.
Predominant age: The incidence of androgenic alopecia increases with increasing age. Tinea capitis and traction alopecia are more common in children.
Predominant sex: Male > Female

SIGNS AND SYMPTOMS
• Hair loss
• Pruritus (in tinea capitis)
• Scaling of the scalp (in tinea capitis)
• Broken hairs (in tinea capitis and traction alopecia)
• Tapered hair at the borders of the patch of alopecia (in alopecia areata)
• Easily removable hairs at the periphery of the patch of alopecia (in alopecia areata)
• Inflammation (in tinea capitis)

CAUSES
Telogen effluvium
  ◊ Postpartum
  ◊ Drugs (oral contraceptives, anticoagulants, retinoids, beta blockers, chemotherapeutic agents, interferon)
  ◊ Stress (physical or psychological)
  ◊ Hormonal (hypo- or hyperthyroidism, hypopituitarism)
  ◊ Nutritional (malnutrition, iron deficiency, zinc deficiency)
  ◊ Diffuse alopecia areata

Anagen effluvium
  ◊ Mycosis fungoides
  ◊ X-ray treatment
  ◊ Drugs (chemotherapeutic agents, allopurinol, levodopa, bromocriptine)
  ◊ Poisoning (bismuth, arsenic, gold, boric acid, thallium)
Cicatricial alopecia
  ◊ Congenital and developmental defects
  ◊ Infection (leprosy, syphilis, varicella-zoster, cutaneous leishmaniasis)
  ◊ Basal cell carcinoma
  ◊ Epidermal nevi
  ◊ Physical agents (acids and alkali, burns, freezing, radiodermatitis)
  ◊ Cicatricial pemphigoid
  ◊ Lichen planus
  ◊ Sarcoidosis
Androgenic alopecia
  ◊ Adrenal hyperplasia
  ◊ Polycystic ovaries
  ◊ Ovarian hyperplasia
  ◊ Carcinoid
  ◊ Pituitary hyperplasia
  ◊ Drugs (testosterone, danazol, ACTH, anabolic steroids, progesterones)
Alopecia areata
  ◊ Unknown, but possibly autoimmune
Traction alopecia
  ◊ Trichotillomania (direct self-pulling of the hair)
  ◊ Tight rollers or braids
Tinea capitis
  ◊ Microsporum species
  ◊ Trichophyton species

RISK FACTORS
• Positive family history of baldness
• Physical or psychological stress
• Pregnancy

DIAGNOSIS

DIFFERENTIAL DIAGNOSIS Search for type of alopecia and then for possible reversible causes

LABORATORY
• Thyroid function tests
• Complete blood count (may reflect an underlying immunologic disorder)
• Free testosterone and dehydroepiandrosterone sulfate (DHEA-S) in women with androgenic alopecia
• Serum ferritin
• VDRL or RPR for syphilis
• Lymphocyte T and B cell number (sometimes low in patients with alopecia areata)
Drugs that may alter lab results:
• Antifungal drugs may make KOH examination falsely negative
• Thyroid drugs will alter the thyroid function tests
Disorders that may alter lab results: N/A

PATHOLOGICAL FINDINGS Scalp biopsy with routine microscopy and direct immunofluorescence will aid in the diagnosis of tinea capitis, diffuse alopecia areata, and the scarring alopecias due to lupus erythematosus, lichen planus, and sarcoidosis

SPECIAL TESTS
• Light hair-pull test (positive in alopecia areata)
• Direct microscopic examination of the hair shaft
• Potassium hydroxide (KOH) examination of the scale, if present (positive in tinea capitis)
• Fungal culture of the scale, if present

IMAGING N/A

DIAGNOSTIC PROCEDURES Scalp biopsy (sometimes)

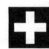

TREATMENT

APPROPRIATE HEALTH CARE
Outpatient

GENERAL MEASURES
• Telogen effluvium - maximum shedding 3 months after the inciting event (medication, stress, nutritional deficiency) and recovery following correction of the cause. Rarely permanent baldness.
• Anagen effluvium - shedding begins days to a few weeks after the inciting event with recovery following correction of the cause. Rarely permanent baldness.
• Cicatricial alopecia - hair follicles are permanently damaged. Only effective treatment is surgical (graft transplantation, flap transplantation, or excision of the scarred area).
• Androgenic alopecia - by 12 months of using topical minoxidil, 39% of subjects reported moderate to marked hair growth. Other treatments for androgenic alopecia are surgical (hair transplantation, scalp reduction, transposition flap, and soft tissue expansion).
• Alopecia areata - usually the disease resolves within three years without treatment. Recurrences are, however, common.
• Traction alopecia - only with discontinuation of the hair pulling will the disorder resolve. Psychologic or psychiatric intervention may be necessary. Successful therapeutic approaches have included medications, behavior modification, and hypnosis.
• Tinea capitis - six to eight weeks of therapy are often necessary

ACTIVITY Fully active

DIET No special diet

PATIENT EDUCATION National Alopecia Areata Foundation, 714 C Street, San Rafael, CA 94901

MEDICATIONS

DRUG(S) OF CHOICE
• Androgenic alopecia - topical minoxidil 2% (Rogaine)
• Alopecia areata - high potency topical steroids
• Tinea capitis - griseofulvin 10 mg/kg per day in children. Ketoconazole 200 mg once daily. Treatment may need continuation for 6-8 weeks.

Contraindications:
• Topical minoxidil - hypersensitivity to minoxidil
• Topical steroids - hypersensitivity to corticosteroids
• Griseofulvin - pregnancy, porphyria, hepatocellular failure, hypersensitivity to griseofulvin
• Ketoconazole - hypersensitivity to ketoconazole

Precautions:
Topical minoxidil
◊ Burning and irritation of the eyes
◊ Salt and water retention
◊ Tachycardia
Topical steroids
◊ Local burning and stinging
◊ Pruritus
◊ Skin atrophy
◊ Telangiectasias
Griseofulvin
◊ Photosensitivity reaction
◊ Lupus-like syndrome
◊ Oral thrush
◊ Granulocytopenia
Ketoconazole
◊ Anaphylaxis
◊ Hepatotoxicity
◊ Oligospermia
◊ Neuropsychiatric disturbances

Significant possible interactions:
• Topical minoxidil - may potentiate orthostatic hypotension
• Griseofulvin - decreases the activity of warfarin. Barbiturates depress the activity of griseofulvin.
• Ketoconazole - may enhance the activity of warfarin. Isoniazid and rifampin decrease the activity of ketoconazole. Concomitant administration with phenytoin may alter the metabolism of either drug.
• H2 blockers decrease absorption of ketoconazole. If concomitant therapy needed, give H2 blocker at least 2 hours after ketoconazole dose.

ALTERNATIVE DRUGS   N/A

FOLLOWUP

PATIENT MONITORING   In patients on ketoconazole, should be monitored closely for possible liver function abnormalities

PREVENTION/AVOIDANCE   N/A

POSSIBLE COMPLICATIONS   N/A

EXPECTED COURSE AND PROGNOSIS
• Telogen effluvium - rarely permanent baldness
• Anagen effluvium - rarely permanent baldness
• Cicatricial alopecia - the hair follicles are permanently damaged
• Androgenic alopecia - depends on treatment
• Alopecia areata - recurrences are common
• Traction alopecia - depends on behavior modification
• Tinea capitis - usually complete recovery

MISCELLANEOUS

ASSOCIATED CONDITIONS   Alopecia areata - Down syndrome, vitiligo, diabetes

AGE-RELATED FACTORS
Pediatric: Tinea capitis only common form of alopecia
Geriatric: Androgenic alopecia more common after 50
Others: N/A

PREGNANCY   Post partum hair loss is due to altered physiology during pregnancy

SYNONYMS
• Androgenic alopecia

ICD-9-CM
• 704.00 Alopecia, unspecified
• 704.01 Alopecia areata
• 704.09 Other
• 110.0 Dermatophytosis of the scalp and beard

SEE ALSO
• Lichen planus
• Tinea capitis
• Anemia
• Syphilis
• Cutaneous T-cell lymphoma
• Acrodermatitis
• Werner's syndrome

OTHER NOTES   N/A

ABBREVIATIONS   N/A

REFERENCES
• Dermatologic Clinics 7/87
• Mitchell, A.V. and Krull, E.A. (eds.): Dermatologic Clinics, 1987. 5(3): 483-603
• Olsen, E.A.: Primary Care, 1989. 16(3): 768-787
• Burke, K.E.: Postgrad Med, 1989. 85(6): 52-77

Author   A. Knight, M.D.

Altitude illness

BASICS

DESCRIPTION Altitude illness is a spectrum of medical problems ranging from mild discomfort to fatal illness that may occur on ascent to higher altitude. It can affect anyone, including the most experienced and fit individual, who ascends to more than about 8,000 feet. Several factors appear to be important in adaptation to altitude: How long the ascent takes, how high, and length of stay. There is a great deal of variation between people and an individual's response may vary from ascent to ascent.
• Acute mountain sickness (AMS): Begins within 4 to 6 hours after arrival at altitude, rare below 8,000 feet, and affects most above 10,000
• High altitude pulmonary edema (HAPE): Abnormal accumulation of fluid in the lungs. Begins 24 to 96 hours after arrival at altitude. Rare below 8,000 feet but affects more than 10% of individuals above 14,500 feet.
• High altitude cerebral edema (HACE): Indicates swelling of the brain. It is the least common but most severe of the high altitude illnesses since it can result in permanent injury or death. Occurs 48 to 72 hours after arrival at altitude. Rare below 12,000 feet.
System(s) affected: Pulmonary, Cardiovascular, Nervous
Genetics: N/A
Incidence/Prevalence: Unknown
Predominant age: Any age (young, well-conditioned climbers have a higher incidence of altitude illness, probably because they push themselves more)
Predominant sex: Male = Female

SIGNS AND SYMPTOMS
AMS mild to moderately severe symptoms:
◊ Headache
◊ Lack of energy and appetite
◊ Mild nausea
◊ Dizziness
◊ Weakness
◊ Insomnia
AMS severe symptoms:
◊ Increased headache
◊ Irritability
◊ Marked fatigue
◊ Shortness of breath with exercise
◊ Nausea and vomiting
◊ Irregular or periodic breathing at night (Cheyne-Stokes)
◊ Breathing apnea
HAPE symptoms:
◊ Excessive shortness of breath on exertion
◊ Severe respiratory distress
◊ Shortness of breath at rest
◊ Dry cough and/or wheezing
◊ Heart rate and respiratory rate increased
◊ Marked periodic breathing present at night
◊ Gurgling breathing
◊ Frothy cough
◊ Wet crackling sounds in the lungs
◊ Confusion
◊ Coma

HACE symptoms:
◊ Progressive headache that is unrelieved by mild pain relievers
◊ Lack of coordination (e.g., unable to perform a heel-to-toe walk)
◊ Confusion and bizarre behavior followed by unconsciousness
◊ Other symptoms of moderate AMS, such as dizziness, vomiting, and irritability, are usually present

CAUSES The physiology of altitude illness is still not completely understood. The fundamental problem results from the fact that with increasing altitude there is a progressive decrease in barometric pressure and a corresponding lower partial pressure of oxygen in inspired air, resulting in less oxygen delivery to the body.

RISK FACTORS
• In general, the faster the ascent and the higher, the more likely a person will experience symptoms of altitude illness
• Chronic illness
• Lack of conditioning

DIAGNOSIS

DIFFERENTIAL DIAGNOSIS
• Viral upper respiratory infection
• Gastroenteritis
• Pneumonia
• Other infections
• Cerebral vascular accident
• Ketoacidosis
• Pulmonary emboli
• Congestive heart failure

LABORATORY
• AMS: Laboratory studies are nonspecific and rarely required for diagnosis
• HAPE: WBC - often slightly elevated, erythrocyte sedimentation rate normal
• Arterial blood gas - may show hypoxia, hypocapnea, alkalosis
Drugs that may alter lab results: N/A
Disorders that may alter lab results: N/A

PATHOLOGICAL FINDINGS N/A

SPECIAL TESTS ECG may show only sinus tachycardia, possibly right heart strain

IMAGING Chest x-ray (in HAPE) shows Kerley's lines and a patchy distribution of edema

DIAGNOSTIC PROCEDURES N/A

TREATMENT

APPROPRIATE HEALTH CARE
Outpatient for mild cases, inpatient for severe cases

GENERAL MEASURES
• Therapy must be tailored to fit severity of disease and may be constrained by the environment
• Definitive treatment is to descend to a lower altitude. Dramatic improvement accompanies even modest reductions in altitude (as little as 1,000 feet).
• Oxygen, given continuously at 1-2 liters per minute helps relieve symptoms. For severe symptoms, continuous oxygen should be administered and descent to a lower altitude is mandatory.
AMS
◊ Descent rarely needed
◊ Fluids, light diet, curtailed activity
HAPE and HACE
◊ Patient must be treated by immediate evacuation to a lower altitude. Occasionally, however, foul weather, lack of transportation or long distances prevent immediate evacuation. In these cases, supportive measures, such as bedrest and oxygen, will help.
◊ Hyperbaric therapy is another effective and practical alternative when descent is not possible. A portable hyperbaric chamber, the "Gamow Bag," made of fabric and weighing only 8 pounds can be inflated to 2 pounds per square inch using a foot pump. This is equivalent to a drop in altitude of about 5,000 feet. Improvement is usually immediate after being placed in the hyperbaric chamber.
◊ If patient is hospitalized, rule out any other pulmonary disease first, provide adequate oxygen (possibly by intubation or positive end-expiratory pressure [PEEP]), bed rest, diuresis if needed and postural drainage

ACTIVITY Rest until symptoms clear

DIET Increased intake of fluids, a light diet, and avoidance of alcohol

PATIENT EDUCATION See guidelines in Prevention/Avoidance

MEDICATIONS

DRUG(S) OF CHOICE
• Aspirin or codeine can be used to relieve the headache. Antibiotics, if infection is present.
• Both dexamethasone and acetazolamide have been used to treat patients with severe symptoms of AMS. Dosage of dexamethasone is 8 mg initially, followed by 4 mg every six hours by mouth. Doses of acetazolamide of up to 1.0 g/day may be required for effective treatment.
• Dexamethasone may be effective in mild cases of HAPE, but this has not been proven
• Diuretics have not been useful
• Corticosteroids should be given even though their effectiveness is questionable
Contraindications: Refer to manufacturer's profile of each drug
Precautions: Refer to manufacturer's profile of each drug
Significant possible interactions: Refer to manufacturer's profile of each drug

ALTERNATIVE DRUGS   N/A

FOLLOWUP

PATIENT MONITORING
• For mild cases, no followup needed
• For more severe cases, follow until symptoms subside
• If underlying cardiopulmonary or cardiovascular disease, follow as needed

PREVENTION/AVOIDANCE
General guidelines
◊ Staged ascent: "Staging" is the process of remaining at an intermediate altitude (6600 to 9800 feet) for a few days before attempting the ultimate altitude
◊ Conventional prescription for avoiding altitude illness is to allow one day to ascend and acclimatize each 1,000 feet from elevations of 10,000 to 14,000 feet (3,048 to 4,267 m). Two days per 1,000 feet at elevations above 14,000 feet.
◊ Sleeping elevation - climber's maximum "climb high and sleep low" is a prudent practice for anyone going above 12,000 feet
◊ Adequate hydration - dehydration increases the likelihood of and worsens the symptoms of AMS
◊ Good physical conditioning
◊ Consider carrying a supply of oxygen
Drug prophylaxis
◊ Acetazolamide (if patient has a history of problems at altitude and/or plans a rapid ascent to above 8,000 feet [in a car or airplane]). Dosage is usually 250 mg orally twice daily, starting 24 hours before ascent and continuing for two to three days while at altitude. Anyone with a known drug allergy to sulfa should avoid acetazolamide.
◊ Dexamethasone may significantly reduce the incidence and severity of acute mountain sickness. The dosage is 2 to 4 mg every six hours, begun the day of the ascent, continued for three days at the higher altitude, then tapered over five days. Adverse side effects are uncommon.

POSSIBLE COMPLICATIONS
• Without treatment, HACE can cause motor and sensory deficits, seizures and coma
• HAPE may progress to cyanosis and respiratory distress syndrome
• Patient may experience high altitude retinal hemorrhage (HARH) - can cause visual changes, but is usually asymptomatic

EXPECTED COURSE AND PROGNOSIS
• Mild to moderate AMS resolves over 1-3 days. Patients may resume ascent once symptoms subside.
• HAPE and HACE patients can expect complete recovery, if there is no underlying disease. Should not resume ascent.
• Problems are more likely to recur in people who have had one or more attacks

MISCELLANEOUS

ASSOCIATED CONDITIONS   N/A

AGE-RELATED FACTORS
Pediatric: Children under 6 are more susceptible than adults
Geriatric: Elderly more likely to have chronic conditions (coronary artery disease, congestive heart failure, chronic obstructive pulmonary disease) that may be exacerbated at altitudes of 6000-8000 feet
Others: Women in premenstrual phase are more vulnerable

PREGNANCY   N/A

SYNONYMS   Mountain sickness

ICD-9-CM   289 mountain sickness acute

SEE ALSO   N/A

OTHER NOTES   N/A

ABBREVIATIONS
• AMS = acute mountain sickness
• HACE = high altitude cerebral edema
• HAPE = high altitude pulmonary edema

REFERENCES
• Zell, S.C. & Goodman, P.H.: Acetazolamide and dexamethasone in the prevention of acute mountain sickness. West J Med, 148:541, 1988
• Johnson, T.S. & Rock, P.B.: Current concepts, acute mountain sickness. New Engl J Med, 319:841, 1988

Author   T. Parikh, M.D. & K. Carmichael, M.D.

Alzheimer's disease

 BASICS

DESCRIPTION A degenerative organic mental disease characterized by progressive brain deterioration and dementia; frequently occurring after age 65. The diagnosis is made on clinical grounds after ruling out treatable disorders with similar characteristics. Long-term care costs to the nation is approximately $40 billion/year.
Usual course - progressive; chronic.
Genetics: Positive family history in 50% of cases. Marker on chromosome 21.
System(s) affected: Nervous
Incidence/Prevalence in USA: 2 million cases/350 million people.
Predominant age: Ages 40-75
Predominant sex: Female > Male

SIGNS AND SYMPTOMS
- Abnormal space perception
- Acalculia
- Amnesia
- Anhedonia
- Anxiety
- Aphasia
- Apraxia
- Confabulation
- Dementia
- Depression
- Extrapyramidal signs
- Intellectual decline
- Loss of interest
- Myoclonus
- Recent memory loss
- Restlessness
- Seizure
- Sleep disturbances
- Stiffness
- Unconcern
- Progressive cognitive impairment

CAUSES
- Unknown, appears to be a familial possibility
- Unsubstantiated possibilities - slow virus, metals (aluminum), acceleration in normal aging

RISK FACTORS Aging

 DIAGNOSIS

DIFFERENTIAL DIAGNOSIS
- Vascular dementia
- Multi-infarct dementia
- Dementia associated with Parkinson's
- Creutzfeldt-Jakob disease
- End-stage multiple sclerosis
- Brain tumor
- Subdural hematoma
- Progressive multifocal leukoencephalopathy
- Metabolic dementia (hypothyroidism)
- Drug reactions
- Alcoholism and other addictions
- Dementia pugilistica
- Other dementias (disorganized thinking, irrelevant speech, inability to maintain attention, sensory misconceptions, sleep-wake cyclical changes, disorientation in time and place, memory impairment)
- Depression (persistent diminished interest and pleasure, insomnia or hyposomnia, psychomotor retardation, feelings of hopelessness and helplessness, thoughts of death, decreased ability to concentrate)
- Toxicity from liver or kidney failure
- Vitamin and other nutritional deficiencies

LABORATORY
To help rule out other causes of dementia:
- ◊ CBC
- ◊ Chemistry panel
- ◊ Thyroid function studies
- ◊ Folate and B-12 levels
- ◊ VDRL
- ◊ Urinalysis
- ◊ ECG (atrial fibrillation)

Drugs that may alter lab results: N/A
Disorders that may alter lab results: N/A

PATHOLOGICAL FINDINGS
- Gross - diffuse cerebral atrophy in association areas, in hippocampus, in amygdala, in some subcortical nuclei
- Micro - pyramidal cell loss
- Micro - decreased cholinergic innervation
- Micro - neuritic senile plaques
- Micro - degeneration of locus ceruleus
- Degeneration of basal forebrain nuclei of Meynert
- Neurofibrillary tangles

SPECIAL TESTS
- EEG - moderate diffuse slowing
- Cerebrospinal fluid (depending on circumstances and clinical information)

IMAGING
- Head CT/MRI - moderate cortical atrophy, ventricular enlargement - to rule out infarcts, subdural hematomas, normal pressure hydrocephalus
- Positive emission tomography (PET) to detect cerebral glucose utilization and/or loss of cells in locus ceruleus

DIAGNOSTIC PROCEDURES This is a clinical diagnosis - history, physical examination, tests (neurological and memory)

 TREATMENT

APPROPRIATE HEALTH CARE
Outpatient, day care, nursing home (when necessary)

GENERAL MEASURES
- Supportive
- Exercises to reduce restlessness
- Occupational therapy
- Music therapy
- Analyze environment for safety and security
- Consider day care centers
- Consider nursing home
Referrals to
- ◊ Visiting nurse
- ◊ Social worker
- ◊ Physical therapist
- ◊ Occupational therapist
- ◊ Speech therapist
- ◊ Lawyer
- ◊ Support groups
- ◊ Alzheimer special care group

ACTIVITY To whatever extent possible

DIET No special diet

PATIENT EDUCATION
- Printed patient information available from: Alzheimer's Association, 70 E. Lake Street, Suite 600, Chicago, IL, (312)853-3060
- Help family understand the progressive nature of the disease
- Arrange durable power of attorney

MEDICATIONS

DRUG(S) OF CHOICE
• No specific drug therapy available. Clinical studies are ongoing.
• Use as few drugs as possible. Alzheimer's patients tolerate them poorly.
• For restlessness - short acting benzodiazepines
• For severe persistent agitation - butyrophenones or phenothiazines
Contraindications: Refer to manufacturer's literature. Avoid anticholinergic drugs, such as antidepressants and antihistamines.
Precautions:
• Refer to manufacturer's literature
Tacrine (Cognex)
◊ Use with caution in persons with a history of neuromuscular disease
◊ Elevation of liver function tests
◊ Use with caution in persons with a history of seizures or asthma
Significant possible interactions: Refer to manufacturer's literature

ALTERNATIVE DRUGS
• Tacrine (Cognex)10-40 mg qid used to treat DAT (doses >100mg/day appear to be associated with increased risk of hepatotoxicity)

FOLLOWUP

PATIENT MONITORING
As often as necessary to treat poor nutrition, medical complications, monitor drug use, provide support for family

EXPECTED COURSE AND PROGNOSIS
Poor; 2-20 year survival; 7 year average survival

PREVENTION/AVOIDANCE
None known

POSSIBLE COMPLICATIONS
• Behavioral - hostility, agitation, wandering, uncooperativeness
• Metabolic - infection, dehydration, drug toxicity
• Others - falls, "sundowning"

MISCELLANEOUS

ASSOCIATED CONDITIONS
• Down syndrome
• Depression
• Insomnia

AGE-RELATED FACTORS
Pediatric: N/A
Geriatric: A frequent and serious problem in this age group
Others: N/A

PREGNANCY
N/A

SYNONYMS
• Presenile dementia
• Senile dementia of the Alzheimer's type (SDAT)
• Primary degenerative dementia

ICD-9-CM
331.0 Alzheimer's disease

SEE ALSO
Disorders listed under Differential diagnosis

OTHER NOTES
N/A

ABBREVIATIONS
N/A

REFERENCES
• Abrams, W.B. & Berkow, R. (eds.): Merck Manual of Geriatrics. Rahway, NJ, Merck & Co., 1990
• Tierney, M.C., et al.: The NINCDS-ADRDA Work Group criteria for the clinical diagnosis of probable Alzheimer's disease: A clinicopathologic study of 57 cases. Neurology 38:359, 1988
• Plum, F. (ed.): Handbook of Physiology: Higher Functions of the Nervous System. Bethesda, MD, American Physiological Society, 1987

Author H. Griffith, M.D. & M. Dambro, M.D.

Amblyopia

 BASICS

 DIAGNOSIS

 TREATMENT

DESCRIPTION Amblyopia describes a reduction in visual acuity that cannot be corrected by eye glasses or contact lenses in the absence of a structural or pathological abnormality of the eye.
System(s) affected: Nervous
Genetics: There is an increased incidence in children where one parent has a history of amblyopia
Incidence/Prevalence in USA:
Approximately 2-2.5% in the general population
Predominant age: May be present from birth or may be detected at any age
Predominant sex: Male = Female

SIGNS AND SYMPTOMS Preschool vision screening is advisable to detect a decrease in visual acuity in one eye

CAUSES
• Strabismic amblyopia is a loss of visual acuity in an individual due to suppression of the images in eye which turns out or in
• Anisometropic amblyopia is present when one eye has a significantly different refractive error than the fellow eye and leads to visual blurring
• Refractive amblyopia is due to uncorrected high refractive error resulting in visual blurring in either or both eyes
• Deprivation amblyopia (amblyopia ex anopsia) is due to relative complete visual deprivation in one eye that can be caused by a congenital abnormality such as a corneal scar or cataract

RISK FACTORS None identified

DIFFERENTIAL DIAGNOSIS The diagnosis of amblyopia can be confused with an organic lesion causing decreased visual acuity and this must always be excluded before the diagnosis of amblyopia is considered

LABORATORY N/A
Drugs that may alter lab results: N/A
Disorders that may alter lab results: N/A

PATHOLOGICAL FINDINGS N/A

SPECIAL TESTS Examination by an ophthalmologist to screen for unequal refractive error, outward turning, or inward turning of the eye (strabismic amblyopia) and proper vision testing of the eye under monocular conditions. A complete slit lamp and dilated funduscopic examination is necessary to exclude an organic cause for the decreased visual acuity.

IMAGING N/A

DIAGNOSTIC PROCEDURES N/A

APPROPRIATE HEALTH CARE All children should have complete visual examinations prior to starting school with each eye tested individually. Those children from families with a known history of amblyopia or strabismus should have special exams by an ophthalmologist.

GENERAL MEASURES
• Correction of the underlying disorder should be instituted at the earliest opportunity
• Full refractive correction and/or patching of the stronger eye to encourage visual development of the amblyopic eye is warranted
• Amblyopia never corrects itself spontaneously and will always require treatment. Children do not outgrow amblyopia.
• Surgical correction of an abnormal eye position may also be required

ACTIVITY No restrictions

DIET No special diet

PATIENT EDUCATION All parents should be made aware of the need to have their children's eyes examined prior to starting school

MEDICATIONS

DRUG(S) OF CHOICE N/A
Contraindications: N/A
Precautions: N/A
Significant possible interactions: N/A

ALTERNATIVE DRUGS N/A

FOLLOWUP

PATIENT MONITORING Once the diagnosis of amblyopia is made, the patient needs to be seen frequently at the discretion of the ophthalmologist until complete resolution of the problem occurs

PREVENTION/AVOIDANCE None

POSSIBLE COMPLICATIONS If there is failure to institute proper therapy early, permanent and profound visual loss can be expected

EXPECTED COURSE AND PROGNOSIS Amblyopia is a treatable condition in most cases if the diagnosis is made early. Patching therapy, eye glasses, and surgical correction of abnormal eye positions can result in near normalcy of vision when instituted early. Visual development occurs during the first several years of life and amblyopia therapy can be effective until approximately age 12.

MISCELLANEOUS

ASSOCIATED CONDITIONS Amblyopia is more common in families with a history of unequal refractive errors, high uncorrected refractive errors, and strabismus

AGE-RELATED FACTORS
Pediatric: More commonly seen in the pediatric age group early in life
Geriatric: When seen in the geriatric population, the diagnosis has usually been made early in childhood
Others: N/A

PREGNANCY N/A

SYNONYMS Lazy eye

ICD-9-CM
368.0

SEE ALSO Strabismus

OTHER NOTES N/A

ABBREVIATIONS N/A

REFERENCES
• Binocular Vision And Ocular Motility. In Ophthalmology Basic and Clinical Science Course. (American Academy of Ophthalmology)
• Harley, R.D.: Pediatric Ophthalmology

Author R. Kershner, M.D., FACS

Amebiasis

 BASICS

 DIAGNOSIS

 TREATMENT

DESCRIPTION Amebiasis is caused by the intestinal protozoan, Entamoeba histolytica. Infection results from ingestion of fecally contaminated food, such as garden vegetables or by direct fecal-oral transmission. Most persons are asymptomatic or have minimal diarrheal symptoms. In a few patients, invasive intestinal or extraintestinal infection results.

Incidence/Prevalence in USA: Probably < 1% overall, but much higher in some risk groups, such as areas with large immigrant populations

System(s) affected: Gastrointestinal

Genetics: N/A

Predominant age: All

Predominant sex: Male > Female; probably because of greater occupational exposure

SIGNS AND SYMPTOMS

Noninvasive infection (up to 99%)
 ◊ Asymptomatic (90%)
 ◊ Mild diarrhea
 ◊ Abdominal discomfort

Invasive intestinal infection
 ◊ Abdominal pain and tenderness
 ◊ Rectal pain
 ◊ Diarrhea
 ◊ Bloody stools
 ◊ Fever (30%)
 ◊ Systemic toxicity

Extraintestinal infection (liver and less commonly lung, skin, brain)
 ◊ Fever
 ◊ Systemic toxicity
 ◊ RUQ abdominal pain and tenderness
 ◊ Nausea and vomiting
 ◊ Diarrhea (50%)

CAUSES Infection is transmitted through contaminated food or water, or through person-to-person contact

RISK FACTORS
• Low socioeconomic status
• Institutional living
• Male homosexuality
• Invasive disease is associated with exposure to more pathogenic strains which are more common in certain geographic locations, some parts of Mexico, South Africa, and India

DIFFERENTIAL DIAGNOSIS
• Other infectious causes of colitis, including shigellosis, Campylobacter infection, pseudomembranous colitis, and occasionally salmonellosis or Yersinia infection
• Noninfectious causes of colitis include ulcerative colitis, Crohn's colitis and ischemic colitis
• Hepatic amebiasis must be distinguished from pyogenic liver abscess or superinfection of amebic abscess

LABORATORY
• Stool for ova and parasites [unfortunately, the sensitivity of this exam is poor]. Diarrheal stool should be examined immediately for trophozoites in addition to fixed stool specimens (repeated as necessary). In invasive intestinal infection, stools are bloody, but fecal leukocytes are frequently absent.
• Serologic tests (especially indirect hemagglutination (IHA), positive in 85% of colitis patients and most patients with extraintestinal disease. Serologic tests should be done in patients with idiopathic inflammatory bowel disease to rule out amebiasis.

Drugs that may alter lab results: Many drugs interfere with stool exams

Disorders that may alter lab results: N/A

PATHOLOGICAL FINDINGS
Colon biopsy
 ◊ Lysis of mucosal cells (flask ulcers)
 ◊ PAS-stained trophozoites
 ◊ Neutrophils at the periphery
Liver biopsy
 ◊ Necrosis surrounded by a rim of trophozoites

SPECIAL TESTS N/A

IMAGING CT scan or ultrasound for hepatic infection

DIAGNOSTIC PROCEDURES
• Rectosigmoidoscopy with biopsy
• Needle aspirate of hepatic lesions may be needed to rule out pyogenic infection or superinfection

APPROPRIATE HEALTH CARE
Outpatient

GENERAL MEASURES
• Fluids and nutrition
• Electrolyte management
• With severe amebic colitis, surgery may be necessary

ACTIVITY In accordance with illness of patient

DIET As tolerated

PATIENT EDUCATION Avoid conditions of re-exposure

MEDICATIONS

DRUG(S) OF CHOICE
• Noninvasive infection - diiodohydroxyquin (also called iodoquinol) 650 mg tid for 20 days
• Invasive infection - metronidazole (Flagyl) 750 mg tid for 5-10 days, followed by a 20 day course of diiodohydroxyquin to eliminate intestinal carriage
Contraindications:
• Use diiodohydroxyquin cautiously in patients with thyroid diseases. Contraindicated in hepatic or renal dysfunction. May cause optic neuritis or peripheral neuropathy.
• Known allergy to given medication
Precautions: None of the agents are proven safe in pregnancy
Significant possible interactions:
Disulfiram reaction with ethanol

ALTERNATIVE DRUGS
Noninvasive infection- diloxanide, paromomycin, metronidazole. Invasive infection- dehydroemetine (as effective as metronidazole, but cardiotoxic), chloroquine (less effective)

FOLLOWUP

PATIENT MONITORING
Patient signs and symptoms, stool for ova and parasite

PREVENTION/AVOIDANCE
Avoid above-mentioned exposures

POSSIBLE COMPLICATIONS
Toxic megacolon with rupture, rupture of hepatic abscess

EXPECTED COURSE AND PROGNOSIS
Untreated invasive amebiasis is frequently fatal. With treatment, improvement usually occurs within a few days. Some patients with amebic colitis have irritable bowel symptoms for weeks after successful treatment.

MISCELLANEOUS

ASSOCIATED CONDITIONS N/A

AGE-RELATED FACTORS
Pediatric: More severe in neonates
Geriatric: More severe in elderly
Others: More severe in patients on corticosteroids and other immunocompromised patients

PREGNANCY
More severe in pregnancy. Most agents are avoided in pregnancy (especially first trimester) because of concerns of teratogenicity. Paromomycin is sometimes recommended for noninvasive disease because it is not absorbed. Infectious disease consultation should be obtained.

SYNONYMS
• Amebic colitis
• Amebic dysentery

ICD-9-CM
006.0 Acute amebic dysentery without mention of abscess
006.3 Amebic liver abscess
006.5 Amebic brain abscess
006.8 Amebic infection of other sites
006.9 Amebiasis, unspecified

SEE ALSO N/A

OTHER NOTES N/A

ABBREVIATIONS N/A

REFERENCES
• Fedorak, R.N. & Rubinoff, M.J.: Basic Investigation of a Patient with Diarrhea. In Diarrheal Diseases. Edited by M. Field. Elsevier Science Publishing Co., Inc., New York, 1991:191-218
• Fedorak, R.N.: Protozoal diarrhea. In Diarrheal Diseases. Edited by M. Field. Elsevier Science Publishing Co., Inc., New York, 1991:319-354.
• Ravdin, J.I. & Petri, W.A., Jr.: Entamoeba histolytica (amebiasis). In Principles and Practice of Infectious Diseases. 3rd Ed. Edited by G.L. Mandell, R.G. Douglas & J.E. Bennett. New York, Churchill Livingstone Inc., 1990:2036-2049

Author R. Adam, M.D.

Amenorrhea

 BASICS

DESCRIPTION The absence of menses
• Primary amenorrhea - occurs when menarche has not occurred by age seventeen
• Secondary amenorrhea - the cessation of menses for three cycles
System(s) affected: Reproductive, Endocrine/Metabolic
Genetics: No known genetic pattern
Incidence/Prevalence in USA: Incidence of secondary amenorrhea 3.3%
Predominant age: Menarche to menopause
Predominant sex: Female only

SIGNS AND SYMPTOMS
• The absence of periods
• Galactorrhea
• Temperature intolerance
• Symptoms of early pregnancy
• Signs of androgen excess

CAUSES
Primary amenorrhea
◊ Imperforate hymen
◊ Agenesis of the uterus and upper 2/3 of the vagina
◊ Turner's syndrome
◊ Constitutional delay
Secondary amenorrhea
◊ Physiological - pregnancy, corpus luteal cyst, breast-feeding, menopause
◊ Suppression of the hypothalamic-pituitary axis - post pill amenorrhea, stress, intercurrent illness, weight loss, low body mass index
◊ Pituitary disease - ablation of the pituitary gland, Sheehan's syndrome, prolactinoma
◊ Uncontrolled endocrinopathies - diabetes, hypo- or hyperthyroidism
◊ Polycystic ovarian disease (POD), (Stein-Leventhal syndrome)
◊ Chemotherapy
◊ Pelvic irradiation
◊ Endometrial ablation (Asherman's syndrome)
◊ Drug therapy - systemic steroids, danazol, GRH-RH analogs
◊ Premature ovarian failure

RISK FACTORS
• Over-training (e.g., long-distance runner, ballet dancer)
• Eating disorders
• Psycho-social crisis

 DIAGNOSIS

DIFFERENTIAL DIAGNOSIS Includes all of the causes listed above. The most common cause of secondary amenorrhea is early pregnancy.

LABORATORY
• Pregnancy test
• Serum prolactin
• FSH
• LH
• T4, TSH
• Blood sugar
Drugs that may alter lab results: N/A
Disorders that may alter lab results:
Pregnancy, menopause, hyperprolactinemia, ovarian suppression, endocrinopathy

PATHOLOGICAL FINDINGS Due to underlying disease

SPECIAL TESTS Laparoscopy - diagnosis of the streak ovaries of Turner's syndrome, or the polycystic ovaries of POD

IMAGING
• Ultrasound may show cysts undetectable on pelvic examination
• Radiologic evaluation of the sella turcica if prolactinomas suspected (elevated serum prolactin)

DIAGNOSTIC PROCEDURES N/A

 TREATMENT

APPROPRIATE HEALTH CARE
Outpatient

GENERAL MEASURES
• Definitive treatment depends on determining the cause of the amenorrhea. May not be necessary to treat all cases especially if just temporary amenorrhea.
• Hymenectomy, done as a day surgery, will be required for those whose primary amenorrhea is due to imperforate hymen

ACTIVITY No restrictions

DIET Correct overweight or underweight by dietary management

PATIENT EDUCATION
• Consists of fully informing the patient of your findings, including the presence or absence of pregnancy, and of the underlying cause
• Specific educational resources can be utilized as necessary, e.g., prenatal classes, menopause support groups
• Specific information should be given about the expected duration of amenorrhea (temporary or permanent), effect on fertility, and the long-term sequelae of untreated amenorrhea (e.g., osteoporosis, vaginal dryness)
• Appropriate contraceptive advice should be given, as fertility returns before menses
• Additional support may be needed if the amenorrhea is associated with a reduction in, or loss of, fertility
• Society for Menstrual Cycle Research, 10559 N. 104th Place, Scottsdale, AZ 85258, (602)451-9731

MEDICATIONS

DRUG(S) OF CHOICE
• Progesterone replacement - medroxyprogesterone (Provera) 5 mg bid for 5 days, will result in a withdrawal bleed if the hypothalamo-pituitary-ovarian axis is intact and there is some endogenous estrogen production
• Estrogen replacement - conjugated estrogen (Premarin) 0.625 mg for 25 days with progesterone added as above for the last 10 days will result in a withdrawal bleed if the uterus and lower genital tract are normal
• Use of hormonal therapies will not correct underlying problem. Other drugs might be required to treat specific conditions, e.g., bromocriptine for hyperprolactinemia.

Contraindications:
• Pregnancy
• Thromboembolic disease
• Previous myocardial infarct, cerebrovascular accident
• Estrogen-dependent malignancy
• Severe hepatic impairment or disease

Precautions:
• Diabetes
• Seizure disorder
• Migraine headache
• Smoker over 35

Significant possible interactions:
Barbiturates, phenytoin, rifampin, corticosteroids, theophyllines, tricyclics, oral anticoagulants (anticoagulant effect may be decreased)

ALTERNATIVE DRUGS
Use of oral contraceptives for hormonal replacement if patient has difficulty following above regimen

FOLLOWUP

PATIENT MONITORING
Depends on the cause, and the treatment chosen. If hormonal replacement is used, discontinuation after six months is advised, to assess spontaneous resumption of menses.

PREVENTION/AVOIDANCE
Maintenance of proper body mass index (BMI)

POSSIBLE COMPLICATIONS
• Estrogen deficiency symptoms, e.g., hot flushes, vaginal dryness
• Osteoporosis, in prolonged hypoestrogenic amenorrhea

EXPECTED COURSE AND PROGNOSIS
Reflects the underlying cause. In secondary amenorrhea from hypothalamo-pituitary suppression, spontaneous resumption of menses with time (99% within 6 months) and correction of body mass index.

MISCELLANEOUS

ASSOCIATED CONDITIONS N/A

AGE-RELATED FACTORS
Pediatric: N/A
Geriatric: N/A
Others: N/A

PREGNANCY One of the primary causes

SYNONYMS N/A

ICD-9-CM
626.0

SEE ALSO Names of individual causes

OTHER NOTES
• Use of hormonal replacement therapy is symptomatic and is discretionary if amenorrhea is temporary (e.g., hypothalamopituitary suppression)
• Patients who are amenorrheic and wish to become pregnant should not be given HRT, but should receive treatment for infertility based on specific cause

ABBREVIATIONS N/A

REFERENCES
Yen, S.S.C. & Jaffe, R.B. (eds.): Reproductive Endocrinology. 2nd Ed. Philadelphia, W.B. Saunders Co., 1986

Author D. Andres, M.D.

Amyloidosis

BASICS

DESCRIPTION A disease characterized by increased deposition of amyloid fibrils in the tissues. Several different proteins may give rise to amyloid. These proteins are present due to their overproduction or decreased clearance. The most common types of amyloidosis are:
Primary amyloidosis: usually associated with the plasma cell disorders multiple myeloma and MGUS (monoclonal gammopathy of undetermined significance)
Secondary amyloidosis: associated with several chronic inflammatory diseases such as rheumatoid arthritis, osteomyelitis, malaria, tuberculosis, and leprosy
Familial amyloidosis: associated with the genetic disease Familial Mediterranean fever
Hemodialysis amyloidosis: associated with renal hemodialysis
Incidence/Prevalence in USA: Not reported
System(s) affected: Endocrine/Metabolic, Cardiovascular, Pulmonary, Renal/Urologic, Musculoskeletal, Gastrointestinal, Nervous, Skin/Exocrine
Genetics: N/A
Predominant Age: 60-70
Predominant Sex: Male > Female (2:1)

SIGNS AND SYMPTOMS
May be highly variable depending upon which organ system is affected and to what degree:
• Fatigue, weight loss, gastroparesis, pseudo-obstruction, malabsorption, diarrhea, macroglossia
• Peripheral neuropathy, carpal tunnel syndrome
• Ascites, hepatomegaly
• Dyspnea, interstitial lung disease, congestive heart failure, arrhythmia, sudden death
• Hilar adenopathy, mediastinal adenopathy
• Symmetrical polyarthritis, rubbery peri-articular soft tissue swelling
• Translucent/waxy skin papules, purpura (especially peri-orbital purpura), edema
• Renal failure, nephrotic syndrome
• Dementia

CAUSES
Primary amyloidosis
The amyloid consists of immunoglobulin light chains (AL) which are overproduced in plasma disorders.
Secondary amyloidosis
The amyloid consists of amyloid fibrillary protein (AA), and its breakdown product, serum amyloid protein (SAA), which are overproduced in chronic inflammatory conditions
Familial amyloidosis
The amyloid consists of amyloid fibrillary protein (AA) which is overproduced in Familial Mediterranean fever
Hemodialysis Amyloidosis
The amyloid consists of beta-2-microglobulin which is normally cleared by the kidney, but cannot be cleared by hemodialysis

RISK FACTORS
• Underlying plasma cell dyscrasia
• Underlying chronic inflammatory disease
• Familial Mediterranean fever
• Hemodialysis

DIAGNOSIS

DIFFERENTIAL DIAGNOSIS
• Peripheral neuropathy - diabetes mellitus, alcoholism, vitamin deficiencies
• Carpal tunnel syndrome - hypothyroidism, trauma, rheumatoid arthritis, etc.
• Restrictive cardiomyopathy: acute viral myocarditis, endomyocardial fibrosis, sarcoidosis, hemochromatosis
• Nephrotic syndrome - glomerulonephritis, renal vein thrombosis
• Renal failure - glomerulonephritis, obstructive uropathy, toxin or drug-induced, acute tubular necrosis
• Symmetric polyarthritis - rheumatoid arthritis, psoriatic arthritis, SLE
• Interstitial lung disease - connective tissue diseases, infectious, sarcoidosis, drug-induced, pneumoconiosis
• Demential - Alzheimer's disease and multi-infarct demential

LABORATORY
• Anemia may be present
• Renal insufficiency will be present in almost 50% at presentation
• Proteinuria will be present in almost 80% at presentation
• In primary amyloidosis, an elevated monoclonal protein level will be found in the serum and/or urine
• In secondary amyloidosis, tests to assess the underlying inflammatory disease will be useful
Drugs that may alter lab results: N/A
Disorders that may alter lab results: N/A

PATHOLOGICAL FINDINGS
• Demonstration of amyloid deposits in tissues
• With Congo Red staining, amyloid produces a green birefringence under polarized light
• Electron microscopy is the definitive diagnostic tool

SPECIAL TESTS N/A

IMAGING Echocardiography (if cardiac involvement is suspected)

DIAGNOSTIC PROCEDURES
• Rectal biopsy (70% positive)
• Bone marrow biopsy (20% positive)
• Abdominal fat pad biopsy
• Endomyocardial biopsy
• Renal biopsy

TREATMENT

APPROPRIATE HEALTH CARE
Outpatient except for serious complications (congestive heart failure, renal failure)

GENERAL MEASURES Change from hemodialysis to peritoneal dialysis, which clears beta-2-microglobulin, in those with hemodialysis amyloidosis

ACTIVITY Fully active as tolerated

DIET
• Low protein, low salt for renal failure patients
• Low salt for congestive heart failure patients

PATIENT EDUCATION N/A

Amyloidosis

 MEDICATIONS

DRUG(S) OF CHOICE
Primary amyloidosis
◊ Treatment of the underlying plasma cell disorder may or may not affect the outcome
◊ Melphalan and prednisone are among the drugs of choice for plasma cell disorders. Colchicine may slow the progression of amyloid deposition.
Secondary amyloidosis
◊ Treatment of the underlying inflammatory process with disease-specific medications usually improves the outcome (i.e., isoniazid and rifampin for M. Tuberculosis)
Familial amyloidosis
◊ Colchicine, 0.6 mg two or three times a day may decrease renal amyloidosis in this condition
Hemodialysis amyloidosis
◊ None
Contraindications: Refer to manufacturer's literature
Precautions: Colchicine - bone marrow depression, including agranulocytosis, pancytopenia, thrombocytopenia, or aplastic anemia, may occur with prolonged administration. Monitor CBC periodically.
Significant possible interactions: Refer to manufacturer's literature

ALTERNATIVE DRUGS N/A

 FOLLOWUP

PATIENT MONITORING
Primary amyloidosis
◊ Regular testing of monoclonal protein levels to assess response to therapy
◊ Regular testing of renal function to assess response to therapy
Secondary and hemodialysis amyloidosis
◊ Follow-up to assess control of the underlying disease process
◊ Regular testing of renal function to assess degree of impairment

PREVENTION/AVOIDANCE N/A

POSSIBLE COMPLICATIONS Despite intervention, worsening renal failure, heart failure, arthropathy, interstitial lung disease, and neuropathy are common

EXPECTED COURSE AND PROGNOSIS
Primary amyloidosis
◊ The prognosis is dependent upon the underlying disease
◊ Once renal failure has developed, the prognosis is usually less than one year
◊ Congestive heart failure has a four month prognosis
◊ Overall prognosis is 12-14 months. Women have better survival than men.
Secondary amyloidosis
◊ The prognosis is much better, depending upon the ability to control the underlying inflammatory process
Familial and hemodialysis amyloidosis
◊ Highly variable

 MISCELLANEOUS

ASSOCIATED CONDITIONS
• Amyloid may bind Factor X leading to bleeding problems
• Splenectomy may ameliorate this condition by decreasing the amount of amyloid produced in the body

AGE-RELATED FACTORS
Pediatric: N/A
Geriatric: In general, older individuals do less well
Others: N/A

PREGNANCY No information available

SYNONYMS N/A

ICD-9-CM
277.3 amyloidosis

SEE ALSO N/A

OTHER NOTES N/A

ABBREVIATIONS N/A

REFERENCES
• Kelley, W.N., ed., Textbook of Internal Medicine, Philadelphia, J.B. Lippincott Co., 1989
• Kyle, R.A., et al.: Primary Systemic Amyloidosis: multivariate analysis for prognostic factors in 168 cases. Blood, 1986, July; 68(1):220-4
• Cohen, A.S., et al.: Survival of patients with primary (AL) amyloidosis. Colchicine-treated cases from 1976-1983 compared with cases seen in previous years (1961-1973). Am J Med 1987, Jun: 82(6):1182-90

Author R. Gorman, M.D.

Amyotrophic lateral sclerosis

BASICS

DESCRIPTION A degenerative disease (or group of diseases) which affects the upper and lower motor neurons.

Amyotrophic lateral sclerosis: the term applied to the sporadic and most common form of the disease. Includes a number of overlapping syndromes such as pseudobulbar palsy, progressive bulbar palsy, progressive muscular atrophy and primary lateral sclerosis.

Familial ALS: an autosomal dominant or recessive disease which is clinically similar to sporadic ALS but probably represents a distinct entity pathologically and biochemically.

ALS-Parkinson-dementia complex of Guam: an ALS like syndrome, often, but not always, associated with Parkinson's syndrome and dementia, which is prevalent amongst the Chamorro Indians of Guam (very rare in the USA).

Incidence in USA: 0.4-1.76/100,000
Prevalence in USA: 5 in 100,000
System(s) affected: Nervous
Genetics: N/A
Predominant age: Rare before age 40 years. Incidence increases with age.
Predominant sex: Male = Female

SIGNS AND SYMPTOMS
Variable combinations of:
◊ Unexplained weight loss
◊ Focal wasting of muscle groups
◊ Limb weakness with variable symmetry and distribution
◊ Difficulty walking
◊ Difficulty swallowing
◊ Slurring of speech
◊ Inability to control affect (emotions)
◊ Atrophy of muscle groups, initially in a myotomal distribution
◊ Fasciculations (other than calves)
◊ Hyperactive deep tendon reflexes (including jaw jerk)
◊ Spares cognitive oculomotor, sensory and autonomic functions

CAUSES
• Sporadic ALS - degeneration of the upper and lower motor neurons with their respective axons. Cause is unknown.
• Familial ALS - a genetically transmitted degenerative disease. Gene locus has been localized to the long arm of chromosome 21 and encodes the enzyme superoxide dismutase (SOD1). At this writing, levels of superoxide dismutase have not yet been proven to be low.
• ALS-Parkinson-dementia complex of Guam - possible relationship to ingestion of the cycad nut

RISK FACTORS
• Age over 40
• Family history of ALS

DIAGNOSIS

DIFFERENTIAL DIAGNOSIS
• Cervical spondylosis
• Lead intoxication
• Plasma cell dyscrasias
• Spinal muscular atrophy (adult form)
• Primary lateral sclerosis
• Familial spastic paraparesis
• Spinal multiple sclerosis
• Tropical spastic paraparesis

LABORATORY
• Possible hexosaminidase deficiency
Drugs that may alter lab results: N/A
Disorders that may alter lab results: N/A

PATHOLOGICAL FINDINGS
• Loss of Betz's cells in the motor cortex
• Atrophic or absent anterior horn cells of spinal cord
• Atrophic or absent neurons within the motor nuclei of the medulla and pons
• Degeneration of the lateral columns of the spinal cord
• Atrophy of the ventral roots
• Grouped atrophy of muscle (motor units)

SPECIAL TESTS   N/A

IMAGING   N/A

DIAGNOSTIC PROCEDURES
• Electromyography - denervation potentials (fibrillations, positive sharp waves) are associated with prominent fasciculations (which suggest anterior horn cell dysfunction). Voluntary motor unit potentials have increased amplitude, long duration and/or polyphasia. The interference pattern is reduced for the force generated and individual motor units have a high rate of discharge.
• Muscle biopsy - will show groups of shrunken angulated muscle fibers (grouped atrophy) amidst other groups of fibers with a uniform fiber type (fiber type grouping).

TREATMENT

APPROPRIATE HEALTH CARE
• Outpatient initially, may ultimately need nursing home placement and/or hospice
• Supportive care for complicating emergencies (aspiration, respiratory failure). Use of a respirator is a major ethical dilemma and is usually not suggested.

GENERAL MEASURES
Prosthetic devices, e.g. wheel chair, etc.

ACTIVITY   As tolerated

DIET   Modify as tolerated. May need tube feedings.

PATIENT EDUCATION
Printed material for patients (and reference lists for physicians) available from The Muscular Dystrophy Association (602-529-2000)

MEDICATION

DRUG(S) OF CHOICE None
Contraindications: N/A
Precautions: N/A
Significant possible interactions: N/A

ALTERNATIVE DRUGS Therapeutic trials of the efficacy of anti-oxidants (vitamins E, C, and B carotene) are expected to be undertaken

FOLLOWUP

PATIENT MONITORING
• Initially every three months, frequency to be increased as need for symptomatic therapy develops

PREVENTION/AVOIDANCE N/A

POSSIBLE COMPLICATIONS
• Aspiration pneumonia
• Decubitus ulcers
• Pulmonary embolism

EXPECTED COURSE AND PROGNOSIS
• ALS usually terminates in death within five years
• Patients predominantly manifesting progressive muscular atrophy have a better prognosis
• There have been reports of spontaneous arrest of the disease

MISCELLANEOUS

ASSOCIATED CONDITIONS None

AGE-RELATED FACTORS
Pediatric: N/A
Geriatric: Symptoms of ALS may inappropriately be attributed to age
Others: N/A

PREGNANCY Pregnancy is uncommon amongst affected individuals. Pregnancy would be unwise in any individual suffering from a disease with so poor a prognosis. If pregnancy did occur, the only foreseeable difficulties would be related to weakness.

SYNONYMS
• Motor neuron disease
• Lou Gehrig's disease
• ALS

ICD-9-CM
• 335.2 motor neuron disease
• 335.20 amyotrophic lateral sclerosis

SEE ALSO N/A

ABBREVIATIONS N/A

OTHER NOTES
• Also referred to as Mill's variant (unilateral involvement)

REFERENCES Rowland, L.P. (ed.): Merritt's Textbook of Neurology. 8th Ed. Philadelphia, Lea and Febiger, 1989

Author C. Bamford, M.D.

Anaerobic and necrotizing infections

BASICS

DESCRIPTION Gangrene is local death of soft tissues due to disease or injury and is associated with loss of blood supply. In this reading, emphasis will be on anaerobic and necrotizing infections which may be associated with development of gas.
Genetics: N/A
Incidence in USA: Infrequent
Prevalence: Rare
Predominant age: Any
Predominant sex: Male = Female

SIGNS AND SYMPTOMS
• Local pain
• Abnormally dark skin and tissues under skin (dark green to black)
• Fever
• Rapid pulse
• Fulminant course leading to death without treatment

CAUSES
• Local injury
• Superimposed infection (surface or deep)

RISK FACTORS
• Poor blood supply (arteriosclerosis)
• Old age
• Trauma
• Diabetes mellitus

DIAGNOSIS

DIFFERENTIAL DIAGNOSIS
Deep infections with muscle involvement and with or without abscess
• Gas gangrene:
◊ Gas gangrene resulting from soft tissue trauma; clostridial myositis; clostridial myonecrosis
◊ Abdominal wall gas gangrene; postoperative clostridial sepsis of the abdominal wall; clostridial myonecrosis of the abdominal wall
◊ Metastatic gas gangrene; gas gangrene without a visible wound; non-traumatic gas gangrene
◊ Uterine clostridial infections
◊ Gas gangrene of the heart
◊ Gas gangrene of the brain
• Streptococcal myositis: anaerobic myonecrosis; anaerobic streptococcal myositis
• Infected vascular gas gangrene; non-clostridial gas gangrene; non-clostridial myositis
• Synergistic necrotizing sepsis; synergistic necrotizing cellulitis‡
Superficial infections with or without abscess
• Hemolytic streptococcal gangrene
• Acute, infectious, staphylococcal gangrene
• Anaerobic cellulitis; crepitant phlegmon; clostridial cellulitis
• Necrotizing fasciitis‡; synergistic gangrene; non-clostridial anaerobic cellulitis; anaerobic cutaneous gangrene; Fournier's gangrene. (Note: If there is extension to the tissues of the abdominal wall below the deep fascia, such as the anterior sheath of the rectus muscle, Fournier's gangrene is a synergistic necrotizing sepsis rather than just a necrotizing fasciitis.)
• Panophthalmitis
Simple clostridial contamination of wounds
Infiltration or injection or aspiration of gas into wounds
• Wounds with gas not produced by bacteria
• Injection of gas into wounds
◊ Therapy (e.g., hydrogen peroxide)
◊ Pranksters' jokes
◊ Malingerers
◊ Psychiatric problems
• Aspiration and dissemination of air into wounds by muscular activity
• Subcutaneous emphysema related to air leak syndrome or trauma
Gas in tissues after industrial accidents
• Magnesiogenous pneumagranuloma
Gas in tissues after injections of chemicals
• Injection of drugs
• Accidental injection of a foreign agent, such as benzene

‡ These are similar infections but are in different locations

LABORATORY
• With severe gangrene, studies will reveal anemia and leukocytosis
• Gram smears for organisms
• Daily serum creatine kinase (CK) determination
Drugs that may alter lab results: Antibiotics prior to culture
Disorders that may alter lab results: N/A

PATHOLOGICAL FINDINGS
• Necrosis of tissues
• Sometimes, gas in tissues

SPECIAL TESTS
Cultures and sensitivity tests for microorganisms reported to produce gas in human tissues: These occur as follows:
◊ Gram-positive anaerobes: Cocci - Peptostreptococcus (anaerobic Streptococcus) (usually with group A Streptococcus [Streptococcus pyogenes, beta-hemolytic Streptococcus] or Staphylococcus aureus)
◊ Gram-positive anaerobes: Bacilli - Clostridium perfringens and other clostridia. Bacilli - Bacteroides fragilis (usually with other anaerobic gram-negative bacilli)
◊ Gram-negative aerobes: Bacilli-Escherichia coli, Klebsiella pneumoniae, Enterobacter species, Proteus species (all usually in mixed infections)

IMAGING
With roentgenograms, gas in tissues

DIAGNOSTIC PROCEDURES
Immediate surgical intervention with longitudinal incisions of skin, superficial fascia, deep fascia, and muscles to look for necrotic tissues

TREATMENT

APPROPRIATE HEALTH CARE
Hospital inpatient

GENERAL MEASURES
• Infectious disease consultation
• Intravenous fluids with glucose, electrolytes, blood, vitamins
• Frequent determinations of CBC and electrolytes
• Immediate surgical intervention for diagnosis and débridement of necrotic tissues
• Prophylaxis for tetanus
• Re-operation if possibility of spreading or unrecognized necrosis (with abnormal daily CK determination)
• Surgical repair for loss of skin and subcutaneous tissues

ACTIVITY
Bedrest

DIET
By mouth, as tolerated

PATIENT EDUCATION
N/A

MEDICATIONS

DRUG(S) OF CHOICE
• Antibiotics: Determined by stained smears, cultures, and sensitivity tests (although anaerobic organisms are difficult to culture and identify). Dosage will vary according to clinical circumstances; refer to manufacturer's literature and suggestions of infectious disease consultant.

```
Gram stain      Presumed organism
----------------------------------
+ cocci         Streptococcus†
+ bacilli       Clostridium spp
- bacilli       Bacteroides spp
- bacilli       Coliforms
----------------------------------
† anaerobic
```
◊ Gram-positive cocci: penicillin G, clindamycin, metronidazole, chloramphenicol or cephalosporins
◊ Gram-positive bacilli: penicillin G, clindamycin, metronidazole, chloramphenicol or cephalosporins
◊ Gram-negative bacilli (Bacteroides): clindamycin, metronidazole, cefoxitin (many B. frag. are resistant) chloramphenicol, ticarcillin or mezlocillin
◊ Gram-negative bacilli (Coliforms): gentamicin, tobramycin, amikacin, cephalosporins, ampicillin, mezlocillin, chloramphenicol or ticarcillin

Contraindications: Sensitivity to drugs

Precautions: Recognize spreading gangrene when patient is receiving sedatives and analgesics

Significant possible interactions: See manufacturer's profile of each drug

ALTERNATIVE DRUGS As above

FOLLOWUP

PATIENT MONITORING
• Monitor effective blood levels of prescribed antibiotics
• Electrolytes
• Nutrition
• CK determination

PREVENTION/AVOIDANCE
• Avoidance of trauma
• Good care of skin

POSSIBLE COMPLICATIONS Failure to recognize spreading gangrene

EXPECTED COURSE AND PROGNOSIS
• Good if gangrene arrested
• Fatality possible

MISCELLANEOUS

ASSOCIATED CONDITIONS
• Diabetes mellitus
• Arteriosclerosis
• Altered immunocompetence: Depressed immunocompetence may require an alteration of treatment

AGE-RELATED FACTORS
Pediatric: N/A
Geriatric: Diseases of the aged with debility and poor blood supply
Others: N/A

PREGNANCY Treatment as for non-pregnant, but consider the pregnancy

SYNONYMS N/A

ICD-9-CM
• 785.4
• 040.0
• 136.9

SEE ALSO Tetanus

OTHER NOTES N/A

ABBREVIATIONS
CBC = complete blood count

REFERENCES
• Centers for Disease Control, Public Health Service, U.S. Department of Health and Human Services: ACIP. Use of vaccines and immune globulin in persons with altered immunocompetence. MMWR 42/RR-4: 1-18, 1993.
• Furste, W., Lobe, T.E. & Botros, N.M: Gangrenous soft tissue infections. Infections in Surgery. 1985;4:837-878
• Furste, W., Dolor, M.C., Rothstein, L.B. & Vest, C.R.: Carcinoma of the large intestine and nontraumatic metastatic clostridial myonecrosis. Diseases of Colon & Rectum. 1986;29:899-904
• Styrt, B. & Gorbach, S.L.: Recent development in the understanding of the pathogenesis and treatment of anaerobe infections. New Engl J Med. 1989;321:240-246 & 298-302

Author W. Furste, M.D.

Anaphylaxis

 BASICS

DESCRIPTION A dramatic, acute, systemic reaction marked by pruritus, flushing, urticaria, respiratory distress, and vascular collapse following antigen exposure in a sensitized person.

System(s) affected: Pulmonary, Cardiovascular, Skin/exocrine, Gastrointestinal, Endocrine/metabolic, Hemic/Lymphatic/Immunologic

Genetics: Genetic predisposition for sensitization to certain antigens

Incidence/Prevalence in USA:
- Major medical problem, but exact figures unknown
- Drug-induced anaphylaxis occurs in 1 of every 2,700 hospitalized patients
- 0.3-0.7 deaths/100,000 per year from anaphylaxis

Predominant age: All ages

Predominant sex: Male = Female

SIGNS AND SYMPTOMS
- Pruritus, flushing, urticaria, angioedema
- Dyspnea, cough, rhonchi
- Rhinorrhea, bronchorrhea, wheezing
- Difficulty swallowing
- Nausea, vomiting, diarrhea, cramps, bloating
- Tachycardia, hypotension, shock, syncope
- Malaise, shivering
- Mydriasis

CAUSES Immunologically mediated process. The majority are IgE mediated, where an antigen causes mast cell degranulation, such as in Hymenoptera stings or the hapten penicillin. Others occur by activating complement, with the anaphylatoxins C3a, C4a, and C5a causing mast cell and basophil degranulation, such as many blood product reactions. Non-immunologic mast cell activators, such as iodinated contrast media or opiates, cause anaphylactoid reactions. Non-IgE, and possibly non-mast cell mediated causes of anaphylaxis-like syndromes include reactions to modulators of arachidonic acid metabolism, sulfiting agents, catamenial anaphylaxis, exercise induced anaphylaxis, and idiopathic recurrent anaphylaxis. Some important causes are:
- Antimicrobials (e.g. penicillin)
- Insect stings (e.g., honeybees, wasps, kissing bugs, deer flies)
- Immunotherapy
- Foods (e.g., peanuts, nuts, fish, crustaceans, mollusks, cow milk, eggs, soybean most common)
- Macromolecules (e.g., chymopapain, insulin, dextran, glucocorticoid, protamine)
- Vaccines
- Blood products
- Diagnostic chemicals (iodinated contrast media)
- Latex rubber (gloves, catheters)
- Ethylene oxide gas (dialysis tubing, other sterilized products)

RISK FACTORS Previous anaphylaxis

 DIAGNOSIS

DIFFERENTIAL DIAGNOSIS
- Anaphylactoid reactions: Occur after the first contact with substance, such as polymyxin, pentamidine, radiographic contrast media, aspirin
- Vasovagal reactions: Bradycardia with hypotension, also does not present with the tachycardia, flushing, urticaria, angioedema, pruritus, or asthma seen in anaphylaxis
- Pseudoanaphylactic reactions: Thought to be caused by release of free procaine
- Systemic mastocytosis: Benign or malignant overgrowth of mast cells. May have leukemia. Urticaria pigmentosa commonly seen in the benign form and is the presence of reddish brown macular-papular cutaneous lesions which urticate after trauma - Darier's sign. Bone marrow biopsy is usually diagnostic. Clinically indistinguishable from anaphylaxis
- Globus hystericus
- Hereditary angioedema: C1q esterase deficiency. In distinction to anaphylaxis there is painless and pruritus-free angioedema without urticaria, flushing or asthma. Usually the onset is slower and if severe airway obstruction is absent, is without hypotension.
- Pheochromocytoma: Paradoxically, because of beta-2 stimulation, some patients with pheochromocytoma present with hypotensive attacks accompanied by tachycardia. Urticaria, angioedema, and asthma are absent.
- Carcinoid syndrome
- Serum sickness

LABORATORY
- Hypoxemia, hypercarbia, acidosis
- Elevated serum and urine histamine (short lived circulation)
- Elevated serum tryptase (hours)

Drugs that may alter lab results: N/A

Disorders that may alter lab results: N/A

PATHOLOGICAL FINDINGS Central hypovolemia associated with peripheral hemostasis

SPECIAL TESTS N/A

IMAGING N/A

DIAGNOSTIC PROCEDURES History and physical findings are diagnostic

 TREATMENT

APPROPRIATE HEALTH CARE
- Outpatient: Those patients with cutaneous angioedema, urticaria, and minimal bronchospasm (with resuscitation equipment available). Released when symptoms and signs have cleared.
- Moderate to severe anaphylaxis or patients who live far from medical facilities should be treated in an emergency room and admitted for overnight observation
- All patients need a prescription at discharge for an emergency epinephrine kit, and should be instructed in its proper use
- Patients should be referred to an allergy specialist if the cause of anaphylaxis is unclear
- Patients with anaphylaxis from insect stings benefit from desensitization immunotherapy after discharge.

GENERAL MEASURES
Treatment depends on severity
- Immediate drug therapy
- Maintain a patent airway - endotracheal intubation and assisted ventilation may be necessary; possibly tracheostomy
- Oxygen
- Tourniquet placed proximal to injected or stung site if possible, to occlude lymphatic and venous drainage (but not arterial flow)
- Rapid desensitization if skin test is positive for a substance that must be given (antisera for botulism, diphtheria or snakebite)
- IV fluids
- Horizontal position with legs elevated
- Monitor vital signs frequently

ACTIVITY Bedrest until anaphylaxis clears

DIET Nothing until anaphylaxis clears

PATIENT EDUCATION Printed patient information available from: Asthma & Allergy Foundation of America, 1717 Massachusetts Avenue, Suite 305, Washington, DC 20036,(800)7-Asthma or American Allergy Association, P.O. Box 7273, Menlo Park, CA 94026, (415)322-1663

MEDICATIONS

DRUG(S) OF CHOICE
Immediate and always
• Epinephrine
◊ Less severe reaction: 0.3-0.5 mg (0.3-0.5 ml of a 1:1000 solution), IM every 20-30 minutes as needed for up to 3 doses
◊ Life-threatening reactions: 0.5 mg (5 ml of a 1:10,000 solution) given IV slowly and repeated every 5-10 minutes as needed. If IV line not possible, intralingual or endotracheal may be effective.
If severe reaction (hypotension)
• Antihistamines (both H1 and H2)
◊ Diphenhydramine (H1) 25-50 mg IV (IM or po) q6h for 24 hours
◊ Cimetidine (H2) 300 mg IV over 3-5 minutes
If persistent hypotension
• Vasopressor (Dopamine)
◊ 200 mg in 500 ml of dextrose in water given by infusion pump.
◊ Titrate to blood pressure.
◊ 3-20 mcg/kg/min commonly used range
◊ Must be given through a high quality IV catheter site, preferably through a central line
For persistent bronchospasm
• Bronchdilators
◊ Aminophylline
(1) 6 mg/kg IV bolus over 10-20 minute period in patients not on theophylline prior to admission
(2) 2.5 mg/kg IV bolus over 10-20 minutes in patients on theophylline prior to admission and without signs or symptoms of toxicity
(3) Follow bolus with infusion at 0.9 mg/kg/min
(4) Maintain blood level of 10-15 mcg/mL
◊ Inhaled beta-2 agonist (albuterol) 2.5 mg (0.5 cc of a 0.5% solution) in 3 cc of normal saline by nebulizer q 1-2 h as needed
Other
• Corticosteroids (hydrocortisone sodium succinate): Does not have an immediate effect but should be administered to prevent prolonged or recurrent anaphylaxis
◊ 250-500 mg IV q 4-6 h (4-8 mg/kg for children)
• Racemic epinephrine: For laryngeal edema
◊ 0.5 cc of a 2.25% solution in 3 cc of normal saline by nebulizer. May repeat every 1-2 hours
• Normal saline or Ringer's lactate: As necessary to maintain tissue perfusion
• Glucagon: May be beneficial for resistant hypotension caused by concurrent beta-blockade therapy
◊ 50 mcg/kg IV bolus over 1 minute, or alternatively, because of short half-life, can give as continuous infusion at 5-15 mcg/min
Contraindications: Refer to manufacturer's literature
Precautions: Refer to manufacturer's literature
Significant possible interactions: Refer to manufacturer's literature

ALTERNATIVE DRUGS   N/A

 FOLLOWUP

PATIENT MONITORING   Vital signs
should be followed closely during treatment and for several hours after anaphylaxis resolved. Symptoms can reoccur for up to 24 hours.

PREVENTION/AVOIDANCE
• Avoid drugs, foods that cause the reaction
• Insect sting anaphylaxis patients should carry a kit containing a pre-filled syringe of epinephrine and an epinephrine nebulizer whenever outdoors, avoid areas where insect exposure is likely, wear shoes outdoors, avoid hair spray, perfume, cologne, aftershave, and brightly colored clothing.
• Carry or wear a medical alerting identification indicating the anaphylaxis causing substance or event
• Clinicians, when administering drugs that may cause anaphylaxis, should be prepared for its occurrence, recognize early signs and have epinephrine available

EXPECTED COURSE AND PROGNOSIS   Favorable if treated

POSSIBLE COMPLICATIONS
• Hypoxemia
• Cardiac arrest
• Death

 MISCELLANEOUS

ASSOCIATED CONDITIONS   N/A

AGE-RELATED FACTORS
Pediatric: N/A
Geriatric: N/A
Others: N/A

PREGNANCY   N/A

SYNONYMS   N/A

ICD-9-CM
• 995.0 anaphylactic shock
• E947 other and unspecified drugs and medicinal substances
• E947.9 unspecified drug or medicinal substance

SEE ALSO
• Food allergy
• Insect bites and stings

OTHER NOTES
• Occasional food or insect sting anaphylaxis patients, if not exposed to the causative antigen in a long time, will lose their sensitivity. Prudence dictates continued carrying of an epinephrine emergency kit.
• Patients needing iodinated contrast studies may be pre-treated with steriods and antihistamines.

ABBREVIATIONS   N/A

REFERENCES
• Braunwald, E., et al. (eds.): Harrison's Principles of Internal Medicine. 12th Ed. New York, McGraw-Hill, 1991
• Callahm, M.L. (ed): Current Therapy in Emergency Medicine. Philadelphia, B.C. Decker Inc., 1987
• Atkinson, T.P, & Kaliner, M.A.: Anaphylaxis. Med Clin NA 76:841, 1992
• Yunginger, J.W.: Anaphylaxis. Ann Aller. 69:87, 1992

Author   S. Knoper, M.D.

Anemia, aplastic

 BASICS

DESCRIPTION An anemia in which the bone marrow fails to produce adequate numbers of peripheral blood elements. Usual course - insidious.
• Pure red cell aplasia is a related syndrome that is caused by a selective failure of the production of erythroid elements. It can be associated with thymomas. Fanconi's anemia is associated with congenital anomalies.
Genetics:
• Genetic pattern undetermined
• Autosomal recessive in Fanconi's anemia
System(s) affected:
Hemic/Lymphatic/Immunologic
Incidence/Prevalence in USA: Not very common
Predominant age:
• Idiopathic - adolescents and young adults
• Pure red cell and Fanconi's anemia - children only
• Secondary - all ages
Predominant sex: Male = Female

SIGNS AND SYMPTOMS
• Cold extremities
• Dyspnea
• Ecchymoses, petechiae
• Fatigue, fever
• Hemorrhage, menorrhagia, occult stool blood, melena, epistaxis
• Pallor
• Palpitations
• Progressive weakness
• Retinal flame hemorrhages
• Systolic ejection murmur
• Weight loss
• Short stature
• Microcephaly
• Thumb anomalies
• Renal anomalies
• Hypospadias

CAUSES
• Idiopathic (about 50% of the cases)
• Injury to pleuripotential stem cells
• Destruction of pleuripotential stem cells
• Immunologic injury
• Toxic exposure, e.g., benzene, inorganic arsenic
• Infectious hepatitis
• Radiation treatment
• Drugs - especially antibiotics, anticonvulsants, gold
• Pregnancy (rare)

RISK FACTORS
• Viral illness
• Stress
• Tumors of thymus

 DIAGNOSIS

DIFFERENTIAL DIAGNOSIS
• Other causes of pancytopenia
• Myelodysplastic disorders
• Acute leukemia
• Hairy cell leukemia
• Systemic lupus erythematosus
• Disseminated infection
• Hypersplenism
• Transient erythroblastopenia of childhood

LABORATORY
• Pancytopenia
• Absence of nucleated RBC in peripheral blood
• Anemia
• Decreased hemoglobin
• Decreased hematocrit
• Leukopenia
• Neutropenia
• Increased bleeding time
• Decreased reticulocytes
• Increased serum iron
• Normal total iron binding capacity (TIBC)
• Borderline high mean corpuscular volume (MCV) > 104
• Hematuria
• Abnormal liver function tests
• Increased chromosomal breaks
Drugs that may alter lab results: N/A
Disorders that may alter lab results: N/A

PATHOLOGICAL FINDINGS
• Normochromic RBC
Bone marrow:
◊ Increased iron stores
◊ Aplastic
◊ Normocytic RBC
◊ Anisocytosis
◊ Decreased myeloblasts
◊ Decreased myelocytes
◊ Macrocytic RBC
◊ Nucleated RBC
◊ Poikilocytosis

SPECIAL TESTS
Bone marrow aspirate, biopsy:
◊ Hypocellular
◊ Decreased erythroid precursors
◊ Decreased megakaryocytes
◊ Lymphocytosis

IMAGING CT of thymus region if thymoma-associated RBC aplasia suspected

DIAGNOSTIC PROCEDURES N/A

 TREATMENT

APPROPRIATE HEALTH CARE
Inpatient. Referral to an institution that has experience in treating these patients is recommended.

GENERAL MEASURES
• Vigorous supportive measures
• Avoid causative agents
• Human leukocyte antigen (HLA) testing on all patients and their immediate families
• Transfusion support (judiciously prescribed)
• Bone marrow transplantation for patients with an HLA-identical donor. Upper age restrictions on transplantations varies (from age 30 up to age 55) among institutions that perform them.
• Immunosuppressive therapy if no suitable donor
• Unrelated donor transplants, if other therapy fails
• Oxygen therapy if needed
• Thymectomy for thymoma
• Good oral hygiene

ACTIVITY Bedrest, reverse isolation

DIET No special diet, but nutritious diet important to improve resistance

PATIENT EDUCATION Printed patient information available from: Aplastic Anemia Foundation of America, P.O. Box 22689, Baltimore, MD 21203, (301)955-2803

Anemia, aplastic

MEDICATIONS

DRUG(S) OF CHOICE
Antithymocyte globulin (ATG)
◊ It is a horse serum containing polyclonal antibodies against human T cells. Skin test patients to determine any hypersensitivity.
◊ Treatment for older patients and patients without a compatible donor
◊ Dosage is 15 mg/kg diluted in 500 mL saline, infused over 4-6 h for 10 consecutive days
◊ May be used as a single agent or in combination with corticosteroids and/or androgenic steroids
Androgens
◊ Clinical trials inconclusive
◊ Useful for some patients lacking other options
◊ Oxymetholone - 3 mg/kg orally per day
◊ 2-3 month trial usually necessary to assess response (Fanconi's anemia)
◊ Prednisone for pure red cell anemia
Contraindications: Refer to manufacturer's literature
Precautions: Refer to manufacturer's literature
Significant possible interactions: Refer to manufacturer's literature

ALTERNATIVE DRUGS
Cyclosporine, prednisone and cyclophosphamide

FOLLOWUP

PATIENT MONITORING
Close monitoring for all treatments. Drugs and other forms of treatment have numerous and severe side effects.

PREVENTION/AVOIDANCE
• Avoid possible toxic agents
• Use safety measures when working with radiation

POSSIBLE COMPLICATIONS
• Hemorrhage
• Infection
• Transfusion hemosiderosis
• Transfusion hepatitis
• Heart failure
• Osteoporosis

EXPECTED COURSE AND PROGNOSIS
Depending on age, treatment available - guardedly favorable

MISCELLANEOUS

ASSOCIATED CONDITIONS N/A

AGE-RELATED FACTORS
Pediatric:
• Pure red cell anemia (Diamond-Blackfan) and Fanconi's anemia are seen more often in children
• Idiopathic aplastic anemia is more common in adolescents
• Secondary aplastic anemia seen in children exposed to ionizing radiation or treated with cytotoxic chemotherapeutic agents
Geriatric: The elderly are more exposed to large numbers of drugs and therefore more susceptible to secondary aplastic anemia
Others: N/A

PREGNANCY Pregnancy may be a cause of aplastic anemia (rare)

SYNONYMS
• Hypoplastic anemia
• Panmyelophthisis
• Refractory anemia
• Aleukia hemorrhagica
• Toxic paralytic anemia

ICD-9-CM
284 aplastic anemia

SEE ALSO N/A

OTHER NOTES N/A

ABBREVIATIONS N/A

REFERENCES Williams, W.J., et al.: Hematology. 4th Ed. New York, McGraw-Hill, 1990

Author M. Dambro, M.D. & Winter, M.D.

Anemia, autoimmune hemolytic

BASICS

DESCRIPTION Acquired anemia induced by binding of autoantibodies and/or complement to the red cells
Three main types
  ◊ Warm antibody (80-90%)
  ◊ Cold reacting antibody (10%)
  ◊ Drug induced
System(s) affected:
Hemic/Lymphatic/Immunologic
Genetics: Unknown
Incidence/Prevalence in USA: Unknown
Predominant age: < 50 years
Predominant sex: Female > Male

SIGNS AND SYMPTOMS
• Weakness
• Fatigue
• Exertional dyspnea
• Dizziness
• Palpitations
• Malaise
• Dyspnea
• Pallor
• Jaundice
• Splenomegaly
• Hepatomegaly
• Tachycardia
• Anemia (may be sudden and life threatening)

CAUSES
Warm antibody
  ◊ Idiopathic (50%)
  ◊ Neoplasia (Leukemia, myeloma, lymphoma, thymoma)
  ◊ Collagen vascular disease
  ◊ Viral infection: e.g., hepatitis
Cold antibody
  ◊ Idiopathic (50%)
  ◊ Infection (Mycoplasma, mononucleosis, viral)
  ◊ Neoplasia (lymphoma)
  ◊ Cold agglutinin diseae
Drug induced
  ◊ Methyldopa, quinidine, penicillin

RISK FACTORS Listed with Causes

DIAGNOSIS

DIFFERENTIAL DIAGNOSIS Other hemolytic anemias

LABORATORY
• Direct Coombs's test - positive
• Anemia
• Increased mean corpuscular volume (MCV)
• Increased mean cell hemoglobin concentration (MCHC)
• Spherocytosis
• Poikilocytosis
• Anisocytosis
• Rouleaux
• Reticulocytosis
• Nucleated RBC
• Large polychromatophilic reticulocytes
• Hyperbilirubinemia
• Decreased haptoglobin
• Hemoglobinemia
• Direct antiglobulin test
Drugs that may alter lab results: N/A
Disorders that may alter lab results: N/A

PATHOLOGICAL FINDINGS
• Bone marrow hyperplasia
• Increased marrow hemosiderin

SPECIAL TESTS
IgG antibody (warm)
IgM antibody (cold)

IMAGING N/A

DIAGNOSTIC PROCEDURES N/A

TREATMENT

APPROPRIATE HEALTH CARE
Inpatient

GENERAL MEASURES
Warm antibody
  ◊ Mild: conservative therapy
  ◊ Moderate: prednisone
  ◊ Severe: high dose prednisone, splenectomy, immunosuppressant, packed red cell transfusion
Cold antibody
  ◊ Supportive
  ◊ Avoid cold
  ◊ Red cell transfusion
  ◊ Consider high dose prednisone
Drug induced
  ◊ Stop the offending drug

ACTIVITY Rest until asymptomatic

DIET No special diet

PATIENT EDUCATION Griffith, H.W.: Instructions for Patients; Philadelphia, 1988 W.B. Saunders Co

MEDICATIONS

DRUG(S) OF CHOICE
• Glucocorticoids - prednisone 1-2 mg/kg each day in divided doses. May need to be adjusted downward if needed for long-term treatment.
Contraindications: Refer to manufacturer's literature
Precautions: Refer to manufacturer's literature
Significant possible interactions: Refer to manufacturer's literature

ALTERNATIVE DRUGS
• Immunosuppressive drugs (if prednisone and splenectomy do not cure)
◊ Azathioprine (Immuran) 125 mg/day for up to 6 months
• Intravenous gamma globulin (IVIG)

FOLLOWUP

PATIENT MONITORING
Monitor carefully if transfusion essential

PREVENTION/AVOIDANCE
No preventive measures known

POSSIBLE COMPLICATIONS
• Shock
• Thromboembolism
• Thrombocytopenic purpura (Evans's syndrome)

EXPECTED COURSE AND PROGNOSIS
• Good with appropriate treatment
• If secondary to an underlying disorder, the prognosis is determined by the course of the primary disease

MISCELLANEOUS

ASSOCIATED CONDITIONS
• Systemic lupus erythematosus
• Chronic lymphocytic anemia
• Diffuse lymphomas

AGE-RELATED FACTORS
Pediatric: May occur in pediatric age group
Geriatric: Unusual in this age group; rule out neoplasia
Others: N/A

PREGNANCY N/A

SYNONYMS N/A

ICD-9-CM
283.0 autoimmune hemolytic anemias

SEE ALSO N/A

OTHER NOTES N/A

ABBREVIATIONS N/A

REFERENCES
• Rosenwasser, L.J. & Joseph, B.Z.: Immunohematologic Disorders. JAMA, 268:2940-5, 1992
• Wheby, M.S. (ed.): Anemia. Medical Clinics of North America. Philadelphia, W.B. Saunders Co., 1992
• Wyngaarden, J.B., Smith, L.H. (eds): Cecil Textbook of Medicine. 18th Ed. Philadelphia, W.B. Saunders Co., 1988

Author B. Murray, M.D.

Anemia, pernicious

BASICS

DESCRIPTION A disorder due to vitamin B12 deficiency. Pernicious anemia is invariably associated with atrophic gastritis and histamine-fast achlorhydria. Vitamin B12 cannot be absorbed in the terminal ileum without intrinsic factor (a secretion of the parietal cells of the gastric mucosa). Usual course - slowly progressive.
Genetics: HLA-DR2; HLA-DR4. Present in the rare form of pernicious anemia that is hereditary. Endemic areas - northern Europe, including Scandinavia.
System(s) affected:
Hemic/Lymphatic/Immunologic, Gastrointestinal, Nervous
Incidence/Prevalence: Unknown
Predominant age: Older adults (> 60 years)
Predominant sex: Male = Female

SIGNS AND SYMPTOMS
• Abnormal reflexes
• Anorexia; weight loss
• Ataxia
• Atrophic glossitis
• Babinski's sign - positive
• Confusion
• Congestive heart failure
• Dementia
• Depression
• Exertional dyspnea
• Extremity numbness
• Extremity paresthesias
• Hepatomegaly
• Pallor
• Palpitations
• Poor finger coordination
• Position sense - decreased
• Prematurely gray-haired
• Purpura
• Romberg's sign, positive
• Skin pigmentation increased
• Sore tongue
• Splenomegaly
• Tachycardia
• Tinnitus
• Vertigo
• Vibration sense - decreased
• Vitiligo
• Weakness

CAUSES
• Atrophic gastric mucosa
• Intrinsic factor deficiency
• Probable autoimmunity against gastric parietal cells
• Autoimmunity against intrinsic factor

RISK FACTORS
• Vegetarian diet, without B12 supplementation
• Gastrectomy
• Blind loop syndrome
• Fish-tapeworm infestation
• Malabsorption syndromes
• Drugs: oral calcium-chelating drugs, aminosalicylic acid, biguanides
• Chronic pancreatitis
• Alcoholism

DIAGNOSIS

DIFFERENTIAL DIAGNOSIS
• Folic acid deficiency
• Myelodysplasia
• Neurological disorders without B12 deficiency
• Liver dysfunction
• Hypothyroidism
• Hemolysis or bleeding
• Drug effects
• Alcoholism

LABORATORY
• Achlorhydria
• Anisocytosis
• Anti-intrinsic poikilocytosis factor antibody
• Anti-parietal cell antibody
• Direct hyperbilirubinemia
• Haptoglobin decreased
• Howell-jolly bodies
• Hypergastrinemia
• Hypersegmented neutrophils
• LDH increased
• Leukopenia
• Macrocytic anemia
• Mean corpuscular volume - 110-140
• Pentagastrin stimulation - stomach pH > 6
• Peripheral blood smear - macro-ovalocytes
• Poikilocytes
• Serum ferritin increased
• Serum vitamin B12 level < 100 pg/mL
• Thrombocytopenia
Drugs that may alter lab results: N/A
Disorders that may alter lab results:
Falsely elevated MCV
  ◊ Cold agglutinins
  ◊ Hyperglycemia
  ◊ Marked hyperleukocytosis
Falsely normal serum vitamin B12 level
  ◊ Myeloproliferitive disorders
  ◊ Liver disease
Falsely low serum B12 level
  ◊ Multiple myeloma
  ◊ Oral contraceptive intake
  ◊ Pregnancy
  ◊ Folate deficiency
  ◊ Transcobalamin I deficiency
  ◊ Recent isotope administration

PATHOLOGICAL FINDINGS
• Bone marrow - hypercellular, macrocytes, iron stores increased
• Nests of megaloblasts
• Giant metamyelocytes
• Macropolymorpholeukocytes
• Hypersegmented neutrophils
• Stomach - atrophic gastritis, goblet cells increased
• Parietal cell atrophy
• Chief cell atrophy
• Gastric cytology - cellular atypia
• Spinal cord - myelin degeneration of the dorsal and lateral tracts
• Peripheral nerve degeneration
• Degenerative changes of the posterior root ganglia

SPECIAL TESTS
• Schilling test plus intrinsic factor - normal vitamin B12 absorption
• Schilling test - decreased vitamin B12 absorption
• Gastric analysis - achlorhydria

IMAGING N/A:

DIAGNOSTIC PROCEDURES
• Bone marrow aspiration
• Detailed history and physical

TREATMENT

APPROPRIATE HEALTH CARE
Outpatient

GENERAL MEASURES
• Treatment must be continued for life
• Identification and treatment of the underlying disorder

ACTIVITY Unlimited

DIET Emphasize meat, animal protein foods, legumes unless contraindicated

PATIENT EDUCATION Griffith, H.W.: Instructions for Patients, p 288, W.B. Saunders Co, Philadelphia (instructions to photocopy for patient)

MEDICATIONS

DRUG(S) OF CHOICE
Parenteral cyanocobalamin (vitamin B12)
◊ 100 micrograms subcutaneously for each dose
◊ Administer daily for the first week
◊ Administer weekly for one month
◊ Monthly injections for remainder of life (patients may be taught to give self-injection)
Contraindications: None
Precautions: Do not give folic acid supplements - may cause fulminant neurological deficit
Significant possible interactions: N/A

ALTERNATIVE DRUGS None

FOLLOWUP

PATIENT MONITORING
• Monthly injections of Vitamin B12
• Endoscopy every 5 years to rule out gastric carcinoma

PREVENTION/AVOIDANCE Early
detection of anemia; workup of anemia

EXPECTED COURSE AND
PROGNOSIS Anemia reversible with parenteral vitamin B12; neurologic effects not reversible with parenteral vitamin B12

POSSIBLE COMPLICATIONS
• Hypokalemia may complicate first week of treatment
• Central nervous system symptoms may be permanent if patient is not treated in less than six months after symptoms begin
• Gastric polyps
• Stomach cancer

MISCELLANEOUS

ASSOCIATED CONDITIONS
• Autoimmune diseases including rheumatoid arthritis, IgA deficiency
• Graves' disease
• Myxedema
• Iron deficiency
• Thyroiditis
• Vitiligo
• Idiopathic adrenocortical insufficiency
• Hypoparathyroidism
• Agammaglobulinemia
• Tropical sprue
• Celiac disease
• Crohn's disease
• Infiltrate disorders of the ileum and small intestine

AGE-RELATED FACTORS
Pediatric:
• Juvenile pernicious anemia occurs in older children and is the same in most respects as in adults
• Congenital pernicious anemia - usually evident before 3 years of age
Geriatric: More common in this age group and often in association with other autoimmune disorders, depression, and dementia
Others: N/A

PREGNANCY N/A

SYNONYMS
• Addison's anemia
• Megaloblastic anemia due to B12 deficiency

ICD-9-CM
• 281.0 pernicious anemia
• 281.1 other vitamin B12 anemia

SEE ALSO Folic acid deficiency

OTHER NOTES
• There is a 3-fold likelihood of developing gastric carcinoma. Suggest endoscopy approximately every 5 years even if asymptomatic.
• Folic acid treatment in patients with pernicious anemia is contraindicated

ABBREVIATIONS N/A

REFERENCES
• Wyngaarden, J.B., Smith, L.H. (eds): Cecil Textbook of Medicine. 18th Ed. Philadelphia, W.B. Saunders Co., 1988
• Williams, W.J., Beutler, E., Erslev, A.J., et al. (eds.): Hematology. 4th Ed. New York, McGraw-Hill, 1990
• Munseys, W. (ed.): The Medical Clinic of North America. V 76; No. 3, May, 1992

Author A. Abyad, M.D.

Anemia, sickle cell

BASICS

DESCRIPTION A chronic hemoglobinopathy transmitted genetically, marked by moderately severe chronic hemolytic anemia, periodic acute episodes of painful "crises", and increased susceptibility to intercurrent infections, especially S. pneumoniae. The heterozygous condition (Hb A/S) is called sickle cell trait and is usually asymptomatic, with no anemia.
System(s) affected:
Hemic/Lymphatic/Immunologic, Musculoskeletal
Genetics: Autosomal recessive, mostly in blacks. Homozygous presence of a variant hemoglobin, HbS or sickle hemoglobin. Heterozygous condition Hb A/S.
Incidence/Prevalence in USA:
Approximately 1 in 500 Black Americans have sickle cell anemia; 8-10% Black Americans have sickle trait
Predominant age: All ages
Predominate sex: Male = Female

SIGNS AND SYMPTOMS
- Often asymptomatic in early months of life
- After 6 months of age, earliest symptoms are pallor and symmetric, painful swelling of the hands and feet (hand-foot syndrome)
- Chronic hemolytic anemia
- Painful "crises" in bones, joints, abdomen, back, and viscera
- Mild scleral icterus
- Increased susceptibility to infections, especially pneumococcal sepsis and Salmonella osteomyelitis
- Functional asplenia
- Delayed physical/sexual maturation, especially boys
- Many multi-system complications, especially in later childhood and adolescence

CAUSES
- At molecular level: Hb S is produced by substitution of valine for glutamic acid in the sixth amino acid position of the beta chains of the hemoglobin molecule. When deoxygenated, Hb S polymerizes and forms long rods that change RBC from biconcave to sickle shape.
- At cellular level: Sickle RBCs are inflexible; odd shape and cell rigidity cause increased blood viscosity, stasis, and mechanical obstruction of small arterioles and capillaries, leading to distal ischemia. Sickle RBCs are also more fragile than normal, leading to hemolytic destruction in blood and reticuloendothelial system.
- At clinical level: Chronic anemia; a variety of "crises"; infections
  ◊ Vaso-occlusive crisis ("painful crisis"): Most common; pain results from tissue necrosis secondary to vascular occlusion and tissue hypoxia. Progressive organ failure and acute tissue damage results from repeated vaso-occlusive episodes.
  ◊ Aplastic crisis: Temporary suppression of RBC production in bone marrow by severe infection
  ◊ Hyperhemolytic crisis: Accelerated hemolysis; increased RBC fragility/shortened life span
  ◊ Sequestration crisis: Splenic sequestration of blood (only in infants/young children)
  ◊ Susceptibility to infection: Impaired/absent splenic function; defect in the alternate pathway of complement activation

RISK FACTORS
Vaso-occlusive crisis
  ◊ Hypoxia
  ◊ Dehydration
  ◊ Infection
  ◊ Fever
  ◊ Acidosis
  ◊ Cold
  ◊ Anesthesia
  ◊ Strenuous physical exercise
Aplastic crisis
  ◊ Severe infections
  ◊ Folic acid deficiency
Hyperhemolytic crisis
  ◊ Acute bacterial infections
  ◊ Exposure to oxidant drugs

DIAGNOSIS

DIFFERENTIAL DIAGNOSIS
- Anemia: Other hemoglobinopathies, e.g., Hb SC disease, HbC disease, Sickle cell-beta thalassemia
- Painful crisis: Other causes of acute pain in bones, joints, and abdomen. Seek infection and other precipitating causes.

LABORATORY
- Hb electrophoresis: Hb S predominates, variable amount Hb F, no Hb A. (In sickle cell trait, both Hb S and A are present).
- Screening tests: Sodium metabisulfite reduction-test; "Sickledex" test
- Anemia; hemoglobin approximately 8 g/dL; RBC indices usually normal but MCV > 75
- Reticulocytosis of 10-20%
- Leukocytosis; bands normal in absence of infection
- Thrombocytosis
- Peripheral smear: few sickled RBC's, polychromasia, nucleated RBC's
- Serum bilirubin mildly elevated (2-4 mg/dL); fecal/urinary urobilinogen high
- ESR low
- Serum LDH elevated
- Haptoglobin absent
Drugs that may alter lab results: N/A
Disorders that may alter lab results:
- Infection
- Other anemias (e.g., iron deficiency)

PATHOLOGICAL FINDINGS
- Variable, dependent on tissue
- Hypoxia/infarction in multiple organs

SPECIAL TESTS N/A

IMAGING.
- Bone scan (to rule out osteomyelitis)
- CT/MRI (to rule out CVA)

DIAGNOSTIC PROCEDURES N/A

TREATMENT

APPROPRIATE HEALTH CARE
- General health care maintenance on outpatient basis should include assessment of growth/development, regular immunizations and Pneumovax, vision/hearing screening, and regular dental care
- Hospitalization required for most crises and complications

GENERAL MEASURES
- Infections/fever - prompt treatment with antibiotics
- Minimize factors that enhance sickling
- Painful crises - hydration (2 X maintenance fluids); analgesics (narcotic and non-narcotic)
- Transfusion needed with aplastic crises, severe complications (i.e., CVA), before surgery, and with recurrent debilitating painful crises

ACTIVITY
- Bedrest with crises. Otherwise, activity level as tolerated.
- Activity may be somewhat limited because of chronic anemia and poor muscular development

DIET Well balanced diet with folic acid supplementation

PATIENT EDUCATION
- Guidelines for prompt management of fever, infections, pain, and specific complications should be reviewed at each visit
- Stress importance of keeping well-hydrated
- Teach early recognition of possible complications, especially education about priapism
- Genetic counseling

MEDICATIONS

DRUG(S) OF CHOICE
• Painful crises (mild, outpatient) - non-narcotic analgesics (ibuprofen, acetaminophen)
• Painful crises (severe, hospitalized) - parenteral narcotics (morphine, Demerol) on fixed schedule; gradually lower dose and replace with oral medication as soon as possible (acetaminophen w/codeine, ibuprofen). Correct dehydration and acidosis.
• Infections - prior to culture results, give antibiotic that covers S. pneumoniae and H. influenzae.
• Prophylactic penicillin controversial but often recommended

Contraindications None
Precautions: Avoid high-dose estrogen oral contraceptives
Significant possible interactions: None

ALTERNATIVE DRUGS   N/A

FOLLOWUP

PATIENT MONITORING
• Frequency determined by number/severity of crises and complications
• Early recognition/early treatment of infections. Parents/patient should be instructed that temperature of 101° F or above requires immediate medical attention.
• All febrile patients require cultures (blood/urine), chest x-ray, CBC/reticulocytes
• For patients who receive chronic transfusions - monitor for hepatitis and hemosiderosis

PREVENTION/AVOIDANCE
Avoid conditions that precipitate sickling (hypoxia, dehydration, cold, infection, fever, acidosis, anesthesia).

POSSIBLE COMPLICATIONS
• Bone infarct
• Aseptic necrosis of femoral head
• Cerebrovascular accidents with neurologic sequellae
• Cardiac enlargement
• Cholelithiasis/abnormal liver function
• Chronic leg ulcers
• Priapism
• Hematuria/hyposthenuria
• Retinopathy
• Acute chest syndrome (infection/infarction), leading to chronic pulmonary disease
• Infections (pneumonia, osteomyelitis, meningitis, pyelonephritis). Increased risk of sepsis with each.
• Hemosiderosis (2° to multiple transfusions)

EXPECTED COURSE AND PROGNOSIS
Anemia is lifelong. In second decade, number of crises diminish but complications more frequent. Some patients die in childhood, of CVA or sepsis. Most patients live to early-mid adulthood; few live > 50 years. Common causes of death are infections, thrombosis, pulmonary emboli, or renal failure.

MISCELLANEOUS

ASSOCIATED CONDITIONS
Psychosocial effects of chronic illness, especially low self-esteem, depression, and dependency. May need counseling, tutoring, and/or vocational training.

AGE-RELATED FACTORS
Pediatric:
• Sequestration crises and hand-foot syndrome seen only in infants/young children
• Functional asplenia in later childhood
<u>Adolescence/young adulthood:</u>
◊ Frequency of complications and secondary organ/tissue damage increase with age
◊ Psychological complications, including body-image and sexual identity problems, interrupted schooling/career training, restriction of activities, stigma of chronic disease, low self-esteem, fear of future
Geriatric: N/A
Others: N/A

PREGNANCY
• Usually complicated and hazardous, especially 3rd trimester and delivery
• Complications include increased number/severity of crises, toxemia, infection, pulmonary infarction, phlebitis
• Fetal mortality 35-40%; abortions/stillbirths, prematurity
• Prophylactic partial exchange transfusion in 3rd trimester reduces maternal morbidity and fetal mortality

SYNONYMS
• Sickle cell disease
• Hb S disease
• S/S disease

ICD-9-CM
• 282.60 sickle cell anemia, unspecified

REFERENCES
• Baehner, R.L. (ed.): Pediatric Clinics of North America: Symposium on Pediatric Hematology; Vol. 27, No. 2, May 1980, 429-447
• Blum, R.W. (ed.): Chronic Illness and Disabilities in Childhood and Adolescence, Grune & Stratton, Orlando, 1984, 265-276

Author   M. Broman, M.D.

Angina

BASICS

DESCRIPTION Symptom complex brought about by myocardial ischemia.
• Classic angina - a heaviness or pressure felt over the precordium, usually triggered by physical exertion or anxiety and relieved by rest
• Angina equivalent - dyspnea, fatigue, nausea, diaphoresis, or pain localized to an atypical location (i.e., jaw) which is brought about by myocardial ischemia and unaccompanied by typical precordial chest pressure
• Variant angina - also referred to as Prinzmetal's angina describes angina occurring at rest or in typical patterns such as after exercise or nocturnally. Prinzmetal's angina is caused by coronary artery spasm and is associated with ECG changes (usually ST elevation) during symptoms
• Unstable angina - pain which is new or which has changed its character to become more frequent, more severe or both. Unstable angina portends myocardial infarction in a certain percentage of patients.
System(s) affected: Cardiovascular
Genetics: Coronary artery disease has genetic implications
Incidence/Prevalence in USA: The presenting symptom of coronary artery disease in 38% of men and 61% of women
Predominant age: Most common in middle age and older men; postmenopausal women
Predominant sex: Male > Female

SIGNS AND SYMPTOMS
• Precordial pressure or heaviness, radiating to the back, neck or arms, brought on by exercise, emotional stress or meals and relieved by rest or nitrates
• Shortness of breath, nausea and diaphoresis often accompany the pain
• Dyspnea may present as the only symptom
• Epigastric pain and symptomatology may masquerade as atypical symptoms

CAUSES
• Atherosclerosis of the coronary arteries
• Coronary artery spasm
• Thrombosis
• Systemic lupus erythematosus
• Polyarteritis nodosa
• Rheumatic myocarditis
• Scleroderma
• Radiation
• Amyloidosis
• Hereditary medionecrosis
• Thrombotic thrombocytopenic purpura
• Aortic stenosis
• Hypertrophic cardiomyopathy
• Primary pulmonary hypertension
• Hypertension
• Aortic insufficiency

RISK FACTORS
• Hypercholesterolemia
• Family history
• Hypertension
• Tobacco abuse
• Alcohol abuse
• Male gender
• Obesity
• Diabetes mellitus
• Hypertension

DIAGNOSIS

DIFFERENTIAL DIAGNOSIS
• Pericarditis
• Aortic dissection
• Mitral valve prolapse
• Pulmonary embolus
• Pulmonary hypertension
• Pneumothorax
• Mediastinitis
• Pleuritis
• Esophagitis
• Esophageal spasm
• Peptic ulcer
• Gastritis
• Cholecystitis
• Costochondritis
• Radiculopathy
• Shoulder arthropathy
• Psychological

LABORATORY
• Total cholesterol - frequently elevated
• HDL cholesterol - frequently reduced
• LDL cholesterol - frequently elevated
Drugs that may alter lab results: N/A
Disorders that may alter lab results: N/A

PATHOLOGICAL FINDINGS
Atherosclerosis of the coronary arteries

SPECIAL TESTS
• ECG - may show evidence of prior myocardial infarction, other findings are nonspecific and tracings are frequently normal. Digoxin and various antiarrhythmic agents may make the ECG uninterpretable. Bundle branch block, Wolff-Parkinson-White syndrome or intraventricular conduction delay may make the ECG uninterpretable.
• Exercise stress testing

IMAGING
• Stress echocardiography
• Stress thallium
• Pharmacological stress or Sestanibi echocardiography
• Coronary angiography

DIAGNOSTIC PROCEDURES As above under Special Tests and Imaging

TREATMENT

APPROPRIATE HEALTH CARE The patient's symptoms should be brought under control medically. If symptoms are unstable, hospitalization is warranted.

GENERAL MEASURES
• Treatment goal - involves reducing myocardial oxygen demand or to increase oxygen supply
• Noninvasive testing is often indicated as a means of stratifying the patient's risk for an event that might seriously compromise myocardial function
• Quit smoking
• Exercise program after physician's approval
• Decrease caffeine intake
• Minimize stress

ACTIVITY As tolerated after consulting physician

DIET
• Low fat, low cholesterol diet
• Weight loss diet, if overweight

PATIENT EDUCATION American Heart Association, 7320 Greenville Avenue, Dallas, TX 75231, (214)373-6300

MEDICATIONS

DRUG(S) OF CHOICE
• Aspirin - 160 mg qd for all patients with coronary disease in which this medication is not contraindicated (i.e., coumadin usage)
• Beta-blockers - metoprolol 25-150 mg bid or atenolol 25-100 mg qd or propranolol 30-120 mg bid-tid. Beta-blockers are effective in reducing the heart rate and thereby decreasing oxygen consumption and reducing angina. Adjust doses according to clinical response. Aim to maintain resting heart rate of 55 - 60 beats per minute. Side effects are frequent and include fatigue, impotence, exacerbation of peripheral vascular and obstructive pulmonary disease, depression and sleep disturbances.
• Nitrates - isosorbide dinitrate (Isordil) 10-60 mg tid. Act through preload reduction and coronary vasodilatation. Tachyphylaxis occurs rapidly and dosing should be no more than 3 times a day with at least 10 hours between the evening and morning doses. Side effects include headaches, which are usually transient, and hypotension especially in volume depleted patients.
• Nitroglycerin 40 mcg sublingually is the most effective therapy for acute anginal episodes. The dose may be repeated several times over a 10-15 minute time period; if the patient does not experience relief he/she should be instructed to seek medical attention immediately.
• Calcium antagonist - long acting formulations of verapamil 160-480 mg qd or diltiazem 90-360 mg qd or nifedipine 30-120 mg qd are available. The various agents have their own individual side effects (i.e., verapamil - constipation; nifedipine - peripheral edema). None of the calcium antagonists should be used in patients with compromised ventricular function (left ventricular ejection fraction < 40%)
• Heparin - intravenously in a dose adequate to increase the PTT to 1.5 x baseline should be initiated in patients diagnosed with unstable angina

Contraindications: Refer to manufacturer's literature
Precautions: Refer to manufacturer's literature
Significant possible interactions:
• Beta-blockers and calcium channel blockers may combine to produce symptomatic heart block although either class of drug may act alone in producing this side effect
• Care must also be taken when combining these classes of drugs (beta-blockers and calcium channel blockers) in patients with even moderately compromised ventricular function

ALTERNATIVE DRUGS
Lipid lowering drugs are often initiated in patients with unfavorable lipid profiles

FOLLOWUP

PATIENT MONITORING
• Depends on the frequency and severity of the complaints
• Hospitalization for initiation of intravenous heparin is indicated in patients diagnosed with unstable angina

PREVENTION/AVOIDANCE
• Discontinue tobacco, adherence to low fat/low cholesterol diet, regular aerobic exercise program
• Consider antilipidemics

POSSIBLE COMPLICATIONS
• Related to myocardial damage occurring during infarction
• Arrhythmia
• Cardiac arrest
• Congestive heart failure

EXPECTED COURSE AND PROGNOSIS
• Variable and depending on the extent of coronary artery disease as well as left ventricular function
• Annual mortality is 3-4% overall

MISCELLANEOUS

ASSOCIATED CONDITIONS
• Hypercholesterolemia
• Claudication
• Crescendo angina
• Mitral regurgitation
• Papillary muscle dysfunction
• Ventricular aneurysm
• Abdominal aortic aneurysm
• Giant cell arteritis
• Pernicious anemia and other high output states
• Polycythemia rubra vera
• Renal artery stenosis
• Takayasu's arteritis
• Graves' disease
• Hypertrophic subaortic stenosis
• Primary hyperthyroidism

AGE-RELATED FACTORS
Pediatric: Suspect familial dyslipidemias in children presenting with manifestations of coronary artery disease
Geriatric: Patients may be very sensitive to the side effects of medications (i.e., beta-blockers - depression)
Others: N/A

PREGNANCY Other diagnosis should be excluded and the patient managed closely by an obstetrician and cardiologist as the metabolic demands of pregnancy will exacerbate symptoms and directly interfere with treatment

SYNONYMS
• Stenocardia
• Heberden's syndrome

ICD-9-CM
• 411.1 angina, unstable
• 413 angina pectoris
• 413.1 Prinzmetal's angina
• 413.9 angina, unspecified

SEE ALSO N/A

OTHER NOTES N/A

ABBREVIATIONS N/A

REFERENCES
• Brandenburg, R.O., Fuster, V., Giuliani, E.R. & McGoon, D.C.: Cardiology: Fundamentals and Practice. Chicago, Year Book Medical Publishers, 1987
• Braunwald, E.: Heart Disease: A Textbook of Cardiovascular Medicine. 3rd Ed. Philadelphia, W.B. Saunders Co., 1988

Author M. Goldberg, M.D.

Angioedema

BASICS

DESCRIPTION Rapid, localized edema of subcutaneous tissues up to several centimeters in diameter. Life threatening if larynx, pharynx is affected. Resolves in hours to days.
• Hereditary angioedema (HAE), type I - recurrent episodes involving both skin and mucous membranes, without urticaria. 25% mortality. Many have abdominal pain from edema of intestinal mucosa. Due to hereditary deficiency of C1-esterase inhibitor (C1-INH).
• Hereditary angioedema (HAE), type II - like type I, but normal levels of non-functional C1-INH
• Acquired angioedema - rare, in some patients with lymphoproliferative malignancies. Successful treatment of malignancy causes resolution of edema. Autoantibody inactivation or consumption of C1-INH.
• Vibratory angioedema - rare, local swelling in response to vibration. May be hereditary.
• Drug induced angioedema - immunologic hypersensitivity, as in penicillin reaction, or non-immunologic, as in aspirin or NSAID
• Angiotensin-converting enzyme (ACE) inhibitor induced angioedema - rare, 0.1% of patients on drug; non-immune; tendency to involve tongue, with life-threatening edema of airway. Can't predict. May occur immediately or after prolonged use of drug.
• Idiopathic angioedema - acute or chronic
System(s) affected: Skin/Exocrine
Genetics: Hereditary angioedema is autosomal dominant
Incidence/Prevalence in USA: About 1 in 5,000. Accompanies urticaria 50% of time.
Predominant age:
• Idiopathic - all ages
• Others - unknown
Predominant sex: Male = Female

SIGNS AND SYMPTOMS
• Occurs alone or with urticaria
• May occur as part of generalized anaphylactic reaction, potentially fatal
• May occur anywhere on body; usually face, extremities, genitalia; often asymmetric (e.g., half of upper lip, one earlobe)
• Rapid onset, usually resolves spontaneously in < 72 hours
• Very little itching in comparison to urticaria. Many have stinging or burning sensation.

CAUSES Allergic or non-allergic, mediated by release of histamine from mast cells in subcutaneous tissues

RISK FACTORS Medications that cause allergic reactions, e.g., penicillins, aspirin

DIAGNOSIS

DIFFERENTIAL DIAGNOSIS
• Anaphylaxis
• Cellulitis
• Erysipelas
• Contact dermatitis
• Lymphedema
• Diffuse subcutaneous infiltrative process
• Localized edema

LABORATORY
• C4 assay (low in HAE). If C4 normal, do urticaria work-up.
• If C4 is low, do C1-INH assay (immunoreactive) for HAE type I, and C1-INH assay (functional) for HAE type II
• If not HAE, do neoplastic work-up to rule out acquired angioedema, vasculitis work-up (CBC, ANA, RA, ESR, skin biopsy) to rule out autoimmune disease
Drugs that may alter lab results:
Antihistamines, H2-blockers, tricyclic antidepressants
Disorders that may alter lab results: N/A

PATHOLOGICAL FINDINGS Edema, vasculitis and/or perivasculitis involving only subcutaneous tissues

SPECIAL TESTS N/A

IMAGING N/A

DIAGNOSTIC PROCEDURES Skin biopsy (correlates poorly with clinical picture)

TREATMENT

APPROPRIATE HEALTH CARE Assure airway patency first! Protect airway if mouth, tongue, throat involved. CPR and transport to emergency room, if necessary.

GENERAL MEASURES Avoidance of known triggers. Cool moist compresses to control itching.

ACTIVITY As desired. HAE patients should avoid violent exercise, trauma.

DIET Avoidance of known trigger foods

PATIENT EDUCATION Educate HAE patients to provide history of disease to health care workers

MEDICATIONS

DRUG(S) OF CHOICE
Antihistamines for acute angioedema:
◊ Adults - hydroxyzine HCl 25 mg tid-qid or diphenhydramine, 25-50 mg q 6h
◊ Children over 6 - hydroxyzine HCl 0.6 mg/kg every 6 hours or diphenhydramine, 25-50 mg q 6h
◊ Children under 6 - diphenhydramine - 5 mg/kg/24 hours divided every 6 hours to a maximum of 300 mg/24 hours
HAE therapy:
◊ Intubation if airway threatened
◊ Epinephrine (1:1000) 0.2-0.3 ml IV or subcutaneous
◊ Fresh frozen plasma. Only effective for 1-12 days; no long term benefit. Risk of hepatitis B. transmission
◊ C1-INH (not yet available in USA)
◊ Danazol (attenuated androgen). For prevention (increases amount of active C1-INH in both types I and II). Give 200-600 mg daily (in 3 divided doses) for 1 month, then 5 days on, 5 days off. Maintenance dose may be determined by decreasing the initial dose approximately 50% every 1-3 months. Increase the dose temporarily if an attack occurs while on the drug. Ineffective in other forms of C1-INH deficiency. Side effects include headaches, weight gain, hematuria, masculinization.
Contraindications: Danazol not for use in childhood, pregnancy, breast feeding, hepatic, cardiac, or renal failure.
Precautions: Antihistamine drowsiness, euphoria (children)
Significant possible interactions: Danazol may potentiate effect of warfarin

ALTERNATIVE DRUGS
• Epsilon-aminocaproic acid (EACA) was used before danazol became available. Prevents activation of plasmin and C1. Rarely can cause thrombophlebitis, embolism, myositis.
• Stanozolol (another androgen, similar to danazol)

FOLLOWUP

PATIENT MONITORING Diagnostic workup if symptoms severe, persistent or recurrent

PREVENTION/AVOIDANCE If etiology known, avoidance. Avoid ACE inhibitors in patients with history of angioedema. Protect airway if mouth, tongue, throat involved.

POSSIBLE COMPLICATIONS
Anaphylaxis, respiratory compromise

EXPECTED COURSE AND PROGNOSIS
Most with idiopathic do well. Chronic forms dependent on nature of defect.

MISCELLANEOUS

ASSOCIATED CONDITIONS
• Urticaria
• Anaphylaxis

AGE-RELATED FACTORS
Pediatric: N/A
Geriatric: N/A
Others: N/A

PREGNANCY N/A

SYNONYMS
• Angioneurotic edema
• Quincke's edema

ICD-9-CM
995.1 angioneurotic edema
(hereditary: 277.6)

SEE ALSO Urticaria

OTHER NOTES
• Same pathophysiology for urticaria and angioedema - localized anaphylaxis causes vasodilatation, vascular permeability of skin (urticaria) or subcutaneous tissue (angioedema)
• Quincke's edema (when it involves uvula)

ABBREVIATIONS
• HAE = hereditary angioedema
• C1-INH = C1 esterase inhibitor

REFERENCES
• Cooper, K.D.: Urticaria and angioedema: Diagnosis and evaluation. J Am Acad Dermatol 25(1):166, 1991
• Greaves, M. & Lawlor, F.: Angioedema: Manifestations and management. J Am Acad Dermatol 25(1):155, 1991

Author J. Perchalski, M.D.

Animal bites

BASICS

DESCRIPTION Bite wounds to humans from dogs, cats, other animals including humans
System(s) affected: Endocrine/Metabolic, Skin/Exocrine, Hemic/Lymphatic/Immunologic, Nervous
Genetics: N/A
Incidence in USA:
• Dog bites: 600/100,000
• Cat bites: 160/100,000
• Snake bites: 15/100,000 non-venomous bites and 3/100,000 venomous bites per year in USA
• Human bites: Often the result of a closed fist injury
• Other animals: Can be domestic or wild
Prevalence in USA: Lifetime prevalence for animal bite 50,000/100,000
Predominant age: All ages, but children more likely to be affected
Predominant sex: Male > Female

SIGNS AND SYMPTOMS
• Bite wounds can be tears, punctures, scratches, avulsions or crush injuries
Dog bites
  ◊ Hands are most commonly affected with up to 68% of bites
  ◊ The face is the site of injury in up to 29% of cases, the lower extremities in 10%, and involvement of the trunk is uncommon
Cat bites
  ◊ Predominantly involve the hands, followed by lower extremities, face and trunk
  ◊ Are more likely to become infected

CAUSES
• Most bite wounds are from a domestic pet known to the victim. Large dogs are the most common source.
• Human bites are often the result of one person striking another in the mouth with a clenched fist

RISK FACTORS
• Dog bites are more common in the early afternoon, especially during warm weather
• Cat bites more common in the morning
• Clenched fist injuries are frequently associated with the use of alcohol

DIAGNOSIS

DIFFERENTIAL DIAGNOSIS The diagnosis is straightforward. What is of concern is judging the risk to the patient from the injury and resulting infection.

LABORATORY
• 85% of bite wounds will yield a positive culture. Gram stain is sensitive but not specific for infecting organism. Wound culture is essential in directing therapy.
• Dog bites - Pasteurella multocida is present in 25% of bites. Streptococcus viridans, Staphylococcus aureus, coagulase-negative Staphylococcus, Bacteroides, EF-2, DF-2, and Fusobacterium can also be found.
• Cat bites - Pasteurella multocida is present in 50% of bites. The wound is often contaminated by other mixed bacteria, including several species of both aerobic and anaerobic organisms.
• Human bites - Streptococcus species, Staphylococcus aureus, Eikenella corrodens and various anaerobic bacteria are common
• Other animal bites - scant information on the pathogens of these
Drugs that may alter lab results: N/A
Disorders that may alter lab results: N/A

PATHOLOGICAL FINDINGS N/A

SPECIAL TESTS N/A

IMAGING
• If bite wound is near a bone or joint, a plain radiograph is needed to check for bone injury and to use for comparison later if osteomyelitis is suspected
• In human bite wounds from clenched fist injuries, order plain film radiographs to check for metacarpal or phalanx fracture

DIAGNOSTIC PROCEDURES Surgical exploration might be needed to ascertain extent of injuries. Exploration should be performed on all serious hand wounds.

TREATMENT

APPROPRIATE HEALTH CARE
• Outpatient setting unless patient has fulminant infection requiring systemic antibiotics, close observation, or surgery

GENERAL MEASURES
• Copious irrigation of the wound with normal saline via a catheter tip is needed to reduce risk of infection
• Devitalized tissue needs débridement
• Consider surgical closure if the wound is clean after irrigation and bite is less than 12 hours old
• Delayed primary closure in 3-5 days is an option for infected wounds
• Splint hand if it is injured
• Human bite wounds on the hands should not be primarily closed due to the high risk of infection
• Elevation of the injured extremity to prevent swelling. Contact the local health department and consult about the prevalence of rabies in the species of animal involved.

ACTIVITY No restriction

DIET No special diet

PATIENT EDUCATION Discussion with parents at "well child checks" should include education on how to avoid animal bites

MEDICATIONS

DRUG(S) OF CHOICE
• Consider anti-rabies therapy
• Use tetanus toxoid in those previously immunized, but more than 5 years since their last dose
• Consider tetanus immune globulin in patients without a full primary series of immunizations

Prophylactic therapy if wound seen in first 12 hours:
◊ Dog bite - penicillin VK 500 mg po qid (child 50 mg/kg/day po given qid) x 3 days
◊ Cat bite - penicillin VK 500 mg po qid (child: 50 mg/kg/day po given qid) x 3 days
◊ Snake bite - if venomous the patient needs rapid transport to facility capable of administering antivenin for definitive therapy. If an envenomation has occurred, prepare to transport the patient to a center specializing in this area or prepare to administer antivenin. Be sure patient is stable for transport; consider measuring and or treating coagulation and renal status along with any anaphylactic reactions before transport.
◊ Others - amoxicillin. Dosage: Adult, 500 mg po tid. Children, 40 mg/kg/day, given tid; or amoxicillin/clavulanate potassium (Augmentin). Dosage: adult, 250-500 mg po tid. Child 20-40 mg/kg/day, given tid

Established infection
◊ Once patient has developed a clinical infection, amoxicillin/clavulanate potassium (Augmentin) can be used pending culture reports

Contraindications: Do not use penicillin-derived antibiotics in those with penicillin allergy
Precautions: Prescribe dosage of antibiotics by body weight and renal function
Significant possible interactions: Antibiotics may decrease efficacy of oral contraceptives

ALTERNATIVE DRUGS
Alternative therapy for penicillin allergic patients:
◊ Approximately 10% cross reactivity with cephalosporins in penicillin allergic patients
◊ Dog bite: tetracyclines if patient is older than 9 years, and in women only if they are not pregnant or breast feeding. Ceftriaxone or erythromycin can also be used.
◊ Cat bite: as for dog bite
◊ Human bite: cefoxitin 80-160 mg/kg/day (up to 12 grams), given in 3 or 4 equally divided doses. Usual dose is 1-2 grams q 6-8 hours. Erythromycin can also be used, 30-40 mg/kg/d in 4 equally divided doses. Usual adult dose is 250 mg qid.

FOLLOWUP

PATIENT MONITORING
• Patient should be rechecked in 24-48 hours if not infected at time of first encounter
• Daily follow up is warranted with active infections
• If antibiotics are used for an active infection, the duration of therapy should be 7-14 days depending on the severity of the infection and the clinical response

PREVENTION/AVOIDANCE
Instruct children and adults about animal hazards

POSSIBLE COMPLICATIONS
Complications from bites can include septic arthritis, osteomyelitis, extensive soft tissue injuries with scarring, sepsis, hemorrhage, death. Gas gangrene can take an exceedingly rapid course and should be treated very aggressively.

EXPECTED COURSE AND PROGNOSIS
Wounds should steadily improve and close over by 7-10 days

MISCELLANEOUS

ASSOCIATED CONDITIONS N/A

AGE-RELATED FACTORS
Pediatric: No special precautions
Geriatric:
• Serious injury from any bite wound is more common in persons greater than 50 years old, those with wounds in the upper extremities or those with puncture wounds
• Increased risk of infection in those greater than 50 years old
Others: N/A

PREGNANCY No special precautions

SYNONYMS N/A

ICD-9-CM
• 879.8 open wound(s) of unspecified site(s) without mention of complications
• 882.0 hand
• 873.40 face

SEE ALSO
• Rabies
• Snake Envenomations: Crotalidae
• Snake Envenomations: Elapidae

OTHER NOTES N/A

ABBREVIATIONS N/A

REFERENCES
• Goldstein, E.J.C.: Management of human and animal bite wounds. Am Acad of Derm. 1989. 6:1275-9
• Anderson, C.R.: Animal bites: Guidelines to current management. Postgrad Med 1992; 134-149

Author G. Bergus, M.D. & S. Meis, M.D.

Ankylosing spondylitis

 BASICS

DESCRIPTION A chronic, usually progressive, condition in which inflammatory changes and new bone formation occurs at the attachment of tendons and ligaments to bone (enthesopathy)
• Sacroiliac joint involvement is the hallmark of ankylosing spondylitis with variable degrees of spinal involvement. However, 20-30% of patients also have larger peripheral joint involvement
System(s) affected: Musculoskeletal
Genetics: Familial clustering and higher than expected frequency of HLA-B27 tissue antigen
Incidence/Prevalence in USA:
• 0.5-5 per 1000 in white males
• Less common in women and Blacks
Predominant age:
• Usually symptoms begin in early twenties
• Onset of symptoms - rarely occurs after age 40
Predominant sex: Male > Female

SIGNS AND SYMPTOMS
• Subgluteal or low back pain and/or stiffness
• Insidious onset
• Onset usually in 3rd decade
• Duration greater than 3 months
• Morning stiffness
• Frequently awaken at night to "walk off" stiffness
• Improvement in stiffness with activity
• Increased symptoms with rest
• Pleuritic chest pain is often an early feature
• Thoracic and cervical spine complaints in advanced disease
• Hip, shoulder, or knee complaints
• Diminished range of motion in the lumbar spine in all three planes of motion
• Loss of lumbar lordosis
• Thoraco-cervical kyphosis (rarely occurs before ten years of symptoms)
• Aortic root dilatation (20%)
• Aortic regurgitation murmur (2%)
• Acute anterior uveitis (20-30%)
• Osteoporosis

CAUSES Unknown

RISK FACTORS
• HLA-B27
• Positive family history
• 10% risk of developing AS (Ankylosing Spondylitis) for HLA-B27 positive child of spondylitic parent

 DIAGNOSIS

DIFFERENTIAL DIAGNOSIS
• Reiter's syndrome
• Psoriatic arthritis
• Diffuse idiopathic skeletal hypertrophy (DISH)
• Spondylitis associated with inflammatory bowel disease
• Rheumatoid arthritis

LABORATORY
• HLA-B27 tissue antigen is present in 90% of patients compared to 5-8% incidence in general population
• Erythrocyte sedimentation rate (ESR) is elevated in 80% of cases, but correlates poorly with disease activity and prognosis
• Absent rheumatoid factor
Drugs that may alter lab results: N/A
Disorders that may alter lab results: N/A

PATHOLOGICAL FINDINGS
• Erosive changes coupled with new bone formation at attachment of tendons and ligaments to bone resulting in ossification of periarticular soft-tissues
• Synovial changes are indistinguishable from rheumatoid arthritis. Erosion of articular cartilage is less severe than in rheumatoid arthritis.

SPECIAL TESTS
• Synovial fluid - mild leukocytosis, decreased viscosity
• Cerebrospinal fluid - increased protein
• EKG - conduction defects
• Measurement of respiratory excursion of chest wall - less than 5 cm maximal respiratory excursion of chest wall measured at fourth intercostal space. Less than 2.5 cm is virtually diagnostic of ankylosing spondylitis.
• Wright-Schober test for lumbar spine flexion is abnormal

IMAGING
• Sacroiliac joint early - sclerosis on both sides of joint not extending more than 1 cm from articular surface
• Sacroiliac joint late - ankylosis of sacroiliac joint
• Spine - "squaring" of vertebral bodies and ossification of annulus fibrosis giving appearance of "bamboo spine". Ankylosis of facet joints.
• Peripheral joint - symmetric erosive changes in larger joints. Pericapsular ossification, sclerosis, loss of joint space.

DIAGNOSTIC PROCEDURES
• Physical examination
• Radiographs - sacroiliac joint films, lumbar spine series

 TREATMENT

APPROPRIATE HEALTH CARE
Outpatient

GENERAL MEASURES
• Posture training and range of motion exercises for spine are essential
• Firm bed
• Sleep in prone position or supine without a pillow
• Breathing exercises 2-3 times/day
• Swimming
• Physical therapy
• Stop smoking, if a smoker

ACTIVITY Encourage active lifestyle

DIET No special diet

PATIENT EDUCATION For patient education materials favorably reviewed on this topic, contact: American Academy of Family Physicians Foundation, P.O. Box 8418, Kansas City, MO 64114, (800)274-2237, ext. 4400

MEDICATIONS

DRUG(S) OF CHOICE
• Nonsteroidal anti-inflammatory drugs provide symptomatic relief
• Selection is empiric, but traditionally indomethacin, 50 mg tid or qid has been used
• Steroids and cytotoxic agents are not effective

Contraindications: See Precautions

Precautions:
• All patients on long term NSAID's should have renal function monitored
• NSAID's may aggravate peptic ulcer disease or cause gastritis
• Don't use NSAID's for patients with a bleeding diathesis or patients requiring anticoagulants

Significant possible interactions: Refer to manufacturer's profile of each drug

ALTERNATIVE DRUGS
Other NSAID's, such as sulindac, naproxen

FOLLOWUP

PATIENT MONITORING Visits every six to twelve months to monitor posture and range of motion

PREVENTION/AVOIDANCE N/A

POSSIBLE COMPLICATIONS
• Spine: Pseudarthrosis, cervical spine fracture (high mortality rate), C1-C2 subluxation, spondylodiscitis, cauda equina syndrome (rare)
• Peripheral joint ankylosis
• Pulmonary: Restrictive lung disease, diaphragmatic breathing, upper lobe fibrosis (rare)
• Cardiac: Conduction defects (20%), aortic insufficiency (2%)
• Uveitis

EXPECTED COURSE AND PROGNOSIS
• Unpredictable course
• Prognosis good if mobility and upright posture maintained. Usually progressive disability.

MISCELLANEOUS

ASSOCIATED CONDITIONS
• Inflammatory bowel disease
• Uveitis
• Iritis

AGE-RELATED FACTORS
Pediatric: N/A
Geriatric: N/A
Others: N/A

PREGNANCY N/A

SYNONYMS
• Rheumatoid spondylitis
• Marie-Strumpell disease

ICD-9-CM
720.0 ankylosing spondylitis

OTHER NOTES
Flexion contractures of the hip and ankylosis may be major contributors to poor posture. Hip arthroplasty should be strongly considered as it may restore upright posture. Heterotopic ossification may occur post operatively and appropriate prophylaxis should be considered.

OTHER NOTES N/A

ABBREVIATIONS N/A

REFERENCES
• Calin, A. (ed.): Spondyloarthropathies. New York, Grune & Stratton, 1983
• Calin, A. and Fries, J.: Ankylosing Spondylitis Discussions in Patient Management. Garden City, New York, Medical Examination Publishing Company, 1978

Author G. Bradbury, M.D. & J. Benjamin, M.D.

Anorectal abscess

BASICS

DESCRIPTION Localized induration and fluctuance due to inflammation of the soft tissue near the rectum or anus. 80% of patients have perianal abscess, the remainder are intrasphincteral or supra levator abscesses

System(s) affected: Gastrointestinal, Skin/Exocrine

Genetics: No known genetic pattern

Incidence/Prevalence in USA: Common

Predominant age: All ages (most common in infants)

Predominant sex: Male > Female (4:1)

SIGNS AND SYMPTOMS
- Perirectal swelling for superficial abscesses
- Perirectal redness
- Perirectal tenderness
- Perirectal throbbing pain
- Fever and other toxic symptoms with deep abscesses
- If abscess is not accompanied by external swelling, digital exam will reveal a swollen tender mass
- Pain on defecation

CAUSES
- Bacterial invasion of the pararectal spaces, originating in an intersphincteric space which may begin with an abrasion or tear in lining of anal canal, rectum or perianal skin
- Organisms: usually mixed, E. coli, Proteus vulgaris, streptococci, staphylococci, bacteroides, pseudomonas aeruginosa

RISK FACTORS
- Inciting trauma
    ◊ Injections for internal hemorrhoids
    ◊ Enema tip abrasions
    ◊ Puncture wounds from eggshells or fish bones
    ◊ Foreign objects
    ◊ Prolapsed hemorrhoid
- Inflammatory bowel disease
- Chronic granulomatous disease
- Immunodeficiency disorders
- Hematologic malignancies (5-8% of these patients will have abscess at some time)

DIAGNOSIS

DIFFERENTIAL DIAGNOSIS
- Carcinoma
- Retrorectal tumors
- Crohn's disease
- Primary lesions of syphilis
- Tuberculous ulceration

LABORATORY CBC - leukocytosis
Drugs that may alter lab results: N/A
Disorders that may alter lab results: N/A

PATHOLOGICAL FINDINGS
- Inflammation of anal mucosa
- Pus
- Inflammatory tissue

SPECIAL TESTS N/A

IMAGING Barium enema

DIAGNOSTIC PROCEDURES
Only indicated if diagnosis in doubt
    ◊ Sigmoidoscopic exam - rule out unusual causes
    ◊ Proctoscopy: redness, induration of anus; tender mass

TREATMENT

APPROPRIATE HEALTH CARE
- Outpatient surgery
- Inpatient surgery with IV antibiotics for supra-levator abscess or toxicity

GENERAL MEASURES
Perianal abscess
    ◊ Abscess incised and drained
    ◊ Local anesthetic frequently appropriate
    ◊ Wound packed with Iodoform gauze (24-48 hours)
Ischiorectal abscess
    ◊ Abscess incised and drained
    ◊ Usually general anesthetic used
    ◊ Wound packed with Iodoform gauze (removed after several days)
    ◊ Fistulectomy may be done at same time in selected cases
After surgery:
    ◊ Sitz baths q 2-4 hours
    ◊ Heating pad, heat lamp or warm compress as needed for pain
    ◊ Encourage moving legs as soon as possible
    ◊ Prevent constipation

ACTIVITY Resume work and normal activity as soon as possible

DIET Increase fiber and fluid intake

PATIENT EDUCATION
- Sitz bath instruction
- Diet instructions
- Dressing change instructions
- Stress length of time to heal
- Stress physical cleanliness
- Possible development of fistula-in-ano
- Stress stool regularity

MEDICATIONS

DRUG(S) OF CHOICE
- Antibiotics - only for toxicity
- Stool softening laxatives

Contraindications: Refer to manufacturer's literature

Precautions: Refer to manufacturer's literature

Significant possible interactions: Refer to manufacturer's literature

ALTERNATIVE DRUGS N/A

FOLLOWUP

PATIENT MONITORING Routine postoperative care with attention to wound healing which should progress from the inside out

PREVENTION/AVOIDANCE
- Avoid constipation
- Don't use enemas
- Avoid rectal temperatures or medicines in immunocompromised patients

POSSIBLE COMPLICATIONS
- Possible anorectal fistula (in 25% of patients)
- Possible rectovaginal fistula
- Incontinence of feces due to rupture through sphincter muscle
- Recurrence of abscess if underlying cause not corrected

EXPECTED COURSE AND PROGNOSIS Slow healing depending on extent of disease, complete healing by 6 months if no complications (much faster in uncompromised patients)

MISCELLANEOUS

ASSOCIATED CONDITIONS
- Crohn's disease
- Other inflammatory disease such as appendicitis, salpingitis, diverticulitis
- Possibly perianal hidradenitis suppurativa, or HIV infection in patients with recurring perianal or ischiorectal abscesses

AGE-RELATED FACTORS
Pediatric: Common in first year of life

Geriatric: In elderly patients, a high pelvirectal abscess may cause no symptoms except lower abdominal pain and fever

Others: N/A

PREGNANCY N/A

SYNONYMS N/A

ICD-9-CM 566

SEE ALSO N/A

OTHER NOTES N/A

ABBREVIATIONS N/A

REFERENCES
- Schwartz, S.I., Shires, G.T., Spences, F.C. & Storer, E.H.: Principles of Surgery. 4th Ed. New York, McGraw-Hill Book Co., 1984
- Ashcraft, K.W. & Holder, T.M.: Pediatric Surgery. 2nd Ed. Philadelphia, W.B. Saunders Co., 1993
- Fazio, V.W.: Anorectal Disorders. In Gastroenterology Clinics of North America. Philadelphia, W.B. Saunders Co., 1987
- Schouten, W.R. & van Vroonhoven, T.J.: Treatment of anorectal abscess with or without primary fistulectomy. Results of a prospective randomized trial. Dis Colon Rectum 1991; 34:60-3

Author T. Black, M.D.

Anorectal fistula

 BASICS

DESCRIPTION
Inflammatory track with one opening in the anal canal and another in perianal skin. Fistulas occur spontaneously or secondary to perirectal abscess. Most fistulas originate in the anal crypts at the anorectal juncture.

Goodsall's rule
◊ If external opening is anterior to an imaginary line drawn horizontally through anal canal, fistula usually runs directly into anal canal
◊ If external opening is posterior to line, the fistula usually curves to posterior midline of anal canal
◊ In children, track is usually straight

Classification
◊ Intersphincteric
◊ Transphincteric
◊ Supra sphincteric
◊ Extrasphincteric

System(s) affected: Gastrointestinal, Skin/Exocrine
Genetics: No known genetic pattern
Incidence/Prevalence in USA: Common
Predominant age: All ages
Predominant sex: Male = Female

SIGNS AND SYMPTOMS
• Constant or intermittent draining or discharge
• Firm tender peri-anal lump
• External anal sphincter pain during and after defecation
• Spasm of external anal sphincter during and after defecation
• Anal bleeding
• Discoloration of skin surrounding the fistula
• Fistulous opening frequently granulose or scarred
• Possible fever

CAUSES
• Erosion of anal canal
• Extension from infection from a tear in lining in anal canal
• Infecting organism is Escherichia coli

RISK FACTORS
• Injection of internal hemorrhoids, puncture wound from eggshells or fish bones, foreign objects, enema tip injuries
• Ruptured anal hematoma
• Prolapsed internal hemorrhoid
• Acute appendicitis, salpingitis, diverticulitis
• Inflammatory bowel disease (chronic ulcerative colitis, Crohn's disease)
• Previous perirectal abscess

 DIAGNOSIS

DIFFERENTIAL DIAGNOSIS
• Pilonidal sinus
• Perianal abscess
• Urethroperineal fistulas
• Ischiorectal abscess
• Submucous or high muscular abscess
• Pelvirectal abscess (rare)
• Rule out: Crohn's disease; carcinoma; retrorectal tumors

LABORATORY
CBC
Drugs that may alter lab results: N/A
Disorders that may alter lab results: N/A

PATHOLOGICAL FINDINGS
• Fistulous tract may be simple or multiple
• Fistulous tract has primary opening in anal crypt, secondary opening in anal skin, para-anal skin perineal skin or in rectal mucus membrane
• Anal sinus - opens in anal crypt
• Termination of sinus is blind and located in para-anal or pararectal tissue

SPECIAL TESTS
N/A

IMAGING
Lower GI series if inflammatory bowel disease suspected

DIAGNOSTIC PROCEDURES
• Proctoscopy
• Sigmoidoscopy
• Probe inserted into tract to determine its course (be careful not to create an artificial opening)

 TREATMENT

APPROPRIATE HEALTH CARE
Outpatient surgery

GENERAL MEASURES
• Fistulotomy - surgical incision of entire length of fistula (unroofing). Mucosal tract may be corrected. Sphincterotomy.
• Fistulectomy - complete excision of tract is usually necessary. Sphincterotomy.
• General anesthesia or regional anesthesia usually required
• Postoperative - hot sitz baths
• Avoid constipation

ACTIVITY
Resume work and normal activity as soon as possible

DIET
Clear liquid diet until gastrointestinal function returns

PATIENT EDUCATION
• Stress peri-anal cleanliness
• Sitz baths

MEDICATIONS

DRUG(S) OF CHOICE
• Broad spectrum antibiotic if active infection
• Stool-softening laxative
Contraindications: Refer to manufacturer's literature
Precautions: Refer to manufacturer's literature
Significant possible interactions: Refer to manufacturer's literature

ALTERNATIVE DRUGS   N/A

FOLLOWUP

PATIENT MONITORING   Frequent followup examinations following surgery to ensure complete healing and assess continence

PREVENTION/AVOIDANCE   N/A

POSSIBLE COMPLICATIONS
• Constipation (urge to defecate may be suppressed due to pain)
• Rectovaginal fistula
• Partial incontinence of fecal material if sphincter is divided
• Delayed wound healing
• Low grade carcinoma may develop in long-standing fistulas
• Recurrent anorectal fistula if fistula is incompletely opened or excised

EXPECTED COURSE AND PROGNOSIS
• Surgical results usually excellent
• Postoperative healing requires 4-5 weeks for perianal fistulas; 12-16 weeks for deeper fistulas

MISCELLANEOUS

ASSOCIATED CONDITIONS
• Possibly associated with penetrating injury, intestinal tuberculosis, ulcerative colitis
• Hidradenitis suppurativa
• Crohn's disease

AGE-RELATED FACTORS
Pediatric: Most common in infants. More frequent in males.
Geriatric: Constipation more likely a complication
Others: N/A

PREGNANCY   N/A

SYNONYMS
• Fistula-in-ano

ICD-9-CM
565.1 Anal fistula

SEE ALSO   N/A

OTHER NOTES   N/A

ABBREVIATIONS   N/A

REFERENCES
• Kirsner, J.B. & Shorter, G. (eds.): Diseases of the Colon, Rectum and Anal Canal. Baltimore, Williams & Wilkins, 1989
• Sleisenger, M.H. and Fordtran, J.S. (eds.): Gastrointestinal Disease: Pathophysiology, Diagnosis, Management. 4th Ed. Philadelphia, W.B. Saunders Co., 1989
• Schwartz, S.I., Shires, G.T., Spences, F.C. & Storer, E.H.: Principles of Surgery. 4th Ed. New York, McGraw-Hill Book Co., 1984
• Welch, K.J., Randolph, J.G., Ravitcl, M.M., O'Neill, J.A. & Rowe, M.L.: Pediatric Surgery. 4th Ed. Chicago, Year Book Medical Publishers, 1986

Author   T. Black, M.D.

Anorexia nervosa

BASICS

DESCRIPTION Intense fear of becoming fat; significant weight loss; amenorrhea (in females), not due to physical disease
Incidence/Prevalence in USA:
Approximately 1% of females; males comprise 5-10% of cases
System(s) affected: Nervous, Gastrointestinal, Cardiovascular, Reproductive
Genetics: N/A
Predominant age: Usually adolescents or young adults
Predominant sex: Female > Male

SIGNS AND SYMPTOMS
- Usually insidious in onset
- Onset may be stress related
- Pronounced weight loss (generally 15% below original or expectable weight)
- Deny that there is a problem
- Claim to feel fat even when emaciated; food refusal
- Preoccupation with body size, weight control
- Reduction in total food intake, especially high calorie foods
- Elaborate food preparation and eating rituals
- Extensive exercise, especially running
- Depression that may be secondary to inanition
- Cracked, dry skin, sparse scalp hair
- Fine, downy lanugo hair on extremities, face, and trunk
- Hypotension and bradycardia
- Hypothermia
- Peripheral edema

CAUSES Unknown; thought to be largely emotional. Co-morbid major depression and/or dysthymia in 50-75% of patients. Obsessive-compulsive disorder in 10-13% of patients.

RISK FACTORS
- Perfectionistic personality
- Low self-esteem
- Achievement pressure; high self-expectations
- Acceptance of the culturally condoned ideal of slimness
- Ambivalence about dependence/independence
- Stress due to multiple responsibilities, tight schedules
- Unstable body image; perceptual distortions

DIAGNOSIS

DIFFERENTIAL DIAGNOSIS Inanition due to physical disorder; brain tumor; bulimia; depressive disorders with loss of appetite; food phobia; conversion disorder; schizophrenic disorder; body dysmorphic disorder

LABORATORY
- Most findings are directly related to starvation, dehydration
- Diminished plasma LH, FSH, T3
- Elevated growth hormone, cortisol
- Positive dexamethasone suppression test
- Diminished plasma tryptophan
- Diminished BUN
- Flat glucose tolerance curve, depressed fasting blood sugar

Drugs that may alter lab results: N/A
Disorders that may alter lab results: N/A

PATHOLOGICAL FINDINGS All are directly related to starvation
- Cracked, dry skin, sparse scalp hair
- Fine, downy lanugo hair on extremities, face, and trunk
- Hypotension and bradycardia
- Hypothermia
- Peripheral edema

SPECIAL TESTS Measure percent body fat

IMAGING Not indicated

DIAGNOSTIC PROCEDURES
- Psychological screening
- Eating Attitudes Test

TREATMENT

APPROPRIATE HEALTH CARE
- Majority can be treated as outpatients
- Hospitalize if weight loss greater than 30% in 6 months; if patient is suicidal; if there is lab or EKG evidence of marked electrolyte imbalance; or if there has been no response to outpatient therapy

GENERAL MEASURES
Inpatient:
◊ If possible admit to specialized eating disorders unit
◊ Bedrest with supervised meals
◊ 300 calorie stepwise increase from 1500 calories or less
◊ Stepwise increase in activity as weight increases
◊ Assess psychological state and nutritional status
◊ Involve patient in establishing target weight
◊ Weigh daily at first, then 3 x per week
◊ Achieve 1-2 pound per week weight gain
◊ Supportive therapy within structured eating disorders program
◊ Tube feeding only as last resort
◊ Medicate for symptom relief
Outpatient:
◊ Build trust, treatment alliance
◊ Assess psychological state and nutritional status
◊ Involve patient in establishing target weight
◊ Achieve gradual weight gain
◊ Weigh weekly at first, monthly when progress is evident
◊ Focus on overall indices of health, rather than weight gain alone
◊ Challenge fear of uncontrollable weight gain
◊ Consider group, cognitive-behavioral, individual, family or couples therapy
◊ Medicate for symptom relief

ACTIVITY
- Stepwise increase as patient gains weight
- Monitor activity; gain patient's cooperation

DIET
- Goal is weight stabilization on a balanced diet with normal eating pattern
- Diminished ruminations about calories, weight

PATIENT EDUCATION
- Provide information on nutrition, metabolic balance
- Provide tools for self monitoring when appropriate
- For patient education materials favorably reviewed on this topic, contact: Anorexia Nervosa & Related Eating Disorders, P.O. Box 5102, Eugene, OR 97405, (503)344-1144

MEDICATIONS

DRUG(S) OF CHOICE
• Short term anxiolytic therapy for starved inpatients (oxazepam 15 mg or alprazolam 0.25 mg before meals) to lessen anxiety about weight gain
• Low dose phenothiazines (Thorazine 10-25 mg/day) useful for inpatients

Contraindications: Refer to manufacturer's literature

Precautions: Starved patients are more sensitive to medication, likely to suffer dangerous or lethal side effects due to compromised liver and kidney function: caution is indicated

Significant possible interactions: Refer to manufacturer's literature

ALTERNATE DRUGS
• When patient is bulimic as well as anorexic and resistant to treatment, consider tricyclics - (imipramine (Tofranil) 10 mg, gradual increase to 200 mg (higher doses in inpatient settings), or desipramine (Norpramin) 25 mg/day, increasing gradually to 150 mg/day. Monitor either with EKG.
• Cyproheptadine (Periactin) 4 mg, increasing gradually if side effects permit to 32 mg/day.
• Clomipramine or fluoxetine (Prozac) 10-40 mg may be considered when obsessive compulsive symptoms predominate
• Metoclopramide (Reglan) 10-15 mg before each meal and at bedtime for abdominal distension due to delayed gastric emptying
• Therapeutic vitamin-mineral supplement

FOLLOWUP

PATIENT MONITORING
• Level of activity
• Weigh weekly until stable, then monthly
• Depression, self-esteem, suicidal ideation
• Ruminations and rituals
• Repeat any abnormal lab values weekly or monthly

PREVENTION/AVOIDANCE
• Encourage rational attitude about weight
• Moderate overly high self-expectations
• Enhance self-esteem
• Diminish stress

POSSIBLE COMPLICATIONS
• Potassium depletion; cardiac arrhythmia; cardiac arrest
• Nitrogen depletion, exhaustion, collapse
• Cardiomyopathy, congestive heart failure
• Delayed gastric emptying
• Convulsions, peripheral neuropathy
• Bone marrow hypoplasia
• Osteoporosis
• Too rapid initial weight gain can cause congestive heart failure or sudden gastric dilatation
• Suicide

EXPECTED COURSE AND PROGNOSIS
• Highly variable
• Poor prognosis indicated by repeated hospitalization, failed treatment, continued low weight, vomiting
• Mortality 6%
• Early age of onset indicates more favorable prognosis
• Many symptoms resolve spontaneously with weight gain

MISCELLANEOUS

ASSOCIATED CONDITIONS
• Major depression
• Bipolar disorder
• Obsessive-compulsive disorder
• Dissociative disorder
• Schizophrenic disorder
• Substance abuse disorder
• Borderline personality disorder

AGE-RELATED FACTORS
Pediatric: Growth can be compromised in preadolescence and early adolescence
Geriatric: Difficult to diagnose in elderly
Others:
• Ballet dancers, gymnasts, models, cheerleaders, and athletes are at relatively high risk
• Ruminations, rituals, and abnormal attitudes toward food and the body often persist even after weight gain

PREGNANCY Unlikely due to amenorrhea

SYNONYMS N/A

ICD-9-CM
307.1 anorexia nervosa

SEE ALSO N/A

OTHER NOTES N/A

ABBREVIATIONS N/A

REFERENCES
• Yates, A.: Current Perspectives on the Eating Disorders: I. History, Psychological and Biological Aspects. J Am Acad Child Adolesc Psychiatry 28(6):813-828, 1989.
• Yates, A.: Current Perspectives on the Eating Disorders: II. Treatment, Outcome, and Research Directions. J Am Acad Child Adolesc Psychiatry 29(1):1-9, 1990.
• Garner, D.M. & Garfinkel, P.: Anorexia Nervosa: A Multidimensional Perspective. New York, Brunner-Mazel, 1982
• Yager, et al.: Practice Guidelines for the Eating Disorders. Am J Psychiatry. 150:207-228, 1993

Author A. Yates, M.D.

Anxiety

BASICS

DESCRIPTION A common acute or chronic, fearful emotion with associated physical symptoms. DSM-III-R recognizes the following sub types:
• Acute situational anxiety: Response to recent stressful event, usually transient symptoms
• Adjustment disorder with anxious mood: Persistent, maladaptive reaction following psychosocial stress and lasting up to six months
• Generalized anxiety disorder: Persistent underlying anxiety or adjustment disorder with anxious mood and significant symptoms of motor tension, autonomic hyperactivity and hypervigilance, lasting more than six months
• Panic disorder: Single panic attack followed by at least a month of anticipatory anxiety or at least four panic attacks in one month; often leads to agoraphobia
• Post-traumatic stress disorder: Recurrent flashbacks or nightmares of catastrophic event by survivors, often associated with autonomic symptoms
• Phobias: Intense recurrent fear of, and avoidance of, an object or situation (simple phobia) or of public embarrassment (social phobia)
• Obsessive-compulsive disorder: Persistent unwanted and disturbing thoughts and recurrent behavioral patterns (i.e., hand washing) which interfere with daily life
System(s) affected: Nervous
Genetics: Panic disorders - increased concordance in monozygotic versus dizygotic twins
Incidence in USA: N/A
Prevalence in USA: 40 million (the most common psychiatric disorder in US)
Lifetime prevalence rate
◊ Panic disorder - female: 1.6-2.1%, male: 0.6-1.2%
◊ Obsessive compulsive disorder - female: 2.6-3.1%, male: 1.1-2.6%
◊ Agoraphobia - female: 5.3-12.5%, male: 1.5-5.2%
Predominant Age: Mainly adults, highest prevalence in 20 to 45 year age group
Predominant Sex: Female > Male

SIGNS AND SYMPTOMS Patterns vary with subtype of anxiety; not all present in each case
• Unrealistic or excessive anxiety or worry
• Sense of impending doom
• Nervousness
• Instability
• Tachycardia; palpitations
• Systolic click murmur
• Hyperventilation, choking sensation
• Labile hypertension
• Sighing respiration
• Nausea or abdominal distress
• Paresthesias
• Diaphoresis
• Dizziness or syncope
• Flushing
• Muscle tension
• Tremulousness
• Restlessness
• Chest tightness, pressure (pseudoangina)
• Headache, backaches, muscle spasm

CAUSES
• Panic disorder and obsessive compulsive disorder are associated with genetic factors
• Psychosocial stressors commonly trigger anxiety disorders and may provoke a genetic diathesis
• Mediated by abnormalities of neurotransmitter systems (serotonin, norepinephrine and gamma-aminobutyric acid [GABA])

RISK FACTORS
• Social and financial problems
• Medical illness
• Family history
• Lack of social support

DIAGNOSIS

DIFFERENTIAL DIAGNOSIS
Cardiovascular:
◊ Ischemic heart disease
◊ Valvular heart disease
◊ Cardiomyopathies
◊ Myocarditis
◊ Arrhythmias
◊ Mitral valve prolapse (most symptomatic cases are associated with panic disorder)
Respiratory:
◊ Asthma
◊ Emphysema
◊ Pulmonary embolism
◊ Hamman-Rich syndrome
◊ Scleroderma
CNS:
◊ Transient cerebral insufficiency
◊ Psychomotor epilepsy
◊ Essential tremor
Metabolic and Hormonal:
◊ Hyperthyroidism
◊ Pheochromocytoma
◊ Adrenal insufficiency
◊ Cushing's syndrome
◊ Hypokalemia, hypoglycemia
◊ Hyperparathyroidism
◊ Myasthenia gravis
Nutritional:
◊ Thiamine, pyridoxine, or folate deficiency
◊ Iron deficiency anemia
Intoxication:
◊ Caffeine
◊ Alcohol
◊ Cocaine
◊ Sympathomimetics
◊ Amphetamines
Withdrawal:
◊ Alcohol
◊ Sedative-hypnotics
Other:
◊ Panic disorder is associated with several physical disorders, including (a) mitral valve prolapse (systolic click-murmur) (b) labile hypertension (c) migraine headaches (d) irritable bowel syndrome
◊ Depression

LABORATORY
• Selective use of laboratory tests, (with minimal to more extensive workup depending on clinical picture). Laboratory tests often normal in anxiety disorders.
• CBC and urinalysis
• Sequential serial multiple analysis (SMA-12 panel)
• Thyroid function studies
Drugs That May Alter Lab Results: N/A
Disorders That May Alter Lab Results: N/A

PATHOLOGICAL FINDINGS N/A

SPECIAL TESTS EEG, ECG, etc.

IMAGING Usually none; chest x-ray possibly

DIAGNOSTIC PROCEDURES
• Psychologic testing (e.g., Zung's anxiety self-assessment, Hamilton's anxiety scale)
• DSM III based interview

TREATMENT

APPROPRIATE HEALTH CARE
Outpatient

GENERAL MEASURES
• Should be based on careful workup and identification of etiology and subtype of anxiety disorders
• Adequate workup
• Identify co-existent substance abuse
• Counseling or psychotherapy along with medications
• Regular exercise program
• Biofeedback in selected cases
• Serial office visits
• Judicious reassurance after other medical disorders ruled out

ACTIVITY Fully active

DIET No special diet

PATIENT EDUCATION
• Printed material available from AAFP Herb L. Huffington Memorial Library: 8880 Ward Parkway
P.O. Box 8418, Kansas City, MO, 1-800-274-2237, ext 4400
• National Institute of Mental Health (NIMH) - National Anxiety Awareness Program, 9000 Rockville Pike, Bethesda, MD 20892

MEDICATIONS

DRUG(S) OF CHOICE

Acute situational anxiety: Short-term (up to 1 month) treatment with benzodiazepines; e.g., alprazolam (Xanax), lorazepam (Ativan), diazepam (Valium). Usual dose of Xanax 0.25 mg two to three times daily, increased if needed in 0.25 mg increments.

Adjustment disorder with anxiety mood: Benzodiazepines as above

Generalized anxiety disorder: Azapirones e.g., buspirone (BuSpar), initially 5 mg bid-tid, increase by 5 mg q2-3days to maximum of 60 mg/day in divided doses

Panic disorder: TCA's, e.g., imipramine (Tofranil). With Tofranil, begin with 10-25 mg qhs; increase by 10-25 mg/day every 2 weeks to maximum of 300 mg/day (100 mg/day maximum in geriatric and adolescent patients). With fluoxetine (Prozac), begin with 4 mg and increase by 4 mg every 5 days to maximum daily dosage of 20-40 mg.

Obsessive-compulsive disorder: Clomipramine (Anafranil), initially 25 mg bid, may increase gradually to 250 mg/day if needed and as tolerated. New serotonergic re-uptake inhibitors (SRI's) also effective (Prozac 40-100 mg/day or sertraline [Zoloft] 100-200 mg/day)

Contraindications:
• Benzodiazepines - acute alcohol intoxication with depressed vital signs, acute angle-closure glaucoma, first-trimester pregnancy, sleep apnea, history of personality disorder or substance abuse. Avoid long-term or prn use.
• Buspirone - concurrent MAO inhibitor therapy
• TCA's - acute myocardial infarction

Precautions:
• Benzodiazepines - advanced age, renal insufficiency, suicidal tendency, open-angle glaucoma on treatment, sudden discontinuation. Sudden discontinuation may increase the risk of developing seizures, especially in patients receiving alprazolam
• Buspirone - hepatic and/or renal dysfunction. Buspirone will not protect against benzodiazepine withdrawal seizures; taper benzodiazepines.
• TCA's - advanced age, glaucoma, benign prostate hypertrophy, hyperthyroidism, cardiovascular disease, liver disease, urinary retention, MAO inhibitor treatment

Significant possible interactions:
• Benzodiazepines
  ◊ cimetidine, oral contraceptives, disulfiram, ethanol, levodopa, rifampin
• Buspirone
  ◊ MAO inhibitors
• TCA's
  ◊ amphetamines, barbiturates, guanethidine, clonidine, epinephrine, norepinephrine, ethanol, MAO inhibitors, propoxyphene
• SRI's
  ◊ MAO inhibitors: may cause fatal serotonin syndrome (confusion, hyperthermia, etc.)

ALTERNATIVE DRUGS
• Generalized anxiety disorder: Short-term use of benzodiazepine or TCA's
• Panic disorder: Although TCA's are the drugs of choice for panic disorder, they are slow in onset of action (two to three weeks). Benzodiazepines may be helpful for initial control of symptoms until the TCA's are effective. Also, 10 to 20% of patients with panic do not tolerate side effects of TCA's. High potency benzodiazepines (alprazolam, clonazepam, lorazepam), fluoxetine (Prozac) or MAO inhibitors are effective alternatives.
• Obsessive-compulsive disorder: Fluoxetine (Prozac) initial dosage 20 mg; may increase by 20 mg each week to a dosage of 40 to 100 mg/day. Sertraline (Zoloft) also effective (initial dose 50 mg, increase by 50 mg every 2 weeks to maximum daily dosage of 150-200 mg).

FOLLOWUP

PATIENT MONITORING
• Followup by regular office visits
• Watch for associated depression and treat if present
• Monitor mental status on benzodiazepines and avoid drug dependence
• Monitor blood pressure, heart rate, anticholinergic side effects on TCA's
• Periodic serum levels, if indicated, for TCA's

PREVENTION/AVOIDANCE
• Management of stress, to extent possible
• Relaxation techniques
• Meditation

POSSIBLE COMPLICATIONS
• Impaired social/occupational functioning
• Drug dependence (benzodiazepines)
• Cardiac arrhythmias (TCA's)

EXPECTED COURSE AND PROGNOSIS
• With active treatment, excellent results can often be obtained, especially with short-term anxiety disorders, including panic disorder
• Obsessive-compulsive disorder, and post-traumatic stress disorder are more difficult to treat, often requiring longer-term psychotherapy and medication (combination treatment)

MISCELLANEOUS

ASSOCIATED CONDITIONS
• Depression (commonly)
• Agoraphobia
• Alcohol or substance abuse
• Somatoform disorders (including somatization disorders, hypochondriasis, and conversion disorder)

AGE-RELATED FACTORS
Pediatric: Reduced dosage of medications in adolescent
Geriatric: Reduced dosage of medications
Others: N/A

PREGNANCY
• Benzodiazepines - contraindicated in first-trimester of pregnancy, and should be used with caution later in pregnancy and during lactation. May cause lethargy and weight loss in nursing infants; avoid breast feeding if mother taking benzodiazepines chronically or in high doses.
• TCA's - there is some evidence of fetal risk, especially in first trimester
• SRI's taper and discontinue, if possible, in first trimester; may be used later in pregnancy

SYNONYMS
• Hyperventilation syndrome
• Panic disorder

ICD-9-CM
300.0 anxiety states

SEE ALSO N/A

OTHER NOTES N/A

ABBREVIATIONS
DSM-III-R = "Diagnostic and Statistical Manual of Mental Disorders", 3rd edition, revised (from the American Psychiatric Association)
TCA = tricyclic antidepressant
SRI = serotonergic re-uptake inhibitor

REFERENCES
• Katon, W. & Geyman, J.P.: Anxiety. In Textbook of Family Practice. Edited by R.E. Rakel. Philadelphia, W.B. Saunders Co., 1990, 1566-1581
• Rakel, R.E. (ed.): Anxiety Profiles: New Perspectives for Diagnosis and Treatment. New York, Science and Medicine, 1991
• Johnson, G.E.: Essentials of Drug Therapy. Philadelphia, W.B. Saunders Co., 1991
• Ellsworth, A.J., Bray, R.F., Bray, B.S. & Geyman, J.P.: The Family Practice Drug Handbook. Chicago, Mosby-Year Book, 1991
• Katon, W.: Panic Disorder in the Medical Setting. Washington, D.C., American Psychiatric Press, 1991
• Roy-Byrne, P.P.: Integrated Treatment of Panic Disorder. Am J Med. Suppl 1A, 495-545, 1992
• Landry, M.J., Smith, D.E., McDuff, D.R. & Baughman, O.L.: Benzodiazepine dependence and withdrawal: Identification and medical management. J AM Bd Fam Prac. 19925:167-171

Author J. Geyman, M.D. & W. Katon, M.D.

Aortic dissection

 BASICS

DESCRIPTION Intimal tear in the aorta propagated via hematoma formation causing further dissection and separation producing a false lumen in the arterial wall.
<u>The Debakey classification:</u>
◊ Type I: Involves the aortic root, aortic arch, and the descending aorta
  ◊ Type II: Involves only the ascending aorta
  ◊ Type III: Involves only the distal aorta beyond the origin of the left subclavian artery
System(s) affected: Cardiovascular
Genetics: N/A.
Incidence/Prevalence in USA:
• 1 in 10,000 patients admitted to hospital; found 1 in 350 patients at autopsy
• 2000 new cases diagnosed annually
Predominant age: Dependent on etiology; Marfan's commonly present in the third and fourth decade; most common between the 6th and 8th decades
Predominant sex: Male > Female (3:1)

SIGNS AND SYMPTOMS
• Abrupt onset of tearing pain
• Shearing anterior chest pain which radiates to the interscapular region
• Back pain
• Syncope
• Symptoms of congestive heart failure
• Stroke
• Limb ischemia
• Abdominal pain
• Acute myocardial infarction
• Spinal cord syndromes/deficits
• Hypotension or hypertension
• Wide pulse pressure
• Murmur of aortic insufficiency
• Features of tamponade
• Dullness in left lung base (effusion)
• Pulse deficits or asymmetry
• Fever

CAUSES
• Pregnancy
• Ehlers-Danlos syndrome
• Relapsing polychondritis
• Chest trauma
• Postcardiovascular surgery
• Cystic medionecrosis
• Hypertension
• Marfan's syndrome
• Aortic stenosis
• Coarctation of aorta
• Bicuspid valve
• Turner's syndrome
• Iatrogenic during arterial catheterization

RISK FACTORS
Hypertension (refer to Causes)

 DIAGNOSIS

DIFFERENTIAL DIAGNOSIS
• Myocardial infarction
• Pulmonary embolism
• Pneumonia
• Pleurisy
• Pericarditis
• Pneumothorax
• Angina
• Acute pancreatitis
• Penetrating duodenal ulcer

LABORATORY No special studies required
Drugs that may alter lab results: N/A
Disorders that may alter lab results: N/A

PATHOLOGICAL FINDINGS
Approximately 60% of intimal tears occur in the proximal ascending aorta. The remainder are found between the origin of the left subclavian artery and ligamentum arteriosum, descending aorta (20%), aortic arch (10%), and the abdominal aorta. Although medionecrosis is found in normal aging aortas, it appears to be more extensive in patients who develop aortic dissection. Cystic medionecrosis is seen in patients with defects in elastin and connective tissue organization i.e. Marfan's, Ehlers-Danlos, etc. Death usually due to rupture and tamponade.

SPECIAL TESTS
• Electrocardiogram - LVH, nonspecific ST-T changes, electrical alternans with associated tamponade
• Echocardiogram - dilated aortic root, increased aortic posterior or anterior wall thickness, pericardial effusion, oscillating intimal flap

IMAGING
• Chest x-ray - widening of the superior mediastinum, left pleural effusion, haziness or enlargement of the aortic knob, double density of the descending aorta, irregular aortic contour, > 5 mm separation of intimal calcification from outer aortic contour, rightward displacement of the trachea, cardiomegaly.

DIAGNOSTIC PROCEDURES
• CT chest - demonstration of two lumens with hematoma formation, detection of intimal flap, differential flow between two lumens, compression of true lumen by false lumen
• Aortogram - demonstration of two lumens, detection of intimal flap, compression of true lumen, ulcer-like projections of contrast, arterial compromise, altered flow patterns, aortic insufficiency (not as sensitive as previous thought)
• Transesophageal echocardiography (TEE) - test of choice for hemodynamically unstable patients
• MRI - if available and patient hemodynamically stable, test of choice since same sensitivity as CT, but higher specificity

 TREATMENT

APPROPRIATE HEALTH CARE
Admission to intensive care unit or transfer to operative suite

GENERAL MEASURES
• Treatment of choice - surgical for all ascending aortic dissections and medical for descending dissections without complications
• Medical therapy is based on decreasing blood pressure and the "shearing" forces of myocardial contractility (dp/dt) to attempt to decrease intimal tear and hematoma propagation
• Arterial blood pressure monitoring is critical
• Careful observation for changes in mentation, neurological signs, or evidence of organ dysfunction
• A Foley catheter should be used to follow urine output
• Swan-Ganz catheterization may be very helpful to monitor cardiac performance and filling pressures during the use of vasoactive and cardiodepressive drugs
• Pain control may be difficult despite use of narcotics

ACTIVITY
Bedrest

DIET
NPO until surgical evaluation is complete and patient classified as medical therapy only

PATIENT EDUCATION
Depending on etiology, emphasis must be placed on risk factors and recurrence of symptoms

MEDICATIONS

DRUG(S) OF CHOICE Propranolol in 1 mg IV doses every 5 minutes until the heart rate is 60-70 beats per minute plus nitroprusside titrated to reduce systolic blood pressure to 100-110 mm Hg

Contraindications:
• Propranolol - in bronchial asthma, diabetes mellitus, Raynaud's disease, sinus bradycardia, A-V heart block greater than first degree, in presence of monoamine oxidase inhibitors, cardiogenic shock, congestive heart failure or right ventricular failure from pulmonary hypertension
• Nitroprusside - In treatment of compensatory hypertension i.e., arteriovenous shunt, in patients with inadequate cerebral circulation, and for use during emergency surgery in moribund patients

Precautions:
• Propranolol should be used cautiously in patients with angina pectoris, cardiac failure, impaired renal or hepatic function, thyrotoxicosis, pre-excitation syndromes, diabetes, hypoglycemia or nonallergic bronchospasm. Propranolol may produce significant bradycardia, heart block or hypotension. Patients should not be suddenly withdrawn from beta blockers.
• Nitroprusside may not lower blood pressure adequately in some patients, so another agent may be required. Excessive nitroprusside or use in patients with renal or hepatic insufficiency may cause cyanide toxicity, through excessive production of serum thiocyanate. Confusion and hyperreflexia are the early signs of thiocyanate toxicity. Because thiocyanate inhibits the uptake and binding of iodine, caution should be exercised in the presence of hypothyroidism. Thiocyanate blood levels should be followed after 48 hours of nitroprusside use. Because of the rapid onset and potency of nitroprusside, administration should be with the use of an infusion pump. Methemoglobinemia may be seen rarely.

Significant possible interactions:
• Propranolol may have interactions with adenosine, albuterol, alfentanil, amiodarone, barbiturates, bromazepam, chlorothiazide, chlorpromazine, chlorpropamide, chlorprothixene, cimetidine, clonidine, dextroamphetamine, diazoxide, dihydroergotamine, diltiazem, disopyramide, tricyclic antidepressants, encainide, epinephrine, flecainide, fluvoxamine, furosemide, glipizide, halofenate, haloperidol, heparin, ibuprofen, indomethicin, insulin, isoniazid, isoproterenol, lidocaine, lidoflazine, methacholine, methyldopa, metoclopramide, naproxen, nifedipine, phenylpropanolamine, procainamide, quinidine, reserpine, rifampin, ritodrine, sulfonylureas, theophylline, thioridazine, tocainide, tubocurarine, verapamil, warfarin.
• Nitroprusside may have interactions with clonidine and other antihypertensives to make their hypotensive effects cumulative

ALTERNATIVE DRUGS
• Labetalol, 10-20 mg IV bolus to a maximum of 300mg total, then titrated to response with an infusion
• Trimethaphan, at an infusion rate of 1-2 mg/min
• Reserpine 0.5-2 mg intramuscularly every 4-8 hours. Onset of action is 1-3 hours
• Methyldopa 250-500 mg every 6 hours. Unfortunately, it has a delayed onset of action of 4 to 6 hours and prolonged duration of 10 to 12 hours.

FOLLOWUP

PATIENT MONITORING
• Systolic blood pressure should be maintained at 120 mm Hg or below as tolerated
• Routine chest x-rays and/or chest CT may be helpful in following the progress of any long-term medically treated patient
• Patients should have a one month follow-up visit, and then at three month intervals. During the follow-up, careful attention should be placed on signs and symptoms of aortic insufficiency, chest or back pain, and development of saccular aneurysms as displayed on chest roentgenogram.

PREVENTION/AVOIDANCE Long-term control of hypertension

POSSIBLE COMPLICATIONS
Redissection, localized saccular aneurysm, aortic valvular insufficiency and progressive aortic enlargement

EXPECTED COURSE AND PROGNOSIS
• Mortality of patients left untreated is approximately 90% in three months
• Hospital survival is estimated at approximately 70% in patients treated both medically and surgically
• Patients with ascending dissection treated early with surgery still have a mortality of 29-38%
• 10 year survival of all operated patients is 40%
• Redissection risk is 13% at 5 years; 23% at 10 years

MISCELLANEOUS

ASSOCIATED CONDITIONS See Causes

AGE-RELATED FACTORS N/A
Pediatric: N/A
Geriatric: N/A
Others: N/A

PREGNANCY Aortic dissection may be associated with cystic medionecrosis of pregnancy and appears to have an increased associated risk with pregnancy. It is still unclear whether pregnancy itself is the originating factor or that it simply contributes to the worsening of an already pre-existing condition.

SYNONYMS
• Dissecting aneurysm

ICD-9-CM
441.0 Dissecting aneurysm (any part)

SEE ALSO N/A

OTHER NOTES N/A

ABBREVIATIONS N/A

REFERENCES
• Hirst, A.E., Jr., Johns, V.J., Jr., Kim, S.W., Jr.: Dissecting aneurysm of the aorta: A review of 505 cases. Medicine 37:217-219, 1958
• Lindsay, J. Jr.: The therapy of dissecting aneurysm of the aorta. Med Concepts Cardiovasc Dis 38:13-19, 1969
• DeSanctis, R.W., Doroghazi, R.M., Austen, W.G., Buckley, M.J.: Aortic dissection. N Engl J Med 317:1060-1067, 1987
• Cigarroa, J.E., Isselbacher, E.M., et al.: Diagnostic imaging in the evaluation of suspected aortic dissection. N Eng J Med, Jan 7, 1993. Vol. 328(1):35-43

Author D. Heiselman, D.O.

Aortic valvular stenosis

BASICS

DESCRIPTION An acquired or congenital obstruction to systolic left ventricular outflow across the aortic valve
System(s) affected: Cardiovascular
Genetics: N/A
Incidence/Prevalence in USA:
• Except for mitral regurgitation due to myocardial disease, valvular aortic stenosis is the most common fatal cardiac valve lesion
• Bicuspid aortic valve has a frequency of 400 per 100,000 live births
Predominant age:
• Age < 30 years - predominantly congenital
• Age 30 to 70 years - most commonly congenital or rheumatic
• Age > 70 years - most commonly degenerative calcification of the aortic valve
Predominant sex:
• Congenital bicuspid valves: Male > Female (4:1)
• Congenital unicuspid valves: Male > Female (3:1)

SIGNS AND SYMPTOMS
• Angina pectoris (most frequent symptom, occurring in 50-70% of patients with severe aortic stenosis)
• Near syncope
• Syncope (often exertional, occurs in 15-30% of patients with severe aortic stenosis)
• Exertional dyspnea
• Orthopnea
• Paroxysmal nocturnal dyspnea
• Palpitations
• Fatigue
• Neurologic events (transient ischemic attack or cerebrovascular accident) due to embolism
• Systolic crescendo-decrescendo murmur, usually best heard at the second right sternal border (may have associated thrill) and may radiate into the carotid arteries
• Ejection (early systolic) click
• Prolonged ejection time
• Delayed, small carotid upstroke
• Delayed/decreased intensity of A2
• Paradoxical splitting of S2
• Left ventricular heave
• A high pitched diastolic blow may be present at the left sternal border (associated aortic regurgitation)

CAUSES
Congenital etiologies
◊ Unicuspid valve
◊ Bicuspid valve (not inherently stenotic, but becomes so as a result of 'wear and tear' thickening and calcification; a calcified bicuspid valve is the most common cause of isolated aortic stenosis in adults)
◊ Three cusped valve with fusion of commissures
◊ Hypoplastic annulus
Acquired etiologies
◊ Rheumatic (or, rarely, other inflammatory disease)
◊ Degenerative calcific aortic stenosis in the elderly

RISK FACTORS History of rheumatic fever

DIAGNOSIS

DIFFERENTIAL DIAGNOSIS
• Mitral regurgitation, either primary or secondary to underlying coronary artery disease or dilated cardiomyopathy. Mitral regurgitation, however, is usually an apical, high frequency, pansystolic murmur, often radiating to the axilla.
• Hypertrophic obstructive cardiomyopathy. This murmur is also a systolic crescendo-decrescendo murmur, but is best heard at the left sternal border and may radiate into the axilla. However, this murmur characteristically is intensified by moving from squatting to standing position and/or Valsalva's maneuver, and lessened by changing from standing to squatting.
• Aortic supravalvular stenosis
• Discrete subaortic stenosis

LABORATORY N/A
Drugs that may alter lab results: N/A
Disorders that may alter lab results: N/A

PATHOLOGICAL FINDINGS
• Left ventricular hypertrophy
• Myocardial interstitial fibrosis
• Aortic valvular calcification in older patients
• 50% incidence of concomitant coronary artery disease

SPECIAL TESTS ECG: Left ventricular hypertrophy, often with associated ST segment depression, conduction defects, left atrial enlargement, ventricular arrhythmias

IMAGING
Chest x-ray
◊ May be normal in compensated, isolated valvular aortic stenosis
◊ Cardiac hypertrophy early, later cardiomegaly
◊ Post stenotic dilatation of the ascending aorta
◊ Calcification of aortic valve cusps (may require fluoroscopy to visualize)

DIAGNOSTIC PROCEDURES
Echocardiography:
◊ Aortic valve morphology, thickening, calcifications
◊ Decreased aortic valve excursion
◊ Planimetry of aortic valve area
◊ Left ventricular hypertrophy
◊ Left ventricular ejection fraction
◊ Chamber dimensions
◊ Presence or absence of wall motion abnormalities suggestive of coronary artery disease
With Doppler echocardiography:
◊ Transvalvular gradient
◊ Valve area
◊ Diastolic function
◊ Associated aortic regurgitation
Cardiac catheterization:
◊ Transvalvular gradient

◊ Valve area
◊ Left ventricle ejection fraction
◊ Concomitant coronary artery disease

TREATMENT

APPROPRIATE HEALTH CARE
Outpatient except for surgical intervention

GENERAL MEASURES
• Aortic stenosis is a progressive disease. The asymptomatic patient with non-critical aortic stenosis can be closely followed with appropriate evaluation.
• All patients with valvular aortic stenosis should receive endocarditis prophylaxis, prior to dental work or invasive procedures regardless of age, etiology or severity of the stenosis (as recommended by the American Heart Association in Circulation, Vol 83, No 3, March, 1991)
• Patients with a rheumatic etiology should receive (in addition to endocarditis prophylaxis prior to dental work or invasive procedures) rheumatic fever prophylaxis, especially if less than 35 years of age, or continue to be in close contact with young children
• Prompt aortic valve replacement is clearly indicated in patients with symptomatic aortic stenosis
• Consider aortic valve replacement in asymptomatic patients with critical aortic stenosis (aortic valve area < 0.8 cm2 or gradient > 50 mm Hg) particularly if there is left ventricular dysfunction, increasing cardiomegaly, and clinical symptoms
• Surgical valve replacement consists of the removal of the stenotic, native valve and placement of a prosthetic mechanical or tissue valve
• Balloon angioplasty of stenotic aortic valves may be of benefit in the pediatric patient with congenital disease. Also feasible (although one must expect suboptimal results) in the elderly, debilitated patient who may not tolerate valve replacement.

ACTIVITY In known or suspected severe aortic stenosis, vigorous physical activity is contraindicated

DIET No restrictions except sodium restriction in presence of congestive heart failure

PATIENT EDUCATION
• Educate the patient about the symptoms of symptomatic aortic stenosis and to report these promptly should they occur
• If moderate or severe aortic stenosis is known or suspected, instruct the patient to avoid vigorous physical activity
• Instruct the patient when prophylactic antibiotics are needed for medical or dental procedures

MEDICATIONS

DRUG(S) OF CHOICE
• None for treatment. Prophylactic antibiotics when needed.
• The use of vasodilators, nitrates, calcium channel blockers, beta blockers as well as diuretics are potentially hazardous in aortic stenosis and should be used very cautiously, if at all
Contraindications: N/A
Precautions: N/A
Significant possible interactions: N/A

ALTERNATIVE DRUGS   N/A

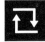
FOLLOWUP

PATIENT MONITORING
• Asymptomatic patients without critical aortic stenosis should be followed with a history and physical examination every 3-6 months
• An echocardiogram should be performed every 6-12 months to assess progression
• Advise the patient to immediately report any symptoms referable to the aortic stenosis

PREVENTION/AVOIDANCE
• Bacterial endocarditis prophylaxis
• Rheumatic fever prophylaxis, where indicated
• Avoidance of vigorous physical activity

POSSIBLE COMPLICATIONS
• Progressive stenosis
• Sudden death
• Congestive heart failure
• Angina
• Syncope
• Hemolytic anemia
• Infective endocarditis

EXPECTED COURSE AND PROGNOSIS
• Mean life expectancy in patients with aortic stenosis is 5 years after the onset of exertional chest discomfort, 3 years after the onset of syncope, 2 years after the development of heart failure
• Sudden death occurs in 15 to 20% of patients with symptomatic aortic stenosis

MISCELLANEOUS

ASSOCIATED CONDITIONS
• Coronary artery disease is present in 50% of patients with aortic stenosis
• Aortic regurgitation (particularly seen in calcified bicuspid valves and rheumatic disease)
• Mitral valve disease (primarily in rheumatic heart disease)

AGE-RELATED FACTORS
Pediatric: N/A
Geriatric: Increased incidence of degenerative calcific aortic stenosis
Others: N/A

PREGNANCY   Severe critical aortic stenosis tolerates poorly the hemodynamic changes in pregnancy, labor and delivery. Pregnancy should be avoided with critical aortic stenosis.

SYNONYMS   N/A

ICD-9-CM   424.1

SEE ALSO   N/A

OTHER NOTES   As the left ventricle is relatively noncompliant in aortic stenosis, atrial contraction is an important component of diastolic filling. The loss of this component with the onset of atrial fibrillation can cause acute clinical and hemodynamic deterioration.

ABBREVIATIONS   N/A

REFERENCES
• Brandenburg, R.O., et al.: Cardiology: Fundamentals and Practice. New York, Year Book Publishers, 1987
• Dalen, J.E. & Alpert, J.S.: Valvular Heart Disease. 2nd Ed. New York, Little Brown & Co
• Hurst, J.W., et al.: The Heart. 7th Ed. New York, McGraw-Hill, 1990
• Braunwald E., et al. (eds.): Harrison's Principles of Internal Medicine. 12th Ed. New York, McGraw-Hill, 1991

Author   J. Galloway, M.D., F.A.C.P.

Appendicitis, acute

BASICS

DESCRIPTION Acute inflammation of the vermiform appendix
• First described by Fitz in 1886
• McBurney described the point of maximal tenderness
System(s) affected: Gastrointestinal
Genetics: Unknown.
Incidence in USA: 10/100,000
Prevalence in USA:
• Most common acute surgical condition of abdomen
• 1 in every 15 persons (7%) at some time in their life
Predominant age:
• Ages 10-30 - Male > Female (3:2)
• Over age 30 - Male = Female
Predominant sex: Slight male predominance

SIGNS AND SYMPTOMS
• Abdominal pain (100%) - periumbilical then right-lower-quadrant (RLQ). Pain lessened with flexion of thigh.
• Muscle guarding
• Anorexia (almost 100%)
• Nausea (90%)
• Vomiting (75%)-mild
• Obstipation
• Diarrhea-mild
• Sequence of symptom appearance (95%)-anorexia, then abdominal pain, then vomiting
• Slight temperature (one degree centigrade) elevation
• Slight tachycardia
• Patient frequently lies motionless with right thigh drawn up
• Maximal tenderness at "McBurney's point"
• Direct and referred RLQ tenderness
• Voluntary and involuntary guarding
• Cutaneous hyperesthesia at T10-12
• Rovsing's sign - RLQ pain with palpatory pressure in LLQ
• Psoas sign-pain with right thigh extension
• Obturator sign-pain with internal rotation of flexed right thigh
• Retrocecal appendix-flank tenderness in RLQ
• Pelvic appendix-local and suprapubic pain on rectal exam

CAUSES
Obstruction of appendiceal lumen
  ◊ Fecaliths (most common)
  ◊ Lymphoid tissue hypertrophy
  ◊ Inspissated barium
  ◊ Vegetable, fruit seeds and other foreign bodies
  ◊ Intestinal worms (ascarids)
  ◊ Strictures

RISK FACTORS
• Adolescent males
• Familial tendency
• Intra-abdominal tumors

DIAGNOSIS

DIFFERENTIAL DIAGNOSIS
• Any cause of the "acute abdomen"
• 75% of erroneous diagnoses accounted for by acute mesenteric lymphadenitis, no organic pathologic condition, acute PID, twisted ovarian cyst, ruptured graafian follicle, acute gastroenteritis
• Also consider urologic causes, inflammatory bowel disease, colonic disorders, and other gynecologic diseases

LABORATORY
• Moderate leukocytosis - 10,000 to 18,000/mm3 in 75%
• Moderate polymorphonuclear predominance
• Urinalysis-elevated specific gravity, hematuria (sometimes), pyuria (sometimes), albuminuria (sometimes)
Drugs that may alter lab results:
• Antibiotics
• Steroids
Disorders that may alter lab results: N/A

PATHOLOGICAL FINDINGS
• Acute inflammation of the appendix
• Local vascular congestion
• Obstruction
• Gangrene
• Perforation with abscess (15 to 30%)

SPECIAL TESTS   N/A

IMAGING   (Used in differential diagnosis and to detect complications).
• KUB: gas-filled appendix; radiopaque fecalith; deformed cecum; fluid level; ileus; free air.
• Barium enema-non-filling appendix; RLQ mass effect
• Ultrasound-appendiceal inflammation; other pelvic pathology, such as inflammatory mass.
• C.T. scan for periappendiceal abscess

DIAGNOSTIC PROCEDURES
• Cornerstone of diagnosis is history and clinical findings
• Diagnostic laparoscopy - consider in young adult females
• Rectal and pelvic examinations
• Intensive in-hospital observation

TREATMENT

APPROPRIATE HEALTH CARE
• Inpatient surgery
• Immediate appendectomy; open or laparoscopic
• Drainage of abscess, if present

GENERAL MEASURES
Preoperative preparation
  ◊ Correction of fluid and electrolyte deficits
  ◊ Consider broad-spectrum antibiotic coverage

ACTIVITY
• Early postoperative ambulation
• Return to full activity by 4 to 6 weeks postop

DIET Regular diet with return of bowel function, usually within 24 to 48 hours postop

PATIENT EDUCATION
• Restricted activity for 4 to 6 weeks postop
• Contact physician for development of postop anorexia, nausea, vomiting, abdominal pain, fever, or chills

MEDICATIONS

DRUG(S) OF CHOICE
• Uncomplicated acute appendicitis - one preoperative dose of broad spectrum antibiotic; cefoxitin (Mefoxin), cefotetan (Cefotan)
• Gangrenous or perforating appendicitis - broadened antibiotic coverage for aerobic and anaerobic enteric pathogens, dosage and choice of antibiotic should be adjusted based on intraoperative cultures. Continue antibiotics for 7 days postop or until patient becomes afebrile with normal white count. Pathogens usually sensitive to ampicillin, gentamicin, and clindamycin.
Contraindications: Documented allergy to specific antibiotic
Precautions: Adjust antibiotic dosages for elderly and renal failure patients
Significant possible interactions: Refer to manufacturer's literature for each drug

ALTERNATIVE DRUGS
• Metronidazole (Flagyl) - anaerobic coverage only
• Ampicillin + sulbactam (Unasyn)
• Ticarcillin + clavulanic acid (Timentin)

FOLLOWUP

PATIENT MONITORING Routine visits at 2 and 6 weeks postoperatively

PREVENTION/AVOIDANCE N/A

POSSIBLE COMPLICATIONS
• Wound infection
• Intra-abdominal abscess, sometimes diaphragmatic
• Fecal fistula
• Intestinal obstruction
• Incisional hernia
• Liver abscess (rare)
• Peritonitis with paralytic ileus

EXPECTED COURSE AND PROGNOSIS
• Generally uncomplicated course in young adults with non-ruptured appendicitis.
• Factors increasing morbidity and mortality are extremes of age and appendiceal rupture.
Morbidity rates:
◊ 3% with non-perforated appendicitis
◊ 47% with perforated appendicitis
Mortality rates:
◊ 0.1% unruptured acute appendicitis
◊ 3% ruptured acute appendicitis
◊ 15% elderly patient with ruptured appendix

MISCELLANEOUS

ASSOCIATED CONDITIONS N/A

AGE-RELATED FACTORS
Pediatric:
• Rare in infancy
• Decreased diagnostic accuracy
• Higher fever, more vomiting
• Rupture earlier
• Rupture rate: 15 to 50%
• May return to full activities earlier
Geriatric:
• Decreased diagnostic accuracy
• Rupture rate: 67 to 90%
• Patients over 60 years of age account for 50% of deaths from acute appendicitis
Others: N/A

PREGNANCY
• Most common extra-uterine surgical emergency
• 1 in 2000 pregnancies
• Difficult diagnosis
• Appendix displaced superolaterally by gravid uterus
• Fetal mortality rate: 2 to 8.5%

SYNONYMS N/A

ICD-9-CM
540.0 appendicitis, with generalized peritonitis
540.9 appendicitis, without mention of peritonitis

SEE ALSO N/A

OTHER NOTES N/A

ABBREVIATIONS

REFERENCES
• Schwartz, S.I. (ed.): Principles of Surgery. 5th Ed. New York, McGraw-Hill, 1989.
• Moody, F.G. (ed.): Surgical Treatment of Digestive Disease. 2nd Ed. Chicago, Year Book Medical Publishers, 1990
• Horattas, M.C., Guyton, D.P. & Wu, D.A.: Reappraisal of appendicitis in the elderly. American Journal of Surgery 1990; 160:291-293

Author A. Fenton, M.D., T. Clark, M.D., & D. Moorman, M.D., F.A.C.S.

Arterial gas embolism

BASICS

DESCRIPTION Air released from an over-pressurized alveolus enters the pulmonary capillaries then travels through the arterial circulation causing occlusion of the cerebral and/or coronary circulation.
• Arterial gas embolism is the most serious and rapidly fatal of all SCUBA diving injuries and is second only to drowning as the leading cause of death associated with sport diving.
• Arterial gas embolism occurs on ascent and the time from alveolar rupture to the manifestation of symptoms is nearly always less than ten minutes.
Incidence in USA: It is estimated (based on injury/mortality reports collected by Divers Alert Network) to occur in approximately 4 per 100,000 sport divers per year.
Prevalence in USA: Unknown, since prevalence is dependent on disease duration
System(s) affected: Cardiovascular, Nervous, Musculoskeletal
Genetics: N/A
Predominant age: Young adult
Predominant sex: Male > Female

SIGNS AND SYMPTOMS
Group 1: Neurologic symptoms only. Divers presenting with neurologic symptoms but without impairment of spontaneous respirations and cardiac function. May be impossible to clinically distinguish from severe decompression sickness.
◊ Asymmetrical multiplegia or paralysis
◊ Tingling or numbness
◊ Blindness or other visual disturbances
◊ Deafness
◊ Vertigo
◊ Dizziness
◊ Headache
◊ Confusion
◊ Convulsions
◊ Aphasia
◊ Personality change; from subtle changes to unconsciousness
Group 2: Loss of consciousness, apnea, and cardiac arrest or dysrhythmia. Divers presenting with both neurologic and cardiac impairments. All of the above signs and symptoms plus those below are possible.
◊ Dysrhythmias
◊ Cardiac arrest

CAUSES
Group 1: Localized obstruction of cerebral blood flow by an embolus of air. Local capillary endothelial damage with vasogenic edema leading to a rise in intracranial pressure and ischemia.
Group 2: This is thought to be due to localized obstruction of both cerebral and coronary blood flow by an embolus of air

RISK FACTORS
• History of a rapid ascent
• History of panic during dive
• History of holding breath while diving
• History of loss of consciousness (or with other noted symptoms) within seconds to minutes after or during a dive

DIAGNOSIS

DIFFERENTIAL DIAGNOSIS
Decompression sickness

LABORATORY
• Hematocrit - increased indicating volume depletion
• Urine analysis - increased specific gravity indicating volume depletion
Drugs that may alter lab results: N/A
Disorders that may alter lab results: N/A

PATHOLOGICAL FINDINGS N/A

SPECIAL TESTS
• ECG

IMAGING
• Chest x-ray to rule out pneumothorax

DIAGNOSTIC PROCEDURES N/A

TREATMENT

APPROPRIATE HEALTH CARE
• Hospital based hyperbaric chamber capable of performing a U.S. Navy Table 6A recompression (165 fsw).

GENERAL MEASURES
• Immediate transport to a suitable hyperbaric chamber for recompression as soon as possible; do not delay with nonessential procedures.
• Transport by aircraft is justifiable if it will save a significant amount of time (aircraft must fly at low altitudes or be capable of maintaining cabin pressure at about one atmosphere)
• Life-saving measures (CPR) must take precedence to sustain life
• Administration of high flow maximum concentration oxygen therapy by a tight fitting mask or by intubation and mechanical ventilation during transport
• Some authorities recommend the Trendelenburg's position for transport if possible
• Maintain hydration with IV fluids
• For assistance and advice in locating the nearest treatment chamber in your area (world-wide) call DIVERS ALERT NETWORK (DAN) at any hour (919) 684-8111

ACTIVITY None until after treatment

DIET None until after treatment

PATIENT EDUCATION DIVERS ALERT NETWORK (DAN) Non-Emergency Information Line (Mon-Fri 9-5 EST) (919) 684-2948

MEDICATIONS

DRUG(S) OF CHOICE None
Contraindications: N/A
Precautions: N/A
Significant possible interactions: N/A

ALTERNATIVE DRUGS None

FOLLOWUP

PATIENT MONITORING
• Frequent neurological checks in the acute pre-treatment and treatment phase
• Complete neurological assessment at one, three, six and twelve at months

PREVENTION/AVOIDANCE
• Strict adherence to diver safety protocols
• No diving after any dive injury or with any medical condition until evaluated and approved by a physician knowledgeable in diving medicine

POSSIBLE COMPLICATIONS
• Long term serious neurologic impairments
• Death

EXPECTED COURSE AND PROGNOSIS
• Complete to partial resolution with adequate treatment

MISCELLANEOUS

ASSOCIATED CONDITIONS
• Pulmonary barotrauma leading to arterial gas embolism, can also cause pneumomediastinum, subcutaneous emphysema, pneumopericardium, pneumothorax, and pneumoperitoneum
• Always consider the possibility of decompression sickness in addition to arterial gas embolism in any SCUBA diver who has recently completed a dive

AGE-RELATED FACTORS
Pediatric: N/A
Geriatric: N/A
Others: N/A

PREGNANCY N/A

SYNONYMS
• Gas embolism
• Air embolism

ICD-9-CM
• 958.0 (any site)

SEE ALSO
• Decompression sickness

OTHER NOTES
• Any diver who has an onset of new symptom(s) or sign(s) after recently completing a SCUBA dive of any type, to any depth, for any period of time - serious consideration must be given as having sustained a dive related injury

ABBREVIATIONS
• DAN = Divers Alert Network
• AGE = arterial gas embolism

REFERENCES
• Shilling, C.W. (ed.): The Physicians Guide to Diving Medicine. New York, Plenum Press, 1984
• Strauss, R.H.: Diving Medicine. Philadelphia, W.B. Saunders Co., 1976

Author J. Bond, M.D.

Arteriosclerotic heart disease

BASICS

DESCRIPTION Arteriosclerosis means thickening of the arterial wall, along with loss of elasticity, that progressively blocks the coronary arteries and their main branches. The process is chronic, occurring over many years, and is the most common cause of cardiovascular disability and death in the USA. Elevated total serum cholesterol and low-density lipoproteins are involved in the development of arteriosclerosis as well as the process of aging and anatomic changes.
System(s) affected: Cardiovascular
Genetics: Tendency is inheritable
Incidence/Prevalence: Common. Causes 35% of deaths in men age 35-50. Death rate age 55-64 - 1:100.
Predominant age: Men 50-60, women 60-70, for peak clinical manifestations
Predominant sex: Male > Female

SIGNS AND SYMPTOMS
• May remain clinically silent, even in advanced stages, and in some instances of ischemia
Clinical manifestations
  ◊ Substernal chest pain
  ◊ Exertional dyspnea
  ◊ Orthopnea
  ◊ Paroxysmal nocturnal dyspnea
  ◊ Extrasystoles
  ◊ Irregular rhythm
  ◊ Tachycardia
  ◊ Systolic murmur
  ◊ Cardiomegaly

CAUSES
• Atherosclerosis
• Narrowing of coronary arteries
• Embolism compromising coronary arteries at orifices
• Subintimal atheromas in large and medium vessels

RISK FACTORS
• Elevated low density lipoprotein (LDL)
• Decreased high density lipoprotein (HDL)
• Elevated triglycerides
• Dissecting aortitis
• Smoking
• Family history of premature arteriosclerosis
• Obesity
• Hypertension
• Stress
• Sedentary life style
• Increasing age
• Male sex
• Female postmenopausal
• Diabetes mellitus

DIAGNOSIS

DIFFERENTIAL DIAGNOSIS N/A

LABORATORY
• Elevated triglycerides
• Elevated total cholesterol
• Elevated low density lipoproteins
• Decreased high density lipoproteins
Drugs that may alter lab results:
Nitroglycerin
Disorders that may alter lab results: N/A

PATHOLOGICAL FINDINGS
• Gross - narrowed coronary arteries
• Micro - cholesterol plaques on intima of coronary vessels
• Fibrotic subendothelial connective tissue of intima with plaque

SPECIAL TESTS
• ECG - ST segment depression, inverted T waves
• Exercise stress test - positive

IMAGING
• Stress thallium test - positive
• Angiography - narrowed coronary arteries
• Echocardiography
• Stress tests with and without contrast

DIAGNOSTIC PROCEDURES N/A

TREATMENT

APPROPRIATE HEALTH CARE
• Outpatient
• Inpatient for acute ischemic syndromes

GENERAL MEASURES
Prevention of further progression of the disease
  ◊ Stop smoking (stop smoking programs, drugs)
  ◊ Treatment of hypercholesterolemia (diet, drugs)
  ◊ Increase high density lipoprotein (diet, exercise)
  ◊ Control of blood pressure
  ◊ Diabetes mellitus treated early and adequately
  ◊ Exercise
  ◊ Prophylactic aspirin
  ◊ Stress reduction
  ◊ Diet changes
  ◊ Weight loss
Treatment of complications
  ◊ Covered elsewhere under the individual topics (e.g., angina pectoris, myocardial infarction, heart failure, stroke, peripheral arterial occlusion, etc.)

ACTIVITY Exercise may be helpful in preventing clinical coronary disease and useful for therapeutic measures

DIET
• Low-fat (20-30 grams of fat/day total intake)
• Weight-loss diet, if obesity a problem
• Increase soluble fiber

PATIENT EDUCATION For patient education materials favorably reviewed on this topic, contact: American Heart Association, 7320 Greenville Avenue, Dallas, TX 75231, (214)373-6300

MEDICATIONS

DRUG(S) OF CHOICE
• Aspirin, one 325 mg tablet/day unless contraindicated
• Stop smoking

Cholesterol-lowering (several regimens available)
◊ Cholestyramine or colestipol, (bile acid sequestrants) 12-32 gm orally in 2-4 divided daily doses
◊ Nicotinic acid 2-6 gm daily in divided doses (may be helpful, but side effects restrict its use)
◊ Gemfibrozil 600 mg twice daily
◊ Probucol 500 mg twice daily
◊ HMG-CoA reductase inhibitors (lovastatin) 20-80 mg daily. Pravastatin and simvastatin recently approved in USA.

Contraindications: Refer to manufacturer's literature
Precautions: SR form of niacin may be linked to hepatotoxicity. Refer to manufacturer's literature.
Significant possible interactions: Refer to manufacturer's literature

ALTERNATIVE DRUGS N/A

FOLLOWUP

PATIENT MONITORING Monitor
cholesterol, triglyceride levels, other preventive programs (weight loss, smoking cessation)

PREVENTION/AVOIDANCE See
General measures

POSSIBLE COMPLICATIONS
• Myocardial infarction
• Ventricular fibrillation
• Congestive heart failure
• Death
• Angina pectoris
• Sudden cardiac death

EXPECTED COURSE AND
PROGNOSIS Guardedly favorable. Many risk factors can be modified.

MISCELLANEOUS

ASSOCIATED CONDITIONS
• Obesity
• Hypertension
• Diabetes
• Hypercholesterolemia

AGE-RELATED FACTORS
Pediatric: Preventive measures can begin early (proper nutrition, exercise, weight control, smoking deterrent programs, etc.)
Geriatric: Greatest incidence in this age group
Others: N/A

PREGNANCY Practically non-existent in
pregnant women

SYNONYMS
• Coronary artery disease (CAD)
• Coronary heart disease
• Coronary arteriosclerosis

ICD-9-CM 414.0 arteriosclerotic heart
disease

SEE ALSO
• Angina pectoris
• Acute myocardial infarction

OTHER NOTES N/A

ABBREVIATIONS N/A

REFERENCES
• Hurst, J.W., et al.: The Heart. 7th Ed. New York, McGraw-Hill, 1990
• Braunwald, E. (ed.): Heart Disease: A Textbook of Cardiovascular Medicine. 3rd Ed. Philadelphia, W.B. Saunders Co., 1988

Author H. Griffith, M.D. & M. Dambro, M.D.

Arthritis, infectious, bacterial

BASICS

DESCRIPTION Invasion of joints by live micro-organisms or their fragments. One of the few curable causes of arthritis. May allow early recognition of systemic infection/disease.
System(s) affected: Musculoskeletal
Genetics: N/A
Incidence/Prevalence in USA:
Neisserial:
   ◊ Responsible for 50% of infectious arthritis
   ◊ Arthritis occurs in 0.6% of the 3% of women with gonorrhea
   ◊ Arthritis occurs in 0.1% of the 0.7% of men with gonorrhea
   ◊ Arthritis occurs in 7% of individuals with N. meningitidis
Non-Neisserial:
   ◊ Perhaps half as frequent as Neisserial
Predominant age:
Neisserial:
   ◊ Especially 15-40, can occur at any age
Non-Neisserial:
   ◊ 50% Prior to age 2: 27% Staphylococcus, 20% Streptococcus, 33% Hemophilus, and 13% other gram negative rods
   ◊ 70% Age 2-14: 34% Staphylococcus, 29% Streptococcus, 13% Hemophilus, and 13% other gram negative rods
   ◊ Adult: 34% Staphylococcus, 38% Streptococcus, 2% Hemophilus, and 26% other gram negative rods
Predominant sex:
• Neisserial: Female > Male (4:1)
• Non-Neisserial: Male > Female (2:1)
• Subacute bacterial endocarditis-related: Male = Female

SIGNS AND SYMPTOMS
• Predominantly monoarticular (90%). (Hemophilus may be pauciarticular and Mycoplasma often presents as a migratory polyarthritis).
• Limited joint use/motion (especially in children)
• Joint effusion, tenderness
• Joint warmth - present in less than 50%
• Joint redness- present in less than 50%
• Loss of joint motion
• Tenosynovitis
• Sudden flare of a single joint in a patient with underlying joint disease
• Fever - in 90% at some time during the course of the infection
• Chills, malaise
• Cutaneous lesions
• Peripheral neuropathy
• Back pain - especially in subacute bacterial endocarditis (SBE)
• Hypertrophic osteoarthropathy - rare, secondary to endocarditis
• Fretfulness - especially in children
• Dermato-arthritis - usually pustular skin lesions in gonorrhea - usually petechial rash in meningococcemia
• Bacteremic phase - migratory polyarthritis, tenosynovitis, high fever, chills, pustules
• Localized phase - usually monoarticular, low grade fever (80%)

CAUSES
• Hematogenous invasion by micro-organisms (80-90%)
• Contiguous spread (10-15%) from adjacent osteomyelitis in children
• Direct penetration of micro-organisms secondary to trauma or joint injection

RISK FACTORS
• Young patient with venereal exposure
• Concurrent extra-articular infection
• Prior arthritis in infected joint
• Rheumatoid arthritis
• Trauma
• Joint puncture or surgery
• Prosthetic joint
• Prior antibiotic, corticosteroid, or immunosuppressive therapy
• Serious chronic illness (e.g., diabetes, liver disease, malignancy, primary immunodeficiency)
• Defective phagocytic mechanisms (e.g., chronic granulomatous disease)
• Intravenous drug abuse
• Travel/habitat history
• Sickle cell anemia

DIAGNOSIS

DIFFERENTIAL DIAGNOSIS
• Gout
• Pseudogout (calcium pyrophosphate deposition disease)
• Spondyloarthropathy (Reiter's syndrome, psoriatic arthritis, ankylosing spondylitis, the arthritis of inflammatory bowel disease)
• Juvenile rheumatoid arthritis
• Type IIa hyperlipoproteinemia
• Foreign body
• Rheumatoid arthritis
• Rheumatic fever
• AIDS
• Cellulitis
• Palindromic rheumatism
• Neuropathic arthropathy
• Lyme arthritis
• Sarcoidosis

LABORATORY
• Synovial fluid usually cloudy with > 50,000 WBC/HPF, but may have fewer white blood cells present or over 100,000. (Caveat - cell count must be performed within 1 hour of obtaining specimen to be valid).
• Synovial fluid white count can be recognized as elevated (in presence of trauma) if RBC:WBC ratio significantly less than 700
• Polymorphonuclear leukocytes usually predominate in synovial fluid
• Synovial fluid glucose often more than 40 mg/dL less than in a simultaneously obtained serum glucose value (in fasting patient). However, arthrocentesis should not be delayed simply to obtain fasting synovial fluid glucose level.
• Westergren erythrocyte sedimentation rate - often elevated, but normal in 20%

• Rheumatoid factor positive in 50% - if endocarditis present and in viral arthritis
• Anti-techoic acid antibodies - with Staphylococcus infection
• Elevated peripheral white blood cell count (in 50-90%)
• Cryoglobulins
• Immune complexes
• Febrile agglutinins (to include Brucella and rickettsial-related titers)
• Antistreptolysin O (ASO) titer is usually normal, exclusive of streptococcal infections
• Depressed synovial fluid and occasionally depressed serum levels of complement
• Microscopic hematuria in subacute bacterial endocarditis (SBE)
• Presence of crystals (e.g., urate or calcium pyrophosphate) does not exclude infectious arthritis
Drugs that may alter lab results:
Antibiotics
Disorders that may alter lab results: N/A

PATHOLOGICAL FINDINGS Synovial biopsy will reveal polymorphonuclear leukocytes and possibly the causative organism

SPECIAL TESTS
• Joint fluid - for gram stain (positive in 50%); culture (positive in 50-70%)
• Serum cidal level assessment of antibiotic adequacy is suggested with virulent organisms or therapeutic unresponsiveness (tenfold margin suggested)
• Blood, orifice, urine cultures. "Bedside culture" is recommended to enhance isolation of fastidious organisms.
• All cultures should be preserved and observed for at least 3 days and preferably 2 weeks. Observing synovial fluid cultures for at least 3 days allows isolation of fastidious organisms such as those of rat bite fever (Streptobacillus moniliformis and Spirillum minus).
• Neisserial infection generally requires use of special agars (e.g., chocolate or Thayer Martin) and relative anaerobic culturing conditions
• Countercurrent immunoelectrophoresis or complement fixation for specific bacterial antigens

IMAGING
X-ray
   ◊ Soft tissue swelling
   ◊ Juxta-articular osteoporosis
   ◊ Radiolucent area (gas) in a joint space from gas forming organisms. (Caveat - may also occur normally as a "vacuum phenomenon").
   ◊ Effacement of the obturator fat pad (with hip involvement)
   ◊ X-ray changes are usually a late phenomenon
   ◊ Rarefaction of subchondral bone may occur as early as 2-7 days
   ◊ Joint space loss (secondary to cartilage destruction) may be seen as early as 4-10 days
   ◊ Erosions
   ◊ Joint destruction with ankylosis may occur as early as 2 weeks

Other imaging techniques
◊ Technetium joint scans - reveal distribution of inflammation
◊ Gallium or WBC-Indium scans - reveal inflammation as well as infection
◊ CT - to identify sequestration
◊ MRI - effusion, perhaps early cartilage damage, osteomyelitis

DIAGNOSTIC PROCEDURES
• Arthrocentesis with gram stain and culture - only positive in 50-70%. Must be done in all patients when possibility of infectious arthritis is considered. Arthrocentesis should probably be performed within 12 hours of suspicion.
• Arthrocentesis approach must avoid contaminated tissue (e.g., overlying cellulitis)

TREATMENT

APPROPRIATE HEALTH CARE
• Hospitalization for parenteral therapy
• Rarely an extremely compliant patient with a very sensitive organism might be treated as an outpatient

GENERAL MEASURES
• Repeat arthrocentesis to drain the joint, as fluid re-accumulates
• Avoid adding anti-inflammatory therapy so as not to compromise assessment of therapeutic response to antibiotic
• Arthrotomy indicated only if fluid accumulated is loculated and/or not amenable to needle drainage
• If a joint prosthesis is present in an infection, the infection is very difficult to eradicate, without removal of the prosthesis
• Treatment is continued for 1-2 weeks after total resolution of all signs of inflammation, 3-4 weeks for gram negative organisms, and 6-8 weeks if the joint was previously diseased (e.g., involved by arthritis)
• Intra-articular antibiotics are not required and may actually aggravate the arthritis

ACTIVITY Limit activity or splint the joint initially. Continuous passive motion may be used as an alternative approach.

DIET No special diet

PATIENT EDUCATION
• Rothschild, B.: Diagnosing and treating infectious arthritis. Geriatric Consultant. 5:14-15, 1986
• Arthritis Foundation pamphlet

MEDICATIONS

DRUG(S) OF CHOICE
Neisserial
◊ If Neisseria is penicillinase-producing (because of rising penicillinase producing

Neisseria gonorrhoeae (PPNG) isolates, penicillin would not be first choice). However the gonorrhea dermato-arthritis-producing organisms usually do not produce penicillinase:
◊ Aqueous penicillin G, 10 million units/day (q4-6h IV) for 3 days, followed by ampicillin (500 mg q 6 h po) for 10 days
◊ In the extremely compliant patient, 1 gm probenecid followed 30 minutes by 3.5 gm ampicillin po, then 500 mg ampicillin po q 6 h (or doxycycline 100 mg bid) for 7 days
◊ 1.5 gm tetracycline po (non-pregnant individual after eruption of permanent teeth), then 500 mg tetracycline q 6 h for 7 days
◊ 500 mg erythromycin intravenously q 6 h for 7 days
Non-Neisserial:
◊ Gram positive cocci in chains or clumps - nafcillin (150 mg/kg/day q 4-6 h IV/IM)
◊ Gram positive diplococci - penicillin 1.4 million units q6h
◊ Gram negative bacilli: In neonates - penicillin and gentamicin; in children age 6 months to 4 years - cefuroxime; in adult - penicillin or cephalosporin plus gentamicin, all at full dose. Clindamycin (at full dose) - in presence of retroperitoneal or pelvic abscess.
◊ Gram negative pleomorphic organisms - clindamycin at full dose (clindamycin has gram negative activity only against anaerobes)
◊ No bacteria seen on smear - penicillin or cephalosporin plus gentamicin, all at full dose
Contraindications: Refer to manufacturer's instructions
Precautions: Observe for allergic reactions/serum sickness
Significant possible interactions: Refer to manufacturer's instructions

ALTERNATIVE DRUGS
Non-Neisserial
◊ In children age 6 months to 4 years - ampicillin (Chloramphenicol may be required to cover resistant Haemophilus)
◊ Infectious disease consult strongly advised to supplement rheumatologist input for Haemophilus infections

FOLLOWUP

PATIENT MONITORING
• Recurrent arthrocentesis, as fluid re-accumulates - to verify sterilization of the joint and to verify reversion of inflammatory signs to normal
• If no definitive improvement within 48 hours, re-evaluate completely
• Complete blood count, liver and kidney function and urinalysis twice a week, while on antibiotics (perhaps with creatinine every other day when gentamicin used)
• Gentamycin levels
• It is essential to followup one week and a month after stopping antibiotics to detect any relapse

PREVENTION/AVOIDANCE
• Prophylaxis in presence of predisposing joint condition
• Condoms and discretion for STD protection

POSSIBLE COMPLICATIONS
• Death (9-33% in elderly, especially with gram negative organisms)
• Limited joint range of motion
• Flail or fused or dislocated joint
• Carpal tunnel syndrome
• Septic necrosis
• Sinus formation
• Ankylosis
• Osteomyelitis
• Postinfectious synovitis
• Shortening of the limb (in children)

EXPECTED COURSE AND PROGNOSIS
• Early treatment should allow cure
• Delayed recognition/treatment complicated by morbidity and mortality

MISCELLANEOUS

ASSOCIATED CONDITIONS
• Systemic infection
• Infection elsewhere
• Immunodeficiency
• Immunosuppression

AGE-RELATED FACTORS
Pediatric: N/A
Geriatric: N/A
Others: N/A

PREGNANCY N/A

SYNONYMS
• Suppurative arthritis
• Septic arthritis

ICD-9-CM 711.9

SEE ALSO Reiter's syndrome

OTHER NOTES N/A

ABBREVIATIONS N/A

REFERENCES
• Rothschild, B.M.: Infectious Arthritis. Fairlawn, CT, Clinical AV, 1982
• Rothschild, B.M. & Martin, L.: Paleopathology: Diseases in the Fossil Record. London, CRC Press, 1993
• Kelly, W.W., Harris, E.D., Jr., Ruddy, S. & Sledge, C.B: Textbook of Rheumatology. Philadelphia, W.B. Saunders Co., 1993
• Gershwin, M.E. and Robbins, D.L.: Musculoskeletal Diseases of Children, New York, Grune & Stratton, 1983

Author B. Rothschild, M.D.

Arthritis, infectious, granulomatous

BASICS

DESCRIPTION Invasion of joints by live micro-organisms or their fragments. One of the few curable causes of arthritis. May allow early recognition of systemic infection/disease.
System(s) affected: Musculoskeletal
Genetics: N/A
Incidence/Prevalence in USA:
• One in three million
• Granulomatous arthritis occurs in 1-3% of patients with tuberculosis infections
Predominant age: Elderly > 75 years
Predominant sex:
• Male > Female (Brucella and mycobacterial)
• Female > Male (fungal)

SIGNS AND SYMPTOMS
• Predominantly monoarticular (90%). Fungal may present as a migratory polyarthritis.
• Joint tenderness
• Limited joint use/motion (especially in children)
• Joint effusion
• Joint warmth - present in less than 50%
• Joint redness - present in less than 50%
• Loss of joint motion
• Tenosynovitis
• Sudden flare of a single joint in a patient with underlying joint disease
• Fever - in 50% at some time during the course of the infection
• Chills
• Malaise
• Cutaneous lesions
• Peripheral neuropathy
• Back pain - especially in tuberculosis and brucellosis
• Hypertrophic osteoarthropathy
• Fretfulness - especially in children
• Doughy swelling, with minimal tenderness
• Dactylitis
• Diaphoresis
• Headache
• Hepatosplenomegaly
• Lymphadenopathy
• Erythema nodosum
• Iritis (with mycobacterial arthritis)

CAUSES
• Hematogenous invasion by microorganisms (80-90%)
• Contiguous spread (10-15%)
• Direct penetration of micro-organisms secondary to trauma

RISK FACTORS
• Concurrent acquired immunodeficiency disease
• Concurrent extra-articular infection
• Prior arthritis in infected joint
• Trauma
• Rheumatoid arthritis
• Joint puncture or surgery
• Prosthetic joint
• Prior antibiotic, corticosteroid, or immunosuppressive therapy
• Serious chronic illness (e.g., diabetes, liver disease, malignancy, primary immunodeficiency)
• Defective phagocytic mechanisms (e.g., chronic granulomatous disease)
• Intravenous drug abuse
• Exposure history (e.g., unpasteurized milk)
• Farmers, butchers, veterinarians
• Travel/habitat history

DIAGNOSIS

DIFFERENTIAL DIAGNOSIS
• Gout
• Pseudogout (calcium pyrophosphate deposition disease)
• Spondyloarthropathy (Reiter's syndrome, psoriatic arthritis, ankylosing spondylitis, the arthritis of inflammatory bowel disease)
• Juvenile rheumatoid arthritis
• Type IIa hyperlipoproteinemia
• Foreign body
• Rheumatoid arthritis
• Rheumatic fever
• AIDS
• Cellulitis
• Palindromic rheumatism
• Neuropathic arthropathy
• Lyme arthritis
• Sarcoidosis

LABORATORY
• Synovial fluid usually cloudy with > 20,000 WBC/HPF, but may have fewer white blood cells present or over 100,000. (Caveat - cell count must be performed within 1 hour of obtaining specimen to be valid).
• Synovial fluid white count can be recognized as elevated (in presence of trauma) if RBC:WBC ratio significantly less than 700
• Polymorphonuclear leukocytes usually predominate in synovial fluid. (Granulomatous and viral arthritis may have a mononuclear cell predominance, but polymorphonuclear leukocytes usually predominate).
• Synovial fluid glucose often more than 40 mg/dL less than in a simultaneously obtained serum glucose value (in fasting patient). However, arthrocentesis should not be delayed simply to obtain fasting synovial fluid glucose level.
• Synovial fluid eosinophilia may occasionally be seen in the healing phase of an infection, but parasitic (e.g., guinea-worm) infection must also be considered
• Westergren erythrocyte sedimentation - often elevated, but normal in 20%
• Rheumatoid factor positive in 50% - if endocarditis present
• Elevated peripheral white blood cell count
• Cryoglobulins
• Immune complexes
• Febrile agglutinins (to include Brucella and rickettsial related titers)
• Antistreptolysin O (ASO) titer is usually normal
• Depressed synovial fluid and occasionally serum levels of complement
• Presence of crystals in urine (e.g., urate or calcium pyrophosphate) does not exclude infectious arthritis

Drugs that may alter lab results: Insulin, antibiotics
Disorders that may alter lab results: Diabetes

PATHOLOGICAL FINDINGS Synovial biopsy may reveal granulomas and possibly the causative organism

SPECIAL TESTS
• Arthrocentesis - bacterial - for silver and acid fast stain and culture
• Arthrocentesis - mycobacterial - acid fast (positive in 20%); culture (positive in 80%)
• Drug sensitivity testing recommended
• Blood, urine cultures
• Sputum cultures
• Gastric lavage for acid fast - increases yield 7%
• Fungal blood cultures
• All cultures should be held for 3 days, preferably 2 weeks. (Observing synovial fluid cultures for at least 3 days allows isolation of fastidious organisms. Acid-fast cultures are held 6 weeks

IMAGING
X-ray
◊ Soft tissue swelling
◊ Osteoporosis
◊ Effacement of the obturator fat pad (with hip involvement) or psoas shadow
◊ X-ray changes are usually a late phenomenon
◊ Rarefaction of subchondral bone may occur as early as 2-7 days
◊ Joint space loss
◊ Erosions
◊ Joint destruction with ankylosis may occur as early as 2 weeks
◊ Subchondral erosion with preservation of joint space is highly suggestive of granulomatous infection
Other imaging techniques
◊ Technetium joint scans - reveal distribution of inflammation
◊ Gallium or WBC-Indium scans - reveal inflammation as well as infection
◊ Computerized tomography - to identify sequestration
◊ Magnetic resonance imaging - perhaps early cartilage damage, osteomyelitis

DIAGNOSTIC PROCEDURES
• Arthrocentesis with gram, silver and acid fast stain, and culture. Must be done in all patients when possibility of infectious arthritis considered.
• Arthrocentesis approach must avoid contaminated tissue (e.g., overlying cellulitis)

TREATMENT

APPROPRIATE HEALTH CARE
• Fungal - initial hospitalization for parenteral therapy
• Mycobacterial - outpatient, once diagnosed
• Brucella - outpatient, once diagnosed

GENERAL MEASURES
• Repeat arthrocentesis to drain the joint, as fluid reaccumulates
• Avoid adding anti-inflammatory therapy so as not to compromise assessment of therapeutic response (to antibiotic)
• Arthrotomy indicated only if fluid accumulated is loculated and/or not amenable to needle drainage
• Infection associated with prosthetic joints may be difficult to eradicate without removal
• For Brucella or fungal infections, treatment is continued for 1-2 weeks after total resolution of all signs of inflammation, and 6-8 weeks if the joint was previously diseased (e.g., involved by arthritis)
• Anti-granulomatous therapy requires a long program (See Tuberculosis)
• Intra-articular antibiotics are not indicated

ACTIVITY Limit/splint joint initially, while pursuing full passive range of motion. Continuous passive motion is an alternative approach.

DIET As tolerated

PATIENT EDUCATION
• Rothschild, B.M.: Diagnosing and treating infectious arthritis. Geriatric Consultant, 5:14-15, 1986
• Arthritis Foundation
1314 Spring Street, NW
Atlanta, GA 30309
(404) 872-7100

 MEDICATIONS

DRUG(S) OF CHOICE
• Medications based on sensitivity of organisms
• Mycobacterial - (use a combination of these three) isoniazid (5 mg/kg, up to 300 mg po qd), rifampin (10 mg/kg, up to 600 mg po qd), and pyrazinamide (15-30 mg/kg up to 2 gm/d). The latter is replaced after 2 months with ethambutol 15 mg/kg. Continue therapy for 9-24 months. Request infectious disease consultation.
• Brucella - tetracycline plus streptomycin or trimethoprim-sulfamethoxazole or rifampin (for dosage, see manufacturer's literature)
• Fungal infection - amphotericin B, ketoconazole, 5-Flurocytosine and even iodide (dependent upon organism) with infectious disease consultation
Contraindications: Refer to manufacturer's information
Precautions: Observe for allergic reactions/serum sickness
Significant possible interactions: Refer to manufacturer's information

ALTERNATIVE DRUGS
• See Tuberculosis
• Infectious disease consultation essential

 FOLLOWUP

PATIENT MONITORING to verify sterilization of the joint and to verify reversion of inflammatory signs to normal
• Treatment of mycobacterial arthritis requires monthly complete blood count, liver and kidney function and urinalysis assessment
• It is essential to followup frequently after stopping antibiotics to detect relapse

PREVENTION/AVOIDANCE Prophylaxis in presence of predisposing joint condition

POSSIBLE COMPLICATIONS
• Limited joint range of motion
• Flail or fused joint
• Carpal-tunnel syndrome
• Septic necrosis
• Sinus formation
• Ankylosis
• Joint dislocation
• Osteomyelitis
• Shortening of the limb (in children)

EXPECTED COURSE AND PROGNOSIS
• Early initiation of treatment should allow cure
• Delayed recognition/treatment complicated by increased morbidity and mortality

 MISCELLANEOUS

ASSOCIATED CONDITIONS
• Systemic infection
• Infection elsewhere
• Immunodeficiency - (medication)
• Immunosuppression

AGE-RELATED FACTORS
Pediatric: Infrequent
Geriatric:
• Grave in elderly
• Tuberculosis much more likely to occur
Others: N/A

PREGNANCY N/A

SYNONYMS
• Fungal arthritis

ICD-9-CM
• 031.8 Mycobacterial arthritis
• 023.9 Brucellosis, unspecified
• 115.99 Fungal arthritis

SEE ALSO
• Brucellosis
• Mycobacteria
• Fungi tuberculosis

OTHER NOTES Infectious arthritis may be caused by many other organisms including bacterial (particularly neisseria), rickettsial, parasitic, fungal, and viral agents. Much of the information contained in this profile applies to these other organisms as well as to granulomatous infections.

ABBREVIATIONS N/A

REFERENCES
• Rothschild, B.M.: Infectious Arthritis. Fairlawn, CT, Clinical AV, 1982
• Gershwin, M.E. and Robbins, D.L.: Musculoskeletal Diseases of Children. New York, Grune & Stratton, 1983
• Rothschild, B.M. & Martin, L.: Paleopathology: Diseases in the Fossil Record. London, CRC Press, 1993
• Kelly, W.W., Harris, E.D., Jr., Ruddy, S. & Sledge, C.B.: Textbook of Rheumatology. Philadelphia, W.B. Saunders Co., 1993

Author B. Rothschild, M.D.

Arthritis, juvenile rheumatoid (JRA)

BASICS

DESCRIPTION Juvenile rheumatoid arthritis (JRA) is the most common form of chronic arthritis in children and a major cause of musculoskeletal disability. There are three subtypes of the disease, determined by the clinical characteristics occurring within the first six months of illness.
• Systemic (sys) JRA - occurs in 10-20% of affected children; usually characterized by a febrile onset with multiple physical and laboratory abnormalities
• Polyarticular (poly) JRA - occurs in 30-40% of affected children; characterized by multiple (> 4) joint involvement and minimal systemic features
• Pauciarticular (pauci) JRA - occurs in 40-50% of affected children; characterized by ≤ 4 joints involved, usually larger joints; a risk for chronic uveitis in young girls and axial skeletal involvement in older boys
System(s) affected: Musculoskeletal, Hemic/Lymphatic/Immunologic
Genetics: HLA-B27 histocompatibility antigen associated with risk of evolving spondyloarthropathy in older boys with pauci JRA. Weaker HLA associations exist for other subtypes (HLA-DR5; HLA-DR8; HLA-DR4).
Incidence/Prevalence in USA: Prevalence approximately 1/1000 children; incidence 1/10,000 children
Predominant age: 1-4 years and 9-14 years
Predominant sex: Female > Male

SIGNS AND SYMPTOMS
Systemic
◊ Arthralgias/arthritis
◊ Chest pain, pericardial friction rub
◊ Dyspnea
◊ Fatigue
◊ Fever
◊ Hepatosplenomegaly
◊ Lymphadenopathy
◊ Myalgias
◊ Rash
◊ Weight loss
Polyarticular
◊ Arthralgia/arthritis
◊ Cold intolerance
◊ Difficulty writing
◊ Fatigue
◊ Growth retardation
◊ Hand weakness
◊ Limitation of motion
◊ Malaise
◊ Morning stiffness
◊ Rheumatoid nodules
◊ Synovial cysts
◊ Synovial thickening
◊ Weight loss
Pauciarticular
◊ Abnormal gait
◊ Eye pain, redness
◊ Joint swelling
◊ Leg length abnormality
◊ Morning stiffness
◊ Photophobia

CAUSES Multifactorial including abnormal immune response, genetic predisposition and environmental triggers, possibly infectious

RISK FACTORS
• HLA-B27 in pauci JRA increases risk for development of spondyloarthopathy
• Rheumatoid factor positivity increases risk for severe arthritis in poly JRA
• ANA positivity increases risk for uveitis in pauci JRA

DIAGNOSIS

DIFFERENTIAL DIAGNOSIS Other rheumatic diseases, especially SLE and dermatomyositis; atypical bacterial or viral infections; hemoglobinopathies; malignancy; vasculitis; rheumatic fever; Lyme disease; post-infectious arthritis; musculoskeletal developmental abnormalities; sympathetic dystrophy

LABORATORY
• WBC normal or markedly elevated (sys)
• Hb normal or low (especially sys)
• Platelet count normal or elevated
• ANA positive approximately 40% (poly or pauci)
• RF positive approximately 10-15% (some polys)
• HLA-B27 positive approximately 70% in pauci boys
• Sedimentation rate (ESR) elevated in most patients with active disease; > 100 ml/hr (Westergren) in active systemic disease
Drugs that may alter lab results: Anti-inflammatory therapy may alter CBC and ESR
Disorders that may alter lab results: Hemoglobinopathies (ESR)

PATHOLOGICAL FINDINGS Synovium shows hyperplasia of synovial cells, hyperemia and infiltration of small lymphocytes and mononuclear cells

SPECIAL TESTS
• Echocardiography (pericarditis)
• Radionuclide scans (infection, malignancy)

IMAGING
• Early radiographic changes - soft tissue swelling, periosteal reaction, juxta-articular demineralization; later changes include joint space loss, articular surface erosions, subchondral cyst formation, sclerosis and joint fusion
• CT and MRI very helpful in delineating early erosions

DIAGNOSTIC PROCEDURES
• Joint fluid aspiration and analysis helpful in excluding infection
• Synovial biopsy occasionally indicated in persistent, atypical monoarthritis

TREATMENT

APPROPRIATE HEALTH CARE
• Outpatient care except for initial diagnostic workup of sys JRA disease and complications for all subtypes
• Pauciarticular patients require ongoing, regular ophthalmic exams to rule out asymptomatic eye disease

GENERAL MEASURES Physical therapy including daily home exercise program required for joints with limited motion; moist heat, sleeping bag or electric blanket to relieve morning stiffness

ACTIVITY
• Full activity as tolerated
• Regular school. May need modified physical education program.

DIET Regular diet with special attention to adequate calcium, iron, protein and caloric intake

PATIENT EDUCATION
• Ongoing education of patients and families needed with special attention to psycho-social needs, behavioral strategies for dealing with pain, and noncompliance, and utilization of health care resources
• Printed and audio-visual information available from local Arthritis Foundation

MEDICATIONS

DRUG(S) OF CHOICE
First-line:
◊ Nonsteroidal anti-inflammatory medications (NSAID's) adequate in approximately 60% of patients. Average of 2-3 trials needed to determine most effective drug for an individual patient; adequate duration of trial for given NSAID 4-6 weeks (if no adverse reaction). FDA approved drugs for children include:
◊ Aspirin 75-90 mg/kg/d
◊ Ibuprofen (Motrin, Advil, Nuprin) 30-50 mg/kg/d (usual dose is 40 mg/kg/d)
◊ Naproxen (Naprosyn) 10-20 mg/kg/d
◊ Tolmetin sodium (Tolmetin) 15-30 mg/kg/d).
Second-line:
◊ 30-40% of patients ultimately require addition of disease-modifying antirheumatic drug (DMARD) e.g., gold, antimalarials, penicillamine, methotrexate
◊ Other agents - corticosteroids for serious cardiac involvement or unresponsive uveitis
Contraindications: Known allergies
Precautions: All (except salicyl salicylate) affect platelet adhesiveness and may worsen a bleeding diathesis. Use caution in renal insufficiency and hypovolemic states.
Significant possible interactions: NSAID's may lower serum levels of digitalis and anticonvulsants, and blunt the effect of loop diuretics. NSAID's may increase serum methotrexate levels.

ALTERNATIVE DRUGS
Other NSAID's; analgesics for pain control

FOLLOWUP

PATIENT MONITORING
• Patients on NSAID's - CBC, urinalysis, minimum every 3-4 months
• Patients on aspirin and/or other salicylates - transaminase and salicylate levels, weekly for first month, then every 3-4 months
• Patients on gold - monthly CBC, urinalysis
• Patient on methotrexate - monthly liver function tests, CBC
• Ophthalmologic monitoring for antimalarials

PREVENTION/AVOIDANCE
• Avoid salicylate therapy during serious viral illness or following varicella exposure due to possible risk for Reye's syndrome
• No known preventive measures for JRA

POSSIBLE COMPLICATIONS
• Blindness
• Band keratopathy
• Glaucoma
• Short stature
• Debilitating joint disease
Patient on NSAID's
◊ Peptic ulcer
◊ Gastrointestinal hemorrhage
◊ Rashes
◊ CNS reactions
◊ Renal disease
◊ Leukopenia
Patient on DMARD's
◊ Bone marrow suppression
◊ Hepatitis
◊ Renal disease
◊ Dermatitis
◊ Mouth ulcers
◊ Retinal toxicity (antimalarials)

EXPECTED COURSE AND PROGNOSIS
• 70-80% ultimately remit, but functional ability depends on adequacy of long-term therapy (disease control and maintaining muscle and joint function)
• Poorest prognosis in polyarticular patients with positive rheumatoid factor (RF); and in systemic juvenile arthritis

MISCELLANEOUS

Associated conditions: Other autoimmune disorders

AGE-RELATED FACTORS
Pediatric: Behavioral and compliance problems frequent in toddlers and teenagers
Geriatric: N/A
Others: N/A

PREGNANCY
Unpredictable effect on disease activity

SYNONYMS
• Juvenile chronic arthritis
• Juvenile arthritis
• Still's disease

ICD-9-CM
• 714 polyarticular juvenile rheumatoid arthritis, chronic
• 714.31 systemic onset JRA
• 714.32 pauciarticular onset
• 714.33 polyarticular onset JRA

SEE ALSO N/A

OTHER NOTES
Treatment goal is to control active disease as well as extra-articular manifestations in order to maintain musculoskeletal function as normal as possible

ABBREVIATIONS
• JRA = juvenile rheumatoid arthritis
• RF = rheumatic factor
• DMARD = disease modifying antirheumatic drug

REFERENCES
• Schaller, J.G.: Juvenile Rheumatoid Arthritis. Pediatrics in Review. 2(6), 163-174, 1980
• Cassidy, J.T. & Petty, R.E.: The Textbook of Pediatric Rheumatology. 2nd Ed. New York, Churchill Livingstone, 1990

Author C. Lindsley, M.D.

Artificial insemination

 BASICS

DESCRIPTION
Sperm are washed free of seminal plasma and placed directly in the uterine cavity. Sperm are washed to remove potentially antigenic proteins, prostaglandins, infectious agents and decapacitation factors reducing the risk of anaphylaxis. Insemination may be with husband's (AIH) or donor semen (AID).

System(s) affected: Reproductive, Endocrine/Metabolic
Genetics: N/A
Incidence/Prevalence in USA: Varies, depending on etiology of infertility, i.e., male factor is responsible for approximately 35% of cases of infertility, and a cervical factor is responsible for approximately 10% of cases
Predominant age: Reproductive age women (18-45 years of age)
Predominant sex: Female only

SIGNS AND SYMPTOMS
Inability to conceive

CAUSES
• Anatomic defects of the vagina or cervix
• Anatomic defects of penis (hypospadias)
• Psychologic/emotional factors (impotence, vaginismus)
• Antisperm antibodies (semen, mucus or serum)
• Cervical mucus abnormalities (diethylstilbestrol exposure or iatrogenic)
• Decreased semen volume
• Oligo-asthenospermia
• Retrograde ejaculation
• Seminal fluid liquefaction defect
• Teratospermia
• Unexplained infertility

RISK FACTORS
• Male factor 35%
• Cervical factor 10%

 DIAGNOSIS

DIFFERENTIAL DIAGNOSIS
• Primary female cervical factor?
• Primary male factor?

LABORATORY
• Semen analysis
• Postcoital test
• Sperm antibody testing
Drugs that may alter lab results:
Clomiphene citrate (Clomid)
Disorders that may alter lab results:
• Abnormal pH of vagina or cervical mucus
• Bacterial infection semen/mucus

PATHOLOGICAL FINDINGS
• Chronic cervicitis
• Chronic prostatitis

SPECIAL TESTS
• Zona free hamster sperm penetration assay
• Bovine cervical mucus sperm penetration test

IMAGING
Hysterosalpingogram

DIAGNOSTIC PROCEDURES
Postcoital test

 TREATMENT

APPROPRIATE HEALTH CARE
Outpatient

GENERAL MEASURES
• Intrauterine insemination should be closely timed with ovulation. Ovulation prediction kits detect the luteinizing hormone (LH) surge which precedes ovulation by 12-36 hours. Intrauterine insemination is performed the day of or the day after the LH surge.
• The volume of inseminate that can be transferred into the uterus is 0.25 to 0.5 ml. Small amounts are used to avoid cramping and flushing the oocyte out of the tube. The volume is also limited by space within the uterus.
• Intrauterine insemination is an office procedure. First, the position of the uterus is determined. A speculum is placed in the vagina and the cervix is visualized. The sample of washed sperm is placed into the uppermost portion of the uterine cavity using an insemination catheter with a disposable tuberculin syringe. Occasionally a tenaculum is needed on the anterior lip of the cervix to straighten the endocervical canal. Cervical dilatation or paracervical block is rarely required. The sample is injected slowly over 30-60 seconds.

ACTIVITY
No restrictions

DIET
No special diet

PATIENT EDUCATION
No vaginal lubricants or douching

MEDICATIONS

DRUG(S) OF CHOICE
• Clomiphene citrate (Clomid) or human menopausal gonadotropins (Pergonal) may be used for controlled ovarian hyperstimulation and ovulation may be initiated by the administration of human chorionic gonadotropin (HCG), an LH-like molecule. Intrauterine insemination is performed 24-36 hours after HCG administration. Clomid predisposes to poor cervical mucus, which can adversely alter sperm/mucus interaction.
Dosages:
◊ Clomiphene: 50 mg daily x 5 days to induce ovulation
◊ Pergonal (menotropins): 75 IU FSH/75 IU LH IM daily x 12 days; then a single dose of chorionic gonadotropin 10,000 IU/day after last dose of menotropins
Contraindications:
• Uncontrolled thyroid and adrenal dysfunction
• An intracranial lesion
• High follicle-stimulating hormone (FSH) level indicating primary ovarian failure
• Abnormal bleeding of undetermined etiology
• Ovarian cysts of unknown origin
• Hypersensitivity
• Pregnancy
Precautions:
• Multiple births - Clomid 8%, Pergonal 25%
• Severe ovarian hyperstimulation (ascites, pleural effusion, dehydration, electrolyte imbalance, pain)
• Ovarian torsion
Significant possible interactions: N/A

ALTERNATIVE DRUGS
• Estrogen in follicular phase of cycle to improve mucus

FOLLOWUP

PATIENT MONITORING
• Those patients on Clomid require a bimanual exam on a monthly basis
• Patients on Pergonal require serum estradiol measurements and pelvic sonography to monitor ovarian response

PREVENTION/AVOIDANCE N/A

POSSIBLE COMPLICATIONS
• Uterine cramping
• Mild vasomotor symptoms
• Infection
• Theoretical but unproven risk is development of antisperm antibodies in response to increase exposure of the immune system to sperm antigens

EXPECTED COURSE AND PROGNOSIS
• Virtually all pregnancies that result, occur within the first six treatment cycles. A 6 month treatment interval usually represents an adequate therapeutic trial.
• There is a documented increase in efficacy with combination of intrauterine insemination and controlled ovarian hyperstimulation (Pergonal)
• The highest success rates are seen with idiopathic or cervical factor problems
• The poorest outcome is with male factor
• Monthly fecundities of 14% have occurred with therapeutic inseminations utilizing fresh semen

MISCELLANEOUS

ASSOCIATED CONDITIONS Causes of infertility

AGE-RELATED FACTORS
Pediatric: N/A
Geriatric: N/A
Others:
• Fecundity is inversely related to maternal age
Contraindications to artificial insemination
◊ Infection (acute cervicitis, endometritis, acute prostatitis, epididymitis, salpingo-oophoritis)
◊ Pregnancy
◊ Unexplained uterine bleeding

PREGNANCY N/A

SYNONYMS
• Therapeutic Insemination
• Intrauterine Insemination

ICD-9-CM 628.4

SEE ALSO N/A

OTHER NOTES For donor insemination, only frozen semen is used and only after a period of "quarantine" to minimize danger of transmission of HIV

ABBREVIATIONS
• LH = leuteinizing hormone
• HCG = human chorionic gonadotropin

REFERENCES Yen, S.S.C. & Jaffe, R.B. (eds.): Reproductive Endocrinology. 2nd Ed. Philadelphia, W.B. Saunders Co., 1986

Author C. Ellis, D.O. & N. Spirtos, D.O.

Asbestosis

 BASICS

DESCRIPTION
A form of pneumoconiosis that can develop 15-20 or more years after regular exposure to asbestos (a heat-resistant and insulating material) has stopped. It is characterized by diffuse interstitial fibrosis. Causes pleural plaques and mesotheliomas of pleura and peritoneum. It increases the risk of tuberculosis and lung cancer in cigarette smokers. Usual course - chronic; progressive.

System(s) affected: Pulmonary
Genetics: No known genetic pattern
Incidence in USA: Less than 10 cases/100,000 people in the U.S. are diagnosed each year
Prevalence in USA: More than a million people have been exposed to significant levels of asbestos
Predominant age: Middle age (40-75 years)
Predominant sex: Male > Female

SIGNS AND SYMPTOMS
- Chest discomfort
- Clubbed fingers
- Crackles
- Cyanosis
- Exertional dyspnea
- Fatigue
- History of asbestos exposure at least 10 years previously
- Malaise
- Nonproductive cough
- Pleural effusion
- Pleuritic pain
- Pulmonary hypertension

CAUSES
- Occupational exposure to asbestos dust or asbestos fibers
- Secondary exposure in families of workers
- Inhalation of asbestos dust
- Macrophage-induced damage to lung parenchyma

RISK FACTORS
- Cigarette smoking
- Asbestos workers
- Mine workers

 DIAGNOSIS

DIFFERENTIAL DIAGNOSIS
Other pneumoconioses (siderosis, stannosis, (due to inhalation of tin oxide), baritosis, coal worker's pneumoconiosis, silicosis, talcosis, shaver's disease)

LABORATORY
- Hypoxemia
- Bronchoalveolar lavage - macrophages, asbestos fibers

Drugs that may alter lab results: N/A
Disorders that may alter lab results: N/A

PATHOLOGICAL FINDINGS
Lung:
◊ Parietal pleural thickening
◊ Parietal pleural calcification
◊ Interstitial inflammation
◊ Interstitial fibrosis
◊ Alveolar wall fibrosis
◊ Extensive pulmonary fibrosis
◊ Alveolar destruction
◊ Cystic changes

SPECIAL TESTS
Pulmonary function test:
◊ Decreased vital capacity
◊ Decreased total lung capacity
◊ Normal FEV1/FVC ratio
◊ Decreased diffusing capacity

IMAGING
Lung scan
◊ Alveolar capillary dysfunction
◊ Small airway narrowing
Chest x-ray
◊ Calcified pleural plaques
◊ Irregular, linear opacities
◊ Bilateral pleural effusion
◊ Pleural thickening
◊ Interstitial fibrosis
◊ Honeycombed lung

DIAGNOSTIC PROCEDURES
Bronchoscopy

 TREATMENT

APPROPRIATE HEALTH CARE
Outpatient

GENERAL MEASURES
- There is no effective treatment once asbestosis has developed
- Malignancy surveillance
- Avoid tobacco smoking
- Relieve respiratory symptoms (chest physiotherapy)
- Manage hypoxia
- Manage cor pulmonale

ACTIVITY
As tolerated. Physical conditioning to the extent possible, conservation of energy when necessary.

DIET
No special diet

PATIENT EDUCATION
Printed patient information available from: Asbestos Victims of America, P.O. Box 559, Capitola, CA 95010, (408)476-3646 or American Lung Association, 1740 Broadway, New York, NY 10019, (212)315-8700

MEDICATIONS

DRUG(S) OF CHOICE
• Supplemental oxygen for advanced disease
• Bronchodilators, if needed
Contraindications: N/A
Precautions: N/A
Significant possible interactions: N/A

ALTERNATIVE DRUGS
• Antibiotics for respiratory infections
• Diuretics
• Digitalis

FOLLOWUP

PATIENT MONITORING
• Chest x-ray
• Occasional pulmonary function tests
• Treat infections promptly

PREVENTION/AVOIDANCE
• Avoid asbestos
• If working with asbestos, strictly follow all safety guidelines
• Avoid tobacco smoke

EXPECTED COURSE AND PROGNOSIS
• Severity depends on duration of exposure and on intensity of exposure
• Lung disease irreversible
• Further increased lung cancer risk with smoking
• Increased risk for mesotheliomas
• Increased risk for tuberculosis

POSSIBLE COMPLICATIONS
• Squamous cell lung carcinoma
• Pulmonary adenocarcinoma
• Pleural mesothelioma
• Peritoneal mesothelioma
• Diffuse interstitial pulmonary fibrosis
• Restrictive lung disease
• Asphyxiation

MISCELLANEOUS

ASSOCIATED CONDITIONS N/A

AGE-RELATED FACTORS
Pediatric: N/A
Geriatric: More likely to have terminal respiratory illness
Others: N/A

PREGNANCY N/A

SYNONYMS Asbestos pneumoconiosis

ICD-9-CM
501 asbestosis

SEE ALSO N/A

OTHER NOTES N/A

ABBREVIATIONS

REFERENCES
• LaDou, J. (ed): Occupational Medicine. Norwalk, CT, Appleton and Lange, 1990
• Rosenstock, L. & Cullen, M.R.: Clinical Occupational Medicine. Philadelphia, W.B. Saunders Co., 1986

Author N. Dambro, M.D.

Ascites

BASICS

DESCRIPTION Effusion and accumulation of serous fluid in the abdominal cavity. Ascites may occur in any condition that causes generalized edema. In children nephrotic syndrome and malignancy are the predominant causes. In adults, cirrhosis, heart failure, nephrotic syndrome and chronic peritonitis are most common.

System(s) affected: Cardiovascular/Gastrointestinal/Hemic/Lymphatic/Immunologic

Genetics: N/A

Incidence/Prevalence: Determined by etiology

Predominant age: Determined by etiology

Predominant sex: Determined by etiology

SIGNS AND SYMPTOMS

- Abdominal pain
- Abdominal fullness
- Abdominal discomfort
- Abdominal distention
- Tight clothing
- Shortness of breath
- Anorexia
- Nausea
- Early satiety
- Pyrosis
- Flank pain
- Weight gain
- Orthopnea
- Flank bulge
- Abdominal fluid wave
- Shifting dullness
- Penile edema
- Scrotal edema
- Umbilical herniation
- Pleural effusion
- Pedal edema
- Rales
- Tachycardia

CAUSES

Peritoneal infection and inflammation
- ◊ Tuberculosis
- ◊ Fungus disease
- ◊ Chronic bacterial due to foreign body, fistula
- ◊ Ruptured viscus
- ◊ Granulomatous peritonitis
- ◊ Vasculitis
- ◊ Eosinophilic gastroenteritis
- ◊ Peritoneal seeding with cancer
- ◊ Ovarian cancers
- ◊ Pancreatic cancers

Metabolic diseases
Hypothyroidism
- ◊ Familial Mediterranean fever
- ◊ Mesenteric or intestinal lymphangiectasia
- ◊ Protein loosing enteropathy
- ◊ Cirrhosis and portal hypertension
- ◊ Cirrhosis
- ◊ Congenital hepatic fibrosis
- ◊ Partial nodular transformation
- ◊ Hepatic vein occlusion (Budd Chiari syndrome)
- ◊ Portal vein occlusion
- ◊ Multiple metastatic tumor nodules in liver

Heart and hepatic congestion
- ◊ Heart failure
- ◊ Constrictive pericarditis
- ◊ Tricuspid stenosis or insufficiency

Traumatic
- ◊ Pancreatic fistula
- ◊ Biliary fistula
- ◊ Lymphatic fistula
- ◊ Hemoperitoneum (trauma, ectopic pregnancy, tumor)
- ◊ Urine

Malignancy
- ◊ Lymphatic obstruction - leukemia, lymphoma
- ◊ Direct peritoneal seeding - ovarian
- ◊ Hepatic replacement - colon, pancreas

Other
- ◊ Nephrotic syndrome
- ◊ Malnutrition with hypoalbuminemia
- ◊ Filariasis

RISK FACTORS Those associated with possible causes

DIAGNOSIS

DIFFERENTIAL DIAGNOSIS
- Obesity
- Air and liquid in distended intestine

LABORATORY

Ascitic fluid
All fluid must have:
- ◊ WBC (>500/mm3)
- ◊ Differential WBC (> 250 PMN)
- ◊ Total protein >2 gm/dl
- ◊ Blood culture bottle inoculated with 10 ml

Useful frequently:
- ◊ Lactic dehydrogenase > 200 IU/Liter
- ◊ Ascites amylase > serum amylase
- ◊ Acid Fast or fungal culture - positive
- ◊ Cytology Positive
- ◊ Gram stain positive for multiple organisms
- ◊ Triglycerides ascites > serum

Infrequently useful:
- ◊ Inspection for scoleces, talcum granules
- ◊ Urea > blood
- ◊ Carcinoma embryonic antigen > 10 ng/ml

Drugs that may alter lab results: Refer to laboratory test reference

Disorders that may alter lab results: Refer to laboratory test reference

PATHOLOGICAL FINDINGS N/A

SPECIAL TESTS
- Diagnostic paracentesis
- Peritoneoscopy
- Others as needed to assist in diagnosis

IMAGING Sonography or CT scan confirm ascites

DIAGNOSTIC PROCEDURES
- Data from laboratory evaluations, clinical findings and other tests used to determine causes

Transudate fluid
- ◊ Protein < 2 gm/dL
- ◊ Lactate dehydrogenase < 200 IU/liter
- ◊ Likely causes include: Congestive heart failure, constrictive pericarditis, inferior vena cava obstruction, Budd-Chiari syndrome, cirrhosis, nephrotic syndrome, hypoalbuminemia

Exudate fluid
- ◊ Protein > 2 gm/dL
- ◊ Lactate dehydrogenase > 200 IU/liter
- ◊ Likely causes include: Neoplasm, tuberculosis, pancreatitis, myxedema, vasculitis

TREATMENT

APPROPRIATE HEALTH CARE May be outpatient or inpatient depending on physical condition

GENERAL MEASURES

For ascites with edema
- ◊ Sodium restriction and diuretics usually initiate diuresis.
- ◊ Sodium restriction that estimated to be obtained at home
- ◊ Water restriction only necessary if sodium levels below 130 mEq/L
- ◊ Maximum weight loss limited to 5 lbs/day

For ascites without edema
- ◊ Sodium, water restriction and diuretics as above
- ◊ Maximum loss of 2 lbs/day

Ascites increasing or failing to respond to treatment
- ◊ Spot specimen urine sodium speeds recognition of response
- ◊ Paracentesis up to 10 L If BUN or creatinine elevated replace IV albumin at 10 gm/L fluid removed
- ◊ Consider in chronic refractory cases peritoneovenous shunt or Transjugular Intrahepatic Portal Shunt (TIPS)

ACTIVITY Activity: Bedrest of benefit in heart failure and when leg edema is prominent, otherwise of limited value.

DIET Sodium restriction needed for several months, so regulate on diet that can be followed outside hospital

PATIENT EDUCATION Diet restrictions

Ascites

 MEDICATIONS

DRUG(S) OF CHOICE
<u>Diuretics are needed in nearly all patients</u>
◊ Spironolactone 100-300 mg/day orally in one dose best for cirrhotic ascites, furosemide 40-120 mg/day orally best for all other etiologies.
◊ Dose should be sufficient to obtain net sodium loss in urine
◊ Spot sodium in mEq/L x estimated urine output (l L if no information) should equal estimated dietary sodium. Increase diuretics daily until this is attained Measure electrolytes before each dose change.
Contraindications: See manufacturer's literature
Precautions: Observe patient daily for changed mental status, oliguria, azotemia, and hyperkalemia
Precautions: Observe patients closely for signs of volume depletion, encephalopathy and renal insufficiency
Significant possible interactions: Avoid concomitant use of potassium supplements if spironolactone is used alone

ALTERNATIVE DRUGS   Other diuretics

 FOLLOWUP

PATIENT MONITORING
• For ascites - changes in body weight and urinary sodium to measure response to therapy
• Monitoring as needed for other therapies

PREVENTION/AVOIDANCE   Dependent upon etiology

POSSIBLE COMPLICATIONS
• Overly aggressive diuresis may lead to hypokalemia, worsening hepatic encephalopathy, intravascular volume depletion, azotemia, and possibly to renal failure and death
• Sympathetic pleural effusion
• Other complications as may be associated with cause of ascites

EXPECTED COURSE AND PROGNOSIS
• Ascites is rarely life-threatening. Conservative therapy usually successful.
• Prognosis variable depending upon the underlying cause

 MISCELLANEOUS

ASSOCIATED CONDITIONS   Listed in Causes

AGE-RELATED FACTORS
Pediatric: N/A
Geriatric: N/A
Others: N/A

PREGNANCY   N/A

SYNONYMS   N/A

ICD-9-CM   789.5 ascites

SEE ALSO   N/A

OTHER NOTES   N/A

ABBREVIATIONS   N/A

REFERENCES   Zakim, D. & Boyer, T. (eds): Hepatology. 2nd Ed. Philadelphia, W.B. Saunders Co., 1989

Author   F. Iber, M.D.

Aspergillosis

 BASICS

DESCRIPTION
Disease caused by a ubiquitous mold that primarily involves the lungs. Disease can be lethal in neutropenic patients. Syndromes include:
- Allergic aspergillosis
  - ◊ Extrinsic allergic alveolitis - hypersensitivity pneumonitis in individuals repeatedly exposed to the fungus.
  - ◊ Allergic bronchopulmonary aspergillosis (ABPA) - pulmonary infiltrates, mucous plugging; secondary to allergic reaction to fungus.
- Aspergillomas - "fungus ball" saprophytic colonization within pre-existing pulmonary cavities.
- Invasive aspergillosis - primarily neutropenic patients; lungs and sometimes other organs involved; frequently lethal.

System(s) affected: Pulmonary. Unusual: Nervous, Gastrointestinal, Cardiovascular, Musculoskeletal
Genetics: No known genetic pattern
Incidence/Prevalence in USA: Rare
Predominant Age: None
Predominant Sex: Male = Female

SIGNS AND SYMPTOMS
- Allergic - cough, wheezing, constitutional symptoms, plug expectoration
- Aspergillomas - hemoptysis; manifestations of underlying disease
- Invasive - fever, cough, rales, rhonchi; toxicity; CNS signs; GI bleeding

CAUSES
Aspergillus species in decreasing order of frequency: fumigatus, flavus, niger

RISK FACTORS
- Allergic - exposure, asthma
- Aspergillomas - COPD, bronchiectasis, TB, malignancy
- Invasive - neutropenia, corticosteroid therapy

 DIAGNOSIS

DIFFERENTIAL DIAGNOSIS
- Allergic - other causes of asthma and hypersensitivity pneumonitis.
- Aspergillomas - neoplasm, TB.
- Invasive - bacterial pneumonia, pulmonary hemorrhage, drug toxicity, malignancy; mucor (sinuses).

LABORATORY
- ABPA - eosinophilia, immediate skin reactivity to aspergillus antigen, precipitating–serum antibodies to aspergillus, elevated serum IgE concentrations.
- Invasive - sputum culture, cultures of bronchoalveolar lavage or bronchial washings; biopsy is definitive; blood cultures almost never positive

Drugs that may alter lab results: None
Disorders that may alter lab results: None

PATHOLOGICAL FINDINGS
Necrotizing pneumonia, hemorrhagic infarcts, blood vessel invasion; branching septate hyphae if organism seen microscopically.

SPECIAL TESTS
- ABPA - immediate skin reactivity to aspergillus antigen, precipitating serum antibodies (precipitins) against aspergillus antigens, elevated serum IgE concentrations, elevated serum IgE and IgG antibodies specific to A. Fumigatus.
- Invasive - none.

IMAGING
Chest x-ray - fleeting infiltrates (ABPA), round intracavity mass (aspergillomas); nodular or patchy infiltrates progressing to diffuse consolidation and cavitation (invasive)

DIAGNOSTIC PROCEDURES
Bronchoscopy, bronchial washings, bronchoalveolar lavage may be helpful in isolating organism in invasive disease; biopsy is diagnostic but often not possible in severely ill, ventilated patients.

 TREATMENT

APPROPRIATE HEALTH CARE
- Allergic - outpatient usually
- Aspergillomas - outpatient usually
- Invasive - inpatient

GENERAL MEASURES
- Allergic
  - ◊ Extrinsic allergic alveolitis - drug therapy, exposure avoidance.
  - ◊ ABPA - corticosteroids
- Aspergillomas - individualized therapy ranging from no therapy to surgical resection of cavities in cases of severe hemoptysis; systemic antifungal therapy is seldom useful.
- Invasive - (prognosis tends to be poor) high dose intravenous antifungal therapy; treatment of underlying disease; ?adjunctive cytokine therapy to reverse neutropenia

ACTIVITY
As tolerated

DIET
No special diet

PATIENT EDUCATION
To specifics of individual circumstances.

MEDICATIONS

DRUG(S) OF CHOICE
• Allergic
  ◊ Extrinsic allergic alveolitis - bronchodilators, cromolyn sodium, steroids.
  ◊ ABPA - steroids.
• Aspergillomas - none.
• Invasive - high dose Amphotericin B (up to 1 mg/kg/day).
Contraindications: Refer to manufacturers literature
Precautions: Amphotericin B can cause significant renal insufficiency and electrolyte abnormalities
Significant possible interactions: Concomitant use of Amphotericin B and other nephrotoxic drugs (aminoglycosides, cyclosporine, etc) can accelerate development of renal insufficiency; likewise, concomitant Amphotericin B and diuretics use can accelerate electrolyte depletion.

ALTERNATIVE DRUGS
Itraconazole may have some utility as alternate to Amphotericin B in invasive disease but is second line.

FOLLOWUP

PATIENT MONITORING
• Allergic
  ◊ Extrinsic allergic, alveolitis - spirometry
  ◊ ABPA - chest x-ray, IgE levels
• Aspergillomas - chest x-ray, symptoms
• Invasive - chest x-ray, CBC

PREVENTION/AVOIDANCE
• Allergic - avoid exposure
• Aspergillomas - treatment of underlying diseases, i.e., COPD, etc.

EXPECTED COURSE AND PROGNOSIS
• Allergic - with treatment prognosis is good; untreated can progress to severe fibrosis, COPD.
• Aspergillomas - prognosis more related to underlying disease.
• Invasive - poor prognosis.

POSSIBLE COMPLICATIONS
• Allergic - bronchiectasis, pulmonary fibrosis, obstructive lung disease.
• Aspergillomas - hemoptyses.
• Invasive - metastatic infection (CNS); death.

MISCELLANEOUS

ASSOCIATED CONDITIONS
• Allergic - asthma.
• Aspergillomas - COPD, TB, pulmonary mycoses, silicosis, sarcoidosis, non-tuberculosis mycobacteria, ankylosing spondylitis, malignancy.
• Invasive - neutropenia

AGE-RELATED FACTORS
Pediatric: N/A
Geriatric: N/A
Others: N/A
• Allergic - Tends to occur in younger patients < 35.
• Aspergillomas - older patients with chronic lung disease
• Invasive - all ages

PREGNANCY N/A

SYNONYMS
• Hypersensitivity pneumonitis
• Fungus ball

ICD-9-CM
484.6 pneumonia in aspergillosis

SEE ALSO N/A

OTHER NOTES N/A

ABBREVIATIONS ABPA = allergic bronchopulmonary aspergillosis

REFERENCES
• Mandell, G.L., et al. (eds.): Principles and Practice of Infectious Diseases. 3rd Ed. Churchill Livingstone, New York, 1990.=
• Levitz, S.M. Aspergillosis. Inf. Dis. Clin. N.A. 3:1:1-18, March, 1989
• Rosenberg, M.,Patterson, R., Mintzer, R., Cooper, B.J., Roberts, M. & Harris, K.E.: Clinical and Immunologic Criteria for the Diagnosis of Allergic Bronchopulmonary Aspergillosis. Ann. Int. Med. 86:405-414, 1977
• Denning, D.W. & Stevens, D.A. Antifungal and Surgical Treatment of Invasive Aspergillosis: Review of 2,121 Published Cases. Rev. Inf. Dis. 12(6):1147-1201, 1990

AUTHOR W. Muth, M.D. & R. Adam, M.D.

Asthma

 BASICS

DESCRIPTION A disorder of the tracheobronchial tree characterized by mild to severe obstruction to airflow. Symptoms vary from coughing to dyspnea, and are generally episodic or paroxysmal, but may be persistent. The clinical hallmark is wheezing, but cough may be the predominant symptom. Commonly misdiagnosed as "recurrent pneumonia" or "chronic bronchitis."
• Acute symptoms are characterized by narrowing of large and small airways due to spasm of bronchial smooth muscle, edema and inflammation of the bronchial mucosa, and production of mucus
• Occurs in a setting in which asthma is likely and other, rarer conditions have been excluded
System(s) affected: Pulmonary
Genetics: No known genetic pattern, although there is a familial association of reactive airway disease (RAD), ectopic dermatitis, and allergic rhinitis
Incidence in USA: 10 million new cases each year, however, there is confusion due to lack of a uniform definition
Prevalence in USA:
• 7-19% of children
• A leading cause of missed school days - 7.5 million/year
Predominant age:
• 50% of cases are children under 10
• Young adult (16-40 years), but may occur at any age
Predominant sex:
• Children under 10: Male > Female
• Puberty: Male = Female
• Adult onset: Female > Male

SIGNS AND SYMPTOMS
Variation in pattern of symptoms; paroxysmal, constant, abnormal pulmonary function tests without symptoms
• Wheezing
• Cough
• Periodicity of symptoms
• Prolonged expiration
• Hyperresonance
• Decreased breath sounds
• Nocturnal attacks
• Pulsus paradoxus
• Cyanosis
• Tachycardia
• Accessory respiratory muscle use
• Flattened diaphragms
• Nasal polyp; seen in cystic fibrosis and aspirin sensitivity
• Clubbing is not seen in asthma
• Growth is usually normal

CAUSES
Allergic factors
◊ Airborne pollens
◊ Molds
◊ House dust (mites)
◊ Animal dander
◊ Feather pillows
Other factors
◊ Smoke and other pollutants
◊ Infections, especially viral
◊ Aspirin, tartrates
◊ Exercise
◊ Sinusitis
◊ Gastroesophageal reflux
◊ Sleep (peak expiratory flow rate [PEFR] lowest at 4 am)
• Current research focuses on inflammatory response (including abnormal release of chemical mediators, eosinophil chemotactic factor, neutrophil chemotactic factor, and others)

RISK FACTORS
• Positive family history
• Viral lower respiratory infection during infancy

 DIAGNOSIS

DIFFERENTIAL DIAGNOSIS
• Foreign body aspiration
• Recurrent pulmonary emboli
• Viral respiratory infections (croup, bronchiolitis)
• Epiglottitis
• Cystic fibrosis
• Congestive heart failure
• Chronic obstructive pulmonary disease
• Hypersensitivity pneumonitis
• Bronchopulmonary aspergillosis
• Tuberculosis
• Hyperventilation syndrome
• Mitral value prolapse
• Habit cough

LABORATORY
• CBC normal
• Nasal eosinophils
• Immunoglobulins
◊ Screen for immunodeficiency
◊ IgE elevated in allergic bronchopulmonary aspergillosis (ABPA)
• Sweat test in chronic childhood asthmatics
• Arterial blood gases in status asthmaticus
Drugs that may alter lab results: N/A
Disorders that may alter lab results: N/A

PATHOLOGICAL FINDINGS
• Smooth muscle hyperplasia
• Mucosal edema
• Thickened basement membrane
• Inflammatory response
• Hyperinflated lungs
• Mucus plugging
• Bronchiectasis is not seen except in association with ABPA
• Increased airway resistance
• Decreased airflow rates
• Ventilation-perfusion mismatching

SPECIAL TESTS
• Home monitoring of peak flow rates - report if drops below 70% of baseline
• Pulmonary function tests - reversible airway obstruction
• Allergy testing
• PPD yearly
• Exercise tolerance testing

IMAGING
Chest x-ray
◊ Hyperinflation
◊ Atelectasis
◊ Airleak

DIAGNOSTIC PROCEDURES
• Bronchoscopy: rarely indicated.
• Spirometry: decreased FEV1
• Chest x-ray: do at least one, but not necessary with each exacerbation

 TREATMENT

APPROPRIATE HEALTH CARE
• Outpatient
• Inpatient for bronchospasm not relieved by beta-agonists and steroids

GENERAL MEASURES
• Eliminate irritants
• Education is essential
• Appropriate prophylactic management with anti-inflammatories such as cromolyn, inhaled steroids
• Increase beta-agonists in response to symptoms
• Consider hyposensitization
The following are NOT recommended:
• Mist
• Large volumes of fluid
• Breathing exercises
• IPPB

ACTIVITY Early diagnosis and appropriate treatment facilitate unrestricted activity.

DIET No special diet

PATIENT EDUCATION
Printed patient information available from:
◊ American Lung Association, 1740 Broadway, New York, NY 10019 (212)315-8700
◊ Asthma and Allergy Foundation of America, Suite 305, Washington, DC 20036, (800)7-ASTHMA, (800-727-8462)

MEDICATIONS

DRUG(S) OF CHOICE
Five major classes of drugs are used:
◊ cromoglycate and nedocromil
◊ steroids (beclomethasone, prednisone, etc)
◊ beta-agonists (albuterol, terbutaline, etc)
◊ methylxanthines (theophylline)
◊ anticholinergics (atropine, ipratropium bromide)
Mild asthma: brief wheezing once or twice a week:
• Intermittent use of beta-agonist (MDI or nebulizer)
• Oral beta-agonist or theophylline may be considered, but have more side effects
Moderate asthma: weekly symptoms interfering with sleep or exercise, occasional ER visits, PEFR 60-80% of predicted
• Regular maintenance schedule
• Cromolyn QID or nedocromil BID
• Consider inhaled steroids (beclomethasone diproprionate) 400µg/day.
• If not controlled with moderate dose inhaled steroid (600 µg/day), consider addition of oral slow-release xanthines or inhaled ipratropium bromide
• Treat exacerbations with inhaled beta-adrenergics and steroid bursts
Severe asthma: frequent symptoms affecting activity, noctural symptoms, frequent hospitalizations, PEFR < 60% predicted, not interfering with growth or development
• Cromolyn as above
• Inhaled steroids; some patients may need alternate day oral steroids
• Theophylline often useful, particularly for nighttime symptoms; therapeutic level 10-20.
Acute exacerbation
• Inhaled beta-agonist (albuterol) to reverse airflow obstruction
• Look for increased work of breathing, air leak syndromes, atelectasis
• Short course of steroids, 2mg/kg p.o. qam for 5-7 days
• IV aminophylline adds toxicity only
• Observe at least one hour
Delivery systems
◊ Children under 2 - nebulizer or MDI with valved spacer and mask
◊ Children 2-4 years - MDI and valved spacer
◊ Over 5 years - MDI or powder inhaler
Hospital management
◊ Steroids IV: solumedrol 2mg/kg once, then 1mg/kg IV q6h
◊ Frequent beta-agonist aerosols
◊ Aminophylline IV drip if not responding well
◊ Rarely: isoproterenol or terbutaline IV; mechanical ventilation

Contraindications:
• Sedatives, mucolytics
• Antibiotics are usually not necessary
• Avoid beta-adrenergic blocking drugs
Precautions: Refer to manufacturer's literature
Significant possible interactions:
Erythromycin and ciprofloxacin slow theophylline clearance and can increase levels 15-20%.

ALTERNATIVE DRUGS
• Ketotifen
• H1-antagonists
• TAO
• methotrexate
• IVIG
• Lasix

FOLLOWUP

PATIENT MONITORING
• PEFR meter at home
• pH and arterial blood gases
• Oximetry
• Electrolytes

PREVENTION/AVOIDANCE
Co-management is essential
◊ Understand medication, inhalers, nebulizers, peak flow meters
◊ Monitor symptoms, peak flows
◊ Pre-arranged action plan for exacerbations
◊ Written guidelines
• Investigate and control triggering factors (pollutants, exercise, house-dust mite, molds, animal dander) if severe
• Annual influenza immunization
• Avoid aspirin
• Avoid sulfites and tartrazine (food additives)

POSSIBLE COMPLICATIONS
• Respiratory failure; mechanical ventilation
• Atelectasis in 25% of hospitalized patients
• Flaccid paralysis after exacerbation (self-limited)
• Death
• Air leak syndromes (pneumothorax, etc.)
• SIADH
• Altered theophylline metabolism

EXPECTED COURSE AND PROGNOSIS
• Excellent, with attention to general health and use of medications to control symptoms
• Less than 50% of children with asthma "outgrow it"
• Mortality risk increases with:
◊ Greater than 3 emergency room visits/year
◊ Nocturnal symptoms
◊ History of ICU admission
◊ Mechanical ventilation
◊ Greater than 2 hospitalizations/year
◊ Steroid dependence (systemic use)
◊ History of syncope with asthma
• Mortality rates are increasing
• If responsive to treatment is poor, review diagnosis and compliance prior to adding more potent therapy

MISCELLANEOUS

ASSOCIATED CONDITIONS
• Reflux esophagitis
• Sinusitis

AGE-RELATED FACTORS
Pediatric: 50% of new cases of asthma occur in children below 10 years
Geriatric: Unusual for initial episode to occur in this age group
Others: N/A

PREGNANCY
• About 50% of asthma patients have no changes, 25% seem to improve and 25% have worse symptoms
• Stress prevention
• Avoid medications with contraindications during pregnancy

SYNONYMS
• Bronchial asthma
• Reactive airway disease

ICD-9-CM
• 493.0 extrinsic asthma
• 493.1 intrinsic asthma
• 493.9 asthma, unspecified

SEE ALSO
• Cystic fibrosis
• Bronchitis
• Immunodeficiency diseases

OTHER NOTES N/A

ABBREVIATIONS
• ABPA = allergic bronchopulmonary aspergillosis
• PFT = pulmonary function test
• RAD = reactive airway disease
• TAO = toleandromycin
• IVIG = IV immunoglobulins
• PEFR = peak expiratory flow

REFERENCES
• Murray, J.F. & Nadel, J.A. (eds.): Textbook of Respiratory Medicine. Philadelphia, W.B. Saunders Co., 1988
• Barnes, P.J.: A new approach to the treatment of asthma. New Engl J Med 321:1517, 1989
• NHLB Guidelines, 1992
• Rachelefsky, G. & Warner, J.: International Consensus on the Management of Pediatric Asthma. Ped Pulmon 15:125-127, 1993

Author N. Dambro, M.D.

Atelectasis

 BASICS

 DIAGNOSIS

 TREATMENT

BASICS

DESCRIPTION Atelectasis (lung collapse) is a portion of lung which is non-aerated, but otherwise normal. May be an asymptomatic finding on chest roentgenogram or associated with symptoms. Pulmonary blood flow to area of atelectasis is usually reduced, thereby limiting shunting and hypoxia. Diagnosis and therapy are directed at basic cause.
System(s) affected: Pulmonary, Cardiovascular
Genetics: Depends on basic condition e.g., cystic fibrosis, asthma, congenital heart disease, etc.
Incidence/Prevalence in USA: Common in general anesthesia and in intensive care with high inspired oxygen concentrations
Predominant age: All ages
Predominant sex: Male = Female

SIGNS AND SYMPTOMS
Small atelectasis
◊ Commonly asymptomatic
◊ Produces no change in the overall clinical presentation
Large atelectasis:
◊ Tachypnea
◊ Cough
◊ Hypoxia which resolves in some cases over 24-48 hours
◊ Dullness to percussion
◊ Absent breath sounds if airway is occluded
◊ Bronchial breathing if airway is patent
◊ Diminished chest expansion
◊ Tracheal or precordial impulse displacement
◊ Wheezing may be heard with focal obstruction

CAUSES
• Increased alveolar surface tension due to cardiogenic or non-cardiogenic pulmonary edema, primary surfactant deficiency, or infection
• Resorptive atelectasis due to airway obstruction from lumenal blockage (mucus, tumor, foreign body), airway wall abnormality (edema, tumor, bronchomalacia, deformation), or extrinsic airway compression (cardiac, vascular, tumor, adenopathy)
• Compression of the lung (lobar emphysema, cardiomegaly, tumor)
• Increased pleural pressure due to fluid or air in the pleural space (pneumothorax, effusion, empyema, hemothorax, chylothorax)
• Chest wall restriction due to skeletal deformity and/or muscular weakness (scoliosis, neuromuscular disease, phrenic nerve paralysis, anesthesia)

RISK FACTORS
• Varies with condition producing atelectasis
• Atelectasis following anesthesia is increased in smokers, obese individuals, and individuals with short, wide thoraces

DIAGNOSIS

DIFFERENTIAL DIAGNOSIS
• Atelectasis is not a specific diagnosis, but rather a result of disease or distorted anatomy. The differential is thus found under Causes.
• The roentgenographic differential includes pneumonia, fluid accumulation, lung hypoplasia, or tumour

LABORATORY N/A
Drugs that may alter lab results: N/A
Disorders that may alter lab results: N/A

PATHOLOGICAL FINDINGS
• Pathology varies with cause
• Obstructive atelectasis - non-aerated lung without inflammation or infiltration

SPECIAL TESTS N/A

IMAGING
Chest roentgenography
◊ May demonstrate linear, round, or wedge shaped densities
◊ Right middle lobe and lingular atelectasis will obscure the ipsilateral heart border
◊ Lower lobe atelectasis will obscure the diaphragm
◊ Air bronchograms are usually absent in obstructive atelectasis
◊ Evidence of possible airway compression, pleural fluid or air should be sought
◊ Diffuse microatelectasis in surfactant deficiency may lead to a ground-glass appearance with striking air bronchograms
◊ Mediastinal structures and the diaphragm move toward the atelectatic region
◊ Adjacent lung may show compensatory hyperinflation

DIAGNOSTIC PROCEDURES
• Bronchoscopy to assess airway patency. (Bronchoscopy as therapy is controversial with the exception of foreign body or other structural causes).
• Echocardiography to assess cardiac status in cardiomegaly
• Chest CT or MRI to visualize airway and mediastinal structures
• Barium swallow to assess mediastinal vascular compression
• Other procedures vary with potential cause

TREATMENT

APPROPRIATE HEALTH CARE Varies with severity

GENERAL MEASURES
• Varies with severity and cause of atelectasis
• Ensure adequate oxygenation and humidification
• Chest physiotherapy with percussion and postural drainage. Consider adding treatments using new airway clearance techniques such as Positive Expiratory Pressure (PEP) mask.
• Incentive spirometry
• Positive pressure ventilation or continuous positive airway pressure in subjects with neuromuscular weakness

ACTIVITY Encourage activity, mobilization as tolerated

DIET No special diet

PATIENT EDUCATION Encourage activity as appropriate. Instruct in basic cause and its therapy.

MEDICATIONS

DRUG(S) OF CHOICE
• Bronchodilator therapy (beta-agonist aerosol)
• Other therapies directed at basic cause - antibiotics, foreign body removal, tumor therapy, cardiac medication, steroids in asthma

Contraindications: Refer to manufacturer's literature

Precautions: Refer to manufacturer's literature

Significant possible interactions: Refer to manufacturer's literature

ALTERNATIVE DRUGS N/A

FOLLOWUP

PATIENT MONITORING
• Varies with cause and patient status
• In simple atelectasis associated with asthma or infection, monthly visits are adequate

PREVENTION/AVOIDANCE
• Avoidance of 100% inspired oxygen (which can rapidly absorb causing atelectasis)
• Foreign body/aspiration precautions
• Postoperative mobilization and/or rotation
• Institute therapies such as chest physiotherapy and incentive spirometry as preventive maneuvers in at-risk patients

POSSIBLE COMPLICATIONS
• Infection with chronic lung damage is an unlikely, but unfortunate complication
• Atelectasis is rarely life-threatening and usually spontaneously resolves

EXPECTED COURSE AND PROGNOSIS
• Resolution with medical therapy
• Surgical therapy needed only for certain causes, or if chronic infection and bronchiectasis supervene

MISCELLANEOUS

ASSOCIATED CONDITIONS N/A

AGE-RELATED FACTORS Very young and very old patients with limited mobility at greater risk
Pediatric: Congenital airway obstruction due to mediastinal cysts, tumor, or vascular rings
Geriatric: Primary and secondary lung tumors sometimes associated
Others: N/A

PREGNANCY Management is similar to non-pregnant and varies with cause

SYNONYMS Lung collapse

ICD-9-CM 518.0

SEE ALSO
• Asthma
• Pneumonia

OTHER NOTES
Round atelectasis:
◊ A pleural based round density on chest roentgenogram with a comet tail of vessel and airway
◊ More common in patients with asbestos exposure
◊ May mimic tumor, but can usually be definitively diagnosed with imaging studies thereby avoiding surgery

ABBREVIATIONS N/A

REFERENCES
• Hazinski, T.H.: Atelectasis. In Kendig's Disorders of the Respiratory Tract in Children. 5th Ed. Edited by V. Chernick. Philadelphia, W.B. Saunders Co., 1990
• Marini, J.J., Pierson, D.J. & Hudson, L.D.: Acute lobar atelectasis: a prospective comparison of fiberoptic bronchoscopy and respiratory therapy. Am Rev Respir Dis 1971; 119:971
• Rickstenste, Sventrik et al.: Effects of Peioric Positive Airway Pressure by Mask on Postoperative Pulmonary Function. CHEST 89:774-781 6/1986

Author N. Dambro, M.D.

Atherosclerosis

 BASICS

DESCRIPTION The common form of arteriosclerosis in which deposits of yellowish plaques (atheromas) containing cholesterol, lipoid material, and lipophages are formed within the intima and inner media of large and medium sized arteries
System(s) affected: Cardiovascular
Genetics: Probable genetic link, but not proven, although a family history of premature atherosclerosis makes the development at a younger age more likely
Incidence in USA: Common, but declining steadily
Prevalence in USA: Extremely common. The effects upon the brain, heart, kidneys, extremities and other vital organs form the leading cause of morbidity and mortality in the USA and most Western countries. Complications of atherosclerosis account for 1/2 of all deaths, and 1/3 of deaths in persons between ages 35-65.
Predominant age: 35 and older
Predominant sex: Male > Female

SIGNS AND SYMPTOMS
Characteristically silent until atheromas produce:
◊ Stenosis
◊ Thrombosis
◊ Aneurysm
◊ Embolus
For lists of possible symptoms see the following titles elsewhere in this book:
◊ Essential hypertension
◊ Coronary arteriosclerosis
◊ Congestive heart failure
◊ Cerebrovascular accident
◊ Atrial arrhythmias
◊ Ventricular arrhythmias
◊ Renal failure, chronic
◊ Dissecting aneurysm
◊ Thrombosis and embolism, arterial

CAUSES
• Biochemical, physiologic, environmental factors that lead to thickening and occlusion of the lumen of arteries
• Aging (some degree of atherosclerosis is universal)
• One or more of the risk factors listed below

RISK FACTORS
• Hypertension
• Elevated serum lipids (especially cholesterol, low-density lipoproteins, accompanied by low concentrations of high-density lipoproteins)
• Tobacco smoking
• Diabetes mellitus
• Obesity
• Male sex
• Physical inactivity
• Increasing age
• Type "A" behavior pattern
• Hard drinking water
• Family history of premature atherosclerosis

 DIAGNOSIS

DIFFERENTIAL DIAGNOSIS N/A

LABORATORY Associated with elevated serum cholesterol; elevated LDL and low HDL
Drugs that may alter lab results: N/A
Disorders that may alter lab results: N/A

PATHOLOGICAL FINDINGS
Early changes (simple) potentially reversible
◊ Accumulation of lipid-laden cells in the intimal layer of the artery (usually monocytes/macrophages from circulating blood)
◊ Lipid streaks in aortas and coronary arteries
Late changes (complicated) usually reversible
◊ Atheromatous plaques with necrosis, fibrosis, calcification
◊ Weakening of elastic lamellae
◊ Neovascularization
◊ Arterial obstruction
◊ Thrombosis

SPECIAL TESTS N/A

IMAGING Calcified atherosclerotic plaques easily identified in major blood vessels on x-ray

DIAGNOSTIC PROCEDURES
• X-ray (often incidental finding)
• Associated with hypercholesterolemia; elevated LDL and low HDL

 TREATMENT

APPROPRIATE HEALTH CARE
Outpatient until complications occur

GENERAL MEASURES
For details see the following titles:
◊ Essential hypertension
◊ Congestive heart failure
◊ Cerebrovascular accident
◊ Renal failure, chronic
◊ Dissecting aneurysm
◊ Thrombosis & embolism, arterial

ACTIVITY Encourage physical fitness

DIET
Initial diet: Step 1
◊ Total fat - < 30% of total calories; saturated fat < 10%
◊ Carbohydrates - 50-60% of total calories
◊ Protein - 10-20% of total calories
◊ Cholesterol - < 300 mg a day
◊ Total calories - amount required to achieve and maintain desirable weight
Initial diet: Step 2
◊ Total fat - < 30% of total calories
◊ Carbohydrates - 50-60% of total calories
◊ Protein - 10-20% of total calories
◊ Cholesterol - < 200 mg a day
◊ Total calories - amount required to achieve and maintain desirable weight

PATIENT EDUCATION
• Crucial parts of preventing and treating atheroscleroses involve nutrition, fitness, and smoking cessation
• Extensive educational materials available from many agencies (e.g., American Heart Association, U.S. Government Printing Office). Use these to help teach patients how to avoid or eliminate risk factors.

Atherosclerosis

MEDICATIONS

DRUG(S) OF CHOICE
See monographs of these topics:
- ◊ Essential hypertension
- ◊ Coronary arteriosclerosis
- ◊ Congestive heart failure
- ◊ Cerebrovascular accident
- ◊ Atrial arrhythmias
- ◊ Ventricular arrhythmias
- ◊ Renal failure, chronic
- ◊ Dissecting aneurysm
- ◊ Thrombosis and embolism, arterial

Contraindications: Refer to manufacturer's literature
Precautions: Refer to manufacturer's literature
Significant possible interactions: Refer to manufacturer's literature

ALTERNATIVE DRUGS See various monographs

FOLLOWUP

PATIENT MONITORING See various monographs

PREVENTION/AVOIDANCE Eliminate risk factors - all or as many as possible

POSSIBLE COMPLICATIONS
- Coronary artery disease
- Renal failure
- Cerebrovascular accidents
- Dissecting or ruptured aneurysms
- Congestive heart failure
- Cardiac arrhythmias
- Sudden death

EXPECTED COURSE AND PROGNOSIS Avoiding risk factors has greatly decreased mortality rates in the past decade

MISCELLANEOUS

ASSOCIATED CONDITIONS
- Essential hypertension
- Coronary arteriosclerosis
- Congestive heart failure
- Cerebrovascular accident
- Atrial arrhythmias
- Ventricular arrhythmias
- Renal failure, chronic
- Aortic dissection
- Thrombosis and embolism, arterial

AGE-RELATED FACTORS
Pediatric: Fatty streaks and deposits in the intima of the aortas of all children begin at age 3 years
Geriatric: Atherosclerosis happens to all who live long enough. Its effects and complications can be minimized and/or delayed by avoiding all risk factors possible.
Others: N/A

PREGNANCY N/A

SYNONYMS N/A

ICD-9-CM 414.0

SEE ALSO
- Essential hypertension
- Congestive heart failure
- Cerebrovascular accident
- Renal failure, chronic
- Dissecting aneurysm
- Thrombosis & embolism, arterial

OTHER NOTES N/A

ABBREVIATIONS N/A

REFERENCES
- Hurst, J.W., et.al.: The Heart. 7th Ed. New York, McGraw-Hill, 1990
- Braunwald, E. (ed): Heart Disease: A Textbook of Cardiovascular Medicine. 3rd Ed. Philadelphia, W.B. Saunders Co., 1988
- Guidelines for cardiopulmonary resuscitation and emergency cardiac care. JAMA, Oct. 28, 1992, Vol. 268, Na16

Author J. Florence, M.D.

Atherosclerotic occlusive disease

 ## BASICS

DESCRIPTION A peripheral arterial disease can be acute or chronic. There is obstruction or narrowing of the lumen of the aorta and its major branches causing interruption of blood flow, usually to feet and legs. Involved arteries may include mesenteric and celiac arteries. Occlusions cause ischemia, discomfort, skin ulceration and gangrene.
System(s) affected: Cardiovascular
Genetics: Family history of early complications of atherosclerosis
Incidence/Prevalence in USA: Increases with age (parallels atherosclerosis)
Predominant age: Older adults
Predominant sex: Male > Female (2:1)

SIGNS AND SYMPTOMS
• Intermittent claudication - exercise induced pain that is relieved by rest is pathognomonic
• Site of occlusion determines site of pain
• Occlusion of abdominal aorta and/or iliac vessels produce claudication in the back, buttocks and hips
• Femoral obstruction causes pain in the calf
• The degree of occlusion determines the exercise tolerance and if severe enough produces pain at rest
• Pulses are diminished or absent
• The limb is cold and pale and typically develops dependant rubor
• Atrophic skin changes often result in shiny hairless skin

CAUSES
• Almost always a complication of atherosclerosis
• Mechanism of occlusion - embolus, thrombosis, fracture, or trauma

RISK FACTORS
• Smoking
• Hyperlipidemia
• Diabetes
• Hypertension
• Physical stress

 ## DIAGNOSIS

DIFFERENTIAL DIAGNOSIS
• Thromboangiitis obliterans (inflammatory disease primarily affecting young male smokers)
• Fibromuscular dysplasia of the peripheral vessels (rare)

LABORATORY N/A
Drugs that may alter lab results: N/A
Disorders that may alter lab results: N/A

PATHOLOGICAL FINDINGS
• Occluding mass in lumen of thrombosed artery
• Calcareous deposits in occluded vessel in medial coat with atheromas

SPECIAL TESTS Doppler ultrasound to compare systolic pressure in upper and lower limbs (ankle: brachial ratio should be higher than 0.95 at rest)

IMAGING Angiography for an individual who may be a candidate for surgery

DIAGNOSTIC PROCEDURES History and physical

 ## TREATMENT

APPROPRIATE HEALTH CARE
Outpatient for conservative management. Inpatient for surgery or more severe cases.

GENERAL MEASURES
• Smoking cessation
• Foot and limb care
• Graduated exercise program
• Weight control
• Pain management
• Cholesterol management
• Appropriate treatment of coexisting disease, i.e., diabetes
• Infection control
• Lifestyle modification
<u>Surgical intervention</u>
◊ Indications for surgery are ischemic pain at rest, or changes likely to lead to amputation, or intolerable symptoms
◊ The procedure depends upon site of lesion. Includes endarterectomy, bypass procedures, transluminal angioplasty, and amputation.
◊ Patients with aorto-iliac disease tend to have good surgical results to a disabling disorder
◊ Surgery should not be performed for femoral popliteal disease unless symptoms are very severe or disabling
◊ Bypass surgery for vessels distal to popliteal artery has little success
◊ Patch grafting
◊ Atherectomy
◊ Laser angioplasty
◊ Stents (wire plastic mesh to stretch and mold to the arterial wall to prevent re-occlusion)
◊ Amputation with failure of arterial reconstructive surgery or with development of gangrene, persistent infection, or intractable pain

ACTIVITY To the degree that symptoms permit

DIET
• Good diet control
• Lose weight, if overweight

PATIENT EDUCATION
• Educate patient regarding symptoms or signs that require early assessment by physician
• Teach careful foot care
• Avoid elevating or applying heat to affected parts
• Urge early ambulation after surgery
• Assist patient with a stop smoking program

MEDICATIONS

DRUG(S) OF CHOICE
• Vasodilator drugs are ineffective
• Pentoxifylline (Trental) for reducing blood viscosity and increasing red cell flexibility may help. Usual dose 400 mg tid.
Contraindications: In patients sensitive to xanthines
Precautions: Most adverse effects are gastrointestinal. Dizziness and headache are also common.
Significant possible interactions: Use cautiously in patients on oral coagulants. Monitor closely for bleeding compilations.

ALTERNATIVE DRUGS Anticoagulants

FOLLOWUP

PATIENT MONITORING
• For acute phase with surgery, closely follow all aspects of postoperative recovery
• For mild chronic cases, follow patient at regular intervals, frequency dependent upon severity of symptoms

PREVENTION/AVOIDANCE
• Periodic health maintenance measures
• Healthy lifestyle including appropriate diet and adequate exercise
• Avoidance of smoking

POSSIBLE COMPLICATIONS
• Necrosis
• Gangrene
• Limb amputation

EXPECTED COURSE AND PROGNOSIS Course varies from slow progression with easily controlled symptoms to rapid deterioration with severe symptoms requiring surgical intervention

MISCELLANEOUS

ASSOCIATED CONDITIONS
• Atherosclerosis
• Arteriosclerosis obliterans
• Fibromuscular dysplasia
• Thromboangiitis obliterans
• Takayasu's arteritis
• Abdominal aortic coarctation
• Radiation injury
• Popliteal artery entrapment syndrome
• Popliteal cystic degeneration
• Arteritis

AGE-RELATED FACTORS
Pediatric: N/A
Geriatric: N/A
Others: N/A

PREGNANCY N/A

SYNONYMS
• Peripheral arterial disease
• Occlusive arterial disease

ICD-9-CM
• 444.22 occlusion, arteries of extremities, lower
• 444.21 occlusion, arteries of extremities, upper

SEE ALSO
• Arteriosclerosis obliterans

OTHER NOTES N/A

ABBREVIATIONS N/A

REFERENCES
• Marcus, M.L.: The Coronary Circulation in Health and Disease. New York, McGraw-Hill, 1983
• Hurst, J.W., et al.: The Heart. 7th Ed. New York, McGraw-Hill, 1990
• Braunwald, E. (ed): Heart Disease: A Textbook of Cardiovascular Medicine. 3rd Ed. Philadelphia, W.B. Saunders Co., 1988

Author S. Smith

Atrial septal defect (ASD)

 BASICS

DESCRIPTION An opening between the left and right atria allowing shunting of blood between the two chambers. The diagnosis is usually made during childhood, even though symptoms and physical signs are not always obvious. One type (ostium secundum) is one of the most prevalent congenital defects among adults. Blood shunts from left to right. There is a resultant right heart volume overload.
Types:
◊ Ostium secundum - occurs in the region of the fossa ovalis (one of the most prevalent congenital defects in adults)
◊ Sinus venosus - occurs in the superior-posterior portion of the atrial septum
◊ Ostium primum - occurs in the inferior portion of the septum primum
System(s) affected: Cardiovascular
Genetics: Congenital defect
Incidence/Prevalence in USA: Accounts for 10% of congenital heart defects
Predominant age: Newborn
Predominant sex: Female > Male (2:1)

SIGNS AND SYMPTOMS
• Early- to mid-systolic murmur at 2nd or 3rd left upper intercostal space
• In large shunts - low-pitched diastolic murmur at lower left sternal border
• Atrial arrhythmias in older patients
• Fixed, split 2nd heart sound
• Easy fatigability
• Frequent respiratory infections
• Failure to thrive (FTT) - children with large shunts
• Finger clubbing
• Cyanosis
• Syncope
• Hemoptysis

CAUSES   Unknown

RISK FACTORS   Congenital heart disease family history

 DIAGNOSIS

DIFFERENTIAL DIAGNOSIS Other congenital heart disease

LABORATORY   N/A
Drugs that may alter lab results: N/A
Disorders that may alter lab results: N/A

PATHOLOGICAL FINDINGS
• Gross defect in atrial septum
• Dilated right atrium
• Enlarged pulmonary artery

SPECIAL TESTS
ECG:
◊ Right bundle branch block
◊ Right ventricular hypertrophy
◊ Atrial fibrillation
◊ Left axis deviation

IMAGING
• X-ray - varying degrees of cardiac enlargement
• Cardiac catheterization (indicated in select patients) demonstrates right ventricle enlargement and location of the shunt
• Echocardiography

DIAGNOSTIC PROCEDURES
• Cardiac angiography
• Echo and Doppler
• Transesophageal echo in adults

 TREATMENT

APPROPRIATE HEALTH CARE
Inpatient for work-up and when surgery is indicated

GENERAL MEASURES
• Surgical repair (particularly when the pulmonary systemic flow ratio is ≥ 2:1)
• Surgical repair delayed until preschool age (3-4) except for large defects to be repaired earlier
• Small atrial septal defect - primary closure with umbrella-like patch via cardiac catheter is an alternative to open heart surgery

ACTIVITY   As tolerated

DIET   No special diet

PATIENT EDUCATION For patient education materials on this topic, contact: American Heart Association, 7320 Greenville Avenue, Dallas, TX 75231, (214)373-6300

MEDICATIONS

DRUG(S) OF CHOICE N/A
Contraindications: N/A
Precautions: N/A
Significant possible interactions: N/A

ALTERNATIVE DRUGS N/A

FOLLOWUP

PATIENT MONITORING Until defect has closed

PREVENTION/AVOIDANCE N/A

POSSIBLE COMPLICATIONS
• Congestive heart failure
• Cyanosis
• Late-onset arrhythmias 10-20 years after surgery (5%)

EXPECTED COURSE AND PROGNOSIS
• Course - chronic
• Favorable in asymptomatic
• Favorable in surgically treated symptomatic patients

MISCELLANEOUS

ASSOCIATED CONDITIONS Mitral stenosis

AGE-RELATED FACTORS
Pediatric: Most frequently appears in this age group
Geriatric: Defects in older persons may still be closed surgically
Others: N/A

PREGNANCY N/A

SYNONYMS N/A

ICD-9-CM 429.71 atrial septal acquired

SEE ALSO Other congenital heart diseases

OTHER NOTES N/A

ABBREVIATIONS N/A

REFERENCES
• Adams, F.H., Emmanouilides, G.C. & Riemenschneider, T.A.: Moss' Heart Disease in Infants and Adolescents. 4th Ed. Baltimore, Williams & Wilkins, 1989
• Perloff, J.K., Child, J.S.: Congenital Heart Disease in Adults. Philadelphia, W.B. Saunders Co., 1991

Author M. Dambro, M.D. & H. Griffith, M.D.

Balanitis

BASICS

DESCRIPTION Inflammation of glans penis
System(s) affected:
Skin/Exocrine, Renal/Urologic
Genetics: N/A
Incidence/Prevalence in USA: N/A
Predominant age: Adult
Predominant sex: Male only

SIGNS AND SYMPTOMS
- Pain, penile
- Dysuria
- Drainage, site of infection
- Erythema
- Prepuce swelling
- Ulceration
- Plaques

CAUSES
- Allergic reaction (condom latex, contraceptive jelly)
- Fungal (Candida albicans) and bacterial infections (Borrelia vincentii, streptococci)
- Fixed drug eruption (sulfa, tetracycline, barbital)
- Plasma cell infiltration (Zoon's balanitis)
- Autodigestion by activated transplant exocrine enzymes

RISK FACTORS
- Presence of foreskin
- Oral antibiotics in male infants can predispose to Candida balanitis

DIAGNOSIS

DIFFERENTIAL DIAGNOSIS
- Leukoplakia
- Lichen planus
- Psoriasis
- Reiter's syndrome
- Lichen sclerosus et atrophicus
- Erythroplasia of Queyrat
- Balanitis Xerotica obliterans

LABORATORY
- Microbiology culture
- Wet mount
- Serology for syphilis
- Serum glucose

Drugs that may alter lab results: None
Disorders that may alter lab results: None

PATHOLOGICAL FINDINGS Plasma cells infiltration with Zoon's balanitis

SPECIAL TESTS Biopsy, if balanitis persistent

IMAGING N/A

DIAGNOSTIC PROCEDURES Biopsy, if persistent

TREATMENT

APPROPRIATE HEALTH CARE
Outpatient

GENERAL MEASURES
- Warm compresses
- Local hygiene
- Consider circumcision as preventative measure

ACTIVITY No limitations

DIET No special diet

PATIENT EDUCATION
- Need for appropriate hygiene
- Avoidance of known allergens

MEDICATIONS

DRUG(S) OF CHOICE
• Fungal - clotrimazole 1% (Lotrimin) bid to affected area or nystatin (Mycostatin) bid to qid to affected area
• Bacterial - Bacitracin qid to affected area or Neosporin qid to affected area. If infection, cephalosporin or sulfa drug by mouth or injection
• Dermatitis - topical steroids qid to affected area
• Zoon's Balanitis - topical steroids qid
Contraindications: Refer to manufacturer's profile of each drug
Precautions: Refer to manufacturer's profile of each drug
Significant possible interactions: Refer to manufacturer's profile of each drug

ALTERNATIVE DRUGS N/A

FOLLOWUP

PATIENT MONITORING Every 1-2 weeks until etiology has been established. Persistent balanitis may require biopsy to rule out malignancy.

PREVENTION/AVOIDANCE
• Proper hygiene and avoidance of allergens
• Circumcision

POSSIBLE COMPLICATIONS
• Meatal stenosis
• Premalignant changes from chronic irritations
• Urinary tract infections

EXPECTED COURSE AND PROGNOSIS With appropriate treatment it should resolve

MISCELLANEOUS

ASSOCIATED CONDITIONS Diabetes mellitus

AGE-RELATED FACTORS
Pediatric: Oral antibiotics predispose infants to candida balanitis
Geriatric: Condom catheters can predispose to balanitis
Others: N/A

PREGNANCY N/A

SYNONYMS N/A

ICD-9-CM
607.1 balanitis
112.2 candida
099.8 venereal

SEE ALSO N/A

OTHER NOTES N/A

ABBREVIATIONS N/A

REFERENCES
• Gillenwater, J.Y., Grayhack, J.T., Howard, S.S., Duckett, J.W. Adult and Pediatric Urology. 2nd Ed. Mosby Year Book, Philadelphia, 1991
• Zoon, J.J.: Balanoposthite chronique cireonscrite benigne à plasmacytes (contra èrythroplasie de Queyrat). Dermatologica. 1952;105:1
• Tom, W.W., Munda, R., First, M.R., et al: Autodigestion of the glans, penis and urethra by activated transplant pancreatic exocrine enzymes. Surgery 1987; 102:99-101

Author J. Miller, M.D. & T. Black, M.D.

Barotitis media

BASICS

DESCRIPTION Acute or chronic traumatic inflammation of the middle ear space secondary to the rapid development of a negative (or less commonly a positive) pressure differential between the surrounding atmosphere of the external canal and the middle ear compartments (tympanic cavity, eustachian tube, and mastoid air cells) This situation is brought about by the inability of the eustachian tube to adequately equilibrate the middle ear air pressure with the moment-to-moment changes in the environmental atmospheric pressures while descending or ascending in air (flight) and/or especially in water (diving). This causes the retraction or protraction of the tympanic membrane with subsequent inflammation and/or rupture. This also may cause asymmetric pressure stimulation of the inner ear and vestibular end-organ.

System(s) affected: Nervous
Genetics: N/A
Incidence/Prevalence in USA: The most common medical disorder experienced by scuba divers. Also highly prevalent among aircraft flight personnel (especially high-performance jet aircraft), passengers, and sky divers.
Predominant age: All ages
Predominant sex: Male = Female

SIGNS AND SYMPTOMS
- Abrupt in onset
- Otalgia (ear pain)
- Feeling of fullness in ear
- Conductive hearing loss
- Dizziness
- Tinnitus
- Vertigo
- Nausea and vomiting
- Transient facial paralysis
- With tympanic membrane rupture the ability to blow air and/or fluid out one's ear while performing a Valsalva maneuver or when sneezing
- Crying in children (which is their only means of autoinflation)

CAUSES
Rapid descent or ascent with eustachian tube obstruction
   ◊ Eustachian tube lock
   ◊ Upper respiratory infections - sinusitis, rhinitis, tonsillitis, and adenoiditis
   ◊ Overzealous forceful Valsalva maneuver (in ascent with vestibular stimulation)
    ◊ Allergic rhinitis
    ◊ Non-allergic rhinitis with eosinophilia
    ◊ Obstructing nasal polyps
    ◊ Deviated nasal septum
    ◊ Congenital abnormalities of inner/middle ear (cleft palate)
    ◊ Nasopharyngeal tumors
Rapid descent or ascent with external ear canal occlusion
   ◊ Otitis externa (swimmer's ear)
   ◊ Impacted cerumen
   ◊ Ear plugs

Trauma to external and middle ear
   ◊ Activities involving external ear trauma - boxing, soccer, water skiing, accidents, etc.
   ◊ Overzealous use of cotton swab in cleaning ear canals

RISK FACTORS
- Participating in high risk activities without adequate eustachian tube autoinflation (Valsalva maneuver, swallowing) and/or with any of the listed causes of eustachian tube and external ear canal dysfunction:
- Scuba diving
- Airplane flight
- Sky diving
- High altitude mountain travelers
- High altitude elevator rides
- Hyperbaric oxygen chamber therapy
- High impact sports
- Infants and young otologically healthy children have difficulty in dilating the eustachian tube (by swallowing) even at small pressure changes and therefore are at higher risk (especially with upper respiratory infection)

DIAGNOSIS

DIFFERENTIAL DIAGNOSIS
- Serous otitis media
- Acute and chronic otitis media
- External otitis
- Myringitis bullosa

LABORATORY N/A
Drugs that may alter lab results: N/A
Disorders that may alter lab results: N/A

PATHOLOGICAL FINDINGS
- Tympanic membrane retraction or protraction with hemotympanum or rupture
- Edema of mucosal lining and capillary engorgement with transudation of middle ear effusion
- Inner ear involvement with rupture of the round or oval windows and leakage of perilymph into the middle ear and perilymphatic fistula development

SPECIAL TESTS N/A

IMAGING Only to rule out suspected nasopharyngeal tumor or sinusitis

DIAGNOSTIC PROCEDURES
- Otoscopic exam
- Audiogram - conductive (middle ear) versus mixed (inner ear) loss
- Surgical exploration to rule out inner ear involvement if suspected

TREATMENT

APPROPRIATE HEALTH CARE
- Outpatient generally
- Inpatient for complicating emergencies, e.g., incapacitating pain requiring myringotomy, large tympanic perforation requiring tympanoplasty

GENERAL MEASURES
- Perform Valsalva method of eustachian tube autoinflation (patient inhales then closes nose with thumb and index finger on nasal alae, then exhales with mouth closed). This will equalize pressures, relieve pain, and restore hearing. This usually needs to be repeated several times during descent or ascent.
- Nasal decongestant spray with repeated applications
- Antihistamines
- If the suggested maneuvers are unsuccessful return to higher altitude if possible and repeat Valsalva
- If ear block occurs, then outpatient politzerization must be performed followed by systemic and oral decongestants
- If associated infection, treat with appropriate antibiotics

ACTIVITY
- No flying or diving until complete resolution of all signs and symptoms and Valsalva maneuver can be performed
- In severe cases, bedrest

DIET Avoid food allergens that cause rhinitis

PATIENT EDUCATION
- Teach Valsalva maneuver
- Educate on how to create allergy-free environment
- Divers Alert Network of Duke University Medical Center, information line (919) 684-2948

Barotitis media

MEDICATIONS

DRUG(S) OF CHOICE
Decongestants:
◊ Oxymetazoline 0.05% (Afrin, Duration, Neo-Synephrine 12-hour, and Dristan-12-hour) two initial sprays 5 minutes apart then q12h
◊ Pseudoephedrine 120 mg (Sudafed 12-hour, Afrinol) q12h po
◊ Phenylpropanolamine 25 mg (Propagest) q12h po
Antihistamines for allergic component:
◊ Diphenhydramine (Benadryl) 25-50mg q6h
◊ Terfenadine (Seldane) 60mg bid
◊ Astemazole (Hismanal) 10mg qday
Contraindications:
• Previous allergic reactions
• Hypertension
• Drowsiness
Precautions:
• All medications must be used on the ground to rule out idiosyncratic reactions that could incapacitate in an airplane or underwater environment
• Elderly are more susceptible to drug side effects, especially Benadryl
Significant possible interactions: Refer to manufacturer's profile of each drug

ALTERNATIVE DRUGS   N/A

FOLLOWUP

PATIENT MONITORING
• Otoscopic until symptoms clear
• In severe cases, audiograms

PREVENTION/AVOIDANCE
• Avoid altitude changes with any risk factors for eustachian tube dysfunction
• Chewing gum while flying especially for children
• Use of recommended medications before the activity

POSSIBLE COMPLICATIONS
• Permanent hearing loss
• Ruptured tympanic membranes
• Serous otitis media

EXPECTED COURSE AND PROGNOSIS
• Ear block - hours to days with complete resolution and return to flight or diving in days to weeks
• Tympanic rupture - weeks to months

MISCELLANEOUS

ASSOCIATED CONDITIONS
• Aerosinusitis
• Aerodontalgia
• Face mask squeeze
• Epistaxis
• Alternobaric vertigo
• Unequal caloric stimulation vertigo
• Anxiety - leading to panic attack
• Temporomandibular joint syndrome
• Inner ear cochlear damage and/or perilymph fistula

AGE-RELATED FACTORS
Pediatric: Healthy children have difficulty in dilating the eustachian tube (by swallowing) even at small pressure changes and therefore are at higher risk (especially with upper respiratory infection)
Geriatric: Drug side effects
Others: N/A

PREGNANCY   Increased nasal congestion

SYNONYMS
• Aerotitis
• Otitic barotrauma
• Middle ear barotrauma
• Middle ear squeeze

ICD-9-CM   993.0

SEE ALSO   N/A

OTHER NOTES   N/A

ABBREVIATIONS   N/A

REFERENCES
• Paparella, M.M., Shumrick, D.A., et al. (eds.): Otolaryngology. 4th Ed. Philadelphia, W.B. Saunders Co., 1991
• Dehart, R.L. (ed.): Fundamentals of Aerospace Medicine. Philadelphia, Lea & Febiger, 1985

Author   S. Johnston III, M.D.

Basal cell carcinoma

 BASICS

DESCRIPTION Malignant tumor of the skin originating from the basal cells of the epidermis and its appendages. Rarely metastasizes but capable of local tissue destruction.
System(s) affected: Skin/Exocrine
Genetics: More common in fair-skin blondes and redheads
Incidence/Prevalence in USA:
Approximately 400,000 cases/year
Predominant age: Generally > 40 but incidence is increasing in younger populations
Predominant sex: Males > Female (although incidence is increasing in females)

SIGNS AND SYMPTOMS
• Begins as a small, smooth surfaced, well defined nodule
• Color pink to red
• "Pearly" translucent border
• Telangiectatic vessels overlying
• May have varying degrees of melanin pigment
• As nodule enlarges, central ulceration and crusting occurs

CAUSES
• Sun exposure
• Inorganic arsenic exposure

RISK FACTORS
• Chronic sun exposure
• Light complexion
• Tendency to sunburn
• Male sex although increasing risk in women due to lifestyle changes e.g., suntan parlors, etc.

 DIAGNOSIS

DIFFERENTIAL DIAGNOSIS Sebaceous hyperplasia, intradermal nevi (pigmented and non-pigmented), molluscum contagiosum

LABORATORY Pathologic examination required to confirm diagnosis
Drugs that may alter lab results: N/A
Disorders that may alter lab results: N/A

PATHOLOGICAL FINDINGS Nidus of basal cells extending into dermis. Characteristic cells resemble normal basal cells with large basophilic, oval nuclei. Rare mitoses. Tumor cells arranged in palisades at periphery.

SPECIAL TESTS N/A

IMAGING N/A

DIAGNOSTIC PROCEDURES Biopsy mandatory to confirm diagnosis

 TREATMENT

APPROPRIATE HEALTH CARE
Outpatient unless extensive lesion

GENERAL MEASURES
• Treatment selection varies with extent and location of lesion, tumor border distinctiveness
• High risk areas - inner canthus, nasolabial sulcus, philtrum, preauricular area, retroauricular sulcus, lip, temple
• Curettage and electrodesiccation - nodular lesion < l cm, in low risk area, if not deeply invasive. Requires specialized training and experience in surgical technique.
• Excision - useful for lesions in high risk areas, not as dependent on lesion size. Poor choice if multiple lesions. Requires appropriate training.
• Cryosurgery - reserved for small lesions in low risk area. Requires specialized training and equipment. May want pre- and post-treatment biopsies.
• Moh's surgery - the preferred microsurgically-controlled surgical treatment for lesions in high risk area, for recurrent lesion, if there is an aggressive growth pattern. Requires referral to appropriately trained dermatologic surgeon.
• Radiation - useful for patients who could not tolerate minor surgical procedures (e.g., elderly patients). Also may be used when preservation of local tissue important such as near lips and eyelids.

ACTIVITY No restrictions except to avoid overexposure to sun

DIET No special diet

PATIENT EDUCATION
• Teach patient appropriate sun avoidance techniques, sunscreens, etc.
• Skin self exam

Basal cell carcinoma

 MEDICATIONS

DRUG(S) OF CHOICE Topical antibiotics after excision for 24 to 48 hours (optional)
Contraindications: N/A
Precautions: N/A
Significant possible Interactions: N/A

ALTERNATIVE DRUGS N/A

 FOLLOWUP

PATIENT MONITORING Every month for 3 months, then twice yearly for 5 years, yearly thereafter

PREVENTION/AVOIDANCE
• Sunscreens
• Hats, long-sleeve shirts
• Avoid excessive tanning

POSSIBLE COMPLICATIONS
• Local recurrence and spread. Usually recurrences will appear within 5 years.
• Metastasis (rare)

EXPECTED COURSE AND PROGNOSIS
• Proper treatment yields 90-95% cure
• Most recurrences happen within 5 years
• Development of new basal cell carcinomas. 36% of patients will develop a new lesion within 5 years.

 MISCELLANEOUS

ASSOCIATED CONDITIONS
• Xeroderma pigmentosum
• Basal cell nevus syndrome

AGE-RELATED FACTORS
Pediatric: Rare in children
Geriatric: Greater frequency in geriatric patients
Others: N/A

PREGNANCY N/A

SYNONYMS
• Basal cell epithelioma
• Rodent ulcer

ICD-9-CM
• 173.3 (face)
• 173.4 (scalp, neck)
• 173.5 (trunk)
• 173.6 (upper limb)
• 173.7 (lower limb)
• 173.9 (site unspecified)

SEE ALSO N/A

OTHER NOTES N/A

ABBREVIATIONS N/A

REFERENCES
• Fitzpatrick, T.N., et al.: Dermatology in General Medicine. New York, McGraw-Hill, 1987
• Friedman, R.J., et al.: Cancer of the Skin. Philadelphia, W.B. Saunders Co., 1991

Author J. Little, M.D.

Behçet's syndrome

 BASICS

DESCRIPTION Rare multisystem, chronic disease characterized by oral and genital mucocutaneous ulcerations, skin rashes, arthritis, thrombophlebitis, uveitis, colitis, and neurologic symptoms.
• Endemic in Japan and Northeastern Mediterranean region.
Genetics:
• One report in a mother and newborn (A. Fam, Ann Rheumatic Dis 1981;40:509-512). Very rarely familial
Incidence/Prevalence in USA:
• 1/100, 000
• 670/100,000 in Japan
Predominant age: 3rd to 4th decades
Predominant sex: Male > Female; as frequently to twice as often

SIGNS AND SYMPTOMS
• Aphthous stomatitis
• Genital ulcers - painful in the male, painless in the female
• Dermal - papulovesicular, erythema nodosum, pathergy, erythema multiforme, vasculitis, pyoderma
• Ocular - iritis, iridocyclitis, chorioretinitis, hypopyon, hemorrhage, papilledema, optic atrophy
• Morning stiffness - in 1/3
• Polyarthritis - self-limited and predominantly affecting lower extremities
• Thrombophlebitis - peripheral, pulmonary, cerebral, Budd Chiari syndrome
• Neurologic - cranial nerve palsy, hemiplegia, intracranial hypertension, meningomyelitis and recurrent meningitis, confusional state
• GI - aphthous ulcers, colitis, melena
• Pulmonary infiltrates - possibly related to thrombosis
• Myopathy/myositis - rare
• Peripheral gangrene - rare
• Epididymitis
• Glomerulonephritis - rare

CAUSES
• Classified as vasculopathy or autoimmune
• HLA-B5 alloantigen relationship
• Possible environmental toxin - heavy metals, pesticides
• Possibly English walnuts or Ginko nuts
• Fibrinolysis abnormality
• One report associated with HIV infection (C. Stein, J Rheumatol 1991;18,1427-8)

RISK FACTORS See Causes

 DIAGNOSIS

DIFFERENTIAL DIAGNOSIS
• Reiter's syndrome and other forms of spondyloarthropathy
• Inflammatory bowel disease (Crohn's disease and ulcerative colitis)
• Syphilis
• Erythema nodosum
• Aphthous stomatitis
• Stevens-Johnson syndrome
• Vasculitis
• Multisystem disease
• Herpes simplex stomatitis
• Thrombophlebitis related to coagulation factor deficiency
• Mollaret's meningitis

LABORATORY
• Erythrocyte sedimentation rate elevation, but can be normal
• Immune complexes detected by Raji cell and C1q solid phase assays
• Cryoglobulin
• Hypergammaglobulinemia
Drugs that may alter lab results: N/A
Disorders that may alter lab results: N/A

PATHOLOGICAL FINDINGS
• May be no recognizable changes
• Mononuclear perivascular infiltration
• Mononuclear infiltrate in synovium
• Endothelial cell swelling
• Partial obliteration of vascular lumen
• Neutrophilic dermatitis (Sweet syndrome) rarely

SPECIAL TESTS
• Depression of plasma antithrombin III levels with active disease
• Increased fibrinolytic activity during attacks
• Anti-neutrophil cytoplasmic antigen antibodies
• Demyelinating antibodies in neuro-Behçet's syndrome
• Anti-cardiolipin antibodies

IMAGING N/A

DIAGNOSTIC PROCEDURES
• Careful history and physical and frequent reevaluation
• Synovial fluid - inflammatory effusion
• Arteriography - for aneurysms or thrombosis

 TREATMENT

APPROPRIATE HEALTH CARE Usually outpatient. Inpatient usually required for neurologic complications

GENERAL MEASURES According to body system involved

ACTIVITY As tolerated

DIET No special diet

PATIENT EDUCATION
• American Behçet's Association, 421 21st Avenue SW, Rochester, MN 55902, (507)281-3059

MEDICATIONS

DRUG(S) OF CHOICE
- Colchicine: 0.6 mg bid
- Topical ocular steroids
- Prednisone: 1mg/kg for severe involvement, especially CNS
- Azathioprine: 2-3mg/kg/day po
- Cyclophosphamide: 50-100mg/day qAM. Patient should drink 8-10 glasses of water/day and report any blood in the urine.
- Methotrexate: use the lowest possible dose; perhaps 7.5mg/week

Contraindications: Refer to manufacturer's literature

Precautions: Refer to manufacturer's literature.
- Absorption of drugs such as amitriptyline, diazepam, carbamazepine, phenytoin, and acetaminophen may be reduced

Significant possible interactions:

ALTERNATIVE DRUGS
- Cyclosporin
- Levamisole - 100-150 mg two days per week
- Chlorambucil - but concern with respect to toxicity
- Thalidomide

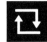 **FOLLOWUP**

PATIENT MONITORING   Dependent on severity of system involvement

PREVENTION/AVOIDANCE   Avoid English walnuts

POSSIBLE COMPLICATIONS
- Death
- Blindness
- Paralysis
- Embolism/thrombosis - pulmonary, vena cava, peripheral
- Aneurysms
- Amyloidosis

EXPECTED COURSE AND PROGNOSIS
- Normal life expectancy, except with neurologic involvement
- Possible vision impairment

 MISCELLANEOUS

ASSOCIATED CONDITIONS
- Amyloid
- Sweet syndrome

AGE-RELATED FACTORS
Pediatric: - rare
Geriatric: - rare
Others: N/A

PREGNANCY   - Possible increase in thrombosis and demise

SYNONYMS
- Mucocutaneous ocular syndrome
- Franceschetti-Valerio syndrome

ICD-9-CM   136.1

SEE ALSO   Vasculitis

OTHER NOTES   N/A

ABBREVIATIONS   N/A

REFERENCES
- International diagnostic study group for Behçet's disease. Evaluation of ('classification') criteria in Behçet's disease -- Towards internationally agreed criteria. Brit J Rheumatol, 1992;31:299-308
- Mizushima, Y.: Behçet's disease. Curr Opin Rheumatol 1991;3:32-35
- Hashimoto, T. & Takeuchi, A.: Treatment of Behçet's disease. Curr Opin Rheumatol 1992;4:31-34
- Shimizu, T., et al.: Behcet disease. Semin Arthritis Rheum 1979; 8:223-260
- K. Chaleby, Clin Chem 1987;33:1679-1681

AUTHOR   BM Rothschild, M.D.

Bell's palsy

 BASICS

DESCRIPTION Paralysis or weakness of the muscles supplied by the facial nerve, typically unilaterally, due to inflammation and swelling of the facial nerve within the facial canal
- Bell's palsy: Idiopathic
- Ramsay Hunt syndrome: Bell's palsy associated with vesicles within the outer ear canal or behind the ear, due to herpes zoster infection (occasionally herpes simplex)
- Facial diplegia: The simultaneous development of bilateral Bell's palsy is highly unusual and conditions such as Guillain-Barré syndrome and chronic meningitis should be considered as possible explanations.

System(s) affected: Nervous
Genetics: There is a familial tendency toward Bell's palsy
Incidence/Prevalence in USA: 25 in 100,000
Predominant age: Affects all ages. Most common in individuals over 30 years of age.
Predominant sex: Male = Female

SIGNS AND SYMPTOMS
- Sudden onset or onset over days
- Unilateral total or partial paralysis of the facial muscles
- Mild "numbness" on the affected side
- Drooling
- Ipsilateral excessive or inadequate tear production
- Ipsilateral loss of taste
- Ipsilateral ear ache

CAUSES
Bell's palsy
  ◊ Inflammation of the facial nerve within the facial canal
    ◊ Exposure to cold
    ◊ Probably viral
Ramsay-Hunt syndrome
  ◊ Herpes zoster
  ◊ Rarely herpes simplex

RISK FACTORS
- Age over 30
- Exposure to cold

 DIAGNOSIS

DIFFERENTIAL DIAGNOSIS
Neoplastic
  ◊ Carcinomatous meningitis
  ◊ Leukemic meningitis
  ◊ Tumors of the parotid gland
  ◊ Tumors of the base of the skull
Infectious
  ◊ Chronic meningitis
  ◊ Bacterial meningitis
  ◊ Osteomyelitis of the base of the skull
  ◊ Otitis media
  ◊ Leprosy
Other
  ◊ Sarcoidosis
  ◊ Melkersson-Rosenthal syndrome (facial paralysis with scrotal tongue)
  ◊ Head injury with fracture of the temporal bone
  ◊ Brainstem stroke (anterior-inferior cerebellar artery)
  ◊ Multiple sclerosis
  ◊ Guillain-Barré syndrome (can initially present as a very typical Bell's palsy)

LABORATORY
- CSF protein - mildly elevated in 1/3 of eases
- CSF cells - mildly elevated in 10% of cases, with a mononuclear cell predominance
Drugs that may alter lab results: N/A
Disorders that may alter lab results: N/A

PATHOLOGICAL FINDINGS
- Edema of the facial nerve
- Occasional hemorrhagic streaks
- Dilatation of the vasa nervorum
- Infiltration of mononuclear cells in some cases
- Atrophy of the facial nerve

SPECIAL TESTS
- Electromyography in the first three weeks after onset of the condition manifests a decreased or absent interference pattern on the affected side, which reflects a reduction or absence of function of the facial motor units. After three weeks, denervation potentials (fibrillations) are typically seen. Eventually, with recovery, low-amplitude, short-duration, polyphasic (nascent) motor units may appear in previously denervated areas. Recovery may be incomplete.
- Nerve conduction velocities may reveal absence or attenuation of the evoked potential, slowing of the conduction velocity or a normal conduction velocity and amplitude
- Blink reflex - the electrophysiological equivalent of the corneal reflex, should be abnormal in all cases

IMAGING MRI to rule out posterior fossa lesions and intracanalicular 8th nerve tumors if clinical suspicion is high

DIAGNOSTIC PROCEDURES Spinal tap may reveal an elevated protein or cell count, however, it is usually not necessary

 TREATMENT

APPROPRIATE HEALTH CARE
Outpatient except for surgical decompression (very controversial and largely abandoned)

GENERAL MEASURES
- Close and patch ipsilateral eye
- Methylcellulose eye drops

ACTIVITY Fully active. Use caution in activities requiring keen depth perception.

DIET No special diet

PATIENT EDUCATION Explanation and reassurance when appropriate

MEDICATIONS

DRUG(S) OF CHOICE
Corticosteroids
• Prednisone: 80 mg po qd for three days, then 60 mg po qd for three days, then 40 mg po qd for three days, then 20 mg po qd for three days, then discontinue use. Course of treatment to begin immediately after onset of Bell's palsy. There is little benefit in starting steroids after four days.
Contraindications: Pre-existing infections including tuberculosis and systemic mycosis
Precautions: Use with discretion in pregnancy, peptic ulcer disease, and diabetes
Significant possible interactions:
• MMR, TOPV, and other live vaccines
• Aspirin in patients with hypoprothrombinemia

ALTERNATIVE DRUGS N/A

FOLLOWUP

PATIENT MONITORING
• Recheck monthly for six to twelve months
• Look for evidence of corneal abrasions. Expect early recovery.

PREVENTION/AVOIDANCE N/A

POSSIBLE COMPLICATIONS
• Unmasking of subclinical infection (such as tuberculosis) by steroid usage
• Steroid induced psychological disturbances
• Corneal abrasion and ulceration

EXPECTED COURSE AND PROGNOSIS
Complete, partial or no recovery of function. Patients with partial denervation typically fully recover. Patients with total denervation usually partially recover, but may exhibit aberrant regeneration (e.g., crocodile tears) or hemifacial spasm as long term complications.

MISCELLANEOUS

ASSOCIATED CONDITIONS N/A

AGE-RELATED FACTORS
Pediatric: N/A
Geriatric: N/A
Others: N/A

PREGNANCY Use steroids cautiously in pregnancy. Consult with obstetrician.

SYNONYMS
• Idiopathic facial paralysis

ICD-9-CM 351.0 Bell's palsy

SEE ALSO N/A

OTHER NOTES N/A

ABBREVIATIONS N/A

REFERENCES
• Dyck, P.J., Thomas, P.K., Lambert, E.H., Bunge, R. (eds.): Peripheral Neuropathy, 2nd Ed. Philadelphia, W.B. Saunders Co., 1984

Author C. Bamford, M.D.

Bladder injury

 BASICS

DESCRIPTION
Due to its well protected location, bladder rupture is unusual. Injury most often secondary to penetrating or blunt trauma and classified as contusion, intraperitoneal or extraperitoneal rupture.
System(s) affected: Renal/Urologic
Genetics: N/A
Incidence/Prevalence in USA: N/A
Predominant Age: N/A
Predominant Sex: N/A

SIGNS AND SYMPTOMS
• History of blow to lower abdomen
• Suprapubic pain
• Urinary retention
• Hematuria (94%)
• Muscle rigidity over lower abdomen
• No peritonitis
• Frequently associated with pelvic fractures

CAUSES
• Forceful blunt or penetrating blow to lower abdomen

RISK FACTORS
• Distended bladder at the time of trauma
• Congenital malformation of bladder
• Prior pelvic or bladder surgery

 DIAGNOSIS

DIFFERENTIAL DIAGNOSIS
• Rupture of the urethra
• Rupture of abdominal viscus
• Pelvic fracture with hematoma

LABORATORY
Hematuria on urinalysis
Drugs that may alter lab results: None
Disorders that may alter lab results: None

PATHOLOGICAL FINDINGS
• Jagged irregular tear in the bladder
• Perforation at the dome of bladder near urachus (blunt trauma)
• Extensive perivesicle hematoma

SPECIAL TESTS
None

IMAGING
• Cystogram with drain out film
• Urethrogram

DIAGNOSTIC PROCEDURES
• Rarely is cystoscopy indicated

 TREATMENT

APPROPRIATE HEALTH CARE
Inpatient

GENERAL MEASURES
• Extraperitoneal rupture, insert foley, admit, comfort care
• Intraperitoneal rupture, immediate surgical repair
• Blunt trauma, contusion, comfort care
• Penetrating injury, exploration, surgical repair
• Antibacterial coverage, broad spectrum
• Anticholinergics for spasm
• Pain medication as required

ACTIVITY
Full activity when associated injuries permit

DIET
No special diet

PATIENT EDUCATION
Printed material available from multiple sources

MEDICATIONS

DRUG(S) OF CHOICE
• Broad spectrum coverage, ciprofloxacin (Cipro) 500 mg bid
• Opium and belladonna suppositories q 6-8 hr prn spasms
• oxybutynin (Ditropan) 5-10 mg tid for spasms
• Adequate pain control as required
Contraindications: Refer to manufacturer's profile of each drug
Precautions: Refer to manufacturer's profile of each drug
Significant possible interactions: Refer to manufacturer's profile of each drug

ALTERNATIVE DRUGS   None

FOLLOWUP

PATIENT MONITORING
• Cystogram repeat in 7-10 days
• Remove catheter when bladder sealed
• Periodic check for infection and stricture formation

PREVENTION/AVOIDANCE
• Use seat belts
• Auto air bag

POSSIBLE COMPLICATIONS
• Infection
• Fistula formation (rare)
• Peritonitis (rare)

EXPECTED COURSE AND PROGNOSIS
• Complete recovery
• Stricture (uncommon) - only long term complication

MISCELLANEOUS

ASSOCIATED CONDITIONS   None

AGE-RELATED FACTORS
Pediatric: Position of bladder makes intraperitoneal rupture more common
Geriatric: N/A
Others: N/A

PREGNANCY   N/A

SYNONYMS   N/A

ICD-9-CM   596.9

SEE ALSO   N/A

OTHER NOTES   N/A

ABBREVIATIONS   N/A

REFERENCES   Walsh, P.C., Gittes, R.F. & Perlmutter, A.D.: Campbell's Urology. Philadelphia, W.B. Saunders Co., 1986

Author   J. Summers, M.D. Ph.D.

Blastomycosis

 BASICS

DESCRIPTION An uncommon, systemic, fungal infection with a broad range of manifestations including pulmonary, skin, bone and genitourinary involvement
System(s) affected: Skin/Exocrine, Pulmonary, Musculoskeletal, Renal/Urologic, Endocrine/Metabolic
Genetics: N/A
Incidence/Prevalence in USA: Ranges from 0.4-4 cases per 100,000 population per year. Higher prevalence in states bordering the Mississippi and Ohio Rivers. Sporadic cases occurring in other areas.
Predominant age: Adults, but 10-20% of cases occur in children
Predominant sex: Male > Female

SIGNS AND SYMPTOMS
Acute infection
◊ Onset may be abrupt or insidious
◊ May be asymptomatic and self-limiting
◊ Incubation period 30-45 days
◊ Fever, chills, myalgias, arthralgias
◊ Cough initially nonproductive, then productive
◊ Hemoptysis (common)
◊ Erythema nodosum
Pulmonary blastomycosis
◊ 60-90% of cases
◊ Three forms - acute, chronic, asymptomatic
◊ Cough - nonproductive to productive
◊ Hemoptysis
◊ Weight loss
◊ Pleuritic chest pain
◊ Pleural effusions - 10%
◊ Respiratory failure in small percentage
◊ Upper lobe fibronodular infiltrates - 50%
◊ Mass lesion - 30%
◊ Diffuse pulmonary infiltrates; cavitation (uncommon)
◊ Pleural thickening
Cutaneous blastomycosis
◊ Most common extrapulmonary manifestation - 40-80%
◊ May occur with or without pulmonary disease
◊ Two types of lesions
◊ Verrucous lesions begin as small papulopustular lesions, slowly spread, become crusted, have sharp borders; central clearing with scar formation and depigmentation; microabscesses noted at periphery of lesion
◊ Ulcerative lesions (initially pustules) form shallow ulcers with raised edges and granulating base
◊ Mucosal lesions may occur
◊ Regional adenopathy (uncommon)
◊ Subcutaneous nodules - cold abscesses

Skeletal blastomycosis
◊ Occurs 25-50% of extrapulmonary cases
◊ Long bones, vertebrae, ribs most commonly involved
◊ Well circumscribed osteolytic lesions
◊ May present with contiguous soft tissue abscesses and/or sinus tracts
◊ Paraspinous abscess may occur in vertebral disease
◊ Acute or chronic arthritis may result from extension of contiguous osteomyelitis
Genitourinary blastomycosis
◊ Occurs in 10-30% of cases
◊ Involves prostate most commonly but also epididymis and testes
◊ Outflow obstruction
◊ Enlarged tender prostate
◊ Involvement of female genitalia uncommon and usually acquired through sexual contact
Other
◊ Central nervous system involvement with acute or chronic meningitis, epidural or cerebral abscesses
◊ Liver, spleen, pericardium, thyroid, gastrointestinal tract, adrenal gland may each be involved

CAUSES
• Inhalation of spores of Blastomyces dermatitidis into lung with spread to other organ systems by lympho-hematogenous dissemination
• Primary inoculation of skin may rarely occur
• Female genital infection may result from sexual transmission

RISK FACTORS
• Occupational or recreational exposure to soil containing spores of B. dermatitidis
• Residence in areas of increased disease prevalence

 DIAGNOSIS

DIFFERENTIAL DIAGNOSIS
• Pulmonary - acute bacterial pneumonia, tuberculosis, other fungal diseases, bacterial lung abscess, empyema, bronchogenic carcinoma
• Cutaneous - bacterial pyoderma, cutaneous mycobacterial infection, other cutaneous fungal infections (sporotrichosis, histoplasmosis, cryptococcosis), squamous cell carcinoma
• Bone - bacterial osteomyelitis, tuberculosis, neoplastic disease
• Genitourinary - bacterial prostatitis, prostate cancer, other fungal infections, tuberculosis

LABORATORY
• Culture of B. dermatitidis from tissue or body secretions on Sabouraud's or other enriched media
• Demonstration of yeast forms (5-15 micrometers in diameter, with refractile cell wall, broad-based budding and no capsule) in tissue or body secretions by wet mount or special stains
• Serologic tests include complement fixation, enzyme-linked immunoassay, immunodiffusion precipitin antibody tests. All have variable sensitivity and low specificity and are not helpful in diagnosis.
• Delayed hypersensitivity skin testing with blastomycin also has low sensitivity and specificity and not useful in diagnosis
Drugs that may alter lab results: N/A
Disorders that may alter lab results:
Histoplasma cross-reacts with serologic tests for blastomycosis

PATHOLOGICAL FINDINGS
• Early inflammatory response with polymorphonuclear leukocytes followed by granuloma formation with lymphocytes and macrophages
• Granulomas do not show caseation necrosis
• Yeast is often found attached to or inside monocytes, macrophages and giant cells

SPECIAL TESTS
• Special staining of tissue with Gomori methenamine silver stain
• Periodic acid-Schiff's stain colors cell wall pink or red
• Mucicarmine stain helps differentiate from encapsulated Cryptococcus

IMAGING
• CT scan of head for CNS lesions
• CT scan of spine for vertebral lesions
• Bone scan for skeletal lesions
• Chest x-ray may show upper lobe fibronodular infiltrates, consolidation, diffuse alveolar infiltrates, mass lesions or pleural thickening

DIAGNOSTIC PROCEDURES
• Aspiration of abscess contents for wet mount and culture
• Needle or surgical biopsy of involved tissue

TREATMENT

APPROPRIATE HEALTH CARE
Inpatient. May be ambulatory but therapy with intravenous antifungal therapy should be instituted as a hospital inpatient with continuation as outpatient once patient is stable.

GENERAL MEASURES
• Systemic antifungal therapy is indicated for all cases of extrapulmonary blastomycosis
• Systemic antifungal therapy is indicated for all but the very mild or asymptomatic pulmonary cases in which a trial of observation may be appropriate
• Surgical débridement of bone lesions if there are areas of devitalized bone
• Surgical drainage of large cutaneous abscesses or pleural empyemas

ACTIVITY   No restrictions, once patient is released from hospital

DIET   No special dietary requirement

PATIENT EDUCATION   Counsel patient and family on potential adverse effects associated with antifungal therapy, duration of therapy required and potential for relapse or chronic infection

MEDICATIONS

DRUG(S) OF CHOICE
Milder forms
• Ketoconazole (Nizoral) 400-800 mg po daily for 6 months
Severe forms
• Amphotericin B (Fungizone): 0.5-0.8 mg/kg IV over 4-6 hours daily for a cumulative dose of 1.5-2 gm
◊ First dose of amphotericin B is given as a test dose of 1 mg in 200 ml dextrose 5% in distilled water intravenously over 2-4 hours
◊ Dose is increased by 10 mg daily until a maintenance dose of 0.5 mg-0.8 mg per kg per day is reached
◊ Rigors can be prevented by pre-infusion dose of meperidine
◊ To reduce infusion-related fever, pre-infusion acetaminophen and diphenhydramine
Contraindications: Life threatening intolerance to amphotericin such as anaphylaxis

Precautions:
• Monitor for hypotension during the infusion
• Monitor renal function, serum sodium, potassium and magnesium, and CBC twice weekly during therapy
• Replace potassium and magnesium as indicated
• When serum creatinine rises to 1.6 mg/dl or greater, dosage interval should be changed to 48 hours
• Watch for phlebitis at infusion site
Significant possible interactions: Avoid use of potentially nephrotoxic drugs such as aminoglycosides which may potentiate nephrotoxicity of amphotericin B

ALTERNATIVE DRUGS
• Efficacy of alternate regimens not well established by controlled studies
• Itraconazole - investigational drug with promise

FOLLOWUP

PATIENT MONITORING
• Monitor closely during early therapy
• Frequency of followup depends on severity of disease
• Monitor serum electrolytes, creatinine and CBC twice weekly during amphotericin B therapy
• Post-therapy followup every 3 months for 2 years then twice yearly

PREVENTION/AVOIDANCE
• Unknown
• Condoms for sexual encounters

POSSIBLE COMPLICATIONS
Treatment-induced nephrotoxicity, electrolyte imbalance, anemia

EXPECTED COURSE AND PROGNOSIS
• Cure in over 90% with appropriate therapy
• Relapse in less than 10% of cases
• Relapse rate higher with ketoconazole therapy
• Adverse reactions with amphotericin B are frequent and significant

MISCELLANEOUS

ASSOCIATED CONDITIONS   N/A

AGE-RELATED FACTORS
Pediatric: Uncommon in children
Geriatric: Prognosis is worse in elderly patients with significant underlying pulmonary or renal disease
Others: N/A

PREGNANCY   Safety of amphotericin B and ketoconazole in pregnancy has not been established

SYNONYMS   North American blastomycosis

ICD-9-CM   116.0

SEE ALSO   N/A

OTHER NOTES   N/A

ABBREVIATIONS   N/A

REFERENCES
• Mandell, G.L. (ed.): Principles and Practice of Infectious Diseases. 3rd Ed. New York, Churchill Livingstone, 1990
• Bradsher,R.W.: Infectious Disease Clinics of North America, Dec. 1988, pg. 877
• Brown, L.R., et al, Mayo Clin Proc 66:29-38, 1991

Author   W. Gardner, M.D.

Blepharitis

BASICS

DESCRIPTION An inflammatory reaction of the eyelid margin. It usually occurs as seborrheic (nonulcerative) or as staphylococcal (ulcerative) blepharitis. Both types may coexist.
System(s) affected: Skin/Exocrine
Genetics: N/A
Incidence/Prevalence in USA: Common (the most frequent ocular disease)
Predominant age: Adult
Predominant sex: Male = Female

SIGNS AND SYMPTOMS
Staphylococcus aureus blepharitis
◊ Itching
◊ Tearing
◊ Burning
◊ Photophobia (light sensitivity)
◊ Usually worse in morning
◊ Recurrent stye (external hordeolum, or internal hordeolum)
◊ Recurrent chalazia (chronic inflammation of meibomian glands)
◊ Fine, epithelial keratitis, lower half of cornea
◊ Ulcerations at base of eyelashes
◊ Broken, sparse, misdirected eyelashes(trichiasis)
Seborrheic blepharitis
◊ Lid margin erythema
◊ Dry flakes, oily secretions on lid margins and/or lashes
◊ Associated dandruff of scalp, eyebrows
◊ Sometimes nasolabial erythema, scaling
Mixed blepharitis (seborrheic with associated Staph aureus)
◊ Most common type of blepharitis
◊ Symptoms and signs of both staph and seborrheic present

CAUSES
Seborrheic
◊ Accelerated shedding of skin cells with associated sebaceous gland dysfunction
◊ P. ovale and P. orbiculare yeasts often colonize
◊ Oil and skin cells foster staph growth
Staphylococcus
◊ Usually part of mixed blepharitis
◊ Colonization of Zeis glands of lid margin and meibomian glands posterior to lashes, with Staphylococcus aureus
◊ Impetigo contagiosa-staph
◊ Infectious eczematoid dermatitis-Staphylococcus is the hapten
◊ Staphylococcus scalded skin syndrome - entire body involved (in young children)
◊ Angular blepharitis-staph - most frequent bacteria involved
Other types of blepharitis
◊ Contact dermatitis with or without secondary Staphylococcus infection
◊ Meibomian gland dysfunction

RISK FACTORS
• Candida
• Seborrheic dermatitis
• Acne rosacea
• Diabetes mellitus
• Immunocompromised state (AIDS, chemotherapy, etc.)

DIAGNOSIS

DIFFERENTIAL DIAGNOSIS
Masquerade syndrome:
◊ Persistent inflammation and thickening of eyelid margin may indicate squamous cell, basal cell, or sebaceous cell carcinoma masquerading as "blepharitis"
◊ These carcinomas may also mimic styes or chalazions
◊ Sebaceous cell carcinoma has a 23% fatality rate (found in one study of eyelid sebaceous cell carcinomas). Up to one half of potentially fatal sebaceous cell carcinomas may resemble benign inflammatory diseases, particularly chalazions and chronic blepharoconjunctivitis.
◊ Any swelling or inflammation of eyelid which does not resolve promptly (within one month) with treatment, is suspect as a possible underlying carcinoma

LABORATORY N/A
Drugs that may alter lab results: N/A
Disorders that may alter lab results: N/A

PATHOLOGICAL FINDINGS Acute or chronic inflammatory cell types

SPECIAL TESTS
• Cultures in atypical blepharitis
• Biopsy in atypical cases that are suspect for carcinoma

IMAGING N/A

DIAGNOSTIC PROCEDURES See Special Tests

TREATMENT

APPROPRIATE HEALTH CARE
Outpatient

GENERAL MEASURES
• Mild seborrheic blepharitis (dry flakes, minimal inflammation) - apply eyelid margin scrubs with eyelid cleanser at least once daily
• If Staphylococcus likely, follow lid scrubs with application of bacitracin, or (second choice), erythromycin ophthalmic ointment, to eyelid margins, using cotton tipped applicator
• Clean lids and apply ointment nightly in mild cases, up to four times daily in severe cases
• Discontinue soft contact lenses until condition cleared
• Chronic recurrent blepharitis requires referral to ophthalmologist for evaluation as to whether patient should continue in lenses

ACTIVITY No restrictions

DIET No restrictions

PATIENT EDUCATION
• Blepharitis "Fact Sheet" from American Academy of Ophthalmology (see References for ordering information)
• Advise patient that blepharitis is a chronic condition, prone to recurrence if hygiene (lid scrubs) are not maintained after antibiotic treatment is discontinued

MEDICATIONS

DRUG(S) OF CHOICE
• Topical treatment, if Staphylococcus likely, application of bacitracin, or (second choice), erythromycin ophthalmic ointment
• In some cases of Staphylococcus blepharitis (e.g., rosacea), systemic tetracycline 250 mg qid x several weeks, tapering to 250 mg daily for one to three months. Alternative is oxacillin 250 mg qid for 1-2 weeks. Used for persistent (despite topical treatment) lid inflammation or recurrent meibomian styes.
Contraindications:
• Allergy to medication
• Oral tetracycline - children less than 8 years, pregnancy
Precautions:
• Avoid medication containing neomycin, as it is sensitizing
• Oral tetracycline may act as a photosensitizer. Patients should use sunscreen with SPF 15 or greater
Significant possible interactions:
Oral tetracyclines
◊ Avoid dairy products, iron preparations or antacids within 2 hours of dose
◊ Oral contraceptives may have reduced efficacy. Use backup contraception.

ALTERNATIVE DRUGS N/A

FOLLOWUP

PATIENT MONITORING Every 2 months

PREVENTION/AVOIDANCE Follow treatment guidelines

POSSIBLE COMPLICATIONS
• Hordeolum (stye)
• Scarring of eyelid margin
• Misdirection of eyelashes (trichiasis)
• Corneal infection

EXPECTED COURSE AND PROGNOSIS Long-term eyelid hygiene required to control

MISCELLANEOUS

ASSOCIATED CONDITIONS See diagnosis section above regarding blepharitis masquerade syndromes

AGE-RELATED FACTORS
Pediatric: N/A
Geriatric: N/A
OTHERS: N/A

PREGNANCY N/A

SYNONYMS N/A

ICD-9-CM 373.00

SEE ALSO N/A

OTHER NOTES N/A

ABBREVIATIONS N/A

REFERENCES
• Tasman,W. (ed.): Duane's Clinical Ophthalmology. Philadelphia, J.B. Lippincott Co., 1991
• Boniuk, M. & Zimmerman, L.E.: Sebaceous carcinoma of the eyelid, eyebrow, caruncle, and orbit. Trans Am Acad Ophthalmol Otolaryngol 72:619, 1968
• Rao, N.A., McLean, I.W. & Zimmerman, L.E.: Sebaceous carcinoma of the eyelids and caruncles: Correlation of clinicopathological features of prognosis. In Ocular and Adnexal Tumors. Edited by F.A. Jakobic. Birmingham, Aesculapius, 1978, p461
• American Academy of Ophthalmology, Department of Patient Education: Blepharitis Fact Sheet. San Francisco, American Academy of Ophthalmology. Available for order as tear-off pads, phone (415)-561-8500 to order or write AAO, P.O. Box 7424, San Francisco, CA 94120-7424.

Author T. Moody, M.D.

Bone tumor, primary malignant

BASICS

DESCRIPTION   Primary malignant bone tumors are rare. Four types make up the majority.
• Malignant fibrous histiocytoma (MFH) - a pleomorphic sarcoma of storiform pattern without differentiation
• Osteosarcoma - similar to malignant fibrous histiocytoma with differentiation to osteoid production
• Chondrosarcoma - cellular cartilaginous lesion with abundant binucleate cells, myxoid areas, and pushing borders
• Ewing's sarcoma - small, blue-round cell neoplasm
System(s) affected: Musculoskeletal
Genetics:
• Unknown (Ewing's has 11/22 chromosomal translocation)
• Osteosarcoma has association with retinoblastoma gene and possible P53
Incidence/Prevalence in USA:
Rare: 5000 bone and soft tissue sarcomas per year, a practicing orthopedic surgeon may see one primary malignant tumor of bone in every five years of practice. Ewing's sarcoma is less common in Blacks.
Predominant age:
• MFH - teens and elderly
• Osteogenic sarcoma - teens and early twenties
• Chondrosarcoma - very young and very old
• Ewing's sarcoma - children, teens, and early twenties
Predominant sex: Male = Female

SIGNS AND SYMPTOMS
• Pain with weight bearing, at rest and at night
• Swelling
• Tenderness
• Fracture with minor trauma
• Minor injury may bring attention to lesion

CAUSES
• Generally unknown
• MFH often follows irradiation or arises in old bone infarct
• Osteosarcoma has association with retinoblastoma gene
• Chondrosarcoma may arise in pre-existing enchondroma or exostosis

RISK FACTORS
• Multiple enchondromatosis (Ollier's disease)–chondrosarcoma
• Multiple hereditary exostosis–chondrosarcoma
• Previous irradiation, risk factor for MFH
• Previous history of bilateral retinoblastoma–osteosarcoma

DIAGNOSIS

DIFFERENTIAL DIAGNOSIS
• Solitary metastatic lesion or myeloma especially in the patient over age 40
• Lymphoma at any age
• Benign bone tumors and benign bone tumors that look aggressive (aneurysmal bone cyst, giant cell tumor, eosinophilic granuloma)
• Infection (osteomyelitis)
• Metabolic bone disease (osteopenia, Paget's, hyperparathyroidism)
• Synovial diseases (pigmented villonodular synovitis, synovial chondromatosis, degenerative or inflammatory synovitis)
• Myositis ossificans and repair reaction to trauma
• Avascular necrosis

LABORATORY
• Generally unhelpful
• 50% of osteosarcomas have an elevated alkaline phosphatase
• Ewing's sarcoma may be associated with an elevated ESR and LDH
• Acid phosphatase, prostatic specific antigen
• Calcium
• Thyroid function tests to exclude thyroid carcinoma
• Elevated ESR
• Serum protein electrophoresis and urine electrophoresis to exclude myeloma
Drugs that may alter lab results: N/A
Disorders that may alter lab results: N/A

PATHOLOGICAL FINDINGS
• Histology in combination with radiographic findings confirms the diagnosis
• PAS staining before and after glycogen digestion with diastase is useful in confirming the diagnosis in 80% of Ewing's sarcomas
• Electron microscopy for glycogen granules is useful in diagnosing Ewing's sarcoma

SPECIAL TESTS
• Open biopsy is preferred over needle biopsy. Needle biopsies run the risk of inadequate tissue for diagnosis.
• Biopsy of associated soft tissue mass may lessen the risk of pathologic fracture
• Biopsy tract should to be excised in continuity with the tumor at the time of resection.

IMAGING
• Plain films provide the most important information regarding the nature of the lesion and guide further testing
• Bone scan - prior to biopsy, looking for other lesions
• CT scan for cortical destruction and internal calcification or ossification. CT scan of the abdomen to exclude hypernephroma.
• MRI scan determines the extent of marrow involvement and associated soft tissue mass
• Chest x-ray and CT for metastatic disease.
• Mammogram to exclude breast carcinoma

DIAGNOSTIC PROCEDURES
• Rectal exam for prostatic nodules
• Laboratory studies for metabolic bone disease

TREATMENT

APPROPRIATE HEALTH CARE
Inpatient surgery

GENERAL MEASURES
• Resection with adequate margin is required to minimize risk of local persistence
• For MFH and osteosarcoma, pre-resection neo-adjuvant chemotherapy treats micrometastatic disease immediately, allows time for ordering replacement prosthesis and bone graft, allows for an in vivo assessment of the chemotherapy responsiveness of the tumor, and may facilitate limb salvage by allowing a "safer" close margin
• Chondrosarcoma in the extremities should be treated exclusively by surgery unless it is of the mesenchymal or de-differentiated high grade variety
• Ewing's sarcoma was traditionally treated with chemotherapy and surgery was limited to those lesions that were extremely large, associated with pathologic fracture, or involved an expendable bone. Most Ewing's sarcoma lesions were irradiated. However, despite irradiation, local recurrence is common up to 25% in pelvic lesions. Therefore, surgery with limb salvage is becoming increasingly popular. A dramatic decrease in size in Ewing's sarcoma occurs after initial chemotherapy and a decision can then be made after restaging as to whether to irradiate or to resect the primary lesion.
• The treatment goal is to minimize local recurrence while preserving function. Limb salvage is employed whenever a safe margin can be obtained.

ACTIVITY   Varies with stage of disease and treatment

DIET   No special diet

PATIENT EDUCATION   Refer to local branch of American Cancer Society for information and support groups

MEDICATIONS

DRUG(S) OF CHOICE
These drugs are administered according to specific protocols. Other protocols may be appropriate.
MFH and osteosarcoma:
◊ Adriamycin
◊ Intra-arterial and intravenous cisplatin
◊ High dose methotrexate with leucovorin rescue
◊ Ifosfamide
◊ Cytoxan
◊ Actinomycin D
◊ Bleomycin
Ewing's sarcoma:
◊ Cytoxan
◊ Vincristine
◊ Actinomycin D
◊ Adriamycin

Contraindications: Refer to manufacturer's literature
Precautions: Left ventricular dysfunction with Adriamycin. Cumulative dose > 550 mg/m2 increases risk. Follow with serial echocardiograms and/or MUGA scans when cumulative dose > 250 mg/m2.
Significant possible interactions:
Myelosuppression

ALTERNATIVE DRUGS   N/A

FOLLOWUP

PATIENT MONITORING
• Patients who require adjuvant chemotherapy are treated after resection of the tumor with maintenance chemotherapy in an adjuvant setting.
• Blood counts for myelosuppression
• Serial echocardiograms when Adriamycin is being used. G-CSF often used to minimize neutropenia risk.
• Chest x-rays obtained every two months for the first year, every three months for the second year, and every four months in the third year
• CT scans of the lungs are initially repeated every four months during first year
• Ewing's sarcoma may recur > 5 years after diagnosis

PREVENTION/AVOIDANCE   None identified

POSSIBLE COMPLICATIONS
• Limb salvage with any primary malignant bone tumor is fraught with potential complications
• Micrometastatic disease occurs at the time of presentation and can appear at any time during the course of treatment or followup
• Local recurrence risk for osteosarcoma with limb salvage is about 10%
• There can be leg length discrepancy, infection, wound dehiscence, skin coverage problems, arterial and nerve injury, non-union of bone grafts, and mechanical loosening of prosthetic implants
• Thoracotomy and continued chemotherapy is often recommended for metastatic disease
• Metastatic Ewing's sarcoma is quite diffuse and is less amenable to thoracotomy

EXPECTED COURSE AND PROGNOSIS
• With amputation alone, 80% of patients with osteosarcoma had pulmonary metastatic disease by two years. With chemotherapy, the five year disease-free survival rate is 50-85%
• Favorable prognostic factors for MFH and osteosarcoma include responsiveness to chemotherapy, distal portions of the extremities, small size, age over ten
• Most chondrosarcomas are of lower grade and have a low risk of metastatic spread and low incidence of local recurrence after adequate surgery
• MFH, osteosarcoma, and Ewing's sarcoma have an overall 50% survival with combined treatment modalities

MISCELLANEOUS

ASSOCIATED CONDITIONS
• A higher incidence of chondrosarcoma is seen in patients with multiple hereditary exostosis, multiple enchondromatosis (Ollier's disease) and patients with enchondromatosis and hemangiomatosis (Maffucci's syndrome)
• Patients with enchondromatosis more often die of GI malignancies than metastatic chondrosarcoma

AGE-RELATED FACTORS
Pediatric: N/A
Geriatric: N/A
Others: N/A

PREGNANCY
• Increased growth of musculoskeletal malignancies during pregnancy
• Soft tissue desmoid tumors have estrogen and progesterone receptors

SYNONYMS   N/A

ICD-9-CM   170.9 (unless otherwise specified)

SEE ALSO   Osteitis deformans (Paget's disease of bone)

OTHER NOTES   Osteosarcoma variants like parosteal, periosteal, and intraosseous osteosarcoma are lower grade lesions with a more favorable prognosis, often not requiring chemotherapy. Other variants, post irradiation, and post-Paget's osteosarcoma metastasize early.

ABBREVIATIONS
ESR = erythrocyte sedimentation rate

REFERENCES
• Enneking, W.F.: Musculoskeletal Tumor Surgery, Volumes I and II. New York, Churchill Livingstone, 1983
• Schajowicz, F. & McGuire, M.H.: Diagnostic difficulties in skeletal pathology. Clinical orthopedics and Related Research. 240:281-310, 1991
• Womer, R.B.: The cellular biology of bone tumors. Clinical orthopedics and Related Research. 262:12-21, 1991
• Simon, M.A.: Limb salvage for osteosarcoma in the 1980's. Clinical orthopedics and Related Research. 270:264-270, 1991

Author I. Harris, M.D.

Botulism

BASICS

DESCRIPTION An intoxication producing paralytic disease, caused by neurotoxins of Clostridium botulinum. The toxin prevents acetylcholine release at presynaptic membranes.
Three forms exist:
◊ Foodborne botulism
◊ Infantile botulism
◊ Wound botulism

System(s) affected: Endocrine/Metabolic, Gastrointestinal, Nervous
Genetics: N/A
Incidence in the USA/Prevalence in USA:
0.034/100,000 with 75% the infantile form.
• Foodborne - 20 to 50 cases per year
• Infantile - 50 to 100 cases per year
• Wound botulism is rare
Predominant age:
• Foodborne - all ages
• Infantile mean age - 3 months
• Wound - usually young adult
Predominant sex:
• Foodborne and infantile - Male = Female
• Wound - Male > Female

SIGNS AND SYMPTOMS
Foodborne
◊ Nonspecific findings early (nausea, vomiting, malaise, dizziness)
◊ Dry mouth
◊ Constipation, urinary retention
◊ Symmetric descending weakness or paralysis
◊ Cranial nerve paralysis (ptosis; extraocular muscle paresis; fixed, dilated pupils; dysphagia)
◊ Postural hypotension
◊ Muscle weakness, respiratory paralysis
◊ Variable deep tendon reflexes
◊ Afebrile
◊ Progression over few days
Infantile
◊ Constipation - early sign
◊ Loss of head control
◊ Loss of suck
◊ Loss of facial expression and verbalization
◊ Symmetric descending weakness and cranial nerve paresis similar to foodborne form
◊ Diminished or absent deep tendon reflexes
◊ Autonomic dysfunction
◊ Afebrile
◊ Usual progression over 2-5 days, can be as short as few hours
Wound
◊ Onset 4-14 days post injury
◊ Findings similar to foodborne botulism
◊ May be febrile

CAUSES
• Ingestion of C. botulinum neurotoxins (A, B, and E most common)
• Foodborne usually from home-canned vegetables or prepared foods
• Infantile from ingestion of spores in environment or occasionally in honey
• Wound due to contamination with toxin-producing C. botulinum

RISK FACTORS
• Foodborne - ingestion of home-canned or prepared foods
• Infantile - ingestion of honey. Breast feeding (controversial).

DIAGNOSIS

DIFFERENTIAL DIAGNOSIS
• Guillain-Barré syndrome
• Encephalitis
• Tick paralysis
• Myasthenia gravis
• Basilar artery stroke
• Congenital neuropathy or myopathy
• Sepsis
• Other poisonings (organophosphate, shellfish, Amanita mushrooms, atropine, aminoglycoside)

LABORATORY Routine tests including CSF exam normal
Drugs that may alter lab results: N/A
Disorders that may alter lab results:
Underlying myoneural disease

PATHOLOGICAL FINDINGS Nonspecific

SPECIAL TESTS
• Stool contains organism and toxin
• Serum toxin present in foodborne form

IMAGING N/A

DIAGNOSTIC PROCEDURES
Electromyogram (EMG) shows characteristic brief, low voltage compound motor-unit, small amplitude, overly abundant action potentials (BSAPs), incremental response to repetitive stimulation

TREATMENT

APPROPRIATE HEALTH CARE
Inpatient, with maximal monitoring capabilities, especially for respiratory failure

GENERAL MEASURES
• Meticulous airway management
• Physical therapy with range of motion exercise and assisted ambulation as tolerated
• Prevention of decubiti
• Wound excision débridement

ACTIVITY Bedrest initially

DIET
• Nasogastric feedings if needed
• Fluid restriction if inappropriate antidiuretic hormone (ADH) syndrome

PATIENT EDUCATION
• When preserving food at home, kill Clostridium botulinum spores by pressure cooking at 250°F (120°C) for 30 minutes
• Toxin can be destroyed by boiling for 10 minutes or cooking at 175°F (80°C) for 30 minutes
• Avoid honey in first year of life

MEDICATIONS

DRUG(S) OF CHOICE
<u>Foodborne</u>
◊ Antitoxin therapy with trivalent A-B-E antitoxin (available at CDC (404) 639-3670 or 639-2888), one vial IV and one vial IM, repeat IV in 2-4 hours if symptoms persist
◊ Penicillin therapy of unclear value
<u>Infantile</u>
◊ Antitoxin therapy not needed
◊ Penicillin therapy of unclear value
◊ Enemas may assist in removal of toxin
<u>Wound</u>
◊ Antitoxin therapy with trivalent A-B-E antitoxin (available at CDC (404) 639-3753 or 639-2888), one vial IV and one vial IM, repeat in 2-4 hours if persistent symptoms
Contraindications: Aminoglycosides - may potentiate paralysis
Precautions: Serum sickness or hypersensitivity reactions in 20% of antitoxin recipients
Significant possible interactions: N/A

ALTERNATIVE DRUGS   N/A

FOLLOWUP

PATIENT MONITORING   Cardiorespiratory monitoring during illness

PREVENTION/AVOIDANCE
• Avoid giving honey to infants
• Do not eat or taste food from bulging cans, or if food is off-smelling, discard it

POSSIBLE COMPLICATIONS
• Aspiration pneumonia
• Nosocomial infection
• Hypoxic tissue damage
• Death

EXPECTED COURSE AND PROGNOSIS
<u>Foodborne and wound</u>
◊ Mortality 25% (< 10% under 20 years of age), usually due to delayed diagnosis and respiratory failure
◊ Full recovery may require months
◊ Sequelae due to hypoxic insults
<u>Infantile</u>
◊ Mortality < 1%
◊ Extended recovery period and sequelae as above

MISCELLANEOUS

ASSOCIATED CONDITIONS   N/A

AGE-RELATED FACTORS
Pediatric: Avoid honey for first year
Geriatric: N/A
Others: N/A

PREGNANCY   N/A

SYNONYMS
• Sausage poisoning
• Kerner's disease

ICD-9-CM   005.1

SEE ALSO   N/A

OTHER NOTES   Organism present in stools of 1-2% of healthy individuals

ABBREVIATIONS   N/A

REFERENCES
• Mandell, G., Douglas, R. & Bennett, J.: Principles and Practice of Infectious Diseases. 3rd Ed. New York, Churchill Livingstone, 1990
• Oski, F., DeAngelis, C., Feigin, R. & Warshaw, J.: Principles and Practice of Pediatrics. Philadelphia, J.B. Lippincott, 1990

Author   B. Wiedermann, M.D.

Brain abscess

BASICS

DESCRIPTION Single or multiple abscesses within the brain, usually occurring secondary to a focus of infection outside the central nervous system. May mimic brain tumor but evolves more rapidly (days to a few weeks). It starts as a cerebritis, becomes an abscess, and subsequently becomes encapsulated.

System(s) affected: Nervous

Genetics: No known genetic pattern

Incidence/Prevalence: Infrequent

Predominant age: All ages

Predominant sex: Male = Female

SIGNS AND SYMPTOMS
• Recent onset of headache becoming severe
• Nausea and vomiting
• Mental changes progressing to stupor and coma
• Afebrile or low-grade fever
• Neck stiffness
• Seizures
• Papilledema
• Focal neurological signs depending on location

CAUSES
• Direct extension from otitis, mastoiditis or sinusitis
• Cranial osteomyelitis
• Penetrating skull trauma
• Prior craniotomy
• Bacteremia from lung abscess, pneumonia
• Bacterial endocarditis
• Fungal infection of the nasopharynx
• Toxoplasma gondii (in AIDS patients)
• Cyanotic congenital heart disease
• Intravenous drug use
• Most common infective organisms - streptococci, staphylococci, and anaerobes (usually same as source of infection)

RISK FACTORS
• AIDS
• Immunocompromised
• IV drug abuse

DIAGNOSIS

DIFFERENTIAL DIAGNOSIS
• Brain tumors
• Stroke
• Resolving intracranial hemorrhage
• Subdural empyema
• Extradural abscess
• Encephalitis

LABORATORY
• WBC may be normal or mildly elevated
• Culture of abscess contents, predominant organisms include Toxoplasma (AIDS), Staphylococcus (trauma), aerobic or anaerobic bacteria, fungi (rare)
• Blood studies - mild polymorphonuclear leukocytosis, elevated sedimentation rate

Drugs that may alter lab results: Prior administration of antibiotics

Disorders that may alter lab results: N/A

PATHOLOGICAL FINDINGS
• Suppuration, liquification, encapsulation, depending on stage of evolution
• Fibrosis

SPECIAL TESTS
Surgical burr hole with aspiration to make a specific bacteriologic diagnosis

IMAGING
• CT or MRI are diagnostic methods of choice - findings are dependent on stages of the abscess
• Radionuclide 117 IN-labeled leucocytes may distinguish abscess from neoplasm

DIAGNOSTIC PROCEDURES
History, physical exam

TREATMENT

APPROPRIATE HEALTH CARE
Inpatient

GENERAL MEASURES
• Palliative and supportive
<u>Medical therapy</u>
◊ For surgical inaccessible, multiple abscesses
◊ For abscesses in early cerebritis stage
◊ Therapy directed toward most likely organism
◊ If abscess does not demonstrate shrinkage in 4 weeks, perform surgical procedure
◊ Small (< 2.5 cm) abscess
<u>Surgical therapy</u>
◊ Mandatory when neurologic deficits are severe or progressive
◊ Used when the abscess is in the posterior fossa
◊ Abscess drainage - (via needle) under stereotactic CT guidance through a burr hole under local anesthesia, is most rapid and effective method. May be repeated if needed.
◊ Craniotomy - if abscess is large or multilocular
◊ Abscess resulting from trauma

ACTIVITY
Bedrest until infection controlled and abscess evacuated or resolving, then up as tolerated

DIET
IV fluids if nausea and vomiting present

PATIENT EDUCATION
For patient education materials favorably reviewed on this topic, contact: Brain Research Foundation, 208 S. LaSalle Street, Suite 1426, Chicago, IL 60604, (312)782-4311

Brain abscess

MEDICATIONS

DRUG(S) OF CHOICE
• Antibiotics according to organism if known
• If organism unknown, begin with penicillin G 4 million units IV every 4 hours, and metronidazole 7.5 mg/kg IV or orally every 8 hours
• Add oxacillin or nafcillin 3 gm IV every 4 hours if trauma or IV drug user
• If infection of otic origin, add third-generation cephalosporin
• Abscess associated with HIV infection assumed to be due to Toxoplasma gondii - daily doses of sulfadiazine 2-8 gm orally and pyrimethamine 50-75 mg orally. (Therapy will be life-long in AIDS patients.)
• Anticonvulsants - phenytoin 100 mg IV or orally every 8 hours, or phenobarbital 30-60 mg IV or by mouth every 6-8 hours. Continue until abscess resolved or perhaps longer. Obtain anticonvulsant levels.
• Following surgical procedure - corticosteroids to reduce edema. Dexamethasone 10 mg IV every 4-6 hours. Taper rapidly. Use usually limited to 1 week. Continue antibiotics for 6-8 weeks.
Contraindications: Sensitivity or allergy to any prescribed medications
Precautions:
• Sulfadiazine poorly water soluble. Patients must maintain adequate hydration or risk developing crystalluria.
• Decrease dosage of penicillins in patients with renal dysfunction
• Monitor serum levels of anticonvulsants
Significant possible interactions: Refer to manufacturer's literature

ALTERNATIVE DRUGS   N/A

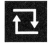
FOLLOWUP

PATIENT MONITORING
• Postsurgical monitoring as needed
• Serial CT or MRI - to confirm progressive resolution, early detection and management of complications

PREVENTION/AVOIDANCE
• Adequate treatment of otitis media, mastoiditis, dental abscess, other predisposing factors
• Prophylactic antibiotics after compound skull fracture or penetrating head wound

POSSIBLE COMPLICATIONS
• Permanent neurological deficits
• Surgical complications
• Recurrent abscess
• Seizures

EXPECTED COURSE AND PROGNOSIS   Survival > 85% with early diagnosis and treatment

MISCELLANEOUS

ASSOCIATED CONDITIONS
• AIDS
• Congenital heart disease

AGE-RELATED FACTORS
Pediatric:
• About one third of cases in pediatric age group. Rarely found in infants under 1 year of age.
• Cyanotic congenital heart disease frequently associated
Geriatric: Age does not affect outcome as much as abscess size and state of neurological dysfunction at presentation
Others: N/A

PREGNANCY N/A

SYNONYMS Cerebral abscess

ICD-9-CM 324.0

SEE ALSO N/A

OTHER NOTES N/A

ABBREVIATIONS N/A

REFERENCES
• Patel, K.S. & Marks, P.V.: Management of focal intracranial infections: Is medical treatment better than surgery? J Neuro Neurosurg Psychiatry 53:472, 1990
• Maniglia, A.J., Goodwin, W.J., Arnold, J.E., et al.: Intracranial abscesses secondary to nasal, sinus, and orbital infections in adults and children. Arch Otolaryngol Head Neck Surg 115:1424, 1989
• Rowland, L.: Merritt's Textbook of Neurology. 8th Ed. Philadelphia, Lea & Febiger, 1989
• Osenbach, R.K. & Loftus, C.M.: Diagnosis and Management of Brain Abscess. Neurosurgery Clinics of North America. 1992;3:403-420

Author D. Levinson, M.D.

Brain injury, traumatic

BASICS

DESCRIPTION Traumatic brain injury (TBI) is a principal cause of death and disability in young adults, at an estimated cost of $25 billion per year in the USA
Several themes underlie discussions of TBI:
◊ TBI comprises a spectrum of disorders in terms of severity and agent of injury
◊ The most common, closed head injury, is most often related to a rapid deceleration of the head, with or without impact, and results in relatively reproducible pathology
◊ TBI is a dynamic process. Not only does the pathologic picture evolve over the first few hours and days after trauma (often with devastating secondary injury), but the physiologic and clinical aspects of recovery continues for years.
◊ The prognosis often requires frequent revision because of the long period of recovery and the multiple, poorly understood variables involved
◊ The outcome from TBI is a composite of neurologic, cognitive, behavioral and psychosocial variables, where the last two variables are probably most important.
◊ The young adult brain has a remarkable ability to compensate for injury; a factor to consider in predicting long-term outcome and in evaluating the value of specific rehabilitation strategies
◊ The TBI patient often manifests a multitude of systemic abnormalities, as a consequence of both brain injury and concomitant trauma outside the brain. Changes in nutrition, cardiopulmonary status, circulating catecholamines, and coagulation are all important.
System(s) affected: Nervous, Cardiovascular, Endocrine/Metabolic
Genetics: N/A
Incidence/Prevalence in USA: Incidence: 200/100,000; 500,000 hospitalizations and 75,000 deaths per year
Predominant age: 15-24
Predominant sex: Male > Female

SIGNS AND SYMPTOMS
• Loss of consciousness
• External signs of head injury
• Labored breathing
• Focal neurologic signs
• Decorticate or decerebrate rigidity
• Bloody cerebrospinal fluid
• Pupils unequal
• Rising blood pressure with increased intracranial pressure
• Posttraumatic amnesia

CAUSES
• Motor vehicle accident (50%)
• Falls
• Assault

RISK FACTORS
• Alcohol
• Prior head injury
• Contact sports

DIAGNOSIS

DIFFERENTIAL DIAGNOSIS Without external evidence or history of head injury other causes of coma should be considered (e.g., drug overdose, infection, metabolic, vascular causes)

LABORATORY N/A
Drugs that may alter lab results: N/A
Disorders that may alter lab results: N/A

PATHOLOGICAL FINDINGS
• Focal injury, including hematoma or contusion, most commonly seen in the orbito-frontal and anterior temporal lobes
• Diffuse axonal injury, which evolves over 12-24 hours and may occur even in mild head injury. A principal cause of long-term disability.
• Superimposed hypoxia/ischemia involving mainly the hippocampus and cortical vascular border zones
• Microvascular injury, also evolves over 6-12 hours and may persist for days. Is probably a major contributor to secondary brain swelling.
• Delayed secondary injury is one of the major determinants of ultimate tissue loss and of mortality. A cascade of biochemical events is set in motion by the trauma, including the generation of oxygen free radicals and the process of lipid peroxidation, release of kinins, excitotoxins, peptides, changes in calcium and magnesium metabolism and activation of the arachidonic acid chain. Acute management is aimed at minimizing this chain of events and protecting the brain from further injury.

SPECIAL TESTS Drug and alcohol screen, diffuse intravascular coagulation panel in severe TBI

IMAGING
• CT scan acutely in all patients with coma, skull fracture, lateralized neurologic signs, or progressive deterioration of Glasgow Coma Scores (GCS)
• Cervical x-ray (associated cervical fracture seen in 5% of severe TBI)
• MRI scan may be useful in post-acute and chronic followup

DIAGNOSTIC PROCEDURES
• Sequential GCS and checks for lateralized neurologic deficit and/or pupillary paralysis
• Intracranial pressure monitoring in comatose patients

TREATMENT

APPROPRIATE HEALTH CARE
Inpatient in intensive care unit for comatose patients

GENERAL MEASURES
Acute management:
◊ Immediate cardiopulmonary resuscitation, avoid hypotension or hypoxia, since the traumatized brain is exquisitely sensitive to hypoxia/ischemia
◊ Intubate the deeply comatose patient, sedate and/or paralyze if necessary
◊ Frequent monitoring with sequential GCS. Beware of the "talk and die" patient, who initially appears well, but deteriorates quickly.
◊ Consider evacuation of intracranial hematomas within 4 hours of injury
◊ Emphasize a "team approach"
◊ Management of systemic metabolic abnormalities. Avoid excessive use of glucose, since hyperglycemia may be detrimental in acute TBI.
Post-acute rehabilitation:
◊ Outcome from TBI is a composite of pre-injury status (intelligence, education) and neurologic, cognitive, behavioral and psycho-social deficits
◊ The most troublesome of these are often the behavioral and psycho-social
◊ The goal of rehabilitation is to aid the natural process of improvement and help the patient return to independent living
◊ While most TBI patients would probably benefit from some level of TBI-specific rehabilitation, the exact type and intensity of treatment for a given patient is debated
◊ Few, if any, rehabilitation strategies have been subjected to the level of scientific scrutiny applied to most other medical therapies
◊ Some over-zealous institutional programs could even be detrimental, particularly if they inadvertently foster continued dependence
◊ Rehabilitation should begin as soon as possible after injury
◊ Essential elements of treatment include proper counseling and support of patient and family, emphasis on training in decision making, behavioral modification, and return to independence

ACTIVITY As tolerated

DIET As tolerated

PATIENT EDUCATION
• National Head Injury Foundation help-line: 1-800-444-6443
• Printed patient information available from: A Chance to Grow, 5034 Oliver Avenue North, Minneapolis, MN 55430, (612)521-2266

MEDICATIONS

DRUG(S) OF CHOICE

Acute management:
◊ Morphine 4-12 mg q 2-4 hours for sedation (if needed)
◊ Paralysis with pancuronium bromide 4 mg q 2-4 hours prn (if needed)
◊ Mannitol, 1 gram/kg/8 hours for increased intracranial pressure
◊ Barbiturate coma for persistent elevation of intracranial pressure
◊ Phenytoin seizure prophylaxis for 2 weeks after severe head injury (GCS < 8 , contusions or hematoma on CT scan)
◊ If seizures occur, then carbamazepine to maintain therapeutic blood level
◊ Use of mega-dose corticosteroids to control acute brain swelling remains very controversial and is generally not recommended.

Chronic management:
◊ Medical control of agitation and aggression remains largely empiric and highly individualized
◊ Avoid neuroleptics such as haloperidol
◊ Consider carbamazepine, lithium, tricyclic antidepressants, beta-adrenergic blockers such as propranolol, or buspirone
◊ "Activating" antidepressants such as amantadine, bromocriptine, desipramine or fluoxetine may be useful in patients who are generally under-aroused with only occasional episodes of agitation

Contraindications: Refer to manufacturer's literature

Precautions: Refer to manufacturer's literature

Significant possible interactions: Refer to manufacturer's literature

ALTERNATIVE DRUGS N/A

FOLLOWUP

PATIENT MONITORING
• Schedule regular follow ups over the first 6-12 months post-injury, but especially over the first month
• Recommend a gradual return to work or school, even after mild to moderate head injury
• The post-concussion syndrome can follow even mild head injury without loss of consciousness and includes headaches, dizziness, fatigue and subtle cognitive or affective changes. Most of these improve markedly over the first 3 months.
• The most important element of mild TBI management, however, is the recognition that initially there is a genuine organic basis for all of these symptoms
• Proper counselling, symptomatic management and gradual return to normal activities is essential to prevent a post-traumatic neurosis which can become refractory to treatment

PREVENTION/AVOIDANCE
• Safety education
• Seat belts, bicycle and motorcycle helmets
• Protective headgear for contact sports

POSSIBLE COMPLICATIONS
• Delayed hematomas
• Maintain high levels of suspicion for chronic subdural hematoma, which may follow even "mild" head injury, especially in the elderly. Often present with headache, decreased mentation.
• Delayed hydrocephalus
• Emotional disturbances and psychiatric disorders resulting from head injury may be refractory to treatment
• Seizure disorders - in about 50% of penetrating head injuries, in about 11% of severe closed head injuries, and in < 5% of head injuries overall. Hematomas significantly increase risk of epilepsy.

EXPECTED COURSE AND PROGNOSIS
• Gradual improvement for many
• 30-50% of severe head injuries may be fatal
• Prolonged coma may be followed by satisfactory outcome

MISCELLANEOUS

ASSOCIATED CONDITIONS Alcohol and drug abuse

AGE-RELATED FACTORS
Pediatric: Outcome for children more positive
Geriatric:
• Poorer prognosis with increasing age
• Subdural hematomas are common after fall or blow; symptoms may be subtle
Others: None

PREGNANCY N/A

SYNONYMS Head injury

ICD-9-CM
• Skull and facial fractures - 800-804
• Concussion - 850
• Cerebral laceration or contusion - 851
• Hematoma - 852
• Other cerebral injury - 854

SEE ALSO
• Spinal cord injury
• Epilepsy

OTHER NOTES N/A

ABBREVIATIONS GCS = Glasgow Coma Score

REFERENCES
• Jennett, B. & Teasdale, G.: Management of Head Injury. Philadelphia, F.A. Davis Co., 1981
• Becker, S. & Gudeman, D.: Textbook of Head Injury. Philadelphia, W.B. Saunders Co., 1989

Author A. Salazar, M.D.

Branchial cleft fistula

 BASICS

DESCRIPTION
A congenital, abnormal tract connecting the skin of neck with an internal structure, resulting from failure of closure of a branchial cleft.
• May involve branchial clefts I-IV
Genetics: 10% have family history
System(s) affected: head and neck
Incidence in USA: Unknown
Prevalence in USA: Unknown
Predominant age: By definition are all present at birth although may remain unnoticed for some time. (Branchial cysts may not present until later childhood).
Predominant sex: Unknown

SIGNS AND SYMPTOMS
• Presence of tiny external opening usually on neck
• Spontaneous mucoid drainage
• External openings may also be marked by a skin tag or cartilage
• Infection may rarely be the presenting sign with erythema, swelling, pain, fever
• 10% are bilateral

CAUSES
• The 1st branchial cleft contributes to the tympanic cavity and eustachian tube. Related fistulae are very rare and tend to be infra or retroauricular. (Preauricular cysts and sinuses are not thought to be of branchial cleft origin).
• The 2nd branchial cleft forms the hyoid bone and tonsillar fossa. Related fistulae course between the internal and external carotid arteries, Internal opening usually at level of tonsillar fossa. External opening along anterior border of sternocleidomastoid muscle.
• 3rd & 4th branchial clefts form parathyroid glands, thymus and portions of thyroid (parafollicular cells). Fistulae are rare, those from 3rd cleft course lateral to carotid artery, both should have external ostia on lower anterior neck.

RISK FACTORS
Positive family history

 DIAGNOSIS

DIFFERENTIAL DIAGNOSIS
• External sinuses
• Branchial cysts must be differentiated from cystic hygroma, dermoid cysts, lymphadenopathy

LABORATORY
culture if signs of infection
Drugs that may alter lab results: N/A
Disorders that may alter lab results: N/A

PATHOLOGICAL FINDINGS
Lined by stratified squamous epithelium, may contain hair follicles, sweat glands, sebaceous glands, cartilage. Some are lined by ciliated columnar epithelium.

SPECIAL TESTS   N/A

IMAGING   N/A

DIAGNOSTIC PROCEDURES
• Sinogram or fistulogram may be done but is of little value

 TREATMENT

APPROPRIATE HEALTH CARE
• Surgical excision
• Outpatient status usually appropriate

GENERAL MEASURES
• Small transverse incision at external ostium with careful dissection of fistula
• Stepladder incisions may be needed
• End of fistula ligated flush with pharyngeal mucosa
• Drains are not used
• Antibiotics only for infection

ACTIVITY   N/A

DIET   N/A

PATIENT EDUCATION   N/A

MEDICATIONS

DRUG(S) OF CHOICE N/A
Contraindications: N/A
Precautions: N/A
Significant possible interactions: N/A

ALTERNATIVE DRUGS N/A

FOLLOWUP

PATIENT MONITORING
• Follow at weekly intervals, if infected, until resolution, than excision
• Postoperative visit at 2 weeks

PREVENTION/AVOIDANCE N/A

EXPECTED COURSE AND PROGNOSIS Good

POSSIBLE COMPLICATIONS
• Facial nerve injury
• Infection
• Carotid artery injury
• Possible recurrence if any epithelium remains
• Neoplastic degeneration of branchial remnants (about 250 reported cases) if not resected

MISCELLANEOUS

ASSOCIATED CONDITIONS Microtia and aural atresia occur with failure of development of 1st branchial cleft.

AGE-RELATED FACTORS
Pediatric: N/A
Geriatric: N/A
Others: N/A

PREGNANCY N/A

SYNONYMS N/A

ICD-9-CM
744.41 branchial cleft sinus or fistula

SEE ALSO N/A

OTHER NOTES Branchial cleft remnants, sinuses, cysts are also the result of failure of branchial cleft to complete its normal development

ABBREVIATIONS N/A

REFERENCES
• Ashcraft, K.W.& Holder, T.M.: Pediatric Surgery. 2nd Ed. Philadelphia, W.B. Saunders Co., 1993
• Welch, K.J., Randolph, J.G., Ravitch, M.M., O'Neill, J.A. & Rowe, M.I.: Pediatric Surgery. 4th Ed. Chicago, Year Book Medical Publishers, Inc., 1986.

Author T. Black, M.D.

Breast abscess

 BASICS

DESCRIPTION
Collection of pus usually localized. Can be associated with lactation or fistulous tracts secondary to squamous epithelial neoplasm or duct occlusion.
System(s) affected: Skin/Exocrine
Genetics: N/A
Incidence/Prevalence in USA: Common
Predominant age:
- Subareolar abscess: post-menopausal
- Puerperal abscess: pre-menopausal

Predominant sex: Female

SIGNS AND SYMPTOMS
- Tender breast lump, fluctuant, usually antilateral
- Erythema
- Draining pus
- Local edema
- Systemic malaise
- Fever
- Nipple and skin retraction
- Proximal lymphadenopathy

CAUSES
- Puerperal abscesses - blocked lactiferous duct
- Subareolar abscess - squamous epithelial neoplasm with keratin plugs or ductal extension with associated inflammation
- Peripheral abscess - stasis of the duct

RISK FACTORS
- Puerperal mastitis 5-11% go on to abscess
- Diabetes
- Rheumatoid arthritis
- Steroids
- Silicone/paraffin implants
- Lumpectomy with radiation
- Heavy cigarette smoking
- Nipple retraction

 DIAGNOSIS

DIFFERENTIAL DIAGNOSIS
- Carcinoma (inflammatory)
- Tuberculosis
- Actinomycosis
- Typhoid
- Sarcoid
- Syphilis
- Hydatid cyst
- Sebaceous cyst

LABORATORY
- Leukocytosis
- Elevated sedimentation rate
- Culture and sensitivity of drainage to identify pathogen, usually staphylococci or streptococcus

Drugs that may alter lab results: None
Disorders that may alter lab results: None

PATHOLOGICAL FINDINGS
- Squamous metaplasia of the ducts
- Intraductal hyperplasia
- Epithelial overgrowth
- Fat necrosis
- Duct ectasia

SPECIAL TESTS   None

IMAGING
- Ultrasound
- Mammogram

DIAGNOSTIC PROCEDURES   Aspiration for culture

 TREATMENT

APPROPRIATE HEALTH CARE
Outpatient unless systemically immunocompromised.

GENERAL MEASURES
- Aspiration
- Cold compresses
- Expression of milk
- Incision and drainage with removal of loculations and biopsy of all non-puerperal abscesses
- Opening all fistulous tracts

ACTIVITY   No restrictions

DIET   No restrictions

PATIENT EDUCATION
- Care of wound
- Breast feeding precautions

MEDICATIONS

DRUG(S) OF CHOICE
- Non-steroidal anti-inflammatory agents
- Erythromycin 250-500mg qid
- First generation, oral cephalosporin
  ◊ cephalexin 500 mg bid
  ◊ cefaclor 250mg tid
- Amoxicillin/clavulanate (Augmentin) 250mg tid

Contraindications: Allergy to antibiotic

Precautions: Refer to manufacturer's profile of each drug

Significant possible interactions: Refer to manufacturer's profile of each drug

ALTERNATIVE DRUGS N/A

FOLLOWUP

PATIENT MONITORING Assure resolution to exclude carcinoma

PREVENTION/AVOIDANCE
- Early treatment of mastitis with milk expression and cold compresses
- Early treatment with antibiotics

POSSIBLE COMPLICATIONS Fistula

EXPECTED COURSE AND PROGNOSIS Good. Complete healing expected in 8 to 10 days, particularly if abscess can be incised and drained.

MISCELLANEOUS

ASSOCIATED CONDITIONS N/A

AGE-RELATED FACTORS
Pediatric: N/A
Geriatric: N/A
Others: N/A

PREGNANCY Most commonly associated with postpartum lactation

SYNONYMS
- Mammary abscess
- Peripheral breast abscess
- Subareolar abscess
- Puerperal abscess

ICD-9-CM
- Acute, chronic, nonpuerperal 611.0
- Puerperal, postpartum 675.1

SEE ALSO N/A

OTHER NOTES N/A

ABBREVIATIONS N/A

REFERENCES
- Benson, E.A.: Management of breast abscesses. World J Surg 1989; 13:753-756
- Dixon, J.M.: Periductal mastitis/duct ectasia. World J Surg 1989; 13:715-720
- Ferrara, J.J., et al.: Non surgical management of breast infections in non lactating women. Am Surg 1990; 56:668-671
- Olsen, C.G. & Gordon, R.E.: Breast disorders in nursing mothers. Am Fam Physician 1990; 41:1509-1515
- Smallwood, J.A.: Benign breast disease. Baltimore, Urban & Schwarzenberg, 1990

Author T. Strigle, M.D. & D. Moorman, M.D.

Breast cancer

BASICS

DESCRIPTION Malignant neoplasm in the breast. Breast cancers are classified as noninvasive (in situ) or invasive (infiltrating) with approximately 70% of all breast cancers possessing a component of invasion.

System(s) affected: Skin/Exocrine

Genetics: Only 20% of patients have a significant family history of breast cancer. This predisposition tends to be autosomal dominant with maternal lineage.

Incidence/Prevalence in USA:
• 1 in 9 women will develop breast cancer within a lifetime
• 150,000 new cases are diagnosed annually, and 50,000 women die annually

Predominant age: 30-80 with peak age 45-65

Predominant sex: Female > Male (1% occurs in male)

SIGNS AND SYMPTOMS
• Palpable mass (55%)
• Abnormal mammogram without a palpable mass (35%)
• Color change (peau d'orange)
• Dimpling
• Nipple retraction
• Breast enlargement
• Axillary mass
• Bone pain (rare)

CAUSES Unknown

RISK FACTORS
• Increased breast cancer risk occurs in first degree relatives (relative risk (RR) = 2.3), with bilateral disease in premenopausal relatives [RR = 10.5], or bilateral disease in postmenopausal relatives (RR = 5.0)
• Increased hormone risks include early menarche, late menopause, nulliparity or first full term pregnancy after age 30
• Women with a prior history of breast cancer or previous breast biopsies revealing atypical changes are at increased risk (5-10 times) for subsequent cancer
• Inconclusive risk factors include exogenous estrogen use, high dietary fat, or high alcohol use

DIAGNOSIS

DIFFERENTIAL DIAGNOSIS
• Differential diagnosis is extensive
• Benign breast disorders such as abscesses, hematomas, or fibroadenomas
• Proliferative breast diseases such as fibrocystic changes, ductal and lobular hyperplasia, or sclerosing adenosis
• Malignant breast diseases including sarcomas, lymphomas, or metastatic disease to breast

LABORATORY Complete blood counts and blood tests of liver and bone function are routinely performed at time of definitive diagnosis

Drugs that may alter lab results: None
Disorders that may alter lab results: None

PATHOLOGICAL FINDINGS
Noninvasive cancers
  ◊ The percentage of non-invasive cancers diagnosed is increasing due to increased mammography screening
  ◊ Usually detected by abnormal mammogram
  ◊ Noninvasive cancers are of two types: Intraductal or intralobular. Intraductal cancers are subdivided by growth patterns: Micropapillary, cribriform, solid, or comedo. The comedo growth pattern is considered more aggressive.
Invasive cancers
  ◊ Tend to present with a breast lump
  ◊ Subdivided into - not-otherwise-specified (50%), lobular (5%), Paget's disease (2%), and miscellaneous (metaplastic, neuroendocrine, or squamous cell carcinomas [1%])
  ◊ Patients with invasive histologies with medullary 6%, colloid 7%, tubular, papillary, and adenoid cystic carcinomas 2%, have improved survival

SPECIAL TESTS
• Assessment of estrogen receptor (ER) and progesterone receptor (PgR) activity on breast cancer tissue has diagnostic and prognostic significance
• Evaluation of HER-2/neu expression, epidermal growth factor receptor (EGF-R), cathepsin D, ploidy analysis, and S phase activity remains investigational
• CA 15-3 and carcinoembryonic antigen (CEA) are investigational blood tests

IMAGING
• Mammography, which detects 80% of breast cancers, is the best technique for the detection of minimal (< 0.5 cm) breast cancer. The most common abnormality representing cancer is an irregular mass. Microcalcifications can occur as the only sign of malignancy in 35% of breast cancers.
• Ultrasound may confirm whether a suspicious lump is solid or cystic
• After diagnosis, baseline bone scan, chest x-ray, and liver imaging (nuclear medicine scan or CT scan) are often performed

DIAGNOSTIC PROCEDURES
• Tissue confirmation of the suspicious mass or abnormal mammogram is essential. Biopsy may be excisional or incisional depending upon the size and location of the abnormality.
• Biopsy of non-palpable lesions is achieved with needle localization
• Cytologic confirmation of a palpable abnormality may be obtained by fine needle aspiration

TREATMENT

APPROPRIATE HEALTH CARE
Patients are usually treated by a team consisting of a medical oncologist, a surgeon, and a radiation oncologist

GENERAL MEASURES
• The decision to treat with hormone or chemotherapy is very complex. Premenopausal women tend to respond more to cytotoxic chemotherapy, and postmenopausal women tend to obtain greater benefit with hormone therapy. Other important factors in the treatment decision include ER and PgR status, nuclear grade, site of metastasis, etc.
Breast cancer treatment for early stage disease (Stage I or II)
  ◊ Consists of local control measures and treatment of micrometastatic disease
  ◊ Either modified radical mastectomy or lumpectomy followed by radiation
  ◊ Axillary nodal sampling should be performed with both procedures to assess probability of disease recurrence
  ◊ Disease-free and overall survival is similar with either procedure
  ◊ The optimal treatment for noninvasive or minimally invasive breast cancer is unclear
Treatment of locally advanced breast cancer (Stage III)
  ◊ Is multidisciplinary with most patients receiving combination cytotoxic chemotherapy and radiation therapy prior to mastectomy
Treatment of metastatic (Stage IV) disease
  ◊ Measures to provide symptom improvement
  ◊ Combinations of chemotherapy, hormone therapy, or radiation therapy

ACTIVITY Minimal activity restrictions exist during treatment

DIET No proven relationship exists between breast cancer and diet

PATIENT EDUCATION
• Patients are instructed in monthly breast self-examination to detect breast lumps, skin or nipple changes and the importance of mammography
• For patient education materials favorably reviewed on this topic, contact: American Academy of Family Physicians Foundation, P.O. Box 8418, Kansas City, MO 64114, (800)274-2237, ext. 4400

Breast cancer

MEDICATIONS

DRUG(S) OF CHOICE
• Adjuvant cytotoxic chemotherapy or hormone therapy is administered to many patients with Stage I or Stage II invasive disease to prevent cancer recurrence
• Therapeutic cytotoxic chemotherapy or hormone therapy is administered to patients with advanced or metastatic disease
• Metastatic disease is considered incurable, but treatable with remissions occurring in 30-40% of patients
• Combination chemotherapy with cyclophosphamide, methotrexate, fluorouracil, or anthracyclines are often used
• Tamoxifen is the most commonly used hormone agent in breast cancer; however, medroxyprogesterone and aminoglutethimide are also active agents
Contraindications: Strict hematologic, renal, hepatic, and cardiac guidelines need to be followed for the administration of cytotoxic chemotherapy
Precautions: Monitoring for infection is important for patients receiving chemotherapy
Significant possible interactions: Drug interactions are common and depend on combinations used. Refer to manufacturer's literature.

ALTERNATIVE DRUGS
Additional efficacious chemotherapy drugs include vinblastine, cisplatin, thiotepa, mitomycin, and etoposide

FOLLOWUP

PATIENT MONITORING
• Up to 60% of patients with invasive disease will relapse within five years despite initial therapy
• The status of the axillary lymph nodes is the most important indicator for disease relapse
• Clinical evaluation and physical examination are most important to detect relapses
• The role of followup blood testing and roentgenographic studies (except mammography) is poorly established

PREVENTION/AVOIDANCE
• Decreasing dietary fat or alcohol has not been shown to alter breast cancer risk
• The synthetic anti-estrogen, tamoxifen, may be a useful prophylactic agent in high risk women
Mammography
◊ In women over 50, mammography screening can reduce mortality by 30%
◊ All women over 35 should have baseline screening mammogram, and it should be repeated every 1-2 years between the ages of 40-49 and annually after 50
◊ Diagnostic mammography should be performed at the advice of the patient's physician

POSSIBLE COMPLICATIONS
• Post-operative: lymphedema (< 5% in modified radical mastectomy), seromas, wound infection, and limited shoulder motion
• Chemotherapy: nausea, vomiting, alopecia, leukopenia, bladder irritation, stomatitis, fatigue, and menstrual abnormalities
•Tamoxifen: hot flushes, menstrual irregularities including menopause, vaginal discharge, hypercalcemia, skin rashes, and possible endometrial carcinoma
• Irradiation: skin reaction, fibrosis (1%), brachial plexopathy (1%), rib fracture (1%), arm edema, pulmonary fibrosis (1%), and rarely second breast malignancy.

EXPECTED COURSE AND PROGNOSIS
10yr Survival
◊ Noninvasive - 95%: Stage I occult: tumors < 1 cm with no axillary node involvement
◊ I occult - 90%: Stage I overt: tumors > 1 cm with no axillary node involvement
◊ II - 40%: Stage II: tumors < 5 cm or axillary node involvement
◊ III - 15%: Stage III: tumors > 5 cm or with chest wall or skin extension, inflammatory changes, or supraclavicular involvement
◊ IV - 0%: Stage IV: metastatic

MISCELLANEOUS

ASSOCIATED CONDITIONS Organ disease at metastatic sites

AGE-RELATED FACTORS Age-specific incidence of breast cancer increases sharply until menopause and continues to increase at a slower rate in the geriatric population
Pediatric: Breast cancer occurs rarely in children with the most common pathology being secretory carcinoma
Geriatric: There is a higher percentage of ER positive tumors (80%) in the geriatric population. This correlates with improved disease-free survival.
Others: N/A

PREGNANCY Breast cancer occurs infrequently during pregnancy (2.8%). Delay in diagnosis is common, and most series report poorer survival related to advanced stage at diagnosis.

SYNONYMS N/A

ICD-9-CM
174 Malignant neoplasm of female breast
175 Malignant neoplasm of male breast

SEE ALSO N/A

OTHER NOTES N/A

ABBREVIATIONS N/A

REFERENCES
• Fisher, B., Redmond, C., Poisson, R., et al.: Eight year results of the NSABP randomized clinical trial comparing total mastectomy and lumpectomy with or without radiation in the treatment of breast cancer. N Engl J Med 320(13):822-828, 1989
• Baker, L.H.: The Breast Cancer Demonstration Project: five-year summary report. CA 32(4):194-198, 1982
• Harris, J.R. & Hellman, S.: The results of primary radiation therapy for early breast cancer at the Joint Center for Radiation Therapy. In Conservation Management of Breast Cancer. Edited by J.R. Harris, S. Hellman & W. Silen. Philadelphia, J.B. Lippincott Co., 1983
• Nolvadex Adjuvant Trial Organization controlled trial of tamoxifen as single adjuvant agent in management of early breast cancer. Lancet 1:836-839, 1985
• Henderson, I.C., Garber, J.E., Breitmeyer, J.B., et al.: Comprehensive management of disseminated breast cancer. Cancer 66(6):1439-48, 1990

Author E. Lower, M.D.

Breast-feeding

 BASICS

DESCRIPTION

Advantages
◊ Fewer respiratory and gastrointestinal infections
◊ Ideal food - easily digestible, nutrients well absorbed, less constipation
◊ Increased contact between mother and baby and, perhaps, added self-esteem for mother
◊ Economical, portable, easy to meet needs quickly
◊ Prolonged breast-feeding (6 months or more) may decrease incidence of allergies in childhood
◊ Mothers often like it more than bottle feeding
◊ More rapid and complete reversion of mother's pelvis and uterus to pre-puerperal state

Contraindications
◊ HIV infection; active TB
◊ Hepatitis is not a contraindication
◊ Substances of abuse will pass into human milk; please see References on drugs in lactation

Physiology
◊ Stimulation of areola causes secretion of oxytocin
◊ Oxytocin is responsible for let-down reflex when milk is ejected from cells into milk ducts
◊ Sucking stimulates secretion of prolactin which triggers milk production. Thus milk is made in response to nursing and increases supply.

Technique
◊ Get in comfortable position, usually sitting or reclining with baby's head in crook of mother's arm (side-lying position often useful following C-Section delivery)
◊ Bring baby to mother to decrease stress on back
◊ Baby's belly and mother's belly should face each other or touch (belly-to-belly)
◊ Initiate the rooting reflex by tickling baby's lips with nipple or finger. As baby's mouth opens wide, mother guides her nipple to back of her baby's mouth while pulling the baby closer. This will ensure that the baby's gums are sucking on the areola, not the nipple.

System(s) affected: Endocrine/Metabolic, Skin/Exocrine

Genetics: N/A

Incidence/Prevalence in USA: A recent paper reported that 52% of women initiated breast-feeding and 18% were still breast-feeding at 6 months. This was a decrease from figures 5 years ago (Peds 88:719-727 10/91).

Predominant age: 16-45

Predominant sex: Female only

SIGNS AND SYMPTOMS   N/A

CAUSES   N/A

RISK FACTORS   N/A

 DIAGNOSIS

DIFFERENTIAL DIAGNOSIS   N/A

LABORATORY   N/A
Drugs that may alter lab results: N/A
Disorders that may alter lab results: N/A

PATHOLOGICAL FINDINGS   N/A

SPECIAL TESTS   N/A

IMAGING   N/A

DIAGNOSTIC PROCEDURES   N/A

 TREATMENT

APPROPRIATE HEALTH CARE
Outpatient

GENERAL MEASURES   See Patient education

ACTIVITY   No restrictions

DIET
• Adequate calorie and protein intake while nursing
• Drink plenty of fluids
• Continue prenatal vitamins
• Fluoride supplement unnecessary if mother drinks fluoridated water

PATIENT EDUCATION

Antepartum
◊ Regular promotion of advantages of breast-feeding
◊ Discuss woman's postpartum plans, i.e., if going to work. Emphasize possibility of nursing part-time after returning to work or nursing until weaning the week before returning to work
◊ For some mothers, you need to explain that an occasional supplemental bottle can be used to give them time away from their baby
◊ Counsel women on technique

Natural history
◊ Colostrum present in breast at birth but may not be seen
◊ Milk will not come in before 3rd day postpartum
◊ Frequent nursing (at least 9 or more times/24 hours) will lead to milk coming in sooner and in greater quantities
◊ Allow baby to determine duration of each nursing; baby will lose weight the first few days and may not get back to birth weight until day 10

Postpartum
◊ Immediate breast-feeding after the birth
◊ Rooming-in to encourage on-demand feeding
◊ Observation of a nursing session by experienced physician or nurse
◊ Avoid formula or water supplementation
◊ Review expectations, techniques. Be very encouraging.
◊ See in office within a few days of discharge, especially if first-time nursing

Signs of adequate nursing
◊ Breasts become hard before and soft after feeding
◊ 6 or more wet diapers in 24 hours
◊ Baby satisfied; appropriate weight gain (average one ounce/day in first few months)
◊ Growth spurts - anticipate these around 10 days, 6 weeks, 3 months, and 4-6 months. Baby will nurse more often at these times for several days. This will increase milk production to allow for further adequate growth.
◊ Supplemental baby vitamins are unnecessary unless the baby has very limited exposure to sun (then needs vitamin D)
Weaning
◊ Breast milk alone is adequate food for first 6 months
◊ Solids may be introduced at 4-6 months
◊ For mothers going to work, start switching the baby to bottle feeding during the hours mother will be gone about a week ahead of time. Do this by dropping a breast-feed every few days and substituting pumped breast milk or formula, preferably given by another caregiver.
◊ To increase the likelihood that baby will take a bottle occasionally, introduce it at 3-4 weeks and give once or twice a week

MEDICATIONS

DRUG(S) OF CHOICE N/A
Contraindications: N/A
Precautions: N/A
Significant possible interactions: N/A

ALTERNATIVE DRUGS N/A

FOLLOWUP

PATIENT MONITORING See mother and baby within a few days of hospital discharge if she is a first-time breast-feeder

PREVENTION/AVOIDANCE N/A

POSSIBLE COMPLICATIONS
Plugged ducts (mother is well except for)
◊ Sore lump in one or both breasts without fever
◊ Use moist hot packs on lump prior to and during nursing; more frequent nursing on affected side; ensure good technique
Mastitis
◊ Sore lump in one or both breasts plus fever and/or redness on skin overlying lump
◊ Use moist hot packs on lump prior to and during nursing; more frequent nursing on affected side; antibiotics covering for Staph Aureus (the most common organism) for at least 7 days
◊ Patients can be quite ill with mastitis
◊ Other possible sources of fever should be ruled out - endometritis, pyelonephritis in particular. Mother should get increased rest, use acetaminophen (Tylenol) as necessary. Fever should resolve within 48 hours or consider changing antibiotics. Lump should also resolve. If it continues, an abscess may be present requiring surgical drainage.
Milk supply inadequate
◊ Check weight gain
◊ Review signs of adequate supply; review technique, frequency and duration of nursing
◊ Check to see if mother has been supplementing, thereby decreasing her own milk production
Sore nipples
◊ Check technique
◊ Baby should be taken off the breast by breaking the suction with a finger in the mouth
◊ Air-dry nipples after each nursing; no breast creams and do not wash nipples with soap and water; check for signs of thrush in baby and mother
Engorgement
◊ Usually develops after milk first comes in (day 3 or 4)
◊ Signs are warm, hard, sore breasts
◊ To resolve, offer baby more frequent nursing; may have to hand express a little milk to soften areola enough to let baby latch on; nurse long enough to empty breasts; generally resolves within a day or two
Flat or inverted nipples
◊ When stimulated, inverted nipples will retract inward, flat nipples remain flat; should check for this on initial prenatal physical
◊ Nipple shells, a doughnut-shaped insert, can be worn inside the bra during the last month of pregnancy to gently force the nipple through the center opening of the shell
◊ Babies can nurse successfully even if the shell does not correct the problem before birth. A lactation consultant or La Leche League member may be a good resource in this situation. Another source: J Human Lactation. 9(1):27-29, 1993.

EXPECTED COURSE AND PROGNOSIS
Healthy baby

MISCELLANEOUS

ASSOCIATED CONDITIONS N/A

AGE-RELATED FACTORS N/A
Pediatric: N/A
Geriatric: N/A
Others: N/A

PREGNANCY N/A

SYNONYMS N/A

ICD-9-CM N/A

SEE ALSO N/A

OTHER NOTES N/A

ABBREVIATIONS N/A

REFERENCES
• Breastfeeding Triage Tool. Seattle-King County Dept of Public Health, 110 Prefontaine South, Suite 500, Seattle, Wash 98104
• Briggs, et al.: Drugs in Pregnancy and Lactation. 3rd Ed. New York, Williams and Wilkins, 1990
• Lawrence, R.A.: Breastfeeding: A Guide for the Medical Profession. 3rd Ed. St. Louis, C.V. Mosby Co., 1989

Author E. Henley, M.D., M.P.H.

Breech birth

BASICS

DESCRIPTION At the time of delivery the fetal buttocks are the presenting part in the maternal pelvis
• Frank breech presentation - the fetal hips are flexed and the knees extended with the feet near the shoulders, accounting for 60-65% of breech presentations at term
• Incomplete breech presentation - one or both of the fetal hips are incompletely flexed, resulting in some part of the fetal lower extremity as the presenting part. Thus the terms single footling, double footling, knee presentation. Accounts for 25-35% of breech presentations.
• Complete breech - similar to frank breech except one or both knees are flexed rather than extended. Accounts for 5% of breech presentations.
System(s) affected: Reproductive
Genetics: N/A
Incidence/Prevalence in USA: 3-4% of singleton term deliveries and up to 15-30% of low birth weight infants (< 2500 grams)
Predominant age: N/A
Predominant sex: Female only

SIGNS AND SYMPTOMS
• Anus palpable on digital vaginal exam
• Leopold's maneuver reveals ballottable head in fundal region

CAUSES Probably a combination of one or more of the risk factors listed below

RISK FACTORS
• Fetal anomalies including anencephaly, hydrocephalus, trisomy 21
• Uterine anomalies
• Uterine relaxation associated with great parity
• Uterine overdistension as in polyhydramnios or multiple gestation
• Placenta previa
• Placental implantation in cornual-fundal region
• Low birth weight or premature infant

DIAGNOSIS

DIFFERENTIAL DIAGNOSIS Diagnosis is made by vaginal exam and confirmed by ultrasound. Can be confused with face presentation on digital vaginal exam.

LABORATORY None
Drugs that may alter lab results: N/A
Disorders that may alter lab results: N/A

PATHOLOGICAL FINDINGS Congenital malformation among term breech infants: Overall incidence 9.0%

SPECIAL TESTS N/A

IMAGING
• Ultrasound - confirms presenting part
• X-ray - flat plate of abdomen and pelvimetry to determine extent of head flexion and pelvic measurements

DIAGNOSTIC PROCEDURES N/A

TREATMENT

APPROPRIATE HEALTH CARE
Inpatient for labor and delivery

GENERAL MEASURES
• Breech delivery is accomplished either vaginally or by cesarean section
• When a patient presents in labor with the fetus in breech position, a decision about a trial of labor or immediate cesarean section must be made
• Obtain a scout film of the abdomen and pelvimetry and estimate fetal weight to assess candidacy for vaginal delivery
• The selection criteria for vaginal delivery are fairly strict to reduce morbidity and mortality for both mother and infant
Cesarean section is recommended in the following circumstances unless the fetus is too immature to survive:
◊ Large (> 3500 grams) or small (< 1500 grams) fetus, estimated by ultrasound or skilled observer
◊ Pelvic contraction or unfavorable pelvic shape (platypelloid and android)
◊ Hyperextended head
◊ Significant fetal heart rate abnormality
◊ Footling breech
◊ Severe fetal growth retardation
◊ Premature fetus greater than 26 weeks with mother in active labor
◊ Previous cesarean section
◊ Abnormal labor including failure to dilate, prolonged second stage, and failure of descent

Cesarean section procedure:
◊ Prepare for cesarean section by starting IV fluids and obtaining blood type and screen, in all patients, in case needed for emergency
◊ A low transverse cesarean section may need to be extended vertically if there is difficulty with head entrapment
◊ General anesthesia with isoflurane can rapidly relax the uterus and allow delivery of an entrapped after-coming head
◊ Cord blood gases should be obtained following delivery
Vaginal delivery procedures:
◊ The candidate for vaginal delivery needs to be attended by a birth attendant skilled in breech delivery, a scrubbed assistant, an anesthesiologist capable of rapid induction of general anesthesia, and an individual skilled in neonatal resuscitation
◊ Leave membranes intact as long as possible to prevent possible cord prolapse
◊ The patient should not push until fully dilated
◊ Cut large episiotomy to allow sufficient room for delivery
◊ The infant should not be touched before the umbilicus crosses the maternal perineum
◊ Traction prior to this point constitutes a complete breech extraction and is associated with higher risk of perinatal morbidity and mortality
◊ With the fetal back anterior, maintain downward traction while grasping the fetal hips until the scapula becomes visible
◊ As one axilla becomes visible rotate the infant until the shoulders are oriented anteriorly and posteriorly allowing their delivery
◊ The fetal head is delivered in a face down position with either piper forceps or manual flexion of the head
◊ Cord blood gases should be obtained following delivery

ACTIVITY Bedrest during labor

DIET Nothing by mouth until delivery accomplished

PATIENT EDUCATION Come to the hospital at the first sign of labor

MEDICATIONS

DRUG(S) OF CHOICE None
Contraindications: N/A
Precautions: N/A
Significant possible interactions: N/A

ALTERNATIVE DRUGS N/A

FOLLOWUP

PATIENT MONITORING
• Continuous fetal heart rate monitoring should be done during labor and delivery
• Six weeks postpartum care is done as with other deliveries

PREVENTION/AVOIDANCE
External version
◊ Conversion to vertex presentation can be attempted from 30-36 weeks gestation
◊ External version can cause abruption, premature rupture of membranes, and feto-maternal hemorrhage
◊ Should only be attempted with continuous fetal heart monitoring in the delivery suite where immediate cesarean section can be done

POSSIBLE COMPLICATIONS
• Trauma to head, soft tissue, brachial plexus and spinal cord - not always prevented by cesarean
• Asphyxia secondary to cord compression or prolapse

EXPECTED COURSE AND PROGNOSIS
• Perinatal morbidity and mortality are much higher in breech births. A large proportion of the deaths are related to congenital abnormalities.
• In patients properly selected for vaginal delivery, potentially perinatal morbidity and mortality, and maternal morbidity are reduced
• For infants less than 1500 grams, there is a much higher rate of cerebral hemorrhage and perinatal death associated with vaginal compared to cesarean delivery

MISCELLANEOUS

ASSOCIATED CONDITIONS See Risk Factors

AGE-RELATED FACTORS
Pediatric: N/A
Geriatric: N/A
Others: N/A

PREGNANCY A problem of pregnancy

SYNONYMS N/A

ICD-9-CM
• Breech extraction (assisted) 72.52
• Above with forceps to after-coming head 72.51
• Total breech extraction 72.54
• Above with forceps to after-coming head 72.53
• Cesarean section lower uterine segment 74.1

SEE ALSO N/A

OTHER NOTES Maneuvers of cesarean breech delivery are similar to vaginal breech extraction and can be associated with severe trauma to the infant

ABBREVIATIONS N/A

REFERENCES Cunningham, F.G., MacDonald, P.C. & Gant, N.F. (eds.): Williams Obstetrics. 18th Ed. Norwalk, CT, Appleton & Lange, 1989

Author K. Vore, M.D.

Bronchiectasis

 BASICS

DESCRIPTION Persistent and irreversible, abnormal dilatation of the bronchi, usually accompanied by infection. Associated with many conditions including some that are congenital or hereditary. Usual course - chronic.

System(s) affected: Pulmonary

Genetics: No single known genetic pattern. See Causes.

Incidence/Prevalence in USA:
• No reliable figures available
• Less common than it once was, probably due to more effective treatment of childhood respiratory infections

Predominant age:
• Middle age (40-75 years)
• Begins most often in early childhood, but symptoms may not appear until later in life

Predominant sex: Male = Female

SIGNS AND SYMPTOMS
• Coarse or moist crackles
• Rhonchi
• Wheezing
• Cough
• Cyanosis
• Decreased breath sounds
• Digital clubbing
• Dyspnea
• Emaciation
• Fatigue
• Fever
• Recurrent pneumonia
• Halitosis
• Hemoptysis
• Orthopnea
• Otitis media, mild deafness
• Pallor
• Sputum, copious, foul-smelling, muco-purulent
• Tachycardia
• Tachypnea
• Weight loss

CAUSES
• Necrotizing pulmonary infections
• Pulmonary abscess
• Bronchial obstruction
• Hypogammaglobulinemia
• Tuberculosis
• Dyskinetic cilia syndrome
• Alpha-1-antitrypsin deficiency
• Aspergillosis
• Kartagener's syndrome (situs in versus, chronic sinusitis, immotile spermatozoa, infertility, bronchiectasis)
• Cystic fibrosis
• Inhaling noxious chemicals
• Severe lung infection in childhood (measles, pertussis, or bronchiolitis)

RISK FACTORS
• Repeated bouts of pneumonia
• Any chronic respiratory illness

 DIAGNOSIS

DIFFERENTIAL DIAGNOSIS
• Chronic bronchitis
• Chronic obstructive pulmonary disease
• Cystic fibrosis
• Pulmonary tuberculosis

LABORATORY
• Anemia
• Positive sputum culture (yields H. influenzae, Streptococcus pneumoniae, staphylococcal or anaerobes)
• Hypoxemia
• Leukocytosis, usually
• Serum immunoglobulins - check for hypogammaglobulinemia, IgE level helpful

Drugs that may alter lab results: N/A

Disorders that may alter lab results: N/A

PATHOLOGICAL FINDINGS
• Bronchi dilatation
• Inflamed bronchi
• Purulent bronchorrhea
• Necrosis of bronchial mucosa
• Peribronchial scarring

SPECIAL TESTS
• Sweat test if cystic fibrosis is suspected
• Skin test for aspergillus
• Respiratory function
• Bronchoscopy useful in locating bleeding site and to exclude adenoma or foreign body
• Ciliary biopsy with electron microscopy (EM)
• Pulmonary function tests

IMAGING
Bronchography
◊ For definitive diagnosis, to help determine extent, and if surgery contemplated
◊ Respiratory function must be optimal (following postural drainage, physiotherapy and bronchodilators)
◊ Performed on only one side at a time
◊ Bronchi dilatation
Fiberoptic bronchoscopy
◊ Recommended when disease is of recent onset or is unilateral
◊ May be combined with bronchography
Chest x-ray
◊ Often normal
◊ Coarse lung markings
◊ Air-fluid level
◊ Cystic lesions
◊ Lung density
CT scan
◊ Less sensitive for diagnosing bronchiectasis in children
◊ Shows dilation of airways
◊ High resolution scans best

DIAGNOSTIC PROCEDURES
• Bronchography
• Bronchoscopy

 TREATMENT

APPROPRIATE HEALTH CARE
Outpatient except for possible surgery

GENERAL MEASURES
• Postural drainage
• Hydration
• Pulmonary resection for severe hemoptysis or destroyed lung (rarely necessary); only if localized
• Bronchial artery embolization may be lifesaving for massive pulmonary hemorrhage
• Physiotherapy to promote drainage
• Avoid cigarette smoking
• Bronchoscopy may be required for extraction of mucus or mycelial plugs, or if physiotherapy has failed

ACTIVITY As fully active as possible

DIET No restrictions

PATIENT EDUCATION Printed patient information available from: American Lung Association, 1740 Broadway, New York, NY 10019, (212)315-8700

MEDICATIONS

DRUG(S) OF CHOICE
Bronchodilators (dependent on pulmonary function tests)
◊ May be helpful for patients with associated asthma or aspergillosis
◊ Beta-adrenergic agonists (e.g., terbutaline) given by metered dose inhaler or with use of a spacer (reservoir device)
Antibiotics
Dependent on culture results, use at intervals
◊ Ampicillin: 250-500 mg orally q 6 hours (50 mg/kg/day in divided doses q 6-8 hours in children less than 20 kg)
or
◊ Tetracycline - 250-500 mg orally q 6 hours (not for use in children under 8, or in pregnancy)
Steroids
Consider for patients with bronchopulmonary aspergillosis. IgE level determines steroid dosing.
Contraindications: Refer to manufacturer's literature
Precautions: Refer to manufacturer's literature
Significant possible interactions: Refer to manufacturer's literature

ALTERNATIVE DRUGS
• For chronic persistent infection, long-term high dose of amoxicillin 3 g every 12 hours is recommended. It does not provide relief for everyone and has more side effects.
• For smokers, use of nicotine replacement (patch system or gum) to aid in smoking cessation. Patients should be counseled not to smoke while on nicotine patches.

FOLLOWUP

PATIENT MONITORING
• Frequent followup for progress of illness, prevention of infection, smoking cessation, and to check on physiotherapy
• At some point in followup, need to discuss with patient the possibility of mechanical ventilation and cardiopulmonary resuscitation in the future. The patient and family should determine if this type of treatment is appropriate.

PREVENTION/AVOIDANCE
• Treat all pneumonias adequately
• Immunizations for viral illnesses (i.e., influenza)
• Immunization for pneumococcal pneumonia
• Routine childhood immunizations, e.g. pertussis, measles.

EXPECTED COURSE AND PROGNOSIS
Chronic. Surgery may be curative if disease localized.

POSSIBLE COMPLICATIONS
• Recurrent pulmonary infections
• Pulmonary hypertension
• Secondary amyloidosis
• Cor pulmonale
• Brain abscess

MISCELLANEOUS

ASSOCIATED CONDITIONS
• Sinusitis
• Cor pulmonale

AGE-RELATED FACTORS
Pediatric: Cystic fibrosis must be ruled out
Geriatric: Elderly more likely to need hospitalization for treatment
Others: N/A

PREGNANCY N/A

SYNONYMS N/A

ICD-9-CM 494 bronchiectasis

SEE ALSO N/A

OTHER NOTES
Conditions that may lead to bronchiectasis include severe pneumonia (especially measles, pertussis, adenoviral infections in children), necrotizing infections due to Klebsiella, staphylococci, influenza virus, fungi, mycobacteria, mycoplasma, bronchial obstruction from any cause (foreign body, carcinoma, enlarged mediastinal lymph nodes

ABBREVIATIONS N/A

REFERENCES N/A

Author K. Hardy, M.D.

Bronchiolitis

 BASICS

DESCRIPTION Inflammation of the bronchioles, usually seen in young children, occasionally in high-risk adults. May be seasonal (winter and spring) and often occurs in epidemics. Usual course: insidious; acute; progressive.
Genetics: N/A
System(s) affected: Pulmonary
Incidence/Prevalence in USA: Medical care provided to 1000-1500/100,000 annually. Estimated incidence is higher.
Predominant age: newborn -2 years (peak age 2-6 months)
Predominant sex: Male > Female

SIGNS AND SYMPTOMS
• Anorexia
• Cough
• Cyanosis
• Expiratory wheezing
• Fever
• Grunting
• Inspiratory crackles
• Intercostal retractions
• Irritability
• Noisy breathing
• Otitis media
• Pharyngitis
• Tachycardia
• Tachypnea
• Vomiting

CAUSES
• Respiratory syncytial virus
• Parainfluenza
• Adenovirus
• Rhinovirus
• Influenza virus
• Chlamydia
• Eye, nose, mouth inoculation
• Exposure to older person with cold
• Day care exposure (significant)
• Idiopathic (most adult cases)

RISK FACTORS
• Contact with infected person
• Children in day care environment
• Heart-lung transplantation patient
• Adults - exposure to toxic fumes, connective tissue disease

 DIAGNOSIS

DIFFERENTIAL DIAGNOSIS
• Asthma
• Vascular ring
• Lobar emphysema
• Foreign body
• Heart disease
• Pneumonia
• Reflux
• Aspiration
• Cystic fibrosis

LABORATORY
• Arterial blood gas - hypoxemia, hypercarbia, acidemia
• Respiratory viral culture - positive
• Respiratory viral antigens - positive
Drugs that may alter lab results: N/A
Disorders that may alter lab results: N/A

PATHOLOGICAL FINDINGS
• Abundant mucous exudate
• Mucosal - hyperemia, edema
• Submucosal lymphocytic infiltrate, monocytic infiltrate, plasmacytic infiltrate
• Small airway debris, fibrin, inflammatory exudate, fibrosis
• Peribronchiolar mononuclear infiltrate

SPECIAL TESTS Pulmonary function studies

IMAGING
Chest x-ray
◊ Focal atelectasis
◊ Air trapping
◊ Flattened diaphragm
◊ Increased anteroposterior diameter
◊ Peribronchial cuffing

DIAGNOSTIC PROCEDURES N/A

 TREATMENT

APPROPRIATE HEALTH CARE
• Most patients can be treated at home
• Inpatient indicated for patient with increased respiratory distress, cyanosis,and dehydration

GENERAL MEASURES
• Most critical phase is first 48-72 hours after onset. Treatment is usually symptomatic.
• Fluid at maintenance
• Mechanical ventilation
• Isolation: contact
• Antiviral agents
• Cardio-respiratory monitoring
• Bronchodilators, especially inhaled
• Steroids not shown to change course

ACTIVITY
• Avoid exposure to crowds, viral illness for 2 months
• Avoid smoke

DIET
• Frequent small feedings of clear liquids
• If hospitalized, may require intravenous fluids

PATIENT EDUCATION Griffith:
Instructions for Patients; Philadephia, W.B. Saunders Co. p 37

MEDICATIONS

DRUG(S) OF CHOICE
• Oxygen
• Bronchodilators effective for acute symptoms. Corticosteroids do not change course.
• For infants and children - ribavirin - inhaled antiviral agent active against RSV. Indicated in patients with underlying cardio-pulmonary disease, young age (< 6 weeks), or with severe RSV (elevated pCO_2; require mechanical ventilation - use with caution via ventilator), Nebulize via small particle aerosol generator (SPAG).
• For adults - corticosteroids and bronchodilators may be effective in some patients
• Antibiotics only if secondary bacterial infection present (rare)
Contraindications: Refer to manufacturer's literature
Precautions: None
Significant possible interactions: None

ALTERNATIVE DRUGS N/A

FOLLOWUP

PATIENT MONITORING
• If patient is receiving home care, follow daily by telephone for 2-4 days
• For hospitalized patient, monitor as needed depending on severity of infection
• Bronchiolitis is associated with apnea.

PREVENTION/AVOIDANCE
• Hand washing
• Contact isolation of infected babies
• Persons with colds should keep contacts with infants to a minimum

EXPECTED COURSE AND PROGNOSIS
• In most cases, recovery is complete within a week
• Mortality statistics differ, but probably under 1%
• High-risk infants (BPD, CHD) may have prolonged course

POSSIBLE COMPLICATIONS
• Bacterial superinfection
• Viral obliterative bronchiolitis
• Apnea
• Respiratory failure
• Death
• Increased incidence of RAD

MISCELLANEOUS

ASSOCIATED CONDITIONS
• Common cold
• Conjunctivitis
• Pharyngitis
• Otitis media
• Diarrhea

AGE-RELATED FACTORS
Pediatric: Most common in infants
Geriatric: N/A
Others: N/A

PREGNANCY N/A

SYNONYMS N/A

ICD-9-CM
466.1 acute bronchiolitis

SEE ALSO N/A

OTHER NOTES N/A

ABBREVIATIONS
• BPD = bronchopulmonary dysplasia
• CHD = congenital heart disease
• RAD = reactive airway disease
• SPAG = small particle aerosol generator

REFERENCES
• Mandell, G.L. (ed.): Principles and Practice of Infectious Diseases. 3rd Ed. New York, Churchill Livingstone, 1990
• Fields, B.N., et al. (eds.): Virology. 2nd Ed. New York, Raven Press, 1990

Author N. Dambro, M.D.

Bronchiolitis Obliterans & Organizing Pneumonia

 BASICS

DESCRIPTION This is a specific reaction of lung tissue to a variety of injuries. The lungs show a pattern of multiple patchy pneumonia. These are seen on chest x-ray as patchy alveolar or ground glass opacifications with or without interstitial infiltrates and may have air bronchograms as well.
System(s) affected: Pulmonary
Genetics: N/A
Incidence/Prevalence in USA: Uncommon
Predominant age: Reported cases range age 0-70, mean age 50's
Predominant sex: N/A

SIGNS AND SYMPTOMS
 • Most cases present with a flu-like illness that lasts 4-10 weeks or longer. Most have been treated with antibiotics without success.
 • Fever
 • Dry cough
 • Weight loss
 • Dyspnea may be severe
 • Crackles and perhaps squeaks over involved area
 • Fatigue

CAUSES Idiopathic. A complex response to a variety of injuries, such as toxic inhalation; post mycoplasma, viral and bacterial infection; aspiration; immunologic factors.

RISK FACTORS
 • AIDS
 • Immunocompromised patients, including transplant patients

 DIAGNOSIS

DIFFERENTIAL DIAGNOSIS
 • Usual interstitial pneumonitis (UIP)
 • Noninfectious diseases
 • Tuberculosis
 • Sarcoidosis
 • Histoplasmosis
 • Berylliosis
 • Goodpasture's syndrome
 • Neoplasm
 • Polyarteritis nodosa
 • Systemic lupus erythematosis
 • Wegener's granulomatosis
 • Sjogren's syndrome
 • Chronic eosinophilic pneumonia

LABORATORY
 • Leukocytosis with a normal differential
 • Elevated ESR, usually quite elevated
 • Negative cultures
 • Negative serology for mycoplasma, Coxiella, Legionella, psittacosis, and fungus
 • Negative viral studies
Drugs that may alter lab results: N/A
Disorders that may alter lab results: N/A

PATHOLOGICAL FINDINGS
 • Intraluminal fibrosis of distal airspaces is the major pathologic feature
 • Fibroblasts and plugs of inflammatory cells and loose connective tissue fill these distal airways
 • The inflammatory cells are mainly lymphocytes and plasma cells
 • Interstitial fibrosis is present
 • The plugs of edematous granulation tissue in the terminal and respiratory bronchioles and alveolar ducts do not cause permanent damage

SPECIAL TESTS
 • Pulmonary function shows a restrictive/obstructive pattern
 • Flow-volume loop shows terminal airway obstruction
 • Chest x-ray may show patchy alveolar opacities often in the mid or upper lung area. A ground glass pattern that may have air bronchograms.
 • V/Q scan: matched patchy defects

IMAGING
 • Chest x-ray - often appears more normal than the physical examination
 • CT scans more accurately define the distribution and extent of the patchy alveolar opacities

DIAGNOSTIC PROCEDURES
 • Open lung biopsy
 • It may be well to use a trial of steroids as a diagnostic trial, though not all would agree
 • If a diagnostic trial is successful, be prepared to treat the patient for at least a year

 TREATMENT

APPROPRIATE HEALTH CARE
Inpatient

GENERAL MEASURES
 • Monitor blood gases or pulse oximetry
 • Oxygen as necessary

ACTIVITY As tolerated

DIET No special diet

PATIENT EDUCATION Followup is especially important. Relapse is common. Treatment is prolonged. If medication tapered too rapidly, relapse may well occur.

MEDICATIONS

DRUG(S) OF CHOICE
Prednisone
◊ 60 mg daily for 1-3 months
◊ Then tapered over a few weeks to 20 mg (this dose may later be given as alternate day therapy). Increase length of taper for patients on long-term therapy to avoid precipitating Addisonian crisis.
◊ Treatment may be needed for one year or more
Contraindications: Refer to manufacturer's literature
Precautions: Be aware of the patient's Mantoux status and history of peptic ulcer disease. Long-term steroid associated with significant adverse effects including Cushing's syndrome, fluid retention, osteoporosis, hyperkalemia, poor wound healing.
Significant possible interactions: Refer to manufacturer's literature

ALTERNATIVE DRUGS
Steroids other than prednisone may be used

FOLLOWUP

PATIENT MONITORING
• Frequent visits, weekly initially
• Emphasize the need to continue the prednisone because of the chance of relapse
• Monitor the lung disease and the side effects of prednisone therapy (Mantoux, monthly CBC, fundoscopic exam every 3-6 months)

PREVENTION/AVOIDANCE   Except for prevention of relapse, none known

POSSIBLE COMPLICATIONS
• Bronchiectasis
• Death, but with proper treatment, recovery is usually complete without permanent sequelae

EXPECTED COURSE AND PROGNOSIS   Complete recovery but individual case management is mandatory

MISCELLANEOUS

ASSOCIATED CONDITIONS
• Rheumatic lung
• Cystic fibrosis
• Bronchopulmonary dysplasia
• Renal failure
• Congestive heart failure
• Adult respiratory distress syndrome
• Drug-induced pneumonitis
• Paraquat poisoning
• Amiodarone toxicity
• Acebutolol toxicity
• Freebase cocaine pulmonary toxicity
• Chronic infectious pneumonia
• Chronic eosinophilic pneumonia
• Hypersensitivity pneumonitis
• Histiocytosis X
• Sarcoidosis
• Pneumoconioses
• Radiation pneumonitis
• Though most were treated with antibiotics only penicillamine and sulfasalazine have been implicated

AGE-RELATED FACTORS
Pediatric: Rare, but has been reported after viral pneumonia (adenovirus influenza). Characteristics include delayed recovery, persistent cough, crackles or wheezing after pneumonia. The laboratory findings are generally not helpful.Imaging shows: V/Qm matched defects; HRCT, bronchiectasis, bronchogram, pruned tree appearance. Diagnosis confirmed by biopsy. Treatment includes steroids (1mg/kg/24hrs for one month, followed by weaning over several months.
Geriatric: Not common
Others: Apparently only seen in adults

PREGNANCY   N/A

SYNONYMS
• Intraluminal fibrosis of distal airways
• Idiopathic BOOP
• Cryptogenic organizing pneumonia (COP)
• Obliterative bronchiolitis

ICD-9-CM
491.8 Other chronic bronchitis

SEE ALSO   N/A

OTHER NOTES   This disease behaves differently than bronchiolitis obliterans (BO). BOOP is a restrictive problem, BO is an obstructive problem. BO causes permanent lung damage and BOOP is completely reversible.

ABBREVIATIONS   N/A

REFERENCES
• Cordier, J.F., Loire, R. & Brune, J.: Idiopathic Bronchiolitis Obliterans Organizing Pneumonia. Chest 1989;96:999-1004
• Mueller, N.L., Staples, C.A. & Miller, R.R.: Bronchiolitis Obliterans Organizing Pneumonia: CT features in 14 patients. In AJR 1990;154:983-987
• Epler, G.R., Colby, T.V., et al.: Bronchiolitis Obliterans Organizing Pneumonia. N Eng J Med 1985;312:152-158
• Hardy KA, Schidlow DV, Zaeri N: Obliterative Bronchiolitis in Children. CHEST 1988; 93; 460-466

Author   D. Pope, M.D.

Bronchitis, acute

 BASICS

DESCRIPTION Inflammation of trachea, bronchi and bronchioles. Generally self-limited with complete healing and full return of function.
System(s) affected: Pulmonary
Genetics: No known genetic pattern
Incidence/Prevalence in USA: Common
Predominant age: All ages
Predominant sex: Male = Female

SIGNS AND SYMPTOMS
• Preceding respiratory tract infection, such as a common cold with coryza, malaise, chills, slight fever, sore throat, back and muscle pain
• Cough, initially dry and unproductive, then productive. Later, mucopurulent sputum
• Fever
• Fatigue, aching
• Hemoptysis
• Chest burning
• Dyspnea (sometimes)
• Rales, rhonchi, wheezing
• No evidence of pulmonary consolidation

CAUSES
• Influenza
• Parainfluenza
• Chlamydia pneumoniae (TWAR agent)
• Bordetella pertussis
• Respiratory syncytial virus
• Coxsackie virus
• Herpes simplex
• Hemophilus influenzae
• Possibly fungi
• Mycoplasma
• Secondary bacterial infection as part of an acute upper respiratory infection
• Streptococcal pneumoniae
• Moraxella catarrhalis
• Mycobacterium tuberculosis

RISK FACTORS
• Fatigue
• Chronic bronchopulmonary diseases
• Chronic sinusitis
• Bronchopulmonary allergy
• Hypertrophied tonsils and adenoids in children
• Immunosuppression
• Air pollutants
• Elderly
• Infants
• Smoking
• Second-hand smoke
• Alcoholism
• Reflux esophagitis
• Tracheostomy
• IgA deficiency

 DIAGNOSIS

DIFFERENTIAL DIAGNOSIS
• Influenza
• Bronchopneumonia
• Bronchiectasis
• Acute sinusitis
• Aspiration
• Cystic fibrosis
• Reactive airways disease
• Bacterial tracheitis
• Retained foreign body

LABORATORY
• Arterial blood gases - hypoxemia
• Leukocytosis
• Sputum culture/gram stain
• Viral titers
• Mycoplasma titers
Drugs that may alter lab results: N/A
Disorders that may alter lab results: N/A

PATHOLOGICAL FINDINGS
• Mucosal hyperemia
• Desquamation of columnar epithelium
• Mucopurulent exudate

SPECIAL TESTS Pulmonary function tests (seldom needed during acute stages) - increased residual volume, decreased maximal expiratory rate

IMAGING Chest x-ray - lungs normal if uncomplicated. Helps rule out other diseases or complications.

DIAGNOSTIC PROCEDURES Symptoms and signs

 TREATMENT

APPROPRIATE HEALTH CARE
Outpatient unless elderly or complicated by severe underlying disease

GENERAL MEASURES
• Steam inhalations
• Vaporizers
• Antibiotics if bacterial etiology suspected
• Stop smoking

ACTIVITY Rest until fever subsides

DIET Increased fluids (up to 3-4 L/day) while febrile

PATIENT EDUCATION For patient education materials favorably reviewed on this topic, contact: American Lung Association, 1740 Broadway, New York, NY 10019, (212)315-8700

MEDICATIONS

DRUG(S) OF CHOICE
• Amantadine therapy if influenza A suspected; most effective if started within 24-48 hours of development of symptoms
• Decongestants if accompanied by sinus condition
• Antipyretic analgesic such as aspirin (in adults) 650 mg q 4-6 hours
• Antibiotics - for more severe symptoms (high fever persists, concomitant COPD, purulent discharge). Best choices are amoxicillin, TMP-SMX (trimethoprim-sulfamethoxazole), or cephalosporin
• Cough suppressant for troublesome cough (not with COPD)
• Bronchodilators (aerosols/steroids)
Contraindications: Refer to manufacturer's literature
Precautions: Refer to manufacturer's literature
Significant possible interactions: Refer to manufacturer's literature

ALTERNATIVE DRUGS
• Other antibiotics if indicated by sputum culture (Moraxella needs different set of antibiotics)
• Antivirals
• Erythromycin or ciprofloxacin (Cipro), if allergic to penicillin

FOLLOWUP

PATIENT MONITORING
• Oximetry until no longer hypoxemic
• Recheck for chronicity

PREVENTION/AVOIDANCE
• Avoid smoking
• Control underlying risk factors (asthma, sinusitis, reflux)
• Avoid exposure

POSSIBLE COMPLICATIONS
• Bronchopneumonia
• Acute respiratory failure

EXPECTED COURSE AND PROGNOSIS
• Usual - complete healing with good return of function
• Can be serious in elderly or debilitated patients
• Cough may persist for several weeks after initial improvement
• Post-bronchitic reactive airways disease (rare)
• Bronchiolitis obliterans with organizing pneumonia (BOOP) (rare)

MISCELLANEOUS

ASSOCIATED CONDITIONS
• Asthma
• Epiglottitis
• Coryza
• Pharyngitis
• Croup
• Influenza
• Smoking
• Pneumonia
• Emphysema
• Sinusitis
• Bronchial obstruction

AGE-RELATED FACTORS
Pediatric:
• Occurrence in this age group usually is in association with other conditions of upper and lower respiratory tract (trachea usually involved)
• Some children seem to be more susceptible than others (if repeated attacks, child should be evaluated for anomalies of the respiratory tract)
• If acute bronchitis is caused by respiratory syncytial virus, may be fatal
Geriatric: Can be a serious illness in this age group, particularly if part of influenza
Others: N/A

PREGNANCY N/A

SYNONYMS N/A

ICD-9-CM 466.0 acute bronchitis

SEE ALSO
• Asthma
• COPD

OTHER NOTES N/A

ABBREVIATIONS N/A

REFERENCES
• Baum, G.L. & Wolinsky, E. (eds): Textbook of Pulmonary Diseases. Boston, Little, Brown & Co., 1983
• Murray, J.F. & Nadel, J.A. (eds.): Textbook of Respiratory Medicine. Philadelphia, W.B. Saunders Co., 1988
• Seaton, A., Seaton, D. & Leitch, A.G.: Crofton and Douglas's Respiratory Diseases. Boston, Blackwell Scientific Publications, 1989

Author A. Cropp, MD & R. Fleming, RN, BSN

Brucellosis

BASICS

DESCRIPTION Systemic bacterial infection caused by Brucella species in infected animal products, or vaccine. Incubation period usually 5-60 days, but highly variable and may be several months. Characterized by intermittent or irregular fevers, with symptoms ranging from subclinical disease to infection of almost any organ system. Bone and joint involvement common. May be chronic or recurrent. Case fatality untreated less than 2%.
System(s) affected: Endocrine/Metabolic, Gastrointestinal, Renal/Urologic, Pulmonary, Nervous, Skin/Exocrine
Genetics: None; some evidence for intrauterine transmission
Incidence in USA: Less than 100/year (85 cases in 1990 - 0.34/100,000); common in developing countries
Prevalence in USA: Not reported.
Predominant age: All ages, but especially 20-60 (occupational exposure), sometimes children (milk-related outbreaks)
Predominant sex:
• Male > Female (occupational exposure)
• Female ≥ Male (milk exposure)

SIGNS AND SYMPTOMS
• Fever (may be undulant, increased in afternoon and evening, maximum 101-104° daily); weakness; headache; sweating; chills; generalized aching; arthralgia (90%)
• Also common - weight loss, depression, irritability, hepatosplenomegaly (20-30%)
• Hepatic dysfunction (abnormal liver function test) 30-60%
• Gastrointestinal symptoms (unusual)
• Lymphadenopathy, especially cervical, inguinal (12-21%)
• Orchitis, epididymitis (normal urinalysis) (2-40%)
• Nephritis, prostatitis (rare)
• Cystitis
• Pulmonary - cough or other pulmonary symptoms, x-ray may be normal (15-25%)
• Cutaneous - many transient, non-specific rashes have been described; also, purpura from thrombopenia (5%)
• Visual disturbances, eye pain
• Chronic fatigue syndrome and various neuro-psychiatric symptoms described. Unclear relationship.
• Also localized suppurative infections (see Complications)

CAUSES
• Brucella ingestion from tissue or milk
• Worst disease: B. melitensis B. suis; also B. canis, B. abortus. Enter through mucous membrane, broken skin, occasionally inhaled. Facultative intracellular parasite, releases endotoxin when destroyed.

RISK FACTORS
• In US, from occupational exposure to infected animals (especially cattle, sheep). Veterinarians, meat processors, farm workers; who may experience accidental exposure to vaccine.
• Consumer exposure to unpasteurized milk products, cheese
• Exposure while traveling in countries where endemic (Mediterranean, N. and E. Africa, central Asia, India, Mexico, Central and South America)
• Worse in chronically ill, immunosuppressed
• Iron deficiency increases susceptibility

DIAGNOSIS

DIFFERENTIAL DIAGNOSIS
• Many non-specific systemic febrile illnesses; a great mimic
• Tularemia
• Psittacosis
• Rickettsial disease
• Visceral leishmaniasis
• Other disease of infected organs
• HIV infection

LABORATORY
• Isolation of organism from blood, discharge, bone or other tissue. Fastidious and slow-growing.
• Acute illness: Blood culture is positive 70%, bone 90%
• May have thrombopenia, disseminated intravascular coagulation; granulopenia, lymphopenia, lymphocytosis. 30-60% with abnormal liver function test.
• Serology: Brucella standard tube agglutination (STA) paired sera, > 1:160 or 4 x rise.
• Recent development of more effective ELISA tests.
• IgM increased initially for several weeks, declines by 3 mos.
• IgG begins rise 2 weeks, may stay up > 1 yr if treated or not treated (though IgM increase may be lower or gone by 6 mos. if treated). IgG rises again with reinfection or reactivation. IgG > 1:160 at 1 year implies ongoing infection.
Drugs that may alter lab results: None
Disorders that may alter lab results: Serologic cross-reaction with F. tularensis, Yersinia enterocolitica, V. cholerae, or vaccinated patients. It has been misdiagnosed in culture as Moraxella phenylpyruvica

PATHOLOGICAL FINDINGS
• Facultative intracellular; can survive inside phagocytic cells, circulate to regional lymph nodes, and into circulation. (Cell-mediated immunity necessary to kill intracellular organism.)
• Macrophages kill, releasing endotoxin that may cause symptoms of acute disease
• Variable tissue reaction depending on site, organisms. Causes local microabscesses; possibly some immune reaction in arthritis.

SPECIAL TESTS Echocardiogram depending on location

IMAGING
• Bone scan, CT, depending on location
• Chest x-ray - pleural effusion, lung cavitation

DIAGNOSTIC PROCEDURES Biopsy, aspiration depending on location

TREATMENT

APPROPRIATE HEALTH CARE
Outpatient in mild cases, hospitalization in severe illness. Cardiac care unit in patients with complicating cardiac disease.

GENERAL MEASURES
• Supportive care
• Specific complications may require surgical drainage, or valve replacement in endocarditis
• In milk-related outbreak, look for other cases

ACTIVITY Bedrest during febrile periods and restricted activity in acute cases

DIET No special diet. May need to provide supplemental foods, e.g., milk shakes, to counter weight loss.

PATIENT EDUCATION Food Safety and Inspection Service, Office of Public Awareness, Dept. of Agriculture, Room 1165-S, Washington, DC 20205, (202)447-9351

MEDICATIONS

DRUG(S) OF CHOICE
• Rifampin 600-900 mg and doxycycline 200 mg given together every day for at least 6 weeks (possible for several months with severe complications). 8.4% relapse rate, not related to drug resistance - use same drugs for relapse.
• Steroids in Herxheimer's reaction, severe illness
Contraindications: Avoid doxycycline in children, pregnant women
Precautions: May get Herxheimer's reaction when therapy initiated
Significant possible interactions:
• Rifampin is a potent inducer for the hepatic P450 enzyme system, and may increase metabolism of many drugs metabolized by the liver including: Acetaminophen, anticoagulants, barbiturates, benzodiazepines, beta-blockers, chloramphenicol, clofibrate, oral contraceptives, corticosteroids, cyclosporine, digoxin, disopyramide, estrogens, hydantoins, methadone, mexiletine, quinidine, sulfones sulfonylureas, theophyllines, tocanide, verapamil, enalapril, ketoconazole, halothane
• Doxycycline: Antacids, anticoagulants, barbiturates, carbamazepine, hydantoins, cimetidine, digoxin insulin, iron salts, lithium, methoxyflurane, oral contraceptives, penicillins, sodium bicarbonate

ALTERNATIVE DRUGS
• Tetracycline orally qid and streptomycin by injection - very effective.(Streptomycin currently not available in the USA except by special request from CDC in Atlanta.)
• Sulfamethoxazole-trimethoprim (Co-trimoxazole) - slightly lower cure, higher relapse rate. Use in children.
• Third generation cephalosporins (being evaluated). Recent study on ceftriaxone showed not as good as doxycycline and streptomycin in acute therapy or in preventing relapse.
• Ciprofloxacin - recent study showed high rate of relapse

 FOLLOWUP

PATIENT MONITORING
Check serology at 6 months and 1 year for chronic disease (difficult to evaluate if continuing exposure). Investigate any evidence of complication, recurrence.

PREVENTION/AVOIDANCE
• Avoid infected milk
• For occupational exposure - caution, possibly vaccination, use of protective goggles, protective gloves

POSSIBLE COMPLICATIONS
• Relapse (5% overall)
• Localized suppurative infections - osteo-articular (20-85%). Includes arthritis (possibly also immune effect), bursitis, tenosynovitis, osteomyelitis, sacroiliitis, vertebral or paraspinous abscess.
• Endocarditis - rare, but main cause of death in brucellosis
• Thrombophlebitis
• Neuro-brucellosis - most are meningeal. Also peripheral neuritis (usually single, bilateral is possible), encephalitis, myelitis, radiculopathy. Possibly neuro-psychiatric symptoms.
• Intrinsic ocular lesions - uveitis, retinal thrombophlebitis, nummular keratitis
• Pneumonitis with pleural effusion
• Hepatitis
• Cholecystitis

EXPECTED COURSE AND PROGNOSIS
• Untreated case fatality < 2%
• Most cases resolve with treatment. 2-3 weeks for acute uncomplicated cases.
• Relapse rate overall, 5%

 MISCELLANEOUS

ASSOCIATED CONDITIONS N/A

AGE-RELATED FACTORS
Pediatric: May be mild, subclinical
Geriatric: N/A
Others: Worse in chronically ill, immunosuppressed

PREGNANCY
May cause miscarriage or abortion, even in subclinical cases

SYNONYMS
• Undulant fever
• Malta fever

ICD-9-CM 023.9

SEE ALSO N/A

OTHER NOTES N/A

ABBREVIATIONS N/A

REFERENCES
• Berenson, A.S.: (ed): Control of Communicable Diseases in Man. 15th Ed. Washington, DC, American Public Health Association, 1990
• Mandell, G.L. (ed.): Principles and Practice of Infectious Diseases. 3rd Ed. New York, Churchill Livingstone, 1990
• Eirian, W. S. (ed): Brucellosis in humans: Its diagnosis and treatment. Acta Pathologica Microbiologica ET Immunologica Scandinavia suppl. 3:21-25, 1988

Author N. Snapp, M.D., M.P.H.

Bulimia nervosa

 BASICS

DESCRIPTION Intense fear of becoming fat; recurrent binge eating, with or without purging by self-induced vomiting, laxatives, diuretics. Alternative pattern: binges followed by sharply restricted diet and/or vigorous exercise.

Incidence/Prevalence in USA:
approximately 2% of females; higher among university women

System(s) affected: Endocrine/Metabolic, Nervous, Gastrointestinal

Genetics: N/A

Predominant age: adolescents and young adults

Predominant sex: Female > Male

SIGNS AND SYMPTOMS
• Patients may switch back and forth between anorexia and bulimia
• Onset may be stress related
• May be average weight or even somewhat obese; most are slightly below average weight but have frequent fluctuations in weight
• Secretive habit, deny that there is a problem
• Gobble high calorie foods during binge
• Claim to feel fat even when below average weight
• Preoccupation with weight control
• Elaborate food collection and hoarding rituals
• Calories expended through vigorous exercise, especially running
• Depressed mood and self-depreciation following the binges
• Vomiting may be effortless
• Abdominal pain
• Parotid swelling
• Eroded teeth
• Scarred hands

CAUSES Unknown; thought to be largely emotional

RISK FACTORS
• Impulsive character traits
• Low self-esteem
• Achievement pressure; high self-expectations
• Acceptance of the culturally condoned ideal of slimness
• Ambivalence about dependence/independence
• Stress due to multiple responsibilities, tight schedules
• Unstable body image; perceptual distortions

 DIAGNOSIS

DIFFERENTIAL DIAGNOSIS
Gastrointestinal disorder; anorexia; psychogenic vomiting, hypothalamic brain tumor; epileptic equivalent seizures; Kluver-Bucy-like syndromes, Kleine-Levin syndrome; schizophrenic disorder; body dysmorphic disorder

LABORATORY
• Elevated BUN
• Hypokalemia
• Metabolic alkalosis
• Hypochloremia
• Elevated basal serum prolactin
• Positive dexamethasone suppression test

Drugs that may alter lab results: N/A
Disorders that may alter lab results: N/A

PATHOLOGICAL FINDINGS
• Eroded tooth enamel
• Esophagitis
• Asymptomatic, non-inflammatory parotid enlargement
• Gastric dilatation
• Infarction and perforation of the stomach

SPECIAL TESTS
• ECG
• Gastric motility
• Thyroid, liver, renal function
• Drug screen

IMAGING Not indicated

DIAGNOSTIC PROCEDURES
Psychological screening: Eating Attitudes Test

 TREATMENT

APPROPRIATE HEALTH CARE Most patients can be treated as outpatients. Hospitalize if patient is suicidal; if there is lab or ECG evidence of marked electrolyte imbalance; marked dehydration; or if there has been no response to outpatient therapy.

GENERAL MEASURES
Inpatient:
◊ If possible, admit to eating disorders unit or unit with structured eating disorders program
◊ Supervised meals and bathroom privileges
◊ No access to the bathroom for 2 hours after meals
◊ Monitor weight and physical activity
◊ Assess psychological state and nutritional status
◊ Involve patient in developing alternatives to purging
◊ Monitor electrolytes
◊ Individual and group therapy
◊ Gradually shift control to patient as she demonstrates responsibility
Outpatient:
◊ Build trust, treatment alliance
◊ Assess psychological state and nutritional status
◊ Involve patient in establishing target goals
◊ Use self-monitoring techniques such as food diary
◊ Identify prodromal states, precipitants
◊ Focus on overall well-being, developing gratifying relationships
◊ Challenge fear of loss of control
◊ Add cognitive restructuring group, individual, family or assertiveness training, relaxation techniques, couples therapy, self-help group

ACTIVITY Monitor excess activity

DIET
• Goal is a balanced diet with adequate calories and a normal eating pattern
• Diminished ruminations about calories, weight
• Reintroduce feared foods

PATIENT EDUCATION
• Seriousness and consequences of bulimic behavior
• Information on nutrition, metabolic balance
• Tools for self monitoring when appropriate

Bulimia nervosa

MEDICATIONS

DRUG(S) OF CHOICE
• Tricyclic medication is indicated for patients who are severely depressed or who have not responded to an adequate trial of therapy. Consider imipramine (Tofranil), 10 mg, gradual increase to 250 mg, monitor with EKG; or desipramine (Norpramin), 25 mg/day, increasing gradually to 150 mg/day, monitor with ECG. Improvement is not necessarily related to blood level.
• Fluoxetine (Prozac) has been found effective in some patients (higher doses 40-60 mg/day are usually necessary).
Contraindications: Refer to manufacturer's literature
Precautions:
• Suicide risk may be high with tricyclics
• Fluoxetine may increase tricyclic levels; monitor levels of TCAs if started after fluoxetine (remember fluoxetine's long half-life)
Significant possible interactions: Lithium and tricyclic medication can be lethal when administered to hypokalemic patients

ALTERNATIVE DRUGS
• If there is an underlying bipolar disorder, patients may benefit from lithium (Eskalith), 300 mg bid, increase gradually to therapeutic blood level (0.6-1.2 mEq/l)
• Some patients respond to monoamine oxidase inhibitors (phenelzine), 60-90 mg/day. Fluoxetine and MAO inhibitor may trigger a serious reaction (serotonin syndrome); allow 5 weeks between fluoxetine and beginning of MAO inhibitor.
• SRI: Other than Prozac (Zoloft, 25-100 mg/day or Paxil, 10-40mg/day may be considered)
• Metoclopramide (Reglan), 10-15 mg before each meal and at bedtime for post-prandial abdominal discomfort
• Note: Non-compliance is common, no drug of proven efficacy

FOLLOWUP

PATIENT MONITORING
• Binge-purge activity
• Level of exercise activity
• Self-esteem, comfort with body and self
• Ruminations and depression
• Repeat any abnormal lab values weekly or monthly until stable

PREVENTION/AVOIDANCE
• Encourage rational attitude about weight
• Moderate overly high self-expectations
• Enhance self-esteem
• Diminish stress

POSSIBLE COMPLICATIONS
• Suicide
• Drug and alcohol abuse
• Potassium depletion; cardiac arrhythmia; cardiac arrest

EXPECTED COURSE AND PROGNOSIS
• Highly variable, tends to wax and wane
• May spontaneously remit
• Patients may drop out of therapy, be lost to follow-up
• Those who stay in therapy tend to improve

MISCELLANEOUS

ASSOCIATED CONDITIONS
• Major depression
• Bipolar disorder
• Obsessive-compulsive disorder
• Schizophrenic disorder
• Substance abuse disorder
• Borderline personality disorder
• Compulsive shoplifting

AGE-RELATED FACTORS
Pediatric: N/A
Geriatric: N/A
Others: Infrequently diagnosed in men or in older women

PREGNANCY
• Poor nutritional status may affect fetus
• Binge-purge may increase or decrease during pregnancy

SYNONYMS N/A

ICD-9-CM
• 783.6 bulimia
• 307.51 nonorganic origin

SEE ALSO N/A

OTHER NOTES
• Anorexic patients may deal with the frustration of chronic food deprivation by converting to bulimia
• Ballet dancers, gymnasts, models, cheerleaders, and athletes are at relatively high risk
• Sub-clinical eating disorders are common in university populations

ABBREVIATIONS
MAO = monoamine oxidase
SRI = serotonergic re-uptake inhibitors
TCA = tricyclic antidepressant

REFERENCES
• Yates, A.: Current Perspectives on the Eating Disorders: I. History, Psychological and Biological Aspects. J Am Acad Child Adolesc Psychiatry 28(6):813-828, 1989.
• Yates, A.: Current Perspectives on the Eating Disorders: II. Treatment, Outcome, and Research Directions. J Am Acad Child Adolesc Psychiatry 29(1):1-9, 1990.
• Garner, D.M. & Garfinkel, P.: Anorexia Nervosa: A Multidimensional Perspective. New York, Brunner-Mazel, 1982
• Yager, et al.: Practice Guidelines for the Eating Disorders. Am J Psychiatry. 150:207-228, 1993

Author A. Yates, M.D.

Burns

BASICS

DESCRIPTION Burns are tissue injuries caused by application of heat, chemicals, electricity, or irradiation to the tissue. Extent of injury (depth of burn) is result of intensity of heat (or other exposure) and the duration of exposure.
- Partial thickness: First degree involves superficial layers of epidermis. Second degree involves varying degrees of epidermis (with blister formation) and part of the dermis.
- Full thickness: Third degree involves destruction of all skin elements with coagulation of subdermal plexus

System(s) affected: Skin/Exocrine
Genetics: N/A
Incidence/Prevalence in USA:
- 2 to 5 million burns/year in USA require assistance, 1,000,000/year require hospitalization, 12,000/year die
- Burns are leading cause of accidental death in children

Predominant age: All ages
Predominant sex: Male = Female

SIGNS AND SYMPTOMS
First degree
  ◊ Erythema of involved tissue
  ◊ Skin blanches with pressure
  ◊ Skin may be tender
Second degree
  ◊ Skin is red and blistered
  ◊ Skin is very tender
Third degree
  ◊ Burned skin is tough and leathery
  ◊ Skin is not tender

CAUSES
- Open flame and hot liquid are most common (heat usually 15-45° C or greater)
- Caustic chemicals or acids (may show little signs or symptoms for the first few days)
- Electricity (may have significant injury with very little damage to overlying skin)
- Excess sun exposure

RISK FACTORS
- Hot water heaters set too high
- Work place exposure to chemicals, electricity or irradiation
- Young children and elderly adults with thin skin are more susceptible to injury
- Carelessness with burning cigarettes
- Inadequate or faulty electrical wiring

DIAGNOSIS

DIFFERENTIAL DIAGNOSIS
- Toxic epidermal necrolysis
- Scalded skin syndrome

LABORATORY
- Hematocrit
- Type and cross
- Electrolytes
- Blood urea nitrogen
- Urinalysis

Drugs that may alter lab results: N/A
Disorders that may alter lab results:
Pre-existing cardiac disease

PATHOLOGICAL FINDINGS
- First degree - devitalization of superficial layers of epidermis, congestion of intradermal vessels
- Second degree - coagulation necrosis of varying depths of epidermis, clefting of epidermis (blister), coagulation of subdermal plexus, skin appendages intact
- Third degree - necrosis of all skin elements, coagulation of subdermal plexus

SPECIAL TESTS
- Children - glucose (hypoglycemia may occur in children because of limited glycogen storage)
- Smoke inhalation - arterial blood gas, carboxyhemoglobin
- Electric burns - electrocardiogram, urine myoglobin, CPK

IMAGING
- Chest x-ray
- Xenon scan may be useful in suspected smoke inhalation

DIAGNOSTIC PROCEDURES
Bronchoscopy may be necessary in smoke inhalation to evaluate lower respiratory tract

TREATMENT

APPROPRIATE HEALTH CARE
Hospitalization for all serious burns
  ◊ Second degree burns over 10% body surface area (BSA), any 3rd degree burn
    ◊ Burns of hands, feet, face or perineum
    ◊ Electrical/lightning burns
    ◊ Inhalation injury
    ◊ Chemical burns
    ◊ Circumferential burn
Transfer to burn center for:
  ◊ 2nd and 3rd degree burns over 10% BSA in patients under 10 years and over 50 years of age
  ◊ 2nd and 3rd degree burns over 20% BSA in any age range
    ◊ Burns of hands, feet, face or perineum
    ◊ Electrical/lightning burns
    ◊ Inhalation injury
    ◊ Chemical burns
    ◊ Circumferential burn
    ◊ Chemical burns with threat of functional impairment

GENERAL MEASURES
Based on depth of burns and accurate estimate of total body surface area (BSA) involved (Rule of nines)
Rule of nines
  ◊ Each upper extremity - adult and child 9%
  ◊ Each lower extremity - adult 18%; child 14%
    ◊ Anterior trunk - adult and child 18%
    ◊ Posterior trunk - adult and child 18%
    ◊ Head and neck - adult 10%; child 18%
- Tetanus prophylaxis
- Remove all rings, watches, etc., from injured extremities to avoid tourniquet effect
- Remove clothing and cover all burned areas with dry sheet
- Flush area of chemical burn
- 100% oxygen administration in all major burns, consider early intubation
- Do not apply ice to burn site
- Nasogastric tube (high risk of paralytic ileus)
- Foley catheter
- Pain relief with Morphine or Demerol-should only be given IV
- ECG monitoring in first 24 hours following electrical burn
- Whirlpool hydrotherapy followed by Silvadene occlusive dressings in severe burns
- Once or twice a day cleansing with dressing changes
- Epilock may be used as dressing in selected patients (especially useful for outpatient treatment of minor burns)

Burn fluid resuscitation

Calculate fluid resuscitation from time of burn, not from time treatment begins.

◊ 2-4 mL Ringer's lactate x body weight (kg) x % BSA burn (1/2 given in first eight hours, 1/4 in second eight hours and 1/4 in third eight hours). In children, this is given in addition to maintenance fluids and is adjusted according to urine output and vital signs.

◊ Colloid solutions are not recommended during the first 12-24 hours of resuscitation

Surgical procedures

◊ Escharotomy may be necessary in constricting circumferential burns of extremities or chest

◊ Tangential excision with split thickness skin grafts

Other

◊ Use of biological membranes or skin substitutes may be indicated for burn coverage

ACTIVITY Early mobilization is the goal

DIET High protein, high calorie diet when bowel function resumes; nasogastric tube feedings may be required in early post-burn period. TPN if NPO expected for > 5 days.

PATIENT EDUCATION
• Use of sunscreen
• Access to electrical cords/outlets
• Isolate household chemicals
• Use low temperature setting for hot water heater
• Household smoke detectors
• Family/household evacuation plan
• Proper storage and use of flammable substances

MEDICATIONS

DRUG(S) OF CHOICE
• Morphine small frequent IV doses (0.1 mg/kg/dose in children)
• Demerol (1 mg/kg/dose in children) IV
• Silver sulfadiazine (Silvadene cream) topically to burn site (can cause leukopenia)
• Electrical burn with myoglobinuria will require alkalinization of urine and mannitol
• No indication for prophylactic antibiotics
• Consider H2 blockers: cimetidine, ranitidine, famotidine, or nizatidine for stress ulcer prophylaxis in severely burned patients

Contraindications: Specific drug allergies

Precautions: Be alert for respiratory depression with narcotics

Significant possible interactions: Refer to manufacturer's profile of each drug

ALTERNATIVE DRUGS
• Sodium mafenide (Sulfamylon)-full thickness burn (caution: metabolic acidosis)
• Silver nitrate 0.5% (messy, leaches electrolytes from burn and causes water toxicity)
• Povidone-iodine (Betadine) Iodine absorption from burn, "tan eschar". Makes débridement more difficult.
• Travase-enzymatic débridement

FOLLOWUP

PATIENT MONITORING According to extent of burn and treatment

PREVENTION/AVOIDANCE Skin grafts or newly epithelialized skin is highly sensitive to sun exposure and thermal extremes

POSSIBLE COMPLICATIONS
• Gastroduodenal ulceration (Curling's ulcer)
• Marjolin's ulcer - squamous cell carcinoma developing in old burn site
• Burn wound sepsis-usually gram negative organisms
• Pneumonia
• Decreased mobility with possibility of future flexion contractures

EXPECTED COURSE AND PROGNOSIS
• First degree burn - complete resolution
• Second degree burn - epithelialization in 10-14 days (deep second degree burns will probably require skin graft)
• Third degree burn - no potential for re-epithelialization, skin graft required
• Length of hospital stay and need for ICU care depends on extent of burn, smoke inhalation and age
• A 50% survival can be expected with a 62% burn in ages 0-14 years, 63% burn in ages 15-40 years, 38% burn in age 40-65 years, 25% burn in patients over 65 years
• 90% of survivors can be expected to return to an occupation as remunerative as their pre-burn employment

MISCELLANEOUS

ASSOCIATED CONDITIONS

Smoke inhalation syndrome
• Occurs within 72 hours of burn
• Suspected in burns occurring in an enclosed space
• Intubation, ventilation with positive end-expiratory pressure (PEEP) assistance

AGE-RELATED FACTORS
Pediatric: N/A
Geriatric: Prognosis poorer for severe burns
Others: N/A

PREGNANCY N/A

SYNONYMS N/A

ICD-9-CM 949.0

SEE ALSO N/A

OTHER NOTES N/A

ABBREVIATIONS BSA = body surface area

REFERENCES
• Gillespie, R.W., Dimik, A.R. & Hallberg, P.W.: Advanced Burn Life Support Course Provider's Manual. Lincoln, Nebraska Burn Institute, 1990
• Schwartz, S.I., Shires, G.T., Spencer, F.C., et al.: Principles of Surgery. 4th Ed. New York, McGraw-Hill Book Co., 1984
• Touloukian, R.J.: Pediatric Trauma. 2nd Ed. St. Louis, Mosby Year Book, 1990

Author T. Black, M.D. & J. Miller, M.D.

Bursitis

BASICS

DESCRIPTION A bursa is a sac that is formed or found in areas subject to friction, such as locations where tendons pass over bony landmarks. Most common sites are subdeltoid olecranon, prepatellar, trochanteric, radiohumeral. They essentially lubricate the region with synovial fluid. Large bursae usually communicate with joints and are responsible for retaining the synovial fluid in place. Bursae are fluid-filled sacs that serve as a cushion between tendons and bones. Bywaters, an English rheumatologist, found at least 78 bursae symmetrically placed on each side of the body.

System(s) affected: Musculoskeletal
Genetics: N/A
Incidence/Prevalence in USA: Common. Traumatic bursitis more likely in patients less than 35 years of age.
Predominant age: 15-50 years (most common in skeletally mature)
Predominant sex: Males > Females

SIGNS AND SYMPTOMS
• Include pain/tenderness/decreased range of motion of affected region
• Erythema
• Swelling
• Crepitus sometimes found

CAUSES
• Bursitis may be acute or chronic, and its etiology is often unknown
• There are many types of bursitis, including infectious, traumatic, inflammatory or gouty
• Less often rheumatoid disease or TB as well as gout and pseudogout

RISK FACTORS Individuals who engage in repetitive and vigorous training or others who suddenly increase their level of activity (e.g., "weekend warriors"). Also, improper or over-zealous stretching may lead to injury.

DIAGNOSIS

DIFFERENTIAL DIAGNOSIS
• Tendonitis, strains and sprains
• Joint pains may be caused by gout, pseudogout, rheumatoid arthritis, osteoarthritis
• Arthritis. Many elderly patients think it is the cause of their pain. (Lars Goran-Larsson, a rheumatologist from Sweden, and John Barn, M.D., reviewed their referrals for a 26-month period and found that 108 of 600 (18%) patients had some form of soft tissue problem rather than arthritis).

LABORATORY CBC, ESR, serum protein electrophoresis, rheumatoid factor (RF), serum uric acid, calcium, phosphorus, alkaline phosphatase, VDRL and joint fluid analysis (when available) will all help in differentiating soft tissue disease from rheumatic and connective tissue disease
Drugs that may alter lab results:
• ESR may be increased with coexistent use of dextran, methyldopa, methysergide, penicillamine, theophylline, vitamin A
• ESR may be decreased with coexistent use of quinine, salicylates, and drugs which cause a high glucose level
Disorders that may alter lab results: N/A

PATHOLOGICAL FINDINGS
• Acute - with early inflammation, bursa is distended with watery or mucoid fluid
• Chronic - bursal wall is thickened and inner surface is shaggy and trabeculated. The space is filled with granular, brown, inspissated blood admixed with gritty, calcific precipitations. Upper extremity tendonitis and bursitis are usually the result of repetitive microtrauma, probably resulting in disruption of fibers leading to pain, spasm and disability.

SPECIAL TESTS ECG (if pain mimics cardiac pain)

IMAGING
• CT or MRI
• Calcific deposits may be seen on plain x-ray

DIAGNOSTIC PROCEDURES
• Aspiration of swollen bursa and evaluation of synovial fluid
• The clinician must differentiate infected from inflammatory bursitis. Fluid analysis and culture help make the diagnosis. If the gram stain and culture yield an infective cause, treat with appropriate antibiotics. If the etiology is inflammatory, give local care.

TREATMENT

APPROPRIATE HEALTH CARE
Outpatient

GENERAL MEASURES
• Conservative therapy consists of rest, ice and local care, elevation, gentle compression (often referred to as RICE therapy (rest-ice-compression-elevation)
• Physical therapy
• Invasive therapy would include aspiration of the bursa, injection of steroids and, in severe cases, surgical excision
• Have patient wear a triangular sling to protect arm and support shoulder
• Treatment of any underlying infection

ACTIVITY Rest and elevation of affected extremity

DIET N/A

PATIENT EDUCATION
• Advice concerning prevention via appropriate warm-up and stretching and avoidance of repetitive injury
• Possible life-style changes to prevent recurrent joint irritation

MEDICATIONS

DRUG(S) OF CHOICE
• Nonsteroidal anti-inflammatories (NSAID's) or aspirin. Injectable steroids and stronger analgesics if needed.
• Antibiotic therapy if infection present
Contraindications: Refer to manufacturer's profile of each drug
Precautions: Refer to manufacturer's profile of each drug
Significant possible interactions: Refer to manufacturer's profile of each drug

ALTERNATIVE DRUGS
• Application of local analgesic balms, injection of a corticosteroid along with lidocaine
• Systemic steroids (if not contraindicated)

FOLLOWUP

PATIENT MONITORING
• Discontinue NSAID's as soon as possible to avoid side effects
• Some patients may require repeated injections (usually no more than three) of a corticosteroid and Lidocaine

PREVENTION/AVOIDANCE
• Appropriate warm-up and cool-down maneuvers, avoidance of overuse or inadequate rest between workouts
• Range of motion exercises
• Maintain high level of fitness and general good health

POSSIBLE COMPLICATIONS
• Acute bursitis may progress to chronic
• Severe long-range limitation of motion

EXPECTED COURSE AND PROGNOSIS
• Most bouts of bursitis heal without sequelae
• Repetitive acute bouts may lead to chronic bursitis necessitating repeated joint/bursal aspirations or eventually surgical excision of involved bursa

MISCELLANEOUS

ASSOCIATED CONDITIONS Tendinitis, sprains, strains, associated stress fractures

AGE-RELATED FACTORS
Pediatric: N/A
Geriatric: More common
Others: N/A

PREGNANCY N/A

SYNONYMS N/A

ICD-9-CM 727.3

SEE ALSO N/A

OTHER NOTES N/A

ABBREVIATIONS N/A

REFERENCES
• Robbins, S.L. & Cotran, R.S.: Pathological Basis of Disease. 2nd Ed. Philadelphia, W.B. Saunders Co., 1989
• Rotstein, B.R.: Soft tissue rheumatism of the upper extremities: diagnosis and management. Medline Professional, Sept, 1991

Author T. Robinson, D.O. & R. Birrer, M.D.

Candidiasis

 BASICS

DESCRIPTION
Candida albicans and related species cause a variety of infections. Cutaneous candidiasis syndromes include erosio interdigitalis blastomycetica, folliculitis, balanitis, intertrigo, paronychia, onychomycosis, diaper rash, perianal candidiasis, and the syndromes of chronic mucocutaneous candidiasis. Mucous membrane infections include oral candidiasis (thrush), esophagitis, and vaginitis. The most serious manifestation of candidiasis is hematogenously disseminated candidiasis (sometimes referred to as systemic candidiasis).

System(s) affected: Skin/Exocrine, Gastrointestinal, Reproductive
Genetics: N/A
Incidence: Approximately 50/100,000. Hematogenously disseminated candidiasis affects at least 120,000 patients annually in the USA.
Prevalence in USA: N/A
Predominant age: All ages are susceptible to hematogenously disseminated candidiasis. Premature neonates are at particularly high risk.
Predominant sex: Male = Female (hematogenously disseminated candidiasis)

SIGNS AND SYMPTOMS
- Fever
- Malaise
- Tachycardia
- Hypotension
- Altered mental status
- Hepatosplenomegaly
- Maculopapular or nodular skin rash

CAUSES
- Most Candida infections are due to Candida albicans. However, other important human pathogens include C. tropicalis, C. krusei, C. stelladtoidea, C. pseudotropicalis, C. guilliermondi, C. parapsilosis, C. lusitaniae, C. lambica, and Torulopsis glabrata.
- Candida species colonize human mucocutaneous surfaces, and most infections are endogenously acquired from this reservoir
- Human-to-human transmission of Candida occurs in some settings

RISK FACTORS
For hematogenously disseminated candidiasis: Neutropenia, antibacterial chemotherapy, indwelling intravascular access devices, prior hemodialysis, mucocutaneous candidiasis

 DIAGNOSIS

DIFFERENTIAL DIAGNOSIS
Includes a variety of cryptic bacterial infections and, in the neutropenic host, multiple opportunistic infections

LABORATORY
N/A
Drugs that may alter lab results: N/A
Disorders that may alter lab results: N/A

PATHOLOGICAL FINDINGS
The characteristic histopathology of lesions of Candida invasion of visceral organs is microabscess formation

SPECIAL TESTS
- The diagnosis is established by isolating the causative organism from blood cultures (lysis/centrifugation blood cultures are superior to broth culture techniques for this purpose) or other normally sterile body sites by demonstration of organisms in histopathologic specimens of normally sterile tissues
- Isolation of Candida from multiple sites should raise the diagnostic suspicion of hematogenously disseminated candidiasis

IMAGING
Imaging techniques are generally not specifically useful in the diagnosis of hematogenously disseminated candidiasis. However, in the syndrome of hepatosplenic candidiasis (chronic systemic candidiasis) imaging of the liver and spleen by liver scan, ultrasound, or CT (the most sensitive) may be useful in suggesting this syndrome as the cause of persistent fever and liver dysfunction.

DIAGNOSTIC PROCEDURES
If blood cultures remain consistently negative, excisional biopsy may be useful in diagnosis. Aspiration and biopsy of skin lesions occasionally seen with hematogenously disseminated candidiasis is also useful.

 TREATMENT

APPROPRIATE HEALTH CARE
Inpatient for hematogenously disseminated candidiasis

GENERAL MEASURES
- Fluid and electrolyte therapy is often required
- Hemodynamic and respiratory support may be required in seriously ill patients
- Removal of potentially infected intravascular access devices

ACTIVITY
As tolerated

DIET
No special diet

PATIENT EDUCATION
Patients should be advised of the nature of the infection and the toxicities associated with therapy

MEDICATIONS

DRUG(S) OF CHOICE Amphotericin B is the drug of choice for all forms of hematogenously disseminated candidiasis. (One exception is hepatosplenic candidiasis, where fluconazole or itraconazole are probably superior to amphotericin B). In some non-neutropenic patients with persistent candidemia, synergistic therapy with amphotericin B and flucytosine may be warranted. Amphotericin B is administered first in a test dose of 1 mg and then in incrementally increasing doses to 0.3 to 0.7 mg/kg/day. (Some authorities administer full dose after the test dose. In a critical ill patient, slow increase in dose is not warranted). Depending on host status and form of hematogenously disseminated candidiasis, total dose requirement ranges from 200 mg to 2.0 gm over a therapeutic duration of 2-10 weeks.

Contraindications: The safety of amphotericin B therapy in pregnant patients has not been established

Precautions:

Amphotericin B

◊ Toxicity is formidable. Acute reactions occur commonly during initiation of therapy, including fever, rigors, and hypotension. These can be ameliorated or eliminated by premedication with acetaminophen, ibuprofen or hydrocortisone, and tend to decline over time with continuing daily therapy. Use meperidine if needed to abort rigors.

◊ Azotemia is a common complication and may be an indication for reducing therapy in some patients (to reduce toxicity, not because of renal elimination of drug). Generally recommended to hold drug if BUN > 40 or creatinine >3.0. Hold until above levels decline, then administer drug every other day. Maintenance of optimal fluid status and prevention of dehydration help minimize risk of azotemia. "Sodium loading" with 77 mEq sodium daily (= 1 L 1/2 normal saline) has been suggested by some authorities to decrease renal toxicity.

◊ Significant hypokalemia (often requires therapy) and renal tubular acidosis (rarely requires therapy) may develop. Significant hypomagnesemia may worsen hypokalemia.

◊ Anemia commonly develops in patients on protracted therapy but is almost always reversible

◊ Headache and phlebitis are common

◊ Leukopenia, thrombocytopenia, and liver function abnormalities are rarely encountered

Significant possible interactions:

Concomitant therapy with cyclosporine or other nephrotoxic agents such as aminoglycoside or vancomycin may increase risk of amphotericin-induced nephrotoxicity

ALTERNATIVE DRUGS Fluconazole 400 mg per day orally or intravenously is a potential alternative agent - especially useful in hepatosplenic candidiasis, where amphotericin B doesn't work well. Clinical experience with fluconazole for hematogenously disseminated candidiasis is inadequate.

FOLLOWUP

PATIENT MONITORING Complete blood count, serum electrolytes, and serum creatinine should be measured at least twice weekly in patients on daily amphotericin B therapy. If blood cultures are positive, they should be repeated until negative.

PREVENTION/AVOIDANCE
Fluconazole 400 mg/day reduces the incidence of candidiasis in patients undergoing induction therapy for acute leukemia or bone marrow transplantation

POSSIBLE COMPLICATIONS
Of hematogenously disseminated candidiasis
◊ Pyelonephritis
◊ Endophthalmitis
◊ Endocarditis, myocarditis, pericarditis
◊ Arthritis, chondritis, osteomyelitis
◊ Pneumonitis
◊ Central nervous system infection

EXPECTED COURSE AND PROGNOSIS Overall mortality for patients with hematogenously disseminated candidiasis is 75%, with mortality attributable to candidemia being 37%

MISCELLANEOUS

ASSOCIATED CONDITIONS See Risk Factors

AGE-RELATED FACTORS
Pediatric: N/A
Geriatric: N/A
Others: N/A

PREGNANCY N/A

SYNONYMS N/A

ICD-9-CM 112.9

SEE ALSO
• Mucocutaneous candidiasis

OTHER NOTES Other candidal infections: Intraperitoneal infection in patients with major abdominal surgery, biliary tract candidiasis, isolated lower urinary tract infection

ABBREVIATIONS N/A

REFERENCES
• Crislip, M.A. & Edwards, J.E., Jr.: Candidiasis. Infect Dis Clinics North America 3:103-133, 1989
• Fraser, V.J., Jones, M., Dunkel, J., Sorfer, S., Medoff, G. & Dunagan, W.C.: Candidemia in a tertiary care hospital: Epidemiology, risk factors, and predictors of mortality. Clin Infect Dis. 15:414-21, 1992

Author R. Greenfield, M.D. & D. Fine, M.D.

Candidiasis, mucocutaneous

BASICS

DESCRIPTION
A mucocutaneous disorder caused by infection with, most commonly, species of Candida. Candida is normally present, in very small amounts, in the oral cavity, gastrointestinal tract, and female genital tract.
- Candida vulvovaginitis - this common form of mucocutaneous candidiasis consists of infections located on the vaginal mucosa, often associated with cutaneous vulvar involvement as well
- Oropharyngeal candidiasis - a candida infection of the oral cavity ("thrush") and/or pharynx. "Thrush" in infants and immunocompromised adult hosts.
- Candida esophagitis - usually associated with an immunosuppressed host
- Gastrointestinal candidiasis - gastritis, sometimes with ulcers, associated with candida infection. The small and large bowel can also be affected.
- Angular cheilitis - fissures formed by candida infection at the corners of the mouth.

System(s) affected: Skin/Exocrine, Gastrointestinal
Genetics: None known
Incidence/Prevalence: Very common, particularly vaginal
Predominant age:
- Infants and older geriatrics predominate for thrush and cutaneous infections
- Women during their child bearing years predominate for vaginitis

Predominant sex: Female > Male (due to the entity of Candida vaginitis)

SIGNS AND SYMPTOMS
In pediatrics
◊ Oral lesions - white, raised, painless, distinct patches
In adults (whether or not immunocompromised)
◊ Vulvovaginal lesions - thin to thick whitish, "cottage cheese" like; erythematous patches in vagina, on labia, on vulva, or other areas of perineum. Range from asymptomatic to intense pruritus with "burning" irritation
◊ Oral lesions - white, raised, painless, distinct patches; erythematous slightly raised patches; thick dark brownish coating; deep fissures
In immunocompromised hosts
◊ Esophagitis - dysphagia, odynophagia, retrosternal pain. May not be associated with thrush.
◊ Gastrointestinal - ulcerations

CAUSES
Species of candida albicans, and less frequently, Candida tropicalis

RISK FACTORS
- Immunosuppression
- Antibacterial therapy
- Douching, chemical irritants, other vaginitides predispose some women to yeast vaginitis
- Dentures
- Chronic steroids (oral or inhaled)
- Birth control pills

DIAGNOSIS

DIFFERENTIAL DIAGNOSIS
- Baby formula can mimic thrush
- Hairy leukoplakia can mimic thrush but does not rub off to an erythematous base, is KOH negative, and is usually on the lateral sides on the tongue.
- Other yeasts may present like candida

LABORATORY
- Potassium hydroxide 10% microscopic slide preparation ("KOH prep"). Breaks down epithelial cell walls allowing yeast forms to be more easily identified.
- Gram stain reveals gram positive yeast forms
- Culture - blood or Sabouraud's agar. A positive may be result of normal flora.

SPECIAL TESTS   N/A
Drugs that may alter lab results:
- Douches and spermicides (intravaginal infection)
- Inadequately dosed antifungal medication
Disorders that may alter lab results:
Other vaginitides (may obscure vaginal slide findings)

PATHOLOGICAL FINDINGS
Slide prep - Mycelia (hyphae) or pseudomycelia (pseudohyphae) yeast forms. A polymorphonuclear leukocyte response is not usually seen.

IMAGING
Esophageal candidiasis will sometimes reveal a "cobblestone" appearance with a barium swallow and, less commonly, fistulas or esophageal dilatation (from denervation)

DIAGNOSTIC PROCEDURES
- For KOH prep, will need sample of discharge or "coating" of infected area
- Esophagitis may need endoscopic biopsy

TREATMENT

APPROPRIATE HEALTH CARE
Outpatient

GENERAL MEASURES
Screen patients with severe immunodeficiency using appropriate history and physical at all routine visits

ACTIVITY   N/A

DIET
A few authorities say rectal colonization may be decreased with active culture yogurt or other live lactobacillus, but no clear correlation

PATIENT EDUCATION
- Advise patients at risk for recurrence about antibacterial therapy overgrowth
- Inform appropriate patients of over-the-counter vaginitis medications
- Cotton underwear may allow for better perineal ventilation and, thus, a less suitable environment for yeast

MEDICATIONS

DRUG(S) OF CHOICE
Vaginal (choose one)
◊ Miconazole (Monistat) 2% cream - one applicator or 100mg suppositories, intravaginally q hs x 7 days
◊ Clotrimazole (Gyne-Lotrimin, Mycelex) - intravaginal suppositories 100mg q hs x 6-7 days or 200mg q hs x 3 days. 1% cream one applicator intravaginally q hs x 6-7 days.
◊ Nystatin (Mycostatin, Nilstat) 100,000 U/gram cream (one applicator) or 100,000 U tablets (one) intravaginally bid x 7 days
Oropharyngeal
◊ Clotrimazole (Mycelex) 10mg troche, slowly dissolve in mouth 5 times per day, preferably over 20 minutes (first choice in most literature)
◊ Nystatin oral suspension - swish and swallow 5-10mL over 20 minutes 4-5 times per day x 14 days. Prophylaxis for relapses consists of above dosages 2-5 times per day.
Esophagitis
◊ Ketoconazole (Nizoral) 200-400mg tablets - one po qd x 14-21 days
or
◊ Fluconazole (Diflucan) 200mg tablet one time, then 100mg po qd x 10-21 days
Gastrointestinal (therapy not well defined)
◊ Fluconazole 200mg tablets - one po qd x 14-21 days
or
◊ Amphotericin B (Fungizone) IV solution - variable dosing, see pharmacology texts for full appropriate administration information

Contraindications:

• Any drug is contraindicated if it causes severe allergic response or a severe adverse reaction
• Ketoconazole or nystatin (if swallow) - severe hepatotoxicity
• Amphotericin B - renal failure

Precautions:

• Vaginal - myconazole is usually drug of choice in pregnancy
• Ketoconazole - rarely, men may have difficulty achieving erections secondary to this drug. May cause light sensitivity. Teratogen in pregnancy and probably excreted in milk. Not well studied in children. Anaphylaxis is reported. Hepatic toxicity has been noted, predominantly with long-term therapy.
• Fluconazole - adjust dose with renal compromise. Hepatotoxicity is rare but reported. Very expensive relative to other oral agents.
• Amphotericin B - renal toxicity and hypokalemia are common. Careful patient monitoring is mandatory. Ketotic diabetics should have well controlled blood sugars prior to administration. Safety during pregnancy is not established.

Significant possible interactions:

• Rarely seen with creams, lotions or suppositories
• Ketoconazole
  ◊ antacids, H2 blockers (achlorhydria): reduce ketoconazole concentration
  ◊ amphotericin: drug antagonism, do not give together.
  ◊ coumadin: potentiates anticoagulation
  ◊ hypoglycemics: enhanced hypoglycemia
  ◊ INH/rifampin: reduce ketoconazole concentration
  ◊ cyclosporine: increased cyclosporine concentration
  ◊ phenytoin: metabolism altered; check levels
  ◊ terfenadine(Seldane), aztemizole: ECG QT abnormalities
  ◊ alcohol: disulfiram reaction possible
• Amphotericin
  ◊ nephrotoxic drugs; enhanced toxicity
  ◊ corticosteroids
  ◊ ketoconazole: drug antagonism, do not give together.
• Fluconazole
  ◊ rifampin: decreased fluconazole concentrations
  ◊ tolbutamide: decreased tolbutamide concentrations
  ◊ warfarin, phenytoin, cyclosporine: metabolism altered; check levels.

ALTERNATIVE DRUGS

Vaginal
◊ Fluconazole 100-200 mg qd x 2-5 days
◊ Terconazole (Terazol) particularly for recurrent cases that may involve imidazole resistance. 0.4% cream - one applicator intravaginally q hs x 7 days; 0.8% cream/80 mg suppositories - one applicator or one suppository intravaginally q hs x 3 days
◊ Any of the antifungal creams or suppositories can be tried every month for a few days near menses to help curb recurrent infections

Oropharyngeal
◊ Ketoconazole 200-400 mg po qd x 14-21 days
◊ Fluconazole 50-200 mg tablets - one po qd x 14-21 days

Esophagitis
◊ Amphotericin B (variable dosing)

FOLLOWUP

PATIENT MONITORING

Immunocompromised persons may need to monitor themselves regularly. Use symptoms to monitor as well as "routine" KOH preps and or visual investigations during vaginal or oral exams.

PREVENTION/AVOIDANCE

• Antibiotics can potentiate candidiasis
• Candida overgrowth is more likely with pH changes from douching, chemicals (such as spermicides) or other vaginitides
• Moist environments are conducive to overgrowth of Candida. Cotton underwear may help deter some Candida infections.

POSSIBLE COMPLICATIONS

• Rarely develops major complications in immunocompetent persons
• With immunocompromised, generally depends on severity of immune status (CD4 count is the most common marker). Moderate immunodepression (CD4 200-500) is often associated with chronic candidiasis. With severe immunodepression (CD4 < 100) thrush can lead to esophagitis and, later, a full systemic infection can involve every organ system, particularly the kidney (candiduria).

EXPECTED COURSE AND PROGNOSIS

• For relative immunocompetent individuals, a benign course and excellent prognosis is the norm. Recurrent vulvovaginitis may be associated with a colonized partner but specifics have not yet been well documented.
• For severely immunosuppressed persons, candida may become an "AIDS defining illness" by CDC criteria and chronicity can cause much morbidity and, less commonly, mortality

MISCELLANEOUS

ASSOCIATED CONDITIONS

• Human immunodeficiency virus
• Other leukopenias
• Diabetes mellitus
• Cancer
• Other immunosuppressive disorders

AGE-RELATED FACTORS

Pediatric: Newborn thrush may be acquired in the birth canal
Geriatric: A common geriatric infection
Others: Vaginitis is common in women of childbearing age. Uncommon to see prepubertal or postmenopausal yeast vaginitis due to hormonal induced changes in the vaginal wall.

PREGNANCY

• No known fetal complications of maternal candida
• See specific "medication precautions" above
• Myconazole is usually drug of choice in pregnancy

SYNONYMS

• Monilia
• Thrush

ICD-9-CM 112.9

SEE ALSO

• Candidiasis

OTHER NOTES

• Most Candida infections are associated with endogenous flora
• Transmission from person to person is rare
• Occasionally Candida vaginitis may be sexually transmitted
• Rarely, oral Candida leukoplakia can be precancerous
• Esophageal candidiasis may occur concurrently with herpes simplex virus esophagitis in severely immunocompromised persons
• Skin testing, often used to diagnose or exclude anergy, is positive in 70-85% of individuals randomly checked in studies
• Thrush (oral candida only)

ABBREVIATIONS N/A

REFERENCES Reese, R.E. & Betts, R.F. (eds.): A Practical Approach to Infectious Diseases. 3rd Ed. Boston, Little, Brown and Co., 1991

Author S. Montauk, M.D.

Cardiac arrest

 BASICS

DESCRIPTION Absence of mechanical cardiac activity
System(s) affected: Cardiovascular
Genetics: N/A
Incidence/Prevalence in USA: 2:1000
Predominant age: Directly correlated with increasing age
Predominant sex: Male > Female

SIGNS AND SYMPTOMS
- Unconscious
- No pulse in large arteries
- Apnea or gasps
- Cyanosis or pallor

CAUSES
- Asystole
- Ventricular fibrillation (VF)
- Pulseless ventricular tachycardia (VT)
- Electromechanical dissociation (EMD)

RISK FACTORS
- Male
- Older age
- Elevated cholesterol
- Hypertension
- Cigarette smoking
- Family history of atherosclerosis

 DIAGNOSIS

DIFFERENTIAL DIAGNOSIS
- Asystole
- Ventricular fibrillation
- Pulseless ventricular tachycardia
- Electromechanical dissociation (cardiac tamponade, pneumothorax, severe hypovolemia, pulmonary embolism)

LABORATORY Arterial Blood Gas to guide bicarbonate treatment, electrolytes as a cause of arrhythmias
Drugs that may alter lab results: N/A
Disorders that may alter lab results:
Hyper- or hypoventilation may alter pH by changing pCO2, so treat bicarbonate or base excess

PATHOLOGICAL FINDINGS Scar tissue from old myocardial infarction

SPECIAL TESTS ECG

IMAGING Fluoroscopy perhaps to guide pacemaker placement (for bradycardia or asystole)

DIAGNOSTIC PROCEDURES
- Pericardiocentesis to diagnose and treat cardiac tamponade
- Thoracostomy (chest tube insertion) or needle aspiration of the chest to diagnose and treat tension pneumothorax

 TREATMENT

APPROPRIATE HEALTH CARE Cardiac arrest team or intensive care setting

GENERAL MEASURES
- Defibrillation
- Intravenous or intra-tracheal epinephrine 1 mg q 5 min
- Closed chest massage (board underneath body)
- Endotracheal intubation
- Intravenous access peripheral or central (preferred, especially if prolonged)
- Monitoring by: Carotid or femoral pulses, pupil size, Capnogram (increasing end-tidal CO2 indicates better lung perfusion and overall cardiac output)

ACTIVITY N/A

DIET N/A

PATIENT EDUCATION N/A

MEDICATIONS

DRUG(S) OF CHOICE
Drug doses for children:
◊ Epinephrine 10 mcg/kg
◊ Atropine 20 mcg/kg
◊ Intraosseous route may be used

In conjunction with CPR:
For ventricular fibrillation and pulseless ventricular tachycardia
◊ Defibrillation X3: 200J, 300J, 360J
◊ Epinephrine (1 mg); repeat every five minutes
◊ Lidocaine 1 mg/kg IV, repeat defibrillation, may repeat .5 mg/kg twice
◊ Bretylium 5 mg/kg, repeat defibrillation, may repeat 10 mg/kg twice
◊ Infusion of the successful anti-arrhythmic (lidocaine or bretylium)
For asystole
◊ Epinephrine 1 mg IV or via endotracheal tube; repeat every five minutes
◊ Atropine 1 mg IV
◊ Pacemaker
◊ Try defibrillation (some ECG leads may look flat, but may show fibrillation in other leads)
For electromechanical dissociation:
◊ Epinephrine 1 mg IV q5min
Contraindications: None
Precautions:
• Bretylium may cause hypotension 15 to 20 minutes after injection
• Epinephrine, atropine, and lidocaine all can be administered intratracheally
• Calcium is not recommended for any standard treatment in cardiac arrest
• Intracardiac epinephrine should not be given if an intravenous or intratracheal route is available
Significant possible interactions: Refer to manufacturer's profile of each drug

ALTERNATIVE DRUGS
Procainamide may be tried as an antiarrhythmic for ventricular fibrillation

FOLLOWUP

PATIENT MONITORING
Intensive care, continuous ECG monitoring, serial cardiac enzymes

PREVENTION/AVOIDANCE
Treat underlying coronary artery disease and potential arrhythmias

POSSIBLE COMPLICATIONS
Ischemia and failure of every organ, especially brain, heart, and kidneys

EXPECTED COURSE AND PROGNOSIS
• About 14% survival for in-hospital arrest
• Outcome of survivors is dependent upon severity of underlying cardiac disease

MISCELLANEOUS

ASSOCIATED CONDITIONS
• Coronary artery disease (including myocardial infarction)
• Ischemic heart disease
• Valvular or congenital heart disease
• Hypertension
• Chest trauma
• Hypovolemia
• Pneumothorax
• Cardiac tamponade
• Pre-excitation syndrome or prolonged QT syndromes

AGE-RELATED FACTORS
Pediatric: Bradyasystole is the most common cause of cardiac arrest, usually from hypoxemia making airway and ventilation management important.
Geriatric: Decreased survival
Others: N/A

PREGNANCY
• Patient should ALWAYS have uterine displacement, by a roll or pad under the right hip. If resuscitation is not effective within 5 to 15 minutes, fetus should be delivered by C-Section to relieve uterine obstruction to maternal blood return, and resuscitation efforts should continue.
• Amniotic fluid embolism or seizures from eclampsia may be precipitating causes of cardiac arrest

SYNONYMS
• Cardiac standstill
• Code Blue

ICD-9-CM
427.5 Cardiac arrest

SEE ALSO
N/A

OTHER NOTES
• Defibrillators maximum output about 360 Joules (Joule = watt-second)

ABBREVIATIONS
N/A

REFERENCES
• Textbook of Advanced Cardiac Life Support, American Heart Association, 1987
• White, R.D.: Cardiopulmonary Resuscitation. In Anesthesia. Edited by R. Miller. New York, Churchill Livingston, 1990
• Safar, P.: Cardiopulmonary Cerebral Resuscitation. In Textbook of Critical Care. Edited by W.C. Shoemaker, et al.: Philadelphia, W.B. Saunders Co., 1988

Author T. Hurd, M.D.

Cardiac tamponade

BASICS

DESCRIPTION Compression of cardiac chambers by acute pressure on the heart from increased volume and pressure of the pericardial fluid
 • As fluid accumulates, pressure primarily affects the compliant cardiac wall and transmits the pressure transmurally, resulting in increased ventricular pressure. This decreases ventricular filling and reduces cardiac output by reducing stroke volume. Contraction is preserved until ventricular diastolic pressures rise enough to limit coronary perfusion.
 • The compensatory mechanisms for tamponade are: Increased peripheral resistance, increased CVP and increased heart rate. All three increase myocardial oxygen denied the heart at a time when perfusion is limited.
 • In some patients, pulsus paradoxus and equalization of pressures may not occur
 • In patients with elevated left ventricular diastolic pressures (as with chronic hypertension), resistance to left ventricle (LV) filling is constant. Throughout the cardiac cycle, equalization of pressures in these patients may only be noted in the right heart chambers with LV pressures being higher than right ventricle (RV) pressures.
 • The absence of pulsus paradoxus and classic hemodynamic finding does not rule out tamponade
System(s) affected: Cardiovascular
Genetics: N/A
Incidence/Prevalence in USA: N/A
Predominant age: N/A
Predominant sex: N/A

SIGNS AND SYMPTOMS
 • Beck's triad - distant heart sounds, hypotension, distended neck veins
 • Most common complaints are of intolerance to minimal activity and dyspnea. Later may develop agitation, CNS depression, coma and cardiac arrest.
 • Decreased systolic blood pressure
 • Narrow pulse pressure
 • Pulsus paradoxus - greater than 15 mm Hg drop in systolic blood pressure between inspiration and expiration
 • Neck veins may be distended and reveal a rapid systolic (X) descent and attenuated or absent diastolic (Y) descent
 • Tachycardia - a compensatory mechanism to maintain output
 • Right upper quadrant tenderness due to hepatic engorgement
 • Increased area of cardiac dullness outside the apical point of maximum impulse

CAUSES
 • Physiology of tamponade depends on size and rapidity of development
 • Uremia
 • Neoplasm - breast, lung, lymphoma, leukemia
 • Postmyocardial infarction (Dressler's)
 • Postoperative - as high as 30% post pericardiotomy
 • Viral Infection - Coxsackie group B, influenza, echo, herpes
 • Bacterial infection - S. aureus, M. tuberculosis, S. pneumoniae (rare)
 • Fungal infection - M. capsulatum
 • Lupus and rheumatologic disease
 • Trauma
 • Placement of central venous catheter, pacer wires
 • Myxedema
 • Drug induced

RISK FACTORS
Cardiac tamponade should be suspected in the hemodynamically unstable patient:
 ◊ With known pericarditis
 ◊ Following blunt or penetrating chest trauma
 ◊ Following open heart surgery or cardiac catheterization
 ◊ With known or suspected intrathoracic neoplasm
 ◊ With suspected dissecting aortic aneurysm
 ◊ Renal failure on dialysis

DIAGNOSIS

DIFFERENTIAL DIAGNOSIS
 • Tension pneumothorax
 • Acute RV failure
 • Chronic obstructive pulmonary disease
 • Constrictive pericarditis
 • Acute acceleration of chronic bronchitis
 • Acute pulmonary emboli
 • Fat emboli
 • Excessive or rapid administration of fluids
 • Abdominal distention from ascites or ileus
 • Increased intrathoracic pressure from pneumothorax, hemothorax, airway obstruction, or mechanical ventilation
 • Administration of vasopressors

LABORATORY
 • CBC
 • Sed rate
 • Cardiac enzymes to rule out acute myocardial infarction
 • Antinuclear antibodies (ANA)
 • Rheumatoid factor
 • BUN/creatinine
 • Pericardial fluid for - culture of bacteria, fungus, mycobacteria, Gram stain, hematocrit, cell count, cytology, glucose, protein, rheumatoid factors, complement levels
Drugs that may alter lab results: N/A
Disorders that may alter lab results: N/A

PATHOLOGICAL FINDINGS Pericardial
blood usually does not clot, but occasionally will

SPECIAL TESTS
ECG
 ◊ May show low voltage QRS complexes, ST segment elevation and PR segment depression of pericarditis
 ◊ Electrical alternans (R wave variation from beat to beat)
 ◊ Electrical alternans is seen in 10-20% of cases of tamponade and 50-60% of these are neoplastic in origin
Right heartl catherization
 ◊ Equalization (within 2-3 mm) of right atrial, pulmonary artery, pulmonary capillary wedge pressure, left atrial and left ventricular diastolic pressure
 ◊ The intracardiac diastolic pressure will approximate the intrapericardial pressure
 ◊ The dip and plateau pattern of constriction or restriction pericardial disease is absent
 ◊ Loss of Y descent on atrial wave form

IMAGING
Chest x-ray:
 ◊ May or may not show enlargement of cardiac shadow (if > 250 cc fluid present)
Echocardiography:
 ◊ Diagnostic cardiac compression
 ◊ Doppler - right sided transvalvular flow greatly exaggerated; left sided flows greatly reduced with inspiration

DIAGNOSTIC PROCEDURES N/A

TREATMENT

APPROPRIATE HEALTH CARE
Inpatient

GENERAL MEASURES
• Maintain hemodynamic stability until definitive correction of the pericardial tamponade
• All patients should have q 15 minute blood pressures, heart rate and at a minimum CVP measurement. Strong consideration should be given to placement of a Swan-Ganz catheter if time allows.
Medical management:
◊ Fluids may be of temporary benefit, but rising filling pressures may further compromise coronary perfusion
Pericardiocentesis surgical treatment:
◊ Indications - when there is rapid deterioration of hemodynamic function, when there is delay in operation for traumatic effusion and for diagnostic reasons
◊ If rapid re-accumulation is anticipated (as in malignancy) it may be helpful to insert a long term drainage catheter. Also consider instillation of sclerosing agents.
◊ Surgery should be performed under the most optimal circumstances available to the operation as the patient's condition allows
◊ Blind pericardiocentesis should be performed only in life threatening emergencies
◊ Ideally echocardiography can be brought to the bedside to assist in needle placement and progress of fluid removal
◊ Invasive monitoring is also helpful to follow decrease in pericardial pressures
◊ Fluoroscopy can also be used
◊ EKG guidance using the "V" lead to avoid contact with the epicardium may be useful
◊ 20% of patients with tamponade will have a negative tap because the pericardial sac contains coagulated material. Hemorrhagic pericardial effusions usually do not clot.

ACTIVITY Bedrest

DIET As tolerated

PATIENT EDUCATION N/A

MEDICATIONS

DRUG(S) OF CHOICE Isoproterenol may temporarily increase cardiac output
Contraindications: Refer to manufacturer's literature
Precautions: Refer to manufacturer's literature
Significant possible interactions: Refer to manufacturer's literature

ALTERNATIVE DRUGS N/A

FOLLOWUP

PATIENT MONITORING Close monitoring until stable

PREVENTION/AVOIDANCE None

POSSIBLE COMPLICATIONS
• Cardiac perforation and/or laceration at time of pericardiocentesis
• Pneumothorax at time of pericardiocentesis
• Constriction of pericardium

EXPECTED COURSE AND PROGNOSIS Good results expected with appropriate treatment

MISCELLANEOUS

ASSOCIATED CONDITIONS
• Myocardial infarction
• Aortic aneurysm

AGE-RELATED FACTORS
Pediatric: N/A
Geriatric: N/A
Others: N/A

PREGNANCY N/A

SYNONYMS N/A

ICD-9-CM 423.9

SEE ALSO N/A

OTHER NOTES N/A

ABBREVIATIONS N/A

REFERENCES
• Heger, J.W., et al.: Cardiology for the House Officer. Baltimore, Williams & Wilkins, 1982
• Civettee, J.M., Taylor, R.W. & Kirby, R.R.: Critical Care. Philadelphia, J.B. Lippincott, 1988
• Rippie, J.M., et al.: Intensive Care Medicine. Boston, Little, Brown and Company, 1991
• Shoemaker, W.C., et al.: Textbook of Critical Care. Philadelphia, W.B. Saunders Co., 1989

Author B. Martin, M.D.

Cardiomyopathy, end stage

 BASICS

DESCRIPTION Congestive heart failure causing symptoms with less than normal activity or at rest and requiring "maximal medical therapy".
Ischemic cardiomyopathy is the product of long standing, severe coronary artery disease, usually associated with multiple myocardial infarctions, often also following multiple coronary bypass operations.
This myopathy and the majority of others share in common four chamber dilatation of the heart, increased wall tension, and wall stress of the left and right ventricles, decreased mechanical efficiency of cardiac function. The tendency to have sub-endocardial ischemia, because of increased wall stress, and increased end diastolic pressures. Markedly decreased ejection fraction of usually in the range of 20% (normal 65%). Because of the abnormal mechanics there is a tendency for these hearts to progressively enlarge with time.

System(s) affected: Cardiovascular
Genetics: Idiopathic hypertrophic subaortic stenosis well known to have a familial distribution
Incidence in USA:
• The number of patients dying from end stage heart disease, per year, under the age of 65, in the US today is approximately 60,000
• 35,000 to 70,000 of the population might benefit from cardiac replacement or chronic support
Prevalence in USA: N/A
Predominant age:
• Ischemic cardiomyopathy is seen predominately in patients from the 5th decade of life and beyond
• Idiopathic and familial cardiomyopathies are seen at an earlier age, as are those related to congenital heart disease, viral cardiomyopathy, alcoholic cardiomyopathy and post partum cardiomyopathy
Predominant Sex: Male > Female (Ischemic cardiomyopathy

SIGNS AND SYMPTOMS
• Shortness of breath at rest
• Dyspnea on minimal exertion
• Paroxysmal nocturnal dyspnea
• Postprandial dyspnea
• Fatigue
• Syncope
• Tachypnea
• Cyanosis, pallor
• Cool vasoconstricted extremities
• Diaphoresis
• Jugular venous distention
• Bi-basilar inspiratory rales
• S3 cardiac gallop
• Liver and spleen enlargement
• Ascites, edema
• Chest pain

CAUSES
• Coronary artery disease
• Idiopathic
• Viral
• Congenital heart disease
• Familial cardiomyopathies, such as "asymmetric septal hypertrophy"
• Postpartum
• Alcoholism
• Cardiac surgery
• Sarcoidosis
• Amyloidosis
• Hemosiderosis
• Radiation

RISK FACTORS
• Hypertension
• Hyperlipidemia
• Obesity
• Diabetes mellitus
• Smoking
• Stress
• Sedentary lifestyle

 DIAGNOSIS

DIFFERENTIAL DIAGNOSIS
• Severe pulmonary disease
• Primary pulmonary hypertension
• Recurrent pulmonary embolism
• Hypothyroidism
• Some advanced forms of malignancy

LABORATORY
• Hyponatremia
• Pre-renal azotemia
• Mild hyperbilirubinemia
• ECG: left ventricular hypertrophy, ventricular strain pattern, left and right atrial enlargement are often seen. In ischemic cardiomyopathies evidence of previous myocardial infarctions indicated by Q-waves and poor R-wave progression in the precordial leads.
Drugs that may alter lab results: Digoxin, Lasix, ACE inhibitors (by improving cardiac function)
Disorders that may alter lab results: N/A

PATHOLOGICAL FINDINGS

SPECIAL TESTS
• Cardiac catheterization may help differentiate between ischemic and other types of cardiomyopathy, elucidate intracavitary pressures, cardiac output, left ventricular function and coronary anatomy. In addition, cardiac catheterization provides an opportunity for assessment for pulmonary artery pressures and pulmonary vascular resistance (mean pulmonary artery wedge pressure in millimeters of mercury divided by cardiac output in liters per minute (normal 1.2)).

• For transplant candidates, the following additional tests are recommended to rule out significant non-cardiac disease: Computed tomographic (CT) scans of the chest and abdomen; 24 hour creatinine clearance; routine pulmonary function studies (including blood gas determination); serologies for hepatitis A, B, C, HIV, Toxoplasma, CMV and EB virus; full panels of renal and liver function; a complete blood count with differential; and a Panorex dental x-ray. Additional diagnostic studies may be indicated if any findings are suspicious for disease which would be a contraindication to transplantation. For instance, any undiagnosed roentgenographic abnormality of the lungs is a contraindication to transplantation.

IMAGING
Chest x-ray
◊ Cardiac enlargement is found in the majority of cardiomyopathies, which are termed dilated cardiomyopathies
◊ Generally, four chamber enlargement is seen and the cardiac silhouette on a posterior-anterior film occupies more than 50% of the transverse diameter
◊ Increased vascular markings to the upper lobes, indicating elevated pulmonary venous pressure
◊ Hazy diffuse densities in the hilar areas, indicating pulmonary edema
◊ Pleural effusions and curly B-lines in the periphery of the lung, indicating engorged pulmonary lymphatics
◊ In hypertrophic cardiomyopathies and cardiomyopathies characterized by normal cardiac size, chest x-ray generally demonstrates pulmonary signs of cardiac failure with a cardiac silhouette which is normal to upper limits in size
Echocardiogram: In the dilated cardiomyopathies, demonstrates four chamber enlargement and global hypokinesias. In hypertrophic cardiomyopathies, severe left ventricular hypertrophy. In ischemic cardiomyopathy, the heart may be normal or enlarged. Usually segmental abnormalities in contraction of the left ventricle can be detected, indicative of previous localized myocardial infarction.
Nuclear multiple gaited acquisition ventriculogram (MUGA): The best study to quantitate ejection fraction, which is often 25% or less.

DIAGNOSTIC PROCEDURES   N/A

TREATMENT

APPROPRIATE HEALTH CARE
Outpatient until time for myocardial transplant or for treatment of severe heart failure

GENERAL MEASURES
• Treatment of heart failure
• Treatment of electrolyte disturbances

ACTIVITY
Limited by varying degrees. Bedrest may be necessary.

DIET
Low fat, low salt, fluid restriction

PATIENT EDUCATION
Careful instructions and precautions for all medications

MEDICATIONS

DRUG(S) OF CHOICE
• Dilated cardiomyopathies, in the usual recommended adult dosage include the following:
  ◊ Digoxin, 0.125-0.25 mg/day
  ◊ Furosemide 40-120 mg two to four times/day
  ◊ Potassium chloride 20 mEq for each 40 mg of furosemide
  ◊ ACE inhibitors - captopril 6.25-50 mg three times/day or enalapril 2.5-25 mg/day
  ◊ Isosorbide dinitrate 20-100 mg four times/day
  ◊ Hydralazine 5-25 mg four times/day (maximum of 300 mg/day divided)
  ◊ Oxygen 2-4 liters/minute by nasal cannula at bedtime

Contraindications:
• Digoxin - 1st or 2nd degree heart block
• Lasix - oliguria, anuria, renal dysfunction

Precautions:
• Digoxin - in patients with renal dysfunction requiring quinidine therapy, the digoxin dosage should be lowered to .125 mg/day and level determined 4 or 5 days later. The potassium level must also be carefully monitored.
• Furosemide - a careful titration of patients with end stage heart disease is necessary when furosemide therapy is employed. Over diuresis may result in dehydration and severe hyponatremia. Potassium therapy is necessary accompaniment to furosemide therapy in order to prevent hypokalemia and hypochloremic alkalosis. A combination of high dose furosemide plus aminoglycoside antibiotics may cause nephrotoxicity or ototoxicity.

• ACE inhibitors - must be used with extreme care. If the patient's blood pressure is already low, it's safest to begin with captopril at a very low dose such as 6.25 mg 3 times/day. The after load reduction or drop in systolic blood pressure, experienced by patients on these drugs may lead to reduction in cardiac size and improved efficiency. Patients survive longer when on ACE inhibitors.
Significant possible interactions: Digoxin - has many potentially significant interactions including antibiotics, amiodarone, verapamil, cholestyramine. Digoxin levels increase in patients on quinidine. Toxicity is more common in this setting.

ALTERNATIVE DRUGS
IV continuous infusion of dobutamine is the only other inotropic support for dilated cardiomyopathy. It may be applicable in an outpatient setting.

FOLLOWUP

PATIENT MONITORING
Once a month followup is usually adequate

PREVENTION/AVOIDANCE
Dietary control of salt and water intake, home blood pressure measurement, daily weight check by the patient are helpful in preventing problems

POSSIBLE COMPLICATIONS
Worsening congestive heart failure, syncope, arrhythmias, sudden death

EXPECTED COURSE AND PROGNOSIS
50% of the patients in New York functional class IV are expected to die within one year. In functional class III, it is probably 25%. With transplant, outlook is brighter.

MISCELLANEOUS

ASSOCIATED CONDITIONS N/A

AGE-RELATED FACTORS
Pediatric: Idiopathic and familial cardiomyopathies are seen at an earlier age, as are those related to congenital heart disease, viral cardiomyopathy, alcoholic cardiomyopathy and postpartum cardiomyopathy
Geriatric: N/A
Others: N/A

PREGNANCY May occur postpartum

SYNONYMS N/A

ICD-9-CM 425.5

SEE ALSO N/A

OTHER NOTES N/A

ABBREVIATIONS
CMV = cytomegalic inclusion virus

REFERENCES
• Copeland, J.G., Cardiac Transplantation. Curr Probl Surg. 25(9):607-72, 1988
• Emery, R.W., et al.: The cardiac donor: A six-year experience. Ann Thorac Surg. 41:356-362, 1986
• Wahlers, T., et al.: Donor heart related variables and early mortality after heart transplantation. J. Heart Transplant. 10:22-27, 1991
• Pickering, J.G., et al.: Fibrosis in the transplanted heart and its relation to donor ischemic time. Circulation. 81:949-958, 1990
• Hosenpud, J.O., et al.: Relation between recipient: Donor body size match and hemodynamics three months after heart transplantation. J. Heart Transplant. 8:241-243, 1989

Author J. Copeland, M.D.

Carotid sinus syndrome

 BASICS

DESCRIPTION
In carotid sinus syndrome (CSS), stimulation of one or both of the hypersensitive carotid sinuses at the bifurcation of the common carotid arteries produces brief episodes of faintness or loss of consciousness. In patients with unexplained recurrent syncope, the incidence of CSS was found to be 28%. Four types are described:
• Cardioinhibitory - the most common form, is vagally-mediated. It causes bradycardia, sinus arrest or atrioventricular block.
• Vasodepressor: a sudden drop of peripheral vascular resistance leads to hypotension without associated cardiac slowing.
• Mixed - combined cardioinhibitory and vasodepressor changes.
• Cerebral - extremely rare, carotid sinus hypersensitivity occurs without bradycardia or hypotension.

System(s) affected: Cardiovascular, Nervous

Genetics: N/A

Incidence/Prevalence in USA: Not known. (In a recent report from the United Kingdom, 32 patients out of 322 (32%) evaluated for recurrent syncope were found to have CSS).

Predominant age: Elderly

Predominant sex: Male > Female

SIGNS AND SYMPTOMS
• Acute onset, usually when standing
• Spontaneous or induced
• Brief faintness or loss of consciousness
• Blurred vision
• Vertigo
• Tinnitus
• Bradycardia
• Pallor
• Sweating
• Tachypnea
• No postictal symptoms

CAUSES
• Stimulation of the hypersensitive baroreceptors in the carotid sinus induces the vagus and sympathetic nerves.
• Carotid body tumors
• Inflammatory and malignant lymph nodes in the neck

RISK FACTORS
• Organic heart disease
• Diffuse atherosclerosis
• Wearing tight collars
• Shaving over region of sinus
• Emotional upheaval
• Turning head to side

 DIAGNOSIS

DIFFERENTIAL DIAGNOSIS
Vasovagal syncope, postural hypotension, primary autonomic insufficiency, hypovolemia, arrhythmias, sick sinus syndrome, syncope secondary to reduced cardiac output, cerebrovascular insufficiency, emotional disturbances, other causes of syncope.

LABORATORY
N/A

Drugs that may alter lab results: N/A

Disorders that may alter lab results: N/A

PATHOLOGICAL FINDINGS
N/A

SPECIAL TESTS
With the patient in the supine position and while the ECG is monitored, manual massage of the carotid sinus causes asystole of more than 3 seconds (cardioinhibitory) and/or a drop in systolic BP of more than 50 mm. Hg (vasodepressor).

IMAGING
N/A

DIAGNOSTIC PROCEDURES
• Electrophysiologic studies have been used in research settings

 TREATMENT

APPROPRIATE HEALTH CARE
Outpatient

GENERAL MEASURES
• Denervation of the carotid sinus by surgery or radiation therapy for selected patients
• Implantation of a permanent pacemaker in selected patients
• Surgery for selected patients with atheromata
• Physiological stimulation of the heart has been used for the treatment of the cardio inhibitory type

ACTIVITY
No restrictions

DIET
No special diet

PATIENT EDUCATION
Avoidance of exacerbating factors that might stimulate the carotid sinus: tight neck collar, shaving, turning of the head to one side, straining at stool.

MEDICATIONS

DRUG(S) OF CHOICE
- Anticholinergics: Atropine
- Sympathomimetics: Ephedrine, theophylline

Contraindications: Refer to manufacturer's instructions

Precautions: Concomitant usage of digitalis, beta-blockers and alpha methyldopa may accentuate response to carotid sinus massage

Significant possible interactions: Refer to manufacturer's instructions

ALTERNATIVE DRUGS N/A

FOLLOWUP

PATIENT MONITORING Follow as an outpatient

PREVENTION/AVOIDANCE Avoidance of pressure on the neck

POSSIBLE COMPLICATIONS Prolonged confusion

EXPECTED COURSE AND PROGNOSIS Serious if syncope associated with atheromatous narrowing of sinus artery or basilar artery

MISCELLANEOUS

ASSOCIATED CONDITIONS
- Sick sinus syndrome
- Atrioventricular block

AGE-RELATED FACTORS
Pediatric: N/A
Geriatric: More likely to occur in elderly. More likely associated with atheromata.
Others: N/A

PREGNANCY N/A

SYNONYMS
- CSS
- Carotid sinus syncope
- Carotid sinus hypersensitivity

ICD-9-CM 337.0

SEE ALSO Atherosclerosis

OTHER NOTES It is clinically important to distinguish CSS from sick sinus syndrome

ABBREVIATIONS CSS (carotid sinus syndrome)

REFERENCES
- Hurst, J.W., et.al.: The Heart. 7th ed. New York, McGraw-Hill, 1990
- Braunwald E., et al. (eds.): Harrison's Principles of Internal Medicine. 12th Ed. New York, McGraw-Hill, 1991
- Braunwald, E. (ed): Heart Disease: A Textbook of Cardiovascular Medicine. 3rd Ed. Philadelphia, W.B. Saunders Co., 1988

Author G. Kikano, M.D.

Carpal tunnel syndrome

 BASICS

DESCRIPTION
This is the most common cause of peripheral nerve compression. The median nerve is compressed as it traverses the carpal tunnel in the wrist and hand. The tunnel is composed of the carpal bones dorsally and the transverse carpal ligament ventrally. It contains flexor tendons and the median nerve. Symptoms tend to effect the dominant hand but over half the patients experience bilateral symptoms.

Genetics: Unknown, however a familial type has been reported

Incidence/Prevalence in USA: Most common entrapment neuropathy

Predominant age: 40 to 60

Predominant sex: Female > Male (3-6:1)

SIGNS AND SYMPTOMS
- Tingling or prickling sensations in the fingers
- Burning pain in the fingers particularly at night (acroparesthesias)
- The symptoms characteristically are relieved by shaking or rubbing the hands
- Arm pain
- Finger sensory loss
- Tinel's sign
- Phalen's sign
- During waking hours symptoms occur when driving the car, reading the newspaper and occasionally when using the hands for repetitive maneuvers
- Symptoms characteristically are confined to the thumb, index and middle finger but many patients do not distinguish this localization and feel the entire hand is affected
- Wasting of the thenar muscles is a late sign
- Weakness of the hand however for such tasks as opening jars is often noted by the patient early on in the disorder

CAUSES
- Causes include disorders which affect the musculoskeletal system in the region of the wrist including trauma or Colles' fracture, degenerative joint disease, rheumatoid arthritis, ganglion cyst, scleroderma
- Hypothyroidism and diabetes are frequently associated with this condition which also occurs with increased frequency during pregnancy
- Other miscellaneous causes includes acromegaly, lupus erythematosus, leukemia, pyogenic infections, sarcoidosis, primary amyloidosis and Paget's disease
- Hyperparathyroidism, hypocalcemia

RISK FACTORS
Repetitive wrist movements such as those of a seamstress or computer operator and occupations which are associated with frequent trauma such as the operation of a pneumatic hammer

 DIAGNOSIS

DIFFERENTIAL DIAGNOSIS
- Cervical spondylosis
- Generalized peripheral neuropathy
- Brachial plexus lesion

LABORATORY
- No one laboratory test is diagnostic
- Normal thyroid function studies and normal glucose metabolism studies may be helpful in excluding these conditions which may be associated with CTS

Drugs that may alter lab results: N/A

Disorders that may alter lab results: N/A

PATHOLOGICAL FINDINGS   N/A

SPECIAL TESTS
- Electromyography will be abnormal in more than 85% of cases; prolonged distal latency of the median motor nerves; the most sensitive indicator is the median sensory distal latency which is prolonged. Furthermore the sensory nerve action potential may be reduced or unobtainable.
- Stimulation of the ulnar nerve should be done as well to exclude generalized polyneuropathy

IMAGING
Special x-ray views of the carpal tunnel may be obtained. These are of limited usefulness unless heterotopic calcification can be identified.

DIAGNOSTIC PROCEDURES
- Tinel's sign - tapping of the wrist proximal to the carpal tunnel may produce electric sensation perceived by the patient, a sign of nerve compression
- Phalen's sign - holding the wrist flexed may precipitate the paresthesias experienced by the patient within a few seconds
- A blood pressure tourniquet to cut off circulation to the arm may precipitate symptoms promptly

 TREATMENT

APPROPRIATE HEALTH CARE
- Outpatient
- Outpatient surgery

GENERAL MEASURES
Non-operative:
◊ Splinting of the wrist in extension may provide significant relief of symptoms. Prolonged use of splinting if possible may allow some symptoms to resolve.
◊ Injection of the carpal tunnel with hydrocortisone (Medrol 40 mg per cc). 1 cc may provide significant temporary relief. This is particularly useful during pregnancy.
Operative:
◊ With few exceptions surgical decompression of the carpal tunnel by dividing the transverse carpal ligament completely provides almost complete relief of symptoms in the overwhelming majority of patients (greater than 95%)
◊ The procedure may be done as an outpatient under local anesthesia in the majority of cases
◊ Healing of the incision generally takes two weeks; an additional two weeks of recuperation may be required before the hand can be fully utilized for tasks requiring strength

ACTIVITY   As tolerated

DIET   No special diet

PATIENT EDUCATION
Carpal Tunnel Syndrome Foundation. For patient education materials favorably reviewed on this topic, contact: American Academy of Family Physicians Foundation, P.O. Box 8418, Kansas City, MO 64114, (800)274-2237, ext.4400

MEDICATIONS

DRUG(S) OF CHOICE Nonsteroidal anti-inflammatory agents such as ibuprofen 400 mg three or four times a day or naproxen sodium 500 mg twice a day will provide significant relief of symptoms in many patients
Contraindications: Gastrointestinal intolerance
Precautions: Gastrointestinal side effects of NSAID's may preclude their use in selected patients
Significant possible interactions: Refer to manufacturer's literature

ALTERNATIVE DRUGS Other NSAID's

FOLLOWUP

PATIENT MONITORING
• Patients treated with wrist splints or other palliative measures such as cortisone injections will require followup in the ensuing 4 to 12 weeks to assess the success of treatment modalities
• Patients treated surgically rarely experience recurrence of the disorder. Routine followup once healing of the incision has occurred is not necessary.

PREVENTION/AVOIDANCE Take a break once an hour when doing repetitive work involving hands

POSSIBLE COMPLICATIONS
• Post-op infection (rare)
• Injury to recurrent branch of the nerve

EXPECTED COURSE AND PROGNOSIS Untreated the condition can be expected to lead to numbness and weakness in the hand with atrophy of hand muscles and permanent loss function of the extremity

MISCELLANEOUS

ASSOCIATED CONDITIONS See Causes

AGE-RELATED FACTORS
Pediatric: N/A
Geriatric: N/A
Others: N/A

PREGNANCY May occur in pregnancy

SYNONYMS N/A

ICD-9-CM 354.0

SEE ALSO N/A

OTHER NOTES N/A

ABBREVIATIONS N/A

REFERENCES
• Joynt; R.J. (ed.): Clinical Neurology. Vol. 4. Philadelphia, J.B. Lippincott Co, 1990
• Seddon, H.: Surgical Disorders of the Peripheral Nerves. Baltimore, Williams and Wilkins Co., 1972

Author F. Wirth, M.D., FACS

Cataract

BASICS

DESCRIPTION Any opacity of the lens, either localized or generalized. Single largest cause of blindness in the world, blinding an estimated 17 million people.
Types include:
◊ Age-related ("senile") - over 90%
◊ Congenital - 1/250 newborns, 10-38% of childhood blindness
◊ Toxic/nutritional
◊ Systemic disease associated e.g., myotonic dystrophy, atopic dermatitis
◊ Metabolic - diabetes (accelerated sorbitol pathway), hypocalcemia, Wilson's disease
◊ "Complicated" - secondary to associated eye disease, e.g., uveitis (juvenile rheumatoid arthritis, sarcoid, etc.). Also secondary to occult tumor (melanoma, retinoblastoma).
◊ Trauma - heat (infrared), electrical shock, radiation, concussion, perforating eye injuries, intraocular foreign body
System(s) affected: Nervous
Genetics:
• Age related cataract has no clear pattern
• Congenital sometimes associated, e.g., heredofamilial systemic disorders (Laurence-Moon-Biedl syndrome), chromosomal disorders (Down syndrome)
Incidence/Prevalence in USA:
• 5% of age 52-62
• 46% of age 75-85 have significant vision loss (20/30 or worse)
• 92% of age 75-85 have some cataract changes
Predominant Age: Depends on type of cataract
Predominant Sex: Male = Female

SIGNS AND SYMPTOMS

Age-related cataract:
◊ Blurred vision, distortion or "ghosting" of images
◊ Problems with visual acuity in bright light or night driving (glare)
◊ Falls or accidents
◊ Injuries (e.g., hip fracture)
◊ Signs on eye examination: A lens opacity consistent with the symptoms
Congenital:
◊ Lens opacity present at birth or within three months after birth
◊ Often asymptomatic or parents notice child's visual inattention or strabismus (lazy eye)
◊ Leukocoria (white pupil reflex), strabismus, nystagmus, associated syndrome signs (as in Down's or Rubella syndromes)
◊ Visual acuity tests abnormal for one or both eyes
◊ Note: Must always rule out ocular tumor. Early diagnosis and treatment of retinoblastoma may be lifesaving.
Other types of cataract:
◊ May present with decreased visual acuity complaint
◊ Appropriate history or signs to help in diagnosis

CAUSES

Age-related cataract:
◊ Continual addition of layers of lens fibers throughout life creates hard, dehydrated lens nucleus which impairs vision (nuclear cataract)
◊ Aging alters biochemical and osmotic balance required for lens clarity, outer lens layers hydrate and become opaque, affecting vision
Congenital:
◊ Usually obscure
◊ Drugs (corticosteroids in first trimester, sulfonamides, etc.)
◊ Metabolic - diabetes in mother, galactosemia in fetus
◊ Intrauterine infection - first trimester (rubella, herpes, mumps)
◊ Maternal malnutrition
Other cataract types:
◊ Have in common that a biochemical/osmotic imbalance disrupts lens clarity
◊ Local changes in lens protein distribution lead to light scattering manifest as lens opacity

RISK FACTORS

• Aging
• Patient with one of the predisposing diseases

DIAGNOSIS

DIFFERENTIAL DIAGNOSIS

• An opaque appearing eye may be due to surface opacities of the cornea (scarring), lens opacities, tumor, retinal detachment, gliotic retinal scar. Biomicroscopic examination (slit lamp) or careful ophthalmoscopic exam should provide diagnosis. A visual acuity worse than 20/30, not easily correctable by glasses, and explainable by the degree of cataract noted on examination makes the diagnosis.
• In the elderly, visual impairment often due to multiple factors, e.g., cataract and macular degeneration both contributing to visual loss
• Age-related cataract - significant if symptoms and ophthalmic exam support cataract as major cause of vision impairment
• Congenital - lens opacity in absence of other ocular pathology such as tumor, nerve glioma, retinopathy of prematurity may be consistent with the visual loss. May cause severe amblyopia.
• Note: No cataract produces an afferent pupillary reaction defect (Marcus Gunn pupil). Abnormal pupillary reactions mandate further evaluation for other pathology.

LABORATORY N/A
Drugs that may alter lab results: N/A
Disorders that may alter lab results: N/A

PATHOLOGICAL FINDINGS Consistent with lens changes found in the type of cataract

SPECIAL TESTS

• Visual quality assessment: Glare testing, contrast sensitivity are sometimes indicated. (Hyperglycemic state as in poor diabetic control creates osmotic change within lens and may alter measurement of visual acuity and refractive state.)
• Retinal/macular function assessment: Potential acuity meter testing, fluorescein retinal angiography sometimes required

IMAGING N/A

DIAGNOSTIC PROCEDURES Noted above in special testing

TREATMENT

APPROPRIATE HEALTH CARE
Outpatient or inpatient surgery

GENERAL MEASURES
Age-related cataract
◊ Surgical removal of the cataract - indicated if visual impairment producing symptoms distressing to the patient, or interfering with lifestyle or occupation, or posing risk of fall or injury
◊ Since significant cataract may develop gradually, patient may not be aware of how it has changed his/her lifestyle. Physician may note a significant cataract and patient reports "no problems". Thus the evaluation requires physician/patient exchange of information.
◊ Surgical technique - cataracts are not removed by laser. Most surgical techniques include implantation of a plastic intraocular lens immediately following cataract extraction.
◊ Anesthesia - usually local, with anesthesiologist monitoring vital signs
◊ Pre-surgical evaluation - by the primary care physician includes physical exam, lab work (CBC, electrolytes, EKG). Patients on anticoagulants may need to temporarily discontinue one week before surgery if possible. Not always necessary, so need to discuss with ophthalmologist.
◊ Postoperative care - usually protective eye shield as directed, topical antibiotic and steroid ophthalmic medications. Avoid lifting, bending over for a few weeks.
Congenital cataract
◊ Treatment is surgical removal of cataract. Newborn may need surgery within days to reduce risk of severe amblyopia. Use of implant lenses controversial.
◊ Postoperative care - long-term patching program for good eye to combat amblyopia. Refractive correction of operative eye, with multiple repeat examinations. Very difficult challenge for physician and parents.

ACTIVITY See above

DIET N/A

PATIENT EDUCATION See above

MEDICATIONS

DRUG(S) OF CHOICE There is no medication at present to prevent or slow the progression of cataracts
Contraindications: N/A
Precautions: N/A
Significant possible interactions: N/A

ALTERNATIVE DRUGS N/A

FOLLOWUP

PATIENT MONITORING
• As cataract progresses, the ophthalmologist may change spectacle correction to maintain vision. When this is no longer practical or successful, surgery is recommended.
• Following surgery, spectacle correction may be required to maximize visual acuity for the patient's need. Usually measured several weeks after surgery.

PREVENTION/AVOIDANCE
• Use of ultraviolet protecting glasses in sunny climates may slow progression of cataract, but this is not proven by controlled studies to date
• Antioxidants (vitamins C, E, etc.) theoretically beneficial, but not proven

POSSIBLE COMPLICATIONS   Blindness

EXPECTED COURSE AND PROGNOSIS
• Ocular prognosis good after cataract removal if no prior ocular disease.
• In congenital cataracts prognosis is often poor because of the high risk of amyblyopia.

MISCELLANEOUS

ASSOCIATED CONDITIONS
• Diabetes
• Ocular diseases

AGE-RELATED FACTORS
Pediatric: See information on congenital cataracts
Geriatric: 92% of people over age 75 have cataracts
Others: N/A

PREGNANCY   See information on congenital cataracts (e.g., rubella syndrome)

SYNONYMS   N/A

ICD-9-CM
• Age-related cataract - 366.19
• Congenital cataract - 743.30

SEE ALSO   N/A

OTHER NOTES   If patient has cataract and symptoms do not seem to support recommended surgery, a second opinion by another ophthalmologist may be indicated

ABBREVIATIONS   N/A

REFERENCES   Tasman, W. (ed.): Duane's Ophthalmology. Philadelphia, J.B. Lippincott Co., 1991

Author   T. Moody, M.D.

Causalgia syndrome

DESCRIPTION Pain syndrome following injury to bone and soft tissue. Pathogenesis is obscure.
System(s) affected: Nervous
Genetics: No known genetic pattern
Incidence/Prevalence in USA: Unknown
Predominant age: No predominant age
Predominant sex: Male > Female

SIGNS AND SYMPTOMS
• Deep aching pain
• Burning pain with superimposed lancinating pain
• Hyperesthesia
• Hyperalgesia
• Pain from a non-noxious stimulus
• Pain most likely in palm or sole, aggravated by minimal physical stimulus such as friction or heat
• Skin - discolored, edematous, cold, hyperesthetic, smooth, glossy
• Stiff joints
• Nails curved and brittle
• Hyperhidrosis

CAUSES
• Partial interruption of nerve conduction by injury, such as gunshot wounds
• Possible shunting of efferent sympathetic impulses into sensory fibers at site of injury in a mixed nerve
• Reflex sympathetic dystrophy

RISK FACTORS Trauma

DIFFERENTIAL DIAGNOSIS Rule out infection, hypertrophic scar, bone fragments, neuroma, central nervous system tumor or syrinx

LABORATORY N/A
Drugs that may alter lab results: N/A
Disorders that may alter lab results: N/A

PATHOLOGICAL FINDINGS
• Partial or complete damage to afferent nerve pathways and probably reorganized central pain pathways
• Most common nerves involved are median and sciatic
• Atrophy in affected muscles
• Incomplete nerve plexus lesion

SPECIAL TESTS N/A

IMAGING Bone scan

DIAGNOSTIC PROCEDURES
Intravenous regional sympathetic block with guanethidine or reserpine (this is a specialized anesthetic technique that may also be therapeutic)

APPROPRIATE HEALTH CARE
Outpatient, except for operative procedures or intravenous sympathetic nerve blockade

GENERAL MEASURES
• Treatment is empiric
• Anesthetic blockade (chemical or surgical) of sympathetic nerve function (transient relief suggests that chemical or surgical sympathectomy will be helpful)
• Intravenous regional sympathetic block with guanethidine or reserpine by pain specialist or anesthetist
• Physical therapy (essential during all phases of treatment)
• Transcutaneous electric nerve stimulation (controversial)
• Inject myofacial painful trigger points
• Briskly rub the affected part several times per day
• Acupuncture can be tried
• Hypnosis
• Relaxation training (alternate muscle relaxing and contracting)
• Biofeedback
• Discourage maladaptive behaviors
• Refer the patient to a specialty pain clinic in difficult cases
• Sympathectomy sometimes necessary

ACTIVITY Maintain as high a level of physical and intellectual activity as possible

DIET No special diet

PATIENT EDUCATION
• Stress staying active physically
• Careful instructions about any prescribed medications

MEDICATIONS

DRUG(S) OF CHOICE
Following agents reported to be of benefit in some cases:
◊ Prazosin (1-8 mg orally in divided doses)
◊ Phenoxybenzamine 40-120 mg daily, orally in divided doses. The initial dose should not exceed 10 mg.
◊ Nifedipine 10-30 mg tid
◊ Prednisone 60-80 mg/day orally, tapered over 2-4 weeks
◊ Tricyclic antidepressants (see manufacturers recommended dose)
Anticonvulsants. (Require serum drug level monitoring, except for clonazepam. Doses must be individualized.):
◊ Carbamazepine 200-1000 mg/day orally
◊ Phenytoin 100-300 mg/day orally
◊ Clonazepam 1-10 mg/day orally
◊ Valproate 750-2250 mg/day orally), maximum of 60 mg/kg
Skeletal muscle relaxant:
◊ Baclofen 10-40 mg/day orally - may act synergistically with carbamazepine and phenytoin
Contraindications: Refer to manufacturer's literature
Precautions: Refer to manufacturer's literature
Significant possible interactions: There are many with this group of drugs. Refer to manufacturer's literature.

ALTERNATIVE DRUGS
Narcotics - only after all non-opioid therapies are exhausted

 ## FOLLOWUP

PATIENT MONITORING
• Watch carefully for adverse reactions to medications
• Several different forms of therapy may need to be tried

PREVENTION/AVOIDANCE
• Mobilization following injury
• Avoidance of nerve damage during surgical procedures
• Splinting of an injured extremity for adequate period of time
• Adequate analgesics during recovery from injuries

POSSIBLE COMPLICATIONS
• Drug mishaps
• Joint contractures
• Contralateral spread of symptoms

EXPECTED COURSE AND PROGNOSIS
• Course - variable; chronic; remitting
• Outlook only satisfactory, may need attempts at several treatment modalities. No one form of therapy is superior to others. Failure to respond to one form does not mitigate against success with another.
• Those patients receiving work compensation for an injury or secondary gain from family or friends are in a separate category and may never get well

 ## MISCELLANEOUS

ASSOCIATED CONDITIONS
• Serious injury to bone and soft tissue
• Herpes zoster

AGE-RELATED FACTORS
Pediatric: N/A
Geriatric: Painful perception is frequently worse in older patients. Start with smaller than usual doses of drugs.
Others:
• Postherpetic neuralgia is a result of partial or complete damage to afferent nerve pathways
• Pain occurring in dermatomes as a sequela of herpes zoster

PREGNANCY Many of the useful drugs are contraindicated in pregnancy

SYNONYMS
• Erythromyalgia, traumatic
• Weir Mitchell causalgia
• Minor causalgia
• Reflex sympathetic dystrophy
• Posttraumatic neuralgia
• Sympathetically maintained pain

ICD-9-CM 354.4

SEE ALSO
• Herpes zoster
• Peripheral neuropathy

OTHER NOTES N/A

ABBREVIATIONS N/A

REFERENCES Bonica, J.J.: The Management of Pain. 2nd Ed. Philadelphia, Lea & Febiger, 1990

Author F. Williams, MD

Celiac disease

BASICS

DESCRIPTION A chronic diarrheal disease characterized by intestinal malabsorption of virtually all nutrients and precipitated by eating gluten-containing foods.
System(s) affected: Gastrointestinal
Genetics: See Risk factors
Incidence/Prevalence in USA: 50-75 in 100,000
Predominant age: Two incidence peaks, age 1 and 60's
Predominant sex: Female > Male (3:2)

SIGNS AND SYMPTOMS
• Diarrhea
• Steatorrhea
• Muscle cramps
• Vertigo
• Nervousness
• Weight loss
• Failure to thrive
• Weakness
• Lassitude
• Fatigue
• Large appetite
• Abdominal distention
• Explosive flatulence
• Abdominal pain, nausea, vomiting are rare

CAUSES Sensitivity to gluten, specifically gliadin fraction

RISK FACTORS
• First order relatives - 10% incidence
• 71% in monozygotic twins

DIAGNOSIS

DIFFERENTIAL DIAGNOSIS Rule out short bowel syndrome, pancreatic insufficiency, Crohn's disease, Whipple's disease, hypogammaglobulinemia, tropical sprue, lymphoma, acquired immune deficiency syndrome, acute enteritis, giardiasis, eosinophilic gastroenteritis

LABORATORY
• Positive anti-gliadin IgA and IgG
• Positive anti-reticulum and anti-endomycial antibodies
• 72 hour fecal fat showing greater than 7% fat malabsorption
• D-xylose test showing malabsorption of this sugar
• Decreased calcium
• Decreased prothrombin time
• Decreased neutral fats
• Decreased cholesterol
• Decreased vitamin A
• Decreased vitamin B12
• Decreased vitamin C
• Decreased folic acid
• Decreased iron
• Decreased total protein
• Anemia
Drugs that may alter lab results: N/A
Disorders that may alter lab results: N/A

PATHOLOGICAL FINDINGS Small bowel biopsy - flattened villi, hyperplasia and lengthening of crypts, infiltration of plasma cells and lymphocytes in lamina propria

SPECIAL TESTS Endoscopy

IMAGING Upper GI series showing flocculation of barium, edema and flattening of mucosal folds

DIAGNOSTIC PROCEDURES Biopsy of the duodenal mucosa with repeat endoscopy and normal biopsy on a gluten-free diet is necessary before a firm diagnosis can be made.

TREATMENT

APPROPRIATE HEALTH CARE
Outpatient

GENERAL MEASURES Removal of gluten from the diet. Rice, corn and soybean flour are safe, palatable substitutes.

ACTIVITY No restrictions

DIET Removal of gluten - wheat, rye, barley and those with gluten additives

PATIENT EDUCATION
• Clinical dietician
• Copy of gluten-free diet
• Possible lay self-help group
• American Celiac Society, 45 Gifford Avenue, Jersey City, New Jersey 07304, (201) 432-1207.

MEDICATIONS

DRUG(S) OF CHOICE
• Usually none
• Prednisone, 40-60 mg/day po in cases of refractory sprue
Contraindications: History of tuberculosis, fungus or herpes infections
Precautions: Use with caution in congestive heart failure, diabetes, peptic ulcer, myasthenia gravis
Significant possible interactions: Diuretics taken concomitantly may lead to potassium depletion

ALTERNATIVE DRUGS
May require supplemental calcium, calcium carbonate, 500 mg po bid, and vitamin D2 (ergo-calciferol, 10-100 micrograms a day; in severe malabsorption, up to 2.5 mg/day may be required)

FOLLOWUP

PATIENT MONITORING
Repeat endoscopy after 6-8 weeks on a gluten-free diet

PREVENTION/AVOIDANCE
Avoid all gluten containing products

POSSIBLE COMPLICATIONS
• Malignancy - less than 10% of patients (50% of which are small bowel lymphoma)
• Refractory sprue - may respond to prednisone 40-60 mg/day po
• Chronic ulcerative jejunoileitis - associated with multiple ulcers, intestinal bleeding, strictures, perforation, obstruction, peritonitis - 7% mortality
• Osteoporosis secondary to decreased vitamin D and calcium absorption
• Dehydration
• Electrolyte depletion
• Death (rare)

EXPECTED COURSE AND PROGNOSIS
Good with correct diagnosis and adherence to gluten free diet. Feel better in seven days. All symptoms usually disappear in four to six weeks. It is unknown whether strict dietary adherence decreases cancer risk.

MISCELLANEOUS

ASSOCIATED CONDITIONS
• May have secondary lactase deficiency
• Extraintestinal manifestation may include marked decrease in bone density
• Dermatitis herpetiformis

AGE-RELATED FACTORS
Pediatric: Children reaching adolescence may outgrow intolerance to wheat but should be cautioned to watch for signs of recurrence in middle age
Geriatric: N/A
Others: N/A

PREGNANCY
No significant effect

SYNONYMS
• Sprue
• Gluten enteropathy
• Celiac sprue

ICD-9-CM
579.0 Celiac disease

SEE ALSO
N/A

OTHER NOTES
N/A

ABBREVIATIONS
N/A

REFERENCES
• McClave, S.: Celiac and Tropical Sprue. In A Manual of Clinical Problems in Gastroenterology. 2nd Ed. Edited by S.J. Chobanian & M.M. Van Ness. 1993
• Stenson, W.F.: Gastrointestinal Diseases. In A Manual of Medical Therapeutics. 25th Ed. Edited by M.J. Orland & R.J. Saltman. 1986
• Trier, J.S.: Celiac Sprue. In Gastrointestinal Disease. 4th Ed. Edited by M.H. Sleisenger & J.S. Fordtran. Philadelphia, W.B. Saunders Co., 1987

Author M. Van Ness, M.D.

Cellulitis (part 1)

BASICS

DESCRIPTION An acute, spreading infection of the dermis and subcutaneous tissue. Several entities are recognized:
• Cellulitis of the extremities - characterized by an expanding, red, swollen, tender or painful plaque with an indefinite border that may cover a wide area
• Recurrent cellulitis of the leg after saphenous venectomy - patients have an acute onset of swelling, erythema of the legs arising months to years after coronary artery bypass. (Surgery using lower extremity veins for by-pass grafts)
• Dissecting cellulitis of the scalp - recurrent painful, fluctuant dermal and subcutaneous nodules
• Facial cellulitis in adults - a rare event. Patients usually develop pharyngitis, followed by high fever, rapidly progressive anterior neck swelling, tenderness and erythema associated with dysphagia
• Facial cellulitis in children - potentially serious. Swelling and erythema of the cheek develop rapidly, usually unilateral
• Cellulitis around the eyes - a potentially dangerous periorbital and orbital infection
• Perianal cellulitis - bright perianal erythema extending from the anal verge approximately 2 to 3 cm onto the surrounding perianal skin
• Pseudomonas cellulitis - may be a localized phenomenon or it may occur during pseudomonas septicemia.
Genetics: No known genetic pattern
Incidence/Prevalence in USA: Unknown
Predominant age:
• Perianal cellulitis - principally in children
• Facial cellulitis - in adults, usually older than 50 years. In children, between 6 months and three years.
Predominant sex: Male = Female (perianal cellulitis more common in boys)

SIGNS AND SYMPTOMS
General
  ◊ Local tenderness
  ◊ Pain
  ◊ Erythema
  ◊ Malaise
  ◊ Fever, chills
  ◊ Involved area is red, hot, and swollen
  ◊ Borders of the area are not elevated and not demarcated
  ◊ Regional lymphadenopathy is common
Recurrent cellulitis
  ◊ Same as above
  ◊ Edema
  ◊ High fever, chills and toxicity
Dissecting cellulitis of the scalp
  ◊ Purulent drainage from burrowing interconnecting abscesses
Facial cellulitis in adults
  ◊ Malaise
  ◊ Anorexia
  ◊ Vomiting
  ◊ Itching
  ◊ Burning
  ◊ Dysplasia
  ◊ Anterior neck swelling

Facial cellulitis in children
  ◊ Irritability
  ◊ Upper respiratory tract infection symptom
Cellulitis around the eye
  ◊ Lid edema
  ◊ Rhinorrhea
  ◊ Orbital pain, tenderness
  ◊ Headache
  ◊ Conjunctival hyperemia
  ◊ Chemosis
  ◊ Ptosis
  ◊ Limitation to occular motion
  ◊ Increase intraocular pressure
  ◊ Disease in corneal sensation
  ◊ Congestion of retinal veins
  ◊ Chorioretinal stria
  ◊ Gangrene and sloughing of lids
Perianal cellulitis
  ◊ Intense perianal erythema
  ◊ Pain on defecation
  ◊ Blood streaked stools
  ◊ Perianal pruritis

CAUSES
Cellulitis of the extremities
  ◊ Group A streptococcus
  ◊ Staphylococcus aureus
  ◊ Human bites: Eikenella corrodens
  ◊ Animal bites (cat and dog): Staphylococci, Pasteurella multocida
Recurrent cellulitis of the leg
  ◊ Non-group A beta hemolytic Streptococci (group C,G,B)
Dissecting cellulitis of the scalp
  ◊ Staphylococcus aureus
Facial cellulitis in adults
  ◊ H. influenza type B
Facial cellulitis in children
  ◊ H. influenza type B
  ◊ Over 3 years with portal of entry staphylococcal and streptococcal
Cellulitis around the eye in adult
  ◊ Staphylococcus aureus most common
  ◊ Streptococcus pyogenes
  ◊ Streptococcus pneumonia
  ◊ Mixed infection
Cellulitis around the eye in children less than five years
  ◊ H. influenza most common
Synergetic necrotizing cellulitis
  ◊ Mixed aerobic-anaerobic flora
Rare causes
  ◊ Anaerobic
  ◊ Clostridium perfringens (gas forming cellulitis)
  ◊ Tuberculosis
  ◊ Syphilitic gumma
Fungal
  ◊ Mucormycosis
  ◊ Aspergillosis
Diabetes mellitus
  ◊ Staphylococcus aureus
  ◊ Streptococci
  ◊ Enterobacteriaceae
  ◊ Anaerobes
Intravenous drug use
  ◊ Staphylococcus aureus
  ◊ Streptococci
  ◊ Enterobacteriaceae
  ◊ Pseudomonas
  ◊ Fungi

Neonates
  ◊ Group B streptococcus
Immunocompromised
  ◊ Bacteria (Serratia, Proteus and other Enterobacteriaceae)
  ◊ Fungi (Cryptococcus neoformans)
  ◊ Atypical mycobacterium
Children with nephrotic syndrome
  ◊ Escherichia coli
Environmental and occupational exposures
  ◊ Erysipelothrix rhusiopathiae
  ◊ Vibrio species
  ◊ Aeromonas hydrophilia

RISK FACTORS
General
  ◊ Previous trauma (laceration, puncture, human or animal bite)
  ◊ Underlying skin lesion (furuncle, ulcer)
  ◊ Surgical wound
  ◊ Recurrent cellulitis
  ◊ Post coronary artery bypass in patients whose saphenous veins have been removed
  ◊ Lower extremity lymphedema secondary to a) radical pelvic surgery b) radiation therapy c) neoplastic involvement of pelvic lymph nodes
  ◊ Mastectomy
  ◊ Diabetes mellitus
  ◊ Intravenous drug use
  ◊ Compromised host
  ◊ Burns
  ◊ Environmental and occupational factors
Periorbital and orbital cellulitis
  ◊ Trauma
  ◊ Chronic sinusitis (anaerobic)
  ◊ Acute sinusitis (aerobic)
  ◊ Retained orbital foreign bodies
  ◊ Puncture wound
  ◊ Surgical procedure: Exploration of orbital tumor, retinal detachment procedure, strabismus operation
  ◊ Acute dacrocystitis
  ◊ Dental or intracranial infection
  ◊ Bacteremia
Synergetic necrotizing cellulitis
  ◊ Mixed aerobic-anaerobic flora

DIAGNOSIS

DIFFERENTIAL DIAGNOSIS
- Acute gout
- Fasciitis/myositis
- Mycotic aneurysm
- Ruptured Baker's cyst
- Thrombophlebitis
- Osteomyelitis
- Retro-orbital cellulitis/abscess
- Herpetic whitlow
- Cutaneous diphtheria
- Pseudogout

Perianal cellulitis
  ◊ Candida intertrigo
  ◊ Psoriasis
  ◊ Pin worm infection
  ◊ Inflammatory bowel disease
  ◊ Behavioral problem
  ◊ Child abuse

LABORATORY
- Aspirates from the point of maximum inflammation. Yield a 45% positive culture rate as compared to a 5% from leading edge culture.
- Blood cultures - potential pathogens isolated in 25% of patients
- Mild leucocytosis with a left shift
- A mildly elevated sedimentation rate
- CBC

Periorbital and orbital cellulitis
  ◊ Aspiration of fluid from the orbit is contraindicated
  ◊ Blood culture more likely to be positive in children < 5 years
  ◊ Culture of discharge from nasal mucosa, nasopharynx and conjunctiva

Drugs that may alter lab results: Previous antibiotic therapy may alter the results
Disorders that may alter lab results: None

PATHOLOGICAL FINDINGS Biopsy of skin shows marked infiltration of the dermis with eosinophils and inflammatory changes

SPECIAL TESTS
- Serial serological testing with antistreptolysin 0, anti-deoxyribonuclease B, and anti hyaluronidase tests may be successful in diagnosing cellulitis caused by group A, C, or G hemolytic streptococci
- Sinus drainage and culture of aspirate

IMAGING
Periorbital and orbital cellulitis
  ◊ B-scan ultrasound
  ◊ Plain orbital and sinus films
  ◊ Computed tomography (CT) is the most accurate and provides the most important information
  ◊ Magnetic resonance imaging is the imaging modality of choice in diagnosing suspected cases of cavernous sinus thrombosis

Gas forming cellulitis
  ◊ Plain x-rays show gas bubbles in the soft tissue
  ◊ CT shows gas and myonecrosis

DIAGNOSTIC PROCEDURES
- Skin biopsy
- Lumbar puncture should be considered for all children with H. influenza type B cellulitis

Cellulitis (part 2)

 TREATMENT

APPROPRIATE HEALTH CARE
Outpatient for mild cases, inpatient for severe infections

GENERAL MEASURES
• Immobilization and elevation of the involved limb to reduce swelling may be needed in H-influenza type B
• Sterile saline dressings to decrease local pain
• Application of moist heat may help in localization of the infection
• Pain may be relieved with cool Burrow's compresses
• Surgical debridement needed in case of gas formation/purulent collections
• Intubation or tracheotomy may be needed for cellulitis of the head or neck
Periorbital and orbital cellulitis
◊ Surgical debridement and/or drainage is needed if abscess develops or if clinical situation deteriorates despite adequate therapy in 24-48 hours or if visual acuity decreases
◊ In orbital mucormycosis, surgical debridement of devitalized tissue is extremely important
Other
◊ In gas gangrene surgical debridement is important
◊ In synergistic necrotizing cellulitis wide filleting incision

ACTIVITY
• Ambulatory in mild infection
• Bedrest in severe infection

DIET Regular diet

PATIENT EDUCATION
• Good skin hygiene
• Avoid skin traumas
• Report early skin changes to health professional

 MEDICATIONS

DRUG(S) OF CHOICE
• Treatment is usually for 12 days with a range of 15-25 days
• Mild early suspected streptococcal etiology - initial injection of aqueous penicillin G (600,000 units) followed by intramuscular procaine penicillin (600,000 units every 8-12 hours)
• Staphylococcal infection or no clues to etiology - use a penicillinase-resistant penicillin (e.g., oxacillin 0.5-1.0 g orally every 6 hours)
• Severe infection - parenteral administration of penicillinase-resistant penicillin (e.g., nafcillin 1.0-1.5 g intravenously every 4 hours)
• Gram negative bacillus as possible etiology - an aminoglycoside (gentamicin) plus a semisynthetic penicillin
• Rapidly progressive cellulitis after a fresh water injury - a penicillinase-resistant penicillin plus gentamicin or chloramphenicol
• Human bites - amoxicillin-clavulanic acid (Augmentin)
• Animal bites (cellulitis at the saphenous site) - initial antibiotic (penicillin or nafcillin) in high dosage by the intravenous route for 6-7 days before switching to other routes of therapy
• Facial cellulitis in adults and children - (H. influenza B) cefotaxime intravenously is the drug of choice
Periorbital and orbital cellulitis
◊ In adults, nafcillin or oxacillin 1.5 g every 4 hours
◊ In children, ampicillin 200 mg/kg/day in divided doses intravenously plus nafcillin or oxacillin (100 mg/kg/day)
◊ Sinus decongestion - nasal sprays, oral decongestants, oral antihistamines
Gas forming cellulitis
◊ Aqueous penicillin G 10-20 million units/day IV
Diabetes mellitus (until culture available)
◊ Cefoxitin
◊ If patient toxic, clindamycin and gentamicin
Intravenous drug abuse (until culture available)
◊ Vancomycin and gentamicin
◊ In compromised hosts (until culture available) - clindamycin and gentamicin
◊ In burn patients - vancomycin and gentamicin
Contraindications:
• Allergies to the antibiotic
• Previous history of allergy to the drug
Precautions: Renal failure, other organ failure
Significant possible interactions: Refer to manufacturer's literature

ALTERNATIVE DRUGS
Mild infection
◊ In patients allergic to penicillin - erythromycin (0.5 g orally every 6 hours)
Severe infection
◊ Vancomycin 1.0-1.5 g/day intravenously
◊ Human bite and animal bites - parenteral cefoxitin
Gas forming cellulitis
◊ Metronidazole 500mg IV q6h
◊ Clindamycin 600mg IV q8h
Periorbital and orbital cellulitis
◊ In adults, cefotaxime or clindamycin or chloramphenicol or vancomycin
◊ In children, if H. influenza resistant to ampicillin - third generation cephalosporin, cefotaxime or chloramphenicol
◊ In immunocompromised - piperacillin and gentamicin

FOLLOWUP

PATIENT MONITORING
• A blood culture at the end of treatment to ensure cure
• Repeat needle aspirate culture
• Repeat blood count if patient was toxic
• Repeat imaging in patients with orbital cellulitis
• Repeat lumbar puncture in case of meningitis

PREVENTION/AVOIDANCE
• Treatment of tinea pedis with antifungal (such as clotrimazole) will prevent recurrent cellulitis of the legs in patients who have had coronary bypass
• Avoid trauma
• Avoid swimming in fresh water or salt water in the presence of skin abrasion
• Avoid human or animal bite
• Use of support stocking in patients with peripheral edema
• Good skin hygiene
• For recurrent cellulitis - prophylactic penicillin G (250-500 mg orally, twice daily)
• In H. influenza cellulitis - rifampin prophylaxis for the entire family of an index case. Rifampin prophylaxis in day-care classroom in which one or two children exposed. Dosage - 20 mg/kg/24 h (maximum of 600 mg a day) for 4 days.

POSSIBLE COMPLICATIONS
• Bacteremia
• Local abscesses
• Super infection with gram negative organisms
• Lymphangitis especially in recurrent cellulitis
• Thrombophlebitis of lower extremities in older patients
Dissecting cellulitis of the scalp
  ◊ Scarring
  ◊ Alopecia
Facial cellulitis in children
  ◊ Meningitis in 8% of patients
Periorbital and orbital cellulitis
  ◊ Osteomyelitis
  ◊ Strabismus
  ◊ Afferent pupillary defect
  ◊ Chronic draining sinus
  ◊ Scarred upper eyelid
  ◊ Profound visual loss
  ◊ Blindness
  ◊ Opthalmoplegia
  ◊ Cavernous sinus thrombosis
  ◊ Meningitis
  ◊ Intracranial abscess
  ◊ Acute infarction of retina and choroid
Gas forming cellulitis
  ◊ Gangrene
  ◊ Amputation
  ◊ 25% mortality

EXPECTED COURSE AND PROGNOSIS
With adequate antibiotic treatment, outlook is good

 MISCELLANEOUS

ASSOCIATED CONDITIONS
Facial cellulitis in children
  ◊ Upper respiratory tract infection
  ◊ Unilateral or bilateral otitis media in 68% of patients
  ◊ Meningitis in 8% of patients
Perianal cellulitis
  ◊ Pharyngitis may precede the infection
Periorbital and orbital cellulitis
  ◊ Sinusitis ethmoiditis in children in 84% of patients
Frontal sinus in adult
  ◊ Subacute bacterial endocarditis
  ◊ Scarlet fever
  ◊ Vaccinia
  ◊ Herpes simplex
  ◊ Herpes zoster

AGE-RELATED FACTORS
Pediatric: Newborn may acquire orbital cellulitis secondary to intrauterine infection
Geriatric: In cellulitis of lower extremities, patients are more prone to develop thrombophlebitis
Others: N/A

PREGNANCY N/A

SYNONYMS N/A

ICD-9-CM 682.9

SEE ALSO
• Erysipelas
• Animal bites

OTHER NOTES N/A

ABBREVIATIONS N/A

REFERENCES
• Habif, T.: Clinical Dermatology. 2nd Ed. St. Louis, C.V. Mosby, 1990
• Mandell, G.L. (ed.): Principles and Practice of Infectious Diseases. 3rd Ed. New York, Churchill Livingstone, 1990

Author A. Abyad, M.D., M.P.H.

Cerebral palsy

 BASICS

DESCRIPTION A term used to describe a group of patients with a non-progressive disorder of movement or posture that is a result of a central nervous system abnormality that occurred prenatally, perinatally, or during the first three years of life
Genetics: Although familial cases have been described, this is not considered a genetic disease
Incidence/Prevalence in USA: 2.1 per 1,000 live births
Predominant age: Because of the definition, this problem is restricted to life. The disease is lifelong, although changes occur as the patient matures.
Predominant sex: Male = Female

SIGNS AND SYMPTOMS
• Slow motor development
• Evidence of central nervous system dysfunction on neurological examination, including exaggerated deep tendon reflexes, and/or clonus, and/or dyskinesias (movement disorders including chorea, athetosis, dystonia), and/or ataxia

CAUSES
• 70% of the time, neither causes nor risk factors can be identified
• In utero infections, malformations, chromosomal abnormalities and strokes are causes

RISK FACTORS
• Prematurity
• Hypoxic ischemia
• Encephalopathy in the perinatal period
• Seizures in the perinatal period
• Interventricular hemorrhage in the perinatal period
• In utero infections
• Meningitis/encephalitis postnatally
• Child abuse

 DIAGNOSIS

DIFFERENTIAL DIAGNOSIS Children with muscle disease will appear floppy; however, most common cause of the floppy baby syndrome is cerebral palsy

LABORATORY To exclude Tay-Sachs metachromatic leukodystrophy, mucopolysaccharidosis
Drugs that may alter lab results: None
Disorders that may alter lab results: None

PATHOLOGICAL FINDINGS Central nervous system abnormalities: CT and MRI might show abnormalities of the brain including cysts, cerebral atrophy, calcification, tumors, malformation, strokes, etc.

SPECIAL TESTS Urine amino acid screening

IMAGING N/A

DIAGNOSTIC PROCEDURES
• History and careful physical
• EEG

 TREATMENT

APPROPRIATE HEALTH CARE Tendon transfers, release of contractures, rhizotomy to decrease spasticity, physical therapy, occupational therapy

GENERAL MEASURES Physical therapy, occupational therapy, orthosis, adaptive equipment

ACTIVITY Full activity depending upon the patient's dysfunction

DIET Normal diet, although constipation is frequent and stool softeners might be considered

PATIENT EDUCATION
• It is very important to educate the patient and parents about the child's disabilities as well as prognosis; cerebral palsy is not always associated with mental retardation
• United Cerebral Palsy Associations, 7 Penn Plaza, Suite 804, New York, NY 10001, (800)USA-1UCP

MEDICATIONS

DRUG(S) OF CHOICE
• Medications to decrease spasticity includes diazepam, dantrolene sodium and baclofen
• Medications for epilepsy might have to be used

Contraindications: Refer to manufacturer's literature

Precautions: Refer to manufacturer's literature

Significant possible interactions: Refer to manufacturer's literature

ALTERNATIVE DRUGS N/A

FOLLOWUP

PATIENT MONITORING Followup visits are important - to determine the development of contractures and to determine the presence of associated problems including epilepsy, learning disabilities, strabismus, hearing loss and mental retardation, are very important

PREVENTION/AVOIDANCE N/A

POSSIBLE COMPLICATIONS Chronicity with permanent disability

EXPECTED COURSE AND PROGNOSIS The patient should improve in function in time

MISCELLANEOUS

ASSOCIATED CONDITIONS
• Epilepsy
• Learning disabilities
• Mental retardation
• Behavioral problems
• Strabismus
• Hearing loss

AGE-RELATED FACTORS
Pediatric: Contractures will increase as a result of growth associated with asymmetrical muscle tone and strength. Scoliosis may develop as a result.
Geriatric: N/A
Others: N/A

PREGNANCY N/A

SYNONYMS
• Little disease
• Cerebral diplegia
• Infantile cerebral paralysis

ICD-9-CM 343.9

SEE ALSO N/A

OTHER NOTES N/A

ABBREVIATIONS N/A

REFERENCES Russman, B.S. & Gage, J.R.: Cerebral Palsy. Current Problems in Pediatrics. 19(2):65-111, 1989

Author B. Russman, M.D.

Cerebrovascular accident (CVA)

 BASICS

DESCRIPTION
The sudden onset of a focal neurological deficit resulting from either infarction or hemorrhage within the brain

Genetics: Inheritance is polygenic with a tendency to clustering of risk factors within families

Incidence/Prevalence in USA: Overall incidence 160/100,000 (age 50-65, 1000/100,000; > 80, 3000/100,000). Prevalence 135/100,000.

Predominant age: Risk increases over age 45 and is highest in the seventh and eighth decades

Predominant sex: Male > Female (3:1)

SIGNS AND SYMPTOMS
- Carotid circulation (hemispheric): Hemiplegia, hemianesthesia, neglect, aphasia, visual field defects; less often headaches, seizures, amnesia, confusion
- Vertebrobasilar (brainstem or cerebellar): Diplopia, vertigo, ataxia, facial paresis, Horner's syndrome, dysphagia, dysarthria
- Impaired level of consciousness
- Cerebellar lesion in patients with headache, nausea, vomiting and ataxia

CAUSES
- Ischemic: Carotid atherosclerotic disease with artery-to-artery thromboembolism
- Cardiac: Cardioembolism secondary to valvular (mitral valve) pathology; mural hypokinesias or akinesias with thrombosis (acute anterior myocardial infarctions or congestive cardiomyopathies); cardiac arrhythmia (atrial fibrillation)
- Hypercoagulable states: Antiphospholipid antibodies, deficiency of protein S, protein C; presence of antithrombin 3, oral contraceptives
- Other causes: Spontaneous and post-traumatic (i.e., chiropractic manipulation) artery dissection, fibromuscular dysplasia, vasculitis, drugs (cocaine, amphetamines)
- Hemorrhagic
- Hypertension: may cause damage to putamen, internal capsule, cerebellum, brainstem, corona radiata
- Amyloid (congophylic) angiopathy: Lobar (cortical) hemorrhages in the elderly
- Vascular malformations: Arteriovenous malformation, cavernous angioma, venous angioma and capillary angioma

RISK FACTORS
- Age
- Hypertension
- Cardiac disease
- Smoking
- Diabetes
- Antiphospholipid antibodies
- Family history

 DIAGNOSIS

DIFFERENTIAL DIAGNOSIS
- Migraine
- Focal seizure
- Tumor
- Subdural hematoma
- Hypoglycemia

LABORATORY N/A
Drugs that may alter lab results: N/A
Disorders that may alter lab results: N/A

PATHOLOGICAL FINDINGS N/A

SPECIAL TESTS
- Duplex carotid ultrasonography
- Cerebral angiography
- ECG
- Transthoracic echocardiogram (TTE); if normal and a cardiac source is suspected, followup with transesophageal echocardiogram
- Holter monitoring
- EEG for suspected seizure
- Prothrombin time (PT) and partial thromboplastin time (PTT). Coumadin prolongs PT.
- Antiphospholipid antibodies

IMAGING
Acute Phase: CT of head to rule out hemorrhage

DIAGNOSTIC PROCEDURES N/A

 TREATMENT

APPROPRIATE HEALTH CARE
- Acute phase: Inpatient care
- Surgical therapy: In medically fit patients with non-disabling stroke, carotid endarterectomy is indicated for stenosis of > 70% on side ipsilateral to stroke; medical therapy for < 30% stenosis
- Best therapy for stenosis of 30-70% is unknown, therefore it is best to refer the patient to a center involved in North American Symptomatic Carotid Endarterectomy Trial (NASCET)

GENERAL MEASURES
- Maintain oxygenation
- Monitor cardiac rhythm for 48 hours
- Control hyperglycemia (keep glucose < 220 mg/dl)
- Control of hypertension pressure if > 200/100 mm Hg
- Prevent hyperthermia
- Early introduction of physiotherapy and ambulation
- Subcutaneous heparin 5,000 units subcutaneously every 12 hours

ACTIVITY
Ambulate as soon as possible

DIET
- Alert with no dysphagia: Diet as tolerated (no added salt if hypertensive)
- Alert with dysphagia: Pureed dysphagia diet or nasogastric feeding tube if indicated

PATIENT EDUCATION
National Stroke Association, 300 East Hampden Ave., Suite 240, Englewood, CO. 80110-2622

MEDICATIONS

DRUG(S) OF CHOICE
• Enteric coated aspirin (EC ASA) 650 mg po bid, or
• Ticlopidine (Ticlid) 250 mg po bid
Contraindications:
• EC ASA - active peptic ulcer disease, hypersensitivity to aspirin, patients who had bronchospastic reaction to ASA or other nonsteroidal anti-inflammatory drugs
• Ticlopidine - known hypersensitivity to the drug, presence of hematopoietic disorders, presence of a hemostatic disorder, conditions associated with active bleeding, severe liver dysfunction
Precautions:
• EC ASA - may aggravate pre-existing peptic ulcer disease, may worsen symptoms in some patients with asthma
• Ticlopidine - 2.4% of patients develop neutropenia (0.8% severe neutropenia) which is reversible with cessation of drug; monitor blood counts every 2 weeks for the first 3 months
Significant possible interactions:
• EC ASA - may potentiate effects of anticoagulants and sulfonylurea, hypoglycemic agents
• Ticlopidine - digoxin plasma levels decreased 15%, theophylline half-life increased from 8.6 to 12.2 hours

ALTERNATIVE DRUGS
• Dipyridamole (Persantine) of no proven benefit
• Sulfinpyrazone (Anturane) of no proven benefit

FOLLOWUP

PATIENT MONITORING
Follow every 3 months for first year then yearly

PREVENTION/AVOIDANCE
• Stop smoking
• Control blood pressure, diabetes, hyperlipidemia
• EC ASA 650 mg bid or ticlopidine 250 mg po bid for patients with prior transient ischemic attack
• Use alcohol in moderation, if at all
• Regular exercise
• Maintain positive psychological outlook
• Maintain weight control

POSSIBLE COMPLICATIONS
• Shoulder subluxation
• Hyperextension knee injury
• Depression
• Sympathetic dystrophy

EXPECTED COURSE AND PROGNOSIS
• Variable depending on severity of stroke
• Posterior circulation strokes have a higher acute mortality rate but generally make a better functional recovery than hemispheric strokes

MISCELLANEOUS

ASSOCIATED CONDITIONS
Major cause of death in first five years after a stroke is cardiac disease

AGE-RELATED FACTORS
Pediatric:
• Cardiac (especially developmental abnormalities)
• Metabolic: Homocystinuria, Fabry's disease
Geriatric: Amyloid (congophylic) angiopathy is most prevalent in elderly, especially if patient also has dementia
Others: Adults < 45 years old most likely to have a cardiac source of embolism

PREGNANCY
• Parturition may increase risk of rupture for aneurysm; amniotic fluid embolism may cause stroke at time of delivery
• Postpartum period associated with increased risk for cerebral venous thrombosis

SYNONYMS
• Stroke
• Reversible ischemic neurological accident
• RIND

ICD-9-CM   436

SEE ALSO
• Transient ischemic attack (TIA)
• Stroke rehabilitation

OTHER NOTES   N/A

ABBREVIATIONS   ET ASA = enteric-coated aspirin

REFERENCES
• Hachinski, V. & Norris, J.W.: The Acute Stroke. Philadelphia, F.A. Davis, 1985
• Barnett, J.H.M., Mohr, J.P., Stein, B.M. & Yatsu, F.M. (eds.): Stroke. New York, Churchill Livingstone, 1986
• Norris, J.W. & Hachinski, V.C.: Prevention of Stroke. Philadelphia, F.A. Davis, 1991

Author   C. Graffagnino, M.D. & V. Hachinski, M.D.

Cervical cancer

 BASICS

DESCRIPTION An invasive process initiated usually at the squamocolumnar junction either by the squamous or adenomatous (glandular) components of the cervical epithelium
Genetics: Not known to be an inherited tendency
Incidence/Prevalence in USA: 17,000 new cases/year; majority of cases confined to cervix (Stage I)
Predominant age: 53 year old women, but possible increasing frequency in younger women
Predominant sex: Female only

SIGNS AND SYMPTOMS
• Irregular vaginal bleeding
• Post-coital vaginal bleeding
• Unusually foul-smelling discharge
• Dyspareunia
• Pelvic pain
• Hematuria
• Rectal bleeding
• Enlarged cervix

CAUSES Probably related to viral infections, including human papilloma virus

RISK FACTORS
• Human papilloma virus infection
• Human immunodeficiency virus infection
• Smoking
• High number of sexual partners
• Early age of first intercourse
• DES daughters

 DIAGNOSIS

DIFFERENTIAL DIAGNOSIS
• Cervicitis, severe
• Cervical polyp
• Carcinoma of endometrium with cervical extension
• Metastatic carcinoma, including choriocarcinoma

LABORATORY
• CBC (question of anemia secondary to chronic blood loss)
• Creatinine (question of ureteral obstruction)
• Liver function tests (question of metastases)
• Papanicolaou smear
Drugs that may alter lab results: N/A
Disorders that may alter lab results: Bleeding or inflammation may obscure presence of cancer cells

PATHOLOGICAL FINDINGS
• Invasive squamous carcinoma most common (80-85%)
• Invasive adenocarcinoma is second most common (15-20%)

SPECIAL TESTS
• Papanicolaou smear (Pap smear) for screening
• Colposcopy and endocervical sampling
• Diagnosis requires cervical tissue biopsy. Needs biopsy large enough to show cervical stroma to diagnose invasive nature.

IMAGING
For advanced disease
  ◊ CT abdomen and pelvis for radiation planning and detection of lymph node metastases
  ◊ Lymphangiogram occasionally for diagnosis of lymph node metastases

DIAGNOSTIC PROCEDURES
Cervical cone biopsy if early invasion or if question of invasion to determine depth of invasion

 TREATMENT

APPROPRIATE HEALTH CARE
Inpatient for complete work-up and treatment

GENERAL MEASURES
Initial disease
  ◊ For lesions with less than 3 mm invasion from basement membrane, no lymphatic or vascular invasion and no confluent tongues
    ◊ Total abdominal hysterectomy
    ◊ Cone biopsy - later hysterectomy
    ◊ Vaginal hysterectomy
    ◊ For cancer confined to the cervix (Stage I) with invasion greater than 3 mm
    ◊ Radical hysterectomy with lymph node dissection
    ◊ Or primary radiation therapy
    ◊ For most lesions greater than Stage I
    ◊ Radiation with or without adjuvant chemotherapy is appropriate
For recurrent disease
    ◊ Pelvic exenteration, if localized
    ◊ Chemotherapy, if metastatic

ACTIVITY As tolerated

DIET If radiation used, may need a lactose restricted diet

PATIENT EDUCATION
• "Sexuality and Cancer" pamphlet. American Cancer Society, 1599 Clifton Rd., Atlanta, GA 30329, (404) 320-3333
• "What You Need to Know About Cancer of the Cervix" and "Cancer Treatments: Consider the Possibilities". National Institutes of Health, Building 31, Room 41-21, 9000 Rockville Pike, Bethesda, MD 20892, (301)496-4236

MEDICATIONS

DRUG(S) OF CHOICE
For adjuvant radiation therapy sensitization
 ◊ 5-FU (Fluorouracil)
 ◊ Hydroxyurea
 ◊ Cisplatin
For recurrent, metastatic disease
 ◊ Bleomycin
 ◊ Etoposide (VP-16)
 ◊ Cisplatin or carboplatin
 ◊ Ifosfamide plus mesna
Contraindications: Each drug has different contraindications and side effects. Refer to manufacturer's profile of each drug.
Precautions: Neutropenia can occur with some combinations
Significant possible interactions: Refer to manufacturer's profile of each drug

ALTERNATIVE DRUGS   None

FOLLOWUP

PATIENT MONITORING
Following initial therapy, evaluation with physical exam and pap smear
 ◊ Every three months for 1-2 years
 ◊ Every six months until five years
 ◊ After five years, yearly evaluations

PREVENTION/AVOIDANCE
• Pap smear may decrease incidence of invasive disease
• Stop smoking
• Decrease exposure to sexually transmitted diseases

POSSIBLE COMPLICATIONS
• Ureteral fistula (less than 2% with treatment)
• Hydronephrosis
• Uremia

EXPECTED COURSE AND PROGNOSIS
• Stage I and II (60% of patients) 50-70% 5 year survival dependent upon risk factors
• Stage III 40% 5 year survival

MISCELLANEOUS

ASSOCIATED CONDITIONS
• Vaginal carcinoma in situ
• Vulvar carcinoma in situ
• Warts

AGE-RELATED FACTORS
Pediatric: N/A
Geriatric: May replace estrogen if ovaries removed
Others: Choice of initial therapy between radiation and radical surgery dependent on activity and general health of individual

PREGNANCY   Can occur in pregnant patients. Choice of therapy and need for therapeutic abortion dependent on stage and gestational age.

SYNONYMS
• Cancer of the uterine cervix
• Cervical malignancy
• Cervical carcinoma

ICD-9-CM   180.0

SEE ALSO   N/A

OTHER NOTES   N/A

ABBREVIATIONS   N/A

REFERENCES
• Cain, J.: Cancer of the Uterine Cervix. In Conn's Current Therapy. Edited by R. Rakel. Philadelphia, W.B. Saunders Co., 1991
• ACOG: Classification and Staging of Gynecologic Malignancies. No.155, May, 1991
• Goodman, J., Bowling, M. & Nelson, J.: Cervical Malignancies. Gynecologic Oncology. New York, Knapp/Berkowitz, 1986

Author   J. Cain, M.D.

Cervical dysplasia

 BASICS

 DIAGNOSIS

 TREATMENT

BASICS

DESCRIPTION Pre-invasive neoplastic epithelial changes in the transformation zone of the uterine cervix often associated with human papilloma virus infections
• Mild dysplasia (CIN I or SIL low grade) - cellular changes are limited to the lower one-third of the squamous epithelium
• Moderate dysplasia (CIN II or SIL high grade) - cellular changes are limited to the lower two-thirds of the squamous epithelium
• Severe dysplasia (CIN III or SIL high grade or carcinoma in-situ) - cellular changes involves the full thickness of the squamous epithelium
Genetics: N/A
Incidence/Prevalence in USA: Difficult to assess due to wide variability in false negative Pap smear reporting and uneven distribution of qualified colposcopists. Prevalence 3,600/100,000 at age 27-28.
Predominant age: The median age for severe carcinoma in-situ is 28 years. Earlier lesions can be expected at younger ages
Predominant sex: Female only

SIGNS AND SYMPTOMS
• Frequently none
• Occasionally there is association with condyloma accuminatum in the vulva, vagina, or anus
• Occasionally there are co-existing sexually transmitted diseases in the lower reproductive tract, e.g., chlamydia, gonorrhea

CAUSES Strong linkage with infections by human papilloma viruses types 6, 11, 16, 18, 31, 33, and 35. Other types of the same virus have also been implicated.

RISK FACTORS
• Multiparity and pregnancy before age 20 years
• Multiple sexual partners
• Early age in first sexual intercourse
• Condyloma accuminatum infection elsewhere in the body
• Cigarette smoking
• Prostitution
• Lower socio-economic status

DIAGNOSIS

DIFFERENTIAL DIAGNOSIS
• Invasive carcinoma of the cervix
• Condyloma acuminatum

LABORATORY N/A
Drugs that may alter lab results: N/A
Disorders that may alter lab results: N/A

PATHOLOGICAL FINDINGS
• Clumping of the nuclear chromatin material
• Reversal of the nuclear/cytoplasmic ratio
• Koilocytosis

SPECIAL TESTS Viral DNA hybridization (Virapap)

IMAGING N/A

DIAGNOSTIC PROCEDURES
• Papanicolaou smear
• Colposcopy and directed cervical biopsies
• Cone biopsy (by cold knife, laser, or loop excision)
• Endocervical curettage
• Loop electrosurgical procedure (LEEP)

TREATMENT

APPROPRIATE HEALTH CARE
• Office evaluation and observation
• Outpatient surgery: cryotherapy, laser ablative or excisional cone, cold knife cone, electro-surgical loop excision of transformation zone

GENERAL MEASURES N/A

ACTIVITY Four weeks of pelvic rest after cone biopsy

DIET No restriction

PATIENT EDUCATION Printed materials on cervical dysplasia

MEDICATIONS

DRUG(S) OF CHOICE
• Treatment is primarily surgical
• 5-fluoro-uracil (Efudex) once or twice daily has been used as vaginal cream for supplemental therapy
Contraindications: Hypersensitivity to Efudex
Precautions:
• If hand is used in application of Efudex, wash hand immediately afterwards
• Avoid contact of Efudex with eyes, nose, or mouth
Significant possible interactions: N/A

ALTERNATIVE DRUGS N/A

FOLLOWUP

PATIENT MONITORING Repeat Pap smears every 4 months during the first year after cone excision for severe dysplasia, every 6 months thereafter. For lesser lesions, repeat Pap smear yearly

PREVENTION/AVOIDANCE
• Monogamy of both sexual partners
• Use of condom during coitus if unable to practice monogamy
• Abstain from smoking
• Yearly Pap smears
• Ability to obtain skilled colposcopy service as needed

POSSIBLE COMPLICATIONS
• Some severe dysplasia will progress to invasive carcinoma of the cervix
Possible complications following cone biopsy of the cervix:
   ◊ Hemorrhage
   ◊ Infection
   ◊ Cervical stenosis
   ◊ Cervical incompetence
   ◊ Infertility
   ◊ Incomplete excision of dysplastic tissue

EXPECTED COURSE AND PROGNOSIS
• Generally excellent
• Persistence of dysplasia can occur due to incomplete excision
• Recurrence of dysplasia can occur due to inability to eradicate the human papilloma virus in the patient's body or prevent new infections

MISCELLANEOUS

ASSOCIATED CONDITIONS
• Condyloma acuminatum
• Carcinoma of the cervix

AGE-RELATED FACTORS
• This is a problem for the women in the reproductive age group. The median age is 28 years for severe dysplasia. For lesser lesions, the median ages tend to be much lower
Pediatric: Very rare
Geriatric: Less frequent
Others: N/A

PREGNANCY
• Dysplasia may progress during pregnancy
• It is important to determine the severity of dysplasia and to exclude the presence of invasive carcinoma during pregnancy
• Dysplasia does not require definitive treatment during pregnancy
• Dysplasia by itself is not an indication for cesarean section

SYNONYMS
• Cervical Intraepithelial Neoplasia (CIN)
• Squamous Intraepithelial Lesion (SIL)

ICD-9-CM 622.1 Dysplasia of cervix (uteri)

SEE ALSO N/A

OTHER NOTES N/A

ABBREVIATIONS N/A

REFERENCES
• Disaia, P.J., Creasman, W.T.: Clinical Gynecologic Oncology. 3rd Ed. St. Louis, The C.V. Mosby Company, 1989
• Wright, T.C., Richart, R.M. & Ferenczy, A.: Electrosurgery for HPV-related diseases of the lower genital tract. New York, Arthur Vision, Inc. & Biovision, Inc., 1992
• Kurman, R.J., (Ed.): Blaustein's Pathology Of The Female Genital Tract. 3rd Ed. New York, Springer-Verlag, 1987
• Novak, E.R., Woodruff, J.D.: Novak's Gynecologic and Obstetric Pathology With Clinical and Endocrine Relations. 8th Ed. Philadelphia, W.B. Saunders Company, 1979
• Herbst, A.L., Mishel, D.R., Stenchever, M.A. & Drogemueller, W.: Comprehensive Gynecology. 2nd Ed. St. Louis, C.V. Mosby Co., 1992

Author A. Shiu, M.D.

Cervical polyps

BASICS

DESCRIPTION Pedunculated masses, usually single, which vary in size from a few millimeters to 3 centimeters and protrude from the cervix; may bleed
Genetics: N/A
Incidence/Prevalence in USA: Common
Predominant age: Most often ages 30-50
Predominant sex: Female only

SIGNS AND SYMPTOMS
• Painless
• Intermenstrual bleeding (slight)
• May cause post-coital spotting

CAUSES
• Unknown for most
• Secondary reaction to cervical infection, erosion, or ulceration

RISK FACTORS   None known

DIAGNOSIS

DIFFERENTIAL DIAGNOSIS
• Prolapsed submucous myoma
• Other causes of intermenstrual bleeding

LABORATORY   N/A
Drugs that may alter lab results: N/A
Disorders that may alter lab results: N/A

PATHOLOGICAL FINDINGS
• Benign hyperplastic endocervical epithelium often with large number of blood vessels
• Size may be increased by edema and inflammation

SPECIAL TESTS
• Diagnosis usually made by pelvic examination
• Perform Pap smear prior to treatment

IMAGING   N/A

DIAGNOSTIC PROCEDURES
Characteristic appearance noted at time of pelvic examination

TREATMENT

APPROPRIATE HEALTH CARE
Outpatient usually. Very large polyps may require removal in operating room.

GENERAL MEASURES
• Simple surgical excision in office with snare, electrocautery, or liquid nitrogen, control bleeding with silver nitrate
• No douching following excision

ACTIVITY   Avoid sexual intercourse until postoperative followup

DIET   General diet

PATIENT EDUCATION   Routine care instructions

MEDICATIONS

DRUG(S) OF CHOICE None
Contraindications: N/A
Precautions: N/A
Significant possible interactions: N/A

ALTERNATIVE DRUGS N/A

FOLLOWUP

PATIENT MONITORING Recheck at routine appointments, 1 and 6 weeks following surgical excision

PREVENTION/AVOIDANCE None known

POSSIBLE COMPLICATIONS
• Bleeding and mild pain with removal
• Spotting for 1 or 2 days

EXPECTED COURSE AND PROGNOSIS Almost always benign. Very rare incidence of dysplasia in polyp. Very rare possibility of malignancy arising.

MISCELLANEOUS

ASSOCIATED CONDITIONS None

AGE-RELATED FACTORS
Pediatric: Very rare
Geriatric: Rare
Others: N/A

PREGNANCY Delay removal until postpartum

SYNONYMS N/A

ICD-9-CM 622.7

SEE ALSO N/A

OTHER NOTES N/A

ABBREVIATIONS N/A

REFERENCES
• Danforth, D.M., Scott, J.R., et al. (eds.): Obstetric and Gynecology. 6th Ed. Philadelphia, J.B. Lippincott, 1990
• Novak, E.R. et al. (eds.): Novak's, Textbook of Gynecology. 11th Ed. Baltimore, Williams & Wilkins, 1988

Author M. Worshtil, M.D.

Cervical spine injury

BASICS

DESCRIPTION
Though an over-simplification, it is best to classify injuries as flexion, extension, compression, or unknown

Flexion injuries
◊ Anterior subluxation - best seen on lateral view of cervical spine as a kyphotic angulation at the point of ligamentous injury. Widening of spinous process at the point of injury may occur.
◊ Facet dislocation - unstable injury, especially when bilateral. Anterior displacement of vertebra (50% of its width) usually indicates bilateral facet dislocation.
◊ Compression fractures - usually associated with disruption of the posterior ligament complex and therefore unstable
◊ Clay-shovelers fracture - avulsion fracture of C7-C6 or T1 spinous process with intact posterior ligaments and therefore stable

Extension injuries
◊ Hangman's fracture - fracture of the pars interarticularis of the axis. It accounts for 10-15% of fractures.
◊ Laminar fracture - difficult to see. Usually in older people who have spondylosis.
◊ Fracture posterior arch atlas - usually stable when an isolated injury
◊ Fracture dislocations - may resemble a flexion injury since the vertebral body is propelled forward and therefore appears as a flexion subluxation

Compression
◊ Jefferson's fracture - a fracture of the arches of C1, best seen on the open mouth view as lateral displacement of C1
◊ Burst fracture - seen on the AP radiograph as a vertical fracture of the body and on the lateral as a commutation of the body with varying degrees of retropulsion of the body

Unknown mechanisms
◊ Odontoid fractures - best seen on the AP view, but lateral views may show a tilt or displacement

System(s) affected: Musculoskeletal, Nervous
Genetics: N/A
Incidence/Prevalence in USA: Cervical injuries account for twelve thousand deaths in the U.S. each year. One-half of these are from motor vehicular accidents.
Predominant age: Most common in ages 16-25
Predominant sex: Male > Female

SIGNS AND SYMPTOMS
• Pain, stiffness, and/or tenderness in an alert patient. If none of these are present the incidence of cervical spine injury is only 1-2%, provided the patient is alert and without alcohol or drug intake. (A lateral cervical spine x-ray should be taken routinely in all severe trauma).
• Head and/or facial trauma/lacerations in patients with altered consciousness

CAUSES Trauma

RISK FACTORS
• Motor vehicle accidents
• Diving accidents

DIAGNOSIS

DIFFERENTIAL DIAGNOSIS
• Joint, muscle or ligament inflammation
• Paresthesias
• Arthritis
• Cervical disk protrusion
• Cervical spondylosis

LABORATORY N/A
Drugs that may alter lab results: N/A
Disorders that may alter lab results: N/A

PATHOLOGICAL FINDINGS N/A

SPECIAL TESTS
Tomograms may be obtained to visualize otherwise obscure fractures, but even these are usually inferior to imaging by CT. MRI is superior in evaluating soft tissue injury.

IMAGING
• The use of CT and MRI scanning has greatly facilitated diagnosis of obscure cervical injuries. The CT may be a little better in some bone injuries, especially in the foramen, while the MRI has the edge with soft tissue evaluation. Both are superior to any previous method.
• X-ray - a lateral view of the cervical spine is only 80-85% accurate in picking up abnormalities. Adding an AP and open mouth odontoid view will increase the accuracy of screening to 90-95%. However, in the presence of pain, tenderness, and/or stiffness, the use of a CT or MRI scan should be considered since 5-10% of cases will have normal radiographs even with a significant cervical injury.

X-rays vary with the type of injury, but a few salient features to be observed are:
◊ Soft-tissue swelling on the lateral view of greater than 5 mm when measured from the inferior border of C3 to the trachea indicates a severe injury (except children)
◊ Widely divergent spinous processes on the lateral view indicates rupture of ligaments
◊ Abnormal widening of either a complete interspace or a portion of the anterior or posterior interspace on lateral view (compare with interspaces above and below)
◊ Malrotation of the spinous processes on the AP view (they should form a straight line)
◊ Inequality of the space on either side of the odontoid on open mouth views

DIAGNOSTIC PROCEDURES N/A

TREATMENT

APPROPRIATE HEALTH CARE
Transportation
◊ 5-15% of spinal cord injuries occur or are made worse during transportation or initial treatment
◊ A carefully applied rigid collar supplemented by sand bags on either side of the head on a rigid backboard is probably the safest method
◊ Oxygen should be given to all patients with injury to the spinal cord. (Patients with high cord lesions die of asphyxiation so assisted ventilation may be needed).
◊ 50% of serious cervical injuries will have associated head, chest, abdominal or major extremity injuries in association. Give first aid to these patients maintaining the "ABC" principle of airway, breathing, and circulation.
◊ Military antishock garment (MASG) can be used in cases of shock
◊ Start an intravenous line if it can be done rapidly. Otherwise, this should not be done as valuable time may be wasted. The principle of "load and go" in cases of ambulance or "swoop and scoop" in the case of helicopters is a good one if an acute care center is close at hand.
Hospital
◊ Prior to dealing with the cervical injury, attention should be directed towards the ABC's (airway, breathing, circulation)
◊ Arterial oxygen should be measured immediately since oxygenation of an injured spinal cord helps prevent further damage and aids in recovery. If the oxygen partial pressure (pO2) is less than 70 mm of mercury, or the cervical lesion is above C5, intubation is indicated. If the patient is breathing, blind nasal intubation can be tried; otherwise the oral approach with a laryngoscope is necessary. Both require careful technique with avoidance of neck extension. If this cannot be done with ease or if there are severe facial injuries, a cricothyroidotomy should be done.
◊ A nasogastric (N-G) tube should always be inserted to prevent vomiting, aspiration. It also prevents gastric dilatation with lung compression and difficult breathing.
◊ In most cases, volume replacement is best accomplished through the femoral route. The subclavian approach risks pneumothorax and further oxygenation problems.
◊ If a pneumothorax is present, a chest tube should always be inserted (first confirmed by X-ray). Needle aspiration is indicated only as a temporary measure to relieve symptoms in a tension pneumothorax prior to insertion of the tube.
◊ In all cord injuries, peritoneal lavage should be done to rule out a severe intra-abdominal injury. This procedure is highly accurate while all physical findings and symptoms are unreliable. (The N-G tube and an indwelling Foley catheter should be done prior to the lavage). In many centers, an abdominal CT has replaced this procedure.

GENERAL MEASURES

• Spinal shock occurs in 25-40% of spinal cord injuries. It is characterized by systolic hypotension and bradycardia. The cause is loss of distal sympathetic tone.
• Head injuries alone do not cause hypotension but can cause hypertension
• Because patients with cervical trauma may sustain other significant injuries, systolic hypotension may be from blood loss and/or spinal shock. Remember that several liters of blood can be lost from a head or perineal wound.
• Shock other than from volume loss or spinal shock can come from pericardial tamponade, tension pneumothorax, or cardiac contusion

ACTIVITY N/A

DIET N/A

PATIENT EDUCATION N/A

MEDICATIONS

DRUG(S) OF CHOICE
Methylprednisolone
◊ If given within 8 hours after the injury, has been shown to not only minimize further injury, but to improve both motor function and sensation for up to six months. This steroid apparently prevents lipid hydrolysis and subsequent destruction of the cell membrane.
◊ Initial dose: 30 mg/kg over a 15 minute period. Then 45 minutes later, 5.4 mg/kg/hr for the next 23 hours. See Bracken 1990, N Engl J Med 322:1405-1411.
Contraindications: None
Precautions: Intravenous Tagamet 300 mg every 6 hours or Zantac 50 mg every 8 hours can be given if a history of ulcer is present. In cases of multiple injuries this is a good way to prevent stress ulcer.
Significant possible interactions: None

ALTERNATIVE DRUGS Naloxone, nimodipine and thyrotropin releasing hormones have been tried with equivocal results. Tests are underway using chemotherapeutic drugs, but these await the outcome of several studies.

FOLLOWUP

PATIENT MONITORING Critical care facilities must be available initially and later physical and occupational therapy units with special skills in spinal cord injuries

PREVENTION/AVOIDANCE N/A

POSSIBLE COMPLICATIONS
• Paresthesia
• Muscle weakness
• Reflex loss
• Sensory loss
• Radiculopathy

EXPECTED COURSE AND PROGNOSIS In cases of significant cord injuries, the prognosis is guarded. With development in newer orthopedic devices, the patients have a much improved lifestyle.

MISCELLANEOUS

ASSOCIATED CONDITIONS N/A

AGE-RELATED FACTORS
Pediatric: N/A
Geriatric: N/A
Others: N/A

PREGNANCY N/A

SYNONYMS Cervical fracture, dislocation

ICD-9-CM 952.0

SEE ALSO N/A

OTHER NOTES N/A

ABBREVIATIONS N/A

REFERENCES
• Summit, et al.: Axial Loading Injuries to Middle Cervical Spine; American Journal of Sports Medicine, 1991, 19(1), pp. 6-20
• Soderstrom & Brumback: Orthopedic Clinics of North American; Vol. 17/. No.1, January 1986; pp. 3-13
• Bracken, M.B. et al.: Efficacy of methylprednisolone in acute spinal cord Injury; JAMA, 1984:251. 45-52
• Bracken, M.B. et al.: A randomized control trial of methylprednisolone or naloxone in the treatment of acute spinal cord injury. Results of the second acute spinal cord Injury study. N Engl J Med 1990; 322:1405-1411
• Jacobs, B.: Cervical Fractures and Dislocations, Clinical Orthopedics. No. 109, June 1975, p. 18

Author F. Johnston, M.D.

Cervical spondylosis

 BASICS

DESCRIPTION
Degenerative changes in the cervical vertebra and/or disk with spur formation and subsequent impingement of neural elements in a narrow cervical canal
Genetics: N/A
Incidence/Prevalence in USA: 30-40% of the population above age 40 years
Predominant age: Above 40 the incidence increases with each passing decade
Predominant sex: Male > Female (3:2)

SIGNS AND SYMPTOMS
• Pain in the posterior neck often associated with radiation into the arms
• Scapular pain
• Pain in the arms is almost always on the outer aspect of the arm at least to elbow level (coronary heart pain is almost always on the inner aspect of the arm)
• Radicular pain into the arms or scapular area may be present without neck pain
• Dysphagia may develop with large anterior osteophytes
• Weakness of extremities - upper and/or lower
• Bladder or bowel incontinence in severe cases
• If an osteophyte develops on a neurocentral joint and extends laterally, it can encroach on the vertebral artery and may cause dizziness, vertigo, tinnitus or interorbital blurring of vision. Symptoms are exacerbated by extremes of movement and even minor neck trauma.
• Loss of neck extension (common)
• Lateral flexion of the cervical spine is limited in the erect position, but greatly increased on lying down. (Functional disorders are not improved by lying down.)
• Long tract signs may develop in severe cases with positive Babinski
• Tenderness of biceps and pectoralis major in C5-6 segment disease
• Tricep tenderness in C6-7 segment disease

CAUSES
Degenerative changes with osteophytes and disk space narrowing

RISK FACTORS N/A

 DIAGNOSIS

DIFFERENTIAL DIAGNOSIS
• Cervical disk disease (the two often co-exist)
• Pancoast tumor of lung
• Rheumatoid arthritis
• Neurological disorders such as multiple sclerosis

LABORATORY N/A
Drugs that may alter lab results: N/A
Disorders that may alter lab results: N/A

PATHOLOGICAL FINDINGS N/A

SPECIAL TESTS N/A

IMAGING
• X-rays of cervical spine, AP, lateral open mouth odontoid and both oblique views should be obtained. Osteophytes and/or joint space narrowing will be evident.
• CT or MRI scans are quite valuable in cases where surgery is contemplated or the diagnosis is in doubt. It is not indicated in the great majority of cases as a careful history and physical examination coupled with routine cervical spine x-rays will make the diagnosis. The decision as to which is better, the CT scan or MRI, is controversial. The MRI depicts cord changes, enlargement, compression, or atrophy better. While the CT, especially in conjunction with myelography, shows the bony changes, especially in foramina involvement. MRI has the obvious advantage of not requiring a myelogram. Postoperatively, the MRI is excellent in evaluation of patients who have failed to obtain relief from surgery or have developed new symptoms. If this does not demonstrate a cause, then a CT scan with contrast can be obtained.

DIAGNOSTIC PROCEDURES N/A

 TREATMENT

APPROPRIATE HEALTH CARE
Outpatient for conservative treatment, inpatient if surgery indicated

GENERAL MEASURES
Medical
◊ Acute phase - moist heat, gentle massage and temporary immobilization with a cervical collar that holds the neck in slight flexion. Intermittent cervical traction may be helpful, but the line of pull should be such that the neck is slightly flexed. Ultrasonic treatments, especially combined with gentle muscle stimulation (US-MS) for 15-20 minutes daily or bid may be helpful in the acute phase.
◊ Chronic - no treatment necessary except for non-narcotic analgesics for symptoms. Any type of activity or work which causes strain of the neck should be avoided.
Surgical
◊ Indications: Severe pain unresponsive to conservative measures, significant or progression of neurologic deficits, long trait signs, vertebral artery syndrome
◊ Most common surgery is anterior interbody fusion with excision of disk and any accessible osteophytes

ACTIVITY
Any activity which does not cause symptoms should be encouraged as the disease is chronic. Needless restrictions can make the patient a medical invalid.

DIET No special diet

PATIENT EDUCATION
• Personally instruct (or have a therapist instruct) in the proper use of orthopedic appliances. Cervical collars should produce a slight flexion of the neck as should traction. Avoid extension in all situations.
• Instruct patients to report any weaknesses, eye symptoms, bladder or bowel incontinence immediately

MEDICATIONS

DRUG(S) OF CHOICE
• Acetaminophen (Tylenol) 500mg qid is the safest regimen. Studies have shown it to be as least as effective as NSAID's.
• NSAID's - aspirin 1.0gm qid is effective in many cases. If this fails, any of the other NSAID's are used with all having about the same success rate. Piroxicam 10mg daily, Tolmentin 600mg tid are some examples. If aspirin therapy is used, salicylate levels should be obtained; therapeutic range is 10-30 mg/dL. Enteric-coated aspirin may be helpful to minimize GI upset.
• Cortisone should not be used in long term management. Occasional injections of trigger zones with 40mg Depo-Medrol may be used, but this should be saved for severe exacerbations.
• Trigger point injection of lidocaine 1%, injected into the "hot areas", especially in the scapular area. Often as effective in relieving symptoms alone as when combined with Depo-Medrol.
Contraindications: NSAID's, except aspirin, should not be used in patients with chronic liver disease. Use with caution in cases of ulcers. If NSAID's are used, misoprostol (Cytotec) 200μg qid should be given concomitantly.
Precautions: Patients on long term NSAID's should be monitored with liver studies 6-8 weeks after initial treatment and then every 3-4 weeks
Significant possible interactions: Refer to manufacturer's profile of each drug

ALTERNATIVE DRUGS
Listed in Drugs of Choice

FOLLOWUP

PATIENT MONITORING
Patients should be seen in 3-4 weeks for evaluation of neurologic status. If this has not changed follow at intervals of 3-6 months, depending on severity of symptoms.

PREVENTION/AVOIDANCE
The midcervical spine is the area usually involved in spondylosis. This portion will develop a flexion deformity causing extension of the upper spine as the body tries to keep the head erect. Avoid any extension strain such as a "spinal manipulation", extension during intubation for a general anesthesia, or cervical strain from auto accidents, especially rear-end collisions. These can cause a basilar artery thrombosis or thrombosis of the posterior inferior cerebellar artery with a subsequent Wallenberg's syndrome. Dysphagia, pain and temperature loss to the same side of the face and opposite side of the body, nystagmus and Horner's syndrome are present in Wallenberg's syndrome.

POSSIBLE COMPLICATIONS
Loss of motion, especially extension, may require adjustments to certain occupations to prevent uncommonly significant muscle loss and instability of gait, bladder or bowel function

EXPECTED COURSE AND PROGNOSIS
Fortunately, the prognosis is for a benign course in the overwhelming majority of cases, though for most of their lives patients will be plagued by pain which exacerbates often with no known cause

MISCELLANEOUS

ASSOCIATED CONDITIONS
Cervical disk disease

AGE-RELATED FACTORS
Pediatric: N/A
Geriatric: N/A
Others: N/A

PREGNANCY
As in the case of rheumatoid arthritis, the symptoms often improve but occasionally are made worse

SYNONYMS
• Cervical arthritis
• Cervical myelopathy
• Cervical osteophyte

ICD-9-CM
756.19. Cervical spondylosis

SEE ALSO
N/A

OTHER NOTES
N/A

ABBREVIATIONS
N/A

REFERENCES
• McNab, Cervical Spondylosis: Clinical Orthopedics, January, 1975, Vol. 109; p.69
• Clifton, et al.: Identifiable causes for poor outcome in surgery for cervical spondylosis, Hans Radiology, November, 1990; 177(2) p. 313-25
• Zarnaze, et al.: American Journal of Roentgenography; February, 1988; 150(2), pp.397-403

Author F. Johnston, .M.D.

Cervicitis

 BASICS

DESCRIPTION An inflammation of the uterine cervix. Infectious cervicitis may be caused by Chlamydia trachomatis, Neisseria gonorrhoeae, Herpes simplex or Trichomonas vaginalis.
• Chronic cervicitis is characterized by inflammation of the cervix without an identified pathogen
Genetics: N/A
Incidence in USA:
• Gonorrhea 190/100,000
• Chlamydia 1040/100,000
• Trichomonas 1200/100,000
Prevalence in USA:
• Gonorrhea 2% of sexually active women under age 30
• Chlamydia 8-40% of women (median 15%)
• Trichomonas 5-25%
Predominant age: Infectious cervicitis is most common in adolescents, but can be seen in women of any age
Predominant sex: Female only

SIGNS AND SYMPTOMS
• Mucopurulent (yellow) discharge from the cervix
• Cervical erosion or erythema
• Easily induced endocervical mucosal bleeding
• Tenderness of cervix
• Frequently asymptomatic

CAUSES
• Chlamydia trachomatis
• Neisseria gonorrhoeae
• Herpes simplex virus
• Trichomonas vaginalis
• Cause of chronic cervicitis unknown

RISK FACTORS
• Multiple sexual partners
• History of sexually transmitted disease
• Postpartum period

 DIAGNOSIS

DIFFERENTIAL DIAGNOSIS
• Vaginal infections with Candida albicans or Trichomonas vaginalis extending onto the cervix
• Carcinoma of the cervix

LABORATORY
• Endocervical gram stain, more than 10 WBC's per high power field (hpf) suggests cervicitis
• Cervical cultures for C. trachomatis, N. gonorrhoeae
• Enzyme assays (Chlamydiazyme and others) sometimes used to screen for chlamydia
• Wet mount for Trichomonas vaginalis
• If ulcerations present, culture for Herpes simplex virus
• Venereal Disease Research Laboratory (VDRL) or rapid plasma reagin (RPR) to rule out concurrent syphilis
Drugs that may alter lab results: Recent antibiotic treatment
Disorders that may alter lab results: N/A

PATHOLOGIC FINDINGS Inflammatory changes on Pap smear

SPECIAL TESTS N/A

IMAGING N/A

DIAGNOSTIC PROCEDURES
Colposcopy is indicated in chronic inflammation, with biopsy of suspicious areas

 TREATMENT

APPROPRIATE HEALTH CARE
Outpatient treatment

GENERAL MEASURES Chronic cervicitis with negative cultures and biopsies may be treated with cryosurgery

ACTIVITY Full activity

DIET No special diet

PATIENT EDUCATION
• Advise patient to use condoms consistently
• If infectious etiology suspected, advise patient to inform her partners

Cervicitis

MEDICATIONS

DRUG(S) OF CHOICE
• If infectious cervicitis suspected, treat without awaiting culture results. Ceftriaxone (Rocephin) 250 mg IM single dose, followed by doxycycline (Vibramycin) 100 mg po bid for 10 days or azithromycin (Zithromax) 1 g single dose
• For Trichomonas, metronidazole 2 g single dose
• For herpes, acyclovir (Zovirax) 200 mg po 5 times daily for 7 days
• Chronic cervicitis with negative cultures is sometimes treated with a sulfonamide containing vaginal cream
• Chronic cervicitis associated with postmenopausal vaginal atrophic changes may respond to topical estrogen creams

Contraindications:
• Doxycycline should not be used in pregnant or nursing mothers
• Metronidazole contraindicated in first trimester of pregnancy

Precautions: Doxycycline should not be taken with milk, antacids, or iron containing preparations

Significant possible interactions:
Doxycycline - warfarin (Coumadin) and oral contraceptives may have their effectiveness reduced

ALTERNATIVE DRUGS
• Spectinomycin 2 g IM can be substituted for ceftriaxone
• Erythromycin base or stearate 500 mg po qid, or erythromycin ethylsuccinate 800 mg po qid can be substituted for doxycycline
• Ofloxacin (Floxin) 300 mg po bid x 7 days

FOLLOWUP

PATIENT MONITORING
• Repeat cultures after treatment for chlamydia or gonorrhea are indicated in pregnant or high risk patients
• Annual Pap smears in sexually active patients screen for chronic cervicitis

PREVENTION/AVOIDANCE
Patients with more than one sexual partner should be advised to use condoms at every encounter

POSSIBLE COMPLICATIONS
• Cervicitis with C. trachomatis or N. gonorrhoeae is associated with an 8-10% risk of subsequent pelvic inflammatory disease
• Moderate to severe inflammation is associated with condyloma acuminatum and cervical carcinoma

EXPECTED COURSE AND PROGNOSIS
• Infectious cervicitis usually responds to systemic antibiotics
• Chronic cervicitis may be resistant to treatment, and should be monitored closely for cervical dysplasia

MISCELLANEOUS

ASSOCIATED CONDITIONS Patients with infectious cervicitis should be screened for other sexually transmitted diseases, syphilis, trichomonas, and possibly human immunodeficency virus (HIV)

AGE-RELATED FACTORS
Pediatric: Infectious cervicitis in children should lead to investigation for possible sexual abuse
Geriatric:
• Chronic cervicitis in postmenopausal women may be related to lack of estrogen
• The possibility of infectious cervicitis should not be overlooked, as many geriatric patients remain sexually active
Others: Adolescents remain a high-risk group for sexually transmitted diseases

PREGNANCY Screen all pregnant women for infectious cervicitis because of the risk of transmission to the fetus

SYNONYMS Mucopurulent cervicitis

ICD-9-CM
• Cervicitis 616.0
• Acute gonococcal cervicitis 098.15
• Chlamydia infection 079.8

SEE ALSO
• Chlamydia sexually transmitted
• Gonococcal infections
• Trichomoniasis
• Cervicitis, ectropion and true erosion
• Cervical dysplasia

OTHER NOTES The presence of Trichomonas does not rule out other concurrent infection

ABBREVIATIONS N/A

REFERENCES
• MMWR 1989;38:S-8
• Pediatr Clin N Am 1989;36(3):489-511
• Danforth, D.M. & Scott, J.R. (eds.): Obstetrics and Gynecology. 4th Ed. Philadelphia, W.B. Saunders, 1983
• The Medical Letter, 1991, 33:119-124

Author B. Majeroni, M.D.

Cervicitis, ectropion, and true erosion

 BASICS

DESCRIPTION
• Cervicitis - inflammatory changes due to infections
• Ectropion - eversion of the cervix in pregnancy
• True erosion - abrupt loss of overlying vaginal epithelium due to trauma, e.g., forceful insertion of vaginal speculum in patient with atrophic mucosa
System(s) affected: Reproductive
Genetics: N/A
Incidence/Prevalence in USA:
• Cervicitis - very common in sexually active women
• Ectropion - very common in pregnant women
• True erosion - occasionally seen in post-menopausal women
Predominant Age: See Prevalence in USA
Predominant Sex: Female only

SIGNS AND SYMPTOMS
• Cervicitis - metrorrhagia, post-coital bleeding, vaginal discharge
• Ectropion - red cervix due to color of the columnar epithelium
• True erosion - vaginal bleeding, sharply defined ulcers of cervix

CAUSES
• Cervicitis - Chlamydia trachomatis, Trichomonas vaginalis
• Ectropion - hormonal changes during pregnancy, especially with progesterone
• True erosion - injury to atrophic epithelium due to estrogen deficiency in menopause

RISK FACTORS
• Cervicitis - sexual contact with infected partner(s), recurrence due to inadequate therapy
• Ectropion - pregnancy
• True erosion - estrogen deficiency, trauma

 DIAGNOSIS

DIFFERENTIAL DIAGNOSIS
• Cervical dysplasia
• Carcinoma of the cervix

LABORATORY
• Saline and potassium hydroxide preparation of cervical/vaginal smears
• Chlamydiazyme or chlamydia cell culture, gonorrhea culture
• Papanicolaou (Pap) smear of the cervix
• Chlamydia DNA probe
Drugs that may alter lab results: N/A
Disorders that may alter lab results: N/A

PATHOLOGICAL FINDINGS
• Cervicitis - acute and chronic inflammatory changes, presence of infective organisms
• Ectropion - none
• True erosion - sharply defined ulcer borders, loss of epithelium

SPECIAL TESTS   None

IMAGING   None

DIAGNOSTIC PROCEDURES
Colposcopy

 TREATMENT

APPROPRIATE HEALTH CARE
Outpatient

GENERAL MEASURES   N/A

ACTIVITY   No restrictions

DIET   No special diet

PATIENT EDUCATION   Provide printed material about sexually transmitted diseases and about estrogen deficiency and estrogen replacement therapy

MEDICATIONS

DRUG(S) OF CHOICE
• Trichomoniasis - metronidazole 500 mg bid for 7 days
• Chlamydial infection - for non-pregnant women, doxycycline 100 mg bid po for 7 days; for pregnant women, erythromycin base 500 mg qid po for 7 days, or erythromycin ethylsuccinate 800 mg qid for 7 days
• Ectropion - none
• True erosion - conjugated estrogen vaginal cream daily for 2 weeks, follow by estrogen replacement therapy
Contraindications:
• Metronidazole - first trimester of pregnancy
• Doxycycline - pregnancy or lactation
• Estrogen - see extended list of contraindications to estrogen use in standard texts
Precautions:
• Metronidazole - possible fetal harm if used in first trimester of pregnancy, disulfiram reaction with alcohol
• Doxycycline - possible fetal harm if used during pregnancy, staining of the infant's teeth if used during breast-feeding, allergy, photosensitization
• Erythromycin - nausea or vomiting
• Estrogens - history of estrogen dependent neoplasms, history of thromboembolic diseases, see extended list of contraindications to estrogen therapy in standard texts
Significant possible interactions:
• Metronidazole & alcohol
• Doxycycline & dairy products, iron preparations, warfarin, and oral contraceptives (use backup contraceptive method)
• Erythromycin & terfenadine (Seldane): may increase terfenadine levels with subsequent ECG changes
• Erythromycin & theophylline (elevated theophylline level)
• Estrogen - N/A

ALTERNATIVE DRUGS
• Metronidazole - AVC cream
• Doxycycline - erythromycin
• Erythromycin - clindamycin
• Estrogen - lubricant, same as that used for vaginal speculum
• Azithromycin 1 gram for one dose only
• Ofloxacin 300mg bid x 7 days
• Amoxicillin 500mg po q8h x 7days

FOLLOWUP

PATIENT MONITORING
• Trichomoniasis - repeat vaginal smear until infection is cleared
• Chlamydial infection - repeat chlamydial culture post antibiotic therapy
• Estrogen deficiency - re-examine in one month to confirm healing

PREVENTION/AVOIDANCE
• Trichomoniasis or chlamydial infection - treatment of sexual partners and use of condom during coitus
• Estrogen deficiency - estrogen replacement therapy

POSSIBLE COMPLICATIONS N/A

EXPECTED COURSE AND PROGNOSIS
• Cervicitis - excellent healing once infection is eradicated
• Ectropion - spontaneous regression post partum
• True erosion - spontaneous healing

MISCELLANEOUS

ASSOCIATED CONDITIONS
• Gonorrhea
• Bacterial vaginosis

AGE-RELATED FACTORS
Pediatric: N/A
Geriatric: Menopause
Others: N/A

PREGNANCY Ectropion

SYNONYMS N/A

ICD-9-CM 616.0

SEE ALSO N/A

OTHER NOTES N/A

ABBREVIATIONS N/A

REFERENCES
• Disaia, P.J., Creasman, W.T.: Clinical Gynecologic Oncology. 3rd Ed. St. Louis, The C.V. Mosby Company, 1989
• Herbst, A.L., Mishell, D.R., Stenchever, M.A. & Droegemueller, W.: Comprehensive Gynecology. 2nd Ed. St. Louis, The C.V. Mosby Co., 1992
• Kurman, R.J., (Ed.): Blaustein's Pathology Of The Female Genital Tract. 3rd Ed. New York, Springer-Verlag, 1987
• Novak, E.R., Woodruff, J.D.: Novak's Gynocologic And Obstetric Pathology With Clinical And Endocrine Relations. 8th Ed. Philadelphia, W.B. Saunders Company, 1979

Author A. Shiu, M.D., FACOG

Chancroid

 BASICS

DESCRIPTION A sexually transmitted disease characterized by painful genital ulcerations and inflammatory inguinal adenopathy. It is uncommon in the United States but found worldwide. Chancroid is endemic in developing countries.
System(s) affected: Reproductive, Skin/Exocrine
Genetics: N/A
Incidence in USA: Approximately 4,700 cases annually (1988,1989, 1990 - CDC data). Actual numbers felt to be greater due to underreporting of cases.
Prevalence in USA: N/A
Predominant age: Teenagers and adults
Predominant sex: Male > Female

SIGNS AND SYMPTOMS
• Tender genital papule that ulcerates after 24 hours
• Irregular edged, painful ulcer(s)
• Ulcers may be 1 mm to 5 cm in size
• Ulcers may occur on the shaft of the penis, glans and meatus in men
• Ulcers in women most commonly occur in labia majora but also seen in labia minora, perineum, thigh, and cervix
• Painful inguinal adenopathy with abscess (bubo) formation in 30% of patients
• Atypical presentations include folliculitis and foreskin abscess

CAUSES Haemophilus ducreyi (gram negative bacterium)

RISK FACTORS
• Multiple sexual partners
• Uncircumcised males
• Prostitutes often are carriers

 DIAGNOSIS

DIFFERENTIAL DIAGNOSIS
• Syphilis
• Herpes Simplex Virus (HSV 1 and 2)
• Lymphogranuloma venereum (LGV)
• Granuloma inguinale

LABORATORY Serologic testing for antibody with ELISA technique. Gram stain; culture of organism on agar and blood medium
Drugs that may alter lab results: Previous antibiotics
Disorders that may alter lab results: None expected

PATHOLOGICAL FINDINGS "School of fish" pattern on gram stain

SPECIAL TESTS N/A

IMAGING N/A

DIAGNOSTIC PROCEDURES
• Gram stain and culture of ulcer exudate
• Aspiration of inguinal bubo (lymph node)

 TREATMENT

APPROPRIATE HEALTH CARE
Outpatient treatment

GENERAL MEASURES
• Saline or Burow's solution soaks to ulcers
• Aspiration of buboes if greater than 5 cm

ACTIVITY Refrain from sexual intercourse until genital lesions fully resolved

DIET N/A

PATIENT EDUCATION
• Sexual counseling
• Use of condoms
• Local wound care
• Treatment of all sexual partners with same regimen as index case

MEDICATIONS

DRUG(S) OF CHOICE Ceftriaxone 250 mg IM once
Contraindications: Allergy to the medication
Precautions: Refer to manufacturer's profile of each drug
Significant possible interactions: Refer to manufacturer's profile of each drug

ALTERNATIVE DRUGS
• Erythromycin 500 mg qid for 7 days
• Ciprofloxacin 500 mg bid for 3 days
• Trimethoprim/sulfamethoxazole double strength bid for 7 days

FOLLOWUP

PATIENT MONITORING
• Patient followed until all clinical signs of infection resolved
• Baseline syphilis serology and at 3 months
• HIV testing at 3 months post-treatment

PREVENTION/AVOIDANCE Avoidance of sexual activity until ulcers resolved

POSSIBLE COMPLICATIONS
• Phimosis
• Balanoposthitis
• Rupture of buboes with fistula formation and scarring

EXPECTED COURSE AND PROGNOSIS
• Full clinical resolution with appropriate treatment
• 5% relapse after treatment

MISCELLANEOUS

ASSOCIATED CONDITIONS
• Syphilis (concurrently in 5% of patients)
• HIV infection

AGE-RELATED FACTORS N/A
Pediatric: N/A
Geriatric: N/A
Others: HIV disease may affect treatment response

PREGNANCY Maternal to infant transmission has not been reported

SYNONYMS
• Soft chancre
• Ulcus molle

ICD-9-CM 0999.O

SEE ALSO N/A

OTHER NOTES Chancroid has been shown to be an established risk factor for acquisition of HIV infection

ABBREVIATIONS N/A

REFERENCES
• Ronald, A.R.: Chancroid and Haemophilus ducreyi. Ann Intern Med, 102:705, 1985
• Ronald, A.R. & Albritton, W.: Chancroid and Haemophilus ducreyi. In Sexually Transmitted Diseases. Edited by K. Holmes, P. Mardh, P.F. Sparling, et al. New York, McGraw-Hill, 1990
• Kirchner, J.T.: The Emerging Clinical Significance of Chancroid. Family Practice Recertification 1990;12:32-44

Author J. Kirchner, D.O

Chickenpox

BASICS

DESCRIPTION A common, highly contagious, childhood exanthem characterized by the development of typical crops of vesicles on the skin and mucous membranes
• Chickenpox is caused by the herpesvirus varicella-zoster virus (VZV). The virus is spread by direct contact or respiratory droplet and outbreaks tend to occur from January to May.
• The usual incubation period is 14-16 days (range 11-21). Patients are infectious from 24 hours before appearance of the rash until the final lesions have crusted. Most people acquire chickenpox during childhood and develop lifelong immunity.
System(s) affected: Skin/Exocrine, Nervous
Genetics: No known genetic pattern
Incidence/Prevalence in USA: Common
Predominant age: Peak incidence 5-9 years, but may occur at any age
Predominant Sex: Male = Female

SIGNS AND SYMPTOMS
• Prodromal symptoms - fever, malaise, anorexia, mild headache
• Characteristic rash - crops of "teardrop" vesicles on erythematous bases
• Lesions erupt in successive crops
• Progress from macule to papule to vesicle, then begin to crust
• Rash present in various stages of development
• Pruritic
• Usually begins on trunk, then spreads to face and scalp
• Minimal involvement of the extremities
• Lesions may be present on mucous membranes, oral and vaginal

CAUSES Transmission to susceptible individuals by respiratory droplet or direct contact with vesicles

RISK FACTORS
• No prior history of varicella
• Immunosuppressed (especially children with leukemia/lymphoma or on high-dose corticosteroids)

DIAGNOSIS

DIFFERENTIAL DIAGNOSIS
• Herpes simplex
• Herpes zoster
• Impetigo
• Coxsackie virus infection
• Papular urticaria
• Scabies
• Dermatitis herpetiformis
• Drug rash

LABORATORY
• Leukocyte count may be normal, low, or mildly increased
• Marked leukocytosis is suggestive of secondary infection
• Multinucleated giant cells on Tzanck smear from scrapings of vesicles
• Isolated virus from human tissue culture
Drugs that may alter lab results: N/A
Disorders that may alter lab results:
• Herpes zoster
• Herpes simplex

PATHOLOGICAL FINDINGS
• Skin lesions histologically identical to herpes simplex virus
• In fatal cases intranuclear inclusions can be found in the endothelium of blood vessels and most organs

SPECIAL TESTS N/A

IMAGING N/A

DIAGNOSTIC PROCEDURES N/A

TREATMENT

APPROPRIATE HEALTH CARE
Outpatient except for complicating emergencies

GENERAL MEASURES
• Supportive/symptomatic treatment
• Good hygiene to avoid secondary infection

ACTIVITY As tolerated. Children may return to school when lesions have scabbed over, temperature is normal and sense of well-being has returned.

DIET No special diet

PATIENT EDUCATION Griffith: Instructions for Patients; Philadephia, 1988 W.B. Saunders Co. p 52

MEDICATIONS

DRUG(S) OF CHOICE
• Antipyretics for fever
• Avoid aspirin because of its link to Reye's syndrome
• Local and/or systemic antipruritic agents for itching
• In immunocompromised host, then varicella-zoster immune globulin (VZIG) available for passive immunization. VZIG must be given within 96 hours after exposure to be beneficial. After 4th day postexposure, wait for rash to develop then give acyclovir 500 mg/m2/day intravenously every 8 hours for 7 days.
• acyclovir, 20 mg/kg/dose, 5 times daily or q4h. Decreases duration of fever and shortens time of viral shedding. Most effective if used within 48 hours of onset of rash.
Contraindications: Hypersensitivity to the drug
Precautions: Possible renal insufficiency with acyclovir
Significant possible interactions:
Concurrent administration of probenecid increases half-life

ALTERNATIVE DRUGS   N/A

FOLLOWUP

PATIENT MONITORING   Usually none in mild cases. If complications occur, intensive supportive care may be required.

PREVENTION/AVOIDANCE
• Isolation of hospitalized patients
• Passive immunization with VZIG for immunocompromised
• A live attenuated vaccine has been developed in Japan and is protective if given before or immediately after exposure

POSSIBLE COMPLICATIONS
• Secondary bacterial infection - cellulitis, abscess, erysipelas, sepsis, septic arthritis/osteomyelitis, staphylococcal pyomyositis
• Pneumonia (20-30% of adults with chickenpox have lung involvement)
• Encephalitis (the most common CNS complication)
• Reye's syndrome
• Purpura
• Lymphadenitis
• Nephritis

EXPECTED COURSE AND PROGNOSIS
• In the healthy child, chickenpox is rarely a serious disease and recovery is complete
• Fatalities rarely occur from complications

MISCELLANEOUS

ASSOCIATED CONDITIONS   N/A

AGE-RELATED FACTORS
Pediatric:
• Neonates born to mothers who develop chickenpox 5 days before or 2 days after delivery are at risk for serious disease. Must give VZIG.
• Varicella bullosa seen mainly in children under two. Lesions appear as bullae instead of vesicles. Clinical course unchanged.
Geriatric: Latent varicella infection may reactivate and cause the exanthem shingles or zoster
Others: N/A

PREGNANCY   Risk of transplacental infection following maternal infection is 25%. Congenital malformations are seen in 5% when the fetus is infected during the 1st or 2nd trimester. There is an increased morbidity for women infected during pregnancy (e.g. pneumonia)

SYNONYMS
• Varicella

ICD-9-CM
052.9 Varicella without mention of complication

SEE ALSO   N/A

OTHER NOTES   N/A

ABBREVIATIONS
VZIG = varicella-zoster immune globulin

REFERENCES   Mandell, G.L. (ed.): Principles and Practice of Infectious Diseases. 3rd Ed. New York, Churchill Livingstone, 1990

Author   L. Olafson, M.D.

Child abuse

BASICS

DESCRIPTION
• Physical abuse - (most frequent type) injury to a child caused by a caretaker for no apparent reason including reaction to unwanted behavior. The use of an instrument on any part of the body is abuse.
• Sexual abuse - contacts or interactions between a child and an adult when the child is being used for sexual stimulation. May be committed by a person less than 18 when that person is significantly older than the victim or in a position of power or control over the victim.
• Neglect - occurs when those responsible for meeting the basic needs of a child fail to do so
System(s) affected: Nervous, Reproductive, Endocrine/Metabolic
Genetics: N/A
Incidence in USA: More than 200,000 per year (National Center on Child Abuse and Neglect)
Prevalence in USA: N/A
Predominant age: 6.1 years average
Predominant sex: Male = Female

SIGNS AND SYMPTOMS
Non-specific symptoms of abuse
◊ Anxiety, depression
◊ Sleep disturbances, night terrors
◊ Increased sex play
◊ School problems
◊ Self-destructive behaviors
Physical abuse
◊ Skin markings (lacerations, burns, ecchymoses, linear contusions)
◊ Contusions with definite shapes (coat hangers, belt buckles)
◊ Circular contusions on trunks or limbs (finger pressure points)
◊ Bites
◊ Cigarette burns on palms, extremities
◊ Immersion injuries with clearly demarcated lines
◊ Oral trauma (torn frenulum, loose teeth)
◊ Ear trauma (ear pulling)
◊ Eye trauma (hyphema, hemorrhage, hematomas)
◊ Abdominal blunt trauma
◊ Fractures
◊ Head trauma
Sexual abuse
◊ Unequivocal abnormalities are found in a small number of children (2-8%)
◊ Abuse often consists of fondling, rubbing and other contacts not likely to produce injuries
◊ Unexplained vaginal injuries or bleeding
◊ Pregnancy
◊ Sexually transmitted diseases
◊ Erythema, localized edema and petechiae of the genitalia
◊ Erythema and increased vascularity of the perihymenal tissues
◊ Increased friability of the posterior fourchette
◊ Hymenal attenuation and asymmetry
◊ Perianal lacerations, scars and fissures
◊ May be no physical signs

Neglect
◊ May be small, scrawny, dirty, with rashes
◊ Fearful or too trusting
◊ Clinging to or avoiding mother
◊ Flat or balding occiput
◊ Abnormal development or growth parameters

CAUSES   Not well-defined

RISK FACTORS
• May be many, but poverty (5 times greater risk), parental substance abuse, lower educational status, maternal history of abuse and negative maternal attitude toward pregnancy appear to be strongly associated

DIAGNOSIS

DIFFERENTIAL DIAGNOSIS
Physical trauma
◊ Bleeding disorders (e.g., classic hemophilia)
◊ Metabolic diseases (e.g., vitamin K deficiency)
◊ Congenital (type I Ehlers-Danlos syndrome)
◊ Salicylate toxicity
◊ Conditions with skin manifestations: Mongolian spots, Schönlein-Henoch purpura, purpura fulminans of meningococcemia, erythema multiforme, hypersensitivity vasculitis, platelet aggregation disorders, disseminated intravascular coagulation (DIC), phytophotodermatitis, car seat burns, staphylococcal scalded skin syndrome, chicken pox, impetigo, osteogenesis imperfecta, congenital syphilis
Neglect
◊ Endocrinopathies (e.g., diabetes mellitus, diabetes insipidus, thyroid disorders, adrenal problems, pituitary problems)
◊ Constitutional
◊ GI (clefts, chalasia, gastroesophageal reflux, celiac disease, inflammatory bowel disease)
◊ Cystic fibrosis
◊ Liver disease
◊ Renal tubular acidosis
◊ CNS abnormalities
Skeletal Trauma
◊ Obstetrical trauma
◊ Prematurity
◊ Nutritional - metabolic defects (scurvy, rickets, mucolipidosis II, secondary hyperparathyroidism)
◊ Infection (congenital syphilis, osteomyelitis)
◊ Osteogenesis imperfecta
◊ Infantile cortical hyperostosis
◊ Leukemia
◊ Histiocytosis X
◊ Metastatic neuroblastoma

LABORATORY
• Urinalysis, urine culture and sensitivity
• CBC
• Electrolytes, creatinine, BUN, glucose
• Some would add PT, PTT, bleeding time, and platelet count.
Drugs that may alter lab results: Usually none
Disorders that may alter lab results: See Differential Diagnosis

PATHOLOGICAL FINDINGS
• Spiral fractures in non-ambulatory patients
• Chip fractures or bucket-handle fractures (classic for abuse)
• Epiphyseal - metaphyseal rib fractures in infants
• Rupture of liver and spleen in abdominal blunt trauma
• Retinal hemorrhages in shaken baby syndrome
• Abnormalities strongly suggesting sexual abuse include: Recent or healed lacerations of the hymen and vaginal mucosa, procto-episiotomy, bite marks
• The presence of sperm is a definitive finding of child abuse

SPECIAL TESTS
Sexual abuse
◊ Wet mount for motile sperm and one fixed for cytopathology exam for sperm
◊ Tests for gonorrhea, chlamydia
◊ Serum pregnancy tests
◊ Rapid plasma reagin (RPR)
◊ Consider HIV testing (needs to be repeated in 6 months)
◊ Acid phosphatase test of secretions for sperm
◊ If the assault occurred within 72 hours of the examination, samples should be collected for the forensic laboratory (contact police investigator for proper protocol)
Neglect
◊ Stool exam
◊ Calorie count
◊ Purifies protein derivative (PPD) and anergy panel
◊ Sweat test
◊ Lead and zinc protoporphyrin levels

IMAGING
• Photographs
• Chest x-ray, skeletal survey (skull frontal and lateral, lateral thoracolumbar spine, frontal upper extremities to include shoulder girdle and hands, frontal lower extremities to include lower lumbar spine, pelvis and feet)
• In some hospitals a standard set of x-rays called a SNAT (suspected non-accidental trauma) series is defined
• Possible bone scan

DIAGNOSTIC PROCEDURES   Possible photo colposcopy in sexual abuse

TREATMENT

APPROPRIATE HEALTH CARE
• Hospital admission for children with moderate to severe injuries, unstable neurologic or cardiovascular exams and those with acute psychological trauma
• If not hospitalized, a child should be sent to another relative or arrange for foster care if the suspected abuser lives with the child
• Counseling is imperative
• Mandatory reporting to Child Protective Authorities

GENERAL MEASURES N/A

ACTIVITY As clinically indicated

DIET As clinically indicated

PATIENT EDUCATION Counsel family not to use negative terms such as "ruined", "violated", or "dirty" in reference to the child. The child's emotional reaction to abuse will be profoundly influenced by the responses of adult caretakers.

MEDICATIONS

DRUG(S) OF CHOICE For prevention of pregnancy in females of reproductive age: Ethinyl estradiol plus norgestrel (Ovral) tablets at once and 2 more tablets after 12 hours. Must be started within 72 hours after unprotected coitus.
Contraindications: Pregnancy
Precautions: 30% of patients experience nausea and vomiting
Significant possible interactions: Refer to manufacturer's profile of each drug

ALTERNATIVE DRUGS None

FOLLOWUP

PATIENT MONITORING Patient must be referred to the appropriate state protective services and followed as closely as clinically and psychologically indicated

PREVENTION/AVOIDANCE Early detection of and intervention in dysfunctional families whenever possible

POSSIBLE COMPLICATIONS Long-term physical and psychological damage

EXPECTED COURSE AND PROGNOSIS Without intervention child abuse is a recurrent and escalating phenomenon

MISCELLANEOUS

ASSOCIATED CONDITIONS
Failure-to-thrive, shortfalls in development, poor school performance, poor social skills, etc.

AGE-RELATED FACTORS
Pediatric: N/A
Geriatric: N/A
Others: N/A

PREGNANCY Use of Ethinyl estradiol and norgestrel reduces rate of pregnancy after rape to under 2% which is one-third the rate that would be expected without intervention

SYNONYMS
• Battered child syndrome
• SNAT

ICD-9-CM 999.5

SEE ALSO N/A

OTHER NOTES When documenting an examination on an allegedly or suspected abused child, especially in cases of possible sexual abuse, never record "findings not consistent with abuse" or "no evidence of abuse." Simply record normal findings and note that the findings neither support nor refute allegations of abuse. The absence of physical findings does not indicate the child's history is incorrect.

ABBREVIATIONS N/A

REFERENCES
• Reece, R.M. (ed.): Pediatric Clinics of North America, Vol 37, No. 4. W.B. Saunders Co. Philadelphia, Harcourt Brace Jovanovich, Inc., August 1990
• Rosenstein, B.J. & Fosarelli, P.D.: Pediatric Pearls. Yearbook Medical Publishers, Inc. Pg 330-334, 1989
• Flaherty, E.G. & Weiss, H.: Medical Evaluation of Abused and Neglected Children. American Journal of Diseases of Children - Vol. 144, March 1990
• Muram, D.: Child Sexual Abuse. Obstetrics and Gynecology Clinics of North America. Vol. 19, No. 1, March 1992
• National Center on Child Abuse and Neglect: Child Sexual Abuse, Incest, Assault and Exploitation. Special Report. HEW Children's Bureau, August, 1992

Author B. Vanderhoff, M.D. & K. Mosser, M.D.

Chlamydia Pneumoniae

 BASICS

DESCRIPTION
Chlamydia pneumoniae, an obligate intracellular bacteria exclusive to humans, has been established as an important cause of adult respiratory disease including pneumonia, bronchitis, sinusitis and pharyngitis. There is no animal reservoir, nor any specific prevention measure.

System(s) affected: Pulmonary

Genetics: No known genetic predisposition

Incidence in USA: The estimated incidence is 100 to 200 cases of pneumonia/100,000/year. Accounts for 6 to 12% of pneumonias and 3 to 6% of bronchitis cases. Studies to date have included relatively few geographic areas. Numbers do not necessarily apply to all areas.

Prevalence in USA: 8-16/100,000. Prevalence of subclinical infection much greater.

Predominant age: Uncommon in children under 5 years. Pneumonia more common in elderly.

Predominant sex: Male > Female (10-25% more)

SIGNS AND SYMPTOMS
• 70% to 90% of infections are mild or subclinical
• Onset often gradual with delayed presentation
• Sore throat and hoarseness may precede cough by a week or more, giving biphasic appearance to illness
• Cough (often prominent with scant sputum)
• Fever (usually early in illness)
• Sore throat
• Rhinitis
• Headache
• Malaise
• Hoarseness
• Sinus congestion
• Rales, rhonchi or wheezing
• Pharyngeal erythema
• Sinus tenderness

CAUSES
Infection with C. pneumoniae

RISK FACTORS
Exposure to a patient with C. pneumoniae

 DIAGNOSIS

DIFFERENTIAL DIAGNOSIS
• Definite diagnosis requires positive serology or culture
• Consider other common bacterial respiratory pathogens, including Streptococcus, Hemophilus, Klebsiella, Mycoplasma and Legionella

LABORATORY
• Leukocyte count usually normal or low
• Sedimentation rate often moderately elevated
• Sputum usually negative by gram stain and routine culture

Drugs that may alter lab results: Early treatment with tetracycline may blunt IgG antibody response

Disorders that may alter lab results: None known

PATHOLOGICAL FINDINGS
Not usually available

SPECIAL TESTS
• Most easily cultured in HL or Hep 2 cells
• Complement fixation (CF) serology for Chlamydia widely available but cannot distinguish C. pneumoniae infection from C. psittaci
• Microimmunofluorescence (MIF) test, which is specific for C. pneumoniae, is available in some settings
• Sera should be obtained at least 3 weeks apart
• Four-fold antibody rise diagnostic of acute infection
• Presence of IgM antibody (> 1:16) or of high IgG antibody titers (> 1:512) by MIF suggests a recent or acute infection

IMAGING
• Chest radiograph may be abnormal even in clinically mild disease
• Infiltrates often subsegmental and unilateral, though bilateral and patch infiltrates suggesting an atypical pneumonia can occur

DIAGNOSTIC PROCEDURES
None

 TREATMENT

APPROPRIATE HEALTH CARE
• Usually outpatient
• Patients with severe pneumonia or coexisting illness may require hospitalization

GENERAL MEASURES
No specific general measures

ACTIVITY
Usually reduced during illness

DIET
No special diet

PATIENT EDUCATION
• Griffith, H.W.: Instructions for Patients; Philadelphia, W.B. Saunders Co.
• For additional patient education materials favorably reviewed on this topic contact:, American Academy of Family Physicians Foundation, P.O. Box 8418, Kansas City, MO 64114, (800)274-2237, ext. 4400

MEDICATIONS

DRUG(S) OF CHOICE
• Tetracycline 500 mg po qid for at least 14 days or
• Doxycycline 100 mg po q 12 hours for at least 14 days
Contraindications: Known allergy to the medication
Precautions: Avoid dairy products, antacids, iron preparations, and sun exposure. Reduce dosage in renal failure. Do not use after first trimester of pregnancy or in children less than 8 years old.
Significant possible interactions:
Tetracyclines may increase the anticoagulant effect of warfarin; may decrease the effectiveness of oral contraceptives

ALTERNATIVE DRUGS
• Erythromycin 250-500 mg qid for 14-21 days
• Beta-lactam (penicillin based) antibiotics and sulfisoxazole not effective

FOLLOWUP

PATIENT MONITORING Weekly until well, for response to treatment and resolution of radiographic abnormalities

PREVENTION/AVOIDANCE
• Transmission presumably via respiratory secretions. Avoid infected persons.
• Hand washing

POSSIBLE COMPLICATIONS
• Erythema nodosum
• Otitis media
• Asthma
• Endocarditis
• Myocarditis
• Pericarditis
• Sarcoidosis

EXPECTED COURSE AND PROGNOSIS
• Resolution of cough and malaise often requires several weeks or longer
• Chronic bronchospastic disease has been reported following acute infection
• Persistent or relapsed symptoms may respond to second course of antibiotics

MISCELLANEOUS

ASSOCIATED CONDITIONS None established

AGE-RELATED FACTORS
Pediatric: Usually milder disease in children
Geriatric: Usually more severe in older adults
Others: None known

PREGNANCY No known special risks

SYNONYMS TWAR

ICD-9-CM None

SEE ALSO
• Pneumonia, Mycoplasma
• Psittacosis

OTHER NOTES
• No seasonal variation
• Most cases occur sporadically, though intrafamilial spread also occurs
• Infection in debilitated or hospitalized patients can be severe
• Reinfection is possible
• Individuals have been reported who are persistently culture positive despite antibiotic treatment
• Country-wide epidemics of C. pneumoniae infections have been documented in the Scandinavian countries

ABBREVIATIONS N/A

REFERENCES
• Grayston, J.T., Campbell, L.A., Kuo, C.C., et al.: A new respiratory tract pathogen: Chlamydia pneumoniae strain TWAR. J Infect Dis. 1990;161:618-25
• Thom, D.H. & Grayston, J.T.: Infections with Chlamydia pneumoniae strain TWAR. Clinics in Chest Medicine. Edited by R.H. Winterbauer 1991;12(2):245-56

Author D.Thom, M.D., Ph.D. & J. Grayston, M.D.

Chlamydial sexually transmitted diseases

 BASICS

DESCRIPTION
The most common STD in USA is caused by Chlamydia trachomatis serovars D-K. Among the smallest prokaryotic organisms, these obligate intracellular, membrane bound organisms cause disease that is often asymptomatic to non-specific in presentation. It is difficult to diagnose both clinically, in the lab, and difficult to provide screening. The infection has serious sequelae. To complicate matters it is most difficult to control in society.

System(s) affected: Reproductive

Genetics: Unknown

Incidence/Prevalence in USA:
- Males 3-5% general medical population, 15-20% STD clinics
- Females 3-5% general medical population, 20% STD clinics

Predominant age: 15-25

Predominant sex: Male = female

SIGNS AND SYMPTOMS
Chlamydia trachomatis has a tropism for columnar or transitional epithelium with subsequent extension to the cervix, uterus, fallopian tubes and peritoneum in females, and epididymis in males, as well as rectal epithelial cells.

Males
- ◊ Urethritis
- ◊ Epididymitis
- ◊ Proctitis
- ◊ Reiter's syndrome

Females
- ◊ Cervicitis
- ◊ Urethral Syndrome
- ◊ Bartholinitis
- ◊ Endometritis
- ◊ Salpingitis/PID
- ◊ Fitz-Hugh-Curtis perihepatitis syndrome

Infants
- ◊ Conjunctivitis
- ◊ Pneumonitis
- ◊ Carriage-pharynx/GI tract

CAUSES
Chlamydia trachomatis serovars D-K

RISK FACTORS
- Sexual promiscuity
- Lower socioeconomic groups
- Prevalence correlates inversely with age

 DIAGNOSIS

DIFFERENTIAL DIAGNOSIS
Neisseria gonorrhea
- ◊ Urethritis
- ◊ Proctitis
- ◊ Epididymitis
- ◊ Cervicitis
- ◊ PID
- ◊ Bartholin's abscess
- ◊ Perihepatitis

Ureaplasma urealyticum
- ◊ Urethritis, epididymitis
- ◊ Reiter's disease
- ◊ PID

Chlamydia trachomatis (Serovars LI-3)
- ◊ Lymphogranuloma venereum
- ◊ Proctitis

LABORATORY
- Chlamydial culture - costly, time consuming, 70-80% sensitive
- Antigen detection - sensitivity 90+%
- Monoclonal antibody direct immunofluorescence
- ELISA determination of eluded chlamydial antigens

Drugs that may alter lab results: N/A

Disorders that may alter lab results: N/A

PATHOLOGICAL FINDINGS N/A

SPECIAL TESTS N/A

IMAGING N/A

DIAGNOSTIC PROCEDURES
- Specimen collection - cell scrapings (obtain with cytology brush) rather than inflammatory discharge will improve yield since this is an epithelial cell disease
- Transport media is imperative - sucrose-phosphate media supplemented with gentamicin, vancomycin, and nystatin

 TREATMENT

APPROPRIATE HEALTH CARE
- Outpatient care for virtually all problems
- Severe pelvic inflammatory disease, Fitz-Hugh-Curtis syndrome, and Reiter's syndrome may need hospitalization

GENERAL MEASURES
- All patients should be evaluated for syphilis and gonorrhea by appropriate gram stains, cultures and serology.
- Empirical therapies may be indicated
- Evaluation and treatment of sex partners - institute empirical treatment of women who are sex partners of men with non-gonococcal urethritis is recommended. Partners of women with mucopurulent cervicitis or salpingitis should also be empirically treated. Since Chlamydial co-infection occurs with gonorrheal disease, anti-chlamydial therapy should be instituted concomitantly.

ACTIVITY
Sexual abstention pending elucidation and treatment of underlying infection

DIET
Avoid dairy products if tetracyclines used for therapy

PATIENT EDUCATION
- Safe sex practices, such as barrier protection
- Offer HIV counseling and testing
- Serious sequelae of Chlamydial disease i.e., tubal infertility
- Behaviors increasing potential to contract other STDs
- Stress need to finish entire course of antibiotics
- For patient education materials favorably reviewed on this topic contact:
American Academy of Family Physicians Foundation, P.O. Box 8418, Kansas City, MO 64114, (800)274-2237, ext. 4400

MEDICATIONS

DRUG(S) OF CHOICE
Urethritis, cervicitis, sexual partners of infected persons
◊ Tetracycline hydrochloride - 500 mg po qid x 7 days
◊ Doxycycline - 100 mg po bid x 7 days
◊ Pregnant females or those intolerant to tetracyclines - erythromycin 500 mg po qid x 7 days
Chlamydial syndromes.
◊ Epididymitis - tetracycline, doxycycline, erythromycin for 10-14 days as above.
◊ Pelvic inflammatory disease - doxycycline for 10-14 days to cover the chlamydial component of PID (gonorrhea and anaerobic organisms must be treated as well; see CDC recommendations: ceftriaxone 250 mg IM once, cefoxitin, other 3rd generation cephalosporin, or a quinolone), erythromycin for 10-14 days may be needed in pregnant or tetracycline intolerant females to treat chlamydial component.
Contraindications: Refer to manufacturer's profile of each drug
Precautions: Refer to manufacturer's profile of each drug
Significant possible interactions: Refer to manufacturer's profile of each drug

ALTERNATIVE DRUGS
• Erythromycin - see above
• Ofloxacin - 300 mg po qid x7 days for cervicitis/urethritis (not to be used in pregnancy)
• Sulfasoxizole - 500 mg po qid x 10 days - urethritis

FOLLOWUP

PATIENT MONITORING
• Test of cure is not routine
• Sexual partners need to be treated to prevent passing the disease back and forth between partners
• Non-resolution or recurrence of symptoms must be immediately reported to the physician
• Severe cases of urethritis/cervicitis as well as the chlamydial syndromes should be seen in follow up after completion of therapy

PREVENTION/AVOIDANCE
Screening evaluation in high prevalence areas

POSSIBLE COMPLICATIONS
Males
◊ Transient oligospermia
◊ Post epididymitis urethral stricture (rare)
Females
◊ Tubal infertility
◊ Tubal pregnancy
◊ Chronic pelvic pain

EXPECTED COURSE AND PROGNOSIS
Prognosis good with compliant therapy

MISCELLANEOUS

ASSOCIATED CONDITIONS
• Pelvic inflammatory disease, epididymitis, cervicitis, urethritis
Other diseases caused by other chlamydial species:
◊ Psittacosis - Chlamydia psittaci
◊ Pneumonia - Chlamydia pneumoniae - Chlamydia trachomatis (infants)
◊ Lymphogranuloma venereum - Chlamydia trachomatis serovars L1-L3
◊ Trachoma - Chlamydia trachomatis serovars A-C

AGE-RELATED FACTORS
Prevalence inversely proportional to age after onset of sexual activity
Pediatric: N/A
Geriatric: N/A
Others: N/A

PREGNANCY
Perinatal acquisition may result in neonatal pneumonia and/or conjunctivitis. Tetracycline is contraindicated in pregnancy. Erythromycin should be used in this situation.

SYNONYMS
N/A

ICD-9-CM
• 615 Inflammatory diseases of uterus, except cervix
• 616 Inflammatory diseases of cervix, vagina, and vulva

SEE ALSO
• Pelvic inflammatory disease
• Epididymitis
• Cervicitis
• Urethritis
• Acquired immune deficiency syndrome

OTHER NOTES
N/A

ABBREVIATIONS
• STD = sexually transmitted disease
• PID = pelvic inflammatory disease
• HIV = human immunodeficiency virus

REFERENCES
• Mardh, R., et al.: Chlamydia. New York, Plenum Medical Book Co., 1989
• Stamm, W.E., Holmes, K.K., et al.: Chlamydia trachomatis Infections in the Adult. In: Sexually Transmitted Diseases. 2nd Ed. New York, McGraw-Hill, 1990

Author R. Mandel, M.D.

Cholangitis

 BASICS

DESCRIPTION
Bacterial inflammation of the bile duct system that is associated with obstructive biliary duct pathology. May be acute or chronic.

System(s) affected: Gastrointestinal

Genetics: N/A

Incidence/Prevalence in USA: N/A

Predominant age: 55-70 years, rare in children, more common in adults

Predominant sex: Female > Male

SIGNS AND SYMPTOMS
May have only one or two symptoms, and the abdominal exam may be unrevealing
- Right upper quadrant pain (RUQ), not severe
- Jaundice
- Chills and fever
- Shock
- CNS depression

CAUSES
Biliary tract obstruction from:
  ◊ Stones
  ◊ Tumor (pancreatic, CBD, metastatic)
  ◊ Benign strictures (postsurgical, PSC)
  ◊ Parasites (Ascaris)
  ◊ Pancreatitis
  ◊ Blood clots
Reflux of small bowel bacteria
  ◊ Choledochoenterostomy
  ◊ "Sump syndrome"
Other
  ◊ Cholecystitis
  ◊ Bacteriemia
  ◊ Surgical, radiographic, endoscopic manipulation

RISK FACTORS
- Cholelithiasis
- Endoscopic or surgical manipulation
- Foreign bodies, such as parasites

 DIAGNOSIS

DIFFERENTIAL DIAGNOSIS
- Acute cholecystitis - pain and tenderness are invariably present. (May be very difficult to distinguish between cholangitis and acute cholecystitis).
- Pyogenic liver abscess
- Hepatitis
- Acute pancreatitis
- Perforated duodenal ulcer
- Pelvic inflammatory disease with peritonitis
- Kidney stones

LABORATORY
- Increasing WBC with left shift
- Hyperbilirubinemia - in 90%
- Alkaline phosphatase - increasing in 90%
- Positive blood culture - in 50% (gram negative aerobes, and some anaerobes)

Drugs that may alter lab results: N/A

Disorders that may alter lab results: N/A

PATHOLOGICAL FINDINGS
In acute toxic disease, pus under pressure in the common bile duct

SPECIAL TESTS
- Need to delineate underlying biliary tract abnormality
- Cholangiography is definitive test
- Percutaneous transhepatic cholangiography (PTC) or endoscopic retrograde cholangiopancreatography (ERCP)

IMAGING
Ultrasound will diagnose gallbladder stones and common bile duct size, but will demonstrate common bile duct calculi in less than 15%

DIAGNOSTIC PROCEDURES
N/A

 TREATMENT

APPROPRIATE HEALTH CARE
Inpatient

GENERAL MEASURES
- Control sepsis, then evaluate with cholangiography and treat underlying biliary tract pathology
- Patients who do not respond to antibiotics and supportive care require emergency decompression of the biliary duct system. This may be accomplished by surgery, endoscopy, or transhepatic cholangiography.
- In case of obstruction secondary to stones, endoscopic papillotomy and stone extraction will drain the duct and may be definitive treatment of the underlying cause and is shown to reduce mortality

ACTIVITY
As tolerated

DIET
Nothing by mouth until acute phase is terminated

PATIENT EDUCATION
For patient education materials favorably reviewed on this topic, contact: National Digestive Diseases Information Clearinghouse, Box NDDIC, Bethesda, MD 20892, (301)468-6344

MEDICATIONS

DRUG(S) OF CHOICE
Antibiotic regimen should cover gram negative aerobes, enterococci, and anaerobes.
◊ Ampicillin 1gm q6h IV (substitute ciprofloxacin in penicillin allergic patient) +
◊ aminoglycoside (e.g., tobramycin, amikacin is an alternative but is expensive) +
◊ metronidazole 500mg q8h IV
Contraindications: Refer to manufacturer's profile of each drug
Precautions: Renal toxicity of aminoglycoside therapy; check peak and trough levels
Significant possible interactions: Refer to manufacturer's profile of each drug

ALTERNATIVE DRUGS N/A

FOLLOWUP

PATIENT MONITORING Requires careful monitoring of hemodynamic parameters

PREVENTION/AVOIDANCE
Cholangiography when indicated at time of cholecystectomy with endoscopic, radiographic, or surgical clearance of retained CBD stones

POSSIBLE COMPLICATIONS
• Most serious is hepatic abscess
• Sepsis
• Secondary sclerosing cholangitis

EXPECTED COURSE AND PROGNOSIS
• Acute cholangitis - good
• Acute toxic cholangitis - mortality high

MISCELLANEOUS

ASSOCIATED CONDITIONS
• Choledocholithiasis
• Malignant tumors
• Benign strictures
• Biliary-enteric anastamosis
• Invasive procedures
• Foreign bodies
• Parasites
• Secondary sclerosing cholangitis

AGE-RELATED FACTORS
Pediatric: N/A
Geriatric: N/A
Others: N/A

PREGNANCY N/A

SYNONYMS N/A

ICD-9-CM 576.1 cholangitis

SEE ALSO Cholelithiasis

OTHER NOTES N/A

ABBREVIATIONS N/A

REFERENCES
• Nahrwold, D.L.: Cholangitis. In Textbook of Surgery. 13th Ed. Edited by D.C. Sabiston. Philadelphia, W.B. Saunders, 1986, pp. 1154-61
• Boeg, J.H. & Way, L.W.: Acute Cholangitis. Ann Surg., 191:264, 1980
• Pitt, H.A. & Longmire, W.P. Jr.: Suppurative Cholangitis. In Critical Surgical Illness. 2nd Ed. Edited by J.M. Hardy. Philadelphia, W.B. Saunders Co., 1980, pp. 380-408

Author E. Saltzstein, M.D. & L. Mercer, M.D

Cholecystitis

BASICS

DESCRIPTION
Inflammation of the gallbladder occurring acutely or chronically, often secondary to previously asymptomatic gallstones.
Genetics: Increased prevalence in Native Americans and Caucasians, less prevalent in African Americans
Incidence/Prevalence in USA:
• Steady increase with age, varies in different ethnic groups. Percentage with gallstones (approximately half will develop symptoms over their lifetime):
  ◊ By age 30, 30% of Native Americans
  ◊ By age 60, 80% of Native Americans
  ◊ By age 60, 30% of Caucasians
  ◊ By age 60, 20% of African Americans
Predominant age: 5th and 6th decade
Predominant sex: Female > Male (2:1)

SIGNS AND SYMPTOMS
• Asymptomatic. 5-10% become symptomatic each year.
Acute cholecystitis
  ◊ Abdominal pain - sudden onset, intense, in epigastrium or right upper quadrant, radiates to shoulder or back. Pathognomic feature is "biliary colic" a pain rising over two to three minutes to a plateau of intensity that is maintained for > 20 minutes.
  ◊ Nausea and vomiting
  ◊ Recurrent attacks following meals by 1-6 hours, lasting > 12 hours until recovered, usually < 3 days
  ◊ Elevated temperature - mild to moderate
  ◊ Local tenderness, rarely diffuse
  ◊ Murphy's sign - inspiratory arrest elicited when palpating right upper quadrant while asking the patient for deep inhalation
  ◊ Palpable gall bladder - 5% of cases
Common duct stone
  ◊ Jaundice in 50%
  ◊ Biliary colic 60%
  ◊ Fever and chills 30%
  ◊ Pruritus 10%
  ◊ Loose bowel movements, light color
  ◊ Mild to marked hepatomegaly > 80%
  ◊ Tenderness infrequent
  ◊ Palpable gall bladder 10%
  ◊ Gallstone ileus (rare)
  ◊ Gallstone > 3 cm fistulizes into bowel and obstructs at ileocecal area
  ◊ Antecedent pain, often over weeks with non-biliary colic
  ◊ Abdominal distension, mild tenderness
  ◊ Air in biliary passages on plain x-ray
  ◊ Intestinal obstruction at level of terminal ileum
Empyema
  ◊ Phlegmon of obstructed gall bladder
  ◊ Insidious weight loss, mild wasting
  ◊ Gradual onset of occult infection signs, fever, anorexia
  ◊ Mass usually present
  ◊ Tenderness usually absent

Chronic cholecystitis
  ◊ Associated with gallstones, often asymptomatic; 20% become symptomatic over 15-20 years
  ◊ Mild dyspepsia following fatty meals

CAUSES
• Gallstones: 90-95% of cases. As they migrate along the biliary passages, they may cause obstruction of cystic duct, leading to acute cholecystitis; obstruction of the common bile duct, causing jaundice, or obstruction of the pancreatic duct, causing pancreatitis.
• Acalculous cholecystitis: 5% of cases. Associated with severe stressful situations including cardiac surgery, multiple trauma. May be associated with ischemic damage to the gall bladder wall.
• Bacteria: usually do not initiate the inflammation but important in the complications of empyema and ascending cholangitis. In emphysematous cholecystitis, clostridia are probably responsible for both initiation and complications.
• Neoplasms and strictures of common bile duct: usually associated with cholangitis and pancreatitis.
• Ischemia: In patients with diabetes, but uncommon
• Torsion: Lost fixation of gallbladder, uncommon

RISK FACTORS
• Cardiac surgery
• Trauma
• Biliary parasites
• Gallstones (see topic Cholelithiasis)

DIAGNOSIS

DIFFERENTIAL DIAGNOSIS
Acute pancreatitis, ulcer, diverticulitis, pyelonephritis, pneumonitis, hepatic abscess, hepatic tumors, Irritable bowel disease, non-ulcer dyspepsia

LABORATORY
Acute cholecystitis
  ◊ Leucocytosis - 12,000-15,000
  ◊ Liver tests usually abnormal; ALT, AST slightly elevated, alkaline phosphatase, GGTP elevated with common duct obstruction
  ◊ Serum amylase may be elevated. If > 1000 units, concomitant pancreatitis should be considered.
Common duct stone
  ◊ High bilirubin in 50%, in 100% after 10 days
  ◊ Elevated alkaline phosphatase and gamma glutamyl transpeptidase (GGT) in 85%
  ◊ Positive blood culture in 15%
  ◊ Barely abnormal ALT, AST
  ◊ Elevated fasting bile salts
  ◊ Elevated WBC if infection

Drugs that may alter lab results:
• Steroids
• Immunosuppressive drugs. These may mask leucocytosis and early signs of inflammation.
Disorders that may alter lab results:
• Old age, malnutrition
• Lymphoma, other immunocompromised states

PATHOLOGICAL FINDINGS N/A

SPECIAL TESTS
99m Tc Imino diacetic acid (HIDA) scan - highly sensitive (97%) for diagnosis of acute cholecystitis. HIDA derivatives are taken up by hepatocytes and excreted in bile and concentrated in gallbladder. Failure to see gallbladder in 1 hour is highly suspicious for acute cholecystitis. Usually abnormal in acalculous cholecystitis.

IMAGING
Plain radiographs (upright)
  ◊ 20% of gallstones are radio-opaque
  ◊ Air cholangiogram if there is gallbladder-gut fistula
  ◊ Emphysematous cholecystitis - air in the gallbladder wall or in lumen
Ultrasonography
  ◊ Best technique to diagnose gallstones (high sensitivity -95% and specificity - 98%)
  ◊ Best noninvasive imaging technique to diagnose acute cholecystitis. Findings include thick gall bladder wall (> 3 mm), gallbladder distension, sludge in lumen, pericholecystic fluid.
Oral cholecystography
  ◊ Used to diagnose gallstones in non-jaundiced patients
  ◊ Cannot be used for acute cholecystitis
  ◊ Intestinal absorption and hepatic function should be intact
CT scan
  ◊ No advantage over ultrasonography in gallstone/acute cholecystitis diagnosis
  ◊ Better than ultrasonography to detect enlargement of pancreas. Helpful in the diagnosis of abscess formation. Shows thickened gall bladder wall in cancer.

DIAGNOSTIC PROCEDURES
• Endoscopic retrograde cholangiopancreatography (ERCP) - to see status of biliary and pancreatic ducts
• Percutaneous transhepatic cholangiography test (PTC) - gives more information about intrahepatic biliary system
• Laparotomy - if unable to make diagnosis by less invasive means

TREATMENT

APPROPRIATE HEALTH CARE
- Outpatient for patients with mild symptoms
- Inpatient - patients with biliary colic lasting for more than 6 hours and showing toxicity, jaundice, rigors, or requiring narcotics for pain
- Ascending cholangitis is a surgical emergency. If laparotomy is inappropriate drainage can be obtained by ERCP or transhepatic cholangiography.

GENERAL MEASURES
- NPO, IV fluids, nasogastric suction
- Surgery (cholecystectomy) is the appropriate treatment for symptomatic cholecystitis. Best performed by laparoscopy if available, but a standard laparotomy is acceptable. If there is jaundice, laparotomy is required. Mortality rate - 0.1% in age < 50 years and 0.8% age > 50.
- In acute cholecystitis - early cholecystectomy is the general practice rather than delayed interval cholecystectomy (delay only if surgery is contraindicated)
- Laparoscopic cholecystostomy - rapidly replacing alternative surgical drainage procedure. If the patient is a poor risk, drainage of the gallbladder or biliary passages can be achieved by radiological or endoscopic techniques. This will allow control of infection and jaundice for several weeks or months.
- Dissolution therapy - infrequently used if laparoscopic cholecystectomy can be performed. Ursodeoxycholic acid (Actigall) in 10 mg/kg is the drug of choice. To be effective there must be a functioning gallbladder on oral cholecystography. Stones must be free of calcium. Many small stones have best prognosis to dissolve. An alternative drug is chenodeoxycholic acid (Chenodiol) 12-15 mg/kg/day.
- Other indications for emergency surgery include - toxic patient, doubtful diagnosis, perforation or abscess

ACTIVITY As tolerated by the patient

DIET
- NPO during acute cholecystitis
- Fatty meals precipitate mild attacks. Avoid if possible.

PATIENT EDUCATION National Digestive Diseases Information Clearinghouse, Box NDDIC, Bethesda, MD 20892, (301) 468-6344

MEDICATIONS

DRUG(S) OF CHOICE
- Mild attack - ampicillin 4-6 gm/day or cefazolin (Ancef) 2-4 gm/day
- Severe attack - gentamicin 3-5 mg/kg/day and clindamycin 1.8-2.7 gm/day. A penicillin could be added if needed.

Contraindications: Hypersensitivity reactions

Precautions:
- Nephrotoxicity, ototoxicity with aminoglycosides
- Adjust the dose according to creatinine clearance

Significant possible interactions: Refer to manufacturer's profile of each drug

ALTERNATIVE DRUGS For acute cholecystitis - 3rd generation cephalosporins

FOLLOWUP

PATIENT MONITORING Post cholecystectomy - follow through postoperative period

PREVENTION/AVOIDANCE Avoid risk factors when possible

POSSIBLE COMPLICATIONS Occur in about 5% cases of acute cholecystitis and include - perforation, abscess formation, fistula formation (intestine, colon, cutaneous), gangrene, empyema, cholangitis, hepatitis, pancreatitis, gallstone ileus, carcinoma

EXPECTED COURSE AND PROGNOSIS
- In general the prognosis is good for gallbladder disease. Those who die during acute episodes are mainly due to other conditions, especially coronary artery disease.
- Symptomatic gallstones usually have recurrent symptoms in 3 to 6 months indicating need for future action
- After cholecystectomy, stones may recur in bile ducts

MISCELLANEOUS

ASSOCIATED CONDITIONS
- Pancreatitis
- Hemolytic anemias such as sickle cell disease, spherocytosis
- Cirrhosis, hypersplenism

AGE-RELATED FACTORS
Pediatric: N/A
Geriatric:
- Sometimes difficult to diagnose
- Complications more likely to occur
- Cholecystectomy mortality rate is higher
Others: N/A

PREGNANCY N/A

SYNONYMS N/A

ICD-9-CM
574.0 Calculus of gallbladder with acute cholecystitis
574.1 Calculus of gallbladder with other cholecystitis
575.0 Acute cholecystitis
575.1 Other cholecystitis (without mention of calculus)

SEE ALSO
- Cholelithiasis
- Cholangitis
- Choledocholithiasis
- See short topics: Adenocarcinoma of the gallbladder; jaundice

OTHER NOTES Lithotripsy - can be used in patients with chronic cholecystitis. Contraindications - stones greater than 25 mm, more than 3 stones, calcified stones, bile duct stones and poor general condition. Largely replaced now by laparoscopic cholecystectomy.

ABBREVIATIONS N/A

REFERENCES
- Gracie, W.A. & Ransohoff, D.F.: The natural history of silent gallstones: the innocent gallstone is not a myth. N Engl J Med 1982 307:798-800
- Sleisenger, M.H. & Fordtran, J.S. (eds.): Gastrointestinal Disease: Pathophysiology, Diagnosis, Management. 4th Ed. Philadelphia, W.B. Saunders Co., 1989

Author A. Verma, M.D., F. Iber, M.D.

Choledocholithiasis

 BASICS

DESCRIPTION Stones in common bile duct (usually composed of cholesterol) that migrate from the gallbladder. Calcium bilirubinate stones may form de novo.
System(s) affected: Gastrointestinal
Genetics: N/A
Incidence/Prevalence in USA: 10-15% of patients with gallbladder stones discovered at time of cholecystectomy
Predominant age: Incidence increases with age
Predominant sex: Females > Males

SIGNS AND SYMPTOMS
- May be asymptomatic
- Biliary colic
- Common bile duct obstruction
- Cholangitis
- Pancreatitis
- Pain can't be differentiated from pain arising from gallbladder
- Epigastric pain
- Abdominal tenderness
- Pain unrelieved by antacids
- Anorexia, vomiting
- Dark urine
- Light colored feces
- Right upper quadrant tenderness
- Palpable gallbladder

CAUSES
- Increased biliary cholesterol secretion
- Chronic hemolytic states
- Hepatobiliary parasitism
- Duct stricture

RISK FACTORS
- Cholelithiasis
- Obesity
- Cirrhosis
- Chronic hemolysis
- Prior cholecystectomy

 DIAGNOSIS

DIFFERENTIAL DIAGNOSIS
- Biliary stricture
- Narrowed biliary - enteric anastomosis
- Sclerosing cholangitis
- Sphincter of Oddi dysfunction
- Biliary parasites
- Papillary stenosis
- Blood clots

LABORATORY
- Increasing WBC
- Increasing alkaline phosphatase
- Hypercholesterolemia (when associated with chronic cholestasis)
- Increased transaminases
- Hyperbilirubinemia
Drugs that may alter lab results: N/A
Disorders that may alter lab results: N/A

PATHOLOGICAL FINDINGS
- Dilated bile ducts
- Bile plugging
- Small bile duct proliferation
- Cholesterol gallstones

SPECIAL TESTS Nuclear medicine (PIPIDA), endoscopic retrograde cholangiopancreatography (ERCP), PTC

IMAGING
- Intraoperative cholangiography - common bile duct filling defects
- Nuclear medicine cholescintigraphy
- Endoscopic cholangiography or PTC - common bile duct filling defects

DIAGNOSTIC PROCEDURES
- Ultrasound will reveal gallbladder stones - not reliable for common bile duct stones, but may reveal ductal dilatation over 75% of the time
- ERCP will visualize the common bile duct and other portions of the upper gastrointestinal tract and will allow for papillotomy plus stone extraction in majority of cases.

 TREATMENT

APPROPRIATE HEALTH CARE
Inpatient

GENERAL MEASURES
- Identification and removal of stones in the course of cholecystectomy
- If the gallbladder has been previously removed, ERCP, papillotomy plus stone extraction
- In the elderly, ERCP and papillotomy with stone removal may prevent or delay the need for cholecystectomy

ACTIVITY As tolerated

DIET Low-fat may be helpful

PATIENT EDUCATION National Digestive Diseases Information Clearinghouse, Box NDDIC, Bethesda, MD 20892, (301)468-6344

MEDICATIONS

DRUG(S) OF CHOICE Antibiotics to treat gram negative aerobes and anaerobes. Selection based on culture and sensitivities. One useful specific regimen, for example: Cefoxitin, 2 grams intravenously perioperatively.
Contraindications: Refer to manufacturer's profile of each drug
Precautions: Refer to manufacturer's profile of each drug
Significant possible interactions: Refer to manufacturer's profile of each drug

ALTERNATIVE DRUGS N/A

FOLLOWUP

PATIENT MONITORING Routine postoperative care

PREVENTION/AVOIDANCE Operative cholangiography at time of cholecystectomy to identify common bile duct stones and then duct exploration or endoscopic sphincterotomy for their removal
• T-tube cholangiogram before removal of tube after operative bile duct exploration

POSSIBLE COMPLICATIONS
• Cholangitis - most frequent (60%)
• Bile duct obstruction
• Pancreatitis
• Biliary enteric fistula
• Hemobilia

EXPECTED COURSE AND PROGNOSIS Good prognosis if treated

MISCELLANEOUS

ASSOCIATED CONDITIONS
• Cholecystitis
• Cholangitis
• Periampullary diverticula

AGE-RELATED FACTORS
Pediatric: N/A
Geriatric: Prognosis guarded
Others: N/A

PREGNANCY Cholestasis of pregnancy may lead to choledocholithiasis

SYNONYMS
• Common bile duct stone
• Common bile duct calculi

ICD-9-CM
547.3 Calculus of bile duct with acute cholecystitis
574.5 Calculus of bile duct without mention of cholecystitis

SEE ALSO
• Cholangitis
• Cholecystitis
• Cholelithiasis
• See short topics: Adenocarcinoma of the gallbladder; jaundice

OTHER NOTES N/A

ABBREVIATIONS ERCP = endoscopic retrograde cholangiopancreatography

REFERENCES
• Nahrwold, D.L.: The Biliary System. In Textbook of Surgery. Edited by D.C. Sabiston. Philadelphia, W.B. Saunders, 1986
• Jordan, G.L., Jr.: Choledocholithiasis. Curr Prob Surg 19:723, 1982

Author E. Saltzstein, M.D., L. Mercer, M.D.

Cholelithiasis

 BASICS

DESCRIPTION
Cholesterol or pigmented stones formed and contained in the gallbladder
System(s) affected: Gastrointestinal
Genetics: N/A
Incidence/Prevalence in USA: 8-10% of population. Increased incidence in American Indians and Hispanics.
Predominant age: Increases with age - peak at sixth decade
Predominant sex: Female > Male (2:1)

SIGNS AND SYMPTOMS
• Mostly asymptomatic. 5-10% become symptomatic each year. Over lifetime, less than half of patients with gallstones develop symptoms.
• Episodic right upper quadrant or epigastric pain radiating to back (biliary colic)
• Nausea
• Vomiting
• Fatty food intolerance (not proven)
• Indigestion

CAUSES
• Production of bile supersaturated with cholesterol
• Decrease in bile content of either phospholipids or bile acids
• Biliary stasis
• Hemolytic diseases
• Biliary infection

RISK FACTORS
• Short gut syndrome
• Inflammatory bowel disease
• Multiparity
• Long term total parenteral nutrition
• Cirrhosis (for pigment stones)
• Hemolytic disorders - hereditary spherocytosis, sickle cell anemia
• Prosthetic cardiac valves
• Biliary parasites
• Rapid weight loss
• Childhood malignancy
• Native American descent
• Diabetes (for complications)
• Female gender

 DIAGNOSIS

DIFFERENTIAL DIAGNOSIS
• Peptic ulcer
• Hepatitis, pancreatitis
• Coronary artery disease
• Appendicitis
• Pneumonia
• Gallbladder cancer
• Renal stones
• Blood clots
• Stricture
• Gallbladder polyps
• Biliary sludge

LABORATORY
None
Drugs that may alter lab results: N/A
Disorders that may alter lab results: N/A

PATHOLOGICAL FINDINGS
Gallstones

SPECIAL TESTS
Hepatobiliary radionuclide scan

IMAGING
• Ultrasound (best technique to diagnose gallstones)
• Oral cholecystogram
• CT scan (no advantage over ultrasound)

DIAGNOSTIC PROCEDURES
N/A

 TREATMENT

APPROPRIATE HEALTH CARE
• Treat all symptomatic gallstones
• Laparoscopic cholecystectomy
• Open cholecystectomy
• Oral dissolution - only if surgery option not available (less than 25% of all patients eligible)
• Direct contact dissolution - only for a small subset of patients - high recurrence rate
• Extracorporeal shock wave lithotripsy - role of this modality unclear and currently under study - not FDA approved
• Percutaneous cholecystostomy in high risk patients

GENERAL MEASURES
• Advise patient of presence of stones
• Observe asymptomatic stones
• Seek treatment if symptoms occur

ACTIVITY
N/A

DIET
Low fat diet may be helpful

PATIENT EDUCATION
• Seek medical attention if signs and symptoms develop
• Additional information available from: National Digestive Diseases Information Clearinghouse, Box NDDIC, Bethesda, MD 20892, (301)468-6344

Cholelithiasis

MEDICATIONS

DRUG(S) OF CHOICE
• Analgesic for symptom relief
• Ursodeoxycholic acid (Actigall) 8-10 mg/kg/day bid-tid - for up to two years - oral dissolution
• Chenodiol (Chenix) 250 mg bid for 2 weeks; then increase by 250 mg increments until a dose of 13-16 mg/kg daily is reached or intolerance develops - oral dissolution
• Methyl tert-butyl ether - contact dissolution

Contraindications:
• Known allergy
• Acute cholecystitis - dissolution agents
• Severe abnormal liver function tests
• Non-functioning gallbladder
• Calcified (radiopaque) stones - relative
• Multiple stones
• Stones greater than 2 cm
• Stones that don't float on oral cholecystogram

Precautions:
• Monitor liver enzymes - may rise in up to 30% of patients
• Monitor serum cholesterol
• Methyl tert-butyl ether should only be used by one experienced with this contact dissolution method
• Observe for severe diarrhea

Significant possible interactions: N/A

ALTERNATIVE DRUGS
NSAID's may have a role in pain relief since prostaglandins are important in the development of pain

NOTES
• Oral dissolution only effective for radiolucent (cholesterol) stones
• Ursodiol probably preferred over chenodiol as it has a lower incidence of adverse effects

FOLLOWUP

PATIENT MONITORING
• Medical attention if asymptomatic stones become symptomatic
• Patients on oral dissolution agents should be followed with liver enzymes, serum cholesterol and imaging studies

PREVENTION/AVOIDANCE
Use of ursodiol (Actigall) with rapid weight loss prevents stone formation

POSSIBLE COMPLICATIONS
• Acute cholecystitis (90-95% secondary to gallstones)
• Gallstone pancreatitis
• Acute cholangitis
• Common bile duct stones with obstructive jaundice
• Gallstone ileus
• Liver abscess
• Biliary-enteric fistula
• Peritonitis
• Gallbladder cancer

EXPECTED COURSE AND PROGNOSIS
• Less than half of patients with gallstones will become symptomatic
• Cholecystectomy - mortality 0.5% elective, 3-5% emergency, morbidity less than 10% elective, 30-40% emergency
• 10-15% will have associated choledocholithiasis
• After cholecystostomy, stones may recur in bile duct

MISCELLANEOUS

ASSOCIATED CONDITIONS
90% of gallbladder carcinomas have gallstones

AGE-RELATED FACTORS
Pediatric:
• Uncommon before 10 years of age
• Associated with blood dyscrasia
Geriatric:
• Incidence increases with age
• Age alone should not alter therapy plan
Others: N/A

PREGNANCY
Attempt conservative therapy but surgery if indicated

SYNONYMS
Gallstones

ICD-9-CM
574.0 Calculus of gallbladder with acute cholecystitis
574.1 Calculus of gallbladder with other cholecystitis
574.2 Calculus of gallbladder without mention of cholecystitis
575.0 Acute cholecystitis
575.1 Other cholecystitis (without mention of calculus)

SEE ALSO
• Cholangitis
• Choledocholithiasis
• Gallstones and cholecystitis
• See short topics: Adenocarcinoma of the gallbladder; jaundice

OTHER NOTES
Laparoscopic cholecystectomy has become most frequently used procedure. (Lithotripsy can be considered in rare circumstances).

ABBREVIATIONS
N/A

REFERENCES
• Hardy, J.D. (ed.): Hardy's Textbook of Surgery. 2nd Ed. Philadelphia, J.B. Lippincott, 1988
• Pitt, H.A. (ed.): The Surgical Clinics of North America. Vol. 70, No. 6. Philadelphia, W.B. Saunders, Dec, 1990

Author G. Williams, M.D.

Cholera

BASICS

DESCRIPTION An acute infectious disease caused by Vibrio cholerae (El Tor type is responsible for current epidemic, the other type, classic, is found only in Bangladesh). Characteristics include severe diarrhea with extreme fluid and electrolyte depletion, and vomiting, muscle cramps and prostration. Usual course: acute; chronic; relapsing.
• Clinical course is 3-5 days, and in the early stages a severely affected patient can lose one liter of fluid per hour
• Endemic areas: India; Southeast Asia; Africa; Middle East; Southern Europe; Oceania; South and Central America
System(s) affected: Gastrointestinal
Genetics: N/A
Incidence/Prevalence in USA: 0.01 cases/100,000. The few cases in the U.S. have been in returning travelers or associated with food brought into the country illicitly.
Predominant age: All ages
Predominant sex: Male = Female

SIGNS AND SYMPTOMS
• Abdominal discomfort
• Anorexia
• Anuria
• Apathy
• Cholera gravis
• Cyanosis
• Decreased skin turgor
• Dehydration
• Diarrhea, painless
• Distant heart sounds
• Diuresis, sudden
• Dysrhythmias
• Fever
• Hypotension
• Hypothermia
• Hypovolemic shock
• Increased or decreased bowel sounds
• Lethargy
• Listlessness
• Malaise
• Non-tender abdomen
• Oliguria
• Rice-water diarrhea
• Seizures
• Sunken eyes
• Tachycardia
• Thirst
• Vomiting
• Washerwoman's fingers
• Weak peripheral pulses
• Weakness

CAUSES
• Enterotoxin elaborated by gram-negative
• Vibrio cholera (O-group 1)
• Human host
• Contaminated food
• Contaminated water
• Contaminated shellfish

RISK FACTORS
• Traveling or living in epidemic areas
• Exposure to contaminated food or water
• Person-to-person transmission (rare)
• In endemic areas, children under age 5
• Attack more severe in blood group O as compared to AB
• Individual with low gastric acid secretion
• Gastrectomy
• Individuals on acid-suppressing medications

DIAGNOSIS

DIFFERENTIAL DIAGNOSIS Other causes of severe diarrhea and dehydration (e.g., Shigella, E. coli, viruses)

LABORATORY
• Stool culture - on selective media (thiosulfate citrate bile salts sucrose [TCBS])
• Typed antisera specific agglutination
• Dark field microscopy - characteristic vibrio motility in stool
• Increased vibriocidal antibodies in unimmunized individual
Laboratory abnormalities of severe dehydration:
◊ Acidemia
◊ Acidosis
◊ Hypokalemia
◊ Hyponatremia
◊ Hypochloremia
◊ Hypoglycemia
◊ Increased specific gravity
◊ Polycythemia
◊ Mild neutrophilic leukocytosis
Drugs that may alter lab results: N/A
Disorders that may alter lab results: N/A

PATHOLOGICAL FINDINGS
• Electron microscopy - organism adherent to mucosa
• Intact mucosa
• Increased cellularity of lamina propria
• Increased cellularity of mucosa
• Vascular congestion
• Lymphoid hyperplasia of Peyer's patches
• Lymphoid hyperplasia of mesenteric lymph nodes
• Lymphoid hyperplasia of spleen
• Cerebral edema
• Acute tubular necrosis
• Vacuolar hypokalemic nephropathy
• Pulmonary edema
• Hyaline membranes
• Bronchopneumonia
• Focal myocardial damage
• Lipid-depleted adrenals
• Tubularization of zona fasciculata

SPECIAL TESTS N/A

IMAGING
• Abdominal film - ileus
• Chest x-ray - microcardia

DIAGNOSTIC PROCEDURES Physical examination and medical history that includes recent travel

TREATMENT

APPROPRIATE HEALTH CARE
Outpatient for mild cases, inpatient for moderate or severe cases

GENERAL MEASURES
• Determination of the amount of fluid loss (may compare patient's previous weight to current weight)
• Rehydration therapy. Oral for mild to moderate cases. Patients with severe dehydration may require intravenous replacement.

ACTIVITY Bedrest until symptoms resolved and strength returns

DIET Small, frequent meals when vomiting stops and appetite returns

PATIENT EDUCATION
• Centers for Disease Control. Traveler's Information Hotline: (404)332-4559 (available 24 hours via a touch-tone telephone).
• International Association for Medical Assistance to Travelers, 417 Center St., Lewiston, NY 14092, (716)754-4883

MEDICATIONS

DRUG(S) OF CHOICE
Oral rehydration therapy
For mild disease:
◊ Oral rehydration solution (ORS) commercial brands available (Pedialyte, Rehydralyte, Resol, Ricelyte) or
◊ ORS formula from World Health Organization (WHO) - per liter: Sodium chloride 3.5 grams, potassium chloride 1.5 grams, glucose 20 grams, trisodium citrate 2.9 grams
Parenteral rehydration
Severely dehydrated patients
◊ IV rehydration (Ringer's lactate) is followed by oral or nasogastric administration of glucose or sucrose-electrolyte solution
Antibiotics
◊ For older children and adults: doxycycline (Vibramycin) - 300mg once or 100mg bid for 3 days or tetracycline 50mg/kg/day for 3 days
◊ For young children: trimethoprim-sulfamethoxazole (SMX/TMP; Bactrim, Septra) 8 mg/kg trimethoprim plus 40 mg/kg sulfamethoxazole per day, divided q12h. This dosage is equivalent to 1 mL/kg of SMX/TMP suspension. Alternatively, furazolidone (Furoxone) 5-10mg/kg/day divided q 6 hours for 3 days.
◊ In pregnancy: furazolidone 100mg qid x7-10 days.
Contraindications:
• Tetracyclines contraindicated in pregnancy and children less than 8 years of age
• Furazolidone and alcohol may cause disulfiram-like reaction. Avoid the mixture.
Precautions: Tetracyclines are photosensitizers. Use sunscreen.
Significant possible interactions: Avoid taking tetracyclines with dairy products, antacids, or iron preparations

ALTERNATIVE DRUGS   N/A

FOLLOWUP

PATIENT MONITORING   Follow patient until symptoms resolved

PREVENTION/AVOIDANCE
• Water purification
• Careful food selection, e.g., no unpeeled raw fruits or vegetables, no raw or undercooked seafood
• Enteric precautions
• Tetracycline for contacts
• Natural infection confers long-lasting immunity
Prophylactic vaccine
◊ 50% effective for 3 to 6 months
◊ Not recommended unless required by destination country, and if so, a single dose is sufficient
◊ Concomitant administration with yellow fever vaccine may result in reduced vaccine response to yellow fever
◊ Invariably associated with local side effects
◊ Systemic side effects of fever and malaise
◊ A new vaccine shows promise, but still in the testing stage

POSSIBLE COMPLICATIONS
• Hypovolemic shock
• Chronic biliary infection
• Up to 50% mortality with untreated shock
• Intermittent stool shedding

EXPECTED COURSE AND PROGNOSIS
• Prompt oral or IV treatment can be lifesaving
• Appropriate disposal of human waste
• Antibiotic treatment reduces duration and infectivity of disease
• Mortality less than 1% with appropriate supportive care
• Increased mortality with untreated hypovolemic shock

MISCELLANEOUS

ASSOCIATED CONDITIONS   Increased risk of disease with gastric achlorhydria

AGE-RELATED FACTORS
Pediatric:
• Breast-feeding is protective against cholera
• Vaccine not recommended for children less than 6 months
Geriatric: N/A
Others: N/A

PREGNANCY   N/A

SYNONYMS
• Asiatic cholera
• Epidemic cholera
• Rice water diarrhea
• Cholera gravis

ICD-9-CM   001.9 cholera, unspecified

SEE ALSO   N/A

OTHER NOTES   Centers for Disease Control does not expect a major outbreak of cholera in the U.S., but it has issued a "Cholera Preparedness Plan", outlining steps for proper surveillance, treatment, laboratory diagnosis, investigation of outbreaks, and public education

ABBREVIATIONS   N/A

REFERENCES)
• Mandell, G.L. (ed.): Principles and Practice of Infectious Diseases. 3rd Ed. New York, Churchill Livingstone, 1990
• Warren, K.S. & Mahmoud, A.A. (eds.): Tropical and Geographical Medicine. New York, McGraw-Hill, 1990
• Dhiman, B.R. & Greenough, C.B., III (eds.): Cholera. New York, Plenum Medical Book Co., 1992

Author   A. Abyad, M.D.

Chronic fatigue syndrome

 BASICS

DESCRIPTION Chronic fatigue syndrome (CFS) is characterized primarily by profound fatigue, in association with multiple systemic and neuropsychiatric symptoms, lasting at least 6 months, severe enough to reduce/impair daily activity.
System(s) affected: Endocrine/Metabolic, Musculoskeletal
Genetics: N/A.
Incidence/Prevalence in USA: 10/100,000
Predominant age: Young adult
Predominant sex: Female > Male (slightly)
Signs and symptoms:
• Fatigue (100%)
• Ability to date onset of illness (100%)
• Unexplained general muscle weakness (90%)
• Arthralgias (90%)
• Forgetfulness (90%)
• Inability to concentrate (90%)
• Emotional lability (90%)
• Myalgias (90%)
• Confusion (90%)
• Mood swings (90%)
• Low-grade fever (37.5-38.6°C) (85%)
• Irritability (85%)
• Prolonged fatigue lasting 24 hours after exercise (80%)
• Depression (80%)
• Headaches (76%)
• Photophobia (76%)
• Difficulty sleeping (76%)
• Allergies (70%)
• Vertigo (40%)
• Adenopathy (40%)
• Shortness of breath (33%)
• Chest pain (33%)
• Nausea (33%)
• Weight loss (30%)
• Hot flushes (30%)
• Palpitations (30%)
• Painful lymph nodes (30%)
• Gastrointestinal complaints (30%)
• Night sweats (25%)
• Weight gain (15%)
• Rash (15%)

CAUSES Unknown. Multiple immunologic abnormalities suggestive of viral reactivation syndrome have been reported, but no one source identified. Attention given most to herpes (EBV and HHV-6) and other enteroviruses, possibly in concert, possibly with environmental factors.

RISK FACTORS Unknown

 DIAGNOSIS

DIFFERENTIAL DIAGNOSIS
• Malignancies
• Autoimmune disease
• Localized infection (occult abscess, etc.)
• Chronic or subacute bacterial disease (endocarditis)
• Lyme disease
• Fungal disease (histoplasmosis, coccidioidomycosis)
• Parasitic disease (amebiasis, giardiasis, helminths)
• HIV related disease
• Psychiatric disease
• Chronic inflammatory disease (sarcoidosis, Wegener's granulomatosis)
• Known chronic viral disease (chronic hepatitis)
• Neuromuscular disease (multiple sclerosis, myasthenia gravis)
• Endocrine disorder (hypothyroidism, Addison's, Cushing's, diabetes mellitus)
• Drug dependency or abuse (including prescription drugs)
• Iatrogenic (as from medication side effects)
• Toxic agent exposure
• Other known or defined systemic disease (chronic pulmonary, cardiac, hepatic, renal, or hematologic disease)
• Physiologic (inadequate or disrupted sleep, menopause, etc.)

LABORATORY :
Initial lab studies
◊ Chemistry panel
◊ CBC
◊ Urinalysis
◊ Thyroid function
Additional studies
◊ ESR
◊ ANA
◊ VDRL
◊ Rheumatoid factor
◊ Purified protein derivative
◊ Serum cortisol
◊ HIV
◊ Immunoglobulin
◊ Epstein-Barr serology
Drugs that may alter lab results: N/A
Disorders that may alter lab results: N/A

PATHOLOGICAL FINDINGS N/A

SPECIAL TESTS None. Diagnosis of exclusion. History, physical exam normal.

IMAGING Experimental at present

DIAGNOSTIC PROCEDURES
• To help establish the diagnosis (guidelines from the Center for Disease Control) - 2 major criteria must be present, along with (1) at least 6 of the other 9 symptoms plus at least 2 of the 3 physical signs; OR (2) at least 8 of the other 9 symptoms
Major criteria:
◊ New onset fatigue lasting longer than 6 months with a 50% reduction in activity
◊ No other medical or psychiatric conditions that could cause symptoms
Symptoms:
◊ Low grade fever
◊ Sore throat
◊ Painful cervical or axillary adenopathy
◊ Generalized muscle weakness
◊ Myalgias
◊ Headaches
◊ Migratory arthralgias
◊ Sleep disturbances (hypersomnia or insomnia)
◊ Neuropsychological complaints (one or more of: photophobia, visual scotomas, forgetfulness, irritability, confusion, difficulty concentrating, depression)
Physical signs:
◊ Low grade fever (37.5-38.6°C)
◊ Pharyngitis (nonexudative)
◊ Cervical or axillary adenopathy

 TREATMENT

APPROPRIATE HEALTH CARE
Outpatient

GENERAL MEASURES
• Because the cause of CFS is unknown and no specific therapy has shown consistent results, the mainstay of therapy is supportive care
• A program of moderate exercise (with rest periods during exacerbations of the disease), a healthy diet, stress reduction, and support groups or counselling is likely to be beneficial and while not necessarily curative will help the patient cope with their disease
• Alternative therapies (chiropractic, homeopathy, acupuncture, enforced rest) helpful for some; no proven efficacy; may be worth trying
• Psychiatric symptoms often prominent but generally felt secondary rather than causative

ACTIVITY As tolerated, but strenuous exercise tends to exacerbate symptoms in most

DIET No restrictions

PATIENT EDUCATION
• Support groups available. Contact CFS Association, 3521 Broadway, Suite 222, Kansas City, MO. 64111; (816) 931-4777
• CFIDS Association. P.O. Box 220398, Charlotte, NC 28222-0398
• International Chronic Fatigue Syndrome Society. P.O. Box 230108, Portland, OR 97223

MEDICATIONS

DRUG(S) OF CHOICE
• None. Ampligen, essential fatty acid therapy, IV immune globulin, vitamin B12, and bovine liver extract (LEFAC) are used experimentally.
• Supportive therapy directed toward symptoms with NSAID's, antidepressants including fluoxetine, others including buspirone.
Contraindications: Refer to manufacturer's literature
Precautions: Refer to manufacturer's literature
Significant possible interactions: Refer to manufacturer's literature

ALTERNATIVE DRUGS   N/A

FOLLOWUP

PATIENT MONITORING   No consensus.
Periodic re-evaluation appropriate for support, symptom relief, assessment for other cause.

PREVENTION/AVOIDANCE   Unknown

POSSIBLE COMPLICATIONS
• Depression
• Socio-economic problems

EXPECTED COURSE AND PROGNOSIS
• Indolent; waxes and wanes
• Generally very slow improvement over months or years

MISCELLANEOUS

ASSOCIATED CONDITIONS
Fibromyalgia (70% reported to meet criteria)

AGE-RELATED FACTORS
Pediatric: Reported in children
Geriatric: Reported in elderly
Others: N/A

PREGNANCY   No information

SYNONYMS
• CFS
• Chronic Epstein-Barr syndrome
• Yuppie flu

ICD-9-CM   300.5 neurasthenia

SEE ALSO   N/A

OTHER NOTES   Controversial topic, data often conflicting

ABBREVIATIONS   N/A

REFERENCES
• Holmes, G.P, Kaplan, J.E., et al.: Chronic Fatigue Syndrome: A Working Case Definition. Annals of Internal Medicine 108, 387-389, Mar. 1988
• Klimas, N.G., et al.: Immunologic Abnormalities in Chronic Fatigue Syndrome. J. Clinical Microbiology 28(6),1403-1410, Jun. 1990
• English, T.: Skeptical of Skeptics. JAMA 265(8), 964, Feb. 27, 1991
• An information packet, for health care providers, is available from the CDC's Viral Diseases Division (404)639-1338

Author   R. Byrd, M.D

Chronic obstructive pulmonary disease and emphysema

BASICS

DESCRIPTION Chronic obstructive pulmonary disease encompasses several diffuse pulmonary diseases including chronic bronchitis, asthma, cystic fibrosis, bronchiectasis, and emphysema. The term usually refers to a mixture of chronic bronchitis and emphysema.
• Chronic bronchitis is defined clinically by increased mucus production and recurrent cough present on most days for at least three months during at least two consecutive years.
• Emphysema is the destruction of interalveolar septa and is thus a pathological definition. The disease occurs in the distal or terminal airways and involves both airways and lung parenchyma.
Genetics:
• Chronic bronchitis is not a genetic disorder although some studies have hinted at a predisposition for development of this condition.
• A rare form of emphysema, antiprotease deficiency (due to alpha 1-antitrypsin deficiency), is an inherited disorder that is an expression of two autosomal codominant alleles.
Incidence in USA: 20-30% of adults, more than 60,000 deaths/year
Prevalence in USA: 8 million people have chronic bronchitis, 2 million people have emphysema
Predominant age: Over 40 years
Predominant sex: Male > Female

SIGNS AND SYMPTOMS
Chronic bronchitis
◊ Cough
◊ Sputum production
◊ Frequent infections
◊ Intermittent dyspnea
◊ Pedal edema
◊ Plethora
◊ Cyanosis
◊ Wheezing
◊ Weight gain
◊ Diminished breath sounds
Emphysema
◊ Minimal cough
◊ Scant sputum
◊ Dyspnea
◊ Often significant weight loss
◊ Occasional infections
◊ Barrel chest
◊ Minimal wheezing
◊ Use of accessory muscles of respiration
◊ Pursed lip breathing
◊ Cyanosis is slight or absent
◊ Breath sounds very diminished

CAUSES
• Cigarette smoking
• Air pollution
• Antiprotease deficiency
• Occupational exposure (i.e., firefighters)
• Infection possibly (viral)

RISK FACTORS
• Passive smoking (especially adults whose parents smoked)
• Severe viral pneumonia early in life
• Aging

DIAGNOSIS

DIFFERENTIAL DIAGNOSIS Acute bronchitis, asthma, bronchiectasis, bronchogenic carcinoma, acute viral infection, normal aging of lungs, occupational asthma, chronic pulmonary embolism, sleep apnea, primary alveolar hypoventilation, chronic sinusitis

LABORATORY
Chronic bronchitis
◊ Hypercapnia
◊ Polycythemia
◊ Hypoxia can be moderate to severe
Emphysema
◊ Normal serum hemoglobin or polycythemia
◊ Normal PaCO2; unless FEV1 < 1L/sec, then can be elevated
◊ Mild hypoxia
Drugs that may alter lab results:
Sedatives including alcohol
Disorders that may alter lab results:
Obesity, concurrent restrictive lung dysfunction, primary pulmonary hypertension, acute infections, anemia, pulmonary embolism

PATHOLOGICAL FINDINGS
Chronic bronchitis
◊ Bronchial mucous gland enlargement
◊ Increased number of secretory cells in surface epithelium
◊ Thickened small airways from edema and inflammation
◊ Smooth muscle hyperplasia
◊ Mucus plugging
◊ Bacterial colonization of airways
Emphysema
◊ Entire lung affected
◊ Bronchi usually clear of secretions
◊ Anthracotic pigment
◊ Alveoli enlarged with loss of septa
◊ Cartilage atrophy
◊ Bullae

SPECIAL TESTS
Pulmonary function testing
◊ Decreased FEV1 with concomitant reduction in FEV1/FVC ratio
◊ FVC may be normal or reduced
◊ Normal or increased total lung capacity
◊ Increased residual volume
◊ Diffusing capacity is normal or reduced

IMAGING
• Chronic bronchitis chest x-ray shows increased bronchovascular markings and cardiomegaly
• Emphysema chest x-ray shows small heart, hyperinflation, flat diaphragms and possibly bullous changes

DIAGNOSTIC PROCEDURES
• Pulmonary function tests
• ABG's
• Chest x-ray

TREATMENT

APPROPRIATE HEALTH CARE
• Outpatient treatment is usually adequate. However, hospitalization may be required for exacerbation, infection, or diagnostic procedures (i.e., transbronchial lung biopsy).
• Acute respiratory failure may require an intensive care unit and possibly a mechanical ventilator to support the patient

GENERAL MEASURES
• Smoking cessation
• Aggressive treatment of infections
• Treat any reversible bronchospasm
• Reduction of secretions through good pulmonary hygiene
• Cor pulmonale may necessitate use of oxygen
• Pulmonary rehabilitation

ACTIVITY As tolerated. Full activity should be encouraged.

DIET A well balanced, high protein diet is suggested. Low carbohydrates may benefit those with hypercarbia.

PATIENT EDUCATION
• Printed material is available from the National Jewish Hospital in Denver, Colorado. The local branch of the American Lung Association also has educational material.
• Coach patients in pulmonary rehabilitation

Chronic obstructive pulmonary disease and emphysema

MEDICATIONS

DRUG(S) OF CHOICE
• Theophylline - (Theo-Dur, Slo-bid, Uniphyl) 400 mg/day. Increase by 100-200 mg in one to two weeks if necessary.
• Sympathomimetics - (Alupent, Proventil, Ventolin, Maxair, Brethaire). 1-2 puffs from the metered dose inhaler every 4-6 hrs. May be increased to every 3 hrs. Use of spacer device (aerochamber, inspirease) may be beneficial. (Up to 4 puffs recommended by some.)
• Anticholinergics - ipratropium (Atrovent). Two puffs (36 mcg) 4 times daily. May take additional inhalations not to exceed 12 in 24 hrs.
• Corticosteroids - prednisone (Deltasone). Given orally 7.5-15 mg/day. Most useful in bronchitis with some reversibility.

Contraindications:
• Theophylline - hypersensitivity
• Sympathomimetics - cardiac arrhythmias associated with tachycardia; hypersensitivity
• Anticholinergics - hypersensitivity to atropine or its derivatives
• Corticosteroids - systemic fungal infections; hypersensitivity

Precautions:
• Theophylline - reduce dosage in patients with impaired renal or liver function; age over 55; CHF. Therapeutic drug level is 10-20 mcg/mL.
Addition of cimetidine, ciprofloxacin, or erythromycin will decrease theophylline clearance causing theophylline levels to rise. Careful monitoring of serum theophylline levels is warranted.
• Rifampin - may cause a decrease in theophylline levels by increasing theophylline metabolism. Monitor serum theophylline level.
• Sympathomimetics - excessive use may be dangerous. May need to reduce dose in patients with cardiovascular disease, hypertension, hyperthyroidism, diabetes or convulsive disorders.
• Anticholinergics - narrow angle glaucoma, prostatic hypertrophy, bladder-neck obstruction
• Corticosteroids - may mask infection or predispose to infection, especially fungal; subcapsular cataracts; glaucoma; adrenocortical insufficiency; psychic derangements; gastrointestinal bleeding; diabetes mellitus, reactivation of tuberculosis

Significant possible Interactions:
• Theophylline - lithium carbonate; propranolol; erythromycin; cimetidine; ranitidine; rifampin; ciprofloxacin
• Sympathomimetics - other sympathomimetics, monoamine oxidase inhibitors or tricyclic antidepressants
• Anticholinergics - refer to manufacturer's profile
• Corticosteroids - NSAID's (indomethacin), aspirin, synthetic thyroid hormone

ALTERNATIVE DRUGS
• Theophylline may be given intravenously or by rectal suppository
• Sympathomimetics may be given as aerosolized solution (albuterol, Metaprel, isoetharine) when mixed with saline; orally (Alupent, Proventil, Brethine, Ventolin) or subcutaneously (terbutaline)
• Anticholinergics - atropine sulfate, glycopyrrolate
• Corticosteroids may be given intravenously (hydrocortisone, methylprednisolone) or inhaled (beclomethasone, flunisolide, triamcinolone acetonide)

FOLLOWUP

PATIENT MONITORING
• Severe or unstable patients should be seen monthly
• When stable, may be seen biannually
• Theophylline level should be checked with each dose adjustment until the desired level (or result) is achieved, then may be checked every 6-12 months
• If home oxygen is required, arterial blood gasses should be checked yearly or with any change in condition. Oxygen saturation (with use of pulse oximetry) should be monitored more frequently.
• Avoidance of travel at high altitude should be encouraged. Air travel with oxygen requires pre-arrangement.

PREVENTION/AVOIDANCE
Avoidance of smoking is the most important preventive measure. Passive smoke also has recently been shown to be harmful.

POSSIBLE COMPLICATIONS
• Infection is common
• Other complications include cor pulmonale, secondary polycythemia, bullous lung disease, acute or chronic respiratory failure, pulmonary hypertension

EXPECTED COURSE AND PROGNOSIS
• The patient's age and post-bronchodilator forced expiratory volume (FEV1) are the most important predictors of prognosis. Those of young age and FEV1 > 50% predicted have a fairly good prognosis. Older patients with more severe lung disease do worse.
• Supplemental oxygen, when indicated, has been shown to increase survival
• Smoking cessation is also important for an improved prognosis
• Malnutrition is a poor prognostic indicator

MISCELLANEOUS

ASSOCIATED CONDITIONS
• Lung cancer
• Coronary artery disease
• Peptic ulcer disease
• Chronic sinusitis
• Malnutrition
• Laryngeal carcinoma

AGE-RELATED FACTORS
Pediatric: Repeated childhood respiratory illnesses make COPD a greater risk
Geriatric: Relative risk is 1.2 to 2.3 times greater than in younger person
Others: Unusual under age 25 unless antiprotease deficiency is present. Incidence increases as age approaches 60.

PREGNANCY N/A

SYNONYMS
• Bronchitis
• COLD (Chronic obstructive lung disease)
• OAD (Obstructive airways disease)
• COPD

ICD-9-CM
• 496 COPD
• 492.8 Emphysema

SEE ALSO
• Asthma
• Bronchitis, acute

OTHER NOTES
Other important considerations for treatment include adequate hydration, supplemental oxygen, antibiotics when indicated, mucolytic agents, pulmonary rehabilitation, good pulmonary hygiene

ABBREVIATIONS
FVC = forced vital capacity
FEV1 = forced expiratory volume at 1 second
COPD = chronic obstructive pulmonary disease

REFERENCES
Fishman, A.: Pulmonary Diseases and Disorders. 2nd Ed. New York, McGraw-Hill Book Co., 1988

Author A. Cropp, M.D., F.C.C.P.

Cirrhosis of the liver

BASICS

DESCRIPTION Histologically cirrhosis is defined by the presence of fibrosis with regenerative nodules. Clinically cirrhosis presents with evidence of portal hypertension, i.e. ascites, variceal bleeding, hepatic encephalopathy.
System(s) affected: Gastrointestinal, Cardiovascular, Endocrine/Metabolic
Genetics: N/A
Incidence/Prevalence in USA: Accounts for over 30,000 deaths per year
Predominant age: Etiology dependent
Predominant sex: Etiology dependent

SIGNS AND SYMPTOMS
The onset of the disease is often insidious with:
◊ Fatigue
◊ Anorexia
◊ Nausea
◊ Abdominal discomfort and distention
◊ Weakness and malaise
Signs and symptoms that are related to cirrhosis are those of complications:
◊ Hematemesis
◊ Encephalopathy
◊ Jaundice
◊ Splenomegaly
◊ Abdominal collateral circulation
◊ Ascites
◊ Gynecomastia
◊ Testicular atrophy
◊ Asterixis (liver flap)
◊ Palmar erythema
◊ Spider angiomas

CAUSES
• Alcoholic cirrhosis
• Chronic viral hepatitis, B (with/without D), C
• Wilson's disease
• Hemochromatosis
• Alpha 1-antitrypsin deficiency
• Cystic fibrosis
• Autoimmune chronic active hepatitis with cirrhosis
• Primary biliary cirrhosis
• Secondary biliary cirrhosis
• Primary sclerosing cholangitis
• Cardiac cirrhosis
• Drug induced (other than alcohol)
• Toxic chemical exposure (e.g., carbon tetrachloride)
Inherited causes that may be present in infancy and childhood:
◊ Glycogen storage disease
◊ Galactosemia
◊ Fructose intolerance
◊ Tyrosinemia
◊ Acid cholesterol ester hydrolase deficiency

RISK FACTORS Included with Causes

DIAGNOSIS

DIFFERENTIAL DIAGNOSIS
• Depends on presentation
• Ascites - increased right heart pressure, hepatic vein thrombosis, peritoneal infection or malignancy, pancreatic disease, thyroid diseas, lymphatic obstructione
• Other causes of UGI bleeding
• Other metabolic encephalopathies - renal, cardiopulmonary, drug.

LABORATORY
• Recognition of liver injury - elevated AST, elevated ALT; elevated alkaline phosphatase. Note: All liver injury tests may be normal.
• Functional impairment of the liver - elevated bilirubin, decreased albumin, elevated globulin, prolonged prothrombin time
Etiologic screen for liver disease
◊ Ceruloplasmin (Wilson's disease)
◊ Iron, iron binding capacity, ferritin (hemochromatosis)
◊ Alpha fetoprotein (hepatocellular cancer)
◊ HBsAg (hepatitis B)
◊ Anti-HCV (hepatitis C)
◊ ANA (autoimmune hepatitis)
◊ Anti-smooth muscle antibody (autoimmune hepatitis)
◊ Anti-mitochondrial antibody (AMA) (primary biliary cirrhosis)
◊ Alpha 1-antitrypsin (deficiency)
◊ Serum protein electrophoresis (SPEP) - increased IgG with any liver disease; increased IgM with primary biliary cirrhosis (PBC)
Drugs that may alter lab results: N/A
Disorders that may alter lab results: N/A

PATHOLOGICAL FINDINGS
• Fibrosis and regenerative nodules; specific findings/patterns may indicate etiology
• Quantitative liver chemistry for iron, copper
• Special stains for iron, copper, bilirubin, collagen, alpha 1-antitrypsin, hepatitis B

SPECIAL TESTS
• Laparoscopic liver biopsy to reduce sampling error
• Cholangiography to rule out common duct obstruction and recognize sclerosing cholangitis
• Doppler ultrasound to indicate direction of flow in portal vein plus patency
• Visceral angiography to determine vascular anatomy, patency and collaterals
• Esophagogastroduodenoscopy to assess varices

IMAGING Ultrasound good for detecting bile duct dilatation and space occupying lesions. Cannot make diagnosis of cirrhosis based on ultrasound alone.

DIAGNOSTIC PROCEDURES
• A liver biopsy establishes the diagnosis of cirrhosis
• Patterns of injury as well as special stains may identify a precise etiology such as alcoholic liver disease, hemochromatosis, alpha 1-antitrypsin deficiency, hepatitis B, primary biliary cirrhosis

TREATMENT

APPROPRIATE HEALTH CARE
Outpatient except for complicating emergencies:
• GI bleeding
• Hepatic encephalopathy
• Spontaneous bacterial peritonitis
• Unexplained decompensation
• Reanl failure

GENERAL MEASURES
• Treatment designed to remove or alleviate underlying cause of cirrhosis, prevent further liver damage and prevent complications
• Phlebotomy for hemochromatosis
• Therapies involve drug treatment, dietary restrictions, rest, other supportive measures Adequate protein intake for liver regeneration
• Possible procedures for portal hypertension include - splenorenal or portacaval anastomosis, transjugular intrahepatic portal-systemic shunt
• Liver transplantation - final stage therapy

ACTIVITY Maintain as active as possible. With peripheral edema, leg elevation necessary.

DIET
• Adequate protein (1 gram/kg) and generous calories to help regenerate the liver
• In the presence of hepatic encephalopathy protein restriction is necessary
• In the presence of ascites salt restriction is necessary (2 gm or less/day)
• In the presence of hyponatremia (Na < 130) fluid restriction is necessary (< 1 liter)
• No alcohol

PATIENT EDUCATION
• Pamphlets are available through: American Liver Foundation, (800)223-0179
• Additional material: National Digestive Diseases Information Clearinghouse, Box NDDIC, Bethesda, MD 20892, (301)468-6344

MEDICATIONS

DRUG(S) OF CHOICE
• Large esophageal varices seen at endoscopy prior to clinical bleeding - Propranolol at a dose to decrease the resting pulse by 25%
• Treatment of ascites - spironolactone 100 mg up to 400 mg every day as a single dose. Takes three days before onset of action. Add furosemide 40-80 mg/day if needed. Loop diuretics may produce a rapid diuresis and subsequent intravascular volume depletion.
• Encephalopathy - lactulose to produce 2-3 soft stools per day. Specific drug based on etiology -penicillamine for Wilson's disease, corticosteroids with or without azathioprine for autoimmune chronic active hepatitis, alfa interferon for chronic hepatitis B and C.
• SBP - ampicillin plus aminoglycoside or cefotaxime alone as initial treatment; norfloxacin 400 mg/day (decreases risk for subsequent development of SBP after treatment)
Contraindications: Refer to manufacturer's literature
Precautions: Refer to manufacturer's literature
Significant possible interactions: Refer to manufacturer's literature

ALTERNATIVE DRUGS   Ursodeoxycholic acid for cholestatic disease

FOLLOWUP

PATIENT MONITORING
• In a stable patient - yearly battery of liver tests. After 10 years, consider alphafetoprotein and imaging to detect hepatocellular carcinoma.
• In an unstable patient - tests may be repeated at weekly intervals
• Have patient monitor weight and maintain a daily diary

PREVENTION/AVOIDANCE
• Limit use of alcohol and other liver toxins
• No sharing of syringes
• Safe sex
• Surveillance of family members when a genetic disease is recognized
• Influenza and pneumococcal vaccines for cirrhosis patients exposed to crowds
• Liver test surveillence while on hepatiotoxic drugs (e.g., INH)

POSSIBLE COMPLICATIONS
• Ascites
• Jaundice
• Coagulopathy
• Hepatic encephalopathy
• Bleeding esophageal varices
• Liver failure
• Carcinoma of the liver (uncommon)
• Susceptibility to infections
• Spontaneous bacterial peritonitis
• Renal failure

EXPECTED COURSE AND
PROGNOSIS A function of ongoing hepatic injury as well as residual hepatic reserve. If a treatable cause is identified and intervention results in cessation of liver destruction, then the prognosis may be good.

MISCELLANEOUS

ASSOCIATED CONDITIONS
• Hepatitis
• Diseases and defects of the bile ducts
• Cystic fibrosis
• Heart failure
• Hepatocellular cancer

AGE-RELATED FACTORS
Pediatric: N/A
Geriatric: Cirrhosis is one of the leading causes of death for people over age 65
Others: N/A

PREGNANCY   Cirrhosis may decompensate during pregnancy. Higher rates of spontaneous abortion, premature birth and perinatal death.

SYNONYMS N/A

ICD-9-CM
• 571.2 Alcoholic cirrhosis of liver
• 571.5 Cirrhosis of liver without mention of alcohol

SEE ALSO N/A

OTHER NOTES N/A

ABBREVIATIONS N/A

REFERENCES
• Sampliner, R.E.: The recognition of early liver disease. Hospital Practice:53-56, March 30, 1989
• Zakim, D. & Boyer, T.D. (eds.): Hepatology, A Textbook of Liver Disease. Philadelphia, W.B. Saunders Co., 1990

Author R. Sampliner, M.D.

Claudication

BASICS

DESCRIPTION The feeling of muscle fatigue after a period of minimal exercise of an extremity. The feeling may progress to a cramp-like pain, usually in the calf muscles. It is always relieved by resting the extremity. It can be reproduced by undergoing a similar exercise pattern. It may occur in the arms, but is more common in the legs, calf > thigh.
System(s) affected: Cardiovascular, Musculoskeletal
Genetics: N/A
Incidence in USA: N/A
Prevalence in USA: Common
Predominant age: Common in males > 55, females > 60
Predominant sex: Male > Female (4:1)

SIGNS AND SYMPTOMS
• May start gradually or suddenly
• Unable to walk distances
• Pain varies from muscle tiredness to a frank cramp in muscle group involved
• May be a loss of hair on toes
• Foot may show rubor on dependency
• Pedal pulses absent
• Popliteal pulse absent
• With thigh claudication, femoral pulse absent

CAUSES
• Lower extremity claudication - blockage of superficial femoral artery, secondary to arteriosclerosis in 95% of cases
• Other causes of arterial blocks - embolus, popliteal entrapment, adventitius cystic disease of popliteal artery, thromboangiitis obliterans
• Thigh and hip claudication - blockage of aortic and iliac vessels
• Upper extremity claudication - similar blocks of subclavian, axillary, and brachial artery

RISK FACTORS
• Smoking
• Diabetes
• Hypertension
• Hyperlipidemia
• Obesity
• Preexisting heart disease

DIAGNOSIS

DIFFERENTIAL DIAGNOSIS
Pseudoclaudication, sometimes secondary to some form of spinal stenosis, usually impinging on the cauda equina portion of the spinal cord. The pain in the legs is characteristically relieved by squatting or sitting. The latter relieves tension on spinal nerve roots. Osteoarthritis of hips and knees sometimes can be confused with claudication, but pain starts immediately on weight bearing.

LABORATORY
Non-invasive vascular monitoring with measurement of blood pressure in the arm compared to pedal arterial pressures before and after exercise establish the diagnosis as well as the severity of occlusion. The patient with one to two block claudication will have an ankle/arm index of 0.7-0.4 with 1.0 being normal. If below 0.4, there is a major threat of losing part of the leg if left untreated. Pseudoclaudication does not affect the pulses in the extremity.
Drugs that may alter lab results: None
Disorders that may alter lab results: Arterial calcinosis, often found in diabetics, will cause a falsely high ankle/arm index

PATHOLOGICAL FINDINGS Absent pulses in the distal extremity, secondary to more proximal arterial occlusion. The occlusion is usually from an arterial plaque.

SPECIAL TESTS Noninvasive vascular tests - pulse volume recordings

IMAGING
• Duplex ultrasound
• Intra-arterial arteriography

DIAGNOSTIC PROCEDURES
Arteriography

TREATMENT

APPROPRIATE HEALTH CARE
Outpatient, except for severe cases or advanced disease

GENERAL MEASURES
• Conservative measures: stop smoking, initiate walking and exercise program, control of hyperlipidemia
• Reduce risk factors
• Surgical treatment with bypass of arterial obstruction may be appropriate in selected cases

ACTIVITY Ambulatory

DIET None

PATIENT EDUCATION Prevention methods

MEDICATIONS

DRUG(S) OF CHOICE
• Aspirin - to reduce platelet aggregation: low dose 80 mg/day
• Pentoxifylline (Trental) - to decrease internal configuration of red cells - 400 mg bid-tid. Administer for at least 6-8 weeks to determine if therapy is effective.
Contraindications: Refer to manufacturer's literature
Precautions: Try to reduce risk factors first
Significant possible interactions: Refer to manufacturer's literature

ALTERNATIVE DRUGS None

FOLLOWUP

PATIENT MONITORING Peripheral vascular studies every 6 months

PREVENTION/AVOIDANCE
• Institute walking program of 4-5 miles
• Avoid smoking

POSSIBLE COMPLICATIONS Only 10% of people without diabetes will progress to some amputation of the involved extremity

EXPECTED COURSE AND PROGNOSIS Gradual improvement in walking distance or progression of problem to gangrene, rest pain and/or tissue necrosis

MISCELLANEOUS

ASSOCIATED CONDITIONS Other manifestations of arteriosclerotic vascular disease - history of myocardial infarction(s), carotid disease, renal vascular hypertension

AGE-RELATED FACTORS
Pediatric: N/A
Geriatric: More common with advancing age
Others: N/A

PREGNANCY N/A

SYNONYMS N/A

ICD-9-CM 443.9

SEE ALSO N/A

OTHER NOTES N/A

ABBREVIATIONS N/A

REFERENCES Rutherford, R.B.: Vascular Surgery, 1984 pp.:4, 33, 64, 88, 113, 683

Author W.V. Sharp, M.D.

Coarctation of the aorta

 BASICS

DESCRIPTION A constriction (discrete or of varying lengths) of the aorta usually located just distal to the left subclavian artery at the junction of the ductus arteriosus
System(s) affected: Cardiovascular
Genetics: No Mendelian inheritance, but common in Turner's syndrome
Incidence/Prevalence in USA: 64/100,000 under 1 year of age
Predominant age: Usually diagnosed in infancy
Predominant sex: Male > Female (1.7:1)

SIGNS AND SYMPTOMS
• Headaches
• Exertional leg fatigue and pain
• Prominent neck pulsations
• Epistaxis
• Hypertension
• Pulse disparity
• Delayed, weak, or absent pulse
• Prominent left ventricular impulse
• Murmur (aortic stenosis or insufficiency, ventricular septal defect, rarely mitral valve)
• S4 systolic ejection click
• Bruit (coarctation, collaterals, patent ductus arteriosus)
• Cyanosis, rarely
• In infancy may also have heart failure, failure to thrive, irritability, tachypnea, and dyspnea
• Extensive collaterals develop from branches of the subclavian, internal mammary, superior intercostal, and axillary arteries

CAUSES Congenital: Takayasu's arteritis, Turner's syndrome, multiple left-sided obstruction

RISK FACTORS
• Turner's syndrome
• Congenital left heart abnormalities

 DIAGNOSIS

DIFFERENTIAL DIAGNOSIS
• Takayasu's arteritis
• Neurofibromatosis
• Pseudocoarctation (with or without hypertension, peripheral vascular disease)

LABORATORY N/A
Drugs that may alter lab results: N/A
Disorders that may alter lab results: N/A

PATHOLOGICAL FINDINGS
• Segmental tubular hypoplasia
• Discrete obstruction with medial thickening
• Distal aneurysm

SPECIAL TESTS
• Doppler examination of pulses reveals disparity
• Electrocardiogram may show left ventricular hypertrophy
• Blood pressures - all 4 extremities

IMAGING
• Chest x-ray may show rib notching, "3" sign, rarely cardiomegaly
• Echocardiography for coarctation and coexisting cardiac anomalies
• Transesophageal echocardiography
• Magnetic resonance imaging (MRI)

DIAGNOSTIC PROCEDURES Cardiac
catheterization and angiography: post-stenotic dilation

 TREATMENT

APPROPRIATE HEALTH CARE
Inpatient surgery

GENERAL MEASURES
• Surgical correction or balloon angioplasty can be done in infancy if urgently needed. Best results when performed age 1-2 years.
• Surgery should be done in childhood and adulthood as soon as coarctation diagnosed to prevent late complications
• Three common surgical procedures for correction of coarctation include 1) end-to-end anastomosis, 2) patch aortoplasty (insertion of dacron patch), and 3) subclavian flap procedure
• Balloon angioplasty of coarctation offers good results for primary treatment and for post-operative re-stenosis

ACTIVITY Exercise may exacerbate
hypertension, but normal activity recommended after correction

DIET No special diet

PATIENT EDUCATION
• Discuss post-coarctation syndrome
• For patient education materials favorably reviewed on this topic, contact: American Heart Association, 7320 Greenville Avenue, Dallas, TX 75231, (214)373-6300

MEDICATIONS

DRUG(S) OF CHOICE
• Prostaglandin E (patency of ductus arteriosus)
• Antibiotic prophylaxis (for dental and/or invasive procedures) for life (even after correction)
• Antihypertensives if needed
• Preload and afterload reduction if heart failure develops
Contraindications: Refer to manufacturer's profile of each drug
Precautions:
• Lowering upper extremity blood pressure may cause hypoperfusion of lower extremities
• Lowering blood pressure not advised in pregnancy unless emergency
Significant possible interactions: Refer to manufacturer's profile of each drug

ALTERNATIVE DRUGS N/A

FOLLOWUP

PATIENT MONITORING Frequent post-operative followup for evidence of re-stenosis (check for hypertension and pulse disparities) and late complications

PREVENTION/AVOIDANCE Patients should be encouraged to have normal lifestyles and activities after coarctation correction

POSSIBLE COMPLICATIONS
• Most common with late or no correction
• Heart failure
• Aneurysm of circle of Willis, rupture possible
• Hypertension
• Rupture or dissection of aortic aneurysm
• Endarteritis or endocarditis (need antibiotic prophylaxis)
• Aortic valve disease (stenosis or insufficiency)
• Post coarctectomy syndrome: recurrence, hypertension, atherosclerotic heart disease, aneurysm at site of coarctectomy, progressive aortic stenosis and/or regurgitation

EXPECTED COURSE AND PROGNOSIS
• Depends on age of repair and presence of other cardiac abnormalities
• Residual or restenosis (6-33%)
• Subsequent cardiac surgery (11%)
• Hypertension (25%)
• Survival after surgery: 10 years (91%), 20 years (84%), 30 years (72%)
• Uncorrected, 80% mortality before age 50

MISCELLANEOUS

ASSOCIATED CONDITIONS
• Bicuspid aortic valve (85%)
• Patent ductus arteriosus (65%)
• Ventricular septal defect (30-35%)
• Aortic stenosis and/or insufficiency
• Subvalvular aortic stenosis
• Mitral valve abnormalities (common)
• Transposition of great vessels or double outlet right ventricle
• Aneurysm of circle of Willis

AGE-RELATED FACTORS Greater risk of complications if correction is delayed beyond early childhood. Often diagnosis is delayed.
Pediatric: N/A
Geriatric: N/A
Others: N/A

PREGNANCY Uncorrected (or restenosis) coarctation carries high risk of aortic rupture or dissection and cerebral hemorrhage (aneurysm of circle of Willis rupture), but lower risk of pre-eclampsia than other forms of hypertension

SYNONYMS N/A

ICD-9-CM 747.1

SEE ALSO N/A

OTHER NOTES N/A

ABBREVIATIONS N/A

REFERENCES
• Hurst, J.W., et al.: The Heart. 7th Ed. New York, McGraw-Hill, 1990
• Adams, F.H., Emmanouilides, G.C. & Riemenschneider, T.A.: Moss' Heart Disease in Infants, Children and Adolescents. 4th Ed. Baltimore, Williams & Wilkins, 1989
• Brandenburg, R.O., et al.: Cardiology: Fundamentals and Practice. Chicago, Year Book Medical Publishers, 1987

Author K. Bellah, M.D.

Coccidioidomycosis

 BASICS

 DIAGNOSIS

 TREATMENT

DESCRIPTION
Pulmonary fungal infection endemic to the Southwest USA. Can become progressive and involve extrapulmonary sites, including bone, CNS, and skin. Known as the "great imitator". Incubation period is 1 to 4 weeks after exposure.

System(s) affected: Pulmonary, Nervous, Musculoskeletal, Skin/Exocrine, Endocrine/Metabolic

Genetics: Unknown

Incidence/Prevalence in USA: 100,000 cases per year. (0.5% extrapulmonary)

Predominant age: All ages

Predominant sex: Male = Female

SIGNS AND SYMPTOMS
• Anorexia
• Arthralgias
• Chest pain
• Chills
• Confusion
• Cough, dry or productive
• Cyanosis
• Dyspnea
• Erythema nodosum
• Fatigue
• Fever
• Headache
• Hepatomegaly
• Hydrocephalus
• Hyperreflexia
• Malaise
• Night sweats
• Pleural friction rub
• Rash
• Sore throat
• Splenomegaly
• Tachycardia
• Tenosynovitis
• Toxic erythema
• Weight loss
• Note: Over half of cases are subclinical

CAUSES
Coccidioides immitis, a soil fungus especially adapted to arid conditions. Liberated spores are inhaled when soil is disturbed: digging, construction sites, archaeological sites, dust storms, spelunking. Soil that lines rodent burrows is worst.

RISK FACTORS
• Certain groups are more prone to dissemination: immunocompromised hosts, pregnant women, African-Americans, Filipinos.
• CNS involvement more common in young white males
• Immunosuppression. Previously infected patients can experience relapse years later through the mechanism of cell-mediated immune deficiency.
• Diabetes mellitus
• AIDS

DIFFERENTIAL DIAGNOSIS
• Pneumonia, all etiologies
• Lung carcinoma
• Sarcoidosis
• Histoplasmosis, other fungi
• Lung abscess
• TB
• Lymphoma
• Meningitis
• Plus all other causes of cough, fever, fatigue
• Old granulomas can be mistaken for tumors

LABORATORY
• Skin test turns positive at 3 weeks to 3 months; may remain positive indefinitely; applying skin test will not interfere with serologies
• Serology - precipitin antibodies (IgM) rise within 2 weeks and disappear after 2 months; complement fixation antibodies (IgG) rise at 1-3 months; patients with mild symptoms may never develop detectable serology
• Culture of sputum, wound exudate, joint aspirate; unlikely to grow fungus in urine, blood, pleural fluid

Drugs that may alter lab results: Steroids may alter ability to react to skin testing

Disorders that may alter lab results: N/A

PATHOLOGICAL FINDINGS
Fungal elements, spherules

SPECIAL TESTS
Biopsy of affected tissue, e.g., lung nodule, skin lesion

IMAGING
Chest x-ray findings include - normal, infiltrate(s), nodule(s), cavity, adenopathy mediastinal or hilar, pleural effusion

DIAGNOSTIC PROCEDURES
If unable to establish diagnosis from skin testing and serologies - bronchoscopy, fine-needle biopsy, open lung biopsy, pleural biopsy, bone/skin/node biopsy

APPROPRIATE HEALTH CARE
• Outpatient except in very severe cases
• Recommend referral to pulmonary or infectious disease specialist if drug treatment becomes imperative. Consider such treatment if IgG titers > 1:16, if disease persists without improvement over 6 weeks, or if skin test remains negative in the face of positive serology.

GENERAL MEASURES
• Cool mist humidifier for dry cough or sore throat
• Rest
• Supportive therapy

ACTIVITY
As tolerated

DIET
No special diet

PATIENT EDUCATION
For patient education materials favorably reviewed on this topic, contact: American Lung Association, 1740 Broadway, New York, NY 10019, (212)315-8700

MEDICATIONS

DRUG(S) OF CHOICE
• In mild cases, treat for symptomatic relief of cough with antitussives plus treat pleuritic pain with nonsteroidal anti-inflammatory agents
For persistent, progressive, or disseminated disease:
◊ Amphotericin B - 0.5-1.0 mg/kg with a total cumulative dose of 2-4 gm
◊ Ketoconazole - 200-400 mg/day
◊ Fluconazole - refer to drug reference for current dosage recommendation
Contraindications: Avoid steroids
Precautions: Amphotericin is highly nephrotoxic.
Significant possible interactions: Refer to manufacturer's profile of each drug. Ketoconazole and H2 blockers (ketoconazole requires an acidic pH for absorption).

ALTERNATIVE DRUGS N/A

FOLLOWUP

PATIENT MONITORING
• If skin test and serology are negative but index of suspicion is high, repeat every 2 weeks. With positive serologies, follow titers every 2 weeks until titers are dropping and patient has clinical improvement or resolution.
• Follow abnormal chest x-rays until findings are resolved or scarring process is complete

PREVENTION/AVOIDANCE
• Not contagious between host and contacts
• Cultures in lab are highly contagious via inhalation and lab personnel must be very cautious when handling specimens
• High risk populations (see Risk factors) should consider avoiding high risk activities, such as construction, archaeological digs, etc.)

POSSIBLE COMPLICATIONS Severe cases are fatal, especially if associated with meningitis. Can cause destruction of pulmonary tissue due to scarring, cavities, etc.
• Hemoptysis

EXPECTED COURSE AND PROGNOSIS
• Most cases are self-limited, resolve within a few months. Progressive and disseminated disease can be difficult to eradicate.
• Prognosis poor if weak cell mediated immunity response or high IgG
• Relapse of extrapulmonary or disseminated disease is common.

MISCELLANEOUS

ASSOCIATED CONDITIONS N/A

AGE-RELATED FACTORS
Pediatric: N/A
Geriatric: N/A
Others: N/A

PREGNANCY Increased risk for dissemination, especially if contracted late in gestation

SYNONYMS
• Cocci
• Desert fever
• Posada-Wernicke disease
• Valley fever
• San Joaquin fever

ICD-9-CM 114.9

SEE ALSO N/A

OTHER NOTES Travel history is essential when working up any pulmonary infection not responding to normal measures

ABBREVIATIONS N/A

REFERENCES
• Braunwald E., et al. (eds.): Harrison's Principles of Internal Medicine. 12th Ed. New York, McGraw-Hill, 1991
• Hedges, E. & Miller, S.: Coccidiomycosis: Office Diagnosis and Treatment. Amer Fam Phys. May, 1990

Author S. Miller, M.D.

Colic, infantile

BASICS

DESCRIPTION Colic is an incompletely understood state of excessive crying seen in young infants who are otherwise well. A working definition - abnormal crying that lasts > 3 hours/day for at least 3 times/week.
Incidence/Prevalence in U.S.A.:
10,000/100,000 in some reports, as high as 25,000/100,000 in others
System(s) affected: Gastrointestinal, Nervous
Genetics: N/A
Predominant Age: 3 weeks of age to 3 months of age
Predominant Sex: Male = Female

SIGNS AND SYMPTOMS
• Rhythmic crying, paroxysmal
• No consolability
• Fist clenching
• Back arching
• Drawing up of infant's legs
• Excessive flatus

CAUSES
• Poorly understood
• Small percentage related to milk allergy

RISK FACTORS Physiologic predisposition in infant

DIAGNOSIS

DIFFERENTIAL DIAGNOSIS
• Any organic cause for excessive crying in infants (i.e. meningitis, sepsis, strangulated hernia, occult fracture)
• Entirely a clinical diagnosis

LABORATORY N/A
Drugs that may alter lab results: N/A
Disorders that may alter lab results: N/A

PATHOLOGICAL FINDINGS N/A

SPECIAL TESTS N/A

IMAGING N/A

DIAGNOSTIC PROCEDURES N/A

TREATMENT

APPROPRIATE HEALTH CARE
Outpatient management

GENERAL MEASURES
• Handling of the colicky infant in a calm and non-stimulating manner should be demonstrated
• Use of pacifier
• Use of gentle rhythmic motion (i.e., car rides)
• Use of music

ACTIVITY N/A

DIET Removal of cow's milk from diet for a one week trial

PATIENT EDUCATION American Academy of Pediatrics, 141 Northwest Point Blvd., P.O. Box 927, Elk Grove Village, IL 60009-0927, (800)433-9016

MEDICATIONS

DRUG(S) OF CHOICE Simethicone may be useful in some cases
Contraindications: N/A
Precautions: N/A
Significant possible interactions: N/A

ALTERNATIVE DRUGS N/A

FOLLOWUP

PATIENT MONITORING Frequent outpatient visits as needed for parental reassurance and education

EXPECTED COURSE AND PROGNOSIS
• Usually subsides by 3 months of age
• Prognosis not sufficiently investigated

PREVENTION/AVOIDANCE N/A

POSSIBLE COMPLICATIONS N/A

MISCELLANEOUS

ASSOCIATED CONDITIONS N/A

AGE-RELATED FACTORS
Pediatric: A problem of infancy
Geriatric: N/A
Others: N/A

PREGNANCY N/A
Others: N/A

SYNONYMS N/A

ICD-9-CM 789.0 abdominal pain

SEE ALSO N/A

OTHER NOTES N/A

ABBREVIATIONS N/A

REFERENCES
• Behrman, R.E. & Kleigman, R.M.: Nelson Textbook of Pediatrics. Philadelphia, W.B. Saunders Co., 1992

Author J. Dansky, M.D.

Colorectal cancer

BASICS

DESCRIPTION A malignant neoplasm arising from the luminal surface of the colon, rectum or anus.
• Adenocarcinoma - by far, most common histologic form, usually arising from benign adenoma. Unequally distributed, with 38% in proximal colon and 62% in distal colon or rectum.
• Carcinoid - uncommon, arising from enterochromaffin cells. Usually located in appendix or rectum; not likely to metastasize unless larger than 2 cm in diameter.
• Squamous cell carcinoma - uncommon form; located in the anal canal. Also called epidermoid or cloacogenic.
• Melanoma - rare; usually presents as pigmented lesion adjacent to dentate line
System(s) affected: Gastrointestinal
Genetics:
• Hereditary autosomal dominant in 5-10%; first-degree relative in 20%
• Ras oncogene mutations seen in 40-50% of adenocarcinoma; alterations of suppressor genes also seen in 75%, especially involving chromosomes 17,18
Incidence/Prevalence in USA: 155,000 new cases/year
Predominant age: Adenocarcinoma usually occurs in individuals > age 50 years with peak incidence in the seventh decade
Predominant sex: Male = Female

SIGNS AND SYMPTOMS
• Vary with location
• Early lesions are frequently asymptomatic
Right-sided adenocarcinoma
  ◊ Anemia
  ◊ Pain and/or mass in right lower quadrant
  ◊ Occult blood in stool
  ◊ Change in appearance of stool (infrequent)
Left-sided adenocarcinoma
  ◊ Change in bowel habits (may be constipation or diarrhea)
  ◊ Reduced caliber of stool
  ◊ Red blood mixed in stool
Rectal adenocarcinoma
  ◊ Bright red rectal bleeding
  ◊ Tenesmus
  ◊ Mass on digital exam
Carcinoid
  ◊ Often incidental finding
  ◊ Appendicitis-like if located in appendix
  ◊ Rectal bleeding
  ◊ Crampy abdominal pain
  ◊ Carcinoid syndrome; occurs with metastases to liver; includes facial flushing, abdominal cramps, diarrhea
Squamous cell carcinoma
  ◊ Painful defecation
  ◊ Rectal bleeding
  ◊ Mass or ulcer in anal canal
  ◊ Non-healing anal fissure

CAUSES
• Undetermined; both genetic and environmental factors may contribute
• Environmental - high dietary animal fat, low dietary fiber

RISK FACTORS
Adenocarcinoma
  ◊ Two-thirds of patients are over 50 years old
  ◊ Pancolonic ulcerative colitis, (2% per year after 10 years active disease)
  ◊ Familial polyposis (100%)
  ◊ Benign adenomas (tubular 3%; villous 9-12%)
  ◊ Coexisting (synchronous) colon cancer (5%)
  ◊ Previous (metachronous) colon cancer (2-5%)
Carcinoid
  ◊ Multiple endocrine adenopathy (MEA), rare
  ◊ Other organs with carcinoid (small bowel, bronchial)
Squamous cell carcinoma
  ◊ Bowen's disease
  ◊ Paget's disease

DIAGNOSIS

DIFFERENTIAL DIAGNOSIS
• Strictures (ischemic, Crohn's, diverticulosis)
• Other neoplasms (prostatic carcinoma, lipoma, leiomyoma, sarcoma, others)
• Infectious/inflammatory lesions (amoeboma, tuberculoma, hemorrhoids)
• Extrinsic masses (abscesses, cysts/pseudocysts, phlegmons)

LABORATORY
• Positive fecal occult blood test
• Anemia
• Urinary 5-Hydroxyindoleacetic acid (5-HIAA); elevated in carcinoid
• Elevated plasma carcinoembryonic antigen (CEA)
Drugs that may alter lab results:
• Aspirin-containing medications and nonsteroidal anti-inflammatory drugs - positive fecal occult blood test
• Smoking - increased carcinoembryonic antigen
Disorders that may alter lab results:
• Peptic ulcer disease, ulcerative colitis, hemorrhoids, benign polyps - positive fecal occult blood test
• Renal failure - increased carcinoembryonic antigen

PATHOLOGICAL FINDINGS
Adenocarcinoma
  ◊ May appear as ulcerated, polypoid, or fungating mass. May extend to local structures or metastasize by blood, lymphatics; staging of tumor reflects level of penetration.
  ◊ Duke's Stage A - mucosal involvement with or without submucosal extension
  ◊ Duke's Stage B1 - to muscularis propria but not through serosa
  ◊ Duke's Stage B2 - extends beyond serosa
  ◊ Duke's Stage C - regional nodes involved
  ◊ Duke's Stage D - distant metastases (liver, lung)
Carcinoid
  ◊ Tend to be multicentric
  ◊ Metastasize by blood, lymphatics
Squamous cell carcinoma
  ◊ Most are ulcerative but may vary greatly in size
  ◊ Metastasize to inguinal lymphatics

SPECIAL TESTS Carcinoembryonic antigen - usually elevated with bulky tumor or metastases

IMAGING
• Barium enema (air-contrast preferred) - may not be necessary if colonoscopy is complete and provides adequate diagnostic information
• Computed tomography - sometimes used to determine extent of pelvic or liver involvement; not usually necessary
• Transrectal ultrasound - may be useful in defining extent of involvement by small rectal lesions

DIAGNOSTIC PROCEDURES
• Anoscopy - useful for anal canal visualization, biopsies
• Proctoscopy/flexible sigmoidoscopy with biopsy - used for distal lesions when complementary barium enema available for proximal colon
• Colonoscopy with biopsy - for primary diagnosis, screening of high-risk patients and post-resection surveillance

TREATMENT

APPROPRIATE HEALTH CARE
Inpatient

GENERAL MEASURES
• Surgical procedures - radical resection of tumor with wide margins; includes segments of normal colon, mesentery, lymph nodes
• Right hemicolectomy for proximal tumors
• Left hemicolectomy for descending colon cancers
• Sigmoid colectomy for sigmoid cancers
• Abdominoperineal resection with colostomy for cancers of distal rectum (within 5-7 cm of dentate line)
• Preoperative or postoperative radiotherapy and chemotherapy: May improve outcome when used for rectal carcinoma
• For carcinoma of anus - combined chemotherapy (5-fluorouracil and mitomycin C) and radiotherapy. Convert to abdominoperineal resection for residual or recurrent tumor.

ACTIVITY
Usually normal; may be slightly modified for patient with stoma

DIET
Usually normal; avoidance of gas-producing foods may be helpful in ostomates (cabbage, beans, onions, alcoholic beverages)

PATIENT EDUCATION
• Facts on Colorectal Cancer, American Cancer Society, 1988
• National Cancer Institute, Dept. of Health And Human Services, Public Inquiries Section, Office of Cancer Communications, Building 31, Room 101-18, 9000 Rockville Pike, Bethesda, MD 20892, (301)496-5583,

MEDICATIONS

DRUG(S) OF CHOICE
• Steroids, somatostatin or methysergide may ameliorate symptoms of carcinoid syndrome
• Stage C adenocarcinoma - 5-FU plus levamisole
Contraindications: Peptic ulcer disease (steroids)
Precautions: Refer to manufacturer's literature
Significant possible interactions: Refer to manufacturer's literature

ALTERNATIVE DRUGS N/A

FOLLOWUP

PATIENT MONITORING
Adenocarcinoma (after remainder of colon is cleared of all lesions)
◊ Colonoscopy - annually x 2 years; then every 3 years
◊ Carcinoembryonic antigen test, liver chemistries, fecal occult blood test - every three months for 2 years; then every 6 months for 2 years; then annually
Carcinoid:
◊ 5-HIAA every 6 months x 2 years, then annually
Squamous cell carcinoma:
◊ Clinical evaluation every 4 months x 1 year, then annually
◊ Biopsy suspicious areas in anus, groin

PREVENTION/AVOIDANCE
Colonic polyps should be removed, examined microscopically. If benign, surveillance colonscopy should be performed every 3 years.

POSSIBLE COMPLICATIONS
Following resections:
◊ Mortality 5-10%
◊ Wound infection 5-15%
◊ Anastomotic stricture/leak/abscess 2-5%
◊ Pneumonia 5-10%
◊ Urinary tract infection 5-20%
During chemotherapy or radiation therapy:
◊ Stomatitis
◊ Proctitis/diarrhea
◊ Temporary loss of hair

EXPECTED COURSE AND PROGNOSIS
Adenocarcinoma:
◊ Overall 5-year survival is 55% but relates to tumor stage in individual patients
◊ Duke's A - 95%
◊ Duke's B1 - 85-90%
◊ Duke's B2 - 60-70%
◊ Duke's C - 15-25%
◊ Duke's D - 5%
Carcinoid:
◊ Overall 5-year survival is 65%
◊ Relates to tumor stage as in adenocarcinoma
Squamous cell carcinoma:
◊ Overall 5-year survival is 79%

MISCELLANEOUS

ASSOCIATED CONDITIONS
Colonic carcinoid - multiple endocrine neoplasia types I, II

AGE-RELATED FACTORS
Pediatric: Adenocarcinoma of colon occurs rarely in children; prognosis is very poor
Geriatric: Coexistence of medical illness may complicate postoperative course
Others: N/A

PREGNANCY N/A

SYNONYMS N/A

ICD-9-CM
• 1540 (colorectal cancer)
• 44144 (colectomy)

SEE ALSO N/A

OTHER NOTES N/A

ABBREVIATIONS N/A

REFERENCES
• Silverman, A.L, Desai, T.K., Dhar, R., et al.: Clinical Features, Evaluation, and Detection of Colorectal Cancer. Gastroenterology Clinics of North America, December 1988. 17:713-25
• Twomey, P., Burchell, M., Strawn, D. Guernsey, J.: Local Control in Rectal Cancer. A Clinical Review and Meta-analysis, Arch Surg, 1989. 124:1174-9
• Vogelstein, B., Fearon, E.R., Hamilton, S.R., et al. Genetic Alterations During Colorectal-tumor Development. N. Engl J. Med, 1988. 319:525-32

Author WH Schwesinger, M.D.

Common cold

BASICS

DESCRIPTION Usually a minor, self-limited, viral infection of the mucosa of the upper respiratory tract, especially the nose, manifested by sneezing, nasal obstruction and discharge, and lasting an average of 6-10 days (range 2-26 days)
System(s) affected: Pulmonary
Genetics: N/A
Incidence/Prevalence in USA: The most frequent illness occurring in humans (41/100 persons per year), accounting for more days of restricted activity than any other
Predominant age: Affects all age groups, but especially children
Predominant sex: Female > Male (slightly)

SIGNS AND SYMPTOMS
General
◊ Coryza (rhinorrhea and sneezing) 50-66%
◊ Sore throat (pharyngitis) almost 50%
◊ Hoarseness and cough 25-50%
◊ Headache 25%
◊ Muscular aches, lethargy, and malaise variable, about 25-45%
◊ Fever and chills variable, about 15-30%
Sequence of symptoms and signs
◊ At the beginning there is loss of sense of well-being, scratchy eyes, burning sensation inside the nose, and discomfort in the nasopharynx
◊ These are soon followed by sneezing, nasal obstruction, and clear nasal discharge
◊ Systemic symptoms (may be worse in children) - malaise, lethargy, headache, chilliness, low grade fever, and aching - are worse during the first two or three days
◊ In the uncomplicated cold, systemic symptoms disappear first, but nasal obstruction and discharge continue and may be accompanied by hoarseness, sore throat, and dry cough
◊ The discharge becomes cloudy or yellowish towards the end of a week and generally disappears within 7-10 days
◊ Nasal mucosa thickened and edematous, usually redder than normal, and covered with a thin watery or cloudy mucous

CAUSES
• Transmission of viruses directly via personal contact, infected droplets of respiratory discharge, and by hand to conjunctiva, nose, and face
Virus types:
◊ Rhinoviruses (100 serotypes) 15-40%
◊ Coronaviruses (at least 3 serotypes) 10-20%
◊ Influenza (A, B, C) 1-5%
◊ Parainfluenza viruses (4 serotypes) 1-5%
◊ Respiratory syncytial virus (one serotype) 1-5%
◊ Adenoviruses (various) 1-5%
◊ Coxsackie viruses (various) 1-2%
◊ Echoviruses (various) 1-2%
◊ Group A beta-hemolytic streptococci 2-10%
◊ No specific agent known (but presumed viral) 30-50%

RISK FACTORS
• Children attending school or daycare
• Parents and siblings of children attending schools or daycare
• Large families
• Secondary attack rate 25% among family members
• Unhygienic family practices
• Cold weather, fatigue, and sleep loss have not been implicated in etiology in experimental studies, even though common colds occur more frequently during winter months

DIAGNOSIS

DIFFERENTIAL DIAGNOSIS
• Influenza (more severe fever, headache, cough and prostration)
• Rubeola (early stages, before rash)
• Rubella (early stages, before rash)
• Mycoplasma pneumoniae infections (more severe and prolonged, patchy pneumonitis not uncommon)
• Concomitant Group A beta-hemolytic streptococcal infection
• Allergic rhinitis (seasonal or perennial)
• Foreign bodies in nose, especially in children
• Secondary bacterial sinusitis and bronchitis
• Secondary bacterial otitis media

LABORATORY
• No specific laboratory tests outside special research labs
• CBC usually normal
Drugs that may alter lab results: N/A
Disorders that may alter lab results: N/A

PATHOLOGICAL FINDINGS
• Histologically, mucosa sparsely infiltrated with neutrophils, lymphocytes, plasma cells, and eosinophils
• Sloughed ciliated epithelial cells in nasal secretions

SPECIAL TESTS
• In office tests for mycoplasma and identification of streptococci
• Bacterial cultures for sinusitis and otitis media are usually not helpful, except in special circumstances
• Nasal smears for leukocytes and eosinophils when allergic rhinitis and sinusitis are being considered

IMAGING
• Radiographs of paranasal sinuses are helpful, but usually unnecessary
• CT and MRI scans useful when serious bacterial complications are suspected

DIAGNOSTIC PROCEDURES
• Fiberoptic nasopharyngoscopy when diagnosis is difficult or complications supervene. Ordinarily not needed.
• Diagnosis is usually entirely clinical, because recovery techniques for viruses are difficult and impractical

TREATMENT

APPROPRIATE HEALTH CARE
Outpatient self-care

GENERAL MEASURES
• Stop smoking
• Limit alcohol intake
• Increase humidity in inspired air by means of steam or cold vaporizers, especially in bedroom (effectiveness of this routine versus stale aerolization of molds ahazard)

ACTIVITY Ambulatory with increased rest first 2-3 days

DIET Regular diet with increased fluid intake

PATIENT EDUCATION
• Teach the expected course, self-care and variations that require physician examination
• Inform about communicability through physical contact, droplet spread
• Discourage inappropriate use of antibiotics
• Advise that immunity to colds is short-lived and that new infections can occur each time there is an exposure
• Additional materials from: American Academy of Family Physicians Foundation, P.O. Box 8418, Kansas City, MO 64114, (800)274-2237, ext. 4400

MEDICATIONS

DRUG(S) OF CHOICE
• There are no preventive or curative drugs, but symptoms can be partially relieved
Oral analgesics:
◊ Aspirin, or acetaminophen (Tylenol and others) 325-650 mg qid for systemic symptoms
◊ Ibuprofen (Motrin, Advil, and others) can be substituted at doses of 400 mg qid
◊ Codeine in small doses, 30 mg bid-qid can be added to aspirin or acetaminophen when systemic symptoms more severe
Oral decongestants:
◊ Pseudoephedrine (Sudafed and others), phenylephrine, and phenylpropanolamine are available over the counter. They are less effective than topical oxymetazoline and may have undesirable side effects.
Antitussives:
◊ Dextromethorphan 10 mg, and codeine 15 mg, are equally effective against cough
◊ Either may be combined in liquid preparations with Guaifenesin 100 mg, (a mucolytic), Robitussin-DM and others. (Note: mucolytic properties not proven.)
Antihistamines:
◊ Limited to control of troublesome rhinorrhea
◊ Caution should be used to prevent over drying of nasal mucosa
Vitamin C:
◊ Does not prevent common colds but might reduce days of disability. Current evidence neither supports nor repudiates its regular use in small or large doses.
Topical decongestants:
◊ Nose drops or sprays containing oxymetazoline 0.05% (Afrin and others) can be used for severe nasal obstruction, but not longer than 3-4 days to avoid rebound hyperemia/congestion. Use generously twice daily.
Antibiotics:
◊ Not indicated in uncomplicated colds
◊ Prescribe towards end of the first week when symptoms are not improving, or getting worse
◊ Patients with concomitant allergic rhinitis and history of repeated bacterial sinusitis might benefit from earlier use, particularly if purulence evolves or emerges. (After 10 days the probability of bacterial secondary infection increases to 80%.)
◊ Choose an antibiotic presumed to be effective against Gram positive cocci, Hemophilus influenzae, B. catarrhalis (Moraxella), and anaerobes
◊ Erythromycin, amoxicillin, and sulfisoxazole-trimethoprim are empiric first line agents for adults
◊ Amoxicillin and erythromycin-sulfisoxazole are useful for children

◊ Alternative drugs, especially for beta lactamase producing organisms, include amoxicillin/clavulanate (Augmentin), cephalosporins, and tetracyclines
◊ There is often an unspoken tug-of-war between patients and physicians about the appropriate use of antibiotics. In the primary care setting scientific dogmatism must be balanced against the patient's previous experience, plus the fact that bacterial sinusitis in its early stages is a clinical diagnosis.
Contraindications: Aspirin should not be given to children because of the association of Reye's syndrome in certain viral infections that might resemble a common cold at the onset, such as influenza or chicken pox
Precautions:
• Oral decongestants, except pseudoephedrine, should not be used in hypertensive patients. They can produce tachycardia and urinary retention. Phenylpropanolamine is the most potent sympathomimetic of the three, stimulates the CNS, and can cause rebound depressive symptoms, hence is subject to abuse in the unwary.
• Aspirin and ibuprofen can cause gastritis and bleeding
• Codeine can cause itching, vomiting and constipation, and in large doses CNS sedation. It may be abused by addicts, but has little addicting potential in others when used in appropriate doses for a few days. Codeine analogs (e.g., hydrocodone) are addicting.
• Antihistamines can be sedating and their anticholinergic effects produce drying of the respiratory mucosa (when it needs to be moist)
• Allergy to antibiotics
• Erythromycin can cause indigestion, abdominal pain and vomiting. The others can facilitate Candida vaginitis.
• Sulfa can produce toxic skin reactions and renal damage
• Broad spectrum penicillins may cause diarrhea
• Tetracyclines should not be prescribed for children because of teeth staining
• Topical decongestants can produce rebound nasal congestion and habituation when used longer than a few days at a time
Significant possible interactions: Syrups should not be used in insulin dependent diabetics

ALTERNATIVE DRUGS
• Interferon nasal sprays may prevent respiratory infections but has no use in treatment
• Virucidal paper handkerchiefs may prove to be helpful in preventing spread of the common cold

FOLLOWUP

PATIENT MONITORING Scheduled followup visits are not necessary if patient education has been appropriate

PREVENTION/AVOIDANCE Careful handwashing

POSSIBLE COMPLICATIONS
• Bacterial infections of paranasal sinuses and middle ears
• Rarely serious bacterial infections of adjacent tissues and structures, e.g., osteomyelitis, cavernous sinus thrombophlebitis, epidural or subdural abscess, meningitis, and brain abscess
• Herpes simplex infections of the nose, lips, and face can become activated

EXPECTED COURSE AND PROGNOSIS
100% recovery expected

MISCELLANEOUS

ASSOCIATED CONDITIONS
• Bronchitis
• Bronchiolitis
• Bronchopneumonia
• Pneumonia
• Croup
• Asthma

AGE-RELATED FACTORS
Pediatric: Highest frequency from ages 1-5 years (about 7-8 colds per year) compared to about 4 per year in older children
Geriatric: N/A
Others: N/A

PREGNANCY N/A

ICD-9-CM 460-

SYNONYMS
• Acute upper respiratory infection
• URI

SEE ALSO N/A

OTHER NOTES N/A

ABBREVIATIONS N/A

REFERENCES
• Wyngaarden, J.B., Smith, L.H. (eds): Cecil Textbook of Medicine. 19th Ed. Philadelphia, W.B. Saunders Co., 1992
• Rachelefsky, G., Katz, R., & Siegel, S.: Pediatric Allergic Disease: Chronic Sinusitis in the Allergic Child. Pediatric Clinic of North America, Vol.35:5, Philadelphia, W.B. Saunders Co., Oct. 1988
• Meyers, B.R.: Antimicrobial Therapy Guide. 4th Ed. Newtown, PA, Antibiotic Prescribing, Inc., 1990

Author G. Stephens, M.D.

Complete atrioventricular (AV) canal

BASICS

DESCRIPTION The central atrioventricular (AV) portion of the cardiac septum and the contiguous mitral and tricuspid valves are abnormal, allowing for an unobstructed atrioventricular canal. Children with Down syndrome and this anomaly rapidly progress to pulmonary vascular obstructive disease (within 3 to 6 months).

Rastelli classification:
◊ Type A: Common anterior AV valve leaflet is divided and attached to the crest of the ventricular septum by chordae
◊ Type B: Common anterior AV valve leaflet is divided and chordae tendineae from the midportions of the divided anterior leaflet are attached to the right ventricular medial papillary muscle
◊ Type C: Common anterior AV valve leaflet is undivided and not attached to the ventricular septum (free-floating leaflet)
System(s) affected: Cardiovascular
Genetics: No known genetic pattern
Incidence/Prevalence in USA: 1 in 250,000 live births; type A being the most common
Predominant age: Congenital, present at birth
Predominant sex: Female > Male

SIGNS AND SYMPTOMS
• Pulmonary congestion
• Congestive heart failure
• Low systemic arterial blood oxygen saturation
• Tachycardia
• Poor feeding
• Growth failure
• Mitral regurgitation
• Pulmonary vascular obstructive disease, and cyanosis (30% in the first 2-3 years)

CAUSES Defective development of the endocardial cushions

RISK FACTORS Unknown

DIAGNOSIS

DIFFERENTIAL DIAGNOSIS
• Atrial septal defect
• Ventricular septal defect
• Incomplete or intermediate AV canal
• Patent ductus arteriosus
• Mitral valve prolapse
• Secondary mitral regurgitation
• Pulmonary vascular obstructive disease
• Anomalous pulmonary venous return

LABORATORY Arterial blood gas
Drugs that may alter lab results: N/A
Disorders that may alter lab results: N/A

PATHOLOGICAL FINDINGS Low oxygen saturation in the arterial blood gas

SPECIAL TESTS
• Cardiac 2-D echo-Doppler showing anatomic defect, increased pulmonary pressures, mitral regurgitation, tricuspid regurgitation, right and left atrial and ventricular enlargements
• EKG - superior QRS axis, right ventricular hypertrophy (RVH), left ventricular hypertrophy (LVH), possibly peaked P waves

IMAGING
• Cardiac angiogram demonstrating AV canal and mitral and tricuspid regurgitation, left and right atrial and ventricular enlargement
• Chest x-ray showing increased pulmonary vasculature, left and right atrial and ventricular enlargement
• MRI offers excellent imaging of crux

DIAGNOSTIC PROCEDURES
• Pulmonary artery catheter showing prominent "V" waves, elevated pulmonary capillary wedge pressures, right atrial "step-up" in oxygen saturations
• Angiography

TREATMENT

APPROPRIATE HEALTH CARE Medical management (lanoxin, diuretics, afterload reducers) either as an inpatient or an outpatient, dependent upon the patient's condition

GENERAL MEASURES
• If pulmonary edema, growth failure and congestive heart failure is refractive in spite of optimal medical therapy, reparative surgery should be pursued as early as possible. Repair should be especially early in children with Down's syndrome (approximately 3 months). Repair should be performed before 2 years of age to avoid the continued progression of pulmonary vascular obstructive disease. Patients more than 2 years of age can undergo repair if the pulmonary vascular resistance (PVR) does not exceed 8-10 units-meters squared. At a minimum, surgical correction includes closure of the interatrial and interventricular septal defects and suspension of the medial aspects of the left and right AV valve leaflets. Pulmonary artery banding might still be a possibility.
• Provide general treatment for congestive heart failure

ACTIVITY As tolerated

DIET High calorie, low salt

PATIENT EDUCATION Instruct regarding travel to altitudes and plane travel causing potential hypoxia

Complete atrioventricular (AV) canal

MEDICATIONS

DRUG(S) OF CHOICE Digoxin, ACE inhibitors or isosorbide dinitrate plus hydralazine, furosemide, potassium supplementation
Doses for term infants
   ◊ Digoxin - oral 30 mcg/kg (digitalizing), then 10 mcg/kg/24 hrs. Adjust to maintain levels within therapeutic range - 0.5-2.0 ng/mL
   ◊ Captopril - 0.05-0.1 mg/kg/dose tid-qid
   ◊ Isosorbide - refer to manufacturer's literature
   ◊ Hydralazine - 0.75-3.0 mg/kg/dose, increase as needed to maximum of 6 mg/kg/dose
   ◊ Furosemide - oral 2 mg/kg, increase as needed to maximum of 6 mg/kg
   ◊ Potassium - supplement patients who require furosemide. Maintenance dose is 2-3 mEq/kg/24 hours.
Contraindications: Profound systemic hypotension, worsening hypoxia and V/Q mismatch with treatment
Precautions: Refer to manufacturer's literature
Significant possible interactions: Refer to manufacturer's literature

ALTERNATIVE DRUGS Dobutamine or amrinone drips

FOLLOWUP

PATIENT MONITORING
 • As indicated by clinical intervention and disease progression
 • Serial measurements of arterial oxygen content
 • Serial measurements of pulmonary vascular resistance

PREVENTION/AVOIDANCE Avoid hypoxic embarrassment in environments of low oxygen tension

POSSIBLE COMPLICATIONS
 • Refractive hypoxia secondary to progressive pulmonary vascular obstructive disease
 • Cyanosis
 • Polycythemia
 • Growth failure
 • Congestive heart failure/pulmonary edema
Complications of surgery:
   ◊ Residual ventricular septal defect
   ◊ Residual left ventricular to right atrial shunting
   ◊ Complete A-V block

EXPECTED COURSE AND PROGNOSIS
PVR less than 5:
   ◊ If undergoing reparative surgery, are at risk for an approximate 10% surgical mortality
   ◊ The majority of those surviving realize complete relief of their symptoms and will need no further treatment
PVR between 5-13 undergoing surgery:
   ◊ Perioperative mortality approachs 33%
   ◊ Survivors realize functional class I or II (New York Heart Association [NYHA] classification)
PVR greater than 5 who do not or can not undergo surgical intervention:
   ◊ Deterioration is progressive with death ranging from 2-16 years of age

MISCELLANEOUS

ASSOCIATED CONDITIONS
 • Down's syndrome. Very high percentage have complete atrioventricular canal lesions.
 • Tetralogy of Fallot
 • Unbalanced canal with left or right dominance

AGE-RELATED FACTORS
Pediatric: Surgical intervention before age 2 or before marked increase in PVR occurs
Geriatric: N/A
Others: N/A

PREGNANCY N/A

SYNONYMS N/A

ICD-9-CM 745.69

SEE ALSO
 • Congenital heart disease
 • Atrioventricular canal defect

OTHER NOTES N/A

ABBREVIATIONS
 AVC = atrioventricular canal
 PVR = pulmonary vascular resistance

REFERENCES
 • Brandenburg, R.O., Fuster, V., Giuliani, E.R. & McGoon, D.C.: Cardiology: Fundamentals and Practice. Chicago, Year Book Medical Publishers, 1987
 • Braunwald, E. (ed): Heart Disease: A Textbook of Cardiovascular Medicine. 3rd Ed. Philadelphia, W.B. Saunders Co., 1988

Author D. Framm, M.D.

Condyloma acuminata

 BASICS

DESCRIPTION
Condyloma acuminata are soft, skin colored, fleshy warts that are caused by the HPV (human papilloma virus). There are at least 60 known types of HPV and types 6, 11, 16, 18, 31, 33 have been associated with condyloma acuminata. The disease is highly contagious, can appear singly or in groups, small or large. They appear in the vagina, on the cervix, around the external genitalia and rectum and occasionally, the throat. The incubation period may be from 1-6 months.
Genetics: N/A
Incidence/Prevalence: Minimum of 10-20% of sexually active women may be infected with HPV. Studies in men suggest a similar prevalence.
Predominant Age: 15-30 years of age
Predominant Sex: Male = Female

SIGNS AND SYMPTOMS
• Tumors, soft, sessile
• Surface smooth to very rough
• Multiple fingerlike projections
• Perianal condylomata acuminatum usually rough and cauliflower-like
• Penile lesions often smooth and papular
• Penile lesions often occur in groups of three or four
• Male sites - frenulum, corona, glans, prepuce, meatus, shaft, scrotum
• Female sites - labia, clitoris, periurethral area, perineum, vagina, cervix (flat lesions)
• Pruritis
• Irritation
• Bleeding (result of trauma)
• Perianal area (both sexes)
• Subclinical HPV infection
• May be detected by Pap test

CAUSES
Human papilloma viruses. These are circular double-stranded DNA molecules. There are over 60 HPV subtypes. The cause of common venereal warts are types 6 and 11. Cervical dysplasia and carcinoma in situ are likely caused by types 16, 18, 31, 33, and 34.

RISK FACTORS
• Young adult
• Sexually active
• Not using condoms
• Possibly subclinical infection
• Young age of commencing sexual activity
• Cigarette smoking
• Poor hygiene
• Pregnancy
• Caucasian
• History of genital warts

 DIAGNOSIS

DIFFERENTIAL DIAGNOSIS
• Condyloma lata (flat warts of syphilis)
• Lichen planus
• Normal sebaceous glands
• Seborrheic keratosis
• Molluscum contagiosum
• Keratomas
• Scabies

LABORATORY
Serologic test for syphilis - negative
Drugs that may alter lab results: N/A
Disorders that may alter lab results: N/A

PATHOLOGICAL FINDINGS
• Possible cervical dysplasia in females
• Benign
• Well organized basal layer
• Underlying infiltration of lymphocytes
• Plasma cells
• Hyperplastic epithelial changes
• Basement membrane intact
• Sometimes difficult to differentiate from squamous cell carcinoma

SPECIAL TESTS
Acetowhitening: Subclinical lesions can be visualized by wrapping the penis with gauze soaked with 5% acetic acid for 5 minutes. Using a IOX hand lens or colposcope, warts appear as tiny white papules. A shiny white appearance of the skin represents foci of epithelial hyperplasia (subclinical infection).

IMAGING
N/A

DIAGNOSTIC PROCEDURES
• Biopsy with highly specialized identification techniques (not clinically useful)
• Colposcopy, androscopy, anoscopy, Pap smear

 TREATMENT

APPROPRIATE HEALTH CARE
Outpatient

GENERAL MEASURES
• Treatment determined by location and size of warts
• Small warts may be treated with topical applications
• Cryotherapy
• Larger warts require laser treatment or electrocoagulation
• Surgical excision for large warts

ACTIVITY
No restrictions

DIET
No special diet

PATIENT EDUCATION
• Explain preventive measures and chronic nature of the infection
• Numerous pamphlets on HPV, STD prevention, condom use
• Emphasize need for women to get regular Pap smears

MEDICATIONS

DRUG(S) OF CHOICE
• Podophyllum in tincture of Benzoin. Apply directly to warts. Leave on for 6 hours, then wash off. Repeat treatment every 7 days until gone
or
• Podofilox (Condylox) - for external warts. Apply to external warts every 12 hours (allowing to dry) for 3 consecutive days. May repeat after 4 days
or
• Cryotherapy - liquid nitrogen is applied to warts in 5-10 second bursts. Usually requires 2-3 weekly sessions.
• Internal warts - topical 5-Fluorouracil or intralesional alpha interferon
Contraindications:
• Podophyllin - do not use during pregnancy or on oral, cervical, urethral or perianal warts. Can use on small number of vaginal warts with careful drying after application.
• Cryotherapy - none
Precautions:
• Podophyllin - to minimize local and systemic reactions, wash treated areas 6-8 hours after application and use ointments to protect surrounding skin from contact with podophyllin
• Cryotherapy - none
Significant Possible Interactions: N/A

ALTERNATIVE DRUGS   N/A

FOLLOWUP

PATIENT MONITORING
• Every 2 weeks for treatment until clear
• Pap test every 1 year for indefinite period
• Biopsy for persistent warts
• Monitor sex partners

PREVENTION/AVOIDANCE
• Use of condoms by infected men
• Use of condoms by male sexual partners of individuals who have been treated for HPV infection
• Abstinence by women until treatment completed
• Circumcision may prevent recurrence in some men

POSSIBLE COMPLICATIONS
• Cervical dysplasia
• Carcinoma - cervical (squamous or adenocarcinoma) penile or rectal
• Male urethral obstruction

EXPECTED COURSE AND PROGNOSIS
• Warts clear with treatment or spontaneous regression
• Recurrence is common with all forms of therapy
• Asymptomatic infection persists indefinitely

MISCELLANEOUS

ASSOCIATED CONDITIONS
• 90% of cervical cancer contains evidence of HPV infection
• Gonorrhea
  Syphilis
• AIDS
• Chlamydia
• Other sexually transmitted disease

AGE-RELATED FACTORS   Young adults, infants and children
Pediatric: N/A
Geriatric: N/A
Others: Venereal warts are increasing in an ever younger population. A recent study of 487 college women showed an infection rate of 48%.

PREGNANCY
• Warts often grow larger in pregnancy and regress spontaneously after delivery. Use cryotherapy.
• HPV can be transmitted to infant at time of delivery and cause laryngeal papillomas

SYNONYMS
• Genital warts
• Venereal warts
• Papilloma acuminatum

ICD-9-CM   078.1 condyloma acuminatum

SEE ALSO   N/A

OTHER NOTES   N/A

ABBREVIATIONS   N/A

REFERENCES
• Connell, E.B. & Tatum, H.J.: Sexually Transmitted Diseases. Durant, OK, Creative Informatives, 1985
• Fitzpatrick, T.B., et al.: Color Atlas and Synopsis of Clinical Dermatology. New York, McGraw-Hill, 1989

Author   R. Daigneault, M.D., F.A.A.P. & K. Bauman, M.D.

Congenital megacolon

 BASICS

DESCRIPTION
Congenital disease of the colon, characterized by functional obstruction and accumulation of feces and massive dilatation of colon

System(s) affected: Gastrointestinal, Nervous

Genetics: Familial 50 times base rate. Sometimes associated with Down's syndrome.

Incidence/Prevalence in USA: 1 in 2000 to 5000 births (Caucasians 91%, Blacks 8%, Oriental 0.5%)

Predominant age: Infancy

Predominant sex:
• Males > Females for short segment (8:2)
• Males > Females for long segment (5:4)

SIGNS AND SYMPTOMS
• Stools in pellets or ribbons with pasty consistency
Early infancy:
  ◊ Onset early in infancy, newborn fails to pass meconium in 24 to 48 hours after birth
    ◊ Obstipation
    ◊ Marked enlargement and distention of abdomen
    ◊ Colonic peristalsis visible
    ◊ Vomiting
    ◊ Palpable fecal mass
    ◊ Growth retardation (possible)
Older infants:
    ◊ Failure to thrive
    ◊ Anorexia
    ◊ Lack of physiologic urge to defecate
    ◊ Empty rectum on digital examination
    ◊ Palpable colon
    ◊ Visible peristalsis
    ◊ Hypoalbuminemia

CAUSES
Congenital absence of Auerbach's and Meissener's autonomic plexuses in bowel wall - usually limited to the colon

RISK FACTORS
• Family history of Hirschsprung's disease
• Offspring risk if parent has short segment - 2%; if parent has long segment - up to 50%
• Sibling risk if male affected - female has 0.6% risk (short segment)
• Sibling risk if female affected - male has 18% risk (long segment)

 DIAGNOSIS

DIFFERENTIAL DIAGNOSIS
• Megacolon, secondary (to Chagas' disease)
• Megacolon, acquired, functional
• Functional constipation
• Hypoganglionosis
• Meconium plug syndrome
• Small left colon syndrome
• Meconium ileus

LABORATORY
Electrolytes, albumin, CBC, urinalysis, thyroid function

Drugs that may alter lab results: N/A

Disorders that may alter lab results: N/A

PATHOLOGICAL FINDINGS
• Congenital absence of Auerbach's and Meissner's autonomic plexuses in myenteric plexus of colon wall
• Obstruction may begin at anus, and may extend proximally to involve varying portions of the colon or terminal ilium
• Enormous dilatation and hypertrophy of all layers of involved colon
• Rectosigmoid aganglionosis
• Submucosal hypertrophied nerve bundles

SPECIAL TESTS
• Proctoscopy: Ampulla empty of feces
• Biopsy: Absence of ganglia in wall of narrowed rectum
• Rectal manometry

IMAGING
X-ray: Barium enema shows:
  ◊ Large ovoid mass mottled by small, irregular gas shadows
  ◊ Dilatation of sigmoid colon above narrowed distal sigmoid or rectum
    ◊ Narrowed portion rippled or segmented
    ◊ Fluid levels within bowel
    ◊ Diaphragm elevated

DIAGNOSTIC PROCEDURES
• Suction aspiration biopsy of bowel wall
• Barium enema
• Proctosigmoidoscopy
• Large bowel wall biopsy
• Laparoscopy: Normal proximal colon dilatation
• Rectal manometry: Internal sphincter relaxation failure

 TREATMENT

APPROPRIATE HEALTH CARE
Early work-up (ambulatory or hospital). Inpatient for surgery.

GENERAL MEASURES
• Treatment may be symptomatic or definitive
• May need emergency correction of fluid and electrolyte imbalance
• Removal of fecal accumulation - retention enemas of 3-4 ounces of mineral oil followed by repeated colonic irrigations with isotonic saline solution. Avoid use of other solutions, e.g., water, soapsuds enemas.
• Surgery (inpatient) for colostomy at site in the colon proximal to aganglionic segment or resection of the aganglionic segment or bypass of the segment. Endorectal pull-through techniques may be utilized.

ACTIVITY
No restrictions

DIET
• Dictated by stage of disease
• Diet will not control the obstipation of Hirschsprung's
• Postoperative diet - standard for age

PATIENT EDUCATION
• After surgery instruct parents to detect and report dehydration, decreased urinary output, sunken eyes, poor skin turgor, vomiting, fever
• Encourage bonding with parents by having parents participate in child's care as much as possible
• Request enterotomy therapist to teach family

MEDICATIONS

DRUG(S) OF CHOICE
• None recommended for treatment
• Preliminary to surgery: Bowel prep with neomycin or nystatin
Contraindications: N/A
Precautions: N/A
Significant possible interactions: N/A

ALTERNATIVE DRUGS N/A

FOLLOWUP

PATIENT MONITORING Closely until recuperated fully from surgical intervention

PREVENTION/AVOIDANCE N/A

POSSIBLE COMPLICATIONS
• Toxic enterocolitis, possibly fatal
• Bleeding and/or perforation

EXPECTED COURSE AND PROGNOSIS Guardedly favorable with surgery prior to onset of complications

MISCELLANEOUS

ASSOCIATED CONDITIONS
• Chagas' disease (secondary aganglionic megacolon may be a late complication of Chagas')
• Megacolon, acquired, functional usually begins in 3rd or 4th year of life
• Down's syndrome
• Septal defects
• Tetralogy of Fallot
• Dandy-Walker syndrome
• Associated with anomalies 22% of the time, especially neurological, cardiovascular, urological, gastrointestinal

AGE-RELATED FACTORS
Pediatric: Occasionally infants have only mild or intermittent constipation with intervening bouts of diarrhea. These cases may not be diagnosed until later in infancy.
Geriatric: N/A
Others: N/A

PREGNANCY N/A

SYNONYMS
• Aganglionic megacolon
• Hirschsprung's disease
• Zer-Wilson's disease (total colonic aganglionosis)

ICD-9-CM 751.3

SEE ALSO N/A

OTHER NOTES Diagnosis must be made as early as possible to prevent toxic enterocolitis

ABBREVIATIONS N/A

REFERENCES
• Ryan, E.T., et al.: J of Ped Surg. Vol. 27, No. 1-76-81, 1992
• Walsh, K., et al. (eds.): Pediatric Surgery. New York, Yearbook Medical Publishers, 1986
• Eastwood, G.L. & Avunduk, C. (eds.): Manual of Gastroenterology. Boston, Little, Brown, 1988
• Barakat, A.Y. (ed.): Renal Disease in Children: Clinical Evaluation & Diagnosis. New York, Springer-Verlag, 1990

Author J. Nard, M.D.

Congestive heart failure

BASICS

DESCRIPTION Congestive heart failure (CHF) is the principal complication of heart disease. It is a pathophysiologic state produced by an abnormality in cardiac function (either transient or prolonged). The heart is unable to transport blood in a sufficient flow to meet the metabolic needs of the peripheral tissues.
• This produces a wide variety of clinical circumstances ranging from acute left ventricular dysfunction (due to tachyrrhythmia, bradyrrhythmia, and acute myocardial infarction) to chronic left ventricular dysfunction (due to chronic volume/pressure overload as seen in valvular heart disease)
• Two physiologic components explain most of the clinical findings of CHF: 1) an inotropic abnormality which results in diminished systolic emptying (systolic failure), and 2) compliance abnormality in which the ability of the ventricles to accept blood is impaired (diastolic failure). Most cases of heart failure have findings consistent with both mechanisms.
System(s) affected: Cardiovascular, Pulmonary
Genetics: N/A
Incidence/Prevalence in USA:
• Occurs at some point in almost all cases of severe heart disease. Frequency and timing of appearance depends on etiology of heart disease.
• Most common inpatient diagnosis for people over 65
Predominant age: Varies according to etiology of heart disease
Predominant sex:
• Male > Female - ages 40-75
• Male = Female - age 75 and over

SIGNS AND SYMPTOMS
Early and mild impairment:
◊ Nocturia
◊ Dyspnea on exertion-cardinal sign of left heart failure
◊ Deteriorating exercise capacity
◊ Fatigue
◊ Difficulty breathing
◊ Weakness
◊ Orthopnea
◊ Tachypnea with mild exertion
◊ Basilar rales
◊ Positive hepatojugular reflux
◊ Faint S3 gallop
Moderate impairment:
◊ Nocturnal cough
◊ Orthopnea
◊ Paroxysmal nocturnal dyspnea
◊ Wheezing, especially nocturnal in absence of history of asthma or infection (cardiac asthma)
◊ Anorexia
◊ Anxiety
◊ Fullness to dull pain in RUQ
◊ Tachypnea at rest
◊ Anxiety
◊ Hepatomegaly with tenderness to palpation

◊ Pallor
◊ Cool extremities due to peripheral vasoconstriction
◊ Prominent rales over bases
◊ Right pleural effusion
◊ Expiratory wheezing
◊ Edema
◊ Quadruple rhythm
◊ Diastolic hypertension
◊ Elevated jugular venous pressure
◊ Cardiomegaly
Severe impairment:
◊ Cerebral dysfunction
◊ Abdominal bloating
◊ Cyanosis
◊ Mild hypotension
◊ Pulsus alternans
◊ Ascites
◊ Anasarca
◊ Frothy sputum and/or pink sputum
◊ Increased P2
◊ Cardiac cachexia
◊ Cheyne-Stokes respirations

CAUSES
• Coronary atherosclerosis (most common)
• Myocardial infarction
• Rheumatic heart disease (mitral and aortic valvular disease)
• Cardiomyopathy - alcohol and non-alcohol related
• Hypertensive heart disease
• Aortic stenosis or regurgitation
• Volume overload
• Beta-blockers or other cardiac depressants

RISK FACTORS
• Iatrogenic inappropriate reduction of intensity of therapy
• Patient non-compliance
• Intercurrent arrhythmia
• Systemic infection
• Pulmonary embolism
• Administration of cardiac agent with negative inotropic effect
• Inappropriate physical, emotional, or environmental stress
• Thyrotoxicosis, pregnancy, or any condition associated with increased peripheral metabolic demand

DIAGNOSIS

DIFFERENTIAL DIAGNOSIS
• Nephrotic syndrome: excluded by absence of history of asymptomatic edema, proteinuria in nephrotic range, and history of renal disease
• Cirrhosis: excluded by absence of stigmata of liver disease, and history of liver disease and its risk factors
• Left heart failure: Findings of pulmonary congestion and diminished cardiac output appearing in patients with myocardial infarction, aortic and mitral valve disease, and hypertensive disease

• Right heart failure: Findings of systemic vascular congestion (edema, ascites) appearing in patients with cor pulmonale, primary tricuspid insufficiency, and most commonly in patients with uncorrected prolonged left heart failure

LABORATORY
Lab findings - early and mild to moderate in severity
◊ Respiratory alkalosis
◊ Mild azotemia
◊ Decreased erythrocyte sedimentation rate
◊ Proteinuria (usually less than 1 gm/24 h that clears with treatment)
◊ Normal serum electrolytes before treatment
Lab findings - severe
◊ Increased creatinine
◊ Hyperkalemia with severe low output state and diuretic therapy
◊ Increased SGOT
◊ Hyperbilirubinemia in severe cases
◊ Dilutional hyponatremia with treatment in severe cases
Drugs that may alter lab results: N/A
Disorders that may alter lab results: N/A

PATHOLOGICAL FINDINGS
Early and acute
◊ Firm lungs with microscopic revealing engorged capillaries with thickening of the alveolar septa with extravasation of red cells and edema fluid
◊ Liver is engorged, firm, and fluid-filled. Microscopic - reveals dilated central hepatic veins and sinusoids.
Late and chronic
◊ Hemosiderin deposits in lungs
◊ "Nutmeg" liver with centrilobular necrosis
◊ Occasionally hemorrhagic nonbacterial enterocolitis with hemorrhagic necrosis secondary to mesenteric vasoconstriction

SPECIAL TESTS N/A

IMAGING
X-ray - mild changes: pulmonary artery wedge pressure = 18-23 mm Hg
◊ Increased heart size
◊ Increased blood flow to the upper lobes
◊ Equalization of flow between the upper and lower lobes
X-ray - moderate severe pulmonary artery wedge pressure = 20-25 mm Hg
◊ Interstitial edema
◊ Kerley's B lines
◊ Perivascular edema
◊ Subpleural edema
X-ray - severe changes: pulmonary artery wedge pressure > 25 mm Hg)
◊ Alveolar edema
◊ Butterfly pattern of pulmonary edema

DIAGNOSTIC PROCEDURES
• Echocardiographic studies and invasive studies, if indicated, when patient stable
• Swan-Ganz catheterization acutely for afterload reduction and inotropic support in the acute setting

TREATMENT

APPROPRIATE HEALTH CARE
Inpatient when severe

GENERAL MEASURES
• Immediate treatment of the heart failure
• Search for underlying correctable conditions
• Eliminate contributing factors when possible
• Supplemental oxygen if required
• Antiembolism stockings
• Heart valve surgery - possibly, if defective heart valve is responsible
• Cardiac transplantation - to be considered in patients (age < 55) without other disqualifying medical problems, who are developing CHF unresponsive to other therapeutic maneuvers, and who are felt to have a life expectancy of less than a year

ACTIVITY
• Bedrest during severe stage, patient sitting up, head of bed elevated
• Increased activity as symptoms subside
• May need to alter life-style to reduce symptoms

DIET
• Salt restriction (initially to 2 grams/day)
• If overweight, consider weight reducing diet

PATIENT EDUCATION
Printed patient information available from:
◊ American Heart Association, 7320 Greenville Avenue, Dallas, TX 75231, (214)373-6300
◊ American College of Cardiology, 911 Old Georgetown Road, Bethesda, MD 20814, (301)897-5400

MEDICATIONS

DRUG(S) OF CHOICE
Digoxin
◊ Given to improve contractility
◊ Loading dose is 0.5 mg IV or po, followed by 0.25 mg q 4-6 hours for 4 doses, then 0.125-0.25 mg po q day
◊ Reduce dosage in elderly patients and patients with renal insufficiency
◊ Of no benefit to patients with mitral stenosis in sinus rhythm
◊ May be harmful to those patients with hypertrophic obstructive cardiomyopathy
Vasodilators
◊ To decrease preload
◊ To decrease afterload and systemic vascular resistance
◊ To improve cardiac output and increase efficiency of left ventricular emptying
◊ Choices include - nitroprusside, nitroglycerin, isosorbide dinitrate, hydralazine, prazosin, enalapril, nifedipine

Sympathomimetic amines
◊ To be used in treatment for severe CHF unresponsive to above measures
◊ Dopamine and dobutamine have been successful for short periods in treatment
◊ Dobutamine has been used on a chronic outpatient basis with intermittent infusion. However, has not been demonstrated to increase survival, and in spite of possibly improving quality of life, has produced reduction in long-term survival.
Others
◊ Diuretics - loop diuretic preferred (e.g., furosemide)
◊ K+ supplementation
Contraindications: Refer to manufacturer's literature
Precautions: Refer to manufacturer's literature
Significant possible interactions: Refer to manufacturer's literature

ALTERNATIVE DRUGS N/A

FOLLOWUP

PATIENT MONITORING
• Variable depending on clinical circumstances. Initially q 2-3 weeks after patient stabilized.
• Closely follow - history and physical findings, chest x-ray, electrolytes, BUN, and creatinine
• Digoxin levels should be checked periodically

PREVENTION/AVOIDANCE Treatment of underlying disorders when possible

POSSIBLE COMPLICATIONS
• Digitalis intoxication
• Electrolyte disturbance
• Atrial and ventricular arrhythmias
• Mesenteric insufficiency
• Protein enteropathy

EXPECTED COURSE AND PROGNOSIS
• Result of initial treatment is usually good, whatever the cause
• Long-term prognosis variable. Mortality rates range from 10% with mild symptoms to 50% with advanced, progressive symptoms.

MISCELLANEOUS

ASSOCIATED CONDITIONS See Causes

AGE-RELATED FACTORS
Pediatric: Usually associated with congenital heart disease
Geriatric: Medications may need dosage adjustment
Others: N/A

PREGNANCY If occurs, will require special care

SYNONYMS
• Heart failure
• Dropsy
• Circulatory failure
• Cardiac failure

ICD-9-CM 428.0 congestive heart failure

SEE ALSO N/A

OTHER NOTES N/A

ABBREVIATIONS N/A

REFERENCES
• Braunwald, E. (ed.): Heart Disease: A Textbook of Cardiovascular Medicine. 3rd Ed. Philadelphia, W.B. Saunders Co., 1988
• Harvey, A.M.: The Principles and Practice of Medicine. 22nd Ed. Norwalk, CT, Appleton & Lange, 1988

Author F. Griff, M.D.

Conjunctivitis

 BASICS

DESCRIPTION Inflammation of palpebral and/or bulbar conjunctiva. Pink eye refers to non-Neisseria bacterial conjunctivitis.
System(s) affected: Nervous, Skin/Exocrine
Genetics: N/A
Incidence/Prevalence in USA: Unknown, but common
Predominant age: Depends on cause
Predominant sex: Male = Female

SIGNS AND SYMPTOMS
General
◊ Conjunctival hyperemia
◊ Burning
◊ Foreign body sensation
◊ Pruritis
◊ Tearing
◊ Exudation and matting
◊ Chemosis
◊ Pseudoptosis
◊ Preauricular adenopathy
◊ Tarsal plate papillary hypertrophy
◊ Tarsal plate lymphoid follicles
◊ Pseudomembranous and membranes
◊ Photosensitivity
◊ Decreased acuity if there is complicating ulcer or keratitis
◊ Granulomas (rare)
Bacterial
◊ Minimal pruritis
◊ Moderate tearing
◊ Profuse exudate, particularly Neisseria species
◊ Usually unilateral (or initially unilateral)
◊ Small tarsal plate papillae
◊ Neisseria species may cause chemosis
◊ Gram and Giemsa stain: Polymorphonuclear neutrophils (PMN's) and bacteria (gram negative intracellular diplococci with Neisseria species)
Viral
◊ Minimal pruritis
◊ Profuse tearing
◊ Minimal exudate
◊ Often bilateral
◊ Preauricular adenopathy common
◊ Associated viral systemic symptom (fever, myalgia, etc.)
◊ Tarsal plate follicles
◊ Pharyngeal follicles if associated pharyngitis
◊ Gram and Giemsa stain: Mononuclear cells (lymphocytes)
◊ Rare chemosis except with epidemic keratoconjunctivitis
◊ Subepithelial corneal opacities with epidemic keratoconjunctivitis
◊ Diffuse punctate corneal fluorescein uptake or dendrites with herpes simplex
◊ Typical zoster rash along ophthalmic branch of trigeminal nerve with varicella-zoster blepharoconjunctivitis
◊ Typical measles rash, Koplik's spots, etc. with measles
Chlamydial
◊ Minimal pruritis
◊ Moderate to profuse tearing
◊ Profuse exudate (sometimes modest)
◊ Often bilateral
◊ Small tarsal plate papillae
◊ Tarsal plate follicles present
◊ Gram and Giemsa stain: PMN's, plasma cells, inclusion bodies, in trachoma large palely- staining lymphoblastic cells
◊ Inclusion conjunctivitis commonly has preauricular adenopathy and large tarsal plate papillae and follicles. Occasionally associated genitourinary symptoms in young adults or history of bilateral conjunctivitis unresponsive to topical antibiotics.
◊ Lymphogranuloma venereum is rare and non-follicular (mostly granulomatous conjunctival) with large preauricular node (visible bubo)
◊ Trachoma rare in the USA (except American Indians of Southwest) and has 4 clinical stages
Allergic
◊ Severe pruritis
◊ Moderate tearing
◊ No exudate
◊ Bilateral
◊ Chemosis very common
◊ Tarsal papillae
◊ Gram and Giemsa's stain: Eosinophils and basophils
◊ Allergic rhinoconjunctivitis has associated sneezing, rhinitis but if not of sufficient duration will not develop papillae
◊ Vernal conjunctivitis is recurrent in warm weather associated with large "cobblestone" papillae in those with history of atopic allergy
◊ Giant papillary conjunctivitis has similar appearance to vernal conjunctivitis with less pruritis and is seen in soft (and occasionally hard) contact lens use
Chemical or irritative
◊ Tarsal follicles with conjunctivitis of topical medications
◊ Tearing and exudation depends on toxicity of chemical
◊ Chemosis common in post therapeutic irrigation
◊ Gram and Giemsa's stain: PMN's if tissue necrosis

CAUSES
Bacterial
◊ Staphylococcus aureus
◊ Streptococcus pneumoniae
◊ Haemophilus influenza
◊ Neisseria gonorrhoeae
◊ Neisseria meningitidis
◊ Rarely other Streptococcal sp., Branhamella catarrhalis, Coliforms, Klebsiella, Proteus, Corynebacterium diphtheriae, Mycobacterium tuberculosis, Treponema pallidum
Viral
◊ Adenoviruses types 3, 4, 7 (pharyngitis with conjunctivitis)
◊ Adenoviruses types 8 and 19 (epidemic keratoconjunctivitis)
◊ Herpes simplex (primary and recurrent)
◊ Enterovirus type 70
◊ Coxsackie virus type A28
◊ Molluscum contagiosum
◊ Varicella
◊ Herpes zoster
◊ Measles virus

Chlamydial
◊ Chlamydia trachomatis (trachoma)
◊ Chlamydia oculogenitalis (inclusion conjunctivitis)
◊ Chlamydia lymphogranulomatis (lymphogranuloma venereum)
Allergic
◊ Rhinoconjunctivitis (hay fever) - humoral
◊ Vernal conjunctivitis
◊ Giant papillary conjunctivitis
◊ Delayed (cellular)
◊ Autoimmune (Sjögren's, pemphigoid, Wegener's granulomatosis)
Chemical or irritative
◊ Topical medication
◊ Home chemicals
◊ Industrial chemicals
◊ Wind
◊ Smoke
◊ Ultraviolet light
Other
◊ Rickettsial, fungal, parasitic, tuberculosis, syphilis, Kawasaki disease
◊ Thyroid disease, gout, carcinoid, sarcoidosis, psoriasis, Stevens-Johnson syndrome, Ligneous conjunctivitis, Reiter's syndrome

RISK FACTORS Numerous, including trauma from wind, cold and heat, chemicals and foreign body

 DIAGNOSIS

DIFFERENTIAL DIAGNOSIS
• Uveitis (iritis, iridocyclitis, choroiditis)
• Acute glaucoma
• Corneal disease or foreign body
• Canalicular obstruction (canaliculitis, dacrocystitis)
• Scleritis and episcleritis

LABORATORY
• Culture from conjunctiva
• Gram and Giemsa stain of the discharge or scrapings
Drugs that may alter lab results: N/A
Disorders that may alter lab results: N/A

PATHOLOGICAL FINDINGS N/A

SPECIAL TESTS
• Cultivation on HeLa cells and neutralization tests for epidemic keratoconjunctivitis
• Bouin fixation and Papanicolaou stain for multinucleated giant cells of herpes simplex conjunctivitis. Also available, viral culture and immunofluorescence test for Herpes simplex.
• Immunofluorescent antibody tests for chlamydia serology
• Frei test for lymphogranuloma venereum

IMAGING N/A

DIAGNOSTIC PROCEDURES
• Culture of exudate
• Smear and stain of exudate

TREATMENT

APPROPRIATE HEALTH CARE
Outpatient

GENERAL MEASURES
• Record acuity
• Fluorescein staining to detect ulcer, keratitis
• No patch
• See Medications
• Culture
• No topical steroids
• Ophthalmologic referral if ulcer, keratitis, suspected herpes or worsens after 24 hours of treatment
• Compresses - warm if infective, cold if allergic or irritative
• Remove purulent material and debris (may require frequent irrigation)
• Giant papillary allergic conjunctivitis requires discontinuing use of contact lenses

ACTIVITY   No restrictions

DIET   No restrictions

PATIENT EDUCATION
• Transmission route of infecting agent if contagious
• Demonstrate eye drop techniques
• Demonstrate ointment techniques

MEDICATIONS

DRUG(S) OF CHOICE
Bacterial
◊ 0.3% tobramycin or gentamicin. As drops (1-2gtts) instilled every 4 hours while awake for 5 days, as ointment qid.
◊ chloramphenicol. As drops (0.5%) instilled every 4 hours while awake for 5 days, as ointment (1%) qid. (Note: Warning - slight hematological risk).
◊ 10% sodium sulfacetamide. As drops (1-2gtts) instilled every 4 hours while awake for 5 days, as ointment qid and hs (stings).
◊ Systemic treatment for Neisseria species as other sites usually involved. Some authorities (with ophthalmology consult) add topical erythromycin.
Viral
◊ 0.1% idoxuridine for herpes simplex. 1 drop qh while awake, then 1 drop every 2 hours during sleeping hours. Treatment should be continued 5-7 days after healing to decrease risk of relapse.
◊ Topical antibiotics to prevent bacterial superinfection or if diagnosis is in doubt
Chlamydial
◊ Oral doxycycline 100 mg bid (3 weeks) for inclusion conjunctivitis
Allergic
◊ Topical vasoconstrictor and/or antihistamine combination such as naphazoline 0.05% /antazoline 0.5% (Albalon-A, Vasocon-A)

◊ Oral antihistamine
◊ Topical cromolyn sodium 2%, 4% (Opticrom) qid starting 2 weeks before season. (Opticrom no longer imported into the U.S. Available in Canada, UK, and Europe in 2% solution.)
Contraindications: Allergy
Precautions:
• Vasoconstrictors make the eye appear less severely affected
• Avoid contamination of medication bottles by touching lids
Significant possible interactions: Refer to manufacturer's profile of each drug

ALTERNATIVE DRUGS
Bacterial
◊ Polymyxin/gramicidin /Polysporin)
◊ Polymyxin/neomycin (Neosporin) (15% of people have hypersensitivity reaction to neomycin)
Viral
◊ Acyclovir for herpes simplex
◊ Consider oral acyclovir in serious viral infections
Chlamydial
◊ Oral tetracycline or erythromycin (3 weeks) for inclusion conjunctivitis. Some authorities recommend topical tetracycline or erythromycin in addition. Tetracyclines contraindicated in pregnancy and in young children less than 8 years old.
Allergic
◊ Numerous topical vasoconstrictors and antihistamines
◊ Numerous oral antihistamines

FOLLOWUP

PATIENT MONITORING   Referral if worse in 24 hours

PREVENTION/AVOIDANCE
• Avoid listed causes when possible
• Wash hands frequently

POSSIBLE COMPLICATIONS
Bacterial
◊ Chronic marginal blepharitis
◊ Conjunctival scar if membrane developed
◊ Corneal ulcer or perforation
◊ Hypopyon
◊ Rare portal of entry for meningococcus
Viral
◊ Corneal scars with herpes simplex
◊ Corneal scars, lid scars, entropion, misdirected lashes with Varicella-zoster
◊ Bacterial superinfection
Chlamydial
◊ Clinical trachoma (not with inclusion conjunctivitis)
Allergic, chemical and others
◊ Bacterial superinfection

EXPECTED COURSE AND PROGNOSIS
Bacterial
◊ 10-14 days without treatment
◊ 2-4 days with treatment
Viral
◊ 10 days for pharyngitis with conjunctivitis
◊ 3-4 weeks for epidemic keratoconjunctivitis
◊ 2-3 weeks for herpes simplex
Chlamydial
◊ 3-9 months for untreated inclusion conjunctivitis
◊ 3-5 weeks for trachoma with treatment

MISCELLANEOUS

ASSOCIATED CONDITIONS   See Causes

AGE-RELATED FACTORS
Pediatric: Neonatal conjunctivitis may be toxic, bacterial (genital tract bacteria or nosocomial) or chlamydial
Geriatric: More likely to have diseases or problems listed in Causes
Others: N/A

PREGNANCY   N/A

SYNONYMS   Pink eye

ICD-9-CM
• 372.5 acute atopic conjunctivitis
• 372.14 other chronic allergic conjunctivitis

SEE ALSO   N/A

OTHER NOTES   N/A

ABBREVIATIONS   N/A

REFERENCES
• Vaughan, D., Asbury, T. & Cook, R.: General Ophthalmology. 11th. Ed. Los Altos, CA, Appleton & Lange, 1986
• Howes, R.: Emergency Clinics of North America. Vol. 6, No. I, Feb., 1988

Author   C. Ricketson, M.D.

Constipation

 BASICS

DESCRIPTION Difficult passage, too infrequently, of feces that are too hard. Because each patient has his or her own concept of constipation, a thorough description of the complaint must be sought from each patient.
System(s) affected: Gastrointestinal
Genetics: Unknown (the condition may be familial)
Incidence in USA: Higher at extremes of life, i.e., among infants/children and the elderly
Prevalence in USA: Common; affects a majority of persons during their lifetimes
Predominant age: All ages can be affected; more frequent at the extremes of life (infancy and old age)
Predominant Sex: Female > Male

SIGNS AND SYMPTOMS
• A lesser frequency of defecation than the patient perceives as "normal"
• Evacuation of a lesser volume of feces, or of feces more inspissated, than the patient perceives as "normal"
• A lack of consistent urgency to stool
• Difficulty expelling feces from the rectum
• Painful evacuation of feces
• A lingering sense of incomplete emptying of the bowel
• Impaction of inspissated feces in the rectum
• A vague malaise, often including lower abdominal fullness and headache, that the patient associates with inadequate bowel evacuation
• Tenesmus

CAUSES
• Electrolyte or hormonal abnormalities
• Congenital impediments, e.g., aganglionic megacolon (Hirschsprung's disease) or excessively elongate, redundant, capacious bowel (dolichocolon)
• Congenital or acquired neuromuscular bowel impairment ("pseudo-obstruction")
• Concomitant illness, injury, or debility
• Mechanical bowel impediment (obstruction or ileus, due to any cause)
• Inadequate fluid intake
• Side-effect of drugs (e.g., anticholinergic agents, opiates)
• Chronic abuse of laxatives or cathartics
• Cultural, emotional, environmental factors
• Painful fecal evacuation from anal disease (e.g., fissures)

RISK FACTORS
• Aging
• Neurosis
• Polypharmacy
• Sedentary life style or condition

 DIAGNOSIS

DIFFERENTIAL DIAGNOSIS The most common and difficult dilemma is to distinguish "functional" disorder from an "organic" lesion

LABORATORY Unrevealing (except when indicative of an associated illness)
• Perform routine CBC to detect anemia that may indicate colorectal malignancy
Drugs that may alter lab results: N/A
Disorders that may alter lab results: N/A

PATHOLOGICAL FINDINGS
• None in common, "functional" constipation
• Paucity or absence of intramural enteric ganglia in certain cases of congenital or acquired megacolon
• Neuromuscular abnormalities in certain cases of "pseudo-obstruction"

SPECIAL TESTS
• In selected cases of long-standing constipation, timed measure of passage of ingested stool markers may help discern differing impediments
• Anorectal motility in patients with suspected Hirschsprung's or anorectal motility disorders
• Defecography may delineate anatomic abnormality

IMAGING
• In severely acute or disturbingly chronic cases, a plain (scout) film of the abdomen may help to discern the extent and nature of the problem
• Barium enema examination and, in selected cases, barium meal examination are indicated in persistent cases
• Cineradiography of passage of barium, instilled in, then expelled from the rectosigmoid segment ("defecography"), may help define evacuation disorders in selected cases

DIAGNOSTIC PROCEDURES
• Digital examination of the anus and rectum is essential in all cases
• Proctosigmoidoscopy is indicated in most cases
• Colonoscopy is seldom required, unless needed to define an abnormality discovered by barium enema or when there is evidence of iron deficiency anemia or either visible or occult blood in the stool

 TREATMENT

APPROPRIATE HEALTH CARE
Outpatient in almost all cases, except when investigation discloses an underlying lesion or obstruction that requires hospitalization

GENERAL MEASURES
• Attempt to eliminate medications that may cause or worsen constipation
• Sparing use of enemas (tepid water in pint volume) can be helpful for some patients
• Avoid the so-called "high colonic irrigation"
• Increase fluid intake

ACTIVITY Encourage adequate exercise

DIET
• When there is no apparent impediment to bowel transit, advise a diet that favors items providing bulk, e.g., fruits, vegetables, whole grain cereals
• Encourage significant increase in fluid intake

PATIENT EDUCATION
• Explanation, in simple terms, of bowel physiology
• Reassurance that the "normal" frequency of bowel evacuation varies widely, and that occasional, mild constipation is in no way deleterious to general well-being
• Instruction in consistent "bowel training" i.e., allowing adequate time for bowel evacuation in a quiet, unhurried environment; instruction in facilitating posture on commode, e.g., thighs flexed toward abdomen

MEDICATIONS

DRUG(S) OF CHOICE
• Bulk-forming agents (hydrophilic colloids) used to supplement diet are not really "drugs" (and the patient should be so informed): these include psyllium (e.g., Konsyl, Metamucil, Perdiem), methylcellulose (e.g., Citrucel), and polycarbophil (e.g., Mitrolan). Dosage must be adjusted to patient's individual need.
• So-called "saline" laxatives are appropriate for short-term use. The usual dose is 15 mL to 30 mL once or twice a day. These include (among many) milk of magnesia, citrate of magnesia, and phosphate of soda; lactulose (Chronulac) produces similar action.

Contraindications:
• Any impediment to bowel transit, such as an obstructing lesion or ileus
• Any acute intra-abdominal inflammatory condition
• Renal failure

Precautions: Advise patient against chronic use of irritant laxatives except for bulk-forming agents

Significant possible interactions: N/A

ALTERNATIVE DRUGS
• Lubricants, such as mineral oil, are unpalatable to many patients, subject to leakage, and impose the risk of aspiration
• Emollient suppositories are useful, if at all, in allaying anorectal soreness
• So-called "stool softeners" probably do little to soften stools but rather induce a sort of secretory diarrhea; they seem to help some patients
• What have been called "irritant cathartics" include ricinoleic acid (castor oil), phenolphthalein (Ex-Lax), and bisacodyl (Dulcolax) and are ill-chosen except for very short-term use
• Osmotic agents (e.g., lactulose) are often used but frequently result in gas and distention and may result in bowel perforation in those with mechanical obstruction
• Cisapride, a newly developed prokinetic agent (not yet available in the US), gives promise of allaying constipation due to hypotonic bowel - especially with pseudo obstruction, "cathartic colon" and irritable bowel syndrome

FOLLOWUP

PATIENT MONITORING What seems to be simple, "functional" constipation, if it persists, should be further investigated for a possible "organic" cause

PREVENTION/AVOIDANCE Because for some patients a tendency to constipation is habitual, instruction in proper diet, bowel training, and use of bulk-forming supplements must be reinforced from time to time

POSSIBLE COMPLICATIONS
• In severe, long-standing cases - acquired megacolon
• With laxative abuse - fluid and electrolyte depletion. Repeated abuse can lead to a damaged "cathartic colon."
• Rectal ulceration ("stercoral ulcer") related to recurrent fecal impaction

EXPECTED COURSE AND PROGNOSIS
Constipation that is only occasional, brief, and responsive to simple measures is harmless. That which is habitual can be a lifelong nuisance.

MISCELLANEOUS

ASSOCIATED CONDITIONS Debility, either general, as in the aged, or that imposed by specific, underlying illness

AGE-RELATED FACTORS
Pediatric: Sometimes it is the misguided, overly punctilious mother who requires primary attention, rather than her constipated infant. Hirschsprung's disease.
Geriatric:
• Elderly persons, who have enjoyed regular bowel action throughout their lives, seldom suffer constipation due to age alone
• Persons with a lifelong tendency to constipation often encounter increasing difficulty with advancing age
• There is an increased incidence of colorectal neoplasms with age that may be associated with constipation.
Others: N/A

PREGNANCY Women with a tendency to constipation may find the condition more troublesome in the third trimester and require dietary adjustment and supplements

SYNONYMS
• Costive bowel
• Locked bowels

ICD-9-CM 564.0 (unless otherwise specified)

SEE ALSO N/A

OTHER NOTES N/A

ABBREVIATIONS N/A

REFERENCES
• Rogers, A.I.: Constipation In Gastrointestinal Symptoms, Clinical Interpretation. Edited by J.E. Berk & W.S. Haubrich. Philadelphia, B.C. Decker Inc., 1991
• Haubrich, W.S.: Constipation. In Bockus Gastroenterology. 4th Ed. Edited by J.E. Berk, et al. Philadelphia, W.B. Saunders Co., 1985
• Devroede, G.: Constipation. In Gastrointestinal Disease. 4th Ed. Edited by M.H. Sleisenger & J.S. Fordtran. Philadelphia, W.B. Saunders Co., 1989
• Wald, A.: Approach to the patient with constipation. In Textbook of Gastroenterology, Vol. I, Edited by T. Yamada. Philadelphia, J.B. Lippincott Co., 1991

Author W. Haubrich, M.D.

Contraception

 BASICS

DESCRIPTION Variety of practices designed to prevent pregnancy in sexually active women. Most are designed to prevent ovulation, to prevent implantation, to be spermicidal or to prevent sperm from reaching egg. Natural family planning aims to avoid coitus at the time of expected ovulation. Failure rates vary among methods. The most effective is permanent sterilization, either tubal sterilization in the female (by electrocautery, loops, clips, or ligation and excision) or vasectomy in the male. Neither should be considered reversible, but either may be reversed under certain circumstances. Surgical attempts at reversal are often unsuccessful.
Commonly used reversible methods and their approximate pregnancy rates per 100 women per year are:
• Implantable hormonal contraception (Norplant) - 1
• Long acting injectable progestogen (Depo-Provera) - 1
• Oral contraception (the pill) - 3
• Condom (rubber) - 12
• Diaphragm - 18
• Sponge - 18
• Periodic abstinence (natural family planning) - 20
• Spermicides alone (foam, suppositories) - 21
Genetics: N/A
Incidence in USA: N/A
Prevalence in USA:
• About two-thirds of women at risk for unwanted pregnancies use contraception
Among individuals of reproductive age having regular coitus
◊ Tubal sterilization 16.6%
◊ Vasectomy 7.0%
◊ Oral contraceptives 18.5%
◊ Condoms 8.8%
◊ Diaphragm 3.5%
◊ Intrauternine device 1.2%
◊ Natural family planning 1.0%
◊ Foam 0.6%
◊ Implantable hormonal contraception N/A
◊ Intramuscular progestogen N/A
Predominant age:
• Female - 11-52 years
• Male - any age after puberty
Predominant sex: Female. However, condom or vasectomy are the common male methods.

SIGNS AND SYMPTOMS N/A

CAUSES N/A

RISK FACTORS Any woman who is ovulating and having intercourse with a fertile male. Contraception is less likely to be used by young adolescents and by those who, because of socioeconomic factors, have less access to medical care, or have limited knowledge about reproduction.

 DIAGNOSIS

DIFFERENTIAL DIAGNOSIS N/A

LABORATORY
Female
◊ Cervical cytology
◊ Cultures for gonorrhea and Chlamydia
◊ Blood lipid studies (with family history of hyperlipidemia or coronary artery disease at a young age)
◊ Blood sugar (if suspected of having diabetes mellitus)
Male
◊ None needed except routine pre-operative studies prior to vasectomy
◊ Semen analysis showing no sperm after vasectomy. (Will require up to 15 ejaculations before aspermia is present for 3 consecutive studies)
Drugs that may alter lab results: None, however, oral contraceptives may increase transport proteins (TBG, SHBG, etc.) and coagulation factors produced by liver, necessitating consideration of the use of oral contraceptives in interpreting results of lab tests. Oral contraceptives may also reduce serum folate. Low dose pills currently in use have practically no effect on either blood sugar or lipid profile as do higher dose pills.
Disorders that may alter lab results: N/A

PATHOLOGICAL FINDINGS Patients on long term oral contraception will often have suppression of growth of endometrial glands. Biopsy of the endometrium will show a thinner mucosa, few glands and stromal edema. This correlates with the reduced menstrual bleeding seen in patients on oral contraception.

SPECIAL TESTS Monitor blood pressure in patients on oral contraceptives - check at 3 months after initiation then annually. Discontinue if hypertension develops on pill

IMAGING N/A

DIAGNOSTIC PROCEDURES N/A

 TREATMENT

APPROPRIATE HEALTH CARE All methods except tubal sterilization are administered outpatient. Tubal sterilization is done as an outpatient surgical procedure.

GENERAL MEASURES Consistent use of method will maximize effectiveness

ACTIVITY N/A

DIET N/A

PATIENT EDUCATION
• Printed materials available from ACOG (1-800-673-8444)
• Oral contraception - take pill daily at approximately same time. If a pill is missed, take two the following day but use an additional method of protection such as a barrier method until next period begins. If two periods are missed, seek medical care to rule out pregnancy. Do not stop pills if a period is missed.
• Intrauterine device - check for the presence of the string in the vagina at least weekly (or at time of each intercourse)
• Condom - check for holes before using. Leave space at tip to act as reservoir for the semen. Withdraw from vagina before penis becomes flaccid. Use a spermicide in addition in order to increase effectiveness.
• Diaphragm - before inserting, place about one tablespoon of spermicidal gel or cream into the dome of diaphragm and line entire rim of the diaphragm with it. Insert the diaphragm and check for proper placement. Leave it in for at least 8 hours after coitus - then remove and clean according to directions. Check for holes. If another act of coitus occurs before 8 hours, insert additional spermicidal gel or cream into vagina without displacing the diaphragm.
• Sponge - leave in for at least 8 hours after coitus. Use additional spermicide for repeat coitus before 8 hours.
• Periodic abstinence - need an accurate record of menstrual cycles for at least 12 months prior to use. The fertile period is calculated as the shortest cycle minus 18 days to the longest cycle minus 11 days. This is a serious problem in the woman with extremely variable cycle length. Additional effectiveness may be attained by observing cervical mucus (for disappearance of clear abundant mucus) and by observing basal temperature rise of about one degree for 3 days. Both usually indicate that ovulation has occurred.
• Depo-Provera - return every 3 months for injection

 MEDICATIONS

DRUG(S) OF CHOICE
• Condoms - latex condom bought over the counter. Do not use with petrolatum which may weaken condom. If lubricant needed, use water-based such as K-Y jelly.
• Spermicides - all contain nonoxynol-9. Over the counter medications - choice depends upon preferences of user and local sensitization to bases. Foam or creams are preferable since they disperse well. Suppositories or tablets first must dissolve, making dispersal unpredictable.
• Sponge - Today sponge (purchased over the counter)
• IUD - 2 currently available: Progestasert (progesterone is the bioactive ingredient. Change annually); Paragard (contains copper - change every 4-6 years). Either are inserted by a practitioner who has been appropriately trained. Insertion is best at time of menses in order to rule out pregnancy.

• Diaphragm - needs fitting by a physician or nurse practitioner. Use the largest size which can be inserted without discomfort or distortion. Refit after childbirth or if weight changes by more than 10%.

• Oral contraception - use sub-50 microgram estrogen dose (30 or 35 micrograms) to minimize side effects and risks. Triphasics contain less total progestogen and therefore are less likely to affect lipid profile adversely by increasing LDL or decreasing HDL. All current pills contain ethinyl estradiol or mestranol as the estrogen. The progestogen varies between manufacturers - all are derivatives of testosterone and slight differences in the molecule produce different biological effects. Generics should be avoided because of uncertain or fluctuating dosage in each batch of pills. Choice of specific pill usually depends upon experiences and preferences of physician. If side effects occur, the pill may be changed. It is impossible to predict any patient's reaction to a particular pill and changing to eliminate side effects is by trial and error. Low dose progestogen-only pills have high pregnancy rates; avoid them.

• Implantable hormonal contraception - 6 silastic tubes implanted into the upper arm. They are effective for up to 5 years and after implantation do not require an active role by the patient.

• Depo-Provera - give 150 mg intramuscular every 3 months. Contraceptive levels of hormone persist for up to 4 months (giving 2-4 week margin of safety).

Contraindications:
• Implantable or intramuscular hormonal contraception - active liver disease, thrombophlebitis, pregnancy, unexplained abnormal uterine bleeding, cholestatic jaundice, hyperlipidemia

• Oral contraception - same as implantable contraception plus noncompliance and estrogen dependent malignancies. Relative contraindications are uterine leiomyomata, hypertension, insulin-requiring diabetes mellitus, and migraine headaches.

• IUD - nulliparity or multiple sexual partners (because of the risk of pelvic inflammatory disease)

• Spermicides - local irritation

• Diaphragm - significant uterine prolapse

• Periodic abstinence - irregular cycles

Precautions: Pregnancy may occur with any method. If it occurs after permanent sterilization, it indicates failure of the procedure and the need for reoperation. In pregnancy with an IUD, remove the device if the string is visible coming from the cervix. If the string is not seen, leave the device in place, although there is slight increase in the risk of spontaneous abortion. In pregnancy, using an oral contraceptive, stop the pill. No increase in rate of birth defects is expected except for a very slight chance of virilization of a female fetus.

Significant possible interactions:
Oral contraceptive effectiveness decreased by:
◊ Dilantin (induces microsomal liver enzymes causing accelerated metabolism of hormones with subsequent reduced blood levels). (The same effect occurs in implantable contraception.)
◊ Antibiotics (changes absorption by altering gastrointestinal passage time)
◊ The above are indications to use a 50 microgram estrogen pill or preferably to use a barrier method in conjunction with a 30 or 35 microgram estrogen pill

ALTERNATIVE DRUGS   N/A

 FOLLOWUP

PATIENT MONITORING   There should be an annual visit for a pelvic exam and Pap smear or whenever side effects or problems occur. An IUD should be checked for its presence one month after insertion. If the string is not found, pelvic ultrasound is used to locate the device in the uterus. Oral contraceptive users should be monitored 3 months after starting for hypertension, following which an annual examination is usually sufficient.

PREVENTION/AVOIDANCE   N/A

POSSIBLE COMPLICATIONS
Serious complications of oral contraception
◊ Thromboembolism - stop method and treat the disorder. Do not resume hormonal contraception.
◊ Hypertension - stop method - do not resume
◊ Myocardial infarction - main risk is in smoker particularly after age 35. Do not use in such patients
Minor side effects of oral contraception
◊ Nausea and vomiting - take pill on full stomach
◊ Breakthrough bleeding - usually self limiting after 3 months. If not, change pill
◊ Amenorrhea - rule out pregnancy - then either change to a different pill or add conjugated estrogen 0.3 mg for the first 10 days of pill package
◊ Cyclic weight gain - use smallest dose of estrogen available
◊ Breast tenderness - rare with low dose pill
◊ Depression - rare with low dose pill
◊ Chloasma - stop pill or cover with makeup
◊ Acne or hirsutism - use triphasic pill to minimize androgen effect or change to a less androgenic progestogen
◊ Cholestatic jaundice - stop pill - do not restart
◊ Weight gain throughout cycle - use triphasic pill to minimize dose of progestogen

Side effects of implantable hormonal contraception
◊ Amenorrhea - about 33% (if it persists for 2 months, rule out pregnancy)
◊ Irregular bleeding - about 33%
Both are self limited after about 1 year and the patient should be informed of side effects before choosing this method
Side effects of intramuscular progestogen (Depo-Provera)
◊ Irregular bleeding during first few months
◊ Amenorrhea - common after 1 year of use
Side effects of IUD
◊ Heavy bleeding and cramps
◊ Salpingitis
◊ All are best managed by removal of device. Salpingitis requires antibiotic therapy in addition.

EXPECTED COURSE AND PROGNOSIS
N/A

 MISCELLANEOUS

ASSOCIATED CONDITIONS   N/A

AGE-RELATED FACTORS
Pediatric: Use of estrogen prior to pubertal growth spurt may lead to a reduction in ultimate height due to epiphyseal closure
Geriatric: After the menopause, oral contraceptives should not be used for estrogen replacement therapy because the hormonal dose is much higher than necessary
Others: Oral contraceptives may be used by healthy non-smokers until after age 50. Ultimately they need to be stopped and the patient observed to see if she is menopausal. Use another method of contraception during the this period until it can be determined that the woman is postmenopausal.

PREGNANCY   See above

SYNONYMS   Birth control

ICD-9-CM   None

SEE ALSO   N/A

OTHER NOTES   Additional benefits of oral contraception include a decrease in the amount of menstrual flow and some protection against both ovarian and endometrial cancer. Relationship to breast cancer is still uncertain due to conflicting data. Some suggest a slight increase in risk in certain groups.

ABBREVIATIONS   N/A

REFERENCES   Speroff, L., Glass, R.H., Kase, N.G.: Clinical Gynecologic Endocrinology and Infertility. 4th Ed. Baltimore, Williams & Wilkins, 1989

Author   A. Langer, M.D.

Cor pulmonale

 BASICS

DESCRIPTION Disturbance in the pulmonary circulation resulting in right ventricular dysfunction
• Acute cor pulmonale - acute dilitation of the right ventricle secondary to pulmonary hypertension usually resulting from massive pulmonary embolism
• Chronic cor pulmonale - hypertrophy and dilitation of the right ventricle resulting from diseases of the pulmonary parenchyma and/or vascular system
System(s) affected: Cardiovascular, Pulmonary
Genetics: No known genetic pattern
Incidence/Prevalence in USA: 5-10% of organic heart diseases
Predominant age: > 45
Predominant sex: Male > Female

SIGNS AND SYMPTOMS
• Dyspnea, cough, sputum production
• Orthopnea, cyanosis
• Distended neck veins with prominent a- and v- waves
• Parasternal heave, palpable P2, right ventricular S3
• Loud pulmonic second sound
• Murmur of tricuspid regurgitation
• Diffuse inspiratory and expiratory rhonchi
• Wheezes
• Hepatomegaly, occasionally the liver is pulsatile
• Ascites, peripheral edema

CAUSES
Disease affecting structure of the pulmonary tree
◊ Chronic obstructive pulmonary diseases
◊ Diffuse interstitial lung diseases: idiopathic pulmonary fibrosis, radiation induced fibrosis
◊ Pulmonary resection
◊ Granulomatous diseases: sarcoidosis, rheumatoid arthritis, systemic lupus erythematosus, eosinophilic granuloma
◊ Bronchiectasis
◊ Cystic fibrosis
◊ Malignant infiltration
Diseases affecting the pulmonary vasculature
◊ Primary pulmonary hypertension
◊ Pulmonary embolism
◊ Pulmonary vascular disease secondary to systemic illness
◊ Intravenous drug abuse
Diseases affecting thoracic cage function
◊ Obesity
◊ Kyphoscoliosis
◊ Neuromuscular diseases
◊ Sleep apnea
Chronic hypoxia at high altitude

RISK FACTORS
• Tobacco abuse
• Living at high altitudes

 DIAGNOSIS

DIFFERENTIAL DIAGNOSIS
• Primary disease of the left side of the heart
• Congenital heart disease

LABORATORY
• Hematocrit - frequently elevated
• pO2 - reduced
Drugs that may alter lab results: N/A
Disorders that may alter lab results: N/A

PATHOLOGICAL FINDINGS
• Evidence of underlying etiology
• Dilated, hypertrophic right ventricle

SPECIAL TESTS ECG - right ventricular hypertrophy (tracings are frequently normal)

IMAGING
• Chest x-ray - evidence of the primary disease, right atrial, ventricular and pulmonary artery enlargement
• Echocardiogram - right ventricular dimensions, assessment of tricuspid regurgitation and Doppler quantitation of pulmonary artery pressure

DIAGNOSTIC PROCEDURES Right heart catheterization for quantitation of ventricular and pulmonary pressures and exclusion of congenital heart disease as etiology of right heart failure

 TREATMENT

APPROPRIATE HEALTH CARE
Outpatient

GENERAL MEASURES
• Vigorous antibiotic treatment of acute respiratory tract infections
• Avoidance of airway irritants (i.e., tobacco smoke) as well as sedatives and tranquilizers which may reduce respiratory effort
• The underlying etiology of cor pulmonale should be adequately treated. Phlebotomy is sometimes useful.

ACTIVITY As tolerated

DIET Moderate salt restriction

PATIENT EDUCATION
• Diet restrictions
• Signs of edema to watch for
• Stress the need for adequate rest
• Referral to social service agency for home care help (oxygen, suctioning, etc.)
• Report any signs of infections to physician
• Avoid use of non-prescription medications, especially sedatives

MEDICATIONS

DRUG(S) OF CHOICE
• O_2 at a flow rate adequate to restore O_2 tensions to > 60 mm Hg in the arterial blood. In patients with CO_2 retention care must be taken not to supply so much O_2 that the patient's hypoxic respiratory drive is inhibited.
• Bronchodilators - (i.e., metaproterenol, albuterol) on a regular dosing schedule of every six hours and more often if necessary
• Diuretics: (i.e., furosemide) for the relief of fluid retention. Dose as necessary.
• Vasodilators: (i.e., hydralazine, nifedipine, diltiazem, prazosin) may be tried if conventional measures fail. Success with these agents can only be measured if they are administered during invasive monitoring and is defined as a > 20% decrease in pulmonary vascular resistance associated with a decreased or unchanged pulmonary artery pressure and an increased or unchanged cardiac output. Monitoring for systemic hypotension during initiation of these medications is necessary.
Contraindications: Vary with the drug being used and the respiratory status and hemodynamics of the particular patient
Precautions: Diuretics - electrolytes should be monitored as excessive loss of potassium and chloride may result in profound metabolic alkalosis
Significant possible interactions: Refer to manufacturer's literature

ALTERNATIVE DRUGS
Digoxin 0.125-0.25 mg/day remains controversial for the treatment of right heart failure. Beneficial effects are not as apparent as in the treatment of left heart failure and electrolyte disturbances with resulting arrhythmias are of concern.

FOLLOWUP

PATIENT MONITORING Depends on the severity of the underlying disease and the extent of right heart failure as well as the medications being used in treatment

PREVENTION/AVOIDANCE Discontinue tobacco use

POSSIBLE COMPLICATIONS N/A

EXPECTED COURSE AND PROGNOSIS Linked to the underlying etiology of cor pulmonale

MISCELLANEOUS

ASSOCIATED CONDITIONS Left heart failure

AGE-RELATED FACTORS
Pediatric: N/A
Geriatric: Metabolism of sedatives and narcotics may be slow, thus the respiratory drive of these patients may be affected for prolonged periods
Others: N/A

PREGNANCY Patient should be seen immediately by a cardiologist as the consequences of an increase in demand for output from the right heart may be quite severe

SYNONYMS N/A

ICD-9-CM
• Cor pulmonale, chronic: 416.9
• Cor pulmonale, acute: 415.0

SEE ALSO N/A

OTHER NOTES N/A

ABBREVIATIONS N/A

REFERENCES
• Brandenburg, R.O., Fuster, V., Giuliani, E.R. & McGoon, D.C.: Cardiology: Fundamentals and Practice. Chicago, Year Book Medical Publishers, 1987
• Braunwald, E.: Heart Disease: A Textbook of Cardiovascular Medicine. 3rd Ed. Philadelphia, W.B. Saunders Co., 1988

Author M. Goldberg, M.D.

Corneal ulceration

 BASICS

DESCRIPTION Corneal ulcers represent an infection of the cornea by bacteria, virus or fungi as a result of breakdown in the protective epithelial barrier. If left untreated, corneal ulcers can result in blindness. Ulcerations may be central or marginal.
Genetics: None
Incidence/Prevalence in USA: Common
Predominant age: None
Predominant sex: Male = Female

SIGNS AND SYMPTOMS
- Eyelid and conjunctiva become inflamed
- Mucopurulent discharge
- The corneal epithelium will be absent with underlying ulceration and infiltration of the corneal stroma with leukocytes
- Foreign body sensation
- Blurred vision
- Light sensitivity
- Pain

CAUSES
- Corneal ulcers are predisposed by the presence of an entry to the external eye. Dry eye, burns, abrasion, contact lenses, inappropriate use of topical anesthetics, antibiotics, or anti-viral drops, immunosuppressant drugs, diabetes, immunodeficiency.
Causative agents for foreign entry:
◊ Gram positive organisms (staphylococci, streptococci, and bacilli)
◊ Anaerobes (cocci, bacilli)
◊ Gram negative organisms (diplococcus, rods, and anaerobes)
◊ Pseudomonas
◊ Viruses such as herpes

RISK FACTORS
- Any abrasive injury
- Contact lenses (especially soft lenses)
- Chronic topical steroid use

 DIAGNOSIS

DIFFERENTIAL DIAGNOSIS Identify infecting organisms

LABORATORY Culture the ulcer
Drugs that may alter lab results:
Pretreatment with topical antibiotics or corticosteroids may delay diagnosis
Disorders that may alter lab results: N/A

PATHOLOGICAL FINDINGS Scrapings for Gram's and Giemsa's stain may demonstrate bacteria, yeast, or intranuclear inclusions which may aid in the diagnosis

SPECIAL TESTS N/A

IMAGING N/A

DIAGNOSTIC PROCEDURES Scrapings of the corneal ulcer may be necessary to identify the underlying organism. The sample should be plated onto the culture media directly.

 TREATMENT

APPROPRIATE HEALTH CARE
- Outpatient or inpatient for severe ulcer or non compliant patient
- All cases of corneal ulceration should be promptly referred to an ophthalmologist

GENERAL MEASURES
- Aggressive topical antibiotic treatment directed toward the causative agent should be instituted immediately while culture studies are pending
- Supplemental topical cycloplegia reduces the inflammation and aids in patient comfort
- Bandaging the eye should be avoided and topical steroids should never be used. Daily evaluation is necessary and prompt consultation with an ophthalmologist or corneal specialist is advised.

ACTIVITY Reduced, until vision returns to normal and healing is complete

DIET No special diet

PATIENT EDUCATION Prevention of abrasions and proper handling of contact lenses can prevent recurrence of corneal ulcers

MEDICATIONS

DRUG(S) OF CHOICE
• Sulfacetamide 10% suspension (bacteriostatic) is only good for low grade conjunctival infections
• Topical gentamicin and tobramycin are effective against Pseudomonas, Enterobacter, Klebsiella, and aerobic gram negative organisms, while cephalosporins (e.g., cefazolin 50 mg/mL) may be effective against many gram negative organisms. The combination aminoglycoside and cephalosporin may be the most appropriate initial therapy.
• Topical quinolones (ciprofloxacin [Ciloxan 0.3%]) were recently introduced for occular use. These may be treatment of choice for Pseudomonas infections.
• Fungal keratitis needs to be treated with parenteral amphotericin B for candida and aspergillus; clotrimazole, miconazole, econazole, and ketoconazole may also be required

Contraindications: Refer to manufacturer's profile of each drug

Precautions: Refer to manufacturer's profile of each drug

Significant possible interactions: Refer to manufacturer's profile of each drug

ALTERNATIVE DRUGS N/A

FOLLOWUP

PATIENT MONITORING The patient should be monitored at least daily

PREVENTION/AVOIDANCE Avoid corneal abrasion or injury and improper contact lens handling

POSSIBLE COMPLICATIONS Scarring of the cornea and loss of vision

EXPECTED COURSE AND PROGNOSIS
• Corneal ulcerations should improve daily and heal with appropriate therapy
• If healing does not occur or the ulcer extends, then consideration should be given to an alternative diagnosis and treatment

MISCELLANEOUS

ASSOCIATED CONDITIONS Chronic ulcerations may be associated with neurotrophic keratitis due to lack of fifth nerve innervation of the cornea. Individuals with thyroid disease, diabetes, immunosuppressive conditions are particularly at risk.

AGE-RELATED FACTORS
Pediatric: N/A
Geriatric: Ring ulceration more common
Others: N/A

PREGNANCY N/A

SYNONYMS N/A

ICD-9-CM 370.0 Corneal ulcer

SEE ALSO N/A

OTHER NOTES N/A

ABBREVIATIONS N/A

REFERENCE None

Author R. Kershner, M.D., F.A.C.S.

Costochondritis

BASICS

DESCRIPTION Anterior chest wall pain associated with pain and tenderness of the costochondral and costosternal regions.
System(s) affected: Musculoskeletal
Genetics: Unknown
Incidence/Prevalence in USA: 10% of chest pain complaints. 15-20% of teenagers with chest pain.
Predominant age: 20-40
Predominant sex: Female

SIGNS AND SYMPTOMS
• Insidious onset
• History of overuse trauma
• History of unusual physical activity
• Often a history of recent upper respiratory infection
• Pain usually sharp in nature, sometimes pleuritic
• Pain involves multiple locations, the second through fifth costal cartilage most often involved
• Pain worse with movement and breathing
• Heat often provides relief of pain
• Chest tightness is often associated with the pain
• Pain sometimes radiates into arm
• Non-suppurative edema and tenderness at rib articulations
• Redness and warmth at sites of tenderness
• Self-limited course
• Often recurs

CAUSES
• Not fully understood
• Trauma
• Overuse

RISK FACTORS Included with causes

DIAGNOSIS

DIFFERENTIAL DIAGNOSIS
Cardiac
 ◊ Coronary artery disease
 ◊ Aortic aneurysm
 ◊ Mitral valve prolapse
 ◊ Pericarditis
 ◊ Myocarditis
Gastrointestinal
 ◊ Gastroesophageal reflux
 ◊ Peptic esophagitis
 ◊ Esophageal spasm
 ◊ Gastritis
Musculoskeletal
 ◊ Fibromyalgia
 ◊ Slipping rib syndrome - involves the lower ribs
 ◊ Costovertebral arthritis
 ◊ Painful xiphoid syndrome
 ◊ Rib trauma with swelling
 ◊ Thoracic disk compression
 ◊ Ankylosing spondylitis
 ◊ Epidemic myalgia
 ◊ Precordial catch syndrome
Psychogenic
 ◊ Anxiety disorder
 ◊ Panic attacks
 ◊ Hyperventilation
Respiratory
 ◊ Asthma
 ◊ Pneumonia
 ◊ Chronic cough
 ◊ Pneumothorax
Other
 ◊ Herpes zoster
 ◊ Spinal tumor
 ◊ Metastatic cancer
 ◊ Substance abuse (cocaine)

LABORATORY The diagnosis of costochondritis is based on a complete and thorough history and physical examination. Laboratory exams should only be utilized if there is concern regarding other elements of the differential Diagnosis. Erythrocyte sedimentation rate inconsistently elevated.
Drugs that may alter lab results: N/A
Disorders that may alter lab results: N/A

PATHOLOGICAL FINDINGS
Costochondral joint inflammation

SPECIAL TESTS None indicated for the diagnosis of costochondritis

IMAGING No imaging is indicated for the diagnosis of costochondritis. Chest x-ray normal.

DIAGNOSTIC PROCEDURES None

TREATMENT

APPROPRIATE HEALTH CARE
Outpatient therapy

GENERAL MEASURES Patient reassurance. Rest and heat.

ACTIVITY As tolerated

DIET Regular

PATIENT EDUCATION Educate the patient in regards to the self-limited nature of the illness. Instruct patient on proper physical activity regimens to avoid overuse syndromes. Also stress the importance of avoiding sudden, significant changes in activity.

MEDICATIONS

DRUG(S) OF CHOICE Nonsteroidal anti-inflammatory drugs (NSAID's) such as aspirin, ibuprofen (Advil, Motrin), naproxen (Anaprox, Naprosyn) or diclofenac (Voltaren). Other analgesics may be used as needed.

Contraindications:
- History of anaphylaxis to aspirin
- Peptic ulcer disease
- Renal insufficiency

Precautions:
- Peptic ulcers may occur with chronic use of non-steroidal anti-inflammatory drugs
- Acute interstitial nephritis
- Drug accumulation with renal insufficiency
- Liver function abnormalities in up to 15% of patients

Significant possible interactions:
NSAID's
  ◊ Albumin-bound drugs - displacement of either drug
  ◊ Warfarin - increased prothrombin time. Monitor prothrombin times closely and adjust warfarin dosage as needed. Monitor lithium levels and adjust lithium dosage as needed. May need to increase lithium dosage when non-steroidal anti-inflammatory drugs have been discontinued.
  ◊ Lithium - increased lithium plasma level
  ◊ Furosemide - decreased natriuretic effect and increased risk of acute renal failure secondary to decreased renal blood flow
  ◊ Propranolol - decreased anti-hypertensive effect

ALTERNATIVE DRUGS Acetaminophen

FOLLOWUP

PATIENT MONITORING Followup in one week

PREVENTION/AVOIDANCE Avoid activity which increases the pain

POSSIBLE COMPLICATIONS
Incomplete attention to differential diagnosis or inappropriate interventions in a desire to ensure that a more life-threatening diagnosis is not missed

EXPECTED COURSE AND PROGNOSIS Self-limited illness

MISCELLANEOUS

ASSOCIATED CONDITIONS Upper respiratory infections

AGE-RELATED FACTORS
Pediatric: Special attention should be paid to psychogenic chest pain with children who perceive family discord
Geriatric: Often present with multiple problems capable of causing chest pain, making a thorough history and physical exam imperative.
Others: N/A

PREGNANCY Unknown

SYNONYMS
- Costosternal syndrome
- Parasternal chondrodynia
- Anterior chest wall syndrome
- Tietze's disease
- Tietze's syndrome
- Chondrocostal junction syndrome

ICD-9-CM 733.99

SEE ALSO N/A

OTHER NOTES N/A

ABBREVIATIONS N/A

REFERENCES
- Fam, A.G.: Approach to musculoskeletal chest wall pain. Primary Care 1988; 15(4):767-782.
- Brucker, F.E., Allard, S.A., Moussa, N.A.: Benign thoracic pain. J. of Royal Society of Medicine 1987; 80:286-289.
- Milov, D.E., Kantor, R.J.: Chest pain in teenagers. Postgraduate Medicine 1990; 88(5):145-154
- A report from ASPN: An exploratory report of chest pain in primary care. J Am Board Fam Prac 1990, 3:143-150

Author S. A. Fields, M.D.

Crohn's disease of the colon

 BASICS

DESCRIPTION An idiopathic inflammatory disease of the small intestine and colon involving all layers of the bowel. It is a slowly progressive and recurrent disease with a tendency to obstruct the bowel, fistulize, and involve adjacent structures in the inflammation. Occasionally occurs at all other sites in the GI tract.

System(s) affected: Gastrointestinal

Genetics:
• 15% of patients have first-degree relatives with inflammatory bowel disease
• All monozygotic twins develop the disease in similar fashion

Incidence in USA:
• 20-100/100,000
• More common in Caucasians than African-Americans or Asians
• More common in Jews

Prevalence in USA: 20-100/100,000

Predominant Age:
• Most cases 15-25 age of onset
• Second smaller peak in ages 55-65

Predominant Sex: Female > Male (slightly)

SIGNS AND SYMPTOMS
All forms of Crohn's
◊ Diarrhea occurs at some time in most patients
◊ Abdominal pain occurs in about two-thirds
◊ Weight loss, pyoderma-gangrenosa
◊ Spondylitis
◊ Symmetrical arthritis
◊ Iritis
◊ Abdominal tenderness often less than expected, in view of symptoms
◊ Abdominal mass (occasionally)
Small bowel disease only
◊ Diarrhea prominent, at any time including nocturnal
◊ Vague abdominal pain frequent. Only half of patients with abdominal pain have associated tenderness, not relieved with evacuation and often aggravated by food.
◊ Intestinal obstruction in one-third. Cramping abdominal pain precedes for months.
◊ Bleeding occurs in 20%, rarely massive
◊ Perianal disease, including fistulae
◊ Internal fistulae
◊ Arthritis 5%
Colon disease only
◊ Diarrhea prominent, at any time including nocturnal
◊ Hematochezia
◊ Abdominal pain in half the patients, often relieved by stooling
◊ Perianal disease in 40%, fistulae
◊ Weight loss prominent
◊ Megacolon occurs in about 10%
◊ Arthritis in 20%
◊ Intestinal obstruction occasional
Colon and small bowel disease
◊ Intestinal obstruction much more common
◊ Arthritis 5%

CAUSES
• Idiopathic
• Aggravated by bacterial infection
• Aggravated by inflammatory cascade

RISK FACTORS More cigarette smokers than expected

 DIAGNOSIS

DIFFERENTIAL DIAGNOSIS
Colon disease
◊ Ulcerative colitis
◊ Ischemic colitis (older age group)
◊ Enteric pathogens
◊ Lymphoma
◊ Tuberculosis
◊ Amebiasis
◊ Adenocarcinoma
◊ Caustic enemas (e.g. H2O2)
Small bowel disease
◊ Tuberculosis
◊ Yersinia
◊ Campylobacter
◊ Chlamydial pelvic inflammation in women
◊ Lymphoma
◊ Actinomycosis
◊ Drugs (e.g., NSAID's)

LABORATORY
• Elevated sedimentation rate
• Anemia common
• Albumin decreased in severe cases
• Serum electrolytes likely to reveal fluid balance problems
• Specific nutrient deficiency - B12, fat soluble vitamins, folate

Drugs that may alter lab results: Sulfa drugs may lower folate after years of administration

Disorders that may alter lab results: All tests are non-specific, similar degrees of disease from other causes produce similar changes

PATHOLOGICAL FINDINGS
• Involvement of all layers of gut wall with inflammation in > 95% cases at least focal areas
• Skip areas in 80% (a normal segment between two involved segments)
• Granuloma in 15%
• Fat hypertrophy following mesenteric vessels in 50% of small bowel disease

SPECIAL TESTS
• Colonoscopy with ileoscopy and biopsy
• Mucosa ulceration, loss, undermining ulcers and distortion, with skip areas

IMAGING
Barium x-rays
◊ Loss of smooth mucosa, undermined ulcers prominent
◊ Narrowed lumen in most involved segments of small bowel
◊ Fistulae from involved segment to other bowel loops, bladder, vagina or external
◊ Skip areas, multiple lesions common

◊ Failure to reflux into ileum on barium enema (not specific)
Plain x-rays
◊ Of painful or distended abdomen (intestinal obstruction)
◊ Toxic patient with colon disease, toxic megacolon
◊ Evaluation of arthritis
◊ Sacroileitis
CT Scans
◊ Define thickening of bowel wall if lumen not narrowed
◊ Define abscess cavities associated with fistulae
◊ Identify extensive perirectal disease

DIAGNOSTIC PROCEDURES
• Ileoscopy and enteroscopy
• The constellation of barium-identified distribution of lesions, endoscopic findings, and biopsies usually establish the diagnosis
• Biopsies of gut mucosa of involved areas are usually compatible with the diagnosis, but not precisely diagnostic. Helpful to rule out other causes.

 TREATMENT

APPROPRIATE HEALTH CARE
• Outpatient management is customary, hospitalization for complications or special treatments
• Disease progresses with average patient requiring surgical treatment each 4 to 7 years

GENERAL MEASURES
• Attention to maintaining weight and nutrition
• Monitor severe cases for fat malabsorption
• Perirectal disease, sitz baths, soap and water after stooling, surgical drainage of perirectal abscesses, surgical treatment of recurrent fistulae if medical management fails
• Extracolonic disease (uveitis, arthritis, dermatitis, sclerosing cholangitis) managed as other diseases in that special area
Indications for surgery:
◊ Severe recurrent hemorrhage
◊ Inability to thrive
◊ Abscess
◊ Total or recurrent intestinal obstruction
◊ Toxicity of megacolon or extensive disease
◊ Symptomatic fistulae other than rectal
◊ Failure of ostomy to function after 1 or more years

ACTIVITY Full activity as tolerated

DIET
• Usually no restrictions
• If fat malabsorption, diminish fat in diet
• If strictures or recurrent obstruction, avoid highly fibrous substances
• If diarrhea prominent, increase dietary fiber (sometimes recommended)

PATIENT EDUCATION An important part of management. Best information from Crohn's and Colitis Foundation of America Inc, 11th floor, Park Ave South, NY 10016, Phone (800)343-3637. Many free pamphlets, local chapters in major metropolitan areas, excellent inexpensive authoritative books. Joining local chapters recommended.

MEDICATIONS

DRUG(S) OF CHOICE
Bringing acute exacerbations or complications under control
◊ Prednisone 20 to 40 mg/day. Response in 1-3 weeks, taper after 4-6 weeks.
◊ Sulfasalazine (or 5-aminosalicylic acid derivative). Increase dose each 4 days from 0.5 gm bid to 1 gm qid if tolerated. Response in 4 to 6 weeks.
Rectal and left sided colon disease
◊ 5-aminosalicylic acid enemas (Rowasa 2 gm) 2-3 times daily
◊ Hydrocortisone enemas (Cortenema) 2-3 times daily or suppositories for proctitis
Predominantly perirectal disease with fistulae
◊ Metronidazole (Flagyl) 250 mg tid for max of 8 weeks
Colon disease in sulfasalazine intolerant patient
◊ Olsalazine (Dipentum) 1 gm/day in two divided doses, increase up to maximum of 2 gm/day (not FDA approved for this indication)
Contraindications: Allergy to prescribed drugs
Precautions:
• Sulfasalazine may not be tolerated by the stomach at necessary dose since it frequently causes nausea, vomiting, and other gastrointestinal distress
• Allergies common
• Male sterility problem with chronic use
• Watch for thrombocytopenia and pancytopenia
Significant possible interactions: Refer to manufacturer's profile of each drug

ALTERNATIVE DRUGS
• Sulfasalazine least costly and well tolerated in 90% of patients. Similar effectiveness but better tolerance with the 5-aminosalicylic acid compounds.
• Metronidazole produces severe peripheral neuritis after months of treatment. Other antibiotics seem similar in action and may be used.

FOLLOWUP

PATIENT MONITORING
• Regular assessment (each 3-6 months if patient is stable) of symptoms, particularly status of weight, pain, diarrhea, hemoglobin and sedimentation rate
• Regular calculation of an activity index based upon:
1) loose stools/day
2) pain
3) general well being
4) systemic manifestations
5) use of antidiarrheal
6) presence of abdominal mass
7) hematocrit
8) change in body weight. Highly useful in following patients and making decisions to increase or diminish medications and/or hospitalize.
• Endoscopy and further images if there are changes in symptoms and signs
• Check liver tests yearly
• Check vitamin B12 level in those with ileal disease or ileal resection

PREVENTION/AVOIDANCE
• Ongoing care with available physician
• Use consultants for review and long term advice

POSSIBLE COMPLICATIONS
• Progression nearly certain - both expansion of old lesions and new lesions occur
• Recurrence after operation nearly certain, usually occurs in gut segment most proximal to anastomoses
• Fistulae may occur
• Extraluminal disease can happen at any time, unrelated to severity or extent of luminal disease
• Limit surgery to essential
• Short bowel syndrome can occur after extensive surgery
• Colon cancer
• Primary sclerosing cholangitis

EXPECTED COURSE AND PROGNOSIS
• Average patient has surgery each 7 years. After 4 surgeries, usually dies.
• Expect disease to recur
• Majority of patients have normal life with work, children, full activities, but overall life is shortened

MISCELLANEOUS

ASSOCIATED CONDITIONS
• Viral gastroenteritis may be much more devastating in Crohn's patients
• Arthritis of two types - similar to rheumatoid and spondylitis
• Variety of skin lesions related, erythema nodosum, non-specific rashes and pyoderma gangrenosum
• Uveal tract disease rare but related
• Sclerosing cholangitis occurs in about 10%, manifest from mild liver test abnormalities including pericholangitis on biopsy to full syndrome

AGE-RELATED FACTORS
Pediatric: Rare
Geriatric: N/A
Others: Occurs at any age

PREGNANCY
• Reversible male sterility after long time on sulfasalazine
• No contraindications to pregnancy for patients with Crohn's disease

SYNONYMS
• Granulomatous colitis
• Regional ileitis

ICD-9-CM 555.9

SEE ALSO N/A

OTHER NOTES N/A

ABBREVIATIONS N/A

REFERENCES
• Farmer, R.G., Hawk, W.A. & Turnbull, R.B.: Clinical patterns in Crohn's disease: a statistical study of 615 cases. Gastroenterology. 68, 627-38, 1975
• Stenson, W.F. & MacDermott, R.P.: Inflammatory Bowel Disease. In Textbook of Gastroenterology. Edited by T. Yamada. Philadelphia, J.B. Lippincott Co., 1991
• Williams, J.G., Wong, W.D., Rothenberger, D.A. & Goldberg, S.M.: Recurrence of Crohn's disease after resection. British Journal of Surgery. 78, 10-19, 1991

Author A. Verma, M.D. & F. Iber, M.D.

Cryptococcosis

 BASICS

DESCRIPTION Cryptococcus neoformans is a fungus which rarely causes disease in hosts with normal immune function. Cryptococcal meningitis is one of the more common AIDS-defining infections in HIV seropositive persons.
System(s) affected: Nervous, Pulmonary, Skin/Exocrine, Endocrine/Metabolic
Genetics: N/A
Incidence/Prevalence in USA: Accounts for 5-8% of opportunistic infections in AIDS patients
Predominant age: Generally adults
Predominant sex: Male > Female

SIGNS AND SYMPTOMS
Cryptococcal meningitis
  ◊ Often insidious onset with subtle findings
  ◊ Frontal or temporal headache (80-95% of patients)
    ◊ Fever (60-80% of patients)
    ◊ Impaired mentation, memory loss
    ◊ Seizures or focal neurologic signs are rare. May occur if cryptococcomas (granulomas) are present
    ◊ Meningismus usually absent (80% of patients)
Pulmonary cryptococcus
    ◊ May be asymptomatic (32% of patients)
    ◊ Cough (54% of patients)
    ◊ Sputum
    ◊ Fever
    ◊ Hemoptysis
    ◊ May disseminate in immunosuppressed patients
Disseminated cryptococcus
    ◊ Painless skin nodules (5-10% of patients). May occur as erythematous papules, vesicles, macules, or ulcers.
    ◊ The heart, bone, kidney, adrenals, eyes, and lymph nodes may harbor infection with symptoms referable to affected organ

CAUSES The cryptococcus fungus is ubiquitous. No person to person transmission has been documented.

RISK FACTORS Immunosuppression which results in reactivation of latent infection (usually foci in lungs). Rarely invasive infection may occur in normal hosts.

 DIAGNOSIS

DIFFERENTIAL DIAGNOSIS
  • In CNS disease - toxoplasmosis, lymphoma, AIDS dementia complex, progressive multifocal leukoencephalopathy, herpes encephalitis, other fungal disease
  • In pulmonary disease - tuberculosis, histoplasmosis, coccidioidomycosis, Kaposi's sarcoma, lymphoma, pneumocystis
  • In disseminated disease - tuberculosis, histoplasmosis, lymphoma, coccidioidomycosis

LABORATORY
  • Latex agglutination assay of cryptococcal antigen in serum, CSF, urine. (False positives and false negatives have occurred but CSF cryptococcal antigen is positive in 95% of culture-proven positive cases.)
  • India ink preparation of CSF (60% positive in non-AIDS patients; 75-85% positive in AIDS patients)
  • Culture of CSF, sputum, blood, urine
Drugs that may alter lab results: N/A
Disorders that may alter lab results: In presence of rheumatoid factor, false positive latex agglutination tests have occurred

PATHOLOGICAL FINDINGS
Inflammation, granuloma formation (may caseate and cavitate), basilar meningitis with mucoid exudate

SPECIAL TESTS Lumbar puncture in cryptococcal meningitis: In non-AIDS patients - elevated opening pressure, elevated CSF protein, decreased glucose and lymphocytic pleocytosis. In AIDS patients - minimal pleocytosis, normal protein and glucose

IMAGING
  • In cryptococcal meningitis - CT of brain is negative unless focal cryptococcomas present
  • In pulmonary cryptococcosis - chest x-ray may show nodules, mass lesions (with occasional cavitation), miliary spread, hilar adenopathy (10%), pleural effusions (less than 5%)

DIAGNOSTIC PROCEDURES Biopsies of skin lesions may be diagnostic

 TREATMENT

APPROPRIATE HEALTH CARE
Inpatient

GENERAL MEASURES N/A

ACTIVITY As tolerated

DIET As tolerated

PATIENT EDUCATION Life-long anti-fungal medication required for suppression

Cryptococcosis

MEDICATIONS

DRUG(S) OF CHOICE
• Amphotericin B at 0.5-0.8 mg/kg/day IV until patient is clinically improving (2-3 weeks). (Some experts add 5-fluocytosine but evidence for increased efficacy is lacking.)
• Fluconazole (Diflucan), an oral (or intravenous) anti-fungal agent is usually given after the patient has improved symptomatically on amphotericin B. Some experts recommend 400 mg/day po until a total of 8-12 weeks of primary therapy has been completed.
• Note: Studies comparing fluconazole vs. amphotericin-B in initial treatment of cryptococcal meningitis are ongoing. Although the initial response is better with amphotericin B, there is some evidence that patients with less severe symptoms (normal mental status) may do well on initial fluconazole (400 mg per day) alone. This course would obviate the need for hospitalization.
Contraindications: Refer to manufacturer's profile of each drug
Precautions: With amphotericin B - permanent renal impairment may occur, hypokalemia, hypomagnesemia; during infusion, fever, chills, headache
Significant possible interactions: Refer to manufacturer's literature

ALTERNATIVE DRUGS   N/A

FOLLOWUP

PATIENT MONITORING
• Monitor clinical status
• Patients who fail treatment (for meningitis) may require intrathecal amphotericin

PREVENTION/AVOIDANCE
• Without suppression, relapse is common (50% in AIDS patients within one year)
• Fluconazole 200 mg po daily is recommended for lifelong suppression
• Avoid bird roosts

POSSIBLE COMPLICATIONS
Cryptococcal infections are fatal unless treated

EXPECTED COURSE AND PROGNOSIS
• Fatal without treatment
• No statistics available on survival

MISCELLANEOUS

ASSOCIATED CONDITIONS
• HIV infection
• AIDS

AGE-RELATED FACTORS
Pediatric: N/A
Geriatric: N/A
Others: N/A

PREGNANCY
Amphotericin contraindicated in pregnancy except when treatment for cryptococcal meningitis becomes imperative

SYNONYMS   Torulosis

ICD-9-CM   117.5

SEE ALSO   N/A

OTHER NOTES   N/A

ABBREVIATIONS
• CSF = cerebrospinal fluid
• AIDS = acquired immunodeficiency syndrome

REFERENCES
• Cohen, P.T., Sande, M., Volberding, P.: The AIDS Knowledge Base. The Medical Publishing Group. A Division of the Massachusetts Medical Society, 1990
• Saag, M., et al.: Comparison of amphotericin B with fluconazole in the treatment of acute AIDS-associated cryptococcal meningitis. New Eng J Med, 1992 Jan 9;326:83-9

Author   C. Carmichael, M.D.

Cryptorchidism

BASICS

DESCRIPTION Incomplete or improper descent of one or both testicles. The condition may be bilateral, but more often, affects the right testis. Normally, descent is in the 7th to 8th month of gestation.
• Ectopic testes - lies outside the usual course of testicle descent prenatally. The ectopic testis may be found within the perineum, above the pubis or along the medial thigh.
• Incomplete descent - mechanical factors prevent passage any farther than the inguinal canal
• Retractile testis (hypermobile testes) - while not true cryptorchidism - is more common. The testis lies within scrotum at times but retracts into inguinal canal.
System(s) affected: Reproductive
Genetics: Occurrence of undescended testes in siblings as well as fathers suggests a genetic etiology
Incidence/Prevalence: 2% of full-term and 10% of premature newborn males
Predominant age: Premature newborns
Predominant sex: Male only

SIGNS AND SYMPTOMS One or both testicles in a site other than the scrotum. May be an isolated defect or associated with other congenital anomalies.

CAUSES
• Unknown
• Impeded by anatomic abnormalities along pathway of descent (e.g., inguinal hernia)

RISK FACTORS Family history of cryptorchidism

DIAGNOSIS

DIFFERENTIAL DIAGNOSIS
• Congenital hemangioma
• Hydrocele

LABORATORY N/A
Drugs that may alter lab results: N/A
Disorders that may alter lab results: N/A

PATHOLOGICAL FINDINGS Higher incidence of carcinoma in undescended testis

SPECIAL TESTS N/A

IMAGING Ultrasonography or CT scan to help locate a nonpalpable testis

DIAGNOSTIC PROCEDURES
Physical exam
◊ Performed with patient in sitting, standing and squatting positions
◊ Observation in warm water may be helpful
◊ Valsalva maneuver and applied pressure to lower abdomen may detect mobile testis (does not require therapy)
◊ Failure to palpate a testis after repeated exams suggests testis is intra-abdominal

TREATMENT

APPROPRIATE HEALTH CARE
Outpatient until surgery performed

GENERAL MEASURES
• Determine type of cryptorchidism if retractile, normal descent generally occurs at puberty
Medical therapy
◊ Administration of chorionic gonadotropin - may cause testicular descent in some boys. Reports of efficacy are inconsistent.
◊ Exact age for initiating therapy is controversial
Surgical therapy
◊ Reasons to consider: Avoids torsion of the cord, averts trauma, decreases risk of malignancy, protects spermatogenesis, may save embarrassment to the patient
◊ Orchiopexy before age 2. Delay in surgery beyond 5 years of age may impair spermatogenesis.

ACTIVITY No restrictions

DIET No special diet

PATIENT EDUCATION Discuss with parents about causes, available treatments, and possible effects on patient's reproduction

MEDICATIONS

DRUG(S) OF CHOICE If medical therapy - chorionic gonadotropin (HCG) 500-1000 international units IM 2 or 3 times/week for a trial period of up to 6 weeks. Other doses - 4000 USP units 3 times a week for 3 weeks; 5000 USP units every other day for 4 doses.
Contraindications: Refer to manufacturer's literature
Precautions: May induce precocious puberty - discontinue drug, effects should reverse in 4 weeks
Significant possible Interactions: Refer to manufacturer's literature

ALTERNATIVE DRUGS N/A

 FOLLOWUP

PATIENT MONITORING Until problem resolved

PREVENTION/AVOIDANCE No preventive measures known

POSSIBLE COMPLICATIONS
• Progressive failure of spermatogenesis if untreated. With orchiopexy, fertility rate still reduced, particularly with bilateral undescended testes.
• Higher incidence of carcinoma (risk may remain despite orchiopexy)
• Hernia development (25%)

EXPECTED COURSE AND PROGNOSIS Disorder usually corrected with medical or surgical therapy, however; possible lifelong consequences

 MISCELLANEOUS

ASSOCIATED CONDITIONS
• Inguinal hernia
• Hemiscrotum
• Hydrocele
• Klinefelter's syndrome
• Hypogonadotropic hypogonadism
• Germinal cell aplasia
• Prune belly syndrome
• Horseshoe kidneys
• Renal agenesis or hypoplasia
• Exstrophy of the bladder
• Ureteral reflux

AGE-RELATED FACTORS
Pediatric: This problem is usually detectable at birth or soon thereafter. If surgery is to be the treatment it should be performed before age 2.
Geriatric: N/A
Others: Puberty: If unilateral cryptorchidism is discovered at or after puberty, treatment of choice is orchiectomy

PREGNANCY N/A

SYNONYMS Undescended testes

ICD-9-CM 752.5

SEE ALSO N/A

OTHER NOTES Delay of surgery beyond age 5 may prevent or impair spermatogenesis, particularly if bilateral cryptorchidism

ABBREVIATIONS N/A

REFERENCE Becker, K.L. (ed.): Principles and Practice of Endocrinology and Metabolism. Philadelphia, J.B. Lippincott Co., 1990

Author E. Lightner, M.D.

Cushing's disease and syndrome

 BASICS

DESCRIPTION Clinical abnormalities associated with chronic exposure to excessive amounts of cortisol (the major adrenocorticoid). The most frequent cause is prolonged use of glucocorticoids.
System(s) affected: Endocrine/Metabolic, Musculoskeletal, Skin/Exocrine, Cardiovascular
Genetics: No known genetic pattern
Incidence/Prevalence in USA: Common
Predominant age: All ages
Predominant sex: Females > Males

SIGNS AND SYMPTOMS
• Moon face (facial adiposity)
• Adipose neck and trunk
• Purple striae on the skin
• Diabetes or glucose intolerance with fasting hyperglycemia and/or glycosuria
• Muscle weakness due to loss of muscle mass from increased catabolism
• Skeletal growth retardation in children

CAUSES
• Prolonged use of glucocorticoids and/or ACTH
• Endogenous ACTH-dependent hypercortisolism
  ◊ ACTH-secreting pituitary tumor
  ◊ Ectopic ACTH production (e.g. oat-cell carcinoma of lung)
• Endogenous ACTH-independent hypercortisolism
  ◊ Adrenal adenoma
  ◊ Adrenal carcinoma
  ◊ Macro/micro nodular hyperplasia

RISK FACTORS
• Any medical problem requiring prolonged use of corticosteroids
• Pituitary tumor
• Adrenal mass

 DIAGNOSIS

DIFFERENTIAL DIAGNOSIS
• Obesity associated with diabetes mellitus
• Adrenogenital syndrome
• Hypercortisolism secondary to alcoholism (Pseudo-Cushing's)

LABORATORY
• Dexamethasone suppresion test
• Urinary 17-Hydroxycorticosteroids and cortisol
• Plasma ACTH concentration
• Corticotropin-releasing factor (CRF) test
• Glycosuria (possible)
• Polycythemia
• Neutrophilia
• Lymphopenia
• Carbohydrate tolerance decreased
• Serum potassium decreased
• Serum sodium decreased
Drugs that may alter lab results: Refer to lab test or drug reference
Disorders that may alter lab results: Refer to lab test reference

PATHOLOGICAL FINDINGS
• Hyalinization of basophilic cells (anterior pituitary)
• Muscular atrophy
• Nephrosclerosis
• Degeneration of pancreatic islet cells

SPECIAL TESTS
• Electrocardiogram - may show signs of hypertension and hypokalemia
• If ACTH-dependent, inferior petrosal sinus sampling for ACTH

IMAGING
• Chest films
• X-rays of the lumbar spine - osteoporosis is common
• If pituitary tumor suspected - visual fields and pituitary CT scan
• If adrenal disease suspected - CT scan

DIAGNOSTIC PROCEDURES Not all tests indicated for every case. Choice of diagnostic procedure dependent on circumstances and judgment. Some tests may need repeating.

 TREATMENT

APPROPRIATE HEALTH CARE
Inpatient for surgical procedures

GENERAL MEASURES
• Depends on etiology. May necessitate radiation, drug therapy, or surgery.
Primary hypersecretion of ACTH
  ◊ Transsphenoidal microsurgery. Radiation therapy as an adjunct for patients not cured.
Adrenocortical tumors
  ◊ Surgical removal when possible
  ◊ If adrenocortical carcinoma, prognosis is poor
Ectopic ACTH production
  ◊ Removal of the neoplastic tissue
  ◊ Metastatic spread makes surgical cure unlikely/impossible
Medical treatment with adrenocortical inhibitors
  ◊ Has not been too successful
  ◊ Should be used when other methods fail
  ◊ In consultation with a clinician having experience in their use

ACTIVITY Determined by patient's symptoms and form of treatment used

DIET
• Potassium supplements
• High protein diet

PATIENT EDUCATION
• Instructions on drug therapy, diet, activity
• Early treatment of infections
• Monitor weight daily
• Emotional lability prevention

MEDICATIONS

DRUG(S) OF CHOICE
• Medications in treatment should be used in consultation with an endocrinologist
Adjunctive management considerations
• Inhibit cortisol production - ketoconazole 400-500 mg twice daily (dosages higher than conventionally recommended)
• Glucocorticoid replacement following surgery. In most cases, can be discontinued by 3-12 months.
Contraindications: Refer to manufacturer's literature
Precautions: Refer to manufacturer's literature
Significant possible interactions: Refer to manufacturer's literature

ALTERNATIVE DRUGS
• Mitotane
• Aminoglutethimide
• Metyrapone

FOLLOWUP

PATIENT MONITORING
• Individualize depending on therapy
• Check regularly for signs of adrenal hypofunction

PREVENTION/AVOIDANCE
• Avoid excessive corticosteroid treatment when possible
• Comprehensive teaching to help patient cope with lifelong treatment

POSSIBLE COMPLICATIONS
• Osteoporosis
• Increased susceptibility to infections
• Virilism
• Pathologic fractures
• Metastases of malignant tumors
• Diabetes insipidus

EXPECTED COURSE AND PROGNOSIS
• Usual course - chronic with cyclic exacerbations and rare remissions
• Guardedly favorable prognosis with surgery

MISCELLANEOUS

ASSOCIATED CONDITIONS Tumors of the pituitary

AGE-RELATED FACTORS
Pediatric: Rare in infancy and childhood. Most cases (under age 8) are due to malignant adrenal tumors.
Geriatric: N/A
Others: N/A

PREGNANCY Can cause exacerbation of Cushing's disease

SYNONYMS N/A

ICD-9-CM 255.0

SEE ALSO N/A

OTHER NOTES Pituitary ACTH excess due to pituitary basophilic or chromophobe tumor causes what is called Cushing's disease

ABBREVIATIONS N/A

REFERENCES
• Kaye, T.B. & Crapo, L.: The Cushing syndrome. An update in diagnostic tests. Ann Intern Med 112:434,1990
• Baxter, J.D. & Tyrell, J.B.: The Adrenal Cortex. In Endocrinology and Metabolism. 2nd Ed. Edited by P. Felig, J.D. Baxter, A.E. Broadus, et al. New York, McGraw-Hill Book Co., 1987

Author W. F. Young, Jr., MD

Cutaneous drug reactions

 BASICS

DESCRIPTION Cutaneous or mucocutaneous eruptions are the most common adverse reactions to oral or parenteral drug therapy. Reactions may be immunologically mediated (either IgE dependent or immune complex dependent and/or other mechanisms not fully appreciated).
• Non-immunologic reactions occur more commonly. The majority of reactions occur within one week of initiation of drug therapy but make occur up to 4 weeks after initiation of therapy.
• Maculopapular and urticarial eruptions are the most common but multiple morphologic types of reactions may occur
Systems affected: Skin, mucus membranes, immunologic
Genetics: No known genetic inheritance pattern
Incidence/Prevalence:
• Three reactions per 1000 drug courses
• Approximately 120 million inpatient drug courses annually in the USA, therefore approximately 144/100,000
• Approximately 125 million Americans regularly use prescription drugs as out patients; overall prevalence in this group is unknown
Predominant age: All ages affected
Predominant sex: Female > Male (specific ratio unknown)

SIGNS AND SYMPTOMS
(note: in order of frequency)
Maculopapular eruptions (exanthems):
  ◊ Most frequent cutaneous reaction
  ◊ Maybe indistinguishable from viral exanthem
  ◊ Erythematous macules and papules
  ◊ Often confluent and symmetrical
  ◊ Pruritus common
  ◊ Mucus membranes, palms and soles maybe involved
  ◊ Onset typically 7-10 days after initiation of drug: may last one to two weeks
Urticaria:
  ◊ Pruritic red wheals distributed anywhere on the body including mucus membranes
  ◊ Individual lesions fade within 24 hours but new urticaria may develop
  ◊ May be mediated by anaphylactic or accelerated IgE reactions, serum sickness or non-immunologic histamine reactions
  ◊ Deep dermal and subcutaneous swelling constitute angioedema and when mucus membranes are involved, maybe life-threatening
Acneform eruptions
  ◊ Pustular lesions but unlike true acne, no comedones
Eczematous reactions
  ◊ Pruritic scale-like erythematous lesions typically on flexor surfaces of arms or legs

Erythema multiforme
  ◊ Target lesions
  ◊ Bullous lesions
  ◊ Mucous membrane involvement (Stevens-Johnson syndrome)
Exfoliative erythroderma
  ◊ Generalized erythema and scaling
  ◊ Potentially life-threatening
Fixed drug eruptions
  ◊ Single or multiple round sharply defined dark red plaques
  ◊ Appear shortly after drug exposure and reappear in the same location after drug ingestion Lesions can occur anywhere: glans penis common in men
  ◊ Onset usually 2 hours after ingestion of drug
  ◊ Some patients have a refractory period during which the drug fails to activate lesions
Lichen planus like eruptions
  ◊ Violaceous papules extensor wrist surfaces
  ◊ Reticular pattern, buccal mucosa
Lupus erythematosus-like reactions
  ◊ Malar erythema
Photosensitivity reaction
  ◊ Phototoxic reactions within 24 hours of light exposure
  ◊ Photoallergic reactions; less common
Vasculitis
  ◊ Petechiae or purpura concentrated on lower legs
Vesiculobullous eruptions
  ◊ Small isolated bullae, erythema multiforme, toxic epidermal necrolysis (potentially fatal)

CAUSES
• Acneform: OCP's, corticosteroids, iodinated compounds, hydantoins, lithium
• Erythema multiforme: Sulfonamides, penicillins, barbiturates, hydantoins, NSAID's, tetracycline, cefaclor
• Erythema nodosum: OCP's, sulfonamides, penicillins
• Fixed drug eruptions: OCP's, barbiturates, salicylates barbiturates, tetracycline, sulfonamides
• Lichenoid: Gold, antimalarials, tetracycline
• Photosensitivity: Phenothiazines, griseofulvin, sulfonamides, tetracycline
• TEN: Hydantoins, NSAID's, sulfonamides
• Vasculitis: Thiazides, gold, sulfonamides, NSAID's, tetracycline
• Bullous: NSAID's, thiazides, barbiturates

RISK FACTORS Drug therapy, especially with sulfonamides, penicillins

 DIAGNOSIS

DIFFERENTIAL DIAGNOSIS
• Viral exanthem: since maculopapular eruptions are the most common form of drug reaction these are often difficult to distinguish from viral exanthems. Presence of fever, lymphocytosis, and other systemic findings may help differentiate.
• Graft versus host disease: In setting of organ transplantation and transfusion of blood

products
• Drug eruptions manifest as many types of dermatosis as previously listed; consider a primary dermatosis in the differential diagnosis. Resolution of the eruption upon withdrawal of a drug will help to clarify.

LABORATORY
• Routine laboratory tests generally nonspecific and usually not helpful
• Eosinophilia: Possible in certain allergic reactions but generally of little value clinically
Drugs that may alter lab results:
Procainamide, hydralazine - positive ANA
Disorders that may alter lab results: N/A

PATHOLOGICAL FINDINGS
• Pathological findings dependent upon type of reaction; may be nonspecific
• Punch biopsy sometimes helpful for fixed drug eruptions which show certain characteristic histological features, i.e. lichenplanus-like or erythma multiforme
• Histologic exam may also be helpful in reactions related to halogen (iodine, bromine) eruptions

SPECIAL TESTS
• Skin testing (useful in IgE mediated reactions)
• IgG and IgM: hemagglutination assays can detect drug-specific antibodies, but not routinely useful

IMAGING N/A

DIAGNOSTIC PROCEDURES
• Detailed drug-use history including all OTC medicines, duration of therapy, medications used within the last four weeks
• Withdrawal of suspected offending agent and observation for resolution of rash
• Selective special testing for suspected IgE mediated reactions

 TREATMENT

APPROPRIATE HEALTH CARE
• Urticaria, angioedema, or bullous lesions are all potentially more serious than other types of reactions therefore these patients should be seen as soon as possible for evaluation
• Consider inpatient treatment for anaphylactic reactions, Stevens-Johnson syndrome, extensive bullous reactions, or toxic epidermal (TEN) necrolysis

Cutaneous drug reactions

GENERAL MEASURES
• Discontinue suspected offending agent. In patients with multiple medications, the decision to discontinue each medication should be based on the likelihood of each individual medication causing the reaction (e.g., 7% for penicillins, sulfonamides) and the risk/benefit ratio of continuing each medication.
• Re-challenge with specific medications thought to have caused urticaria, angioedema, anaphylaxis, erythema multiforme, or other bullous lesions is potentially dangerous

ACTIVITY
• No specific restrictions in general
• For acute eczematous or urticarial reactions with intense pruritus, tepid bathing and avoidance of activities resulting in perspiration may be helpful
• For toxic epidermal necrolysis, admit to burn unit

DIET No dietary restrictions

PATIENT EDUCATION Printed patient information is available from American Academy of Dermatology, 930 N. Meacham Rd., P.O. Box 4014, Schaumberg, IL 60168-4014 (708)330-0230

MEDICATIONS

DRUG(S) OF CHOICE
• Specific therapy depends on the type of drug eruption. Most require no specific therapy.
• Symptomatic therapy helpful for pruritus, xeroses, urticaria and angioedema
• For pruritus - antihistamines (Benadryl, Atarax)
• Anaphylaxis or wide spread urticaria - epinephrine 1:1000, 0.01 mL per kilogram (0.3 mL maximum) subcutaneous
• For anaphylaxis, severe urticaria, erythema multiforme - corticosteroids parenterally as indicated by patient's condition; or on tapering po schedule (10-14 days). Therapy of epidermal necrolysis contraversial; majority do not favor use of systemic corticosteroids
• Topical lubricants, emollients for eczematous reactions
• Topical corticosteroids for limited eczematous type eruptions, or for lichenoid eruptions
Contraindications: Refer to manufacturer's information
Precautions: Refer to manufacturer's information
Significant possible interactions: Refer to manufacturer's information

ALTERNATIVE DRUGS N/A

FOLLOWUP

PATIENT MONITORING
• For urticarial, bullous, or erythema multiforme-like lesions, close patient followup is indicated to insure there is no progression
• Patients with systemic anaphylaxis or wide spread bullous lesions, including toxic edidermal necrolysis, should be admitted to hospital until condition improves
• Maintain at least telephone follow-up until eruption has completely cleared
• Label patient's chart with the suspected agent and the specific type of reaction

PREVENTION/AVOIDANCE
• Future avoidance of specific drugs and any analogs
• Be aware of any potential cross over reactions [i.e. 8-10% incidents of reactions of cephalosporins in patient's sensitized to penicillins and the cross-over for the anticonvulsive drugs hydantoin, barbiturates, and carbamazepine (Tegretol)]
• Always question patient's about prior drug reactions, specific type of reaction, and use of OTC medicines

EXPECTED COURSE AND PROGNOSIS
• Eruptions generally fade within days after removing offending agent
• Urticaria, angioedema, bullous reactions, are potentially more serious, even life-threatening

POSSIBLE COMPLICATIONS
• Anaphylaxis
• Laryngeal edema
• Possible associated bone marrow suppression
• Possible cross reaction to chemically similar agents with future exposure

MISCELLANEOUS

ASSOCIATED CONDITIONS N/A

AGE-RELATED FACTORS
Pediatric: May occur in this age group
Geriatric:
• Possibly more likely in this age group due to greater number of medications
• Severe systemic reactions less well tolerated
Others: N/A

PREGNANCY N/A

SYNONYMS
• Drug eruptions
• Dermatitis medicamentosa

ICD-9-CM 693 0

SEE ALSO N/A

OTHER NOTES N/A

ABBREVIATIONS N/A

REFERENCES
• Bigby, M., et al.: Drug-induced cutaneous reactions. J Amer Med Assn 256 3358, 1986
• Habif, T: Clinical Dermatology. 2nd Ed. St Louis, C V Mosby, 1990
• Fitzpatrick, T.B, et al. (eds): Dermatology in General Medicine. 3rd Ed. New York, McGraw-Hill, 1987
• Arndt, K.A.: Manual of Dermatologic Therapeutics. 4th Ed. Boston, Little, Brown & Co, 1989

Author J. R. Richard, MD

Cutaneous squamous cell carcinoma

 BASICS

 DIAGNOSIS

 TREATMENT

DESCRIPTION Malignant epithelial tumor arising from keratinocytes
System(s) affected: Skin/Exocrine
Genetics: N/A
Incidence in USA: N/A
Prevalence in USA: Varies within geographic U.S. 32.3/100,000 for Caucasian males; 14.3/100,000 for Caucasian females
Predominant age: Elderly population
Predominant sex: Male > Female

SIGNS AND SYMPTOMS
• Occurs most commonly in chronically sun-exposed areas in light-skinned people e.g., scalp, neck, upper extremities, back of hands, superior surface of pinna
• Often develops in previously damaged skin, e.g., solar keratoses, actinic cheilitis
• In African Americans - equal frequency in sun-exposed and unexposed
• Tumors present often as small, firm nodules with indistinct margins or as plaques
• Surface may be smooth, verrucous or papillomatous
• Varying degrees of ulceration, erosion, crust, scale
• Color often red to red-brown to tan
• May appear white in areas of moisture
• May arise in chronic skin ulcers, e.g., venous stasis ulcers
• May arise in scars
• Can arise in skin damaged by radiation, x-rays, etc.
• Varies from slowly growing, locally invasive to aggressive tumor with propensity to metastasis
• On lip, often arises in patch of leukoplakia

CAUSES
• Exact mechanism not established, epidemiologic and experimental evidence suggests the following as causative agents
• Sunlight (solar radiation)
• Radiation exposure
• Inorganic arsenic exposure
• Exposure to coal tar, other oil and tar derivatives
• Immunosuppression by medications or disease

RISK FACTORS
• Older age
• Male
• Outdoor actinic exposure
• Irish-Scottish-British descent
• Fair complexion, fair hair
• Light blue or green eyes
• Poor tanning ability with tendency to burn

DIFFERENTIAL DIAGNOSIS
Keratoacanthoma, basal cell carcinoma, actinic keratosis, malignant melanoma

LABORATORY Requires biopsy for precise pathologic diagnosis
Drugs that may alter lab results: N/A
Disorders that may alter lab results: N/A

PATHOLOGICAL FINDINGS Abnormal epithelial cells extending into the dermis from the epidermis. Varying degrees of atypical appearance can be noted.

SPECIAL TESTS N/A

IMAGING N/A

DIAGNOSTIC PROCEDURES Surgical biopsy mandatory to ensure proper and precise diagnosis

APPROPRIATE HEALTH CARE All outpatient unless extensive lesion

GENERAL MEASURES
• Excisional surgery - appropriate for almost all squamous cell lesions
• Electrodesiccation and curettage - used for small lesions (generally < 1.0 cm) on flat surfaces, e.g., forehead, cheek. Requires training and expertise in electrosurgery.
• Indications for Moh's chemosurgery include: Recurrent tumor; larger, ill-defined lesions; presence of bone or cartilage invasion; multiple carcinomas; lesion in area of late radiation change. Requires referral to appropriately trained dermatologic surgeon.
• Radiation therapy - suitable for larger advanced lesions. Requires specialized training.

ACTIVITY Full activity

DIET No restrictions

PATIENT EDUCATION
• Instruct patient in skin self exam
• Appropriate sun avoidance measures, e.g., sunscreens, protective clothing
• Patient education materials available from American Cancer Society

MEDICATIONS

DRUG(S) OF CHOICE N/A
Contraindications: N/A
Precautions: N/A
Significant possible interactions: N/A

ALTERNATIVE DRUGS N/A

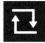

FOLLOWUP

PATIENT MONITORING After therapy, skin exam every month for 3 months, 6 months post-treatment, then yearly

PREVENTION/AVOIDANCE
• Sun-avoidance measures - sunscreens, hats, etc.
• Avoid contact with known carcinogenic compounds

POSSIBLE COMPLICATIONS
• Recurrence locally
• Metastatic disease

EXPECTED COURSE AND PROGNOSIS
• About 90-95% cure rate with appropriate treatment
• Lesion equal to or greater than 2 cm more prone to recur
• Head and neck lesions have better prognosis

MISCELLANEOUS

ASSOCIATED CONDITIONS
• Xeroderma pigmentosum
• Albinism
• Chronic skin ulcers of the leg
• Chronic thermal burns
• Actinic keratosis (cutaneous horn)
• Bowen's disease

AGE-RELATED FACTORS
Pediatric: N/A
Geriatric: N/A
Others: N/A

PREGNANCY N/A

SYNONYMS
• Squamous cell carcinoma of the skin
• Epidermoid carcinoma
• Prickle cell carcinoma

ICD-9-CM
Code varies with location
173.3 (face)
173.4 (scalp, neck)
173.5 (trunk)
173.6 (upper limb)
173.7 (lower limb)
173.9 (site unspecified)

SEE ALSO N/A

OTHER NOTES N/A

ABBREVIATIONS N/A

REFERENCES
• Fitzpatrick, T.N., et al.: Dermatology in General Medicine. New York, McGraw-Hill Book Company, 1987
• Friedman, R.J., et al.: Cancer of the Skin. Philadelphia, W.B. Saunders Co., 1991

Author J. Little, M.D.

Cutaneous T cell lymphoma

 BASICS

DESCRIPTION Cutaneous T-cell lymphoma (mycosis fungoides) is an uncommon chronic lymphoma characterized by a malignant proliferation of T-helper cells in the skin. In the late stage, the lymph nodes and viscera are affected.
Genetics: Evidence suggests increased frequency of HLA antigens Aw31 and Aw32
System(s) affected: Skin/Exocrine, Hemic/Lymphatic/Immunologic
Incidence/Prevalence in USA: 0.29 cases per 100,000 per year
Predominant age: Most cases occur in fifth and sixth decades, incidence increases with age
Predominant sex: Male > Female

SIGNS AND SYMPTOMS
Skin eruption
   ◊ Patches (eczema-like rash)
   ◊ Plaques
   ◊ Tumors
   ◊ Pruritus
   ◊ Exfoliative erythroderma
   ◊ Ulcers of the skin
   ◊ Lymphadenopathy
   ◊ Hepatomegaly (late)
   ◊ Splenomegaly (late)

CAUSES Unknown

RISK FACTORS
• HTLV-I
• Exposure to petrochemicals, metals and solvents

 DIAGNOSIS

DIFFERENTIAL DIAGNOSIS
Patches:
   ◊ Parapsoriasis
   ◊ Atopic eczema
   ◊ Nummular eczema
Plaques:
   ◊ Parapsoriasis
   ◊ Psoriasis
Tumors:
   ◊ Other primary skin cancers
   ◊ Internal malignancies metastatic to skin
Exfoliative erythroderma:
   ◊ Psoriasis
   ◊ Atopic dermatitis
   ◊ Drug eruption

LABORATORY
• CBC with differential and platelets
• Total lymphocyte count
• Automated chemical profile
Drugs that may alter lab results: N/A
Disorders that may alter lab results: N/A

PATHOLOGICAL FINDINGS
Skin biopsy:
   ◊ Epidermotropism
   ◊ Pautrier's microabscesses
   ◊ Widened, fibrotic papillary dermis
   ◊ Superficial band-like dermal infiltrate

SPECIAL TESTS
• Sézary's cell preparation
• Electron microscopy
• HTLV-I serology
• Enzyme histochemistry
• DNA flow cytometry
• Immunophenotyping
• Immunogenotyping
• Molecular cytogenetics
• Polymerase chain reaction

IMAGING
• Chest x-ray
• CT scan of abdomen

DIAGNOSTIC PROCEDURES
• Skin biopsy - diagnostic procedure of choice
• Lymph node biopsy
• Bone marrow biopsy
• Liver biopsy

 TREATMENT

APPROPRIATE HEALTH CARE The majority of patients can be managed on an outpatient basis

GENERAL MEASURES
• No disease-specific special measures
• Treatment should be individualized for each patient as in most cases this is a chronic slowly progressive disease

ACTIVITY Fully active

DIET No special diet

PATIENT EDUCATION By physician on individual basis

MEDICATIONS

DRUG(S) OF CHOICE
• Therapy must be individualized. There is no universally accepted standard approach to treatment of this disease.
• Topical nitrogen mustard (Mustargen) (for early disease) in aqueous or ointment preparation applied once daily to entire skin surface avoiding genitalia
Contraindications: See manufacturer's profile of each drug
Precautions:
• Delayed hypersensitivity occurs in 50%
• Radiometric - patients should practice prudent sun avoidance
• Maintenance treatment required after clearing
Significant possible interactions: See manufacturer's profile of each drug

ALTERNATIVE DRUGS
• PUVA (psoralen and ultraviolet A light)
• Topical carmustine (BCNU)
• Total body electron beam therapy
• Localized orthovoltage x-ray therapy
• Interferon
• Retinoids (e.g., etretinate)
• Extracorporeal photochemotherapy
• Systemic chemotherapy

FOLLOWUP

PATIENT MONITORING Must be individualized

PREVENTION/AVOIDANCE N/A

POSSIBLE COMPLICATIONS Metastatic spread to organs other than skin

EXPECTED COURSE AND PROGNOSIS
• The development of lymphadenopathy, tumors or cutaneous ulcerations during the course of the disease is associated with a median survival of 4 years
• The appearance of the third sign (irrespective of the order developed) is associated with a median survival of 1 year

MISCELLANEOUS

ASSOCIATED CONDITIONS N/A

AGE-RELATED FACTORS
Pediatric: N/A
Geriatric: N/A
Others: N/A

PREGNANCY N/A

SYNONYMS
• Mycosis fungoides
• Sézary's syndrome

ICD-9-CM
202.8 Other lymphomas

SEE ALSO N/A

OTHER NOTES Sézary's syndrome is the leukemic variant of cutaneous T cell lymphoma. Characteristics include erythroderma, pruritus, adenopathy and circulating atypical cells with cerebriform nuclei.

ABBREVIATIONS N/A

REFERENCES
• Edelson, R.L.: J. Am Acad Derm 2: 89-106, 1980
• Braverman, I.M : Curr Prob Derm 3 (6): 184-227, 1991

Author V. Soong, M.D.

Cystic fibrosis

BASICS

DESCRIPTION Generalized, autosomal recessive disorder of infants, children and young adults with widespread dysfunction of the exocrine glands. Characteristics include chronic pulmonary disease, pancreatic insufficiency, abnormally high levels of electrolytes in the sweat and less frequently biliary cirrhosis, diabetes mellitus.
System(s) affected: Pulmonary, Gastrointestinal, Endocrine/Metabolic, Reproductive
Genetics: Autosomal recessive, gene on chromosome 7. Linkage detection in families with known disease. Probes for direct detection available.
Incidence/Prevalence: The most common lethal genetic disease. Caucasians: 1 in 2000 births, lower in African-Americans, Native Americans and Asian ancestry.
Incidence in USA: In 1992: 20,333.
Predominant age: Infants, children and young adults (oldest patient at time of diagnosis was 65)
Predominant sex: Male = Female

SIGNS AND SYMPTOMS
Endocrine sweat gland:
◊ Increased concentrations of sodium and chloride leading to hyponatremia, hypochloremia, arrhythmias
◊ Dehydration with heat and infections
Respiratory:
◊ Wheezing
◊ Chronic cough
◊ Dyspnea
◊ Tachypnea
◊ Barrel chest
◊ Cyanosis
◊ Recurrent bronchitis and pneumonia leading to bronchiectasis
◊ Predominant flora - Staphylococcus aureus and Pseudomonas
◊ Digital clubbing
◊ Nasal polyposis
Gastrointestinal:
◊ Meconium ileus
◊ Failure to thrive
◊ Distal intestinal obstruction syndrome (DIOS)
◊ Chronic, recurrent abdominal pain
◊ Gastroesophageal reflux
◊ Voracious appetite prior to diagnosis
◊ Abdominal distension
◊ Hypoelectrolytemia and alkalosis
◊ Characteristically frequent, bulky, foul - smelling, pale stool with a high fat content
◊ Vitamin deficiencies (A,D,E,K)
◊ Rectal prolapse
Others:
◊ Delayed weight gain during growth and development
◊ Retarded bone growth
◊ Delayed sexual development
◊ Males infertile

CAUSES Autosomal recessive genetic defect

RISK FACTORS Positive family history (rarely seen due to recessive nature)

DIAGNOSIS

DIFFERENTIAL DIAGNOSIS
• RAO
• Recurrent pneumonias
• Brinchiectasis
• Infertility

LABORATORY
• Elevation of sodium and chloride concentrations in sweat (quantitative pilocarpine iontophoresis sweat test)
• Stool trypsin and chymotrypsin absent or diminished
• 72 hour fecal fat excretion - increased fat in stool
• Decreased albumin, fat soluble vitamins
• CF gene screen (reference lab)
• Pseudomonas in respiratory secretions
Drugs that may alter lab results: N/A
Disorders that may alter lab results:
• Edema
• Hypoproteinemia
• Inadequate quantities of sweat to study

PATHOLOGICAL FINDINGS
• Lungs (major problem) - chronic inflammation, inspissated mucus, bronchiectasis with areas of fibrosis and atelectasis
• Pancreas - obstructed ducts, acini replaced by fibrotic tissue, cysts, amorphous eosinophilic concretions and thick mucus
• Liver - secretions obstruct biliary ducts; focal biliary cirrhosis
• Intestine - hypertrophied mucous glands
• Males - hypoplastia or atrophy of vas deferens

SPECIAL TESTS
• Pulmonary function studies (2-3 times a yesr)
• Sputum culture and sensitivity
• Exercise testing
• Response to bronchodilators - may show paradoxical drop
• In newborns - serum concentration of immunoreactive trypsin reported to be elevated and used as a means of newborn screening. Radioimmune assay developed for use with dried blood spots that are routinely collected for newborn metabolic screening.
• Genetic testing to identify patient defect and analyze family for carrier status or prenatal diagnosis

IMAGING
Chest x-ray - hyperaeration, hilar adenopathy, occasional pneumothorax, bronchiectasis, blebs

DIAGNOSTIC PROCEDURES
Diagnosis made in presence of clinical symptoms and positive sweat test, gene screen

TREATMENT

APPROPRIATE HEALTH CARE
• Outpatient usually
• Inpatient during infections or other crisis

GENERAL MEASURES
• Care by experienced physician and team (respiratory therapist, nurse, nutritionist, physical therapist, counsellor, social worker)
• Goals are to prevent and treat respiratory failure and pulmonary complications
• Postural drainage and chest physiotherapy
• Pancreatic enzyme replacement
• Regular exercises for fitness
• Press for adequate growth through good nutrition - supplements may be needed
• Aerosol B2 agonists
• Antibiotics
• Oxygen therapy when needed
• Barium enemas or surgery for unrelieved meconium ileus (newborn)
• For fecal accumulation and intussusception in adults - enemas of diatrizoate sodium or Golytely per NG
• Surgery may be indicated for some complications
• Insulin, if diabetes develops
• Organ transplants possible for lung, liver, endocrine pancreas

ACTIVITY
Physical conditioning to the extent possible for cardiorespiratory fitness (does not improve pulmonary function)

DIET
• Allow salting of foods per patient preference
• High protein
• High calories (1.5 x recommended for general population)
• High fat (previously not recommended)
• Vitamin supplements (double RDA)

PATIENT EDUCATION
Written information and support: Cystic Fibrosis Foundation, 6931 Arlington Road, Ste. 2000, Bethesda, MD 20814, (800)344-4823

MEDICATIONS

DRUG(S) OF CHOICE
IV antibiotics
◊ According to culture and sensitivity studies when ill with respiratory infections
◊ For pseudomonas infections - IV tobramycin, start with 10 mg/kg/24 hrs; peak 8-12 µg/mL; trough 1-2 µg/mL plus IV ceftazidime, antipseudomonas penicillin. Newer option for pseudomonas - tobramycin inhaled 80 mg tid.
◊ For staphylococcal infections - IV Keflin, cephalosporin, based on sensitivity
Other therapies
◊ Pancreatic enzyme replacements (Pancrease, Creon)
◊ Bronchodilators
◊ Oxygen therapy for severe pulmonary insufficiency or hypoxemia
◊ Occasional assisted ventilation, controversial
◊ IPPB contraindicated
◊ Routine administration of annual influenza vaccine

Contraindications: Refer to manufacturer's literature

Precautions: Refer to manufacturer's literature. Higher dosages for shorter administration intervals usually required.

Significant possible interactions: Refer to manufacturer's literature

ALTERNATIVE DRUGS N/A

FOLLOWUP

PATIENT MONITORING   At least 3 times a year; cystic fibrosis center if possible

PREVENTION/AVOIDANCE
In prenatal situations
◊ Genetic counseling
◊ Prenatal diagnosis for future pregnancies
For complications
◊ For respiratory infections - maintain pertussis and measles immunity; annual influenza immunization
◊ Avoid general anesthetics. Consider epidural, spinal, or local.
◊ Good medical teamwork in the management of the multifaceted problems of the disease

POSSIBLE COMPLICATIONS
- Atelectasis
- Pneumothorax
- Hemoptysis
- Right heart failure
- Pulmonary hypertension
- Pulmonary emphysema
- Digital clubbing
- Hypertrophic pulmonary osteoarthropathy
- Diabetes
- Metabolic alkalosis
- Volume depletion
- Bleeding esophageal varices
- Symptomatic biliary cirrhosis
- Intestinal obstruction
- Females anovulatory (fertility rate about 80%)
- Numerous psychosocial aspects
- Malnutrition
- Retarded growth

EXPECTED COURSE AND PROGNOSIS
- Largely dependent on pulmonary involvement
- Prognosis improving due to early detection and aggressive treatment
- Median survival is to age 29

MISCELLANEOUS

ASSOCIATED CONDITIONS See Complications

AGE-RELATED FACTORS
Pediatric: Diagnosis usually confirmed in infancy or early childhood but some go undetected until adolescence. Newborn screening methods are in development. Psychosocial considerations
Geriatric: N/A
Others: N/A

PREGNANCY   If cystic fibrosis patient's condition (pulmonary and nutrition) good at start of pregnancy, usually returns to that level following birth. If these conditions are compromised before pregnancy, they deteriorate following birth.

SYNONYMS N/A

ICD-9-CM   277.0 cystic fibrosis

SEE ALSO N/A

OTHER NOTES
- Advise genetic counseling for at-risk individuals
- Encoded protein on long arm of chromosome 7 contains 1480 amino acids
- Multiple types of gene defects are possible (>200 defined)

ABBREVIATIONS N/A

REFERENCES
- Tizzano, F. & Buchwald, M.: Cystic fibrosis: Beyond the gene to therapy. Jour of Pediatrics; 1992;120;337-343
- Tizzano, F. & Buchwald, M.: Recent advances in cystic fibrosis research. Jour of Pediatrics; 1993;122:985-988
- Schidlow, D.V., Taussig, L.M. & Knowles, M.R.: Cystic Fibrosis Foundation Conference Report on Pulmonary Complications of Cystic Fibrosis; Pediatric Pulmonology; 15:187-198 (1993)
- Taussig, L.M.: Cystic Fibrosis. New York, Thieme-Stratton Inc., 1984

Author N. Dambro, M.D.

Cytomegalovirus inclusion disease

BASICS

DESCRIPTION Infection with cytomegalovirus, a DNA virus belonging to the herpes family. All cytomegaloviruses have a propensity for remaining latent in man. They cannot be propagated in laboratory animals or in most cell cultures.
• The disease occurs world-wide and may be transferred in several ways, including by human contact. Approximately four out of five people over age 35 have been infected with cytomegalovirus, usually during childhood or early adulthood. In most of these, the disease is mild and overlooked.
• CMV infection during pregnancy can be hazardous to the fetus and may lead to stillbirth, brain damage, birth defects or to severe neonatal illness
• The name derives from the infected cells that are large and bear intranuclear inclusions
• Infection may be in almost any organ, but the salivary glands are the most common site in children and the lungs in adults. This infection can occur congenitally, postnatally, or at any age
Categories of CMV infections include:
◊ Congenital: These infections vary greatly from cytomegaloviremia in a normal infant to the cause of abortion, stillbirth, postnatal death from hemorrhage, anemia, liver or CNS damage.
◊ Acute infection in a normal host
◊ Infections in bone marrow transplant patients - usually pneumonia
◊ Infection in patients with AIDS - usually retinitis
◊ Infections in other immunocompromised patients - pulmonary, gastrointestinal, or renal disease
System(s) affected: Pulmonary, Skin/Exocrine, Nervous
Genetics: May be passed from mother to fetus
Incidence/Prevalence in USA:
• Common, but frequently asymptomatic
• Up to 90% of adults have been infected, almost all with inapparent disease. Infection seems to be more common in homosexual males.
Predominant age: All ages, peaks at < 3 months; 16-40 years, and 40-75 years
Predominant sex: Male > Female

SIGNS AND SYMPTOMS
Congenital:
• Abortion
• Asymptomatic cytomegaloviremia
• Hemorrhage
• Anemia
• Jaundice
• Signs of CNS damage
Acquired:
(Acute infection in a normal or immunocompromised host)
• May be asymptomatic
• Fatigue
• Nausea
• Vomiting
• Bone pain
• Chills
• Fever
• Diarrhea
• Jaundice
• Hepatomegaly
• Splenomegaly
• Dyspnea
Infections in bone marrow transplant patients:
• Pneumonitis with cough, fever, chills, chest pain
Infections in AIDS patients:
• Retinitis
• Esophageal, gastric, small bowel and colonic ulcerations
• Pneumonitis

CAUSES
• Infection with cytomegalovirus
• Reactivation of a latent process in patients who are immunosuppressed

RISK FACTORS
• HIV infection
• AIDS
• Organ transplantation (50% attack rate, depending on serologic status)
• Blood transfusion. A postperfusion syndrome may develop in 2 to 4 weeks in patients having fresh blood transfusions. Characteristics include fever lasting 2 to 3 weeks, hepatitis, with or without jaundice, atypical lymphocytosis similar to that of infectious mononucleosis, and a skin rash.
• Immunocompromised host
• Living in closed population
• Corticosteroid therapy
• Day care environment - infant or geriatric

DIAGNOSIS

DIFFERENTIAL DIAGNOSIS
• Congenital: Bacterial, viral, and protozoan infections, such as toxoplasmosis, rubella, syphilis
• Acquired: Viral hepatitis, infectious mononucleosis

LABORATORY
• Human fibroblastic cell culture inoculation may isolate the virus from urine, blood, other body fluids, or tissues
• Leukopenia
• Thrombocytopenia
• Increased lymphocytes
• Demonstration of CMV in secretions or tissues by immunofluorescence with commercially available monoclonal antibodies or by in situ hybridization
Drugs that may alter lab results: N/A
Disorders that may alter lab results: N/A

PATHOLOGICAL FINDINGS Giant cells with basophilic inclusion bodies

SPECIAL TESTS
• Human fibroblastic tissue cultures to isolate the virus
• Immunofluorescence techniques for virus demonstrations

IMAGING Skull film - intracranial calcifications

DIAGNOSTIC PROCEDURES
• Bronchoscopy in bone marrow transplant patients if suspicious of CMV pneumonia
• Buffy coat culture
• Endoscopic biopsy of gastrointestinal tract

TREATMENT

APPROPRIATE HEALTH CARE
Inpatient for disseminated infection or CMV reactivation syndrome

GENERAL MEASURES Isolation

ACTIVITY Bedrest

DIET No special diet

PATIENT EDUCATION

MEDICATIONS

DRUG(S) OF CHOICE
• CMV immunoglobulin
• Antivirals, such as ganciclovir (relatively resistant to acyclovir)
Contraindications: Refer to manufacturer's literature
Precautions: Refer to manufacturer's literature
Significant possible interactions: Refer to manufacturer's literature

ALTERNATIVE DRUGS N/A

FOLLOWUP

PATIENT MONITORING Close followup in ICU (isolated) during infection with disseminated form

PREVENTION/AVOIDANCE Avoid immunosuppression (when possible)

POSSIBLE COMPLICATIONS
• Chorioretinitis
• Encephalitis
• Mononucleosis
• Colitis
• Deafness
• Mental retardation

EXPECTED COURSE AND PROGNOSIS Disseminated form often fatal

MISCELLANEOUS

ASSOCIATED CONDITIONS
• Acquired immune deficiency syndrome (AIDS)
• Corticosteroid therapy
• Leukemia
• Lymphoma

AGE-RELATED FACTORS
Pediatric: May occur congenitally or postnatally
Geriatric: N/A
Others: N/A

PREGNANCY N/A

SYNONYMS
• Giant cell inclusion disease
• CID
• CMV
• Salivary gland virus disease

ICD-9-CM 078.5

SEE ALSO N/A

OTHER NOTES N/A

ABBREVIATIONS N/A

REFERENCES
• Mandell, G.L. (ed.): Principles and Practice of Infectious Diseases. 3rd Ed. New York, Churchill Livingstone, 1990
• Onorato, I.M. et al: Epidemiology of Cytomegaloviral Infection: Recommendations for Prevention & Control. In Rev Infect Dis. 1985;7:479
• Cohen, J.I. & Corey, G.R.: Cytomegalovirus Infection in the Normal Host. Medicine. 1985;64:100-114

Author V. D. Rodgers, M.D.

Decompression sickness

BASICS

DESCRIPTION Metastatic dissolution of gas bubbles (usually nitrogen) into tissues caused by a relatively rapid decrease in the environmental pressure. Five types based on symptomatology:
• Limb bends - gas deposition in tissues causes a poorly-localized "pain-only" syndrome; may herald more serious disease.
• Cerebral bends - stroke-like picture due to paradoxical arterial gas embolism (via A-V or intracardiac shunt), de-novo arterial gas formation, and/or cerebral edema.
• Spinal cord bends - transverse paresis caused by retrograde venous thrombosis with patchy necrosis and edema of the spinal cord; predilection for high lumbar nerve roots due to lack of collateral circulation.
• Inner ear bends - development of bubble formation and hemorrhage in labyrinthine fluid spaces and vasculature.
• Lung bends ("chokes") - excessive venous bubbles develop and release vasoactive substances causing pulmonary irritation and bronchoconstriction. The primary symptoms are substernal chest pain (worse with inspiration), dyspnea, and cough.
System(s) affected: Cardiovascular, Nervous, Musculoskeletal, Pulmonary
Genetics: N/A
Incidence/Prevalence in USA: Uncommon, even in high-density diving areas and areas of caisson work
Predominant age: 20-29
Predominant sex: 95% males, although there is no evidence to suggest increased susceptibility based on sex.

SIGNS AND SYMPTOMS
• 95% present in 3-4 hours, but may be delayed for 24 hours or more
• Burning blebs (skin bends)
• Painful pruritic red rash
• Vague, poorly-localized pain
• Headache
• Ataxia
• Delirium
• Coma
• Convulsions
• Confusion
• Patchy numbness
• Respiratory "chokes" in 2%
• Behnke's sign
• Arrhythmia
• Bradycardia or tachycardia
• Hypotension
• Tachypnea
• Subcutaneous emphysema along tendon sheaths (rare)

CAUSES
• Rapid ascent from scuba diving (depth > 33 feet)
• Rapid ascent/decompression in an airplane
• Tunnel work = caisson disease
• Inadequate pressurization/denitrogenation when flying
• Flying to altitude too soon after scuba diving

RISK FACTORS
• Prolonged dive at depth over 33 feet
• Obesity
• Multiple, repetitive scuba dives
• Cold water diving
• Poor physical conditioning
• Vigorous physical activity
• Dehydration
• Local injury
• Patent foramen ovale (for neurologic symptoms)

DIAGNOSIS

DIFFERENTIAL DIAGNOSIS Arterial gas embolism, traumatic injury to extremity, musculoskeletal strains, urticaria, malingering

LABORATORY
• ABG - may show decreased pO2, decreased pCO2, and metabolic acidosis.
• CBC - increased hematocrit in severe cases due to dehydration. Thrombocytopenia.
• Coagulation tests - may see increased fibrin split products and increased prothrombin time
Drugs that may alter lab results: N/A
Disorders that may alter lab results: N/A

PATHOLOGICAL FINDINGS
• Skin lesions: painful, pruritic, blotchy red rash on torso, burning blebs on skin, lymphedema
• Joints: erythema and edema on the periarticular surfaces

SPECIAL TESTS EEG - irregular slowing with cerebral bends

IMAGING
• Chest x-ray - pneumothorax, mediastinal emphysema; +/- right heart enlargement. Plain x-ray or ultrasound - gas bubbles in joints, tendons, bursae muscles.
• CT scan - should be performed on all patients with history of trauma or neurologic signs

DIAGNOSTIC PROCEDURES "Test of pressure" = trial of recompression to 2.8 ATA/100% oxygen/10'

TREATMENT

APPROPRIATE HEALTH CARE Referral through Divers' Alert Network [DAN (919)684-8111] to nearest hyperbaric facility for recompression test. The specific treatment may vary from institution to institution, but is based on the procedures first established in the Armed Services (e.g., US Navy Table 6). Patients may be sent home when cutaneous symptoms only are present, if the appropriate response to therapy is observed in the emergency department.

GENERAL MEASURES
• 100% oxygen via tight nonbreathing mask
• Fluid resuscitation (avoid D5W or hypotonic IV solutions with cord injury). Despite the theoretical advantages of volume expanders (dextran, albumin, etc.), no experimental or clinical studies support their use since they are not without risk.
• Rapid referral to hyperbaric chamber facility
• Position recumbent or Trendelenburg (for cerebral symptoms)
• Transport via ground, low-altitude airplane, or aircraft pressurized to sea level

ACTIVITY Bedrest when neurologic involvement present

DIET As tolerated

PATIENT EDUCATION Anyone who desires to perform scuba diving should be certified by an appropriate diving agency: NAUI, PADI, SSI, or YMCA. Sport divers who have not been diving for > 6 months should review diving principles/skills via a refresher course.

MEDICATIONS

DRUG(S) OF CHOICE 100% oxygen; diazepam 5-15 mg IV (IM absorption unpredictable) for inner ear decompression sickness. Symptoms of vertigo, nausea and vomiting may get significant relief. The use of steroids has been advocated by some for the assumed vasogenic edema seen in decompression sickness. This form of therapy remains controversial and not proven in controlled clinical trials. If steroids are prescribed, they should not be used for more than 4-5 days for neurological symptoms.
Contraindications: Hypersensitivity to benzodiazepines and acute narrow-angle glaucoma
Precautions: Administration of diazepam requires monitoring of the respiratory status, blood pressure and heart rate. Dosage reductions are required in the elderly and patients with hepatic dysfunction.
Significant possible interactions: Benzodiazepines potentiate the effects of other CNS depressants.

ALTERNATIVE DRUGS
Adjunctive therapy:
   ◊ Digitalization for CHF/tachycardia
   ◊ Aminophylline NOT useful for "chokes"
   ◊ Roles of steroids and heparin not determined

FOLLOWUP

PATIENT MONITORING Symptomatic assessment for relapse/progression which occurs in 25%

PREVENTION/AVOIDANCE
• Follow decompression tables (Navy, NAUI, PADI) for diving to depth (> 33 feet) or use dive computers that calculate nitrogen content of various tissues
• Allow adequate time between diving and flying to altitude (24 hours)

POSSIBLE COMPLICATIONS
• Oxygen toxicity with seizures (infrequent and unpredictable)
• Neurologic sequelae for non-responders
• Long-term risk of aseptic necrosis

EXPECTED COURSE AND PROGNOSIS
• Excellent for early symptomatic presentation, referral and treatment
• Related to duration and severity of symptoms prior to treatment
• Although recompression therapy is best administered early as possible, some patients may still benefit even at six to nine days after the incident, referral is critical, even if symptoms resolve, since 25% of patients will relapse

MISCELLANEOUS

ASSOCIATED CONDITIONS N/A

AGE-RELATED FACTORS
Pediatric: N/A
Geriatric: N/A
Others: N/A

PREGNANCY Pregnant patient with DCS a priority as fetus may also be affected; no contra-indication to recompression

SYNONYMS
• Bends
• Paretic bends

ICD-9-CM 993.3

SEE ALSO Arterial gas embolism

OTHER NOTES
• The diagnosis may be difficult due to the variable clinical manifestations. The most important clue is recent decompression.
• 71% of nervous system DCS present as skin or limb bends
• Limb bends with musculoskeletal complaints frequently diagnosed as malingering due to vague nature
• Only way to exclude the diagnosis in patient at risk is a negative test of pressure

ABBREVIATIONS N/A

REFERENCES
• Bove, A. & Davis J.C.: Diving Medicine. 2nd Ed. Philadelphia, W.B. Saunders; 1990
• Catron P.W. & Flynn E.T.: Adjuvant drug therapy for decompression sickness: A review. Undersea Biomed Res 1982; 9:161-173

Author J. Welko, M.D., & D. Heiselman, D.O.

Dementia

BASICS

DESCRIPTION A pathologic process defined as a persistent impairment of a prior level of intellectual functioning
• Dementia of the Alzheimer's type (DAT) is the most common form and characterized by a relentless deterioration of higher cortical functioning. The rate of deterioration is variable.
• Multi-infarct dementia (MID) occurs as a result of clinical or subclinical cerebral infarcts secondary to atherosclerosis. Deterioration is stepwise with periods of clinical plateaus.
• Sub-cortical dementia is accompanied by movement and gait disorders and characterized by psychomotor slowing
• Secondary dementias - also referred to as "reversible dementias" because the cognitive impairment may reverse with treatment of the primary disorder
System(s) affected: Nervous
Genetics:
• At least 15% of patients with DAT will report a positive family history
• Persons with Trisomy 21 (Down's syndrome) who survive into their 20's and 30's will inevitably develop a progressive dementia
Incidence in USA: 0.5% between ages 60-64; 3.2% between ages 80-90
Prevalence in USA:
• 1480/100,000
• 1.2 million people in the U.S. have severe dementia and another 2.5 million have moderate illness; 10% of all persons over the age of 65 have clinically important dementia
Predominant age: Increasing incidence with increasing age. Can occur in younger persons secondary to Trisomy 21 or AIDS.
Predominant sex: Male = Female

SIGNS AND SYMPTOMS
• Impaired short- and long-term memory
• Impaired abstract thinking
• Impaired judgment
• Aphasia
• Apraxia
• Agnosia
• Anomia
• Personality change, emotional outbursts, wandering, restlessness, hyperactivity
• Sleep disturbances
• Mood disturbances
• Urinary incontinence (usually late in DAT or normal pressure hydrocephalus)
• Fecal incontinence (late)
• Rigidity (especially with subcortical dementias)
• Tremor (especially with subcortical dementias)
• Hallucinations
• Delusions
• Overt paranoid behavior
• Weight loss
• Seizures

CAUSES
• DAT - genetic predisposition in 15%
• MID - due to cerebral atherosclerosis or emboli with clinical or subclinical infarcts
• Cortical dementias - causes include Parkinsonism, progressive supranuclear Palsy, and Huntington's disease
• Secondary dementias - causes include hypothyroidism, vitamin B deficiency, normal pressure hydrocephalus, AIDS, syphilis, and various medications. The dementia will be accompanied by the other signs and symptoms characteristic of the primary disorder.

RISK FACTORS
• Increasing age
• Prevalence of atherosclerotic disease (MID)
• Trisomy 21 (Down's syndrome)
• History of head trauma
• History of CNS infection

DIAGNOSIS

DIFFERENTIAL DIAGNOSIS
• Delirium
• Normal aging (Age-associated memory impairment)
• Depression
• Schizophrenia
• Sensory deprivation states
• Chronic alcoholism
• Heat stroke
• Postsurgical and/or postanesthesia state

LABORATORY
Done primarily to rule out potentially reversible causes
• Thyroid function tests
• Syphilis serology
• Serum B12 and folate
• Complete blood count and screening metabolic profile
Drugs that may alter lab results: Thyroid hormone replacement may affect the thyroid function tests
Disorders that may alter lab results: False positive syphilis serology with acute infections, leprosy, subacute bacterial endocarditis, and autoimmune disorders

PATHOLOGICAL FINDINGS
• DAT - granulovesicular degeneration, neurofibrillary tangles, senile neuritic plaques, microvascular amyloid
• MID - old infarcts, atherosclerotic disease
• Cortical dementia - degeneration of nigrostriatal neurons

SPECIAL TESTS
• Mental status testing
• Neuropsychologic testing
• Electroencephalogram for patients with altered consciousness or associated seizures

IMAGING
• Head computed tomography if history suggestive of a mass, or focal neurologic signs or in patient with dementia of brief duration
• Magnetic resonance imaging (MRI) is more sensitive than computed tomography for detection of soft tissue lesions (small infarcts, mass lesions, atrophy of the brainstem, and other subcortical structures). MRI may also clarify ambiguous computed tomography findings.
• Isotope cisternography if suspicious of normal pressure hydrocephalus

DIAGNOSTIC PROCEDURES N/A

TREATMENT

APPROPRIATE HEALTH CARE
• Outpatient except when complications warrant hospitalization
• Nursing home - if disease progresses to the point that long-term care becomes necessary

GENERAL MEASURES
• Daily schedules and written directions
• Support and education of caregivers
• Emphasis on nutrition, personal hygiene, personal safety (accident-proofing the home) and supervision
• Discussions with the family concerning advanced directives
• Socialization (adult day care)
• Sensory stimulation (prominent displays of clocks and calendars)
• Improvement in sleep hygiene
• Pharmacotherapy should be reserved for specific behavioral symptoms after nonpharmacologic therapy has failed

ACTIVITY Fully active with direction and supervision

DIET No special diet

PATIENT EDUCATION
• The 36-Hour Day by Mace and Rabins
• Printed material available from the Alzheimer's Association; 1-800-621-0379

Dementia

MEDICATIONS

DRUG(S) OF CHOICE
• Appropriately treat secondary causes, such as hypothyroidism or Vitamin B12 deficiency
• With other causes, drugs are used to treat behavioral symptoms after nonpharmacologic therapy has failed
• Sun-downing, aggressive behavior - antipsychotics such as haloperidol (Haldol) 0.5-1.0 mg at bedtime or thioridazine (Mellaril) 10-25 mg twice a day are reasonable choices in a non-emergency situation
• Depression - nortriptyline (Pamelor) 20-50 mg or desipramine (Norpramin) 25 mg bid
• Sleep disturbance - hypnotics should not be used on a regular basis. Intermittent use of triazolam (Halcion) 0.125 mg, lorazepam (Ativan) 0.5 mg, or chloral hydrate 500 mg at bedtime is occasionally warranted
• Tacrine (Cognex)10-40 mg qid used to treat DAT (doses >100mg/day appear to be associated with increased risk of hepatotoxicity)

Contraindications:
• Antipsychotics (haloperidol, thioridazine) - severe depression; Parkinson's disease; hypo- or hypertension
• Tricyclic antidepressants (nortriptyline, desipramine) - acute recovery phase following myocardial infarction, acute narrow-angle glaucoma
• Acute active liver disease, active untreated peptic ulcers

Precautions:
• In the elderly, begin with small doses and increase slowly

Antipsychotics
◊ Use with caution in patients with severe cardiovascular disorders because of the possibility of severe hypotension
◊ Tardive dyskinesia
◊ Neuroleptic malignant syndrome
◊ Lowered seizure threshold
◊ Monitor bone marrow function with CBC

Tricyclic antidepressants (TCA)
◊ Anticholinergic effects
◊ Sedation, increased confusion
◊ May produce arrhythmia, sinus tachycardia, and prolong conduction time
◊ Lowered seizure threshold

Benzodiazepines
◊ Dependence
◊ Sedation, increased confusion
◊ Respiratory depression
◊ Withdrawal symptoms

Tacrine (Cognex)
◊ Use with caution in persons with a history of neuromuscular disease
◊ Elevation of liver function tests
◊ Use with caution in persons with a history of seizures or asthma

Significant possible interactions:
• Antipsychotics - lithium may induce extrapyramidal symptoms and disorientation
• Tricyclic antidepressants (TCA) - monoamine oxidase inhibitors should not be administered with TCA. Antipsychotic administration, cimetidine and estrogens may increase the TCA concentration
• Benzodiazepines - increased serum phenytoin concentration. Cimetidine may increase the benzodiazepine concentration
• THA (Cognex) decrease theophylline dose by 50%. Use with caution with anticholinergic medications and NSAID's

ALTERNATIVE DRUGS
• Lithium carbonate
• Carbamazepine (Tegretol)

FOLLOWUP

PATIENT MONITORING
• Periodic mental status testing to assess progression and predict prognosis
• Periodic monitoring of nutritional status
• Periodic monitoring of the caregiver status to assess for caregiver stress
• Periodic assessment of the environment for safety
• Liver function tests with Tacrine therapy

PREVENTION/AVOIDANCE N/A

POSSIBLE COMPLICATIONS
• Antipsychotic-induced extrapyramidal effects
• Falls
• Pressure sores
• Malnutrition
• Constipation
• Various infections

EXPECTED COURSE AND PROGNOSIS
• DAT - a progressive disease with variable rates of progression, but inevitably leading to profound cognitive impairment
• MID - less likely to be progressive but cognitive improvement is unlikely
• Cortical dementias - treatment of the disease rarely has an effect on the cognitive deficit as cognitive impairment is generally a late component
• Secondary dementias - treatment of the underlying condition may lead to remarkable cognitive improvement

MISCELLANEOUS

ASSOCIATED CONDITIONS N/A

AGE-RELATED FACTORS
Pediatric: N/A
Geriatric: N/A
Others: N/A

PREGNANCY N/A

SYNONYMS Senility

ICD-9-CM
290.10 DAT
290.40 MID

SEE ALSO Alzheimer's disease, Parkinson's disease, Huntington's chorea, cerebrovascular accident, Down's syndrome, hypothyroidism, syphilis, Creutzfeldt-Jakob disease, juvenile amaurotic familial idiocy, pellagra, Pick's disease, Wilson's disease

OTHER NOTES N/A

ABBREVIATIONS
DAT = dementia of Alzheimer's type
MID = multi-infarct dementia

REFERENCES
• NIH Consensus Conference on Differential Diagnosis of Dementing Diseases. JAMA, 1987, 258(23): 3411-3416
• American Psychiatric Association Diagnostic and Statistical Manual of Mental Disorders (Third Edition-Revised). Washington, D.C., 1987
• Van Horn, G.: The American Journal of Medicine. 1987, 83:101-110

Author A. Knight, M.D

Depression

BASICS

DESCRIPTION Depression results when a person experiences more frustration and anger than he or she can handle. Each person is capable of handling a different amount of frustration or anger. The result is an abnormal receptor-neurotransmitter relationship at the synapse mainly in the limbic system in the brain. The presynaptic receptors deal primarily with the storage, release and uptake of the neurotransmitter. The primary neurotransmitters, both monoamines, are serotonin and norepinephrine. The available antidepressants, according to the latest theory, may increase the sensitivity of the post-synaptic receptor sites and decrease the presynaptic receptor sites. It is thought by some that the antidepressants may work by blocking the uptake of the neurotransmitters, thereby upgrading the synapse by having more available.
• Bipolar - mood disorders in which both manic and depressive episodes occur
• Unipolar - mood disorders in which only depressive episodes occur
System(s) affected: Nervous
Genetics: Possible defect on chromosome II or X
Incidence/Prevalence in USA: Estimated that 5-20% of population will experience a significant depression at some time
Predominant age:
• Bipolar - mean, 30 years
• Unipolar - mean, 40 years
Predominant sex: Female > Male

SIGNS AND SYMPTOMS
• Depressed mood
According to DSM III, major depression is probable when at least four of the following exist in addition to a disturbance in mood:
◊ Poor appetite - either weight gain or loss (may eat or drink out of boredom or reasons other than appetite)
◊ Sleep disorder - either insomnia or hypersomnia
◊ Fatigue - tiredness is out of proportion to the amount of energy expended
◊ Psychomotor retardation or agitation (restlessness, irritability or withdrawal)
◊ Anhedonia - lack of interest in pleasure, decreased sexual appetite, lack of pleasure in those things the person used to enjoy
◊ Poor self image - self reproach, excessive guilt
◊ Difficulty in concentrating, poor memory, unable to make decisions
◊ Suicidal ideation. Sometimes when people begin to recover they gain enough energy to think about and sometimes to attempt suicide.

CAUSES
• Impaired synthesis of the neurotransmitters
• Increased breakdown or metabolism of the neurotransmitters
• Increased pump uptake of the neurotransmitters. When a person experiences anger or frustration these chemicals are released at the synapse. The action potential is passed on from neuron to neuron. Following this the neurotransmitter is 1) reabsorbed into the neuron where it is either destroyed by an enzyme or actively removed by a reuptake pump and stored until needed or 2) destroyed by monoamine oxidase (MAO) located in the mitochondria.
• Lack of these neurotransmitters causes certain types of depression, e.g., decreased norepinephrine causes dullness and lethargy, while decreased serotonin causes irritability, hostility and suicide ideation

RISK FACTORS
• Females more likely to develop depressive illness than males
• Strong family history (depression, suicide, alcoholism, other substance abuse)
• Presence of chronic disease, especially multiple diseases
• Migraine headaches
• Back pain
• Chronic pain
• Recent myocardial infarction
• Peptic ulcer disease
• Insomnia
• Stressful situations
• Adolescence
• Advancing age
• Retirement
• Children with behavioral disorders, especially hyperactivity

DIAGNOSIS

DIFFERENTIAL DIAGNOSIS
• Organic brain diseases
• Endocrine diseases, such as hypothyroid and hyperthyroid diseases
• Diabetes mellitus
• Liver failure
• Renal failure
• Chronic fatigue syndrome
• Vitamin deficiency (pernicious anemia, pellagra)
• Medication side effects (many drugs cause or worsen depression)
• Medication overdose
• Medication abuse
• Withdrawal from medication
• Alcohol abuse
• Substance abuse
• Withdrawal from abused substance (alcohol, cocaine, marijuana)

LABORATORY
• Unfortunately there is no good test for depression
• Methoxyhydroxyphenylglycol (MHPG), the metabolite of norepinephrine, can be measured in urine and in some laboratories in the CSF. Similarly the major CNS metabolite of serotonin, 5-hydroxyindoleacetic acid (5-HIAA), can be measured in the urine and CSF. These tests are not a good reflection of the levels in the central nervous system, but rather in the peripheral nervous system.
• Decadron suppression test
• Complete blood count

• SMA-18
• Urinalysis
• Erythrocyte sedimentation rate
• B12, folate levels
• Rapid plasma reagin (RPR)
• Thyroid function studies, including TSH
Drugs that may alter lab results: All psychoactive drugs
Disorders that may alter lab results: Thyroid disease

PATHOLOGICAL FINDINGS N/A

SPECIAL TESTS
• ECG, (diagnosis of arrhythmia, especially heart block)
• EEG

IMAGING CT or MRI of brain, if organic brain syndrome (OBS) included in differential

DIAGNOSTIC PROCEDURES
• SDS (Self-rating Depression Scale—Zung's)
• BDI (Beck's depression inventory)
• Other screening instruments (GDS-General Health Questionnaire, CRSD-Carroll's Rating Scale for Depression, CDI-Children's Depression Inventory)
• Depression is primarily a clinical diagnosis that depends on skillfully eliciting family, social and psychosocial factors

TREATMENT

APPROPRIATE HEALTH CARE
Outpatient

GENERAL MEASURES
• Psychotherapy is good in helping the patient solve the problems caused by depression. Also, counselling is helpful in dealing with suicide, interpersonal problems, and problems dealing with society.
• Use the correct medication
• Use the correct dosage
• Use the correct medication long enough

ACTIVITY No restrictions

DIET No special diet

PATIENT EDUCATION
• Carefully teach about medications
• Consider referral to support groups
• Stress need for long-term treatment and followup
• Recommend reading for patients, e.g., How to Cope With Depression by DePaulo and Ablow
• Contact local support groups through National Depression Manic Depression Association (DMDA), 800-82-MDMDA

Depression

MEDICATIONS

DRUG(S) OF CHOICE
Therapy may be initiated based on predominate symptoms:

Anxiety, restlessness, irritability or sleeplessness:

◊ Amitriptyline (Elavil, Endep) 150-300 mg/day qhs

◊ Nortriptyline (Pamelor, Aventyl) 75-150 mg/day qhs (a metabolite of amitriptyline)

◊ Doxepin (Adapin, Sinequan) 150-300 mg/day qhs

◊ Trazodone (Desyrel) 150-300 mg/day qhs

◊ Trimipramine (Surmonti1) 75-250 mg/day qhs

Fatigue, hypersomnia, indecisiveness or difficulty in concentration:

◊ Imipramine (Tofranil, Tipramine) 150-300 mg/day

◊ Desipramine (Norpramin, Pertofrane) 150-300 mg/day (metabolite of imipramine)

◊ Fluoxetine (Prozac) 20 mg/day q am

◊ Sertraline (Zoloft) 50-100 mg/day q am

◊ Paroxetine (Paxil) 10-30 mg/day q am

◊ Protriptyline (Vivactil) 30-60 mg/day

◊ Bupropion (Wellbutrin) 100-450 mg/day

Contraindications: Refer to manufacturer's profile of each drug

Precautions:
• All of these medications have anticholinergic, orthostatic, and sedating side effects
• Decrease beginning dose by half for children and elderly
• Most common side effects are dry mouth, constipation and sleepiness. Frequently people sweat profusely. Most side effects decrease or disappear in 2-3 weeks.
• Fluoxetine, sertraline, paroxetine best given in the morning
• Write prescriptions for small total amounts initially to prevent suicide (TCAs fatal with doses > 1-1.5 gm in adults)
• TCAs may produce arrhythmias and lower seizure threshold.

Significant possible Interactions:
• Refer to manufacturer's profile of each drug
• Avoid nonprescription drugs containing pseudoephedrine, phenylephrine, or phenylpropanolamine (cold medicines)

ALTERNATIVE DRUGS
• Clomipramine (Anafranil) 100-250 mg/day (Although primarily used to treat obsessive-compulsive disorder)
• MAO Inhibitors - significant drug and food interactions limit their use by primary care physicians

FOLLOWUP

PATIENT MONITORING
• See patient within 2 weeks after starting medication. The patient will probably not feel greatly improved at this visit.
• During followup visits evaluate side effects, dosage and effectiveness of the medication
• Follow about every 2 weeks until improvement begins. If treatment is adequate, the depression should improve within 4 weeks of initiating treatment.
• Follow every three months thereafter
• Explain to the patient that the treatment must continue even after improvement
• Plan to treat at least six months to two years. Longer in patients with family history of depression and the very young.

PREVENTION/AVOIDANCE See
Causes and Risk factors

POSSIBLE COMPLICATIONS
• Suicide
• Failure to improve

EXPECTED COURSE AND
PROGNOSIS This is one of the most rewarding conditions to treat because, once you find the right drug and the right dose, you can almost guarantee the patient that he or she will improve

MISCELLANEOUS

ASSOCIATED CONDITIONS
• Manic depression (bipolar)
• Schizophrenia
• Schizo-affective disorders
• Psycho-physiological disorders
• Physical disorders
• Cyclothymic and grief reactions
• Alcoholism

AGE-RELATED FACTORS
Pediatric: Depression occurs in children
Geriatric: More common in elderly and difficult to precisely diagnose
Others: N/A

PREGNANCY Caution in using
psychoactive medications in pregnancy. Rely on psychotherapy and support groups until pregnancy is completed.

SYNONYMS Unipolar affective disorder

ICD-9-CM
• 311 Depressive disorder, not elsewhere classified
• 296.2 Major depressive disorder, single episode
• 296.3 Major depressive disorder, recurrent episode

SEE ALSO N/A

OTHER NOTES
• Depression is the fourth most common reason to visit the family physician
• Like so many other medical illnesses with psychological symptoms, family, doctors and patients tend to try to overlook this condition because they feel they should be able to control it themselves

ABBREVIATIONS
TSH = thyroid stimulating hormone

REFERENCES
• Davis, R.E. & Wengert, J.W.: Biochemical Theories of Depression. Physician Assistant, Dec, 1987
• Kavan, M.G.: Screening for Depression. In AFP, Mar 1990
• Cohn, J., et al.: Choosing the Right Antidepressant. Patient Care, July 15, 1990
• Stewart, A., et al.: Functional Status and Well-being of Patients With Chronic Conditions. JAMA, Aug 18, 1990

Author L. Masters, M.D.

Dermatitis herpetiformis

 BASICS

DESCRIPTION Dermatitis herpetiformis is an intensely pruritic papulovesicular disease on extensor skin surfaces
System(s) affected: Skin/Exocrine
Genetics: High incidence of HLA B8/Dw3
Incidence/Prevalence in USA: Uncommon. Prevalence not known and most likely varies with the race and ethnicity of the population studied.
Predominant age: 15-60, mean age of onset is in the fourth decade
Predominant sex: Male > Female (1.5:1)

SIGNS AND SYMPTOMS
• Symmetrical intensely pruritic, papulovesicular eruption
• Elbows and extensor forearms are the most common site of involvement
• Buttocks, knees, upper back, posterior neck and scalp also frequent
• Oral lesions in 33%
• Secondary excoriations may be prominent
• Burning or stinging feeling may be prominent

CAUSES Unknown

RISK FACTORS
• Gluten-sensitive enteropathy
• Family history of dermatitis herpetiformis

 DIAGNOSIS

DIFFERENTIAL DIAGNOSIS
• Scabies
• Erythema multiforme
• Bullous pemphigoid
• Transient acantholytic dermatosis
• Subcorneal pustular dermatosis
• Erythema elevatum diutinum
• Papular urticaria
• Eczema
• Excoriations

LABORATORY Abnormal thyroid function tests in 32%
Drugs that may alter lab results:
• Thyroid
• Steroids
Disorders that may alter lab results: N/A

PATHOLOGICAL FINDINGS
• Papillary dermal neutrophilic microabscesses
• Subepidermal vesicles

SPECIAL TESTS Direct immunofluorescence reveals granular IgA deposition in the dermal papilla

IMAGING Thyroid scan if indicated by physical exam

DIAGNOSTIC PROCEDURES Skin biopsy

 TREATMENT

APPROPRIATE HEALTH CARE
Outpatient

GENERAL MEASURES No special measures

ACTIVITY Fully active

DIET Clinical improvement occurs with gluten-free diet

PATIENT EDUCATION Contact American Academy of Dermatology, 930 N. Meacham Rd., P.O. Box 4014, Schaumber, IL 60168-4014, (708)330-0230

MEDICATIONS

DRUG(S) OF CHOICE Dapsone 50 mg per day will usually improve symptoms within 24 to 48 hours in adults. Average maintenance dose is 100 to 200 mg per day.
Contraindications: See manufacturer's profile of each drug
Precautions:
Side effects of dapsone include:
◊ Hemolytic anemia
◊ Methemoglobinemia
◊ Toxic hepatitis
◊ Cholestatic jaundice
◊ Hypoalbuminemia
◊ Sensory and motor neuropathy
◊ Psychosis
◊ Infectious mononucleosis syndrome with fever and lymphadenopathy
◊ Agranulocytosis
◊ Aplastic anemia
◊ Exfoliative dermatitis
◊ Erythema multiforme
◊ Erythema nodosum
◊ Urticaria
◊ Dapsone is secreted in breast milk and will produce hemolytic anemia in infants
◊ Dapsone will produce a severe hemolytic anemia in patients with glucose-6-phosphate dehydrogenase (G6PD) deficiency
Significant possible interactions: See manufacturer's profile of each drug

ALTERNATIVE DRUGS Sulfapyridine

FOLLOWUP

PATIENT MONITORING
• Baseline CBC and liver function studies should be obtained
• G6PD should be obtained in Asians, blacks and those of southern Mediterranean descent
• CBC should be checked weekly for first month, monthly for the next five months and semi-annually thereafter
• Chemistry profile should be checked every six months
• Patient should be made aware of potential hemolytic anemia and the blue-gray discoloration associated with methemoglobinemia

PREVENTION/AVOIDANCE N/A

POSSIBLE COMPLICATIONS N/A

EXPECTED COURSE AND PROGNOSIS
• Patients respond dramatically to dapsone
• Strict adherence to a gluten-free diet will produce improvement of clinical symptoms and a decrease in dapsone requirement in the majority of patients
• Occasional new lesions (2-3 per week) are to be expected and are not an indication for altering daily dosage

MISCELLANEOUS

ASSOCIATED CONDITIONS
• Gluten-sensitive enteropathy
• Hyperthyroidism
• Hypothyroidism
• Thyroid nodules
• Multi-nodular goiter
• Thyroid carcinoma
• Pernicious anemia
• Gastrointestinal lymphoma
• Immunologic disorders including systemic lupus erythematosus, Addison's disease, rheumatoid arthritis, ulcerative colitis, Raynaud's phenomenon, atopy, Sjögren's syndrome, vitiligo, and dermatomyositis have been reported to be associated with dermatitis herpetiformis

AGE-RELATED FACTORS
Pediatric: Dapsone dose must be adjusted
Geriatric: N/A
Others: N/A

PREGNANCY Data is inconclusive but suggests that dapsone is safe during pregnancy. It is recommended that adherence to a strict gluten-free diet, preferably for 6-12 months before conception be instituted in the hope of eliminating the need for dapsone during pregnancy.

SYNONYMS Duhring's disease

ICD-9-CM 694.0

SEE ALSO N/A

OTHER NOTES N/A

ABBREVIATIONS N/A

REFERENCES
• Zone, J.J.: Prob. in Derm. Vol. 3, No. 1:6-41
• Hall, R.P.: J. Am Acad. Derm 16:1129-44, 1987

Author V. Soong, M.D.

Dermatitis, atopic

 BASICS

DESCRIPTION Chronic pruritic eczematous condition affecting characteristic sites. Associated with family history of atopy (asthma, allergic rhinitis, atopic dermatitis).
Genetics: Genetic predisposition - family history positive in two-thirds of cases
Incidence/Prevalence in USA: Common; incidence 7-24/1000
Predominant age: Mainly childhood disease. Affects 5% of all children, usually starting after 2 months of age. Atopic dermatitis is present by age 5 in 90% of patients.
Predominant sex: Male = Female (females tend to have somewhat worse prognosis)

SIGNS AND SYMPTOMS
• Pruritis is the most common symptom
Distribution of lesions
◊ Infants - trunk, face, and extensor surfaces
◊ Children - antecubital and popliteal fossae
◊ Adults - face, neck, upper chest, and genital areas
◊ In adults with limited distribution of lesions a history of childhood eczema is a clue to diagnosis
Morphology of lesions
◊ Infants - erythema and papules; may develop oozing, crusting vesicles
◊ Children and adults - lichenification and scaling are typical with chronic eczema
◊ Family history of atopic dermatitis may be more useful than morphology in making the diagnosis
Associated features
◊ Facial erythema, mild to moderate
◊ Perioral pallor
◊ Infraorbital fold (Dennie's sign/Morgan line)
◊ Dry skin
◊ Increased palmar linear markings
◊ Pityriasis alba (hypopigmented asymptomatic areas on face and shoulders)
◊ Keratosis pilaris

CAUSES Unknown. Genetically determined, non-allergic disease.

RISK FACTORS
• Skin infections
• Emotional stress
• Irritating clothes and chemicals
• Excessively hot or cold climate
• Food allergy in children (controversial)

 DIAGNOSIS

DIFFERENTIAL DIAGNOSIS
• Photosensitivity rashes
• Contact dermatitis (especially if only the face is involved)
• Scabies
• Seborrheic dermatitis (especially in infants)
• Psoriasis or lichen simplex chronicus if only localized disease is present in adults
• Rare conditions of infancy: Histiocytosis X, Wiskott-Aldrich syndrome, ataxia-telangiectasia syndrome

LABORATORY Serum IgE levels are frequently elevated
Drugs that may alter lab results: N/A
Disorders that may alter lab results: N/A

PATHOLOGICAL FINDINGS Epidermis is thickened and hyperkeratotic. Dermis shows perivascular inflammation.

SPECIAL TESTS None

IMAGING None

DIAGNOSTIC PROCEDURES Skin biopsy shows nonspecific eczematous changes. (Biopsy is rarely required since diagnosis is made on clinical grounds.)

 TREATMENT

APPROPRIATE HEALTH CARE
Generally outpatient, using topical corticosteroids

GENERAL MEASURES
• Decrease stress if possible
• Avoid agents that may cause irritation (e.g., wool, perfumes)
• Minimize sweating
• Lukewarm (not hot) baths
• Minimize use of soap
• Frequent systemic lubrication with oil baths, moisturizers, etc.
• Phototherapy may be useful

ACTIVITY No restrictions

DIET There is controversy regarding the role of food allergies and exacerbations of atopic dermatitis. Food allergies do not play a role in adult eczema. In infants and children the most common suspicious foods are eggs, milk, wheat and peanuts. Consider elimination diets (e.g., for 3-4 weeks) and food challenges. Also consider delaying introduction of the common suspicious foods until an infant is 6 months old.

PATIENT EDUCATION
• Eczema is not caused by nerves
• Eczema is not caused by an allergy
• Goal is control, not cure (although many patients will outgrow their disease)
• See also Epstein, E.: Common Skin Disorders. 3rd Ed. Medical Economics, 1988

Dermatitis, atopic

 MEDICATIONS

DRUG(S) OF CHOICE
• Topical steroids achieve good control in 90% of patients
• In infants and children, use 1% topical hydrocortisone
• In adults, may use higher potency (over 1%) topical corticosteroids in areas other than face and skin folds
• Use short courses of higher potency corticosteroids for flares, then return to the lowest potency that will control dermatitis
Contraindications: None
Precautions: Beware chronic use of potent fluorinated corticosteroids, as it may cause striae or atrophy, especially in children. High potency topical corticosteroids may produce systemic effects if used for prolonged periods.
Significant possible interactions: None

ALTERNATIVE DRUGS
• Coal tars (e.g., tar-oil baths, topical tar at bedtime, etc.)
• Antihistamines for pruritis (e.g., hydroxyzine, 10-25 mg at bedtime and prn)
• Plastic occlusion - in combination with topical medication, this promotes absorption and may be useful for secondary infection (e.g., erythromycin or dicloxacillin)
• For stubborn localized eczema, may use intralesional steroids
• For severe atopic dermatitis, consider systemic steroids for 1-2 weeks, e.g., prednisone 60-80 mg/day po initially, tapered over 7-14 days. Start topical steroids simultaneously to assist in rapid taper of oral steroids.

 FOLLOWUP

PATIENT MONITORING
Individualize, depending on severity of disease

PREVENTION/AVOIDANCE
• See General Measures
• Smallpox vaccine should be avoided because of risk of eczema herpeticum (see Possible Complications)

POSSIBLE COMPLICATIONS
• Cataracts are more common in patients with atopic dermatitis
• Skin infections (usually staphylococcus aureus); sometimes subclinical
• Eczema herpeticum - generalized vesiculopustular eruption caused by infection with herpes simplex or vaccinia virus. Patients are acutely ill and require hospitalization.
• Atrophy and/or striae if fluorinated corticosteroids are used on face or skin folds
• Systemic absorption may occur if large areas of skin are treated, particularly if high-potency medications and occlusion are combined

EXPECTED COURSE AND PROGNOSIS
• Chronic disease that tends to burn out with age. 90% of patients have spontaneous resolution by puberty.
• Some adults may continue to have localized eczema, e.g., chronic hand or foot dermatitis, eyelid dermatitis, or lichen simplex chronicus

 MISCELLANEOUS

ASSOCIATED CONDITIONS
• Asthma
• Allergic rhinitis
• Hyper-IgE syndrome (Job's syndrome) which is characterized by atopic dermatitis, elevated IgE, recurrent pyodermas, and decreased chemotaxis of mononuclear cells

AGE-RELATED FACTORS
Pediatric: More frequent
Geriatric: Relatively rare
Others: N/A

PREGNANCY N/A

SYNONYMS
• Eczema
• Disseminated neurodermatitis
• Atopic eczema
• Atopic neurodermatitis
• Constitutional dermatitis
• Besnier's prurigo

ICD-9-CM 691.8

SEE ALSO N/A

OTHER NOTES If very resistant to treatment, search for a coexisting contact dermatitis

ABBREVIATIONS

REFERENCES Habif, T.: Clinical Dermatology. 2nd Ed. St. Louis, C.V. Mosby, 1990

Author E. Lackermann, M.D.

Dermatitis, contact

BASICS

DESCRIPTION The cutaneous reaction to an external substance
• Primary irritant dermatitis is due to direct injury of the skin. It affects individuals exposed to specific irritants and generally produces discomfort immediately after exposure.
• Allergic contact dermatitis (ACD) affects only individuals previously sensitized to the contactant. It represents a delayed hypersensitivity reaction, requiring several hours for the cascade of cellular immunity to be completed to manifest itself.
Genetics: Increased frequency of ACD in families with allergies
Incidence/Prevalence in USA: N/A
Predominant age: All ages
Predominant sex: Male = Female. Variations due to differences in exposure to offending agents as well as normal cutaneous variations between male and female (eccrine and sebaceous gland function and hair distribution).

SIGNS AND SYMPTOMS
Acute
◊ Papules, vesicles, bullae with surrounding erythema
◊ Crusting and oozing may be present
◊ Pruritus
Chronic
◊ Erythematous base
◊ Thickening with lichenification
◊ Scaling
◊ Fissuring
Distribution
◊ Where epidermis is thinner (eyelids, genitalia)
◊ Areas of contact with offending agent (e.g., nail polish)
◊ Palms and soles more resistant
◊ Deeper skinfolds spared
◊ Linear arrays of lesions
◊ Lesions with sharp borders and sharp angles - pathognomonic

CAUSES
Plants
◊ Rhus-urushiol (poison ivy, oak, sumac)
◊ Primary contact - plant (roots/stems/leaves)
◊ Secondary contact - clothes/fingernails (not blister fluid)
Chemicals
◊ Nickel - jewelry, zippers, hooks, watches
◊ Potassium dichromate - tanning agent in leather
◊ Paraphenylenediamine - hair dyes, fur dyes, industrial chemicals
◊ Turpentine - cleaning agents, polishes, waxes
◊ Soaps, detergents

Topical medicines
◊ Neomycin - topical antibiotics
◊ Thimerosal (Merthiolate) - preservative in topical medications
◊ Anesthetics - benzocaine
◊ Parabens - preservative in topical medications
◊ Formalin - cosmetics, shampoos, nail enamel

RISK FACTORS
• Occupation
• Hobbies
• Travel
• Cosmetics
• Jewelry

DIAGNOSIS

DIFFERENTIAL DIAGNOSIS
• Based on clinical impression - appearance, periodicity, localization
• Groups of vesicles - herpes simplex
• Diffuse bullous or vesicular lesions - bullous pemphigoid
• Photo-distribution - phototoxic/allergic reaction to systemic allergen
• Eyelids - seborrheic dermatitis
• Scaly eczematous lesions - atopic dermatitis, nummular eczema, lichen simplex chronicus, stasis dermatitis, xerosis

LABORATORY N/A
Drugs that may alter lab results: N/A
Disorders that may alter lab results: N/A

PATHOLOGICAL FINDINGS
• Intercellular edema
• Bullae

SPECIAL TESTS Patch tests for allergic contact dermatitis (systemic corticosteroids or recent, aggressive use of topical steroids may alter results)

IMAGING N/A

DIAGNOSTIC PROCEDURES Patch test

TREATMENT

APPROPRIATE HEALTH CARE
Outpatient

GENERAL MEASURES
• Removal of offending agent
• Topical soaks with cool tap water, Burow's solution (1:40 dilution), or saline (1 tsp/pint water), or silver nitrate solution (25.5%)
• Lukewarm water baths - antipruritic
• Aveeno (oatmeal) baths
• Chronic - emollients (white petrolatum, Eucerin)

ACTIVITY Stay active, but avoid overheating

DIET No special diet

PATIENT EDUCATION
• Avoidance of irritating substance
• Cleaning of secondary sources (nails, clothes)
• Fallacy of blister fluid spreading disease

MEDICATIONS

DRUG(S) OF CHOICE
<u>Topical</u>
◊ Shake lotion of zinc oxide, talc, menthol 0.25%, phenol 0.5%
◊ Corticosteroids - high potency steroids, fluocinonide 0.05% ointment (Lidex) 3-4 times daily. Caution regarding face/skinfolds - use lower potency steroids and avoid prolonged usage.
◊ Calamine lotion
◊ Topical antibiotics for secondary infection (bacitracin, gentamicin, erythromycin)
<u>Systemic</u>
◊ Antihistamine - hydroxyzine 25-50 mg qid, diphenhydramine 25-50 mg qid
◊ Corticosteroids - prednisone. Taper starting at 60-80 mg/d, tapered over 10-14 days.
◊ Antibiotics - erythromycin 250 mg qid if secondarily infected
Contraindications: N/A
Precautions:
• Drowsiness from antihistamines
• Local skin effects - atrophy, stria, telangiectasia from prolonged use of potent topical steroids
Significant possible interactions: N/A

ALTERNATIVE DRUGS   N/A

FOLLOWUP

PATIENT MONITORING
• As necessary for recurrence
• Patch testing for etiology after resolved

PREVENTION/AVOIDANCE   Avoid causative agents. Use of protective gloves (with cotton lining) may be helpful.

POSSIBLE COMPLICATIONS
• Generalized eruption secondary to autosensitization
• Secondary bacterial infection

EXPECTED COURSE AND PROGNOSIS   Self-limited, benign

MISCELLANEOUS

ASSOCIATED CONDITIONS   N/A

AGE-RELATED FACTORS
Pediatric: Younger individuals - increased incidence of positive patch testing due to better delayed hypersensitivity reactions
Geriatric: Increased incidence of irritant dermatitis secondary to skin dryness
Others: N/A

PREGNANCY   Usual cautions with medications

SYNONYMS   Dermatitis Venenata

ICD-9-CM
• 692 Contact dermatitis and other eczema
• 692.9 Unspecified cause

SEE ALSO   N/A

OTHER NOTES   N/A

ABBREVIATIONS   ACD = allergic contact dermatitis

REFERENCES
• Bondi, E., Jegasothy, B. & Lazarus, G.: Dermatology, Diagnosis and Therapy. Norwalk, CT, Appleton & Lange, 1991
• Abel, E. & Farber, E.: Scientific American Inc., New York, 1985

Author   J. Stearns, M.D.

Dermatitis, diaper

 BASICS

 DIAGNOSIS

 TREATMENT

DESCRIPTION Diaper dermatitis is a rash occurring under the covered area of a diaper. The rash may be an irritant contact dermatitis, candidiasis, atopic dermatitis or seborrheic dermatitis.
System(s) affected: Skin/Exocrine
Genetics: N/A
Incidence/Prevalence in USA: Common
Predominant age: Infants
Predominant sex: Male = Female

SIGNS AND SYMPTOMS
Irritant contact diaper dermatitis
◊ Prominent rash on buttocks and pubic skin
◊ Creases of skin are relatively spared
◊ Rash is dusky red and shiny
◊ Skin seems chapped
◊ Weeping, crusting, and excoriations are not prominent
Candidiasis diaper rash
◊ Initial involvement of creases with rapid extension
◊ Color: bright red
◊ Accompanying edema
◊ Isolated satellite papules and pustules at margins of inflammatory plaques
◊ Excoriations are prominent
◊ Positive KOH preparation
◊ Positive cultures
Atopic diaper dermatitis
◊ Distribution spares creases
◊ Genitalia frequently involved
◊ Itch-scratch cycle with excoriations are prominent
◊ Child scratches vigorously at night
◊ Weeping, crusting, excoriations sometimes present; secondary bacterial infection can occur
Seborrheic diaper dermatitis
◊ Dusky-red patches and plaques deep within skin creases
◊ Non-interginous skin is relatively spared
◊ Weeping, crusting, excoriations - not prominent
◊ Other sites of seborrheic dermatitis are frequently present: retroauricular, axillary folds, scalp

CAUSES Irritation to skin from retained urine. (Ammonia and/or detergents probably do not play a prominent role.)

RISK FACTORS
• Infrequent diaper changes
• Waterproof diapers
• Improper laundering
• Family history of dermatitis
• Hot, humid weather
• Recent treatment with oral antibiotics

DIFFERENTIAL DIAGNOSIS
• Contact dermatitis
• Seborrheic dermatitis
• Candidiasis
• Atopic dermatitis
• Acrodermatitis enteropathica
• Letter-Siwe's disease

LABORATORY Culture will reveal candida, if present
Drugs that may alter lab results: N/A
Disorders that may alter lab results: N/A

PATHOLOGICAL FINDINGS Varying inflammation is the most prominent finding

SPECIAL TESTS
• KOH preparation
• Culture pustules if present

IMAGING N/A

DIAGNOSTIC PROCEDURES
• Culture lesions
• KOH preparation

APPROPRIATE HEALTH CARE
Outpatient

GENERAL MEASURES
• Expose the buttocks to air as much as possible
• Don't use waterproof pants during treatment - day or night. They keep skin wet and subject to rash or infection.
• Change diapers frequently - even at night if the rash is extensive
• Don't use soap or boric acid to wash the rash area. Cleanse with cotton dipped in mineral oil.
• Discontinue using baby lotion, powder, ointment or baby oil (except zinc oxide)
• Zinc oxide ointment to the rash at the earliest sign of diaper rash, and 2 or 3 times a day thereafter

ACTIVITY Protect from overheating

DIET No special diet

PATIENT EDUCATION Information in General Measures

MEDICATIONS

DRUG(S) OF CHOICE
• If candidiasis suspected or diaper rash persistent, use antifungal such as miconazole nitrate 2% cream, miconazole powder, econazole (Spectazole), clotrimazole (Lotrimin), or ketaconazole (Nizoral) cream, at each diaper change.
• Miconazole powder, imidazole or ketaconazole creams are all effective
• If inflammation is prominent, consider very low potency steroid cream, such as hydrocortisone 1% tid along with an antifungal cream or and combination product such as Vioform-hydrocortisone cream
• If a secondary bacterial infection is suspected, use an anti-Staphylococcal oral antibiotic or mupirocin (Bactroban) ointment topically

Contraindications: N/A

Precautions: Avoid high or the moderate potency steroids often found in combination steroid-antifungal mixtures

Significant possible interactions: N/A

ALTERNATIVE DRUGS   N/A

FOLLOWUP

PATIENT MONITORING   Recheck weekly until clear, then at times of recurrence

PREVENTION/AVOIDANCE   See General Measures

POSSIBLE COMPLICATIONS
Secondary bacterial infection

EXPECTED COURSE AND PROGNOSIS   Quick complete clearing with appropriate treatment

MISCELLANEOUS

ASSOCIATED CONDITIONS
• Contact (allergic or irritant) dermatitis
• Seborrheic dermatitis
• Psoriasis
• Candidiasis
• Atopic dermatitis

AGE-RELATED FACTORS
Pediatric: Problem confined to this age group
Geriatric: N/A
Others: N/A

PREGNANCY   N/A

SYNONYMS   Diaper rash

ICD-9-CM   691.0

SEE ALSO
• Contact dermatitis
• Candidiasis
• Atopic dermatitis
• Psoriasis

OTHER NOTES   Two or more types of diaper dermatitis can exist concomitantly. If so, treat each accordingly.

ABBREVIATIONS   N/A

REFERENCES
• Fitzpatrick, T.B, et al. (eds.): Dermatology In General Medicine, 3rd Ed. New York, McGraw-Hill, 1987
• Sams, W.M. & Lynch, P.J. (eds.) Principles and Practices of Dermatology. New York, Churchill Livingstone, Inc., 1990
• Oski, F.A., et al. (eds): Principals and Practice of Pediatrics. Philadelphia, J.P. Lippincott, 1990

Author   C. Zucker, M.D.

Dermatitis, exfoliative

 BASICS

DESCRIPTION A generalized scaling eruption of the skin, either idiopathic in nature or secondary to underlying cutaneous or systemic disease
System(s) affected: Skin/Exocrine
Genetics: No known genetic pattern
Incidence/Prevalence in USA: Rare; estimated 1% of hospitalizations for skin disease
Predominant Age: 75% of patients are over age 40
Predominant sex: Male > Female (2:1)

SIGNS AND SYMPTOMS
• Fine generalized scales with mild erythema and lichenification of skin
• With acute onset and in early stages of exudative dermatitis, may have thin epidermis, erythema, and exudation with subsequent development of crusting
• Initial distribution is that of any underlying cutaneous disease, Subsequently, as exfoliative dermatitis further develops, this distribution is lost and the scaling is generalized.
• With no underlying cutaneous disease, the distribution initially favors the genital region, trunk, and head before generalizing
• Sensation of skin tightness
• Nail dystrophy
• Hair loss, with alopecia in up to 25%
• Pruritis
• Fever in 40-50%
• Chills
• Malaise/weakness
• Mucous membranes spared
• Anemia (both microcytic and macrocytic) in up to 65%
• Eosinophilia
• Nontender generalized lymphadenopathy
• Steatorrhea
• Hepatomegaly in 20-35%
• Splenomegaly when underlying lymphoma/leukemia present
• Gynecomastia
• Hypoproteinemia
• Dehydration
• High output cardiac failure
• Tachycardia

CAUSES
• Idiopathic in up to 25% of cases
• 75% may occur in response to one of the following:
  ◊ Atopic dermatitis
  ◊ Colon carcinoma
  ◊ Contact dermatitis (10%)
  ◊ Drug eruptions (10%)
  ◊ Fungal disease with id reaction
  ◊ Ichthyosiform dermatoses
  ◊ Leukemia
  ◊ Lichen planus
  ◊ Lung carcinoma
  ◊ Lymphoma - 15% of cases overall and 35-50% of patients over age 40
  ◊ Medications - sulfonamides and sulfones, penicillins, cephalosporins, anticonvulsants, NSAID's, codeine, heavy metals, INH, quinidine, captopril, iodine, antimalarials
  ◊ Multiple myeloma
  ◊ Mycosis fungoides
  ◊ Pemphigus foliaceus
  ◊ Pityriasis rosea
  ◊ Pityriasis rubra pilaris
  ◊ Psoriasis
  ◊ Pyoderma with id reaction
  ◊ Reiter's syndrome
  ◊ Scabies
  ◊ Seborrheic dermatitis
  ◊ Sezary syndrome
  ◊ Staphylococcal scalded skin syndrome
  ◊ Stasis dermatitis
  ◊ Toxic epidermal necrolysis

RISK FACTORS
• Underlying diseases as noted above
• Male sex
• Age greater than 40

 DIAGNOSIS

DIFFERENTIAL DIAGNOSIS Acutely eczematous dermatoses such as contact dermatitis and drug eruptions should be considered

LABORATORY None diagnostic. May have elevated WBC with eosinophilia, elevated ESR, and decreased albumin.
Drugs that may alter lab results: N/A
Disorders that may alter lab results: N/A

PATHOLOGICAL FINDINGS May have characteristics of the underlying cutaneous disease. Other changes are nonspecific: Hyperkeratosis, parakeratosis, acanthosis in the epidermis; and edema, vasodilation, perivascular infiltrates with lymphocytes, histiocytes, and eosinophils in the dermis.

SPECIAL TESTS None

IMAGING Chest x-ray and other imaging procedures as indicated to investigate any underlying disease process

DIAGNOSTIC PROCEDURES
• Careful history and physical
• Skin biopsy; lymph node biopsy and bone marrow biopsy as indicated to investigate an underlying disease process

 TREATMENT

APPROPRIATE HEALTH CARE Outpatient except in those cases with complications of secondary infection, dehydration, or heart failure

GENERAL MEASURES
• Withdrawal of any implicated medications or treatment of any identified underlying infection/disease
• Protection from development of hypothermia
• Cool colloid baths with Aveeno (1 cup in 10 inches water)
• Local moisturizing ointments/lotions

ACTIVITY As tolerated

DIET High protein. Increased fluid intake should be encouraged in those with more extensive skin involvement.

PATIENT EDUCATION
• Patients should avoid any identified etiologic agents
• Patients with underlying diseases that have caused exfoliative dermatitis can be educated regarding symptomatic treatment of the dermatitis and be advised that successful treatment of the underlying disease will usually also be successful for the exfoliative dermatitis
• Protection against hypothermia and dehydration and identification of signs of infection should be part of the education process
• Advise those patients, without an identified cause for the exfoliative dermatitis, that many cases spontaneously remit (exact number uncertain) and that medical therapy to control symptoms can be provided
• American Academy of Dermatology (708)330-0230

MEDICATIONS

DRUG(S) OF CHOICE
• Systemic corticosteroids initial dosage equivalent to prednisone 40 mg/day with increases in dosage by 20 mg/day if there is no response after 3-4 days at a given dose. Subsequently, dosage should be tapered to control symptoms.
• In addition, treatment specific to any underlying infection or disease should be provided
Contraindications: Psoriasis as the underlying cause of the exfoliative dermatitis
Precautions: Atopic dermatitis and seborrheic dermatitis as underlying causes
Significant possible interactions: Refer to manufacturer's literature

ALTERNATIVE DRUGS
• Antihistamines can be useful for pruritis and topical steroids can be used for more localized disease
• When psoriasis is the underlying cause, methotrexate, etretinate, phototherapy, or other treatments specific to this disease should be provided
• Photochemotherapy may be useful therapy for treating exfoliative dermatitis associated with mycosis fungoides
• Isotretinoin has been used when pityriasis rubra pilaris is the underlying cause

FOLLOWUP

PATIENT MONITORING Patients should be monitored for response to therapy, development of complications, and for adverse effects related to therapy

PREVENTION/AVOIDANCE Known or suspected etiologic agents should be avoided

POSSIBLE COMPLICATIONS
• Infection
• Hypothermia
• Dehydration/electrolyte disturbances
• Heart failure

EXPECTED COURSE AND PROGNOSIS
• In patients with an identified underlying cause, the course and prognosis will parallel the primary disease
• For patients with idiopathic exfoliative dermatitis, the prognosis is poor with frequent recurrences or chronic symptoms requiring chronic steroid therapy

MISCELLANEOUS

ASSOCIATED CONDITIONS Any of the infections or diseases listed under causes

AGE-RELATED FACTORS
Pediatric: Less common, but may occur, associated with atopic dermatitis medications or the inherited dermatoses
Geriatric: N/A
Others: N/A

PREGNANCY N/A

SYNONYMS
• Erythroderma
• Pityriasis rubra

ICD-9-CM 695.89

SEE ALSO N/A

OTHER NOTES N/A

ABBREVIATIONS N/A

REFERENCES
• Fitzpatrick, T.B., et al. (eds.): Dermatology In General Medicine. 3rd Ed. New York, McGraw-Hill, 1987
• Moschella, S.L., Hurley, H.J.: Dermatology. 2nd Ed. Philadelphia, W.B. Saunders Co., 1985
• Domonkos, A.N., Arnold, H.L. & Odom, R.B.: Andrews' Diseases of the Skin. 8th Ed. Philadelphia, W.B. Saunders Co., 1990
• Sauer, G.C.: Manual of Skin Diseases. Philadelphia, J.B. Lippincott Co., 1991

Author M. King, M.D. & M. LeDuc, M.D.

Dermatitis, seborrheic

 BASICS

DESCRIPTION Chronic, superficial, inflammatory condition affecting hairy regions of the body, especially scalp, eyebrows, and face. Mechanism of disease unknown.
Genetics: Positive family history common
Incidence/Prevalence in USA: Common
Predominant age: Infancy, adolescence, and adulthood
Predominant sex: Male = Female

SIGNS AND SYMPTOMS
Infants
◊ Cradle cap - greasy scaling of scalp, sometimes with associated mild erythema
◊ Diaper and/or axillary rash
◊ Onset typically about age one month
◊ Usually resolves by age 8-12 months
Adults
◊ Red, greasy, scaling rash in most locations, consisting of patches and plaques with indistinct margins
◊ Red, smooth, glazed appearance in skin folds
◊ Minimal pruritis
◊ Chronic waxing and waning course
◊ Bilateral and symmetrical
◊ Most commonly located in hairy skin areas with numerous sebaceous glands, e.g., scalp and scalp margins, eyebrows and eyelid margins, nasolabial folds, ears and retroauricular folds, presternal area and mid-upper back

CAUSES
• Pityrosporum ovale (the cause of tinea versicolor) may be a contributing factor
• Genetic and environmental factors also contribute to disease, i.e., disease flares are common with any stress or illness
• Disease also seems to parallel increased sebaceous gland activity in infancy and adolescence or as a result of some acnegenic drugs

RISK FACTORS
• Parkinson's disease
• AIDS (disease severity correlated with progression of immune deficiency)
• Emotional stress

 DIAGNOSIS

DIFFERENTIAL DIAGNOSIS
• Dandruff - scaling of the scalp only, without the inflammation of seborrheic dermatitis. (Treatment of mild seborrhea and dandruff are the same anyway.)
• Atopic dermatitis - (distinction may be difficult in infants)
• Psoriasis - usually knees, elbows, nails will be involved. Scalp psoriasis will be more sharply demarcated than seborrhea, with crusted, infiltrated plaques rather than mild scaling and erythema.
• Candida
• Tinea cruris or capitis - suspect these when usual medications fail, or if there is hair loss
• Eczema of auricle or otitis externa
• Rosacea
• Discoid lupus erythematosus
• Histiocytosis X - may appear as seborrheic type eruption. Consider biopsy if usual therapies fail and especially if petechiae are noted.

LABORATORY N/A
Drugs that may alter lab results: N/A
Disorders that may alter lab results: N/A

PATHOLOGICAL FINDINGS Nonspecific changes of eczematous dermatitis. (Biopsy unnecessary unless there is a suspicion of Histiocytosis X).

SPECIAL TESTS N/A

IMAGING N/A

DIAGNOSTIC PROCEDURES N/A

 TREATMENT

APPROPRIATE HEALTH CARE
Outpatient

GENERAL MEASURES
• Increase frequency of shampooing
• Sunlight in moderate doses may be helpful

ACTIVITY Full activity

DIET No special diet

PATIENT EDUCATION Goal of treatment is control, rather than cure, of disease. Seborrheic dermatitis does not cause hair loss.

Dermatitis, seborrheic

 MEDICATIONS

DRUG(S) OF CHOICE
• Cradle cap: Frequent shampooing with salicylic and sulfur shampoos (e.g., Sebulex), and 1% hydrocortisone lotion. Remove thick scale by applying warm olive or mineral oil and then wash off several hours later with Dawn dishwashing detergent.
• Scalp involvement in adults: Start with over the counter anti-seborrheic shampoos. (These contain sulfur, coal tar, salicylic acid, selenium sulfide, or zinc pyrithione). For thick scalp scale, apply coal tar topical solution (e.g., 10% Liquor Carbonis Detergens (LCD) in Nivea oil, a prescription item) at bedtime, then shampoo with Dawn detergent each morning. (Removing thick scalp may require 1 to 3 weeks). If shampoos fail, add topical steroid solutions, or gels, applied sparingly 2 to 3 times per week and massaged in thoroughly.
• Face: 1% hydrocortisone cream applied thinly, 2 to 4 times per day
• Ears and scalp margin: Fluorinated corticosteroid cream or ointment once or twice per day (e.g., 0.1% triamcinolone cream)
• Eyelids: 1% hydrocortisone in opthalmic ointment base once per day. For eyelid crusting, may cleanse with dilute Johnson's Baby Shampoo on a cotton swab.
• Chest/back: Low strength fluorinated corticosteroid cream or anti-seborrheic shampoo
• Skin folds: 1% hydrocortisone cream. If candida is also present, add miconazole, nystatin, or clotrimazole.
• For secondary infections: Short course of erythromycin or dicloxacillin
Contraindications: None
Precautions: Fluorinated corticosteroids and higher concentrations of hydrocortisone (e.g., 2.5%) may cause atrophy or striae if used on the face or on skin folds
Significant possible interactions: None

ALTERNATIVE DRUGS
For difficult or diffuse cases, ketoconazole (Nizoral) cream once per day may be useful

 FOLLOWUP

PATIENT MONITORING Every 2 to 12 weeks as necessary, depending on disease severity and degree of patient sophistication

PREVENTION/AVOIDANCE N/A

POSSIBLE COMPLICATIONS
• Skin atrophy or striae possible from fluorinated corticosteroids, especially if used on the face
• Glaucoma - can result from use of fluorinated steroids around the eyes
• Photosensitivity - occasionally caused by tars
• Herpes keratitis - rare complication of herpes simplex. Instruct patient to stop eyelid steroids if herpes simplex develops.

EXPECTED COURSE AND PROGNOSIS
• In infants, seborrheic dermatitis usually remits after 6 to 8 months
• In adults, seborrheic dermatitis is usually chronic and unpredictable, with exacerbations and remissions. Disease is usually easily controlled with shampoos and topical steroids.

 MISCELLANEOUS

ASSOCIATED CONDITIONS Parkinson's disease, AIDS (disease severity correlated with progression of immune deficiency)

AGE-RELATED FACTORS
Pediatric: Common in infants
Geriatric: N/A
Others: N/A

PREGNANCY N/A

SYNONYMS
• Seborrhea
• Cradle cap

ICD-9-CM 690

SEE ALSO N/A

OTHER NOTES N/A

ABBREVIATIONS N/A

REFERENCES Habif, T.: Clinical Dermatology. 2nd Ed. St. Louis, C.V. Mosby, 1990

Author E. Lackermann, M.D.

Dermatitis, stasis

 BASICS

DESCRIPTION Chronic, noninflammatory edema of the lower leg accompanied by cycle of scratching, excoriations, weeping, crusting, and inflammation
System(s) affected: Skin/Exocrine
Genetics: Familial link probable
Incidence in USA: Common in older patient
Prevalence in USA: Common over 50 years of age
Predominant age: Adult, geriatric
Predominant sex: Female > Male

SIGNS AND SYMPTOMS
• Violaceous (sometimes brown) colored lesions - due to deoxygenation of venous blood (postinflammatory hyperpigmentation)
• Distribution - medial aspect of ankle with frequent extension onto the foot and lower leg
• Noninflammatory edema precedes the skin eruption
• Stasis ulcers (frequently accompanies stasis dermatitis) secondary to cuts, bruises, excoriations to the weakened skin around the ankle
• Mild pruritis, pain (if ulcer present)

CAUSES
• Continuous presence of edema in ankles, usually present because of venous valve incompetency (varicose veins)
• Trauma to edematous, eczematized skin

RISK FACTORS
• Atopy
• Superimposition of itch-scratch cycle
• Trauma
• Previous deep vein thrombosis
• Previous pregnancy
• Prolonged medical illness
• Obesity
• Secondary infection
• Low-protein diet
• Old age

 DIAGNOSIS

DIFFERENTIAL DIAGNOSIS
Other eczematous diseases such as:
◊ Atopic dermatitis
◊ Contact dermatitis (due to topical agents used to self-treat)
◊ Neurodermatitis

LABORATORY Culture stasis ulcers if you decide to use antibiotics (use of antibiotics topically or systemically is controversial)
Drugs that may alter lab results: N/A
Disorders that may alter lab results: N/A

PATHOLOGICAL FINDINGS Chronic inflammation

SPECIAL TESTS Culture ulcer base or prurient crusted areas to determine whether secondary infection is present

IMAGING N/A

DIAGNOSTIC PROCEDURES N/A

 TREATMENT

APPROPRIATE HEALTH CARE
• Outpatient
• Inpatient for vein stripping or skin grafts

GENERAL MEASURES
• Leg elevation - heels higher than knees, knees higher than hips
• Compression stockings (Jobst or non-fitted type)
• Elastic wraps such as Ace bandages
• Unna's paste boot (zinc gelatin) - only when lesions are dry
• When there is weeping and crusting - bedrest, soaks, and intermittently wrapped elastic bandages. (Soaks may be wet wraps with normal saline.) Apply topical steroids after each soak. Apply lubricants over the topical steroids.
• Place non-stick bandages (e.g., Telfa) over the eczematous areas)
• Fill ulcers with Gelfoam or Debrisan particles
• Re-wrap with gauze strips and Ace
• Technique: Moist zinc oxide bandages (Gelocast) in overlapping strips from toes to knee. Re-apply once a week.

ACTIVITY
• Avoid standing still
• Stay active
• Elevate foot of bed unless contraindicated

DIET No special diet. Lose weight, if overweight.

PATIENT EDUCATION
• Stress staying active to keep circulation and leg muscles in good condition. Walking is ideal.
• Keeping legs elevated while sitting or lying
• Don't wear girdles, garters, or pantyhose with tight elastic tops
• Don't scratch
• Elevate foot of bed with 2-4 inch blocks

MEDICATIONS

DRUG(S) OF CHOICE
• Burow's wet dressings and cooling pastes
• Topical triamcinolone 0.1% (Kenalog, Aristocort) cream/ointment tid or topical betamethasone
• Valerate 0.1% (Valisone) cream/ointment/solution tid
• Topical antipruritic - pramoxine, camphor, menthol
Contraindications: N/A
Precautions: Refer to manufacturer's literature
Significant possible interactions: N/A

ALTERNATIVE DRUGS
• Consider antibiotics on basis of culture results of exudate from ulcer craters
• Lubricants when dermatitis is quiescent

FOLLOWUP

PATIENT MONITORING
If Unna's boot is used - cut off and reapply boot once a week (restricts edema and prevents scratching)

PREVENTION/AVOIDANCE
• Avoid recurrence of edema with compression stockings
• Topical lubricants twice daily to prevent fissuring and itching

POSSIBLE COMPLICATIONS
• Secondary bacterial infection
• Deep vein thrombus
• Bleeding at dermatitis sites
• Squamous cell carcinoma in edges of long standing stasis ulcers
• Scarring, which in turn leads to further compromise to blood flow and increased likelihood of minor trauma

EXPECTED COURSE AND PROGNOSIS
Chronic course with intermittent exacerbations and remissions

MISCELLANEOUS

ASSOCIATED CONDITIONS
• Varicose veins
• Other eczematous disease

AGE-RELATED FACTORS
Pediatric: N/A
Geriatric: Common in this age group
Others: N/A

PREGNANCY N/A

SYNONYMS
• Gravitational eczema
• Varicose eczema
• Venous dermatitis

ICD-9-CM 454.1

SEE ALSO Varicose veins

OTHER NOTES N/A

ABBREVIATIONS N/A

REFERENCES
• Moschella, S.L., Hurley, H.J.: Dermatology, 2nd Ed. Philadelphia, W.B. Saunders, 1985
• Fitzpatrick, T.B, et al. (eds.): Dermatology In General Medicine, 3rd Ed. New York, McGraw-Hill, 1987
• Sauer, G.C.: Manual of Skin Diseases. 6th Ed. Philadelphia, J.B. Lippincott, 1991

Author J. Florence, M.D.

Diabetes insipidus

 BASICS

DESCRIPTION Defective regulation of water balance secondary to decreased secretion of vasopressin or failure of response to vasopressin
• Inadequate secretion of vasopressin may be due to loss of or malfunction of the neurosecretory neurons that make up the neurohypophysis (posterior pituitary)
• Insensitivity to vasopressin - a disorder of renal tubular function resulting in inability to respond to vasopressin in absorption of water
• Excessive water intake - (primary polydipsia) usually of functional origin

System(s) affected: Endocrine/Metabolic
Genetics: Familial cases of vasopressin deficiency have been reported (commonly autosomal dominant) but the disease is usually isolated, and often secondary to other disorders.
• Nephrogenic diabetes insipidus (insensitivity to vasopressin)- usually inherited (sex linked recessive), expressed in males, rarely in females
Incidence/Prevalence in USA: N/A
Predominant age:
• Vasopressin deficiency may occur at any age including infancy and childhood
• Nephrogenic diabetes insipidus is usually manifest in infancy
Predominant sex: Central or vasopressin-deficient diabetes insipidus is encountered in males with rare exception, reflecting its x-linked recessive mode of inheritance

SIGNS AND SYMPTOMS
• Thirst
• Polyuria
• Dehydration
• Headache
• Visual disturbance
• Head trauma

CAUSES
• Inadequate secretion of vasopressin - a variety of pathologic lesions may produce damage including tumors (craniopharyngioma, lymphoma, metastasis); infections (meningitis, encephalitis), trauma, granulomas (sarcoid, histiocytosis), or vascular disorders. Some are idiopathic or familial.
• Excessive water intake (psychogenic)
• Insensitivity to vasopressin - genetic defect in resorption of water in renal tubule (collecting ducts)
Lithium, demeclocycline, and methoxyflurane may produce nephrogenic diabetes insipidus

RISK FACTORS N/A

 DIAGNOSIS

DIFFERENTIAL DIAGNOSIS
• Diabetes mellitus and other causes of polydipsia and polyuria
• Increased solute load for excretion as occurs with high salt intake
• Psychogenic polydipsia (ultimately impairs vasopressin secretion)
• Nephrogenic diabetes insipidus (differentiate from vasopressin deficiency by clinical trial of desmopressin [DDAVP])

LABORATORY
• Hypernatremia (presenting manifestation, particularly in infants and children)
• Inability to concentrate urine (measure by osmolality, rather than specific gravity)
• Urinary glucose (to rule out diabetes mellitus)
• Plasma vasopressin or urinary vasopressin following osmotic stimulus, such as fluid restriction or administration of hypertonic saline
Drugs that may alter lab results: Lithium, demeclocycline and methoxyflurane may produce vasopressin insensitivity
Disorders that may alter lab results: Hypokalemia and hypercalcemia alter ability to concentrate urine

PATHOLOGICAL FINDINGS
Degeneration and death of neurosecretory neurons in the neurohypophysis

SPECIAL TESTS
Testing ability to concentrate urine in face of water deprivation should be done by measuring urine and plasma osmolality before and after a six hour period of thirst. This should be done during the day. It is not wise to do overnight thirst tests, particularly in children. The most valuable measurement is the urine/plasma osmolal ratio. The results are sometimes difficult to interpret since low ratios may be found in patients with primary polydipsia. If results support the diagnosis, DDAVP should be administered to test renal concentrating ability.

IMAGING If the diagnosis of diabetes insipidus is made, appropriate studies for cause including imaging of the brain must be performed
N/A

DIAGNOSTIC PROCEDURES Fluid deprivation to concentrate urine

 TREATMENT

APPROPRIATE HEALTH CARE Often, but not always, initial diagnosis and management requires hospitalization. Continuing care may be provided on an outpatient basis with self-medication.

GENERAL MEASURES
• Control of fluid balance and prevent dehydration
• Check weight daily
• Provide good skin and mouth care

ACTIVITY Not restricted

DIET Normal with free access to fluids except that young infants with nephrogenic diabetes insipidus may benefit from low solute formula

PATIENT EDUCATION
• Administration and dosage of intranasal DDAVP
• Importance of having access to fluids as thirst dictates
• Wear a medical identification neck tag or bracelet

Diabetes insipidus

 MEDICATIONS

DRUG(S) OF CHOICE
• Central (vasopressin deficient) diabetes insipidus - desmopressin (DDAVP) (a derivative of vasopressin) given intranasally two times daily in dosage necessary to control polyuria or polydipsia usually (10-25 µg) or 2 - 4 µg parenterally in 2 divided doses
• Nephrogenic diabetes insipidus - thiazide diuretics
Contraindications: DDAVP should be used with caution in the immediate postoperative period for intracranial lesions because of possible cerebral edema
Precautions: Overdose of DDAVP may produce water intoxication in patients with excessive water intake
Significant possible interactions: See manufacturer's profile of each drug

ALTERNATIVE DRUGS
• Chlorpropamide (Diabinese) 250-500 mg/day reduces polyuria and polydipsia
• Clofibrate (Atromid S) at a maximum dose of 1 gm tid also has an antidiuretic effect
• Hydrochlorothiazide 50 mg/day
Note: The effects of these alternate drugs are not as predictable as DDAVP

 FOLLOWUP

PATIENT MONITORING
• Requires regular followup at intervals of 2-3 weeks initially and 3-4 months later
• Adjustment of treatment based on the urine and electrolyte concentrations and patient's symptoms

PREVENTION/AVOIDANCE
Avoid situations of marked increase in water loss. Take fluids as dictated by thirst with no water restriction.

POSSIBLE COMPLICATIONS
• Dilatation of urinary tract has been observed (probably secondary to large volume of urine)
• Complications of primary disease (tumor histiocytosis, etc.) should be anticipated
• In nephrogenic diabetes, there is an associated retardation of mental development in some patients (cause undetermined)

EXPECTED COURSE AND PROGNOSIS
• Condition is usually permanent, although an occasional case following trauma or tumor goes into permanent remission
• Prognosis of diabetes insipidus per se is good depending on underlying disorder
• Without treatment, dehydration can lead to confusion, stupor and coma

 MISCELLANEOUS

ASSOCIATED CONDITIONS
• Infection (e.g., encephalitis, tuberculosis, syphilis)
• Tumors
• Xanthomatosis
• Pyelonephritis
• Renal amyloidosis
• Potassium depletion
• Sjögren's syndrome
• Sickle cell anemia
• Chronic hypercalcemia

AGE-RELATED FACTORS
Pediatric: Nephrogenic diabetes insipidus is usually manifest in infancy
Geriatric: N/A
Others: N/A

PREGNANCY N/A

SYNONYMS N/A

ICD-9-CM
253.5 Diabetes insipidus

SEE ALSO N/A

OTHER NOTES N/A

ABBREVIATIONS
DDAVP = brand name of desmopressin

REFERENCES Robertson, G.L.: Posterior Pituitary Hormones. In Endocrinology and Metabolism. Edited by P. Felig, J.D. Baxter, A.E. Broadus & L.A. Frohman. New York, McGraw-Hill, 1987, p 340

Author W. Cleveland, M.D.

Diabetes mellitus, insulin-dependent (IDDM or Type I)

BASICS

DESCRIPTION Absolute deficiency of endogenous insulin production that leads to inappropriate elevated blood glucose levels and end-organ complications such as accelerated atherosclerosis, neuropathy, nephropathy, and retinopathy

Genetics: 95% of white patients express either DR3 or DR4 [or both] HLA gene product compared to 45-50% in control groups

Incidence/Prevalence in USA:
• Type I and type II (NIDDM or non-insulin dependent diabetes) affect 1 to 2% of population
• Type I is 26 per 1000 by age 20

Predominant age:
• The majority falls below the age of 40
• 2 peaks of incidence - around puberty and in 6th to 7th decade

Predominant sex: Male = Female

SIGNS AND SYMPTOMS
• Weight loss from dehydration and wasting
• Polyuria
• Polydipsia
• Increased appetite unless in diabetic ketoacidosis
• Diabetic ketoacidosis can be the presenting event
• Monilial vaginitis and itching
• Proteinuria

CAUSES Destruction of beta cells in the pancreas as they are perceived by the cytotoxic T lymphocyte as non self. A viral infection may cause them to be perceived as such.

RISK FACTORS
• Being a sibling or a monozygotic twin of the patient
• Expressing HLA B8-B15
• Expressing HLA DR3\DR4

DIAGNOSIS

DIFFERENTIAL DIAGNOSIS The diabetic ketoacidosis is easily differentiated from the hyperosmolar coma by the absence of ketoacidosis and the higher reading of glycemia and osmolarity in the latter

LABORATORY Fasting plasma glucose should be greater or equal to 140 mg/dl on at least 2 separate occasions

Drugs that may alter lab results:
• Amphetamines
• Argine
• Benzodiazepines
• Beta-adrenergic blockers
• Chlorthalidone
• Clofibrate
• Corticosteroids
• Dextrothyroxine
• Diazoxide
• Epinephrine
• Furosemide
• Glucose IV
• Insulin
• Lithium
• MAO inhibitors
• Nicotinic acid (large doses)
• Oral contraceptives (estrogen-progestogen combinations)
• Oral hypoglycemics
• Phenolphthalein
• Phenothiazines
• Phenytoin
• Thiazide diuretics
• Triamterene
• Caffeine
• Ethanol

Disorders that may alter lab results:
• Recent infection
• Fever
• Pregnancy
• Acute illness
• Cushing's disease, hemochromatosis, pheochromocytoma, injury to central nervous system, tumor of pancreas islet cells, malabsorption, Addison's disease, hypothyroidism, hypopituitarism
• Reduced carbohydrate several days before test

PATHOLOGICAL FINDINGS
• Pancreatic islets are infiltrated by T lymphocytes and show loss of beta cells
• In target organs such as blood vessels, kidneys, nerves and retina, there are basement membrane lesions which can be seen by electron microscopy

SPECIAL TESTS
• HbA1c, if high, means that the plasma glucose was high over the preceding 2 to 3 months
• HLA typing and anti-beta-cell antibodies are usually not ordered. Those antibodies are rarely positive after one year of onset of the disease because beta cells are not present any longer.
• Oral glucose tolerance test (OGTT)

IMAGING N/A

DIAGNOSTIC PROCEDURES N/A

TREATMENT

APPROPRIATE HEALTH CARE
Outpatient

GENERAL MEASURES
• Initiate a team support system that includes physician, dietician /nurse/patient educator, family and patient
• Patients should follow a diet that will meet several objectives: Control blood sugar, maintain a fair lipid profile and achieve ideal body weight
• Educate patient and family about insulin use and about complications as well as a perspective of the nature of their illness and its implications

ACTIVITY
• Should not be restricted. Obtain and maintain a good level of physical conditioning.
• Teaching should emphasize how to manipulate the insulin dose according to the planned physical activity

DIET Long term compliance is the important element

PATIENT EDUCATION
• Specific instructions for diet and exercise
• Insulin injection technique
• Insulin dose adjustment according to level of activity and food intake
• Blood sugar monitoring technique
• Foot inspection
• Regular ophthalmologist followup
• Recognition of symptoms of ketoacidosis and hypoglycemia

Diabetes mellitus, insulin-dependent (IDDM or Type I)

MEDICATIONS

DRUG(S) OF CHOICE

Insulin: Conventional therapy is one to two subcutaneous injections per day with NPH and regular insulin
◊ Multiple subcutaneous injections are used when a tight control of blood sugar is needed
◊ Usually the action of regular insulin peaks at 2.5-5 hours and that of NPH at 8-12 hours
◊ Pregnancy and renal transplantation are the two absolute indications for multiple subcutaneous injections or continuous subcutaneous insulin injection, i.e., insulin pump
Contraindications: Insulin allergy manifested by anaphylaxis, which is very rare, contraindicates the resumption of treatment before desensitizing the patient with a special one day technique
Precautions: Tight control of glycemia predisposes to more frequent episodes of hypoglycemia
Significant possible interactions: Sulfa drugs, beta blockers, corticosteroids, diuretics

ALTERNATIVE DRUGS
Majority of experts now advise against use of oral hypoglycemics since these patients lack insulin

FOLLOWUP

PATIENT MONITORING
Monitor monthly for complications until insulin regulated

PREVENTION/AVOIDANCE
There is no firm evidence to show that late complications can be prevented by near normalization of blood sugar over long time

POSSIBLE COMPLICATIONS
• Diabetic ketoacidosis: An acute complication resulting from the absence of insulin which fails to suppress glucagon, which in turn releases free fatty acid (FFA) from the adipose tissue and at the same time raises the blood sugar. The former causes ketoacidosis by transforming the FFA to ketones in the liver. The latter will cause diuresis and dehydration results in diabetic ketoacidosis.

Late complications:
◊ Atherosclerosis: Low density lipoprotein (LDL) becomes glycosylated and easily trapped by the collagens predisposing to all manifestations of atherosclerosis
◊ Retinopathy: the leading cause of blindness in United States. Yearly exam by ophthalmologist is a minimum requirement beginning 5 years after onset of the disease.
◊ Nephropathy: A leading cause of death and a major cause of end stage renal disease in United States. It starts by microalbuminimia (30 to 550 mg/24 hours), initially intermittent, then persistent. Macroalbuminuria follows, which once begun causes renal function to steadily decline. Treatment includes managing the hypertension, following a low protein diet, and eventually renal dialysis.
◊ Neuropathy: Peripheral (bilateral) with symptoms ranging from numbness to severe pain and/or autonomic neuropathy with slow gastric emptying, nocturnal diarrhea, orthostatic hypotension. Treatment is symptomatic.
◊ Foot ulcers: Neuropathy decreases pain perception. Repetitive trauma can be followed by ulcers. Increased risk for infection and osteomyelitis in the underlying bone.
◊ Hypoglycemia from overdose of insulin or relative hyponutrition

EXPECTED COURSE AND PROGNOSIS
Complications take years to start and may remain asymptomatic for years

MISCELLANEOUS

ASSOCIATED CONDITIONS
Other auto immune endocrinopathies may coexist, e.g., Addison's disease

AGE-RELATED FACTORS
Pediatric: See juvenile diabetes mellitus
Geriatric: Tight control of glycemia with old age and late onset of diabetes mellitus type I is unwarranted because dangerous hypoglycemia is more frequent with tight control
Others: N/A

PREGNANCY
• At the time of embryogenesis, hyperglycemia increases the incidence of congenital malformations. Hence, planning the pregnancy and tightly controlling the blood sugar before conception is important.
• Hyperglycemia increases the perinatal morbidity and mortality, especially macrosomia and respiratory distress syndrome. Tight control of glycemia is very important and method used to achieve it is either multiple subcutaneous insulin injections or insulin pump.

SYNONYMS
• IDDM
• Type I diabetes mellitus

ICD-9-CM 250.00 Adult-onset type diabetes mellitus without mention of complication

SEE ALSO
• Diabetic Ketoacidosis
• Diabetes mellitus, juvenile

OTHER NOTES
• Insulin resistance: Defined as the need for more than 200 units of insulin per day to prevent ketosis and control hyperglycemia. It is mainly due to IgG production as insulin antibodies. It is rare - 1 per 1000 of patients. Treatment is prednisone.
• Somogyi effect: A morning hyperglycemia resulting from an early morning hypoglycemia misleading to increase the PM dose of insulin. This causes a vicious circle of more hypoglycemia/reactive hyperglycemia. The treatment is to reduce the PM insulin dose instead of increasing it.
• Insulin allergy: Due to IgE, manifests by local inflammatory reaction, generalized urticaria or anaphylaxis. Mild symptoms treated by antihistamines; severe ones by desensitization.
• Dawn phenomenon: Physiologic increase in morning insulin requirement resulting in morning hyperglycemia despite optimal insulin doses. Treatment: small dose of NPH at bedtime.
• Hypoglycemia: Results from insulin overdosing, skipping a meal or increase in physical activity without reducing the insulin dose. Manifested by tremulousness, tachycardia, sweating, hunger (due to epinephrine secretion) and confusion, stupor, coma, seizure, and focal neurological findings (due to central nervous system effect of hypoglycemia). Treatment is glucose IV or orally, or glucagon injection.

ABBREVIATIONS
N/A

REFERENCES
• Braunwald E., et al. (eds.): Harrison's Principles of Internal Medicine. 12th Ed. New York, McGraw-Hill, 1991
• Becker, K.L. (ed.): Principles and Practice of Endocrinology and Metabolism. Philadelphia, J.B. Lippincott, 1990

Author K. Deeb, M.D.

Diabetes mellitus, juvenile

BASICS

DESCRIPTION
Insulin-dependent juvenile diabetes mellitus is a chronic disease caused by pancreatic insufficiency (deficiency) of insulin, resulting in hyperglycemia. Features include:
• Patients insulinopenic and require injected insulin
• Prone to ketosis
• Usually of rapid onset
• Nutritional status - normal or thin
• Stability of disease is labile
• Response to oral drugs uncommon
• Seasonability - January-April are peak onset periods (children less than 6 years old have greater degree of seasonability)

System(s) affected: Endocrine/Metabolic

Genetics:
• Mode of genetic expression not clear
• Genes located on major histocompatibility complex on chromosome 6
• HLA DR3 and DR4 are individually associated with increased risk factor of 4; if carrying both susceptibility genes, relative risk factor increases to 12
• HLA B8 and B15 also associated with increased risk

Incidence/Prevalence: Incidence of 15 out of 100,000 per year. Racial predilection for Caucasian American. African-Americans have lowest overall incidence of Type I diabetes.

Predominant age: Mean age of onset 8-12 years, peaking in adolescence; onset about 1.5 years earlier in girls than boys. Rapid decline in incidence after adolescence.

Predominant sex: Male = Female

SIGNS AND SYMPTOMS
• Polyuria and polydipsia
• Polyphagia is classic, but not common
• Anorexia is commonly observed
• Weight loss (usually from 10-30%, and often almost devoid of body fat at time of diagnosis)
• Increased fatigue
• Decreased energy levels and lethargy
• Muscle cramps
• Irritability and emotional lability
• Vision changes, such as blurriness
• Altered school and work performance
• Headaches
• Anxiety attacks
• Chest pain and occasional difficult breathing
• Abdominal discomfort and pain
• Nausea
• Diarrhea or constipation

CAUSES
• The inherited defect causes an alteration in immunologic integrity, placing the beta cell at special risk for inflammatory damage. The mechanism of damage is autoimmune.

Environmental factors include:
• Viruses (such as mumps, coxsackie, CMV, and hepatitis viruses)
• Dietary factors - breast feeding may provide a degree of protection against the disease while diets high in dairy products are associated with increased risk

• Possible risk in diets high in nitrosamines
• Environmental toxins
• Emotional and physical stress

RISK FACTORS
• Certain HLA types (see above)
• Presence of a specific 64K protein which may be responsible for antibody formation
• Increased risk when either insulin-dependent or non-insulin dependent diabetes present in any first-degree relatives

DIAGNOSIS

DIFFERENTIAL DIAGNOSIS
• Benign renal glycosuria
• Type II (non-insulin-dependent) diabetes mellitus - a small number of children might have MODY (maturity-onset diabetes of the young)

Secondary diabetes
◊ Some with just glucose intolerance, while others may have true clinical diabetes
◊ Pancreatic disease (pancreatitis, cystic fibrosis)
◊ Hormonal disorders (pheochromocytoma, multiple endocrine adenomatosis)
◊ Inborn errors of metabolism (glycogen storage disease, Type I)
◊ Genetic disorders with insulin resistance (acanthosis nigricans)
◊ Hereditary neuromuscular disease
◊ Progeroid syndromes
◊ Obesity (Prader-Willi syndrome)
◊ Cytogenetic syndromes (Trisomy 21, Klinefelter's and Turner's syndromes)
◊ Miscellaneous (such as infantile-onset diabetes mellitus)
• Drug or chemical-induced glucose intolerance (see list below)
• Acute poisonings (salicylate poisoning can be associated with hyperglycemia and glycosuria, and may mimic diabetic ketoacidosis)

LABORATORY
• Blood glucose
• Electrolytes
• Venous pH
• U/A for glucose and ketones
• CBC (WBC may be elevated)
• Hemoglobin AIC level
• C-peptide insulin level
• Islet-cell antibodies
• T4 and thyroid antibodies

Drugs that may alter lab results:
The following may cause hyperglycemia (particularly in a patient who is prone to diabetes)
◊ Hormones - glucagon, glucocorticoids, growth hormone, epinephrine, estrogen and progesterone (oral contraceptives), thyroid preparations
◊ Drugs - thiazide diuretics, furosemide, acetazolamide, diazoxide, beta-blockers, alpha-agonists, calcium channel blockers, phenytoin, phenobarbital sodium, nicotinic acid, cyclophosphamide, l-asparaginase, epinephrine-like drugs (decongestants and diet pills), nonsteroidal anti-inflammatory agents,

nicotine, caffeine, sugar-containing syrups, fish oils

Disorders that may alter lab results: See under Differential Diagnosis above

PATHOLOGICAL FINDINGS
Inflammatory changes with lymphocytic infiltration around the Islets of Langerhans, or islet cell destruction

SPECIAL TESTS
• Oral glucose tolerance test (possibly with insulin levels, if diagnosis is questionable)
• Intravenous glucose test (for possible early detection of subclinical diabetes)
• Consider HLA-typing

IMAGING
None indicated

DIAGNOSTIC PROCEDURES
None, except laboratory studies

TREATMENT

APPROPRIATE HEALTH CARE
• Initial care - inpatient stabilization versus outpatient management, preferably in a diabetes unit where a team approach is used
• If in diabetic ketoacidosis (DKA), initial therapy of IV fluids and IV insulin till stable, then usual management - restore electrolyte and acid-base balance, correct hyperglycemia, prevent hypoglycemia and hyperkalemia, risk of cerebral edema
• Rest of health care is done by the family at home. Encourage the child to do as much self-care as possible, based on age.

GENERAL MEASURES
Overall "control" of carbohydrate metabolism for the very young child:
◊ Normoglycemia (adjusted for age) "tight" control with striving for blood glucose levels in range of 80-150 mg/dL all the time, might be dangerous (risk of repeated hypoglycemia)
◊ Hemoglobin AIC level as close to the normal (nondiabetic) range as possible
Overall good health
◊ Asymptomatic
◊ Normal appearance
◊ Try to keep lipid profile normal
Normal growth and development
◊ Reach optimal height for genetic potential
◊ Appropriate and timely pubertal maturation
◊ Coping psychosocial development - normal school or work attendance and performance. Normal future goals and career plans.
Prevent acute complications
◊ Hypoglycemic insulin reactions
◊ Diabetic ketoacidosis
◊ Delay or prevent chronic complications

ACTIVITY
• All normal activities, including full participation in any sports activities desired
• Regular, rather than periodic, aerobic exercise is preferable

DIET Appropriate diabetes exchange (ADA) diet for age (carbohydrate-50%, protein-20%, fat-30%)

PATIENT EDUCATION
• Complete initial education and ongoing education for patient and family. Team approach is ideal, if available
• For patient education materials favorably reviewed on this topic contact: American Academy of Family Physicians Foundation; P.O. Box 8418; Kansas City, MO 64114; (800)274-2237, ext 4400

MEDICATIONS

DRUG(S) OF CHOICE
Insulin (U-100)
◊ Source: Human or pure pork
◊ Type: NPH, Lente, Regular, Ultralente, 70/30 premixture
◊ Brand: Novolin, Humulin, Nordisk
Insulin regimens (given subcutaneously)
◊ NPH/Lente and Regular often in a 2:1 ratio, given twice daily (pre-breakfast and pre-supper). AM dose usually 1/2 to 2/3 of total daily insulin dose.
◊ 3 dose regimen consists of pre-breakfast dose of NPH/Lente and regular; supper dose of just regular; and bedtime dose of NPH/Lente (this regimen may prevent the dawn or Somogyi phenomenon)
◊ 4 dose regimen of regular insulin only before breakfast, lunch, and supper, and NPH/Lente at bedtime
◊ Insulin pump (external) therapy - in select patients, giving basal hourly insulin, 50% of total daily needs; pre-meal boluses, before 3 meals and bedtime snack; all insulin given is regular insulin
Contraindications: None
Precautions: Avoid hypoglycemia, the dawn phenomenon, and Somogyi syndrome (rebound hyperglycemia)
Significant possible interactions: None

ALTERNATIVE DRUGS
• Oral hypoglycemics usually not indicated in Type I diabetes (unless an obese patient, who may have MODY; or a combination of Type I and Type II)
Pharmacologic intervention (non-insulin therapy):
◊ Cyclosporine A: reduces rate of autoimmune beta cell destruction, must be started in initial weeks after the diagnosis of diabetes is made (studies: at 1 year, 20% of cyclosporine-treated patients on no insulin, compared to 12-15% of placebo controls; after 1 year, progressive decline in beta cell function and loss of remission. Toxic side effects include renal disease, hypertension, lymphoma formation.
◊ Other interventional drugs being studied: Azathioprine, steroids, nicotinamide

FOLLOWUP

PATIENT MONITORING
• Initially, frequent outpatient followup visits till stable; every 2-3 months thereafter. Monitor height growth, weight gain, sexual maturation.
• Daily home blood glucose monitoring with home blood glucose meter (One-Touch, Accuchek, Glucometer, Exactech, Answer, etc.) 3-4 times daily, with adjustment/supplementation of insulin dose based on blood glucose levels
• Periodic measurement of hemoglobin AIC to assess overall glycemic control (about every 3 months)
• Yearly measurement of serum lipids and thyroid function
• Regular review and update of dietary management. Adjust for increased caloric needs for age, level of physical activity, pubertal growth spurt, changes in weight.

PREVENTION/AVOIDANCE
• Hypoglycemia
• Diabetic ketoacidosis
• Excessive weight gain
• Psychologic problems related to chronic disease

POSSIBLE COMPLICATIONS
• Chronic/long-term
• Microvascular disease (retinopathy, nephropathy)
• Neuropathy
• Hyperlipidemia
• Macrovascular disease (coronary artery disease and cerebral artery disease)
• Foot problems

EXPECTED COURSE AND PROGNOSIS
• Initial remission or "honeymoon" phase with decreased insulin needs and easier overall control, usually lasts 3-6 months and rarely beyond a year
• Progression to "total diabetes" when endogenous insulin is insignificant; usually is gradual, but a major stress or illness may bring it on more acutely
Late history:
◊ Increasing longevity and "quality of life" with careful blood glucose monitoring and improvement in insulin delivery regimens and systems
◊ At this time, probable reduced life expectancy, but this has improved dramatically over the past 20 years
◊ Continue to be optimistic about advances being made in diabetes treatment and research that may prevent or at least minimize the complications of diabetes

MISCELLANEOUS

ASSOCIATED CONDITIONS
• Diabetes is associated with other autoimmune diseases such as hypothyroidism and Addison's Disease (screening regularly for hypothyroidism particularly important in females, who have a much higher incidence of this already)
• Diabetes mellitus can also be seen as part of multiple endocrine adenomatosis

AGE-RELATED FACTORS
Pediatric: Type I Diabetes mellitus is much more prevalent in the pediatric age groups. Over the past 10 years, a larger percentage of very young children (less than 5 years of age) present with diabetes.
Geriatric: N/A
Others: N/A

PREGNANCY It is now possible to have a safe pregnancy, with vaginal delivery of a term baby (but with intensive monitoring and care by an endocrinologist skilled in managing pregnant diabetic patients)

SYNONYMS
• Childhood diabetes
• Brittle Diabetes

ICD-9-CM 250.01

SEE ALSO
• Diabetes mellitus, insulin-dependent (IDDM or Type I)

OTHER NOTES None

ABBREVIATIONS
MODY = maturity-onset diabetes of the young

REFERENCES
• Travis, L. et al.: Diabetes Mellitus in Children and Adolescents. Philadelphia, W.B. Saunders Co., 1987
• Pediatric and Adolescent Endocrinology, Pediatric Clinics of North America, Volume 34, Number 4, W.B. Saunders Company, August 1987
• Lebovitz, H.E. (ed): Therapy for Diabetes Mellitus and Related Disorders. American Diabetes Association, Inc., 1991

Author R. Schultz, M.D.

Diabetes mellitus, non-insulin dependent (NIDDM)

 BASICS

DESCRIPTION Non-ketosis prone hyperglycemia and glucose intolerance due to defects in insulin secretion and peripheral insulin action. Accounts for 80% of diabetic cases.

System(s) affected: Endocrine/Metabolic

Genetics: Strong polygenic familial susceptibility. Concordance is nearly complete in identical twins.

Incidence in USA: 300/100,000 (males 230/100,000, females 340/100,000)

Prevalence in USA:
• 5,000/100,000
• 3.5% in general population. NIDDM is more common in some groups such as Pima Indians with 35% prevalence.

Predominant age: Typically occurs after age 40

Predominant sex: Female > Male in Caucasian populations

SIGNS AND SYMPTOMS
• Related to hyperglycemia and complications including nephropathy, neuropathy, and retinopathy
• Polyuria
• Polydipsia
• Polyphagia
• Weight loss
• Weakness
• Fatigue
• Frequent infections

CAUSES Genetic factors and obesity are important

RISK FACTORS
• Family history
• Gestational diabetes

 DIAGNOSIS

DIFFERENTIAL DIAGNOSIS
• Insulin-dependent diabetes mellitus
• Pancreatic insufficiency
• Pheochromocytoma
• Cushing's syndrome
• Corticosteroid use
• "Stress" hyperglycemia

LABORATORY
• Fasting blood sugar greater than 140 on two occasions
• Random plasma glucose ≥ 200 mg/dL plus classic symptoms of DM (e.g., polydipsia, polyuria, polyphagia, weight loss)
• FBS < 140 plus sustained elevated plasma glucose during at least 2 oral glucose tolerance tests. The 2 hour sample and at least one other between 0 and 2 hours after 75 gram glucose dose should be ≥ 200 mg/dL. Do not do if FBS > 140.
• Hemoglobin A1C is elevated

Drugs that may alter lab results: Corticosteroids can cause hyperglycemia

Disorders that may alter lab results: Cushing's syndrome

PATHOLOGICAL FINDINGS N/A

SPECIAL TESTS Glucose tolerance test usually not necessary, except when diagnosing gestational diabetes

IMAGING N/A

DIAGNOSTIC PROCEDURES N/A

 TREATMENT

APPROPRIATE HEALTH CARE Regular outpatient follow-up except for complicating emergencies such as severe hyperglycemia, hyperosmolar coma, and severe infections

GENERAL MEASURES
• Home monitoring of blood or urine glucose
• Regular examination for complications: retinopathy, neuropathy, nephropathy

ACTIVITY Regular aerobic exercise can improve glucose tolerance and decrease medication requirements

DIET
• American Diabetes Association (ADA) provides dietary recommendations for NIDDM. The most important part of this diet is weight loss in obese patients. The diet is similar to that recommended by the American Heart Association and includes increased complex carbohydrate, decreased fat and moderation in salt and alcohol.
• Dietary treatment alone can often result in adequate metabolic control in NIDDM

PATIENT EDUCATION
• Education is critical for patients with NIDDM. Include information on the disease, medication treatment, self-monitoring, foot care, physical activity and diet management
• Support groups and classes certified by the ADA are recommended
• The ADA has prepared numerous patient education materials (430 North Michigan Ave. Chicago, IL 60611 or contact local ADA affiliate listed in white pages of telephone directory)

Diabetes mellitus, non-insulin dependent (NIDDM)

MEDICATIONS

DRUG(S) OF CHOICE
• First generation oral agents - tolbutamide, tolazamide, chlorpropamide
• Second generation oral agents - glyburide, glipizide
• Insulin - regular, NPH, Lente, Ultralente
Contraindications:
• To oral agents: Insulin dependent diabetes mellitus, ketotic patient, pregnancy, history of allergy
• Use caution in liver or renal disease and acute infection or stress
Precautions: Warn patients of signs of hypo- and hyperglycemia
Significant possible interactions: Drugs which potentiate oral hypoglycemics e.g., salicylates, clofibrate, coumadin, chloramphenicol, ethanol

ALTERNATIVE DRUGS N/A

FOLLOWUP

PATIENT MONITORING
• Frequency of followup depends on compliance and degree of metabolic control. Every two to four months is typical.
• Review of symptoms and home blood glucose levels
• Blood glucose (consider Hemoglobin A1C)
• Funduscopy
• Cardiopulmonary exam
• Foot exam for ulcers, arterial insufficiency, neuropathy
• After five years, perform yearly: Ophthalmologist exam, monitor for proteinuria and renal insufficiency

PREVENTION/AVOIDANCE Avoidance
of weight gain and obesity and maintenance of regular physical activity may prevent or delay NIDDM

POSSIBLE COMPLICATIONS
• Appear to be due to effects of diabetes mellitus on arterial walls in one form or another
• Peripheral neuropathy
• Proliferative retinopathy
• Nephropathy and chronic renal failure
• Atherosclerotic cardiovascular and peripheral vascular disease
• Hyperosmolar coma
• Gangrene of extremities
• Blindness
• Glaucoma
• Cataracts
• Skin ulceration
• Charcot joints

EXPECTED COURSE AND PROGNOSIS
• Maintenance of normal blood sugar levels may delay or prevent complications of diabetes
• In susceptible individuals, complications begin to appear 10-15 years after onset, but can be present at time of diagnosis since NIDDM may go undetected for years

MISCELLANEOUS

ASSOCIATED CONDITIONS
• Hypertension is common
• Strict control may retard renal complications
• Hyperlipidemia
• Impotence

AGE-RELATED FACTORS
Pediatric: Occasional cases of nonketosis-prone diabetes mellitus have been seen in children
Geriatric: NIDDM is common in the elderly and is a significant contributing factor to blindness, renal failure, and lower limb amputations
Others: NIDDM is generally of adult onset, appearing after age 40

PREGNANCY Diabetes can cause
significant maternal complications and fetal wasting. Intensive management by those skilled in this area has improved the outcome dramatically.

SYNONYMS
• Adult onset diabetes mellitus
• Type II diabetes mellitus
• Nonketotic diabetes mellitus
• NIDDM

ICD-9-CM 250.0, 250.2, 250.4, 250.5, 250.6, 250.7, 250.8, 250.9

SEE ALSO N/A

OTHER NOTES N/A

ABBREVIATIONS
• NIDDM = Non-insulin dependent diabetes mellitus
• ADA = American Diabetic Association

REFERENCES
• Beigelman, P. & Kumar, D.: Diabetes Mellitus for the House Officer. Baltimore, Williams and Wilkins, 1986
• Krall, L.P. & Beaser, R.S. (eds.): Joslin Diabetes Manual. 12th Ed. Philadelphia, Lea and Febiger, 1989
• Yhi-Järvin, H. et al.: Comparison of insulin regimens in patients with NIDDM. NEJM 1992; 327:1426-33

Author D. Gray, M.D.

Diabetic ketoacidosis

 BASICS

DESCRIPTION
A true medical emergency secondary to absolute or relative insulin deficiency characterized by hyperglycemia, ketonemia, metabolic acidosis, and electrolyte depletion

System(s) affected: Endocrine/Metabolic

Genetics: N/A

Incidence/Prevalence in USA: 46 episodes/10,000 diabetic patients

Predominant age: 0-19 years of age

Predominant sex: Male = Female

SIGNS AND SYMPTOMS
- Polyuria
- Polydipsia
- Generalized weakness
- Malaise/lethargy
- Nocturia
- Nausea/vomiting
- Abdominal pain and tenderness
- Decreased bowel sounds
- Decreased perspiration
- Hypotension
- Hypothermia
- Decreased reflexes
- Coma
- Confusion
- Tachycardia
- Tachypnea
- Fever +/-
- Breath fruity, with acetone smell
- Dry mucous membranes
- Anorexia or increased appetite

CAUSES
- Insulin dependent diabetes mellitus
- Infarction (myocardial) 5-7%
- Infection (30-40%) usually respiratory or urinary
- Idiopathic (20-30%)
- Medication non-compliance
- CVA
- Trauma
- Surgery
- Emotional stress

RISK FACTORS
- Any condition that leads to an absolute or relative insulin deficiency
- History of corticosteroid therapy

 DIAGNOSIS

DIFFERENTIAL DIAGNOSIS
- Hyperosmolar non-ketotic coma
- Alcoholic ketoacidosis
- Lactic acidosis
- Acute hypoglycemic coma
- Uremia

LABORATORY
- Blood sugar elevated (usually 250-800 range)
- Serum ketosis
- Urine ketosis
- Glycosuria
- Hyponatremia
- Hyperamylasemia
- Hypertriglyceridemia
- Hypercholesterolemia
- Increased BUN
- HCO3 <15
- Decreased calculated total body K+
- Metabolic acidosis on ABG
- Increased serum osmolality
- Increased anion gap

Drugs that may alter lab results: N/A

Disorders that may alter lab results:
- With concomitant lactic acidosis, acetoacetate production may be inhibited in presence of high levels of beta hydroxybutyrate. The nitroprusside reaction, which measures only acetoacetate, may not be strongly positive.
- A very low serum sodium (< 110 mmol/L) suggests an artifact due to severe hypertriglyceridemia
- Severe acidosis gives artificially high K+ level
- Markedly increased serum ketones may cross react and cause a falsely high serum creatinine

PATHOLOGICAL FINDINGS   N/A

SPECIAL TESTS
- ECG (especially if MI suspected). May also assist in evaluation of K+ status. Usually shows sinus tachycardia.
- Urine and blood cultures

IMAGING
Chest x-ray to rule out pulmonary infection

DIAGNOSTIC PROCEDURES   N/A

 TREATMENT

APPROPRIATE HEALTH CARE
- Inpatient intensive care. This is a life threatening emergency.
- Goals are to increase rate of glucose utilization by insulin-dependent tissues, to reverse ketonemia and acidosis, and to correct the depletion of water and electrolytes.

GENERAL MEASURES
- IV Fluids adults: 1L normal saline over 30 minutes, 1L normal saline over next hour, then 500 cc/hr (approximately 7 cc/kg/hr) x 4 hrs or until dehydration improves, then 250 cc/hour (3.5 cc/kg/hr). Switch to D5 in 1/2 normal saline when serum glucose < 300. Expect to give 4-8 L/ first 24 hrs. (Some do not recommend initial IV bolus).
- Pediatric maintenance requirements: 100 cc/kg for first 10 kg, 50 cc/kg for second 10 kg and 20 cc/kg thereafter. Fluid deficit: (Multiply patient's body weight by percentage dehydration). Replace maintenance and deficit evenly over 48 hours.

ACTIVITY   Bedrest

DIET
Nothing by mouth initially. Advance to pre-ketotic diet when nausea and vomiting are controlled.

PATIENT EDUCATION
- For prevention, careful control of blood glucose
- Monitor glucose carefully during periods of stress, infection, trauma etc.

MEDICATIONS

DRUG(S) OF CHOICE
- Insulin-initiate infusion at 0.1U/kg/hr
- Potassium
- Bicarbonate
- Phosphate

Contraindications:
- No demonstrable clinical benefit from bicarbonate with a pH > 7.0.
- Hold K+ if > 5.5

Precautions:
- Double insulin if no response in serum glucose over first 2 hours
- Must continue insulin until serum bicarbonate and anion gap normalize
- Add dextrose to IV fluid when blood sugar < 300
- If using bicarbonate, add 50 mg NaHCO3 to 1L 1/2 NS and give over 2 hours
- Delay K+ administration in patients with inadequate urine output or evidence of diabetic nephropathy
- If blood sugar does not fall by approximately 75 mg % q 2 hrs, increase insulin rate
- Taper IV insulin and start NPH/Reg insulin after acidosis clears and patient is eating

Significant possible interactions: For each 0.1 unit of pH, serum K+ will change by approximately 0.6 meq K in the opposite direction

ALTERNATIVE DRUGS N/A

FOLLOWUP

PATIENT MONITORING
- Monitor mental status, vital signs, urine output q 30-60 minutes until improved, then q 2-4 hrs x 24 hrs
- Blood sugar q 1 hr until < 300 mg/dL, then q 2-6 hrs
- K+, HCO3, Na+, anion gap, q 2 hrs
- Phosphate, Ca++, Mg++, q 4-6 hrs

PREVENTION/AVOIDANCE
- Monitor glucose closely during stressful situations
- Careful insulin control

POSSIBLE COMPLICATIONS
- Cerebral edema
- Pulmonary edema
- Venous thrombosis
- Hypokalemia
- Myocardia infarction
- Acute gastric dilatation
- Late hypoglycemia
- Erosive gastritis
- Infection
- Respiratory distress
- Hypophosphatemia
- Mucormycosis

EXPECTED COURSE AND PROGNOSIS
- DKA accounts for 14% of all hospital admissions for diabetes and for 16% of all diabetic related fatalities
- Overall mortality of 5-15%
- In children < 10 years old, DKA causes 70% diabetes related fatalities

MISCELLANEOUS

ASSOCIATED CONDITIONS Look for complications of chronic diabetes (nephropathy, neuropathy, retinopathy, etc.)

AGE-RELATED FACTORS
Pediatric:
- Occasionally children or adolescents with DKA exhibit marked mental deterioration, including development of coma 4-6 hrs after therapy has begun. Mortality is high.
- Diagnose by CT scan
- Treat with IV bolus of 1 gram mannitol/kg in 20% solution
- If no response, hyperventilation to a pCO2 of 28 mm Hg

Geriatric: Must be careful with renal status or congestive heart failure
Others: N/A

PREGNANCY Risk of fetal death with DKA during pregnancy is nearly 50%

SYNONYMS N/A

ICD-9-CM 250.1

SEE ALSO
- Diabetes mellitus, insulin-dependent (IDDM or Type I)
- Diabetes mellitus, juvenile

OTHER NOTES N/A

ABBREVIATIONS N/A

REFERENCES
- Braunwald E., et al. (eds.): Harrison's Principles of Internal Medicine. 12th Ed. New York, McGraw-Hill, 1991
- Wyngaarden, J.B., Smith, L.H. (eds): Cecil Textbook of Medicine. 19th Ed. Philadelphia, W.B. Saunders Co., 1992

Author S. Abercrombie

Diarrhea, acute

 BASICS

DESCRIPTION Diarrhea of abrupt onset in a healthy individual is most often related to an infectious process. A variety of symptoms are often observed, including frequent passage of loose or watery stools, fever, chills, anorexia, vomiting and malaise.
• Acute viral diarrhea - the most common form, usually occurs for 1-3 days, and is self-limited. It causes changes in the small intestine cell morphology such as villous shortening and an increase in the number of crypt cells.
• Bacterial diarrhea - may be suspected if there is a history of a similar and simultaneous illness in individuals who have shared contaminated food with the patient. Diarrhea developing within 12 hours of the meal is most likely due to ingestion of a preformed toxin.
• Protozoal infections - such as Giardia lamblia cause prolonged, watery diarrhea that often afflicts travelers returning from endemic areas where the water supply has been contaminated.
• Traveler's diarrhea - typically begins three to seven days after arrival in a foreign location and is generally quite acute
System(s) affected: Gastrointestinal, Endocrine/Metabolic
Genetics: N/A
Incidence/Prevalence: N/A
Predominant age: All ages
Predominant sex: N/A

SIGNS AND SYMPTOMS
• Loose liquidy stools +/- blood or mucus
• Fever
• Abdominal pain and distension
• Headache
• Anorexia
• Malaise
• Vomiting
• Myalgia
• With Giardia - cramping, pale-greasy stools, fatigue, weight loss, chronicity

CAUSES
Bacterial
  ◊ E. coli
  ◊ Salmonella
  ◊ Shigella
  ◊ Campylobacter jejuni
  ◊ Vibrio parahaemolyticus
  ◊ Vibrio cholerae
  ◊ Yersinia enterocolitica
Viral
  ◊ Rotavirus
  ◊ Norwalk virus
Parasitic
  ◊ Giardia lamblia
  ◊ Cryptosporidium
  ◊ Entamoeba histolytica

RISK FACTORS
• Individual from an industrialized country visiting a developing country
• Immunocompromised host

 DIAGNOSIS

DIFFERENTIAL DIAGNOSIS
• Ulcerative colitis
• Crohn's disease
• Drugs (cholinergic agents, magnesium-containing antacids)
• Pseudomembranous colitis secondary to antibiotic use
• Diverticulitis
• Spastic (irritable) colon
• Fecal impaction
• Malabsorption
• Zollinger-Ellison syndrome
• Ischemic bowel
• Gastrinoma

LABORATORY
• CBC - increased WBC with a left shift may indicate an infectious process; decreased hemoglobin/hematocrit may indicate anemia from blood loss
• Serum electrolytes - increased sodium from dehydration, decreased potassium from diarrhea
• BUN, creatinine - elevated in dehydration
• PH - hyperchloremic acidosis
• Stool sample - occult blood (present in IBD, bowel ischemia, bacterial infections), fecal leukocytes (present in diarrhea caused by Salmonella, Campylobacter, Yersinia), bacterial culture and sensitivity (for Salmonella, Yersinia, Shigella, Campylobacter), ova and parasites, C. difficile toxin, Ziehl-Neelsen stain (for Cryptosporidium)
Drugs that may alter lab results: N/A
Disorders that may alter lab results: N/A

PATHOLOGICAL FINDINGS
• Viral diarrhea - changes in small intestine cell morphology that include villous shortening, increased number of crypt cells and increased cellularity of the lamina propria
• Bacterial diarrhea - bacterial invasion of colonic wall leads to mucosal hyperemia, edema and leukocytic infiltration

SPECIAL TESTS N/A

IMAGING Abdominal x-rays (flat plate and upright) are indicated in patients with abdominal pain or evidence of obstruction to rule out toxic megacolon and bowel ischemia

DIAGNOSTIC PROCEDURES
Sigmoidoscopy indicated in patients with bloody diarrhea or suspected pseudomembranous colitis

 TREATMENT

APPROPRIATE HEALTH CARE
Outpatient except for complicating emergencies (dehydration)

GENERAL MEASURES
• Replacement of lost fluid and electrolytes
• Clear liquids such as tea, broth, carbonated beverages (without caffeine) and rehydration fluids (e.g., Gatorade) to replace lost fluid
• Packets of rehydration salts (one packet to be diluted in one quart of water); drink until thirst is quenched; will help in replacing lost electrolytes

ACTIVITY Bedrest

DIET
• During periods of active diarrhea, avoid coffee, alcohol, dairy products, most fruits, vegetables, red meats, and heavily seasoned foods
• After 12 hours with no diarrhea, begin by eating clear soup, salted crackers, dry toast or bread, and sherbet
• As stooling rate decreases, slowly add to diet, rice, baked potato, and chicken soup with rice or noodles
• As stool begins to retain shape, add to diet baked fish, poultry, applesauce, and bananas

PATIENT EDUCATION See guidelines in Prevention/Avoidance

MEDICATIONS

DRUG(S) OF CHOICE
• Loperamide (4 mg followed by 2 mg capsule after each formed stool) or bismuth subsalicylate (30 mL every half hour until 8 doses) may be helpful in mild diarrhea
• If diarrhea persists and a bacterial or parasitic organism is identified, antibiotic therapy should be started:
  ◊ Giardia - metronidazole 250 mg tid for 5-10 days
  ◊ E. Histolytica - metronidazole 500-750 mg tid for 10 days
  ◊ Shigella - TMP/SMX 160 mg and 800 mg, respectively, bid for five days, or ciprofloxacin (Cipro) 500 mg bid for 10 days
  ◊ Campylobacter - erythromycin 250 mg qid for 5 days or ciprofloxacin (Cipro) 500 mg bid for 7 days
  ◊ C. difficile - metronidazole 250 mg tid for 10-14 days
  ◊ Traveler's diarrhea - TMP/SMX one double strength tablet bid for 3 days or ciprofloxacin (Cipro) 500 mg bid for 3 days

Contraindications:
• Antibiotics are contraindicated in Salmonella infections unless caused by S. typhosa or the patient is septic
• Avoid alcoholic beverages with metronidazole due to possibility of disulfiram reaction

Precautions:
• Antiperistaltic agents (e.g., loperamide) should be used in caution with patients suspected of having infectious diarrhea or antibiotic associated colitis
• Doxycycline, TMP/SMX, ciprofloxacin - may cause photosensitivity. Use sunscreen.

Significant possible interactions:
• Salicylate absorption from bismuth subsalicylate can cause toxicity in patients already taking aspirin containing compounds and may alter anticoagulation control in patients taking coumadin
• Ciprofloxacin and erythromycin increase theophylline levels

ALTERNATIVE DRUGS
Doxycycline 100 mg bid for 3 days

FOLLOWUP

PATIENT MONITORING
If diarrhea continues for three to five days with or without blood or mucus then consult physician

PREVENTION/AVOIDANCE
• Frequent oversights during foreign travel include brushing teeth with contaminated water, ingesting ice cubes, or eating cold salads or meats
• Avoid uncooked or undercooked seafood or meat, buffet meals left out for several hours, or food served by street vendors

POSSIBLE COMPLICATIONS
• Dehydration
• Sepsis
• Shock
• Anemia

EXPECTED COURSE AND PROGNOSIS
A common problem that is rarely life-threatening if attention is given to maintaining adequate hydration

MISCELLANEOUS

ASSOCIATED CONDITIONS
• Diabetes mellitus
• Ileal resection
• Gastrectomy
• Hyperthyroidism

AGE-RELATED FACTORS
Pediatric:
• Rotavirus is a common cause of viral diarrhea in the winter months and is accompanied with vomiting
• Other etiologies include overfeeding, medications, cystic fibrosis and malabsorption
Geriatric: Watery diarrhea in elderly patient with chronic constipation may be caused by fecal impaction or obstructing carcinoma
Others: N/A

PREGNANCY
Avoid dehydration since this may lead to preterm labor

SYNONYMS
N/A

ICD-9-CM
558.9

SEE ALSO
N/A

OTHER NOTES
N/A

ABBREVIATIONS
N/A

REFERENCES
• Hirschhorn, N. & Greenough, W.B.: Progress in oral rehydration therapy. Scientific American, 264:5, 1991
• Dupont, H.L. & Edelman, R.: Infectious diarrhea: From E.Coli to Vibrio. Patient Care, May 30,1991

Author T. Parikh, M.D.

Diarrhea, chronic

 BASICS

DESCRIPTION The too frequent passage of stools that are too loose for too long. (Greater than 200 g/day stool for > 1 month, in Western societies.) Because each patient has their own concept of diarrhea, a thorough description of the complaint must be sought
System(s) affected: Gastrointestinal
Genetics:
• Adult disaccharide (usually lactose) intolerance is common in populations whose ethnicity is other than Central or Northern European
• Celiac sprue may be familial
Incidence in USA: N/A
Prevalence in USA: Fairly common, especially as diarrhea that alternates with constipation as a protracted functional bowel disorder
Predominant age: All ages can be affected; more frequent in middle or advanced age
Predominant Sex: Female > Male

SIGNS AND SYMPTOMS
• More frequent defecation than the patient perceives as "normal"
• Evacuation of stools of lesser consistency than the patient perceives as "normal"
• Repeated urgency to defecate
• In some cases, occasional incontinence of stools
• Fear of incontinence (common)
• Weight loss (rare)
• Depletion of fluid and electrolytes (rare)
• Often, lower abdominal cramping before and during defecation

CAUSES
• Motility disturbance, as in functional bowel disorder, especially when alternating with constipation
• Osmosis of fluid into the enteric lumen, by poorly absorbed solutes (e.g., Mg++, sorbitol) and as in malassimilation states
• Secretory "drive" of electrolytes and fluid from enterocytes into the intestinal lumen, as activated by certain drugs and various humoral factors
• Injury to enterocytes, as in chronic inflammatory bowel disease, neoplastic infiltration, radiation enteritis
• Persistent enteric infection is seldom a cause of chronic diarrhea, except in giardiasis and conditions marked by bacterial overgrowth in the small bowel

RISK FACTORS
• Chronic use of laxatives or cathartics
• Chronic drinking of alcohol
• Long-standing, severe diabetes mellitus
• Previous surgery, such as cholecystectomy, gastric resection, vagotomy, small bowel resection or by-pass
• Emotional turmoil
• AIDS/HIV infection
• Use of dietary aids (e.g., containing sorbitol or mannitol)

 DIAGNOSIS

DIFFERENTIAL DIAGNOSIS The most common and difficult dilemma is to distinguish "functional" disorder from an "organic" lesion.

LABORATORY
• Hemogram and blood chemistry panel are usually unrevealing except when indicative of associated illness or electrolyte depletion such as in hypokalemia
• Microscopic examination of stool specimen for ova and parasites
• Equally informative is the clinician's own gross inspection of representative stools
• Stool culture for pathogenic bacteria
• If secretory diarrhea is suspected, determination of certain serum peptides (e.g., gastrin, vasoactive intestinal peptide) may be helpful
• 24 hour stool collection to document volume
• Measure fecal fat after 100 gram/day fat diet
• Measure stool Na+ plus K+.
Serum osmality - 2x(Na+ plus K+) = osmotic gap. High osmotic gap suggests ingested osmotically active material (e.g., sorbitol) while low osmotic gap suggests secretory cause.
Drugs that may alter lab results: N/A
Disorders that may alter lab results: N/A

PATHOLOGICAL FINDINGS
• None in common "functional" diarrhea
• When present, findings are those of the associated or underlying disease

SPECIAL TESTS
• To distinguish between osmotic and secretory types of diarrhea, have the patient fast; osmotic diarrhea will subside, but secretory diarrhea will be unabated
• If cathartic abuse is suspected, test stools for phenolphthalein and anthroquinones
• Hydrogen breath test can be useful in detecting disaccharide intolerance and enteric bacterial overgrowth
• If intestinal malabsorption is suspected, duodenal mucosal biopsy (usually by endoscopy). This is usually not done unless there is evidence of steatorrhea.
• If collagenous or microscopic colitis is suspected (especially in an elderly woman), colonoscopy and serial mucosal biopsy are essential

IMAGING
Barium enema or barium meal examinations may reveal evidence of occult chronic inflammatory bowel disease or other enteric lesion

DIAGNOSTIC PROCEDURES
• Proctosigmoidoscopy is always well-advised
• Colonoscopy if diarrhea is associated with occult blood in stool or with iron deficiency
• Full colonoscopy is seldom required unless needed to seek a specifically suspected condition
• Finding of melanosis coli on endoscopy suggests anthrocine cathartic abuse (e.g., senna)

 TREATMENT

APPROPRIATE HEALTH CARE
Outpatient in almost all cases. An exception is when severe, protracted diarrhea has resulted in fluid and electrolyte depletion that requires parenteral correction.

GENERAL MEASURES When fluid or electrolyte depletion is only slight, oral supplementation of electrolyte solution will suffice

ACTIVITY Restricted only for the debilitated patient

DIET
• Usually no restriction required, except for avoidance of "diarrheogenic" items, such as prunes, etc. Avoid lactose-containing products for 2 weeks after viral gastroenteritis
• Reduction or avoidance of lactose-containing dairy products in cases of lactose intolerance
• A low-gluten diet, strictly adhered to, is essential in correction of diarrhea due to celiac sprue
• In cases of chronic diarrhea alternating with constipation, the dietary supplement of hydrophilic colloids (e.g., psyllium or synthetic analogs) may help to "normalize" bowel action

PATIENT EDUCATION
• Explanation, in simple terms, of bowel physiology
• Reassurance that "normal" frequency of bowel evacuation varies widely, and that occasional, mild "diarrhea" is in no way deleterious

MEDICATIONS

DRUG(S) OF CHOICE
• Selection depends on recognition, if possible, of the underlying cause. Dosages given below apply to adults.
For nonspecific suppression of diarrhea:
◊ Liquid stools can be given substance by use of nonabsorbable hydrophilic colloids, such as psyllium or synthetic analogs; especially helpful in reducing incontinence. Diphenoxylate (Lomotil) 5 mg to 20 mg daily or loperamide (Imodium) 4 mg to 16 mg daily, in doses calculated and timed according to the patient's individual need. (Opiates, e.g., codeine, paregoric, etc., also are effective, but their use has been largely superseded).
◊ Kaolin/pectin (e.g., Kaopectate, Donnagel) 1 to 8 tablespoons daily, divided and timed according to individual need
◊ Bismuth (e.g., Pepto-Bismol) 2 to 16 tablespoons daily, divided and timed according to individual need
More specific agents include:
◊ For lactose intolerance, supplemental lactase (Lactaid, Lactrase)
◊ For "bile salt diarrhea," cholestyramine (Questran, Cholybar), psyllium
◊ For peptide-induced diarrhea, octreotide acetate (Sandostatin)
◊ For gastric hypersecretion, H2-receptor antagonists (e.g., cimetidine or ranitidine)
Contraindications: Any impediment to bowel transit, obstruction, ileus
Precautions: Excessive dosage may lead to obstipation
Significant possible interactions: N/A

ALTERNATIVE DRUGS
Selection depends on underlying cause

FOLLOWUP

PATIENT MONITORING
What seems to be simple "functional" diarrhea, if it persists, should be further investigated for possible discovery of an underlying cause

PREVENTION/AVOIDANCE
Persons subject to chronic diarrhea should refrain from an excess of "diarrheagenic" foods and beverages containing sorbitol

POSSIBLE COMPLICATIONS
In severe cases, fluid and electrolyte depletion

EXPECTED COURSE AND PROGNOSIS
Passage of loose stools that is only occasional, brief, and responsive to simple measures is harmless. That which is habitual can be a lifelong nuisance.

MISCELLANEOUS

ASSOCIATED CONDITIONS
Chronic inflammatory bowel disease (ulcerative colitis, Crohn's disease), malassimilation syndromes, diabetes, and others

AGE-RELATED FACTORS
Pediatric: Infants and children may be subject to diarrhea of dietary origin, which they often "grow out of"
Geriatric: Elderly persons who have enjoyed regular bowel action throughout their lives, seldom suffer chronic diarrhea due to age alone; those with a lifelong tendency to diarrhea may encounter increasing difficulty with advancing age
Others: N/A

PREGNANCY N/A

SYNONYMS
• Loose bowels
• The runs

ICD-9-CM
558.9 Other and unspecified noninfectious gastroenteritis

SEE ALSO N/A

OTHER NOTES N/A

ABBREVIATIONS N/A

REFERENCES
• Krejs, G.J.: Diarrhea. In Cecil Textbook of Medicine. 18th Ed. Vol. 1. Edited by J.B. Wyngaarden & J.B. Smith. Philadelphia, W.B. Saunders Co., 1988. pp. 725-732
• McHardy, G.G., Haubrich, W.S. & Berk, J.E.: Diarrhea. In Gastrointestinal Symptoms; Clinical Interpretation. Edited by J.E. Berk and W.S. Haubrich. Philadelphia, B.C. Decker Inc., 1991. pp. 138-149
• Powell, D.W.: Approach to the Patient with Diarrhea. In Textbook of Gastroenterology, Vol. 1. Edited by T. Yamada, et al.: Philadelphia, J.B. Lippincott Co., 1991. pp. 722-778

Author W. Haubrich, M.D.

Digitalis toxicity

BASICS

DESCRIPTION A condition that may result from digitalis overdosage, hypokalemia, advanced degenerative heart disease with conduction disturbances, or a combination of factors. Toxicity may develop even when serum levels are within normal range. Usual course - acute; chronic.
Genetics: No known genetic pattern
System(s) affected: Cardiovascular, Nervous
Incidence/Prevalence in USA: Occurs in 5-23% of patients sometime during therapy
Predominant age: Middle age to elderly (40-75 years)
Predominant sex: Male = Female

SIGNS AND SYMPTOMS
- Abdominal pain
- Anorexia
- Bilateral central scotomata
- Bizarre mental symptoms in elderly patients
- Blurred vision
- Bradycardia
- Confusion
- Delirium
- Depression
- Diarrhea
- Disorientation
- Drowsiness
- Fatigue
- Hallucinations
- Halos around lights
- Headache
- Hypotension
- Impaired color vision
- Irregular pulse
- Lethargy
- Loss of visual acuity
- Mydriasis
- Nausea
- Neuralgia
- Nightmares
- Personality changes
- Photophobia
- Restlessness
- Vertigo
- Vomiting
- Weakness

CAUSES
- Alkalosis
- Cor pulmonale
- Hemodialysis
- Hypernatremia
- Hypokalemia
- Hypomagnesemia
- Hypothyroidism
- Myocarditis
- Overdosage
- Poisoning with plants containing cardiac glycosides, such as oleander, foxglove
- Procaine
- Quinidine
- Reserpine
- Steroids

RISK FACTORS
- Anoxia
- Catecholamines
- Diuretics
- Hypercalcemia
- Myocardial infarction
- Recent cardiac surgery
- Renal failure
- Suicide attempt

DIAGNOSIS

DIFFERENTIAL DIAGNOSIS
- Heart block
- Renal disease
- Other causes of life-threatening arrhythmia

LABORATORY
- Eosinophilia
- Increased digitalis level, especially if ≥ 4 ng/mL
- Potassium - hyperkalemia with acute ingestion; hypokalemia with chronic ingestion of excess or chronic renal failure
Drugs that may alter lab results: Any digitalis drug
Disorders that may alter lab results: Many cardiac abnormalities

PATHOLOGICAL FINDINGS N/A

SPECIAL TESTS
EKG:
◊ Accelerated junctional rhythms
◊ Atrial flutter
◊ Atrial premature contractions
◊ Atrial tachycardia with AV block
◊ Bidirectional tachycardia
◊ Bundle branch block
◊ Junctional premature beats
◊ Sinus bradycardia
◊ Sinus bradycardia with junctional tachycardia
◊ Ventricular fibrillation
◊ Ventricular premature contractions
◊ Wenckebach's block with junctional premature beats
◊ P-R changes
◊ Q-T changes
- Note that no arrhythmia is unique to digitalis toxicity, thus any sudden change in cardiac rhythm suggests possible toxicity

IMAGING N/A

DIAGNOSTIC PROCEDURES N/A

TREATMENT

APPROPRIATE HEALTH CARE
Inpatient - coronary care unit

GENERAL MEASURES
- Discontinue digitalis
- Pacemaker insertion for heart block
- Check serum electrolytes
- Correst calcium and magnesium abnormalities
- Avoid quinidine, which may increase serum digoxin levels by displacing digoxin from its binding sites and by decreasing renal and nonrenal excretion
- Avoid beta-adrenergic blocking drugs and isoproterenal
- Procainamide may be used
- If the patient is hemodynamically stable with primarily enhanced vagal activity (1st or 2nd degree AV block) and if the peak digitalis effect has been reached, no acute therapy is required

ACTIVITY Bedrest with monitoring

DIET Low salt, low fat

PATIENT EDUCATION Griffith, H.W.: Instructions for Patients; Philadelphia, W.B. Saunders Co. p117

MEDICATIONS

DRUG(S) OF CHOICE
• Fluid plus electrolyte therapy. If serum potassium is low, give 80 mEq KCl in 1 liter 5% D/W at rate of 6 mL/min (0.5 mEq/min). (Note - patient must be on a cardiac monitor when receiving potassium at rates greater than 10 mEq/hr. Also monitor serum potassium frequently, since hyperkalemia may develop.)
• Correct acidity

Digoxin Immune Fab (Digibind)
◊ Indicated only for treatment of severe, life-threatening arrhythmias due to digoxin or digitoxin overdosage
◊ Obtain a digoxin level before administration - be aware that the digoxin level may be falsly high if measured < 6 hours after ingestion
◊ Do not draw another digoxin level for 4 days after Digibind administration given drugs half-life of up to 20 hours in patients with normal renal function
◊ For adults and children ingesting an unknown amount of digoxin, administer 10 vials of Digibind in 50 mL of NSS IV over 30 minutes. Observe response and administer an additional 10 vials if clinically indicated. Watch for volume overload in children
◊ For toxicity during chronic therapy: Adults, 15 vials Digibind in 50 mL NSS IV over 30 minutes; children, < 20 kg, 1 vial should suffice
• Lidocaine 50 to 100 mg IV (for ventricular arrhythmias), repeated in 3-5 minutes if needed, up to a total of 300 mg. Give no more than 300 mg in 1 hour. One protocol calls for an initial bolus of lidocaine followed by 20-50 mcg/kg/min infusion for maintenance.

Contraindications: Refer to manufacturer's literature
Precautions: Refer to manufacturer's literature
Significant possible interactions: Refer to manufacturer's literature

ALTERNATIVE DRUGS
• Phenytoin as alternative to lidocaine - 100 mg q 3-5 minutes up to 1000 mg
• Consider atropine, cholestyramine

FOLLOWUP

PATIENT MONITORING
• Close EKG monitoring, potassium and digitalis levels throughout total treatment
• Monitor kidney function

PREVENTION/AVOIDANCE
• Store digitalis safely
• Monitor for toxicity
• Fluid plus electrolyte therapy according to need as determined by periodic studies, particularly of potassium level
• If there is a documentable recent exposure, consider gastric decontamination by lavage and administer activated charcoal
• Symptomatic overdose patients might best be managed by a poison control center or toxicologist

EXPECTED COURSE AND PROGNOSIS
Recovery likely if patient survives 24 hours

POSSIBLE COMPLICATIONS
• Death
• Conduction defects
• Life threatening rhythm disturbances

MISCELLANEOUS

ASSOCIATED CONDITIONS
• Chronic heart failure
• Acute pulmonary edema

AGE-RELATED FACTORS
Pediatric: N/A
Geriatric: Morbidity and mortality greater
Others: N/A

PREGNANCY N/A

SYNONYMS N/A

ICD-9-CM 972.1 poisoning by cardiotonic glycosides

SEE ALSO Ventricular arrhythmias

OTHER NOTES N/A

ABBREVIATIONS N/A

REFERENCES
• Carter, B.L., et al.: Monitoring digoxin therapy in two long-term facilities. J Am Genatr Soc. 29:263, 1981
• Beller, G.A., et al.: Digitalis intoxication: a prospective clinical study with serum level correlations. N Engl J Med. 284:989, 1971
• Duhme, D.W., et al.: Reduction of digoxin toxicity associated with measurement of serum levels. Ann Int Med. 80:516, 1974
• Marcus, F.I.: Diagnosing digitalis intoxication. Hospital Med. P 75, Jul, 1990
• Burroughs Wellcome Co: Digibind product information. Research Triangle Park, NC., 1991

Author B. Vanderhoff, M.D.

Diphtheria

BASICS

DESCRIPTION Acute respiratory tract infection caused by Corynebacterium diphtheriae, usually producing a membranous pharyngitis
• Incubation period 2 to 5 days. Infection usually occurs in fall and winter in temperate regions. In the tropics, seasonal trends are less distinct.
• Transmission by respiratory route from infected person or carrier. Man is the only reservoir.
Several forms occur:
◊ Membranous pharyngotonsillar diphtheria - the membrane is gray, adheres to the pharynx and is surrounded by erythema. The underlying mucosa bleeds when the membrane is removed.
◊ Nasal diphtheria - unilateral discharge
◊ Obstructive laryngotracheitis - complication when membrane descends into larynx or bronchial tree. When it breaks up, total obstruction of the airway may occur. Primarily in young children.
◊ Cutaneous diphtheria - punched-out ulcer covered by gray membrane (particularly in tropics and among homeless). Peaks August to October in southern United States.
System(s) affected: Pulmonary, Skin, Cardiac, Nervous
Genetics: N/A
Incidence/Prevalence in USA: 1.6 in 100,000,000 for non-cutaneous form
Predominant age: Children less than 15 and poorly immunized adults. Diptheria is a very rare condition in the U.S. today and has not been observed in children in recent years.
Predominant sex: Male = Female

SIGNS AND SYMPTOMS

Membranous pharyngotonsillar diphtheria:
◊ Initially, white to yellow membrane which is easily removed
◊ Adherent, whitish-gray, leathery membrane on tonsils or pharynx
◊ Removing membrane causes bleeding of mucosa
◊ Injected pharynx
◊ Membrane may become black due to hemorrhage
◊ Sore throat
◊ Cervical adenopathy with swelling
◊ Malaise and prostration
◊ Enlarged, tender cervical and submandibular lymph nodes
◊ May progress to edematous, swollen neck (bull neck)
◊ Paralysis of soft palate
◊ Low grade fever of 37.8-38.8°C (100-100.9°F)
◊ Thrombocytopenia and purpura
Nasal diphtheria:
◊ Serosanguineous or seropurulent discharge and excoriations
◊ Often discharge is unilateral
◊ Often chronic, mild course

Obstructive laryngotracheitis:
◊ Hoarseness
◊ Croupy cough
◊ Progresses to dyspnea and stridor
◊ Labored breathing
◊ Thick speech
Cutaneous diphtheria:
◊ On skin, conjunctiva, vulva, vagina, penis
◊ Primary cutaneous diphtheria - starts as tender pustule on lower extremity and becomes deep, round, punched-out ulcer covered by grayish membrane
◊ Secondary infection of preexisting wound - purulent exudate, partial membrane

CAUSES Corynebacterium diphtheriae

RISK FACTORS
• Crowded living conditions
• Inadequate immunization. In the U.S.A., 22-62% of people age 18 to 39 years and 41-84% of people over 60 years of age lack protective levels of antibody.
• Lower socioeconomic status
• Native Americans
• Alcoholism
• Travelers: outbreaks have occurred in the Ukraine

DIAGNOSIS

DIFFERENTIAL DIAGNOSIS
• Bacterial pharyngitis including group A streptococcus
• Viral pharyngitis
• Mononucleosis
• Oral syphilis
• Candidiasis
• Vincent's angina
• Acute epiglottitis

LABORATORY
• Gram-positive rods in the pathognomonic Chinese character configuration
• Moderate leukocytosis
• Thrombocytopenia
• Transient albuminuria
• Methylene-blue stains can assist in a presumptive diagnosis in experienced hands
• Culture from nose and throat beneath membrane and have plated on special media
• Should test for toxigenicity of strain
Drugs that may alter lab results: If an antibiotic was used, then 5 or more days may be required for the culture to grow on Loeffler's medium
Disorders that may alter lab results: N/A

PATHOLOGICAL FINDINGS
• Pleomorphic gram-positive rods
• Necrotic epithelium
• Hyaline degeneration

SPECIAL TESTS
• Serial ECG's and cardiac enzymes to detect myocarditis
• Delayed peripheral nerve conduction velocities
• Culture on Loeffler's or tellurite medium is positive in 8 to 12 hours if not previously treated with an antibiotic. Laboratory must be alerted to use one of the special media.

IMAGING N/A

DIAGNOSTIC PROCEDURES
• Culture throat or lesions
• Smear of exudate for gram stain

TREATMENT

APPROPRIATE HEALTH CARE
• Inpatient, initially hospitalized in unit which can monitor cardiac and respiratory status. (Must act on presumptive diagnosis because therapy cannot wait for culture confirmation).
• Isolation unit until cultures on two consecutive days are negative. The first culture must be taken at least 24 hours after the cessation of antibiotic therapy.

GENERAL MEASURES
• Have intubation or tracheostomy readily available. For laryngeal disease, laryngoscopy is desirable. Intubation or tracheostomy should be considered early for laryngeal disease.
• Avoid hypnotics and sedatives while monitoring respiratory status
• Physical therapy in convalescence for range of motion exercises to prevent contractions

ACTIVITY Bedrest (for at least 3 weeks until risk of developing myocarditis has passed)

DIET Liquid to soft as tolerated

PATIENT EDUCATION Explain aspects of illness and complications

MEDICATIONS

DRUG(S) OF CHOICE
Both antitoxin and antibiotics are needed for non-cutaneous diptheria.
• Equine antitoxin: Use 20,000 to 40,000 units of antitoxin for laryngeal or pharyngeal disease of less than 48 hours duration, 40,000 to 60,000 units for nasopharyngeal lesions, 80,000 to 120,000 units for extensive disease of 3 or more days duration or swelling of the neck (bull neck). Administer antitoxin by IV infusion over 60 minutes and/or by intramuscular injection. Some experts recommend treating cutaneous disease with 20,000 to 40,000 units of antitoxin while others doubt its value when there are no signs of systemic disease.
• Erythromycin parenterally or orally, 40-50 mg/kg/day; maximum of 2 grams/day for 14 days
Contraindications: See Precautions
Precautions: Equine antitoxin: 7% of patients are sensitive to equine antitoxin and need desensitization. Always test for hypersensitivity to antitoxin with intradermal or conjunctival tests, preferably both. Intradermal skin test with a 1:100 dilution of antitoxin. A positive reaction is the development of urticaria within 20 minutes of injection. For conjunctival testing, place one drop of a 1:10 dilution of antitoxin into the conjunctival sac of one eye and 0.1 mL of normal saline in the other as a control. A positive response is itching, watering and diffuse redness.
Significant possible interactions: N/A

ALTERNATIVE DRUGS
Penicillin G intramuscularly, 100,000 to 150,000 units/kg/day in four divided doses up to 600,000 units per day

FOLLOWUP

PATIENT MONITORING
• ECG, cardiac enzymes and respiratory status. Serial ECG 2-3 times per week for 4-6 months to detect myocarditis.
• Elimination of the organism should be documented by three negative cultures at least 24 hours apart. The first culture should be at least 24 hours after the completion of antimicrobial therapy.
• During convalescence, patients should be immunized against diphtheria because infection does not necessarily confer immunity

PREVENTION/AVOIDANCE
<u>Prevention is by immunization:</u>
◊ Children 6 weeks up to 7 years of age should receive doses at 2, 4, 6 and 15 months of age with 0.5 mL of DTP vaccine IM If the pertussis component is contraindicated then pediatric DT should be used. A booster dose should be given at 4-6 years of age.
◊ Unimmunized persons 7 years of age or older should receive two doses of Adult TD 4-8 weeks apart with a third dose 6-12 months later. 0.5 mL of TD should be given IM
◊ Subsequently, booster doses with TD should be given every 10 years to all individuals without a contraindication
◊ Immunized individuals may develop diphtheria but their course is milder; immunization protects against the toxin, not infection or microbial carriage in the nose, pharynx or skin
◊ Disinfect all articles in contact with patient
◊ Close contacts should be cultured and given antibiotic prophylaxis. Previously immunized contacts should receive a booster of diphtheria toxoid. Unimmunized contacts should begin the series. Prophylaxis is best with erythromycin for 7 days.

POSSIBLE COMPLICATIONS
• Myocarditis (10-25% of patients) may occur early
• Cranial and peripheral neuropathy (2 - 6 weeks after onset)
• ECG abnormalities in two-thirds of patients, including: bundle branch block, tachycardia, atrial or ventricular fibrillation, extrasystoles
• Right sided heart failure
• Local paralysis of soft palate and posterior pharynx demonstrated by regurgitation of fluids through the nares
• Peripheral and cranial neuropathy affecting primarily motor nerve functions. Motor dysfunction starts proximally and extends distally. Usually slowly resolves.
• Guillain-Barré-like syndrome

EXPECTED COURSE AND PROGNOSIS
• 5%-10% mortality rate
• Prognosis guarded until recovery
• 5-10% chronicity

MISCELLANEOUS

ASSOCIATED CONDITIONS N/A

AGE-RELATED FACTORS
Pediatric: N/A
Geriatric: N/A
Others: N/A

PREGNANCY N/A

SYNONYMS N/A

ICD-9-CM
032 Diphtheria
032.0 Faucial diphtheria
032.1 Nasopharyngeal diphtheria
032.2 Anterior nasal diphtheria
032.3 Laryngeal diphtheria
032.8 Other specified diphtheria
032.81 Conjunctival diphtheria
032.82 Diphtheritic myocarditis
032.83 Diphtheritic peritonitis
032.84 Diphtheritic cystitis
032.85 Cutaneous diphtheria
032.89 Other
032.9 Diphtheria, unspecified

SEE ALSO N/A

OTHER NOTES N/A

ABBREVIATIONS N/A

REFERENCES
• Rakel, R.E. (ed.): Conn's Current Therapy 1993. Philadelphia, W.B. Saunders Co., 1993
• Report of the Committee on Infectious Diseases, 1991. Elk Grove Village, American Academy of Pediatrics, 1991.
• Immunization Practices Advisory Committee: Diphtheria, Tetanus, and Pertussis: Recommendations for Vaccine Use and Other Preventative Measures. MMWR, 1991; 40 (RR-10)

Author R. Zimmerman, M.D. & G. Poland, M.D.

Disseminated intravascular coagulation (DIC)

 BASICS

DESCRIPTION Generation of fibrin in the blood, occurring in complications of obstetrics, (e.g., abruptio placenta), infection (especially gram-negative), malignancy
System(s) affected:
Hemic/Lymphatic/Immunologic
Genetics: Homozygous protein C or protein S deficiency
Incidence/Prevalence in USA: Unknown
Predominant age: None
Predominant sex: Male = Female

SIGNS AND SYMPTOMS
- Epistaxis
- Gingival bleeding
- Mucosal bleeding
- Hemoptysis
- Hematemesis
- Metrorrhagia
- Cough
- Dyspnea
- Confusion
- Disorientation
- Stool blood
- Hematuria
- Oliguria
- Fever
- Skin petechiae
- Purpura
- Ecchymosis
- Skin hemorrhagic necrosis
- Localized rales
- Tachypnea
- Pleural friction rub
- Retinal hemorrhages
- Anuria
- Thrombophlebitis
- Stupor
- Peripheral cyanosis

CAUSES
- Coagulation disorder due to widespread activation of clotting mechanism
- Obstetric complications
- Infection
- Neoplasms
- Intravascular hemolysis
- Vascular disorders; thrombosis
- Snake bite
- Massive tissue injury
- Trauma
- Hypoxia
- Liver disease
- Infant and adult RDS
- Purpura fulminans

RISK FACTORS
- Pregnancy
- Prostatic surgery
- Head injury

 DIAGNOSIS

DIFFERENTIAL DIAGNOSIS
- Massive hepatic necrosis
- Vitamin K deficiency
- Thrombocytopenic purpura
- Hemolytic-uremic syndrome
- Hexomonophosphate shunt

LABORATORY
- Thrombocytopenia
- Increased partial thromboplastin time
- Increased prothrombin time
- Increased thrombin time
- Decreased fibrinogen
- Increased fibrin degradation product (FDP)
- Decreased antithrombin III
- Increased bleeding time
- Schizocytosis
- Anemia
- Leukocytosis
- Increased lactate dehydrogenase (LDH)
- Increased BUN
- Decreased factor V
- Decreased or increased factor VIII
- Decreased factor X
- Decreased factor XIII
- Hemoglobinemia
- Hematuria
- Guaiac-positive
- Decreased protein C

Drugs that may alter lab results: N/A
Disorders that may alter lab results: N/A

PATHOLOGICAL FINDINGS N/A

SPECIAL TESTS N/A

IMAGING Chest x-ray Bilateral perihilar soft density

DIAGNOSTIC PROCEDURES N/A

 TREATMENT

APPROPRIATE HEALTH CARE
Inpatient

GENERAL MEASURES
- Treat underlying condition e.g., evacuation of uterus in abruptio placenta. Broad-spectrum antibiotics for gram-negative sepsis.
- Replacement of blood loss
- Platelet concentrates
- Fresh frozen plasma
- Cryoprecipitate

ACTIVITY As tolerated

DIET No special diet

PATIENT EDUCATION Griffith, H.W.: Instructions for Patients; Philadelphia, W.B. Saunders Co. p115

Index

ORDER ADDITIONAL COPIES OF THE WORLD'S BEST CURRENT THERAPY BOOK!

To order either this year's edition (1994) or next year's edition (1995) of **Griffith & Dambro: THE 5-MINUTE CLINICAL CONSULT**, return the postage-paid card below to receive the book on a 90-day approval, **or order from your local medical bookstore.**

ALSO

Take advantage of the **standing order offer** for **Griffith & Dambro: THE 5-MINUTE CLINICAL CONSULT** to receive annual revisions each year as published. Don't miss this opportunity to obtain future editions automatically, available either direct from the publisher **or through your local medical bookstore.**

YES! Please send me additional copies of the books checked below. If not completely satisfied, I may return the books with the invoice within 90 days at no further obligation.

☐ Send me _____ copies of **Griffith & Dambro: THE 5-MINUTE CLINICAL CONSULT, 1995** ISBN#1773-5, approx. $49.50

☐ Send me _____ copies of **Griffith & Dambro: THE 5-MINUTE CLINICAL CONSULT, 1994** ISBN#1753-0, $49.50

☐ Send me **Griffith & Dambro: THE 5-MINUTE CLINICAL CONSULT** every year upon publication beginning with the 1995 edition.

☐ Check enclosed (plus $4.00 handling)

☐ Bill me (plus postage & handling)

☐ Charge my credit card (plus postage & handling)
Card No. _____

☐ VISA   ☐ MasterCard   ☐ American Express
Exp. Date _____
CA, IL, MD, & PA residents add state sales tax.
Prices are subject to change without notice.

Name _____

Address _____

City/State/Zip _____

Phone No. (___) _____

☐ Send me information on a CD-ROM version.

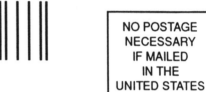

NO POSTAGE
NECESSARY
IF MAILED
IN THE
UNITED STATES

BUSINESS REPLY MAIL
FIRST CLASS PERMIT NO. 313 MALVERN, PA

POSTAGE WILL BE PAID BY ADDRESSEE

LEA & FEBIGER
200 CHESTER FIELD PARKWAY
MALVERN, PA 19355-9895

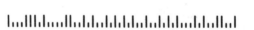

MEDICATIONS

DRUG(S) OF CHOICE
• Anticoagulants (heparin) if clinical findings suggest developing thrombotic complications, but never after head injury
• Broad-spectrum antibiotics for sepsis
Contraindications:
• Head injury
• Hemorrhagic stroke
Precautions: Refer to manufacturer's literature
Significant possible interactions: Refer to manufacturer's literature

ALTERNATIVE DRUGS
For DIC associated with metastatic prostatic carcinoma, consider heparin, aminocaproic acid (Amicar)

FOLLOWUP

PATIENT MONITORING
Closely until much improved

PREVENTION/AVOIDANCE
No preventive measures known

POSSIBLE COMPLICATIONS
• Acute renal failure
• Shock
• Cardiac tamponade
• Hemothorax
• Intracerebral hematoma
• Gangrene and loss of digits

EXPECTED COURSE AND PROGNOSIS
Poor, mortality about 60%

MISCELLANEOUS

ASSOCIATED CONDITIONS
Thromboembolic phenomena associated with venous thrombosis, thrombotic vegetations on the aortic heart valve, arterial emboli, neonatal purpura fulminans (homozygous protein C or protein S deficiency)

AGE-RELATED FACTORS
Pediatric: N/A
Geriatric: N/A
Others: N/A

PREGNANCY
N/A

SYNONYMS
• Consumptive coagulopathy
• Defibrination syndrome
• DIC

ICD-9-CM
286.6 Defibrination syndrome

SEE ALSO
N/A

OTHER NOTES
N/A

ABBREVIATIONS
N/A

REFERENCES
• Braunwald E., et al. (eds.): Harrison's Principles of Internal Medicine. 12th Ed. New York, McGraw-Hill, 1991
• Stites, D.P., Stobo, J.D., Wells, J.V.(eds): Basic and Clinical Immunology, 6th Ed. New York, Appleton & Lange, 1987

Author SG Smith

Dissociative disorders

BASICS

DESCRIPTION The key symptoms of dissociative disorders are a sudden change in one's state of consciousness, identity, motor behavior, thoughts, feelings and perception of external reality to such an extent that these functions do not operate congruently. Many pathologic symptoms can be found, but the patient experiences dysphoria, suffering, and maladaptive functioning. These disorders, according to DSM-III-R, include:
◊ Psychogenic amnesia
◊ Psychogenic fugue
◊ Multiple personality disorder
◊ Depersonalization disorder
◊ Dissociative disorder (not otherwise specified). Some authors also include - somnambulism (sleep-walking), conversion reactions, pseudo-epilepsy and (in some cultures) a variety of possession syndromes.
System(s) affected: Nervous
Genetics: N/A
Incidence/Prevalence in USA: 8-10% of the general population
Predominant age:
• Adolescents and young to middle age adults
• Rare to begin as a new illness in the elderly. However, if untreated, may linger from childhood into adult and old age.
Predominant sex: Female > Male (2:1)

SIGNS AND SYMPTOMS
Psychogenic amnesia:
• Sudden inability to recall important personal information not explained by ordinary forgetfulness or black-outs during intoxication with alcohol or other drugs
Psychogenic fugue:
• Sudden unexpected travel away from home or customary place of work with an inability to recall one's past
• Assumption of a new identity (partial or complete)
• Above symptoms are not related to the presence of multiple personality disorder, partial complex seizures, or temporal lobe epilepsy
Multiple personality disorder:
• The existence within one person of two or more distinct personality states which recurrently take control of the person's behavior
• Reports of time distortion, lapses and discontinuities
• Experiencing voices from inside one's head
• Chronic headaches
• History of severe emotional or physical abuse as a child
• Spontaneously referring to self as "he/she," "we," "us"
• Eating disorders
• Flashbacks
• Feelings of derealization
• Feelings of depersonalization
• Amnesia about important childhood events
• Personal objects and belongings that cannot be accounted for
• Disowning unrecalled behaviors
• Different handwriting styles

• Different signatures and names found in personal diary
• Sudden mood changes
• Sudden behavioral changes, i.e., from adult to young child
• Épisodes of déjà vu
• Feeling controlled by "another person" from within
• Self-inflicted violence such as wrist cutting
Depersonalization disorder:
• Recurrent experience of feeling detached from one's body as if one is an outside observer of one's mental processes and physical existence
• Recurrent experience of feeling like an automaton or as if being in a dream
• Reality testing remains intact
• Symptoms cause marked distress in the patient
• Other disorders such as schizophrenia, panic disorder, agoraphobia, temporal lobe epilepsy, and multiple personality disorder must be ruled out to qualify for this diagnosis
Dissociative disorder NOS:
• Predominant features are dissociative symptoms and the clinical picture does not meet the criteria for a specific dissociative disorder as mentioned above
• Derealization without depersonalization
• Sudden unexpected travel with dissociative features without the assumption of a new identity, partial or complete
• Trance-like states - altered states of consciousness with markedly diminished focused responsiveness to environmental stimuli. The patient appears to be day-dreaming.
• Cases in which secondary personalities never assume complete executive control of the individual's behavior

CAUSES
• Physical, emotional, verbal, or sexual abuse in childhood
• Sudden and severe trauma or threat to one's psychological or physical integrity
• Sudden and unexpected exposure to watching others being killed or severely injured (as in an industrial or car accident)
• A preponderance of coping with trauma and internal or inter-personal conflicts by the use of dissociation

RISK FACTORS
Exposure to neglect, abuse and trauma in one's childhood

DIAGNOSIS

DIFFERENTIAL DIAGNOSIS
• Other mental or CNS disorder: Schizophrenia, depression, anxiety disorder, mania, obsessive/compulsive disorder, identity disorder, phobic disorders, eating disorders
• Extreme sensory deprivation
• Epilepsy
• Early phases of dementia
• Encephalitis
• Head trauma
• Migraine

• Cerebral vascular disease
• Brain tumors
• Endocrinopathy: Hypoglycemia, hypothyroidism, hyperthyroidism
• Miscellaneous: Huntington's disease, carbon monoxide poisoning, mescaline intoxication, botulism, hyperventilation

LABORATORY
• Toxicology screening has significant importance to rule out the influence of alcohol or other psychotropic drugs
Drugs that may alter lab results: Lithium carbonate may produce hypothyroidism
Disorders that may alter lab results: Patients with dissociative disorders (especially multiple personality disorder) may present with medical oddities such as fast healing of broken bones, radiologic pictures resembling other conditions such as brain atrophy, brain infarcts, lupus, or abnormal pulmonary function tests. Any of these may lead to an erroneous diagnosis.

SPECIAL TESTS EEG to rule out epilepsy and sleep disorders.

IMAGING CT scan and MRI of the head to rule out multiple infarct dementia, brain tumors, and some forms of encephalopathy

DIAGNOSTIC PROCEDURES
• Neuro-psychological testing is helpful in ruling out learning disabilities and cognitive deficits due to early dementia or borderline mental retardation
• Psychological testing helps in the identification of specific psychiatric disorders, personality structure and dynamics
• Dissociation scales help in the assessment of the patients' tendency to dissociate in day-to-day living activities
• Sodium amytal interviews (Narcoanalysis) and special interviews under hypnosis have been found useful in the uncovering of underlying trauma, internal conflicts, and hidden personality states
• Some patients are instructed to keep a personal diary and write in it at least once per day. The diary is reviewed by the clinician for changes in the patient's handwriting and signature.

TREATMENT

APPROPRIATE HEALTH CARE
• Treatment of choice is individual psychotherapy delivered on an outpatient basis
• At times of crisis, patients need intensive treatment in a hospital setting. Hospitalization is used for protective reasons in patients with suicidal or homicidal impulses and in patients with self-inflicted violence.
• Intensive care in the hospital is used to verify the diagnosis with special tests and to begin the treatment program that continues on an outpatient basis

Dissociative disorders

GENERAL MEASURES
• Individual psychotherapy plus behavior modification, narcoanalysis and narcosynthesis, hypnoanalysis and hypnotherapy, teaching the patient self-hypnosis, relaxation therapy, and guided imagery
• Support groups, group therapy, expressive art therapy, occupational and recreational therapy are useful adjuncts
• Bibliotherapy and graphotherapy are useful

ACTIVITY
Restrictions are based on the individual condition of the patient

DIET N/A

PATIENT EDUCATION
• Instruct patients in the use of self-hypnosis, relaxation exercises and guided imagery
• Bibliotherapy in selected cases. Patients are encouraged to read about their condition and be inspired by others who have been diagnosed, treated, and helped. An example is the book, "A Mind of My Own" by Chris Sizemore, published by W. Morrow, New York, 1989.

 MEDICATIONS

DRUG(S) OF CHOICE
No medications are specifically curative. The following have been helpful:
• Antidepressants when depression is present
• Benzodiazepines for anxiety and insomnia
• Propranolol, 80-400mg/day may help control flashbacks and other dissociative symptoms
• Neuroleptics (in low doses) have shown limited success in patients with a propensity for self-abusive behavior. Thioridazine, 10-200mg/day; haloperidol, 2-10mg/day; chlorprothixene, 3-200mg/day.
• In severe agitation, Droperidol 1-5mg IM is effective in producing calm sleep and stopping agitation
• Mood swings, in dissociative disorders, do not respond to the use of lithium carbonate, carbamazepine or divalproex as well as in bipolar or unipolar mood disorders
Contraindications: Short acting benzodiazepines that produce a "high" - use caution in patients with drug abuse/dependence history
Precautions:
• Be aware of suicide potential with TCAs
• Avoid long-term use of neuroleptics if moderate to high doses are required. Very low doses of neuroleptics have been successfully used for periods of two years or more without producing tardive dyskinesia or other extra-pyramidal side effects.
Significant possible interactions: Avoid MAO inhibitors with TCAs

ALTERNATIVE DRUGS
• Buspirone, for control of anxiety 30 - 80 mg/day
• Clomipramine, 75 - 200 mg/day for control of obsessive-compulsive symptoms

 FOLLOWUP

PATIENT MONITORING
• Outpatients require a minimum of one hour of psychotherapy per week and up to 3-4 sessions per week to avoid frequent and long hospitalizations
• Hospitalized patients require more intensive treatment, including daily psychotherapy

PREVENTION/AVOIDANCE
• Prevention of child abuse through parent education, and forceful intervention by community agencies
• Effective crisis intervention following individual trauma and natural, or man-made disasters are crucial in the prevention of chronic morbidity and disability

POSSIBLE COMPLICATIONS
• Self-inflicted violence
• Suicide attempts
• Substance abuse and chemical dependency

EXPECTED COURSE AND PROGNOSIS
• Without treatment the natural history of dissociative disorders ranges from spontaneous improvement, or recovery in cases of psychogenic amnesia, psychogenic fugue, and depersonalization disorder, to acute and chronic morbidity in others
• Patients with multiple personality disorder, without treatment, may go through life disguised with the facade of healthy functioning, although suffering from episodes of depression, confusion, mood swings, etc. As they get older, the intensity and frequency of the dissociative experiences may decrease and they tend to crystallize around one or two major personality states.
• Effective treatment may produce partial or full recovery for many patients

 MISCELLANEOUS

AGE-RELATED FACTORS
Pediatric:
• Children and adolescents have more day-dreaming compared to adults; however, when this day-dreaming is associated with a change in academic functioning in a child who is not mentally retarded, child abuse or neglect should be suspected

Geriatric:
• Propensity to dissociate decreases and so do the incidence and prevalence of dissociative disorders
• Elderly more likely to experience side effects with psychotropic medications
Others: N/A

PREGNANCY N/A

SYNONYMS
• Hysterical neurosis; (dissociative type)
• Hysteria
• Ganser's syndrome

ICD-9-CM
300.15 Dissociative disorder or reaction unspecified
301.50 Histrionic personality disorder, unspecified

SEE ALSO N/A

OTHER NOTES
The fourth edition of the American Psychiatric Association's Diagnostic and Statistical Manual of Mental Disorders (DSM-IV) is to be published and implemented in 1994. In includes the following changes for Dissociative Disorders:
◊ The diagnostic name, psychogenic amnesia, has been changed to dissociative amnesia.
◊ The diagnostic name, psychogenic fugue, has been changed to dissociative fugue.
◊ The diagnostic name of multiple personality disorder has been change to dissociative identity disorder (multiple personality disorder) to convey the idea that the essence of this disorder is an absence of integration of the patient's identity, rather than the existence of multiple "persons" in one individual.

ABBREVIATIONS
MAO = monamine oxidase
TCA = tricyclic antidepressant

REFERENCES
• American Psychiatric Association: Diagnostic and Statistical Manual of Mental Disorders, 3rd Ed., Revised. Washington, DC, American Psychiatric Association,1987 pp. 269-277
• Kluft, R.P.: The Dissociative Disorders. In Textbook of Psychiatry. J.A. Talbott, R.E. Hales and S.C. Yudofsky (Eds.) American Psychiatric Press, pp. 557-585, 1988
• Ross, C.A.: Multiple Personality Disorder: Diagnosis. Clinical Features and Treatment, New York, John Wiley & Sons, Inc, 1989
• Kluft, R.P. & Fine, C.G.: Clinical Perspectives on Multiple Personality Disorder. Washington, DC, American Psychiatric Press, Inc., 1993

Author M. Torem, M.D

Diverticular disease

BASICS

DESCRIPTION Diverticulosis of the colon and its varied clinical consequences. It is considered to be a deficiency disease of western societies.
• Diverticula of colon: Herniation of the colon mucosa through the muscular layer, usually at the site of a perforating artery, lying between two layers of serosa in the mesentery. They are more common in the sigmoid and distal colon and increase in numbers with age.
• Diverticulitis: An abscess or peridiverticular inflammation initiated by the rupture of a mucosal microscopic abscess into the mesentery. Such infection may progress, fistulize into the genitourinary system, obstruct, or spontaneously resolve. Develops in about 5% of subjects with diverticulosis each year. Over a lifetime about half of patients with diverticulosis develop inflammation.
System(s) affected: Gastrointestinal
Genetics: No known genetic pattern
Incidence in USA: 2200-3000/100,000 (diverticulitis)
Prevalence in USA: Up to 20% in general population but increases progressively with age reaching up to 40%-50% in 6th-8th decade
Predominant age: Rare below 40 years, most common in 6th-8th decade
Predominant sex: Male = Female

SIGNS AND SYMPTOMS
Diverticulosis
◊ Only 10-25% of subjects harboring diverticula will develop symptoms (possibly related to coexistent irritable bowel disease)
◊ Pain - due to tension in colonic wall, mostly in left lower quadrant, worse after eating, some relief following bowel movement or passage of flatus
◊ Diarrhea or constipation
◊ Palpable mass in left iliac fossa - firm, tender
◊ Abdomen may be distended and tympanitic
◊ Absent signs of peritoneal inflammation
◊ Melena, hematochezia if diverticula bleed
Diverticulitis
◊ Pain - acute onset, mostly localized in left lower quadrant. Prominently associated with tenderness in same region.
◊ Fever with chills as severity increases
◊ Anorexia, nausea, vomiting
◊ Constipation or diarrhea
◊ Rebound tenderness, involuntary guarding, board-like rigidity
◊ Palpable mass - tender, firm, fixed
◊ Abdomen distended and tympanitic
◊ Bowel sounds depressed or could be exaggerated if obstruction ensues
◊ Dysuria, frequency if bladder involved
◊ Pneumaturia, fecaluria if colovesical fistula develops
◊ Rectal exam may reveal tenderness, induration, mass in the cul-de-sac

CAUSES
• Causes are speculative/not clearly proven
• Defects in colonic motility and increased intraluminal pressure, partially brought about by too little fecal volume
• Colonic segmentation - nonpropulsive contractions producing isolated segments or little chambers with high pressure in them
• Low fiber diet - increases segmentation and causes higher intraluminal pressure
• Defects in colonic wall strength
• Cause of bleeding unclear, not related to diverticulitis. Right sided diverticula, though less common, account for 50% of all bleeding from diverticula.

RISK FACTORS
• Age over 40
• Low residue diet
• Previous diverticulitis

DIAGNOSIS

DIFFERENTIAL DIAGNOSIS
• Irritable bowel syndrome
• Lactose intolerance
• Carcinoma of distal colon
• Ulcerative colitis, Crohn's disease
• Angiodysplasia (for rectal bleed)
• Ischemic or infectious colitis
• Appendicitis
• Other gynecologic and urologic disorders

LABORATORY
• WBC count normal in diverticulosis, elevated with immature polymorphs in diverticulitis
• Hemoglobin low if bleeding is a symptom
• Sedimentation rate elevated in diverticulitis
• Urine analysis may reveal WBC's, RBC's, pus cells in fistula formation
• Urine culture - persistent infection in colovesical fistula
• Blood culture - positive in diverticulitis with generalized peritonitis
Drugs that may alter lab results:
• Steroids
• Other immunosuppressive drugs
Disorders that may alter lab results:
• Elderly patient
• Lymphomas, other immunocompromised states
• Severe malnutrition

PATHOLOGICAL FINDINGS
• Prediverticular state - myochosis (thickening of circular layer of muscle, shortening of tenia, restriction of lumen)
• Multiple diverticula - spastic colon diverticulosis, simple massed diverticulosis, right sided diverticulosis
• Solitary diverticulum - giant sigmoid diverticulum
• Diverticulitis - inflammation, necrosis, perforation
• Diverticulitis - earliest stage, rupture of a mucosal abscess into mesentery. Does not start with obstruction of the neck as does appendicitis.

SPECIAL TESTS
• 99mTc labeled RBC scan for bleeding (rarely used) and/or angiography
• Gallium or indium labeled leukocytes to localize abscess (rarely used)

IMAGING
• Plain film abdomen supine and upright - useful in peritonitis and perforation
• Barium enema - best means for diagnosis of diverticulosis. Less useful in diagnosis of diverticulitis.
• Diverticuli may be seen on endoscopy, but less sensitive than Barium enema.
• CT scan with or without rectal contrast - diagnostic for abscess, fistula, size and location of inflammatory mass
• Angiography - diagnostic as well as therapeutic in diverticular bleeding
• Fistulograms

DIAGNOSTIC PROCEDURES
• Colonoscopy and flexible sigmoidoscopy - helpful in diagnosis of diverticulosis and extremely valuable in differential diagnosis to prove or rule out cancer. Ulcerative or ischemic colitis can uniformly be diagnosed by these modalities.
• Cystoscopy - in colovesical fistula

TREATMENT

APPROPRIATE HEALTH CARE
• Outpatient diverticulitis (pain, tenderness, leukocytosis, but no toxicity or peritoneal signs)
• About 2% subjects require hospitalization for toxicity, septicemia, peritonitis or failure to resolve in a few days. About half of these will require surgery.
• Toxic patients require hospitalization and intravenous antibiotics at least until response

GENERAL MEASURES
• IV fluids, analgesics, nasogastric suction
• Indications for surgery - severe diverticulitis, perforation, abscess, fistula, severe diverticular bleeding (requiring more than 2,000 mL of blood in 24 hours), recurrent episodes
• Surgical procedures - resection of the portion of the colon involved (usually sigmoid, or sigmoid and descending colon and direct anastomosis). If there is abscess or fistula, drainage or more extensive surgery and a diverting colostomy required.

ACTIVITY Fully active in diverticulosis, restricted activity in diverticulitis

DIET
• NPO during acute diverticulitis, progress to fluids, then to high fiber as normal bowel function returns
• All patients with diverticula should increase dietary fiber to high level through foods, and/or fiber supplement if appropriate

PATIENT EDUCATION
• Importance of high fiber diet and recognizing the symptoms of complications at early stage
• Additional material from:
National Digestive Diseases Information Clearinghouse, Box NDDIC, Bethesda, MD 20892, (301)468-6344

MEDICATIONS

DRUG(S) OF CHOICE
Diverticulosis
◊ Pain syndromes - may be treated with antispasmodics, buspirone (BuSpar) 15-30 mg/day or meperidine (Demerol) 100-150 mg/day along with high fiber diet
◊ Constipation and diarrhea, manage as indicated for irritable bowel disease
Diverticulitis
◊ Oral treatment for mild disease - metronidazole (Flagyl) 250-500 mg every 8 hours and amoxicillin (500 mg every 8 hours) combination, or ciprofloxacin 500 mg bid. Expect response within 3 days. Continue oral therapy for one week.
◊ More severe cases in hospital - gentamicin 3-5 mg/kg/day plus clindamycin 1.8-2.7 gm/day along with analgesic. Aminoglycoside dose varies with creatinine clearance.
Diverticular bleeding
◊ Vasopressin 0.2-0.3 units/minute through selective intra-arterial catheter. Used when bleeding demonstrated at angiography.
Contraindications: Hypersensitivity reaction
Precautions:
• Avoid morphine and other opiates except for Demerol
• Watch for renal toxicity and ototoxicity with aminoglycosides
Significant possible interactions: Refer to manufacturer's profile of each drug

ALTERNATIVE DRUGS Tobramycin and metronidazole, 3rd generation cephalosporins

FOLLOWUP

PATIENT MONITORING
• Some physicians would not do any invasive studies; others have recommended repeat barium enema every 3 years if symptoms infrequent or absent, or following corrective surgery.
• Colonoscopy, if needed based on above results

PREVENTION/AVOIDANCE High fiber diet, psyllium, agar, methylcellulose

POSSIBLE COMPLICATIONS
• Hemorrhage
• Perforation
• Peritonitis
• Bowel obstruction
• Abscess - paracolic, subhepatic, subphrenic
• Fistula - colovesical, colovaginal, colocutaneous

EXPECTED COURSE AND PROGNOSIS
• Prognosis is good with early detection and treatment of the complications
• Of those with a first episode of diverticulitis who are successfully managed medically, up to 67% will not have subsequent attacks requiring hospitalization; 33% will recur. Two or three recurrences in 1-2 years is an indication to electively remove the involved segment of colon.
• Of those with diverticular bleeding, up to 20% will rebleed in a period of months to years

MISCELLANEOUS

ASSOCIATED CONDITIONS Often occurs in conjunction with spastic colon

AGE-RELATED FACTORS
Pediatric:
• Very rare
• When present, it is more aggressive and recurrent in young age
Geriatric:
• More common
• May sometimes be difficult to diagnose
Others: N/A

PREGNANCY Differentiate from ectopic pregnancy

SYNONYMS N/A

ICD-9-CM
• 562.10 Diverticulosis of colon without mention of diverticulitis
• 562.11 Diverticulitis of colon without mention of diverticulitis

SEE ALSO Irritable bowel syndrome

OTHER NOTES N/A

ABBREVIATIONS N/A

REFERENCES
• Rege, R.V., et al.: Curr Probl Surg. 26, 133-89, 1989
• Sleisenger, M.H. & Fordtran, J.S. (eds.): Gastrointestinal Disease. 4th Ed. Philadelphia, W.B. Saunders Co., 1989

Author A. Verma, M.D. & F. Iber, M.D.

Down's syndrome

 ## BASICS

DESCRIPTION A common form of mental retardation whose cause is unknown. All patients have extra chromosome 21 material; chromosome non-disjunction usually occurs in female meiosis. The syndrome occurs in all races with equal frequency.
Trisomy 21: 90% of patients, an extra chromosome 21 is found in all cells
Translocation 21: 5% of patients, extra chromosome 21q material is translocated to another chromosome, usually 13 or 15. For the 5% of translocation trisomies, 1/2 are new, 1/2 have a parental carrier.
Mosaic 21: 5% of patients, 2 or more cell populations found, usually normal and trisomy 21. Clinical manifestations milder.
System(s) affected: Nervous, Cardiovascular, Skin/Exocrine
Genetics: As above. Extra chromosome comes from mother in > 90% of the cases.
Incidence/Prevalence in USA: 1 in 800 births
Predominant age: Most identified at birth. Life-span shortened.
Predominant sex: Male = Female

SIGNS AND SYMPTOMS
Infants and children
◊ Brachycephaly (100%)
◊ Hypotonia (80%)
◊ Posterior 3rd fontanel
◊ Small ears, +/- superior ear folds, +/- low set ears
◊ Mongoloid slant, eyes (90%)
◊ Epicanthic folds (90%)
◊ Brushfield's (speckled) spots of iris (50%)
◊ Esotropia (50%)
◊ Depressed nasal bridge
◊ Enlarged tongue (75%)
◊ Small chin
◊ Short neck
◊ Cardiac murmur (50%)
◊ Abnormal dermatoglyphics, including single palmar crease, distal palmar triradius, and absence of plantar whorl (ball of foot)
◊ Developmental delay, which may not be apparent in 1st year
In adults
◊ Most findings milder, but brachycephaly remains
◊ Patients are retarded (IQ = 40-45) but usually personable and cooperative
◊ Most adults can care for their personal needs. Some have jobs, but all require a sheltered environment.

CAUSES Genetic

RISK FACTORS
Increases with mother's age:
◊ 1/2000, age 20
◊ 1/200, age 35
◊ 1/100, age 37
◊ 1/20, age 45

 ## DIAGNOSIS

DIFFERENTIAL DIAGNOSIS
• Minor familial anomalies such as Mongoloid slant, epicanthic folds and depressed nasal bridge, particularly in a child with hypotonia
• The presence of a whorl on the ball of the foot usually indicates a normal child

LABORATORY A chromosome test is definitive and should always be done because of the chance of translocation
Drugs that may alter lab results: N/A
Disorders that may alter lab results: N/A

PATHOLOGICAL FINDINGS Alzheimer's plaques found in 100% of brains after age 20

SPECIAL TESTS N/A

IMAGING Abdominal ultrasound for urinary tract anomalies in children with pyuria or fevers of unknown origin

DIAGNOSTIC PROCEDURES Cardiac echo in all children with a murmur

 ## TREATMENT

APPROPRIATE HEALTH CARE
• Genetic evaluation and counseling
• Cardiac evaluation and ECG
• Appropriate pediatric health care

GENERAL MEASURES
• Parents can usually adapt to a special child
• Most important is to address parental fears and treat the infant normally
• Infant stimulation programs recommended, but definitive proof of effectiveness is lacking

ACTIVITY
• Fully active unless heart disease
• A controlled environment is needed for older children and adults

DIET No special diet. Programs suggesting megavitamin therapy has been disproved.

PATIENT EDUCATION
◊ National Down Syndrome Congress, 1800 Dempster St., Park Ridge, IL 60068-1146, (800) 232-NDSC
◊ National Organization of Rare Disorders (NORD) Conn.
◊ March of Dimes (local agency)

MEDICATIONS

DRUG(S) OF CHOICE N/A
Contraindications: N/A
Precautions: N/A
Significant possible interactions: N/A

ALTERNATIVE DRUGS N/A

FOLLOWUP

PATIENT MONITORING
• 1 or 2 subsequent genetic visits to complete counseling and a visit at 1-2 years
• Follow cardiac status carefully

PREVENTION/AVOIDANCE
• Prenatal chorion villus biopsy at 9-10 weeks and amniocentesis at 13-15 weeks
• A low screening maternal serum alpha-fetoprotein (MSAFP) at 14-16 weeks gestation finds 1/3 of cases
• Prenatal testing recommended for all pregnant females over 35, but this only impacts 25% of cases
• Recurrence is one-fifth to one-sixth for parents with a balanced translocation. There is no increased recurrence in families with mosaic Down's.

POSSIBLE COMPLICATIONS
• Bowel obstruction (fistula, intestinal anomalies [10%])
• Hirschsprung's disease (3%)
• Thyroid disease (hypo-and hyperthyroidism 5-8%)
• Leukemia (0.5%)
• Congenital heart disease (50%) especially endocardial cushion defect, ventricular septal defect
• Alzheimer's disease

EXPECTED COURSE AND PROGNOSIS
• Development is normal in the first year in about one-third of cases and mildly delayed in the rest
• Development slows after age 1 and language and cognition are moderately delayed
• The outcome and longevity may be dependent on congenital heart disease
• Some adult individuals can work in protected situations but none are independent
• Intestinal complications and congenital heart disease may be of immediate concern
• Hypothyroid disease occurs after 6 months when found, and diminished growth is the principal sign
• Clinical Alzheimer's disease in 1/3 of patients after age 35
• There is premature aging. Most patients die at 50-60, earlier if there is heart disease.

MISCELLANEOUS

ASSOCIATED CONDITIONS N/A

AGE-RELATED FACTORS
Pediatric: N/A
Geriatric: Seldom survive to geriatric age
Others: N/A

PREGNANCY Pregnancy is possible in patients with Down's syndrome. The risk for Down's syndrome in her infant is 50%.

SYNONYMS
• Trisomy 21
• Trisomy G

ICD-9-CM 758.0

SEE ALSO N/A

OTHER NOTES Mongolism is a term no longer used

ABBREVIATIONS N/A

REFERENCES
• Behrman, R.E. & Kliegman, R.M. (eds.): Nelson Textbook of Pediatrics. 14th Ed. Philadelphia, W.B. Saunders Co., 1992
• Smith, D.: Recognizable Patterns of Human Malformation. 4th Ed. Philadelphia, W.B. Saunders Co., 1988

Author P. Benke, M.D.

Dumping syndrome

 BASICS

DESCRIPTION Gastrointestinal symptoms resulting from rapid gastric emptying. Usually occurs following gastric surgery (gastrectomy, vagotomy, pyloroplasty).
System(s) affected: Gastrointestinal
Genetics: N/A
Incidence in USA: After vagotomy: 0.9% of proximal gastric vagotomy; 10-22% truncar vagotomy
Prevalence in USA: Unknown
Predominant age: Middle age to elderly
Predominant sex: Male = Female

SIGNS AND SYMPTOMS
Most common to least common:
• Diarrhea
• Nausea, vomiting
• Early satiety
• Abdominal discomfort
• Flushing
• Tachycardia
• Diaphoresis
• Syncope or near syncope
• Orthostasis

CAUSES Introduction of hyperosmolar food into intestine following surgery

RISK FACTORS Surgical drainage procedures, particularly gastrectomy

 DIAGNOSIS

DIFFERENTIAL DIAGNOSIS
• Mechanical obstruction
• Gastroenteric fistula
• Celiac sprue
• Crohn's disease
• Pancreatic exocrine insufficiency

LABORATORY
• Postprandial hypoglycemia
• Anemia
• Hypoalbuminemia
Drugs that may alter lab results: Insulin
Disorders that may alter lab results:
Diabetes mellitus

PATHOLOGICAL FINDINGS N/A

SPECIAL TESTS N/A

IMAGING
• Upper GI series - barium rapidly emptying from stomach
• Nuclear medicine gastric emptying study

DIAGNOSTIC PROCEDURES N/A

 TREATMENT

APPROPRIATE HEALTH CARE
Outpatient

GENERAL MEASURES
• Frequent small meals
• Surgery only if dietary and medical management unsuccessful and symptoms debilitating

ACTIVITY
• No restrictions
• Lying down after eating or when symptoms occur

DIET
• Low carbohydrate
• Frequent small meals
• Drink fluids between meals only
• High protein diet
• Adequate caloric intake
• Some patients may be sensitive to milk

PATIENT EDUCATION National Digestive Diseases Information Clearinghouse, Box NDDIC, Bethesda, MD 20892, (301)468-6344

MEDICATIONS

DRUG(S) OF CHOICE
<u>Antimuscarinic agents:</u>
◊ Atropine 0.4-0.6mg
◊ Cyproheptadine 30 minutes before meals
<u>New agents</u>
◊ Octreotide (Sandostatin) 200-600 mcg/day subcutaneous or IV, given in divided doses q8h. Can be very expensive.
<u>Others</u>
◊ Pectin/guar gum
Contraindications:
• Hypersensitivity
• Closed angle glaucoma
• Bladder neck obstruction
Precautions: Atropine-like effects include blurred vision, dry mouth, urinary retention, tachycardia, constipation
Significant possible interactions: Refer to manufacturer's literature

ALTERNATIVE DRUGS   N/A

FOLLOWUP

PATIENT MONITORING   Follow to be sure of adequate nutrition

PREVENTION/AVOIDANCE
• Eating frequent, small, dry meals that contain no refined carbohydrates
• Restrict fluids to between meals

POSSIBLE COMPLICATIONS
• Hypoglycemia
• Malnutrition
• Electrolyte disturbances including hypokalemia

EXPECTED COURSE AND PROGNOSIS   Favorable

MISCELLANEOUS

ASSOCIATED CONDITIONS
• Peptic ulcer disease
• Reactive hypoglycemia
• Gastrectomy/vagotomy

AGE-RELATED FACTORS
Pediatric: N/A
Geriatric: N/A
Others: N/A

PREGNANCY   N/A

SYNONYMS   Early postgastrectomy syndrome

ICD-9-CM
564.2 Postgastric surgery syndromes

SEE ALSO
• Gastric ulcer disease
• Duodenal ulcer disease
• Diarrhea
• Hypoglycemia

OTHER NOTES   N/A

ABBREVIATIONS   N/A

REFERENCES
• Sleisenger, M.H. & Fordtran, J.S. (eds.): Gastrointestinal Disease: Pathophysiology, Diagnosis, Management. 4th Ed. Philadelphia, W.B. Saunders Co., 1989
• Spiro, HW (ed): Clinical Gastroenterology, 4th ed., New York, McGraw-Hill, 1993.

Author   P. Jaffe, M.D.

Dupuytren's contracture

 BASICS

DESCRIPTION Contracture of the palmar fascia due to fibrous proliferation resulting in flexion deformities and loss of function. Similar change may rarely occur in plantar fascia. It usually appears simultaneously.

System(s) affected: Musculoskeletal

Genetics:
• Autosomal dominant with variable penetrance
• 10% of patients have a positive family history

Incidence/Prevalence in USA:
• Unknown
• Norway - 9% males and 3% females

Predominant age: 50

Predominant sex: Male > Female (ranges from 2:1 to 10:1)

SIGNS AND SYMPTOMS
• Unilateral or bilateral (50%)
• Right hand more frequent
• Ring finger more frequent
• Ulnar digits more affected than radial
• Mild pain early
• Later painless plaques or nodules in palmar fascia
• Extends into a cord-like band in the palmar fascia
• Skin adheres to fascia and becomes puckered
• Nodules can be palpated under the skin
• Digital fascia becomes involved as disease progresses
• Web space contractures
• Dupuytren's diathesis can involve plantar (Ledderhose's - 10%) and penile (Peyronies's - 2%) fascia
• Knuckle pads

CAUSES
• Unknown
• Ischemia to the fascia with oxygen free radical formation
• Possibly related to release of angiogenic basic fibroblast growth factor

RISK FACTORS
• Smoking
• Alcohol intake
• Increasing age
• Male/Caucasian
• Diabetes mellitus
• Epilepsy
• Chronic illness (e.g., pulmonary tuberculosis, liver disease)
• Hypercholesterolemia
• Liver disease
• HIV infection

 DIAGNOSIS

DIFFERENTIAL DIAGNOSIS
• Early for callosity
• Tendon abnormalities

LABORATORY N/A

Drugs that may alter lab results: N/A

Disorders that may alter lab results: N/A

PATHOLOGICAL FINDINGS
• Myofibroblasts
• First stage (proliferative) - increased myofibroblasts
• Second stage (residual) - dense fibroblast network
• Third stage (involutional) - myofibroblasts disappear

SPECIAL TESTS N/A

IMAGING N/A

DIAGNOSTIC PROCEDURES N/A

 TREATMENT

APPROPRIATE HEALTH CARE
• Outpatient monitoring and physical therapy
• Inpatient if surgery indicated

GENERAL MEASURES
• Steroid injection for acute tender nodule
• Physiotherapy is ineffective
• Isolated involvement of palmar fascia can be followed
• Metacarpo-phalangeal (MP) joint involvement can be followed if flexion contracture is < 30 degrees

Surgery - selective fascial ray release
◊ Indications: Any involvement of the proximal interphalangeal (PIP) joints. Hueston's table-top test, if positive, consider surgery (when the palm is placed on a flat surface, the digits can not be simultaneously placed fully on the same surface as the palm because of flexion contractures).
◊ May require skin grafts for wound closure with severe cutaneous shrinkage
◊ 80% have full range of movement if operated on early
◊ Amputation of little finger, if severe and deforming

ACTIVITY
• No restrictions
• Physical therapy after surgery - started 3-5 days postsurgery (passive and active exercises, posterior dynamic extension splints)

DIET No special diet

PATIENT EDUCATION
• Avoid risk factors especially with a strong family history
• Regular follow-up by physician every 6 months-1 year

MEDICATIONS

DRUG(S) OF CHOICE Steroid injection for an acute tender nodule
Contraindications: N/A
Precautions: N/A
Significant possible interactions: N/A

ALTERNATIVE DRUGS N/A

FOLLOWUP

PATIENT MONITORING Follow patient in early stages of disease

PREVENTION/AVOIDANCE None known. Avoid risk factors when possible.

POSSIBLE COMPLICATIONS
- Postsurgery development of reflex sympathetic dystrophy
- Postoperative recurrence or extension 46-80%
- Postoperative hand edema and skin necrosis
- Digital infarction

EXPECTED COURSE AND PROGNOSIS
- Unpredictable, but usually slowly progressive
- Earlier in life it starts or diasthesis - more rapidly progressive and destructive
- Reports of clinical regression with continuous passive skeletal traction in extension and under a skin graft
- Recurrence rate after surgery is 10-34%

MISCELLANEOUS

ASSOCIATED CONDITIONS
- Alcoholism
- Epilepsy
- Diabetes mellitus
- Chronic lung disease
- Occupational hand trauma (vibration white finger)
- Shoulder-hand syndrome
- Status post myocardial infarction
- Hypercholesterolemia

AGE-RELATED FACTORS
Pediatric: N/A
Geriatric: Primarily in this age group
Others: N/A

PREGNANCY N/A

SYNONYMS N/A

ICD-9-CM
728.6 Contracture of palmar fascia (Dupuytren's)

SEE ALSO N/A

OTHER NOTES N/A

ABBREVIATIONS N/A

REFERENCES
- Attali, P., Ink, O., et al.: Dupuytren's Contracture, Alcohol Consumption and Chronic Liver Disease. In Arch Intern Med 147:1065-1067, 1987
- Hill, N. & Hurst, L.: Dupuytren's Contracture. Hand Clinics. 5(3):349-357, 1989
- Way, L.W.: Current Surgical Diagnosis & Treatment. 8th Ed. Los Altos, CA, Lange, 1989
- Hueston, J.T.: Repression of Dupuytren's contracture. J of Hand Surg. 17(4):453-7, Aug., 1992

Author J. Minteer, M.D.

Dysfunctional uterine bleeding (DUB)

BASICS

DESCRIPTION Abnormal uterine bleeding, usually associated with anovulatory cycles, in the absence of other detectable organic lesions. This unit will deal only with women of reproductive age. Three major categories are:
• Estrogen breakthrough bleeding
• Estrogen withdrawal bleeding
• Progestin breakthrough bleeding
System(s) affected: Reproductive, Endocrine/Metabolic
Genetics: Unclear; tendency to have familial characteristics
Incidence/Prevalence in USA: Exact numbers not available, widespread prevalence, without specific geographic variation
Predominant age: 12-45
Predominant sex: Female only

SIGNS AND SYMPTOMS
Uterine bleeding:
◊ Unrelated to menses
◊ In excess of normal menstrual flow
◊ Occurring in an irregular pattern
◊ Rarely painful
Absence of:
◊ Other systemic symptoms
◊ Unusual bleeding from other areas
◊ Urinary or gastrointestinal irregularities
◊ Sustained aspirin or anticoagulant use
◊ Use of hormonal preparations
◊ Evidence of thyroid disease
◊ Galactorrhea
◊ Pregnancy (especially ectopic)
◊ Evidence for reproductive tract malignancy

CAUSES
After Eisenberg:
◊ Midcycle spotting - caused by a decrease in estrogen at midcycle following ovulation
◊ Frequent menses - due to short follicular phase as a result of inappropriate feedback at pituitary/hypothalamic level
◊ Deficiency of luteal phase - associated with premenstrual spotting or polymenorrhea when luteal phase is suddenly shortened by prematurely decreased progesterone; due to corpus luteum insufficiency
◊ Prolonged corpus luteum activity - caused by persistent progesterone production - results in prolonged cycles or protracted episodes of bleeding
◊ Anovulation - production of estrogen unaccompanied by cyclic surges of leuteinizing hormone (LH) or secretion of progesterone from the corpus luteum. 90% of all DUB is anovulatory. Usually seen at extremes of reproductive life.
◊ Other - uterine lesions, leiomyomata, polyps, carcinoma, vaginal infection, foreign body, ectopic pregnancy, hydatid mole, endocrine dysfunction (especially thyroid), blood dyscrasias

RISK FACTORS Listed with Causes

DIAGNOSIS

DIFFERENTIAL DIAGNOSIS
• Advanced liver disease
• Anabolic steroids
• Hematological disease (von Willebrand's, leukemia, thrombocytopenia)
• Hormonal imbalance
• Iatrogenic causes
• Intrauterine devices
• Medications (oral contraceptives, corticosteroids, hypothalamic depressants, anticholinergics, digitalis, anticoagulants
• Pregnancy (ectopic, incomplete miscarriage
• Thyroid disease
• Trauma
• Uterine cancer
• Uterine leiomyomas

LABORATORY
• Rarely necessary unless clinical picture suggests other endocrine or hematological disease, or if patient is perimenopausal
• Consider thyroid function tests, CBC, PT, PTT, workup for hirsutism, HCG (to rule out pregnancy and/or hydatid mole), prolactin (pituitary dysfunction)
Drugs that may alter lab results: N/A
Disorders that may alter lab results: N/A

PATHOLOGICAL FINDINGS Variable, depending on the disease process present. Pathological review of endometrial sampling specimens is mandatory in all patients.

SPECIAL TESTS Basal body temperature to document anovulation

IMAGING
• Ultrasound may be helpful in identifying ovarian cysts and uterine tumors
• transvaginal ultrasound (TVUS) recently developed and may be useful in many circumstances. Consider TVUS if you suspect pregnancy, anatomic problems, polycystic ovarian syndrome. The ultrasonographer should have a great deal of experience with the technique.

DIAGNOSTIC PROCEDURES
• Careful history of bleeding, with graphic display of cycles often helpful
• Pelvic examination
• Pap smear
• Endometrial biopsy in selected patients:
◊ All patients over 35 years of age
◊ Obese patients
◊ Patients with diabetes mellitus
◊ Patients with hypertension
◊ Patients with suspected polycystic ovary syndrome
• Dilatation and curettage in those who have higher risk for endometrial hyperplasia and carcinoma (consider D&C more strongly over endometrial biopsy if the suspected diagnosis is endometritis, atypical hyperplasia, or carcinoma):
◊ Heavy, uncontrolled bleeding
◊ Histological examination is necessary, but biopsy is contraindicated
◊ Medical curettage fails

TREATMENT

APPROPRIATE HEALTH CARE Almost always outpatient; may need hospitalization for profuse bleeding and hemodynamic instability

GENERAL MEASURES
Acute (profuse bleeding, hemodynamic instability):
◊ Dilatation and curettage
◊ Hysterectomy in selected (rare) cases
Nonacute:
◊ Hysterectomy in selected patients if medical therapy fails
◊ Endometrial ablation in selected patients if medical therapy fails

ACTIVITY As tolerated

DIET Normal; include adequate iron

PATIENT EDUCATION
• Thorough yet easily comprehended explanation of diagnostic approach and plan of treatment is important. Many questions regarding fertility, cancer, and infectious disease.
• Discuss ways for patient to avoid prolonged stress or emotional turmoil
• American College of Obstetricians & Gynecologists (ACOG), 409 12th St., SW, Washington, DC 20024-2188, (800)762-ACOG

MEDICATIONS

DRUG(S) OF CHOICE

Acute:
◊ Conjugated equine estrogens (25 mg intravenously) every 4 hours for a maximum of six doses
◊ When bleeding has stopped, induce shedding of the endometrium with 10 mg medroxyprogesterone qd for 10-13 days, or with oral contraceptive medication containing 35 mcg of ethinyl estradiol or equivalent
◊ Correct anemia with supplemental iron therapy

Nonacute:
◊ Progestin (if patient not bleeding when seen:) Medroxyprogesterone acetate 10 mg each day for 10-13 days
◊ Estrogen and progesterone (if bleeding when seen or bleeding continues with progesterone or with OCP's): Add 1.25 mg conjugated estrogens daily for days 1-25
◊ Oral contraceptives: Any preparation is usually adequate; initial therapy is one pill qid for five to seven days. After bleeding, withdrawal may begin normal regimen, usually for at least 3 months or give medroxyprogesterone, 10 mg every 30 days to induce menses. Can add conjugated estrogens (Premarin) 1.25 mg daily for 7 days during and in addition to regimen in order to stop intermenstrual bleeding.
◊ Prostaglandin synthetase inhibitors (e.g., Naproxen sodium, Mefenamic acid): Can decrease amount of blood loss
◊ Gonadotropin-releasing hormone agonists (induce hypoestrogenism and amenorrhea): Leuprolide acetate, nafarelin, goserelin
◊ Correct anemia with supplemental iron therapy

Contraindications: Therapy should not be instituted until a reasonable attempt at diagnosis has been made, and other causes of uterine bleeding have been considered. "Blind" hormonal therapy is ill-advised and potentially dangerous.

Precautions: Absence of withdrawal bleeding requires workup. Estrogens should not be administered to perimenopausal women or those at risk for endometrial cancer until endometrial hyperplasia and carcinoma have been excluded. Failure of a particular regimen should prompt thorough review of the diagnostic pathway before further steps are taken.

Significant possible interactions: Refer to manufacturer's profile of each drug

ALTERNATIVE DRUGS

• 100 mg IM progesteron in oil (an alternate to oral methylprogesterone). This works well for active bleeding. Not appropriate for cyclic therapy.
• Vaginal suppositories due to leakage and uncertain amount of effective medication should not be used.
"Natural" progesterone lozenges (sublingual/oral) have not be adequately studied for use with with DUB and have questionable safety.
• Danazol (unlabeled use): 200-400 mg/day. Much more expensive and may cause masculinization. Usually reserved for women planning to undergo endometrial ablation soon.

FOLLOWUP

PATIENT MONITORING All women treated for DUB with estrogens should maintain a menstrual calendar to document the pattern of bleeding abnormalities and their relation to therapy

PREVENTION/AVOIDANCE N/A

POSSIBLE COMPLICATIONS

• Anemia
• Adenocarcinoma of the uterus if prolonged unopposed estrogen stimulation in women with intact uterus
• Significant side effects of individual preparations. See manufacturer's printed information.

EXPECTED COURSE AND PROGNOSIS

• Varies with pathophysiologic process
• In young women, most anovulatory cycles can be treated confidently and successfully with physiologically sound therapeutic regimens, without surgical intervention

MISCELLANEOUS

ASSOCIATED CONDITIONS Listed with Causes

AGE-RELATED FACTORS
Pediatric: N/A
Geriatric: Uterine bleeding in a postmenopausal female must be pursued as if there were carcinoma or other significant pathology present
Others: Early postpubertal females and those in their later reproductive years most often affected

PREGNANCY May confuse with ectopic pregnancy, hydatidiform mole

SYNONYMS N/A

ICD-9-CM
626.8 Disorders of menstruation and other abnormal bleeding from female genital tract, other

SEE ALSO Ectopic pregnancy, dysmenorrhea, menorrhagia

OTHER NOTES If DUB cannot be controlled with medical treatment, options besides hysterectomy are available. Among these are the ND:YAG laser or electrocautery of the endometrium with a ball-end recsectoscope.

ABBREVIATIONS N/A

REFERENCES
• Anderson, A.B.M., Haynes, P.J., Guilleband, J. & Turnbull, A.C.: Reduction of menstrual blood loss by prostaglandin synthetase inhibitors. Lancet 1:774,1976
• DeVore, G.R., Owens, O. & Kase, N.: Use of intravenous Premarin in the treatment of dysfunctional uterine bleeding - a double-blind randomized control study. Obstet Gynecol 59:285, 1982
• Speroff, L., Glass, R.H. & Kase, N.G. (eds.): Clinical Gynecologic Endocrinology and Infertility. 4th Ed. Baltimore, Williams and Wilkins, 1989
• Cowan, B.D. & Morrison, J.C.: Management of abnormal genital bleeding in girls and women. N Engl J Med 324:1710, 1991
• Eisenberg, E.: Obstetrics and Gynecology (National Medical Series for Independent Study). Edited by W.W. Beck. New York, John Wiley & Sons, 1986
• Goldfarb: H.A.: A review of 35 endometrial ablations using ND:YASG laser for recurrent menorrhagia. Obstet Gynecol Clin 1990; 79 (5pt1):833-835

Author K. Elward, M.D., M.P.H.

Dyshidrosis

 BASICS

DESCRIPTION
• Dyshidrotic eczema: Recurrent vesicular eruption primarily of the palms, soles and interdigital areas. The term pompholyx (Greek "bubble") is generally reserved for the cases of deep-seated pruritic vesicles (the so-called "sago grain" appearance). Generally associated with, but not caused by, hyperhidrosis (excessive sweating).
• Lamellar dyshidrosis: A fine spreading exfoliation of the superficial epidermis in the same distribution as described above. Hyperhidrosis may or may not be associated.

System(s) affected: Skin/Exocrine
Genetics: N/A
Incidence/Prevalence in USA: 20/100,000
Predominant age: Usually < age 40
Predominant sex: Male = Female

SIGNS AND SYMPTOMS
Dyshidrotic eczema
◊ Small superficial vesicles of the palms and soles and between the fingers and toes
◊ Scaling, fissures and lichenification may follow vesicle formation
◊ Burning and itching are common
◊ Bilateral and frequently symmetrical lesions
◊ Vesicles may sometimes coalesce to form larger vesicles or even bullae
◊ Vesicles may rupture leading to a fine scaling similar to tinea
Lamellar dyshidrosis
◊ Small white macules which spread peripherally
◊ Central area begins to scale
◊ Desquamation of the horny layer of the skin that continues to spread

CAUSES
• Exact cause is not known
• May represent an id reaction especially to a dermatophyte infection
• Stress may play a role since dyshidrosis is more frequent in anxious individuals, and those with psychosocial stress
• Hyperhidrosis is not a cause, but is often associated with the disease

RISK FACTORS
• Atopic dermatitis
• Contact dermatitis
• Dermatophytosis
• Bacterial infections
• Foods
• Drugs such as aspirin or other salicylates

 DIAGNOSIS

DIFFERENTIAL DIAGNOSIS
• Tinea manuum or pedis
• Id reaction
• Contact dermatitis
• Atopic dermatitis
• Drug reaction
• Dermatophytid
• Pustular psoriasis
• Seborrheic dermatitis
• Acrodermatitis continua
• Pustular bacterid

LABORATORY   N/A
Drugs that may alter lab results: N/A
Disorders that may alter lab results: N/A

PATHOLOGICAL FINDINGS
• Dyshidrotic eczema: Reveals fine 1-2 mm spongiotic vesicles intraepidermally. Sweat ducts are not involved.
• Lamellar dyshidrosis: Exfoliation of the horny layer of the epidermis

SPECIAL TESTS   N/A

IMAGING   N/A

DIAGNOSTIC PROCEDURES
• Diagnosis is usually based on clinical exam
• Skin biopsy

 TREATMENT

APPROPRIATE HEALTH CARE
Outpatient

GENERAL MEASURES
• Avoidance of possible causative factors (see Risk factors)
• Though hyperhidrosis is not a cause, excessive sweating may increase pruritis and burning
• Moisturizers will give symptomatic relief of dry scaly lesions
• If feet involved, wear shoes with leather soles rather than rubber (e.g., sneakers). Wear socks made of cotton instead of synthetic materials. Remove shoes and socks whenever possible to allow sweat evaporation and to apply lubricants.

ACTIVITY   Avoid, when possible, stress or excessive sweating (may be psychological or thermal sweating). Avoid excess detergents and water.

DIET   No restrictions

PATIENT EDUCATION
• Instructions on self-care, complications and avoidance
• Explain the association between stress and dyshidrosis and suggest counseling if appropriate

MEDICATIONS

DRUG(S) OF CHOICE
<u>Dyshidrotic eczema-mild cases</u>
◊ Topical steroids (medium to high potency), or
◊ 5% salicylate in alcohol (provided salicylates are not a cause), or
◊ 3% Vioform
<u>Dyshidrotic eczema-moderate to severe cases</u>
◊ A systemic corticosteroid such as short course of oral prednisone
◊ Intramuscular ACTH or triamcinolone acetonide (40 mg)
◊ PUVA (psoralens and ultraviolet A) therapy is effective therapy (including mild cases)
<u>Lamellar dyshidrosis</u>
◊ Application of tar preparations (Estar)
◊ Intramuscular corticosteroids
◊ Keratolytics and moisturizers are sometimes helpful
Contraindications: Refer to manufacturer's profile of each drug
Precautions: Refer to manufacturer's profile of each drug
Significant possible interactions: Refer to manufacturer's profile of each drug

ALTERNATIVE DRUGS   N/A

FOLLOWUP

PATIENT MONITORING   As needed

PREVENTION/AVOIDANCE
• Control of emotional stress, avoid sweating
• Treatment for psychological factors, if appropriate

POSSIBLE COMPLICATIONS   Bacterial secondary infections

EXPECTED COURSE AND PROGNOSIS
• Benign and without scarring
• Lesions will often resolve spontaneously, though faster with appropriate treatment
• Recurrence is the rule rather than the exception

MISCELLANEOUS

ASSOCIATED CONDITIONS   N/A

AGE-RELATED FACTORS
Pediatric: N/A
Geriatric: N/A
Others: N/A

PREGNANCY   N/A

SYNONYMS
• Pompholyx
• Cheiropompholyx
• Keratolysis exfoliativa

ICD-9-CM
705.81 Dyshidrosis

SEE ALSO   N/A

OTHER NOTES   N/A

ABBREVIATIONS   N/A

REFERENCES
• Domonkos, A.N., Arnold, H.L. & Odom, R.B.: Andrew's Diseases of the Skin. 8th Ed. Philadelphia, W.B. Saunders Co., 1990
• Fitzpatrick, T.B., et al. (eds.): Dermatology in General Medicine. 3rd Ed. New York, McGraw-Hill, 1987
• Fitzpatrick, T.B.: Color Atlas and Synopsis of Clinical Dermatology. New York, McGraw-Hill, 1983
• Sauer, R.: Manual of Skin Diseases. Philadelphia, J.B. Lippincott, 1985

Author   S. Kincaid, M.D.

Dysmenorrhea

 BASICS

DESCRIPTION Pelvic pain occurring at or around the time of menses. Is a leading cause of absenteeism for women under age 30
• Primary dysmenorrhea - without pathological physical findings
• Secondary dysmenorrhea - pain occurring prior to or during menses, often more severe than primary, having a secondary pathologic (structural) cause
System(s) affected: Reproductive
Genetics: Not well studied
Incidence/Prevalence in USA:
• 40% of adult females have menstrual pain
• 10% are incapacitated for 1-3 days each month
Predominant age:
• Primary - teens to early 20's
• Secondary - 20's to 30's
Predominant sex: Female only

SIGNS AND SYMPTOMS
• Mild - pelvic discomfort or cramping or heaviness on first day of bleeding with no associated symptoms
• Moderate - discomfort occurring on first 2-3 days of menses and accompanied by mild malaise, diarrhea and headache
• Severe - intense, cramp-like pain lasting 2-7 days; often with gastrointestinal upset, back pain, thigh pain, and headache

CAUSES
Primary:
◊ Elevated production (2-7 times normal) of prostaglandins and other mediators in the uterus which produce uterine ischemia through:
  ◊ Platelet aggregation
  ◊ Vasoconstriction
  ◊ Dysrhythmic contractions with pressures higher than the systemic blood pressure
Secondary:
◊ Congenital abnormalities of uterine or vaginal anatomy
  ◊ Cervical stenosis
  ◊ Pelvic infection
  ◊ Adenomyosis
  ◊ Endometriosis
  ◊ Pelvic tumors - especially leiomyomata

RISK FACTORS
Primary:
  ◊ Nulliparity
  ◊ Positive family history
Secondary:
  ◊ Pelvic infection
  ◊ Sexually transmitted diseases
  ◊ Endometriosis

 DIAGNOSIS

DIFFERENTIAL DIAGNOSIS
Primary:
  ◊ History is characteristic
Secondary:
  ◊ Pelvic or genital infection
  ◊ Complication of pregnancy
  ◊ Missed or incomplete abortion
  ◊ Ectopic pregnancy
  ◊ Uterine or ovarian neoplasm
  ◊ Endometriosis
  ◊ Urinary tract infection

LABORATORY Noncontributory except in case of acute infection, in which case white blood cell count may be elevated and blood cultures positive
Drugs that may alter lab results:
Antibiotics
Disorders that may alter lab results: N/A

PATHOLOGICAL FINDINGS
Primary:
  ◊ None
Secondary:
  ◊ Uterine enlargement
  ◊ Leiomyomata
  ◊ Ligamentous thickening
  ◊ Fixation of pelvic structures
  ◊ Endometritis
  ◊ Salpingitis

SPECIAL TESTS
• Primary - ultrasound to rule out secondary
• Secondary - ultrasound or laparoscopy to define anatomy

IMAGING N/A

DIAGNOSTIC PROCEDURES
Primary:
  ◊ History is characteristic
  ◊ Physical examination should be normal
Secondary:
  ◊ History of onset more than 18-24 months after menarche
  ◊ Physical examination may reveal anatomic abnormalities or tenderness
  ◊ Laparoscopy (rarely needed)

 TREATMENT

APPROPRIATE HEALTH CARE
• Primary - outpatient
• Secondary - usually outpatient

GENERAL MEASURES
• Secondary dysmenorrhea - treatment of infections or suppression of endometrium if endometriosis is suspected. May be surgical, if due to severe endometriosis (presacral neurectomy), adenomyosis (hysterectomy) depending on cause.
• General physical conditioning
• Transcutaneous electrical nerve stimulator (TENS)

ACTIVITY Normal

DIET Normal

PATIENT EDUCATION
• Reassure patient that primary dysmenorrhea is treatable with use of nonsteroidal anti-inflammatory agents prior to menses and/or oral contraceptives, and will usually abate with age and parity
• Booklet: Painful Periods (Dysmenorrhea). Warner Lambert, Inc. PR-06-R-0457-P-2A (11-82)
• Primary Health Care Handbook. Edited by Shamansky, Cecere & Shellenberger. Boston, Little, Brown, 1984. Dysmenorrhea, pp. 229-30

MEDICATIONS

DRUG(S) OF CHOICE
• Ibuprofen (Motrin, Advil, Nuprin, etc.) 400-600 mg every 4-6 hours,
or
• Naproxen sodium (Anaprox) 550 mg every 12 hours,
or
• Aspirin 650 mg every 4-6 hours,
or
• Other nonsteroidal anti-inflammatory drugs
• Oral contraceptives

Contraindications:
• Platelet disorders
• Gastric ulceration or gastritis
• Thromboembolic disorders
• Vascular disease
• Contraindications to oral contraceptives

Precautions:
• GI irritation
• Lactation
• Coagulation disorders
• Impaired renal function
• Congestive heart failure
• Liver dysfunction

Significant possible interactions:
• Coumarin-type anticoagulants
• Aspirin with other NSAID's
• Methotrexate
• Furosemide
• Lithium

ALTERNATIVE DRUGS
Nifedipine (Procardia XL) 30 mg (not approved for this use)

FOLLOWUP

PATIENT MONITORING N/A

PREVENTION/AVOIDANCE
• Primary - none known
• Secondary - reduce risk of sexually-transmitted diseases

POSSIBLE COMPLICATIONS
• Primary - anxiety and/or depression
• Secondary - infertility from underlying pathology

EXPECTED COURSE AND PROGNOSIS
• Primary - improves with age and parity
• Secondary - likely to require therapy based on underlying cause

MISCELLANEOUS

ASSOCIATED CONDITIONS N/A

AGE-RELATED FACTORS N/A
Pediatric: Onset with first menses raises probability of genital tract anatomic abnormality such as transverse vaginal septum, uterine anomalies
Geriatric: N/A
Others: N/A

PREGNANCY
Consider ectopic pregnancy in differential diagnosis of pelvic pain with vaginal bleeding

SYNONYMS Menstrual cramps

ICD-9-CM
625.3 Dysmenorrhea

SEE ALSO Endometriosis

OTHER NOTES N/A

ABBREVIATIONS N/A

REFERENCES
• Dawood, M.Y.: Dysmenorrhea. In Clin Obstet Gynecol. Mar:33(1):168-78, 1990
• Coupey, S.M. & Ahlstrom, P.: Common menstrual disorders. Pediatr Clin North Am. Jun:36(3):551-71, 1989
• Benedetto, C.: Eicosanoids in primary dysmenorrhea, endometriosis and menstrual migraine. In Gynecol Endocrinol. 3(1):71-94, 1989

Author J. Daugherty, M.D.

Dyspareunia

BASICS

DESCRIPTION Recurrent and persistent genital pain associated with intercourse, in either the male or female. Dyspareunia may be due to organic, emotional or psychogenic causes.
• Primary: Present throughout one's sexual history
• Secondary: Arising from some specific event or condition, e.g., menopause, drugs
• Superficial: Difficulty or pain at or near the introitus or vaginal barrel associated with penetration
• Deep: Pain after penetration located at the cervix or lower abdominal area
• Complete: Present under all circumstances
• Situational: Occurring selectively with specific situations
System(s) affected: Reproductive
Genetics: N/A
Incidence/Prevalence in USA:
• Most women who are sexually active will experience dyspareunia at some time in their lives. Approximately 15% (4-40%) of adult women will have dyspareunia on a few occasions during a year. About 1% to 2% of women will have painful intercourse on a more than occasional basis.
• Male prevalence unknown
Predominant age: All ages
Predominant sex: Female > Male

SIGNS AND SYMPTOMS Varying degrees of pelvic/genital pressure, aching, tearing and/or burning

CAUSES
Disorders of vaginal outlet
◊ Hymenal ring abnormalities
◊ Postmenopausal atrophy
◊ Decreased lubrication
◊ Episiotomy scars
◊ Infections
◊ Trauma
◊ Adhesions
◊ Clitoral irritation
Disorders of vagina
◊ Infections
◊ Decreased lubrication
◊ Pelvic relaxation resulting in rectocele, uterine prolapse or cystocele
◊ Inflammatory or allergic response to foreign substance
◊ Abnormality of vault due to surgery or radiation
◊ Congenital malformations
Disorders of pelvic structures
◊ Pelvic inflammatory disease
◊ Endometriosis
◊ Malignant or benign tumors of the uterus
◊ Ovarian pathology
◊ Pelvic adhesions
Disorders of the gastrointestinal tract
◊ Inflammatory bowel disease
◊ Crohn's disease
◊ Diverticulitis
◊ Constipation
◊ Hemorrhoids
◊ Fistulas

Disorders of the urinary tract
◊ Ureteral or vesical lesions
Male
◊ Genital muscle spasm
◊ Infection and irritation of penile skin
◊ Cancer of penis
◊ Penile anatomy disorders
◊ Prostate infections and enlargement
◊ Infection of seminal vesicles
◊ Testicular disease
◊ Torsion of spermatic cord
◊ Musculoskeletal disorders of pelvis and lower back
Psychologic disorders
◊ Fear
◊ Anxiety
◊ Phobic reactions
◊ Conversion reactions
◊ Hostility towards partner
◊ Psychological trauma

RISK FACTORS
• Diabetes
• Estrogen deficiency
• Alcohol/marijuana consumption
• Menopause

DIAGNOSIS

DIFFERENTIAL DIAGNOSIS
• Vaginismus

LABORATORY
• Gonorrhea culture
• Wet mount
• Chlamydia culture
• Urine analysis
• Urine culture
• Pap smear to assess estrogen status
Drugs that may alter lab results: N/A
Disorders that may alter lab results: N/A

PATHOLOGICAL FINDINGS Dependent on etiology

SPECIAL TESTS N/A

IMAGING
• Voiding cystourethrogram if urinary tract involvement
• Gastrointestinal contrast studies if GI symptoms

DIAGNOSTIC PROCEDURES
• Colposcopy and biopsy if vaginal/vulvar lesions
• Laparoscopy if complex deep penetration pain
• Cystoscopy if urinary tract involvement
• Sigmoidoscopy if GI involvement

TREATMENT

APPROPRIATE HEALTH CARE
Outpatient

GENERAL MEASURES
• Education and reassurance of both partners is the foundation of any treatment plan
• Organic causes should be identified during the evaluation and treated appropriately. Once organic causes have been ruled out, individual and/or couple therapy should be initiated.

ACTIVITY Routine

DIET Regular

PATIENT EDUCATION Patient education models, information on sexual arousal techniques, Kegel exercise information (Instructions for Patients, Griffith, H.W., W.B. Saunders Co., Philadelphia; Our Bodies, Ourselves, Boston Women's Health Collective, Simon & Schuster, New York)

MEDICATIONS

DRUG(S) OF CHOICE Dependent on the etiology. May include antibiotics for infection, estrogen for vaginal atrophy, analgesics for pain, and lubricants for dryness.
Contraindications: N/A
Precautions: N/A
Significant possible interactions: N/A

ALTERNATIVE DRUGS N/A

FOLLOWUP

PATIENT MONITORING Dependent on therapy. Every 6-12 months once resolved.

PREVENTION/AVOIDANCE Avoidance of alcohol and tobacco products

POSSIBLE COMPLICATIONS N/A

EXPECTED COURSE AND PROGNOSIS The majority of cases will respond to treatment

MISCELLANEOUS

ASSOCIATED CONDITIONS Vaginismus

AGE-RELATED FACTORS
Pediatric: N/A
Geriatric: The incidence increases dramatically in the postmenopausal woman who is not receiving HRT primarily because of vaginal atrophy. Over half of all sexually active women will report dyspareunia.
Others: N/A

PREGNANCY The episiotomy has been associated with dyspareunia. Some studies show the incidence is decreased in women who have had midline episiotomy when compared with those who have had a mediolateral episiotomy.

SYNONYMS N/A

ICD-9-CM
• 302.76 Psycho-sexual dysfunction with functional dyspareunia
• 625.0 Pain and other symptoms associated with female genital organs, dyspareunia
• 608.89 Male

SEE ALSO
• Endometriosis
• Pelvic inflammatory disease
• Sexual dysfunction
• Vaginismus
• Vulvovaginitis, estrogen deficient
• Vulvovaginitis, monilial

OTHER NOTES N/A

ABBREVIATIONS N/A

REFERENCES Sciarra, J.: Obstetrics and Gynecology. Philadelphia, J.B. Lippincott Co., 1991

Author S. Henderson, M.D.

Dyspepsia, functional

BASICS

DESCRIPTION Condition characterized by the presence of chronic intermittent symptoms of epigastric pain, often associated with epigastric fullness, early satiety, bloating, nausea and/or vomiting without mucosal lesions or other structural abnormalities of the gastrointestinal tract.
System(s) affected: Gastrointestinal
Genetics: N/A
Incidence/Prevalence in USA: Common, affecting 15% to 20% of patients referred to gastroenterologists
Predominant Age: Middle-aged adults, but can be seen in children
Predominant Sex: Females > Males

SIGNS AND SYMPTOMS
- Belching
- Aerophagia, gaseousness, abdominal distension
- Borborygmus
- Epigastric pain, gnawing or burning eating may improve or worsen
- Substernal pain, gnawing or burning
- Intermittent dysphagia
- Anorexia, nausea, or vomiting
- Change in bowel habits
- Abdominal tenderness
- No anatomic abnormalities

CAUSES
- Often unknown, may be of several different etiologies
- Evanescent ulcers (20% to 30% go on to develop ulcers)
- Gastric motility disorder or lower pain threshold to gastric distention
- Adverse drug effects (NSAID's, antibiotics, acetaminophen, iron, theophylline, potassium)
- Increased sensitivity to caffeine
- Increased sensitivity to gastric acid
- Helicobacter pylori has not been shown to play a role
- No association with moderate alcohol intake or cigarette smoking
- Not primarily a psychosomatic disorder
- Not associated with increased basal acid secretion

RISK FACTORS
- Other functional disorders
- Anxiety
- Depression

DIAGNOSIS

DIFFERENTIAL DIAGNOSIS
- Gastroesophageal reflux
- Cholecystitis
- Peptic ulcer disease
- Gastric cancer
- Esophageal spasm
- Malabsorption syndromes
- Pancreatic disease
- Irritable bowel syndrome
- Aerophagia
- Ischemia heart disease
- Diabetes mellitus
- Thyroid disease
- Connective tissue disorders
- Conversion disorder

LABORATORY
- Recommended in all patients
- CBC
- Chemistry panel
- Stool for occult blood
- Erythrocyte sedimentation rate

Drugs that may alter lab results: Too many to list
Disorders that may alter lab results: N/A

IMAGING
Recommended in:
◊ Patients over 45 years of age at onset or symptoms
◊ Patients with symptoms and signs suggesting more serious disease
◊ Patients who need added reassurance
◊ Younger patients who do not respond rapidly to empiric treatment or have rapid recurrence of symptoms after treatment
Usual
◊ Endoscopy (recommended)
◊ Upper GI series
Sometimes
◊ Barium enema
◊ Gallbladder studies (e.g., ultrasound or oral cholecystogram)

SPECIAL TESTS
- Esophageal manometry (rarely needed)
- 24-hour intra-esophageal pH monitoring (rarely needed)
- Electrogastrography (research tool)

PATHOLOGICAL FINDINGS None (by definition)

DIAGNOSTIC PROCEDURES Careful history and physical. Normal studies of esophagus, stomach, duodenum, pancreas and gallbladder.

TREATMENT

APPROPRIATE HEALTH CARE
Outpatient

GENERAL MEASURES
- Supportive measures
- Reassurance
- Do not over investigate
- Dietary changes (see below)
- Avoid tight clothing
- Elevate head of bed
- Maintain ideal body weight
- Explore psychological issues

ACTIVITY
- Stress reduction
- Relaxation techniques
- Physical exercise
- Reflux precautions where applicable

DIET
- Avoid foods known to exacerbate symptoms
- Frequent small meals low in fat
- Avoid regular and decaffeinated coffee
- Avoid tea, cocoa, chocolate
- Avoid heavy alcohol use
- Avoid cigarette smoking
- Avoid aspirin containing compounds and NSAID's (and possibly acetaminophen)

PATIENT EDUCATION Items in Diet and Activity sections

MEDICATIONS

DRUG(S) OF CHOICE
• 60% of patients improve with placebo
• No FDA approved medications
• Acid reduction drugs - H2 antagonists, Proton pump inhibitors (Omeprazole), antacids

Precautions:
• Differ with each treatment
• H2 antagonist dosage should be adjusted in patients with renal disease
• Calcium containing antacids have been known to precipitate the formation of kidney stones after long-term usage.

Contraindications:
• Differ with each treatment
• Magnesium containing antacids should be avoided in patients with significant renal dysfunction

Significant possible interactions:
• Differ with each treatment
• H2 blockers interact with drugs metabolized by and affecting the liver
• Antacids compete with digoxin, iron salts, tetracycline, fluoroquinolones, and other drugs for absorption
• Refer to manufacturer's literature for more details on each drug

ALTERNATIVE DRUGS
• Prokinetic drugs - metoclopramide, erythromycin
• Mucosal protectant drugs - sucralfate (Carafate)
• Bismuth subsalicylate (Pepto-Bismol)

FOLLOWUP

PATIENT MONITORING
• Usual duration of medication is 4 weeks, then 2 weeks intermittently for exacerbations. If chronic medication use is needed, should have drug holidays to assess continued need.
• Continuing observation to provide support and reassurance
• Minimize diagnostic studies unless disabling symptoms persist or new problems

PREVENTION/AVOIDANCE
Continued health habits suggested under TREATMENT (i.e., avoid activities known to exacerbate problems, maintain healthy life style, continue stress reduction techniques)

POSSIBLE COMPLICATIONS
Undiagnosed serious pathology

EXPECTED COURSE AND PROGNOSIS
• Long-term or chronic symptoms with periods that are symptom free
• Some percentage may develop true ulcer disease

MISCELLANEOUS

ASSOCIATED CONDITIONS
Other functional GI disorders

AGE-RELATED FACTORS
Pediatric: Look for family system dysfunction
Geriatric: Cancer risk is higher
Others: N/A

PREGNANCY
May exacerbate

SYNONYMS
• Non-ulcer dyspepsia
• X-ray negative dyspepsia
• Moynihan's dyspepsia
• Pseudo-ulcer dyspepsia
• Non-organic dyspepsia
• Nervous dyspepsia

ICD-9-CM
536.8 Dyspepsia and other specified disorders of function of stomach

SEE ALSO
N/A

OTHER NOTES
N/A

ABBREVIATIONS
N/A

REFERENCES
Talley, N.J.: Non-ulcer Dyspepsia: Current Approaches to Diagnosis and Management. Am Fam Phys 47;1993:1407-1416

Author P. McGann, M.D. & V. Morell, M.D.

Dysphagia

 BASICS

DESCRIPTION The sensation of a food bolus lodging in the esophagus. This is a disorder of esophageal transport and is a symptom of an underlying process. The problem is commonly divided into oropharyngeal and esophageal types.
System(s) affected: Gastrointestinal
Genetics: N/A
Incidence/Prevalence in USA: N/A
Predominant age: All ages
Predominant sex: Male = Female

SIGNS AND SYMPTOMS
• Food "stuck" in esophagus - patient may localize to specific area, usually behind the sternum or to suprasternal area (if localized behind the sternum, there is a good correlation with anatomic site)
• Choking
• Pressure sensation in mid-chest
• If total obstruction - salivation, vomiting, choking
• Symptoms should distinguish whether dysphagia is for solids or liquids or both
• Pneumonia
• Weight loss
• Symptoms of gastroesophageal reflux disease
• Longer time required to eat meals due to unconsciously chewing food more thoroughly

CAUSES
In Children
  ◊ Malformations - congenital (esophageal atresia, choanal atresia)
  ◊ Malformations - acquired (corrosive or herpetic esophagitis)
  ◊ Neuromuscular/neurologic - delayed maturation, cerebral palsy, muscular dystrophy
  ◊ Gastroesophageal reflux disease
In Adults
  ◊ Structural - tumors (cancer or benign), strictures (peptic, chemical, trauma, radiation, drugs), rings & webs, extrinsic compression (goiter)
  ◊ Gastroesophageal reflux disease
  ◊ Neuromuscular - achalasia, diffuse esophageal spasm, scleroderma, myasthenia gravis

RISK FACTORS
• Children - hereditary and/or congenital malformations
• Adults - age > 50 years, when cancer of esophagus is more likely
• Smoking
• Long history of gastroesophageal reflux
• Medications (quinine, potassium chloride, vitamin C, tetracycline, non-steroidal antiinflammatory drugs, and others)

 DIAGNOSIS

DIFFERENTIAL DIAGNOSIS
• Cardiac chest pain
• Globus hystericus

LABORATORY   See Special tests
Drugs that may alter lab results:
Esophageal manometry
  ◊ Anticholinergics (propantheline)
  ◊ Calcium channel blockers (nifedipine)
  ◊ Nitrates (nitroglycerin)
  ◊ Prokinetics (metoclopramide)
  ◊ Sedatives (diazepam)
Disorders that may alter lab results: N/A

PATHOLOGICAL FINDINGS
• Squamous cell adenocarcinoma
• Barrett's metaplasia
• Fibrous tissue of a ring, web or stricture
• Acute or chronic inflammatory change
• Heterotopic gastric mucosa (inlet patch)

SPECIAL TESTS
In infants and children
  ◊ Observe sucking/eating
  ◊ Attempt to pass nasogastric tube to assess esophageal patency
  ◊ Endoscopy
  ◊ Esophageal manometry
In adults
  ◊ Endoscopy
  ◊ Esophageal manometry
  ◊ Barium cine/video esophagram
  ◊ Ambulary 24 with pH testing

IMAGING
• X-ray - chest, neck, abdomen
• Contrast x-ray - esophagram, cine-esophagram, modified cine-esophagram (cookie swallow)
• CT scan of chest

DIAGNOSTIC PROCEDURES
• Endoscopy with biopsy
• Esophageal manometry
• Esophageal pH monitoring

 TREATMENT

APPROPRIATE HEALTH CARE
• Outpatient for those conditions where the patient is able to maintain nutrition and where there is little risk of complication
• Hospitalization may be required for either infants or adults where dysphagia is associated with total or near total obstruction of the esophageal lumen
• Endoscopy and/or esophageal dilatation may be needed for stenoses
• Surgery may be needed in either benign or malignant processes

GENERAL MEASURES
• Determine esophageal patency
• Assure airway and pulmonary function
• Exclude cardiac disease
• Assess nutritional status
• Esophageal dilatation (pneumatic or bougie)
• Surgery - esophageal stent; laser for late cancer

ACTIVITY   No restriction

DIET   Varies from nothing by mouth to near normal, depending on the degree of obstruction

PATIENT EDUCATION
• Counsel on avoiding irritating drugs
• Counsel on chewing, consistency of food
• In infants and children - discuss underlying problem and therapy for recurrent aspiration
• In adults - discuss etiology and therapy (need for repeat dilatations). Speech therapy may be helpful in teaching swallowing techniques.

MEDICATIONS

DRUG(S) OF CHOICE
For spasms:
◊ Nitrates
◊ Calcium channel blockers (nifedipine 10-30 mg tid)
For esophagitis:
◊ Antacids
◊ H2-blockers (cimetidine, ranitidine, nizatidine, famotidine)
◊ Proton pump inhibitors (omeprazole), in case of H2-blocker failure
◊ Prokinetic agents (metoclopramide)
Contraindications:
• Anticholinergics - obstructive uropathy, glaucoma, myasthenia gravis, achalasia
• Nitrates - early myocardial infarction, severe anemia, increased intracranial pressure
Precautions: May need to use liquid forms of medications
Significant possible interactions: Refer to manufacturer's profile of each drug

ALTERNATIVE DRUGS N/A

FOLLOWUP

PATIENT MONITORING The type of reassessment and frequency of follow-up is related to the specific etiology of the dysphagia

PREVENTION/AVOIDANCE
• Very hot or very cold foods may worsen
• Observe feeding of infants closely for aspirations - have suction available
• Advice for correction of poorly fitting dentures in adults or elderly

POSSIBLE COMPLICATIONS
• Aspiration
• Esophageal "asthma"
• Pneumonia
• Barrett's esophagus
• Death

EXPECTED COURSE AND
PROGNOSIS Course and prognosis varies with the specific diagnosis (cancer - poor; esophageal peptic stricture - good)

MISCELLANEOUS

ASSOCIATED CONDITIONS
• Esophageal carcinoma
• Gastroesophageal reflux
• Dysphagia lusoria
• Achalasia
• Symptomatic diffuse esophageal spasm
• Scleroderma
• Myasthenia gravis
• CVA

AGE-RELATED FACTORS
Pediatric: Congenital malformations
Geriatric:
• Poor dentition and/or dentures
• Drug induced
Others: N/A

PREGNANCY N/A

SYNONYMS N/A

ICD-9-CM 787.2

SEE ALSO ICD-9-CM code for specific etiology

OTHER NOTES This is a symptom of an abnormal process. A search for the etiology is of great importance.

ABBREVIATIONS N/A

REFERENCES
• Silverman, A., Roy, C.C.: Pediatric Clinical Gastroenterology. New York, C.V. Mosby Co, 1983
• Kahrilas, P.J.: Oropharyngeal Causes of Dysphagia. Pract Gastro., 14(1):29, 1990
• Pope, C.E.: Motor Disorders. In Gastrointestinal Disease. 4th Ed. Edited by M.H. Sleisenger & J.S. Fordtran. Philadelphia, W.B. Saunders Co., 1989
• Goyal, R.K.: Dysphagia. In Harrison's Principles of Internal Medicine. 12th ed. Edited by E. Braunwald. New York, McGraw-Hill, 1991

Author D. Roe, M.D

Eclampsia (toxemia of pregnancy)

BASICS

DESCRIPTION The presence of seizure activity in an obstetric patient with the syndrome of hypertension, edema, and proteinuria (pre-eclampsia), in a patient without underlying neurological disease. Nearly all postpartum cases occur within 24 hours of delivery.

System(s) affected: Reproductive, Nervous, Hemic/Lymphatic/Immunologic

Genetics: There does seem to be some genetic predisposition. The single-gene model best explains the frequency of about 25%, but multifactorial inheritance is also possible.

Incidence/Prevalence IN USA:
• Unclear; incidence varies, but preeclampsia has been reported to complicate 5% of all deliveries
• 0.5-2% of preeclamptic patients will progress to eclampsia. With improved monitoring and prepartum care, this number has decreased in recent years.

Predominant age: Most of the cases occur in younger women because of the higher incidence of preeclampsia in younger (nulliparous) women. However, older (> 40 years), preeclamptic patients have 4 times the incidence of seizures compared with patients in their 20's.

Predominant sex: Female only

SIGNS AND SYMPTOMS
• Tonic-clonic seizure activity (focal or generalized)
• Headache, visual disturbance and epigastric or right upper quadrant pain often precedes seizure
• Seizures may occur once or repeatedly
• Postictal coma, cyanosis (variable)
• Temperatures > 39°C consistent with CNS hemorrhage
• Disseminated intravascular coagulation (DIC), thrombocytopenia, liver dysfunction, renal failure associated
• Proteinuria
• Up to 30% may not have edema, 20% may not have proteinuria
• Normal blood pressure, even in "response" to treatment, does not rule out potential for seizures
• Hemoconcentration - predisposition to pulmonary and or cerebral edema with fluid therapy. There is actually an excess of extracellular fluid that is inappropriately distributed to the extracellular spaces.

CAUSES
• Exact cause of seizures remains unclear
• Trophoblastic tissue seems to be required, and somehow results in widespread vasospasm
• Severe cerebral vasoconstriction; hemorrhages occur due to failure of the constriction to limit perfusion pressure in the capillaries, with consequent rupture and vasogenic cerebral edema and ring hemorrhages

RISK FACTORS
• Young nulliparous woman
• Nulliparity age > 35
• Obstetric conditions associated with abundance of chorionic villi (multifetal gestation, trophoblastic disease, erythroblastosis)
• Preexisting hypertension or renal disease
• Strong family history of preeclampsia-eclampsia
• Poor prenatal care prevents early detection and treatment of preeclampsia, thereby increasing the risk of progression to eclampsia

DIAGNOSIS

DIFFERENTIAL DIAGNOSIS
• Epilepsy
• Cerebral tumors
• Ruptured cerebral aneurysm
• Until other causes are proven, however, all pregnant women with convulsions should be considered to have eclampsia

LABORATORY
• CBC/platelets
• 24 hour urine for protein/creatinine
• Liver function testing (LDH, AST)
• Uric acid
• Electrolytes
• BUN

Drugs that may alter lab results:
Concurrent treatment with Dilantin, barbiturates (not with magnesium)

Disorders that may alter lab results: N/A

PATHOLOGICAL FINDINGS Cerebral edema, hyperemia, focal anemia, thrombosis, and hemorrhage; cerebral lesions account for 40% of eclamptic deaths

SPECIAL TESTS EEG, cerebral spinal fluid studies (CSF) - rarely useful in management

IMAGING Computed tomography can evaluate for mass lesions, infarct, hemorrhages, but is rarely used when usual clinical picture is present. Should be considered if focal findings persist or uncharacteristic signs/symptoms present.

DIAGNOSTIC PROCEDURES
• No additional procedures generally applicable
• EEG may vary from posterior slow waves to status epilepticus, but is rarely useful
• Cerebral spinal fluid studies are of no value unless other causes (e.g., meningitis) are seriously considered in differential diagnosis

TREATMENT

APPROPRIATE HEALTH CARE
• Inpatient, with parenteral access for medications and availability for invasive monitoring if necessary
• Adequacy of newborn care facilities should be considered and transport arranged for newborn if needed

GENERAL MEASURES Control of convulsions, correction of hypoxia and acidosis, lowering blood pressure, steps to effect delivery as soon as convulsions are controlled

ACTIVITY Bedrest

DIET Nothing by mouth until stable, then usual seizure precautions; low salt diet commonly recommended

PATIENT EDUCATION
• Explain to the patient and partner/family what has happened and the need for the prompt actions necessary to ensure the safety of the mother and infant
• Additional materials from: American College of Obstetricians & Gynecologists, 409 12th St., SW, Washington, DC 20024-2188, (800)762-ACOG

Eclampsia (toxemia of pregnancy)

MEDICATIONS

DRUG(S) OF CHOICE
• Protocol of Parkland Hospital as described in Williams' Obstetrics (1989): Control of convulsions with magnesium sulfate, 4 grams as a 20% solution intravenously at a rate of 0.5-1 gram per minute. Follow with 10 grams of 50% magnesium sulfate solution, one-half injected into each buttock. If convulsions persist after 15 minutes, give up to 2 grams additional intravenously as a 20% solution at a rate not to exceed 1 gram/minute. Every four hours thereafter, repeat 5 grams of 50% solution IM Prior to administration, must assure that
a) patellar reflex is present; b) respirations are not depressed; c) urine output has been at least 25 cc/hr.
• Many others give magnesium intravenously (as proposed by Zuspan et al.). One method is to provide the initial 4-6 grams intravenously, followed by an infusion of 1-3 grams/hour, with the amount given gauged on the basis of the neurological exam, particularly the patellar reflex. Levels of 6-8 mEq/L are felt to be "therapeutic". There is little evidence that any one route is preferable, although one advantage may be that intravenous administration can be immediately discontinued if necessary.
• Fluid therapy: Ringer's lactate with 5% dextrose at 60-120 mL/hr, with careful attention to fluid-volume status. Invasive monitoring may be needed. Earlier transfusion may be considered due to attenuated intravascular volume and hemoconcentration.
Contraindications:
• Previous sensitivity/intolerance to a specific drug
• Avoid diuretics which can decrease the already lowered intravascular volume
• Hyperosmotic agents are dangerous due to capillary leakage
Precautions: Careful monitoring of neurological status, urine output, respirations, and fetal status
Significant possible interactions:
Combinations of medications may cause respiratory depression. Calcium carbonate (1 gram administered slowly IV) can reverse magnesium-induced respiratory depression.

ALTERNATIVE DRUGS
Other drugs popular in Europe include benzodiazepines, e.g., diazepam 2 mg/min until resolution or 20 mg given, or lorazepam 1-2 mg/min up to total of 10 mg, or phenytoin 18-20 mg/kg at a rate of 20-40 mg/min, or phenobarbital 100 mg/min to a total of 20 mg/kg given

FOLLOWUP

PATIENT MONITORING
Blood pressure, neurological examination, condition of fetus

PREVENTION/AVOIDANCE
• Adequate prenatal care
• Good control of preexisting hypertension
• Recognition and treatment of preeclampsia

POSSIBLE COMPLICATIONS
• 56% have transient deficits including cortical blindness
• Most women do not have long-term sequelae from eclampsia
• Death from toxemia or its complications
• Death of fetus

EXPECTED COURSE AND PROGNOSIS
• 25% of eclamptic women will have hypertension in subsequent pregnancies, but only 5% of these will be severe, and only 2% will be eclamptic again
• Eclamptic, multiparous women may be at higher risk for subsequent essential hypertension
• Multiparous women with eclampsia have higher mortality in subsequent pregnancies than primiparous women
• Racial factors are unclear, since the higher incidence of essential hypertension in blacks may predispose them to higher rates of hypertension postpartum, rather than a history of eclampsia

MISCELLANEOUS

ASSOCIATED CONDITIONS
None

AGE-RELATED FACTORS
Pediatric: Essential for adequate neonatal care/facilities
Geriatric: N/A
Others: Younger patients have highest incidence, but most likely related to the fact that younger patients represent largest numbers of primigravidas

PREGNANCY
By definition, a complication of pregnancy

SYNONYMS
• Pregnancy-associated seizures
• Toxemic seizures

ICD-9-CM
• 642.4 Mild or unspecified pre-eclampsia
• 642.5 Severe pre-eclampsia
• 642.6 Eclampsia
• 642.9 Unspecified hypertension complicating pregnancy, childbirth, or the puerperium
• 780.3 Convulsions

SEE ALSO
Preeclampsia

OTHER NOTES
N/A

ABBREVIATIONS
N/A

REFERENCES
• Cunningham, F.G., MacDonald, P.C. & Gant, N.F. (eds.): Williams' Obstetrics. 18th Ed. Norwalk CT, Appleton and Lange, 1989
• Chesley, L.C., Annitto, J.E. & Cosgrove, R.A.: Long-term follow-up study of eclamptic women: sixth periodic report. Am J Obst Gynecol. 124: 446,1976
• American College of Obstetrics and Gynecology. Technical bulletin, Number 91, 1986

Author K. Elward, M.D.

Ectopic pregnancy

BASICS

DESCRIPTION Extrauterine pregnancy - any pregnancy existing outside the confines of the uterine cavity
• Tubal pregnancy - pregnancy existing within the different portions of the fallopian tubes, i.e., ampullary (55%), isthmic (25%), fimbrial (17%), interstitial (cornual) (2%)
• Ovarian pregnancy - pregnancy existing within the confines of an ovary
• Abdominal pregnancy - pregnancy existing in the abdominal (peritoneal) cavity, most commonly within the cul-de-sac. Occasionally it may implant on the intestines, pelvic side-walls, omentum, or even on the surfaces of the liver or spleen.
• Cervical pregnancy - pregnancy is implanted in the substance of the cervix below the level of the internal os
• Intraligamentary pregnancy - after a tubal pregnancy ruptures, the surviving embryo secondarily implants within the confine of the anterior and posterior leaves of the broad ligament
System(s) affected: Reproductive
Genetics: N/A
Incidence/Prevalence in USA:
• 88,000 cases in 1987
• 16.8 per 1000 pregnancies (live birth, legally induced abortions, and ectopic pregnancies)
Predominant age: Over 40% occurred in women between ages 20 and 29
Predominant sex: Female only

SIGNS AND SYMPTOMS
Tubal pregnancy:
◊ Pelvic pain
◊ Amenorrhea followed by irregular vaginal bleeding
◊ Abdominal tenderness
◊ Adnexal tenderness or mass
◊ Tenesmus
◊ Shoulder pain
◊ Syncope
◊ Passage of decidual cast
Ovarian pregnancy:
◊ Pain and cramps
◊ Pelvic mass
◊ Vaginal bleeding after a period of amenorrhea
◊ Clinical shock after rupture
Abdominal pregnancy:
◊ History suggestive of tubal abortion or rupture
◊ Pregnancy complicated by unusual gastrointestinal symptoms
◊ Fetal movements very marked or painful
◊ Easy palpation of the fetal parts or movements
◊ Pregnancy described by a multipara as "different"
◊ False labor near term
◊ High lying fetus in abnormal presentation, often transverse
◊ Displacement of a firm, long cervix
◊ Palpation of the fetal parts through the vaginal fornix
◊ Unusually loud vascular souffle

Cervical pregnancy:
◊ A soft and disproportionately enlarged cervix equal to or greater than the uterine corpus (hourglass effect)
◊ Extrusion of dark tissue through the external os
◊ Continuous vaginal bleeding after amenorrhea
Intraligamentary pregnancy:
◊ History suggestive of tubal abortion or rupture
◊ Unilateral pelvic mass associated with pain

CAUSES
Tubal pregnancy:
◊ Previous tubal pregnancy
◊ Pelvic inflammatory disease
◊ Endometriosis
◊ Previous tubal surgery
◊ Salpingitis isthmica nodosa
◊ Pelvic adhesions
◊ Pelvic tumors
Ovarian pregnancy:
◊ Implantation of the fertilized ovum on the ovarian surface
◊ Tubal abortion with secondary implantation of the embryo on the tubal surface
Abdominal pregnancy:
◊ Tubal abortion with secondary implantation
◊ Uteroperitoneal fistula following rupture of cesarean section or myomectomy scars
◊ External transmigration theory
◊ Menstrual regurgitation of a fertilized ovum theory
Cervical pregnancy:
◊ Unreceptive endometrium to implantation due to infection
◊ Uterine myomas
◊ Atrophic endometrium
◊ Septate uterus
◊ Presence of intrauterine device (IUD)
◊ Scarring of the endometrium
◊ Oral contraceptive use
Intraligamentary pregnancy:
◊ Rupture of a tubal pregnancy and secondary implantation between the anterior and posterior leaves of the broad ligament

RISK FACTORS
• Previous tubal surgery
• Previous pelvic inflammatory disease
• Pelvic adhesions
• Previous tubal pregnancy
• Previous uterine surgery
• Use of an intrauterine device
• History of endometritis

DIAGNOSIS

DIFFERENTIAL DIAGNOSIS
• Uterine abortion
• Appendicitis
• Salpingitis
• Ruptured corpus luteum cyst
• Cornual myoma or abscess
• Ovarian tumor
• Endometrioma
• Cervical cancer
• Cervical phase of uterine abortion
• Placenta previa

LABORATORY
• Urine pregnancy test
• Human chorionic gonadotropin (HCG) - serial quantitative serum beta
• Serial blood counts to quantify blood loss
Drugs that may alter lab results: N/A
Disorders that may alter lab results: N/A

PATHOLOGICAL FINDINGS
Tubal pregnancy:
◊ Presence of chorionic villi within the tubal wall
Ovarian pregnancy (Spiegelberg's criteria):
◊ The pregnancy must occupy the position of the ovary
◊ The pregnancy must be connected to the uterus by the utero ovarian ligament
◊ The ipsilateral oviduct must be normal
◊ The pregnancy sac must show the presence of ovarian tissue
Abdominal pregnancy - primary form:
◊ Both ovaries and oviducts must be normal
◊ There is no uteroperitoneal fistula
◊ Attachment of the conceptus is exclusively to the peritoneal surface
Abdominal pregnancy - secondary form:
◊ Fetal or placental tissue is found within the abdominal cavity beyond the ovaries or oviducts
Cervical pregnancy:
◊ Chorionic villi are implanted within the substance of the uterine cervix below the level of the internal os
◊ The uterine cavity above the internal os is free of the products of conception
Intraligamentary pregnancy:
◊ The products of conception is within the confine of the broad ligament

SPECIAL TESTS
• Culdocentesis
• Endometrial biopsy and/or dilatation and curettage

IMAGING
• Pelvic and abdominal ultrasonography
• CT scan
• MRI

DIAGNOSTIC PROCEDURES
• Laparoscopy
• Laparotomy

TREATMENT

APPROPRIATE HEALTH CARE
- Outpatient for most evaluation and treatment
- Outpatient surgery for unruptured tubal pregnancy
- Inpatient surgery for unstable hemodynamic conditions after resuscitation

GENERAL MEASURES
- Laparotomy is required for ovarian, abdominal, and intraligamentary pregnancy
- Careful curettage, packing of the cervix and uterine cavity, bilateral internal iliac artery ligations, or even hysterectomy may be necessary as treatment for cervical pregnancy
- Unruptured tubal pregnancy may be treated by salpingostomy
- Unruptured tubal pregnancy of less than 4 cm. diameter may be treated through laparoscopy or with Methotrexate

ACTIVITY Variable

DIET Variable

PATIENT EDUCATION American College of Obstetricians & Gynecologists (ACOG), 409 12th St., SW, Washington, DC 20024-2188, (800)762-ACOG

MEDICATIONS

DRUG(S) OF CHOICE
- Methotrexate as primary treatment for unruptured tubal pregnancy and for persistent disease after salpingostomy
- Methotrexate as supplementary treatment for retained placenta after delivery of the fetus in abdominal pregnancy
- Dosage: Methotrexate 1 mg/kg IM every other day with leucovorin 0.1 mg/kg IM in between. Maximum of 4 doses of methotrexate or 25-30 mg methotrexate x 1 without leucovorin

Contraindications: Pregnant women with psoriasis

Precautions: Methotrexate has toxic effects on the hematologic, renal, gastrointestinal, pulmonary, and neurologic systems

Significant possible interactions: Refer to manufacturer's profile of each drug

ALTERNATIVE DRUGS Actinomycin-D

FOLLOWUP

PATIENT MONITORING
- Serial serum quantitative B-HCG until level drops to near zero
- Followup pelvic ultrasonogram for persistent or recurrent masses
- Followup imaging studies for retained placenta in abdominal pregnancy, e.g., ultrasonography, CT scan, and MRI

PREVENTION/AVOIDANCE
- Reliable contraception
- Repeat tubal pregnancies occur in about 12%. For patient who becomes pregnant again, use ultrasound to verify intrauterine pregnancy.

POSSIBLE COMPLICATIONS
- Hemorrhage and hypovolemic shock
- Infection
- Loss of reproductive organs after complicated surgery
- Infertility
- Urinary and/or intestinal fistulas after complicated surgery
- Need for blood transfusions with its hazards
- Disseminated intravascular coagulation

EXPECTED COURSE AND PROGNOSIS With early diagnosis and treatment, rupture unlikely to occur

MISCELLANEOUS

ASSOCIATED CONDITIONS N/A

AGE RELATED FACTORS
Pediatric: N/A
Geriatric: N/A
Others: N/A

PREGNANCY N/A

SYNONYMS
- Extrauterine pregnancy
- Tubal pregnancy
- Ovarian pregnancy
- Abdominal pregnancy
- Cervical pregnancy
- Intraligamentary pregnancy

ICD-9-CM 633 Ectopic pregnancy

SEE ALSO N/A

OTHER NOTES N/A

ABBREVIATIONS N/A

REFERENCES
- Herbst, A.L., Mishell, D.R., Stenchever, M.A. & Droegemueller, W.: Comprehensive Gynecology. 2nd Ed. St. Louis, The C.V. Mosby Co., 1992
- Durfee, R.B., Pernoll, M.L.: Early Pregnancy Risks, Current Obstetric and Gynecologic Diagnosis and Treatment. 7th Ed. Norwalk, CT, Appleton and Lange, 1991
- Kurman, R.J. (ed.): Blaustein's Pathology of the Female Genital Tract. 3rd Ed. New York, Springer-Verlag, 1987
- Novak, E.R,, Woodruff, J.D.: Novak's Gynecologic and Obstetric Pathology With Clinical and Endocrine Relations. 8th Ed. Philadelphia, W.B. Saunders Co., 1979

Author A. Shiu, M.D., FACOG

Ejaculatory disorders

 BASICS

DESCRIPTION Premature ejaculation: Inability to constantly control the ejaculatory reflex is a common sexual disorder affecting all age groups. Definition criteria vary, e.g., inability to maintain an erection of sufficient duration to satisfy a partner, or ejaculation that occurs before individual wants it to. Natural biological response is to ejaculate within 2 minutes after vaginal penetration. Ejaculatory control is an acquired behavior that increases with experience.
• Retarded ejaculation: A rare condition in which erection is normal, or prolonged, but ejaculation does not occur
• Retrograde ejaculation: The valve at the base of the bladder fails to close during ejaculation and the ejaculate is forced backward into the bladder. Erection and sexual pleasure are usually not diminished.
System(s) affected: Reproductive, Nervous
Genetics: No known genetic pattern
Incidence/Prevalence: Premature ejaculation is common (particularly in the adolescent)
Predominant age: All age groups
Predominant sex: Male only

SIGNS AND SYMPTOMS
• Ejaculation occurring before individual wishes
• Ejaculation does not occur following normal erection (including masturbation)

CAUSES
• Peripheral neuropathy
Premature ejaculation
  ◊ Adolescence
  ◊ Fear of sexually transmitted disease
  ◊ Anxiety
  ◊ Psychological factors
  ◊ Guilty feelings about sex
  ◊ Interpersonal maladaptation (marital problems, unresponsiveness of mate)
  ◊ Close proximity of other persons in the household (e.g., mother-in-law)
Retarded ejaculation
  ◊ Rarely may be due to underlying painful disorder, e.g., prostatitis, seminal vesiculitis
  ◊ Usually psychogenic
  ◊ Diabetes mellitus
  ◊ Some drugs may impair ejaculation, e.g., thioridazine, mesoridazine, antihypertensives, beta-blockers, certain antidepressants
Retrograde ejaculation
  ◊ Prostatectomy
  ◊ Surgery on the neck of the bladder
  ◊ Extensive pelvic surgery
  ◊ Retroperitoneal lymph node dissection for testicular cancer (also can produce failure of emission)
  ◊ Neurologic disorders, e.g., multiple sclerosis
  ◊ Drugs, e.g., amoxapine, desipramine, imipramine

RISK FACTORS Listed with Causes

 DIAGNOSIS

DIFFERENTIAL DIAGNOSIS N/A

LABORATORY
• Laboratory test results are usually normal
• Post-ejaculate urinalysis will confirm retrograde ejaculation when infertility is a concern
Drugs that may alter lab results: N/A
Disorders that may alter lab results: N/A

PATHOLOGICAL FINDINGS N/A

SPECIAL TESTS N/A

IMAGING N/A

DIAGNOSTIC PROCEDURES Detailed sexual history

 TREATMENT

APPROPRIATE HEALTH CARE
Outpatient

GENERAL MEASURES
• Identification of any medical cause (even if not reversible) helps patient accept condition
• Improve partner communication
• Reduce performance pressure
• Use sensate focus therapy
• Techniques to learn ejaculatory control, e.g., coronal squeeze technique or start-and-stop technique
• Use of a variety of resources may be necessary, e.g., psychiatrists, psychologists, sex therapists, vascular surgeons, urologists, endocrinologists, neurologists
• If drugs are a possible cause, consider discontinuing or changing dosage
• Retrograde ejaculation may be helped if intercourse occurs when bladder is full

ACTIVITY No restrictions

DIET No special diet

PATIENT EDUCATION Reassurance reduces anxiety and speeds recovery

MEDICATIONS

DRUG(S) OF CHOICE None
Contraindications: N/A
Precautions: N/A
Significant possible interactions: N/A

ALTERNATIVE DRUGS N/A

 FOLLOWUP

PATIENT MONITORING As needed depending on type of therapy

PREVENTION/AVOIDANCE N/A

POSSIBLE COMPLICATIONS
Psychological impact on some males - signs of severe inadequacy, self-doubt, additional anxiety and guilt

EXPECTED COURSE AND PROGNOSIS Usually curative with therapy

 MISCELLANEOUS

ASSOCIATED CONDITIONS
• Neurological disorders, e.g., multiple sclerosis
• Prostatitis
• Psychological disorders
• Interpersonal disorders

AGE-RELATED FACTORS
Pediatric: N/A
Geriatric: Age alone does not cause ejaculation problems
Others: N/A

PREGNANCY N/A

SYNONYMS
• Premature ejaculation
• Retarded ejaculation
• Retrograde ejaculation
• Inhibited orgasm in males

ICD-9-CM
• 608.89 ejaculation painful
• 306.59 ejaculation psychogenic
• 302.75 ejaculation premature

SEE ALSO N/A

OTHER NOTES N/A

ABBREVIATIONS N/A

REFERENCES
• Yaffe, M. & Fenwick, E.: Sexual Happiness: A Practical Approach. New York, H. Holt & Co., 1988
• Stine, C.C. & Collins, M.: Male sexual dysfunction. Prim Care. 16:1031, 1989
• Walsh, P.C., Gittes, R.F. & Perlmutter, A.D.: Campbell's Urology. Philadelphia, W.B. Saunders Co., 1986
• Segraves, RT.: Effects of Psychotropic Drugs on Human Erection and Ejaculation. Arch Gen Psych 46:275-284, 1989.

Author M. Thomas, M.D.

Encopresis

 BASICS

DESCRIPTION The regular passage of fecal material into clothes or other inappropriate places by a child older than four years of age
System(s) affected: Gastrointestinal
Genetics: Unknown
Incidence/Prevalence in USA: 1.3% of all children > 4 years of age
Predominant age: 70% have onset before 5 years of age
Predominant sex: Males:Females 1.5:1.

SIGNS AND SYMPTOMS
• Constipation usually accompanies encopresis
• Unrecognized constipation and/or stool retention often precedes the symptom presented to the care provider
• Large amount of fecal material on abdominal, pelvic or rectal exam
• Pasty stool found on underclothes
• Fecal or foul odor surrounds the child
• Often intermittent periumbilical pain
• Occasional passage of a voluminous stool
• History of painful bowel movements
• Some children seem shy, withdrawn, acting out or aggressive behavior
• Some have had psychotherapy
• Some have had recurrent urinary tract infections

CAUSES
Many events precipitate constipation and hence encopresis
Psychologic
  ◊ Resistance to using toilet facilities, such as school bathrooms or outdoor toilets during camping trips
Anatomic
  ◊ Anal fissure or painful defecation
  ◊ Muscle hypotonia
  ◊ Slow intestinal motility
  ◊ Aganglionic megacolon or Hirschsprung's disease
  ◊ Spinal cord defects or injuries
  ◊ Anal stenosis
  ◊ Anterior displacement of the anus: anogenital index (the distance from the posterior aspect of the vagina or scrotum to the anus divided by the full distance to the tip of the coccyx) >0.34 females/>0.45 males
  ◊ Post surgical stricture of anus or rectum
  ◊ Pelvic mass
  ◊ Neurofibromatosis
Dietary or metabolic
  ◊ Lack of fiber
  ◊ Excessive protein or milk intake
  ◊ Inadequate water intake
  ◊ Hypothyroidism

RISK FACTORS
• Boys are more often affected
• Difficulty with bowel training
• Unresolved fecal retention and impaction

 DIAGNOSIS

DIFFERENTIAL DIAGNOSIS
• Not difficult when brought to provider's attention
• Suspect when exam detects soiling of underclothes as the problem is often not mentioned by mother or child
• Must look for underlying treatable causes of the constipation

LABORATORY
• Urinalysis and urine culture may be indicated
• Thyroid function studies
Drugs that may alter lab results: N/A
Disorders that may alter lab results: N/A

PATHOLOGICAL FINDINGS N/A

SPECIAL TESTS N/A

IMAGING Abdominal plain films are occasionally necessary if an impaction is suspected but not detected by abdominal or rectal examination

DIAGNOSTIC PROCEDURES N/A.
• Detailed history and complete physical including neurological examination of lower extremities and genital area and a digital rectal examination usually is sufficient for a diagnosis
• History of constipation prior to one month of age is almost always present with aganglionic megacolon and that history would warrant a barium enema and/or rectal biopsy

 TREATMENT

APPROPRIATE HEALTH CARE
Hospital admission and abdominal x-ray may be necessary to insure complete removal of impaction

GENERAL MEASURES
• The impaction must be eliminated before starting maintenance treatment
• Avoid redevelopment of an impaction
• Avoid frequent and repeated digital examinations, enemas, and suppositories
• Biofeedback training as alternate therapy
• Child to sit on toilet twice a day at the same times each day for 10-15 minutes and 10-15 minutes after a meal

ACTIVITY Unrestricted

DIET
• Avoid excessive milk, bananas, apples, gelatin
• Increase fiber

PATIENT EDUCATION
• Your Child's Health by Barton D. Schmitt, M.D.
• Education and demystifying the process
• Careful and full explanation of the treatment plan
• Allay the guilt and avoid punishment for soiling

MEDICATIONS

DRUG(S) OF CHOICE
• Give 1-3 enemas the first day of treatment: hypophosphate (Fleet's) 1 ounce per 20 pounds of body weight or normal saline (2 tsp table salt per quart of warm water) 2 ounces per year of age to maximum of 16 ounces
• Insert bisacodyl (Dulcolax) suppositories twice on day 2 and once on day 3 of treatment
• Mineral oil (at least 2 tablespoons per day) for at least 6 months (mix in cold orange juice to help it go down)
• Multiple vitamins daily, given between mineral oil doses
• Stool softeners and bulk producers are helpful (Kondremul, Citrucel, Metamucil, Mitrolan, Maltsupex and fiber wafers)
Contraindications: Refer to manufacturer's profile of each drug
Precautions: Avoid bedtime doses of mineral oil to decrease risk of aspiration. Refer to manufacturer's profile of each drug
Significant possible interactions: Refer to manufacturer's profile of each drug

ALTERNATIVE DRUGS N/A

FOLLOWUP

PATIENT MONITORING
• Continue the maintenance treatment program for at least 6 months and maybe for as long as 1-2 years
• Visits every 4-10 weeks for support and to ensure compliance
• Telephone availability to prevent problems and adjust doses
• Redevelopment of impaction must be removed as above
• Counselling and/or referral for associated psychosocial issues

PREVENTION/AVOIDANCE
• Optimal feeding practices
• Normal bowel function and recommendations for bowel training
• Early detection of problems
• Use of dark Karo syrup and fiber for hard stools
• Prompt treatment of perianal dermatitis to avoid painful defecation
• Look for signs of relapse which include large caliber stools, decrease in frequency of defecation, soiling

POSSIBLE COMPLICATIONS
• Excessive enemas or suppositories may cause colitis
• Perianal dermatitis
• Anal fissure

EXPECTED COURSE AND PROGNOSIS
• Usually responds well though relapses may occur
• Children with psychosocial or emotional problems which preceded the encopresis are more recalcitrant to treatment

MISCELLANEOUS

ASSOCIATED CONDITIONS Perianal dermatitis

AGE-RELATED FACTORS
Pediatric: N/A
Geriatric: N/A
Others: N/A

PREGNANCY N/A

SYNONYMS
Soiling

ICD-9-CM
787.6 Incontinence of feces

SEE ALSO Constipation

OTHER NOTES N/A

ABBREVIATIONS N/A

REFERENCES
• Hatch, T.F.: Encopresis and constipation in children. Pediatric Clinics of N Am 1988; 35(2):257-78
• Schmitt, B.D.: Soiling with constipation. Parent handout in Clinical Reference Systems, Ltd. 1989
• Olness, K., McParland, F. & Piper, L.: Biofeedback: A new modality in the management of children with fecal soiling. J Pediatrics 1980; 96:505-509

Author B. Duncan, M.D

Endocarditis, infective (part 1)

BASICS

DESCRIPTION A disease resulting from infection primarily of the valvular endocardium and occasionally the mural endocardium
• Acute endocarditis: Aggressive course, usually caused by more virulent organisms, such as Staphylococcus aureus, group B streptococcus, may not have underlying valve lesion
• Subacute endocarditis: indolent course, usually caused by alpha-hemolytic streptococci, enterococci, Haemophilus species, etc.
• Endocarditis in intravenous drug abusers: Commonly involves the tricuspid valve. Staphylococcus aureus is the most common infecting organism.
• Early prosthetic valve endocarditis: Occurs within 60 days of valve implantation. Staphylococci, gram-negative bacilli and Candida are common infecting organisms.
• Late prosthetic valve endocarditis: Occurs 60 days or longer after valve implantation. Staphylococcus epidermidis, alpha-hemolytic streptococci and enterococci are common infecting organisms.
System(s) affected: Cardiovascular and others
Genetics: Unknown
Incidence in USA: 1.7-4.2/100,000
Prevalence in USA: 0.32-1.3/1000 hospital admissions
Predominant age: All ages
Predominant sex: Male > Female (slightly)

SIGNS AND SYMPTOMS
• Fever, may be high, low or absent. May be only symptom in prosthetic valve endocarditis.
• Night sweats, chilly sensation
• Malaise, myalgia, joint pain
• Back pain, may be severe
• Anorexia, weight loss
• Stiff neck
• Delirium, headache
• Paralysis, hemiparesis, aphasia
• Numbness, muscle weakness
• Cold extremity with pain
• Bloody urine, may be gross or microscopic
• Bloody sputum, from septic pulmonary emboli
• Petechiae
• Conjunctival hemorrhage
• Hemorrhagic or necrotic pustule
• Pain of finger tip, or toe tip (subjective symptom of Osler node)
• Chest pain, shortness of breath, cough
• Pallor
• Roth spot
• Osler node
• Janeway lesion
• Heart murmur, may be absent
• Neck vein distention
• Gallops
• Rales
• Cardiac arrhythmia
• Pericardial rub
• Pleural friction rub
• Splenomegaly

CAUSES
• Staphylococcus aureus is a causative organism in all types of endocarditis, especially acute endocarditis and endocarditis seen in IV drug abusers
Acute endocarditis
  ◊ Staphylococcus aureus
  ◊ Streptococcus groups A,B,C,G
  ◊ Haemophilus influenzae
  ◊ Haemophilus parainfluenza
  ◊ Streptococcus pneumoniae
  ◊ Enterococcus species
  ◊ Neisseria gonorrhea
Subacute endocarditis
  ◊ Alpha-hemolytic streptococci (viridans streptococci)
  ◊ Streptococcus bovis
  ◊ Enterococcus species (E. faecalis, E. faecium, E. durans)
  ◊ Haemophilus aphrophilus and paraphrophilus
  ◊ Actinobacillus actinomycetemcomitans
  ◊ Cardiobacterium hominis
  ◊ Eikenella corrodens
  ◊ Kingella kingae
  ◊ Staphylococcus aureus
Endocarditis in intravenous drug-abusers
  ◊ Staphylococcus aureus
  ◊ Pseudomonas aeruginosa
  ◊ Pseudomonas cepacia
  ◊ Other gram-negative bacilli
  ◊ Enterococcus species
  ◊ Candida species
Early prosthetic valve endocarditis
  ◊ Staphylococcus aureus
  ◊ Staphylococcus epidermidis
  ◊ Gram-negative bacilli
  ◊ Candida species
  ◊ Aspergillus species
Late prosthetic valve endocarditis
  ◊ Alpha-hemolytic streptococci (viridans streptococci)
  ◊ Enterococcus species
  ◊ Staphylococcus epidermidis
  ◊ Candida species
  ◊ Aspergillus species

RISK FACTORS
Conditions predisposed to development of endocarditis
  ◊ Prosthetic cardiac valves, including bioprosthetic and homograft valves
  ◊ Previous bacterial endocarditis, even in the absence of heart disease
  ◊ Most congenital cardiac malformations
  ◊ Rheumatic and other acquired valvular dysfunction, even after valvular surgery
  ◊ Hypertrophic cardiomyopathy
  ◊ Mitral valve prolapse with valvular regurgitation
  ◊ Indwelling intravascular devices
Dental or surgical procedures that may cause transient bacteremia leading to endocarditis in susceptible hosts
  ◊ Dental procedures known to produce gingival irritation, including professional cleaning
  ◊ Tonsillectomy and/or adenoidectomy
  ◊ Surgical operations that involve intestinal or respiratory mucosa
  ◊ Bronchoscopy with a rigid bronchoscope
  ◊ Sclerotherapy for esophageal varices
  ◊ Esophageal dilatation
  ◊ Gallbladder surgery
  ◊ Cystoscopy
  ◊ Urethral dilatation
  ◊ Urethral catheterization if urinary tract infection is present
  ◊ Urinary tract surgery if urinary tract infection is present
  ◊ Prosthetic surgery
  ◊ Incision and drainage of infected tissue
  ◊ Vaginal hysterectomy
  ◊ Vaginal delivery in the presence of infection

DIAGNOSIS

DIFFERENTIAL DIAGNOSIS
• Brain abscess
• Cerebral embolus especially in a young person
• Cerebral hemorrhage with fever
• Connective tissue diseases
• Fever of unknown origin
• Glomerulonephritis
• Intra-abdominal infections
• Meningitis
• Myocardial infarction
• Osteomyelitis
• Pericarditis
• Purulent meningitis
• Rheumatic fever
• Salmonellosis
• Tuberculosis
• Septic pulmonary infarcts

LABORATORY
• Positive blood cultures taken at different times
• 2-dimensional echocardiography, not always positive for vegetations (trans-esophageal echocardiography has high sensitivity)
• Leukocytosis in acute endocarditis
• Anemia in subacute endocarditis
• Elevated erythrocyte sedimentation rate
• Decreased C3, C4, CH50 in subacute endocarditis
• Hematuria, microscopic or macroscopic
• Rheumatoid factor in subacute endocarditis

Drugs that may alter lab results:
Antibiotics may make blood cultures falsely negative

Disorders that may alter lab results:
• Endocarditis caused by fungi, Chlamydia trachomatis, Chlamydia psittaci, Coxiella burnetii may be associated with negative blood cultures
• Prolonged incubation of blood cultures is needed in endocarditis caused by fastidious organisms, e.g., Haemophilus species, Actinobacillus actinomycetemcomitans, Cardiobacterium hominis, Eikenella corrodens, Kingella species, Brucella species

PATHOLOGICAL FINDINGS
• Vegetations on the affected endocardium are composed of platelets, fibrin and colonies of micro-organisms. Destruction of valvular endocardium, perforation of valve leaflets, rupture of chordae tendinae, abscesses of myocardium, rupture of sinus of Valsalva, pericarditis may occur.
• Emboli and/or infarction may be found in different body organs. Abscesses and micro-abscesses may be found in different organs. Kidneys may show embolic and/or immune-complex glomerulonephritis.

SPECIAL TESTS   N/A

IMAGING
• Pulmonary ventilation perfusion scan may be done in right-sided endocarditis
• Computerized axial tomographic scan may be useful in locating abscesses

DIAGNOSTIC PROCEDURES
• Transesophageal echocardiography may be useful, especially in prosthetic or bioprosthetic valve endocarditis
• Cardiac catheterization may be indicated to ascertain the degree of valvular damage
• Aortic root injection may be useful when aortic root abscess or rupture of sinus of Valsalva is suspected

Endocarditis, infective (part 2)

 TREATMENT

APPROPRIATE HEALTH CARE
• Initial hospitalized care
• Intensive care may be needed in critically ill patients
• Outpatient home intravenous antibiotic therapy may be utilized in selected patients who are stable and reliable

GENERAL MEASURES
• Treatment for congestive heart failure if it occurs
• Oxygen treatment may be indicated
• Hemodialysis may be used in patients who develop renal failure

ACTIVITY
• Bedrest is indicated initially
• Ambulation when clinically improved

DIET No special diet

PATIENT EDUCATION
• Instruct patient regarding importance of dental hygiene
• Emphasize to patient that it is important to take antibiotic prophylaxis when undergoing certain dental/surgical procedures
• Give the patient an AHA wallet card listing antibiotic regimens for prophylaxis. Obtain the AHA wallet card, 78-1003 (CP), from local chapters of American Heart Association.

 MEDICATIONS

DRUG(S) OF CHOICE
• Endocarditis due to penicillin-susceptible viridans streptococci and Streptococcus bovis: Aqueous crystalline penicillin G 10-20 million U/24 h IV in 4-6 equally divided doses, plus gentamicin 1 mg/kg IM or IV (not to exceed 80 mg) every 8 h for 2 weeks (6 weeks for prosthetic valve endocarditis). In patients with native valve endocarditis: Those older than 65 years of age, those with impairment of the eight nerve or of renal function, or those with central nervous system involvement, use aqueous crystalline penicillin G only, in the same dosage alone for 4 weeks.
• Endocarditis due to enterococci: Aqueous crystallin penicillin G 20-40 million U/24 h in 6 equally divided doses, plus gentamicin 1 mg/kg IM or IV (not to exceed 80 mg) every 8 h for 4-6 weeks (6 weeks for prosthetic valve endocarditis)
• Endocarditis due to Staphylococcus aureus: Oxacillin or nafcillin 2 g IV every 4 h. For the first 3-5 days, gentamicin 1 mg/kg IM or IV (not to exceed 80 mg) every 8 h may be added. Treat for 6 weeks for both native valve and prosthetic valve endocarditis.
• Prosthetic valve endocarditis due to coagulase-negative staphylococci: Vancomycin 15 mg/kg (not to exceed 1 g) IV infused over 1 h every 12 h, plus rifampin 300 mg po every 8 h, both for 6 weeks, plus gentamicin 1 mg/kg IM or IV (not to exceed 80 mg) every 8 h for the first 2 weeks

Contraindications: For patients who are allergic to penicillin, use alternative drugs

Precautions:
• In patients with renal impairment, dosage adjustment should be made for penicillin G, oxacillin, gentamicin, cefazolin, vancomycin
• Rapid infusion of vancomycin (less than one hour) may cause "red-neck syndrome", an intense redness or rash over the upper half of the body. This is due to histamine release and not an allergic reaction. It will disappear when the rate of infusion is reduced.

Significant possible interactions:
• The combination of vancomycin and gentamicin may cause increased incidence of renal toxicity
• Rifampin may increase the requirement for coumarin oral anticoagulant and oral hypoglycemic agents

ALTERNATIVE DRUGS
For patients who are allergic to penicillin
◊ Endocarditis due to penicillin-susceptible viridans streptococci and Streptococcus bovis: Cefazolin 1 g IM or IV every 8 h (not to be used in patients with immediate type hypersensitivity to penicillin), or vancomycin 15 mg/kg (not to exceed 1 g) IV infused over 1 h every 12 h for 4 weeks (6 weeks for prosthetic valve endocarditis)
◊ Endocarditis due to enterococci: Desensitization to penicillin should be considered. Vancomycin 15 mg/kg (not to exceed 1 g) IV infused over 1 h every 12 h, plus gentamicin 1 mg/kg IM or IV (not to exceed 80 mg) every 8 h for 4-6 weeks (6 weeks for prosthetic valve endocarditis).
◊ Endocarditis due to Staphylococcus aureus: Cefazolin 2 g IV every 8 h (not to be used in patients with immediate-type hypersensitivity to penicillin), or vancomycin 15 mg/kg (not to exceed 1 g) IV infused over 1 h every 12 h, for 6 weeks (native valve and prosthetic valve endocarditis)

FOLLOWUP

PATIENT MONITORING
• Gentamicin blood levels should be performed if used for more than 5 days, and in patients with renal dysfunction. Peak gentamicin level should be around 3 mcg/mL and trough less than 1 mcg/mL.
• Vancomycin blood levels should be performed in patients with renal dysfunction. Desired peak level is 30-45 mcg/mL and trough less than 10 mcg/mL.
• Twice weekly BUN and serum creatinine should be performed while the patient is receiving gentamicin

PREVENTION/AVOIDANCE
• Dental caries should be treated while the patient is being treated for endocarditis
• Patients should maintain good oral hygiene
• Antibiotic prophylaxis should be given to the patient who is undergoing dental and surgical procedures that may cause transient bacteremia
Standard antibiotic regimen for dental/oral/upper respiratory tract procedures: (May be used in patients with prosthetic valves)
◊ Amoxicillin 3 g orally one h before procedure, then 1.5 g 6 h after initial dose
◊ For patients who are allergic to penicillin: Erythromycin ethylsuccinate 800 mg or erythromycin stearate 1.0 g orally 2 h before a procedure, then one-half the dose 6 h after the initial administration; or clindamycin 300 mg orally 1 h before a procedure and 150 mg 6 h after initial dose
Alternate antibiotic regimens for dental/oral/upper respiratory tract procedures
◊ For patients unable to take oral medications: Ampicillin 2.0 g IV (or IM) 30 minutes before procedure, then ampicillin 1.0 g IV (or IM) or amoxicillin 1.5g po 6h after initial dose
◊ For patients who are allergic to penicillin: Clindamycin 300mg IV 30 minutes before a procedure and 150mg IV (or orally) 6h after initial dose
For patients considered to be high risk and are not candidates for standard regimen
◊ Ampicillin 2.0g IV (or IM) plus gentamicin 1.5mg/kg IV (or IM) (not to exceed 80mg) 30 minutes before procedure, then amoxicillin 1.5g po 6h after initial dose; alternatively, the parenteral regimen may be repeated 8h after initial dose
◊ For patients who are allergic to penicillin: Vancomycin 1.0g IV infused over one hour, starting one hour before procedure and no repeat dose

Standard antibiotic regimen for genitourinary/gastrointestinal procedures
◊ Ampicillin 2.0 g IV (or IM) plus gentamicin 1.5 mg/kg IV (or IM) (not to exceed 80 mg) 30 minutes before procedure, then amoxicillin 1.5 g orally 6 h after initial dose (alternatively, the parenteral regimen may be repeated once 8 h after initial dose)
◊ For patients who are allergic to penicillin: Vancomycin 1.0 g IV infused over one h plus gentamicin 1.5 mg/kg IV (or IM) (not to exceed 80 mg) one hour before procedure and may be repeated once 8 h after initial dose
Alternate oral regimen for low-risk patients undergoing genitourinary/gastrointestinal procedures
◊ Amoxicillin 3.0 g orally one h before procedure, then 1.5 g 6 h after initial dose

POSSIBLE COMPLICATIONS
• Congestive heart failure
• Ruptured valve cusp
• Sinus of Valsalva aneurysm
• Aortic root abscesses
• Myocardial abscesses
• Myocardial infarction
• Pericarditis
• Cardiac arrhythmia
• Meningitis
• Cerebral emboli
• Brain abscesses
• Ruptured mycotic aneurysm
• Septic pulmonary infarcts
• Splenic infarcts
• Arterial emboli and infarcts
• Arthritis
• Myositis
• Glomerulonephritis
• Acute renal failure
• Mesenteric infarct

EXPECTED COURSE AND PROGNOSIS
• In staphylococcal endocarditis, fever and positive blood cultures may persist up to 10 days after appropriate treatment started
• In streptococcal endocarditis, there should be clinical response within 48 hours of antibiotic treatment and blood cultures should be negative soon after antibiotic treatment is started
• Prognosis depends largely on the possible complications

MISCELLANEOUS

ASSOCIATED CONDITIONS
Most patients who have tricuspid valve endocarditis are intravenous drug abusers or have indwelling IV lines

AGE-RELATED FACTORS
Pediatric: N/A
Geriatric: Prognosis is worse in elderly people
Others: N/A

PREGNANCY
Use of gentamicin should be used with caution; avoid use if possible

SYNONYMS
• Bacterial endocarditis
• Infectious endocarditis
• Subacute bacterial endocarditis
• Subacute infective endocarditis

ICD-9-CM
• Infective endocarditis: 421.0
• Prosthetic valve endocarditis: 996.61

SEE ALSO N/A

OTHER NOTES
Cardiac surgery to replace infected valve may be performed before antibiotic treatment course is completed when:
◊ There is evidence of congestive heart failure due to valve incompetence, or
◊ Multiple major systemic emboli have occurred, or
◊ The infection is caused by resistant organisms, e.g., fungus, Pseudomonas aeruginosa, or
◊ There is relapse of prosthetic valve endocarditis or
◊ There is persistent bacteremia despite antibiotic treatment

ABBREVIATIONS N/A

REFERENCES
• Watanakunakorn, C. & Burkert, T.: Infective endocarditis at a large community teaching hospital, 1980-1990. A review of 210 episodes. Medicine 1993;72:90-102
• Bisno, A.L., Dismukes, W.E., Durack, D.T., et al.: Antimicrobial treatment of infective endocarditis due to viridans streptococci, enterococci, and staphylococci. JAMA 1989; 261: 1471-1477
• Dajani, A.S., Bisno, A.L., Chung, K.J., et al.: Prevention of bacterial endocarditis. Recommendations by the American Heart Association. JAMA 1990; 264: 2919-2922

Author C. Watanakunakorn, M.D.

Endometriosis

BASICS

DESCRIPTION Heterotopic islands of uterine mucosa (endometrium) found in many locations.
• Pelvic sites - peritoneal surfaces (bladder, cul-de-sac, pelvic side walls, broad ligaments, uterosacral ligaments, fallopian tubes, and uterus), lymph nodes, ovaries, bowel
• Distant sites - vagina, cervix, abdominal wall, arm, leg, pleura, lung, diaphragm, kidneys, spleen, gallbladder, nasal mucous membranes, spinal canal, stomach, breast
System(s) affected: Reproductive
Genetics: N/A
Incidence in USA: 8-30/100,000
Prevalence in USA: Unknown, but, may be as high as 50% in women of reproductive age (probable range 8-30%)
Predominant age: Women of reproductive age
Predominant Sex: Female only

SIGNS AND SYMPTOMS
• Infertility (30-40% of patients with endometriosis)
• Dyspareunia
• Dysmenorrhea
• Dyschezia
• Chronic pelvic pain
• Premenstrual spotting
• Spontaneous abortion
• Luteinized unruptured follicle syndrome

CAUSES
• Retrograde menstruation (Sampson's theory)
• Lymphatic/vascular metastases (Halban's theory)
• Direct implantation
• Coelomic metaplasia (coelomic epithelium undergoes metaplasia forming functioning endometrium)

RISK FACTORS
• Hereditary/genetic predisposition
• Personality traits (achieving, egocentric, overanxious, perfectionist, intelligent, underweight - but validity of these observations lacking)
• Delayed childbearing
• Luteinized unruptured follicle syndrome (granulosa/theca cells undergo luteinization but actual follicular rupture fails to occur, thereby predisposing to limited progesterone secretion into peritoneal cavity thus allowing refluxed endometrial cells to implant and proliferate)

DIAGNOSIS

DIFFERENTIAL DIAGNOSIS Differential diagnosis of pelvic pain include all causes of acute abdomen including complications of intrauterine pregnancy and extrauterine, urinary tract infection, irritable bowel syndrome, ulcerative colitis, Crohn's disease, pelvic adhesions, acute salpingitis, ruptured ovarian cyst, and other conditions

LABORATORY No special value, but CA-125 levels may be elevated
Drugs that may alter lab results: N/A
Disorders that may alter lab results: N/A

PATHOLOGICAL FINDINGS Biopsy of endometriotic lesions usually demonstrate both endometrial glands and stroma

SPECIAL TESTS CA-125

IMAGING Vaginal/abdominal ultrasound (identify only endometriomas of ovaries)

DIAGNOSTIC PROCEDURES
Laparoscopy

TREATMENT

APPROPRIATE HEALTH CARE
Diagnose and treat "early" to prevent sequelae such as infertility and pelvic pain

GENERAL MEASURES
• At the time of laparoscopy, attempt laser vaporization or fulguration of implants, drainage/resection of ovarian endometriomas, and lysis of pelvic adhesions
• Consider uterosacral ligament laser vaporization/fulguration for presacral neurectomy for severe pelvic pain or dysmenorrhea. Microsurgery or in-vitro fertilization (IVF) or gamete intrafallopian tube transfer (GIFT) may be necessary in cases where laparoscopic surgery followed by superovulation induction with human menopausal gonadotropins (Pergonal) and artificial intrauterine insemination have failed to achieve pregnancy.

ACTIVITY Activity may be limited depending upon severity of pelvic pain

DIET No special diet

PATIENT EDUCATION
• Prevention of disease difficult but may be maintained in quiescent state with oral contraceptive agents
• Printed materials available from The American Fertility Society, 2140 11th Ave South, Suite 200, Birmingham, AL 35205-2800, (205) 933-8494

Endometriosis

MEDICATIONS

DRUG(S) OF CHOICE
Gonadotropin-releasing hormone (GnRH) agonists such as
◊ Nafarelin (Synarel) intranasal 400 mcg/day divided as 2 inhalations/day, one in each nostril. If patient continues with menses after 2 months of treatment, dose may be increased to 800 mcg
◊ Leuprolide acetate (Lupron or Depo Lupron) 0.5-1.0 mg/day or 3.75-7.5 mg/month, respectively
Maintenance:
◊ 6-9 months of therapy followed by "active" attempts at pregnancy or maintenance therapy with oral contraceptive agents
◊ Calcium supplementation 1000-1500 mg/day is recommended when using GnRH analog therapy to prevent calcium loss as women become severely hypoestrogenic
Contraindications: Any contraindication to the drug itself or of hypoestrogenemia
Precautions:
• Calcium loss secondary to hypoestrogenemia
• Hot flashes secondary to hypoestrogenemia
• Paresthesias of face and upper extremities
Significant possible interactions: Refer to manufacturer's literature

ALTERNATIVE DRUGS
• Danazol (Danocrine) 400-800 mg/day for 6-9 months
• Medroxyprogesterone acetate (Provera) 30 mg/day for 6-9 months
• Megestrol acetate (Megace) 40 mg/day for 6-9 months
• "Continuous" oral contraceptives (Lo/Ovral or Ovral) until childbearing is desired

FOLLOWUP

PATIENT MONITORING
• Monitor serum estradiol levels until less than 10 pg/mL when using GnRH analogs
• Monitor patients pain response with history and physical exams every 8-12 weeks
• Monitor size of ovarian endometriomas with ultrasound every 8-12 weeks
• May need additional surgery depending upon patient's fertility and/or pelvic pain

PREVENTION/AVOIDANCE
• Pregnancy seems to have a temporary ameliorating effect upon the course of the disease
• Endometriosis is generally a recurring disorder that may persist even into early menopause

POSSIBLE COMPLICATIONS
• Infertility/subfertility
• Sterility
• Chronic pelvic pain
• Total abdominal hysterectomy and bilateral salpingo-oophorectomy

EXPECTED COURSE AND PROGNOSIS
• Pregnancy should occur, but depends upon the severity of the disease
• Signs and symptoms generally regress with the onset of the menopause, but can usually be controlled during the reproductive years

MISCELLANEOUS

ASSOCIATED CONDITIONS
• Pelvic endometriosis is rarely associated with endometrioid carcinoma of the ovary
• Hematuria with bladder involvement
• Rectal bleeding with bowel involvement
• Hemoptysis with lung involvement

AGE-RELATED FACTORS
Pediatric: N/A
Geriatric: Endometriosis may persist even during early menopause and may be exacerbated with estrogen replacement therapy
Others:
• Endometriosis of the intramural portion of the fallopian tube may cause isthmic proximal tubal obstruction and infertility
• Infertility may not only be related to anatomical disruption of pelvic structures but to liberation of peritoneal macrophages which can predispose to gamete phagocytosis
• Immune disorders such as production of anti-endometrial antibodies can also be associated with reproductive dysfunction

PREGNANCY Refer to board certified reproductive endocrinologist or gynecologist with expertise in infertility

SYNONYMS Endometriosis externa

ICD-9-CM
• 617.1
• 617.3

SEE ALSO N/A

ABBREVIATIONS N/A

OTHER NOTES Educate female patients of reproductive age as to the signs and symptoms of pelvic endometriosis

REFERENCES Speroff, L., Glass, R.H. & Kase, N.G.: Endometriosis and Infertility. In Clinical Gynecologic Endocrinology and Infertility. 4th Ed. Edited by C.L. Brown. Baltimore, Williams & Wilkins, 1989, p. 547

Author N. Spirtos, D.O. & M. Attaran, M.D.

Enuresis

BASICS

DESCRIPTION
Involuntary urination
- Nocturnal enuresis: involuntary urination during sleep more than once a month in girls over 5 and in boys over 6 years of age
- Day-time enuresis: involuntary urination during wakeful hours
- Primary enuresis: the child who has never been completely continent for an extended (3-6 month) period
- Secondary enuresis: the return of the involuntary loss of urinary control after an extended period of urinary continence.

System(s) affected: Renal/Urologic, Nervous

Genetics: N/A

Incidence/Prevalence in USA:
Approximately 10% of children

Predominant age: Occurs in 40% of three year olds, 10% of six year olds, 3% of 12 year olds, and 1% of 18 year olds

Predominant sex: Male > Female

SIGNS AND SYMPTOMS
- Important historical information includes age, primary or secondary incontinence, nocturnal or diurnal or both, voiding pattern (intermittently continent or wet all the time), any delay in developmental milestones, toilet training techniques
- Inability to keep from urinating while asleep at least once per month
- Diurnal enuresis may be associated with frequency, dysuria, or activities that cause an increase in intra-abdominal pressure
- Some children may be withdrawn and shy and some may show aggressive behaviors; both may be secondary to the enuresis and not primary behaviors
- Stress factors such as intrafamilial discord, significant life events, psychosocial or emotional problems may be present

CAUSES
Primary enuresis
◊ Nocturnal enuresis alone rarely has a psychiatric, neurologic or anatomic basis (reduced bladder capacity is usually functional, not anatomic)
◊ Reduced bladder capacity (normal capacity is 2 oz at birth and increases 1 oz per year of age up to 12 oz) and/or frequent uninhibited contractions (maturational lag or persistent infantile pattern)
◊ Some suggestion that food allergies may influence bladder capacity
◊ Spinal cord malformations are rarely found

Secondary enuresis and/or Diurnal enuresis
◊ Bacteriuria
◊ Inability to concentrate urine due to insufficient anti-diuretic hormone or to renal tubular defect
◊ Glucosuria
◊ Pelvic mass such as pregnancy
◊ Spinal cord malformations are still rare but a careful examination of the lower back for signs of spinal dysrhaphia and a thorough neurologic examination of lower extremities and genital area is mandatory

RISK FACTORS
- History of one parent having been enuretic gives 44% occurrence rate in offspring
- History of both parents having been enuretic gives a 77% occurrence rate in their offspring
- First born child

DIAGNOSIS

DIFFERENTIAL DIAGNOSIS
- Diabetes insipidus
- Diabetes mellitus
- Renal tubular defects
- Spinal cord malformations or tumors

LABORATORY
- Urinalysis including specific gravity, glucose, protein, microscopic exam
- Urine culture
- Tests for pregnancy if history indicates

Drugs that may alter lab results: N/A
Disorders that may alter lab results: N/A

PATHOLOGICAL FINDINGS
Usually none

SPECIAL TESTS
Estimation of bladder size: Have the child hold urine until the urge is unbearable. Then measure urine in a measuring cup.

IMAGING
- Renal ultrasound, intravenous pyleogram, or voiding cystourethrogram are necessary only if urinary tract infections are associated with the enuresis
- Historical information and/or abnormal physical findings may suggest the need for spinal x-rays or imaging studies of the cord

DIAGNOSTIC PROCEDURES
Observation of the child's urinary stream for caliber and projectile force may be helpful

TREATMENT

APPROPRIATE HEALTH CARE
Outpatient

GENERAL MEASURES
- Counseling and behavior modification
- Anticipatory guidance relative to toilet training
- Treatments which are free from side effects can be started when child is toilet trained
- Secondary or diurnal enuresis needs more investigation and other treatments appropriate to the identified etiology
- Encourage daytime fluids and encourage less frequent urination to help increase bladder size
- Discourage any fluids during the 2 hours prior to bedtime
- Protect the bed from urine by having the child wear extra thick underwear (not diapers), put a towel on the bed in the area of the child's bottom, and cover the mattress with plastic
- Encourage the child to take responsibility for the problem
- Encourage the child to get up to urinate during the night but parents should not awaken the child to urinate
- When enuresis occurs, the child should rinse pajamas and underwear and the towel
- Do not punish the child for wet nights, but act sympathetically
- Heap praise on the child for dry nights. A calendar for gold stars or happy faces can be used as an incentive.
- Bladder stretching exercises may be helpful
- Self-awakening or hypnotherapy programs may be helpful
- Bed-wetting alarms have the greatest rate of success (70%) and the lowest rate of relapse (30%)

ACTIVITY
No restrictions

DIET
No fluids for 2 hours prior to bedtime

PATIENT EDUCATION
- Inform parents that most children overcome the problem between 6 and 10 years of age
- Since enuresis is self-limiting, potential harmful treatments should be avoided

MEDICATIONS

DRUG(S) OF CHOICE Tricyclic antidepressants - such as imipramine (1-2 mg/kg hs to maximum of 50 mg) or desipramine. Initial success is offset by a high relapse rate resulting in an overall success rate after withdrawal of only 40%.
Contraindications: Refer to manufacturer's profile of each drug
Precautions:
• Imipramine can cause arrhythmias or conduction blocks. Obtain an EKG prior to starting this drug.
• Imipramine is one of the leading causes of childhood drug-related deaths in the US; usually from accidental overdose
Significant possible interactions: Refer to manufacturer's profile of each drug

ALTERNATIVE DRUGS Desmopressin (20-40 mcg hs), an analogue of vasopressin, has a high success rate but also high rate of relapse on withdrawal of the drug. Safety is controversial. Be sure to obtain informed consent if you decide to try this drug.

FOLLOWUP

PATIENT MONITORING Frequent visits are necessary for support and encouragement

PREVENTION/AVOIDANCE No preventive measures known

POSSIBLE COMPLICATIONS Urinary tract infection

EXPECTED COURSE AND PROGNOSIS
• Self-limiting problem
• By age 4.5 years, only 12% of children will not have complete urinary control. These 12% convert to complete control at a rate of 15% per year. By puberty, only 2-3% have not achieved complete control.

MISCELLANEOUS

ASSOCIATED CONDITIONS
• Psychosocial problems
• Institutionalization

AGE-RELATED FACTORS
Pediatric: N/A
Geriatric: N/A
Others: N/A

PREGNANCY N/A

Synonyms
• Bed-wetting
• Primary nocturnal enuresis

ICD-9-CM 307.6, 788.3

SEE ALSO N/A

OTHER NOTES N/A

ABBREVIATIONS N/A

REFERENCES
• McLorie, G.A., Husmann, D.A.: Incontinence and enuresis. Pediatr Clinics of N Am. 34:1159—1174, 1987
• Rutherford, A.: Enuresis: its diagnosis and management. A general practice perspective. Aust Fam Phys. 17(9):749-754, 1988
• Starfield, B.: Enuresis: its pathogenesis and management. Clin Pediatr. 11(6):343-350, 1972

Author B. Duncan, M.D.

Eosinophilic pneumonias

 BASICS

 DIAGNOSIS

 TREATMENT

DESCRIPTION Group of diseases characterized by eosinophilic pulmonary infiltration, plus eosinophilia in the peripheral blood. The diseases are of both known and unknown etiology. Usual course: acute; benign.

Classifications:
◊ Löffler's syndrome (simple pulmonary eosinophilia)
◊ Asthmatic pulmonary eosinophilia (allergic bronchopulmonary aspergillosis)
◊ Drug-induced pulmonary eosinophilia
◊ Tropical pulmonary eosinophilia
◊ Chronic or prolonged pulmonary eosinophilia
◊ Hypereosinophilic syndrome
◊ Churg-Strauss syndrome (polyarteritis nodosa)

System(s) affected: Pulmonary
Genetics: No known genetic pattern
Incidence/Prevalence in USA: Unknown
Predominant age: Young adult (16-40 years); middle age (40-75 years)
Predominant sex: Male = Female (ratio differs among the various classifications)

SIGNS AND SYMPTOMS
• Mild fever
• Symptoms may be mild or life-threatening
• Cough
• Dyspnea
• Wheezing
• Anorexia
• Decreased localized breath sounds
• Localized crackles
• Diffuse rhonchi
• Mucoid sputum
• Tachycardia

CAUSES
• Idiopathic (though hypersensitivity suspected)
• Drugs/toxins (penicillin, nitrofurantoin, isoniazid, chlorpropamide, sulfonamides, antituberculosis therapy (PAS), gold, aspirin, hydralazine)
• Parasites
• Toxocara larvae
• Filariae
• Nematodes (Stronglyloides, Ascaris, Ancylostoma
• Aspergillus fumigatus (asthmatic pulmonary eosinophilia)

RISK FACTORS
• Patients with chronic disorders, e.g., asthma
• Living or traveling in certain geographical areas, e.g., India, Ceylon, Burma, Malaysia, Indonesia, tropical Africa, South America, South Pacific

DIFFERENTIAL DIAGNOSIS
• Tuberculosis
• Sarcoidosis
• Hodgkin's disease
• Other lymphoproliferative disorders
• Eosinophilic granuloma of the lung
• Desquamative interstitial pneumonitis
• Collagen vascular disease
• Hypereosinophilic syndrome
• Wegener's granulomatosis

LABORATORY
• Findings determined by etiology
• Leukocytosis
• Eosinophilia
• A. fumigatus found in sputum
• Positive filarial complement fixation
• Elevated IgE levels
• Increased WBC
• Elevated ESR
• Stool examination for parasites

Drugs that may alter lab results: N/A
Disorders that may alter lab results: N/A

PATHOLOGICAL FINDINGS
Lung
◊ Alveolar eosinophilic filling
◊ Septal eosinophilic infiltration
◊ Septal plasma cell infiltration

SPECIAL TESTS
• Lung biopsy when diagnosis uncertain or clinical course is severe (rare)
• Pulmonary function studies

IMAGING Chest x-ray - migratory infiltrates, small pleural effusion; transient infiltrates

DIAGNOSTIC PROCEDURES History and physical with particular emphasis on drug intake, recent travel to tropical areas, and systemic symptoms

APPROPRIATE HEALTH CARE
Outpatient for milder cases. More severe cases may require inpatient care.

GENERAL MEASURES
• Mild cases (Löffler's) may require no specific therapy
• Coughing and deep breathing exercises to clear secretions
• Discontinuing offending drug
• Treatment of underlying parasite infestation

ACTIVITY As tolerated.

DIET High calorie, high protein, soft diet

PATIENT EDUCATION Information about activity, diet, symptoms of recurrence to watch for

MEDICATIONS

DRUG(S) OF CHOICE
• Corticosteroid therapy. In chronic pulmonary eosinophilia, 20-40 mg prednisone daily. In Churg-Strauss syndrome may require large doses e.g., 40-60 mg of prednisone daily. Withdrawal should be possible after recovery.
• Treat asthma, if present
• Piperazine for Ascaris infestation
• Diethylcarbamazine (available only from the manufacturer) 6-8 mg/kg orally in 3 divided doses a day for 10-14 days for tropical pulmonary eosinophilia
• Appropriate vermifuges for helminthic infections
Contraindications: Refer to manufacturer's literature
Precautions: Refer to manufacturer's literature
Significant possible interactions: Refer to manufacturer's literature

ALTERNATIVE DRUGS
In Churg-Strauss syndrome, cases resistant to corticosteroid therapy, adding azathioprine or cyclophosphamide may be helpful

 FOLLOWUP

PATIENT MONITORING
Physical examinations and chest x-rays until resolved

PREVENTION/AVOIDANCE
None

EXPECTED COURSE AND PROGNOSIS
• Excellent in the milder forms
• Corticosteroid therapy is dramatically effective in more severe cases and may be life saving in idiopathic chronic pulmonary eosinophilia

POSSIBLE COMPLICATIONS
• Recurrence which may require reinstitution of steroid therapy
• Some patients may show evidence of small airways dysfunction
• Delay in treatment of tropical pulmonary eosinophilia amy result in irreversible pulmonary fibrosis

 MISCELLANEOUS

ASSOCIATED CONDITIONS
• Asthma
• Hypersensitivity pneumonitis
• Wegener's granulomatosis

AGE-RELATED FACTORS
Pediatric:
Geriatric: More morbidity, probably due to decreased lung capacity and likelihood of concomitant diseases
Others: N/A

PREGNANCY
N/A

SYNONYMS
• Löffler's syndrome
• Pulmonary infiltrates with eosinophilia syndrome

ICD-9-CM
518.3 eosinophilic pneumonia

SEE ALSO
N/A

OTHER NOTES
N/A

ABBREVIATIONS
N/A

REFERENCES
Nutman, T.B., Ottesen, E.A. & Cohen, S.G.: The Eosinophil, eosinophilia, and eosinophil-related disorders, III & IV. Allergy Proc 10:33 & 10:47, 1989

Author R. Taraszewski, MD

Epididymitis

BASICS

DESCRIPTION Inflammation of the epididymis resulting in scrotal pain, swelling and induration of the posterior-lying epididymis, and eventual scrotal wall edema, involvement of the adjacent testicle, and hydrocele formation

System(s) affected: Reproductive

Genetics: N/A

Incidence/Prevalence in USA: Common

Predominant age: Usually younger sexually active men or older men with urinary infection, but may also rarely occur in prepubertal boys

Predominant sex: Male only

SIGNS AND SYMPTOMS
- Scrotal pain, sometimes extending to the groin region, may begin relatively acutely over several hours
- Urethral discharge or symptoms of urinary tract infection, such as frequency of urination, dysuria, cloudy urine, or hematuria
- Initially, only the posterior-lying epididymis, usually the lowermost tail section, will be very tender and indurated
- Elevation of the testes/epididymis improves the discomfort
- Entire hemiscrotum becomes swollen, the testis becomes indistinguishable from the epididymis, the scrotal wall becomes thick and indurated, and reactive hydrocele may occur
- Fever and chills occur with severe infection and abscess formation

CAUSES
Younger than age 35
  ◊ Usually chlamydia or Neisseria gonorrhea
  ◊ Look for serous urethral discharge (chlamydia) or purulent discharge (gonorrhea)
Older than age 35
  ◊ Coliform bacteria usually, but sometimes Staphylococcus aureus or epidermidis
  ◊ Often associated with distal urinary tract obstruction
  ◊ Tuberculosis, if sterile pyuria and nodularity of vas deferens
  ◊ Sterile urine reflux after transurethral prostatectomy
  ◊ Granulomatous reaction following bacillus Calmette-Guerin (BCG) intravesical therapy for superficial bladder cancer
Prepubertal boys
  ◊ Usually coliform bacteria
  ◊ Evaluate for underlying congenital abnormalities, such as vesicoureteral reflux or ectopic ureter

RISK FACTORS
- Urinary tract infection, particularly prostatitis
- Indwelling urethral catheter
- Urethral instrumentation or transurethral surgery
- Urethral stricture

DIAGNOSIS

DIFFERENTIAL DIAGNOSIS
- Epididymal congestion following vasectomy
- Testicular torsion
- Torsion of appendix testis
- Mumps orchitis
- Testicular tumor
- Testicular trauma
- Epididymal cyst
- Spermatocele
- Hydrocele
- Varicocele

LABORATORY Pyuria on urinalysis, leukocytosis, gram stain urethral discharge

Drugs that may alter lab results: N/A

Disorders that may alter lab results: N/A

PATHOLOGICAL FINDINGS
- Gross and microabscesses
- Organisms reach the epididymis through the lumen of the vas deferens
- Interstitial congestion
- Fibrous scarring

SPECIAL TESTS N/A

IMAGING Ultrasound of scrotum, radionuclide scan

DIAGNOSTIC PROCEDURES Scrotal exploration or aspiration of epididymis (rarely performed)

TREATMENT

APPROPRIATE HEALTH CARE
- Outpatient, usually
- Inpatient, if septic or if surgery is scheduled

GENERAL MEASURES
Medical
  ◊ Scrotal elevation
  ◊ Ice pack
  ◊ Spermatic cord block with local anesthesia in severe cases
Surgical procedures
  ◊ Aspiration of hydrocele to assist examination of scrotal contents and relieve discomfort
  ◊ Vasostomy to drain infected material
  ◊ Scrotal exploration, if uncertain whether this is epididymitis or testicular torsion
  ◊ Drainage of abscesses, epididymectomy, or epididymo-orchiectomy in severe cases not responding to antibiotics

ACTIVITY Bedrest for minimum of 1-2 days

DIET No restrictions, but force fluids

PATIENT EDUCATION
- Limit activity, immobilize scrotal contents
- Stress completing course of antibiotics, even when asymptomatic

Epididymitis

MEDICATIONS

DRUG(S) OF CHOICE
<u>Younger than age 35 for chlamydia</u>
◊ Doxycycline (Doryx) 100 mg orally bid for 10 days --OR--
◊ Tetracycline 500 mg orally qid for 10 days
<u>Older men with bacteriuria</u>
◊ Trimethoprim/sulfamethoxazole (Bactrim or Septra) double strength orally bid for 10-14 days
◊ Ciprofloxacin (Cipro) 500 mg orally bid for 10-14 days
◊ Norfloxacin (Noroxin) 400 mg orally bid for 10-14 days
<u>Analgesia</u>
◊ Non-steroidal anti-inflammatory drug (e.g., naproxen or ibuprofen) for mild to moderate pain
◊ Acetaminophen with codeine or oxycodone for moderate to severe pain
<u>Septic or toxic patient</u>
◊ Third generation cephalosporin (ceftriaxone 1-2 gm IV/IM every 24 hours)
◊ Aminoglycoside (gentamicin 1 mg/kg IV/IM every 8 hours, adjusted for renal function) after a loading dose of 2 mg/kg
Contraindications: None
Precautions: Refer to manufacturer's profile of each drug
Significant possible interactions: Refer to manufacturer's profile of each drug

ALTERNATIVE DRUGS N/A

FOLLOWUP

PATIENT MONITORING Office visits until all signs of infection have cleared

PREVENTION/AVOIDANCE
• Vasectomy or vasoligation during transurethral surgery
• Antibiotic prophylaxis for urethral manipulation
• Early treatment of prostatitis
• Avoid vigorous rectal examination with acute prostatitis

POSSIBLE COMPLICATIONS
• Recurrent epididymitis
• Infertility
• Fournier's gangrene (necrotizing synergistic infection)

EXPECTED COURSE AND PROGNOSIS
• Pain improves within 1-3 days, but induration may take several weeks/months to completely resolve
• If bilateral involvement, sterility may result

MISCELLANEOUS

ASSOCIATED CONDITIONS
• Prostatitis
• Urethritis

AGE-RELATED FACTORS
Pediatric:
• Bacteremia from Haemophilus influenzae infection may produce acute epididymitis
• In adolescent males, must rule out acute testicular torsion
Geriatric: Diabetic patients with sensory neuropathy may have little pain despite severe infection/abscess
Others: N/A

PREGNANCY N/A

SYNONYMS
Epididymo-orchitis

ICD-9-CM
604 orchitis and epididymitis

SEE ALSO N/A

OTHER NOTES
• Syphilis, brucellosis, blastomycosis, coccidioidomycosis, and cryptococcosis are rare causes of epididymitis
• Non-bacterial epididymitis and epididymo-orchitis are not rare. Cause is not clear, but may be secondary to retrograde extravasation.

ABBREVIATIONS N/A

REFERENCES Berger, R.E. Urethritis and epididymitis. Semin Urol 1983;1:139

Author P. Nieh, M.D.

Epiglottitis

 BASICS

DESCRIPTION
Acute inflammation of the supraglottic structures with inflammation of the epiglottis, vallecula, aryepiglottic folds and arytenoids
Genetics: N/A
Incidence/Prevalence in USA:
• 0.1% of all pediatric hospital admissions
• 8% of all pediatric admissions for upper airway obstruction
• 55% of all pediatric intensive care unit admissions for upper airway obstruction
Predominant age:
• 3-7 years most common, though any age can be affected
• Generally older than typical croup patient
• Infrequent in adults
Predominant sex: Male = Female

SIGNS AND SYMPTOMS
• Sudden onset and fulminating course
• Fever
• Dysphagia, drooling
• Sore throat
• Cervical adenopathy
• Respiratory distress
• "Tripod" position (sitting propped up on hands with head forward and tongue out)
• Muffled voice/cry (vs. hoarseness in croup)
• Minimal cough (vs. barky cough in croup)
• Toxic appearance/shock (occasionally, due to associated septicemia)
• Stridor softer and less prominent than croup
• Usually no history of prodromal upper respiratory infection (vs. positive history in croup)
• Bacteremia
• Hypoxia. A late symptom usually not present unless totally obstructed.

CAUSES
• Haemophilus influenza in children
• Haemophilus influenza and Group A Streptococcus in adults

RISK FACTORS
Underlying chronic pulmonary pathology

 DIAGNOSIS

DIFFERENTIAL DIAGNOSIS
• Viral croup (laryngotracheobronchitis)
• Sepsis
• Aspirated foreign body
• Bacterial tracheitis (pseudomembranous croup)
• Peritonsillar abscess
• Retropharyngeal abscess
• Diphtheria in an unimmunized patient

LABORATORY
• Blood culture (positive in over 90%)
• Epiglottic swab culture (positive in 70%)
Drugs that may alter lab results: N/A
Disorders that may alter lab results: N/A

PATHOLOGICAL FINDINGS N/A

SPECIAL TESTS N/A

IMAGING
• Neck radiographs are contraindicated if epiglottitis is suspected, due to danger of sudden complete airway obstruction
• Chest radiographs are indicated for endotracheal tube placement. Pneumonia can occur as a complication.

DIAGNOSTIC PROCEDURES
• Visualization of epiglottis with tongue depressor is contraindicated due to danger of sudden complete airway obstruction
• Controlled visualization of epiglottis at intubation in operating room is diagnostic
• Lumbar puncture is indicated if there is clinical suspicion of meningitis
• In adult, indirect laryngoscopy is generally safe

 TREATMENT

APPROPRIATE HEALTH CARE
Hospitalize during acute illness

GENERAL MEASURES
• Each institution should have emergency protocol involving a team of emergency room physicians, pediatricians, anesthesiologists, surgeons, pediatric intensivists, and pediatric ICU nurses (principles are similar for pediatric and adult patients)
• Call anesthesiologist to bedside
• Have equipment for intubation and needle cricothyrotomy or percutaneous tracheostomy at bedside
• Notify OR
• Notify pediatric surgery or ENT for standby in OR in case tracheostomy becomes necessary
• Keep patient quiet, calm, sitting up (in parent's arms)
• Avoid venipuncture, blood gases, oxygen masks, intravenous lines, injections, monitors, and radiographs
• Avoid sedation
• Avoid racemic epinephrine
• Avoid examining the pharynx
• Transport patient and parent together to OR in a wheelchair
• Intubate all patients, preferably in OR under controlled circumstances by experienced anesthesiologist with surgery or ENT on standby for emergency tracheostomy
• Tracheostomy not indicated unless intubation unsuccessful
• Tape airway securely in place and use a bite block if indicated
• Splint elbows and restrain arms to avoid self-extubation
• Use humidity in a tent and avoid T-piece (traction increases risk of accidental extubation)
• CPAP, mechanical ventilation, and sedation usually unnecessary
• Pay attention to supervision and pulmonary toilet/suctioning to minimize risk of endotracheal tube plugs

ACTIVITY N/A

DIET
IV fluid initially, then nasogastric feedings while intubated

PATIENT EDUCATION
Reassurance about treatment and outcome

MEDICATIONS

DRUG(S) OF CHOICE Cefuroxime (150 mg/kg/day divided q 6 hours). Start promptly after blood and epiglottic cultures are obtained.
Contraindications: Refer to manufacturer's profile
Precautions: Refer to manufacturer's profile
Significant possible interactions: Refer to manufacturer's profile

ALTERNATIVE DRUGS
• Chloramphenicol (100 mg/kg/day divided q 6 hours). Follow levels.
• Steroids and racemic epinephrine of no benefit
• Antipyretics if necessary

FOLLOWUP

PATIENT MONITORING
• Serial exams to detect secondary foci of infection
• Follow swallowing ability and presence of an air leak around endo/nasotracheal tube
• Followup laryngoscopy prior to extubation (advocated by some)
• Observe in ICU for 24 hours following extubation

PREVENTION/AVOIDANCE
• H. Influenza vaccine is effective though not 100% protective
• Rifampin prophylaxis (20 mg/kg once daily for 4 days, maximum daily dose 600 mg) for all household and day care contacts. Family and close contacts may be asymptomatic carriers of H. influenza

POSSIBLE COMPLICATIONS
• Pneumonia, meningitis, cervical adenitis, septic arthritis, pericarditis, cellulitis (rare)
• Septic shock (in about 1%)
• Pneumothorax, pneumomediastinum (very rare)
• Death from asphyxia

EXPECTED COURSE AND PROGNOSIS
• Most can be extubated after 24 to 48 hours
• Morbidity and mortality is low with appropriate intervention

MISCELLANEOUS

ASSOCIATED CONDITIONS N/A

AGE-RELATED FACTORS
Pediatric: N/A
Geriatric: N/A
Others: N/A

PREGNANCY N/A

SYNONYMS Supraglottitis

ICD-9-CM
• 464.30 Acute Epiglottitis without mention of obstruction
• 464.31 Acute Epiglottitis with mention of obstruction

SEE ALSO N/A

OTHER NOTES N/A

ABBREVIATIONS N/A

REFERENCES
• Gerber, A.C. & Pfenningerm, J.: Acute epiglottitis: Management during intubation and hospitalization. Intensive Care Med, 1986; 12:407-411
• Vernon, D.D. & Ashok, P.S.: Acute epiglottitis in children: A conservative approach to diagnosis and management. Crit Care Med, 1986;14: 23-25
• Blanc, V.F., Duquenne, P. & Charest, J.: Acute epiglottitis: An overview. Acta Anaesthesial Belg, 1986; 37: 171-178

Author D. Neddenriep, M.D.

Epistaxis

BASICS

DESCRIPTION Hemorrhage from nostril, nasal cavity or nasopharynx
• Anterior bleed: Originates from anterior nasal cavity, usually Little's area (Kiesselbach's plexus) on septum just above posterior end of nasal vestibule. Second most common is anterior end of inferior turbinate.
• Posterior bleed: Originates from posterior nasal cavity or nasopharynx usually under the posterior half of the inferior turbinate or the roof of the nasal cavity
System(s) affected: Pulmonary
Genetics: N/A
Incidence/Prevalence in USA: Unknown
Predominant age: Less than 10 years and over 50 years
Predominant sex: Male = Female

SIGNS AND SYMPTOMS Usually nostril hemorrhage, however cases of posterior bleed may be asymptomatic or present with hemoptysis, nausea, hematemesis or melena

CAUSES
• Idiopathic (most common)
• Traumatic/blunt - nose picking (epistaxis digitorum), low humidity, foreign body
• Infection - upper respiratory, acute/chronic rhinitis, acute/chronic sinusitis
• Vascular abnormalities - sclerotic vessels of age, hereditary hemorrhagic telangiectasia, arteriovenous malformation
• Neoplasm
• Hypertension (usually in combination with another cause)
• Coagulopathy - hereditary (e.g., hemophilia), therapeutic or adverse effect of drugs, blood dyscrasias, leukemias, thrombocytopenia or platelet dysfunction
• Septal perforation
• Septal deviation (one side is overexposed to dry air)
• Bleeding originating in a sinus (fracture, tumor)
• Endometriosis (nasal ectopic endometrium)

RISK FACTORS Included in Causes

DIAGNOSIS

DIFFERENTIAL DIAGNOSIS Epistaxis is a symptom or a sign, not a disease. Less than 10% are caused by neoplasm or coagulopathy.

LABORATORY CBC, crossmatch for hypovolemic shock or anemia
Drugs that may alter lab results: N/A
Disorders that may alter lab results: N/A

PATHOLOGICAL FINDINGS N/A

SPECIAL TESTS As indicated for unusual causes

IMAGING Sinus films

DIAGNOSTIC PROCEDURES
Angiography (rarely)

TREATMENT

APPROPRIATE HEALTH CARE
• Outpatient (usually). Inpatient for severe hemorrhage.
• Elderly patient with posterior bleeds and balloons or packing usually requires admission

GENERAL MEASURES
• Resuscitation as indicated
• Sedation, analgesic, antihypertensive or anticoagulant reversal as needed
• Patient should be gowned and sitting, if stable. Gown, gloves, and eye protection for examiner.
• Attempt to locate bleeding site using headlamp, suction, nasal speculum and help of assistant. Clear nasal cavity of blood with suction, forceps withdrawal of clot or patient blowing nose. If bleeding has stopped, rub suspicious areas with wet cotton tipped applicator to identify site. Diffuse ooze or multiple sites suggests systemic cause. In cases of posterior bleed try to identify as either roof or low posterior site since each has different arterial supply (will be important if arterial ligation is necessary).
• Locating the bleeding site may be difficult if patient presents with bilateral bleed. Usually there is only one bleeding site and the blood appears on the other because of 1-septal perforation, 2-obstruction of the affected side by pinching or packing or 3-there is a posterior bleed and blood passes behind the nasal septum. Clues are the side on which bleeding started and a careful examination using suction, headlamp and speculum.

Anterior bleed:
◊ Place pledget soaked in vasoconstrictor and local anesthetic in cavity and pinch nostril for several minutes to stop bleeding by direct pressure
◊ Remove pledget and visualize vessel. Cauterize with silver nitrate stick directly on vessel with firm pressure for 30 seconds.
◊ Alternative chemical cautery includes bead of chromic acid or 25% trichloracetic acid. Larger vessels respond better to thermal cautery or bipolar electrocautery. Avoid indiscriminate cauterization of a large area.
◊ If unsuccessful, apply second dose of anesthetic and place anterior pack using 1/2 x 72 inch ribbon gauze impregnated with petroleum jelly (Vaseline). Use bayonet forceps and nasal speculum to insert in folding layers as far back as possible. Press each layer firmly down on the last in one continuous strip with the folded ends alternating front and back. The average nasal cavity will accommodate the full length if properly placed. Tape 2x2 gauze over nostril as drip catch and to prevent packing end from falling out nostril.
Posterior bleed:
◊ Traditional posterior packing as described in ENT texts has been replaced by various balloon systems. However it is very effective if balloon systems fail to control bleeding.
◊ Balloon systems include single large balloon with or without central tube for airway. They usually come in 3 or 4 sizes and right or left. Other systems provide a small (10 cc) posterior balloon and larger (30 cc) anterior balloon. After local anesthesia, the tube is placed in the affected nostril and is passed to the nasopharynx as one would a nasogastric tube. Then inflate the posterior balloon with air or water (see manufacturer's directions) and pull forward to press upon the posterior area. Then inflate the anterior balloon. A very effective method uses a 10 to 14 Fr foley catheter. Place tip of foley through the nostril to nasopharynx or upper oropharynx. Visualize through mouth avoiding placement in hypopharynx. Inflate balloon 7 to 15 cc. Pull forward until balloon wedges in posterior passage. Have assistant maintain gentle traction and place catheter along mid-section of lateral wall of nasal cavity. Insert anterior pack described above. Maintain catheter traction and stretch slightly. Place umbilical cord clamp on catheter across nostril against anterior pack so that elasticity of catheter compresses balloon against anterior pack. Protect facial skin from clamp by padding with 2x2 gauze. Drape rest of catheter over ear and tape in place.
Intractable bleed:
◊ Bilateral packing is sometimes required to achieve adequate compression
◊ Bleeding from roof may be controlled by placing double balloon system with small anterior pack placed above anterior balloon. Inflation then raises pack to place pressure on roof.
◊ Intractable bleed will require surgical arterial ligation (ideally after visual identification of bleeding site to define appropriate arterial supply). Alternative is angiographic selective arterial embolization.

ACTIVITY Bedrest with head at 45 to 90 degrees

DIET No alcohol or hot liquids

PATIENT EDUCATION Demonstrate proper pinching pressure techniques

MEDICATIONS

DRUG(S) OF CHOICE
• Vasoconstrictor: Cocaine (4%), phenylephrine (0.25%), xylometazoline (0.1%), epinephrine (I:1000)
• Anesthetic: Cocaine (4%), lidocaine laryngeal spray, lidocaine jelly (2%), lidocaine solution (4%), lidocaine viscous (2%)
• Some experts suggest systemic antibiotics and decongestants to prevent sinusitis with packs or balloons
• Consider iron supplementation for patients with considerable blood loss
Contraindications: Allergy to any component
Precautions:
• Hypertension, coronary artery disease with epinephrine
• Large doses of cocaine in children
Significant possible interactions: Refer to manufacturer's profile of each drug

ALTERNATIVE DRUGS Numerous other topical anesthetics and vasoconstrictors

FOLLOWUP

PATIENT MONITORING Hemodynamics and blood loss as indicated. Packs or balloons removed in 24 to 36 hours.

PREVENTION/AVOIDANCE Liberal application of petroleum jelly (Vaseline) to nostril to prevent drying and picking. Humidification at night. Cut fingernails.

POSSIBLE COMPLICATIONS
• Sinusitis
• Double balloon systems tend to migrate posteriorly, if anterior balloon breaks, patient may obstruct airway with migrated posterior balloon. Prevent by placing umbilical cord clamp across end of tubing at nostril after inflation.
• Septal hematoma or abscess from excessive trauma during packing
• Septal perforation secondary to aggressive cauterization
• External nasal deformity secondary to pressure necrosis from the anterior component of posterior packing
• Mucosal pressure necrosis secondary to high balloon inflation pressures
• Cocaine, lidocaine toxicity
• Vasovagal episode during packing

EXPECTED COURSE AND PROGNOSIS Good results with proper treatment

MISCELLANEOUS

ASSOCIATED CONDITIONS In the elderly - hypertension, atherosclerosis and conditions that decrease platelets and clotting functions

AGE-RELATED FACTORS
Pediatric: More likely anterior bleed
Geriatric: More likely posterior bleed
Others: N/A

PREGNANCY N/A

SYNONYMS Nosebleed

ICD-9-CM 784.7 Epistaxis

SEE ALSO N/A

OTHER NOTES N/A

ABBREVIATIONS N/A

REFERENCES
• Votey, Dudley. Emerg. Clin. N.A. 7(1) Feb. 1989
• Perretta et al. Emerg. Clin. N.A. 5(2) May 1987
• Wong, Jafek. Pediatric Otorhinolaryngology. Appleton-Century-Crofts, 1989

Author C. Ricketson, M.D.

Epstein-Barr virus infections

BASICS

DESCRIPTION Epstein-Barr virus (EBV) is a member of the herpesvirus (DNA virus) group. EBV is tropic for B lymphocytes apparently are infected in the oropharynx through salivary exchange; infected B cells then circulate in the blood and are distributed to the bone marrow and lymphoreticular system. The virus can also be found in infected epithelial cells of the buccal mucosa, salivary glands, tongue and ectocervix. Within the oropharynx both parotid ductal epithelium and pharyngeal squamous epithelial cells harbor EBV DNA and are sites of viral replication and release. This suggests that chronic epithelial replication brings about continuous reinfection of B lymphoid cells. Immune T cell responses to latently infected B cells account for the clinical findings.
• Epstein-Barr virus (EBV) infections acquired early in life are asymptomatic or associated with non-specific symptoms suggesting upper respiratory infections.
EBV-associated disorders include:
◊ Infectious mononucleosis (IM): the symptomatic primary EBV infection seen in otherwise healthy older children, adolescents and young adults. Clinical features are variable in severity and duration; in children the disease is generally mild, whereas in adults it is more severe and protracted. The incubation period is 30-50 days.
◊ X-linked lymphoproliferative syndrome (Duncan's disease)
◊ Lymphoproliferative syndromes due to EBV infections in transplant patients
◊ Lymphomas (B cell lymphoblastic, T cell)
◊ Lymphocytic interstitial pneumonitis
◊ Hairy leukoplakia of the tongue and central nervous system lymphomas in AIDS patients
◊ Burkitt's lymphoma
◊ Nasopharyngeal carcinoma
◊ Parotid carcinoma
◊ Hodgkin's disease
System(s) affected:
Hemic/Lymphatic/Immunologic
Genetics: N/A
Incidence in USA:
• Incidence is about 60/100,000 persons
• College students: 5,000/100,000 persons
Prevalence in USA: Worldwide in distribution, but clinical IM is observed predominantly in countries with advanced socio-hygienic conditions
Predominant Age:
• Older children, adolescents and young adults
• By young adult life, 60-90% of persons are antibody positive
Predominant Sex: Male = Female

SIGNS AND SYMPTOMS
• May begin abruptly or insidiously
• In adults, the temperature may rise to 103° F and gradually falls over a variable period of 7-10 days; in severe cases temperature elevations of 104-105° F may persist for 2 weeks
• Children usually have a low-grade fever or may be afebrile
• Diffuse hyperemia and hyperplasia of oropharyngeal lymphoid tissue
• Gelatinous, grayish-white exudative tonsillitis persists for 7-10 days in 50%
• Petechiae develop at the border of the hard and soft palates in 33%
• Tender lymphadenopathy (cervical nodes are most commonly enlarged)
• Axillary, epitrochlear, popliteal, inguinal, mediastinal and mesenteric nodes may be affected
• Lymph node enlargement subsides over days or weeks
• Splenomegaly in 50%
• Abnormal hepatic enzymes in 80% of patients for several weeks after onset. Hepatomegaly in 10-15%.
• Pneumonitis
• Chest pain (myocarditis and pericarditis)
• Hilar adenopathy may be observed in IM cases having extensive lymphoid hyperplasia
Neurologic (rare)
◊ Aseptic meningitis
◊ Bell's palsy
◊ Meningoencephalitis
◊ Guillain-Barré syndrome
◊ Transverse myelitis
◊ Cerebellar ataxia
◊ Acute psychosis
Hematologic (rare)
◊ Hemolytic anemia with marked neutropenia during early weeks of disease
◊ Aplastic anemia
◊ Agammaglobulinemia
Skin manifestations (3-16%)
◊ Erythematous macular or maculopapular rash
◊ Petechial and purpuric exanthems have been reported
◊ Rash location - trunk and upper arms; occasionally the face and forearms involved
◊ Urticarial lesions on the abdomen, arms, legs

CAUSES The Epstein-Barr virus

RISK FACTORS
• Age
• Socio-hygienic level
• Geographic location

DIAGNOSIS

DIFFERENTIAL DIAGNOSIS
• Streptococcal pharyngitis and tonsillitis
• Diphtheria
• Blood dyscrasias
• Rubella
• Measles
• Viral hepatitis
• Cytomegalovirus
• Toxoplasmosis

LABORATORY
Lymphocytes and atypical lymphocytes
◊ Essential to the diagnosis of IM is the presence of increased numbers of lymphocytes and atypical lymphocytes in peripheral blood. Total lymphocyte counts may constitute 60-70% of peripheral blood leukocytes.
◊ In the first week after onset of illness, the white blood cell count is normal or moderately decreased. By the second week, lymphocytosis develops with more than 10% atypical lymphocytes. Such cells vary in size and shape with indented, oval or horseshoe-shaped nuclei and basophilic, vacuolated, foamy cytoplasm.
◊ During early illness, atypical lymphocytes are B cells transformed by EBV; later, the atypical cells are primarily T cells having immunoregulatory function
Antibodies
◊ Heterophile antibodies in 80-90% of adults. Most sera from such patients cause sheep red cells to agglutinate after absorption with guinea pig kidney antigens, but not after absorption with beef red blood cells
◊ The heterophile antibody responsible for the differential absorption is an IgM response which usually appears during the first or second week of illness and persists for 3 to 6 months. Sheep cell agglutinins are not specific for IM and may occur in other conditions including serum sickness, infectious hepatitis, rubella, leukemia and Hodgkin's disease; low titers may also be found in normal healthy individuals.
◊ Differential absorption techniques distinguish these agglutinins from EBV heterophile antibodies. In general, the agglutinin titer is higher in IM than in other disorders; an unabsorbed heterophile titer greater than 1:128 and 1:40 or higher after absorption is significant.
Specific antibodies to EBV-associated antigens
◊ Develop regularly in IM
◊ Viral capsid (VCA)-specific IgM and IgG are present early in illness; VCA-IgM responses disappear after several months whereas VCA-IgG antibodies persist for life.
◊ Antibodies to EBV early antigen (EA) complexes, associated with viral replication, are present in 70-80% of patients during acute disease and usually disappear after 6 months
◊ Antibodies to the EBV nuclear antigen complex (EBNA) appear slowly and develop 1-6 months after onset
Drugs that may alter lab results: N/A
Disorders that may alter lab results:
• Atypical lymphocytes are not specific for Epstein-Barr infections and may be present in other clinical conditions including rubella, infectious hepatitis, allergic rhinitis, asthma and primary atypical pneumonia. In IM, increased numbers of atypical forms are present in peripheral blood whereas in other disorders the quantitative percentage is usually less.
• Results of VCA-IgM antibody assays may be false-positive due to the presence of rheumatoid factors in the blood

PATHOLOGICAL FINDINGS
- Widespread focal and perivascular aggregates of mononuclear cells are found throughout the body
- Mononuclear infiltrations involve lymph nodes, tonsils, spleen, lungs, liver, heart, kidneys, adrenal glands, skin and central nervous system
- Bone marrow hyperplasia develops regularly and small granulomas may be present; these are non-specific and have no prognostic significance
- A polyclonal B cell proliferative response is characteristic of IM. Relatively few circulating lymphocytes are infected by EBV and represent less than 0.1% of circulating mononuclear cells in acute illness.

SPECIAL TESTS N/A

IMAGING Ultrasound, splenomegaly

DIAGNOSTIC PROCEDURES See under Laboratory

TREATMENT

APPROPRIATE HEALTH CARE
Outpatient usually

GENERAL MEASURES
- The treatment is chiefly supportive
- During acute stage, rest in bed

ACTIVITY
- Decided on an individual basis during convalescence
- Excess exertion, heavy lifting and participation in contact sports are prohibited during acute illness and also in the presence of splenomegaly. Rupture of the spleen may be fatal if not recognized and requires blood transfusions, treatment for shock, and splenectomy.

DIET
- Maintain adequate fluid intake
- Low fat, high carbohydrate diet
- Avoid alcohol for 5-6 months

PATIENT EDUCATION Reassurance and support

MEDICATIONS

DRUG(S) OF CHOICE
- Antimicrobial agents (usually a penicillin) if throat culture is positive for Group A, beta-hemolytic streptococci. Avoid ampicillin because of rash that occurs with ampicillin in mononucleosis.

- Use aspirin and warm saline gargles to relieve the pain of pharyngeal involvement and enlarged lymph nodes
- In severe cases, codeine or meperidine

Corticosteroid therapy
◊ In patients who have severe pharyngo-tonsillitis with oropharyngeal edema and airway encroachment, a short course of corticosteroids may be utilized. Prednisone or its equivalent. Start with an initial dosage of 10-15 mg QID for 2 days. Decrease by 5 mg daily so that steroid treatment is discontinued in approximately 10 days.
◊ Considered for patients with marked toxicity or major complications (e.g., hemolytic anemia, thrombocytopenic purpura, neurologic sequelae, myocarditis, pericarditis and severe generalized dermatologic lesions). With profound thrombocytopenia, refractory to corticosteroid therapy, splenectomy may be necessary.

Contraindications: Steroids are not recommended in the treatment of mild, uncomplicated IM
Precautions: Refer to manufacture's literature
Significant Possible Interactions: Refer to manufacture's literature

ALTERNATIVE DRUGS N/A

FOLLOWUP

PATIENT MONITORING
- Avoid contact sports, heavy lifting, and excess exertion until the spleen and liver have returned to normal size.
- Eliminate alcohol or exposure to other hepatotoxic drugs until liver function studies return to normal
- Patients should be monitored closely on an outpatient basis during the first 2-3 weeks after onset of symptoms. Thereafter patients may be followed for an additional month or so, until all symptoms have subsided.
- Rarely, laboratory results resolve more slowly and symptoms including malaise, fatigue, intermittent sore throat and lymphadenopathy may persist for several months

PREVENTION/AVOIDANCE N/A

POSSIBLE COMPLICATIONS
- Airway obstruction
- Hematologic or neurologic complications
- Toxemia
- Splenic rupture (rare)

Hypersensitivity skin rash
◊ Develops 7-10 days after initiation of ampicillin treatment; this generalized erythematous maculopapular eruption occurs mainly over the trunk and extremities, including palms and soles

◊ Rash persists for approximately one week and desquamation may continue for several days
◊ Hypersensitivity skin rashes may also develop in IM cases with the use of ampicillin analogues such as amoxicillin and certain other penicillins, including methicillin.

EXPECTED COURSE AND PROGNOSIS
- Most IM cases in older age groups are mild or moderate in severity
- Acute symptoms usually last 2-3 weeks and patients usually recover uneventfully over 4-8 weeks

MISCELLANEOUS

ASSOCIATED CONDITIONS N/A

AGE-RELATED FACTORS
Pediatric:
- Infection during infancy and childhood usually subclinical
- Clinical IM more common in older children and young adults
Geriatric: Heterophile positive IM has been reported in an elderly patient 5 weeks following blood transfusion
Others: N/A

PREGNANCY One large prospective study of pregnant women failed to demonstrate evidence of any intrauterine EBV infection. However, rare birth defects considered to be due to congenital EBV infection have been reported; such defects include cataracts, hypotonia, cryptorchidism and micrognathia.

SYNONYMS N/A

ICD-9-CM 075 infectious mononucleosis

SEE ALSO N/A

OTHER NOTES N/A

ABBREVIATIONS N/A

REFERENCES
- Niederman, J.C., McCollum, R.W., Henle, G. & Henle, W.: Infectious mononucleosis: clinical manifestations in relation to EB virus antibodies. JAMA 1968;203: 205-208
- Miller, G., Niederman, J.C. & Andrews, L.L.: Prolonged oropharyngeal excretion of Epstein-Barr virus after infectious mononucleosis. New Engl J Med. 1973; 288: 229-232
- Rickinson, A.B., Yao, Q.Y. & Wallace, L.E.: The Epstein-Barr virus as a model of virus-host interactions. Br Med Bull 1985;41:75-79
- Miller, G., Katz, B.Z. & Niederman, J.C.: Some recent developments in the molecular epidemiology of Epstein-Barr virus infection. Yale J Biol Med. 1986;60:307-316

Author J. Niederman, M.D.

Erysipelas

 BASICS

DESCRIPTION Bacterial cellulitis involving the superficial skin lymphatics usually due to group A streptococcus. Usually acute, but a chronic recurrent form also exists
Genetics: N/A
Incidence/Prevalence in USA: Unknown
Predominant age: Usually infants and adults over 40. Greatest in elderly (> 75 years).
Predominant sex: Male = Female

SIGNS AND SYMPTOMS
• Prodrome of malaise, fever and chills
• Headache, vomiting are prominent
• Arthralgias
• Pruritis
• Skin discomfort
• Vesicles
• Facial redness
• Acute onset of erythema
• Begins as erythematous patch
• Sharply demarcated raised border
• Center of lesion defervesces as periphery spreads
• Desquamation and vesicle formation can occur
• Face is the most common area involved, especially nose and ears
• Chronic form may recur hours to years after initial episode
• Chronic form usually recurs at site of the previous infection
• Fever is usually the differentiating factor among similar skin manifestations

CAUSES Group A beta-hemolytic streptococcus

RISK FACTORS
• Operative wounds
• Fissured skin (especially at the nose and ears)
• Any inflamed skin
• Traumatic wounds/abrasions
• Leg ulcers/stasis dermatitis
• Chronic diseases (diabetes, malnutrition, nephrotic syndrome)
• Immunocompromised or debilitated individual

 DIAGNOSIS

DIFFERENTIAL DIAGNOSIS
• Erysipeloid (little toxicity)
• Contact dermatitis (no fever)
• Angioneurotic edema (no fever)
• Scarlet fever (usually more widespread without edema)
• Lupus (of the face, less fever, positive antinuclear antibodies)
• Polychondritis (of the ear)
• Dermatophytid
• Tuberculoid leprosy

LABORATORY
• Leukocytosis (usually > 15,000)
• Strep may be cultured from exudate or from non-involved sites
• Antistreptolysin (ASO), streptozyme, anti-DNAse may be helpful
• Blood culture
Drugs that may alter lab results: N/A
Disorders that may alter lab results: N/A

PATHOLOGICAL FINDINGS
• Edema
• Vasodilation and enlarged lymphatics
• Infiltration of polymorphonuclear leukocytes, lymphocytes and other inflammatory cells
• Endothelial cell swelling
• Gram positive cocci

SPECIAL TESTS N/A

IMAGING N/A

DIAGNOSTIC PROCEDURES None

 TREATMENT

APPROPRIATE HEALTH CARE
Outpatient

GENERAL MEASURES
• Symptomatic treatment of aches and fever
• Adequate fluid intake
• Local treatment with cold compresses

ACTIVITY Bedrest with activity based on severity of illness

DIET No special diet

PATIENT EDUCATION Importance of completing medication regimen prescribed

MEDICATIONS

DRUG(S) OF CHOICE
• Penicillin for at least ten days (improvement in 24-48 hours). Dose Pen VK: Children - 25-50mg/kg/day divided q6h; Adults - 250-500mg/dose q6h.
• Parenteral antibiotics are recommended for severe or complicated cases (1-2 million units every 4-6 hours)
• In chronic recurrent infections some authors recommend lower dose daily maintenance/prophylactic treatment after the acute infection resolves

Contraindications: Penicillin allergy

Precautions: Refer to manufacturer's profile of each drug

Significant possible interactions: Refer to manufacturer's profile of each drug

ALTERNATIVE DRUGS
• Erythromycin. Dose: Children - 30-40mg/kg/day divided q6h; Adults - 250mg/dose q6h.
• Cephalosporins

FOLLOWUP

PATIENT MONITORING
Patients should be treated until all symptoms and skin manifestations have resolved

PREVENTION/AVOIDANCE
• Maintenance antibiotics for chronic recurrent cases
• Men who shave within five days of facial erysipelas are more likely to have a recurrence
• In recurrent cases, search for other possible source of streptococcal infection (e.g., tonsils, sinuses, teeth, toenails, etc.)

POSSIBLE COMPLICATIONS
• Bacteremia
• Scarlet fever
• Pneumonia
• Abscess
• Embolism
• Gangrene
• Meningitis
• Sepsis
• Death

EXPECTED COURSE AND PROGNOSIS
• Adequate treatment results in full recovery
• Chronic edema/scarring can result from chronic recurrent cases
• Rarely elephantiasis may result from chronic recurrent cases
• Untreated cases sometimes will resolve spontaneously

MISCELLANEOUS

ASSOCIATED CONDITIONS N/A

AGE-RELATED FACTORS
Pediatric:
• Group B strep may be a cause in neonates/infants
• Abdominal involvement more common in infants
• Face, scalp, and leg common in older children
Geriatric:
• Fever may not be as prominent
• More prone to complications
• High output cardiac failure may occur in debilitated patients with underlying cardiac disease
• Face and lower extremity most common areas
Others: N/A

PREGNANCY N/A

SYNONYMS
• Saint Anthony's fire
• Ignis sacer

ICD-9-CM 035

SEE ALSO N/A

OTHER NOTES
Patients on systemic steroids may be more difficult to diagnose since signs and symptoms of the infection may be masked by anti-inflammatory action of the steroids

ABBREVIATIONS N/A

REFERENCES
• Fitzpatrick, T.B., et al.: Color Atlas and Synopsis of Clinical Dermatology. New York, McGraw-Hill, 1983
• Sauer, R: Manual of Skin Diseases. Philadelphia, J.B. Lippincott, 1985
• Domonkos, A.N., Arnold, H.L., & Odom, R.B.: Andrew's Diseases of the Skin. 8th Ed. Philadelphia, W.B. Saunders Co., 1990
• Wherle, P.F. & Tops, F.H., Sr.: Communicable and Infectious Diseases. St. Louis, C.V. Mosby, 1981
• Fitzpatrick, T.B., et al. (eds.): Dermatology in General Medicine. 3rd Ed. New York, McGraw-Hill, 1987

Author S. Kincaid, M.D.

Erythema multiforme

BASICS

DESCRIPTION An acute, self-limited hypersensitivity reaction involving the skin and mucous membranes
• Erythema multiforme minor - milder form characterized by a pleomorphic rash with or without involvement of one mucous membrane site
• Erythema multiforme major - severe, with extensive skin and mucous membrane involvement. It may involve multiple organ systems as complications of the disease, and is commonly referred to as Stevens-Johnson Syndrome.
System(s) affected: Skin/Exocrine
Genetics: Possible association with HLA-B15
Incidence in USA: Uncertain; estimated 1% of outpatient visits
Prevalence in USA: N/A
Predominant Age: Peak incidence in 20's and 30's; rare under age 3 and over age 50
Predominant sex: Male > Female (3:2)

SIGNS AND SYMPTOMS
• Variable and nonspecific prodrome, often with features of upper respiratory tract infection
• Sudden onset, rapidly progressive, symmetrical pleomorphic rash on palms, soles, dorsum of hands and extensor surface of extremities and face
• Mucous membrane vesicles/ulceration in 20-45% of cases
• Classic skin rash is "target lesion" consisting of central erythema or purpura, with or without vesiculation, surrounded by normal appearing skin and an outer ring of erythema
• Burning sensation to skin/mucous membranes
• Pruritus usually absent
• Corneal ulcerations

CAUSES
Idiopathic in up to 50% of cases. The remaining 50% may represent a hypersensitivity response to one of the following:
• Viral infections - particularly herpes simplex; also Epstein-Barr, Coxsackie, echovirus, varicella, mumps and poliovirus
• Bacterial infections - especially Mycoplasma pneumoniae; also brucellosis, diphtheria, Yersinia, tuberculosis, tularemia, and gonorrhea
• Protozoan infections
• Collagen vascular disease
• Medications - especially sulfonamides, penicillins, anticonvulsants, salicylates
• Vaccines - tetanus/diphtheria (Td), bacillus Calmette-Guerin (BCG), oral polio vaccine (OPV)
• Malignancy
• Pregnancy
• Premenstrual hormonal changes
• Consumption of beer
• Reiter's syndrome
• Sarcoidosis

RISK FACTORS
• Previous history of erythema multiforme
• Male sex

DIAGNOSIS

DIFFERENTIAL DIAGNOSIS
• Urticaria
• Necrotizing vasculitis
• Drug eruptions
• Contact dermatitis
• Pityriasis rosea
• Secondary syphilis
• Ringworm
• Pemphigus vulgaris
• Pemphigoid
• Dermatitis herpetiformis
• Herpes gestationis
• Septicemia
• Serum sickness
• Viral exanthems
• Rocky Mountain spotted fever
• Collagen vascular diseases
• Mucocutaneous lymph node syndrome
• Meningococcemia
• Lichen planus
• Behcet's syndrome
• Recurrent aphthous ulcers
• Herpetic gingivostomatitis
• Granuloma annulare

LABORATORY None
Drugs that may alter lab results: N/A
Disorders that may alter lab results: N/A

PATHOLOGICAL FINDINGS Epidermal necrolysis is characteristic. Spongiosis, intracellular edema, vacuolar changes at the dermal-epidermal junction, edema and extravasated erythrocytes in the dermis may also be seen on biopsy specimen.

SPECIAL TESTS None

IMAGING N/A

DIAGNOSTIC PROCEDURES Skin biopsy

TREATMENT

APPROPRIATE HEALTH CARE
Outpatient, except in those cases with severe extensive skin involvement (see Stevens-Johnson syndrome) or with oral involvement precluding oral intake, in whom dehydration may occur

GENERAL MEASURES
• Withdrawal of any implicated medications or treatment of any identified underlying infection/disease
• For mild cases, symptomatic treatment is sufficient. For more severe cases, meticulous wound care and use of Burow's solution or Domeboro solution dressings.
• Oral lesions can be treated with mouthwashes with warm saline, or a solution of diphenhydramine, Xylocaine, and Kaopectate to provide symptomatic relief and oral hygiene, and to facilitate oral intake

ACTIVITY As tolerated

DIET As tolerated. Increased fluid intake should be encouraged in those with more extensive skin involvement.

PATIENT EDUCATION Patients should be reassured that the disease is self-limited. Recurrences are possible. Encourage avoidance of any identified etiologic agent.

MEDICATIONS

DRUG(S) OF CHOICE Systemic corticosteroids, initial dosage equivalent to prednisone 1-2 mg/kg/day with subsequent tapering. (Particularly useful in rapidly evolving or more severe cases). Treatment specific to any underlying infection or disease should be provided.

Contraindications: Any infectious process in which use of steroids would be contraindicated

Precautions: Refer to manufacturer's profile of each drug

Significant possible interactions: Refer to manufacturer's profile of each drug

ALTERNATIVE DRUGS Acyclovir may be given to suppress recurrent herpetic disease if this is identified as the underlying cause

FOLLOWUP

PATIENT MONITORING The disease is self-limited, however, during the course of the illness patients should be followed closely for development of severe disease or complications

PREVENTION/AVOIDANCE
• Known or suspected etiologic agents should be avoided
• Acyclovir may help prevent herpes-related erythema multiforme
• Tamoxifen has been shown to prevent premenstrual related disease

POSSIBLE COMPLICATIONS
• Progression to Stevens-Johnson syndrome or toxic epidermal necrolysis
• Secondary infections
• Dehydration/electrolyte disturbances
• Ophthalmic complications of corneal ulcerations or iritis

EXPECTED COURSE AND PROGNOSIS
• Rash evolves over 1-2 weeks and subsequently resolves within 2-3 weeks, generally without scarring or sequelae
• Following resolution there may be some post-inflammatory hyperpigmentation
• Risk of recurrence may be as high as 37%

MISCELLANEOUS

ASSOCIATED CONDITIONS
• Any of the infections or diseases listed under Causes
• Stevens-Johnson syndrome and toxic epidermal necrolysis are more severe forms of the disease

AGE-RELATED FACTORS
Pediatric: More severe forms of the disease tend to occur in younger males. Rare under age 3 years.
Geriatric: Rare over age 50 years
Others: N/A

PREGNANCY Reported as a possible etiologic condition

SYNONYMS Erythema exudativum multiforme

ICD-9-CM 695.1 erythema multiforma

SEE ALSO
• Stevens-Johnson syndrome
• Urticaria
• Contact dermatitis
• Pityriasis rosea
• Tinea corporis
• Pemphigus vulgaris
• Herpes gestationis
• Dermatitis, herpetiformis
• Serum sickness

OTHER NOTES Because it is an immunologic reaction, drug related erythema multiforme will not occur until 7-14 days after exposure to the offending agent, unless the patient has had the medication previously

ABBREVIATIONS N/A

REFERENCES
• Fitzpatrick, T.B., et al. (eds.): Dermatology. In General Medicine. 3rd Ed. New York, McGraw-Hill, 1987
• Moschella, S.L. & Hurley, H.J.: Dermatology. 2nd Ed. Philadelphia, W.B. Saunders Co., 1985
• Domonkos, A.N., Arnold, H.L. & Odom, R.B.: Andrews' Diseases of the Skin. 8th Ed. Philadelphia, W.B. Saunders Co., 1990

Author M. LeDuc, M.D. & M. King, M.D.

Erythema nodosum

BASICS

DESCRIPTION Clinical pattern of multiple, bilateral, cutaneous, inflammatory, non-ulcerating, non-scarring eruptions that undergo characteristic color changes ending in temporary bruise-like areas. Occurs most commonly on the extensor surface of the shins, less common on thighs and forearms. It is often idiopathic, but may be seen as a response to a variety of clinical entities. Will usually subside in 3 to 6 weeks without scarring or atrophy.
System(s) affected: Skin/Exocrine
Genetics: N/A
Incidence/Prevalence in USA: Unknown
Predominant age: 20-30 years
Predominant sex: Female > Male (3:1)

SIGNS AND SYMPTOMS
• Raised, warm, tender, brightly erythematous nodules located on anterior shins
• Can also occur on any area with subcutaneous fat
• Diameter 1-15 cm
• Fever, malaise, chills
• Arthralgias
• Bluish discoloration late in course
• Hilar adenopathy
• Episcleral lesions

CAUSES
• Idiopathic
• Bacterial - streptococcal infections, tuberculosis, leprosy, Yersinia enterocolitica, tularemia, Campylobacter, salmonella, Shigella, gonorrhea
• Sarcoid
• Drugs - sulfonamides, oral contraceptives, bromides
• Pregnancy
• Deep fungal - dermatophytes, coccidioidomycosis, histoplasmosis, blastomycosis
• Viral/chlamydial - infectious mononucleosis, lymphogranuloma venereum, paravaccinia
• Enteropathies - ulcerative colitis, Crohn's disease
• Malignancies - lymphoma/leukemia, sarcoma, post radiation therapy

RISK FACTORS Listed with Causes

DIAGNOSIS

DIFFERENTIAL DIAGNOSIS
• Superficial thrombophlebitis
• Cellulitis
• Septic emboli
• Erythema induratum (cold, ulcerating nodules on calves)
• Nodular vasculitis (warm, ulcerating nodules)
• Weber-Christian disease (violaceous, scarring nodules)
• Lupus panniculitis
• Cutaneous polyarteritis nodosa
• Sarcoidosis granulomata
• Lymphoma

LABORATORY
• Elevated erythrocyte sedimentation rate
• CBC: mild leukocytosis
• Throat culture, ASO titers
• Stool culture and leukocytes if indicated
• Skin testing for mycobacteria if indicated
Drugs that may alter lab results:
Antecedent antibiotics may affect cultures
Disorders that may alter lab results: N/A

PATHOLOGICAL FINDINGS
• Septal panniculitis
• Neutrophilic infiltrate in septa of fat tissue, early in course
• Mononuclear cells and histiocytes predominate, late in course
• Lower dermis/subcutis involvement and septal fibrosis may occur

SPECIAL TESTS N/A

IMAGING Chest x-ray for hilar adenopathy or infiltrates

DIAGNOSTIC PROCEDURES Deep skin biopsy including subcutaneous fat. Not often essential.

TREATMENT

APPROPRIATE HEALTH CARE
Outpatient

GENERAL MEASURES
• Wet dressings (hot soaks and topical medications are not useful)
• Discontinue potentially causative drugs
• Treat underlying disease

ACTIVITY
• Bedrest, keep legs elevated
• Elastic wraps or support stockings may be helpful if patients want to be up and around

DIET No restrictions

PATIENT EDUCATION
• Lesions will resolve over a few months
• No scarring is anticipated
• Joint aches and pains may persist
• Less than 20% recur

MEDICATIONS

DRUG(S) OF CHOICE
Non-steroidal anti-inflammatory drugs (NSAID):
◊ Aspirin 325mg 8-12 per day; use enteric coated to decreased GI upset. Titrate to blood levels.
◊ Indomethacin - 75-150 mg per day, divided tid
◊ Naproxen (Naprosyn) - 500-1000 mg per day, divided bid

Contraindications:
• Active or recent peptic ulcer disease
• History of NSAID hypersensitivity

Precautions:
• Gastrointestinal upset/bleeding
• Fluid retention
• Dose reduction in elderly, especially those with renal disease, diabetes, heart failure
• May mask fever
• NSAIDs may elevate liver function tests

Significant possible interactions:
• May blunt antihypertensive effects of diuretics and beta-blockers
• NSAID's can elevate plasma lithium levels
• Caution advised with naproxen or any highly protein-bound drug since it may compete for albumin binding and elevate levels
• NSAID's can cause significant elevations in and prolongation of methotrexate levels

ALTERNATIVE DRUGS
• Potassium iodide 400-900 mg daily, divided bid-tid
• Corticosteroids only in very severe, refractory cases

FOLLOWUP

PATIENT MONITORING Monthly followup or as dictated by underlying disorder

PREVENTION/AVOIDANCE N/A

POSSIBLE COMPLICATIONS Vary according to underlying disease. None expected from lesions of erythema nodosum.

EXPECTED COURSE AND PROGNOSIS
• Individual lesions resolve over 3-6 week course
• Total time course of 6-12 weeks, but may vary with etiologic disease if present
• Joint aches and pains may persist for years
• Lesions do not scar
• One or more recurrences in 12-14% of cases; these occur over variable periods, averaging several years, seen most often with sarcoid, streptococcal infection, pregnancy, and oral contraceptives

MISCELLANEOUS

ASSOCIATED CONDITIONS See Causes

AGE-RELATED FACTORS N/A
Pediatric: Incidence equal male and female
Geriatric: N/A
Others: N/A

PREGNANCY May have repeat outbreaks during pregnancy

SYNONYMS Dermatitis contusiformis

ICD-9-CM 695.2

SEE ALSO N/A

OTHER NOTES
• Lofgren's syndrome (erythema nodosum and hilar adenopathy) is seen with multiple etiologies and does not exclusively indicate sarcoid
• Clinical variant of erythema nodosum migrans (subacute nodular migratory panniculitis) is often unilateral with nodules fewer in number, smaller in size and longer lasting, often extending radially by division into smaller nodules

ABBREVIATIONS N/A

REFERENCES
• Kannuksela, M.: Clinics in Dermatology. October-December, 1986; pp 88-95
• Fitzpatrick, T.B., et al. (eds.): Dermatology in General Medicine. 3rd Ed. New York, McGraw-Hill, 1987

Author K. Mosser, M.D. & B. Vanderhoff, M.D.

Erythroblastosis fetalis

BASICS

DESCRIPTION Hemolytic anemia of the fetus or newborn, caused by transplacental transmission of maternal antibody. Usually triggered by maternal and fetal blood group incompatibility.

System(s) affected:
Hemic/Lymphatic/Immunologic

Genetics: 13% of marriages have pairings of an Rh-positive man and Rh negative woman

Incidence/Prevalence in USA: Uncommon

Predominant age: Newborn

Predominant sex: Male = Female

SIGNS AND SYMPTOMS
- Hepatomegaly
- Splenomegaly
- Pallor
- Respiratory distress
- Anasarca
- Jaundice
- Icterus
- Edema
- Shock
- Hypotension
- Pulmonary edema
- Petechiae
- Purpura

CAUSES
- Maternal antibody (Anti-A, Anti-B, Kell, Duffy, etc)
- Maternal isoimmunization by Rh antigens

RISK FACTORS
- Zygocity of father (if heterozygous, 50% of his offspring will have the Rh antigen, if homozygous, 100% of his offspring will have the Rh antigen)
- Pairing of Rh positive father and Rh negative mother. 1:27 of these couples will have erythroblastotic children.
- Pregnancy if mother becomes sensitized

DIAGNOSIS

DIFFERENTIAL DIAGNOSIS N/A

LABORATORY
- Increased indirect bilirubin
- Hyperbilirubinemia
- Anemia
- Hypoglycemia
- Positive direct or indirect Coomb's test
- Polychromasia
- Increased nucleated RBC
- Increased reticulocytes
- Thrombocytopenia

Drugs that may alter lab results: N/A
Disorders that may alter lab results: N/A

PATHOLOGICAL FINDINGS Erythroid hyperplasia

SPECIAL TESTS N/A

IMAGING N/A

DIAGNOSTIC PROCEDURES N/A

TREATMENT

APPROPRIATE HEALTH CARE
- Severe neonatal infusion care unit.
- Mild: close observation in normal nursery

GENERAL MEASURES
- Exchange transfusion immediately, if required
- Phototherapy
- High titer anti-Rh-gamma globulin (1 vial standard dose) should be given to mothers within 72 hours following delivery if there is Rh incompatibility
- All Rh negative mothers even with no apparent sensitization should be treated with a standard 300 mg dose of anti-Rh antibody at about week 28 of pregnancy

ACTIVITY No restrictions

DIET No restrictions

PATIENT EDUCATION Griffith: Instructions for Patients; Philadelphia, W.B. Saunders Co. Fourth ed, p283, to photocopy and hand out to patient.

MEDICATIONS

DRUG(S) OF CHOICE None except maternal anti-RH-factor immunoglobulin
Contraindications: Rh positive individuals
Precautions: N/A
Significant possible interactions: N/A

ALTERNATIVE DRUGS N/A

FOLLOWUP

PATIENT MONITORING Closely following exchange transfusion

PREVENTION/AVOIDANCE
• Maternal anti-Rh-factor immunoglobulin administration after each pregnancy
• If bilirubin levels remain elevated in amniotic fluid: Intrauterine transfusions to fetus abdominal cavity at 10 day to 2 week intervals until 32 to 34 weeks gestation

POSSIBLE COMPLICATIONS
• Death in utero
• Pulmonary edema
• Anemia
• Congestive heart failure
• Shock
• Asphyxia
• Disseminated intravascular coagulation (DIC)
• Kernicterus (poor feeding, flaccidity, opisthotonus, seizures, apnea, neonatal death)

EXPECTED COURSE AND PROGNOSIS Cure with appropriate early treatment

MISCELLANEOUS

ASSOCIATED CONDITIONS N/A

AGE-RELATED FACTORS
Pediatric: A problem of newborns exclusively
Geriatric: N/A
Others: N/A

PREGNANCY
• Chronic viral hepatitis B, (with/without D), C.

SYNONYMS
• Erythroblastosis neonatorum
• Hemolytic disease of the newborn
• Congenital anemia of the newborn
• Icterus gravis neonatorum
• Hydrops fetalis

ICD-9-CM
773 hemolytic disease of fetus or newborn, due to isoimmunization

SEE ALSO N/A

OTHER NOTES N/A

ABBREVIATIONS N/A

REFERENCES
• Cunningham, F.G., MacDonald, P.C. & Gant, N.F. (eds.): Williams' Obstetrics. 18th Ed. Norwalk CT, Appleton and Lange, 1989
• Danforth, D.M., Scott, J.R., et al. (eds.): Obstetrics and Gynecology. 6th Ed. Philadelphia, J.B. Lippincott, 1990

Author M. Dambro, M.D. & H. Griffith, M.D.

Esophageal tumors

 BASICS

DESCRIPTION
• Carcinomas - begin in the esophagus (primary) and usually occur in the lower third of the esophagus and pass through the chest. Types: Squamous cell carcinoma; adenocarcinoma (new data suggest marked rise in incidence of adenocarcinoma may now account for more than 25% of esophageal cancer). At the time of diagnosis, 80% have metastases to the lymph nodes in the neck, mediastinum, or celiac region of the abdomen.
• Benign neoplasms - rare. Types: Leiomyoma (most common, may be multiple, but has an excellent prognosis), papilloma, and fibrovascular polyps.

System(s) affected: Gastrointestinal

Genetics: No known genetic pattern

Incidence in USA:
• Squamous cell: 3-15/100,000 males; 3-4/100,000 females (highest incidence in Blacks)
• Adeno: Rising incidence (vast majority have Barrett's esophagus)

Prevalence in USA: 5-7/100,000 (squamous cell)

Predominant age: > 50 years (peak incidence 50-60)

Predominant sex: Male > Female (2.6:1)

SIGNS AND SYMPTOMS
• Progressive dysphagia from solids over weeks to months
• Rapid weight loss
• Regurgitation and aspiration are common (especially at night)
• Cachexia
• Supraclavicular lymphadenopathy
• Esophageal obstruction
• Hiccups
• Cough
• Hoarseness
• Nail bed clubbing

CAUSES
Unknown. Most esophagus cancers are primary, but some spread from other body parts.

RISK FACTORS
• Smoking
• Excess alcohol consumption
• Head and neck tumors
• Nitrates in foods
• Lye stricture
• Achalasia
• Tylosis
• Plummer-Vinson syndrome (anemia and esophageal web)
• Coexisting primary oral, pharyngeal carcinoma
• Esophageal webs
• Barrett's metaplasia (develops in 10-40% of patients with chronic gastroesophageal reflux)
• Celiac sprue
• Exposure to radiation

 DIAGNOSIS

DIFFERENTIAL DIAGNOSIS
• Benign causes of dysphagia, achalasia
• Benign tumors of esophagus
• Motility disorders of the esophagus

LABORATORY
• Esophageal biopsy/brushing
• Anemia

Drugs that may alter lab results: N/A

Disorders that may alter lab results: N/A

PATHOLOGICAL FINDINGS
• Location - 20% in upper third, 30% in middle third, 50% in lower third
• Elevated plaques
• Ulceration
• Strictures

SPECIAL TESTS
Esophagoscopy

IMAGING
• Barium swallow - stenosing lesion
• CT scan - valuable for staging the lesion
• X-ray of the upper-intestinal tract may show pneumonitis, pleural effusion, lung abscess
• Endoscopy ultrasound - staging (most accurate)

DIAGNOSTIC PROCEDURES
• Esophagoscopy with biopsy - for accurate tissue diagnosis
• Brush cytology (> 95% positive)
• Bronchoscopy - distortion of the bronchial lumen, blunting of the carina, or intrabronchial tumor
• Once tumor is identified, liver function studies and ultrasonography and/or CT scan for evidence of liver metastases
• Endoscopy ultrasound is most sensitive and specific test to determine local spread

 TREATMENT

APPROPRIATE HEALTH CARE
• Inpatient
• Home care or extended-care facility following definitive treatment

GENERAL MEASURES
• Palliative therapeutic options include: surgery, radiotherapy, chemotherapy, laser photocoagulation, photodynamic therapy, dilation. placement of endoluminal prosthesis (stent) or combination of these methods. The specific choice will depend on the extent of the tumor and symptoms and the individual patient's state of health.
• Majority of tumors are not resectable for cure at time of presentation
• Important to stage the lesion before determining treatment plan
• Strictures may be dilated
• Prior to surgery - average patient requires nutritional and pulmonary preparation, e.g., feeding tube with formula diet and respiratory therapy
• Tube prosthesis may be attempted for patients who have failed other methods of palliation

ACTIVITY
Adjusted to patient's ability

DIET
• Soft to liquid
• High calorie supplements (usually liquid)

PATIENT EDUCATION
For patient education materials favorably reviewed on this topic, contact: National Cancer Institute, Dept. of Health And Human Services, Public Inquiries Section, Office of Cancer Communications, Building 31, Room 101-18, 9000 Rockville Pike, Bethesda, MD 20892, (301)496-5583

MEDICATIONS

DRUG(S) OF CHOICE
• Anxietolytics in selected patients
• Chemotherapy
• Analgesics
• Antacids, H2 receptor antagonist, or proton pump inhibitors when gastroesophageal reflux symptoms co-exist
• Metoclopramide or cisapride if gastric emptying problems coexist (frequently paraneoplastic)
Contraindications: Refer to manufacturer's literature
Precautions: Refer to manufacturer's literature
Significant possible interactions: Refer to manufacture's literature

ALTERNATIVE DRUGS N/A

FOLLOWUP

PATIENT MONITORING Individualized to follow results of preoperative and postoperative treatment

PREVENTION/AVOIDANCE
• Avoid tobacco, excess alcohol, corrosive chemicals
• Endoscopic surveillance of those at high risk (Barrett's, esophagus, head and neck cancer)

EXPECTED COURSE AND PROGNOSIS
• Overall 5-year survival 5%; in squamous cell carcinoma with uninvolved lymph nodes 15-20%
• Death rate following resection or bypass is 10-15%

POSSIBLE COMPLICATIONS
• Metastases to anterior jugular, supraclavicular, subdiaphragmatic lymph nodes, liver, lungs
• Complications from surgical procedures (anastomotic leak, fistula formation, empyema, malnutrition)
• Radiation can cause esophageal perforation, fistula, esophagitis, pneumonitis, myelitis, and pulmonary fibrosis
• Toxicities of chemotherapy - nausea, vomiting, hair loss, gastroenteritis, hematopoietic and immune depression
• Tubes can become blocked or dislodged
• Aspiration from esophageal obstruction

MISCELLANEOUS

ASSOCIATED CONDITIONS
• Barrett's metaplasia
• Head and neck cancer
• Achalasia

AGE-RELATED FACTORS
Pediatric: N/A
Geriatric: Most common in males over 60
Others:
• Uncommon under age 50
• Definitive treatment is standard regardless of age
• Symptomatic therapy requires dose adjustment for very old and very young

PREGNANCY N/A

SYNONYMS
• Esophagus squamous cell carcinoma
• Esophagus adenocarcinoma

ICD-9-CM 150 malignant neoplasm of esophagus

SEE ALSO Gastroesophageal reflux

OTHER NOTES N/A

ABBREVIATIONS N/A

REFERENCES
• Chabner, B.A. & Collins, J.M.: Cancer Chemotherapy: Principles and Practice. Philadelphia, J.B. Lippincott Co., 1990
• Livstone, E.M.: General considerations of tumors of the esophagus. In Bockus' Gastroenterology. 4th Ed. Edited by J.E. Berk. Philadelphia, W.B. Saunders Co., 1985

Author P. Jaffe, M.D.

Failure to thrive (FTT)

 BASICS

DESCRIPTION Failure to thrive is a symptom (rather than a disease) characterized by disproportionate failure to gain weight in comparison to height due to caloric insufficiency (or under utilization of ingested food) without obvious etiology.

Genetics: No consistent genetic pattern

Incidence/Prevalence in USA:
• Not known
• 3-5% of pediatric in-patient admissions are for evaluation of failure to thrive (FTT). It is a common and difficult diagnostic problem.

Predominant age: Usually 6-12 months; almost all are under 3-5 years

Predominant sex: Male = Female

SIGNS AND SYMPTOMS
• Weight low for age
• Growth chart shows significant deceleration of weight gain
• Difficult personality, feeding and sleep problems
• Apathetic and withdrawn, or watchful and alert
• Poor hygiene
• Signs of inflicted trauma
• Primary caretaker characteristics - psychosocial problems, often depressed
• Family characteristics - unstable, disturbed

CAUSES
• Organic etiology: less than 20%, usually gastrointestinal or neurologic
• Environmental deprivation: about 70%, of which one-third are simple educational problems, such as incorrect feeding
• Normal, small children (about 10%) not truly FTT

RISK FACTORS
• Parent with psychosocial problems
• Premature or sick newborn
• Infant with physical deformity
• Unstable, disturbed family

 DIAGNOSIS

DIFFERENTIAL DIAGNOSIS Any condition of sufficient severity to cause failure to gain weight adequately, including child abuse

LABORATORY
• Routine laboratory work-up should be kept to a minimum
  • CBC
  • Sedimentation rate
  • Urinalysis
  • Urine culture
  • Chemical profile, including BUN, calcium, phosphorus
  • Other studies dictated by results of history and physical examination, such as thyroid profile, pituitary studies

Drugs that may alter lab results: NA

Disorders that may alter lab results: Various blood chemistries may be altered by malnutrition regardless of cause

PATHOLOGICAL FINDINGS N/A

SPECIAL TESTS Dictated by results of history and physical

IMAGING
• Skeletal survey if there is suspicion or evidence of physical abuse
• X-rays for bone age (wrist film)

DIAGNOSTIC PROCEDURES
• Careful, detailed history and physical examination are most important
• Observation of infant and his or her interaction with caretakers and environment essential
• If suspicious of Turner's Syndrome, a karyotype is indicated. Buccal smears were previously the test of choice but are no longer considered appropriate.

 TREATMENT

APPROPRIATE HEALTH CARE Outpatient, except inpatient when all other attempts to improve have failed

GENERAL MEASURES
• Admission to inpatient setting
• Use of few sympathetic primary caretakers in hospital
• Provision of stimulation, cuddling, affection as inpatient or outpatient

ACTIVITY No restrictions

DIET Provision of balanced, high caloric diet on both a scheduled and ad lib basis, 150-200 kcal/kg/day

PATIENT EDUCATION Depends on etiology of FTT. When environmental deprivation is established, attempts to re-educate in a non-punitive way is essential.

MEDICATIONS

DRUG(S) OF CHOICE None; routine vitamin supplementation
Contraindications: N/A
Precautions: N/A
Significant possible interactions: N/A

ALTERNATIVE DRUGS N/A

FOLLOWUP

PATIENT MONITORING
• When etiology is organic, followup depends on particular disease involved
• When environmental deprivation is established, extremely close followup, both at home and in office is essential. If family fails to comply, child protection authorities must be notified and foster care may be necessary.

PREVENTION/AVOIDANCE Stable home life with caring parents

POSSIBLE COMPLICATIONS N/A

EXPECTED COURSE AND PROGNOSIS Long-term prognosis of children with FTT due to environmental deprivation is not encouraging. Many children remain small, most demonstrate developmental and educational deficiencies and personality disorders. Only one-third are ultimately normal.

MISCELLANEOUS

ASSOCIATED CONDITIONS N/A

AGE-RELATED FACTORS N/A
Pediatric: N/A
Geriatric: N/A
Others: N/A

PREGNANCY N/A

SYNONYMS N/A

ICD-9-CM 783.4

SEE ALSO
• Turner's syndrome
• Trisomies

OTHER NOTES N/A

ABBREVIATIONS FTT = failure to thrive

REFERENCES
• Sills, R. H.: Failure to Thrive. In Difficult Diagnosis in Pediatrics. Edited by J.A Stockman. Philadelphia, W.B. Saunders Co., 1990

Author K. Wegner, M.D.

Fecal impaction

 BASICS

DESCRIPTION Incomplete evacuation of feces, leading to formation of a large, firm, immovable mass of stool in the rectum (70%), sigmoid flexure (20%) or proximal colon (10%). The rectosigmoid colon dilates to accommodate the mass, which, in turn, is not pliable enough to pass through the disproportionately small anal canal by the patient's weak defecation effort. Impacted stool may exist as a single mass (stercolith) or as a composite of small, rounded fecal particles (scybalum).
Genetics: Fecal impaction of the cecum may be seen in cystic fibrosis
Prevalence in USA:
• General population - 1% (1000/100,000)
• Children - 1.5%
• Nursing home residents - 30%
Predominant age: Over age 60
Predominant sex: No sex preponderance in adults. Among children, 75% are boys.

SIGNS AND SYMPTOMS
• Fecal incontinence, interpreted as "diarrhea"
• Postprandial abdominal pain
• Tenesmus
• Colic
• Nausea, vomiting
• Anorexia, weight loss
• Dehydration
• Headache
• General malaise
• Agitation; confusion
• Fever to 39.5°C (103°F)
• Tachycardia
• Tachypnea
• Urinary frequency, incontinence
• Large mass of stool palpable in lower left quadrant and rectal vault

CAUSES
• Diet lacking in fiber
• Drugs (stimulant laxatives, opiates, benzodiazepines, tricyclic antidepressants, phenothiazines, antihypertensives, sucralfate, iron, aluminum-containing antacids)
• Local or generalized neurogenic bowel disorders (e.g., stroke, parkinsonism, spinal cord lesions)
• Painful rectal conditions inhibiting voluntary defecation, (e.g., anal fissure, hemorrhoids)
• Neoplastic or inflammatory obstructing lesions
• Hypothyroidism
• Hypokalemia
• Hypercalcemia
• Excess of gastrointestinal inhibitory hormones (prolactin, endorphins, glucagon, secretin)

RISK FACTORS
• Institutionalization
• Psychogenic illness
• Immobility, inactivity
• Pica
• Chronic renal failure; renal transplant recipients

 DIAGNOSIS

DIFFERENTIAL DIAGNOSIS
• Irritable bowel syndrome
• Gastroenteritis, colitis
• Diverticulitis
• Appendicitis
• Carcinoma of the colon

LABORATORY
• Leukocytosis to 15,000 WBC/cu.mm
• Hyponatremia
• Hypokalemia
• Stool may be positive for occult blood
• Anemia, due to blood loss
Drugs that may alter lab results: N/A
Disorders that may alter lab results: N/A

PATHOLOGICAL FINDINGS N/A

SPECIAL TESTS Sigmoidoscopy may be used to clarify the nature of a rectosigmoid mass beyond digital reach

IMAGING
• Plain abdominal radiography identifies masses of stool or signs of obstruction if digital exam unrevealing
• Barium enema can differentiate feces from tumor

DIAGNOSTIC PROCEDURES N/A

 TREATMENT

APPROPRIATE HEALTH CARE
Outpatient

GENERAL MEASURES
• Manual fragmentation and extraction of fecal mass (after lubrication with lidocaine jelly) by physician or nurse
• More proximal masses can be disimpacted with water jet directed through fiberoptic sigmoidoscope
• Enemas - containing 20% water soluble contrast material (Gastrografin, Hypaque) may further fragment stool bolus
• Laparotomy - necessary only in extreme cases
• For complete evacuation after partial fragmentation - bisacodyl suppositories or enemas with mineral oil, tap water or sodium phosphate
• Ensure minimum fluid intake of 1.5-2.0 liters/day (may use poorly absorbed isosmotic solution of polyethylene glycol, e.g., Golytely, Colyte)

ACTIVITY Increased activity important

DIET High fiber

PATIENT EDUCATION
• Avoid catharsis
• No hot water, soap or hydrogen peroxide enemas! They may burn or irritate rectal mucosa, causing bleeding.

MEDICATIONS

DRUG(S) OF CHOICE None
Contraindications: Avoid lactulose, since colonic distention can result from its bacterial fermentation
Precautions: N/A
Significant possible interactions: N/A

ALTERNATIVE DRUGS N/A

FOLLOWUP

PATIENT MONITORING
• Less than one bowel movement every other day suggests impaction
• Periodic rectal exam

PREVENTION/AVOIDANCE
• Establish regular, consistent toilet time by evoking gastrocolic reflex
• Maintain high fiber diet
• Reinforce exercise
• Install user-friendly commodes
• Use hydrophilic mucilloids (Metamucil) or stool-wetting agents (Colace) as needed
• Consider biofeedback; bowel training
• Periodic enemas, if indicated

POSSIBLE COMPLICATIONS
Complications of impaction
◊ Urinary tract obstruction
◊ Recurrent urinary tract infections
◊ Intestinal obstruction
◊ Spontaneous perforation of colon
◊ Stercoral ulceration
◊ Hernia
◊ Volvulus
◊ Megacolon
◊ Rectal prolapse
◊ Pneumothorax
◊ Hepatic encephalopathy
◊ Hypoxia
◊ Hypovolemic shock
Complications of disimpaction
◊ Sepsis
◊ Hypotension
◊ Instrumental perforation
◊ Bleeding
◊ Postoperative obstruction

EXPECTED COURSE AND PROGNOSIS
• Reimpaction likely, if bowel program not followed
• Prognosis poor for perforation with peritonitis
• Mortality with impaction and obstruction highest in very young and very old (up to 16%)

MISCELLANEOUS

ASSOCIATED CONDITIONS Pulmonary aspiration

AGE-RELATED FACTORS
Pediatric: Habitual neglect of defecation urge, because of interference with play, may promote impaction
Geriatric:
• Measure thyroid function, electrolyte activity and urea nitrogen levels in elderly patients presenting with impaction
• Much more likely to occur in patients over 80
Others: N/A

PREGNANCY Impaction can produce dysfunctional labor, dystocia

SYNONYMS Terminal reservoir syndrome

ICD-9-CM 560.39

SEE ALSO
• Constipation
• Encopresis

OTHER NOTES Electrohydraulic lithotripsy has been used to safely remove large calcified fecaliths

ABBREVIATIONS N/A

REFERENCES Sleisenger, M.H., Fordtran, J.S. (eds.): Gastrointestinal Disease. 5th Ed. Philadelphia, W.B. Saunders, 1993

Author R. Viken, M.D

Femoral neck fracture

BASICS

DESCRIPTION Fracture of the head or neck of the femur, usually as the result of a fall
Types
◊ Neck, subcapital or transcervical
◊ Intertrochanteric
◊ Subtrochanteric; usually caused by more severe trauma and has higher incidence in males than the other types
System(s) affected: Musculoskeletal
Genetics: No known genetic factor
Incidence/Prevalence in USA:
• 200,000 patients per year over the age of 65 have fracture of hips
• In women over age 75, there is a 1% incidence per year
Predominant age: 80% occur in those over age 60
Predominant sex: Female > Male

SIGNS AND SYMPTOMS
• Pain in hip. If severe, it usually indicates a displaced fracture. Mild pain usually occurs in non-displaced fractures.
• Pain in knee. Pain is referred from hip and may occur in absence of hip pain.
• External rotation of leg
• Shortening of leg

CAUSES
• Falls
• Motor vehicle trauma
• Spontaneous in pathologic conditions

RISK FACTORS
• Osteoporosis, usually post menopausal
• Metastatic cancer
• Neurological disease
• Severe renal disease with secondary hyperparathyroidism

DIAGNOSIS

DIFFERENTIAL DIAGNOSIS Rule out primary or metastatic malignancy

LABORATORY Routine pre-operative laboratory including CBC, chemical profile, electrolytes
Drugs that may alter lab results: N/A
Disorders that may alter lab results: N/A

PATHOLOGICAL FINDINGS
Osteoporosis

SPECIAL TESTS N/A

IMAGING
• X-rays - AP and "frog leg" lateral of hip
• X-ray Ap pelvis to rule out pelvis fracture as cause of pain. Also provides information regarding appearance of opposite side.
• X-ray remainder of femur to include knee
• X-ray any other tender or painful area as other fractures are common and symptoms may be ignored with severe pain of hip fracture
• CT or MRI scans are not routinely indicated as the diagnosis is usually obvious from plain radiographs

DIAGNOSTIC PROCEDURES N/A

TREATMENT

APPROPRIATE HEALTH CARE
• Treat as semi-emergency
• During transportation to hospital, gentle traction of the leg, especially Buck's traction 5# will help relieve discomfort. This can be maintained in bed, but requires close observation of circulation and skin changes.

GENERAL MEASURES
• Medical evaluation to have patient in best possible condition before surgery
• Surgery is almost always indicated. Older patients do not tolerate long periods of bed confinement.
• A hip prosthesis or pins are used in neck fractures. Nails or screws with side plates are used in intertrochanteric fractures. For subtrochanteric fractures, a nail with a long side plate, or intermedullary hip screws, or reconstructive rods may be used.
• Protect pressure points to avoid decubitus ulcers, especially on the sacrum, heels and malleoli

ACTIVITY
• Patients should be up (for toilet, and prevention of deep vein thrombosis and decubiti) as soon as possible after surgery, usually the next day
• Ambulate as soon as possible after surgery, e.g., with use of a walker. Close supervision by an experienced therapist necessary.

DIET No special diet

PATIENT EDUCATION Refer to physical therapy for walking instructions; usually non-weight bearing for several weeks at least

MEDICATIONS

DRUG(S) OF CHOICE Analgesics, as indicated. Drug of choice might be morphine sulfate 2-10 mg q3h prn with change to oral opioids as soon as possible.
Contraindications: Associated head injury or severe respiratory disease
Precautions: Dosage should be lower in older people to avoid respiratory problems
Significant possible interactions: Refer to manufacturer's literature

ALTERNATIVE DRUGS N/A

FOLLOWUP

PATIENT MONITORING
• X-rays of the hip taken prior to discharge from the hospital and every 8-12 weeks afterward until healed
• Monitor postoperative physical therapy for full recovery

PREVENTION/AVOIDANCE
• Prophylactic treatment for osteoporosis
• Use walking canes or walkers if patient has unsteady gait
• Have older people use proper chair for sitting. Should not allow hip flexion greater than 90 degrees since rising from this position requires external rotation of the extremity with subsequent torsional forces which can cause fracture.
• Use sturdy rails in showers, bathrooms, stairs, or ramps

POSSIBLE COMPLICATIONS
• Mental deterioration. Present in 90% of older patients for varying periods of time after surgery. Usually subsides, but may persist due to pre-existing arteriosclerosis.
• Infection. More common in comminuted fractures and patients with diabetes. Surgical implants should be left in place and antibiotics given as indicated by culture and sensitivity. Some require the wound to be opened and drained.
• Aseptic necrosis of femoral head. Occurs in 25-30% of femoral neck fractures. Treatment requires a prosthetic replacement in older patients.
• Phlebitis. Prophylaxis with aspirin 5 gm daily or dipyridamole (Persantine) 25 mg tid.
Nonunion
◊ In case of neck fractures, a prosthetic replacement is indicated
◊ In the intertrochanteric fracture, a bone graft, usually with replacement of the nail and plate, is indicated

EXPECTED COURSE AND PROGNOSIS
• Hip fractures remain a serious injury in older people. There is a 15-20% three month mortality in trochanteric fractures and 10% in neck fractures.
• Sixty-five percent of patients can be expected to return to their former state of health

MISCELLANEOUS

ASSOCIATED CONDITIONS
• Osteoporosis
• Metastatic malignancy

AGE-RELATED FACTORS
Pediatric: N/A
Geriatric: Hip fractures common in geriatric age group
Others: N/A

PREGNANCY N/A

SYNONYMS
• Subcapital fracture
• Trochanteric fracture
• Hip fracture

ICD-9-CM 820. (use appropriate modifier)

SEE ALSO Osteoporosis

OTHER NOTES None

ABBREVIATIONS N/A

REFERENCES
• Clinical Orthopedics #218, May, 1987; Symposium of hip fractures; pp. 2-104
• Bentley, G.: Impacted Fracture of the Neck of the Femur. Bone & Joint Surgery 1968, 50:B:551
• Sarmiento, A., et al.: Avoidance of Complications. Clinical Orthopedics 53:47, 1967

Author F. Johnston, M.D.

Fertility problems

BASICS

DESCRIPTION Failure to conceive after one year of unprotected intercourse
System(s) affected: Reproductive, Endocrine/Metabolic
Genetics: N/A
Incidence/Prevalence in USA: 10-15% of all couples
Predominant age: Increases with age, e.g., ages 30-34: 14% infertile, ages 35-39: 20% infertile, ages 40-45: 25% infertile
Predominant sex: N/A

SIGNS AND SYMPTOMS
• Thorough history and physical should be performed on each partner
• Genital/pelvic infection (e.g., pelvic inflammatory disease) often associated with an obstruction of reproductive tract
• Endocrine dysfunction (e.g., hypothyroidism, hypogonadism, abnormal puberty) often associated with abnormalities of ovulation or spermatogenesis
• Sexual dysfunction (e.g., premature ejaculation) may contribute to the problem
• Anovulatory cycles are frequently irregular, without premenstrual symptoms nor dysmenorrhea. Some patients may have features (e.g., hirsutism) suggestive of polycystic ovarian syndrome.
• Endometriosis is often associated with cyclic premenstrual pain and dysmenorrhea

CAUSES
• Most couples have more than one factor
• Male factors 30-40%
• Ovulation factors 15%
• Cervical/uterine factors 10%
• Tubal/peritoneal factors 25-30%
• Immunologic factors 5%
• Psychogenic/nutritional/metabolic factors 5%

RISK FACTORS Multiple - see under Causes

DIAGNOSIS

DIFFERENTIAL DIAGNOSIS Only basic elements of evaluation and diagnosis will be discussed here. Most of the tests of spermatogenesis and ovulation should be repeated at least once if abnormal.

LABORATORY
Semen analysis, normal values are:
  ◊ Volume 2-6 mL
  ◊ pH 7-8
  ◊ Viscosity - liquefies within one hour
  ◊ Count - 20 million or greater
  ◊ Motility - 50% or more
  ◊ Morphology - 60% or more
Post coital test
  ◊ Evaluates sperm/cervical mucous interaction
  ◊ Cervical mucus is aspirated with a tuberculin syringe from the os after intercourse during the fertile period
  ◊ If 10 or more sperm with directional movement are seen per high-power field of a microscope, the result is good. Sperm with shaking motion suggest sperm antibody.
Basal body temperature charting
  ◊ Assesses ovulation and adequacy of the luteal phase
  ◊ Morning temperature should rise about one degree Fahrenheit at the time of ovulation and remain elevated for 13-14 days
Serum progesterone
  ◊ Assesses ovulation and corpus luteum function
  ◊ A level of 15 or greater correlates with normal corpus luteum function
  ◊ Should be obtained on approximately day 21 of a 28 day menstrual cycle
Endometrial biopsy
  ◊ Obtain on day 25-27 of a 28 day cycle
  ◊ Assesses ovulation, function of the corpus luteum, and normalcy of the endometrium
The following tests are useful to evaluate underlying causes of anovulation or low sperm counts:
  ◊ Thyroid stimulating hormone and prolactin (elevations associated with suppressed gonadal function)
  ◊ Testosterone (decreased in primary gonadal failure)
  ◊ Follicle stimulating hormone (FSH) and luteinizing hormone (LH) (elevated in primary gonadal failure, decreased in hypopituitarism)
Drugs that may alter lab results:
Semen abnormalities can be caused by:
  ◊ Cimetidine
  ◊ Spironolactone
  ◊ Furadantin
  ◊ Sulfasalazine
  ◊ Marijuana
  ◊ Chemotherapeutic agents
  ◊ Cocaine
  ◊ Occupational/environmental hazards
Disorders that may alter lab results:
• Polycystic ovarian disease
• Endometriosis
• Severe hypospadias
• Retrograde ejaculation (often associated with diabetes)
• Varicocele

• Testicular injury (e.g., surgery, mumps, trauma)
• Occupational/environmental hazards

PATHOLOGICAL FINDINGS N/A

SPECIAL TESTS Multiple tests (e.g., hamster egg penetration assay) are available to study specific aspects of reproduction, but are used only by fertility specialists, and available in only specialized labs

IMAGING Hysterosalpingogram (HSG) - evaluates tubal patency and uterine contour. This procedure may have some therapeutic benefit.

DIAGNOSTIC PROCEDURES
Laparoscopy - should be deferred until basic evaluation is complete

TREATMENT

APPROPRIATE HEALTH CARE
Outpatient evaluation, with attention to the emotional support of the couple

GENERAL MEASURES
• Dispel myths and provide accurate information
• Simultaneously evaluate and counsel both partners
• Find and correct causes of infertility
• Provide information on adoption when appropriate
• Consider varicocele repair for abnormal semen analysis
• Consider donor insemination for refractory abnormalities of semen analysis
• Consider laparotomy for tubal anastomosis, lysis of adhesions, and correction of tubal obstruction

ACTIVITY
• Males with low sperm counts should avoid hot tubs/saunas (decreased spermatogenesis with elevated scrotal temperature)
• If the male has low sperm counts, intercourse should be timed to occur approximately every 36 hours during the fertile period. Delay of intercourse beyond 7 days also adversely affects semen quality.

DIET N/A

PATIENT EDUCATION
Printed patient information available from:
  ◊ RESOLVE, 5 Water St, Arlington, MA 02174
  ◊ Fertility Research Foundation, 1430 Second Avenue, Suite 103, New York, NY 10021, (212)744-5500
  ◊ American College of Obstetricians & Gynecologists, 409 12th St, SW, Washington, DC 20024-2188, (800)762-ACOG

MEDICATIONS

DRUG(S) OF CHOICE
• Clomiphene citrate (indicated for induction of ovulation). Typical dose - 50 mg daily x 5 days. This estrogen antagonist binds to receptors in the hypothalamus and stimulates increased release of gonadotropin releasing hormone (GnRH), leading to increased secretion of follicle stimulating hormone (FSH) and luteinizing hormone (LH) from the pituitary.
• Bromocriptine (indicated for treatment of anovulation associated with hyperprolactinemia and normal head CT scan or microadenomas). Dose - 1.25-2.5 mg/day. Increase slowly as tolerated to maximum of 15 mg/day.

Contraindications:
• Clomiphene - hyperprolactinemia, pituitary failure, ovarian cysts
• Bromocriptine - pituitary macroadenomas

Precautions:
• Clomiphene - hyperstimulation syndrome, multiple pregnancy, blurred vision, diplopia. Pelvic exams are useful to rule out ovarian enlargement. Cervical mucus may be scant and require estrogen supplementation.
• Bromocriptine - headaches, visual field defects, and diabetes insipidus may occur during pregnancy of patients with macroadenomas

Significant possible interactions:
• Clomiphene - none
• Bromocriptine - alcohol, antihypertensives, tricyclic antidepressants, phenothiazines

ALTERNATIVE DRUGS
Human chorionic gonadotropin, human menopausal gonadotropin (hMG), GnRH analogs (all used for induction of ovulation)

FOLLOWUP

PATIENT MONITORING
See under Diagnosis

PREVENTION/AVOIDANCE
Prevention of sexually transmitted disease and subsequent pelvic inflammatory disease

POSSIBLE COMPLICATIONS
• Pleural gestation with ovulation induction
• Ectopic pregnancy following tubal re-anastomosis

EXPECTED COURSE AND PROGNOSIS
• Prognosis is generally good
• About half of couples conceive during the second year of unprotected intercourse
• If the couple has been infertile for four or more years, the prognosis tends to be poor

MISCELLANEOUS

ASSOCIATED CONDITIONS
Increasing tubal damage associated with pelvic inflammatory disease and IUD use

AGE-RELATED FACTORS
• Increasing anovulation with increasing age
• Increased disease burden with age from diseases like endometriosis, and cumulative exposure to environmental/occupational hazards
Pediatric: N/A
Geriatric: N/A
Others: N/A

PREGNANCY
N/A

SYNONYMS
N/A

ICD-9-CM
• Male infertility 606.9
• Female infertility 628.9

SEE ALSO
N/A

OTHER NOTES
N/A

ABBREVIATIONS
N/A

REFERENCES
Speroff, L., Glass, R. & Kase, N.: Clinical Gynecologic Endocrinology and Infertility. 4th Ed. Baltimore, Williams & Wilkins, 1989

Author E. Lackermann, M.D.

Fever of unknown origin (FUO)

BASICS

DESCRIPTION Defined in 1961 by Petersdorf and Beeson as: Temperature greater than 38.3°C on several occasions during a period of at least 3 weeks and having an uncertain diagnosis after 1 week's evaluation in a hospital
 • In light of the fact that technologic advances have been made and more diagnostic tests are available on an outpatient basis, new criteria have been proposed: Fever greater than 38.3°C on at least four occasions over a 14 day period and illness of 14 days duration without an obvious cause.
Genetics: N/A
Incidence/Prevalence in USA: No data on actual incidence
Predominant age: All ages
Predominant sex: Dependent on etiology

SIGNS AND SYMPTOMS
 • Fever does not present as the only manifestation of a disease. The type and pattern of fever is of little help in making the diagnosis.
 • Constitutional symptoms that almost always accompany a fever: headache, myalgia, malaise

CAUSES
Infection
 ◊ Abdominal abscesses
 ◊ Mycobacterial infection
 ◊ Cytomegalovirus
 ◊ Renal
 ◊ Osteomyelitis
 ◊ Catheter infections
 ◊ Amebic hepatitis
 ◊ Wound infections
 ◊ Other miscellaneous infections
Neoplasms
 ◊ Lymphoma
 ◊ Leukemia
 ◊ Solid tumors (hypernephroma)
 ◊ Hepatoma
 ◊ Atrial myxoma
 ◊ Colon cancer
Collagen vascular disease
 ◊ Temporal arteritis
 ◊ Polyarteritis nodosa
 ◊ Rheumatic fever
 ◊ Systemic lupus erythematosus
 ◊ Rheumatoid arthritis
 ◊ Polymyalgia rheumatica
Other causes
 ◊ Granulomatous diseases
 ◊ Pulmonary emboli
 ◊ Drug fever
 ◊ Thermoregulatory disorders
 ◊ Endocrinologic diseases
 ◊ Occupational causes
 ◊ Periodic fever
 ◊ Factitious/fraudulent fever
 ◊ Other

RISK FACTORS
 • Recent travel
 • Exposure to biologic or chemical agents
 • Persons in AIDS risk group
 • Elderly persons
 • Drug abuse
 • Immigrants

DIAGNOSIS

DIFFERENTIAL DIAGNOSIS See Causes

LABORATORY
 • CBC - leukopenia, anemia, thrombocytopenia/thrombocytosis
 • Sedimentation rate - elevated
 • Liver function tests (especially alkaline phosphatase) - evidence of inflammation, obstruction or infiltrative disease
 • Blood cultures (not to exceed 6)
 • Urinalysis and urine culture
Drugs that may alter lab results: N/A
Disorders that may alter lab results: N/A

PATHOLOGICAL FINDINGS Dependent on etiology

SPECIAL TESTS
 • Tuberculin skin test - may not be helpful if anergic or acute infection. If test negative, repeat in 2 weeks.
 • Sputum and urine cultures for tuberculosis
 • Gastric washing for tuberculosis
 • Serologic tests - Epstein-Barr, hepatitis, syphilis, Lyme disease, Q fever, cytomegalovirus, amebiasis/coccidiomycosis
 • HIV antibody test
 • Serum protein electrophoresis - if immunologic etiology suspected
 • Thyroid function tests - if thyroiditis suspected
 • Rheumatoid factor and antinuclear antibody test - if collagen vascular disease suspected

IMAGING
 • Chest x-ray
 • Abdominal films
 • Sinus x-rays - if clinically indicated
 • Bone scan - if osteomyelitis or metastatic disease suspected
 • CT scan or MRI of abdomen and pelvis (plus directed biopsy, if indicated) - if infectious process or mass lesions suspected
 • 67-gallium or Tc-sulfur colloid scan - if infectious process or tumor suspected
 • Ultrasound of abdomen and pelvis (plus directed biopsy, if indicated) - if mass lesions, renal obstruction or gallbladder/biliary tree pathology suspected
 • Echocardiogram - if cardiac valve lesions, atrial myxomas or pericardial effusion suspected
 • Ventilation/perfusion scan - if pulmonary emboli suspected

DIAGNOSTIC PROCEDURES
 • Bone Marrow - if granulomatous disease, infection or malignancy suspected
 • Liver biopsy - if granulomatous disease suspected
 • Temporal artery biopsy - if giant cell arteritis suspected
 • Lymph node, muscle or skin biopsy - if clinically indicated
 • Spinal tap - if clinically indicated
 • Exploratory laparotomy - if otherwise unsuccessful in determining etiology

TREATMENT

APPROPRIATE HEALTH CARE
 • Outpatient
 • Hospitalization reserved for ill and debilitated and also in those in which factitious fever has been ruled out or an invasive procedure is indicated

GENERAL MEASURES
 • Attempt to determine etiology before initiating therapy
 • Avoid therapeutic trials unless as a last resort and only if therapy is reasonably specific
 • "Shotgun" approaches are condemned since they do not solve the problem, obscure the clinical picture and have effects

ACTIVITY Ambulatory primarily

DIET N/A

PATIENT EDUCATION Maintain an open line of communication between physician and patient/family as the workup progresses; the extended time required in establishing a diagnosis can be frustrating for all parties

MEDICATIONS

DRUG(S) OF CHOICE Dependent on diagnosis
Contraindications: N/A
Precautions: N/A
Significant possible interactions: N/A

ALTERNATIVE DRUGS N/A

FOLLOWUP

PATIENT MONITORING If the etiology of the fever continues to elude the physician, a history and physical examination along with screening laboratory studies should be repeated

PREVENTION/AVOIDANCE N/A

POSSIBLE COMPLICATIONS
Dependent on etiology

EXPECTED COURSE AND PROGNOSIS Dependent on etiology and age. One year survival rates reflecting deaths due to all causes: 91% age < 35, 82% age 35-64, 67% age > 64.

MISCELLANEOUS

ASSOCIATED CONDITIONS N/A

AGE-RELATED FACTORS
Pediatric:
 • Infections and collagen-vascular diseases most likely etiology
 • Inflammatory bowel disease common etiology in older children and adolescents
 • Has a better prognosis than in non-pediatric cases
Geriatric:
 • Most common causes are acute leukemia, Hodgkin's lymphoma, intra-abdominal infections, tuberculosis and temporal arteritis
 • Signs and symptoms in the elderly are much more nonspecific
 • Mortality rates are higher in the elderly
Others: Consider factitious fever in young female health care workers

PREGNANCY N/A

SYNONYMS N/A

ICD-9-CM 780.6

SEE ALSO Specific etiologies

OTHER NOTES N/A

ABBREVIATIONS N/A

REFERENCES
 • Brusch, J. & Weinstein L.: Fever of Unknown Origin. Medical Clinics of North America. 72:1247-1261, 1988
 • Wakefield, K,. Henderson, S. & Streit, J.: Fever of Unknown Origin in the Elderly. Primary Care.16:501-513, 1989
 • Knockaert, D.C., et al.: Fever of unknown origin in the 1980's: an update of the diagnostic spectrum. Arch Int Med. 1992;152:511-55

Author S. Henderson, M.D.

Fibrocystic breast disease

BASICS

DESCRIPTION Fibrocystic breast disease is a generalized term for benign breast disorders such as lumps and pain. It is, however, a misnomer since it has neither a well-defined set of symptoms, nor a clear etiology. The term benign breast disease is preferred. Benign lumps are usually smooth, regular, and mobile. The following classifications are useful:

Lumps:
◊ Physiologic nodularity - lumps vary with the phase of the menstrual cycle, common in young women
◊ Mastoplasia - a ropy, thickening of the breast tissue, most common in the upper outer quadrant, persists throughout the menstrual cycle
◊ Cysts - distended, fluid filled masses caused by an imbalance between secretion and absorption in the breast lobule, common in the decade preceding menopause
◊ Fibroadenoma - benign solid tumor, smooth margins, mobile, most common tumor in teenagers and young women, may occur at any age after thelarche
◊ Phyllodes tumors - painless, solid, smooth, lobular, bulky; stromal hyperplasia; 10% are malignant

Nipple discharge
◊ Although considered one of the warning signs for breast cancer, 90% of patients with nipple discharge have benign disease
◊ Bilateral duct ectasia - most common cause of nipple discharge; benign inflammatory condition; bilateral, sticky, multicolored discharge; usually has to be expressed
◊ Bilateral galactorrhea (prolactin-secreting pituitary tumors) - usually in association with amenorrhea; drugs (isoniazid, methyldopa, thiazides, reserpine, tricyclic antidepressants); trauma
◊ Unilateral intraductal papilloma - spontaneous discharge from one duct. Carcinoma must be excluded.

Pain
◊ Cyclical mastodynia - hormonal, an exaggeration of the normal premenstrual tenderness
◊ Non-cyclical - sclerosing adenosis, cysts, chest wall muscle spasm, costochondritis, neuritis, stress, referred pain

Inflammatory conditions
◊ Fat necrosis - a solid lump with or without pain that can mimic carcinoma
◊ Superficial phlebitis of the thoracoepigastric vein (Mondor's disease) - local tenderness and induration
◊ Abscess - exquisite pain and tenderness, erythema (common), not always a definite mass, common with lactation and squamous metaplasia of lactiferous ducts (Zuska's disease), usually caused by staphylococcal organisms

Growth disorders
◊ Accessory nipples (polythelia)
◊ Absence of the breast (amastia)
◊ Absence of the nipple (athelia)
◊ Hypoplasia (often associated with hypoplasia of the thorax and pectoral muscles, and abnormalities of the hand, i.e., Poland's syndrome)
◊ Gigantomastia - occurs during puberty and pregnancy
◊ Gynecomastia - occurs in men in association with puberty, senescence, liver disease, and testicular tumors, and medications such as digoxin and cimetidine

Genetics:
• Little is known about the genetic aspects of benign breast disease
• Family history of cysts common
• Epithelial hyperplasia with atypia increases relative risk 4 times for the subsequent development of breast cancer
• Family history of breast cancer in a first degree relative plus atypia increases relative risk 9 times

Incidence/Prevalence in USA: Unknown. It is estimated that at least 50% of women have benign breast symptoms during their lifetime.

Predominant age:
• Symptoms tend to occur in menstruating women
• Mastoplasia - most common in women from mid 20's to 55 years of age
• Cysts - usually seen in women in their 40's
• Cyclical mastodynia - common in menstruating women
• Non-cyclical pain - can occur at any age after breast development

Predominant sex: Female > Male (almost exclusively)

SIGNS AND SYMPTOMS
• Asymptomatic
• Breast pain
• Breast tenderness
• Pain subsides after menses
• Smooth masses
• Tense masses
• Fluctuant masses
• Bilateral masses
• Breast engorgement
• Breast thickening
• Nipple discharge

CAUSES
• The etiology of benign breast disease is unknown

Possible causes
◊ Luteal phase defect in progesterone
◊ Increased estrogen (17 beta estradiol)
◊ Hyperprolactinemia
◊ End organ hypersensitivity to estrogen
◊ Sensitivity to methylxanthines
◊ Dietary fat intake

RISK FACTORS
• Unknown
• The effect of consumption of methylxanthine-containing substances, e.g., coffee, tea, cola, and chocolate is controversial

DIAGNOSIS

DIFFERENTIAL DIAGNOSIS
• Lumps - breast cancer
• Skin changes - breast cancer, eczema
• Pain - costochondritis, chest wall muscle spasm, neuralgia, anxiety, depression, breast cancer, angina pectoris, gastroesophageal reflux, Pancoast tumor

LABORATORY Cytology of nipple discharge
Drugs that may alter lab results: N/A
Disorders that may alter lab results: N/A

PATHOLOGICAL FINDINGS Hyperplasia of breast epithelium or stroma, adenosis, microcysts, macrocysts, duct ectasia (plasma cell mastitis), apocrine metaplasia

SPECIAL TESTS N/A

IMAGING
Mammography
◊ Signs of malignancy include irregular mass, clustered masses, calcifications, architectural distortion, dilated duct
◊ May be normal in presence of malignancy
Ultrasonography
◊ Useful for differentiating cystic from solid lesions

DIAGNOSTIC PROCEDURES
• Fine needle aspiration and biopsy - allows differentiation of cystic and solid lesion. Cells sent for cytology can diagnose cancer with a high degree of accuracy. Low morbidity.
• Core needle biopsy - usually not indicated for fibrocystic disease. Useful in diagnosis of a large cancer.
• Excisional biopsy - indicated for all solid lumps that are not clearly benign

TREATMENT

APPROPRIATE HEALTH CARE
Outpatient. May be inpatient for biopsy or surgery.

GENERAL MEASURES
• Evaluate to be certain there is no malignancy by means of imaging and diagnostic procedures
• Pain rarely severe or disabling
• Frequently resolves spontaneously
• Reassure patient there is no malignancy
• Cold compresses may be helpful
• Well fitting, supportive brassiere (worn night and day)
• Possibly excision (under local anesthesia) of benign fibroadenoma or phyllode tumors, and fat necrosis lesions

ACTIVITY
No restrictions. Avoid activities that may cause trauma to the breasts.

DIET
Abstention from methylxanthines (coffee, tea, chocolate)

PATIENT EDUCATION
• American College of Obstetricians & Gynecologists, 409 12th St., SW, Washington, DC 20024-2188, (800)762-ACOG
• Booklet on Breast Self Examination from Primary care and Care and Cancer, 17 Prospect St., Huntington, NY 11743, (516)424-8900
• National Cancer Institute (800)4-CANCER

MEDICATIONS

DRUG(S) OF CHOICE
• For cyclical pain and swelling unresponsive to general measures - vitamin B6 50 mg per day and spironolactone (Aldactone) 10 mg bid premenstrually may be helpful or iodine (kelp tablets) 150 mcg daily for 3 months
• For more severe disease - danazol (Danocrine) 100-200 mg per day or bromocriptine 2.5 mg bid x 3 months may be useful, but side effects and expense limit their usefulness
Contraindications: Refer to manufacturer's literature
Precautions: Refer to manufacturer's literature
Significant possible interactions: Refer to manufacturer's literature

ALTERNATIVE DRUGS N/A

FOLLOWUP

PATIENT MONITORING
• Patients with fibrocystic change may have an increased risk of malignancy
• If there is no atypia on biopsy the risk is only minimally increased
• Patients with atypical ductal or lobular hyperplasia have a relative risk of cancer about five times that of the average woman
• Atypical hyperplasia and a family history of cancer in a first degree relative raises the risk to 8 or 9 times normal
• Patients need to be assessed with clinical examination, radiological studies, and, sometimes, biopsy to be certain a given lump is not malignant
• Followup times are variable depending on the clinical situation. A young patient in whom physiological nodularity is suspected should be observed through one menstrual cycle.
• Mammograms should be obtained at age 35, at least every 1-2 years after age 40, and yearly after age 50
• Ultrasound is useful to differentiate cysts from solid lesions, but is not used for screening
• Aspiration cytology is useful for diagnosis of cysts and solid lesions. The false positive rate ranges from 0-5.8%, and the false negative rate from 1.7-22%.
• When physical examination, mammography, and needle aspiration are used in combination, detection rates for breast cancer range from 93-100%
• Patients at high risk (8 or 9 times normal) may need to be seen every six months, and may warrant a discussion regarding prophylactic mastectomy

PREVENTION/AVOIDANCE
Avoiding caffeine may reduce breast pain

POSSIBLE COMPLICATIONS
• Fibrocystic change can make physical examination and mammograms difficult to interpret
• Atypical hyperplasia may lead to cancer

EXPECTED COURSE AND PROGNOSIS
Benign, chronic, recurring, intermittent

MISCELLANEOUS

ASSOCIATED CONDITIONS
Breast carcinoma

AGE-RELATED FACTORS
Pediatric: Biopsy in children should be avoided since a developing breast bud may be inadvertently removed
Geriatric: Not as common in this age group
Others: Prophylactic mastectomy for pain is rarely indicated since many patients have underlying psychiatric problems

PREGNANCY N/A

SYNONYMS
• Chronic cystic mastitis
• Adenosis
• Benign breast disease
• Mammary dysplasia
• Fibrocystic disease

ICD-9-CM
610.1 diffuse cystic mastopathy

SEE ALSO N/A

OTHER NOTES N/A

ABBREVIATIONS N/A

REFERENCES
• Grundfest-Broniatowski, S. & Esselstyn, C.B.E., Jr.: Controversies in Breast Disease: Diagnosis and Management. New York, Marcel Dekker, Inc., 1988
• Harris, J.R., Hellman, S., Henderson, I.C. & Kinne, D.W.: Breast Diseases. Philadelphia, J.B. Lippincott Co., 1987

Author S. Grundfest-Broniatowski, M.D., F.A.C.S.

Fibrositis

BASICS

DESCRIPTION Extremely common pain phenomenon occurring in a defined pattern, reproduced by pressure on "trigger points"
System(s) affected: Musculoskeletal
Genetics: N/A
Incidence/Prevalence in USA: 3 in 100
Predominant age: 18-70
Predominant sex: Female > Male

SIGNS AND SYMPTOMS
<u>Pressure manually applied to specific sites, referred to as "trigger points" reproduce the patient's symptoms:</u>
◊ Temporalis - above the ear
◊ Anterior to tragus of ear
◊ Scalenus capitis
◊ Sternocleidomastoid
◊ Low anterior neck
◊ Pectoralis minor
◊ Manubriosternal
◊ Anterior and posterior axillary folds
◊ Trapezius ridge
◊ Upper rhomboids
◊ Lower rhomboids
◊ Iliac crest
◊ Mid-buttocks
◊ Mid-rectus femoris
◊ Mid-vastus lateralis
◊ Quadriceps insertion - at the patella
◊ Humeral epicondyles (many investigators would diagnose fibromyalgia, while some prefer epicondylitis)
<u>Other signs and symptoms</u>
◊ Typically insidious in onset
◊ Pain is increased in the morning, with weather changes, anxiety, stress
◊ Pain improved by mild physical activity or vacations (stress-relieving situations)
Non-restorative sleep, with early morning awakening in an unrefreshed state.
◊ Abnormal non-rapid eye movement (non-REM) stage IV sleep
◊ Generalized fatigue or tiredness
◊ Anxiety
◊ Chronic headache
◊ Irritable bowel syndrome
◊ Subjective, non-confirmable complaints of swelling or numbness, not associated with objective neurologic findings
◊ Depression
◊ Reduced physical endurance
◊ Decreased social interaction

CAUSES
• Loss of non-REM stage IV sleep
• Stress
• Trauma

RISK FACTORS
• Sleep disturbance
• Trauma
• Depression
• Weather changes

DIAGNOSIS

DIFFERENTIAL DIAGNOSIS
• Hypothyroidism
• Psychogenic rheumatism
• Muscle strain/sprain
• Muscle disease
• Polymyalgia rheumatica
• Temporal arteritis

LABORATORY
• Normal Westergren erythrocyte sedimentation rate
• Normal creatinine phosphokinase and aldolase
• Normal TSH, T3 resin uptake and T4
• Normal complete blood count, renal and liver function
Drugs that may alter lab results: Steroids
Disorders that may alter lab results: N/A

PATHOLOGICAL FINDINGS None

SPECIAL TESTS Thermography

IMAGING Thermography

DIAGNOSTIC PROCEDURES The clinical history and physical examination

TREATMENT

APPROPRIATE HEALTH CARE
Outpatient

GENERAL MEASURES
Electroprobe, electrical stimulation, ultrasound, hot packs, conditioning, increasing social interactions and general conditioning exercises

ACTIVITY
Fully active. However, the pain of fibrositis may be so distracting as to reduce attentiveness, predisposing to error and accident.

DIET No restrictions

PATIENT EDUCATION
Printed material: Rothschild, B.: Diagnosing and treating fibrositis and fibromyalgia. Geriatric Consultant, 9(5/6):26-28, 1990

MEDICATIONS

DRUG(S) OF CHOICE
• Nonsteroidal anti-inflammatory drugs (NSAID's) may provide non-narcotic symptomatic pain relief
<u>Sleep restorative without interfering with stage IV sleep:</u>
Reinforce discontinuation if paradoxical effect, memory loss, thought process changes, or behavior changes.
◊ Amitriptyline (Elavil) 10 mg 2 po hs prn, increased gradually to 50 mg
◊ Cyclobenzaprine (Flexeril) 10 mg tid prn
◊ Triazolam (Halcion) 0.125 mg po hs po increased gradually to 0.5 mg (for short-term use only at higher dose)
◊ Temazepam (Restoril) 15 mg po hs prn, increased to 30 mg
◊ Flurazepam (Dalmane) 15 mg po hs prn, increased to 30 mg (note: Significant "hangover" potential secondary to long half-life)
Contraindications: Drug allergy, suicide potential
Precautions:
• NSAID's - refer to manufacturer's literature
• Others - observe for grogginess or aberrant behavior, discontinue if it occurs. Benzodiazepines should be used only for short periods. Psychological and/or physical dependence may occur. However, if the patient is nonfunctional without them, long-term use is reasonable.
Significant possible interactions:
• NSAID's - refer to manufacturer's literature
• Others - digoxin, phenytoin, MAO inhibitors

ALTERNATIVE DRUGS
Trazodone (Desyrel) 50 mg po hs prn

FOLLOWUP

PATIENT MONITORING
• For efficacy at 2-4 weeks
• For medication side effects every 3-6 months

PREVENTION/AVOIDANCE
• Adequate sleep
• General conditioning exercises

POSSIBLE COMPLICATIONS
• Chronicity
• Fibromyalgia is allegedly a greater source of work loss and dysfunction than rheumatoid arthritis

EXPECTED COURSE AND PROGNOSIS
• With resolution of sleep disturbance, may resolve totally
• Aggressive physical therapy is critical in those who do not respond
• Approximately 5% do not respond to any form of therapeutic intervention. Hypnosis may be attempted in that group.

MISCELLANEOUS

ASSOCIATED CONDITIONS
So common almost any disease can be associated with it

AGE-RELATED FACTORS
Pediatric: Uncommon
Geriatric: Common; polypharmacy may be part of the problem
Others: N/A

PREGNANCY
Limits therapeutic approach to physical therapy modalities

SYNONYMS
• Fibromyalgia
• Myofascial pain syndrome

ICD-9-CM
729.1

SEE ALSO
• Irritable bowel syndrome
• Chronic fatigue syndrome

OTHER NOTES
Perhaps the most common cause of neck or back pain in this patient population and most common rheumatologic problem in general

ABBREVIATIONS
N/A

REFERENCES
• Rothschild, B.M. & Martin, L.: Paleopathology: Diseases in the Fossil Record. London, CRC Press, 1993
• Rothschild, B.M.: Fibromyalgia: An explanation for the aches and pains of the 90's. Comprehensive Therapy, 1991; 17(6): 9-14
• Rothschild, B.M.: Diagnosing and treating fibrositis and fibromyalgia. Geriatric Consultant, 9(5/6):26-28, 1990
• Yunus, M., Masi, A.T., Calabro, J.J., Miller, K.A. & Feigenbaum, S.L.: Primary fibromyalgia (fibrositis): Clinical study of 50 patients with matched normal controls. Semin Arthritis Rheum, 11:151-171, 1981
• Wolfe, F., Smythe, H.A., Yunus, M.B. & Bennett, R.M., et al.: The American College of Rheumatology criteria for the classification of fibromyalgia. Arthritis Rheum. 33:160-172, 1990

Author B. Rothschild, M.D.

Folliculitis

 BASICS

DESCRIPTION Inflammation of hair follicles, often due to microbes or chemical irritation. May be superficial or deep.
System(s) affected: Skin/Exocrine
Genetics: No known genetic pattern
Incidence/Prevalence in USA: Common (no statistics available)
Predominant age: All ages
Predominant sex: Male > Female

SIGNS AND SYMPTOMS
• Characteristic lesions are yellow or gray pustules surrounded by erythema and pierced by a hair
• Lesions are commonly grouped
• Lesions may occur on any body surface. Common on scalp, beard area, and limbs.
• Patients are usually afebrile and without systemic symptoms
• Nontender or slightly tender
• May be pruritic

CAUSES
• Staphylococcus aureus - most common agent
• Pseudomonas aeruginosa - occurs in bathing suit areas of users of hot tubs and saunas
• Candida albicans - occurs in patients on immunosuppressants or long-term antibiotic therapy. May also occur on the back of hospitalized, febrile patients.
• Dermatophyte fungi - uncommon, but may occur in beard area
• Exposure to various agents - such as hydrocarbons, and some drugs (such as iodides)

RISK FACTORS
• Abrasion
• Injury
• Nearby surgical wounds or draining abscesses
• Tight clothing (jeans folliculitis)
• Poor hygiene
• Exposure to hydrocarbons
• Use of hot tubs or saunas
• Immunodeficiency
• Diabetes mellitus

 DIAGNOSIS

DIFFERENTIAL DIAGNOSIS
• Ingrown hairs (especially in the beard area of black males who shave)
• Keratosis pilaris (follicular papules on extensor surfaces of extremities in atopic individuals)
• Contact dermatitis
• Tinea
• Acne
• Pustular miliaria
• Flat warts
• Molluscum contagiosum

LABORATORY
• Gram stain - look for gram positive cocci
• KOH preparation - look for budding yeast or hyphae
• Culture
Drugs that may alter lab results: N/A
Disorders that may alter lab results: N/A

PATHOLOGICAL FINDINGS Suppurative inflammation

SPECIAL TESTS N/A

IMAGING N/A

DIAGNOSTIC PROCEDURES Biopsy may be required in resistant cases, or if diagnosis is in doubt

 TREATMENT

APPROPRIATE HEALTH CARE
Outpatient

GENERAL MEASURES
• Cleanse area bid with antibacterial soap (e.g., Dial)
• Shampoo daily with Selsun Blue for lesions on scalp
• Apply moist heat to allow the lesion to drain
• Change razor blade daily
• Avoid use of topical oils
• Avoid exposure to causative factors

ACTIVITY Fully active

DIET No special diet

PATIENT EDUCATION As listed under General Measures

MEDICATIONS

DRUG(S) OF CHOICE
Staphylococcus aureus
◊ Dicloxacillin (Dycill, Dynapen, Pathocil) 250 mg po every 6 hours for 10 days
◊ Erythromycin, 250 mg po every 6 hours for 10 days
Pseudomonas aeruginosa
◊ Ciprofloxacin (Cipro) 500 mg po twice daily for 10 days (Other quinolones may be used alternatively)
◊ Ofloxacin (400 mg bid)
Contraindications:
• History of hypersensitivity to the antibiotic
• Quinolone antibiotics are contraindicated in pregnancy and pediatrics
Precautions: Refer to manufacturer's literature
Significant possible interactions:
• Ciprofloxacin and norfloxacin - antacids, sucralfate, oral anticoagulants, theophylline, caffeine, probenecid
• Erythromycin - theophylline, oral anticoagulants, carbamazepine, corticosteroids, digoxin, ergot alkaloids, cyclosporine, phenytoin

ALTERNATIVE DRUGS
Mupirocin (Bactroban) topical therapy to affected area three times a day

FOLLOWUP

PATIENT MONITORING
• One return visit in 2 weeks if symptoms abate
• Resistant cases should be followed every 2 weeks until cleared

PREVENTION/AVOIDANCE
• Good personal hygiene, avoid sharing towel or washcloth. Discard any dressings carefully.
• Avoidance of causative factors
• Find and treat family members or friends who may be a source of reinfection

POSSIBLE COMPLICATIONS
May occasionally progress to furuncles

EXPECTED COURSE AND PROGNOSIS
• Usually resolves with treatment
• May recur in Staph. carriers. Mupirocin may be required on nares of patient to treat carrier state. Family carriers may also need to be treated.
• Resistant or severe cases may warrant testing for diabetes mellitus or immunodeficiency

MISCELLANEOUS

ASSOCIATED CONDITIONS
• Diabetes mellitus
• Immunodeficiency

AGE-RELATED FACTORS
Pediatric: N/A
Geriatric: N/A
Others: N/A

PREGNANCY
Pruritic folliculitis of pregnancy is a rare disorder that resolves spontaneously after delivery

SYNONYMS
Sycosis

ICD-9-CM
704.8

SEE ALSO
N/A

OTHER NOTES
N/A

ABBREVIATIONS
N/A

REFERENCES
Habif, T.: Clinical Dermatology: A Color Guide to Diagnosis and Therapy. 2nd Ed. St. Louis, C.V. Mosby, 1990

Author M. Kimmel, M.D.

Food allergy

BASICS

DESCRIPTION Food allergy is a hypersensitivity reaction which is caused by certain foods. Adverse reactions after food ingestion may be caused by immunologic mechanisms, such as the classic IgE allergic response, or by non-immunologic mediated mechanisms.
System(s) affected:
Hemic/Lymphatic/Immunologic, Gastrointestinal, Skin/Exocrine, Pulmonary, Nervous
Genetics: In family members with a history of food hypersensitivity, the probability of food allergy in subsequent siblings may be as high as 50%
Incidence in USA:
• The incidence of IgE mediated food allergy has been estimated to range from 1-7% of the population
• In children up to 4 years of age the incidence is between 8-16%
• Only about 3-4% of children over 4 years of age have persisting food allergy. Therefore, it is frequently a transient phenomena.
Prevalence in USA: 1-3%
Predominant age: All ages, but more common in infants and children
Predominant sex: Male > Female (2:1)

SIGNS AND SYMPTOMS
Gastrointestinal (system usually affected)
  ◊ More common: Nausea, vomiting, diarrhea, abdominal pain, occult bleeding, flatulence, bloating
  ◊ Less common: Malabsorption, protein losing enteropathy, eosinophil-gastroenteritis, and colitis
Dermatologic
  ◊ More common: Urticaria/angioedema, atopic dermatitis, pallor or flushing
  ◊ Less common: Contact rashes
Respiratory
  ◊ More common: Allergic rhinitis, asthma and bronchospasm, cough, serous otitis media
  ◊ Less common: Pulmonary infiltrates (Heiner's syndrome), pulmonary hemosiderosis
Neurologic
  ◊ Less common: Hyperkinesis, tension-fatigue syndrome, migraine headaches, syncope
Other symptoms:
  ◊ Systemic anaphylaxis, vasculitis
  ◊ Suspected manifestations include enuresis, proteinuria and arthropathy
  ◊ Behavioral disturbances, irritability, disinterest
  ◊ Growth retardation

CAUSES
• Any food or ingested substance can cause allergic reactions. Most commonly implicated foods include cow's milk, egg whites, wheat, soy, peanut, fish, tree nuts (walnut and pecan), shellfish, melons, sesame seeds, sunflower seeds, chocolate.
• Several food dyes and additives can elicit allergic-like reactions

RISK FACTORS
• Persons with allergic or atopic predisposition are at increased risk of hypersensitivity reaction to foods
• Family members with a history of food hypersensitivity

DIAGNOSIS

DIFFERENTIAL DIAGNOSIS
• A careful history is necessary to document a temporal relationship with the manifestations of suspected food hypersensitivity
• The gastrointestinal, dermatologic, respiratory, neurologic or other systemic manifestations may mimic a variety of clinical entities

LABORATORY
• Eosinophilia in either blood or tissue suggests atopy
• Epicutaneous (prick or puncture) allergy skin tests are useful in documenting IgE mediated immunologic hypersensitivity. In most clinical situations, the allergy skin tests are good for screening. An oral challenge should be completed to accurately determine the clinical hypersensitivity. The overall agreement between allergy skin testing and oral food challenge is approximately 60% (i.e., a positive skin test showing a positive challenge reaction to a particular food).
• Radioallergosorbent (RAST) test can also detect specific IgE antibodies to offending foods. In certain laboratories, the RAST test was almost as accurate as a skin test in predicting positive oral challenges.
• Leukocyte histamine release and assays for circulating immune complexes are predominantly research procedures and are of limited use in clinical practices. Assays for IgG and IgG 4 subclass antibodies are commercially available. There are no convincing data that these tests are reliable for the diagnosis of food allergy.
• The provocative injection and sublingual provocative tests are both highly controversial and have been proven to be useless for the diagnosis of food allergy
• The leukocytotoxic assay is an unproven diagnostic procedure and is not useful for the diagnosis of allergy
Drugs that may alter lab results: N/A
Disorders that may alter lab results: N/A

PATHOLOGICAL FINDINGS Acute and chronic rectal inflammation

SPECIAL TESTS Stool exam, mucus, eosinophilia

IMAGING Upper GI series for gastric antral inflammation, in rare cases

DIAGNOSTIC PROCEDURES
Elimination and challenge test
  ◊ The best procedure for confirming food allergy
  ◊ First, the suspected food is eliminated from the diet for 1-2 weeks
  ◊ The patient's symptoms are monitored. If the patient's symptoms disappear or substantially improve, an oral challenge with the suspected food should be performed under medical supervision.
  ◊ Optimally, this challenge should be performed in a double-blind, placebo controlled manner
  ◊ Most allergic reactions will occur within 30 minutes to 2 hours after the challenge, although late reactions have also been described, which may occur from 12-24 hours

TREATMENT

APPROPRIATE HEALTH CARE
Outpatient

GENERAL MEASURES
• Avoidance of the offending food is the most effective mode of treatment for patients with food allergies
• Those patients with exquisite and severe allergy hypersensitivity to a food should be more cautious in their avoidance of that food. They should carry epinephrine for self-administration in the event that the offending food is ingested unknowingly, and a subsequent immediate reaction develops.
• Immunotherapy or hyposensitization with food extracts by various routes, including subcutaneous immunotherapy or sublingual neutralization are not recommended since the success with these methods have not been proven in controlled scientific studies

ACTIVITY No restrictions

DIET As determined by tests

PATIENT EDUCATION Patients should be counselled by a dietician to be sure that they maintain a nutritionally sound diet, in spite of avoiding those foods to which patient is sensitive

MEDICATIONS

DRUG(S) OF CHOICE
• The use of cromolyn has been suggested, but is not practical for use in most patients with food allergy
• Recent studies have suggested the use of ketotifen, which is a mast cell stabilizer. This drug is not available in the United States.
Contraindications: N/A
Precautions: N/A
Significant possible interactions: N/A

ALTERNATIVE DRUGS   N/A

FOLLOWUP

PATIENT MONITORING   As needed

PREVENTION/AVOIDANCE   Avoidance
of offending food

POSSIBLE COMPLICATIONS
• Anaphylaxis
• Angioedema
• Bronchial asthma
• Enterocolitis
• Eczematoid lesions

EXPECTED COURSE AND PROGNOSIS
• Most infants will outgrow their food hypersensitivity by 2-4 years. It may be possible to reintroduce the offending food cautiously into the diet (particularly helpful when the food is one that is difficult to avoid).
• Adults with food hypersensitivity (particularly to milk, fish, shellfish or nuts) tend to maintain their allergy for many years

MISCELLANEOUS

ASSOCIATED CONDITIONS   N/A

AGE-RELATED FACTORS
Pediatric: N/A
Geriatric: N/A
Others: N/A

PREGNANCY   N/A

SYNONYMS
• Allergic bowel disease
• Dietary protein sensitivity syndrome

ICD-9-CM   693.1

SEE ALSO
• Celiac disease
• Irritable bowel syndrome
• Pyloric stenosis
• Acute epiglottitis

OTHER NOTES   N/A

ABBREVIATIONS   N/A

REFERENCES
• Sampson, H.A.: Adverse Reactions to Foods. In Allergy Principles and Practice. 4th Ed. New York, C.V. Mosby Co., 1993
• Chiaramonte, L.T., et al. (eds.): Food Allergy. Philadelphia, Marcel Dekker, 1988
• Metcalf, D.D., et al. (eds.): Food Allergy, Adverse Reactions to Foods and Food Additives. New York, Blackwell Scientific, 1991

Author   S. Fineman, M.D.

Food poisoning, bacterial

BASICS

DESCRIPTION A variety of related illnesses resulting from ingestion of food contaminated with bacteria capable of causing disease. The illness may be produced by bacterial infection itself (salmonellosis, shigellosis) or by toxins produced by the bacteria (Staphylococcus aureus, Clostridium perfringens, Bacillus cereus).

Genetics: N/A

Incidence/Prevalence in USA: Poor reporting overall. Estimated 6.3 million cases/year. 1 in 10 Americans with foodborne diarrhea/year. Approximate incidence is 2,500/100,000.

Predominant age: All ages

Predominant sex: Male = Female

SIGNS AND SYMPTOMS
Suspect when multiple persons become ill after eating the same meal. Timing and type of clinical presentation can aid in establishing etiology.
- Nausea, vomiting 1-8 hours after meal (S. aureus, B. cereus)
- Cramps, diarrhea 8-16 hours after meal (C. perfringens, B. cereus)
- Fever, cramps, diarrhea 18-72 hours after meal (Campylobacter jejuni, Yersinia enterocolitica, E. coli, Vibrio parahaemolyticus, Shigella and Salmonella species)
- Bloody diarrhea without fever 3-5 days after meal (verotoxigenic E. coli, occasionally C. jejuni)
- Pseudoappendicitis (Y. enterocolitica)
- Sepsis, meningitis (Listeria monocytogenes, Shigella and Salmonella species)
- Occasional metastatic foci of infection (arthritis, L monocytogenes, Salmonella, etc.)

CAUSES
- S. aureus (preformed enterotoxin)
- B. cereus (preformed enterotoxin)
- C. perfringens (enterotoxin elaborated in gut)
- C. jejuni (tissue invasion)
- Y. enterocolitica (tissue invasion)
- E. coli (enterotoxigenic, verotoxigenic [hemorrhagic], and tissue invasive forms)
- V. parahaemolyticus (toxin elaboration, possibly invasion)
- Shigella species (tissue invasion)
- Salmonella species (tissue invasion)
- L. monocytogenes (tissue invasion)

RISK FACTORS
Ingestion of:
- High protein foods: egg salad, cream-filled pastries, poultry, ham - S. aureus
- Cereals, fried rice, dried foods and herbs, meats, vegetables - B. cereus
- Meats, gravies, dried foods, vegetables - C. perfringens
- Under-cooked poultry, meat, raw dairy products - C. jejuni
- Under-cooked pork, other meat and dairy products - Y. enterocolitica
- Raw vegetables and other foods, contaminated water - E. coli
- Raw and cooked seafood - V. parahaemolyticus
- Raw vegetables, egg salads, contaminated water - Shigella
- Under-cooked eggs, poultry, dairy products, meat - Salmonella
- Under-cooked meat, dairy products, and many other foods - L. monocytogenes

DIAGNOSIS

DIFFERENTIAL DIAGNOSIS
- Infectious gastroenteritis of any kind
- Inflammatory bowel disease
- Appendicitis and other acute surgical abdominal processes
- Hepatitis

LABORATORY Culture of stool most reliable. Laboratory must be specifically notified of diagnostic considerations for most pathogens except Salmonella and Shigella.

Drugs that may alter lab results: Prior or concomitant antibiotic therapy may eliminate pathogen from stool

Disorders that may alter lab results: N/A

PATHOLOGICAL FINDINGS Only present in invasive or colitic syndromes

SPECIAL TESTS Sigmoidoscopy (occasionally needed)

IMAGING N/A

DIAGNOSTIC PROCEDURES
- Stool culture
- Epidemiologic investigation
- Culture of suspected food source if available

TREATMENT

APPROPRIATE HEALTH CARE Usually outpatient management sufficient. Hospitalization for septicemias or focal infections, severe electrolyte imbalance or dehydration.

GENERAL MEASURES
- Most are self-limited syndromes and do not require specific therapy
- Oral solutions for rehydration. Intravenous fluid and electrolyte replacement if necessary for more severe dehydration (particularly in the elderly).
- For infants, rehydration product (e.g., Pedialyte) provides adequate fluid and electrolyte replacement. Don't use for more than 1 to 2 days without clinical reassessment for nutritional needs.

ACTIVITY Bedrest for comfort if needed during the acute phase

DIET Eliminate contaminated food. Bland diet during recovery. Nothing by mouth, if needed, for excessive vomiting or diarrhea.

PATIENT EDUCATION
- Avoidance of raw or under-cooked foods
- Proper food storage and preparation techniques such as refrigeration
- Instruction on prevention if patient traveling to foreign countries

MEDICATIONS

DRUG(S) OF CHOICE For septicemias and focal infections, antibiotic therapy may be indicated (e.g., ampicillin plus aminoglycoside for listeriosis):

Contraindications:
• Avoid antiperistaltic agents in colitic (bloody diarrhea) syndromes since they may increase the chance of dissemination
• Antiemetics may be given but are usually unnecessary

Precautions: N/A

Significant possible interactions: Digoxin toxicity with electrolyte imbalance, exacerbation of diuretic effects

ALTERNATIVE DRUGS N/A

FOLLOWUP

PATIENT MONITORING Individualized based on degree of dehydration and electrolyte imbalance, or signs of sepsis. Serious disturbances require hospitalization, frequent vital signs, strict recording of input and output with appropriate fluid replacement.

PREVENTION/AVOIDANCE
• No ingestion of raw seafood, meats, or poultry
• Avoid any unpasteurized dairy products
• Clean thoroughly any food preparation area in contact with causative items
• Ensure proper cooling of any prepared foods not immediately consumed

POSSIBLE COMPLICATIONS
• Cardiovascular collapse
• Arrhythmias from electrolyte disturbance
• Septicemias or other metastatic infections
• Hypoglycemic seizures or coma

EXPECTED COURSE AND PROGNOSIS Resolution of signs and symptoms over a few days in most cases

MISCELLANEOUS

ASSOCIATED CONDITIONS N/A

AGE-RELATED FACTORS
Pediatric:
• Day care center outbreaks may occur. Perhaps at higher risk of complications from antiperistaltic drugs.
• Newborns and infants are a high risk for mortality and complications
• Shigellosis is a rare cause of chronic vaginal discharge in young girls
Geriatric:
• Nursing home outbreaks may occur
• Significant cause of mortality
Others: N/A

PREGNANCY Perinatal salmonellosis, listeriosis, and campylobacteriosis may secondarily infect newborn with severe consequences of sepsis and meningitis

SYNONYMS N/A

ICD-9-CM
• 003 other salmonella infections
• 005 other food poisoning (bacterial)

SEE ALSO
• Diarrhea, acute
• Gastroenteritis infectious
• Intestinal parasites
• Salmonella infections
• Typhoid fever
• Brucellosis
• Botulism
• Dehydration
• Hypokalemia
• Appendicitis

OTHER NOTES N/A

ABBREVIATIONS N/A

REFERENCES
• Mandell, G.L., Douglas, R.G., Jr. & Bennett, J.E.: Principles and Practice of Infectious Diseases. 3rd Ed. New York, Churchill Livingstone, 1990
• Roberts, D.: Sources of infection: Food. Lancet 336:859, 1990

Author BL Wiedermann, M.D.

Fragile X syndrome

BASICS

DESCRIPTION Fragile X syndrome is the second most common cause of mental retardation (after Down's syndrome), associated with a cytogenetic abnormality, and is thus, the most common form of familial mental retardation. This condition received its name from the cytogenetic marker in which a "fragile site" is seen on the long arm of the X chromosome (Xq27.3). That is associated with abnormal increase in CGG repeat in DNA of carrier and affected individual.

System(s) affected: Nervous, Reproductive, Musculoskeletal

Genetics:
• The pattern of inheritance is X-linked, however, this condition is seen in both sexes. Males are usually more severely affected than females.
• The specific factors controlling the expression of genes at the fragile X site are not fully understood
• 80% of males with the fragile X chromosome will be affected with moderate to severe mental retardation, with 20% unaffected and defined as transmitting males
• Only one third of the female carriers will have mental retardation, and their degree of handicap usually is less severe. Females may demonstrate emotional problems.

Incidence/Prevalence in USA: Affected males = 1/1250 and transmitting males 1/5000 which gives an overall male prevalence of 1/1000. Affected females = 1/2000 and an overall female carrier rate of 1/700. Based on these estimates, 1/850 people carry the fragile X chromosome.

Predominant age: Life-long condition

Predominant sex: Males usually more severely affected, but females demonstrate a higher carrier rate

SIGNS AND SYMPTOMS
The signs and symptoms seen in the "classical" case of fragile X syndrome may be diagnostic; however, the clinical presentation is extremely varied, is age-dependent, and sex-influenced. Blacks are also less likely to show the characteristic features.

Early childhood:
◊ Global developmental delay with speech severely affected
◊ Overgrowth
◊ Autistic behaviors

Postpubertal males (affected)
◊ Mental retardation (100%)
◊ Macro-orchidism (> 95%)
◊ Long, thin face (60-65%)
◊ Prominent jaw (60-65%)
◊ Large ears (> 7.0 cm) (60-65%)
◊ Midface hypoplasia (50-60%)
◊ Prominent forehead (40%)
◊ Large, fleshy hands (30%)

CAUSES Transmission of affected X chromosome

RISK FACTORS
• Transmitting males are intellectually normal and pass the affected chromosome to all of their daughters who often show no effects but have affected sons
• Affected females transmit the affected chromosome to their offspring on a 50/50 chance basis
• No affected males are reported to father children

DIAGNOSIS

DIFFERENTIAL DIAGNOSIS
• Fragile X syndrome should be considered in patients (male or female) with mental retardation of unknown etiology
• Many male children will present primarily with speech delay or overgrowth and have been misdiagnosed as having cerebral gigantism (Soto's) syndrome
• Data indicates that perhaps 7% of children diagnosed as autistic have fragile X syndrome

LABORATORY
• Detection of the fragile X marker chromosome requires specialized cytogenetic testing in an experienced laboratory. Chromosome analysis should be requested in all mentally retarded patients without a diagnosis.
• Molecular genetic testing (DNA) is currently the diagnostic test of choice. Molecular studies can identify carrier states in intellectually normal patients.

Drugs that may alter lab results: N/A
Disorders that may alter lab results: N/A

PATHOLOGICAL FINDINGS See Signs and Symptoms

SPECIAL TESTS See laboratory. Affected patients are in need of educational and psychological evaluation for the development of learning programs.

IMAGING N/A

DIAGNOSTIC PROCEDURES See Differential diagnosis and Laboratory

TREATMENT

APPROPRIATE HEALTH CARE
Affected individuals will usually require life-long adult supervision and should be referred to the local mental retardation board for case management

GENERAL MEASURES Early detection allows initiation of pre-school intervention programs

ACTIVITY Full activity

DIET No special diet

PATIENT EDUCATION
• The patient and the family should receive genetic evaluation and counseling
• Patient and family could contact: The National fragile X Foundation, Denver, CO. 800-688-8765

MEDICATIONS

DRUG(S) OF CHOICE Folic acid 20 mg qd, has been reported anecdotally to improve behavior and attention span in prepubertal males. No statistical benefit has been observed in children or adults during double-blind studies.
Contraindications: N/A
Precautions: N/A
Significant possible interactions: N/A

ALTERNATIVE DRUGS N/A

FOLLOWUP

PATIENT MONITORING General health maintenance

PREVENTION/AVOIDANCE Genetic counseling and evaluation of at-risk family members and pregnancies. Prenatal diagnosis is available.

POSSIBLE COMPLICATIONS Learning and/or behavioral problems (which are more frequent among female patients)

EXPECTED COURSE AND PROGNOSIS
• Affected individuals may require life-long adult supervision
• Life-span is generally not affected
• Several studies have shown a slow progressive decline in intelligence and adaptive behavior with increasing age

MISCELLANEOUS

ASSOCIATED CONDITIONS
• Speech problems
• Developmental delay
• Mental retardation
• Maladaptive behavior
• Attention deficit disorder/hyperactivity disorder (ADHD) is found with greater frequency among individuals with neuropsychological dysfunction. Treatment for ADHD among the mentally retarded is not unlike that for the "normal" population. Data indicates overuse of psychoactive substances to aid caretakers.

AGE-RELATED FACTORS
Pediatric: N/A
Geriatric: N/A
Others: N/A

PREGNANCY Patient and family should receive genetic evaluation and counseling as prenatal diagnosis is available

SYNONYMS
• Martin-Bell Syndrome
• Marker X Syndrome
• X-linked Mental Retardation

ICD-9-CM 758.9

SEE ALSO N/A

OTHER NOTES Extensive family history is mandatory

ABBREVIATIONS ADHD = Attention deficit disorder/hyperactivity disorder

REFERENCES
• Simensen, R.J. & Rogers, R.C.: Fragile X Syndrome. American Family Physician, 39(5): 185-193, 1989
• Hagerman, R.J. & McKenare, P.: 1992 Fragile X Conference Proceedings: The National Fragile X Foundation. Dillon, CO, Spectra Publishing Co., 1992

Author R. Simensen, Ph.D. & R. Rogers, M.D.

Frostbite

 BASICS

DESCRIPTION A localized complication of exposure to the cold, resulting in diminished blood flow to the affected part (especially hands, face or feet). Dehydration, enzymatic destruction and ultimately cell death occurs. In severe cases, deep tissue freezing may occur with damage to underlying blood vessels, muscles and nerve tissue.

System(s) affected: Endocrine/Metabolic, Skin/Exocrine

Genetics: N/A

Incidence/Prevalence in USA:
Approximately 4,800/year

Predominant age: All ages

Predominant sex: Male = Female

SIGNS AND SYMPTOMS

• Injured area first appears cold, hard, white and is anesthetic to touch. Progresses to blotchy-red, swollen and painful regions after rewarming.
• Loss of cutaneous sensation
• Numbness
• Throbbing pain
• Paresthesia
• Excessive sweating
• Joint pain
• Pallor
• Subcutaneous edema
• Hyperemia
• Blistering
• Blue discoloration
• Skin necrosis
• Gangrene

CAUSES

• Prolonged exposure to cold
• Refreezing thawed extremities

RISK FACTORS

• Impaired cerebral function
• Under the effects of alcohol or drug abuse
• Underlying psychiatric disturbance
• Ambient temperature less than 0°F
• Smoker
• Elderly
• Raynaud's phenomenon

 DIAGNOSIS

DIFFERENTIAL DIAGNOSIS Frostnip - superficial damp cold injury

LABORATORY

• Hemoconcentration
• Decreased hepatic function

Drugs that may alter lab results: N/A

Disorders that may alter lab results: N/A

PATHOLOGICAL FINDINGS

• Ice crystallization in the intravascular extracellular space
• Atrophy
• Fibroblastic proliferation
• Skin necrosis

SPECIAL TESTS ECG - bradycardia, atrial fibrillation, atrial flutter, ventricular fibrillation, diffuse T wave inversion

IMAGING N/A

DIAGNOSTIC PROCEDURES N/A

 TREATMENT

APPROPRIATE HEALTH CARE
Outpatient or inpatient, depending on severity

GENERAL MEASURES

• Emergency measures for patient without pulse or respiration. Such measures may include CPR and internal warming with warm IV's and warm oxygen (see hypothermia)
• Prevent refreezing. May be necessary to keep frostbitten part frozen until patient can be transported to a care facility.
• Treat for hypothermia
• Cautious rewarming. May immerse frozen body part for several minutes in water no hotter than 40-42°C (104-107°F).
• Keep patient dry. If conscious, give warm fluids with high sugar content.
• Amputation not to be considered until it is definite that tissues are dead. May take about 3 weeks to know if the tissue is permanently injured.
• Prevention of infection, once treatment begins
• Ongoing whirlpool therapy for cleansing and debridement

ACTIVITY

• As tolerated, protect injured body parts
• Initiate physical therapy once healing progresses sufficiently

DIET

• As tolerated
• Warm oral fluids

PATIENT EDUCATION

• Local library
• Exposure protection
• Early signs and symptoms of frostbite

MEDICATIONS

DRUG(S) OF CHOICE
• Warm IV fluids via central venous pressure (CVP) line
• Heated oxygen
• For myxedema coma - L Thyroxine 500 mcg IV plus 300 mg hydrocortisone
• Tetanus toxoid
• For severe pain - analgesics or narcotics
• Antibiotics may be required for infection
• Maintenance - gastric lavage, peritoneal dialysis, hemodialysis, and mediastinal lavage if needed

Contraindications: Refer to manufacturer's profile of each drug
Precautions: Refer to manufacturer's profile of each drug
Significant possible interactions: Refer to manufacturer's profile of each drug

ALTERNATIVE DRUGS N/A

FOLLOWUP

PATIENT MONITORING
• Preferably electronic probe for temperature monitoring
• Followup for physical therapy progress, infection, other complications

PREVENTION/AVOIDANCE
• Dress in layers with appropriate cold weather gear. Cover exposed areas and extremities appropriately.
• Proper preparation for trips to cold climates. Avoid alcohol.

POSSIBLE COMPLICATIONS
• Hyperglycemia
• Acidosis
• Refractory arrhythmias
• Tissue loss. Distal parts of an extremity may undergo spontaneous amputation.
• Gangrene
• Death

EXPECTED COURSE AND PROGNOSIS
• Anesthesia and bullae may occur
• The affected areas will heal or mummify without surgery. The process may take 6-12 months for healing. Patient may be sensitive to cold and experience burning and tingling.

MISCELLANEOUS

ASSOCIATED CONDITIONS Alcohol and/or drug abuse

AGE-RELATED FACTORS
Pediatric: Loss of epithelial growth centers
Geriatric:
• Associated disease states increase mortality
• Periarticular osteoporosis complicates
• More prone to hypothermia
Others: N/A

PREGNANCY Acidosis

SYNONYMS Dermatitis congelationis

ICD-9-CM 991.3

SEE ALSO N/A

OTHER NOTES N/A

ABBREVIATIONS N/A

REFERENCES
• Rakel, R.E.: Textbook of Family Practice. 3rd Ed. Philadelphia, W.B. Saunders Co., 1989
• Berkow, R., et al. (eds.): Merck Manual. 14th Ed. Rahway, NJ, Merck Sharp & Dohme, 1986
• Kelly, K.J., Glaeser, P., Rice, T.B. & Wendelberger, K.J.: Profound accidental hypothermia and freeze injury of the extremities in a child. In Critical Care Medicine. Baltimore, Williams & Wilkins, 1990
• Urschel, J.D.: Frostbite: Predisposing factors and predictors of poor outcome. In Trauma. Baltimore, Williams & Wilkins, 1990

Author T. Robinson, D.O. & R. Birrer, M.D.

Frozen shoulder

BASICS

DESCRIPTION Adhesive capsulitis which restricts shoulder motion in all directions. The disorder may complicate other inflammatory shoulder disorders.
System(s) affected: Musculoskeletal
Genetics: N/A
Incidence/Prevalence: Unknown
Predominant age: Middle aged and elderly
Predominant sex: Female > Male

SIGNS AND SYMPTOMS
• Decreased range of motion in all directions sometimes bilaterally
• Diffuse shoulder tenderness

CAUSES Alteration in the axillary fold of the shoulder capsule

RISK FACTORS
• Sedentary workers
• Immobilization
• Diabetes
• Peripheral vascular disease

DIAGNOSIS

DIFFERENTIAL DIAGNOSIS
• Infection
• Degenerative arthritis
• Pancoast's tumor
• Chronic posterior dislocation

LABORATORY   N/A
Drugs that may alter lab results: N/A
Disorders that may alter lab results: N/A

PATHOLOGICAL FINDINGS Morphologic changes of fibrosis and fibroplasia without inflammation

SPECIAL TESTS N/A

IMAGING Arthrogram (if used) - decreased redundancy in axillary folds and obliteration of the space in axillary region

DIAGNOSTIC PROCEDURES   N/A

TREATMENT

APPROPRIATE HEALTH CARE
Outpatient

GENERAL MEASURES
• Prophylactic physiotherapy
• Passive manipulation under general anesthesia and injection of steroids (controversial)
• Wearing a sling
• Application of heat
• Lastly, operative arthrotomy of the anterior inferior hanging axillary fold and subscapularis tendon
• Gentle passive and active assisted range-of-motion to tolerance

ACTIVITY No restrictions. Passive exercise of the shoulder. Avoid forceful manipulation of the shoulder joint during exercises.

DIET No restrictions

PATIENT EDUCATION Techniques for passive exercise

MEDICATIONS

DRUG(S) OF CHOICE
• NSAID's
• Corticosteroid injections (controversial)
Contraindications: Those of NSAID's
Precautions: Refer to manufacturer's literature
Significant possible interactions: Refer to manufacturer's literature

ALTERNATIVE DRUGS N/A

 FOLLOWUP

PATIENT MONITORING As needed

PREVENTION/AVOIDANCE Stretching, both active and passive

POSSIBLE COMPLICATIONS N/A

EXPECTED COURSE AND PROGNOSIS Persistence in exercise program shows improvement in motion and decreased pain over 6-18 months

 MISCELLANEOUS

ASSOCIATED CONDITIONS N/A

AGE-RELATED FACTORS
Pediatric: N/A
Geriatric: N/A
Others: N/A

PREGNANCY N/A

SYNONYMS Adhesive capsulitis

ICD-9-CM 726.0

SEE ALSO N/A

OTHER NOTES N/A

ABBREVIATIONS N/A

REFERENCES
• Rakel, R.E (ed.): Textbook of Family Practice, 4th Ed. Philadelphia, W.B. Saunders Co., 1990
• Parker, R.D., et al.: Frozen Shoulder Part I, Orthopedics, Volume 12, No.6, June, 1989

Author S. Jackson, M.D.

Furunculosis

 BASICS

DESCRIPTION
Acute abscess of a hair follicle due to infection by Staphylococcus aureus. Spreads away from hair follicle into surrounding dermis.
System(s) affected: Skin/Exocrine
Genetics: Unknown
Incidence in USA:
• Uncommon in children unless immunodeficiency state present (i.e., can appear in young girls with hyperimmunoglobulin E-Staphylococcal syndrome (Job's syndrome)
• Increase in frequency after puberty
Prevalence in USA: Common (exact numbers unknown)
Predominant age: Adolescents and young adults. Uncommon in young children unless immunodeficiency state present (i.e., can appear in young girls with hyperimmunoglobulin E-staphylococcal syndrome [Job's syndrome]).
Predominant sex: Males = Females

SIGNS AND SYMPTOMS
• Painful erythematous papules/nodules (1-5 cm) with central pustulation
• Located only in hirsute sites of body, especially areas prone to friction or minor trauma (i.e., underneath belt, anterior thighs)
• May be singular or multiple
• No fever or systemic symptoms
• Tender red perifollicular swelling, terminating in discharge of pus and necrotic plug
• Pus usually drains spontaneously

CAUSES
Pathogenic strain of Staphylococcus aureus

RISK FACTORS
• Carriage of pathogenic strain of Staphylococcus in nares, skin, axilla, and perineum
• Rarely, polymorphonuclear leukocyte defect or hyperimmunoglobulin-E/Staphylococcus abscess syndrome
• Diabetes mellitus, malnutrition, alcoholism
• Primary immunodeficiency disease (chronic granulomatous disease, Chediak-Higashi syndrome, C3 deficiency, C3 hypercatabolism, transient hypogammaglobulinemia of infancy, immunodeficiency with thymomoa, Wiskott-Aldrich syndrome)
• Secondary immunodeficiency (leukemia, leukopenia, neutropenia, therapeutic immunosuppression)

 DIAGNOSIS

DIFFERENTIAL DIAGNOSIS
• Folliculitis
• Pseudofolliculitis
• Carbuncles
• Ruptures Epidermal cyst

LABORATORY
Culture of abscess material
Drugs that may alter lab results:
Antibiotics
Disorders that may alter lab results: N/A

PATHOLOGICAL FINDINGS
Histopathologically - perifollicular necrosis containing fibrinoid material and neutrophils. At deep end of necrotic plug, in subcutaneous tissue, is a large abscess with a gram stain positive for small collections of staph aureus.

SPECIAL TESTS
None except for immunoglobulin levels in rare cases

IMAGING
N/A

DIAGNOSTIC PROCEDURES
Culture of abscess material

 TREATMENT

APPROPRIATE HEALTH CARE
Outpatient

GENERAL MEASURES
• Moist, warm compresses (provides comfort, encourages localization/pointing/drainage) 30 minutes, 4 times a day
• If pointing or large, incise and drain
• Consider packing to promote drainage
• Routine culture not necessary for localized abscess in non-diabetic patients with normal immune system
• Systemic antibiotics usually unnecessary, unless extensive surrounding cellulitis or fever
• If recurrent, problem usually related to chronic skin carriage of particular strain of Staphylococcus in nares or on skin. Treatment goals are to 1) decrease or eliminate pathogenic strain or 2) in very difficult cases, implant less aggressive strain.
<u>Suppression of pathogenic strain</u>
◊ Culture nares, skin, axilla, perineum
◊ Begin therapeutic antibiotic doses
◊ Wash entire body and fingernails (with nailbrush) daily for 1-3 weeks with Betadine, Hibiclens, or Phisohex soap (all can cause dry skin)
◊ After shower ointments
◊ Sanitary practices - change towels, washcloths and sheets daily; clean shaving instruments; avoid nose-picking; change wound dressings frequently
<u>Replacement of pathogenic strain with nonpathogenic strain (502A bacterial interference)</u>
◊ Culture nose and lesions to document pathogenic strain
◊ Culture family members if disease involves them
◊ Treat patient and infected household members with antibiotics
◊ Discontinue topical/oral antibiotics 48 hours then inoculate anterior nares with Staphylococcus aureus 502A (stock bacteria) (tilt head back, swab each anterior nares with 2 soaked cotton swabs of culture while patient sniffs material into nares and nasopharynx)
◊ Followup 1 month later; repeat process if abscesses not controlled

ACTIVITY
Avoid contact sports (i.e., wrestling) if active lesions. Otherwise no restrictions.

DIET
Unrestricted

PATIENT EDUCATION
Refer to: Habif, T.: Clinical Dermatology. 2nd Ed. St. Louis, C.V. Mosby, 1990

MEDICATIONS

DRUG(S) OF CHOICE

If abscesses multiple, if lesions have marked surrounding inflammation, or if immunocompromised
◊ Obtain culture and place on antibiotics for at least 14 days
◊ Cloxacillin (Tegopen) or dicloxacillin (Dynapen, Pathocil) 250 mg qid, or
◊ Erythromycin (E-mycin, PCE) 250-500 tid

Suppression of pathogenic strain
◊ Dicloxacillin or cloxacillin 250 mg qid x 21 days
◊ Erythromycin 250-500 mg tid (if penicillin allergic) x 21 days
◊ If above fails - begin 1-3 month course of antibiotics. May need to add rifampin 600 mg q day x 10 days
◊ After showering - bacitracin ointment or mupirocin to both anterior nares with cotton swab tid-qid x > 14 days

Replacement of pathogenic strain
◊ Treat patient and infected household members with dicloxacillin 250 mg qid or if child/infant with 50 mg/kg/day qid x 7-10 days

Contraindications:
• Cloxacillin and dicloxacillin - penicillin allergy
• Erythromycin, mupirocin - hypersensitivity

Precautions:
• Cloxacillin and dicloxacillin - anaphylactic reaction
• Erythromycin - cautious use in patients with impaired hepatic function; GI side effects especially abdominal cramping; pregnancy category B

Significant possible interactions:
Erythromycin - increases theophylline/carbamazepine levels; decreases warfarin clearance

ALTERNATIVE DRUGS N/A

FOLLOWUP

PATIENT MONITORING Instruct patient to see physician if compresses unsuccessful

PREVENTION/AVOIDANCE Patient education regarding self care (see General Measures section. Treatment and prevention are interrelated.)

POSSIBLE COMPLICATIONS
• Scarring
• Bacteremia
• Metastatic seeding (i.e., septal/valve defect, arthritic joint)

EXPECTED COURSE AND PROGNOSIS
• Self-limited (usually drains pus spontaneously and will heal with or without scarring within several days)
• Recurrent/chronic lasting for months or years

MISCELLANEOUS

ASSOCIATED CONDITIONS
• Usually normal immune system
• Diabetes mellitus
• Polymorphonuclear leukocyte defect (rare)
• Hyperimmunoglobulin-E/staphylococcal abscess syndrome (rare)
• See Risk factors for others

AGE-RELATED FACTORS
Pediatric: N/A
Geriatric: N/A
Others: Most common after puberty. Clusters have been reported in teenagers living in crowded quarters.

PREGNANCY N/A

SYNONYMS Boils

ICD-9-CM 680.9

SEE ALSO Folliculitis

OTHER NOTES
• If abscess culture grows gram negative bacteria or fungus then consider polymorphonuclear neutrophil (PMN) leukocyte function defect
• Hydradenitis suppurativa is a particular form of furunculosis
• Can order Staphylococcus aureus 502A from American Type Culture Collection, Rockville, Md.

ABBREVIATIONS N/A

REFERENCES
• Sams, Jr., W.M. & Lynch, P.: Principles and Practice of Dermatology. New York, Churchill Livingstone, 1990
• du Vivier, A.: Dermatology in Practice. Philadelphia, J.B. Lippincott Co., 1990
• Habif, T.: Clinical Dermatology. 2nd Ed. St. Louis, C.V. Mosby, 1990

Author P. Slomiany, M.D.

Galactorrhea

 BASICS

DESCRIPTION Milky nipple discharge. Galactorrhea technically does not include serous, purulent, or bloody nipple discharge.
System(s) affected: Endocrine/Metabolic
Genetics: N/A
Incidence/Prevalence in USA: 1-50% of non-pregnant, reproductive-aged women (studies vary widely)
Predominant age: Reproductive ages (15-50)
Predominant sex: Almost exclusively female

SIGNS AND SYMPTOMS
• Milky nipple discharge
• May also have signs/symptoms of associated conditions (e.g., hypothyroidism, Cushing's disease, acromegaly, fibrocystic breast disease)
• May also have signs/symptoms of pituitary enlargement (e.g., headache, visual field loss)

CAUSES
• Physiologic (pregnancy and up to 6 months after delivery or after stopping breast-feeding)
• Prolactin producing pituitary adenoma
• Medications (e.g., opioids, tricyclics, metoclopramide, verapamil, phenothiazines, alpha-methyldopa, isoniazid, estrogens, reserpine, butyrophenones)
• Oral contraceptive pill withdrawal
• Hypothyroidism
• Chest wall conditions (e.g., herpes zoster, post-thoracotomy, fibrocystic changes)
• Postoperative state (any major surgery, but especially oophorectomy)
• Chiari-Frommel (idiopathic galactorrhea more than 6 months postpartum)
• Idiopathic
• Miscellaneous causes (e.g., sarcoid, renal failure, Cushing's disease, cirrhosis, and head trauma)

RISK FACTORS Listed with Causes

 DIAGNOSIS

DIFFERENTIAL DIAGNOSIS
• Non-milky discharge (e.g., serous) - consider fibrocystic disease
• Purulent discharge - consider mastitis
• Bloody discharge - rule out breast malignancy

LABORATORY
• Check prolactin level and thyroid functions in all galactorrheic patients
• Check FSH/LH if also amenorrheic
• Check growth hormone (GH) and adrenal steroids, if clinically suspect acromegaly or Cushing's disease
Drugs that may alter lab results: See medications listed under Causes. Most of these cause galactorrhea by causing hyperprolactinemia.
Disorders that may alter lab results: N/A

PATHOLOGICAL FINDINGS N/A

SPECIAL TESTS Formal visual field testing if pituitary adenoma suspected

IMAGING
• Pituitary MRI if prolactin even minimally elevated, or if any other reason to suspect pituitary disease clinically
• CT only if MRI not available. Avoid "coned-down" or plain tomograms of pituitary as they are relatively insensitive.

DIAGNOSTIC PROCEDURES N/A

 TREATMENT

APPROPRIATE HEALTH CARE
Outpatient unless pituitary resection needed (very rare)

GENERAL MEASURES
• Treat underlying causes as indicated; galactorrhea by itself is not harmful
• Other reasons to treat include symptom management (if symptoms cause patient anxiety), fertility restoration (if amenorrheic), to cause growth retardation or regression of adenoma, or to prevent osteoporosis (if estrogen deficient)
• "Watchful waiting" is often most appropriate
• Large adenomas may be treated with x-ray therapy (variable success, 50% risk of panhyperpituitarism at 5 years) or transsphenoidal adenoma removal (90% success, 5% major complications)
• Discontinue offending medications, if any

ACTIVITY No restrictions

DIET No restrictions

PATIENT EDUCATION
• Discussion of treatment rationale and risks
• Discussion of symptoms of complications of growing pituitary adenoma (e.g., central headache, visual field loss)

MEDICATIONS

DRUG(S) OF CHOICE Bromocriptine (Parlodel). Start low at 2.5 mg daily, then increase as tolerated over several weeks to 2.5 mg tid.
Contraindications: Uncontrolled hypertension, sensitivity to any ergot alkaloids, preeclampsia
Precautions:
• Nausea (often dose limiting)
• Orthostasis
• Drowsiness
• Lightheadedness and syncope
• Hypertension (rare)
• Seizures (rare)
Significant possible interactions:
Dopamine agonists (e.g., phenothiazines, butyrophenones, others listed under Causes)

ALTERNATIVE DRUGS N/A

FOLLOWUP

PATIENT MONITORING
• Depends on etiology
• If hyperprolactinemic, check prolactin level every 6-12 months, formal visual field testing yearly, and MRI every 2-5 years, depending on clinical course

PREVENTION/AVOIDANCE N/A

POSSIBLE COMPLICATIONS
• Depends on underlying cause
• If pituitary adenoma, there is risk of permanent visual field loss

EXPECTED COURSE AND PROGNOSIS
• Depends on underlying cause
• Symptoms tend to recur after discontinuation of bromocriptine

MISCELLANEOUS

ASSOCIATED CONDITIONS See Causes

AGE-RELATED FACTORS
Pediatric: N/A
Geriatric: N/A
Others: N/A

PREGNANCY Adenomas can grow dramatically during pregnancy. Most galactorrhea during pregnancy is physiologic.

SYNONYMS
• Disordered lactation
• Nipple discharge

ICD-9-CM 676.6

SEE ALSO Hyperprolactinemia, pituitary adenoma

OTHER NOTES Can occur in males, but usually not unless/until they are extremely hyperprolactinemic

ABBREVIATIONS N/A

REFERENCES
• Kleinberg, D.L., Noel, G.H. & Frantz, A.G.: Galactorrhea: A study of 235 cases including 48 with pituitary tumors. N Engl J Med 296:589,1977
• Yen, S.S.C. & Jaffe, R.B. (eds.): Reproductive Endocrinology: Physiology, Pathophysiology, and Clinical Management Philadelphia, W.B. Saunders Co.,1986

Author G. Swain, M.D.

Gastric malignancy

 BASICS

DESCRIPTION Gastric malignancy may occur anywhere in the stomach, and the greater curvature. Infiltration to lymph nodes, omentum, lungs and liver is rapid. Uncommon in U.S. natives.
System(s) affected: Gastrointestinal
Genetics:
• 2 to 4 times more common in first degree relatives
• More common in people with blood group A
Incidence in USA: 9.6/100,000 (24,400 new cases per year)
Prevalence in USA: N/A
Predominant age: Over 55
Predominant sex: Male > Female (2:1)

SIGNS AND SYMPTOMS
• Chronic non-colicky abdominal pain (especially in epigastrium)
• Anorexia
• Pain unrelieved by antacids
• Pain exacerbated by food
• Pain relieved by fasting
• Dysphagia
• Nausea and vomiting
• Constipation
• Early satiety

CAUSES Unknown. Possible association with H. pylori infection.

RISK FACTORS
• Diet rich in additives (smoked, pickled or salted foods; highly spiced oriental foods)
• Achlorhydria
• Atrophic gastritis/intestinal metaplasia
• Pernicious anemia
• Prior gastric resection
• Smoking/tobacco abuse
• Ethnic background: Hispanic, Japanese, Chilean, Costa Rican. First or second generation Japanese, Chilean or Costa Rican in the United States.
• Polyps or dysplasia anywhere in alimentary canal
• Helicobacteria pylori infection
• Familial polyposis

 DIAGNOSIS

DIFFERENTIAL DIAGNOSIS
• Gastric lymphoma
• Peptic ulcer with or without hemorrhage
• Eosinophilic gastroenteritis
• Giant hypertrophic gastritis (Ménétrier's disease)
• Carcinoma of the colon
• Functional dyspepsia
• Carcinoma of body or tail of the pancreas
• Angiodysplasia of the colon
• GI sarcoidosis
• Small intestinal lymphoma
• Crohn's disease

LABORATORY
• Positive stool guaiac for blood
• Hemoglobin less than 12
• Hematocrit less than 35
• Albumin less than 3 gram/dl
Drugs that may alter lab results: N/A
Disorders that may alter lab results:
Pernicious anemia may cause a false positive pentagastrin test

PATHOLOGICAL FINDINGS
• Adenocarcinomas 90% (75% ulcerative gastric carcinomas, 10% polypoid, 15% diffuse infiltrative scirrhous [linitis plastica])
• Gastric lymphomas 6%
• Gastric sarcomas less than 4%

SPECIAL TESTS Pentagastrin test - stomach pH less than 6

IMAGING Double contrast upper GI study - barium filling defect

DIAGNOSTIC PROCEDURES Upper endoscopy for direct visualization, cytology and biopsy

 TREATMENT

APPROPRIATE HEALTH CARE
Inpatient

GENERAL MEASURES
• Surgical excision of the tumor with resection of the local lymph nodes offers the only chance for cure. Even patients who are not felt to have a curable lesion should be offered an attempt at surgical reduction of the tumor since it offers the best form of palliation and improves the likelihood of benefit if chemotherapy and/or radiation therapy is administered. Exception is a carcinoma of the gastric cardia.
Surgical procedures
◊ Radical subtotal gastrectomy with gastrojejunostomy or gastroduodenostomy is the usual treatment of choice. A large part of the stomach along with the greater and lesser omentum is removed en bloc. At times a splenectomy and distal pancreatectomy are also performed. Direct extensions are also excised.
◊ Total gastrectomy is indicated only if necessary to remove the local lesion
◊ Local excision for palliation of incurable lesion by resection of bleeding area or area of obstruction

ACTIVITY As tolerated

DIET Dependent on the surgical procedure. Supplemental feedings or total parenteral nutrition (TPN) may be necessary to insure adequate caloric intake.

PATIENT EDUCATION Contact local American Cancer Society
Cancer Research Institute Helpbook: What to Do If Cancer Strikes. FDR Station, Box 5199, New York, NY 10150-5199.

MEDICATIONS

DRUG(S) OF CHOICE Combination therapy of 5-fluorouracil and doxorubicin with mitomycin-C or cisplatin. Dosing of these drugs is very patient specific; refer to AHFS Drug Information, American Society of Hospital Pharmacists, 1990.

Contraindications:
• 5-fluorouracil: Poor nutritional state, depressed bone marrow function, serious infections, major surgery in last month
• Doxorubicin: Preexisting myelosuppression, impaired cardiac function
• Mitomycin-C: Platelet count less than 75,000/mm3, leukocyte count less than 3000/mm3, serum creatinine greater than 1.7 mg/dL, coagulation disorders, serious infections

Precautions:
• Myelosuppression can occur with any of these agents
• 5-fluorouracil: Stomatitis, gastrointestinal injury, alopecia
• Doxorubicin: Stomatitis, gastrointestinal injury, alopecia, cardiac toxicity
• Mitomycin-C: Renal toxicity, hypercalcemia, gastrointestinal injury, cardiac toxicity
• Cisplatin: Ototoxicity, renal tubular damage, hypomagnesemia, hypokalemia, hypocalcemia, hemorrhagic cystitis

Significant possible interactions:
• Cisplatin: Aminoglycosides may potentiate nephrotoxicity and ototoxicity
• Loop diuretics may potentiate ototoxicity

ALTERNATIVE DRUGS Radiation therapy is of little benefit due to the radioresistancy of gastric tumors and the high doses of radiation required. It does have use in the palliation of pain.

FOLLOWUP

PATIENT MONITORING Routine, frequent followup is necessary to monitor disease state, assess treatments, monitor for recurrence/metastasis, and assess nutritional status

PREVENTION/AVOIDANCE N/A

POSSIBLE COMPLICATIONS
• Metastatic disease (especially hepatic, cerebral and pulmonary)
• Anemia (especially pernicious)
• Pyloric stenosis

EXPECTED COURSE AND PROGNOSIS
• The prognosis for gastric carcinoma is not optimistic. Since most lesions do not produce symptoms until late in their course, gastric carcinomas are usually advanced at the time of diagnosis. Surgery offers the only chance for a cure.
• Overall 5 year survival rate 16% (if local disease only 53%, regional spread 16%, distant spread 2%)

MISCELLANEOUS

ASSOCIATED CONDITIONS
• Predisposed by giant hypertrophic gastritis (Ménétrier's disease)
• Predisposed by intestinal metaplasia of the stomach
• Atrophic gastritis

AGE-RELATED FACTORS
Pediatric: Rare
Geriatric: Prevalence greater
Others: N/A

PREGNANCY N/A

SYNONYMS Linitis plastica

ICD-9-CM 151.0-9

SEE ALSO Esophageal carcinoma

OTHER NOTES
• Patients in lower socioeconomic classes are at greater risk of developing gastric tumors
• Migrants from high incidence areas (such as Iceland, Chile or Japan) to low incidence areas maintain an increased risk while their offspring have an occurrence rate that corresponds to the new location

ABBREVIATIONS N/A

REFERENCES
• Braunwald, E., et al. (eds.): Harrison's Principles of Internal Medicine. 12th Ed. New York, McGraw-Hill, 1991
• Rubin, P.: Clinical Oncology for Medical Students and Physicians: A Multidisciplinary Approach. 6th Ed. New York, American Cancer Society, 1987

Author S. Henderson, M.D.

Gastritis

 BASICS

DESCRIPTION Inflammatory reaction in the stomach; typically involves the mucosa, seldom the full thickness of the stomach wall
• Patchy erythema of gastric mucosa: a common endoscopic finding; usually insignificant
• Erosive gastritis: a reaction to mucosal injury by a noxious chemical agent, e.g., drugs (especially NSAIDs) or alcohol
• Reflux gastritis: a reaction to protracted reflux exposure to bile and pancreatic juice, usually associated with a defective pylorus; typically limited to the prepyloric antrum
• Hemorrhagic gastritis (stress ulceration): a reaction to hemodynamic disorder, viz., hypovolemia or hypoxia (as in shock). Also, very common in intensive care units (ICU).
• Infectious gastritis: commonly associated with Helicobacter pylori (whether infection by this organism is opportunistic or an actual cause of gastritis is uncertain); viral infection, usually as a component of systemic infection, is common; significant infection by other specific microbes is rare
• Gastric mucosal atrophy, sometimes called atrophic gastritis: frequent, in varying degrees, in the elderly; invariable in primary (pernicious) anemia
System(s) affected: Gastrointestinal
Genetics: Unknown (except, probably, for gastric mucosa atrophy)
Incidence/Prevalence in USA: N/A
Predominant age: All ages can be affected; an estimated 60% of persons older than 60 years harbor H. pylori in their gastric mucosa, but in only a small fraction is this a significant infection
Predominant sex: Male = Female

SIGNS AND SYMPTOMS
• Nondescript epigastric distress, often aggravated by eating
• Anorexia
• Nausea, with or without vomiting
• Significant bleeding is unusual except in hemorrhagic gastritis

CAUSES
• Alcohol
• Aspirin and other nonsteroidal anti-inflammatory drugs
• Bile reflux
• Pancreatic enzyme reflux
• Stress (hypovolemia or hypoxia)
• Radiation
• Staphylococcus aureus exotoxins
• Bacterial infection
• Viral infection
• Pernicious anemia
• Gastric mucosal atrophy

RISK FACTORS
• Age over 60
• Exposure to potentially noxious drugs or chemical agents
• Hypovolemia, hypoxia (shock)

 DIAGNOSIS

DIFFERENTIAL DIAGNOSIS
• Functional gastrointestinal disorder
• Peptic ulcer disease
• Linitis plastica

LABORATORY Usually unremarkable, except when blood loss results in anemia
Drugs that may alter lab results: N/A
Disorders that may alter lab results: N/A

PATHOLOGICAL FINDINGS Acute or chronic inflammatory infiltrate in gastric mucosa, often with distortion or erosion of adjacent epithelium. Presence of H. pylori may be confirmed.

SPECIAL TESTS
• 13C-urea breath test (for H. pylori)
• ELISA for anti-H. pylori immunoglobulin G
• Gastric acid analysis may be abnormal but is not a reliable indicator of gastritis

IMAGING Radiography is not a reliable indicator of gastritis

DIAGNOSTIC PROCEDURES
Gastroscopy, usually with biopsy, is essential for a precise diagnosis

 TREATMENT

APPROPRIATE HEALTH CARE
Outpatient, except for severe hemorrhagic gastritis

GENERAL MEASURES
• No specific therapy for gastritis (with the exception of C. pylori infection)
• Parenteral fluid and electrolyte supplements required if vomiting prevents food intake

ACTIVITY Usually no restriction

DIET Restriction, if any, depends on severity of symptoms (e.g., light, soft diet)

PATIENT EDUCATION Explanation, reassurance

MEDICATIONS

DRUG(S) OF CHOICE
• Antacids - best given in liquid form, 30mL 1 hour after meals and at bedtime; useful mainly as an emollient
• H-2 receptor antagonists e.g., cimetidine (Tagamet) - "priming" dose of 300mg IV, then a steady infusion of 37.5-75mg per hour, dissolved in the running fluid. Patients less severely ill - oral cimetidine 300mg q6h (or ranitidine [Zantac] or famotidine [Pepcid] or nizatidine [Axid]). Not shown to be clearly superior to antacids.
• Sucralfate (Carafate) 1 g q4-6h on an empty stomach. Rationale uncertain, but empirically helpful.
• Prostaglandins (e.g., misoprostol [Cytotec]), can help allay gastric mucosal injury, suggested dosage of 100-200mcg qid
• To eradicate H. pylori, "triple therapy" is advised, viz., bismuth (as Pepto-Bismol) 30mL liquid or 2 tablets qid for 4 weeks) plus metronidazole 250mg qid for the first week, plus tetracycline 250mg qid or amoxicillin 250mg tid for 2-4 weeks
Contraindications: Hypersensitivity to the drug(s)
Precautions:
• If bismuth is prescribed, warn patient of black stools
• Refer to manufacturer's profile of each drug
Significant possible interactions: Refer to manufacturer's profile of each drug

ALTERNATIVE DRUGS   N/A

FOLLOWUP

PATIENT MONITORING   Gastroscopy
should be repeated after 6 weeks if gastritis has been severe or if symptomatic response to treatment has not been achieved

PREVENTION/AVOIDANCE
• Patients should be warned of known or potentially injurious drugs or chemical agents
• Patients liable to hypovolemia or hypoxia (especially patients confined to an intensive care ward) should receive prophylactic therapy

POSSIBLE COMPLICATIONS   Bleeding
from extensive mucosal erosion or ulceration

EXPECTED COURSE AND PROGNOSIS
• Most cases clear spontaneously when the cause has been identified and allayed
• Recurrence of H. pylori infection may require a repeated course of treatment

MISCELLANEOUS

ASSOCIATED CONDITIONS
• Gastric or duodenal peptic ulcer
• Primary (pernicious) anemia

AGE-RELATED FACTORS
Pediatric: Gastritis rarely occurs in infants or children
Geriatric: Persons over 60 often harbor apparently harmless H. pylori infection
Others: N/A

PREGNANCY   N/A

SYNONYMS
• Erosive gastritis
• Reflux gastritis
• Hemorrhagic gastritis
• Gastritis, acute

ICD-9-CM   535.5 (unless otherwise specified)

SEE ALSO   N/A

OTHER NOTES   N/A

ABBREVIATIONS
NSAIDs = nonsteroidal anti-inflammatory drugs

REFERENCES
• Richardson, C.T.: Gastritis. In Cecil Textbook of Medicine. Edited by J.B. Wyngaarden, and L.H. Smith, Jr. Philadelphia, W. B. Saunders Co., 1988; pp 689-692
• Graham, D.Y., Malaty, H.M., Evans, D.G., et al.: Epidemiology of Helicobacter pylori in an asymptomatic population in the US. Gastroenterology. 100:1495-1501, 1991
• Zinner, M.J., Rypins, E.B., Martin, L.R., et al.: Misoprostol versus antacid titration for preventing stress ulcers in postoperative surgical ICU patients. Ann Surg. 210:590-595, 1989

Author   W. Haubrich, M.D.

Gastroesophageal reflux disease

BASICS

DESCRIPTION Reflux of gastroduodenal contents into the esophagus with or without esophageal inflammation
System(s) affected: Gastrointestinal
Genetics: N/A
Incidence in USA: Increasing
Prevalence in USA: Recent Gallup surveys reveal 65% of adults have suffered heartburn and 24% have had symptoms for more than 10 years. 17% of adults use indigestion aids at least once weekly, and only 24% of sufferers have consulted a physician. Children affected 1/300-1000; 30-80% of pregnant women report heartburn.
Predominant age: All ages
Predominant sex: Male = Female

SIGNS AND SYMPTOMS
• Heartburn (pyrosis) 70-85%
• Regurgitation 60%
• Dysphagia (suggests possible stricture) 15-20%
• Angina-like chest pain 33%
• Bronchospasm 15-20%
• Laryngitis (dysphonia)
• Globus sensation
• In infants: Recurrent emesis, failure to thrive, apnea syndrome

CAUSES
• Inappropriate relaxation of lower esophageal sphincter (LES) (idiopathic, food- or drug-related)
• Pregnancy (progestational hormones cause decreased LES pressure)
• Scleroderma (reduced esophageal motility and incompetent LES)
• Chalasia of infancy
• Delayed gastric emptying (impaired acid clearance)
• Acid hypersecretion (e.g., Zollinger-Ellison syndrome)
• Heller's myotomy for achalasia (30% develop reflux)

RISK FACTORS
• Foods that lower LES pressure (high-fat content, yellow onions, chocolate, peppermint)
• Foods that irritate esophageal mucosa (citrus fruits, spicy tomato drinks)
• Hiatal hernia - acid trapping
• Cigarette smoking
• Excessive alcohol
• Coffee
• Medications that lower LES pressure (e.g., theophylline, anticholinergics, progesterone, calcium channel blockers (nifedipine, verapamil), alpha adrenergic agents, diazepam, meperidine
• Indwelling nasogastric tube
• Chest trauma
• In children: Down's syndrome, mental retardation, cerebral palsy, repaired tracheoesophageal fistula

DIAGNOSIS

DIFFERENTIAL DIAGNOSIS
• Infectious esophagitis (candida, herpes, cytomegalovirus)
• Chemical esophagitis (lye ingestion)
• Radiation injury
• Crohn's disease
• Angina pectoris
• Esophageal carcinoma
• Pill-induced esophagitis (e.g., doxycycline, quinidine, potassium chloride, etc.)
• Achalasia
• Ulcer disease

LABORATORY N/A
Drugs that may alter lab results: N/A
Disorders that may alter lab results: N/A

PATHOLOGICAL FINDINGS
• Acute inflammation
• Hyperplasia (thickening) of the basal zone of the epithelium seen in 85%
• Lengthening of vascular channels within vascular papillae so that they approach the luminal surface
• Barrett's epithelial change - gastric columnar epithelium (intestinal metaplasia) migrates upward into the distal esophagus; may be associated with strictures and peptic ulceration; dysplasia and malignant transformation

SPECIAL TESTS
• Esophageal pH monitoring (antacids, H2 blockers, proton pump inhibitors and other antisecretory agents can give false negative pH monitoring)
• Esophageal manometry (anticholinergics, theophylline, calcium channel blockers, meperidine, diazepam may give falsely low LES pressure on manometry)
• Acid perfusion (Bernstein) test
• Gastric analysis

IMAGING
• Barium swallow: Presence of a sliding hiatal hernia appears to be a predictor of reflux esophagitis; mucosal irregularity due to inflammation and edema; prominent longitudinal folds, erosions, ulcers; smoothly tapered strictures; pseudodiverticula
• Radionuclide scintigraphy

DIAGNOSTIC PROCEDURES
• Endoscopy:

Grade	Finding
0	normal
I	erythema, friability
II	nonconfluent erosions
III	confluent erosions, exudate
IV	ulceration, stricture

Grade	% pts with grade
0	22
I	32
II	30
III	12
IV	4

• Barrett's change suspected when salmon-colored mucosa extends > 2 cm above normal squamocolumnar junction (seen in up to 10%).
• Mucosal biopsy
• Cytology for Barrett's dysplasia. (flow cytometry useful adjunct when available)
• Metoclopramide may give falsely negative gastric emptying results

TREATMENT

APPROPRIATE HEALTH CARE
• Outpatient diagnosis (typical heartburn history has a positive predictive value of >80% and warrants empiric therapy in absence of alarm symptoms)
• Inpatient if surgery indicated.

GENERAL MEASURES
• Elevate head of bed, avoid lying down directly after meals
• Avoid stooping, bending, tight-fitting garments
• Avoid drugs causing decreased LES pressure
• Weight loss
• Avoid voluntary eructation
Stepped therapy
  ◊ Phase I - lifestyle and diet modifications plus antacids
  ◊ Phase II - H2 blockers
  ◊ Phase III - 1) high-dose H2 blocker or omeprazole or 2) H2 blockers plus cisapride, metoclopramide or sucralfate
  ◊ Phase IV - surgery

ACTIVITY Full activity

DIET Avoid chocolate, peppermint, onions, high-fat foods, alcohol, tobacco, coffee, citrus juices

PATIENT EDUCATION Patient educational materials available from Digestive Diseases Clearinghouse, Suite 600, 1555 Wilson Blvd., Rosslyn, VA 22209. (212)685-3440

Gastroesophageal reflux disease

MEDICATIONS

DRUG(S) OF CHOICE
• Mild to moderate disease: H2 blockers in equipotent oral doses, e.g., cimetidine (Tagamet) 800 mg bid or 400 mg qid, or ranitidine (Zantac) 150 bid, or famotidine (Pepcid) 20 mg bid - 40 mg q hs, or nizatidine (Axid) 150 mg bid. Expected endoscopic healing rates 30-50% at 6 weeks, 50-80% at 12 weeks.
• Erosive esophagitis: Zantac 150 qid, Pepcid 40 mg bid, Tagamet 800 bid or 400 qid for up to 12 weeks
• Severe disease (refractory to initial therapy): Omeprazole (Prilosec) 20-40 mg daily or higher-dose H2 blockers (e.g., ranitidine 150 mg qid)
Contraindications: Known hypersensitivity to H2 blockers, omeprazole
Precautions:
• Use half-strength therapy for renal failure
• Avoid cimetidine when potentially interacting drugs are co-administered (or closely monitor prothrombin time or serum levels)
• Omeprazole approved only for short-term use (6-12 weeks)
Significant possible interactions:
• Cimetidine interacts with > 60 drugs (e.g., theophylline, warfarin, phenytoin, lidocaine). Refer to manufacturer's profile.
• Omeprazole may prolong the elimination of diazepam, warfarin and phenytoin

ALTERNATIVE DRUGS
• Antacids; alginates (Gaviscon)
• Metoclopramide (Reglan) 5-10 mg before meals used adjunctively with H2 blockers (neuropsychiatric side effects in 30%)
• Bethanechol (Urecholine) used adjunctively with H2 blocker (cholinergic side effects common)
• Cisapride 10 mg qid

FOLLOWUP

PATIENT MONITORING Follow symptomatically; repeat endoscopy at 6-12 weeks for poor symptomatic response; annual endoscopy and biopsy for Barrett's esophagus (to detect dysplasia)

PREVENTION/AVOIDANCE
• Long-term maintenance therapy with H2 blockers along with lifestyle and diet modifications to prevent symptomatic relapse
• Annual endoscopy, biopsy and cytology to detect dysplasia in Barrett's epithelium
• Peptic strictures may require periodic dilatation
• Omeprazole 10-20mg daily is very effective but long-term safety remains controversial
• Antireflux surgery should be considered for patients with severe disease in lieu of chronic drug therapy

POSSIBLE COMPLICATIONS
• Peptic stricture (10-15%)
• Hemorrhage (3%)
• Barrett's esophagus (10%)
• Pulmonary or ear, nose, throat complications (5-10%)
• Noncardiac chest pain
• Adenocarcinoma from Barrett's epithelium

EXPECTED COURSE AND PROGNOSIS
• Majority of patients respond well to BID H2 blocker therapy
• Symptoms and esophageal inflammation often return promptly when treatment withdrawn
• Relapse prevention therapy with H2 blockers/omeprazole often requires the acute healing dose be maintained
• Antireflux surgery (e.g., fundoplication) for complications or "refractory" disease; excellent short-term results but long-term followup is relatively limited
• Regression of Barrett's epithelium does not routinely occur despite adequate medical or surgical therapy

MISCELLANEOUS

ASSOCIATED CONDITIONS
• Reflux-induced asthma
• Pulmonary aspiration
• Chronic cough/throat clearing
• Loss of dental enamel
• Halitosis
• Laryngitis
• Globus sensation
• Vocal cord granulomas

AGE-RELATED FACTORS
Pediatric:
• Reflux symptoms generally resolve by age 18 months
• Vomiting, weight loss, failure to thrive more common than heartburn
• Positional treatment = use of infant seat for 2-3 hours after meals; thickened feedings
• Drug treatment = antacids or liquid H2 blockers (e.g., Zantac syrup)
• Surgical therapy for severe symptoms (apnea, choking, persistent vomiting) is successful in 85-95%
Geriatric: Complications more likely
Others: N/A

PREGNANCY
• Heartburn (when first experienced): 52% in first trimester, 24% in second trimester, and 9% in third trimester
• Tends to recur in subsequent pregnancies
• Symptomatic therapy includes multiple small meals, avoid lying down for 2-3 hours after meals, elevating the head of the bed at night
• Antacids or H2 blockers are probably safe in the 3rd trimester

SYNONYMS
• Reflux esophagitis
• Peptic esophagitis
• Barrett's esophagus
• Symptomatic hiatal hernia

ICD-9-CM
• Esophagitis 530.1
• Hiatal hernia 750.6
• Heartburn 787.1

SEE ALSO
• Peptic ulcer disease
• Esophageal tumors

OTHER NOTES Alkaline (bile) reflux accounts for up to 15% of Barrett's esophagus and severe esophagitis

ABBREVIATIONS
LES = lower esophageal sphincter
GER = Gastroesophageal reflux
GERD = Gastroesophageal reflux disease

REFERENCES
• McCallum, R.W. & Mittal, R.K., (eds.): Gastroesophageal reflux disease. In Gastroenterology Clinics of North America, September 1990; 19:3
• Tytgat, G.N.J., Bianchi-Porro, G., Feussner, H., et al.: Long-term strategy for the treatment of gastro-oesophageal reflux disease. In Gastroenterology International, 1991; 4:21-32
• Koufman, J.A.: The otolaryngologic manifestations of gastroesophageal reflux disease (GERD). In Laryngoscope, 1991; 101(Suppl. 53):1-78
• Sontag SJ. Rolling review: gastroesophageal reflux disease. Aliment Pharmacol Ther 1993; 7:293-312.

Author J. Lewis, M.D.

Giant cell arteritis

 BASICS

DESCRIPTION
A systemic granulomatous large vessel arteritis, most commonly affecting the branches of the cranial arteries, (but may involve other aortic branches), seen primarily in the elderly. Frequently associated with polymyalgia rheumatica (PMR).

System(s) affected:
Hemic/Lymphatic/Immunologic, Cardiovascular

Genetics: May be important, several family clusters have been identified

Incidence/Prevalence in USA: More common in northern latitudes: 15-30/100,000 person over 50/year, vs. southern latitudes (less than 2/100,000 in some series). Primarily Caucasians.

Predominant age: 60 years or older (very rare under 50). Incidence increases with age.

Predominant sex: Female > Male (4:1)

SIGNS AND SYMPTOMS
• Onset may be abrupt or insidious over months

Local
◊ Headache - usually unilateral temporal, may be generalized or occipital
◊ Jaw/tongue "claudication" upon mastication
◊ Visual disturbances (i.e., amaurosis, scotoma, diplopia, blindness)
◊ Scalp tenderness
◊ Ischemic optic neuritis
◊ Swollen, red temporal artery
◊ Decreased temporal artery pulse (may be increased early)

Systemic
◊ Polymyalgia rheumatica - seen in 40-60%
◊ Fever (low grade)
◊ Fatigue/malaise
◊ Weight loss
◊ Anorexia
◊ Arthralgias

CAUSES
• Etiology unknown
• Possibly immunologic mechanism

RISK FACTORS
• Age over 50
• Presence of polymyalgia rheumatica

 DIAGNOSIS

DIFFERENTIAL DIAGNOSIS
• Cerebral vasculitides
• Other causes of headache (tumor, sinusitis, cervical or temporomandibular joint arthritis)
• Cerebral vascular insufficiency
• Other connective tissue disease

LABORATORY
• ESR (Westergren) usually greater than 50
• ESR may be normal in 10% of patients
• Elevated alkaline phosphatase over 1.5 x normal (unusual)
• Elevated aspartate aminotransferase (AST) over 1.5 x normal (unusual)
• Anemia - mild to moderate, normochromic/normocytic
• Mild leukocytosis
• Mild thrombocytosis

Drugs that may alter lab results:
Prednisone

Disorders that may alter lab results: N/A

PATHOLOGICAL FINDINGS
Inflammatory infiltrate (either mononuclear cells or granulomas with giant multinucleated cells) seen in the intima and media of large vessels with resultant disruption of the internal elastic lamina. Lesions may be isolated (i.e., skip lesions).

SPECIAL TESTS   N/A

IMAGING
Temporal arteriography (in a few selected cases)

DIAGNOSTIC PROCEDURES
Temporal artery biopsy
◊ Minimum 2.5 cm segment of vessel with serial sections
◊ Within 72 hours of starting steroids
◊ If negative, must consider biopsy of contralateral artery

 TREATMENT

APPROPRIATE HEALTH CARE
• Inpatient (or outpatient surgery) initially for temporal artery biopsy. Outpatient subsequently.
• If there is a high index of suspicion, immediately institute corticosteroid therapy while arranging temporal artery biopsy

GENERAL MEASURES   N/A

ACTIVITY   Ambulatory ad lib

DIET
• Appropriate salt restriction
• Adequate calcium intake
• Watch serum glucose

PATIENT EDUCATION
• Precautions regarding steroid use
• Exacerbation of disease with medication dose adjustment

MEDICATIONS

DRUG(S) OF CHOICE
Prednisone - early:
◊ 60 mg prednisone/d; divided dose initially, then single morning dose (never use every other day steroids)
◊ Begin slow taper after 4 weeks if asymptomatic and ESR decreased (occasionally patient may not normalize ESR)
Prednisone - taper:
◊ Taper initially by 5 mg every 2 weeks to dose of 10-15 mg if above guidelines are met. (Must be individualized).
◊ Continue 10-15 mg daily for several months-year, with periodic attempts to taper (i.e., every 3-6 months) by 1 or 2 mg
◊ Use symptoms and ESR to help guide taper
◊ Average time to disease remission 3-4 years, range 1-10 years
Contraindications: Systemic fungal infections.
Relative contraindications: Avoid if possible in patients with congestive heart failure, diabetes mellitus, systemic fungal or bacterial infection (must treat infection concurrently if steroids are necessary).
Precautions:
Long term steroid use
◊ Associated with several potentially severe adverse effects, including: Increased susceptibility to infection, glucose intolerance, adrenal suppression, muscle wasting, osteoporosis, peptic ulcer disease, sodium and water retention, cataracts, avascular necrosis, GI bleeding, psychosis, weight gain
◊ Use lowest possible dose for shortest duration
◊ Upon discontinuing, if the patient has received long-term therapy, taper slowly to avoid Addisonian crisis
Significant possible interactions: Refer to manufacturer's literature

ALTERNATIVE DRUGS
Cytotoxic agents only if patient cannot use steroids (brittle diabetes mellitus, severe osteoporosis, congestive heart failure etc.) or fails to respond to steroids

FOLLOWUP

PATIENT MONITORING
• ESR - repeat at monthly intervals initially and while tapering, then every 3 months
• Follow visual/constitutional symptoms monthly initially, then as needed

PREVENTION/AVOIDANCE N/A

POSSIBLE COMPLICATIONS
• Complications related to steroids
• Exacerbation of disease during therapy or taper

EXPECTED COURSE AND PROGNOSIS
• With early treatment, resolution of symptoms and preservation of vision
• Average length of disease 3-4 years
• With no treatment, high risks of blindness and stroke

MISCELLANEOUS

ASSOCIATED CONDITIONS
Polymyalgia rheumatica

AGE-RELATED FACTORS
Pediatric: Does not occur in this age group
Geriatric: Incidence increases with age (twice as common in patients over 80 as it is in 50-59 age group)
Others: N/A

PREGNANCY N/A

SYNONYMS N/A

ICD-9-CM 446.5 giant cell arteritis

SEE ALSO Polymyalgia rheumatica

OTHER NOTES Westergren ESR is preferable. If other ESR used (i.e. Wintrobe or ZSR) then cannot use the listed guidelines for abnormalities

ABBREVIATIONS GCA=Giant cell arteritis
• TA = temporal arteritis

REFERENCES
• Hunder, G.G.: Giant Cell Arteritis and Polymyalgia Rheumatica. In Textbook of Rheumatology. 3rd Ed. Edited by W.N. Kelly, E.D. Harris, S. Ruddy & C.B. Sledge. Philadelphia, W.B. Saunders Co., 1989
• Hunder, G.G. et al.: The American College of Rheumatology 1990 Criteria for the Classification of Giant Cell Arteritis. In Arthritis Rheum,1990;33:1122-1128

Author B. Walsh, D.O. & E. Gall, M.D.

Giardiasis

BASICS

DESCRIPTION Intestinal infection caused by the protozoan parasite, Giardia lamblia. Infection results from ingestion of the cysts that excyst into trophozoites which colonize the small intestine and cause the symptoms. The cycle is continued when the trophozoites encyst in the small intestine and water, food, or hands are contaminated by feces of the infected person. Most infections result from fecal-oral transmission or ingestion of contaminated water, less commonly from contaminated food.
System(s) affected: Gastrointestinal
Genetics: N/A
Incidence/Prevalence in USA: 5% of patients with stools submitted for ova and parasite exams. Overall prevalence is lower and variable.
Predominant age: All ages, but most common in early childhood
Predominant sex: Slightly more common in males

SIGNS AND SYMPTOMS
• Approximately 25-50% of infected persons are symptomatic
• Chronic diarrhea (lasting more than 5-7 days and frequently weeks)
• Abdominal bloating
• Flatulence
• Loose, greasy, foul-smelling stools
• Weight loss
• Nausea
• Lactose intolerance

CAUSES Protozoan parasite (Giardia lamblia) infection acquired through fecal-oral transmission or ingestion of contaminated water, less commonly from contaminated food

RISK FACTORS
• Day care centers
• Male homosexuality
• Wilderness camping

DIAGNOSIS

DIFFERENTIAL DIAGNOSIS
• Includes other etiologies of small intestinal diarrhea
• Infectious causes include cryptosporidiosis, isosporiasis
• Other causes of malabsorption includes celiac sprue, tropical sprue, bacterial overgrowth syndromes, Crohn's ileitis
• Irritable bowel is suspected when diarrhea is not accompanied by weight loss

LABORATORY
• Stool for ova and parasites, repeated 3 times if necessary. Cysts are seen in fixed or fresh stools and occasionally, trophozoites are found in fresh diarrheal stools.
• Fluorescent antibody and ELISA tests are available
Drugs that may alter lab results: A number of drugs interfere with stool exams
Disorders that may alter lab results: N/A

PATHOLOGICAL FINDINGS Intestinal biopsy shows flattened, mild lymphocytic infiltration and trophozoites on the surface.

SPECIAL TESTS String test (Enterotest). A gelatin capsule on a string is swallowed and left in the duodenum for several hours or overnight.

IMAGING N/A

DIAGNOSTIC PROCEDURES
Esophagogastroduodenoscopy with biopsy and sample of small intestinal fluid.

TREATMENT

APPROPRIATE HEALTH CARE
Outpatient for mild cases, inpatient if symptoms are severe

GENERAL MEASURES
• Medical therapy for all infected individuals
• Fluid replacement if dehydrated

ACTIVITY As tolerated

DIET Good nutrition, low lactose, low fat

PATIENT EDUCATION Avoidance of risk factors

Giardiasis

MEDICATIONS

DRUG(S) OF CHOICE Quinacrine (Atabrine) 100 mg tid for 5-7 days, or metronidazole (Flagyl) 250 mg tid for 5-7 days
Contraindications: Both are relatively contraindicated in pregnancy, especially first trimester
Precautions:
• Rare toxic psychosis with quinacrine
• Theoretical risk of carcinogenesis with metronidazole
Significant possible interactions: Occasional disulfiram reaction with metronidazole

ALTERNATIVE DRUGS
• Furazolidone 8 mg/kg/day tid for 10 days (slightly less effective, but commonly used in pediatrics because it is well tolerated)
• Paromomycin (Humatin), a nonabsorbable aminoglycoside which is probably less effective, but commonly recommended in pregnancy because of theoretical risk of teratogenicity of other agents

FOLLOWUP

PATIENT MONITORING Symptoms, weight, stool exams

PREVENTION/AVOIDANCE Good hand washing when caring for diapered children, water purification when camping

POSSIBLE COMPLICATIONS Those of malabsorption and weight loss

EXPECTED COURSE AND PROGNOSIS Untreated giardiasis lasts for weeks. Patients usually (90%) respond to treatment within a few days and most of the non-responders or relapses respond to a second course with the same or a different agent.

MISCELLANEOUS

ASSOCIATED CONDITIONS Hypogammaglobulinemia and possibly IgA deficiency. The diarrhea is more severe and prolonged in these patients.

AGE-RELATED FACTORS
Pediatric: Most common in early childhood
Geriatric: N/A
Others: N/A

PREGNANCY Concern for potential teratogenicity of medications. Consult infectious disease specialist or gastroenterologist for symptomatic disease.

SYNONYMS N/A

ICD-9-CM 007.1 Giardiasis

SEE ALSO N/A

OTHER NOTES G. lamblia is also called G. duodenalis, G. intestinalis

ABBREVIATIONS N/A

REFERENCES
• Fedorak, R.N. & Rubinoff, M.J.: Basic Investigation of a Patient with Diarrhea. In Diarrheal Diseases. Edited by M. Field. New York, Elsevier Science Publishing Co., Inc., 1991
• Adam R. D.: The Biology of Giardia spp. Microbiol, Rev 1991; 55:706-732
• Hill, D.R.: Giardia lamblia. In Principles and Practice of Infectious Diseases. 3rd Ed. Edited by G.L. Mandell, R.G. Douglas & J.E. Bennett. New York, Churchill Livingstone, 1990

Author R. Adam, M.D.

Gilbert's disease

 BASICS

DESCRIPTION Mild chronic or intermittent unconjugated hyperbilirubinemia (not due to hemolysis) with otherwise normal liver function
System(s) affected:
Hemic/Lymphatic/Immunologic
Genetics: Data suggests an autosomal dominant inheritance with variable expression
Incidence/Prevalence in USA: About 7% of the population
Predominant age: Present from birth, but most often presents in the second or third decade of life; heterozygous for single abnormal gene
Predominant sex: Male > Female (2-7:1)

SIGNS AND SYMPTOMS No significant symptoms have been attributed to this disorder, although a variety of nonspecific symptoms have been described. There are no abnormal physical findings other than occasional mild jaundice

CAUSES The hyperbilirubinemia results from impaired hepatic bilirubin clearance (approximately 30% of normal). Hepatic bilirubin conjugation (glucuronidation) is reduced, though this is likely not the only defect.

RISK FACTORS None

 DIAGNOSIS

DIFFERENTIAL DIAGNOSIS Hemolysis, ineffective erythropoiesis (megaloblastic anemias, certain porphyrias, thalassemia major, sideroblastic anemia, severe lead poisoning, congenital dyserythropoietic anemias), cirrhosis, chronic persistent hepatitis, pancreatitis or biliary tract disease

LABORATORY
• Bilirubin: less than 6 mg/dL and usually less than 3 mg/dL, virtually all unconjugated
• CBC with peripheral smear is normal
• Reticulocyte count is normal
• Liver function tests (SGOT, SGPT, alkaline phosphatase, GGT) are normal
• Fasting and postprandial serum bile acids are normal
• Up to 60% of patients have clinically insignificant mild hemolysis which frequently can only be detected with sophisticated red cell survival studies
Drugs that may alter lab results: Bilirubin level may be raised by nicotinic acid and lowered by phenobarbital
Disorders that may alter lab results: Bilirubin levels increase during fasting, and may increase during a febrile illness

PATHOLOGICAL FINDINGS None

SPECIAL TESTS None

IMAGING N/A

DIAGNOSTIC PROCEDURES
• A liver biopsy is not usually needed to exclude other diagnoses
• Some clinicians recommend confirming the diagnosis by reducing daily caloric intake to 400 kcal for 48 hours, which results in a two to threefold increase in unconjugated bilirubin

 TREATMENT

APPROPRIATE HEALTH CARE
Outpatient. The most important treatment is to make a positive diagnosis of Gilbert's disease to reassure the patient and prevent further unnecessary procedures

GENERAL MEASURES None

ACTIVITY Full activity

DIET Normal

PATIENT EDUCATION Reassure the patient that the condition is benign with no known sequelae

MEDICATIONS

DRUG(S) OF CHOICE N/A
Contraindications: N/A
Precautions: N/A
Significant possible interactions: N/A

ALTERNATIVE DRUGS N/A

FOLLOWUP

PATIENT MONITORING If history, physical examination, and laboratory tests are normal, see the patient on two or three further occasions during the ensuing 12 to 18 months. If the patient develops no symptoms, reticulocytosis or new liver function abnormalities, make the diagnosis of Gilbert's disease.

PREVENTION/AVOIDANCE N/A

POSSIBLE COMPLICATIONS No known complications

EXPECTED COURSE AND PROGNOSIS The disorder is benign with an excellent prognosis

MISCELLANEOUS

ASSOCIATED CONDITIONS Gilbert's disease may be part of a spectrum of hereditary disorders which includes types I and II Crigler-Najjar syndrome

AGE-RELATED FACTORS
Pediatric: It is rare for the disorder to be diagnosed before puberty
Geriatric: N/A
Others: N/A

PREGNANCY The relative fasting that may occur with morning sickness can elevate the bilirubin level

SYNONYMS Gilbert's syndrome

ICD-9-CM 277.4

SEE ALSO N/A

OTHER NOTES N/A

ABBREVIATIONS N/A

REFERENCES
• Okolicsanyi, L., Fevery, J., Billing, B., et al.: How should mild, isolated unconjugated hyperbilirubinemia be investigated? Sem Liver Dis., 3(1):36-41, 1983
• Watson, K.J.R., Gollan, J.L.: Gilbert's syndrome. Bailliere's Clin Gastroenterol. 3(2):337-55, 1989

Author R. Marlow, M.D.

Gingivitis

BASICS

DESCRIPTION Inflammation of the gingiva, one of the forms of significant oral infections

Others forms of oral infection:

◊ Periodontitis - progression of gingivitis to connective tissue and alveolar bone

◊ Vincent's angina (trench mouth, necrotizing ulcerative gingivitis, fusospirochetosis) - fusiform bacillus or spirochete infection

◊ Glossitis - inflammation of the tongue (see separate title on this subject)

System(s) affected: Gastrointestinal

Genetics: No known genetic pattern

Incidence/Prevalence: Pandemic, 90% of the population affected

Predominant age: Mostly adult

Predominant sex: Male = Female

SIGNS AND SYMPTOMS
- Mouth odor (bad breath)
- Gum swelling (painless)
- Gum redness
- Change of normal gum contours
- Gum bleeding when flossing or brushing
- Periodontal pockets
- Edema of interdental papillae
- Narrow band of bright red inflamed gum surrounding neck of tooth
- Vincent's angina - ulcers, fever, malaise, regional lymphadenopathy, pain

CAUSES
- Noncontagious
- Inadequate plaque removal
- Blood dyscrasias
- Reaction to oral contraceptives
- Vincent's - fusiform bacillus or spirochete infection
- Allergic reactions
- Endocrine disturbances, i.e., pregnancy, menses
- Chronic debilitating disease

RISK FACTORS
- Diabetes mellitus
- Malocclusion
- Poor dental hygiene
- Mouth breathing
- Faulty dental restoration

DIAGNOSIS

DIFFERENTIAL DIAGNOSIS
- Gingivitis of diabetes mellitus
- Gingivitis of pregnancy
- Desquamative gingivitis
- Gingivitis in leukemia
- Phenytoin gingivitis
- Pericoronitis
- HIV

LABORATORY Smear to identify causative agent

Drugs that may alter lab results: N/A

Disorders that may alter lab results: N/A

PATHOLOGICAL FINDINGS
- Acute or chronic inflammation
- Broken crepuscular epithelium
- Hyperemic capillaries
- Polymorphonuclear infiltration
- Papillary projections in subepithelial tissue
- Fibroblasts

SPECIAL TESTS N/A

IMAGING N/A

DIAGNOSTIC PROCEDURES N/A

TREATMENT

APPROPRIATE HEALTH CARE
Outpatient

GENERAL MEASURES
- Remove irritating factors (plaque, calculus, faulty dentures)
- Good oral hygiene
- Regular dental check-ups
- Vigorous chewing
- Periodontal surgery (sometimes)
- No smoking
- Warm saline rinses twice daily

ACTIVITY No restrictions

DIET Assure adequate vitamins and minerals

PATIENT EDUCATION Printed patient information available from: American Dental Association, 211 E. Chicago Avenue, Chicago, IL 60611, (800)621-8099

MEDICATIONS

DRUG(S) OF CHOICE
• Antibiotics - e.g., penicillin, pediatric dose 25-50 mg/kg/day divided q6h; adult dose 250-500 mg q6h, or
• Erythromycin - pediatric dose: 30-40 mg/kg/day divided q6h; adult dose 250 mg q6h
• Topical corticosteroids (i.e., triamcinolone in orabase)

Contraindications: Allergy to antibiotics

Precautions: Erythromycin frequently causes significant gastrointestinal upsets

Significant possible interactions: Refer to manufacturer's literature

ALTERNATIVE DRUGS
Other antibiotics according to culture or smear

FOLLOWUP

PATIENT MONITORING
Until clear

PREVENTION/AVOIDANCE
• Good oral hygiene, daily brushing and flossing
• Cleaning by a dentist or hygienist every 6 months or sooner

POSSIBLE COMPLICATIONS
Severe periodontal disease

EXPECTED COURSE AND PROGNOSIS
• Usual course - acute; relapsing; intermittent; chronic
• Prognosis - generally favorable, responds well to appropriate treatment

MISCELLANEOUS

ASSOCIATED CONDITIONS
• Periodontitis
• Glossitis

AGE-RELATED FACTORS
Pediatric: Mild cases common in children and usually requires no treatment

Geriatric: More frequent in this age group (due more to lifelong accumulation, rather than increased susceptibility)

Others: N/A

PREGNANCY
Characteristics - hyperplasia, pedunculated gingival growths, pyogenic granuloma

SYNONYMS
Denture sore mouth

ICD-9-CM
523.1

SEE ALSO
Glossitis

OTHER NOTES
N/A

ABBREVIATIONS
N/A

REFERENCES
Berkow, R., et al. (eds.): Merck Manual, 15th Ed. Rahway, NJ, Merck Sharp & Dohme, 1987

Author T. Lewis, D.D.S.

Glaucoma, chronic open-angle

 BASICS

DESCRIPTION A precise definition of "glaucoma" is difficult to find. It is believed that if the intraocular pressure (IOP) is sufficiently high that it will result in damage to the optic nerve tissue and ultimately loss of visual field and visual acuity. (There remains debate as to the cause and effect relationship of increased IOP and optic nerve damage. Clearly, increased IOP is associated with optic nerve damage).
• In chronic open-angle glaucoma (COAG), aqueous secretion by the ciliary body is normal, and its flow between the lens and the iris through the pupil into the anterior chamber is normal; however, the trabecular meshwork (TM) does not permit as rapid egress of aqueous from the eye with the result that the pressure becomes elevated
System(s) affected: Nervous
Genetics: N/A
Incidence/Prevalence: Glaucoma affects approximately 4% of the population above the age of 40, with over 90% of these glaucomas being COAG
Predominant age: Over age 40 (affects all ages)
Predominant sex: Male = Female

SIGNS AND SYMPTOMS None until far advanced; then, gradual painless visual loss

CAUSES
• Obstruction to outflow through the trabecular meshwork (TM) (most common)
• Obstruction to the outflow from Schlemm's canal and the aqueous veins created by elevated orbital venous pressure (as in A-V malformations, orbital congestion due to thyroid disease, etc.)
• Too much aqueous secretion (extremely rare)

RISK FACTORS
• Positive family history
• Diabetes mellitus
• African American Ancestry

 DIAGNOSIS

DIFFERENTIAL DIAGNOSIS
• Vascular occlusive disease
• Severe anemia
• Hemodynamic crisis in past

LABORATORY N/A
Drugs that may alter lab results: N/A
Disorders that may alter lab results: N/A

PATHOLOGICAL FINDINGS
Ophthalmoscopic - optic nerve head damage

SPECIAL TESTS N/A

IMAGING N/A

DIAGNOSTIC PROCEDURES
• IOP recording - elevated
• Visual field testing - loss
• Characteristic optic nerve damage

 TREATMENT

APPROPRIATE HEALTH CARE
Outpatient

GENERAL MEASURES
• Treatment of COAG is directed at lowering the intraocular pressure so that a healthy IOP to optic nerve perfusion pressure gradient is restored
• The disease cannot be cured, it can only be controlled. Control can be obtained by decreasing the rate of aqueous secretion, by increasing the rate of aqueous outflow, or by a combination of the two.
• For the most part, medical therapy is able to lower the IOP sufficiently to protect the optic nerve and visual field from progressive damage and ultimate visual field damage and visual loss
• When medical therapy not successful, laser or conventional surgery is indicated.

ACTIVITY No limitations

DIET No special diet

PATIENT EDUCATION
• Necessity for periodic IOP checks and eye exams
For patient education materials favorably reviewed on this topic, contact:
◊ Foundation for Glaucoma Research, 490 Post Street, Suite 830, San Francisco, CA 94102, (415)986-3162
◊ American Academy of Ophthalmology, 655 Beach Street, San Francisco, CA 94109, (415)561-8500

MEDICATIONS

DRUG(S) OF CHOICE
Medications can be used singly or in combination to achieve the desired reduction of IOP. Begin with a single agent, then add a 2nd or 3rd in a stepwise fashion.
Topical
• Reduction of aqueous secretion
◊ beta-adrenergic blocking agents (timolol, betaxolol, levobunolol, carteolol)
◊ adrenergic agents (epinephrine, and dipivefrin, the "pro-drug" of epinephrine)
• Increase aqueous humor outflow (cholinergic agents)
◊ direct-acting cholinergic agents (pilocarpine, carbamylcholine) "fool" the eye into believing that acetylcholine has been administered
◊ indirect acting cholinergic agents (physostigmine, demecarium bromide, echothiophate iodide, and isoflurophate [DFP]) are all cholinesterase inhibitors
Systemic
• Reduction of aqueous secretion
◊ acetazolamide (Diamox, the prototype)
◊ dichlorphenamide (sulfonamide)
◊ methazolamide (sulfonamide)
Contraindications:
• The non-selective beta-adrenergic blocking agents (timolol, levobunolol) are relatively contraindicated for patients with obstructive airway disease
• Carbonic-anhydrase inhibitors are contraindicated with history of sensitivity to sulfonamides
Precautions:
• Sympathomimetic agents - used with caution in patients with cardiovascular disease
• Carbonic anhydrase inhibitors - used with caution in patients with a history of nephrolithiasis, myeloproliferative disorders, respiratory acidosis, severely compromised lung capacity, diabetes mellitus, hepatic disease (especially cirrhosis)
• Beta-adrenergic antagonists must be used with caution in patients with marginal cardiac output, diabetes mellitus, bradycardia, or patients receiving oral beta-blockers

Significant possible interactions:
• Cholinesterase inhibitors - with the administration of general anesthesia. Should a depolarizing agent such as succinylcholine be used for intubation, these patients will not be able to metabolize this agent and will be respirator-dependent until the systemic activity of cholinesterase is restored, i.e., 3 weeks. Deaths have been reported from this unfortunate complication.
• Carbonic anhydrase inhibitors - may decrease excretion of some drugs (e.g., amphetamines, procainamide, quinidine, tricyclic antidepressants). May potentiate salicylate toxicity secondary to systemic acidosis.
• Beta-adrenergic antagonists have been associated with death in patients also on calcium channel blockers

ALTERNATIVE DRUGS N/A

FOLLOWUP

PATIENT MONITORING
• Every 3-4 months for life
• Chronic carbonic anhydrase inhibitor therapy requires periodic monitoring of the blood count for evidence of reduction in the hemoglobin, hematocrit, and white blood cell count as well as K+ wasting

PREVENTION/AVOIDANCE N/A

POSSIBLE COMPLICATIONS N/A

EXPECTED COURSE AND PROGNOSIS
• Lifetime IOP control
• Excellent visual prognosis, unless diagnosis delayed until disorder far advanced or in end-stages

MISCELLANEOUS

ASSOCIATED CONDITIONS Diabetes mellitus

AGE-RELATED FACTORS
Pediatric: N/A
Geriatric: N/A
Others: N/A

PREGNANCY N/A

SYNONYMS Chronic simple glaucoma

ICD-9-CM 365.11; 377.14

SEE ALSO N/A

OTHER NOTES N/A

ABBREVIATIONS
COAG = chronic open-angle glaucoma
IOP = intraocular pressure

REFERENCES Hoskins, H.D. & Kass, M. (eds.): Becker-Shaffer's Diagnosis and Therapy of the Glaucomas. 6th Ed. St. Louis, C.V. Mosby, 1989

Author B. Hodes, M.D.

Glaucoma, primary angle-closure

BASICS

DESCRIPTION Primary angle-closure glaucoma results from obstruction of aqueous humor outflow through the trabecular meshwork by peripheral iris apposition with consequent elevation in intraocular pressure (IOP). The underlying mechanism is pupillary block, in which aqueous egress through the pupil is limited causing forward iris displacement. Angle-closure glaucoma can occur in subacute, acute, and chronic forms and is associated with an anatomically narrow anterior chamber angle; the angle comprises the peripheral iris, anterior ciliary body, trabecular meshwork, and peripheral cornea and can only be observed with a special examination technique called gonioscopy. In its acute form, primary angle-closure glaucoma is an ophthalmic emergency with a natural history of severe visual loss.

System(s) affected: Nervous
Genetics: Polygenic inheritance; first degree relatives have a 2-5% lifetime risk
Incidence in USA: 100 cases/100,000 population
Prevalence in USA: 500/100,000 (Blacks and Asians more common than Causacians)
Predominant Age: 55-70
Predominant Sex: Female > Male

SIGNS AND SYMPTOMS

Subacute
 ◊ Dull ache in or around one eye
 ◊ Mildly blurred vision
 ◊ Symptoms occur when watching TV or movies in dark room, reading, or when fatigued. Relieved by sleep or rest.
 ◊ Normal intraocular pressure (10-23 mmHg)
 ◊ Shallow anterior chamber
 ◊ Iris bombé
 ◊ Intermittent peripheral anterior synechiae
 ◊ Enlarged pupil
Acute
 ◊ Ocular pain
 ◊ Blurred vision
 ◊ Lacrimation
 ◊ Halos around lights
 ◊ Frontal headache
 ◊ Nausea and vomiting
 ◊ Symptoms likely to occur with times of emotional stress and with activities as for subacute form
 ◊ Elevated intraocular pressure (usually 40-80 mmHg)
 ◊ Corneal microcystic edema
 ◊ Lid edema, conjunctival hyperemia, and circumcorneal injection
 ◊ Fixed mid-dilated pupil, often oval
 ◊ Shallow anterior chamber often with inflammatory reaction
Chronic
 ◊ May have symptoms of subacute form or may be asymptomatic
 ◊ Multiple peripheral anterior synechiae
 ◊ Normal or elevated intraocular pressure
 ◊ Increased cup to disc ratio
 ◊ Normal pupil

CAUSES Predisposing ocular anatomy

RISK FACTORS
• Small cornea
• Hyperopia
• Shallow anterior chamber
• Eskimo ancestry
• Female sex
• Use of antidepressants or other drugs with cholinergic inhibition
• Cataract

DIAGNOSIS

DIFFERENTIAL DIAGNOSIS
• Neovascular glaucoma
• Absolute glaucoma
• Malignant glaucoma
• Plateau iris syndrome
• Miotic induced glaucoma
• Phacomorphic glaucoma
• Anterior uveitis

LABORATORY None
Drugs that may alter lab results: N/A
Disorders that may alter lab results: N/A

PATHOLOGICAL FINDINGS
• Corneal stromal and epithelial edema
• Endothelial cell loss
• Iris stromal necrosis
• Anterior subcapsular cataract (glaukomflecken)
• Optic disc congestion, cupping
• Atrophy

SPECIAL TESTS Gonioscopy

IMAGING N/A

DIAGNOSTIC PROCEDURES Careful ophthalmic examination including indentation gonioscopy and tonometry

TREATMENT

APPROPRIATE HEALTH CARE
• For acute form - inpatient admission from office or emergency room
• Other forms - outpatient

GENERAL MEASURES
For acute form
 ◊ Intravenous access for administering medications is helpful, antiemetics may be necessary
 ◊ Definitive treatment is laser iridotomy once the attack is broken, intraocular pressure has normalized, and intraocular inflammation has subsided
Other forms - surgical procedures
 ◊ Peripheral iridectomy
 ◊ Argon or Nd:YAG laser iridotomy (procedure of choice for subacute and chronic forms)

ACTIVITY For acute form - bedrest until attack broken

DIET Usual for patient

PATIENT EDUCATION
• Usually patients need bilateral treatment since second eye is at risk for same disease process
For patient education materials favorably reviewed on this topic, contact:
 ◊ Foundation for Glaucoma Research, 490 Post Street, Suite 830, San Francisco, CA 94102, (415)986-3162
 ◊ American Academy of Ophthalmology, 655 Beach Street, San Francisco, CA 94109, (415)561-8500

MEDICATIONS

DRUG(S) OF CHOICE
For acute form:
◊ Hyperosmotic agents - oral 50% glycerin 0.1-1.5 g/kg or oral isosorbide 1.5-2.0 g/kg, and/or intravenous mannitol 20% 1-2 g/kg over 45 minutes
◊ Carbonic anhydrase inhibition - acetazolamide (Diamox) 500 mg IV plus 500 mg po, then 250 mg po q6h prn
◊ Beta-blockers - timolol 0.5% (Timoptic) q12h or levobunolol 0.5% (Betagan) q12h or betaxolol 0.5% (Betoptic) q12h
◊ Miotics - pilocarpine 2-4% one dose. In complicated cases with multiple mechanisms, miotics may paradoxically worsen the condition. Hence, they must be used with caution.
◊ Corticosteroid - prednisolone acetate 1% (Pred Forte) q4-6h
For subacute and chronic forms:
◊ Treatment is surgical
Contraindications: With history of recent intraocular surgery, possibility of malignant glaucoma is increased and miotics may be contraindicated
Precautions:
• Timolol, levobunolol, and betaxolol, use with caution in patients with chronic heart failure or chronic obstructive pulmonary disease
• Mannitol, use with caution in patients with chronic heart failure or renal failure
• Acetazolamide, use with caution in patients with history of nephrolithiasis or metabolic acidosis
Significant possible interactions:
Acetazolamide may accelerate potassium loss and metabolic acidosis in patients on other diuretics

ALTERNATIVE DRUGS   As above

FOLLOWUP

PATIENT MONITORING
• Subacute and chronic forms, check tonometry and gonioscopy initially every 3 months after laser iridotomy, follow visual fields every 6-12 months
• Acute form, discharge after laser iridotomy and intraocular pressure are controlled and follow as with the chronic form
• Consider frequent serum electrolytes while on mannitol
• Semi-annual CBC while on acetazolamide

PREVENTION/AVOIDANCE
Prophylactic laser treatment of second eye

POSSIBLE COMPLICATIONS
• Chronic corneal edema
• Corneal fibrosis and vascularization
• Iris atrophy
• Cataract
• Lens subluxation
• Optic atrophy
• Malignant glaucoma
• central retinal vein occlusion

EXPECTED COURSE AND PROGNOSIS
• Varies with delay of patient presentation and severity of attack
• Preceding chronic angle-closure may have caused optic atrophy
• Recurrence is quite rare following peripheral iridotomy or iridectomy and implies a rare variant known as the iris plateau syndrome

MISCELLANEOUS

ASSOCIATED CONDITIONS
• Cataract
• Microphthalmos
• Hyperopia

AGE-RELATED FACTORS
Pediatric: Rare
Geriatric: Secondary angle closure glaucoma can be caused by many common eye conditions in the elderly including cataract, ocular surgery and diabetes
Others: N/A

PREGNANCY   N/A

SYNONYMS
• Acute glaucoma
• Narrow angle glaucoma

ICD-9-CM
• Acute: 365.20
• Subacute: 365.02

SEE ALSO   Chronic open angle glaucoma

OTHER NOTES
Medications (higher risk) that may exacerbate angle-closure glaucoma:
◊ Systemic or topical anticholinergics
◊ Topical sympathomimetics
◊ Antihistamines
◊ Phenothiazines
◊ Antidepressants
Medications (lower risk) that may exacerbate angle-closure glaucoma:
◊ Benzodiazepine
◊ Carbonic anhydrase inhibitors
◊ CNS stimulants (including cocaine)
◊ MAO inhibitors
◊ Systemic sympathomimetics
◊ Theophylline
◊ Vasodilators

ABBREVIATIONS   N/A

REFERENCES
• Ritch, R., Shields, M.B. & Krupin, T.: The Glaucomas. St. Louis, C.V. Mosby, 1989
• Fraunfelder, F.T. & Roy, F.H.: Current Ocular Therapy 3. 3rd Ed., Philadelphia, W.B. Saunders Co., 1990

Author   R. Fante, M.D.

Glomerulonephritis, acute

BASICS

DESCRIPTION An immunologic response to an infection (usually streptococcal) which damages the renal glomeruli. It can be initiated also by a variety of other bacterial and viral infections. This is an immune complex, hypocomplementemic glomerulonephritis. Most common in children. Characterized by diffuse inflammatory changes in the glomeruli and clinically by the abrupt onset of hematuria with red blood cell casts, and mild proteinuria. Accompanied in many cases by hypertension, edema, and azotemia.
System(s) affected: Renal/Urologic
Genetics: No known genetic pattern
Incidence in USA: 20/100,000/year (1-2% of pyoderms and 8% of streptococcal infections in children; occurs with impetigo in the late summer and with staphlococcal pharyngitis in the winter)
Prevalence in USA: N/A
Predominant age:
• 60% of cases in children 2-12 years old
• Only 10% older than 40 years of age
Predominant sex: Male > Female

SIGNS AND SYMPTOMS
Classic findings of acute nephritis
◊ Hematuria (100%)
◊ Oligoanuria (52%)
◊ Edema (85%)
◊ Hypertension (82%)
◊ Hypocomplementemia (C3) (83%)
◊ Gross hematuria (30%), tea-colored urine
◊ Edema of face and eyes in the am and feet and ankles in the afternoons and evenings
◊ Fever (rare)
Other signs and symptoms
◊ Pharyngitis
◊ Respiratory infection
◊ Scarlet fever
◊ Dark urine
◊ Weight gain
◊ Abdominal pain
◊ Anorexia
◊ Back pain
◊ Pallor
◊ Impetigo

CAUSES
• Follows group A beta-hemolytic streptococcus infection
• "Nephrogenic" strains of strep - groups 1, 4, 11, 12, 49, "Red Lake" 55, 60
• Unusual to have a second attack - protective immunity to nephritogenic antigen
• Cases of "postinfective" glomerulonephritis have been reported from pneumococcus, meningococcus, chickenpox, and hepatitis
• Streptococcal infection precedes renal lesions by 1-3 weeks
• Pharyngitis precedes renal lesions by 1-2 weeks (1, 2, 4, 12)
• Impetigenesis - (types 49, 55, 57) usually precedes throat or otitis media infection by 2-4 weeks

RISK FACTORS
• 15% occurrence rate after infection with nephritogenic strain
• Endemic with cyclic epidemics
• Subclinical cases 20 times more common
• Streptococcal infection (e.g., scarlet fever or erysipelas) can be associated with rheumatic fever or acute glomerulonephritis but not both

DIAGNOSIS

DIFFERENTIAL DIAGNOSIS
• Membranoproliferative glomerulonephritis
• Other postinfective glomerulonephritis
• Systemic lupus erythematosus
• IgA nephropathy
• Anaphylactoid purpura

LABORATORY
• Streptococcal tests that include many antigens are most sensitive (+ or -) for screening but not quantitative (Streptozyme)
• Antistreptolysin O (ASO) - quantitative titer is obtained. Increased in 60-80% of cases. Increase begins 1-3 weeks, is highest 3-5 weeks, normal in 6 months. ASO titer is unrelated to severity, duration or prognosis of renal disease.
• Red blood cells casts on urinalysis - 1) destroyed by centrifugation. 2) disintegrate in urine, particularly alkaline urine.
• Morphologically, red blood cells from glomerular bleeding are distorted while those from lower urinary tract have normal morphology
• U/P creatinine > 40, decreased renin
• Culture throat and skin lesions for streptococcus
• C3 and C4 complements are best for evaluation
• Hyaluronidase antibody
• Hypertriglyceridemia
• Proteinuria
• Red blood cell casts
• Decreased glomerular filtration rate
• Uremia
• Increased serum creatinine
• Anemia
Drugs that may alter lab results: N/A
Disorders that may alter lab results: N/A

PATHOLOGICAL FINDINGS
On renal biopsy
◊ Diffuse proliferative glomerulonephritis
◊ Electron microscopy - subepithelial deposits
◊ Immunofluorescence - C3 in almost all cases, some with IgG and IgM

SPECIAL TESTS N/A

IMAGING N/A

DIAGNOSTIC PROCEDURES N/A

TREATMENT

APPROPRIATE HEALTH CARE
Inpatient usually

GENERAL MEASURES
• Decrease salt - no-added salt diet until edema and hypertension clear
• Decrease fluids to insensible losses - plus 2/3 of the urine output until diuresis
• Dialysis - peritoneal dialysis or hemodialysis for symptomatic azotemia, unresponsive hyperkalemia, intractable acidosis, diuretic resistant pulmonary edema

ACTIVITY Can return to full activity after clinically improved

DIET
• "No-added" salt diet until edema, hypertension, and azotemia clear
• Restrict protein in presence of azotemia and metabolic acidosis

PATIENT EDUCATION National Kidney Foundation, 30 E. 33rd Street, Suite 1100, New York, NY 10016, (212)889-2210

MEDICATIONS

DRUG(S) OF CHOICE
Hyperkalemia
◊ No potassium in IV fluids until hyperkalemia resolves
◊ Kayexalate resin 1 gm/kg in 10% sorbitol, pr or p.o.
◊ Correct acidosis 2 mEq/kg sodium bicarbonate (NaHCO3)
◊ Correct hypocalcemia - 0.5 cc/kg 10% calcium gluconate IV over 30 minutes for symptomatic hyperkalemia. For non-symptomatic hyperkalemia use oral calcium carbonate 1 gm Ca++/day.
Pulmonary edema
◊ Oxygen
◊ Furosemide
◊ Digitalization is not effective
Edema
◊ Furosemide 1-2 mg/kg/dose given bid po or IV
◊ Treatment with diuretics decreases the duration and severity of edema and hypertension
Acidosis
◊ Sodium bicarbonate 2 mEq/kg/dose IV over 30 minutes to correct acidosis
Strep infection
◊ Give penicillin IM or po for 10 days
Hypertension
◊ Hydralazine 0.25 to 1.0 mg/kg/dose given pm or q 6 hours
Contraindications: Refer to manufacturer's literature
Precautions: Refer to manufacturer's literature
Significant possible interactions: Refer to manufacturer's literature

ALTERNATIVE DRUGS   N/A

FOLLOWUP

PATIENT MONITORING
• Depends on severity of disease
• Urinalysis at 2, 4 and 8 weeks and 4, 6 and 12 months
• Stop followup when urinalysis is clear
• Monitor blood pressure each visit
• Monitor serum creatinine at 2, 6, and 12 months
• C3 complement should be normal by 6 weeks

PREVENTION/AVOIDANCE   Treat streptococcal infections aggressively

POSSIBLE COMPLICATIONS
• Hypertensive retinopathy
• Hypertensive encephalopathy
• Rapidly progressive glomerulonephritis
• Abnormal urinalysis may persist for years
• Chronic renal failure (rare)
• Nephrotic syndrome
• Marked decline in glomerular filtration rate

EXPECTED COURSE AND PROGNOSIS
• Immediate mortality - 0.5% or less
• Long-term - excellent in children. Almost all patients recover completely.
• May have more morbidity in adults or in those with pre-existing renal lesions
• Microscopic hematuria persisting for up to 24 months
• Proteinuria persists for up to 3 months
• Symptoms can be exacerbated by a intercurrent illness but rarely after 12 months
• Urine may be darker after strenuous exercise

MISCELLANEOUS

ASSOCIATED CONDITIONS   N/A

AGE-RELATED FACTORS
Pediatric: Common in children age 2 years to 16 years
Geriatric: N/A
Others: N/A

PREGNANCY   N/A

SYNONYMS
• Acute nephritic syndrome
• Postinfectious glomerulonephritis
• Acute post-streptococcal glomerulonephritis

ICD-9-CM   580 glomerulonephritis, acute

SEE ALSO   Goodpasture's syndrome

OTHER NOTES   N/A

ABBREVIATIONS   N/A

REFERENCES
• Brenner, B. & Rector, F.: The Kidney. Philadelphia, W.B. Saunders Co., 1991
• Holliday, M., Barratt, T. & Vernier, R.: Pediatric Nephrology. 2nd Ed. Baltimore, Williams & Wilkins, 1986

Author   W. Arnold, M.D.

Glossitis

BASICS

DESCRIPTION Acute or chronic inflammation of the tongue either as a primary disease or symptom of systemic disease
System(s) affected: Gastrointestinal
Genetics: N/A
Incidence/Prevalence in USA: Common
Predominant age: All ages
Predominant sex: Male > Female

SIGNS AND SYMPTOMS
• Reddened tip and edges of tongue (with pellagra, anemia, excess smoking)
• Fiery red, swollen, ulcerated tongue (pellagra)
• Tongue smooth and pale (anemias)
• Ulcers (herpetic or aphthous lesions, streptococcal infection, erythema multiforme, pemphigus)
• White patches (candidiasis, syphilis, leukoplakia, lichen planus, mouth breathing)
• Denuded smooth areas (geographic tongue)
• Painful tongue (anemia or pellagra)
• Hairy tongue (follows antibiotic therapy, fever or excessive use of mouthwashes with peroxide)
• Tenderness, pain, swelling of the tongue (infections or trauma)
• Burning, painful tongue (candidiasis, anemia, diabetes, malignancies)
• Non-painful solitary ulcerations (malignancy)

CAUSES
Systemic:
  ◊ Avitaminosis (particularly B group, e.g., pellagra)
  ◊ Anemia (pernicious, iron deficiency)
  ◊ Skin diseases (e.g., lichen planus, erythema multiforme, aphthous lesions, Behcet's syndrome, pemphigus vulgaris, syphilis)
Local:
  ◊ Infections (viral, candidiasis, tuberculosis, streptococcal)
  ◊ Trauma (ill-fitting dentures, burns, convulsive seizures)
  ◊ Primary irritants (alcohol, tobacco, hot foods, spices)
  ◊ Sensitization (chemical irritants, e.g., dyes, mouth wash, toothpaste, systemic drugs)
  ◊ Malignancy

RISK FACTORS
• Low socioeconomic status
• Poor nutrition
• Dentures
• Smoking
• Alcoholism
• Anxiety
• Depression
• Advancing age

DIAGNOSIS

DIFFERENTIAL DIAGNOSIS
Systemic:
  ◊ Avitaminosis (particularly B group, e.g., pellagra)
  ◊ Anemia (pernicious, iron deficiency)
  ◊ Skin diseases (e.g., lichen planus, erythema multiforme, aphthous lesions, Behcet's syndrome, pemphigus vulgaris, syphilis)
Local:
  ◊ Infections (viral, candidiasis, tuberculosis, streptococcal)
  ◊ Trauma (ill-fitting dentures, burns, convulsive seizures)
  ◊ Primary irritants: alcohol, tobacco, hot foods, spices
  ◊ Sensitization (chemical irritants, e.g., dyes, mouth wash, toothpaste, systemic drugs)
  ◊ Malignancy
  ◊ Geographic tongue - a normal varient

LABORATORY
• CBC
• Serologic tests for syphilis
• Chemical profile
• Tests for vitamin B12 deficiency
• Postprandial glucose
• Smear and culture lesions when indicated
Drugs that may alter lab results: N/A
Disorders that may alter lab results: N/A

PATHOLOGICAL FINDINGS Varies
according to underlying causes

SPECIAL TESTS
•Biopsy solitary lesions that do not respond to treatment in one week
• 10% KOH scrapings for suspected candidiasis

IMAGING N/A

DIAGNOSTIC PROCEDURES
• Biopsy
• KOH scrapings

TREATMENT

APPROPRIATE HEALTH CARE
Outpatient

GENERAL MEASURES
• Avoid any possible sensitizing irritants or agents
• Specific therapy for oral infections (see Medications)
• Local treatment (see Medications)
• Analgesics when needed
• Request dental evaluation
• Scrupulous oral hygiene

ACTIVITY No restrictions unless there is a systemic infection

DIET Bland or liquid diet

PATIENT EDUCATION Griffith:
Instructions for Patients; Philadephia, W.B. Saunders Co. 4th ed., 1989 p.303

Glossitis

MEDICATIONS

DRUG(S) OF CHOICE
• For Candidiasis: Nystatin oral suspension 400,000 u (4 mL) to 600,000 u qid for 10 days as an oral rinse, then swallowed
• For oral infections: Oral penicillin V, see manufacturer's literature for dosage

Local treatment:
◊ Mouth rinse with 2% lidocaine viscous, 1 tablespoon before each meal and every 3 hours if needed for pain
◊ Mouth wash of 1/2 teaspoon sodium bicarbonate in 8 oz warm water qid
◊ Mouth rinse with carbamide peroxide 10% (Gly-Oxide) 1/2 cc qid for irritation, apthous ulcers
◊ Triamcinolone 0.1% in emollient dental paste applied to specific lesions, especially aphthous ulcers

Contraindications: Refer to manufacturer's literature
Precautions: Refer to manufacturer's literature
Significant possible interactions: Refer to manufacturer's literature

ALTERNATIVE DRUGS
For candidiasis:
◊ Clotrimazole - 10 mg oral lozenges 5 times a day for 10 days. Or
◊ Ketoconazole - one 200 mg tablet (for children 1/4 tablet) orally once a day

FOLLOWUP

PATIENT MONITORING
• Re-visits periodically when needed until healing occurs
• If lesions do not heal, biopsy is indicated

PREVENTION/AVOIDANCE   N/A

POSSIBLE COMPLICATIONS
• Lymphadenopathy
• Chronicity

EXPECTED COURSE AND PROGNOSIS
• Prompt improvement when cause can be identified and treated
• Aphthous ulcers, erythema multiforme and hairy tongue often recur

MISCELLANEOUS

ASSOCIATED CONDITIONS
• Diabetes mellitus
• HIV infection

AGE-RELATED FACTORS
Pediatric: Median rhomboid glossitis is a developmental lesion causing a rhomboid-shaped, smooth, reddish, nodular area on the dorsal surface of the back portion of the middle third of the tongue. This type of glossitis is innocuous and requires no treatment.
Geriatric: Many patients with glossitis are postmenopausal or elderly
Others: N/A

PREGNANCY   N/A

SYNONYMS   N/A

ICD-9-CM   529

SEE ALSO   N/A

OTHER NOTES   Some symptoms of glossitis have no organic cause. Treat symptoms and reassure regarding malignancy.

ABBREVIATIONS   N/A

REFERENCES
• Dreizen, S.: The Telltale Tongue. Postgrad Med. March, 1984;75:150
• Pondborg, J.J.: Atlas of Diseases of the Oral Mucosa. 4th Ed. Philadelphia, W.B. Saunders Co., 1986

Author   J. R. Richard, MD

Gonococcal infections

BASICS

DESCRIPTION Gonorrhea is a purulent inflammation of mucous membrane surfaces caused by a sexually transmitted microorganism, the gonococcus. Virtually any mucous membrane may be infected. Occasionally the organism may become blood-borne causing a characteristic syndrome of fever, skin lesions and arthralgias/tenosynovitis or septic arthritis.
• Hematogenous dissemination may also lead to endocarditis, or rarely, meningitis
• Salpingitis, in women, local extension from the endocervical canal to the fallopian tubes is common. The ovaries may be involved with abscess formation. The entire complex of upper genital tract infection in women is referred to as pelvic inflammatory disease (PID).
• In men, the epididymis may become infected with extension to the testicle
• An asymptomatic carrier state can occur in both sexes

System(s) affected: Reproductive, Musculoskeletal, Skin/Exocrine, Nervous, Cardiovascular

Genetics: Individuals with congenital absence of the late components of the complement cascade (C 7,8,9) are prone to develop dissemination of local gonococcal infections

Incidence/Prevalence in USA:
1400/100,000 people in USA

Predominant age: 15-29

Predominant sex: Male > Female (symptomatic disease)

SIGNS AND SYMPTOMS

In males, adolescent and adult:
◊ Scant to copious purulent urethral discharge (98%)
◊ Dysuria (98%)
◊ Testicular pain (1%)
◊ Asymptomatic urethral infection (incidence of about 1%)
◊ Urethral Stricture

Homosexual male:
◊ Rectal discharge: purulent or bloody
◊ Tenesmus
◊ Rectal burning or itching
◊ Asymptomatic rectal infection

Female without PID:
◊ Endocervical discharge (on pelvic exam) (96%)
◊ Vaginal discharge
◊ Dysuria
◊ Bartholin's gland abscess
◊ Asymptomatic cervical infection
◊ Vaginal discharge
◊ Asymptomatic cervical infection (approximately 20%)

Female with PID:
◊ Dysmenorrhea
◊ Metromenorrhagia
◊ Lower abdominal pain and tenderness
◊ Fever
◊ Cervical traction tenderness
◊ Palpable, tender fallopian tubes and/or ovaries

◊ Abdominal rebound tenderness
◊ Infertility
◊ Chronic pelvic pain

Both sexes:
◊ Pharyngeal infection - asymptomatic infection (98%), sore throat, exudative pharyngitis (< 1%)
◊ Eye Infection (rare) - purulent discharge, conjunctivitis, chemosis, eyelid edema, corneal ulceration
◊ Disseminated syndromes - fever; chills; arthralgias (small joints); synovial sheath tenderness and swelling (hands and/or feet); painful skin lesions (pustular, red, tender); septic arthritis
◊ Endocarditis - rapid cardiac valve destruction, high fevers
◊ Meningitis - meningeal signs, headache, skin lesions, fever, altered mental status

Infants and children:
◊ Eye Infection (rare - because of routine ocular prophylaxis in the USA) - purulent discharge, conjunctivitis, chemosis, eyelid edema, corneal ulceration
◊ Pneumonia (of the newborn) - fever, infiltrate on chest x-ray
◊ Meningitis - meningeal signs, headache, skin lesions, fever, altered mental status
◊ Vulvovaginitis - vaginal discharge
◊ Rectal Infection
◊ Pharyngeal infection - asymptomatic infection (98%), sore throat, exudative pharyngitis (< 1%)
◊ Disseminated syndromes - fever; chills; arthralgias (small joints); synovial sheath tenderness and swelling (hands and/or feet); painful skin lesions (pustular, red, tender); septic arthritis

CAUSES Neisseria gonorrhoeae

RISK FACTORS
• Sexual exposure to an infected individual without barrier protection (condom)
• Multiple sexual partners
• Infant - passage through the infected birth canal of the mother
• Children - sexual abuse by infected individual
• Auto-inoculation (finger to eye)
• For PID - use of intrauterine devices

DIAGNOSIS

DIFFERENTIAL DIAGNOSIS
• Chlamydial infections (may mimic all aspects of gonococcal infections except disseminated syndromes)
• Urinary tract infections
• Other infectious vaginitides (yeast, trichomonas, bacterial vaginosis)

LABORATORY
• Gram stain of exudate from infected mucosal surface
• Demonstration of pairs or clumps of gram-negative kidney-shaped diplococci within the cytoplasm of polymorphonuclear leukocytes. The adjacent surfaces are slightly concave.
• Sensitivity of urethral smear in symptomatic male - 95%
• Sensitivity of endocervical smear in infected woman - 60-70%
• Culture of exudate on selective medium (Thayer-Martin or Martin-Lewis, containing antibiotics to inhibit other micro-organisms). Demonstration of typical organisms by gram-stain morphology and growth on selective media constitutes a "presumptive" diagnosis of gonococcal infection. Should always be done in women because of low sensitivity of the smear, and in suspected cases of child abuse.
• Sensitivity of blood culture in disseminated disease - 50%
• Sensitivity of joint fluid culture in septic arthritis - 50%

Drugs that may alter lab results: Prior administration of even small amounts of many commonly available antibiotics may render a culture falsely negative

Disorders that may alter lab results: N/A

PATHOLOGICAL FINDINGS
• Exudate consisting of polymorphonuclear leukocytes is typical
• In PID - loss of ciliated columnar epithelium from the fallopian tubes. Tubes, pelvic mesentery and ovaries may be bound together with dense fibrosis and abscess formation.

SPECIAL TESTS
• Testing for antimicrobial susceptibility. B-lactamase production and chromosomally mediated resistance to penicillin and/or tetracycline are becoming more common. B-lactamase testing should be routine in the laboratory.
• Confirmation of the isolate as the gonococcus by standard sugar fermentation tests, enzymatic tests or DNA probes. Important in medicolegal situations such as rape or child abuse since other Neisseria, which are normal inhabitants of mucous surfaces, may look like the gonococcus.

IMAGING Pelvic ultrasound or CT scan may demonstrate thick, dilated fallopian tubes or abscess formation

DIAGNOSTIC PROCEDURES
• Culdocentesis may demonstrate free purulent exudate, and provide material for gram staining and culture
• Gram staining material from unroofed skin lesions of disseminated disease may sometimes show typical organisms

Gonococcal infections

TREATMENT

APPROPRIATE HEALTH CARE
• Outpatient with a followup visit for repeat examination and culturing for uncomplicated infection in adults
• Hospitalization for suspected hematogenous infection
• Hospitalization for pneumonia or eye infection in infants
• Hospitalization for women with PID if they cannot take oral medications, if significant tubo-ovarian abscess is present or if the patient is pregnant

GENERAL MEASURES
• Abstain from sexual activity until after followup examination, plus testing and treatment of partner(s)
• Blood test for syphilis
• Encouragement to obtain testing for HIV infection

ACTIVITY
Fully active for uncomplicated disease

DIET
No special diet

PATIENT EDUCATION
• Discuss sexually transmitted diseases and methods of prevention
• Discuss HIV infection and risks; encourage patient and partner(s) to be tested

MEDICATIONS

DRUG(S) OF CHOICE
• Uncomplicated ano-genital gonorrhea in adults: An injectable 3rd generation cephalosporin - ceftriaxone 250 mg IM or ceftizoxime 500 mg IM. Note: All regimens should be followed by tetracycline 500 mg po qid for 7 days or doxycycline 100 mg po bid for 7 days. In the pregnant patient, erythromycin 500 mg po qid for 7 days should be substituted for a tetracycline.
• Disseminated gonococcal infections: Ceftriaxone 1 gm IV once daily for 7 days followed by cefaclor 500 mg given every 8 hours for 4-5 days, or cefuroxime axetil 250 mg po bid for 4-5 days, or ciprofloxacin 750 mg po bid for 4-5 days
• PID (out patient schedule): Ceftriaxone 500 mg IM on day 1 and on day 5, plus doxycycline 100 mg po bid for 14 days. Metronidazole 250 mg po qid for 14 days may be added if a mixed anaerobic infection is suspected.
• Infections in infants: Ceftriaxone 25-50 mg/kg IV or IM every 12 hours for 7 days
• Infections in children: Children weighing 100 pounds (45 kg) or more should receive ceftriaxone 125 mg IM

Contraindications: Refer to manufacturer's profile of each drug
Precautions: Refer to manufacturer's profile of each drug
Significant possible interactions: Refer to manufacturer's profile of each drug

ALTERNATIVE DRUGS
If organisms are not penicillin resistant, aqueous crystalline penicillin G may be substituted for IV cephalosporins in complicated disease. (Note: only some penicillin resistance is now due to penicillinase production). Ampicillin or amoxicillin plus probenecid may be substituted for cephalosporins in uncomplicated disease.

FOLLOWUP

PATIENT MONITORING
Repeat cultures from mucosal sites one week after completing therapy

PREVENTION/AVOIDANCE
• For recurrence: No sexual intercourse until culture results known/partner(s) tested and treated
• For prevention of initial infection: Condoms offer partial protection

POSSIBLE COMPLICATIONS
• Urethral stricture in men
• Infertility in women
• Corneal scarring after eye infections
• Destruction of joint articular surfaces
• Destruction of cardiac valves, particularly aortic
• Death from congestive failure or meningitis

EXPECTED COURSE AND PROGNOSIS
With adequate, early therapy complete cure and return to normal function is the rule

MISCELLANEOUS

ASSOCIATED CONDITIONS
Other sexually transmitted infections such as syphilis, HIV infection, hepatitis B, herpes and vaginal infections in women

AGE-RELATED FACTORS
Pediatric: N/A
Geriatric: N/A
Others: N/A

PREGNANCY
PID during pregnancy may be associated with fetal loss, or premature labor and delivery

SYNONYMS
N/A

ICD-9-CM
098 Gonococcal infections

SEE ALSO
Chlamydial infection

OTHER NOTES
N/A

ABBREVIATIONS
N/A

REFERENCES
• Dallabetta, G. & Hook, E.W.: Gonococcal Infections. In Infectious Disease Clinics of North America. March 1987, pp25-54
• Mardh, P.A. & Danielsson, D.: Diagnostic testing for selected sexually transmitted diseases: Guidelines for Clinicians: Neisseria gonorrhoeae. In Sexually Transmitted Diseases. Edited by K.K. Holmes, et al. 2nd Ed. New York, McGraw-Hill, 1984

Author S. Thompson, M.D., M.P.H.

Gout

BASICS

DESCRIPTION Inflammatory reaction to urate crystals in joints, bones and subcutaneous structures. Initially, a hyperacute arthritis which may progress to a chronic arthritis. Rarely it may present as a chronic arthritis. Recognition of the crystals in fluid is pathognomonic.
• Primary gout - the most common: underexcretion or overproduction of uric acid
• Secondary gout - related to myeloproliferative diseases or their treatment, therapeutic regimens producing hyperuricemia, renal failure, renal tubular disorders, lead poisoning, hyperproliferative skin disorders, enzymatic defects (e.g., deficient hypoxanthine guanine phosphoribosyltransferase, glycogen storage diseases)
System(s) affected: Musculoskeletal, Endocrine/Metabolic, Renal/Urologic
Genetics: N/A
Incidence in USA: 100/100,000
Prevalence in USA:
• Under age 18: Rare
• Age 18-44: 3
• Age 45-64: 21
• Age over 65: 35
Predominant age: 30-60
Predominant sex: Male > Female (20:1)

SIGNS AND SYMPTOMS
• Hyperacute onset (within 24 hours) of severe pain, swelling, redness, and warmth in one or two joints (75% are monoarticular)
• Soft tissue redness, swelling, warmth
• Exquisite tenderness
• Propensity for first MTP joint, symptomatic in 50% of initial attacks; eventually in 75%
• Acute untreated attacks last 2-21 days
• Attack may be isolated, more often repetitive, 2nd attack may not occur for years
• Recurrent attacks last longer and occur more frequently with each recurrence
• Intracritical period - absence of inflammation (until the chronic or tophaceous phase occurs)
• Rarely polyarticular - proximal interphalangeal, distal interphalangeal, metacarpal phalangeal, wrist, knee, ankle, midtarsal joints, heel
• Migratory polyarthritis is a rare presentation
• 50% of untreated patients develop a chronic arthritis within 3-42 years
• Inflammatory synovial effusion
• Subcutaneous or intraosseous nodules (20%), referred to as tophi - may affect ears (antihelix), extensor aspects of peripheral joints (e.g., olecranon), rarely fingertips, cornea, aorta, spine or even intracranial
• Subcutaneous nodules may have a creamy (urate) discharge
• Fever, chills
• Carpal tunnel syndrome
• Kidney stones

CAUSES
• Hyperuricemia
• Dietary excess (e.g., anchovies, sardines, sweetbreads, kidney, liver and meat extracts)
• Inborn errors of metabolism
• Lead poisoning (Saturnine gout from moonshine)

RISK FACTORS
• Ethanol ingestion
• Family history
• Polynesian extraction (e.g., Samoan gout)
• Medications - aminophylline, caffeine, corticosteroids, cytotoxic drugs, diazepam, diphenhydramine, diuretics, L-dopa, dopamine, epinephrine, ethambutol, methaqualone, alpha-methyl dopa, nicotinic acid, probenecid (low dose), pyrazinamide, salicylates (< 10/dL blood levels), sulfinpyrazone (low dose), vitamins B12 and C.
• Diuretics may be responsible for 20% of secondary gout
• Ketosis
• Surgery or trauma
• Obesity (50%)
• Hypertension (50%)
• Vascular disease
• Diabetes
• Renal failure
• Hypothyroidism
• Hyperparathyroidism; hypoparathyroidism
• Hyperlipidemia types II, IV, V
• Paget's disease
• Hyperproliferative skin disorders (e.g., psoriasis)
• Lymphoproliferative disorders
• Calcium pyrophosphate deposition disease
• Sarcoidosis
• Hemolytic anemia
• Hemoglobinopathies
• Pernicious anemia
• Radiation treatment
• Type I glycogen storage disease
• Down's syndrome
• Gut sterilization by antibiotics

DIAGNOSIS

DIFFERENTIAL DIAGNOSIS Infectious arthritis, pseudogout (calcium pyrophosphate deposition disease), type IIa hyperproteinemia, amyloidosis, multicentric reticulohistiocytosis, hyperparathyroidism, spondyloarthropathy, rheumatoid arthritis (rarely)

LABORATORY
• WBC usually elevated with left shift during acute attacks
• ESR usually elevated during acute attacks
• Hyperuricemia may be present, although not diagnostic
Drugs that may alter lab results:
• Intra-articular steroids - many have inherent birefringence, which will cause confusion on synovial fluid analysis
• Hyperuricemia - induced by drugs that reduce effective circulating blood volume (induced by low dose aspirin, probenecid or sulfinpyrazone)

• Cyclosporine - induced renal insufficiency
Disorders that may alter lab results: N/A

PATHOLOGICAL FINDINGS
• Urate crystals in synovial membrane (98% of specimens processed entirely anhydrously [urate is water soluble])
• Tophus in 29% of individuals with untreated gout of 5 years duration, in 74% of individuals with untreated gout of 40 years duration

SPECIAL TESTS
• Synovial fluid white blood cell count is usually inflammatory (10,000-70,000 cells/dL), but may have as few as 1,000 WBC/dL
• Wet mounts of synovial fluid reveal negatively birefringent urate crystals on polarizing exam
• Gout crystals may be identified in asymptomatic joints

IMAGING
• X-ray is usually normal in the first year of uncontrolled disease.
• X-ray in chronic gout reveals "punched-out" erosions (lytic areas) often with periosteum overgrowing the erosion ("overhanging edge" sign). This is highly suggestive, but may also be caused by amyloidosis, type IIa hyperlipoproteinemia, and by multicentric reticulohistiocytosis.
• X-ray erosions with preservation of joint space is similarly characteristic. X-ray rarely reveals intraosseous lytic areas (tophi).
• Bone scan reveals increased nuclide concentration at affected sites

DIAGNOSTIC PROCEDURES
• Arthrocentesis with polarizing optical examination
• Biopsy of synovial membrane or subcutaneous nodule, processing the specimen anhydrously (urate is water soluble) and examining with polarizing optics

TREATMENT

APPROPRIATE HEALTH CARE
Outpatient, except for consideration of associated joint infection or for therapeutic unresponsiveness

GENERAL MEASURES Two components must be addressed: Controlling the acute attack of gout; addressing the underlying cause

ACTIVITY Affected joint(s) at rest until hyperacute phase is controlled

DIET Reduce ingestion of fat, alcoholic beverages, sardines, anchovies, liver, sweetbreads

PATIENT EDUCATION
• Arthritis Foundation pamphlet on gout
• Rothschild, B.M.: Hyperuricemia in the elderly. Geriatric Consultant, 4:14-16, 31, 1985.

MEDICATIONS

DRUG(S) OF CHOICE

Acute attack
◊ A NSAID at full dosage for 2-5 days
◊ When acute attack is controlled, reduce dose by 1/4 - 1/2

Hyperuricemia
◊ Initiate when acute attack controlled (unless kidneys at risk because of unusual uric acid load)
◊ Generally not pursued unless recurrent attacks or evidence of tophaceous or renal disease
◊ Any contributing medication regimens are first altered and any predisposing medical conditions/habits addressed
◊ Patient is tested for uric acid excretion (< 600 mg/day while on purine free diet or < 800 mg/day on unrestricted diet implies hypoexcretor)
◊ Hypoexcretor: probenecid is initiated at 500 mg qd and increased by 500 mg at monthly intervals, until the uric acid is lowered to normal range or at least 2 mg/dl less than the levels during which attacks are noted. (Maximum dose 2-3 g/day.) Urinary alkalinization and recommendation of ingestion of copious amounts of fluid are adjunctive.
◊ Hyperexcretor, tophaceous or renal disease are present: allopurinol, initiated at 100 mg qd and increased by 100 mg weekly, to a maximum of 600 mg per day.

Contraindications:

Related to medicinal control of the acute attack:
◊ Peptic ulcer disease
◊ Psychosis
◊ Severe headache
◊ Pregnancy
◊ Concomitant anticoagulant use
◊ Presence of a blood dyscrasia

Related to probenecid control of the underlying hyperuricemia:
◊ Uric acid overproduction
◊ Uric acid stones
◊ Renal impairment
◊ Concomitant salicylates

Related to allopurinol control of the underlying hyperuricemia:
◊ Bone marrow suppression
◊ Liver disease
◊ Concomitant cytotoxic drugs
◊ Diuretics may require increased amount of allopurinol

Precautions:

• Probenecid and allopurinol may themselves predispose to acute gouty attacks. Low dose NSAID is used for 6-24 months to reduce this risk.
• Reduce NSAID dosage in presence of renal or liver disease
• Reduce cytotoxic drug dose in presence of allopurinol
• With allopurinol there is a possibility of skin rashes

Significant possible interactions:

Related to medicinal control of the acute attack:
◊ Anticoagulants
◊ Anti-diabetic agents
◊ Anticonvulsants
◊ Lithium

Related to probenecid control of the underlying hyperuricemia:
◊ Antibiotics
◊ Antidiabetic agents
◊ Thiopental
◊ Ketamine
◊ NSAID's
◊ Lorazepam
◊ Rifampin
◊ Antagonized by pyrazinamide, salicylates

Related to allopurinol control of the underlying hyperuricemia:
◊ Mercaptopurine (requires reduction of chemotherapy dose to 1/3 of usual dose)
◊ Azathioprine
◊ Methotrexate
◊ Possibly cyclophosphamide
◊ Anticoagulants
◊ Antidiabetic agents

ALTERNATIVE DRUGS

Related to control of the acute attack:
◊ Colchicine (a controversial toxic agent) which must be taken within 24 hours of onset of the acute attack to be effective
◊ Intra-articular long-acting (depot) corticosteroid (if infection definitely ruled out)

Related to control of the underlying hyperuricemia in the hypoexcretor:
◊ Sulfinpyrazone, initiated at 400 mg qd

FOLLOWUP

PATIENT MONITORING

Related to medicinal control of the acute attack and suppressing attacks:
◊ Adjusting therapeutic regimen if no significant clinical response to therapy within 3 days of its initiation.
◊ CBC, renal and hepatic blood testing and urinalysis at one week, six weeks and every three months

Related to control of the underlying hyperuricemia:
◊ CBC, uric acid level, renal and hepatic blood testing, and urinalysis at monthly intervals (with dosage/regimen modification) until desired serum uric acid level achieved

PREVENTION/AVOIDANCE

Avoidance of exacerbating medications/diets/habits where possible

POSSIBLE COMPLICATIONS

• Increased susceptibility to infection
• Urate nephropathy
• Uric acid nephropathy
• Renal stones
• Nerve/spinal cord impingement

EXPECTED COURSE AND PROGNOSIS

• With early treatment, total control
• If recurrent attacks, successful uric acid adjustment (requiring lifelong use of uricosuric or allopurinol medication) usually suppresses further activity
• During the first 6-24 months of uricosuric or allopurinol therapy, acute gout may occur

MISCELLANEOUS

ASSOCIATED CONDITIONS

• Myeloproliferative disorders
• Lymphoproliferative disorders
• Ethanolism
• Hyperlipidemia
• Obesity
• Hypertension
• Diabetes
• Lesch-Nyhan syndrome - chorea, spasticity, self-mutilation in childhood

AGE-RELATED FACTORS

Pediatric: Onset in this age group identifies gout secondary to an inborn error of metabolism or underlying disease process
Geriatric: Usually related to medications
Others: N/A

PREGNANCY   Usual pregnancy precautions

SYNONYMS   N/A

ICD-9-CM

• Gout or tophus 274.0
• Ear tophus or renal 274.1
• Lead related 984.9

SEE ALSO

• Alcoholism
• Sickle cell anemia

OTHER NOTES   N/A

ABBREVIATIONS

MP = metatarsal phalangeal
NSAID = nonsteroidal anti-inflammatory drug

REFERENCES

• Yu, T.F.: Gout. In Diagnosis and Management of Rheumatic Diseases. Edited by W. Katz. Philadelphia, J.B. Lippincott, 1988
• Kelley, W.N., Harris, E.D., Jr., Ruddy, S. & Sledge, C.B.: Textbook of Rheumatology. Philadelphia, W.B. Saunders Co., 1993
• Rothschild, B.M.: Crystalline Arthritis: Gout. Fairlawn, CT, Clinical AV, 1982

Author   B. Rothschild, M.D.

Granuloma annulare

 BASICS

DESCRIPTION Chronic, self-limited inflammation of the skin exhibited by annularly arranged papules
• Localized granuloma annulare - the more common form consists of a solitary group of flesh colored papules that gradually involute centrally to form circles or semi-circles
• Disseminated granuloma annulare - occurs less often and consists of widespread lesions with the same characteristics as localized type
System(s) affected: Skin
Genetics: Not specified, although a familial incidence has been noted among siblings, twins, and successive generations
Incidence/Prevalence in USA: Not specified
Predominant age:
• Localized granuloma annulare - children and young adults
• Disseminated granuloma annulare - adults in 4th to 7th decades
Predominant sex: Females > Males (2:1)

SIGNS AND SYMPTOMS
• Papular, circular or semi-circular lesions
• Papules usually found on dorsal surface of hands, fingers, feet, extensor aspects of arms and legs, trunk
• Subcutaneous nodules seen on palms, legs, buttocks, scalp
• Lesions may be pruritic on rare occasions

CAUSES Unknown

RISK FACTORS
• Diabetes mellitus
• Positive family history

 DIAGNOSIS

DIFFERENTIAL DIAGNOSIS
• Papular lesions - necrobiosis lipoidica, cutaneous amyloidosis, annular elastolytic granuloma, papular sarcoid, lichen planus, tinea, tuberculoid (TT) or borderline tuberculoid (BT) leprosy
• Subcutaneous nodules - rheumatoid nodules

LABORATORY If disseminated form, check blood sugar
Drugs that may alter lab results: N/A
Disorders that may alter lab results: N/A

PATHOLOGICAL FINDINGS Palisading granuloma with histiocytes and epithelial cells surrounding a central zone of altered collagen in the mid to upper dermis

SPECIAL TESTS N/A

IMAGING N/A

DIAGNOSTIC PROCEDURES Inspection of skin usually reveals diagnosis. Skin scraping to rule out fungi can be done. If diagnosis is in doubt skin biopsy can be performed.

 TREATMENT

APPROPRIATE HEALTH CARE
Outpatient

GENERAL MEASURES Treatment is not always satisfactory.

ACTIVITY Full activity

DIET American Diabetic Association guidelines when associated with diabetes

PATIENT EDUCATION If patient has disseminated form, papules may be accentuated by sun exposure

MEDICATIONS

DRUG(S) OF CHOICE
• Localized form - intralesional triamcinolone acetonide, 5 mg/mL injected into the elevated border only. A 30 gauge needle is used. May be repeated at monthly intervals.
• Topical steroids with occlusion or incorporated in tape are occasionally useful for localized form
• Disseminated form - dapsone 100 mg qd or bid; PUVA or REPUVA

Contraindications: Dapsone should not be given to patients with G6PD deficiency
Precautions: See manufacturer's profile of each drug
Significant possible interactions: See manufacturer's profile of each drug

ALTERNATIVE DRUGS
• For disseminated form isotretinoin 80 mg qd is used in refractive cases
• Niacinamide 1.5 gm qd or potassium iodide is recommended by some

FOLLOWUP

PATIENT MONITORING Depends on nature of treatment; generally two week intervals while undergoing treatment

PREVENTION/AVOIDANCE Avoid sun-exposure in patients with disseminated form if association with light

POSSIBLE COMPLICATIONS None

EXPECTED COURSE AND PROGNOSIS Lesions disappear without scarring in 75% of patients in two years. 40% of patients experience recurrences

MISCELLANEOUS

ASSOCIATED CONDITIONS Diabetes mellitus is mainly associated with disseminated granuloma annulare but the frequency is unknown

AGE-RELATED FACTORS
Pediatric: N/A
Geriatric: Disseminated form is more common in older patients
Others: N/A

PREGNANCY N/A

SYNONYMS N/A

ICD-9-CM 695.89

SEE ALSO N/A

OTHER NOTES N/A

ABBREVIATIONS N/A

REFERENCES
• Habif, T.: Clinical Dermatology. 2nd Ed. St. Louis, C.V. Mosby, 1990
• Domonkos, A.N., Arnold, H.L., & Odom, R.B.: Andrew's Diseases of the Skin. 8th Ed. Philadelphia, W.B. Saunders Co., 1990

Author G. Silko, M.D.

Granuloma, pyogenic

BASICS

DESCRIPTION Benign, solitary mass involving the oral cavity, most frequently the gingiva (70%)
Systems affected: Oral cavity
Genetics: N/A
Incidence/Prevalence: Unknown
Predominant age: Any, most frequently second to fifth decades
Predominant sex: Slight predilection for females

SIGNS AND SYMPTOMS
• Sessile or pedunculated
• Granular, smooth or slightly nodular
• Soft
• May be ulcerated, bleeding easily
• Red, purple, or brown in color
• Ranges from a few millimeters to 2-3 centimeters in diameter

CAUSES
• Thought to be an over-reaction to minor trauma
• May be related to hormonal changes in pregnancy

RISK FACTORS
• Pregnancy
• Intraoral trauma or surgery

DIAGNOSIS

DIFFERENTIAL DIAGNOSIS
• Peripheral ossifying granuloma
• Giant cell granuloma
• Odontogenic fibroma
• Kaposi's sarcoma
• Malignant melanoma
• Angiolymphoid hyperplasia with eosinophilia
• Metastatic carcinoma

LABORATORY N/A
Drugs that may alter lab results: N/A
Disorders that may alter lab results: N/A

PATHOLOGICAL FINDINGS
• Micro-small, endothelial lined vascular spaces
• Micro- loose or dense connective tissue stroma
• Micro- acute and chronic inflammatory cells
• Micro- no true granuloma formation
• Micro- abundant mitotic activity

SPECIAL TESTS N/A

IMAGING N/A

DIAGNOSTIC PROCEDURES Excisional biopsy

TREATMENT

APPROPRIATE HEALTH CARE
Outpatient

GENERAL MEASURES
• Surgical excision of lesion (with cleaning of adjacent teeth if lesion is gingival)
• May recur if inadequately excised
• Occasional spontaneous resolution
• Good oral hygiene

ACTIVITY As tolerated

DIET As tolerated

PATIENT EDUCATION Patient should avoid trauma to the area following excision

MEDICATIONS

DRUG(S) OF CHOICE None
Contraindications: N/A
Precautions: N/A
Significant possible interactions: N/A

ALTERNATIVE DRUGS N/A

FOLLOWUP

PATIENT MONITORING As needed

PREVENTION/AVOIDANCE Good oral hygiene

POSSIBLE COMPLICATIONS
Recurrence

EXPECTED COURSE AND PROGNOSIS Complete resolution expected with adequate excision.

MISCELLANEOUS

ASSOCIATED CONDITIONS N/A

AGE-RELATED FACTORS N/A
Pediatric: N/A
Geriatric: N/A
Others: N/A

PREGNANCY Lesion also occurs in pregnant women, and is known as "pregnancy tumor"

SYNONYMS
• Pregnancy tumor
• Granuloma gravidum

ICD-9-CM
• Pyogenic granuloma 686.1
• Maxillary alveolar ridge 522.6
• Oral mucosa 528.9

SEE ALSO N/A

OTHER NOTES N/A

ABBREVIATIONS N/A

REFERENCES
• Wood, N.K. & Goaz, P.W.: Differential Diagnosis of Oral Lesions. St. Louis, C.V. Mosby, 1985
• Ash, M.M.: Oral Pathology. Philadelphia, Lea & Febiger, 1986

Author G. Suits, M.D. & L. Howell, M.D.

Guillain-Barré syndrome

BASICS

DESCRIPTION Acute onset of progressive motor weakness usually beginning distally. Symmetric and often accompanied by sensory loss. Follows antecedent infection by eight weeks in 65% of cases.

Incidence/Prevalence in USA: 0.6-1.9 cases per 100,000 annually, non-seasonal, non-epidemic in nature

System(s) affected: Nervous, Endocrine/Metabolic

Genetics: Recurrent form - chronic relapsing polyneuropathy shows correlation with HLA-Aw30 and HLA-Aw31

Predominant age: Occurs at all ages

Predominant sex: Male = Female

SIGNS AND SYMPTOMS
• Symmetrical distal muscle weakness beginning in legs, ascends rapidly (in a few days) to the arms (accompanied by paresthesia, which may be evanescent)
• Hypotonia
• Reduced reflexes, then loss of deep tendon reflexes - 100%
• "Stocking" distribution sensory loss (variable)
• Bulbar involvement - bilateral facial and oropharyngeal paresis
• Difficulty swallowing
• Urinary retention
• Respiratory muscle paralysis
• Blood pressure fluctuation
• Inappropriate ADH secretion

CAUSES
• Thought to be autoimmune. Triggered by antecedent infection. Described after URI, infectious mononucleosis, cytomegalovirus infections, herpes zoster, influenza A, mycoplasma, mumps, AIDS, Lyme disease, lymphoma (especially Hodgkin's), serum sickness, and postsurgical.
• 1976-77 swine flu vaccine triggered a rash of cases (1/100,000 receiving vaccine). Not seen with subsequent flu vaccines.

RISK FACTORS Antecedent infection

DIAGNOSIS

DIFFERENTIAL DIAGNOSIS
• Neuropathy of many other causes - heavy metals (lead, arsenic), industrial agents acrylamide, carbon disulfide, trichlorethylene, rapeseed oil, hexacarbons, organophosphate esters
• Secondary to other organic disease - diabetes, uremia, porphyria, amyloidosis, lupus, polyarteritis nodosa, rheumatoid arthritis, carcinoma, lymphoma, multiple myeloma, polio
• Secondary to deficiency states - alcoholism, B12, folic acid
• Drugs - gold, sulindac, hydralazine, nitrous oxide, disulfiram, glutethimide, phenytoin, nitrofurantoin, dapsone, metronidazole, isoniazid, pyridoxine dose greater than 2 grams/day
• Hereditary causes of polyneuropathy - Charcot-Marie-Tooth, Roussy-Levy, metachromatic leukodystrophy, adrenoleukodystrophy, Anderson-Fabry disease, porphyria polyneuropathy, Krabbe disease, Déjérine-Sottas, Refsum's disease, Andrade's indicator, abetalipoproteinemia

LABORATORY
• CSF - elevation of CSF protein without accompanying cellular response. Elevation begins within a week of symptoms and peaks at 4-6 weeks. Protein elevation may be very high (> 1000 mg/dl).
• CBC - can see early leukocytosis with left shift which resolves during course of illness
Drugs that may alter lab results: N/A
Disorders that may alter lab results: N/A

PATHOLOGICAL FINDINGS
• Segmental demyelination of peripheral nerves, axonal degeneration
• Inflammatory lesion - lymphocyte and macrophage invasion of myelin sheath

SPECIAL TESTS Electromyography - finding sharp waves or fibrillations indicate axonal degeneration. Nerve conduction is slowed due to demyelination. Usually not necessary to establish diagnosis.

IMAGING N/A

DIAGNOSTIC PROCEDURES Lumbar puncture - CSF opening pressure normal, usually no cellular response (see lab, above), glucose normal, protein increased, sometimes greatly (> 1000 mg/dl). When very high, elevation in oncotic pressure can increase CSF volume and lead to an increase in CSF pressure and papilledema.

TREATMENT

APPROPRIATE HEALTH CARE
• Hospitalization with ICU available in anticipation of respiratory support by mechanical ventilation. Respiratory support may be needed for prolonged periods in some patients. May necessitate tracheostomy.
• Hospital capable of performing plasmapheresis

GENERAL MEASURES
• Measurement of vital capacity and arterial blood gases. Vital capacity < 1000 mL and PaO2 < 70 indicate need for assisted ventilation.
• Blood pressure support
• Plasmapheresis (blood exchange) in severe cases (those requiring mechanical ventilation or who cannot walk). Shortens course and reduces time on ventilator.
• Encourage fluid intake to maintain urine volume of 1 to 1.5 L/day
• Monitor serum electrolytes to prevent water intoxication
• Cradles for bedclothes to protect patient from trauma and pressure
• Moist heat to help relieve pain and permit early physical therapy

ACTIVITY No limitation. Physical therapy to prevent contractures.

DIET No special diet

PATIENT EDUCATION Guillain-Barré Foundation International, P.O. Box 262, Wynnewood, PA 19096, (215)667-0131

MEDICATIONS

DRUG(S) OF CHOICE
• No drug therapy recommended. Steroids not shown to be of benefit in GBS.
• Prednisone used in the chronic form of the disease "chronic relapsing polyneuropathy"
• Pressors such as dopamine for blood pressure support
Contraindications: See manufacturer's profile of each drug
Precautions: See manufacturer's profile of each drug
Significant possible interactions: See manufacturer's profile of each drug

ALTERNATIVE DRUGS N/A

FOLLOWUP

PATIENT MONITORING Patient will require physical rehabilitation to regain strength

PREVENTION/AVOIDANCE N/A

POSSIBLE COMPLICATIONS
<u>During course:</u>
◊ Diabetes insipidus
◊ Syndrome of inappropriate ADH (SIADH)
◊ Autonomic involvement
◊ Rebound of symptoms after stopping plasmapheresis if begun too early in the course of the disease
<u>Subsequent development of chronic course:</u>
◊ Chronic inflammatory demyelinating polyradiculoneuropathy (CIDP). This has an insidious onset following GBS, and continues for years. Plasmapheresis benefits 1/3 of these patients.

EXPECTED COURSE AND PROGNOSIS
• In pure or predominant demyelination - weakness and paralysis progresses over a two week period, stabilizes, and then gradually improves
• 10-23% require ventilatory support
• 7-22% are left with mild disability-mild weakness or reflex loss
• About 10% have severe residual. These are the patients who had a more prolonged course, longer time on ventilator or significant axonal degeneration. Axonal regeneration requires 6-18 months.
• Mortality is about 3%

MISCELLANEOUS

ASSOCIATED CONDITIONS
• Neurofibromatosis
• Development of chronic relapsing polyneuropathy

AGE-RELATED FACTORS
Pediatric: N/A
Geriatric: N/A
Others: N/A

PREGNANCY No data

SYNONYMS
• Ascending paralysis
• Acute idiopathic polyneuritis
• Acute immune mediated polyneuritis (AIMP)
• Landry-Guillain-Barré
• Acute polyneuropathy
• Infectious idiopathic polyneuropathy
• Landry's ascending paralysis
• Acute segmentally demyelinating polyradiculoneuropathy

ICD-9-CM
357.0

SEE ALSO N/A

OTHER NOTES N/A

ABBREVIATIONS N/A

REFERENCES
• Adams, R.D. & Victor, M.: Principles of Neurology. 4th Ed. New York, McGraw-Hill, 1989

Author K. Hall, M.D.

Gynecomastia

 BASICS

DESCRIPTION
A benign glandular enlargement of the male breast that is generally bilateral (may be asymmetric, or rarely, unilateral)
Type I: Benign adolescent hypertrophy
  ◊ Physiologic distoid subacute mass
  ◊ Resolves spontaneously
Type II: Physiologic gynecomastia
  ◊ Generalized enlargement to greater degree
Type III:
  ◊ Obesity simulates gynecomastia
Type IV:
  ◊ Pectoral muscle hypertrophy
System(s) affected: Skin/Exocrine, Endocrine/Metabolic
Genetics: Some instance of familial gynecomastia may be inherited as a male-limited autosomal trait
Incidence in USA: 38-64% of pubertal males
Prevalence in USA: Rare except when drug-induced
Predominant age: Puberty; and over the age of 65 (especially with a weight gain)
Predominant sex: Male only

SIGNS AND SYMPTOMS
• Usually asymptomatic
• May be painful and tender if it has developed rapidly (drug-induced, refeeding gynecomastia)

CAUSES
• Physiologic - transient in neonatal boys and at puberty
• Exposure to a high level of estrogen compared to testosterone concentration
• Tumors - estrogen secreting, gonadotropin secreting
• Drug-induced (hormones, marijuana, digitalis, spironolactone, cimetidine, ketoconazole, cytotoxic drugs, antihypertensives, sedatives, antidepressants, amphetamine)
• Systemic disorders - cirrhosis, thyrotoxicosis, renal failure
• Androgen production deficiency
• Androgen resistant syndromes
• Trauma
• Idiopathic

RISK FACTORS
• Klinefelter's syndrome
• Obesity
• Testicular failure
• Recovery from prolonged severe illness associated with malnutrition and weight loss (refeeding gynecomastia)
• Family history
• Peutz-Jeghers syndrome
• Male pseudohermaphroditism

 DIAGNOSIS

DIFFERENTIAL DIAGNOSIS
• Obesity with increase in adipose tissue
• Carcinoma of the male breast
• Lipomas
• Neurofibromas

LABORATORY
• Laboratory evaluation rarely indicated
• Human chorionic gonadotropin levels - high levels may lead to finding a choriocarcinoma or other hCG-secreting tumor
• Plasma testosterone and leuteinizing hormone measurements - help diagnose hypogonadism
• Serum estradiol
• Serum prolactin
• Liver function
• Others if clinically indicated e.g., thyroid function, chromosomal analysis
Drugs that may alter lab results: N/A
Disorders that may alter lab results:
• Cirrhosis
• Thyrotoxicosis
• Renal failure

PATHOLOGICAL FINDINGS
• Dense, periductal hyaline, collagenous connective tissue
• Hyperplastic ductal lining
• Plasma cell infiltrate

SPECIAL TESTS
Full endocrine investigations may be indicated

IMAGING
CT, ultrasonography or x-ray (rarely indicated)

DIAGNOSTIC PROCEDURES
• History and physical exam to determine possible etiology
• Biopsy, if suspicious

 TREATMENT

APPROPRIATE HEALTH CARE
Outpatient

GENERAL MEASURES
Non-operative
  ◊ Correct underlying disorder
  ◊ Withdrawal of causative drug if feasible
  ◊ Observation with reassurance that problem is transient
Operative
  ◊ Biopsy if suspicious of cancer
  ◊ Subcutaneous mastectomy for severe, persistent cases or those with psychological concerns

ACTIVITY
No restrictions

DIET
• No special diet
• If obesity a problem, weight loss diet

PATIENT EDUCATION
N/A

MEDICATIONS

DRUG(S) OF CHOICE None
Contraindications: N/A
Precautions: N/A
Significant possible interactions: N/A

ALTERNATIVE DRUGS N/A

FOLLOWUP

PATIENT MONITORING
• Every 3-6 months for physiologic gynecomastia
• Until well for non-physiologic gynecomastia

PREVENTION/AVOIDANCE In men taking estrogen for prostate cancer - low dose radiation prior to institution of diethylstilbestrol

POSSIBLE COMPLICATIONS None expected

EXPECTED COURSE AND PROGNOSIS
• Physiologic gynecomastia clears without treatment (may take up to 2 years)
• Drug withdrawal cures
• Other causes - outcome depends on etiology
• Little change in Type III without substantial weight loss
• Good results with subcutaneous mastectomy

MISCELLANEOUS

ASSOCIATED CONDITIONS Listed with Causes

AGE-RELATED FACTORS
Pediatric:
• Transient gynecomastia seen in neonatal boys
• At puberty, may be observed in 38-64% of boys
Geriatric: Drug induced form more common
Others: N/A

PREGNANCY N/A

SYNONYMS Male breast hypertrophy

ICD-9-CM 611.1

SEE ALSO N/A

OTHER NOTES N/A

ABBREVIATIONS N/A

REFERENCES
• Becker, K.L. (ed.): Principles and Practice of Endocrinology and Metabolism. Philadelphia, J.B. Lippincott Co., 1990
• Holder, T.M. & Ashcroft, K.W. (eds.): Pediatric Surgery. 2nd Ed. Philadelphia, W.B. Saunders Co., 1993
• Mahoney, C.P.: Adolescent gynecomastia. Differential diagnosis and management. Pediatr Clin North Am 37:1389, 1990

Author T. Black, M.D.

Headache, cluster

BASICS

DESCRIPTION Attacks of severe, unilateral headache around the eye and temple with ipsilateral lacrimation, rhinorrhea, ptosis, miosis and nasal stuffiness. Attacks last approximately 30-120 minutes and occur 1-3 times per day (often waking the patient) at the same time of day for up to 12 weeks typically followed by 1-24 months without an attack.
System(s) affected: Nervous
Genetics: Unknown
Incidence/Prevalence in USA: 69 per 100,000 population
Predominant age: Mean age at onset - 30 years in men, later in women
Predominant sex: Male > Female (6:1)

SIGNS AND SYMPTOMS
• Sudden onset of headache
• Headache reaches crescendo within 15 minutes, lasts < 2 hours
• Pain is unilateral, oculotemporal or oculofrontal
• Severe, piercing or boring (rarely throbbing) pain
• Homolateral Horner's syndrome
• Retro-orbital pain
• Lacrimation (84%)
• Infected conjunctiva (58%)
• Ptosis (57%)
• Nasal stuffiness (48%)
• Rhinorrhea (43%)
• Bradycardia (43%)
• Nausea (40%)
• Perspiration (26%)
• Restlessness
• Characteristic timing of episodes of headache at same time(s) on consecutive days, and of "clusters" of these days separated by attack-free weeks or months

CAUSES
• Actual cause unknown
• Disorder of arterial tone in cerebral arteries
• Disturbance of circadian rhythm based in hypothalamus
• Disorder of serotonin metabolism or transmission in CNS
• Disorder of histamine concentrations or receptors

RISK FACTORS
• Male sex
• Age > 30 years
• Possible relationship to previous head injury or surgery
• Attacks triggered by nitroglycerine, alcohol

DIAGNOSIS

DIFFERENTIAL DIAGNOSIS Headache secondary to other pathology in head and neck, migraine, trigeminal or other facial neuralgias, temporal arteritis, pheochromocytoma, Raeder's syndrome

LABORATORY Not used except to rule out differential diagnoses
Drugs that may alter lab results: N/A
Disorders that may alter lab results: N/A

PATHOLOGICAL FINDINGS N/A

SPECIAL TESTS N/A

IMAGING MRI for atypical presentations or for those unresponsive to treatment

DIAGNOSTIC PROCEDURES N/A

TREATMENT

APPROPRIATE HEALTH CARE
Outpatient

GENERAL MEASURES
• During cluster periods, avoid bright light or glare, alcohol, excessive anger, stressful activity or excitement. These will precipitate attacks.
• Tobacco may make cluster refractory to drug treatment

ACTIVITY
• Avoid self-injury during bouts of excruciating pain
• Vigorous physical activity at first symptoms may abort attack
• Ipsilateral carotid compression may reduce pain
• Ipsilateral compression of superficial temporal artery relives pain in 40%, but increases in 40%

DIET
• During clusters, alcohol precipitates attacks
• Rarely, specific foods (chocolate, eggs, dairy products) trigger attacks

PATIENT EDUCATION
• Focus on nature of condition and how to avoid precipitants
• Assist patient in learning self-treatment methods

MEDICATIONS

DRUG(S) OF CHOICE
Acute attack:
◊ Sumatriptan 6 mg subcutaneous, repeat in one hour if necessary, maximum 12 mg/24 hr
◊ Ergotamine aerosol (Medihaler Ergotamine) 0.36-1.08 mg (1-3 inhalations). Maximum 6 inhalations or 4 mg in 24 hours.
◊ Oxygen 100% at 8-10 L/min for 10-15 minutes administered by tight-fitting mask. Up to 5 sessions per day.
◊ Lidocaine intranasal instillation of 1 ml of 4% topical solution slowly on same side as symptoms. Position patient supine with head extended 45° and rotated 40° to side of pain. May need to premedicate with 1-2 drops intranasal 0.5% phenylephrine for nasal stuffiness.
◊ Dihydroergotamine mesylate (D.H.E.45) 1 mg IM or IV
◊ Methoxyflurane 10-15 drops inhaled from tissue
Prophylaxis (to shorten cluster period or prevent expected attacks)
◊ Ergotamine timed to provide peak dose at anticipated time of attack, e.g., 2 mg rectal suppository 1 hour before, or 1-2 mg orally 2 hours before
◊ Prednisone - various dosages suggested, e.g., 80 mg/day for 7 days followed by rapid tapering over 6 days or 40 mg/day for 5 days tapering over 3 weeks
◊ Methysergide (Sansert) 4-10 mg/day in divided doses tid or qid for 4-6 weeks
◊ Lithium carbonate (Eskalith) 300 mg 2-4 times daily. Use concurrently with ergotamine (2-4 mg/day) if necessary.
Contraindications: Specific to drugs - myocardial or peripheral ischemia, pregnancy, peptic ulceration, diarrhea, thyroid suppression
Precautions:
• Specific to drugs - vasoconstriction, adrenal or thyroid suppression, retroperitoneal fibrosis, increased nausea, hypertension
• Screen individual patients for potential drug abuse risk
• Avoid alcohol and tobacco during clusters
Significant possible interactions: Refer to manufacturer's profile of each drug

ALTERNATIVE DRUGS
• Indomethacin up to 150 mg daily
• Nifedipine 40-120 mg/day
• Nimodipine up to 240 mg/day
• Sumatriptan 6 mg subcutaneous

FOLLOWUP

PATIENT MONITORING
• To anticipate cluster bouts and initiate early prophylaxis
• Monitor for side effects of medications
• Education for patient and family

PREVENTION/AVOIDANCE
• Nitroglycerine, alcohol and some foods can induce cluster
• Tobacco slows response to medication
• Disturbances of sleep cycle induce attacks
• Emotion, anger, excessive physical activity induce attacks

POSSIBLE COMPLICATIONS
• Self-injury during attack
• Side effects of drugs
• Potential for drug abuse

EXPECTED COURSE AND PROGNOSIS
• Recurrent attacks
• Prolonged remissions

MISCELLANEOUS

ASSOCIATED CONDITIONS
• Significantly higher incidence of peptic ulcer, coronary artery disease (males)
• Prior history of migraine frequent (significant in females)

AGE-RELATED FACTORS
Women more likely to begin around menopause or later
Pediatric: N/A
Geriatric: N/A
Others:
• Characteristic appearance: "Leonine" face, thickened skin, above average height, more likely to have hazel eye color and be heavier smokers. No evidence of specific psychological type.
• Consider surgical treatments to trigeminal nerve if refractory to drug therapy

PREGNANCY
Very rare in pregnancy age groups

SYNONYMS
• Migrainous neuralgia
• Sphenopalatine neuralgia
• Histamine cephalalgia

ICD-9-CM
784.0

SEE ALSO
Other causes of headaches

OTHER NOTES
N/A

ABBREVIATIONS
N/A

REFERENCES
• Raskin, N.H.: Headache. 2nd Ed. New York, Churchill Livingstone, 1988
• Dalessio, D.J.: Wolff's Headache and Other Head Pain. 5th Ed. New York, Oxford University Press, 1987
• Sumatriptan Cluster Headache Study Group. N Engl J Med, 1991;325:322-6
• Dechant, K.C. & Clissold, S.P.: Sumatriptan (Review). Drugs, 1992; 43:776-98

Author A. Walling, M.D.

Headache, tension

 BASICS

DESCRIPTION Tension headache can be divided into two types:
• Episodic - usually associated with some stressful event, is of moderate intensity, self-limited, and usually responds to non-prescription preparations
• Chronic - often recurring daily, bilateral location, usually occipito-frontal and associated with contracted muscles of the neck and scalp
System(s) affected: Musculoskeletal
Genetics: 40% have a positive family history for headache
Incidence/Prevalence in USA: Common
Predominant age: 60% have onset after age 20 (unusual to begin after age 50)
Predominant sex: Female > Male

SIGNS AND SYMPTOMS
• Bilateral headache in 90%
• Located fronto-occipital or generalized
• Dull, pressing or band-like
• Intensity varies throughout the day
• Often present upon arising or shortly thereafter
• Chronic headaches have a duration greater than 5 years in 75% of patients
• Insomnia
• Teeth grinding
• Not aggravated by physical activity
• Difficulty concentrating
• Muscular tightness or stiffness in neck, occipital and frontal regions

CAUSES
• Poor posture
• Stress and/or anxiety
• Depression (found in 70% of those with daily headache)
• Low platelet serotonin
• Cervical osteoarthritis
• Intramuscular vasoconstriction

RISK FACTORS
• Risk of addiction to analgesics
• Risk of epilepsy is four times that of the general population
• Obstructive sleep apnea
• Medications
• Excess caffeine

 DIAGNOSIS

DIFFERENTIAL DIAGNOSIS
• Cervical spondylosis
• TMJ syndrome
• Caffeine-dependency
• Non-prescription analgesic dependency
• Depression
• Head injury
• Severe anemia or polycythemia
• Uremia and hepatic disorders
• Toxic effects from drugs or fumes
• Dental disease
• Paget's disease of bone
• Chronic sinusitis
• Refractive error
• Hypertension
• Hypoxia
• Temporal arteritis
• Migraine
• Lesions of the eye or middle ear
• Lesions of the oral cavity

LABORATORY
• CBC
• SMAC-20
• Thyroid studies
• ESR in anyone over 50 years of age
Drugs that may alter lab results: N/A
Disorders that may alter lab results:
Chronic hepatitis, renal and thyroid conditions

PATHOLOGICAL FINDINGS Normal neurological examination, furrowed brow, tense masseter muscle, tight muscles in the scalp and neck

SPECIAL TESTS N/A

IMAGING
• X-rays of cervical spine
• Head CT or MRI necessary only when headache pattern has recently changed or there is a positive finding on neurological exam

DIAGNOSTIC PROCEDURES NA

 TREATMENT

APPROPRIATE HEALTH CARE
Outpatient setting

GENERAL MEASURES Relief measures - use relaxation routines; rest in quiet, dark room with cold washcloth over eyes; hot bath or shower; massaging back of neck and temples

ACTIVITY Encourage physical fitness, range of motion and strengthening exercises for the neck

DIET No demonstrated link between diet and tension headache

PATIENT EDUCATION
• Life style changes to minimize stress. Suggest patient seek counseling, if appropriate.
• Encourage relaxation techniques, aerobic exercise, assertiveness training
• Patient information available from the National Headache Foundation, 5252 N. Western Ave., Chicago, IL 60625 1-800-843-2256

MEDICATIONS

DRUG(S) OF CHOICE
Acute attack - nonsteroidal anti-inflammatory drugs (NSAID's):
◊ Naproxen sodium (Naprosyn) 500 mg/bid
◊ Fenoprofen calcium (Nalfon) 600 mg/day (200 mg q 4-6 hours)
◊ Ibuprofen (Motrin, Advil) 400 mg/tid
◊ Ketoprofen (Orudis) 50 mg/tid
Prophylaxis for chronic tension headache - antidepressants
◊ Amitriptyline (Elavil) 50-100 mg/day
◊ Desipramine (Norpramin) 50-100 mg/day
◊ Imipramine (Tofranil) 50-100 mg/day
◊ Nortriptyline (Pamelor) 25-50 mg/day
Contraindications:
• NSAID's and antidepressants, in general, not suitable for use in children
• Antidepressants should not be used concomitantly with MAO inhibitors
Precautions:
• Do not use antidepressants in presence of acute myocardial infarction
• Avoid over dependance on non-prescription caffeine containing preparations
• Use NSAID's with precaution in patients with history of previous peptic disease
Significant possible Interactions:
Antidepressants and alcohol create accentuated depression

ALTERNATIVE DRUGS
Beta blockers - prophylaxis (select one):
◊ Propranolol (Inderal LA) 80 mg/daily
◊ Nadolol (Corgard) 40 mg/daily
◊ Atenolol (Tenormin) 50-100 mg/daily
Combination agent - prophylaxis
◊ Acetaminophen and isometheptene (Midrin) one capsule tid

FOLLOWUP

PATIENT MONITORING
A warm, nonjudgmental, understanding relationship with the physician is the best predictor for a successful treatment program

PREVENTION/AVOIDANCE
• Physical therapy
• Biofeedback and relaxation therapy
• Cervical traction
• Injection of trigger points

POSSIBLE COMPLICATIONS
• Undue reliance on non-prescription caffeine-containing analgesics
• Dependance/addiction to narcotic analgesics
• GI bleed from NSAID use

EXPECTED COURSE AND PROGNOSIS
• Usually follows a chronic course when life stressors are not changed
• Most cases are intermittent and should not interfere with work or normal life span

MISCELLANEOUS

ASSOCIATED CONDITIONS
10% of patients with tension headache also have migraine headache

AGE-RELATED FACTORS
Pediatric: 15% will have onset at age less than 10 years
Geriatric: Onset of new headache in the elderly is always worrisome and cause for careful study
Others: Unusual for tension-type headaches to begin after age 50

PREGNANCY
No documented relationship

SYNONYMS
• Muscle contraction headache
• Cephalgia

ICD-9-CM
307.81

SEE ALSO
N/A

OTHER NOTES
N/A

ABBREVIATIONS
N/A

REFERENCES
• Bonica, J.J.: The Management of Pain, 2nd Ed. Philadelphia, Lea and Febiger, 1990

Author D. McHard, M.D.

Hearing loss

BASICS

DESCRIPTION Complete or partial hearing loss that may involve the middle ear (mechanical, conductive) or the inner ear (nerve, sensorineural)
Genetics: Both types may be on a genetic basis
Incidence in USA: 140/100,000/year (134 adults, 6 school age children)
Prevalence in USA: 3,494 (cases/100,000), with 3,333 for adults and 161 for school age children.
Predominant age: All ages, but more common in elderly
Predominant sex: Male = Female

SIGNS AND SYMPTOMS Obvious difficulty hearing, with possible association of other symptoms such as tinnitus, dizziness, pain, and blockage

CAUSES
Conductive
◊ Cerumen impaction
◊ Perforation of tympanic membrane
◊ Middle ear fluid (serous otitis media)
◊ Acute otitis media
◊ Adhesive otitis media
◊ Damage to ossicles (trauma, infection, etc.)
◊ Tympanosclerosis (thickening of drum that may produce fixation)
◊ Otosclerosis (new bone growth that produces stapes fixation)
◊ Cholesteatoma (growth of skin into middle ear)
◊ Middle ear tumor (glomus, etc.)
◊ Congenital problems (atresia, ossicular fixation, etc.)
◊ Temporal bone fracture, injuries
Sensorineural
◊ Acoustic tumor
◊ Meniere's disease
◊ Noise induced (industrial, recreational, occupational)
◊ Hereditary
◊ Congenital
◊ Viral (relatively common, esp. mumps)
◊ Ototoxicity (ASA, quinine, gentamicin, kanamycin, etc.)
◊ Syphilis - hearing loss, tinnitus, dizzy
◊ Presbycusis (hearing loss related to aging)
◊ Temporal bone injury, fracture
◊ Metabolic (hypothyroid, etc.)
◊ Perilymphatic (inner ear) fistula (usually secondary to pressure changes or trauma)

RISK FACTORS Nasal allergy and other causes of eustachian tube obstruction; exposure to loud noise levels; use of ototoxic antibiotics; prematurity; heredity (otosclerosis)

DIAGNOSIS

DIFFERENTIAL DIAGNOSIS
• In conductive loss, must rule out cholesteatoma
• In sensorineural loss, must rule out acoustic tumor

LABORATORY N/A
Drugs that may alter lab results: N/A
Disorders that may alter lab results: N/A

PATHOLOGICAL FINDINGS N/A

SPECIAL TESTS
• Audiometry including pure tone and speech testing, and impedance (middle ear pressure) testing. Both types of hearing loss may fluctuate, making audiometric results variable from test to test. Marked conductive loss in one ear may be difficult to exclude (mask) when testing opposite ear.
• Otoscopy with operating microscope (sometimes necessary to see small superior, attic perforation, indicating a cholesteatoma)

IMAGING
• CT scan (not routinely needed) is useful to demonstrate tumors and cholesteatoma of the temporal bone
• MRI scan is more useful to show acoustic and other cerebellopontine angle tumors (usually produce a sensorineural hearing loss)

DIAGNOSTIC PROCEDURES
• Exploratory tympanotomy sometimes necessary to confirm presence of middle ear fluid, tumor, etc.
• Underlying conditions are identified primarily on basis of history of hearing loss, otoscopy, and hearing test (audiometry)

TREATMENT

APPROPRIATE HEALTH CARE
Outpatient

GENERAL MEASURES
Conductive (mechanical)
◊ Cerumen: Remove with suction and irrigation (not if perforation is present). Don't direct water against drum but rather against canal wall. Manipulation with wire curette (ear canal skin very delicate in elderly) may be helpful.
◊ Tympanic membrane perforation: Surgical correction
◊ Serous otitis (primarily in children). Treat underlying conditions. Use decongestants, antibiotics. Urge inflation of eustachian tube (hold nose and blow).
◊ Adhesive otitis: Looks like perforation. Treat eustachian tube problem. May need surgery.

◊ Damage to ossicles: Don't manipulate. Refer to otolaryngologist.
◊ Tympanosclerosis: Drum has white plaques. Treat only if hearing loss is present.
◊ Otosclerosis: Suspect on basis of history of onset, early in life, that is progressive, with positive family history of hearing loss. Consider surgery.
◊ Cholesteatoma: Identify by perforation that is located near margin of drum
◊ Middle ear tumor: May see through drum. Most commonly will be glomus tumor, which has red color and may cause pulsation. Significant problem, needs prompt referral to otolaryngologist.
◊ Congenital deformity: Don't attribute all hearing loss in children to infections and middle ear fluid. Refer to otolaryngologist.
◊ Temporal bone injury: If limited, may only involve middle ear. Drum likely to appear blue. Refer to otolaryngologist.
Sensorineural (nerve)
◊ Acoustic tumor: Most significant type of hearing loss. Very important to diagnose promptly. Suspect when hearing loss, dizziness, and/or tinnitus are present. Needs much higher degree of suspicion on part of primary care physician. Refer.
◊ Meniere's disease: See chapter on this subject
◊ Noise damage: The most common cause of hearing loss in this country. Very frequent on occupational basis, and has the attention of federal government (OSHA regulations). Also occurs secondary to sports and recreation (hunting, use of guns, loud music, chain saws, shop tools). Needs much greater level of recognition at primary care level. Refer.
◊ Hereditary/congenital: Needs immediate recognition early in life, so that if significant, hearing aids can be placed.
◊ Viral: A relatively common cause of permanent hearing loss, frequently unilateral, e.g., mumps
◊ Ototoxic (medication): Needs much more recognition at primary care level. Suspect when hearing loss, and perhaps dizziness and tinnitus come on during course of treatment with certain antibiotics (and many other medications). See Medications.
◊ Syphilis: Treat with high dose penicillin given intravenously, as well as steroids
◊ Presbycusis: No specific treatment available, but important to provide hearing rehabilitation. This includes counseling patient to avoid factors that may cause further loss (noise exposure, ototoxic drugs). Emphasize development of lip reading skills, and counseling family to pronounce words clearly, face patient when speaking, etc. Offer hearing aid trial when patient is a suitable candidate.
◊ Temporal bone injury: No treatment available specifically for hearing loss
◊ Metabolic: Treatment of specific problem (e.g. hyperlipidemia, hypothyroid)
◊ Perilymphatic fistula: Diagnosis based on history of injury to ear including barotrauma during diving. Treatment is early exploration to confirm fistula in round or oval window of middle ear, with repair of fistula.

ACTIVITY
• Patients having perforation of the ear drum or ventilation tube in place should be advised not to swim or allow water to enter the ear
• Patients having hearing loss secondary to noise exposure should be advised to avoid loud noise, or to use suitable protection (ear plugs or ear muffs)

DIET Patients whose hearing loss is due to Meniere's disease should avoid excessive use of salt

PATIENT EDUCATION See information under other headings

MEDICATIONS

DRUG(S) OF CHOICE
• Cerumen impaction - it is frequently helpful to soften the wax prior to removing it. Cerumenex is popular, but should not be used in the presence of a perforation, and may produce a skin reaction. A good alternative is simply to place, or have the patient place hydrogen peroxide in the ear canal prior to wax removal. pHisoHex and topical Colace are also useful to soften very hard wax.
• Acute otitis media - erythromycin or amoxicillin
• Chronic otitis media with purulent drainage - Cortisporin otic drops (or an equivalent) placed into the ear canal (3-6 drops tid)
• Serous otitis media - decongestant (Entex) and erythromycin
• Sudden sensorineural hearing loss with no apparent cause - steroid therapy in high dosage form (80 mg/day of prednisone, or equivalent steroid) may be helpful
Contraindications: History of sensitivity to any of the antibiotics referred to above
Precautions: Avoid the temptation of over-diagnosing "red ear" and using antibiotics without a well thought out diagnosis
Significant possible interactions: Refer to manufacturer's literature

ALTERNATIVE DRUGS
• Acute otitis media - cefaclor
• Chronic ear infection with drainage - ear drops and powder containing ciprofloxacin. Gentamicin drops is another alternative.

FOLLOWUP

PATIENT MONITORING Hearing testing (audiometry) as the primary means of monitoring patient progress

PREVENTION/AVOIDANCE
• Impaired eustachian tube function (serous otitis media, acute otitis media) - improve tubal function with treatment of allergic and sinus disease. Treat upper respiratory infections (URI) promptly and aggressively if ear problems are frequent.
• Sensorineural hearing loss due to noise exposure (or any type of nerve deafness) - advise against excessive noise exposure; recommend ear plugs/ear muffs
• Nerve deafness due to ototoxic medications may be prevented by the avoidance, or careful use of drugs known to be ototoxic (consider audiometric monitoring if used). The most frequently implicated antibiotics are gentamicin, kanamycin, neomycin, vancomycin, and streptomycin. Implicated drugs include lidocaine, morphine, digitalis, quinidine, and furosemide. Use of these drugs cannot always be avoided. Be more suspicious of the possibility that a given medication might be ototoxic, and when hearing loss is a problem, to prescribe with care.
• Serious nerve deafness resulting from CNS disease (meningitis, lues) may be prevented by thorough treatment of the primary problem
• If URI present, avoid flying or diving

POSSIBLE COMPLICATIONS
• Middle ear problems may progress to chronic ear problems (perforations, cholesteatoma)
• Cholesteatoma is capable of producing major complications including permanent loss of hearing, balance problems, facial nerve paralysis, meningitis, lateral sinus thrombosis, and brain abscess. Glomus tumors and acoustic tumors must be identified, or major CNS complications may result.
• Meniere's disease may proceed to total and permanent hearing loss if not treated, and may occur in spite of treatment
• Severe nerve deafness, particularly associated with tinnitus may produce such an emotional impact on the patient that suicide may occur. Treat the patient with empathy and understanding, offer help even if it seems limited. Encouragement and followup care are extremely helpful in managing these patients.

EXPECTED COURSE AND
PROGNOSIS Sensorineural hearing loss is usually permanent. Other types may be improved, cured or have progression halted.

MISCELLANEOUS

ASSOCIATED CONDITIONS Noise, allergy, sinus disease, trauma, heredity, ototoxicity, CNS infections (meningitis, lues), age, hyperlipidemia, hypothyroid, and barotrauma

AGE-RELATED FACTORS
Pediatric: Eustachian tube problems and secondary middle ear problems are more common in infants and small children, usually becoming less frequent by approximately age 10
Geriatric: Presbycusis is common and is made worse by noise exposure and other factors
Others: N/A

PREGNANCY Otosclerosis may become active during pregnancy

SYNONYMS N/A

ICD-9-CM Cerumen: 380.4; perforation: 389.02 and 384.21; serous otitis media: 381.10 and 389.03; acute otitis media: 382.00 and 389.03; adhesive otitis media: 389.03 and 385.13; ossicular damage: 389.03 and 872.72; tympanosclerosis:385.03 and 389.03; otosclerosis: 387.0; cholesteatoma: 384.22; glomus tumor of middle ear: 212.0; congenital conductive loss: 744.04, 744.02, and 389.03; temporal bone fracture with conductive hearing loss: 384.21, 389.02, and 801.01; acoustic neuroma: 225.1; Meniere's disease: 386.01; noise related sensorineural hearing loss (SNHL): 388.12; hereditary SNHL:389.8, V19.2; congenital SNHL: 389.18 and 744.3; viral SNHL: 389.18 and 079.9; ototoxic SNHL: 389.18 and 960.6; luetic SNHL: 094.86; age related SNHL (presbycusis): 388.01; temporal bone injury with SNHL: 951.5; perilymphatic fistula with SNHL: 386.41 and 389.18

SEE ALSO N/A

OTHER NOTES N/A

ABBREVIATIONS SNHL = sensorineural hearing loss

REFERENCES DeWeese, D.D., Saunders, W.H., Schuller, D.E. & Schleuning, A.J.: Otolaryngology-Head and Neck Surgery. 7th Ed. St. Louis, C.V. Mosby Company, 1988. Chapter 39, pp. 445-477

Author G. Gardner, M.D.

Heat exhaustion & heat stroke

 BASICS

 DIAGNOSIS

 TREATMENT

DESCRIPTION
A continuum of increasingly severe heat illnesses caused by dehydration, electrolyte losses, and failure of the body's thermoregulatory mechanisms
• Heat exhaustion is an acute heat injury with hyperthermia due to dehydration
• Heat stroke is extreme hyperthermia with thermoregulatory failure and profound central nervous system dysfunction

System(s) affected: Endocrine/Metabolic, Nervous

Genetics: N/A

Incidence/Prevalence In USA: Dependent on predisposing conditions in combination with environmental factors

Predominant age: More likely in children or elderly

Predominant sex: Male = Female

SIGNS AND SYMPTOMS
Heat Exhaustion
◊ Fatigue and lethargy
◊ Weakness
◊ Dizziness
◊ Nausea, vomiting
◊ Myalgias
◊ Headache
◊ Profuse sweating
◊ Tachycardia
◊ Hypotension
◊ Lack of coordination
◊ Agitation
◊ Intense thirst
◊ Hyperventilation
◊ Paresthesias
◊ Core temperature elevated but < 103°F
Heat Stroke
◊ Exhaustion
◊ Confusion, disorientation
◊ Coma
◊ Hot, flushed, dry skin
◊ Core temperature > 105°F

CAUSES
Failure of heat-dissipating mechanisms or an overwhelming heat stress leading to a rise in core temperature, dehydration and salt depletion

RISK FACTORS
• Poor acclimatization to heat or poor physical conditioning
• Salt or water depletion
• Obesity
• Acute febrile or gastrointestinal illnesses
• Chronic illnesses - uncontrolled diabetes or hypertension, cardiac disease
• Alcohol and other substance abuse
• High heat and humidity, poor air circulation in environment
• Heavy, restrictive clothing

DIFFERENTIAL DIAGNOSIS
Other causes of elevated temperature, dehydration or circulatory collapse
◊ Febrile illnesses, sepsis
◊ Drug-induced fluid loss
◊ Cardiac arrhythmia or infarction
◊ Acute cocaine intoxication
◊ Malignant hyperthermia (an autosomally inherited disorder of skeletal and cardiac muscle in which patients have abnormal muscle metabolism on exposure to halothane or skeletal muscle reactants)

LABORATORY
• Used primarily to detect end-organ damage
• Electrolytes, urinalysis
• Creatinine, blood urea nitrogen
• Liver enzymes
• Complete blood count
• Increased urine specific gravity
• Results of above studies yield hypernatremia, hyperchloremia, hemoconcentration

Drugs that may alter lab results: Diuretics

Disorders that may alter lab results: N/A

PATHOLOGICAL FINDINGS
Only those associated with major organ system failure

SPECIAL TESTS N/A

IMAGING N/A

DIAGNOSTIC PROCEDURES
Rectal temperature monitoring

APPROPRIATE HEALTH CARE
Emergency treatment - best in a hospital setting

GENERAL MEASURES
• Rapid cooling - remove clothing, wet patient down, ice packs
• Fluid and electrolyte replacement with hypotonic oral fluids or IV 0.5-1.0 liter normal saline

ACTIVITY Rest with legs elevated

DIET
• Cool or cold clear liquids only (non-carbonated)
• Avoid caffeine
• Unrestricted sodium

PATIENT EDUCATION
• Stress the importance of proper conditioning and acclimatization
• Instruct patients to recognize heat stress signs and symptoms
• Maintain as much skin exposure as possible in hot, humid conditions, while using proper sun block protection
• Avoid dehydration with proper fluids during activity or exercise - 8 oz fluid intake for every 15 minutes of moderate exercise

MEDICATIONS

DRUG(S) OF CHOICE No medications are required in the initial management. Use isotonic saline solution to rehydrate.
Contraindications: N/A
Precautions: N/A
Significant possible Interactions: N/A

ALTERNATIVE DRUGS N/A

FOLLOWUP

PATIENT MONITORING
 • Rectal temperature monitoring - cooling may be discontinued when the core temperature drops to 102°F and stabilizes
 • Heat stroke patients may require airway management, hemodynamic monitoring and careful fluid and electrolyte administration and monitoring

PREVENTION/AVOIDANCE Most important factor in preventing heat stress is adequate fluid replacement. Allow acclimatization to hot weather through proper conditioning and activity modification. Dress appropriately with loose-fitting, open weave, light-colored clothing.

POSSIBLE COMPLICATIONS
 • May involve failure of any major organ system
 • Cardiac arrhythmias or infarction
 • Pulmonary edema, adult respiratory distress syndrome
 • Coma, seizures
 • Acute renal failure
 • Rhabdomyolysis
 • Disseminated intravascular coagulation
 • Hepatocellular necrosis

EXPECTED COURSE AND PROGNOSIS
 • Good when mental function is not altered and when serum enzymes are not elevated. Recovery is within 24-48 hours in most cases.
 • The mortality rate for heat stroke (10-80%) is directly related to the duration and intensity of hyperthermia as well as to the speed and effectiveness of diagnosis and treatment

MISCELLANEOUS

ASSOCIATED CONDITIONS N/A

AGE-RELATED FACTORS
Pediatric: Children are more susceptible
Geriatric: Elderly are more susceptible
Others: N/A

PREGNANCY May be more prone to volume depletion with heat stress

SYNONYMS
 • Heat illness
 • Heat injury
 • Hyperthermia
 • Heat collapse
 • Heat prostration

ICD-9-CM
 • Heat exhaustion 992.5
 • Heat stroke 992.0

SEE ALSO Hyperthermia, malignant

OTHER NOTES N/A

ABBREVIATIONS N/A

REFERENCES)
 • Mellion, M.B. & Shelton, G.L.: Safe exercise in the heat and heat injury. In The Team Physician's Handbook. Edited by Mellion M.B., Walsh, A.R. & Shelton, G.L., Philadelphia, Hanley & Belfus, 1990, pp 59-69
 • Hubbard, R.W. & Armstrong, L.E.: Hyperthermia: new thoughts on an old problem. Phys Sportsmed. 17(6):97-113, 1989

Author P. Eiff, M.D. & S. Fields, M.D.

Hemochromatosis

 BASICS

DESCRIPTION A hereditary disorder in which the small intestine absorbs excessive iron. Since the body lacks any way to excrete iron, the excess is stored in glands and muscle, such as the liver, pancreas, and heart. Over the years, the involved organs begin to fail.

System(s) affected: Endocrine/Metabolic

Genetics: Autosomal recessive; acquired; HLA-A3; HLA-B14; HLA-B7

Incidence/Prevalence in USA:
3 cases/1000 people (heterozygote frequency 1 in 10) - the most common abnormal gene in the US population

Predominant age: Present from birth, but symptoms usually present in the fifth and sixth decades

Predominant sex: Male = Female (clinical signs are more frequent in men (8:1 male to female ratio)

SIGNS AND SYMPTOMS
- Weakness (83%)
- Abdominal pain (58%)
- Arthralgia (43%)
- Loss of libido or potency (38%)
- Amenorrhea (22%)
- Dyspnea on exertion (15%)
- Neurologic symptoms (6%)
- Hepatomegaly (83%)
- Increased skin pigmentation (75%)
- Loss of body hair (20%)
- Splenomegaly (13%)
- Peripheral edema (12%)
- Jaundice (10%)
- Gynecomastia (8%)
- Ascites (6%)
- Testicular atrophy
- Hepatic tenderness
- Diabetes mellitus symptoms

CAUSES
- The mechanism for increased iron absorption in the face of excessive iron stores is unknown. Iron metabolism appears normal in this disease except for a higher level of circulating iron.
- Iron overload may be due to thalassemia, sideroblastic anemia, liver disease, excess iron intake, chronic transfusion

RISK FACTORS
- The disease is a genetic disorder. Some variables influence the age of onset and severity of symptoms
- Intake of iron, especially from vitamin supplements. These may contain large amounts of iron as well as vitamin C, which enhances iron absorption
- Alcohol increases the absorption of iron (as high as 41% of patients with symptomatic disease are alcoholic)
- Loss of blood delays the onset of symptoms, such as blood loss in women because of menstruation and pregnancy.

 DIAGNOSIS

DIFFERENTIAL DIAGNOSIS
- Repeated transfusions
- Hereditary anemias with ineffective erythropoiesis
- Alcoholic cirrhosis
- Porphyria cutanea tarda
- Atransferrinemia
- Excessive ingestion of iron (rare)

LABORATORY
- Transferrin saturation (serum iron concentration divided by total iron-binding capacity x 100): greater than 70% is virtually diagnostic of iron overload; 50% or higher warrants further evaluation
- Serum ferritin: greater than 300 mcg/L for men and 120 mcg/L for women
- Urinary iron
- Increased urine hemosiderin
- Hyperglycemia
- Decreased FSH
- Decreased LH
- Decreased testosterone
- Increased SGOT
- Hypoalbuminemia

Drugs that may alter lab results: Iron supplements, transfusions may elevate serum iron

Disorders that may alter lab results: Inflammatory reactions, other forms of liver disease, certain tumors (e.g., acute granulocytic leukemia), rheumatoid arthritis may elevate serum ferritin

PATHOLOGICAL FINDINGS
- Increased hepatic parenchymal iron stores
- Hepatic fibrosis and cirrhosis with hepatomegaly
- Pancreatic enlargement
- Excess hemosiderin in liver, pancreas, myocardium, thyroid, parathyroid, joints, skin
- Cardiomegaly
- Joint deposition of iron

SPECIAL TESTS
After diagnosis established, consider oral glucose tolerance test to rule out diabetes and echocardiogram to rule out cardiomyopathy

IMAGING
CT scan, MRI, and magnetic susceptibility measurement (MSM) are being studied for measuring body iron, but have not yet reached validation and general availability

DIAGNOSTIC PROCEDURES
Liver biopsy for stainable iron is the standard for diagnosis. Presence or absence of cirrhosis can also be ascertained.

 TREATMENT

APPROPRIATE HEALTH CARE
Outpatient

GENERAL MEASURES
- Removal of excess iron by repeated phlebotomy once or twice weekly to establish and maintain a mild anemia (hematocrit of 37-39%)
- When the patient finally becomes iron deficient, a lifelong maintenance program of 4-6 phlebotomies a year to keep storage iron normal

ACTIVITY Full activity unless significant heart disease

DIET
- An iron-poor diet is not of significant benefit
- Avoid alcohol, iron-fortified foods, and iron-containing supplements
- Restrict vitamin C to small doses between meals
- Tea chelates iron and may be drunk with meals

PATIENT EDUCATION Updated information available from the Hemochromatosis Research Foundation, Inc., P.O. Box 8569, Albany, NY 12208

MEDICATIONS

DRUG(S) OF CHOICE None. Only when phlebotomy is not feasible or in the presence of severe heart disease should the iron-chelating agent deferoxamine (Desferal) be considered.
Contraindications: N/A
Precautions: N/A
Significant possible interactions: N/A

ALTERNATIVE DRUGS None

FOLLOWUP

PATIENT MONITORING
• Measure hematocrit before each phlebotomy - skip phlebotomy if hematocrit is less than 36%
• Schedule an additional phlebotomy when hematocrit is greater than 40%
• When anemia becomes refractory, repeat transferrin saturation and serum ferritin to confirm depletion of iron stores
• When iron stores are depleted, 4 to 6 phlebotomies a year should keep iron stores normal
• During maintenance therapy, measure transferrin saturation and serum ferritin yearly
• Liver biopsy to assess iron stores when serum and ferritin results have not normalized

PREVENTION/AVOIDANCE Family members should be screened

POSSIBLE COMPLICATIONS
• Cirrhosis
• Hepatoma (only in patients with cirrhosis)
• Diabetes mellitus
• Cardiomyopathy
• Arthritis
• Hypogonadism

EXPECTED COURSE AND PROGNOSIS
• Patients diagnosed before cirrhosis develops and treated with phlebotomy have a normal life expectancy
• Life expectancy is reduced in patients with cirrhosis, diabetes mellitus, and patients that require longer than 18 months of phlebotomy therapy to return iron stores to normal

MISCELLANEOUS

ASSOCIATED CONDITIONS See Possible complications

AGE-RELATED FACTORS
Pediatric: Although rare, iron overload can occur even as early as 2 years of age. The disorder can be diagnosed before iron overload is clinically apparent
Geriatric: N/A
Others: N/A

PREGNANCY Avoid iron supplements

SYNONYMS
• Bronze diabetes
• Troisier-Hanot-Chauffard syndrome

ICD-9-CM 275.0

SEE ALSO N/A

OTHER NOTES Most patients with hemochromatosis go undiagnosed. Since treatment with phlebotomy will prevent all complications when begun early, the diagnosis of hemochromatosis should be considered much more frequently by physicians

ABBREVIATIONS N/A

REFERENCES
• Crosby, W.H.: Hemochromatosis: Current concepts and management. Hosp Pract (Off) 22(2):173-7,181-92, 1987
• Smith, L.H.: Overview of hemochromatosis. West J Med.,153:296-308, 1990

Author R. Marlow, M.D.

Hemophilia

BASICS

DESCRIPTION
• Hemophilia A and hemophilia B are clinically indistinguishable, inherited bleeding disorders due to a deficiency of coagulant factor VIII (hemophilia A) or factor IX (hemophilia B)
• Disease severity is determined by percent of coagulant factor present. Less than 1% factor activity is severe, 1-5% factor activity is moderate, 5-25% factor activity is mild. Those with greater than 25% factor activity rarely may fail to clot after major trauma or surgery.
System(s) affected:
Hemic/Lymphatic/Immunologic
Genetics: Both hemophilia A and hemophilia B are X-linked, recessive
Incidence/Prevalence in USA:
• Hemophilia A - 10 in 100,000 males
• Hemophilia B - 2 in 100,000 males
Predominant age:
• Both are congenital conditions
• Severe disease generally noted at birth or in first year
• Mild disease may not be diagnosed until young adulthood
Predominant sex: Females are generally asymptomatic carriers. Rare exceptions occur from consanguinity within families, concomitant Turner's syndrome, or extremely disproportionate lyonization resulting in the preponderance of cells in the carrier female containing the X chromosome with the hemophilic gene.

SIGNS AND SYMPTOMS
• Bleeding into soft tissues, muscles, and weight-bearing joints
• Bleeding occurs hours to days after injury, can involve any organ, and can continue for hours to days
• Compartment syndromes and ischemic nerve damage from large hematomas
• Repeated bleeding into a joint causes osteoarthritis, articular fibrosis, and joint ankylosis
• Hematuria

CAUSES Congenital

RISK FACTORS Positive family history. Can predict risk to offspring using simple Mendelian genetics for an X-linked recessive disorder.

DIAGNOSIS

DIFFERENTIAL DIAGNOSIS
• Von Willebrand's disease
• Vitamin K deficiency (factor IX is vitamin K dependent)
• Other factor deficiencies, afibrinogenemia, dysfibrinogenemia, fibrinolytic defects, platelet disorders

LABORATORY
• Activated partial thromboplastin time (PTT) is prolonged while platelet count, and prothrombin time are normal
• Bleeding time is prolonged in 15-20% of patients with hemophilia A
• PTT is corrected when mixed with normal plasma
• Hemophilia A - diagnostic test is low factor VIII.
• Hemophilia B - diagnostic test is low factor IX
Drugs that may alter lab results: Recent aspirin use will increase bleeding time, leading to confusion with Von Willebrand's disease
Disorders that may alter lab results: N/A

PATHOLOGICAL FINDINGS
• Synovial hemosiderosis
• Articular cartilage degeneration
• Thickening of periarticular tissues
• Bony hypertrophy

SPECIAL TESTS Hemophilia A - carrier detection compares the ratio of factor VIII to von Willebrand's factor protein and is predictive in up to 95% of cases

IMAGING N/A

DIAGNOSTIC PROCEDURES N/A

TREATMENT

APPROPRIATE HEALTH CARE
• Outpatient
• Home transfusion therapy
• Inpatient for infusions following significant bleeding episodes

GENERAL MEASURES
• Avoid aspirin or aspirin-containing drugs
• Treat early. Symptoms often precede obvious bleeding.
• An uncomplicated, soft tissue bleeding or an early hemarthrosis requires a single infusion to 15-20% activity
• More extensive hemarthrosis or retroperitoneal bleeding requires bid infusions for 72 or more hours to 25-50% activity
• Life-threatening bleeding into the CNS requires maintaining levels greater than 50% activity for 2 weeks
• Major surgery requires greater than 50% activity preoperatively, continued for 2 weeks postoperatively
• Orthopedic care and physical therapy to prevent contractures and maintain joint mobility
• Vaccinate against hepatitis B at time of diagnosis
• Maintain good dental care

ACTIVITY
• Attempt to lead as normal a life as possible
• Restrict activities in proportion to the degree of factor deficiency, but maintaining a trim physical condition is important

DIET No special diet

PATIENT EDUCATION
• Teach patient and family about signs and symptoms to watch for
• Genetic counseling
• Home care with self administered replacement therapy is often used
• Printed patient information available from: National Hemophilia Foundation, 110 Green Street, Room 406, New York, NY, 10012, (212)219-8180

Hemophilia

MEDICATIONS

DRUG(S) OF CHOICE
Hemophilia A:
◊ Requires plasma products enriched in factor VIII (cryoprecipitate, factor VIII concentrate)
◊ 1 unit of factor VIII (the amount in 1 mL of plasma) will raise the plasma level of the recipient by 2% per kilogram of body weight. (Ask blood bank how many units are in the preparation you will be using. Typically about 100 units factor VIII in one bag of cryoprecipitate.)
◊ To calculate amount of factor VIII needed: Number units needed = [(desired percent activity minus current percent activity) times (body weight in kilograms)] divided by 2% per unit per kilogram
◊ For example: 70 kg man with 5% activity needs to be taken to 25% activity. Equation for number units needed: [(25% - 5%) x (70 kg)] / 2% per kg = [(25 - 5) x (70)] / 2 = 700 units needed (or approximately 7 bags of cryoprecipitate needed).
◊ Half-life of factor VIII is 8-12 hours, therefore need to infuse at least bid to maintain a chosen factor VIII level, and tid when tight control of the level is needed
Hemophilia B:
◊ Fresh frozen plasma for mild to moderate bleeding. Generally requires about 500 mL bid. There is danger of volume overload.
◊ Factor IX concentrate for moderate to severe hemorrhage and patients to undergo surgery. One unit/kg will raise levels 1%
Contraindications: None
Precautions: Hemophilia B - Factor IX concentrates contain trace amounts of activated vitamin K-dependent factors and therefore are thrombogenic and carry a risk for thromboembolism
Significant possible interactions: N/A

ALTERNATIVE DRUGS
• Desmopressin should be used in mild situations to transiently raise factor VIII levels
• Epsilon-aminocaproic acid can be used for minor dental work following a single factor VIII infusion. Epsilon-aminocaproic acid greatly enhances the risk of thromboembolism and should be used with caution with factor IX concentrates.
• Patients with inhibitors to factor VIII may require intensive plasmapheresis, large doses of concentrate, infusion of prothrombin complex concentrates (by-passing products), or porcine factor VIII

FOLLOWUP

PATIENT MONITORING
Regular evaluations every 6 to 12 months include a musculoskeletal evaluation, an inhibitor screen, liver tests, and tests for antibodies to hepatitis viruses and human immunodeficiency virus (HIV)

PREVENTION/AVOIDANCE
Genetic counseling

POSSIBLE COMPLICATIONS
• Factor VIII and IX preparations and transfusions result in viral hepatitis, chronic liver disease, and acquired immunodeficiency syndrome (AIDS). However, recent advances in factor VIII concentrate preparation should prevent future HIV infection and hepatitis B and C.
• Hemophilia A - 10-20% of patients develop inhibitors to factor VIII, typically those with severe disease receiving multiple transfusions. Type I (high responders) inhibitors to factor VIII rapidly neutralize factor VIII and prevent effective transfusion therapy. Type II (low responders) inhibitors are low-titer and may respond to higher than normal doses of factor VIII.

EXPECTED COURSE AND PROGNOSIS
• Repeated hemarthroses result in eventual deformity and crippling
• Survival is normal for those with mild disease, and mortality is increased 2 to 6 fold in those with moderate to severe disease, primarily due to complications of infection
• Median life expectancy with this condition peaked in late 1970's at 68 years, and is now declining due to the AIDS epidemic
• Up to 70% are HIV seropositive, especially those with severe disease, and 4% with severe disease develop AIDS

MISCELLANEOUS

ASSOCIATED CONDITIONS None

AGE-RELATED FACTORS
Pediatric: Mean age of onset of symptoms is 1.5 years for severe disease (often noted in first year), 3.0 years for moderate disease, and 5.0 years for mild disease
Geriatric: N/A
Others: N/A

PREGNANCY
• The vast majority of females are asymptomatic carriers, although an occasional carrier will bleed at time of surgery. They require no specific treatment during pregnancy or delivery.
• Prenatal diagnosis previously required sampling fetal blood for coagulant activity. Newer prenatal detection schemes detect an identifiable restriction fragment length polymorphism or a gene deletion or rearrangement in a sample of chorionic villus or from fluid obtained at amniocentesis.

SYNONYMS N/A

ICD-9-CM
286.0 Hemophilia A
286.1 Hemophilia B

SEE ALSO N/A

OTHER NOTES
• Recombinant factor VIII is available. It has biologic activity and clinical efficacy comparable to plasma factor VIII, while posing no risk of transmitting hepatitis viruses or HIV. There are factor VIII and factor IX concentrates prepared from human plasma using a monoclonal antibody method plus either heat or detergent treatment of the concentrate. These monoclonal-prepared concentrates have the lowest risk for hepatitis B and essentially no risk for HIV infection.
• Hemophilia A; Factor VIII deficiency, classic hemophilia
• Hemophilia B; Factor IX deficiency, Christmas disease

ABBREVIATIONS N/A

REFERENCES
• Jones, P.K. & Ratnoff, O.D.: The Changing Prognosis of Classic Hemophilia (Factor VII "Deficiency"). Ann Int Med 1991; 114(8):641-8
• Schwartz, R.S., et al.: Human Recombinant DNA-Derived Antihemophilic Factor (Factor VIII) in the Treatment of Hemophilia A. N Engl J Med 1990; 323(26):1800-5

Author R. Dolin, M.D.

Hemorrhoids

BASICS

DESCRIPTION Varicosities of the hemorrhoidal venous plexus. Usual course - acute; chronic; relapsing.
• External hemorrhoids are located below the dentate line and covered by squamous epithelium
• Internal hemorrhoids are located above the dentate line
System(s) affected: Gastrointestinal, Cardiovascular
Genetics: No known genetic pattern
Incidence/Prevalence in USA: Common
Predominant age: Adults, although may occur at any age
Predominant sex: Male = Female

SIGNS AND SYMPTOMS
• Rectal bleeding
• Anal protrusion
• Anal pain (with ulceration or thrombosis)
• Pruritis
• Constipation
• Straining with defecation
• Bowel incontinence
• Dilated hemorrhoidal vein
• Hematochezia
• Stool mucus
• Sensation of incomplete evacuation of the rectum
• Anal fissure
• Anal infection
• Anal ulceration
• Hemorrhoidal prolapse
• Hemorrhoidal strangulation
• Anemia
• Hemorrhoidal thrombosis

CAUSES Dilated veins of hemorrhoidal plexus

RISK FACTORS
• Pregnancy
• Colon malignancy
• Liver disease
• Portal hypertension
• Constipation
• Occupations that require prolonged sitting
• Loss of muscle tone in old age, rectal surgery, episiotomy, anal intercourse
• Obesity

DIAGNOSIS

DIFFERENTIAL DIAGNOSIS N/A

LABORATORY N/A
Drugs that may alter lab results: N/A
Disorders that may alter lab results: N/A

PATHOLOGICAL FINDINGS N/A

SPECIAL TESTS
• Anoscopy
• Sigmoidoscopy

IMAGING N/A

DIAGNOSTIC PROCEDURES
• Inspection of the rectum
• Inspection following straining at stool

TREATMENT

APPROPRIATE HEALTH CARE
Outpatient. Inpatient possibly for surgery.

GENERAL MEASURES
• Dependent on type and severity of hemorrhoids
• Warm sitz baths
• Manual reduction of prolapse
• Ligation (rubber band, 1 every 2 weeks for 3-6 treatments)
• Injection therapy
• Cryosurgery (for external hemorrhoids)
• Surgical resection (for combined hemorrhoids or internal hemorrhoids with major prolapse) in patients with severe bleeding, intolerable pain, pruritis and large prolapse. Contraindicated for patients with blood dyscrasias, gastrointestinal carcinoma, and during first trimester of pregnancy.
• Correction of constipation

ACTIVITY
• No restrictions
• Encourage physical fitness
• Avoid prolonged sitting on the toilet

DIET High fiber (roughage)

PATIENT EDUCATION Explain usual benignity

MEDICATIONS

DRUG(S) OF CHOICE
- Analgesics
- Stool softeners
- Witch hazel compresses
- Topical anesthetic ointments

Contraindications: Refer to manufacturer's literature

Precautions: Refer to manufacturer's literature

Significant possible interactions: Refer to manufacturer's literature

ALTERNATIVE DRUGS N/A

FOLLOWUP

PATIENT MONITORING As needed, depending on treatment

PREVENTION/AVOIDANCE
- Avoid constipation
- Lose weight, if overweight
- Avoid prolonged sitting on the toilet
- Avoid prolonged sitting at work. Get up and move around periodically.

POSSIBLE COMPLICATIONS
- Thrombosis
- Secondary infection
- Ulceration
- Anemia
- Incontinence
- Carcinoma (rare)

EXPECTED COURSE AND PROGNOSIS
- Cure
- Spontaneous resolution

MISCELLANEOUS

ASSOCIATED CONDITIONS
- Liver disease
- Pregnancy
- Portal hypertension
- Constipation

AGE-RELATED FACTORS
Pediatric:
- Uncommon in infants and children. Look for underlying cause, e.g., venacaval or mesenteric obstruction, cirrhosis, portal hypertension.
- Occasionally, as in adults, hemorrhoids may result from chronic constipation, fecal impaction and straining at stool. Surgery is rarely required.

Geriatric: Common in elderly along with rectal prolapse

Others: N/A

PREGNANCY Common in pregnancy. Usually resolves after pregnancy. No treatment required, unless extremely painful.

SYNONYMS Piles

ICD-9-CM
455.6 hemorrhoids, nos

SEE ALSO
- Carcinoma of colon
- Rectal carcinoma
- Portal hypertension

OTHER NOTES N/A

ABBREVIATIONS N/A

REFERENCES
- Fazio, V.W.: Anorectal Disorders. In Gastroenterology Clinics of North America, Philadelphia, W.B. Saunders Co., 1987
- Guthrie, J.F.: The Current Management of Hemorrhoids. In Pract Gastroenterol. 1987;11:56

Author F. Iber, M.D.

Hepatic encephalopathy

 BASICS

DESCRIPTION Altered mental and neuromotor functioning associated with acute or chronic liver disease and/or portal systemic shunting of blood. The prominent features are mild to marked forgetfulness, impaired arousability, and a "flapping tremor" (asterixis).
System(s) affected: Gastrointestinal, Nervous
Genetics: Unknown
Incidence/Prevalence in USA:
• Occurs in 1/3 cases of cirrhosis
• Occurs in all cases of fulminant hepatic failure
• Present in nearly half of patients who reach the stage of liver disease requiring transplantation
Predominant age: Parallels that of fulminant liver disease with peak in the 40's, and cirrhosis with peak in late 50's. May occur at any age.
Predominant sex: Male = Female (reflecting the underlying liver disease)

SIGNS AND SYMPTOMS
Ages 10-60
◊ Prominent signs of underlying liver disease (50%), jaundice most common, ascites second most common
◊ Gastrointestinal hemorrhage with hematemesis or melena (20%)
◊ Systemic infection, urinary tract or pulmonary (20%)
◊ Four stages of confusion and obtundity described. 1) is forgetfulness, disturbance in nocturnal sleep, daytime drowsiness, 2) is mild confusion but arousability, 3) is arousable, but markedly confused, limited orientation and thought content, 4) is unarousable.
◊ Asterixis prominent in stages 2, 3
◊ Handwriting and hand coordination deteriorated in stages 1, 2
◊ Tremor prominent in stage 2
◊ Psychotic thoughts infrequent
◊ Reflexes symmetrically hyperactive
◊ Tremor and asterixis not observed in ocular muscles
◊ Mental and neurological signs change rapidly (over 6 to 12 hours)
Age over 60
◊ Signs of underlying liver disease diminished (25%)
◊ Confusion more prominent
◊ Precipitating gastrointestinal hemorrhage or infection less often identified
◊ Remains in stage 1 or 2 for many days
◊ Progression slower
Age under 10
◊ Signs of underlying liver disease prominent, usually fulminant hepatic failure or extremely advanced cirrhosis
◊ Progression through the stages very rapid, often 6 to 12 hours
◊ Precipitating cause frequently not identified

CAUSES
• Shunting of intestinal blood through the severely diseased liver without the intervention of viable liver cells
• Shunting of such blood through collateral circulation or surgically constructed portacaval shunts
• Thus hepatic coma may occur in extremely advanced acute liver disease (fulminant hepatic failure) or following portacaval shunting. However, it is most common in long standing cirrhosis of the liver with spontaneous shunting of intestinal blood through collaterals.

RISK FACTORS
• Advancing age is the most prominent risk factor
• Viral hepatitis
• Drug hepatotoxicity (acetaminophen, halothane, carbon tetrachloride, yellow phosphorus)
• Pregnancy
• Herpes virus

 DIAGNOSIS

DIFFERENTIAL DIAGNOSIS
• Head trauma, concussion, subdural hematoma
• Alcohol withdrawal syndrome
• Toxic confusion due to medication
• Toxic confusion due to illicit drug use
• Meningitis
• Metabolic encephalopathy related to anoxia, hypoglycemia, hypokalemia, hypo- or hypercalcemia, uremia

LABORATORY
• Screening blood, sputum and urine cultures to identify infection
• Hematology to identify anemia and signs of infection
• Standard biochemistry profile to identify hypokalemia, bilirubinemia, altered calcium status, hypomagnesemia, urea, hypoglycemia
• Arterial blood gases
• Liver tests to evaluate severity of underlying liver disease
• Prothrombin and partial thromboplastin time
• Venous ammonia (elevated in 70% of liver coma)
• Toxicology screen for illicit drugs
Drugs that may alter lab results:
• Infusion of amino acid solutions may affect ammonia level
• Opiate administration - producing severe constipation may affect ammonia level
Disorders that may alter lab results:
• Uremia may affect ammonia level
• Rapid and severe tissue breakdown, massive burns, trauma or infection may affect ammonia level

PATHOLOGICAL FINDINGS
• Brain edema in 100% of fatal cases
• Glial hypertrophy in chronic encephalopathy

SPECIAL TESTS
• Electroencephalogram shows symmetrical slowing of basic (alpha) rhythm in common with other forms of metabolic encephalopathy
• Visually-evoked potential specific in stages 2, 3 and 4

IMAGING
• Useful only to rule out other diagnoses
• CT scan of head most useful

DIAGNOSTIC PROCEDURES
• Clinical setting and findings adequate in 80% of cases
• Venous ammonia of great aid in patients with chronic liver disease when the clinical findings are confusing
• EEG is useful to a limited extent, but findings are similar in other forms of metabolic encephalopathy
• Response to treatment often confirms the diagnosis

 TREATMENT

APPROPRIATE HEALTH CARE
• Outpatient for stages 1 and 2 when diagnosis is clear and if recurrent can be managed satisfactorily
• Stages 3 or 4 require inpatient management
• Stage 3 or 4 in fulminant hepatic failure is a strong indication for evaluation for liver transplantation. Transfer to a transplant center should be considered.

GENERAL MEASURES
• Identify and treat vigorously precipitating causes - gastrointestinal bleed, infection, sedative drugs, or electrolyte imbalance are most common
• Stage 2 or higher - attention to adequate fluid intake, and at least 1000 kcal of food daily
• Give Fleet's enema to all patients without diarrhea
• Clumsiness and poor judgment prominent. Be sure patient has the care needed to avoid falls, cuts on broken glass, smoking burns, machinery or auto accidents.
• Avoid sedative or opiate medications. Benzodiazepine sedatives and opiate derivatives such as Lomotil have caused liver coma.

ACTIVITY
• As tolerated
• Avoid driving and machinery

DIET
• Integrate with needs of underlying liver disease
• Lower total protein. Stage 1 - avoid protein gluttony. Stage 2 - limit red meat and consume small portions of all other protein foods, total protein for day 50-60 grams. Stage 3 - consume 40 gram protein or vegetable protein diet (about 20 grams). Stage 4 - consume 10 or fewer grams of protein. For all stages at least 1000 kcal ingested daily.
• As coma improves, increase dietary protein as tolerated

PATIENT EDUCATION
• Include family in education
• Dietician instruction in eating lower protein diets, avoid protein binging
• Avoid unnecessary sedative or antianxiety medications and opiates
• Recognition of early signs and to get treatment promptly
• Pamphlets of the American Association for the Study of Liver Diseases (6900 Grove Road, Thorofare, NJ 08086. Ph. 609-848-1000) are quite good for family

 MEDICATIONS

DRUG(S) OF CHOICE
• Lactulose syrup (Cephulac) 30 ml of 50% solution four times daily. Diminish to bid, when 3 or more bowel movements a day occur daily.
• If stage 4 is present, worsening occurs, or no improvement in 2 days, add antibiotics. Amoxicillin 4 gm/day is suitable. Neomycin 1-4 gm/day in 4 divided doses may be used if renal status is good.
• Antacids as needed
Contraindications:
• Total ileus
• Hypersensitivity reaction
Precautions:
• Potassium depletion
• Electrolyte imbalance
• Renal failure
Significant possible interactions: Refer to manufacturer's profile of each drug

ALTERNATIVE DRUGS Any antibiotic affecting intestinal flora

 FOLLOWUP

PATIENT MONITORING
• To optimize treatment a trail-making test should be followed (provided by Cephulac makers). Apply to Stage 1 and 2 patients to determine how much maintenance treatment and diet needed. Should be run daily at first and then at each office visit when changes in drugs and diet are made.
• Patients with changed findings should be seen twice weekly
• Stable patients should be seen monthly
• Trail-making test performed at each office visit

PREVENTION/AVOIDANCE
• Avoid unessential medications, particularly opiates, sedatives
• Avoid protein binges

POSSIBLE COMPLICATIONS
• Recurrence
• Stable, chronic, impaired status
• With many recurrences, permanent basal ganglion injury (non-Wilsonian hepatolenticular degeneration)
• Hepatorenal syndrome
• Acute tabular necrosis
• Bleeding
• Disseminated intravascular coagulation
• Bacteremia
• Shock

EXPECTED COURSE AND PROGNOSIS
In acute or fulminant
  ◊ With adequate aggressive treatment, disappears without residue or recurrence
In chronic liver disease
  ◊ Coma returns
  ◊ With each recurrence it becomes more and more difficult to treat
  ◊ Plateau of maximum improvement shows a decrement over several years, such that the degree of improvement with treatment is less and less. Eventual 80% mortality.

 MISCELLANEOUS

ASSOCIATED CONDITIONS
• Liver disease
• Rarely with portacaval shunt with normal liver function

AGE-RELATED FACTORS See under Signs and symptoms
Pediatric: N/A
Geriatric: N/A
Others: N/A

PREGNANCY May occur as a complication of pregnancy

SYNONYMS
• Hepatic coma
• Liver coma

ICD-9-CM 572.2

SEE ALSO N/A

OTHER NOTES N/A

ABBREVIATIONS N/A

REFERENCES
• Gammal, S.H., et al.: Hepatic encephalopathy. Med Clin North Am. 73, 793-813, 1989
• Jones, E.A., et al.: Ann Intern Med. 110, 532-46, 1989
• Chapman, R.W., et al.: Liver transplantation for acute liver failure. Lancet. 335 (8680), 32-5, 1990

Author A. Verma, M.D. & F. Iber, M.D.

Hepatitis, viral

BASICS

DESCRIPTION A group of systemic infections (involving the liver) with common clinical manifestations, but caused by different viruses with typically distinctive epidemiological patterns; hepatitis A (HAV), hepatitis B (HBV), hepatitis C (HCV), hepatitis D (HDV), hepatitis E (HEV)
System(s) affected: Gastrointestinal
Genetics: N/A
Incidence/Prevalence in USA:
• HAV: In major US population centers, 50% over age 49 have serum hepatitis A antibodies. Of cases of acute hepatitis, HAV is found in 25%; however, this percentage is decreasing
• HBV: Approximately 200,000 young adults become infected with HBV each year; there are over 500,000 HBV carriers (10% of those infected). Post-transfusion HBV infection now less than 2% of blood recipients. 5% of the world's population estimated to be infected with HBV (300 million). HBV may be second only to tobacco among human carcinogens.
• HCV: Responsible for 20% of sporadic hepatitis, becoming the most common cause of acute viral hepatitis. It is estimated that 150,000 new HCV infections occur annually.
• HDV: Unknown
• HEV: Unknown
Predominant age: Unknown for most
• HAV occurs in all ages; rare in infants. Susceptibility increases linearly with age.
Predominant sex: Unknown for most
• Fulminant HBV infection: Male>Female (2:1)

SIGNS AND SYMPTOMS
Common for the different viral agents; severity varies to some degree with the infecting agent
• Fatigue (> 80%), malaise (67%), nausea, vomiting (80%), anorexia (54%), dark urine (84%)
• Jaundice (in adults, 62%)
• Fever (60%); unusual with HBV and HCV
• Abdominal pain (56%)
• Headache, meningismus (occasional)
• Two thirds of HCV infections anicteric and associated with mild symptoms
• The majority of hepatitis A patients have subclinical or flu-like illness

CAUSES
• Multiple viruses
• There may be simultaneous infection with more than one virus
• HAV and HEV transmitted enterically (fecal-oral route) including contaminated food sources; parenteral route rare
• Maximum infectivity (fecal shedding) 2 weeks prior to visible jaundice
• May be endemic in institutions
• HBV transmitted sexually, through contaminated blood or blood products including infection acquired perinatally; also fecal-oral route. Co-infection, superinfection or chronic infection with HDV markedly increases severity, morbidity and mortality of HBV

• HCV transmitted through blood transfusions, other exposures from contaminated blood or its products (e.g., patients with hemophilia receiving factor VIII or IX concentrates, patients on hemodialysis). In 50%, mode of transmission of HCV unknown.
• HDV identified only with HBV infection

RISK FACTORS
• Health care workers/other occupational risks
• Hemodialysis patients
• Recipients of blood and/or blood products
• Intravenous drug users
• Sexually active homosexual males
• Household exposure
• Adopted children from areas of high exposure
• Intimate exposure
• Positive needlestick

DIAGNOSIS

DIFFERENTIAL DIAGNOSIS
• Infectious mononucleosis
• Primary or secondary hepatic malignancy
• Ischemic hepatitis
• Drug-induced hepatitis
• Alcoholic hepatitis

LABORATORY
• Marked elevation of AST/ALT (particularly ALT, 400-several thousand IU)
• Mild to moderate elevation of alkaline phosphatase
• Bilirubin from normal to markedly elevated; with elevation, conjugated and unconjugated fractions usually increased
• Serological markers to identify specific viruses (See Table)
• For more severe hepatitis, measure prothrombin and partial thromboplastin times, serum albumin, electrolytes and glucose, CBC and platelets

```
------------------------------
Diagnosis    Biochemical markers
HAV:
  A, R       Anti-HAV IgM
  P          Anti-HAV IgG
HBV:
  A, E       HBsAg
  A          Anti-HBc IgM,
               HBsAg, HBeAg
  C          HBsAg, +/- HBeAg
HCV:
  A,C,Rcv    Anti-HCV
HDV:
  A          HDAg, Anti-HDV IgM
  P          Anti-HDV IgG
HEV:         Test not available
------------------------------
A-acute infection
R-recent infection
C-chronic infection
P-previous infection
E-early/carrier state
Rcv-Recovered
```

• Patients with severe HBV infection should be tested for co-infection with HDV
• HBeAg indicates high infectivity (horizontal and vertical transmission)
• Persistence > 10 weeks indicates probable chronic liver disease

• Present rate of false positive Anti-HCV (ELISA) tests high; particularly in patients with hypergammaglobulinemia; recombinant immunoblot assay-2 (RIBA-2) better
• In early acute HCV infection, anti-HCV may be negative; retesting in 3-6 months may be necessary
Drugs that may alter lab results: N/A
Disorders that may alter lab results: N/A

PATHOLOGICAL FINDINGS Liver biopsy in persistent or chronic disease shows wide range of histologic changes including variable inflammation and/or necrosis, cholestasis, steatosis, fibrosis, cirrhosis or chronic active hepatitis. Clinical course does not predict severity of histopathologic changes.

SPECIAL TESTS Liver biopsy usually necessary for determination of type and extent of liver injury in clinically persistent disease and to exclude other diseases

IMAGING Usually not of diagnostic importance. Ultrasound may demonstrate ascites or exclude obstruction.

DIAGNOSTIC PROCEDURES
• Careful history and search for possible source of exposure; exclude drugs
• Tenderness on fist percussion over the liver; may be hepatomegaly
• Jaundice may or may not be present
• Serum "liver function tests" often elevated before bilirubin increases; measure aminotransferases in acute illnesses when there is no evident cause
• Serum biochemical markers for each virus indicate present or previous infection; satisfactory for diagnosis in 90% of patients

TREATMENT

APPROPRIATE HEALTH CARE
• Outpatient care unless patient requires intensive clinical and lab monitoring
• Segregation from others not necessary except for food handlers with hepatitis A, or health care workers with hepatitis B or C
• Consider liver transplantation in fulminant acute hepatitis. HCV patients do relatively well following transplantation.

GENERAL MEASURES
• Correct coagulation defects
• Correct abnormal fluid and electrolyte concentrations
• Correct acid-base imbalance
• Correct hypoglycemia
• Correct any impairment of renal function

ACTIVITY
• As tolerated
• Limitation of activity does not affect recovery from HAV

DIET Adequate caloric intake and balanced nutrition

PATIENT EDUCATION
• Proper use and disposal of needles by medical staff, drug users (both non-IV and IV drug users at risk)
• Proper hygiene, particularly food handlers
• HBV sexually transmitted; sexual transmission of HCV low

MEDICATIONS

DRUG(S) OF CHOICE
• Interferon Alfa-2b (Intron A) and possibly ribavirin (Virazole) (only for HCV) shown to induce remission (25-50%, HBV; 40%, HCV) and to decrease abnormal aminotransferase concentrations in chronic HBV and HCV infection. With discontinuance, values often return to previous levels. Relapse reversed in responders with reinstitution of treatment. 40-50% of patients with HCV treated with interferon (6 month's course) continued remission after therapy stopped.
• In HCV infection, treatment for aggressive hepatitis or progressive course
• In cholestatic HAV, short course of corticosteroids may shorten illness
Contraindications:
• For interferon, platelet count < 75,000. Mouse immunoglobulin, egg protein or neomycin allergy
• Corticosteroid therapy may contribute to morbidity and increased mortality
Precautions: Other disorders of coagulation, myelosuppression, seizures, pregnancy, fertile age group, lactation
Significant possible interactions: Refer to manufacturer's profile of each drug

ALTERNATIVE DRUGS   N/A

FOLLOWUP

PATIENT MONITORING
• Serial measurement of serum AST/ALT
• Appropriate serum viral biochemical markers useful for evaluation of recovery or progression
• Chronic disease may require multiple liver biopsies
• Monitoring of symptomatic patients needed for metabolic complications
• Monitoring of WBC, platelets necessary with interferon-alpha treatment

PREVENTION/AVOIDANCE
• Screening of blood products
• Proper disposal of needles both in medical facilities and among intravenous drug abusers
HAV
◊ Good sanitation, hygiene to control HAV
◊ Prevention by immune globulin (passive immunization) - 0.02 mL/kg IM in those exposed to HAV (given 1-2 weeks after exposure prevents illness in 80-90%)
◊ For prolonged exposure (travelers), immune globulin given as 0.02-0.05 mL/kg IM every 5 months
◊ Administration of immune globulin also for close contacts of patients. Day care staff/children (when a case occurs), those associated with an institution with multiple cases, and those traveling to areas of high prevalence.
◊ Routine prophylaxis not otherwise indicated
HBV
◊ Now can immunize for HBV with three IM injections of hepatitis B vaccine - 0.5 mL/dose for children under 11 years, 1.0 mL for adults, 1 month and 6 months apart
◊ For individuals from high risk groups (see Risk factors), use HBV human immune globulin within 24 hr after exposure (0.06 mL/kg IM) for prophylaxis
◊ In addition, the CDC has recommended screening of all pregnant women for the disease and vaccination of all infants at birth. The schedule is 3 injections - at birth, 2 months, and 6 to 18 months.
HCV: No specifics on prevention/avoidance
HDV: Preventing HBV will prevent HDV
HEV: No specifics on prevention/avoidance

POSSIBLE COMPLICATIONS   Acute or subacute necrosis, chronic active or chronic persistent hepatitis, cirrhosis, hepatic failure; hepatocellular carcinoma; autoimmune phenomena with hepatitis B (e.g., nephritis, and others)

EXPECTED COURSE AND PROGNOSIS
• Varies with causative virus
• Severity of hepatic encephalopathy best predictor of poor survival in hepatic failure
• HAV may cause mild disease, often without jaundice (usual in children); does not result in chronic liver disease; mortality < 1%. With recovery, usually lifetime immunity. Three unusual variants; relapsing (10%), cholestatic, fulminant.
• HBV (mortality 1%) and HDV (with icterus, mortality 2-20%) usually more severe symptoms; often progresses to persistent or chronic liver disease, cirrhosis, liver failure or hepatocellular carcinoma (HCC)
• In HCV, regardless of severity of illness, > 50% of patients progress to chronic hepatitis, 20% to cirrhosis, and in some, liver failure
• With chronic HDV, 70% develop cirrhosis; low incidence of HCC
• HEV does not result in chronic disease

MISCELLANEOUS

ASSOCIATED CONDITIONS   Viral hepatitides sometimes associated with arthritis, urticaria, immune complex nephritis (particularly membranous glomerulopathy), anemias (including aplastic anemia), dermatitis and cardiomyopathy (usually with HBV, rare with HCV)

AGE-RELATED FACTORS
Pediatric:
• HAV milder in children than adults; usually anicteric and may be unrecognized unless AST/ALT measured in systemic infections
• HBV infection in children more acute than in adults, less prolonged, less frequent complications, usually complete recovery
Geriatric: N/A
Others:
• Alcohol abuse a major contributing factor for chronic liver disease from HBV and HCV. Measure viral biochemical markers in patients with alcoholic liver disease (especially anti-HCV).
• Patients with impaired immune function may have more severe problems with HBV infection

PREGNANCY
• Test, in later gestation, for HBsAg
• HBV transmitted vertically (< 10%) as well as perinatally and produces carrier state in approx 30%. Give HBIg and HBV vaccine within 12 hours of birth followed by HBV vaccine, 0.5 mL IM at ages 1 and 6 months. Measure HBsAg and HBsAb at age 1 year to know prophylaxis successful (> 95%).
• HEV has high mortality (40%) in pregnant women in developing world

SYNONYMS   N/A

ICD-9-CM   070 viral hepatitis

SEE ALSO   N/A

OTHER NOTES   Cases of acute hepatitis to be reported to public health authorities

ABBREVIATIONS   HAV = hepatitis A; HBV = hepatitis B; HCV = hepatitis C; HDV = hepatitis D; HEV = hepatitis E

REFERENCES
• Edmond, J.C., et al.: Liver transplantation in the management of fulminant hepatic failure. Gastroenterology. 96:1583-1589, 1989
• Davis, G.L., Balart, L.A., Schiff, E.R., et al.: Treatment of chronic hepatitis C with recombinant interferon alpha: a multicenter randomized, controlled trial. N Engl J Med. 321:1501-506, 1989
• Schiff, E.: Immunoprophylaxis of viral hepatitis: A practical guide. Am J Gastroenterology. 82:287-91, 1987

Author   D. Sandberg, M.D.

Hepatoma

BASICS

DESCRIPTION Primary malignant tumor of liver arising from hepatic parenchymal cells (hepatocytes), blood vessels or cholangioles within the liver, excluding gallbladder and biliary passages. With the exception of fibrolamellar type almost always associated with an underlying liver disease, usually cirrhosis.

System(s) affected: Gastrointestinal
Genetics: No known genetic pattern
Incidence/Prevalence in USA:
 • 1-5 new cases per 100,000 of population per year
 • Among known cirrhotics, 2-5 cases/100/year
Predominant age: 6th-8th decade (mean age 55-62 years) in USA and western countries. Among immigrants from Asia and Africa occurs 2-3 decades earlier.
Predominant sex: Male > Female (3-4:1)

SIGNS AND SYMPTOMS
Early curable stage
 ◊ Paraneoplastic syndrome - feminization, precocious puberty
 ◊ Palpable nodule on liver
 ◊ Age 2 to 6 years - abdominal mass in liver, abdominal pain, irregular hepatomegaly
Usual adult manifestations
 ◊ Known cirrhosis or prominent clinical signs of cirrhosis - 80%
 ◊ Abdominal pain - 80%, right upper quadrant, dull ache to severe, aggravated by jolting
 ◊ Hepatomegaly - 80-90%, irregular, nodular, firm to hard, tender
 ◊ Weight loss, 30%
 ◊ Hepatic arterial bruit, 20%
 ◊ Friction rub - rare, more common in metastatic liver disease
 ◊ Nausea, vomiting
 ◊ Fever - 10-50%, low grade, intermittent
 ◊ Paraneoplastic manifestations - hypertrophic osteoarthropathy, carcinoid syndrome, feminization, polycythemia
 ◊ Hemoperitoneum, most common tumor cause
 ◊ Unexplained deterioration of stable cirrhosis
 ◊ Budd-Chiari syndrome
 ◊ Blockage of portal vein, inferior vena cava, renal veins

CAUSES
 • Cirrhosis - accounts for 60 to 80% of cases. Alcoholic cirrhosis most important in western world. Reported risk of hepatoma in alcoholic cirrhosis is 3-10% with micronodular pattern.
 • Hepatitis B virus infection - associated with > 70% of cases worldwide. Most important factor in Africa and Asia but less important in western countries. In USA, HBsAg is positive in 20% cases of this tumor.
 • Hepatitis C virus infection - 50-70% of HBsAg negative patients are positive for anti-HCV antibody, an important factor in hepatoma patients not due to HBV infection. Particular problem in orientals.
 • Mycotoxins (aflatoxins) - metabolite of fungus Aspergillus flavus that contaminates foods. Two series, B1 and derivatives and G1 and derivatives. B1 being the most potent carcinogen, important in Sub-Saharan Africa and Southeast Asia, no significant role in USA.
 • Vinyl polymer, but not the finished product, produces angiosarcoma

RISK FACTORS
 • Primary liver disease - cirrhosis, chronic active hepatitis
 • HBsAg positivity, anti-HCV antibody
 • Chronic use of oral contraceptives
 • Hemochromatosis
 • Alpha-1-antitrypsin deficiency
 • Primary biliary cirrhosis
 • Metabolic disorders (tyrosinemia, Niemann-Pick disease)
 • Clonorchiasis, gallstones, choledochal cysts - cholangiocarcinoma

DIAGNOSIS

DIFFERENTIAL DIAGNOSIS
 • Early asymptomatic tumor - underlying liver conditions, e.g., cirrhosis, chronic hepatitis; benign liver nodules, hamartoma, hemangioma, metastatic adenocarcinoma, gallstones, or gallbladder polyp
 • Late symptomatic tumor with hepatomegaly - hepatic cyst, adenoma, hemangioma, abscess, metastatic malignancy of liver, cirrhosis with activity, infarction of liver, fatty infiltration, thrombosis of hepatic veins, portal vein, inferior vena cava, active viral hepatitis, alcoholic hepatitis
 • Ruptured tumor - all causes of acute abdomen, traumatic hemoperitoneum

LABORATORY
 • Erythrocytosis, elevated Ca, low glucose
 • Liver function test abnormalities
Tumor markers
 ◊ Alphafetoprotein (AFP) - single most important lab test for screening and diagnosis of hepatoma - 70%. Negative in angiosarcoma, cholangiocarcinoma and fibrolamellar carcinoma. Level > 400 ng/mL is diagnostic, level does not correlate with prognosis.
 ◊ Other markers - des-gamma-carboxyprothrombin, gamma glutamyl transferase, carcinoembryonic antigen (CEA), variant alkaline phosphatase, isoferritins
Drugs that may alter lab results:
Hypoglycemic agents, calcitonin, vitamin D
Disorders that may alter lab results:
Acute or chronic hepatitis, germ cell tumors, pregnancy. All cause slight elevation of AFP.

PATHOLOGICAL FINDINGS
 • Nodular - 75%, usually in cirrhotic liver
 • Massive - common in children and non-cirrhotic livers, more prone to rupture
 • Diffuse - rare, a large part of liver is involved
 • Hepatocellular origin - most commonly multicentric, well differentiated, usually superimposed on underlying cirrhosis. Almost always produces bile. Anaplastic form often difficult to be certain of cell of origin or differentiate from metastatic malignancy.
 • Fibrolamellar - single nodule, non-cirrhotic, extensive fibrous stroma
 • Cholangiocarcinoma - multicentric, most often mixed with hepatocellular elements
 • Angiosarcoma
 • Liver biopsy of possible tumor nodule
 • Skinny needle cytoaspiration of nodule

IMAGING
 • Plain x-ray - Useful to demonstrate metastatic involvement to lung and bone
 • Ultrasound - best diagnostic imaging technique, capable of detecting tumor < 1 cm, and may be positive when AFP is normal. Has been useful in serially following cases of cirrhosis to identify hepatocellular cancer when under 2 cm and curable.
 • CT scan - valuable in determining extrahepatic spread of the disease
 • MRI - helpful in delineating the details of tumor, and invasion of vessels
 • Hepatic arteriography - mostly done to see the anatomy of hepatic vessels and extent of tumor while considering resection, embolization, dearterialization or intra-arterial infusion of cytotoxic agents. Most useful in detecting angiosarcoma.
 • Lipiodal angiography and CT - lipiodal is readily taken up by tumor cells, this technique can detect even millimeter sized lesions. Lipiodal also serves as a vehicle to deliver chemotherapeutic or radioactive agents to the tumor.
 • Gallium scans - 90% of hepatocellular carcinoma and 60% of other types of liver cell tumors take up and retain gallium for up to 48 hours

DIAGNOSTIC PROCEDURES
 • Liver biopsy - recommended for all tumors and particularly small nodules detected on serial ultrasound
 • Fine needle aspiration - under ultrasonography, may be difficult to determine cell origin when anaplastic, unable to diagnose fibrolamellar and angiosarcoma due to too small a sample of tissue
 • Laparoscopy - to visualize the extent of tumor, to see whether non-tumorous liver is cirrhotic, peritoneal spread, and obtain diagnostic biopsy
 • Exploratory laparotomy with operative biopsy, commonly used in children

Hepatoma

TREATMENT

APPROPRIATE HEALTH CARE
• Surgery is the best treatment offering the only chance of curing hepatoma, highly effective in children when even large tumor masses, usually of the fibrolamellar type are identified, cure rate > 70%
• Surgery could be done in the form of lobectomy, hepatectomy, liver transplantation
• Criteria for resection: No distant spread, involvement of one lobe, no invasion of surrounding vessel, no cirrhosis in non-tumorous liver, medical fitness, in children no size limitation. 5 year survival rate is 70% in children and 20% in adults.
• Liver transplantation: Can be done if both lobes are involved and no spread beyond the liver. Recurrence rate is 90% in transplanted liver, 2 year survival rate 25-30%.
• Cases with unresectable hepatoma can be treated in an extended care facility, hospice, inpatient or as outpatient depending on their clinical status

GENERAL MEASURES   Precautions to avoid falls, attention to nutrition

ACTIVITY   Usually as tolerated

DIET   High calorie, low protein diet

PATIENT EDUCATION   Important for prevention; abstinence from alcohol and IV drugs, vaccination against HBV

MEDICATIONS

DRUG(S) OF CHOICE   Only for unresectable hepatoma patients. Doxorubicin (Adriamycin) 60-75 mg/sq meter every 3 weeks. Dose can be repeated depending on the response. Only partial response in 25% cases.
Contraindications:
• Cardiomyopathy
• Poor hepatic reserves (bilirubin > 2.0)
Precautions: Neutropenia with nadir at 10-14 days, septicemia, cardiotoxicity (25%) if cumulative dose > 550 mg/sq meter, hepatotoxicity
Significant possible interactions: N/A

ALTERNATIVE DRUGS
• Fluorouracil (5-FU), cyclophosphamide, methotrexate have been used but no promising results
• Immunotherapy: Radiolabeled antibodies like 131-I-antiferritin have been used. Can be used in conjunction with doxorubicin (Adriamycin), still experimental.
• Intra-arterial injection of 131-I Lipiodol or Lipiodol/Adriamycin, not in common use

FOLLOWUP

PATIENT MONITORING
• After successful resection there is high risk for recurrence
• Check AFP every 1-2 months
• Ultrasound every 4-6 months

PREVENTION/AVOIDANCE
Prevention against HBV infection/cirrhosis
◊ General education regarding risks of exposure to HBV and precautions to avoid this
◊ Vaccination in high risk individuals - nurses, doctors, dialysis unit staff, lab technicians
◊ Abstinence from alcohol, IV drugs, homosexual behavior
◊ Persistent HBV and HCV infections eradicated with alpha interferon
Screening and early diagnosis
◊ Early diagnosis to detect asymptomatic tumor (< 3 cm) at a potentially curable stage has been emphasized. The only screening test available so far is AFP testing which can detect 70-80% of tumors < 3 cm when used in conjunction with serial high resolution sonography.
◊ AFP should be done every 6 months in high risk individuals (cirrhosis, chronic active hepatitis) along with annual ultrasound. In moderate risk subjects (HBsAg positive but asymptomatic), AFP should be done yearly followed by ultrasound if it is abnormal.
◊ Patients exposed to 10 or more years of vinyl chloride polymerization should have q 6 months sonography. New nodules should be promptly biopsied.

POSSIBLE COMPLICATIONS   Rupture, hemoperitoneum, liver failure, cachexia, metastases to other organs

EXPECTED COURSE OF PROGNOSIS
Unresectable symptomatic tumors
◊ Grave prognosis, seldom live more than 6 months
◊ After liver transplantation - 2 year survival rate 25-30%
◊ After chemotherapy or chemoimmunotherapy, only partial remission in one quarter of cases
Resectable asymptomatic tumors
◊ Better prognosis, 5 year survival rate 25% and 2 year survival rate 50-60%
◊ Results are even better after resection if hepatoma is in a non-cirrhotic liver

MISCELLANEOUS

ASSOCIATED CONDITIONS
• Infections - chronic hepatitis B, Hepatitis C, Delta hepatitis, clonorchiasis and schistosomiasis
• Primary liver diseases - alcoholic cirrhosis, primary biliary cirrhosis
• Metabolic Diseases - Alpha-1-antitrypsin deficiency, hemochromatosis, Wilson's disease, tyrosinemia

AGE-RELATED FACTORS   Can occur in all age groups
Pediatric: Second most common tumor in first year of life following Wilms tumor. High cure rate.
Geriatric: N/A
Others: N/A

PREGNANCY   N/A

SYNONYMS
• Hepatocellular Carcinoma
• Liver cancer
• Fibrolamellar carcinoma
• Cholangiocarcinoma

ICD-9-CM   155.0

SEE ALSO   N/A

OTHER NOTES
In Africa and Southeast Asia
◊ Incidence of hepatoma is high - 15-20 cases/100,000/year
◊ Age group is younger - 3rd and 4th decade
◊ Male to female ratio is high - 6:1 to 7:1
◊ Aflatoxin and HBV are the major factors and cirrhosis is less important
◊ Course is more progressive and fulminant
◊ Tumors are mostly at unresectable stage at first presentation

ABBREVIATIONS
• HBsAg = hepatitis B surface antigen
• HCV = hepatitis C virus
• HBV = hepatitis B virus
• AFP = alpha-fetoprotein

REFERENCES
• Zakim, D. & Boyer, T.D.: Hepatology, A Textbook of Liver Disease. 2nd Ed. Philadelphia, W.B. Saunders Co., 1990
• Regan, L.S.: Screening for hepatocellular carcinoma in high-risk individuals: A clinical review. Arch Intern Med. 149, 1741-44, 1989

Author A. Verma, M.D. & F. Iber, M.D.

Herpangina

BASICS

DESCRIPTION Infectious disease caused by Coxsackievirus group A. Characteristics - fever of short duration, typical vesicular or ulcerated lesions in the post pharynx or on the soft palate. Usual course - acute.
System(s) affected: Metabolic/digestive
Genetics: N/A
Incidence/Prevalence: N/A
Predominant age: 3 months-16 years
Predominant sex: Male = Female.

SIGNS AND SYMPTOMS
- Anorexia
- Drooling
- Sore throat
- Fever
- Malaise
- Irritability
- Listlessness
- Local pain
- Emesis
- Backache
- Headache
- Coryza
- Diarrhea
- Bilateral discrete vesicles, gray base
- Erythematous periphery
- Vesicles may rupture ulcers
- Posterior pharynx location - pharynx, tonsils, soft palate, little involvement of anterior 2/3 of mouth

CAUSES
- Coxsackievirus A
- Coxsackievirus B

RISK FACTORS Contact with infected person

DIAGNOSIS

DIFFERENTIAL DIAGNOSIS Herpes simplex - multiple ulcers, lips, anterior mouth are more common. diagnose with herpes culture.

LABORATORY
- Slight leukocytosis (<50%)

Drugs that may alter lab results: Cutaneous lesions also present (uticaria, erythema multiforme)
Disorders that may alter lab results: N/A

PATHOLOGIC FINDINGS Positive viral culture - mouth washings, stool

SPECIAL TESTS
- Complement fixation
- Hemaglutton inhibition tests

IMAGING N/A

DIAGNOSTIC PROCEDURES N/A

TREATMENT

APPROPRIATE HEALTH CARE
Outpatient

GENERAL MEASURES
- Self-limited
- Palliative and support
- Hydration

ACTIVITY No restrictions

DIET Clear liquids

PATIENT EDUCATION N/A

MEDICATIONS

DRUG(S) OF CHOICE
- Analgesics
- Topical anesthetics
- 2% (UISCVS xylocaine solution)

Contraindications: N/A
Precautions: N/A
Significant possible interactions: N/A

ALTERNATIVE DRUGS N/A

FOLLOWUP

PATIENT MONITORING Hydration

PREVENTION/AVOIDANCE Avoid contact with infected individual

POSSIBLE COMPLICATIONS
- Exanthem
- Meningitis
- Myocarditis
- Encephalitis

EXPECTED COURSE AND PROGNOSIS Excellent

MISCELLANEOUS

ASSOCIATED CONDITIONS N/A

AGE-RELATED FACTORS
Pediatric: N/A
Geriatric: N/A
Others: N/A

PREGNANCY N/A

SYNONYMS N/A

ICD-9-CM
074.0 herpangina

SEE ALSO N/A

OTHER NOTES N/A

ABBREVIATIONS N/A

REFERENCES Bondi, J., Jegasothy, B. & Lazarus, G.: Dermatology, Diagnosis and Therapy. Norwalk, CT, Appleton & Lange, 1991

Author J. Stearns, M.D.

Herpes gestationis

 BASICS

DESCRIPTION
A rare dermatopathic, immune-mediated and self-limited eruption most often occurring during mid-pregnancy
• Onset is in second trimester of pregnancy with remission after delivery except for some postpartum flares. May recur in subsequent pregnancies.
• Characterized by pruritic polymorphous vesicles, papules, and/or bullae often located in peri-umbilical or other truncal areas. May affect the buttocks, forearms, palms, or soles; less frequently scalp and face may be involved. Clustered vesicles may coalesce to form bullae, rupture to form crusts, then heal with hyperpigmentation.
• Mucous membranes are spared but intestinal mucosa may have celiac-like lesions without significant clinical malabsorption

System(s) affected: Skin/Exocrine, Reproductive
Genetics: Genetic predisposition possible, suggested by increased HLA-A1, -B8, and -DR3 antigens in affected women
Incidence in USA: Rare; 1 per 4000-50,000 pregnancies
Prevalence in USA: See Incidence
Predominant age: Child-bearing years
Predominant sex: Female only

SIGNS AND SYMPTOMS
Intensely pruritic papules and/or vesicles, occurring first in peri-umbilical area and spreading more generally

CAUSES
• Unknown but immune alterations suspected
• Not caused by herpes virus

RISK FACTORS
• Episode in prior pregnancy
• Herpes simplex does not increase risk

 DIAGNOSIS

DIFFERENTIAL DIAGNOSIS
Other pruritic conditions of pregnancy
◊ Besnier's prurigo gestationis with excoriated papules and no vesicles; usually limited to extensor surface of extremities
◊ Papular urticarial papules and plaques of pregnancy (PUPPP syndrome) which has urticarial plaques and small papules with a narrow, pale halo and no vesicles
◊ Impetigo herpetiformis has sterile pustules, not vesicles, and may involve mucous membranes, groin, and inner thighs
◊ Papular dermatitis of pregnancy
Non-pregnancy conditions to consider
◊ Dermatitis herpetiformis (much more chronic and more often in middle-aged males)
◊ Bullous pemphigoid
◊ Toxic drug eruption including erythema multiforme

LABORATORY
• Tzanck smear negative
• Herpes simplex virus culture negative
• Peripheral eosinophilia may be present
Drugs that may alter lab results: N/A
Disorders that may alter lab results: N/A

PATHOLOGICAL FINDINGS
• Subepidermal vesicle often with eosinophils and edema of dermal papillae
• Acantholysis is rare
• Inflammation surrounds superficial and deep dermal vessels

SPECIAL TESTS
Biopsy with direct immunofluorescence shows intense deposition of C3 (100%) and IgG (30-40%) along basement membrane. Serum may have circulating IgG antibasement membrane autoantibodies (10-20%) by indirect immunofluorescence; if not, half have herpes gestationis (HG) factor (a protein that fixes complement to basement membrane in-vitro human skin preparations).

IMAGING
N/A

DIAGNOSTIC PROCEDURES
Biopsy

 TREATMENT

APPROPRIATE HEALTH CARE
Outpatient

GENERAL MEASURES
• Differentiate from herpes virus infection
• Relieve pruritus
• Prevent secondary infection
• Soothing compresses such as Domeboro or Burrow's solution may help relieve itching

ACTIVITY
As tolerated

DIET
No special diet

PATIENT EDUCATION
• Educate about difference between this and herpes virus infection
• Inform of possible fetal risks and possibility of limited disease in newborn

MEDICATIONS

DRUG(S) OF CHOICE
• Topical steroids and antihistamines for mild pruritus
• Most will require systemic corticosteroids in doses of 20-60 mg/day (at the minimum effective dose) through first month postpartum
Contraindications: Weigh risk of aggravating hyperglycemia, potential effects on maternal and fetal bone, increased susceptibility to infections versus benefit of relieving pruritus, and resolving the lesions
Precautions:
• Use prednisone cautiously in patients with immune impairment, diabetes, or thrombophlebitis
• If prednisone has been used over several weeks, taper when discontinuing to prevent cortisol deficiency
Significant possible interactions:
Methylprednisolone may enhance toxicity of erythromycin

ALTERNATIVE DRUGS   Pyridoxine

FOLLOWUP

PATIENT MONITORING   Watch for secondary bacterial infection

PREVENTION/AVOIDANCE
• Avoid other people with infections, since there is susceptibility of open skin lesions and decreased resistance secondary to corticosteroids
• Some authorities recommend cesarean section when mother is known to be infected
• Avoid scalp monitors if disease involves maternal genitalia
• Use of estrogens or progesterone may trigger flare-up

POSSIBLE COMPLICATIONS
• Secondary bacterial infection
• Excess systemic medication in pregnancy
• Fetal deaths
• Premature births
• Fetal growth retardation
• Conjunctivitis
• Keratitis
• Cataracts
• Shock
• Transient herpes gestationis in the neonate

EXPECTED COURSE AND PROGNOSIS
• Spreads during 2nd-3rd trimester
• Remits after delivery
• Often flares in puerperium
• Tends to recur in subsequent pregnancies
• Systemic steroids may suppress new lesions, relieve pruritus, and dampen course; fetal outcome may be worsened

MISCELLANEOUS

ASSOCIATED CONDITIONS
• Pregnancy
• Hydatidiform mole
• Choriocarcinoma

AGE-RELATED FACTORS
Pediatric:
• Has been associated with preterm birth (22%) and still birth (< 10%)
• Rare cases of transient neonatal herpes gestationis are usually mild and resolve spontaneously; these are probably from passive transfer of antibasement membrane antibodies and HG factor
Geriatric: N/A
Others: N/A

PREGNANCY   By definition, a condition of pregnancy and puerperium

SYNONYMS   Dermatitis gestationis

ICD-9-CM
• 646.80 (unspecified relation to delivery)
• 646.83 (antepartum)

SEE ALSO   N/A

OTHER NOTES   Uncommon intrauterine infections are associated with microcephaly intracranial calcification and chorioretinitis

ABBREVIATIONS   N/A

REFERENCES
• DeGarmo, B.H.: Drug Master. St. Louis, Rapha Group Software, 1991
• Gabbe, S.G., Niebyl, J.R. & Simpson, J.L. (eds.): Obstetrics: Normal and Problem Pregnancies. New York, Churchill Livingstone, 1980
• Pritchard, J.A., MacDonald, P.C. & Gant, N.F. (eds.): Williams Obstetrics. Norwalk, CT, Appleton-Century-Crofts, 1985
• Zone, J.J. & Provost, T.T.: Bullous Disease. In Dermatology. Edited by S.L. Moschella. Philadelphia, W.B. Saunders Co., 1985

Author   A. Slaughter, M.D.

Herpes simplex

BASICS

DESCRIPTION Viral disease with many manifestations, usually seen as painful vesicles that often occur in clusters on skin, cornea, or mucous membranes; may occur as encephalitis, pneumonia, or disseminated infection.
Usual course of primary disease is 2 weeks; duration of recurrences varies; viral shedding in recurrence is briefer than with primary disease. Newborns or individuals with immune compromise are at risk for major morbidity or mortality.
System(s) affected: Skin/Exocrine, Nervous
Genetics: N/A
Incidence in USA: 29.2/100,000 office visits/year
Prevalence in USA:
 • Widespread; 0.65-20% of adults may be excreting HSV1 or HSV2 at any given time
 • Prevalence of antibodies varies from 30% in higher socioeconomic strata to 100% in lower socioeconomic strata; 20,000-70,000/100,000
Predominant age: All ages
Predominant sex: Male = Female

SIGNS AND SYMPTOMS
 • Vesicles - usually cluster and open as painful ulcerated lesions, often with erythematous base
Primary disease classic variations include:
 ◊ Herpetic whitlow - localized primary infection on a finger with intense itching and pain, followed by vesicles that may coalesce with swelling, erythema, and may mimic pyogenic paronychia; neuralgia and axillary adenopathy sometimes; heals over 2-3 weeks without incision. Primary inoculation of other abraded skin can occur (e.g., herpes gladiatorum in wrestlers).
 ◊ Primary herpetic gingivostomatitis and pharyngitis - first infection with HSV1 usually in early childhood; incubation from 2-12 days, then fever, sore throat, pharyngeal edema and erythema; small vesicles develop on pharyngeal and oral mucosa, rapidly ulcerate and increase in number to involve soft palate, buccal mucosa, tongue, floor of mouth, and often lips and cheeks; tender gums may bleed; fetid breath, cervical adenopathy; fever, general toxicity, poor oral intake, and drooling contribute to dehydration; autoinoculation of other sites may occur; resolves in 10-14 days with slower resolution of adenopathy
 ◊ Primary genital herpes -see Herpes, genital topic
 ◊ Primary herpes keratoconjunctivitis - by HSV1 usually; can present as unilateral conjunctivitis with regional adenopathy, as blepharitis with vesicles on lid margin, as keratitis with dendritic lesions or with punctate opacities; lasts 2-3 weeks but systemic involvement prolongs process
 ◊ Eczema herpeticum - diffuse pox-like eruption complicating atopic dermatitis; one cause of Kaposi's varicelliform eruption; sudden appearance of lesions in typical atopic areas (upper trunk, neck, head); high fever,

local edema, adenopathy, umbilicated vesicles develop hemorrhagic crust or become pustular; appear in crops for up to a week; significant fluid or blood loss and secondary bacterial infections can cause fatality; similar serious inoculations can occur with severe burn patients and go unrecognized under the eschar.
 ◊ Neonatal herpes simplex - perinatal primary infection is life-threatening and usually acquired by vaginal birth of infected mother; fetal risk and neonatal risk are greater in mothers with primary genital herpes infection since shedding is more prolonged and the inoculum is greater; incubation from 5-7 days usually (rarely 4 weeks); cutaneous, mucous membrane, or ocular signs in only 70%; congenital infection via prenatal transplacental virus transfer may present with jaundice, hepatosplenomegaly, DIC, encephalitis, seizures, temperature instability, chorioretinitis, and/or conjunctivitis with or without skin vesicles; neurologic morbidity worse with HSV2 than with HSV1 in neonates; fatal hepatic or adrenal necrosis may occur
Recurrent diseases from endogenous reactivation include:
 ◊ Herpes labialis - recurrent lesions on lips with HSV1, usually less than one recurrence per six months, but 5-25% may have more than one attack per month; precipitating events may be sunlight, fever, trauma, menses, stress; prodrome of pain, burning, itching may last 6-48 hrs before vesicles appear, often at vermilion border with increased pain; will ulcerate and crust within 48 hrs; heals within 8-10 days generally; may have local adenopathy
 ◊ Ocular herpes - may recur as keratitis, blepharitis, or keratoconjunctivitis; may have dendritic ulcers, decreased corneal sensation, less visual acuity; uveitis may cause permanent visual loss
 ◊ Recurrent genital herpes (herpes progenitalis) - see Herpes, genital topic

CAUSES Herpes simplex virus, a DNA virus of two major types: HSV1 and HSV2; most often HSV1 is associated with oral lesions and HSV2 with genital lesions but reverse occurs also

RISK FACTORS
 • Immune compromise (brief as with occurrence of other illness or stress, or more chronic as with chemotherapy, malignancy, or AIDS)
 • Newborns - if exposed to actively infected mother via birth canal or if exposed to case in nursery (insufficient maternal passive antibody transfer); risk greatest for neonate of mother with active primary H. simplex infection
 • Prior HSV infection
 • Sexual intercourse with infected person (condoms can help prevent but location of some lesions may permit spread even with condoms)
 • Occupational exposure (medical/dental risk more for HSV1 whitlow and general community to HSV2 whitlow)

DIAGNOSIS

DIFFERENTIAL DIAGNOSIS
 • Impetigo - straw-colored vesicles that crust
 • Aphthous stomatitis - grayish, shallow erosions with ring of hyperemia, usually only anterior in mouth and lips
 • Herpes zoster - unilateral dermatome distribution
 • Syphilitic chancre - usually painless ulcer
 • Herpangina - vesicles predominate on anterior tonsillar pillars, soft palate, uvula and oropharynx but not more anteriorly on lips or gums (usually caused by group A Coxsackievirus)
 • Stevens-Johnson syndrome
 • Other causes of Kaposi's varicelliform eruption are varicella and Coxsackievirus A16

LABORATORY
 • Tzanck smear shows multinucleated giant cells often with Cowdria type A intranuclear inclusions (scrape material from lesion onto slide, fix with ethanol or methanol, stain with Giemsa or Wright preparation; alternatively spray slide with cytological fixative and stain as for Pap smear)
 • Herpes simplex virus culture - only half of true positives available in 2 days; rest may take 6 days or longer to be positive; not considered as reasonable means to follow activity of recurrent disease near labor and delivery
Drugs that may alter lab results: N/A
Disorders that may alter lab results:
Varicella (herpes zoster) has identical findings on Tzanck smear

PATHOLOGICAL FINDINGS
Multinucleated giant cells with 2-15 nuclei per cell with eosinophilic inclusion bodies within nuclei; intraepithelial edema (ballooning degeneration) and intracellular edema; brain biopsy (in encephalitis) has hemorrhagic necrosis of gray and white matter with acute and chronic inflammation, thrombosis and fibrinoid necrosis of parenchymal vessels, and intranuclear inclusions in astrocytes, oligodendroglia, and neurons

SPECIAL TESTS
 • Specific HSV antibody titers show fourfold or greater rise between acute and convalescent sera with primary infection; not helpful with recurrences generally
 • IgM HSV antibodies may appear in first 4 weeks of life in infected infants

IMAGING N/A

DIAGNOSTIC PROCEDURES
Occasionally biopsy is needed

TREATMENT

APPROPRIATE HEALTH CARE
Outpatient

GENERAL MEASURES
• Limited skin lesions (as in recurrent herpes labialis) may benefit from early unroofing of vesicles and application of Campho-Phenique
• Intermittent cool moist dressings with Domeboro or Burow's solution
• Inability to void from severe periurethral lesions may be remedied by pouring a cup of warm water over genitals while urinating or sitting in a warm bath to urinate
• Children with gingivostomatitis may require IV hydration
• Extensive skin disease (as with neonates or with eczema herpeticum) may require vigorous volume replacement
• Screen for other sexually transmitted diseases with primary genital herpes

ACTIVITY   No restrictions

DIET   Avoid acidic foods with gingivostomatitis

PATIENT EDUCATION
• Avoid contact with immune compromised persons including neonates
• Prevent both spread to others and autoinoculation
• For genital herpes - avoid sexual contact while disease is active; stress protective benefits and limits of condoms and reinforce benefits of mutually monogamous sexual relations. See Herpes, genital topic also.

MEDICATIONS

DRUG(S) OF CHOICE
Analgesics (non-narcotic)
Acyclovir: Has specific indications in immune compromised persons with either primary or recurrent disease, in encephalitis, or in others with significant genital disease; doses should be adjusted downward for renal insufficiency
◊ Neonatal herpes simplex - 10 mg/kg IV over 1 hr q 8 hr x 10-14 days
◊ Encephalitis - 10 mg/kg IV over 1 hr q 8 hr x 10 days (for ages 6 months-12 years give 500 mg/m2)
◊ Primary genital - see Herpes, genital topic
◊ Recurrent genital herpes - see Herpes, genital topic
◊ Recurrent herpes labialis - generally not an indication, but anecdotal reports claim benefit
Contraindications: Hypersensitivity or intolerance

Precautions:
• Reduce dosage in renal insufficiency
• May get some nausea, vomiting, or headache; some encephalopathic reactions
• Pregnancy - use only if benefits exceed risk to fetus; can be passed in breast milk
Significant possible interactions:
Probenecid can elevate intravenous acyclovir half-life and reduce renal clearance

ALTERNATIVE DRUGS
Vidarabine: Has indications for herpes simplex encephalitis, neonatal infections, and keratitis. However, it is poorly soluble. One liter of IV solution will solubilize at most 450 mg of vidarabine. The drug should be used cautiously in patients with renal dysfunction.
◊ Encephalitis - 15 mg/kg/day x 10 days (age < 30 years and higher levels of consciousness do better)
◊ Neonatal - 30 mg/kg/day x 10 days
◊ Keratitis - ophthalmic (Vira-A) 3% ointment 1/2 inch 5 times daily for 7-21 days or longer. Other topicals - idoxuridine and trifluorothymidine (refer to ophthalmologist).

FOLLOWUP

PATIENT MONITORING   Observe for disappearance of lesions and resolution of systemic manifestations

PREVENTION/AVOIDANCE   See Patient Education

POSSIBLE COMPLICATIONS
• Herpes encephalitis - brain biopsy may be needed for diagnosis
• Herpes pneumonia
• Aseptic meningitis
• Herpes septicemia

EXPECTED COURSE AND PROGNOSIS
• Good for treatment of recurrent episodes
• Expect frequent recurrences

MISCELLANEOUS

ASSOCIATED CONDITIONS   Erythema multiforme

AGE-RELATED FACTORS
Pediatric: Previously described
Geriatric: Decreased immunological competence of old age may increase risk
Others: N/A

PREGNANCY
• Decision whether or not to perform cesarean section to reduce contact of neonate with virus is based on observation of active or clinically suspicious lesions on the cervix or in birth canal at time of labor and delivery. Duration of shedding and risk to fetus or newborn is greatest with primary disease.
• Infection in utero can cause significant fetal mortality and morbidity (prematurity and growth retardation). Research is needed to determine feasibility/safety of intravenous acyclovir for primary disease during pregnancy.

SYNONYMS   N/A

ICD-9-CM
• 054.0 Eczema herpeticum
• 054.10 Genital herpes (unspecified)
• 054.2 Herpetic gingivostomatitis
• 771.2 Neonatal herpes simplex
• 054.9 Herpes labialis

SEE ALSO   Herpes, genital

OTHER NOTES   N/A

ABBREVIATIONS   N/A

REFERENCES
• Brown, Z.A., et al.: Effects on infants of a first episode of genital herpes during pregnancy. N Engl J Med. 1987;317:1246-1251
• Arvin, A.M.: Antiviral treatment of herpes simplex in neonates and pregnant women. J Am Acad Derm. 1988;.18:200-202
• Brown, Z.A. & Baker, D.A.: Acyclovir therapy during pregnancy. Obstet Gynecol. 1989;73:526-531
• Centers for Disease Control. 1989 Sexually transmitted diseases treatment guidelines. MMWR 1989;38(No S-8)16-18
• Hirsch, M.S.: Herpes simples virus. In Principles and Practice of Infectious Diseases. Edited by G.L. Mandell, et al. New York, Churchill Livingstone, 1990
• Waldron, C.A.: Face, lips, tongue, teeth, oral soft tissues, jaws, salivary glands and neck. In Anderson's Pathology. Edited by J.M. Kissane. St Louis, C.V. Mosby Co.,1990

Author   A. Slaughter, M.D.

Herpes zoster

 BASICS

DESCRIPTION
An illness commonly presenting as a painful unilateral dermatomal eruption. Zoster results from reactivation of varicella-zoster (chicken pox) virus that has been dormant in the dorsal root ganglia.
System(s) affected: Skin/Exocrine, Nervous
Genetics: N/A
Incidence in USA: 200/100,000/year
Prevalence in USA:
 • Occurs in 10% to 20% of the population at some time
 • Active herpes zoster 16.7/100,000
 • Post herpetic neuralgia 60/100,000
Predominant age: Increasing incidence with aging. 80% of cases occur in persons over age 20 years (2-3 per 1000 age 20 to 50; 10 per 1000 > 80 years).
Predominant sex: Male = Female

SIGNS AND SYMPTOMS
Prodromal phase (sensations over involved dermatome prior to rash)
 ◊ Tingling
 ◊ Itching
 ◊ Boring or knifelike pain
Acute phase
 ◊ Constitutional symptoms
 ◊ Fatigue
 ◊ Malaise
 ◊ Headache
 ◊ Low-grade fever
 ◊ Dermatomal rash
 ◊ Weakness (1% may have weakness in distribution of rash; herpes zoster motoricus)
 ◊ Initially erythematous and maculopapular that evolves rapidly to grouped vesicles
 ◊ Vesicles become pustular and/or hemorrhagic in 3 to 4 days
 ◊ Resolution of rash with crusts separating. by 14 to 21 days
 ◊ Possible sine herpete (zoster without rash)
Chronic phase
 ◊ Postherpetic neuralgia (15% overall; increases dramatically with age)

CAUSES
Reactivation of dormant varicella-zoster (chicken pox) virus in dorsal root ganglia

RISK FACTORS
 • Increasing age
 • Compromised cell-mediated immunity in immunosuppressed patients or patients with malignancy
 • Spinal surgery
 • Spinal cord radiation
 • Leukemia
 • Lymphoma

 DIAGNOSIS

DIFFERENTIAL DIAGNOSIS
 • Rash - herpes simplex virus, Coxsackievirus, contact dermatitis, superficial pyoderma
 • Pain - cholecystitis, pleuritis, myocardial infarction

LABORATORY
 • Rarely necessary
 • Viral culture
 • Tzanck smear (does not distinguish from herpes simplex and false negatives occur)
 • Monoclonal antibody tests
 • Acute and convalescent antibody titers
Drugs that may alter lab results: N/A
Disorders that may alter lab results: N/A

PATHOLOGICAL FINDINGS
 • Multinucleated giant cells with intralesional inclusion
 • Lymphatic infiltration of sensory ganglia with focal hemorrhage and nerve cell destruction

SPECIAL TESTS N/A

IMAGING N/A

DIAGNOSTIC PROCEDURES
Biopsy for direct immunofluorescence testing (rarely done)

 TREATMENT

APPROPRIATE HEALTH CARE
Outpatient unless disseminated or occurring as complication of serious underlying disease requiring hospitalization

GENERAL MEASURES
 • Wet dressings with tap water or 5% aluminum acetate (Burow's) applied 30 to 60 minutes 4-6 times per day
 • Lotions such as calamine

ACTIVITY No restrictions

DIET No special diet

PATIENT EDUCATION
 • Duration of rash is 2-3 weeks
 • Potential for dissemination and worrisome signs (constitutional illness signs and spreading rash)
 • Potential postherpetic neuralgia

Herpes zoster

MEDICATIONS

DRUG(S) OF CHOICE
• Pain medications (acetaminophen, codeine, nonsteroidal anti-inflammatory drugs)
• Silver sulfadiazine (Silvadene) topically for secondarily infected rash
• Acyclovir (Zovirax) IV 5 mg/kg every 8 hours or po 800 mg every 4 hours (5 doses per day). Clearly indicated for zoster associated with serious underlying condition and in ophthalmic zoster. For ophthalmic zoster 600 mg q 4 h (5 times daily).
• Acyclovir in others if initiated early (within 48 hours of rash) is of benefit in relieving symptoms and speeding resolution of rash, but cost and side effects make benefits marginal
• Data is conflicting regarding acyclovir in acute phase reducing incidence/severity of post herpetic neuralgia
Contraindications: Refer to manufacturer's profile of each drug
Precautions:
• Monitor renal function when using acyclovir
• Refer to manufacturer's profile of each drug
Significant possible interactions:
• Probenecid may inhibit excretion of acyclovir
• Refer to manufacturer's profile of each drug

ALTERNATIVE DRUGS Vidarabine, topical idoxuridine in DMSO

FOLLOWUP

PATIENT MONITORING Symptom dependant

PREVENTION/AVOIDANCE
• None at present
• Zoster patients may transmit virus causing varicella (chickenpox) to susceptible persons
• Varicella vaccines under investigation have not eliminated zoster

POSSIBLE COMPLICATIONS
• Postherpetic neuralgia
• Meningoencephalitis
• Cutaneous dissemination
• Superinfection of skin lesions
• Visceral involvement
• Peripheral motor weakness
• Segmental myelitis
• Cranial nerve syndromes especially ophthalmic and facial (Ramsay Hunt syndrome)
• Corneal ulceration
• Guillain-Barré syndrome

EXPECTED COURSE AND PROGNOSIS
• Resolution of rash within 14 to 21 days
• Postherpetic neuralgia defined as pain persisting at least one month after rash has healed
• Postherpetic neuralgia incidence increases with age (4% age 30-50; 34% over age 80 years)

MISCELLANEOUS

ASSOCIATED CONDITIONS
Immunocompromise including HIV infection, transplant recipients, and malignancies

AGE-RELATED FACTORS
Pediatric:
• Occurs rarely in children (primarily immunosuppressed)
• Has been reported in infants primarily infected in utero
Geriatric:
• Increased incidence and prevalence
• Increased incidence of postherpetic neuralgia
Others: Consider HIV infection in young patients with zoster

PREGNANCY Can occur during pregnancy

SYNONYMS Shingles

ICD-9-CM 053.9 (site specific codes not listed preferred by Medicare)

SEE ALSO
• Chickenpox
• Herpes simplex
• Herpes zoster ophthalmic

OTHER NOTES Corticosteroid efficacy to prevent postherpetic neuralgia remains inconclusive. Capsaicin, transcutaneous electrical nerve stimulation (TENS) and low dose amitriptyline are the current treatment(s) of choice. Treatment with acyclovir may prevent or reduce postherpetic neuralgia.

ABBREVIATIONS DMSO = dimethyl sulfoxide

REFERENCES
• Carmichael, J.K.: Treatment of Herpes Zoster and Postherpetic Neuralgia. Am Fam Phys. July 1991
• Huff, J.C., et al.: Therapy of herpes zoster with oral acyclovir. Am J Med 85 (suppl 2A):84, 1988

Author L. Halverson, M.D.

Herpes, genital

BASICS

DESCRIPTION Herpes simplex virus (usually HSV-2) infection involving the genital organs
• Primary genital herpes - initial infection with herpes simplex. No previous antibodies to HSV, involves genitalia.
• First-episode (non-primary) genital herpes - prior infection with a herpes simplex serotype, first genital involvement
• Recurrent (secondary) genital herpes - reactivation of latent herpes virus infection, usually previous genital involvement
System(s) affected: Nervous, Skin/Exocrine, Reproductive
Genetics: N/A
Incidence in USA: 50-200/100,000 (300,000 - 700,000 cases/year)
Prevalence in USA: 10,000-30,000/100,000 people
Predominant age: 18-40
Predominant Sex: Female > Male

SIGNS AND SYMPTOMS

Primary genital herpes
◊ Fever
◊ Headache
◊ Malaise
◊ Myalgia
◊ Burning genital pain
◊ Dysuria (female)
◊ Dyspareunia
◊ Elevated temperature
◊ Inguinal adenopathy
◊ Aseptic meningitis in 30%
◊ Vesicles, on an edematous erythematous base, which ulcerate, crust over, and resolve spontaneously within 21 days
◊ Bilateral lesions, primarily affecting the external genitalia: Female - labia majora/minora, inner thighs, vaginal mucosa, cervix, perianal skin; male - penile glans, penile shaft, urethra
Non-primary - first episode genital herpes
◊ Burning genital pain
◊ Vesicles, on a non-edematous erythematous base, which ulcerate, crust over, and resolve spontaneously within 14-17 days
Non-primary - recurrent genital herpes
◊ Prodromal symptoms - burning, numbness, tingling, paresthesia of genitals at site of previous lesions which occur approximately 24 hours prior to the eruption of new vesicles
◊ Burning genital pain
◊ Vesicles, on a non-edematous erythematous base, which ulcerate, crust over, and resolve spontaneously within 7-10 days
◊ Unilateral lesions

CAUSES
• Herpes simplex virus
• Type 1 (HSV-1) - 10-30%
• Type 2 (HSV-2) - 70-90%

RISK FACTORS
Primary inoculation
◊ Sexual activity
◊ Fomites - wet towels (rare)
Triggers (recurrent)
◊ Genital trauma
◊ Menses
◊ Intercurrent infection
◊ Emotional stress

DIAGNOSIS

DIFFERENTIAL DIAGNOSIS
• Syphilis
• Chancroid
• Lymphogranuloma venereum
• Atypical genital warts
• Scabies
• Molluscum contagiosum
• Allergic contact dermatitis
• Trauma

LABORATORY
• Viral tissue culture - swab vesicle fluid or ulcer
• Tzanck prep. Sensitivity = 40-50% compared to culture; multinucleated giant cells.
• Pap smear
• ELISA, direct fluorescent assay (DFA), radioimmunoassay (RIA) and complement fixation. Sensitivity = 80% compared to culture. Primary herpes - 4 x increase acute/convalescent titer; recurrent herpes - no increase in acute/convalescent titer.
Drugs that may alter lab results: Calcium agglutinate swabs not recommended for culture
Disorders that may alter lab results: Varicella-zoster will give identical Tzanck prep results

PATHOLOGICAL FINDINGS
Histopathologic-cytopathic changes
◊ Intracellular edema of epithelial cells
◊ Nuclear margination of chromatin
◊ Formation of Cowdry type A intranuclear inclusions
◊ Cell fusion into multinucleated giant cells

SPECIAL TESTS   N/A

IMAGING   N/A

DIAGNOSTIC PROCEDURES   N/A

TREATMENT

APPROPRIATE HEALTH CARE
Outpatient, self-care

GENERAL MEASURES
• Analgesics - NSAID's
• Topical anesthetics - lidocaine
• Cool compresses - Burow's solution 4-6 times a day
• Ice packs to perineum
• Sitz baths
• Local perineal hygiene

ACTIVITY
• Avoid intercourse in the presence of symptomatic genital lesions
• Appropriate rest if systemic manifestations (primary) are present

DIET   N/A

PATIENT EDUCATION Pamphlets and telephone information available from - Herpes Resource Center ASHA/HRC, P.O. Box 13827, Research Triangle Park, North Carolina 27709-9940, HRC Hotline (919)361-8488

MEDICATIONS

DRUG(S) OF CHOICE
Acyclovir (Zovirax)
◊ Primary or 1st episode: 200 mg po 5 times per day for 7-10 days
◊ Severe local or disseminated disease: 5 mg/kg IV q 8 hrs for 7 days
◊ Encephalitis: 10 mg/kg IV, q 8 hours hours for 10 days
◊ Recurrent episodes: 200 mg po 5 times/day x 5 days
◊ Chronic suppression: 400 mg po bid or 200 mg po 2-5 times/day
Contraindications: Documented allergy to acyclovir
Precautions:
• Not approved for routine use in pregnancy
• Drug is excreted in breast milk
• Modify dose in patients with significant renal insufficiency
Significant possible interactions:
Acyclovir (Zovirax)
◊ Methotrexate - use with caution in patients who have had a neurologic reaction to intrathecal methotrexate
◊ Interferon - acyclovir is synergistic in vitro with interferon. Clinical significance is unknown. Use with caution in patients with prior neurological reactions to interferon.
◊ Probenecid - will decrease renal excretion, increase serum concentration

ALTERNATIVE DRUGS
Acyclovir topical ointment - less effective than oral administration

FOLLOWUP

PATIENT MONITORING
• Acute episode - followup (usually outpatient) advisable if symptoms suggest the presence of complications
• Latent infection - annual pap smear; careful exam of pregnant women during prenatal visits and at onset of labor

PREVENTION/AVOIDANCE
• Condoms/spermicide advised in sexual activity
• Avoid multiple sexual partners
• Avoid stress when possible

POSSIBLE COMPLICATIONS
• Vaginal discharge
• Secondary bacterial infection
• Urinary retention
• Aseptic meningitis
• Transmission to neonate
• Increased risk for HIV infection

EXPECTED COURSE AND PROGNOSIS
• Primary - resolution of signs/symptoms in 14-21 days
• First episode - non-primary - resolution of signs/symptoms in 14-17 days
• Recurrent - resolution of signs/symptoms in 7-10 days
• Latent infection - recurrences in > 50% of individuals (with variable frequency)
• Infection in immunocompromised individual - prolonged severe local or disseminated disease is common

MISCELLANEOUS

ASSOCIATED CONDITIONS
• Herpes labialis
• Syphilis
• Gonorrhea
• Non-gonococcal urethritis/cervicitis
• Genital warts (HPV)
• AIDS (HIV)
• Trichomoniasis

AGE-RELATED FACTORS
Pediatric:
• Genital lesions in prepubertal child is suggestive of sexual abuse
• Neonatal infection occurs in 1/5,000 live births and results in death or significant neurologic impairment in 85% of individuals. Most neonatal infections result from asymptomatic viral shedding from past maternal infection.
Geriatric: N/A
Others: N/A

PREGNANCY
• Greatest risk for neonatal infection occurs with primary genital infection of mother at time of delivery
• Cesarean section is indicated if herpetic genital lesions are present during labor
• Any lesion suspicious for genital herpes during pregnancy should be cultured
• Routine surveillance cultures for women with a history of genital herpes are indicated only at the time of labor
• Acyclovir is not approved for routine use during pregnancy, but is used by some clinicians during the last 1-2 weeks of pregnancy to avoid activation of lesions

SYNONYMS
Herpes genitalis

ICD-9-CM
054.10

SEE ALSO
N/A

OTHER NOTES
N/A

ABBREVIATIONS
N/A

REFERENCES
• Bernstein, D.I.: Effects of prior HSV-1 infection on genital HSV-2 infection. Prog Med Virol. 1991; 38:109-127
• Dawkins, B.J.: Genital herpes simplex infections. Primary Care Clinics of North America. 1990; 17:95-113
• Stone, K.M. & Whittington, W.L.: Treatment of genital herpes. Rev Infect Dis. 1990; pp: s610-s619
• Drugs for Sexually Transmitted Diseases. The Medical Letter on Drugs and Therapeutics. 1991, Vol 33;119-124
• Prober, C.C.: Herpetic Vaginitis in 1993. Clinical Obstetrics and Gynecology. 1993; vol 36, No. 1,177-187

Author G. Levine, M.D.

Hiccups

BASICS

DESCRIPTION Sudden, involuntary, contraction of the inspiratory muscles (predominantly the diaphragm) terminated by abrupt closure of the glottis stopping the inflow of air and producing the characteristic sound.
System(s) affected: Pulmonary, nervous
Genetics: N/A
Incidence in USA: Self limited hiccups are extremely common; intractable hiccups are rare
Prevalence in USA: N/A
Predominant age: All ages (including fetus)
Predominant sex: Male (4:1)

SIGNS AND SYMPTOMS Hiccup attacks usually occur at brief intervals and last only a few seconds or minutes. Bouts lasting more than 48 hours often imply an underlying physical or metabolic disorder. Intractable hiccups may occur continuously for months or years. Hiccups usually occur with a frequency of 4 to 60 per minute.

CAUSES
• Pathophysiologic significance is unknown; hiccups have been associated with more than 100 underlying disorders.
• Results from stimulation of one or more limbs of the hiccup reflux arc (vagus and phrenic nerves) with a "hiccup center" located in the upper spinal cord
• In men greater than 90% have an organic basis while in women a psychogenic cause is more likely
• Specific underlying causes include:
  ◊ Alcoholism
  ◊ CNS lesions (brainstem tumors, vascular lesions, Parkinson's disease)
  ◊ Diaphragmatic irritation (tumors, pericarditis, eventration, splenomegaly, hepatomegaly, peritonitis)
  ◊ Hair, insect or foreign body irritating tympanic membrane
  ◊ Pharyngitis, laryngitis
  ◊ Mediastinal and other thoracic lesions (pneumonia, aortic aneurysm, tuberculosis, myocardial infarction, lung cancer)
  ◊ Esophageal lesions (reflux esophagitis, achalasia, Candida esophagitis, carcinoma, obstruction)
  ◊ Gastric lesions (ulcer, distention, cancer)
  ◊ Hepatic lesions (hepatitis, hepatoma)
  ◊ Pancreatic lesions (pancreatitis, pseudocysts, cancer)
  ◊ Inflammatory bowel disease
  ◊ Cholelithiasis, cholecystitis
  ◊ Prostatic disorders
  ◊ Appendicitis
  ◊ Postoperative, abdominal procedures
  ◊ Toxic metabolic causes (uremia, hyponatremia, gout, diabetes)
  ◊ Drug induced (dexamethasone, methylprednisolone, benzodiazepines, alpha methyldopa)
  ◊ Psychogenic causes (hysterical neurosis, grief, malingering)
  ◊ Idiopathic

RISK FACTORS
• General anesthesia
• Post-operative state
• Irritation of the vagus nerve branches
• Structural, vascular, infectious or traumatic CNS lesions

DIAGNOSIS

DIFFERENTIAL DIAGNOSIS See Causes (burping [eructation] may be confused with hiccups)

LABORATORY N/A
Drugs that may alter lab results: N/A
Disorders that may alter lab results: N/A

PATHOLOGICAL FINDINGS N/A

SPECIAL TESTS N/A

IMAGING Fluoroscopy is useful to determine if one hemidiaphragm is dominant

DIAGNOSTIC PROCEDURES N/A

TREATMENT

APPROPRIATE HEALTH CARE
• Outpatient (usually)
• Inpatient (if elderly, debilitated or intractable hiccups)

GENERAL MEASURES
Treat any specific underlying cause when identified.
• Dilate esophageal stricture or obstruction
• Remove hair or foreign body from ear canal
• Angostura bitters for alcohol induced hiccups
• Catheter stimulation of pharynx for operative and post-operative hiccups
• Anti-fungal treatment for Candida esophagitis
• Correct electrolyte imbalance
Simple home remedies
• Swallowing a spoonful of sugar
• Sucking on a hard candy
• Holding breath and increasing pressure on diaphragm (Valsalva maneuver)
• Tongue traction
• Lifting the uvula with a cold spoon
• Drinking from the far side of a glass
• Inducing fright
• Smelling salts
• Rebreathing into a paper (not plastic) bag
• Sipping ice water
Medical measures
• Relief of gastric distention (gastric lavage, nasogastric aspiration, induced vomiting)
• Counterirritation of the vagus nerve (supraorbital pressure, carotid sinus massage, digital rectal massage)
• Respiratory center stimulants (breathing 5% carbon dioxide)
• Phrenic nerve block of dominant hemidiaphragm; phrenic crush, transection
• Psychiatric (hypnosis, behavioral modification)
• Miscellaneous (cardioversion, acupuncture)

ACTIVITY As tolerated

DIET Avoid gastric distension from overeating, carbonated beverages, aerophagia

PATIENT EDUCATION See General Measures

MEDICATIONS

DRUG(S) OF CHOICE
Possible drug remedies:
• Baclofen (GABA analog) 5-10 mg tid (best bet)
• Chlorpromazine 25-50 mg IV
• Haloperidol 2-12 mg IM
• Phenytoin 200 mg IV then 100 mg qid
• Metoclopramide 5-10 mg qid
• Nifedipine 10-20 mg qd-tid
• Amitriptyline 10 mg tid

Contraindications: Refer to manufacturer's literature (Baclofen is not recommended in patients with stroke or other cerebral lesions).
Precautions: Refer to manufacturer's literature (abrupt withdrawal of Baclofen should be avoided)
Significant possible interactions: Refer to manufacturer's literature

ALTERNATIVE DRUGS
• Amantadine, Levodopa/Carbidopa in Parkinson's disease
• Steroid replacement in Addison's disease
• Antifungal agent in Candida esophagitis
• Ondansetron in carcinomatosis with vomiting

FOLLOWUP

PATIENT MONITORING   Until hiccups cease

PREVENTION/AVOIDANCE
• Correct underlying cause
• Maintenance drug therapy (e.g. Baclofen 5-10 mg TID.; Phenytoin 100 mg QID.; Valproic acid 15 mg/kg undivided doses; Nifedipine 10-20 mg qd.-TID.; Metoclopramide 10 mg QID.)

POSSIBLE COMPLICATIONS
• Inability to eat
• Weight loss
• Exhaustion, debility
• Insomnia
• Cardiac arrhythmias
• Wound dehiscence
• Death (rare)

EXPECTED COURSE AND PROGNOSIS
• Hiccups often cease during sleep
• Most acute benign hiccups resolve with home remedies or spontaneously
• Intractable hiccups may last for years and decades
• Hiccups have persisted despite bilateral phrenic nerve transection

MISCELLANEOUS

ASSOCIATED CONDITIONS   See Causes

AGE-RELATED FACTORS
Pediatric: May persist from fetal state
Geriatric: Can be a serious problem among the elderly
Others: See possible complications

PREGNANCY   Fetal hiccups noted as rhythmic fetal movements (confirmed sonographically), fetal hiccups often recur in subsequent pregnancies

SYNONYMS
• Hiccoughs
• Singultus

ICD-9-CM
786.8

SEE ALSO   N/A

OTHER NOTES   N/A

ABBREVIATIONS   N/A

REFERENCES   Lewis, J.H.. Hiccups-Causes and Cures. Journal of Clinical Gastroenterology, 1985; 7:539-552.

Author   J. Lewis, M.D.

Hidradenitis suppurativa

BASICS

DESCRIPTION Acute, tender, cyst-like abscesses in apocrine gland bearing skin (axillae, anogenital area, pubes, areolae (mammary), also apocrine glands scattered around umbilicus, scalp, trunk and face). In chronic cases there develops fibrotic sinus tracts with intermittent drainage and periodic acute abscesses.
Genetics: Unknown
System(s) affected: Skin/Exocrine
Incidence/Prevalence in USA: Common
Predominant age: Late puberty through age 40, commonly 30-40.
Predominant sex: Female (perianal) > Male (axillary)

SIGNS AND SYMPTOMS
• Papules (dome-shaped) 1-3 cm in size
• Nodules (dome-shaped) 1-3 cm in size
• Larger lesions fluctuate
• Distribution - Apocrine glands as above with axillae and groin most common
• Multiple recurrences at the same site
• Healing sites accompanied by scarring and sinus tracts
• Comedones may be present

CAUSES
• Blockage of pilosebaceous units to which apocrine glands are attached. This activity occurs (acne-like) after hormone stimulation beginning with puberty.
• Blockage of apocrine follicles may possibly be caused by embryologic malformation of apocrine duct, compression of the duct due to sweat retention, or bacterial infection
• May be part of "follicular occlusive triad"; acne conglobata, dissecting cellulitis of scalp, hidradenitis suppurativa)

RISK FACTORS
• Obesity
• African American
• Female
• Acne
• Diabetes Mellitus
• Hypercholesterolemia
• Low basal metabolic rate

DIAGNOSIS

DIFFERENTIAL DIAGNOSIS
• Furunculosis. Differentiate by specific culture and also by the response to specific antibiotics.

LABORATORY Culture of exudate from lesion: Staphylococci, Streptococci, E. Coli, Proteus with chronic condition, usually not anaerobes, increase antibiotic resistance. Normocytic anemia with chronic cases.
Drugs that may alter lab results: N/A
Disorders that may alter lab results: N/A

PATHOLOGICAL FINDINGS Acute and chronic inflammation, multiple comedones, sinus tracts when recurrent

SPECIAL TESTS Culture discharge from lesion(s)

IMAGING N/A

DIAGNOSTIC PROCEDURES Incision and drainage of lesion(s) and biopsy

TREATMENT

APPROPRIATE HEALTH CARE
• A) Symptomatic treatment acute lesions (See General Measures)
• B) Surgery: remove sinus tracts, exteriorization with curettage and electrodesiccation, treatment for severe, intractable cases- excision and skin graft
• C) Prevent new lesions

GENERAL MEASURES
• Local cleansing (germicidal soap)
• Improve environmental factors that cause follicular blockage
• Minimize heat exposure and sweating
• Lose weight if overweight
• Avoid constrictive clothing/frictional trauma
• Avoid underarm antiperspirants and deodorants
• 2 months trial with antibiotic (See Medications)
• Birth control pills (female only), if antibiotic therapy fails
• Injection of lesions with depot-type steroids (e.g., triamcinolone)
• Incision and drainage of lesions
• Consider excisional surgery (draining lesions are not contraindications for surgery)
• Consider oral retinoids
• Consider brief course of systemic corticosteroids

ACTIVITY Fully active

DIET No restrictions

PATIENT EDUCATION
• Minimize heat exposure and sweating
• Reduce weight if obese
• Avoid constrictive clothing
• Medication precautions

MEDICATIONS

DRUG(S) OF CHOICE
• Tetracycline 250mg qid or 500mg tid for 2 or more months, or
• Minocin 100mg bid po, or
• Clindamycin 2% lotion or neomycin cream topically to control odor.
• Erythromycin 1-1.5gm qd po
• Doxycycline 100mg bid 7-14 days
• Other antibiotics depending on culture
Contraindications: Tetracycline - pregnancy, children < 8 years
Precautions: Tetracycline - do not take dairy products, antacids, or iron preparations within 2 hours of tetracycline dose. Use sunscreen (SPF 15 or better) to avoid phototoxicity.
Significant possible interactions: Refer to manufacturer's literature

ALTERNATIVE DRUGS
• Birth control pills with low-dose progesterone (e.g., Norinyl, Ortho-Novum, Enovid). Female patients only.
• Isotretinoin (Accutane) 40-80 mg/day po for 4 months. No Accutane during pregnancy (highly teratogenic). Still frequent recurrences.
• Review professional literature before prescribing birth control pills or Accutane

FOLLOWUP

PATIENT MONITORING Revisits monthly, or more often if needed

PREVENTION/AVOIDANCE N/A

POSSIBLE COMPLICATIONS
• Lymphedema
• Contracture formation at the sites of lesions
• Squamous cell carcinoma my develop in indolent sinus tracts
• Disseminated infection - unusual
• Restricted limb mobility
• Urethral/rectal fistula
• Anemia
• Arthritis
• Amyloidosis
• Renal Failure
• Interstitial Keratitis

EXPECTED COURSE AND PROGNOSIS
• Individual lesions (with or without drainage) heal slowly in 10-30 days
• Recurrences may last for several years
• Rare spontaneous resolution
• Relentlessly progressive

MISCELLANEOUS

ASSOCIATED CONDITIONS
• Acne
• Perifolliculitis capitis (dissecting cellulitis of scalp)
• Obesity with associated diabetes mellitus, atopy, acanthosis nigrans

AGE-RELATED FACTORS
Pediatric: Rarely occurs before puberty (1 case reported in a 2 year old)
Geriatric: Rare after menopause
Others: Common late puberty through age 40

PREGNANCY No Accutane treatment during pregnancy

SYNONYMS N/A

ICD-9-CM 705.83 Hidradenitis

SEE ALSO N/A

OTHER NOTES
• Some patients develop only two or three papules per year. Others develop new lesions and drain as rapidly as old ones resolve.
• Although 50% of patients receiving Accutane, in doses similar to those for acne, obtain appreciable improvement, relapse occurs quickly upon discontinuing

ABBREVIATIONS N/A

REFERENCES
• Moschella, S.L. & Hurley, H.J.: Dermatology, 2nd Ed. Philadelphia, W.B. Saunders, 1985
• Lynch, P.J.: Dermatology for the House Officer. Baltimore, Williams & Wilkins, 1987
• Bell, B.A. & Ellis, H.: Hydradenitis Suppurativa. Journal of the Royal Society of Medicine. Vol. 71, pg. 511-515, 1978
• Sauer, G.C.: Manual of Skin Diseases. 6th Ed. Philadelphia, J.B. Lippincott, 1991
• Orkin M. (ed.): Dermatology. Lange, 1991

Author P. Jaster, M.D.

Histoplasmosis

BASICS

DESCRIPTION Fungal infection with Histoplasma capsulatum, a dimorphic soil-dwelling saprophyte that has multiple clinical manifestations. Initial infection in the normal host is often asymptomatic. Other manifestations include a self-limiting flu-like syndrome, mediastinal fibrosis, scar tissue residual, chronic cavitary disease in individuals with obstructive lung disease and disseminated histoplasmosis in the immunocompromised host and infants.
• H. capsulatum has worldwide distribution; the most endemic region in North America is the central United States. The fungus exists in mycelial form in nature and in yeast phase when exposed to mammalian temperatures. Spores may remain active for up to ten years. Exposure to bird or bat excrement promotes growth of the fungus for unexplained reasons.
• Chronic pulmonary histoplasmosis - usually occurs in white males with obstructive lung disease and apical bullous lung pathology. These patients exhibit evidence of an indolent infectious process.
• Disseminated histoplasmosis infection in the immunocompromised is a rare opportunistic infection which may mimic sepsis syndrome and progress to multiple organ system failure

System(s) affected: Pulmonary, Gastrointestinal

Genetics: There is no known genetic predisposition or inheritance

Incidence/Prevalence in USA:
• Infection in endemic areas is virtually 100%; few patients develop active disease. There are approximately 500,000 new infections in the United States per year.
• Occurrence in AIDS patients is 2%-5%
• Disseminated histoplasmosis occurs in < 0.05% of infections, one-third of these are infants < 1 year old, in adults there is an increased prevalence with age > 60 years

Predominant age:
• None in acute histoplasmosis
• Infants < 1 year old are at higher risk for disseminated histoplasmosis

Predominant sex:
• Acute histoplasmosis - Male = Female
• Disseminated histoplasmosis -
Male > Female (5:1-10:1)

SIGNS AND SYMPTOMS
• Primary infection in the normal host is usually asymptomatic
• Exposure to a heavy inoculum of spores is likely to produce a flu-like syndrome: Headache, fever, chills, nonproductive cough, myalgias and arthralgias

CAUSES Dimorphic fungus Histoplasma capsulatum

RISK FACTORS
• Spelunking
• Cleaning chicken coops
• Excavation near bird roosts
• Demolition or remodeling of old buildings
• Exposure to decayed wood or dead trees
• Performing routine activities in areas with high accumulation of bird droppings
• Immunosuppression

DIAGNOSIS

DIFFERENTIAL DIAGNOSIS
• Atypical pneumonia and viral pneumonitis
• Other fungal diseases such as blastomycosis, coccidioidomycosis
• Other granulomatous diseases such as M. tuberculosis and sarcoidosis
• Pneumoconiosis
• Lymphoma
• Malignancies associated with hilar lymphadenopathy

LABORATORY
• Complement fixation antibodies at titers 1:8 or 1:16 are presumptive for diagnosis, > 1:32 is strongly supportive as is an acute 4-fold titer rise. Determining the presence of H and M bands may be helpful.
• For chronic histoplasmosis and disseminated disease, cultures of sputum, bronchoalveolar lavage, bone marrow, lymph nodes, blood, liver and cerebrospinal fluid may be positive. Demonstration of characteristic organisms by silver stain on biopsy and bronchoalveolar lavage and bronchial washing specimens is diagnostic.

Drugs that may alter lab results: None known

Disorders that may alter lab results:
• Serologic tests may be falsely negative early in infection or in the immunocompromised patient
• False positive results may occur with tuberculosis and other fungal diseases
• Slow clearance of antibodies may identify patients with past Histoplasmosis infection who now present with a different disease
• False positive complement fixation titers may occur after histoplasmin skin antigen testing

PATHOLOGICAL FINDINGS Poorly formed caseating granulomas on biopsy or bronchoscopy specimens with identification of characteristic yeast forms by methenamine silver stain

SPECIAL TESTS
• Determine the presence of urinary H. capsulatum antigen
• Bronchoscopy
• Liver and bone marrow biopsies

IMAGING
• Routine chest roentgenogram which may reveal calcified hilar adenopathy
• If indicated, computerized axial tomogram of the chest to differentiate mediastinal fibrosis from mediastinal granuloma

DIAGNOSTIC PROCEDURES
• Serologic blood work
• Bronchoscopy with bronchoalveolar lavage and transbronchial biopsy
• Liver and bone marrow biopsies for suspected disseminated disease
• Mediastinoscopy for lymph node biopsy

TREATMENT

APPROPRIATE HEALTH CARE
• Acute primary and chronic cavitary histoplasmosis are treated outpatient
• Disseminated histoplasmosis requires hospitalization for initial treatment

GENERAL MEASURES 99% patients with acute primary histoplasmosis resolve spontaneously and require only symptomatic treatment

ACTIVITY Avoid potential high risk exposures which may lead to reinfection

DIET No restrictions

PATIENT EDUCATION Reinforce need for extended treatment in chronic cavitary histoplasmosis and the need for maintenance therapy in patients with AIDS

MEDICATIONS

DRUG(S) OF CHOICE
Disseminated histoplasmosis
◊ Amphotericin B - test dose is 1 mg followed by 0.25 mg/kg/dose, which may be slowly increased to 0.5 mg/kg/dose. Cumulative dose to 1-2 gm.
◊ Ketoconazole, 400 mg daily, has been used in selected cases with good results
AIDS patients
◊ The infection is rarely eradicated by treatment, therefore therapy should involve amphotericin B 1.0-1.5 g over 6-8 weeks
◊ Maintenance therapy with ketoconazole 400 mg daily or amphotericin B 50-100 mg weekly
Chronic cavitary histoplasmosis
◊ Amphotericin B 2.0-2.5 grams cumulative, or
◊ Ketoconazole 400 mg daily for 6-12 months
Mediastinal granuloma
◊ Can mimic fibrosing mediastinitis, may respond to treatment with amphotericin B
Fibrosing mediastinitis
◊ Has no active infection present and is not treatable
Contraindications: No contraindications to treatment in patients with progressive cavitary disease or disseminated histoplasmosis. The latter has a mortality rate of 80% if untreated.
Precautions:
Amphotericin B
◊ Dosage probably does not need to be adjusted for creatinine clearance
◊ It is nephrotoxic. Renal function must be monitored closely. Monitor electrolytes, especially potassium and magnesium.
◊ Rigors can be prevented by pre-infusion meperidine. Fever and chills can be diminished by pre-infusion dose of acetaminophen plus diphenhydramine.
Ketoconazole
◊ Is associated with gastrointestinal upset
◊ May inhibit testosterone synthesis and should be used with caution in patients with underlying hepatic dysfunction
Significant possible interactions:
• Expected benefits outweigh possible risks.
Ketoconazole
◊ Requires an acid environment for dissolution. If the patient requires antacid or H2 blockade, administer at least 2 hours after dose of ketoconazole
◊ Co-administration of terfenadine may cause cardiac arrhythmias
◊ May increase cyclosporine levels

ALTERNATIVE DRUGS Fluconazole has shown in vitro activity against H. capsulatum and may be an alternate therapy in selected cases

FOLLOWUP

PATIENT MONITORING
Patients receiving chronic therapy should have renal function and liver chemistries evaluated every 1-2 months. Chest roentgenograms should be obtained to evaluate response to therapy at regular intervals.

PREVENTION/AVOIDANCE
Maintenance therapy is required in AIDS patients

POSSIBLE COMPLICATIONS
• Bronchial, tracheal and virgult or esophageal obstruction secondary to adenopathy, broncholithiasis
• Pulmonary, splenic and hepatic calcifications, rarely pericarditis, pleurisy or effusion
• Fibrosing mediastinitis can cause stenosis of vascular and bronchial structures within the mediastinum causing pulmonary hypertension, superior vena cava syndrome and bronchial obstruction
• Acute renal failure and hepatic dysfunction secondary to medications
• Amphotericin induced hypokalemia
• Relapse occurring in the immunocompromised or inadequately treated patient with disseminated histoplasmosis

EXPECTED COURSE AND PROGNOSIS
• Excellent for primary histoplasmosis with 99% resolving spontaneously
• The prognosis for chronic cavitary pulmonary histoplasmosis is determined by the loss of lung parenchyma and pulmonary function
• Treatment of disseminated disease in AIDS/non-AIDS cases does improve outcome with ketoconazole having > 80% success rate and amphotericin B being 60-100% successful. Despite maintenance therapy in AIDS patients, there is a 10% to 50% relapse rate.

MISCELLANEOUS

ASSOCIATED CONDITIONS
• Disseminated histoplasmosis is an opportunistic infection in the immunocompromised host
• HIV infection

AGE-RELATED FACTORS
Pediatric: 1/3 of cases of disseminated histoplasmosis occurs in infants < 1 year old
Geriatric: Increased incidence of disseminated histoplasmosis in males during 6th and 7th decades
Others: N/A

PREGNANCY No increased incidence

SYNONYMS N/A

ICD-9-CM 115.9

SEE ALSO N/A

OTHER NOTES N/A

ABBREVIATIONS N/A

REFERENCES
• Dismukes, W.E., Cloud, G., Bowles, C., et al.: Treatment of blastomycosis and histoplasmosis with ketoconazole. Ann Intern Med 1985;103:861-872
• Wheat, L.J., Slama, T.G., Eitzen, H.E., et al.: A Large Urban Outbreak of Histoplasmosis: Clinical Features. Ann Intern Med 1981;94:331-337
• Wheat, L.J., Kohler, R.B. & Tewari, R.P.: Diagnosis of Disseminated Histoplasmosis by Detection of Histoplasma capsulatum Antigen in Serum and Urine Specimens. In N Engl J Med 1986;314:83-88
• Wheat, L.J., Connolly-Stringfield, P.A., Baker, R.L., et al.: Disseminated Histoplasmosis in the Acquired Immune Deficiency Syndrome: Clinical Findings, Diagnosis and Treatment, and Review of the Literature. In Medicine 1990;69:361-374

Author M. Connolly, Jr., M.D. & R. Baughman, M.D.

HIV infection and AIDS

BASICS

DESCRIPTION The human immunodeficiency virus is a retrovirus which infects cells with CD4 receptors, most notably the CD4 lymphocytes (also called T-4 or T-helper cells). Infection causes cell death in these lymphocytes and therefore a decline in immune function. Secondary immunodeficiency caused by the human immunodeficiency results in opportunistic infections, malignancies, and neurologic lesions in individuals in whom there is no prior history of immunologic abnormality. These opportunistic infections define the acquired immunodeficiency syndrome (AIDS). As of 1/1/93 all HIV infected persons with <200 CD4 cells are categorized as AIDS.

Our understanding of HIV infection is still limited. Apart from opportunistic infections due to immune suppression, the HIV virus also appears to have direct effects on the central nervous system, the GI tract and other systems. Autoimmune phenomena also may contribute to the clinical spectrum in HIV infection.

Genetics: None
Incidence/Prevalence: Greater than 250,000 infected persons
Predominant age: Young adults - 25-44
Predominant sex: Male > Female

SIGNS AND SYMPTOMS
• Chronic infection with variable course (about 10 years from the time of infection for 50% of infected persons to develop AIDS)
CDC classification system:
◊ Acute infection: Mononucleosis-like syndrome with fever, rash, myalgia, and malaise (this is a self-limited syndrome occurring about 6-8 weeks postinfection, associated with the development of HIV antibody)
◊ Asymptomatic infection: Follows initial infection; variable duration
◊ Persistent generalized lymphadenopathy: Characteristics - lymph node enlargement 1 cm or greater in two or more extra-inguinal sites. Adenopathy persists longer than three months. No other illness to explain the adenopathy.
◊ Other diseases: A) Constitutional: Fever lasting more than one month, involuntary weight loss of more than ten percent baseline weight, persistent diarrhea, skin rash, severe chronic fatigue. B) Neurologic disease: Dementia, myelopathy or peripheral neuropathy not explained by other illness. C) Secondary infectious disease: 1) AIDS-defining opportunistic infections: Pneumocystis carinii pneumonia; chronic cryptosporidial diarrhea; cerebral toxoplasmosis; extra -intestinal Strongyloides; isosporiasis; esophageal. bronchial or pulmonary candidiasis; cryptococcosis; histoplasmosis; coccidioidomycosis, disseminated mycobacterial disease; cytomegalovirus disease; chronic mucocutaneous or disseminated herpes simplex; progressive multifocal

leukoencephalopathy. 2) Other specified infections: Oral hairy leukoplakia, multidermal zoster, nocardioses, tuberculosis (pulmonary), recurrent salmonella bacteremia, oral candidiasis. D) Secondary cancers: Kaposi's sarcoma, non-Hodgkin's lymphoma, and primary brain lymphoma.
◊ Other conditions: These represent clinical findings or diseases not classified above that may be attributed to HIV infection. They include idiopathic thrombocytopenic purpura, seborrheic dermatitis, chronic lymphoid interstitial pneumonitis, alopecia, and renal disease.

CAUSES Human immunodeficiency virus infection (HIV)

RISK FACTORS
• Sexual activity: Homosexual men are at greatest risk but all sexually active people are at some degree of risk, dependent on the risk factors of, and number of, sexual partners
• Intravenous drug use (sharing of contaminated needles)
• Blood transfusions or recipients of blood products: Highest risk from 1975 to March 1985 when HIV screening of blood was instituted. Transmission outside this time period is possible but less likely.
• Hemophiliacs who have received pooled plasma products are at high risk. (Neither gamma globulin nor Hepatitis B vaccine produced in the United States have been identified with HIV transmission.)
• Children of HIV-infected women: About 30% of the children of women with HIV infection during pregnancy will be infected. Breast feeding is a possible route of transmission and therefore not recommended for infected mothers.
• Health care workers: Greatest risk is inadvertent needle stick (risk estimate 1 in 250)

DIAGNOSIS

DIFFERENTIAL DIAGNOSIS (See CDC classification under signs and symptoms). Many illnesses mimic HIV infection. Screen any patient for HIV infection when there is prolonged illness without ready explanation.

LABORATORY
ELISA (enzyme-linked immunosorbent assay)
◊ Reported as reactive or non-reactive. Reactive tests should be repeated. Confirm repeatedly reactive tests by another type of test (most commonly the Western Blot).
◊ The sensitivity and specificity of the ELISA test is greater than 98% and may approach 100%
Western blot (WB)
◊ Test results are positive, negative, or indeterminate (indeterminate tests result from non-specific reactions of HIV-negative sera with some HIV proteins)
◊ Currently the CDC recommends reaction with two of the following three bands as criteria for positivity: P24; gp41, and gp 120/160. If the

WB is indeterminate, perform follow-up testing at three and six months.
Tests for HIV antigen (HIV p24 antigen) or HIV nucleic acids (the polymerase chain reaction)
◊ Are available but expensive and of limited usefulness at this time
Drugs that may alter lab results: None
Disorders that may alter lab results: None

SPECIAL TESTS As indicated by suspicion of opportunistic infection or HIV-associated condition.

IMAGING As indicated by suspicion of opportunistic infection or HIV-associated condition.

TREATMENT

APPROPRIATE HEALTH CARE
Primary care provider in an outpatient setting. Consultation with infectious disease or HIV specialist prior to onset of acute situations.

GENERAL MEASURES
The initial visit work-up:
◊ Past medical history including STD's and TB with dates and treatment
◊ Review of systems to include fever, chills, diarrhea, weight loss, fatigue, adenopathy, cough, shortness of breath, dyspnea on exertion, visual changes, headaches, neurologic changes, skin rash, oral sores, sinusitis, odynophagia
◊ Social history
◊ Complete physical examination, including PAP smear
◊ Immunization review (pneumococcal, influenza, and Td recommended in adults, only. OPV contraindicated in children [use IPV]).
◊ Studies: CBC with differential and platelets; SMAC; UA; FTA and RPR; CD4 absolute count and %lymphocytes CD4; hepatitis B sAg and sAb; chest x-ray; PPD with control Coccidioides titer if in, or from, endemic area.
• Patients with less than 500 CD4 cells have been shown to benefit from antiretroviral treatment with zidovudine and presumably from other antiretroviral agents
• Patients with less than 200 CD4 cells or with oral candidiasis or other signs of significant immune suppression should receive Pneumocystis carinii prophylaxis
• Patients with less than 100 CD4 cells should receive prophylaxis against Mycobacterium avium complex.

ACTIVITY Encourage regular exercise. Many community HIV groups have organized "wellness" activities.

DIET
• Encourage good nutrition
• Avoid raw eggs, unpasteurized milk and other potentially contaminated foods
• Many patients require vitamin supplementation

PATIENT EDUCATION
• Provide frank, complete, non-judgmental information on the routes of transmission (primarily sexual and needle sharing). Teach infected persons how to minimize risk to others.
• Pre-printed and additional information material is available from a wide variety of sources including: National AIDS Hotline - (800)342-2437 [Spanish (800)342-7432]
• National Institute of Health AIDS Clinical Trials Group (800)874-2572. Information on AIDS/HIV clinical trials.
• American Foundation for AIDS Research: (212)719-0033. Information on new treatments and research.

MEDICATIONS

DRUG(S) OF CHOICE
There are four anti-retroviral agents and considerable controversy surrounds the optimal usage of these drugs; consultation with knowledge experts is recommended.
• Didanosine
• Stavudine
• Zalcitabine
• Zidovudine
Contraindications: N/A
Precautions: Side effects - granulocytopenia and anemia (dose limiting toxicities), headaches, nausea and vomiting, muscle weakness, nail discoloration and fatigue. Early side effects may abate over first month.
Significant possible interactions: Refer to manufacturer's literature
• TMP/SMX may cause increased hematologic toxicity. Monitoring - CBC and SMAC should be checked at two and four weeks; then monthly for three months; then every three months.

ALTERNATIVE DRUGS
• Didanosine (ddl) - in failure or intolerance of zidovudine
• Zalcitabine - in combination with zidovudine

FOLLOWUP

PATIENT MONITORING
• Frequency determined largely by the patient's clinical and psychological status and by the need to monitor drug toxicity and immune function
• CD4 counts should be rechecked every 3 months
Check at subsequent visits:
  ◊ Complete, careful physical exam
  ◊ Complete review of systems especially focused on neurologic symptoms (CNS infection, malignancy, or dementia), visual changes (CMV retinitis), diarrhea, fever, night sweats, shortness of breath, dyspnea on exertion (early Pneumocystis carinii pneumonia), and odynophagia (esophageal candidiasis)

PREVENTION/AVOIDANCE
When possible: avoid unscreened blood products; avoid unprotected sexual intercourse; use condoms; avoid intravenous drug abuse; avoid contact with bodily fluids of HIV carriers

POSSIBLE COMPLICATIONS
• Immunodeficiency
• Opportunistic infections (see Associated Conditions)
• Kaposi's sarcoma
• AIDS meningoencephalitis
• Neuropsychiatric symptoms
• Thrombocytopenia

EXPECTED COURSE AND PROGNOSIS
• When HIV infection leads to AIDS, life expectancy is two to three years. AIDS defining opportunistic infections usually do not develop until CD4 counts are less than 200. In HIV infection, CD4 counts decline at a rate of 50 to 80 per year with more rapid decline as counts drop below 200.

MISCELLANEOUS

ASSOCIATED CONDITIONS
• AIDS-related complex, acalculous cholecystitis, Epstein-Barr virus, hepatitis B infection, hepatitis non-A non-B infection, plus those listed in Signs and Symptoms as AIDS defining opportunistic infections
• Syphilis: Much more aggressive in HIV-infected persons. The definitive treatment for syphilis in HIV infected persons is controversial at this time; consult with an STD specialist.
• Tuberculosis: TB is becoming co-epidemic with HIV. HIV infection changes the management of TB and thus all persons with TB should be tested for HIV, or if not tested, should be treated with three drugs as if HIV-infected

AGE-RELATED FACTORS
Pediatric: Progresses more rapidly in infants
Geriatric: Progresses more rapidly in those over 50
Others: N/A

PREGNANCY Consistent standards of care not yet evolved. There appears to be an increased risk of bacterial pneumonia during pregnancy and some increased risk of premature birth in HIV-infected women. Cause still not understood.

SYNONYMS
• Acquired immune deficiency syndrome

ICD-9-CM
042 Human immunodeficiency virus infection with specified conditions
042.0 With specified infections
042.1 Causing other specified infections
042.9 Acquired immunodeficiency syndrome, unspecified
043 Human immunodeficiency virus causing other specified conditions
043.0 Causing lymphadenopathy
043.1 Causing diseases of the central nervous system
043.2 Causing other disorders involving the immune mechanism
043.3 Causing other specified conditions
043.9 ARC, unspecified
044 Other HIV infection
044.0 Causing specified acute infections
044.9 HIV infection, unspecified

OTHER NOTES
• Increased risk of cervical cancer in HIV-infected women. Perform pap smears every 6 months or more often.
• Health care workers: Greatest risk is inadvertent needle stick (risk: 1 in 250).

SEE ALSO
• Pneumonia, pneumocystis carinii
• Kaposi's sarcoma
• Candidiasis
• Candidiasis, mucocutaneous
• Atypical mycobacterial infection
• Cytomegalovirus inclusion disease
• Tuberculosis
• Lymphoma

ABBREVIATIONS N/A

REFERENCES
• Cohen, P., Sande, M. & Volberding, P.: The AIDS Knowledge Base. Waltham, Massachusetts, The Medical Publishing Group, 1990
• Abrams, D., Grieco, M. & McMeeking, A.: AIDS/HIV Treatment Directory. New York, American Foundation for AIDS Research, (quarterly)

Author K. Carmichael, M.D.

Hodgkin's disease

BASICS

DESCRIPTION Malignant disease of the lymphoid tissue, caused by malignant transformation of an uncertain progenitor cell to the pathognomonic Reed-Sternberg cell. Disease spreads to the contiguous lymphoid tissue, and eventually to non-lymphoid tissue. The Rye classification is based on pathologic findings:
  ◊ Nodular sclerosis - most common
  ◊ Mixed cellularity - 2nd most common
  ◊ Lymphocyte depletion
  ◊ Lymphocyte predominance
Incidence/Prevalence: 3.5/100,000. Incidence 7,500/year in US.
System(s) affected:
Hemic/Lymphatic/Immunologic
Genetics: No known genetic pattern
Predominant age: Bimodal, with peaks at ages 20 and 70
Predominant sex: Male > Female

SIGNS AND SYMPTOMS
• Enlarged lymph nodes (painless)
• Fever (Pel-Ebstein fever)
• Night sweats
• Weight loss > 10%
• Fatigue
• Anorexia

CAUSES Unknown

RISK FACTORS
• Immunodeficiency (acquired and inherited)
• Autoimmune diseases

DIAGNOSIS

DIFFERENTIAL DIAGNOSIS
• Other lymphomas
• Infectious lymphadenopathy
• Other solid tumor metastases
• Sarcoidosis
• Autoimmune diseases
• AIDS
• Drug reaction

LABORATORY
• CBC with differential
• Chemistry profile
• ESR
• Liver function tests
• Renal function tests
Drugs that may alter lab results:
Phenytoin may produce pseudolymphoma
Disorders that may alter lab results: N/A

PATHOLOGICAL FINDINGS
• Reed-Sternberg cell (RS cell) - bilobed or multi-lobed with prominent inclusion nucleoli
• Diffuse infiltrate of lymphocytes with obliteration of lymph nodes
• Large round reticular cells

SPECIAL TESTS N/A

IMAGING
• Chest x-ray
• CT of chest, abdomen, and pelvis
• Role of MRI still evolving
• Lymphangiogram
• Gallium scan, bone scan (used infrequently)
• Abdomen ultrasound

DIAGNOSTIC PROCEDURES
• Lymph node biopsy - needle aspiration not sufficient
• Exploratory laparotomy with splenectomy in individual cases
• Bone marrow biopsy - especially if stage B
• Liver biopsy in individual cases

TREATMENT

APPROPRIATE HEALTH CARE
• Inpatient or outpatient for staging
Initial staging is critical to therapy
  ◊ Stage I - single node group
  ◊ Stage II - two or more node groups on same side of diaphragm
  ◊ Stage III - node groups on both sides of diaphragm
  ◊ Stage IV - dissemination involving extra-lymphatic organs (not the spleen which is considered lymphoid tissue)
  ◊ Subclassified "A" - asymptomatic disease in any stage
  ◊ Subclassified "B" - symptomatic disease in any stage with: 10% weight loss, night sweats, or fever not otherwise explained
  ◊ Subclassified "X" - bulky disease (widening of mediastinum by more than one-third or > 10 cm nodal mass)

GENERAL MEASURES
• Treatment is aimed for cure with minimum toxicity
• Treatment can be radiation alone, chemotherapy alone, or combination therapy based on staging and tumor burden
• Stages I and II - typically radiation therapy alone, unless bulky disease
• Stage III A - mainly with radiation therapy
• Stage III B , and IV - chemotherapy, and also radiation if bulky disease
• Autologous bone marrow transplant for patients who fail chemotherapy

ACTIVITY As tolerated

DIET No restrictions

PATIENT EDUCATION
• Discuss gonadal side effects of therapy, and consider sperm banking for males
• Risks of secondary malignancy
• For patient education materials on this topic, contact: Leukemia Society of America, 733 3rd Avenue, New York, NY 10017, (212)573-8484

MEDICATIONS

DRUG(S) OF CHOICE
• Note: Must be monitored by experienced oncologist
MOPP chemotherapy - 4 week cycles
◊ Mechlorethamine (nitrogen mustard) 6.0 mg/m2 IV on days 1 and 8
◊ Vincristine (Oncovin) 1.4 mg/m2 IV on days 1 and 8
◊ Procarbazine 100 mg/m2 po on days 1 through 14 (avoid vanilla, cheese and wine when taking procarbazine)
◊ Prednisone 40 mg/m2 po on days 1 through 14. Use in cycles 1 and 4.
ABVD chemotherapy - 4 week cycles
◊ Doxorubicin (Adriamycin) 25 mg/m2 IV days 1 and 15
◊ Bleomycin 10 mg/m2 IV days 1 and 15
◊ Vinblastine 6.0 mg/m2 IV days 1 and 15
◊ Dacarbazine 375 mg/m2 IV days 1 and 15
• Note: Recently people have advocated alternating cycles with MOPP/ABVD to minimize toxicity. Repeat cycles at least 6 times if blood counts permit.
Contraindications: As in general for chemotherapy
Precautions: Chemotherapy toxicity, bone marrow suppression
Significant possible Interactions: Refer to manufacturer's literature

ALTERNATIVE DRUGS N/A

FOLLOWUP

PATIENT MONITORING CBC, hydration status

PREVENTION/AVOIDANCE
• Pneumovax if splenectomy is planned for staging

POSSIBLE COMPLICATIONS
• After chemotherapy and radiation therapy, may develop secondary malignancies
• Sterility, and gonadal dysfunction
• Hypothyroidism
• Bone marrow suppression
• Immunosuppressed infections
• Anemia
• Idiopathic thrombocytopenic purpura and thrombotic thrombocytopenic purpura
• Coronary artery disease
• Pulmonary fibrosis

EXPECTED COURSE AND PROGNOSIS
• 75% overall survival
• Stage I - 90% 5 year
• Stage II - 90% 5 year
• Stage III - 75% 10 year
• Stage IV - 66% 10 year
• Symptomatic (class B) - prognosis worse
• Asymptomatic (class A) - prognosis better

MISCELLANEOUS

ASSOCIATED CONDITIONS T-cell infections

AGE-RELATED FACTORS
Pediatric: Increased risk for males
Geriatric: N/A
Others: Increased incidence of nodular-sclerosis pathologic classification in younger groups

PREGNANCY Following treatment, if fertility is maintained, pregnancy can be normal

SYNONYMS Malignant lymphoma

ICD-9-CM
201.9x Hodgkin's disease, unspecified
201.7x Hodgkin's disease, lymphocyte depletion
201.6x Hodgkin's disease, mixed cellularity
201.5x Hodgkin's disease, nodular sclerosis
201.4x Hodgkin's disease, lymphocyte predominance
Fifth digit:
0 - Unspecified site
1 - Head, face, neck nodes
2 - Intra-thoracic nodes
3 - Intra-abdominal nodes
4 - Axillary and arm nodes
5 - Inguinal and leg nodes
6 - Pelvic nodes
7 - Spleen involved
8 - Multiple site nodes

SEE ALSO N/A

OTHER NOTES N/A

ABBREVIATIONS N/A

REFERENCES Urba, W.J. & Longo, D.L.: Review in N Engl J Med 326(10), p678-87, Mar 92

Author R. Ram, M.D.

Hordeolum (Stye)

 BASICS

DESCRIPTION The common term "stye" refers to any inflammation or infection of the eyelid margin involving the hair follicles of the eyelashes (external hordeolum), meibomian glands (internal hordeolum), or granulomatous infection of the meibomian glands (chalazion)
System(s) affected: Skin/Exocrine
Genetics: No known genetic pattern
Incidence/Prevalence in USA: Extremely common
Predominant age: None
Predominant sex: Male = Female

SIGNS AND SYMPTOMS
• Redness of the margin of the eyelid with scaling, collection of discharge
• Localized inflammation of the eyelashes
• Patients may experience itching or scaling of the eyelids, chronic redness, eye irritation leading to localized tenderness and pain

CAUSES
• The most common causes of eyelid infections are staphylococcal, although other organisms may also be involved
• Seborrhea can predispose to infections of the eyelid

RISK FACTORS
• Predisposing blepharitis (low grade infections of the eyelid margin)
• Poor eyelid hygiene
• Contact lens wearers
• Application of make-up

 DIAGNOSIS

DIFFERENTIAL DIAGNOSIS
• Blepharitis
• Eyelid neoplasms

LABORATORY Culture of the eyelid margins is usually not necessary
Drugs that may alter lab results: None
Disorders that may alter lab results: None

PATHOLOGICAL FINDINGS Bacterial contamination and white cells in eyelid discharge

SPECIAL TESTS None

IMAGING None

DIAGNOSTIC PROCEDURES History and eye examination

 TREATMENT

APPROPRIATE HEALTH CARE
Outpatient

GENERAL MEASURES
• Warm compresses to the area of inflammation can help increase blood supply and potentiate spontaneous drainage
• Good personal hygiene with attention to cleansing the eyelids on a daily basis to prevent recurrent infections
• Application of an antibiotic ointment (such as erythromycin) to the margin of the eyelid after proper cleansing. (Except children under 12, where there is a risk of blurred vision and amblyopia.) Helps reduce bacterial proliferation.
• If the infection becomes localized to a single gland, incision, drainage, and curettage is sometimes necessary. This is an in-office procedure with a local anesthetic.

ACTIVITY No restrictions

DIET No special diet

PATIENT EDUCATION
• The patient should be instructed in proper cleansing of the eyelids using a solution of tap water and baby shampoo or a commercially prepared hypoallergenic cleanser
• The stye should not be squeezed

MEDICATIONS

DRUG(S) OF CHOICE
• Erythromycin ophthalmic ointment
• Occasionally use of an aminoglycoside ophthalmic ointment such as gentamicin may be necessary if refractory to simpler treatment
Contraindications: None
Precautions: None
Significant possible interactions: None

ALTERNATIVE DRUGS None

 FOLLOWUP

PATIENT MONITORING The patient should be seen within several weeks to assess the effectiveness of therapy

PREVENTION/AVOIDANCE Eyelid hygiene

POSSIBLE COMPLICATIONS None expected. An internal hordeolum, if untreated, may lead to generalized cellulitis of the lid.

EXPECTED COURSE AND PROGNOSIS Responds well to treatment, but tends to recur in some patients

 MISCELLANEOUS

ASSOCIATED CONDITIONS
• Acne
• Seborrhea

AGE-RELATED FACTORS
Pediatric: N/A
Geriatric: N/A
Others: N/A

PREGNANCY N/A

SYNONYMS
• Internal hordeolum
• External hordeolum
• Chalazion hordeolum
• Zeisian sty
• Meibomian sty

ICD-9-CM
• Hordeolum 373.1
• Chalazion 373.2
• Blepharitis 373.0

SEE ALSO N/A

OTHER NOTES N/A

ABBREVIATIONS N/A

REFERENCES None

Author R. Kershner, M.D., F.A.C.S.

Horner's syndrome

 BASICS

DESCRIPTION
Horner's syndrome is caused by interruptions of the sympathetic nerve supply to the eye and results in miosis, ptosis, and absence of sweating of the ipsilateral face and neck
 • Peripheral lesion - distal to superior cervical ganglion
 • Central lesion - proximal to superior cervical ganglion
Genetics: Some autosomal dominant familial incidence
System(s) affected: Nervous, Skin/Exocrine
Incidence/Prevalence in USA: Unknown
Predominant age: May occur at any age
Predominant sex: Male = Female

SIGNS AND SYMPTOMS
 • Ptosis (drooping of the eyelid)
 • Miosis (narrowing of the pupil of the eye)
 • Anhidrosis
 • Enophthalmos is sometimes found
 • Iris (in congenital Horner's) - pigmentation, blue-gray, mottled

CAUSES
 • Interruption of the sympathetic nerve fibres that originate in the hypothalamus and travel down to the lateral part of the brain stem to exit in the thoracic area. These fibers synapse in the cervical sympathetic ganglia and the postganglionic fibers travel to the eye along the wall of the carotid and ophthalmic arteries.
 • Idiopathic

RISK FACTORS
 • Apical bronchogenic carcinoma
 • Aneurysm of the carotid or subclavian artery
 • Injuries to the carotid artery high in the neck
 • Congenital Horner's syndrome
 • Dissection of the aorta
 • Cluster headaches, approximately 20% which have an accompanying homolateral Horner's syndrome. The syndrome may outlast the headaches.
 • Carotid artery occlusion, approximately 15% of patients with carotid artery occlusion develop ipsilateral Horner's syndrome - may occur without evidence of cerebral ischemia, neck injuries or operative procedures
 • Syringomyelia
 • Inflammatory process

 DIAGNOSIS

DIFFERENTIAL DIAGNOSIS
Neurological diseases

LABORATORY   N/A
Drugs that may alter lab results: N/A
Disorders that may alter lab results: N/A

PATHOLOGICAL FINDINGS
 • Brainstem lesion
 • Massive hemisphere lesion
 • Cervical cord lesion
 • Root lesion
 • Sympathetic chain lesion

SPECIAL TESTS
 • Instillation of 4% solution of cocaine into conjunctival sac produces dilatation of the pupil in Horner's syndrome caused by a central sympathetic pathways lesion. (Response is absent in peripheral sympathetic lesion.)
 • Instillation of 1:1000 solution of epinephrine into conjunctival sac produces dilatation of the pupil in Horner's syndrome caused by a peripheral sympathetic lesion

IMAGING   CT/MRI of the brain, chest, spinal cord

DIAGNOSTIC PROCEDURES
 • Spinal tap - occasionally indicated in addition to above.

 TREATMENT

APPROPRIATE HEALTH CARE
Inpatient or outpatient, depending upon cause

GENERAL MEASURES
 • Search for tumor or other compressive lesion is indicated for any patient who develops Horner's syndrome
 • Horner's syndrome in itself does not produce any disability or require treatment
 • Treatment is management of the underlying condition

ACTIVITY   Disease dependent

DIET   Disease dependent

PATIENT EDUCATION   N/A

MEDICATIONS

DRUG(S) OF CHOICE Therapy appropriate for the underlying disease
Contraindications: N/A
Precautions: N/A
Significant possible interactions: N/A

ALTERNATIVE DRUGS N/A

FOLLOWUP

PATIENT MONITORING Disease dependent

PREVENTION/AVOIDANCE None known

EXPECTED COURSE AND PROGNOSIS Variable with cause

POSSIBLE COMPLICATIONS Chronic pupillary constriction

MISCELLANEOUS

ASSOCIATED CONDITIONS
• Wallenberg's syndrome
• Pancoast's tumor

AGE-RELATED FACTORS
Pediatric: N/A
Geriatric: N/A
Others: N/A

PREGNANCY N/A

SYNONYMS
• Bernard-Horner syndrome
• Bernard's syndrome
• Cervical sympathetic syndrome
• Oculosympathetic syndrome

ICD-9-CM 337.9 Horner's syndrome

SEE ALSO N/A

OTHER NOTES N/A

ABBREVIATIONS N/A

REFERENCES Pryce-Phillips, W. & Murray, T.J.: Essential Neurology. New York, Scientific American Medicine, 1991

Author S. Smith

Huntington's chorea

BASICS

DESCRIPTION An inherited disease characterized by dementia and chorea that has a gradual onset and slow progression. Symptoms usually don't develop until after 30 years of age. By the time of diagnosis the patient has usually reproduced and passed the disease to another generation.
System(s) affected: Nervous
Genetics: Autosomal dominant; genetic marker on chromosome 4
Incidence/Prevalence in USA: 4-8 cases/100,000 people in the U.S.
Predominant age: Young adult (16-40); middle age (40-75)
Predominant sex: Male = Female

SIGNS AND SYMPTOMS
• Chorea
• Dysphagia
• Dysarthria
• Impaired recent memory
• Impaired judgment
• Intellectual decline
• Emotional disturbances
• Depression
• Anxiety
• Delusions
• Aggressiveness
• Urinary incontinence
• Bowel incontinence
• Weight loss
• Hypotonia
• Gait disturbance
• Postural instability
• Hyperkinesia
• Abnormal eye movements
• Facial twitching
• Emotional lability
• Apathy
• Withdrawal
• Dementia
• Bradykinesia
• Rigidity
• Hypertonia
• Clonus
• Mania
• Hallucinations
• Delusions
• Paranoia
• Schizophrenia
• Impulsiveness
• Hostility
• Agitation
• Primitive reflexes

CAUSES Hereditary genetic defect on short arm of chromosome number 4

RISK FACTORS Family history

DIAGNOSIS

DIFFERENTIAL DIAGNOSIS
• Other causes of dementia
• Other causes of dyskinesia, including drug induced

LABORATORY
• Decreased endogenous gamma-aminobutyric acid (GABA)
• Decreased glutamic acid decarboxylase
• Decreased choline-acetyltransferase
Drugs that may alter lab results: N/A
Disorders that may alter lab results: N/A

PATHOLOGICAL FINDINGS
• Gross - cerebral atrophy
• Gross - atrophic caudate nucleus
• Gross - atrophic putamen
• Gross - ventricular enlargement
• Gross - atrophic globus pallidus
• Gross - atrophic frontal lobes
• Gross - atrophic parietal lobes
• Gross - cortical atrophy
• Micro - loss of small neurons of striatum with fibrillary gliosis
• Micro - loss of small neurons with fibrillary gliosis in ventrolateral thalamic nucleus
• Micro - loss of small neurons with fibrillary gliosis in substantia nigra
• Electron microscopy - membranous whorls
• Electron microscopy - increased numbers of dense synaptic vesicles in presynaptic nerve terminals

SPECIAL TESTS N/A

IMAGING
• CT or MRI - cerebral atrophy and atrophy of caudate nucleus
• Positron emission tomography (PET) - reduced glucose utilization
• Head CT - enlarged lateral ventricle

DIAGNOSTIC PROCEDURES N/A

TREATMENT

APPROPRIATE HEALTH CARE
Outpatient

GENERAL MEASURES
• Genetic counseling
• Symptomatic treatment (dopamine receptor blocking drugs), such as phenothiazines or haloperidol

ACTIVITY Full activity as long as possible

DIET No special diet, but mechanical soft with liquid supplements may be needed.

PATIENT EDUCATION Counseling for offspring

MEDICATIONS

DRUG(S) OF CHOICE For dyskinesia and/or behavioral problems: Haloperidol (Haldol) 1 mg bid and increased every 3 or 4 days until satisfactory response
Contraindications: Refer to manufacturer's literature
Precautions: Extrapyramidal reactions, tardive dyskinesia may occur. Can be treated with anticholinergic medication.
Significant possible interactions: Do not administer with meperidine due to possibility of serotonin syndrome.

ALTERNATIVE DRUGS
- Presynaptic dopamine - depleting agents
- Reserpine
- Tetrabenazine
- Postsynaptic dopamine antagonists
- Tricyclic antidepressants
- Antipsychotics

FOLLOWUP

PATIENT MONITORING Periodically for behavioral changes

PREVENTION/AVOIDANCE Genetic counseling

POSSIBLE COMPLICATIONS
- Choking
- Subdural hematoma
- Chorea
- Personality changes
- Dementia
- Death

EXPECTED COURSE AND PROGNOSIS Poor, progressive impairment, fatal outcome within 20 years

MISCELLANEOUS

ASSOCIATED CONDITIONS N/A

AGE-RELATED FACTORS
Pediatric: Usually does not occur until after puberty
Geriatric: Usually fatal before geriatric age group
Others: N/A

PREGNANCY N/A

SYNONYMS Chronic progressive hereditary chorea

ICD-9-CM 333.4

SEE ALSO N/A

OTHER NOTES N/A

ABBREVIATIONS N/A

REFERENCES
- Rowland, L.: Merritt's Textbook of Neurology. 8th Ed. Philadelphia, Lea & Febiger, 1989
- Meissen, G.J., et al.: Predictive Testing for Huntington's Disease With Use of a Linked DNA Marker. N Engl J Med. 1988;318:535

Author R. Viken

Hydrocele

 BASICS

DESCRIPTION
Hydrocele is a collection of fluid within the scrotum.
- Communicating hydrocele: Associated with a patent processus vaginalis, has associated indirect inguinal hernia
- Non-communicating hydrocele: Infantile type - no communication, frequent spontaneous resolution. Adult type - no communication, infrequent resolution.
- Hydrocele of the cord: Distal portion of processus vaginalis has closed, mid-portion patent and fluid filled, proximal portion may be open or closed
- Acute hydrocele: Acute fluid collection resulting from an acute process within the tunica vaginalis

System(s) affected: Reproductive
Genetics: Unknown
Incidence in USA: Not known but estimated to be 1% of adult males
Prevalence in USA: 1000/100,000
Predominant age: Childhood
Predominant sex: Male only

SIGNS AND SYMPTOMS
- Swelling in scrotum or inguinal canal
- Demonstrated fluctuation in size (communicating hydrocele)
- Usually not painful
- Sensation of heaviness in scrotum
- Pain radiating to back (occasionally)
- Fluid collection in scrotum that transilluminates

CAUSES
- Closure of processus vaginalis trapping peritoneal fluid (non-communicating)
- Closure of distal processus, trapping fluid in mid portion of processus vaginalis (hydrocele of cord)
- Failure of closure of processus vaginalis (communicating hydrocele)
- Infection
- Tumors
- Trauma
- Ipsilateral renal transplantation

RISK FACTORS
- Ventriculoperitoneal shunt
- Exstrophy of the bladder
- Ehlers-Danlos syndrome
- Peritoneal dialysis

 DIAGNOSIS

DIFFERENTIAL DIAGNOSIS
- Indirect inguinal hernia
- Orchitis
- Epididymitis
- Traumatic injury to testicle
- Torsion of testicle or torsion of appendix testes

LABORATORY N/A
Drugs that may alter lab results: N/A
Disorders that may alter lab results: N/A

PATHOLOGICAL FINDINGS Patent processus vaginalis in communicating hydroceles

SPECIAL TESTS N/A

IMAGING
- Abdominal x-ray - may be useful to distinguish incarcerated hernias from hydrocele (rarely needed)
- Inguino-scrotal ultrasound - should be able to distinguish presence or absence of bowel
- Testicular nuclear scan - to distinguish testicular torsion

DIAGNOSTIC PROCEDURES N/A

 TREATMENT

APPROPRIATE HEALTH CARE
- Outpatient surgery
- Observation in early infancy until definite communication demonstrated or until 1-2 years of age

GENERAL MEASURES
- Inguinal approach with ligation of processus vaginalis and drainage of hydrocele sac in children. (In hydrocele of cord, sac can be completely removed).
- Scrotal approach with drainage of hydrocele and resection of tunica vaginalis in adults
- In adults no therapy is needed unless hydrocele causes discomfort or unless there is a significant underlying cause such as tumor
- Jaboulay-Winkelmann procedure (for thick hydrocele sac) - hydrocele sac wrapped posteriorly around cord structures
- Lord procedure (for thin hydrocele sac) - radial sutures used to gather hydrocele sac posterior to testis and epididymis
- Aspiration of hydrocele should not be done (with possible exception of postoperative hydrocele)

ACTIVITY Full activity after surgery

DIET for age

PATIENT EDUCATION N/A

MEDICATIONS

DRUG(S) OF CHOICE N/A
Contraindications: N/A
Precautions: N/A
Significant possible interactions: N/A

ALTERNATIVE DRUGS N/A

FOLLOWUP

PATIENT MONITORING
• Follow at 3 month intervals until decision for/against surgery made
• Postoperative, follow up at 2-4 weeks and then at 2-3 month intervals until resolution of any post-operative (traumatic) hydrocele

PREVENTION/AVOIDANCE N/A

POSSIBLE COMPLICATIONS
• Post-operative traumatic hydrocele common. Usually resolves spontaneously.
• Injury to vas deferens or spermatic vessels
• Suture granuloma
• Hematoma
• Wound infection

EXPECTED COURSE AND PROGNOSIS Recovery should be rapid and complete

MISCELLANEOUS

ASSOCIATED CONDITIONS
• Ehlers-Danlos syndrome
• Exstrophy of bladder
• Indirect inguinal hernia
• Hydrocephalus with ventriculo-peritoneal shunt
• Peritoneal dialysis

AGE-RELATED FACTORS
Pediatric: In communicating hydrocele consider contralateral inguinal exploration
Geriatric: N/A
Others: N/A

PREGNANCY N/A

SYNONYMS N/A

ICD-9-CM 603.9

SEE ALSO N/A

OTHER NOTES N/A

ABBREVIATIONS N/A

REFERENCES
• Gillenwater, J.Y., Grayhach, J.T., Howards, S.S., Duckett, J.W.: Adult & Pediatric Urology. 2nd Ed. Philadelphia, Marby Year Book, 1991
• Holder, T.M. & Ashcraft, K.W.: Pediatric Surgery. 2nd Ed. Philadelphia, W.B. Saunders Co., 1993
• Kelalis, P.P., King, L.R. & Belman, A.B.: Pediatric Urology. 2nd Ed. Philadelphia, W.B. Saunders Co., 1985
• Resnick, M.I. & Kursh, E.D.: Current Therapy in Genito-Urinary Surgery. 2nd Ed. St. Louis, Mosby-Year Book, 1992

Author T. Black, M.D. & J. Miller, M.D.

Hydronephrosis

BASICS

DESCRIPTION
Unilateral or bilateral dilatation of the urinary tract at any level secondary to intrinsic and/or extrinsic obstruction to urine flow. May also be functional.

System(s) affected: Renal/Urologic

Genetics: Unknown

Incidence/Prevalence in USA:
- Children 2 in 100
- Adults 3.8 in 100

Predominant age: All ages. Bimodal peaks: congenital and over age 60.

Predominant sex:
- Age 0 - 20 years: Male = Female
- Age 20 to 60 years: Female > Male
- Age greater than 60 years: Male > Female

SIGNS AND SYMPTOMS
- Varies with acute or chronic presentation
- Chronic hydronephrosis may be completely asymptomatic
- "Colic" referred to vulva or to testicle (lithiasis) with acute obstruction
- Change in urine output (anuria, polyuria, intermittent variation in urine volume)
- Hesitancy
- Dribbling
- Urinary tract infections
- Decreased force of urine
- Nocturia
- Abdominal mass
- Frequency and urgency
- Thirst
- Hypertension (may be accelerated)
- Edema
- After relief - post obstructive diuresis
- Abdominal mass
- Epididymitis

CAUSES
Intrinsic, congenital
  ◊ Stenosis (ureteral or urethral)
  ◊ Adynamic ureter
  ◊ Spinal cord defects
Intrinsic, acquired◊
  ◊ Renal lithiasis
  ◊ Neoplasm (renal, ureteral or bladder)
  ◊ Papillary necrosis with sloughed papilla
  ◊ Ureterocele
  ◊ Trauma
  ◊ Blood clot
  ◊ Fungus ball
  ◊ Granuloma (tuberculosis)
  ◊ Neurogenic bladder
  ◊ Other nervous system diseases - tabes dorsalis, multiple sclerosis, diabetes mellitus, traumatic spinal cord injury
  ◊ Anticholinergics
  ◊ Phimosis
  ◊ Ureteral valve
  ◊ Polyp or stricture
  ◊ Schistosomiasis (hematobium)
Extrinsic
  ◊ Retroperitoneal-neoplasm, blood, abscess, fibrosis, aneurysm
  ◊ Crohn's disease
  ◊ Lymphocele, hydrocele

  ◊ Gynecologic - Gravid uterus, endometriosis, pelvic inflammatory disease, abscess, cyst, iatrogenic-ureteral injury during surgery, gynecologic malignancy, uterine prolapse
  ◊ Sjogrens syndrome (pseudolymphoma)
Functional or non-mechanical - congenital
  ◊ Mega-ureter
  ◊ Prune belly syndrome
  ◊ Extra renal pelvis
Functional or non-mechanical - other
  ◊ Diabetes insipidus
  ◊ Diuretics
  ◊ Pregnancy
  ◊ Vesico-ureteral reflux
  ◊ Post obstructive residual
  ◊ Post surgical: post ureteral anastomosis
  ◊ Progestational agents

RISK FACTORS
- Radiation
- Prostatic hypertrophy and/or malignancy
- Renal lithiasis
- Methysergide
- Analgesic abuse (papillary necrosis, transitional cell carcinoma)
- Sickle cell anemia (papillary necrosis)
- Diabetes mellitus (papillary necrosis)
- Bleeding diathesis
- Anticholinergics
- See causes

DIAGNOSIS

DIFFERENTIAL DIAGNOSIS See causes

LABORATORY
- May be completely normal
- Azotemia
- Hyperkalemia
- Metabolic acidosis (with and without anion gap)
- Hypernatremia (diabetes insipidus)
- Urine analysis - hematuria, crystals, bacteriuria
- Decreased urine concentrating ability
- Polycythemia (rare)
- Anemia of chronic renal disease

Drugs that may alter lab results:
Nephrotoxins may aggravate azotemia (nonsteroidal anti-inflammatory drugs, immunosuppressants, aminoglycosides, iodinated contrast, anticholinergics)

Disorders that may alter lab results: N/A

PATHOLOGICAL FINDINGS
- Thin renal cortex
- Renal tubular atrophy
- Medullary destruction
- See causes

SPECIAL TESTS
- Kidney and urinary bladder (KUB)
- Voiding cystourethrogram
- Measurement post void residual
- Ultrasound prostate with rectal transducer
- Prostatic specific antigen, acid phosphatase (malignancy)

IMAGING
- Ultrasound - abnormal renal function, cortical thinning, ureteral dilatation
- IVP with tomograms (normal renal function): Renal pelvis dilatation
- Renal flow scan, diuretic renogram
- CT scan
- MRI
- Pulsed and color Doppler

DIAGNOSTIC PROCEDURES
To determine location, etiology of hydronephrosis :
  ◊ Cystoscopy/retrograde pyelography
  ◊ Antegrade pyelography
  ◊ Loopography (obstruction with ureteral diversion)

TREATMENT

APPROPRIATE HEALTH CARE
Outpatient

GENERAL MEASURES
- Females: Pelvic pap smear for potential gynecologic malignancy. Appropriate work-up for recurrent urinary tract infections.
- Males: Anatomic study of the urinary tract for any urinary tract infection, appropriate review of systems and digital rectal exam for prostatic hypertrophy. Prostatic specific antigen, acid phosphatase, rectal transducer ultrasound of prostate for prostatic enlargement.
Relief of obstruction for preservation of renal function
  ◊ Foley catheter for prostatic hypertrophy
  ◊ Transurethral resection of the prostate gland for prostatic hypertrophy
  ◊ Nephrostomy tube
  ◊ Pyeloplasty
  ◊ Surgical diversion of ureters
  ◊ Ureteral stents
  ◊ Percutaneous nephrolithotomy (lithiasis)
  ◊ Basket capture (lithiasis)
  ◊ Lithotripsy (lithiasis with or without stent and percutaneous nephrolithotomy)
  ◊ Nephrectomy
Neurogenic hydronephrosis
  ◊ Frequent voiding
  ◊ Double voiding
  ◊ Suprapubic pressure
  ◊ Intermittent catheterization
  ◊ Cholinergics
  ◊ Surgical reimplantation of ureters
  ◊ Antibiotics, when needed for infection
Uremia
  ◊ Dialysis
  ◊ Hyperkalemia (calcium, Kayexalate, insulin and glucose)
  ◊ Treat acidosis
  ◊ Treat hypocalcemia

ACTIVITY Fully active

DIET
• If not uremic, no restriction
• When uremic - protein, salt, potassium restriction as needed

PATIENT EDUCATION
Printed material available from National Kidney Foundation, 30 East 33rd St., Ste. 1100, New York, New York, 10016 (800)622-9010. "What Everyone Should Know About Kidneys and Kidney Disease" (Order #01-01 BP English, #01-02 BP Spanish)

MEDICATIONS

DRUG(S) OF CHOICE Lithiasis - treatment specific for stone
Contraindications: Allergy to drug
Precautions: N/A
Significant possible interactions: N/A

ALTERNATIVE DRUGS N/A

FOLLOWUP

PATIENT MONITORING
• Imaging procedure of choice depending on etiology of hydronephrosis (IVP, renal scan, cystoretrogrades, ultrasound)
• Metabolic studies for nephrolithiasis
• Appropriate cancer screening if applicable

PREVENTION/AVOIDANCE
• Avoid anticholinergics when obstruction present
• Avoid dehydration with lithiasis

POSSIBLE COMPLICATIONS
• Urinary tract infection from instrumentation
• Fibrosis from radiation for pelvic malignancy
• Obstruction from stone fragments on lithotripsy
• Postoperative bleeding

EXPECTED COURSE AND PROGNOSIS
• Contingent on relief of obstruction and residual renal function
• Excellent course and prognosis with relief of obstruction and restoration of normal renal function

MISCELLANEOUS

ASSOCIATED CONDITIONS See causes

AGE-RELATED FACTORS
Pediatric: Hydronephrosis most often congenital
Geriatric: In males, most often due to prostatic enlargement
Others: N/A

PREGNANCY Frequent temporary cause of hydronephrosis

SYNONYMS
• Urinary tract obstruction
• Obstructive uropathy
• Obstructive nephropathy
• Post-renal insufficiency
• Caliectasis
• Pyelectasis
• Ureterectasis

ICD-9-CM
• Congenital 753.2
• Other 591

SEE ALSO
• Chronic Renal Failure
• Acute Renal Failure

OTHER NOTES N/A

ABBREVIATIONS N/A

REFERENCES Obstructive Nephropathy: Pathophysiology and Management. In Renal and Electrolyte Disorders. 4th Ed. Edited by R.W. Schrier. Boston, Little Brown & Co., p. 581, 1992

Author G. Rutecki, M.D.

Hypercalcemia associated with malignancy

BASICS

DESCRIPTION The most common cause of hypercalcemia diagnosed in a hospital setting is malignancy, often heralding the patient's demise. Because of the extremely poor prognosis, it must be differentiated from other, more treatable, entities.
System(s) affected: Endocrine/Metabolic, Musculoskeletal, Nervous, Gastrointestinal
Genetics: N/A
Incidence in USA: N/A
Prevalence in USA: Occurs in 5-10% of cancer patients
Predominant age: N/A
Predominant sex: N/A

SIGNS AND SYMPTOMS
• Severity of symptoms depends on calcium level, rapidity of onset of hypercalcemia, state of hydration, and underlying malignancy
• Anorexia, nausea
• Polyuria, dehydration
• Lethargy, stupor, coma

CAUSES
Solid tumors:
◊ 80% have increased levels of nephrogenous cyclic AMP, reflecting activity of ectopic parathormone-related peptide(s). True ectopic PTH production is exceedingly rare.
◊ Lung cancer (25% of cases usually squamous, less common are adenocarcinoma and large cell, rarely small cell)
◊ Squamous carcinoma of head, neck, esophagus, female genital tract (20% of cases)
◊ Renal cell carcinoma (8% of cases)
Myeloma, lymphoma, breast cancer with osseous metastases, and others:
◊ Nephrogenous cyclic AMP is reduced, reflecting suppression of PTH by nonparathyroid hypercalcemia
◊ Factors implicated include interleukin-1, prostaglandins (E series), transforming growth factors alpha and beta, tumor necrosis factor, lymphotoxin, colony stimulating factor
◊ Direct resorption of bone by metastatic tumor (controversial)
◊ 1-alpha hydroxylase activity of some lymphomas, causing tumoral production of 1,25-dihydroxyvitamin D

RISK FACTORS
• Dehydration
• Immobilization

DIAGNOSIS

DIFFERENTIAL DIAGNOSIS
(not including benign familial hypercalcemia)
• Vitamins A and D
• Immobilization
• Thyrotoxicosis
• Addison's disease
• Milk alkali syndrome
• Inflammatory disorders
• Neoplastic-related disorders
• Sarcoidosis, TB, and other granulomatous diseases
• Thiazides, lithium; theophylline and aspirin toxicity
• Rhabdomyolysis
• AIDS
• Paget's disease, parenteral nutrition, parathyroid disease

LABORATORY
• Serum calcium: Total calcium level depends on binding proteins. Adjusted calcium can be estimated by:
Ca(adj) = Ca(tot) −0.8 x (albumin −4)
• Ionized calcium: Physiologically most important, affected by pH. May be measured directly if specimen is collected under anaerobic conditions and analyzed promptly.
• PTH assay: "Intact" molecule (especially two-site, noncompetitive) methods have greatest specificity, almost always suppressed, in malignancy. If elevated in a cancer patient, suspect concomitant hyperparathyroidism.
• PTH-related peptide: Assays now are clinically available; often elevated in hypercalcemia of malignancy (see above)
• 25-hydroxyvitamin D: May be elevated in vitamin D intoxication
• 1,25-dihydroxyvitamin D: Elevated in up to 50% of hypercalcemic patients with lymphoma
Drugs that may alter lab results: N/A
Disorders that may alter lab results: N/A

PATHOLOGICAL FINDINGS N/A

SPECIAL TESTS Staging techniques as necessary to determine extent of malignancy

IMAGING If there is laboratory evidence of primary hyperparathyroidism, imaging (such as ultrasound, CT, MRI, or nuclear thallium-technetium subtraction scans) may be required in patients with previous neck surgery, prior to re-exploration

DIAGNOSTIC PROCEDURES N/A

TREATMENT

APPROPRIATE HEALTH CARE
Inpatient

GENERAL MEASURES
• Treatment of underlying malignancy
• Maintain hydration, encourage oral fluids; intravenous saline diuresis

ACTIVITY Avoid bed rest or immobilization as much as possible

DIET No special diet

PATIENT EDUCATION N/A

MEDICATIONS

DRUG(S) OF CHOICE
• Loop diuretics - use only after adequate hydration
• Calcitonin - 4-8 IU/kg SC or IM every 8-12 hours. Intramuscular route preferred if patient is dehydrated. Nontoxic, acts in 12-24 hours, minor but uncomfortable side effects include nausea, flushing, cramps. "Escape" phenomenon may be antagonized by steroids.
• Plicamycin (mithramycin) - 25 µg/kg IV over several hours. Very effective. Onset < 12 hours, peak effect 48-72 hours, duration 3-9 days. Toxicity - nausea, thrombocytopenia, hepatic and renal toxicity.
• Biphosphonates currently available - disodium etidronate. 7.5 mg/kg IV daily for 3-7 days. Efficacy similar to plicamycin but less toxic. Long-term use over several months may cause osteopenia and fractures. Newer agents being developed and tested. Pamidronate (Aredia) recently approved; 60 mg IV.
• Glucocorticoids - (40-60 mg/day prednisone or equivalent). Most effective in vitamin D intoxication, may be helpful in myeloma, lymphoma and other granulomatous disorders. Usually not effective in solid tumors.
• Oral phosphates - 1-2 gm/day neutral phosphates, 4 divided doses. Modest hypocalcemic effect, but significant GI distress.
• Intravenous phosphate - should be avoided because of calcium-phosphate precipitation in tissues, risk of severe hypotension
• Gallium nitrate - 100-200 mg/M2/day for 5-7 days. Dilute in 1000 mL 5% dextrose and infuse continuously over 24 hours.

Contraindications: Refer to manufacturer's literature
Precautions: Refer to manufacturer's literature
Significant possible interactions: Refer to manufacturer's literature

ALTERNATIVE DRUGS   Listed above

FOLLOWUP

PATIENT MONITORING   Frequent serum calcium and electrolyte determinations, expect relapse

PREVENTION/AVOIDANCE   Encourage adequate hydration and activity, especially in multiple myeloma

POSSIBLE COMPLICATIONS   N/A

EXPECTED COURSE AND PROGNOSIS   Median survival after diagnosis of tumoral hypercalcemia is approximately 30 days

MISCELLANEOUS

ASSOCIATED CONDITIONS   N/A

AGE-RELATED FACTORS   N/A
Pediatric: N/A
Geriatric: N/A
Others: N/A

PREGNANCY   N/A

SYNONYMS   Tumoral hypercalcemia

ICD-9-CM
275.4 Disorders of calcium metabolism

SEE ALSO   N/A

OTHER NOTES   N/A

ABBREVIATIONS   N/A

REFERENCES   Marcus, R., (ed.): Endocrinology and Metabolism Clinics of North America-Vol. 18, No. 3, September 1989, pp 778-828

Author   J. Rudick, M.D.

Hypercholesterolemia

 BASICS

DESCRIPTION Serum cholesterol > 200 mg/dL. High risk 240 mg/dL or more.
• High density lipoprotein fraction of cholesterol (HDL) - protective, low density lipoprotein (LDL) - atherogenic
System(s) affected: Endocrine/Metabolic, Gastrointestinal, Cardiovascular
Genetics: Heterozygous familial. Hypercholesterolemia, 1 in 500 cases. Autosomal dominant hypercholesterolemia 1 in 1 million.
Incidence/Prevalence in USA: 120 million people with cholesterol 200 mg/dL or more, 60 million with 240 mg/dL or more
Predominant age: Prevalence increases with age
Predominant sex: Male > Female

SIGNS AND SYMPTOMS
• Corneal arcus before 50
• Xanthomata
• Xanthelasma
• Arterial bruits
• Claudication
• Angina pectoris
• Stroke
• Myocardial infarction

CAUSES
Primary
  ◊ Diet
  ◊ Heredity
  ◊ Obesity
  ◊ Sedentary life-style
  ◊ Stress
Secondary
  ◊ Hypothyroidism
  ◊ Diabetes mellitus
  ◊ Nephrotic syndrome
  ◊ Obstructive liver disease
  ◊ Progestins
  ◊ Anabolic steroids
  ◊ Diuretics except indapamide (Lozol)
  ◊ Beta blockers except those with intrinsic sympathomimetic activity (ISA)
• Some immunosuppressants

RISK FACTORS
• Obesity
• Heredity

 DIAGNOSIS

DIFFERENTIAL DIAGNOSIS N/A

LABORATORY
• High density lipoprotein fraction of cholesterol (HDL), low density lipoprotein (LDL), triglycerides must be checked fasting
• Cholesterol is considered elevated if > than 200 mg/dL
• T7 and TSH initially hyperthyroidism may cause hypercholesterolemia
Drugs that may alter lab results: Caffeine may increase cholesterol
Disorders that may alter lab results: Hypothyroidism, nephrotic syndrome, obstructive liver disease

PATHOLOGICAL FINDINGS N/A

SPECIAL TESTS N/A

IMAGING N/A

DIAGNOSTIC PROCEDURES N/A

 TREATMENT

APPROPRIATE HEALTH CARE
Outpatient, except for complicating emergencies, e.g., myocardial infarction

GENERAL MEASURES
• Requires intervention: HDL less than 30, LDL greater than 160. Triglycerides may be over 200.
• Cholesterol 200-240 without coronary artery disease or two risk factors (male, smoking, HDL less than 35, severe obesity, diabetes, hypertension, strong family history) - prudent diet and recheck in one year
• Cholesterol 200-240 with coronary artery disease or two or more risk factors (male, smoking, HDL less than 35, severe obesity, diabetes, hypertension, strong family history) - lipoprotein analysis with further action based on HDL and LDL
• Cholesterol over 240 - lipoprotein analysis with further action based on HDL and LDL

ACTIVITY Aerobic exercise at least 30 minutes, three times weekly. Important for increasing HDL, lowering total cholesterol, and losing weight.

DIET Reduce saturated fat, reduce dietary cholesterol, increase fiber, increase intake of fruits, vegetables, whole grains. Emphasize, vegetarian, meatless, eggless, cheeseless meals, with poultry, fish, and nonfat milk or yogurt. Minimal daily alcohol use may increase HDL.

PATIENT EDUCATION American Heart Association publications

MEDICATIONS

DRUG(S) OF CHOICE
• Cholestyramine (Questran), or Colestipol (Colestid) bile acid binding resins. One to six packets per day taken qd, bid, or tid. Effect: 15-30% fall in LDL.
• Nicotinic acid: 500 mg to 3 gm taken one to three times daily with meals in timed release formulation to minimize side effects. Effect: 15-30% LDL lowering, decreases triglycerides. Hepatic dysfunction more common in patients who take sustained release niacin than in those who take immediate release form. Best to start with low doses and increase as tolerated.
• Lovastatin (Mevacor), an HMG-CoA reductase inhibitor: 20-80 mg per day, taken in single or divided doses with meals. Most suggest taking with evening meal. Effects: 25-45% LDL decrease, decreases triglycerides.

Contraindications:
• Cholestyramine (Questran) - complete biliary obstruction
• Nicotinic acid - hepatic dysfunction, acute peptic ulcer, diabetes mellitus.
• Lovastatin (Mevacor) - active liver disease, pregnancy

Precautions:
• Cholestyramine (Questran) - gradually increase dose on weekly basis to minimize GI side effects (particularly constipation, flatulence)
• Colestipol or cholestyramine should be mixed with fruit juice or stirred into a pulpy fruit before administration. The powder should not be taken in its dry form since it may cause esophageal or GI blockage.
• Nicotinic acid - blood glucose and liver function tests must be monitored during early stages of therapy to insure no deleterious effect. Generalized flushing after dosage may be blocked by a concomitant aspirin.
• Lovastatin (Mevacor) - liver function tests every three months during the first 15 months and periodically thereafter. Myositis with markedly elevated creatine kinase (CK) may occur. Cataract formation in excess has not been proven.

Significant possible interactions:
• Cholestyramine (Questran) - other drugs taken less than one hour before or within six hours after may be bound and not absorbed as well. Fat soluble vitamins A, D, E and K absorption may be impeded.
• Nicotinic acid - none
• Lovastatin (Mevacor) - concomitant gemfibrozil, niacin, or immunosuppressives increase possibility of myositis

ALTERNATIVE DRUGS
Other HMG-CoA reductase inhibitors - pravastatin, simvastatin

 FOLLOWUP

PATIENT MONITORING
• While on medication, monitor cholesterol, HDL, LDL, triglycerides 2-4 times yearly depending on medication
• Cholesterol less than 200 - repeat in 5 years

PREVENTION/AVOIDANCE
Prudent diet and weight control for all

POSSIBLE COMPLICATIONS
Coronary heart disease

EXPECTED COURSE AND PROGNOSIS
1% decrease in cholesterol results in 2% decreased risk of coronary heart disease

 MISCELLANEOUS

ASSOCIATED CONDITIONS
• Hypertension
• Obesity
• Diabetes mellitus
• Smoking

AGE-RELATED FACTORS
Pediatric:
Screening every five years beginning as early as six. (Childhood screening is controversial because no studies have shown a clear link between hypercholesterolemia in childhood to hypercholesterolemia in adulthood. Furthermore, the risks of reducing cholesterol in childhood are not known.)
If total cholesterol greater than 170, check HDL and LDL levels. If LDL is 110-125 = moderate risk, if LDL is greater than 125 = high risk.
Geriatric: Elevated cholesterol is a coronary heart disease risk factor over age 65 and should be treated as well
Others: N/A

PREGNANCY
Fetal nutritional demands may alter diet and drug treatment

SYNONYMS
N/A

ICD-9-CM
272.0

SEE ALSO
N/A

OTHER NOTES
N/A

ABBREVIATIONS
N/A

REFERENCES
• National Cholesterol Education Program. Arch Intern Med. 148:36-69, 1988
• Peters, W.: Drug Therapy to Lower Cholesterol. In Practical Cardiology. May, 1988, 38-47

Author J. Carter, M.D.

Hyperemesis gravidarum

 BASICS

DESCRIPTION Persistent vomiting in a pregnant woman that interferes with fluid and electrolyte balance, as well as nutrition. Usually associated with the first 8 to 20 weeks of pregnancy. Believed to have biomedical and behavioral aspects. Associated with high estrogen levels. Symptoms usually begin about 2 weeks after first missed period.

System(s) affected: Gastrointestinal, Reproductive, Endocrine/Metabolic
Genetics: Unknown
Incidence/Prevalence in USA:
• 2% of pregnancies have electrolyte disturbances
• 50% of pregnancies have at least some gastrointestinal disturbance
Predominant age: 21-31
Predominant sex: Female only

SIGNS AND SYMPTOMS
• Hypersensitivity to smell
• Alteration in taste
• Nausea
• Vomiting with retching
• Acidosis
• Decreased urine output
• Volume depletion
• Fatigue
• Starvation

CAUSES
• Unknown
• May be psychological factors
• Hyperthyroidism
• Hyperparathyroidism
• Gestational hormones
• Liver dysfunction
• Autonomic nervous system dysfunction

RISK FACTORS
• Trophoblastic activity
• Gonadotropin production stimulated
• Altered gastrointestinal function
• Various odors
• Taste or sight of food
• Hyperthyroidism
• Hyperparathyroidism

 DIAGNOSIS

DIFFERENTIAL DIAGNOSIS
Other common causes of vomiting must be considered:
◊ Gastroenteritis
◊ Gastritis
◊ Reflux esophagitis
◊ Peptic ulcer disease
◊ Cholelithiasis
◊ Cholecystitis
◊ Pyelonephritis
◊ Anxiety

LABORATORY
• Electrolytes decreased
• Urinalysis - glucosuria, albuminuria, granular casts and hematuria (rare)
• Increased uric acid
• Reduced protein
Drugs that may alter lab results: None likely
Disorders that may alter lab results: N/A

PATHOLOGICAL FINDINGS Fatty degeneration of the liver; renal tubular damage; heart damage; petechial brain hemorrhages

SPECIAL TESTS None indicated for the diagnosis of hyperemesis gravidarum

IMAGING No imaging is indicated for the diagnosis of hyperemesis gravidarum

DIAGNOSTIC PROCEDURES Only indicated if it is necessary to rule out other diagnoses

 TREATMENT

APPROPRIATE HEALTH CARE
• Outpatient therapy
• In some severe cases, inpatient parenteral or enteral volume and nutrition repletion may be indicated

GENERAL MEASURES
• Patient reassurance
• Bedrest
• If dehydrated, IV fluids. Repeat if there is a recurrence of symptoms following initial improvement.

ACTIVITY As tolerated after improvement

DIET
• Nothing by mouth for first 24 hours if patient is ill enough to require hospitalization
• For outpatient: A diet rich in carbohydrates and protein, such as fruit, cheese, cottage cheese, eggs, beef, poultry, vegetables, toast, crackers, rice. Limit intake of butter. Patients should avoid spicy meals and high fat foods.

PATIENT EDUCATION
• Attention should be given to psychosocial issues such as possible ambivalence about the pregnancy
• Patients should be instructed to take small amounts of fluid frequently to avoid volume depletion

MEDICATIONS

DRUG(S) OF CHOICE
• Pyridoxine 10-30 mg daily IV. Not always effective, but not harmful.
• Antihistamines (e.g., diphenhydramine [25-50 mg Q 4-6 hours] or dimenhydrinate, or doxylamine)
• Phenothiazines (e.g., promethazine or prochlorperazine)
• Meclizine 25 mg every six hours
Contraindications: All medications taken during pregnancy should balance the risks and benefits both to the mother and the fetus
Precautions:
• Phenothiazines - associated with prolonged jaundice, extrapyramidal effects, hyper- or hyporeflexia in newborns
• Meclizine - associated with cleft palate in newborns
Significant possible interactions: Refer to manufacturer's profile of each drug

ALTERNATIVE DRUGS
Avoid all drugs if possible

FOLLOWUP

PATIENT MONITORING
• Follow up on a daily basis for weight monitoring in severe cases
• Special attention should be given to monitoring for ketosis, hypokalemia, or acid-base disturbances due to hyperemesis

PREVENTION/AVOIDANCE
Anticipatory guidance in first and second trimester regarding dietary habits in hopes of avoiding volume and nutritional depletion

POSSIBLE COMPLICATIONS
• Patients with greater than a five percent weight loss are associated with intrauterine growth retardation and fetal anomalies
• Hemorrhagic retinitis
• Liver damage
• CNS deterioration, sometimes to coma

EXPECTED COURSE AND PROGNOSIS
• Self-limited illness with good prognosis if patient's weight is maintained at greater than 95% of the pre-pregnancy weight
• With complication of hemorrhagic retinitis, mortality rate is 50%

MISCELLANEOUS

ASSOCIATED CONDITIONS
Hyperthyroidism

AGE-RELATED FACTORS N/A
Pediatric: N/A
Geriatric: N/A
Others: N/A

PREGNANCY
Problem is confined to early pregnancy

SYNONYMS Morning sickness

ICD-9-CM
• 643.0 for uncomplicated hyperemesis gravidarum less than 22 weeks
• 643.1 for severe hyperemesis gravidarum with metabolic disturbance

SEE ALSO N/A

OTHER NOTES N/A

ABBREVIATIONS N/A

REFERENCES
• Gross, S., Librach, C. & Cecetti, A.: Maternal weight loss associated with hyperemesis gravidarum: A predictor of fetal outcome. Am. J. Obstet. Gynecol. 160:906-909, 1989
• Mori, M., Amino, N., Tamaki, H., Miyai, K. & Tanizawa, O.: Morning sickness and thyroid function in normal pregnancy. Obstet. and Gynecol. 72(3):355-359, 1988
• Andolsek, K.M. (ed.): Obstetric Care: Standards of Prenatal Intrapartum and Postpartum Management. Philadelphia, Lea & Febiger, 1989
• Abell, T. & Riely, C.: Hyperemesis gravidarum. Gastrointestinal Clinics NA. 21(4):835-849, 1992

Author S. Fields, M.D. & P. Eiff, M.D.

Hyperkalemia

BASICS

DESCRIPTION A common electrolyte disorder with plasma potassium concentration > 5.0 mEq/L. Four major causes:
• Increased load - either endogenous from tissue release or exogenous from a high intake which is usually in association with impaired excretion
• Decreased excretion - due to decreased glomerular filtration rate
• Cellular redistribution - shifting of intracellular (which is the major store of potassium) to extracellular space
• Factitious - related to improper collection or transport of blood sample
System(s) affected: Endocrine/Metabolic, Cardiovascular, Nervous
Genetics: N/A
Predominant age: N/A
Incidence/Prevalence in USA: Common
Predominant sex: Male = Female

SIGNS AND SYMPTOMS
Cardiac - most important, dominating, and frequent symptom
◊ Peaked T wave
◊ Flattened p wave
◊ Prolonged p-Q interval
◊ Widened QRS complex
◊ Sine wave
◊ Ventricular fibrillation
◊ Cardiac arrest
Neuromuscular
◊ Numbness
◊ Weakness
◊ Flaccid paralysis

CAUSES
Pseudohyperkalemia
◊ Hemolysis (most common)
◊ Thrombolysis
◊ Leukocytosis
◊ Infectious mononucleosis
◊ Familial
◊ Procedural technical error (ischemic blood draw due to tight, prolonged tourniquet application)
Redistribution
◊ Acidosis
◊ Insulin deficiency
◊ Beta blockade due to beta blocking drugs
◊ Digitalis intoxication
◊ Succinylcholine
◊ Arginine hydrochloride/lysine hydrochloride
◊ Periodic paralysis
◊ Fluoride intoxication
◊ Exercise with heavy sweating
Excessive endogenous potassium load
◊ Hemolysis
◊ Rhabdomyolysis
◊ Internal bleeding
Excessive exogenous potassium load
◊ Parenteral administration
◊ Excess in diet
◊ Overdose of potassium supplements

Diminished potassium excretion
◊ Decreased glomerular filtration rate (acute or far-advanced chronic renal failure)
◊ Decreased mineral corticoid activity
◊ Defect in tubular secretion (renal tubular acidosis II and IV)
◊ Drugs - nonsteroidal anti-inflammatory agents, cyclosporine, potassium sparing diuretics

RISK FACTORS
• Impaired urinary excretion
• Acidemia
• Massive cell breakdown
• Use of potassium sparing diuretics
• Excess potassium supplementation

DIAGNOSIS

DIFFERENTIAL DIAGNOSIS
• Cardiac arrhythmias
• Hypocalcemia

LABORATORY Potassium greater than 5.0 meq/L
Drugs that may alter lab results: N/A
Disorders that may alter lab results:
• Acidemia - potassium shifts from intracellular to extracellular space in effort to buffer acid load. Once acidemia is corrected, the potassium may return to normal or even become decreased.
• Insulin deficiency

PATHOLOGICAL FINDINGS N/A

SPECIAL TESTS
• Cortisol and aldosterone levels to check for mineralocorticoid deficiency when other causes are ruled out
• ECG changes usually evolve as potassium rises above 6.0 meq/L

IMAGING N/A

DIAGNOSTIC PROCEDURES N/A

TREATMENT

APPROPRIATE HEALTH CARE
Inpatient with cardiac monitoring if ECG changes are present or potassium is greater than 6.0 meq/L

GENERAL MEASURES
• Discontinue any K-sparing drugs or dietary K
• Major goal is to find the cause of hyperkalemia
• If hyperkalemia is severe, treat first, then do diagnostic investigations

ACTIVITY Bedrest

DIET 80 mEq or less of potassium per 24 hours

PATIENT EDUCATION Consult with dietician

MEDICATIONS

DRUG(S) OF CHOICE
• Dextrose (1 ampule of D50) and insulin (10 units of regular subcutaneous). Temporary shift of potassium intracellularly taking effect in the first 30 minutes but only lasting a short while.
• Sodium bicarbonate (50-100 mEq) dosage in conjunction with the pH. Effects are temporary.
• Sodium polystyrene sulfonate (Kayexalate) 30-60 grams by mouth or by rectum. Effective in 1-4 hours and is a definitive treatment. May repeat q6h if necessary.
• Calcium gluconate (1 ampule) which is cardio-protective only and should only be used when ECG changes are present
• Hemodialysis when other measures are not effective

Contraindications: None

Precautions: Sodium bicarbonate and Kayexalate provide a sodium load that may exacerbate fluid overload in cardiac or renal failure patients

Significant possible interactions: See manufacturer's profile of each drug

ALTERNATIVE DRUGS   N/A

FOLLOWUP

PATIENT MONITORING   Serial renal panels until correction complete

PREVENTION/AVOIDANCE   Diet and oral supplement compliance

POSSIBLE COMPLICATIONS
• Life threatening cardiac arrhythmias
• Hypokalemia

EXPECTED COURSE AND PROGNOSIS   Full resolution with correction of the underlying etiology. Reduction of plasma potassium should begin within the first hour of initiation of treatment.

MISCELLANEOUS

ASSOCIATED CONDITIONS
• Renal failure
• Mineralocorticoid deficiency

AGE-RELATED FACTORS
Pediatric: N/A
Geriatric: Increased risk for hyperkalemia in this age group due to decreases in renin and aldosterone
Others: N/A

PREGNANCY   N/A

SYNONYMS   N/A

ICD-9-CM   276.7

SEE ALSO   N/A

OTHER NOTES   N/A

ABBREVIATIONS   N/A

REFERENCES
• Braunwald, E., et al. (eds.): Harrison's Principles of Internal Medicine. 12th Ed. New York, McGraw-Hill, 1991
• Brenner, B.M. & Rector, F.C., Jr.: The Kidney. 4th Ed. Philadelphia, W.B. Saunders Co., 1990

Author   S. Kant, M.D. & P. Anderson, M.D.

Hypernatremia

BASICS

DESCRIPTION Water content of body fluid is deficient compared to sodium content (serum Na > 150 mEq/L)
• Significant hypernatremia (serum Na > 160 mEq/L) - may not indicate total body sodium content
• Hypertonicity - increased solutes in extracellular fluid (ECF) which do not cross cell membranes, e.g., sodium, mannitol or glucose. Shifts water from intracellular fluid (ICF) to ECF.
• Hyperosmolality - increased solutes e.g., urea or alcohol, which freely cross all membranes or sodium which does not cross cell membranes. May be present without hypertonicity.
System(s) affected: Endocrine/Metabolic
Genetics: No known genetic pattern. Some diabetes insipidus (DI) may be hereditary.
Incidence in USA: Common in the elderly (e.g. 1% of hospitalized patients over age 65); also may occur with diarrhea in infants
Prevalence in USA: N/A
Predominant age: N/A
Predominant sex: Male = Female

SIGNS AND SYMPTOMS
• Severity of symptoms usually correlate with the extent of hyperosmolality
• Primary neurological - thirst, restlessness, irritability, disorientation, delirium, coma, convulsions
• Dry mouth and mucous membranes
• Lack of tears and decreased salivation
• Flushed skin
• Fever
• Oligo/anuria
• Hyperventilation
• Hyperreflexia
• Brain hemorrhage
• Thirst is the primary protection against hypertonicity

CAUSES
Sodium excess - total body sodium increased
◊ Oral - improperly mixed infant formula, salt given as "punishment" or as a prank, sea water ingestion
◊ IV - NaCl or Na2CO3 during cardiopulmonary resuscitation, intrauterine NaCl for abortion
Water deficit - total body sodium normal
◊ Decreased intake: e.g., thirst, decreased access to water
◊ Increased urine water loss, e.g., diabetes insipidus
◊ Increased insensible water loss, e.g., fever, hyperventilation, hypermetabolic state
Hypotonic fluid loss - total body sodium decreased
◊ Loss of fluid containing sodium - without adequate water replacement
Urinary loss
◊ Osmotic diuretics
◊ Diabetes mellitus
◊ Diuresis from acute tubular necrosis (ATN) or from relief of acute urinary obstruction

GI loss
◊ Diarrhea, especially in children
Insensible loss
◊ Sweat
◊ Newborns under radiant warmers

RISK FACTORS
• Children
• Elderly
• Comatose patients

DIAGNOSIS

DIFFERENTIAL DIAGNOSIS
• Diabetes insipidus
• Hyperosmotic coma
• Salt ingestion
• Hypertonic dehydration

LABORATORY
• Serum Na > 150 to 170 - usually dehydration
• Serum Na > 170 - usually diabetes insipidus
• Serum Na > 190 - usually chronic salt ingestion
Diabetes insipidus
◊ Urine osmolality less than serum osmolality
◊ Urine sodium usually low
◊ Polyuria
◊ Neurogenic vs. nephrogenic diabetes insipidus
Hyperosmolar coma
◊ Blood sugar elevated
◊ Decreased urine output
◊ Increased urine osmolality
Salt ingestion
◊ Increased urine Na
◊ Increased urine osmolality
Hypertonic dehydration
◊ Decreased urine sodium
◊ Increased urine osmolality
Drugs that may alter lab results: A variety of medications may raise or lower sodium levels. Refer to a laboratory test reference.
Disorders that may alter lab results: N/A

PATHOLOGICAL FINDINGS N/A

SPECIAL TESTS
• Water deprivation (diabetes insipidus does not increase urine osmolality when hypernatremic)
• Antidiuretic hormone (ADH) stimulation (nephrogenic diabetes insipidus does not increase urine osmolality after ADH or DDAVP)

IMAGING CAT scan or MRI in diabetes insipidus - to rule out craniopharyngioma, tumor or median cleft syndrome

DIAGNOSTIC PROCEDURES History, physical, laboratory studies, family history for NDI

TREATMENT

APPROPRIATE HEALTH CARE
Inpatient (many patients are already hospitalized and hypernatremia develops after admission)

GENERAL MEASURES
• Water replacement orally, if patient conscious
• Treat hypovolemia first, then treat hypernatremia
• Calculated water deficit = 1 + (140 - current serum Na) x wt (kg) x 0.55
• Dialysis - especially with serum Na > 200 mEq/L

ACTIVITY Bedrest until stable or underlying condition resolved or controlled

DIET
• Assure proper nutrition during acute phase
• After resolution of acute phase, may want to consider sodium restricted diet for patient
• Severe salt restriction in nephrogenic diabetes insipidus

PATIENT EDUCATION Patients with diabetes insipidus must avoid salt and drink large amounts of water

Hypernatremia

 MEDICATIONS

DRUG(S) OF CHOICE
Hypovolemia
◊ Isotonic saline (normal saline or Ringer's lactate) 10-20 mL/kg IV over 1-2 hrs. May repeat if 10% or greater dehydration.
◊ Isotonic fluids: 5% dextrose with half-normal saline until urine output established
Hypernatremia
◊ Hypotonic fluids (NaCl or dextrose 5% in water)
◊ Decrease serum Na by 0.5 mEq/L/hour or by no more than 20 mEq/L/day. Allows idiogenic osmoles to resolve (mostly taurine in brain cell water).
◊ Potassium and phosphate, if needed
Neurogenic diabetes insipidus (DI)
◊ Desmopressin acetate (DDAVP) 0.01 mcg/kg/dose given intranasally bid
◊ May use 2.5 dextrose in water if giving large volumes of water in DI or NDI to avoid glycosuria
Nephrogenic diabetes insipidus (NDI)
◊ Chlorothiazide, 10 mg/kg/dose given bid
◊ Chlorpropamide 100-250 mg each morning
Contraindications: Refer to manufacturer's literature
Precautions:
• Rapid correction of hypernatremia can cause pulmonary edema. Hypocalcemia often occurs during correction.
• In diabetes insipidus - high rates of dextrose 5% in water can cause hyperglycemia and glucose induced diuresis
Significant possible interactions: Refer to manufacturer's literature

ALTERNATIVE DRUGS
Consider nonsteroidal anti-inflammatories in nephrogenic diabetes insipidus

 FOLLOWUP

PATIENT MONITORING
• For patient in an acute setting, frequent re-examinations
• Electrolytes frequently
• Urine osmolality and urine output in DI
• Ensure adequate calories are ingested
• Daily weights

PREVENTION/AVOIDANCE
• Treatment or prevention of underlying cause
• Avoid preparing infant formula at home, and never add salt to any commercial infant formula

POSSIBLE COMPLICATIONS
• CNS thrombosis or hemorrhage
• Seizures
• Mental retardation
• Hyperactivity
• Chronic hypernatremia - over two days duration has higher mortality
• Serum sodium > 180 mEq/L - often have residual CNS damage

EXPECTED COURSE AND PROGNOSIS
Most recover but rate of neurological impairment is high

 MISCELLANEOUS

ASSOCIATED CONDITIONS Disorders listed under Causes

AGE-RELATED FACTORS N/A
Pediatric:
• May occur in low birth weight newborns
• May result from incorrect preparation of infant formula
Geriatric:
• More common in the elderly hospitalized patient, resulting in a higher morbidity or mortality
• Hypernatremia may be caused by administration of loop diuretics
Others: N/A

PREGNANCY N/A

SYNONYMS N/A

ICD-9-CM 270.6 disorders of urea cycle metabolism

SEE ALSO N/A

OTHER NOTES N/A

ABBREVIATIONS DI = diabetes insipidus

REFERENCES
• Brenner, B.M. & Rector, F.C., Jr.: The Kidney. 4th Ed. Philadelphia, W.B. Saunders Co., 1991
• Holliday, M., Barrett, T. & Vernier, R.: Pediatric Nephrology. 2nd Ed. Baltimore, Williams & Wilkins. 1986
• Kokko, J. & Tannen, R.: Fluid and Electrolytes. 2nd Ed. Philadelphia, W.B. Saunders Co., 1990

Author W. Arnold, M.D.

Hyperparathyroidism

 BASICS

DESCRIPTION Hyperparathyroidism represents a loss in control of the body's normal regulatory feedback mechanism on the parathyroid glands and their ability to maintain a normal serum calcium
• Primary hyperparathyroidism - direct hyperfunction of the parathyroid glands due to either glandular hyperplasia or adenoma
• Secondary hyperparathyroidism - usually found in chronic renal disease or vitamin D deficient states which cause hyperplasia of all four glands and associated increase in activity
• Multiple endocrine neoplasia (MEN syndromes) - disease states with associated endocrine malfunctions with parathyroid gland hyperplasia leading to a hyperparathyroid state
• Parathyroid carcinoma - extremely rare
System(s) affected: Endocrine/Metabolic
Genetics: N/A
Incidence/Prevalence in USA:
• Rare in children
• Male adults 60 years or older - 100 cases/100,000
• Female adults 60 years or older - 300-400 cases/100,000
• All-age adjusted incidence - 42 cases/100,000
• Prevalence all ages - 250 cases/100,000 population
Predominant age: Age greater than 50
Predominant sex: Females > Males (4:1)

SIGNS AND SYMPTOMS
• "Painful bones, renal stones, abdominal groans and psychic moans." You must think of it to diagnose it.
Renal:
◊ Nephrolithiasis
◊ Nephrocalcinosis
◊ Reduced glomerular filtration rate
◊ Thirst
◊ Polydipsia
◊ Polyuria
Gastrointestinal:
◊ Abdominal distress
◊ Gastroduodenal ulcer
◊ Pancreatitis
◊ Pancreatic calcification
◊ Constipation
◊ Vomiting
◊ Anorexia
◊ Weight loss
Skeletal:
◊ Bone pain and tenderness
◊ Cystic bone lesions
◊ Skeletal demineralization
◊ Spontaneous fracture
◊ Vertebral collapse
◊ Osteoporosis
Mental:
◊ Fatigue
◊ Apathy
◊ Anxiety
◊ Depression
◊ Psychosis

Neurologic:
◊ Somnolence
◊ Coma
◊ Diffuse EEG abnormalities
Neuromuscular:
◊ Muscle fatigue
◊ Weakness
◊ Hypotonia
Cardiovascular:
◊ Hypertension
◊ Short QT interval
Articular/periarticular:
◊ Arthralgia
◊ Gout
◊ Pseudogout
◊ Periarticular calcification
Ocular:
◊ Band keratopathy
◊ Conjunctivitis
◊ Conjunctival calcium deposits

CAUSES
Primary hyperparathyroidism
◊ Caused by usually one but sometimes multiple parathyroid gland hyperplasia or adenomatous changes which cause an unregulated increase of parathyroid hormone (PTH) production and release, causing increase in serum calcium
Secondary hyperparathyroidism
◊ Seen most often in chronic renal failure because of adaptive parathyroid gland hyperplasia and hyperfunction
◊ Renal parenchymal loss resulting in hyperphosphatemia
◊ Impaired calcitriol production leading to hypocalcemia
◊ General skeletal and renal resistance to PTH for reasons unknown

RISK FACTORS
• Age greater than 50
• Female
• Occurs more frequently in temperate than tropical climates
• Higher incidence in people exposed to therapeutic low dose radiation

 DIAGNOSIS

DIFFERENTIAL DIAGNOSIS
• Other causes of elevated serum calcium level must be excluded
Due to increased PTH:
◊ Ectopic hyperparathyroidism
◊ Bronchogenic carcinoma
◊ Carcinoma of the kidney
Nonparathyroid causes:
◊ Malignancy - breast carcinoma, multiple myeloma, lymphoma, leukemia, prostate cancer, Paget's disease
◊ Granulomatous disease - sarcoidosis, tuberculosis, berylliosis, histoplasmosis, coccidiomycosis
◊ Drugs - thiazide diuretics, furosemide, vitamin D intoxication, vitamin A excess, lithium, milk alkali syndrome, exogenous calcium intake
◊ Endocrine - hyperthyroidism, hypothyroidism, acute adrenal insufficiency, vipoma, pheochromocytoma
◊ Familial hypocalciuric hypercalcemia
◊ Immobilization

LABORATORY
• Elevated serum calcium greater than 10.2 mg/dL on 3 successive measurements
• Elevated serum immunoreactive parathyroid hormone (iPTH) levels
• Low serum phosphate levels, less than 2.5 mg/dL
• Elevated serum chloride levels
• Decreased serum CO2
• Hyperchloremic metabolic acidosis
• Increase in urinary cyclic AMP
Drugs that may alter lab results: N/A
Disorders that may alter lab results: N/A

PATHOLOGICAL FINDINGS
• Parathyroid hyperplasia - all parathyroid glands with cellular changes
• Parathyroid adenoma - only one gland usually with cellular changes
• Parathyroid carcinoma - cellular changes consistent with malignancy, i.e., cellular atypia, lymph node changes

SPECIAL TESTS Immunoassay directed against intact PTH molecule

IMAGING
• Neck ultrasonography
• Thallium technetium scanning
• Magnetic resonance imaging
• CT scanning with and without contrast

DIAGNOSTIC PROCEDURES
• Percutaneous needle biopsy aspiration for cytology and PTH determination
• Open surgical removal with frozen section diagnosis

TREATMENT

APPROPRIATE HEALTH CARE
Outpatient usually. Inpatient for surgery or for treatment of underlying cause.

GENERAL MEASURES
• Surgical removal of diseased gland is only proven curative therapy for hyperparathyroidism (subtotal resection)
• A few patients with mild asymptomatic hypercalcemia due to hyperparathyroidism may not be candidates for surgery and may be managed conservatively. Avoiding dehydration is most important treatment.
Surgical
• In preoperative and immediately postoperative patients, large fluid intake is indicated to help prevent formation of renal stones
• Open neck surgical exploration advocated approach
• Removal of obviously diseased gland with biopsies of other glands to make sure physiologically viable
• Total resection of all four glands with transplantation of normal gland to forearm advocated by some
• Special attention must be made during exploration and removal of parathyroid glands for ectopic gland in the neck area
• Postoperative course needs special attention paid to airway and risk of airway compromise
• Monitoring renal functions closely

ACTIVITY   As tolerated

DIET   As indicated by condition of patient

PATIENT EDUCATION
• Educate about medications
• Importance of periodic lab exams

 MEDICATIONS

DRUG(S) OF CHOICE
• Furosemide diuretics (Lasix) may be helpful in well hydrated individuals who are hypercalcemic
• Estrogens (Premarin, Estrace, Estraderm) are indicated in postmenopausal females with hyperparathyroidism
Contraindications: Avoid diuretics in individuals who are hypercalcemic
Precautions: Refer to manufacturer's literature
Significant possible interactions: Refer to manufacturer's literature

ALTERNATIVE DRUGS   N/A

 FOLLOWUP

PATIENT MONITORING
Postoperatively
◊ Monitor renal function closely
◊ Potential precipitous fall in serum calcium resulting in development of transient tetany

PREVENTION/AVOIDANCE   N/A

POSSIBLE COMPLICATIONS
• Skeletal damage (pathologic fractures)
• Renal damage
• Urinary tract infections
• "Parathyroid poisoning"
• Hypertension
From surgery:
◊ Hypoparathyroidism
◊ Recurrent laryngeal nerve damage
◊ Bleeding
◊ Infection
◊ Unsuccessful surgery (5%)

EXPECTED COURSE AND PROGNOSIS
• Postoperative course requires following of serum calcium to make sure hyperparathyroid state does not redevelop
• Prognosis is excellent in primary hyperparathyroidism with resolution of many of the preoperative symptoms
• Secondary hyperparathyroidism carries a poor prognosis because of the primary disease state of chronic renal failure

 MISCELLANEOUS

ASSOCIATED CONDITIONS   Multiple
endocrine neoplasia (MEN) syndromes

AGE-RELATED FACTORS
Pediatric: N/A
Geriatric:
• Common in the elderly
• More likely to have a secondary disease
• May cause confusion and be interpreted as senile dementia
Others: N/A

PREGNANCY   Rarely occurs during
pregnancy

SYNONYMS   N/A

ICD-9-CM
• Primary hyperparathyroidism - 252.0
• Ectopic - 259.3
• Secondary hyperparathyroidism in chronic renal disease - 588.8

SEE ALSO   N/A

OTHER NOTES   N/A

ABBREVIATIONS   PTH = parathyroid
hormone

REFERENCES
• Arnaud, C.D.: The parathyroid glands, hypercalcemia, and hypocalcemia. In Cecil Textbook of Medicine. 18th Ed. Edited by J.B. Wyngaarden & J.B. Smith. Philadelphia, W.B. Saunders Co., 1988
• Clark, O. & Quan-Yank, D.: Primary hyperparathyroidism: a surgical perspective. In Endocrinology and Metabolism Clinics of North America 1989;18(3):701-715

Author   P. McCarville, M.D.

Hypersensitivity pneumonitis

 BASICS

DESCRIPTION
Hypersensitivity pneumonitis (extrinsic allergic alveolitis) is a diffuse inflammatory disease of the lung caused by repeated inhalation of dust constituted of animal proteins, plant proteins or reactive inorganic compounds. Regardless of the etiologic inhalant, most forms share common features:
• Involvement of peripheral airways, alveoli and interstitium
• Mononuclear cell infiltration of interstitium with granuloma formation and increased alveolar macrophage activity
• Precipitating antibodies against offending dust without complement activation
• Normal IgE and eosinophil levels in chronic form. May present as either acute or sub-acute to chronic progressive pneumonitis.
System(s) affected: Pulmonary
Genetics:
Not related to:
◊ Atopic predisposition
◊ Blood type
◊ HLA type
Incidence/Prevalence in USA:
• National prevalence unknown
• 1-8% of farmers and 6-15% of pigeon breeders develop related pneumonitis
Predominant age: All ages, but tends to occur in adults because of occupation related exposure
Predominant sex: Male = Female

SIGNS AND SYMPTOMS
Acute hypersensitivity pneumonitis:
◊ The following occur within 6 hours of exposure to the offending antigen and may mimic an acute infectious pneumonia:
◊ Fever up to 40°C
◊ Cough
◊ Dyspnea
◊ Malaise
◊ Body aches
◊ Rare hemoptysis or sputum production
◊ Hypoxia
◊ Fine, mid-to end-inspiratory crackles in chest
Chronic hypersensitivity pneumonitis:
◊ Chronic progressive condition without acute exacerbation:
◊ Chronic cough
◊ Dyspnea and exercise limitation
◊ Anorexia and weight loss
◊ Fatigue
◊ Progressive hypoxia and cyanosis
◊ Clubbing
◊ Fine, mid-end inspiratory crackles in chest
◊ Cor pulmonale with right heart failure

CAUSES
• Exposure to dust capable of inciting immune response
Some examples:
◊ Farmer's lung (Thermophilic actinomycetes)
◊ Air conditioner lung (Thermophilic actinomycetes)
◊ Bagassosis (Thermophilic actinomycetes)
◊ Bird breeder's lung (Avian protein and blood)
◊ Rat handler's lung (rat urine and protein)
◊ Isocyanate lung (toluene diisocyanate [TDI], methylene diisocyanate [MDI] exposure)
◊ Washing powder lung (Bacillus subtilis enzymes)

RISK FACTORS
• Intensity of exposure
• Size (1-5 micron particles reach deep into lung)
• Smokers at lower risk than non-smokers

 DIAGNOSIS

DIFFERENTIAL DIAGNOSIS
Acute hypersensitivity pneumonia:
◊ Acute infectious pneumonia
◊ Influenza
◊ Adenovirus
◊ Mycoplasma
◊ Pyogenic bacteria
◊ Pneumocystis carinii
◊ Fungus
Chronic hypersensitivity pneumonia:
◊ Tuberculosis
◊ Sarcoidosis
◊ Pneumoconiosis
◊ Scleroderma
◊ Rheumatoid lung
◊ Lupus erythematosis
◊ Eosinophilic granuloma
◊ Lymphangitic carcinomatosis
◊ Fungal infections
◊ Pneumocystis carinii pneumonia
◊ Drug reactions
◊ Hemosiderosis
◊ Idiopathic pulmonary fibrosis

LABORATORY
• Leukocytosis with polymorphonuclear predominance in acute form
• Non-specific elevation of immunoglobulins and erythrocyte sedimentation rate
• Positive rheumatoid test and mononucleosis spot test
• Negative blood, sputum, throat cultures
Drugs that may alter lab results:
Bronchodilators alter lung function
Disorders that may alter lab results:
Asthma or atopy may lead to eosinophilia or increased IgE levels and confuse picture

PATHOLOGICAL FINDINGS
Acute hypersensitivity pneumonitis:
◊ Alveolar walls infiltrated by polymorphs, lymphocytes, macrophages, plasma cells
◊ Eosinophils are rare
◊ Alveolar space contains proteinaceous exudate and edema
◊ Alveolar capillaries with fibrin/platelet thrombi, but no vasculitis

Chronic hypersensitivity pneumonitis:
◊ Alveolitis and interstitial inflammation with lymphocytes, plasma cells and histiocytes with non-caseating granulomas
◊ Focal granulomatous inflammation of bronchioles
◊ Interstitial fibrosis and honeycombing in severe cases

SPECIAL TESTS
• Serum IgG precipitating antibodies to offending agent. Note: 40-50% of non-hypersensitive individuals with high exposure have positive precipitating antibodies.
• Skin testing: Standardized agents poorly available and of limited use
• Inhalation challenge testing can cause severe reactions and therefore is usually not performed except in specialized, in-hospital units
Pulmonary function studies demonstrate:
◊ Reduced lung volume
◊ Impaired gas transfer
◊ Forced expiratory volume (FEV) 1, forced vital capacity (FVC) and FEV1/FVC ratio may be normal early on and then drop with the development of chronic airway obstruction
◊ Forced expiratory flow (FEF) 25-75 and flows near residual volume may be reduced
◊ Decreased lung compliance
Bronchoalveolar lavage
◊ Acute form with neutrophils and lymphocytes
◊ Chronic form with high lymphocytes (60%) mostly T-cells of CD-8 type
◊ Differentiate from sarcoid which has mostly T-cells of CD-4 type
Lung biopsy
◊ Rarely needed if treatment and avoidance of exposure results in improvement (see Pathological Findings)

IMAGING
Acute hypersensitivity pneumonitis on chest roentgenography:
◊ 30-40% abnormal chest roentgenogram
◊ Diffuse interstitial infiltrate with hazy background
◊ Fine nodular shadows from 1-3 mm in size
◊ Linear striated shadows
◊ Occasional lower lobe consolidation
◊ Resolution between attacks
Chronic hypersensitivity pneumonitis on chest roentgenography:
◊ Reticulonodular pattern
◊ Linear shadows and nodules change from fine to coarse pattern with progression of disease
◊ No hilar adenopathy, pleural effusion, or pneumothorax
◊ Upper lobe predominance in 40-50% of cases with ring shadows and bronchiectasis

DIAGNOSTIC PROCEDURES
• Lung biopsy rarely needed for diagnosis
• Role of CT scan is unclear

TREATMENT

APPROPRIATE HEALTH CARE
Outpatient except for acute pneumonitis cases and admission for workup (bronchial alveolar lavage (BAL), lung biopsy, challenge studies)

GENERAL MEASURES
Avoidance of offending antigen

ACTIVITY
Full activity, unless advanced disease

DIET
Normal

PATIENT EDUCATION
• Stress pathogenesis and critical importance of avoidance of allergen
• Stress risk of irreversible lung damage with continued exposure
• Note that chronic exposure may lead to a loss of acute symptoms with exposure, i.e., patient may lose awareness of exposure-symptom relationship
• Printed patient information available from: American Lung Association, 1740 Broadway, New York, NY 10019, (212)315-8700

MEDICATIONS

DRUG(S) OF CHOICE
• Avoidance is primary therapy
• Corticosteroids: Prednisone (2 mg/kg/day or 60 mg/m2/day) or other comparable corticosteroid medication. Initial course of one to two weeks with progressive withdrawal of medication. Alternate day therapy if exposure cannot be discontinued may help, but may not prevent progression.
Contraindications: Refer to manufacturer's literature
Precautions:
Observation for side effects:
◊ Immunosuppression
◊ Salt and water retention
◊ Osteoporosis
◊ Acne
◊ Hirsutism
◊ Behavioral changes
◊ Weight gain/appetite increase
Significant possible interactions: In patients with renal or cardiovascular disease a corticosteroid with minimal sodium retention should be chosen

ALTERNATIVE DRUGS
• Bronchodilators may symptomatically improve patients
• Oxygen may be needed in advanced cases

FOLLOWUP

PATIENT MONITORING
Initial followup should be weekly to monthly depending upon severity and course

PREVENTION/AVOIDANCE
Antigens must be avoided to stop process

POSSIBLE COMPLICATIONS
• Progressive interstitial fibrosis with end-stage lung disease
• Cor pulmonale and right heart failure

EXPECTED COURSE AND PROGNOSIS
• Excellent prognosis with reversal of pathologic findings with effective treatment of early disease
• Stabilization of severe, advanced disease with avoidance and anti-inflammatory medication

MISCELLANEOUS

ASSOCIATED CONDITIONS
N/A

AGE-RELATED FACTORS
Pediatric: N/A
Geriatric: N/A
Others: N/A

PREGNANCY
Avoidance of antigen in early pregnancy. Avoidance and medication in later pregnancy.

SYNONYMS
• Extrinsic allergic alveolitis
• Allergic interstitial pneumonitis

ICD-9-CM
495.9

SEE ALSO
N/A

OTHER NOTES
In acute form, consider other toxic, non-hypersensitivity related conditions such as silo-filler's lung

ABBREVIATIONS
N/A

REFERENCES
• Sharma, O.P.: Hypersensitivity pneumonitis. Disease-a-Month. July 1991; 37(7): 409-71
• Krumpe, P.E., Lum, C.C.Q. & Cross, C.E.: Approach to the patient with diffuse lung disease. Med Clin North Am. September 1988; 72(5): 1225-1246

Author NN Dambro, MD

Hypertension, essential

BASICS

DESCRIPTION Hypertension is defined as a sustained elevated blood pressure (systolic blood pressure of 140 mm Hg or greater and/or diastolic blood pressure of 90 mm Hg or greater). Also conceptually includes the blood pressure level at which the benefits of action exceed those of inaction. Hypertension is a strong risk factor for cardiovascular disease.
System(s) affected: Cardiovascular
Genetics: Blood pressure levels are strongly familial but no clear genetic pattern has been discerned. The strong familial risk for cardiovascular diseases should be concomitantly considered.
Incidence/Prevalence in USA: 58 million in 1983 (20-25% of population)
Predominant age: Essential (primary, benign, idiopathic) hypertension usually has its onset in the 20's to 30's
Predominant sex: Males > Females (males tend to run higher pressures than females but more importantly have a significantly higher risk of cardiovascular disease at any given blood pressure)

SIGNS AND SYMPTOMS
• Hypertension should be considered asymptomatic except in extremes or after related cardiovascular complications develop
• Headache can be seen especially with higher blood pressures. This is often present on awakening and occipital in nature.
• Retinopathy - narrowed arteries, AV nicking, copper or silver wiring of retinal arterioles
• Increased A2 heart sound

CAUSES
• Over 90% of hypertension has no identified cause. These can be labeled essential or primary hypertension.
• Secondary causes of hypertension include four areas:
Renal parenchymal
  ◊ Glomerulonephritis
  ◊ Pyelonephritis
  ◊ Polycystic kidneys
Endocrine
  ◊ Primary hyperaldosteronism
  ◊ Pheochromocytoma
  ◊ Hyperthyroidism
  ◊ Cushing's syndrome
Vascular
  ◊ Coarctation
  ◊ Renal artery stenosis
Chemical
  ◊ Oral contraceptives
  ◊ NSAID's
  ◊ Decongestants
  ◊ Antidepressants
  ◊ Sympathomimetics
  ◊ Many industrial chemicals
  ◊ Corticosteroids
  ◊ Ergotamine alkaloids
  ◊ Lithium
  ◊ Cyclosporine

RISK FACTORS
• Family history
• Obesity
• Alcohol
• Excess dietary sodium
• Stress
• Physical inactivity

DIAGNOSIS

DIFFERENTIAL DIAGNOSIS Secondary hypertension (because of the low incidence of reversible secondary hypertension, special tests should be considered only if the history, physical, or basic laboratory evaluation indicates the possibility)

LABORATORY
• Hemoglobin and hematocrit or CBC
• Complete urinalysis (sometimes reveals proteinuria)
• Potassium, calcium and creatinine
• Cholesterol
• Fasting blood glucose
• Uric acid
Drugs that may alter lab results:
Numerous drugs and foods interfere with catecholamine measurements in considering pheochromocytoma
Disorders that may alter lab results: N/A

PATHOLOGICAL FINDINGS
Late complications include
  ◊ Stroke
  ◊ Retinal vascular narrowing, hemorrhages, exudates, papilledema
  ◊ Left ventricular hypertrophy
  ◊ Congestive heart failure
  ◊ Ischemic heart disease
  ◊ Proteinuria and nephrosclerosis

SPECIAL TESTS
Only if history, physical or lab indicates
  ◊ IVP and renal arteriogram
  ◊ Plasma catecholamines, urinary metanephrines/vanillylmandelic acid
  ◊ Plasma renin
  ◊ Aortogram
  ◊ ECG

IMAGING
If history or physical indicate
  ◊ Chest X-ray
  ◊ Ultrasonography
  ◊ IVP
  ◊ Digital subtraction arteriography
  ◊ Angiogram

DIAGNOSTIC PROCEDURES
• Renal biopsy if renal parenchymal disease is suspected
• A presumptive diagnosis of hypertension can be made if the average of at least three blood pressure measurements exceeds either 90 mm Hg diastolic or 160 mm Hg systolic, assuming proper resting conditions, cuff size and application are maintained

The Joint National Committee on Detection, Evaluation, and Treatment of High Blood Pressure (JNC) recommends a good history and physical exam with emphasis on:
  ◊ Family history of hypertension and cardiovascular disease
  ◊ Personal past history of cardiovascular, cerebrovascular and renal disease as well as diabetes
  ◊ Previous elevated blood pressures
  ◊ Previous treatments
  ◊ History of weight gain, exercise activities, sodium intake, fat intake and alcohol use
  ◊ Symptoms suggesting secondary hypertension
  ◊ Psychosocial and environmental factors affecting blood pressure
  ◊ Other cardiovascular risk factors such as obesity, smoking, hyperlipidemia, and diabetes
  ◊ Fundoscopic exam for arteriolar narrowing, arteriovenous compression, hemorrhages, exudates, and papilledema
  ◊ Complete cardiac and peripheral pulse exam. Compare radial and femoral pulse for differences in volume and timing.
  ◊ Abdominal exam for masses and bruits. Listen high in the flanks over the kidneys.

TREATMENT

APPROPRIATE HEALTH CARE
Outpatient

GENERAL MEASURES
• Goal blood pressures should be individualized based on risk factors but generally treat to diastolic < 90 mm Hg and systolic < 160 mm Hg
• Weight reduction for obese patients may significantly lower blood pressures
• Smoking cessation is an important part of a comprehensive cardiovascular risk reduction program
• Biofeedback and relaxation exercises have been shown to reduce blood pressures

ACTIVITY Normal activity with an appropriate aerobic fitness program

DIET
• Some patients will respond to to a reduced salt diet
• Alcohol consumption should be reduced to less than 1 ounce per day
• Decrease saturated fats and increase polyunsaturated fats
• Potassium and calcium should be considered although absolute effect uncertain

PATIENT EDUCATION
• Emphasize asymptomatic nature of hypertension and importance of lifetime treatment
• Review risk factors for cardiovascular disease with emphasis on comprehensive preventive program
• Printed Aids for High Blood Pressure Education: A Guide to Evaluated Publications, NIH Publication No. 85-1244

MEDICATIONS

DRUG(S) OF CHOICE
• First line choices include the following four categories and their representatives

Diuretics
◊ Hydrochlorothiazide 12.5-50 mg qd
◊ Chlorthalidone 12.5-50 mg qd
◊ Indapamide 2.5-5 mg qd

ACE inhibitors
◊ Captopril 25-300 mg bid
◊ Enalapril 2.5-20 mg qd
◊ Fosinopril 10-80 mg qd
◊ Lisinopril 5-20 mg qd
◊ Ramipril 2.5-20 mg qd
◊ Quinapril 10-80 mg qd
◊ Benazepril 10-40 mg qd
◊ Cilazapril 2.5-5 mg qd
◊ Perindopril 1-16 mg qd
◊ Spirapril 12.5-50 mg qd

Calcium channel blockers
◊ Diltiazem (sustained release) 180-360 mg qd
◊ Felodipine 5-20 mg qd
◊ Isradipine 2.5-10 mg bid
◊ Nicardipine 20-40 mg tid
◊ Nifedipine (slow release system) 30-120 mg qd
◊ Nitrendipine 5-40 mg qd
◊ Verapamil (sustained release) 120-480 mg qd

Beta blockers
◊ Acebutolol 400-800 mg qd
◊ Atenolol 25-100 mg qd
◊ Metoprolol 50-200 mg qd
◊ Nadolol 40-320 mg qd
◊ Penbutolol 20-40 mg qd
◊ Pindolol 5-30 mg bid
◊ Propranolol 40-240 mg/day, divided bid
◊ Timolol 10-40 mg daily, divided bid
◊ Betaxolol 5-40 mg qd

Contraindications:
• See manufacturer's insert for complete contraindications
• Diuretics may worsen gout and diabetes
• Beta blockers are contraindicated in reactive airway disease, heart failure, and heart block. Diabetes and peripheral vascular disease are relative contraindications.
• Diltiazem and verapamil should be used cautiously with heart failure or block
Precautions: See manufacturer's profile of each drug
Significant possible interactions: See manufacturer's profile of each drug

ALTERNATIVE DRUGS
Many may be added to the above for combination therapy

Alpha adrenergic agents
◊ Prazosin 1-10 mg bid
◊ Terazosin 1-20 mg qd
◊ Doxazosin 1-16 mg qd

Centrally acting adrenergic inhibitors
◊ Clonidine 0.1-1.2 mg bid or weekly patch 0.1 mg/day to 0.3 mg/day
◊ Guanabenz 4-32 mg bid
◊ Guanfacine 1-3 mg qd
◊ Methyldopa 250-2000 mg bid

Peripherally acting adrenergic inhibitors
◊ Guanadrel 5-75 mg daily, divided bid
◊ Guanethidine 10-50 mg qd
◊ Reserpine 0.1-0.25 mg qd
◊ Labetalol 100-900 mg bid

Vasodilators
◊ Hydralazine 25-150 mg bid
◊ Minoxidil (rarely used due to adverse effects)

Loop diuretics
◊ Furosemide 20-320 mg qd
◊ Bumetanide 0.5-2 mg qd
◊ Ethacrynic acid 25-100 mg qd

Potassium sparing diuretics
◊ Generally used in patients who have developed hypokalemia with thiazide diuretics
◊ Amiloride 5-10 mg qd
◊ Spironolactone 25-100 mg qd
◊ Triamterene 50-150 mg qd

FOLLOWUP

PATIENT MONITORING
• Once stable, patients should be reevaluated at least every 3 to 6 months
• Review compliance, effectiveness and adverse reactions
• Quality of life issues should be considered, including sexual function
• At least annual evaluation of urinalysis, creatinine and potassium are appropriate, generally as part of a screening laboratory panel

PREVENTION/AVOIDANCE   Diet, exercise, reduce stress, stop smoking, little or no alcohol, compliance in taking medications

POSSIBLE COMPLICATIONS
• Congestive heart failure
• Renal failure
• Myocardial infarction
• Stroke
• Hypertensive heart disease

EXPECTED COURSE AND PROGNOSIS   Good with adequate control

MISCELLANEOUS

ASSOCIATED CONDITIONS   See list in Causes

AGE-RELATED FACTORS
Pediatric:
• Blood pressure should be measured during routine examinations
• Hypertension can accompany a wide variety of acute and chronic illnesses in this age group
Geriatric: Isolated systolic hypertension more common in this group. Therapy has been shown to be effective although adverse reactions to medications are more frequent.
Others: N/A

PREGNANCY   Elevated blood pressures during pregnancy may be either chronic hypertension or pregnancy induced preeclampsia. Maternal and fetal mortality benefit from treatment. See topic on preeclampsia. Some medications may adversely affect the fetus.

SYNONYMS
• Benign hypertension
• Idiopathic hypertension
• Familial hypertension
• High blood pressure
• Chronic hypertension
• Genetic hypertension

ICD-9-CM   401.1

SEE ALSO
• Hypertension, malignant
• Hypertension, emergency

OTHER NOTES   N/A

ABBREVIATIONS   N/A

REFERENCES
• Kaplan, N.M.: Clinical Hypertension. Baltimore, Williams & Wilkins, 1990
• McMahon, F.G.: Management of Essential Hypertension. New York, Futura Publishing, 1990
• The Fifth Report of the Joint National Committee on the Detection, Evaluation, and Treatment of High Blood Pressure. In Arch Intern Med 153: 154-183 Jan, 1993

Author   D. Burtner, M.D.

Hypertension, malignant

BASICS

DESCRIPTION Severe hypertension characterized by retinopathy with or without papilledema, associated with necrosis of small arteries and arterioles. The diastolic pressure is generally greater that 130 mm Hg.
System(s) affected: Cardiovascular, renal
Genetics: No genetic pattern
Incidence/Prevalence in USA: Incidence: Approximately 1% of hypertensive patients
Predominant age: Average age 40 years
Predominant sex: Male > Female

SIGNS AND SYMPTOMS
- Headache 40%
- Blurred vision 40%
- Cardiac symptoms (chest pain, dyspnea) 25%
- Nausea and vomiting 15%
- Focal neurologic signs < 5%
- Hypertension > 90%
- Retinopathy, grade III or IV (exudates, hemorrhages) with or without papilledema > 90%
- Pulmonary edema 50-90%
- Stupor or coma 50-90%
- Restlessness 50-90%
- Seizures 50-90%

CAUSES
- Hypertension - ten times more frequent in secondary hypertension than essential hypertension
- Noncompliance with antihypertensive medication
- Pathophysiology related to autoregulatory failure in the presence of high arterial pressures

RISK FACTORS
- African American
- Tobacco use
- Secondary hypertension

DIAGNOSIS

DIFFERENTIAL DIAGNOSIS
- Severe hypertension without retinopathy - consider pheochromocytoma, clonidine withdrawal, tyramine ingestion with MAO-inhibitor use
- Thrombotic thrombocytopenic purpura

LABORATORY
- Red cell casts (> 90%)
- Hematuria (> 90%)
- Proteinuria (> 90%)
- Azotemia (> 90%)
- Decreased creatinine clearance (> 90%)
- Hypokalemic alkalosis (> 90%)
- Microangiopathic hemolytic anemia (50-90%)
- Thrombocytopenia (50-90%)
- Disseminated intravascular coagulation (50-90%)
Drugs that may alter lab results: N/A
Disorders that may alter lab results: N/A

PATHOLOGICAL FINDINGS
- Fibrinoid arteriolar necrosis (> 90%)
- Glomerular onion skin lesion (50-90%)
- Renal tubular degeneration (50-90%)

SPECIAL TESTS N/A

IMAGING
- Renal ultrasound: small kidneys
- Renal scan: decreased isotope uptake

DIAGNOSTIC PROCEDURES N/A

TREATMENT

APPROPRIATE HEALTH CARE
Hospitalization, intensive care with hemodynamic monitoring as dictated by clinical status

GENERAL MEASURES Goal is to resolve symptoms, reduce diastolic blood pressure to 100 mm Hg (or mean arterial pressure to < 120 mm Hg), and maintain urine output greater that 20 mL/hr. Too rapid lowering of BP can lead to cerebral ischemia.

ACTIVITY Bed rest

DIET Low sodium

PATIENT EDUCATION
- Emphasis on compliance with treatment
- American Heart Association, 7320 Greenville Avenue, Dallas, TX 75231, (214)373-6300

MEDICATIONS

DRUG(S) OF CHOICE
• Nitroprusside (Nipride): 0.3 mcg/kg/min (25-50 mcg/min) IV infusion and titrate in a very few minutes to a maximum of 10 mcg/kg/min. Immediate onset of action; ideal for patients with ischemia, CHF, aortic dissection (use with beta blocker), or intracranial hemorrhage. Contraindicated in pregnancy.
• Trimethaphan (Arfonad): 0.5-1 mg/min (500 mg/500 mL D5W) and titrate. Immediate onset of action; second line therapy when nitroprusside cannot be used.
• Labetalol (Trandate, Normodyne): Initial dose of 20 mg IV over 2 min, then follow with increasingly higher doses (40-80 mg) at 10 minute intervals until desired blood pressure is reached or a cumulative dose of 300 mg has been given. Experience limited in malignant hypertension, but beneficial with combined alpha- and beta-blocking effect. Avoid in CHF, asthma, heart block.
• Diazoxide (Hyperstat): 1-3 mg/kg IV push to maximum of 150 mg q 5-15 minutes. Contraindicated in patients with ischemic heart disease, dissection, intracranial hemorrhage, or AV shunts.
• Nifedipine (Procardia): 10-20 mg sublingual. Intermediate onset; drug of choice when invasive monitoring not required. Contraindicated in aortic dissection.
• Hydralazine: 5-15 mg IV. Repeat doses as needed. Preferred treatment in pregnant women.
• Phentolamine (Regitine): 2-5 mg IV. Drug of choice in suspected pheochromocytoma crisis, clonidine withdrawal, CNS trauma, MAO-I crisis.
Contraindications: See above with individual drugs
Precautions: Beware of cyanide and thiocyanate toxicity with nitroprusside, especially in presence of renal dysfunction or prolonged administration (>3 days)
Significant possible Interactions: Refer to manufacturer's literature

ALTERNATIVE DRUGS
Dopamine-1 receptor agonists (still investigational) may preserve renal function better than other agents. Oral therapy should be started after blood pressure is controlled with emergency parenteral therapy.

FOLLOWUP

PATIENT MONITORING
Follow blood pressure, renal function, urinalysis

PREVENTION/AVOIDANCE
Appropriate management of hypertension

POSSIBLE COMPLICATIONS
• Renal failure
• Encephalopathy
• Congestive heart failure
• Stroke
• Retinopathy

EXPECTED COURSE AND PROGNOSIS
• With treatment, > 70% survival at 5 years, 50% renal failure
• Without treatment, > 90% mortality

MISCELLANEOUS

ASSOCIATED CONDITIONS
• Chronic renal failure
• Renovascular hypertension
• Acute glomerulonephritis
• Renal vasculitis
• Pheochromocytoma
• Preeclampsia

AGE-RELATED FACTORS
Pediatric: May manifest encephalopathy at lower blood pressures than adults
Geriatric: Higher mortality
Others: N/A

PREGNANCY
Hydralazine drug of choice. Treat eclampsia.

SYNONYMS
• Accelerated hypertension
• Hypertensive emergency

ICD-9-CM
401.0

SEE ALSO
• Hypertension, essential
• Hypertensive emergencies
• Pheochromocytoma

OTHER NOTES
N/A

ABBREVIATIONS
N/A

REFERENCES
• Haber, E. & Slater, E.E.: Hypertensive Emergencies in High Blood Pressure, In Scientific American Medicine, Edited by E. Rubenstein & D.D. Federman. 1978-1992; Scientific American Inc.
• Williams, G.H.: Hypertensive Vascular Disease. In Harrison's Principles of Internal Medicine, 12th Ed. Edited by E. Braunwald, et al. New York, McGraw-Hill, 1991

Author A. Warner, M.D.

Hypertensive emergencies

 BASICS

DESCRIPTION
Terminology describing hypertensive emergencies can be confusing. Terms such as "hypertensive crisis", "malignant hypertension", "hypertensive urgency", "accelerated hypertension" and "severe hypertension" are all used in the literature and often overlap. Some definitions include a specific diastolic or systolic blood pressure reading, while others emphasize an acute change in the blood pressure or the presence of specific clinical syndromes.
• Severe hypertension is defined as a diastolic blood pressure of 115 mm Hg or greater. Patients with severe hypertension may or may not have a hypertensive emergency. A hypertensive emergency occurs when an acute elevation of blood pressure causes rapid and progressive end-organ damage, particularly in the cardiovascular, renal and central nervous systems.

Genetics: N/A

Incidence/Prevalence: Less than 1% of patients with hypertension

Predominant age: Young or middle-aged patients with known hypertensive disease

Predominant sex: Male > Female

SIGNS AND SYMPTOMS
• Headache
• Seizure
• Visual disturbances
• Chest pain
• Shortness of breath
• Orthopnea and dyspnea on exertion
• Focal deficits
• Acute myocardial ischemia
• Unstable angina
• Infarction
• Pulmonary edema
• Cerebrovascular accident
• Hemorrhage
• Thrombosis
• Embolus
• Subarachnoid hemorrhage
• Acute renal failure

CAUSES
• Drugs that elevate blood pressure - decongestants, appetite suppressants, steroids (including oral contraceptives), monoamine oxidase inhibitors (MAOI's) in combination with certain foods or drugs, and drugs of abuse such as cocaine or amphetamine
• Withdrawal from antihypertensives, especially clonidine (Catapres)
• Withdrawal from CNS depressants
• Antihypertensive withdrawal
• Eclampsia/preeclampsia

RISK FACTORS
• History of hypertension
• Drug abuse
• Non-compliance with medications

 DIAGNOSIS

DIFFERENTIAL DIAGNOSIS
Other CNS pathology

LABORATORY
• Urinalysis and renal function tests
• Urine drug screen in selected patients
• Blood count and smear may indicate microangiopathic hemolytic anemia
• Serum electrolytes can be measured to check for hypokalemia
• Calcium, glucose, uric acid and lipid profiles
• Subsequent work-up for renal artery stenosis or pheochromocytoma in selected patients

Drugs that may alter lab results: N/A

Disorders that may alter lab results: N/A

PATHOLOGICAL FINDINGS
Extreme blood pressure elevations can overwhelm the autoregulatory mechanisms for organ blood flow resulting in damage to the arteriolar and capillary beds. This process produces organ hemorrhages and edema from the leakage of blood and fluid.

SPECIAL TESTS
• Electrocardiography may reveal ischemia or left ventricular hypertrophy
• Funduscopic examination may reveal papilledema, exudates or hemorrhages

IMAGING
Chest radiographs:
◊ May show pulmonary edema and cardiomegaly due to congestive heart failure
◊ Mediastinal widening and blunting of the aortic knob consistent with a dissecting aneurysm

DIAGNOSTIC PROCEDURES
• Blood pressure - measured with an appropriately sized cuff, and two or more readings from both arms should be averaged before the blood pressure is accepted as elevated
• Sphygmomanometer is recommended

 TREATMENT

APPROPRIATE HEALTH CARE
Patients should be managed in an intensive care unit

GENERAL MEASURES
• Place the patient in a comfortable environment, which in itself may help lower the blood pressure
• While treatment must be individualized, a general goal is to lower the mean arterial pressure by approximately 20-25% or reduce diastolic pressure to 100-110 mm Hg over one hour
• If ongoing end-organ damage is thought to be secondary to the hypertensive state, prompt treatment with intravenous medication is indicated. Monitor patient closely so that a rapid fall in blood pressure can be avoided.
• Optimally, an arterial catheter is used to continuously monitor blood pressure
• Antihypertensive medications should be delivered by an intravenous infusion pump
• Mean arterial pressure is approximately one-third of the sum of twice the diastolic pressure plus the systolic pressure

ACTIVITY Restricted in intensive care setting. A quiet environment without excess stimulation is preferred.

DIET No diet ordered until blood pressure under control, then, low sodium diet for hypertension

PATIENT EDUCATION
• Importance of medication compliance
• Lack of symptoms with hypertension until organ damage occurs

MEDICATIONS

DRUG(S) OF CHOICE

• The specific drug used for management of hypertensive emergencies depends on the end organs affected and the patient's overall clinical status. All medications are administered IV unless otherwise indicated. Dosages listed below.

Hypertensive encephalopathy
◊ Nitroprusside (Nipride, Nitropress) infusion 0.5-10.0 mcg per kg per minute
or
◊ Diazoxide (Hyperstat) infusion 7.5-30.0 mg per minute
or
◊ Labetalol (Normodyne, Trandate) bolus 20-80 mg every 10-15 minutes; infusion 0.5-2.0 mg per minute

Central nervous system events
◊ Nitroprusside (treat only if diastolic pressure > 130 mm Hg) infusion: 0.5-10.0 mcg per kg per minute

Myocardial ischemia
◊ Nitroglycerin infusion 5-100 mcg per minute
or
◊ Labetalol (Normodyne, Trandate) bolus 20-80 mg every 10-15 minutes; infusion 0.5-2.0 mg per minute or
◊ Oral nifedipine (Adalat, Procardia) 10 or 20 mg nifedipine capsule. Patient bites the capsule and then swallows it. If the desired blood pressure response is not achieved in 20-30 minutes, a repeat dose of 10 mg can be administered.

Congestive heart failure
◊ Nitroprusside (Nipride, Nitropress) infusion 0.5-10.0 mcg per kg per minute
or
◊ Nitroglycerin infusion 5-100 mcg per minute

Aortic dissection
◊ Nitroprusside (Nipride, Nitropress) infusion 0.5-10.0 mcg per kg per minute and propranolol (Inderal) 2-4 mg/hr or
◊ Trimethaphan (Arfonad) infusion 0.5 to 5.0 mg per minute and propranolol (Inderal) 2-4 mg/hr

Renal failure
◊ Nitroprusside (Nipride, Nitropress) infusion 0.5-10.0 mcg per kg per minute
◊ Labetalol (Normodyne, Trandate) bolus 20-80 mg every 10-15 minutes; infusion 0.5-2.0 mg per minute

Pheochromocytoma
◊ Phentolamine (Regitine) bolus 5-10 mg every 5-15 minutes or
◊ Labetalol (Normodyne, Trandate) bolus 20-80 mg every 10-15 minutes; infusion 0.5-2.0 mg per minute or
◊ Nitroprusside infusion 0.5-10.0 mcg per kg per minute

Antihypertensive withdrawal
◊ Labetalol (Normodyne, Trandate) bolus 20-80 mg every 10-15 minutes; infusion 0.5-2.0 mg per minute or
◊ Phentolamine (Regitine) bolus 5-10 mg every 5-15 minutes

Interactions between monoamine oxidase inhibitors and foods or drugs
◊ Phentolamine (Regitine) bolus 5-10 mg every 5-15 minutes or
◊ Labetalol (Normodyne, Trandate) bolus 20-80 mg every 10-15 minutes; infusion 0.5-2.0 mg per minute

Eclampsia/preeclampsia
◊ Hydralazine (Apresoline) bolus 5-20 mg every 20 minutes

Severe hypertension (hypertensive urgencies) without acute end-organ damage
◊ Oral nifedipine (Adalat, Procardia) 10 or 20 mg nifedipine capsule. Patient bites the capsule and then swallows it. If the desired blood pressure response is not achieved in 20-30 minutes, a repeat dose of 10 mg can be administered or
◊ Clonidine - give an oral loading dose of 0.2 mg followed by 0.1 mg per hour until blood pressure has been lowered or a total dose of 0.8 mg has been administered

Contraindications:
• Diazoxide - not recommended for patients with suspected myocardial ischemia, congestive heart failure or aortic dissection
• Labetalol, because of its beta-blockade property, should not be used in patients with asthma, chronic obstructive lung disease, congestive heart failure, heart block, cardiogenic shock or severe bradycardia

Precautions:
• Nitroprusside - when intravenous nitroprusside is continued for more than 48-72 hours, or the patient has compromised renal function, plasma thiocyanate levels should be monitored so that cyanide toxicity can be prevented
• Diazoxide - may produce reflex tachycardia with increased myocardial oxygen consumption (can be prevented by pretreatment with intravenous propranolol [Inderal])
• Hydralazine may produce reflex tachycardia and increase myocardial oxygen consumption (response can be mitigated by using a beta blocker before administration of hydralazine). Hydralazine should be used with caution when myocardial insufficiency is suspected.

Significant possible interactions: N/A

ALTERNATIVE DRUGS   Listed above

FOLLOWUP

PATIENT MONITORING   Monitor closely to avoid a rapid fall in blood pressure

PREVENTION/AVOIDANCE   Counsel patient on importance of compliance with antihypertensive treatment and dangers of abrupt stopage of medication

POSSIBLE COMPLICATIONS
• Abrupt lowering of the blood pressure may result in inadequate cerebral or cardiac blood flow, leading to stroke or myocardial ischemia
• Authorities have questioned whether the benefits of aggressive treatment outweigh the risks in patients with severe hypertension but no end-organ damage. No studies have proven that aggressive treatment reduces the risk of long-term morbidity or mortality from hypertensive urgencies.

EXPECTED COURSE AND PROGNOSIS
• The blood pressure should return to normal levels within 24 hours
• Begin chronic oral antihypertensives (see chapter on hypertension)

MISCELLANEOUS

ASSOCIATED CONDITIONS   N/A

AGE-RELATED FACTORS
Pediatric: Usually associated with renal disease
Geriatric: N/A
Others: N/A

PREGNANCY   See eclampsia and preeclampsia

SYNONYMS
• Hypertensive crisis
• Severe hypertension

ICD-9-CM   437.2

SEE ALSO
• Hypertension, essential
• Hypertension, malignant

OTHER NOTES   N/A

ABBREVIATIONS   N/A

REFERENCES
• Gifford, R.W.: Management of Hypertensive Crisis. J Amer Med Soc, 1991; 226:829-835
• Calhoun, D.A. & Oparil, S.: Treatment of hypertensive crisis. N Engl J Med, 1990;323:1177-83
• The 1988 report of the Joint National Committee on Detection, Evaluation, and Treatment of High Blood pressure. Arch Intern Med, 1988;148:1023-38

Author   A. Sanders, M.D.

Hyperthyroidism

 BASICS

DESCRIPTION
The reaction to excess production of thyroid hormone. Types of hyperthyroidism include:
• Graves' disease (GD) - the most common form - an autoimmune disease. Thyroid stimulating immunoglobulins (TSI's) of the IgG class are produced and bind to thyrotropin (TSH) receptors on the thyroid gland. The TSI's mimic the action of TSH and cause excess secretion of thyroxine (T4) and triiodothyronine (T3). Goiter and ophthalmopathy are common characteristics.
• Spontaneously resolving hyperthyroidism (SRH) - uncommon disorder which is a variant of lymphocytic thyroiditis. Goiter and eventual hypothyroidism are important features
• Toxic multinodular goiter - occurs late in life. Nodules are insidious and almost never malignant. No ophthalmopathy or localized myxedema present.
• Toxic uninodular goiter - solitary nodule with autonomous function. Almost always benign.
• Other causes are rare and include TSH-secreting, pituitary tumors, surreptitious ingestion of T4 or T3, functioning trophoblastic tumors, and iodine-induced hyperthyroidism
System(s) affected: Endocrine/Metabolic
Genetics: Unknown
Incidence/Prevalence in USA: 1:1000 in women, 1:3000 in men
Predominant age: Any age, peaks in 3rd and 4th decades
Predominant sex: Female > Male

SIGNS AND SYMPTOMS
In adults
◊ Nervousness (85%)
◊ Increased sweating (70%)
◊ Heat intolerance (70%)
◊ Palpitations and tachycardia (75%)
◊ Dyspnea (75%)
◊ Fatigue and weakness (60%)
◊ Weight loss (0%)
◊ Increased appetite (40%)
◊ Ophthalmopathy (25%)
◊ Goiter (95%)
◊ Tremor (65%)
◊ Warm and moist skin (72%)
◊ Emotional lability
In children
◊ Linear growth acceleration
◊ Ophthalmic abnormalities more common

CAUSES
• Graves' disease - autoimmune disease
• Spontaneously resolving hyperthyroidism - autoimmune disease, with increased risk during pregnancy
• Toxic uninodular goiter - unknown

RISK FACTORS
• Positive family history
• Female sex
• Other autoimmune disorders

 DIAGNOSIS

DIFFERENTIAL DIAGNOSIS
• Anxiety
• Malignancy
• Diabetes
• Pregnancy
• Menopause
• Pheochromocytoma

LABORATORY
• T3 - Radioimmunoassay (RIA) > 200 ng/mL
• T4 - RIA >12.5 mcg/dl
• Free thyroxine index (FTI) >12
• TSH - RIA undetectable
• Radioiodine uptake (RIU) - high in Graves' disease, low in spontaneously resolving hyperthyroidism, high or normal in toxic nodules
Drugs that may alter lab results:
• Anabolic steroids
• Androgens
• Estrogens
• Heparin
• Iodine containing compounds
• Phenytoin
• Rifampin
• Salicylates
• Thyroxine
Disorders that may alter lab results:
• A variety of non-thyroidal illnesses can alter T4 and T3 with little effect on TSH
• FTI permits correction of misleading results caused by pregnancy and estrogens

PATHOLOGICAL FINDINGS
• Graves' disease - hyperplasia
• Spontaneously resolving hyperthyroidism - lymphocytic infiltration
• Toxic nodules - nodule formation

SPECIAL TESTS
Immunoradiometric assays

IMAGING
Thyroid scans using radioiodine: diffuse in GD, patchy in SRH, focal in toxic nodule

DIAGNOSTIC PROCEDURES   N/A

 TREATMENT

APPROPRIATE HEALTH CARE
• Outpatient except for treatment of thyroid storm, a life-threatening condition which may cause heart failure, mania, or coma
• Inpatient when subtotal thyroidectomy is the mode of treatment

GENERAL MEASURES
Antithyroid drugs, therapeutic radioiodine, and rarely, subtotal thyroidectomy

ACTIVITY
Modify activity according to disease severity

DIET
Sufficient calories to prevent weight loss

PATIENT EDUCATION
Importance of compliance with drug therapy

Hyperthyroidism

MEDICATIONS

DRUG(S) OF CHOICE
Initial treatment
- Propylthiouracil (PTU)
  ◊ Adults (preferred in elderly, those with cardiac disease, thyroid storm, and pregnant and lactating women) 100-900 mg/day po given tid
  ◊ Children > 10, 150-300 mg/day po given tid or 5-7 mg/kg/day. Radioiodine often first choice
  ◊ Children 6-10, 50-150 mg/day po given tid or 5-7 mg/kg/day. Radioiodine often first choice.
- Methimazole (MMI) (Tapazole)
  ◊ Adults 15-60 mg/day po given once daily
  ◊ Children 6-10, 0.4 mg/kg/day po given daily
Maintenance with antithyroids
- PTU
  ◊ Adults 50-600 mg/day given bid po
  ◊ Children 50 mg bid po (or 1/2-2/3 of initial dose)
- MMI
  ◊ Adults 5-30 mg/day po given daily
  ◊ Children 0.2 mg/kg/day po given daily
Thyrotoxic crisis
- PTU (preferred over MMI)
  ◊ Adults 15-20 mg po q4h during the first day (as an adjunct to other therapies)
  ◊ Neonates 10 mg/kg/day po given q4h
Additional drugs:
  ◊ Radioiodine therapy - Sodium iodine131 (Iodotope I-131). Dosage calculation: (80uCi/g thyroid tissue x thyroid weight) divided by 24 hour radioactive iodine uptake
  ◊ Beta blocker - propranolol (Inderal) 40-240 mg daily po
Contraindications:
- Radioiodine therapy - pregnancy and nursing
- Propranolol - congestive heart failure, asthma, chronic bronchitis, pregnancy, hypoglycemia
Precautions:
- PTU and MMI - may cause dermatitis agranulocytosis or hepatotoxicity
- Radioiodine therapy - may cause fetal hypothyroidism or malformation if administered during pregnancy
Significant possible interactions: Oral anticoagulants may be potentiated by PTU

ALTERNATIVE DRUGS
Ipodate sodium (Oragrafin) - 0.5 g qid po

FOLLOWUP

PATIENT MONITORING
- Repeat thyroid tests twice a year
- CBC and liver function tests when appropriate
- Therapy with antithyroids continues 3-12 months
- After radioiodine therapy, thyroid function tests at 6 weeks, 12 weeks, 6 months and annually thereafter if euthyroid

PREVENTION/AVOIDANCE   N/A

POSSIBLE COMPLICATIONS
- Hypoparathyroidism, recurrent laryngeal nerve damage, and hypothyroidism with subtotal thyroidectomy
- Development of hypothyroidism after radioiodine treatment
- Visual loss or diplopia due to severe ophthalmopathy
- Localized pretibial myxedema at any time
- Thyroid acropachy
- Cardiac failure in the elderly with underlying heart disease
- Osteoporosis
- Muscle wasting
- Nephrocalcinosis

PREVENTION/AVOIDANCE   N/A

EXPECTED COURSE AND PROGNOSIS
With precise diagnosis and adequate treatment, prognosis is good

MISCELLANEOUS

ASSOCIATED CONDITIONS
Other autoimmune diseases and Down syndrome

AGE-RELATED FACTORS
Pediatric: Neonates treated with antithyroids 2-3 months. Most children treated with antithyroids.
Geriatric:
- Characteristic symptoms and signs may be absent in elderly
- Harder to diagnose
- Cardiac failure more likely
Others: N/A

PREGNANCY
- Treat with small doses of PTU due to increased risk of spontaneous abortion and premature delivery in hyperthyroid pregnant women
- Avoid treatment induced hypothyroidism
- Symptoms may be confusing
- Thyrotoxicosis often improves during pregnancy and relapses postpartum
- Radioiodine therapy absolutely contraindicated

SYNONYMS   Thyrotoxicosis

ICD-9-CM
- 242.0 toxic diffuse goiter
- 242.9 thyrotoxicosis without mention of goiter or other cause

SEE ALSO   N/A

OTHER NOTES   N/A

ABBREVIATIONS
- TSI = thyroid stimulating immunoglobulins
- TSH = thyroid stimulating hormone
- T4 = thyroxine
- T3 = triiodothyronine
- RIA = radioimmunoassay
- FTI = free thyroxine index
- RIU = radioiodine uptake
- PTU = propylthiouracil
- MMI = methimazole

REFERENCES
- Bardin, C.W., (ed.): Current Therapy in Endocrinology and Metabolism. 4th Ed. Philadelphia, B.C. Decker, 1991
- Becker, K.L. (ed.): Principles and Practice of Endocrinology and Metabolism. Philadelphia, J.B. Lippincott, 1990
- Degroot, L.J. (ed.): Endocrinology. 2nd Ed. Philadelphia, W.B. Saunders Co, 1989

Author   R. Levy, M.D.

Hypertriglyceridemia

BASICS

DESCRIPTION The hypertriglyceridemias are a heterogenous family of disorders due to disturbances in synthesis or degradation of triglycerides rich plasma lipoprotein.
• Normal triglycerides is less than 100 in children and less than 150 mg/dL in adults.
• Borderline hypertriglyceridemia: 250-500 mg/dL
• Distinct hypertriglyceridemia: More than 500 mg/dL
<u>Physiology:</u> The major triglycerides containing lipoproteins are:
◊ Chylomicron: In post prandial state from absorption of dietary fat from the gut.
◊ Vary low density lipoprotein (VLDL): In fasting state endogenous synthesis from carbohydrates and fatty acid in the liver.
◊ Intermediate density lipoprotein (IDL): From degradation of chylomicron and VLDL
<u>Classification:</u> Hypertriglyceridemia falls into one of the following groups based on the lipoprotein pattern:
◊ Type I Elevated chylomicron
◊ Type II-b Elevated LDL and VLDL
◊ Type III Elevated IDL
◊ Type IV Elevated VLDL
◊ Type V Elevated VLDL and chylomicrons
Note: This classification is only descriptive and provides little insight into the mechanism of the disorders. A single disease state can lead to several different lipoprotein patterns, the pattern can change with time and a single lipoprotein phenotype can be caused by multiple disease states.
Genetics:
• Familial combined hyperlipidemia - autosomal dominant
• Polygenic hyperlipidemia - polygenic
• Familial hypertriglyceridemia - autosomal dominant
• Familial dyslipoproteinemia - autosomal recessive
Incidence/Prevalence in USA:
• Familial combined hyperlipidemia - 1/200
• Polygenic hyperlipidemia - unknown
• Familial hypertriglyceridemia - 1/500
• Familial dyslipoproteinemia - 1/10,000
Predominant age: N/A
Predominant sex: Male > Female

SIGNS AND SYMPTOMS
• Very high triglycerides (over 1,000)
◊ Abdominal pain/acute pancreatitis
◊ Eruptive xanthoma
◊ Lipemia retinalis
◊ Hepatosplenomegaly
◊ Memory loss/dementia
◊ Peripheral neuropathy/paresthesia
• Atherosclerosis

CAUSES
<u>Primary</u>
◊ Sporadic
◊ Genetic
<u>Secondary</u>
◊ Condition associated with hypertriglyceridemia: Obesity, diabetes mellitus, pregnancy, uremia/dialysis, hypothyroidism, nephrotic syndrome, acromegaly, Cushing's syndrome, systemic lupus erythematosis, dysgammaglobulinemias, glycogen storage Type I, lipodystrophy
◊ Drugs associated with hypertriglyceridemia: Alcohol, estrogen, birth control pill, beta blockers, diuretics, glucocorticoid, isotretinoin/retinoid, bile acid binding resins cause a modest (<10%) elevation in some patients with Type II hyperlipidemia.

RISK FACTORS
• Genetic susceptibility
• Obesity
• Diabetes
• Alcoholism
• Exacerbated by medical illness and/or drug (see secondary causes)

DIAGNOSIS

DIFFERENTIAL DIAGNOSIS N/A

LABORATORY N/A
Drugs that may alter lab results: N/A
Disorders that may alter lab results: N/A

PATHOLOGICAL FINDINGS N/A

SPECIAL TESTS N/A

IMAGING N/A

DIAGNOSTIC PROCEDURES N/A

TREATMENT

APPROPRIATE HEALTH CARE
Outpatient usually. Inpatient, if underlying disorder warrants.

GENERAL MEASURES
• A thorough search for correctable secondary causes and treating an underlying illness or removing an incriminated drug
• In case of primary hypertriglyceridemia, screening the other family members
• Treatment is indicated in distinct hypertriglyceridemia to prevent acute pancreatitis and in mild hypertriglyceridemia to prevent CAD in patients with high risk, strong family or personal history of atherosclerosis.
• Treatment of severe hypertriglyceridemia associated with pancreatitis - hospitalization, elimination of dietary fat; if diabetic, continuous IV infusion of insulin

ACTIVITY Usually no restrictions. Exercise is important.

DIET Weight reduction to ideal body weight with AHA Step I Diet (55-60% carbohydrate, less than 30% fat, and 10-15% protein)

PATIENT EDUCATION
• Smoking cessation
• Elimination of alcohol.

MEDICATIONS

DRUG(S) OF CHOICE
Gemfibrozil
   ◊ Drop triglycerides by 20-70%
   ◊ Decrease hepatic VLDL synthesis and increase VLDL metabolism
   ◊ Dosage: 600 mg bid
Nicotinic acid
   ◊ Drop triglycerides by 20-50%
   ◊ Inhibit hepatic VLDL synthesis
   ◊ Dosage: 1-3 g/day
Contraindications: Refer to manufacturer's literature
Precautions:
Gemfibrozil
   ◊ Side effects - upper and lower GI side effects (usually mild and are the most frequent adverse effects), cholelithiasis, myalgia, hepatotoxicity
   ◊ May increase the incidence of myopathy/rhabdomyalisis if given with HMG-CoA reductase inhibitors
Nicotinic acid
   ◊ Side effects - flushing and pruritus (prostaglandin mediated and alleviated by ASA)
   ◊ Upper GI discomfort and peptic ulcer disease (PUD)
   ◊ Hepatotoxicity (more with sustained release preparation)
   ◊ Hyperuricemia and gout, hyperglycemia, toxic amblyopia
Significant possible interactions:
• Gemfibrozil/coumadin: enhance anticoagulation effect; monitor PT closely following addition or withdrawal of gemfibrozil.

ALTERNATIVE DRUGS
• HMG-CoA reductase inhibitors (lovastatin, pravastatin, simvastatin): lower triglycerides 10-20%
• Fish oil

FOLLOWUP

PATIENT MONITORING
• Fasting lipid profile
• Liver function test, CPK, CBC diff

PREVENTION/AVOIDANCE   Covered in other headings

POSSIBLE COMPLICATIONS
• Acute pancreatitis
• Atherosclerosis

EXPECTED COURSE AND PROGNOSIS
• Good in secondary disorder if the underlying causes are eliminated
• In primary, may need life long treatment

MISCELLANEOUS

ASSOCIATED CONDITIONS
• Mostly associated with low HDL cholesterol
• May be associated with hypercholesterolemia

AGE-RELATED FACTORS
Pediatric: In severe cases only diet is recommended
Geriatric: N/A
Others: N/A

PREGNANCY   All drugs are contraindicated during pregnancy

SYNONYMS
• Hyperlipidemia
• Chylomicronemia syndrome

ICD-9-CM
• 272.4 hyperlipidemia
• 272.3 Type I or V hyperlipidemia (chylomicronemia syndrome)
• 272.1 hypertriglyceridemia
• 272.2 Type III, Type II-b, hyperlipoproteinemia

SEE ALSO   N/A

OTHER NOTES   N/A

ABBREVIATIONS
• VLDL = very low density lipoprotein
• IDL = intermediate density lipoprotein
• LDL = low density lipoprotein
• CAD = coronary artery disease
• AHA = American Heart Association
• PUD = peptic ulcer disease

REFERENCES
• NIH consensus conference, triglycerides, HDL and coronary heart disease, JAMA: 505-510, 269:1993
• LaRosa, J.C.: Lipid disorders. In Endocrinology and Metabolism Clinics of North America. Vol. 19:2. Philadelphia, W.B. Saunders Co., 1990

Author   R. Moattari, M.D.

Hypoglycemia, diabetic

 BASICS

DESCRIPTION An abnormally low concentration of glucose in the circulating blood of a diabetic. A side effect of insulin and/or sulfonylurea treatment in the course of normal treatment of diabetes mellitus.
System(s) affected: Endocrine/Metabolic
Genetics: No known genetic pattern
Incidence in USA:
• Most type I diabetics experience hypoglycemia. Tightly controlled type I often experience hypoglycemia weekly.
• Type II diabetics experience hypoglycemia much less frequently than type I diabetics
Prevalence in USA:
• Most common in type I diabetics
• Common in type II diabetic patients treated with oral agents and/or insulin
• Uncommon in diabetics treated with diet and exercise alone
Predominant age: All ages
Predominant sex: Male = Female

SIGNS AND SYMPTOMS
Adrenergic hypoglycemia signs and symptoms include:
  ◊ Pallor
  ◊ Tremulousness
  ◊ Nervous anxiety
  ◊ Irritability
  ◊ Tachycardia
  ◊ Diaphoresis
  ◊ Weakness
Neuroglycopenic hypoglycemia signs and symptoms include:
  ◊ Diplopia
  ◊ Lethargy
  ◊ Inability to concentrate or remember
  ◊ Confusion
  ◊ Behavior change
  ◊ Paresthesias
  ◊ Hunger
  ◊ Seizure
  ◊ Coma

CAUSES
• Loss of the hormonal counter-regulatory mechanism in glucose metabolism
• Diet - too little food (skipping a meal)
• Medication - too much insulin (improper dose or timing)
• Erratic absorption of insulin or oral hypoglycemics
• Adverse reaction from other medications
• Exercise - unplanned or excessive exercise
• Alcohol consumption
• Vomiting or diarrhea

RISK FACTORS
• Two or three times more common in the "tight control" patient (according to data from the Diabetes Control and Complications Trial)
• Greater than 5 years duration of diabetes
• Elderly patient
• Renal disease
• Liver disease
• Congestive heart failure
• Hypothyroidism
• Hypoadrenalism
• Gastroenteritis
• Starvation
• Alcoholism

 DIAGNOSIS

DIFFERENTIAL DIAGNOSIS
• Gastrointestinal dysfunction causing postprandial hypoglycemia or alimentary reactive hypoglycemia
• Hormonal deficiency states (hormonal reactive hypoglycemia)
• Idiopathic reactive hypoglycemia
• Hypoglycemia of sepsis
• Islet cell tumors
• Factitious hypoglycemia from surreptitious injection of insulin

LABORATORY
• Plasma glucose ≤ 45 mg/dL or less
• "Suspect" low when plasma glucose is between 45 and 60 mg/dL
• In children plasma glucose ≤ 40 mg/dL
Drugs that may alter lab results: N/A
Disorders that may alter lab results: N/A

PATHOLOGICAL FINDINGS N/A

SPECIAL TESTS Chronic hypoglycemia is evidenced by a low glycohemoglobin level

IMAGING N/A

DIAGNOSTIC PROCEDURES
• History
• Physical exam
• Plasma, or whole blood glucose

 TREATMENT

APPROPRIATE HEALTH CARE
• Outpatient except for complicating emergencies (coma, unapparent cause, long acting oral hypoglycemic)
Admit the patient if:
  ◊ There is any doubt of the cause
  ◊ Expectation of prolonged hypoglycemia
  ◊ Inability of the patient to drink

GENERAL MEASURES
• Education is the mainstay of prevention
• Any sugar-containing food or beverage which can be rapidly absorbed e.g., unsweetened juices, Lifesavers candies, glucose tabs

ACTIVITY Rest until glucose is normal

DIET Avoid extra calories without changing the source of the problem - excess insulin or oral hypoglycemic

PATIENT EDUCATION
• Most important measure is prevention
• Educate patients, their relatives and close friends
• Teach home glucose monitoring and self-adjustment for insulin therapy, diet control, and exercise regimen

MEDICATIONS

DRUG(S) OF CHOICE
General
   ◊ Oral administration of small molecule sugars (saccharose/glucose)
   ◊ Approximately 60-90 calories repeated every 15 minutes until blood sugar is 100 mg/dL or more
   ◊ It takes about 15 minutes for the carbohydrates to be digested and to enter the blood stream as glucose
In patients with loss of consciousness at home
   ◊ Administer glucagon IM or subcutaneous in the deltoid or anterior thigh:
     ◊ If under 5 years old, give 0.25 to 0.50 mg
     ◊ Older child (5-10 years old) give 0.50 to 1 mg
     ◊ Over 10 years old, give 1 mg
If emergency medical personnel are present or patient hospitalized
   ◊ Give one-half amp 50% dextrose every 5-10 minutes until the patient awakens
   ◊ Then feed orally and/or administer 5% dextrose intravenously
Contraindications: None
Precautions: Refer to manufacturer's literature
Significant possible interactions:
Treatment may cause hyperglycemia (called somogyi phenomenon)

ALTERNATIVE DRUGS
Acarbose, a potent alpha-glucosidase inhibitor slows the absorption kinetics of dietary carbohydrates by reversible competitive inhibition of alpha-glucosidase activity, and so reduces the post-prandial blood glucose increment and insulin response

FOLLOWUP

PATIENT MONITORING
Home glucose monitoring

PREVENTION/AVOIDANCE
• Educating patients, family and close friends
• Maintaining a routine schedule of diet, medication and exercise
• Regular blood-glucose testing
• Wearing a medical alert identification bracelet or necklace

POSSIBLE COMPLICATIONS
• Diabetic shock
• Permanent neurological damage

EXPECTED COURSE AND PROGNOSIS
Full recovery is usual depending on the rapidity of diagnosis and treatment

MISCELLANEOUS

ASSOCIATED CONDITIONS
• Autonomic dysfunction
• Neuropathies
• Cardiomyopathies

AGE-RELATED FACTORS
Pediatric: Significance of hypoglycemia in infants of diabetic mothers remains to be defined
Geriatric: Often not diagnosed in the elderly
Others: N/A

PREGNANCY
With hypoglycemic reactions during pregnancy the fetus is less likely to be hypoglycemic because of active transport of glucose across the placenta

SYNONYMS
• Low blood sugar
• Insulin reaction
• Insulin shock
• Reactive hypoglycemia

ICD-9-CM
Hypoglycemia (spontaneous) 251.2; coma 251.0; reactive 251.2

SEE ALSO
Diabetes, type I and II

OTHER NOTES
• The tighter the diabetic control the greater the importance of home glucose monitoring to avoid hypoglycemia
• In patients receiving beta blockers, the drug will mask tachycardia, but not the sweating

ABBREVIATIONS
N/A

REFERENCES
• Schwartz, S.: Management of Diabetes Mellitus. 2nd Ed. Oklahoma, Essential Medical Information Systems, Inc., 1991
• Cahill, G.: Hypoglycemia. New York, Scientific American Medicine, 1991
• American Diabetes Association Clinical Education Program

Author J. Florence, M.D.

Hypoglycemia, nondiabetic

BASICS

DESCRIPTION Hypoglycemia is an abnormally low blood glucose level. Occurs often in diabetic patients (covered under a separate topic) and has a less common appearance in nondiabetic patients
• Reactive hypoglycemia - in response to a meal, specific nutrients, or drugs. May occur within 2-3 hours after a meal, or later. Also seen after gastrointestinal surgery (in association with dumping syndrome in some patients).
• Spontaneous (fasting) hypoglycemia - may be associated with a primary condition, e.g., hypopituitarism, Addison's disease, myxedema, or in disorders related to liver malfunction, and renal failure. If hypoglycemia presents as a primary manifestation, other disorders to consider include hyperinsulinism and extrapancreatic tumors.
System(s) affected: Endocrine/Metabolic
Genetics: Some aspects may involve genetics (e.g., hereditary fructose intolerance)
Incidence/Prevalence in USA: Unknown
Predominant age: Older adult
Predominant sex: Female > Male

SIGNS AND SYMPTOMS
Central nervous system (CNS)
◊ Headache
◊ Confusion
◊ Visual disturbances
◊ Palsy
◊ Changes in personality
◊ Convulsions
◊ Coma
Heart
◊ Palpitations
◊ Hypotension
Gastrointestinal
◊ Hunger
◊ Nausea
◊ Belching
Adrenergic
◊ Sweating
◊ Anxiety
◊ Tremulousness
◊ Dizziness
◊ Diaphoresis
◊ Nervousness

CAUSES
Reactive
◊ Meals (high in refined carbohydrates)
◊ Certain nutrients - e.g., fructose, galactose, leucine
◊ Drugs or alcohol - (e.g., sulfonylureas, salicylates) can cause excess glucose utilization or deficient glucose production
◊ Gastrointestinal surgery
◊ Unknown
Spontaneous
◊ Hepatic disease
◊ Islet cell tumor
◊ Extrapancreatic tumor
◊ Drugs (surreptitious use - injection of insulin or taking oral hypoglycemics)
◊ Exercise
◊ Fever
◊ Pregnancy
◊ Renal glycosuria
◊ Large tumor
◊ Ketotic hypoglycemia of childhood

RISK FACTORS Listed with Causes

DIAGNOSIS

DIFFERENTIAL DIAGNOSIS
• CNS disorders
• Psychogenic

LABORATORY
• Measurement of blood and plasma glucose
• C-peptide measurement
Drugs that may alter lab results: Many drugs can affect levels. Refer to a drug or laboratory reference.
Disorders that may alter lab results: N/A

PATHOLOGICAL FINDINGS N/A

SPECIAL TESTS
• Plasma glucose overnight fasting - < 60 mg/dl
• Plasma glucose 72-hour fasting - < 45 mg/dl for females and < 55 mg/dl for males
• Oral glucose tolerance - < 50 mg/dl
• IV tolbutamide test - normal
• Insulin radioimmunoassay - elevated insulin levels if islet cell tumor present

IMAGING N/A

DIAGNOSTIC PROCEDURES
• Over/interpretation of glucose tolerance tests may lead to an overdiagnosis of hypoglycemia. More than 1/3 of normal patients have hypoglycemia with or without symptoms during a 4 hour tolerance test.
• For definitive diagnosis - patient should have 1) documented occurrence of low blood glucose levels; 2) symptoms that occur when the blood glucose is low; 3) evidence that the symptoms are relieved specifically by the ingestion of sugar or other food; 4) identification of the particular type of hypoglycemia

TREATMENT

APPROPRIATE HEALTH CARE
Outpatient except for severe cases. May also be inpatient for testing.

GENERAL MEASURES
• Oral carbohydrate for alert patient without drug overdose (2-3 tablespoons of sugar in glass of water or fruit juice, 1-2 cups of milk, a piece of fruit, soda cracker)
• If patient unable to swallow, glucagon IM or subcutaneously
• In hypoglycemia caused by drugs or certain nutrients, avoid or control the causative agents
• In hypoglycemia following meals - try high protein diet with restricted carbohydrates
• Avoid stress
• If islet cell tumor (insulinoma) - correct surgically. If it is inoperable, drug therapy may relieve symptoms
"Non-hypoglycemic hypoglycemia" or "pseudohypoglycemia"
◊ Many patients (often females, ages 20-45) present with the diagnosis of reactive hypoglycemia (self-diagnosed or over/interpretation of tests)
◊ Symptoms usually pertain to chronic fatigue and somatic complaints (stress usually has a role in these symptoms)
◊ Management is difficult. Listening is important. Dietary changes, e.g., 120 gm carbohydrate diet, low in simple sugars can be recommended.
◊ Counseling - for stress or other problems may be useful

ACTIVITY May need to revise exercise routine

DIET
• High protein, low carbohydrate
• Frequent (6), small feedings instead of 2-3 larger meals

PATIENT EDUCATION
• Instructions about fasting tests and interpretations of results
• Dietary instruction
• Stress counseling, if appropriate
• Recognition of early symptoms of hypoglycemia and how to take corrective action

MEDICATIONS

DRUG(S) OF CHOICE
• Once an established diagnosis is made, drug therapy appropriate to the underlying disorder
• In patient unable to swallow - glucagon IM or subcutaneously. If no response, give IV glucose.
• For inoperable insulinoma - hypoglycemia may be controlled with diazoxide, verapamil, or streptozocin. May require diuretic therapy concomitantly.
• Postsurgical gastrectomy patients unresponsive to diet changes may benefit from propantheline which delays gastric emptying
Contraindications: Refer to manufacturer's literature
Precautions: Refer to manufacturer's literature
Significant possible interactions: Refer to manufacturer's literature

ALTERNATIVE DRUGS N/A

FOLLOWUP

PATIENT MONITORING Dependent on type and severity of symptoms, and treatment of underlying cause

PREVENTION/AVOIDANCE
• Follow dietary and exercise guidelines
• Patient recognition of early symptoms and taking corrective action

POSSIBLE COMPLICATIONS If tumor removed (insulinoma), some surgical risk involved

EXPECTED COURSE AND PROGNOSIS Favorable, with recognition and appropriate treatment

MISCELLANEOUS

ASSOCIATED CONDITIONS
• Insulinoma
• Severe liver disease
• Alcoholism
• Adrenocortical insufficiency
• Myxedema
• Malnutrition (patients with renal failure)
• Gastrointestinal surgery
• Panhypopituitarism
• Addison's disease

AGE-RELATED FACTORS
Pediatric: Usually divided into 2 syndromes - 1) transient neonatal hypoglycemia and 2) hypoglycemia of infancy and childhood
Geriatric: More likely to have underlying disorders or using causative drugs
Others: N/A

PREGNANCY N/A

SYNONYMS
• Postprandial hypoglycemia
• Functional hypoglycemia
• Idiopathic hypoglycemia
• Alimentary hypoglycemia
• Postgastrectomy hypoglycemia
• Alcohol-induced hypoglycemia
• Factitious hypoglycemia
• Iatrogenic hypoglycemia
• Exogenous hypoglycemia

ICD-9-CM 251.2

SEE ALSO N/A

OTHER NOTES N/A

ABBREVIATIONS N/A

REFERENCES
• Braunwald E., et al. (eds.): Harrison's Principles of Internal Medicine. 12th Ed. New York, McGraw-Hill, 1991
• Krause, M.V. & Mahan, L.K.: Food, Nutrition, and Diet Therapy. 8th Ed. Philadelphia, W.B. Saunders Co., 1990

Author M. Dambro, M.D. & W. Griffith, M.D.

Hypokalemia

BASICS

DESCRIPTION Hypokalemia is defined as a state in which serum potassium (K) concentration is below the normal range, commonly 3.5-5.0 mEq/L. It can occur as a result of depletion of total body stores when associated with decreased intake or excessive gastrointestinal (GI) or renal losses. However, only 2% of total body K is extracellular, and hypokalemia can occur in the presence of normal total body K in those conditions that favor translocation of K from the extracellular to the intracellular compartment.

System(s) affected: Endocrine/Metabolic, Nervous, Musculoskeletal, Renal/Urologic

Genetics:
Some familial disorders are rare causes of hypokalemia
◊ Familial hypokalemic periodic paralysis
◊ Congenital adrenogenital syndromes
◊ Liddle's syndrome
◊ Familial interstitial nephritis

Incidence/Prevalence in USA: Common

Predominant age: N/A

Predominant sex: Male = Female

SIGNS AND SYMPTOMS
• Neuromuscular (most prominent manifestations) - skeletal muscle weakness (may range from mild weakness to total paralysis, including respiratory muscles); may lead to rhabdomyolysis in severe cases. Smooth muscle involvement may lead to gastrointestinal hypomotility producing ileus and constipation.
• Cardiovascular - ventricular arrhythmias, hypotension, cardiac arrest
• Renal - polyuria, nocturia due to impaired concentrating ability
• Metabolic - hyperglycemia

CAUSES
General causes
◊ Decreased intake (uncommon) - anorexia nervosa, deficient diet in alcoholics
◊ Gastrointestinal K loss - vomiting, diarrhea, laxative abuse, fistulas, villous adenoma, ureterosigmoidostomy
◊ Intracellular shift of K - metabolic alkalosis, insulin excess, beta adrenergic catecholamine excess (acute stress, intake of B2 agonists), hypokalemic periodic paralysis, intoxications (theophylline, barium, toluene)
Renal K loss
◊ Drugs - diuretics, penicillin antibiotics, aminoglycosides
◊ Mineralocorticoid excess states - primary hyperaldosteronism, secondary hyperaldosteronism (congestive heart failure, cirrhosis, nephrotic syndrome, malignant hypertension, renin-producing tumors), Bartter's syndrome, congenital adrenogenital syndromes, exogenous mineralocorticoids (glycyrrhizic acid in licorice, carbenoxolone, steroids in nasal sprays), Liddle's syndrome
◊ Glucocorticoid excess states - Cushing's syndrome, exogenous steroids, ectopic ACTH production

◊ Renal tubular acidosis (RTA)
◊ Leukemia
◊ Magnesium depletion

RISK FACTORS Any disorder or medication regimen requiring potassium supplementation

DIAGNOSIS

DIFFERENTIAL DIAGNOSIS Spurious hypokalemia which occurs when blood with a high WBC count (> 100,000/mm3) is allowed to stand at room temperature (WBC's extract K from plasma)

LABORATORY Serum potassium < 3.5 mEq/L.

Drugs that may alter lab results: N/A

Disorders that may alter lab results: Leukemia and other conditions with high WBC

PATHOLOGICAL FINDINGS
• Vacuolization of proximal and distal renal tubular cells
• In severe hypokalemia, necrosis of cardiac and skeletal muscle

SPECIAL TESTS
• ECG - flattening or inversion of T waves, increased prominence of U waves, depression of ST segment, ventricular ectopia
• Work-up for etiology - excessive renal K loss is present when urinary K is in excess of 20 meq/day in the presence of hypokalemia. In the patient with excessive renal K loss and hypertension (HTN), plasma renin and aldosterone levels should be determined to differentiate adrenal from non-adrenal causes of hyperaldosteronism. If HTN is absent and the patient is acidotic, RTA should be considered. If HTN is absent and serum pH is normal to alkalotic, a high urine chloride (> 10 meq/day) suggests hypokalemia secondary to diuretics or Bartter's syndrome and a low urine chloride (< 10 meq/day) suggests vomiting as the probable cause.

IMAGING If there is evidence of mineralocorticoid excess (see Special tests), proceed with CT scan of adrenal glands

DIAGNOSTIC PROCEDURES N/A

TREATMENT

APPROPRIATE HEALTH CARE
• Hypokalemia is usually not an emergency. For asymptomatic patients being treated with oral replacement, outpatient followup is sufficient.
• Patients with cardiac manifestations will require intravenous replacement with cardiac monitoring in an intensive care setting

GENERAL MEASURES
• Treatment of the underlying cause, if hypokalemia is mild
• When hypokalemia is severe, potassium replacement is necessary

ACTIVITY No restrictions

DIET In mild hypokalemia (K=3.0-3.5 meq/L.) not caused by GI losses, dietary supplementation may be sufficient. Potassium-rich foods include oranges, bananas, cantaloupes, prunes, raisins, dried beans, dried apricots, and squash.

PATIENT EDUCATION
• Instructions for diet
• If potassium supplementation is necessary, stress need for compliance

MEDICATIONS

DRUG(S) OF CHOICE
• For non-emergent conditions (serum K > 2.5 mEq/L., no cardiac manifestations), oral therapy is preferred and doses of 40-120 mEq/day are usually adequate. Potassium chloride is suitable for all forms of hypokalemia. Other K salts may be indicated if there is a coexisting disorder: Potassium bicarbonate or bicarbonate precursor (gluconate, acetate, or citrate) in metabolic acidosis or phosphate in phosphate deficiency.
• For emergent situations (serum K < 2.5 mEq/L., arrhythmias), intravenous replacement is indicated. The rate of administration should not exceed 20 mEq/hour and maximum recommended concentration is 60 mEq/L. of saline for peripheral administration. Central may give higher concentration.
• In non-emergent situations, intravenous K should be given only when oral administration is not feasible (e.g., vomiting, postoperative state). In this setting, rate should not exceed 10 mEq/hour and concentration should not exceed 40 mEq/L.

Contraindications: None
Precautions:
• Any form of K replacement carries the risk of hyperkalemia
• Serum K should be checked more frequently in groups at higher risk: Elderly, diabetics, and patients with renal insufficiency
• Patients receiving digitalis and patients with diabetic ketoacidosis in whom intracellular shift in K is expected after insulin therapy is initiated must have more aggressive replacement

Significant possible interactions:
Concomitant administration of K sparing diuretics (spironolactone, triamterene, amiloride) magnify the risk of hyperkalemia

ALTERNATIVE DRUGS   None

FOLLOWUP

PATIENT MONITORING
• Patients receiving intravenous therapy should have their serum K level checked frequently (q 4-6 hours)
• Patients requiring potassium supplements should have serum potassium studied at intervals dictated by calculation of patient compliance

PREVENTION/AVOIDANCE   Patients
being started on diuretics should be advised to increase their dietary K intake (see Diet)

POSSIBLE COMPLICATIONS
Hyperkalemia

EXPECTED COURSE AND
PROGNOSIS   The ease of correction of hypokalemia and the need for prolonged treatment rests on the primary cause. If this can be eliminated (e.g., resolution of diarrhea, discontinuation of diuretics, removal of adrenal tumor), hypokalemia is expected to resolve and no further treatment is indicated.

MISCELLANEOUS

ASSOCIATED CONDITIONS   N/A

AGE-RELATED FACTORS   N/A
Pediatric: Not common in this age group, but may occur in chronic gastrointestinal loss or secondary to hyperadrenalism
Geriatric:
• Diuretic therapy, diarrhea and chronic laxative abuse are most common causes for hypokalemia in this age group
• May need to correct magnesium depletion
Others: N/A

PREGNANCY   Treatment is same

SYNONYMS   N/A

ICD-9-CM   276.8

SEE ALSO   N/A

OTHER NOTES   N/A

ABBREVIATIONS   RTA = renal tubular acidosis

REFERENCES
• Raymond, K.H. & Kunau, R.T., Jr.: Hypokalemic states. In Clinical Disorders of Fluid and Electrolyte Metabolism. Edited by M.H. Maxwell, C.R. Kleeman & R.G. Narins. New York, McGraw-Hill, 1987, pp. 519-546
• Gabow, P.A. & Peterson, L.N.: Disorders of potassium metabolism. In Renal and Electrolyte Disorders. Edited by R.W. Schrier. Boston, Little, Brown and Company, 1986, pp. 207-250

Author   S. Kant, M.D. & B. Padilla, M.D.

Hypokalemic periodic paralysis

BASICS

DESCRIPTION Episodic weakness associated with low serum potassium (K+) levels
Two forms exist:
◊ Familial hypokalemic periodic paralysis-the more common form (FHPP) is usually inherited as an autosomal dominant trait
◊ Hypokalemic periodic paralysis with thyrotoxicosis (HPPT)-rarer, usually affects Oriental males.
Genetics: Autosomal dominant (FHPP)
Incidence in USA: Not known (rare)
Prevalence in USA: Not known (rare)
Predominant age: Onset of disease in late childhood or adolescence (FHPP), early adulthood (HPPT). Onset of disease after age 35 extremely rare.
Predominant sex:
• Male > Female (3:1) (FHPP)
• Male > Female (20:1) (HPPT)

SIGNS AND SYMPTOMS
• Episodic attacks of limb muscle weakness which last from a few hours to several days
• Typical attack comes on during sleep which was preceded by strenuous exercise
• Attacks also provoked by high carbohydrate or high sodium (Na+) meals
• Cold, stress, alcohol, diuretics, insulin, or epinephrine may also exacerbate attack
• Strength between attacks usually normal
• After years of prolonged, frequent attacks patient may develop persistent proximal weakness
• Myalgias
• Proximal weakness greater than distal weakness
• Muscles of the eyes, face, tongue, pharynx, larynx, diaphragm, and sphincters rarely involved
• Deep tendon reflexes hypoactive
• Sensibility preserved

CAUSES
• Exact pathogenesis unknown
• Abnormality is in the muscle membrane
• Contractile apparatus normal
• Defect may be related to increased Na+ "leak" across membrane into cell
• Na+ leak reduces electrical potentials across muscle membrane, muscle will not propagate action potential and will not contract
• As cell membrane Na+,K+-ATPase pump tries to move Na+ out of cell, extracellular K+ brought into cell due to K+-Na+ exchange

RISK FACTORS
• Male
• Age under 35
• Family history (FHPP)
• Oriental race (HPPT)

DIAGNOSIS

DIFFERENTIAL DIAGNOSIS
• Hyperkalemic periodic paralysis (adynamia episodica)
• Paramyotonia congenita
• Normokalemic periodic paralysis
• Barium poisoning
• Hyperventilation
• Secondary hypokalemia (laxative or diuretic use, diarrhea, vomiting, renal or adrenal disease, clay ingestion)
• Myasthenia gravis
• Guillain-Barré syndrome
• Tick paralysis
• Cataplexy
• Sleep paralysis
• Presyncope
• "Drop attacks"
• Akinetic epilepsy

LABORATORY
• Hallmark is low serum K+-as low as 1.8 meq/l
• Urine K+ normal
• Elevated T3, T4, Free thyroid index, and decreased TSH (HPPT only)
Drugs that may alter lab results: N/A
Disorders that may alter lab results: N/A

PATHOLOGICAL FINDINGS
• Muscle biopsy may show atrophy, centrally placed vacuoles of sarcoplasm
• Electron-microscopy studies show vacuoles are due to progressive dilatation of sarcoplasmic reticulum

SPECIAL TESTS
• With mild hypokalemia electrocardiogram (ECG) may show S-T depression, flattened T waves, presence of U waves
• With severe hypokalemia ECG may show peaked P waves, prolonged P-R interval, widened QRS
• Electromyography not helpful

IMAGING Thyroid scans using radioiodine (HPPT only)

DIAGNOSTIC PROCEDURES
Provocative testing (50 to 100 g oral glucose with 2 to 4 g oral sodium followed by exercise, or 50 to 100 g oral glucose with 10-20 IU subcutaneous insulin) may be required. Patient should have cardiac monitoring during testing.

TREATMENT

APPROPRIATE HEALTH CARE
• Severe hypokalemia or weakness-inpatient with cardiac monitoring
• Mild hypokalemia or weakness-outpatient with close follow up

GENERAL MEASURES May rarely need respiratory support

ACTIVITY As tolerated

DIET
• Avoid high carbohydrate, high sodium foods
• K+ rich fruit of dubious benefit

PATIENT EDUCATION N/A

MEDICATIONS

DRUG(S) OF CHOICE
Acute attack
◊ Oral potassium chloride (KCl), 0.2 to 0.4 meq/kg, repeated every 15 to 30 min depending on response of ECG, serum K+, muscle strength
◊ In life-threatening situation or if vomiting give intravenous (IV) KCl in mannitol (5% glucose or normal saline IV may worsen situation). Bolus 0.1 meq/kg every 5 to 10 min, monitor ECG, serum K+.
Prevention of attacks in FHPP
◊ Oral KCl
◊ Acetazolamide (Diamox), 125 to 1000 mg/d divided qd to bid
Prevention of attacks in HPPT
◊ Treat underlying thyrotoxicosis with beta-adrenergic blocking agents (propranolol [Inderal] and others)
◊ Acetazolamide contraindicated
Contraindications:
• Marked hepatic or renal dysfunction, hypersensitivity, adrenal failure, hyperchloremic acidosis, low serum Na+, K+ (acetazolamide)
• Cardiogenic shock, sinus bradycardia, 2nd or 3rd degree AV block, congestive heart failure, bronchial asthma (propranolol)
Precautions:
• Infusion of IV KCl must be monitored to avoid inadvertent infusion of large and potentially fatal doses
• Peripheral intravenous KCl infusion rates greater than 10 meq/h may be painful
• Drowsiness or paresthesias at high doses (acetazolamide)
• Impaired hepatic or renal function (propranolol)
Significant possible interactions:
• High dose aspirin (acetazolamide)
• Reserpine, verapamil, aluminum hydroxide, phenytoin, rifampin, chlorpromazine, cimetidine, theophylline (propranolol)

ALTERNATIVE DRUGS
Acute attack
◊ None
Prevention of attacks in FHPP
◊ Triamterene (Dyrenium) 25 to 100 mg/d
◊ Spironolactone (Aldactone) 25 to 100 200 mg/d
Prevention of attacks in HPPT
◊ Propylthiouracil, radioactive ablation of the thyroid

FOLLOWUP

PATIENT MONITORING
Follow serum K+, electrolytes (if on acetazolamide), follow thyroid function tests (if on propranolol or propylthiouracil)

PREVENTION/AVOIDANCE
See medication prevention of attacks, diet

POSSIBLE COMPLICATIONS
Cardiac arrhythmias, respiratory collapse

EXPECTED COURSE AND PROGNOSIS
• Frequency of attacks usually lessens with age
• After years of prolonged, frequent attacks patient may develop persistent proximal weakness

MISCELLANEOUS

ASSOCIATED CONDITIONS
• Hyperthyroidism with hypokalemic periodic paralysis with thyrotoxicosis, HPPT

AGE-RELATED FACTORS
Pediatric: Onset of disease in late childhood or adolescence
Geriatric: Onset of disease after age 25-35 extremely rare, frequency of attacks usually lessens with age
Others: N/A

PREGNANCY N/A

SYNONYMS
• Paroxysmal myoplegia (familial hypokalemic periodic paralysis)

ICD-9-CM
359.3 hypokalemic familial periodic paralysis

SEE ALSO
• Hypokalemia
• Hyperthyroidism
• Myasthenia gravis
• Guillain-Barré syndrome

OTHER NOTES N/A

ABBREVIATIONS
• K+ = potassium
• Na+ = sodium
• ATPase = adenosine triphosphatase
• FHPP = Familial hypokalemic periodic paralysis
• HPPT = Hypokalemic periodic paralysis with thyrotoxicosis

REFERENCES
• Furman, R.E, & Barch, R.: Pathophysiology of Myotonia and Periodic Paralysis. In Diseases of the Nervous System, Clinical Neurobiology. Edited by A.K. Asbury, G.M. McKhann, & W.I. McDonald. Philadelphia, W.B. Saunders Co., 1986
• Griggs, R.C.: Periodic Paralysis. In Harrison's Principles of Internal Medicine. 12th ed. Edited by J.D. Wilson, et al. New York, McGraw Hill,1991
• Stedwell R., Allen, K.M. & Binder, L.S.: Hypokalemic Paralysis: A Review of the Etiologies, Pathophysiology, Presentation, and Therapy. Am J Emerg Med 1992;10:143-8
• Sterns, R.H. & Narins, R.G.: Disorders of Potassium Balance. In Internal Medicine. 3rd Ed. Edited by J.H. Stein. Boston, Little Brown & Co, 1990

Author C. Vincent, M.D.

Hyponatremia

BASICS

DESCRIPTION
Defined as a plasma sodium concentration < 135 mEq/L
- Hypovolemic hyponatremia - there is a decrease in total body water (TBW) and a greater decrease in total body sodium. The extracellular fluid (ECF) volume is decreased. Orthostatic hypotension and other changes consistent with hypovolemia are present.
- Euvolemic hyponatremia - there is an increase in TBW with a normal total body sodium. The ECF volume is minimally to moderately increased but there is no edema.
- Hypervolemic hyponatremia - there is an increase in total body sodium and a greater increase in TBW. The ECF is increased markedly and there is edema.
- Redistributive hyponatremia - there is a shift of water from the intracellular compartment to the extracellular compartment with a resultant dilution of sodium. TBW and total body sodium are unchanged. This occurs with hyperglycemia.
- Pseudohyponatremia - there is a dilution of the aqueous phase by excessive proteins or lipids. TBW and total body sodium are unchanged. This occurs in hypertriglyceridemia or multiple myeloma.

System(s) affected: Endocrine/Metabolic
Genetics: N/A
Incidence/Prevalence in USA: Described as the most common electrolyte disorder seen in a general hospital population. A recent study of hospitalized patients found an incidence of 1% and a prevalence of 2.5%.
Predominant age: All ages
Predominant sex: Male = Female

SIGNS AND SYMPTOMS
- Lethargy
- Disorientation
- Generalized weakness
- Muscle cramps
- Anorexia
- Hiccups
- Nausea and vomiting
- Agitation or delirium
- Stupor
- Coma
- Depressed deep tendon reflexes
- Hypothermia
- Positive Babinski responses
- Cheyne-Stokes respiration
- Pseudobulbar palsy
- Seizures
- Orthostatic hypotension
- Cranial nerve palsies

CAUSES
Hypovolemic hyponatremia (extrarenal loss of sodium)
- ◊ Gastrointestinal loss - vomiting, diarrhea
- ◊ Third spacing - peritonitis, pancreatitis, burns, rhabdomyolysis
- ◊ Skin loss - burns, sweating, cystic fibrosis
- ◊ Lung loss - bronchorrhea
Hypovolemic hyponatremia (renal loss of sodium)
- ◊ Salt losing nephritis

- ◊ Mineralocorticoid deficiency
- ◊ Diuretic
- ◊ Bicarbonaturia - renal tubular acidosis, metabolic alkalosis
- ◊ Ketonuria or anion gap acidosis
- ◊ Partial urinary tract obstruction
- ◊ Osmotic diuresis
Euvolemic hyponatremia
- ◊ Hypothyroidism
- ◊ Pure glucocorticoid deficiency
- ◊ Drugs
- ◊ Stress
- ◊ Syndrome of inappropriate antidiuretic hormone release (SIADH). Causes include pulmonary and central nervous system disorders.
Hypervolemic hyponatremia
- ◊ Nephrotic syndrome
- ◊ Cirrhosis
- ◊ Congestive heart failure
- ◊ Renal failure
Redistributive hyponatremia
- ◊ Hyperglycemia
- ◊ Mannitol infusion
Pseudohyponatremia
- ◊ Hypertriglyceridemia
- ◊ Multiple myeloma

RISK FACTORS
Excessive fluid intake

DIAGNOSIS

DIFFERENTIAL DIAGNOSIS
See Causes

LABORATORY
- Serum sodium less than 135
- Plasma osmolality
- Urine sodium
- BUN
- Creatinine
Hypovolemic hyponatremia
- ◊ Plasma osmolality low
- ◊ BUN/creatinine ratio greater than 20/1
- ◊ Urine sodium > 20 mEq/L - renal loss
- ◊ Urine sodium < 10 mEq/L - extrarenal loss
- ◊ Serum potassium > 5.0 - consider mineralocorticoid deficiency
Euvolemic hyponatremia
- ◊ Plasma osmolality low
- ◊ BUN/creatinine ratio less than 20/1
- ◊ Urine sodium > 20 mEq/L
Hypervolemic hyponatremia
- ◊ Plasma osmolality low
- ◊ Urine sodium < 10 mEq/L in nephrotic syndrome, CHF, cirrhosis
- ◊ Urine sodium > 20 mEq/L in acute and chronic renal failure
Redistributive hyponatremia
- ◊ Plasma osmolality normal or high
- ◊ Glucose or mannitol levels elevated
Pseudohyponatremia
- ◊ Plasma osmolality normal
- ◊ Triglyceride or protein levels elevated
Drugs that may alter lab results: N/A
Disorders that may alter lab results: N/A

PATHOLOGICAL FINDINGS
N/A

SPECIAL TESTS
For euvolemic hyponatremia a thyroid stimulating hormone (TSH) to rule out hypothyroidism and a one-hour cosyntropin stimulation test to rule out adrenal insufficiency

IMAGING
- CT of head if pituitary problem suspected or if SIADH from CNS problem suspected
- Chest x-ray to rule out pulmonary pathology if SIADH diagnosed

DIAGNOSTIC PROCEDURES
N/A

TREATMENT

APPROPRIATE HEALTH CARE
- Inpatient treatment mandatory if acute hyponatremia or symptomatic
- Inpatient treatment advised if asymptomatic and serum sodium less than 125 mEq/dl

GENERAL MEASURES
- Assess all medications patient is taking
- Institute seizure precautions

ACTIVITY
Varies according to patient mental status

DIET
- Euvolemic hyponatremia - water restriction to 1000 cc/day
- Hypervolemic hyponatremia - water and sodium restriction
- Hypovolemic hyponatremia - isotonic saline
- Redistributive or pseudohyponatremia - treat underlying cause

PATIENT EDUCATION
N/A

MEDICATIONS

DRUG(S) OF CHOICE
• Severe symptomatic hyponatremia: The use of hypertonic saline (3%) is clearly indicated only in patients who are both severely symptomatic and have sodium concentrations less than 120 mEq/L. Three percent saline should be used at a rate of 1 cc/kg/hr. This will raise the serum sodium level by approximately 1 mEq/L/hr. The hypertonic saline infusion should only continue until a serum sodium of 120 mEq/dL is reached or the patient becomes asymptomatic. Avoid correction by more than 12 mEq/L/day.
• Chronic hyponatremia: If hyponatremia does not improve with fluid restriction or other appropriate treatment, consider using demeclocycline. In doses of 600-1200 milligrams per day, the drug produces a nephrogenic diabetes insipidus.
• Maintenance: Clinical judgment

Contraindications: Demeclocycline can cause nephrotoxicity in patients with liver disease

Precautions:
• Demeclocycline - photosensitivity and nausea can occur
• Three percent saline-rapid correction of severe symptomatic hyponatremia has been associated with central pontine myelinolysis (CPM). This neurologic disorder induces loss of myelin and supportive structures in the pons and occasionally in other areas of the brain. CPM is seen one to several days after rapid correction of serum sodium and is characterized by gradual neurologic deterioration.

Significant possible interactions:
Demeclocycline - oral anticoagulants, oral contraceptives, penicillin

ALTERNATIVE DRUGS   N/A

FOLLOWUP

PATIENT MONITORING
• Serum sodium level should be monitored when clinically indicated. If three percent saline is used the sodium level should be checked hourly.
• Volume status should be monitored if 3% or 0.9% saline is used

PREVENTION/AVOIDANCE   Dependent on underlying condition

POSSIBLE COMPLICATIONS
• Occult tumor may present with SIADH
• Hypervolemia if saline used
• Central pontine myelinolysis

EXPECTED COURSE AND PROGNOSIS   With recognition and proper treatment a return to normal serum sodium and resolution of neurologic symptoms is expected. Prognosis is dependent on underlying condition.

MISCELLANEOUS

ASSOCIATED CONDITIONS
• Hypothyroidism
• Hypopituitarism
• Adrenocortical hormone deficiency

AGE-RELATED FACTORS   N/A
Pediatric: N/A
Geriatric: N/A
Others: N/A

PREGNANCY   N/A

SYNONYMS   N/A

ICD-9-CM   276.1

SEE ALSO   N/A

OTHER NOTES   N/A

ABBREVIATIONS
• TBW = total body weight
• ECF = extracellular fluid
• SIADH = syndrome of inappropriate antidiuretic hormone

REFERENCES   Schrier, R.W.: Renal and Electrolyte Disorders. 3rd Ed. Boston, Little brown and Co., 1986

Author   C. Zucker, M.D. & G. Erbstoesser, M.D.

Hypoparathyroidism

 BASICS

DESCRIPTION Deficiency of parathyroid hormone (PTH) from disease, injury or congenital malfunction of the parathyroid glands. Manifested as hypocalcemia producing neuromuscular symptoms ranging from paresthesia to tetany.
Classifications:
◊ Hypoparathyroidism (follows accidental removal or damage to parathyroid glands during surgery; may be transient or permanent)
◊ Idiopathic (parathyroids absent or atrophied)
◊ Pseudohypoparathyroidism (no PTH deficiency, but target organs do not respond to its action)
System(s) affected: Endocrine/Metabolic, Nervous, Musculoskeletal
Genetics: Idiopathic hypoparathyroidism may have a genetic component
Incidence/Prevalence in USA: All forms are rare
Predominant age: All ages
Predominant sex: Male = Female

SIGNS AND SYMPTOMS
• Neuromuscular excitability as carpopedal spasm
• Increased deep tendon reflexes
• Chvostek's sign: hyperirritability of the facial nerve when tapped
• Traousseau's sign: carpopedal spasm within 2 minutes of inflating a blood pressure cuff over systolic pressure
• Dysphagia
• Organic brain syndrome
• Psychosis
• Mental deficiency (children)
• Tetany (paresthesias, pain, difficulty walking, laryngospasm, stridor, cyanosis, seizures)
• Dry hair
• Brittle fingernails
• Dry, scaly skin
• Cataracts
• Cardiac arrhythmias

CAUSES
• Idiopathic: An autoimmune genetic disorder or congenital absence of the parathyroid glands
• Acquired: Results from accidental removal of or injury to one or more parathyroid glands during neck surgery or irradiation

RISK FACTORS
• Neck surgery
• Neck trauma
• Head and neck malignancies

 DIAGNOSIS

DIFFERENTIAL DIAGNOSIS
• Rickets and osteomalacia
• Candidiasis
• Pseudohypoparathyroidism
• Addison's disease
• Pernicious anemia

LABORATORY
• Serum calcium - decreases
• Serum phosphorus - increased (> 5.4 mg/100 mL)
• RIA (radioimmunoassay for parathyroid hormone - decreased
• Urinary calcium (Sulkowitch's test) - decreased urine calcium (in 70% of patients)
Drugs that may alter lab results:
Corticosteroids
Disorders that may alter lab results:
Other hormonal disorders

PATHOLOGICAL FINDINGS
• Complete or almost complete replacement of parathyroid gland parenchymal tissue by fat
• Brain blood vessels calcified

SPECIAL TESTS
• ECG - increased Q-T and S-T intervals (due to hypocalcemia)
• Serum carotene (normal)
• D-xylose absorption
• 72 hour stool fat
• Slit-lamp - may show early posterior lenticular cataract formation

IMAGING
X-ray:
◊ Increased bone density
◊ Tooth roots absent
◊ Calcification of cerebellum, choroid plexus, cerebral basal ganglia

DIAGNOSTIC PROCEDURES N/A

 TREATMENT

APPROPRIATE HEALTH CARE
• Inpatient for work-up
• Inpatient for tetany
• Outpatient followup

GENERAL MEASURES
• Transient forms of hypoparathyroidism may not require treatment
Acute attack hypoparathyroid tetany
◊ Is life-threatening and requires immediate IV treatment to raise calcium levels
◊ Verify adequate airway is present
◊ If patient is awake, breathing into paper bag can help raise serum calcium levels also
◊ Seizure prevention
◊ May require tracheostomy
Maintenance
◊ Lifelong calcitriol and calcium
◊ Maintain serum calcium in the low normal range 8.5-9 mg/dL
◊ Skin softeners for scaly skin
◊ Adequate control is difficult and requires careful attention to avoid overtreatment or undertreatment

ACTIVITY As tolerated

DIET No special diet

PATIENT EDUCATION
• Careful and detailed instructions about maintenance therapy
• Importance of periodic blood chemical evaluations
• Signs and symptoms of over treatment and under treatment to watch for

MEDICATIONS

DRUG(S) OF CHOICE
For tetany:
◊ Immediate IV calcium gluconate 10-20 mL of 10% solution given slowly until tetany ceases
◊ Calcium salts orally as soon as possible, 1-2 g daily
◊ Oral vitamin D (ergocalciferol [400 IU/day])
or
◊ Dihydrotachysterol - pediatric dose: 0.1-0.5 mg/day. Adult dose: 0.5-1.0 mg/day. Adjust based on serum calcium and phosphate levels.
or
◊ Calcitriol - pediatric dose: 10-50 mg/kg/24hr. Adult dose: 0.25 mcg/24hr. Then 0.25 mcg qod. Adjust based on calcium and phosphorous levels.
Maintenance:
◊ Calcium - 1-2 g daily in divided doses
◊ Oral vitamin D (ergocalciferol or dihydrotachysterol or calcitriol)
◊ If associated endocrinopathies - appropriate hormone replacement
◊ Thiazide diuretic - for some patients to increase phosphate excretion and decrease calcium excretion
Contraindications: Refer to manufacturer's literature
Precautions: Refer to manufacturer's literature
Significant possible interactions: Refer to manufacturer's literature

ALTERNATIVE DRUGS N/A

FOLLOWUP

PATIENT MONITORING
• Outpatient after tetany
• Periodic blood chemical evaluations

PREVENTION/AVOIDANCE Care in surgical procedure that may cause damage to parathyroid

POSSIBLE COMPLICATIONS
• Neuromuscular symptoms (reversible)
• Cataracts
• Basal ganglia calcifications
• If condition starts early in childhood - stunting of growth, malformation of teeth, mental retardation
• Hypothyroidism
• Parkinsonian symptoms
• Ossification of the paravertebral ligaments
• Complications of overtreatment or undertreatment
• Institutionalized due to permanent mental damage

EXPECTED COURSE AND PROGNOSIS
• Course - acute, chronic
• Transient hypoparathyroidism following surgery is reversible
• Fair outlook with diagnosis and treatment

MISCELLANEOUS

ASSOCIATED CONDITIONS
• DiGeorge's syndrome
• Addison's disease
• Mucocutaneous candidiasis

AGE-RELATED FACTORS
Pediatric:
• May occur in premature infants
• Congenital absence of parathyroids
• May appear later in childhood as idiopathic
Geriatric: Hypocalcemia fairly common in the elderly and may be due to multiple abnormalities
Others: N/A

PREGNANCY N/A

SYNONYMS Parathyroid tetany

ICD-9-CM 252.1 Hypoparathyroidism

SEE ALSO N/A

OTHER NOTES N/A

ABBREVIATIONS N/A

REFERENCES
• Wilson, J.D. & Foster, D.W. (eds): Williams Textbook of Endocrinology. 7th Ed. Philadelphia, W.B. Saunders Co., 1985
• Scriver, C.R., Beuadet, A.L., Sly, W.S., et al.: The Metabolic Base of Inherited Disease. 6th Ed. New York, McGraw-Hill, 1989

Author R. P. Levy, MD

Hypopituitarism

 BASICS

DESCRIPTION Generalized condition caused by partial or total failure of the pituitary gland's vital hormones - ACTH, TSH, LH, FSH, HGH, prolactin
System(s) affected: Endocrine/Metabolic, Reproductive, Skin/Exocrine, Nervous, Gastrointestinal, Musculoskeletal
Genetics: Some pituitary defects are congenital
Incidence/Prevalence in USA: Relatively rare
Predominant age: Occurs in adults and children. In children it causes dwarfism and pubertal delay.
Predominant sex: Male = Female

SIGNS AND SYMPTOMS
- Usually starts in pattern of hypogonadism or gonadotropin failure (decreased FSH and LH)
- Signs of hypofunction of target organs
- Secondary amenorrhea
- Impotence
- Infertility
- Decreased libido
- Diabetes insipidus
- Lethargy
- Tiredness
- Sensitivity to cold
- Hypoglycemia
- Anorexia
- Nausea
- Abdominal pain
- Lactation failure
- Retarded growth
- Failure of secondary sexual characteristics to develop
- Mental aberrations
- Headache
- Hemianopia
- Blindness

CAUSES
- Lesions or tumors of the anterior pituitary gland (intrasellar or extrasellar)
- Congenital defects
- Pituitary infarction (postpartum)
- Hypophysectomy (surgical, chemical, irradiation)
- Granulomatous disease
- Sometimes idiopathic
- Accidental or surgical trauma

RISK FACTORS
- Trauma
- Pregnancy and delivery

 DIAGNOSIS

DIFFERENTIAL DIAGNOSIS
- Primary hypothyroidism
- Anorexia nervosa
- Chronic liver disease
- Myotonia dystrophica
- Addison's disease
- Primary myxedema
- Primary psychosis

LABORATORY
- Confirms hormonal deficiencies
- Radioimmunoassay of all pituitary hormones
- Provocative tests
Drugs that may alter lab results: Any hormone
Disorders that may alter lab results:
- Cushing's syndrome
- Addison's disease
- Hyperthyroidism
- Hypothyroidism

PATHOLOGICAL FINDINGS
- Destruction of anterior pituitary
- Atrophy of adrenal cortex, thyroid, gonads

SPECIAL TESTS
- Careful testing for smell
- Visual field examination by quantitative perimetry

IMAGING
- X-rays - chest, skull, hands, wrists (for bone age)
- CT scan or MRI (head)

DIAGNOSTIC PROCEDURES N/A

 TREATMENT

APPROPRIATE HEALTH CARE
- Outpatient
- Inpatient for surgery when hypopituitarism is due to a pituitary tumor and/or irradiation

GENERAL MEASURES
- Hormonal replacement
- Exercise program to rehabilitate
- Wear medical identification
- Surgery or x-ray radiation (or both) for pituitary tumor

ACTIVITY Encourage active physical exercise program

DIET High calorie, high protein

PATIENT EDUCATION
- Wear medical identification bracelet
- Stress need for additional cortisone at time of any major physical stress (e.g., fever above 101°, acute illness)

MEDICATIONS

DRUG(S) OF CHOICE
Replacement of hormones secreted by the target glands:
- ◊ Cortisol
- ◊ Thyroxine
- ◊ Androgen or cyclic estrogen
- ◊ Human growth hormone (for treating dwarfism)
- ◊ Dosages and administration schedule vary according to age and sex, refer to manufacturer's literature

Contraindications: Refer to manufacturer's literature
Precautions: Refer to manufacturer's literature
Significant possible interactions: Refer to manufacturer's literature

ALTERNATIVE DRUGS N/A

FOLLOWUP

PATIENT MONITORING 3 and 12 month evaluations for post-treatment hormonal status. For patients with pituitary tumors include visual fields, thyroid and adrenal function, sellar computerized imaging.

PREVENTION/AVOIDANCE None

POSSIBLE COMPLICATIONS
- Blindness
- Adrenal crisis
- Long-term medications

EXPECTED COURSE AND PROGNOSIS
- Course - acute, chronic
- Variable, but guardedly favorable with replacement therapy
- If due to postpartum necrosis, may have complete or partial recovery

MISCELLANEOUS

ASSOCIATED CONDITIONS
- Childhood hypopituitarism
- Sheehan's syndrome
- Hypothyroidism

AGE-RELATED FACTORS
Pediatric: Hypopituitarism in this age group leads to dwarfism due to lack of growth hormone
Geriatric: More difficult to diagnose
Others: N/A

PREGNANCY Severe postpartum hemorrhage can lead to hypopituitarism

SYNONYMS
- Pituitary cachexia
- Hypopituitarism syndrome
- Simmond's syndrome or disease
- Panhypopituitarism

ICD-9-CM
253.2 panhypopituitarism

SEE ALSO N/A

OTHER NOTES N/A

ABBREVIATIONS N/A

REFERENCES
- Sheehan, H.L. & Summers, V.K.: The syndrome of hypopituitarism. Q.J. Med 42:319, 1949
- Foster, D.W. & Wilson, J.D. (eds.): Williams Textbook of Endocrinology. 8th Ed. Philadelphia, W.B. Saunders Co., 1991

Author William F. Young, Jr., MD

Hypothermia

BASICS

DESCRIPTION Hypothermia occurs when a core (rectal, tympanic or esophageal) temperature falls below 35°C (95°F). It may take several hours or several days to develop. As the body temperature falls, all organ system are effected; cerebral blood flow decreases and the metabolic rate declines rapidly. Patients who have been immersed for as long as 45 minutes in very cold water and appear to be dead have still been resuscitated.
System(s) affected: Endocrine/Metabolic, Cardiovascular, Nervous, Skin/Exocrine
Genetics: N/A
Incidence/Prevalence in USA: Estimates vary widely due to lack of pathological evidence, and that hypothermia is usually considered a secondary cause in diagnosing disorders
Predominant age: Very young and the elderly
Predominant sex: Male = Female

SIGNS AND SYMPTOMS
Mild
Lethargy
  ◊ Mild confusion
  ◊ Shivering
  ◊ Loss of fine motor coordination
  ◊ Increased pulse and blood pressure
  ◊ Peripheral vasoconstriction
Moderate
Delirium
  ◊ Bradycardia
  ◊ Hypotension
  ◊ Hypoventilation
  ◊ Cyanosis
  ◊ Arrhythmias
  ◊ Semicoma and coma
  ◊ Muscular rigidity
  ◊ Generalized edema
  ◊ Slowed reflexes
Severe
Very cold skin
  ◊ Rigidity
  ◊ Apnea
  ◊ No pulse - ventricular fibrillation or asystole
  ◊ Areflexia
  ◊ Unresponsive
  ◊ Fixed pupils

CAUSES
• Cold water immersion
• Cold weather exposure
• Subacute cold stress in persons with impaired thermoregulatory function

RISK FACTORS
• Malnutrition
• Homeless
• Outdoor workers
• Trauma victims
• Alcohol consumption
• Drug intoxication (barbiturates, phenothiazines, cyclic antidepressants, parasympatholytics, benzodiazepines, narcotics)
• Endocrinopathies (hypothyroidism, hypopituitarism, hypoadrenalism, hypoglycemia)
• Hypothalamic and CNS dysfunction
• Sepsis
• Cardiovascular disease
• Bronchopneumonia

DIAGNOSIS

DIFFERENTIAL DIAGNOSIS
• Cerebrovascular accidents
• Intoxication
• Drug overdose
• Complications of diabetes, hypothyroidism, hypopituitarism

LABORATORY
• Arterial blood gases (reported in the uncorrected form)
• Complete blood and platelet counts
• Toxicology screen
• Serum electrolytes
• Prothrombin time
• Partial thromboplastin time
• Fibrinogen levels
• BUN/creatinine
• Glucose
• Amylase
• Liver function studies
Drugs that may alter lab results: Refer to laboratory test reference
Disorders that may alter lab results: Refer to laboratory test reference

PATHOLOGICAL FINDINGS
• Moderate dilation of right heart
• Pulmonary edema

SPECIAL TESTS
• Temperature measure - with special thermometers that can record low temperatures and measure core temperatures. Oral temperatures are of no value.
• Electrocardiogram - slowing of sinus rate with T-wave inversion, QT-interval prolongation, hypothermic J waves (Osburn waves) characterized by a notching of the QRS complex and ST segment
• Thyroid and pituitary function tests

IMAGING
X-rays of the cervical spine, chest, abdomen, if appropriate

DIAGNOSTIC PROCEDURES
History of prolonged exposure to cold may make the diagnosis obvious, but hypothermia may be overlooked, especially if patient is comatose

TREATMENT

APPROPRIATE HEALTH CARE
Inpatient (emergency room or intensive care)

GENERAL MEASURES
• Establish ABC's of basic life support; establish airway, intubate if necessary. Give warm humidified oxygen. Correct metabolic acidosis.
• Evaluate for frostbite
Rewarming
  ◊ Dependent on severity of hypothermia
  ◊ Rate of rewarming should be 0.5 2°C/hour. More rapid rewarming can cause ventricular fibrillation and hypovolemic shock.
With all patients
  ◊ Remove wet garments
  ◊ Protect against heat loss and wind chill
  ◊ Maintain horizontal position
  ◊ Monitor core temperature and cardiac rhythm
Mild hypothermia
  ◊ Passive rewarming (wrap in heated blanket or clothing)
  ◊ Administration of heated (45°) intravenous solutions
  ◊ Warm fluids may be given if fully alert
Moderate hypothermia
  ◊ Active external rewarming
  ◊ Heated blankets
  ◊ Heating pads
  ◊ Radiant heat sources
  ◊ Alcohol-circulating blankets
Severe hypothermia
  ◊ Active internal (core) rewarming
  ◊ Peritoneal dialysis
  ◊ Gastrointestinal, colonic, or bladder lavage with warm fluids
  ◊ Heated intravenous fluids
  ◊ Heated humidified oxygen
  ◊ Thoracic cavity lavage
  ◊ Extracorporeal blood rewarming
Cardiac arrhythmias
  ◊ Atrial fibrillation and sinus bradycardia are common, but patients usually convert to normal sinus rhythm with rewarming
  ◊ Transient type ventricular arrhythmias should not be treated. If treatment is required, bretylium is recommended.
  ◊ If cardiac pacing required, preferable to use external noninvasive pacemaker
Sepsis bacterial infections
  ◊ In infants - signs may not be evident, initiate treatment with broad-spectrum antibiotic until culture results are available
  ◊ Older children and adults - if no signs, can usually wait for culture results

ACTIVITY Bedrest. Because of the cold, heart is irritable and susceptible to arrhythmias. Special care should be taken in moving and transporting.

DIET Warm fluids only, if alert and able to swallow

PATIENT EDUCATION
• Preventive measures to avoid recurrence
• If due to inadequate clothing or housing, refer patient to a social service agency

Hypothermia

 MEDICATIONS

DRUG(S) OF CHOICE
• For sepsis or bacterial infection, antibiotics
• If ventricular fibrillation requires treatment, bretylium may be helpful
• For hypoglycemia, IV glucose
• Steroid use is controversial

Contraindications: Refer to manufacturer's literature

Precautions: Refer to manufacturer's literature

Significant possible interactions: Refer to manufacturer's literature

ALTERNATIVE DRUGS N/A

 FOLLOWUP

PATIENT MONITORING
During acute episode
◊ Lab work repeated frequently (with particular attention to changes in electrolyte and glucose levels)
◊ Continuous cardiac monitoring
◊ Urinary output monitoring
◊ Temperature monitoring
◊ Follow blood gases, both corrected and uncorrected
Following acute episode
◊ Continued therapy for any underlying disorder

PREVENTION/AVOIDANCE
• Appropriate clothing for cold weather, with particular attention to head, feet and hand coverings
• If walking or climbing in cold climate, carry survival bags lined with space blankets for use if stranded or injured
• Avoid alcohol, especially if anticipating exposure to cold weather
• Alertness to early symptoms and initiating preventive steps, e.g., drinking warm fluids
• Adequate heat in the home
• Review patient's medications that may predispose to hypothermia (e.g., neuroleptics, sedatives, hypnotics, tranquilizers) and decrease dosage or discontinue if appropriate and feasible
• Referral of patient to social service agency for help with adequate housing, heat or clothing

POSSIBLE COMPLICATIONS
• Cardiac arrhythmias
• Hypotension secondary to marked vasodilatation of rewarming
• Pneumonia (aspiration and broncho)
• Pulmonary edema
• Pancreatitis
• Peritonitis
• Gastrointestinal bleeding
• Acute tubular necrosis
• Intravascular thromboses
• Metabolic acidosis
• Gangrene of extremities

EXPECTED COURSE AND PROGNOSIS
• Mortality rates are decreasing for hypothermia due to increased recognition and advanced therapy. Mortality usually dependent upon the severity of underlying cause of hypothermia.
• In previously healthy individuals, recovery is usually complete
• Mortality rate in healthy patients - < 5%
• Mortality rate in patients with co-existing illness - >50%

MISCELLANEOUS

ASSOCIATED CONDITIONS
• Congestive heart failure
• Hypothyroidism
• Hypopituitarism
• Uremia
• Addison's disease
• Ketoacidosis
• Pulmonary infection
• Sepsis
• Brain injury, tumor
• Diabetes

AGE-RELATED FACTORS
Pediatric: All infants are at increased risk of hypothermia because of their limited ability to produce heat when placed in a cold environment. This is particularly true during the first 12 hours of life and in asphyxiated infants. Newborns should be placed under a radiant heat source and the amniotic fluid dried off.

Geriatric:
• Older adults have a lower metabolic rate and it is more difficult for them to maintain normal body temperature when environmental drop below 18°C
• Aging also impairs the ability to detect temperature changes
• This population also has increased incidence of diseases that decrease heat production, increase or impair thermoregulation

Others: N/A

PREGNANCY N/A

SYNONYMS Accidental hypothermia

ICD-9-CM
• 991.6 accidental
• 995.89 anesthetic
• 778.2-778.3 newborn
• 780.9 not associated with low environmental temperature

SEE ALSO Frostbite

OTHER NOTES N/A

ABBREVIATIONS N/A

REFERENCES
• Cassel, C.K., Riesenberg, D.E., Sorensen, L.B. & Walsh, J.R. (eds): Geriatric Medicine. 2nd Ed. New York, Springer-Verlag, 1990
• Callahm, M.L. (ed): Current Therapy in Emergency Medicine. Philadelphia, B.C. Decker Inc., 1987

Author S. Henderson, M.D.

Hypothyroidism, adult

BASICS

DESCRIPTION A clinical state resulting from decreased circulating levels of free thyroid hormone or from resistance to hormone action. Myxedema connotes severe hypothyroidism.
System affected: Endocrine/metabolic
Genetics:
• No known genetic pattern for idiopathic primary hypothyroidism
• Hypothyroidism may be associated with Type II autoimmune polyglandular syndrome, which is associated with HLA-DR3, DR4
• Secondary hypothyroidism frequently results from treatment for Graves disease, which may be familial
Incidence/Prevalence in USA:
• 1-2/1000 women, Less common in men.
• 5-10/1000 in general population
• Over age 65, increases to 6-10% of women, 2-3% of men
Predominant age: Over 40
Predominant sex: Women > Men, 5-10:1

SIGNS AND SYMPTOMS
Symptoms
◊ Onset may be insidious, subtle
◊ Weakness, fatigue, lethargy
◊ Cold intolerance
◊ Decreased memory
◊ Hearing impairment
◊ Constipation
◊ Muscle cramps
◊ Arthralgias
◊ Paresthesias
◊ Modest weight gain (10 pounds)
◊ Decreased sweating
◊ Menorrhagia
◊ Depression
◊ Hoarseness
◊ Carpal tunnel syndrome
Signs
◊ Dry, coarse skin
◊ Dull facial expression
◊ Coarsening or huskiness of voice
◊ Periorbital puffiness
◊ Swelling of hands and feet
◊ Bradycardia
◊ Hypothermia
◊ Reduced systolic blood pressure
◊ Increased diastolic blood pressure
◊ Reduced body and scalp hair
◊ Delayed relaxation of deep tendon reflexes
◊ Macroglossia
◊ Dilutional hyponatremia
◊ Anemia (usually normochromic, normocytic)
◊ Enlarged heart on chest x-ray (often due to pericardial effusion)

CAUSES
• Post-ablative (most common) follows radioactive iodine therapy or thyroid surgery. Delayed hypothyroidism may develop in patients treated with thioamide drugs (propylthiouracil, methimazole) 4 to 25 years later.
• Primary hypothyroidism may develop as a result of autoimmune thyroiditis, or be idiopathic
• With goiter, most commonly due to autoimmune disease, such as Hashimoto's thyroiditis; or heritable biosynthetic defects, iodine deficiency (rare in the U.S.), or drug induced (iodides, lithium, phenylbutazone, aminosalicylic acid)
• Suprathyroid hypothyroidism, may be due to due to deficiency of thyrotropin-releasing hormone (TRH) from the hypothalamus or thyroid-stimulating hormone (TSH) from the pituitary
• Transient hypothyroidism may result from silent thyroiditis (most common in post partum period) and subacute granulomatous thyroiditis

RISK FACTORS
• Risk increases with increasing age
• Autoimmune diseases

DIAGNOSIS

DIFFERENTIAL DIAGNOSIS
• Nephrotic syndrome
• Chronic nephritis
• Neurasthenia
• Depression
• Euthyroid sick syndrome
• Congestive heart failure
• Primary amyloidosis
• Dementia from other causes

LABORATORY
• Total serum thyroxine (T4) - decreased
• T3 resin uptake - increased
• TSH (radioimmunoassay)- elevated
• Free T4 index (= T3 resin uptake x total serum T4) - low
• In severe hypothyroidism, anemia, elevated cholesterol, CPK, LDH, AST, hyponatremia
Drugs that may alter lab results:
• Thyroid supplement
• Cortisone
• Dopamine
• Phenytoin
• Estrogen or androgen therapy in excess of replacement
Disorders that may alter lab results:
• Any severe illness
• Pregnancy
• Chronic protein malnutrition
• Hepatic failure
• Nephrotic syndrome

PATHOLOGICAL FINDINGS
Thyroid may be small, atrophic or enlarged

SPECIAL TESTS Radioimmunoassay

IMAGING None necessary

DIAGNOSTIC PROCEDURES
Combination of low T4 (and/or a low free T4 index) and an elevated TSH (greater than 20 μU per mL) is virtually diagnostic of primary thyroid failure

TREATMENT

APPROPRIATE HEALTH CARE
Outpatient except for complicating emergencies (coma, hypothermia)

GENERAL MEASURES Goals of treatment are to restore and maintain a euthyroid state

ACTIVITY As tolerated

DIET
• High-bulk diet may be helpful to avoid constipation
• Low fat diet for obese patients

PATIENT EDUCATION
• Importance of compliance with thyroid replacement therapy
• Need for lifelong treatment
• Report to physician any signs of infection, heart problems
• Signs of thyrotoxicity

MEDICATIONS

DRUG(S) OF CHOICE
Levothyroxine (Synthroid, Levothroid, others)
◊ 50-100 µg/day. Increase by 25 µg/day every 4-6 weeks until TSH is in normal range.
◊ Dosage requirements may vary with age, sex, residual secretory capacity of thyroid gland, other drugs being taken by patient, intestinal function
◊ Elderly patients may require lower dose because clearance is decreased

Contraindications:
• Thyrotoxic heart disease
• Uncorrected adrenocorticoid insufficiency

Precautions:
• Start with lower doses in the elderly and patients with heart disease
• Diabetic patients may need readjustment of hypoglycemic agents with institution of thyroxine
• Dosage of oral anticoagulants may need adjustment; monitor prothrombin time while initiating treatment

Significant possible interactions:
• Oral anticoagulants
• Insulin
• Oral hypoglycemics
• Estrogen
• Oral contraceptives
• Cholestyramine
• Ferrous sulfate may decrease absorption when taken concomitantly

ALTERNATIVE DRUGS   None currently recommended

FOLLOWUP

PATIENT MONITORING
• Every 6 weeks until stabilized, then every 6 months
• Follow cardiac status closely in older patients

PREVENTION/AVOIDANCE   N/A

POSSIBLE COMPLICATIONS
• Treatment induced congestive heart failure in people with coronary artery disease
• Myxedema coma - life threatening complication of hypothyroidism
• Increased susceptibility to infection
• Megacolon
• Organic psychosis with paranoia
• Adrenal crisis with vigorous treatment of hypothyroidism
• Infertility
• Hypersensitivity to opiates
• Overtreatment over long periods can lead to bone demineralization

EXPECTED COURSE AND PROGNOSIS
• With early treatment, striking transformations in approved appearance and mental function. Return to normal state is the rule.
• Relapses will occur if treatment is interrupted
• If untreated, may progress to myxedema coma

MISCELLANEOUS

ASSOCIATED CONDITIONS
• Hyponatremia
• Anemia
• Idiopathic adrenocorticoid deficiency
• Diabetes mellitus
• Hypoparathyroidism
• Myasthenia gravis
• Vitiligo
• Hypercholesterolemia
• Mitral valve prolapse
• Depression
• Rapid cycling bipolar disorder

AGE-RELATED FACTORS
Pediatric: N/A
Geriatric:
• Characteristic sign and symptoms frequently changed or absent. Hypothyroidism is common in elderly. Diagnosis based on laboratory criteria.
• Replacement therapy is usually about two thirds of the dose used in young adults.
Others: N/A

PREGNANCY
• Replacement therapy may need adjustment. TSH levels should be monitored monthly during first trimester.
• Postpartum - check TSH levels at about 6 weeks
• Painless subacute thyroiditis may occur in the post partum period leading to transient hypothyroidism lasting about 3 months. Treatment with replacement therapy may be warranted. Up to 30% of these individuals develop permanent hypothyroidism.

SYNONYMS   Myxedema

ICD-9-CM
• 244 acquired hypothyroidism
• 244.0 postsurgical hypothyroidism
• 244.2 iodine hypothyroidism

SEE ALSO   Thyroiditis

OTHER NOTES
Surgical procedures:
◊ Hypothyroid patients (mild to moderate) tolerate surgery with mortality and complications similar to euthyroid patients
◊ If surgery is elective, render patient euthyroid prior to procedure
◊ If surgery is urgent, proceed with the procedure with individualized replacement therapy preoperatively and postoperatively

ABBREVIATIONS   N/A

REFERENCES
• Wolf, P.G. & Meek, J.C.: Practical approach to the treatment of hypothyroidism. Am Fam Phys 1992;45:722-31
• Kelly, W.N. (ed.): Textbook of Internal Medicine. 2nd Ed. Philadelphia, J.B.Lippincott Co., 1992
• Branch, W.T.: Office Practice of Medicine. Philadelphia, W.B. Saunders Co., 1987

AUTHOR   B. Majeroni, M.D.

Id reaction

BASICS

DESCRIPTION A localized or generalized autosensitization skin reaction to a primary infection (fungi most often, sometimes unknown) at a site distant to a primary infection
• Most commonly the "id" reaction occurs on the hands with an acute dermatophytosis of the feet
System(s) affected: Skin/Exocrine
Genetics: N/A
Incidence/Prevalence in USA: Unknown, but common
Predominant age: All ages beyond infancy
Predominant sex: Male = Female

SIGNS AND SYMPTOMS
• Dyshidrotic-like, pruritic vesicular eruptions most commonly involving the sides of the fingers
• May occur as generalized eruptions
• May be accompanied by generalized adenopathy, splenomegaly, anorexia, and fever
• Generalized reaction may be seen with tinea capitis

CAUSES Autosensitization to blood-borne circulating antigens at sensitized areas of skin

RISK FACTORS
• Tinea of the feet or hands
• Fungal infection elsewhere on the skin

DIAGNOSIS

DIFFERENTIAL DIAGNOSIS Dyshidrotic eczema

LABORATORY
• Absence of fungal infection at site of reaction
• Definite fungal infection at a distant site
Drugs that may alter lab results: N/A
Disorders that may alter lab results: N/A

PATHOLOGICAL FINDINGS
• Vesicles in the upper dermis
• Lack of inflammation
• Acanthosis
• Increased granular cell layer

SPECIAL TESTS Positive trichophytin skin test. Not very useful.

IMAGING N/A

DIAGNOSTIC PROCEDURES Potassium hydroxide (KOH) prep

TREATMENT

APPROPRIATE HEALTH CARE
Outpatient

GENERAL MEASURES "Id" reaction will resolve with appropriate treatment of underlying primary infection

ACTIVITY Fully active

DIET No special diet

PATIENT EDUCATION N/A

MEDICATIONS

DRUG(S) OF CHOICE Appropriate medications to treat primary infection
Contraindications: Refer to manufacturer's profile of each drug
Precautions: Refer to manufacturer's profile of each drug
Significant possible interactions: Refer to manufacturer's profile of each drug

ALTERNATIVE DRUGS Systemic steroids bring about prompt clearing of the autoeczematous lesions, but will cause the underlying, original disease to heal more slowly

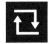

FOLLOWUP

PATIENT MONITORING Followup until original infection is resolved

PREVENTION/AVOIDANCE Prompt treatment of infections

POSSIBLE COMPLICATIONS
Secondary bacterial infection may occur

EXPECTED COURSE AND PROGNOSIS
• Resolution, with adequate treatment of primary disorder
• Recrudescence if treatment is inadequate

MISCELLANEOUS

ASSOCIATED CONDITIONS Primary fungal infection

AGE-RELATED FACTORS
Pediatric: N/A
Geriatric: N/A
Others: N/A

PREGNANCY N/A

SYNONYMS
• Dermatophytid
• Trichophytid

ICD-9-CM 692.89

SEE ALSO N/A

OTHER NOTES Not all dyshidrotic eruptions are "id" reactions

ABBREVIATIONS N/A

REFERENCES Habif, T.: Clinical Dermatology. 2nd Ed. St. Louis, C.V. Mosby, 1990

Author J. Parker, M.D.

Idiopathic hypertrophic subaortic stenosis (IHSS)

BASICS

DESCRIPTION This entity was the first instance of the larger entity of hypertrophic cardiomyopathy (HCM) with the characteristic finding being that of inappropriate myocardial hypertrophy disproportionate to the hemodynamic load
• Idiopathic hypertrophic subaortic stenosis (IHSS) is a subgroup of HCM recognized by, or characterized by, the findings of a dynamic pressure gradient in the subaortic area
• IHSS is therefore characterized clinically by the findings of both diastolic dysfunction (producing impaired ventricular filling with elevated atrial filling pressures producing dyspnea) and systolic dysfunction (producing limitation of cardiac output response to exercise, exertional syncope, and increasing secondary left ventricular hypertrophy)
• Diagnosis usually is made by recognition of signs associated with outflow obstruction, but symptoms are predominantly characterized by diastolic dysfunction
System(s) affected: Cardiovascular
Genetics:
• Autosomal dominant with > 50% penetrance
• Evidence of disease (usually milder) is found in 25% of first degree relatives. Relatives usually do not have outflow obstruction, exhibit only localized hypertrophy, and are asymptomatic.
Incidence/Prevalence in USA: Uncommon
Predominant age: Most commonly presents in third decade (disease of young adulthood), but occurs from newborns to elderly
Predominant sex: Male = Female

SIGNS AND SYMPTOMS
• Dyspnea - mainly a result of diastolic dysfunction and initially exertional in onset (50-90%)
• Angina pectoris (50-90%)
• Syncope - exertional (50-90%)
• Presyncope - exertional (50-90%)
• Fatigue (50-90%)
• Palpitations (50-90%)
• Sudden death (50%)
• Congestive heart failure (50%)
• Paroxysmal nocturnal dyspnea (50%)
• Double apical impulse due to prominent atrial system
• Point of maximal impulse (PMI) displaced laterally
• Rapidly rising bifid carotid pulse
• Prominent S4
• S2 variable splitting (depending on degree of outflow obstruction)
• Harsh systolic crescendo-decrescendo murmur best heard between apex and left sternal border
• Murmur - increases and lengthens with Valsalva strain, standing, amyl nitrite; decreases with sudden squatting, lying down, passive leg raising, isometric handgrip

CAUSES Thickened septum that impinges on the anterior leaflet of the mitral valve during systole and causes outflow obstruction

RISK FACTORS Family history of HCM

Diagnosis

DIFFERENTIAL DIAGNOSIS Differential is between fixed outflow obstruction such as aortic stenosis (AS) and IHSS. Can be determined at bedside by difference in character of carotid pulse. In AS it is slow-rising and reduced in volume versus the rapid-rising bifid pulse of IHSS. Bedside hemodynamic maneuvers (Valsalva, etc.) also help to differentiate.

LABORATORY N/A
Drugs that may alter lab results: N/A
Disorders that may alter lab results: N/A

PATHOLOGICAL FINDINGS
• Distinctive pattern of left ventricular hypertrophy - localized disproportionate hypertrophy of the left ventricular septum with the ratio of septal to free wall thickness being greater than 1.3:1 without anatomic evidence of pressure overload
• Dilated atria
• Increased left ventricle mass and small chamber sizes
• Mural plaque of left ventricular outflow tract
• Mitral valve thickening
• Anatomic variants - apical form not associated with intraventricular gradients and localized mid-ventricular obstruction form
• Disorganization and disarray septal muscle bundles
• Abnormal intramural coronary arteries

SPECIAL TESTS
Electrocardiogram: Common findings (50-90%)
◊ Non-specific ST-T wave abnormalities
◊ Left ventricular hypertrophy
Electrocardiogram: Less common findings (<50%)
◊ Prominent and abnormal Q waves in anterior precordial and lateral limbs lead, simulating myocardial infarction
◊ P-wave abnormalities indicating left atrial enlargement
◊ Short PR interval with QRS morphology suggestive of pre-excitation without clear evidence of pre-excitation (rare in IHSS)
◊ Holter findings - frequent ventricular arrhythmias with up to 25% revealing ventricular tachycardia
◊ Atrial fibrillation - late finding and poor prognostic sign

IMAGING Chest x-ray - variable findings from normal cardiac size to cardiomegaly, none of which is pathognomonic

DIAGNOSTIC PROCEDURES
Echocardiography
◊ Asymmetric septal hypertrophy with septal to free wall ratio greater than 1.3:1
◊ Abnormal systolic anterior leaflet motion of the mitral valve
◊ Left ventricular hypertrophy

◊ Left atrial enlargement
◊ Small ventricular chamber size with increased contractility
◊ Partial systolic closure of aortic valve in mid-systole
◊ Mitral valve prolapse
◊ Mitral regurgitation by Doppler
◊ Decreased mid-aortic flow coincident with systolic anterior leaflet motion of mitral valve by Doppler
Radionuclide
◊ Thallium scintigraphy with stress at times reveals positive defects in setting arteriographically normal coronary arteries
Cardiac catheterization and angiocardiography
◊ Hemodynamic measurement documents degree and lability of outflow obstruction, and diastolic characteristics of left ventricle
◊ Angiocardiography documents left and right ventricular anatomy and coronary arterial anatomy

TREATMENT

APPROPRIATE HEALTH CARE
Outpatient usually. Inpatient for studies and/or surgery.

GENERAL MEASURES
• Therapy based on pathophysiology, namely interventions to reduce ventricular contractility or increase ventricular volume, ventricular compliance, and outflow tract dimensions
• Digitalis glycosides are contraindicated except for atrial fibrillation with uncontrolled response
• Nitrates and sympathomimetic amines (e.g., isoproterenol) are contraindicated except with concomitant coronary heart disease
• Diuretics are relatively contraindicated because of their effect on ventricular volume or left ventricular myotomy
• Surgical: Left ventricular myomectomy - done only in setting of severe symptoms refractory to therapy in those patients with outflow gradient > 50 mm Hg, either at rest or with provocation. 95% successful in abolishing gradient with 70% of patients having marked symptomatic improvement for at least 5 years.

ACTIVITY
• Strenuous exercise, especially competitive sports, should not be undertaken because of high risk of sudden death. Younger patients with little or no functional impairment have the greatest risk of sudden death.
• Sports participation in patients with IHSS is not permitted if any of the following are present: Marked left ventricle hypertrophy, significant outflow gradient, significant supraventricular and/or ventricular arrhythmias, or history of sudden death in relatives with hypertrophic cardiomyopathy

Idiopathic hypertrophic subaortic stenosis (IHSS)

DIET No special diet, but may need to reduce caloric intake, due to reduced activity

PATIENT EDUCATION
• Activity restrictions
• Refer for psychosocial counseling if appropriate (patient and family may suffer from restricted life-style and chronic disease problems)
• Recommend family learn cardiopulmonary resuscitation methods

MEDICATIONS

DRUG(S) OF CHOICE
Propranolol (Inderal)
  ◊ May decrease outflow obstruction: Some evidence suggests that it may increase ventricular compliance. No clear evidence that it reduces incidence of sudden death.
  ◊ 1/3 to 2/3 of patients experience symptomatic improvement
  ◊ May titrate up to dose of 320 mg/day to obtain clinical effect provided patient tolerates dose
Verapamil (Calan, Isoptin)
  ◊ Alternative to therapy with propranolol
  ◊ May have better effect on exercise performance
  ◊ Decrease in outflow gradient due to depression of cardiac contractility
  ◊ Improves diastolic filling by improved diastolic relaxation
Amiodarone (Cordarone)
  ◊ Limited use in treating ventricular arhythmias because of documented pro-arrhythmic effects in HCM
  ◊ Only to be used in patients with ventricular tachycardia associated with hemodynamic compromise. Use of drug is to be guided by initial and followup electrophysiological studies.
Contraindications:
Verapamil:
  ◊ Major side effects include depression of impulse formation and A-V block, negative inotropism, and vasodilatation - all of which can result in hypotension, shock, pulmonary edema, and death
  ◊ Therefore, relatively contraindicated for use in patients with increased left ventricle end diastolic pressure (LVEDP), paroxysmal nocturnal dyspnea (PND), orthopnea, and/or in patients with sinus node disease and A-V block (unless there is an appropriate pacing device)
Precautions: See manufacturer's profile of each drug
Significant possible interactions: See manufacturer's profile of each drug

ALTERNATIVE DRUGS N/A

FOLLOWUP

PATIENT MONITORING Yearly when symptoms and pharmacologic regimens become stable

PREVENTION/AVOIDANCE
• Avoid strenuous exercise, especially competitive sports
• Avoid rapid standing
• Avoid inotropic drugs and diuretics
• Use antitussives for infections that are accompanied by a cough

POSSIBLE COMPLICATIONS
• Sudden death
• Congestive heart failure
• Arrhythmia
• Atrial fibrillation with mural thrombosis formation
• Infective mitral endocarditis

EXPECTED COURSE AND PROGNOSIS
• Annual mortality rate - 4% a year (sudden death most common reason)
• Chronic illness with restricted life-style

MISCELLANEOUS

ASSOCIATED CONDITIONS
• Mitral regurgitation
• Essential hypertension
• Mitral valve prolapse
• Angina pectoris

AGE-RELATED FACTORS
Pediatric:
• IHSS being recognized with increasing frequency
• Children may be asymptomatic. Evaluation of a heart murmur may disclose IHSS.
Geriatric: Occurrence is more frequent with increasing age. Female prevalence is greater in this age group.
Others: N/A

PREGNANCY N/A

SYNONYMS
• Hypertrophic obstructive cardiomyopathy (HOCM)
• Muscular subaortic stenosis

ICD-9-CM 425.1

SEE ALSO N/A

OTHER NOTES Genetic counseling may be appropriate

ABBREVIATIONS
• HCM = hypertrophic cardiomyopathy
• AS = aortic stenosis

REFERENCES
• Braunwald, E. (ed.): Heart Disease: A Textbook of Cardiovascular Medicine. 3rd Ed. Philadelphia, W.B. Saunders Co., 1988
• Maron, B.J. et al.: Sudden death in hypertrophic cardiomyopathy. A profile of 78 patients. Circulation 65. 1388, 1982

Author F. Griff, M.D.

Idiopathic thrombocytopenic purpura (ITP)

 BASICS

DESCRIPTION
A decrease in the circulating number of platelets (< 100,000 per microliter) in absence of toxic exposure or a disease associated with a low platelet count. It occurs as a secondary effect of peripheral platelet destruction as well as decreased platelet production. It is a disease of exclusion.
- Acute ITP - a disease of childhood which usually follows an acute infection and has spontaneous resolution within 2 months. Platelet counts < 20,000. This is a common disorder.
- Chronic ITP - a disease which persists after 6 months without a specific cause. Usually seen in adults and persists for months to years. Platelet count typically 30,000-80,000.

System(s) affected:
Hemic/Lymphatic/Immunologic
Genetics: No known genetic pattern
Incidence/Prevalence in USA: 1 in 10,000
Predominant age:
- Acute ITP - children ages 2-9 years old
- Chronic ITP - 20-50 years old
Predominant sex:
- Acute ITP - Male = Female
- Chronic ITP - Female > Male (3:1)

SIGNS AND SYMPTOMS
- Post traumatic bleeding at 40,000-60,000 platelet count
- Petechial hemorrhages
- Purpura
- Bruising tendency
- Gingival bleeding
- Gastrointestinal bleeding
- Mucocutaneous hemorrhages
- Menometrorrhagia
- Menorrhagia
- Recurrent epistaxis
- Neurological symptoms secondary to intracerebral bleeding
- Non-palpable spleen (absence of splenomegaly is an essential diagnostic criterion)
- Spontaneous bleeding < 20,000 platelet count

CAUSES
IgG autoantibodies on platelet surface

RISK FACTORS
- Acute infection
- Age
- Cardiopulmonary by-pass
- Hypersplenism
- Autophospholipid antibody syndrome
- Preeclampsia
- HIV infection

 DIAGNOSIS

DIFFERENTIAL DIAGNOSIS
- Drug induced immune thrombocytopenia. Over 150 drugs have been implicated
- Infections
- Acute leukemia
- Thrombotic thrombocytopenia purpura (TTP)
- Hemolytic uremic syndrome
- Factitious: "platelet clumping on the peripheral smear"
- Thrombocytopenia secondary to sepsis
- Myelodysplastic syndrome, particularly in the older patient
- Decreased production in marrow: malignancy, drugs, viruses, megaloblastic anemia
- Post transfusion
- Isoimmune neonatal purpura
- Disseminated intravascular coagulation (DIC)

LABORATORY
- Decreased platelet count: 5,000-75,000
- Relative lymphocytosis and slight eosinophilia
- Prolonged bleeding time (not useful in the presence of thrombocytopenia)
- Anemia
- PT, PTT normal
Drugs that may alter lab results: N/A
Disorders that may alter lab results: N/A

PATHOLOGICAL FINDINGS
- Peripheral smear shows normal red and white cells with diminished but large platelets
- Marrow reveals abundant megakaryocytes with normal erythroid and myeloid precursors

SPECIAL TESTS
- Peripheral smear
- Platelet associated antibody (PA-IgG)

IMAGING
CT of head to rule out intracranial bleeding

DIAGNOSTIC PROCEDURES
Bone marrow aspiration/biopsy

 TREATMENT

APPROPRIATE HEALTH CARE
- Outpatient management unless patient at risk for bleeding (platelet count < 20,000)
- Admit patients with active bleeding

GENERAL MEASURES
- Specific treatment usually not necessary unless count is < 100,000
- Splenectomy in patients who fail medical therapy. Be sure to administer pneumococcal vaccine 1 month prior to splenectomy.

ACTIVITY
Minimal activity to prevent injury or bruising. Avoid contact sports.

DIET
No special diet

PATIENT EDUCATION
Avoidance of ASA and other platelet inhibiting drugs

Idiopathic thrombocytopenic purpura (ITP)

MEDICATIONS

DRUG(S) OF CHOICE
• Acute ITP: prednisone 1-2 mg/kg/day for 4 weeks, then taper. If refractory, consider splenectomy.
• Chronic ITP: prednisone 60 mg/day for 4-6 weeks, then taper. May require repetition. If ineffective at non-toxic doses, consider splenectomy. Prednisone may then be effective. If still refractory, consider alternate drugs.
Contraindications: Do not administer gamma globulin if patient has IgA deficiency
Precautions: Refer to manufacturer's literature
Significant possible interactions: Anaphylaxis in patients with IgA deficiency who have IgA auto-antibodies

ALTERNATIVE DRUGS
• Acute ITP: IV gamma globulin 1-2 gm/kg single dose or 400 mg/kg/day for 5 days. Minor adverse reactions - chills, nausea, headache, joint pains in 2-7%. If this occurs, slow the rate of infusion. Gamma globulin may be effective alone or as a pretreatment to facilitate platelet transfusion. May delay need for splenectomy.
• Chronic ITP: high doses of intravenous gamma globulin in emergencies
• Danazol: 200-400 mg bid. There is decreased efficiency in young patients who have not had splenectomy.
• Immunosuppressive agents (vincristine, cyclophosphamide, azathioprine)
• Plasmapheresis
• Interferon alfa 2b

FOLLOWUP

PATIENT MONITORING
• Frequent platelet counts, daily to weekly, depending on severity and treatment
• Follow clinical status of hemostasis

PREVENTION/AVOIDANCE
Avoid medications (when feasible) that inhibit platelet function (such as aspirin), or those that suppress bone marrow

POSSIBLE COMPLICATIONS
• 1% mortality due to intracranial hemorrhage
• Severe blood loss
• Corticosteroid adverse effects
• Pneumococcal infections if patient must have splenectomy. Use pneumococcal vaccine.

EXPECTED COURSE AND PROGNOSIS
Acute ITP:
  ◊ 80-85% completely recover within 2 months
  ◊ 15% proceed to chronic ITP
Chronic ITP:
  ◊ 10-20% recover spontaneously
  ◊ Remainder with diminished platelets for months to years
  ◊ May see remissions and relapses

MISCELLANEOUS

ASSOCIATED CONDITIONS
Acute ITP:
  ◊ Varicella
  ◊ Other viral infections
Chronic ITP:
  ◊ HIV
  ◊ Graves' disease
  ◊ Hashimoto's thyroiditis
  ◊ Sarcoidosis
  ◊ Systemic lupus erythematosus
  ◊ Autoimmune hemolytic anemia (Evans' syndrome)

AGE-RELATED FACTORS
Pediatric:
• The acute form is primarily a childhood disease
• Better prognosis than adults
Geriatric: ITP is uncommon in this age group; look for other cause of low platelet count
Others: N/A

PREGNANCY
• Patient in labor should receive intravenous gamma globulin due to risk to the infant
• Platelet autoantibodies cross the placenta and may cause neonatal thrombocytopenia. Consider prednisone 10-20 mg/day for 10-14 days prior to delivery.
• Preeclampsia may cause thrombocytopenia unrelated to ITP

SYNONYMS
• Postinfectious thrombocytopenia
• Immune thrombocytopenic purpura
• Werlhof's disease

ICD-9-CM 287.3

SEE ALSO N/A

OTHER NOTES N/A

ABBREVIATIONS N/A

REFERENCES
• Schrier, S.L.: Disorder of hemostasis and coagulation. Scientific American Medicine. New York, Scientific American Inc., 5(6):13-17, 1988
• Aster, R.H., George, J.M.: Hemostasis. In Hematology. Edited by W.J. Williams, et al. New York, McGraw-Hill, 1990
• Kirchner, J.T.: Acute and chronic immune thrombocytopenic purpura. Post Grad Med 92:112-126;1992

Author J. Kirchner, D.O. & R. Scott, M.D.

Immunizations

 BASICS

DESCRIPTION For the prevention of certain diseases.
Specific indications:
<u>Hepatitis B</u>
• Healthcare workers
• Male homosexuals
• Newborns
• Travelers to endemic areas
• Laboratory personnel who might be exposed to the virus
• Intravenous drug users
• Patient's with a sexually transmitted disease
<u>Pneumococcal</u>
• All persons over age 65
• All patients prior to splenectomy
• Patients with chronic liver, heart, lung or renal disease
• Patients with diabetes mellitus, HIV
<u>Influenza</u>
• All persons over age 65
• Healthcare workers
• Patients with chronic heart, lung or renal disease (may begin at 6 months of age)
• Patients with diabetes mellitus, HIV
<u>Diphtheria, tetanus, pertussis (pediatric)</u>
• All children starting at age 2 months
• May be given up to the 7th birthday
<u>Diphtheria and tetanus (pediatric)</u>
• Children who cannot take DTP
• Children less than 7 years of age
<u>Tetanus and diphtheria (adult)</u>
• Children age 7 or over and adults
<u>Measles, mumps and rubella</u>
• Children at age 15 months and again between 4 and 6 years
• Adults (especially medical personnel and daycare workers) without prior immunization or uncertain immunizations born after 1957
• International travelers
• College students
<u>Polio</u>
• All children starting at 2 months of age
• Adults previously immunized who will travel to areas where polio is prevalent
• Unimmunized adults should receive the inactivated form of the vaccine
Genetics: N/A
Incidence/Prevalence in USA: N/A
Predominant age: N/A
Predominant race: N/A
Predominant sex: N/A

SIGNS AND SYMPTOMS N/A

CAUSES N/A

RISK FACTORS N/A

 DIAGNOSIS

DIFFERENTIAL DIAGNOSIS N/A

LABORATORY
• HBv: 95% develop adequate antibody to Hepatitis B (anti-HBs) after 3 immunizations.
Drugs that may alter lab results: N/A
Disorders that may alter lab results: N/A

PATHOLOGICAL FINDINGS N/A

SPECIAL TESTS N/A

IMAGING N/A

DIAGNOSTIC PROCEDURES N/A

 TREATMENT

APPROPRIATE HEALTH CARE N/A

GENERAL MEASURES
• Informed patient consent should discuss consequences of specific diseases and risks of immunizations
• Antipyretics (acetaminophen) are useful for the mild fever which may accompany immunizations

ACTIVITY No restrictions after immunization

DIET No specific restrictions after immunization

PATIENT EDUCATION Report adverse effects promptly. Minor redness, swelling, and or soreness at the site of injections can be expected; ice packs may be helpful.

```
---IMMUNIZATION SCHEDULE------------------------------------------------------
Age              Every  Immunization
------------------------------------------------------------------------------
Birth                   HBv
1-2 months              HBv
2 months                DTP, Polio, HbCV#1
4 months                DTP, Polio, HbCV#2
6 months                DTP, HBv, HbCV#3 (if HbOC used)
12 months               HbCV#3 (if PRP-OMP used)
15 months               DTP/DTaP, Polio, MMR, HbCV#4 (if HbOC used)
4-6 years               DTP/DTaP†, Polio†, MMR
16 years        10yrs   Td
65 yrs          yr      Influenza
65 yrs          once    Pneumococcal
------------------------------------------------------------------------------
†Not needed if previous vaccine given after the 4th birthday.
```

MEDICATIONS

DRUG(S) OF CHOICE

```
--IMMUNIZATION DOSES----------
Agent          Dose (ml)   Route
-----------------------------------
DTP              0.5         IM
MMR              0.5         SQ
Polio (TOPV)     0.5         PO
Polio (eIPV)     0.5         SQ
HBv†             ††          IM
HbCV             0.5         IM
Influenza        0.5         IM
Td and DT        0.5         IM
Pneumococcal     0.5         IM
-----------------------------------
```

```
†Newborns of mothers who are
hepatitis B surface antigen
positive should also receive
HBIG
††Variable. See manufacturer's
directions.
```

```
--TETANUS WOUND PROPHYLAXIS---
                 Prior Tetanus
Type of          immunizations
wound         -------------------
              |           |
              | Uncertain | ≥3
              | or <3 doses |doses
              |   Td   TIG |  Td‡
-----------------------------------
Clean†    |    Yes   No  |  10
Dirty††   |    Yes   Yes |  5
Puncture  |    Yes   Yes |  5
Major†††  |    Yes   Yes |  5
-----------------------------------
```

```
For example, an adult with a
puncture wound and 2 prior
doses of tetanus toxoid should
receive both Td and TIG.
---
‡TIG not needed; give Td if
years indicated have passed
since last immunization
  †Clean: Minor wound
  ††Dirty: Contaminated with
dirt, feces, or saliva
  †††Major: Burn, frostbite,
crush injury
```

Contraindications:
• Anaphylaxis to thimerosal: Avoid giving DTP, DT, TD, PRP-OMP, multi-dose vials of HbOC, influenza, and some brands of pneumococcal vaccine
• Anaphylaxis to neomycin: Avoid giving MMR, TOPV, eIPV
• Anaphylaxis to streptomycin: Avoid giving TOPV, eIPV, MMR, DTP, HbCV
• Anaphylaxis to immunization
• Encephalopathy within 7 days after DTP: Give DT on next immunization

Precautions:
DTP
• Suspected neurologic disease: Delay immunization until clarified
• Fever of ≥ 40.5ºC (105ºF) within 48 hours after previous DTP
• Collapse or shock-like state (hypotonic-hyporesponsive episode) within 48 hours after DTP
• Seizure within 3 days after DTP
• Persistent, inconsolable crying lasting ≥3 hrs within 48 hours after DTP

• The following are not contraindications and DTP may be given if present:
  ◊ Family history of convulsions: Pre-treat with acetaminophen and after DTP q4h for 24 hrs
  ◊ Family history of SIDS
  ◊ Family history of adverse event following DTP
  ◊ Temperature <40.5ºC (105ºF) following a prior DTP
Other
• Immunocompromised patients should, in general, not receive live viral vaccines (MMR and TOPV), although patients with HIV may receive MMR and eIPV.
• Persons with unavoidable (e.g. household) contact with the immunocompromised should not receive TOPV (give eIPV).

Significant possible interactions:
• Avoid MMR within 3 months after gamma globulin
• Administer influenza and DTP at least 3 days apart

ALTERNATIVE DRUGS None

FOLLOWUP

PATIENT MONITORING None routinely needed.
• Hepatitis: May measure antibody (anti-HBs) response after HBv if protection is very important (e.g., healthcare workers and immuno-compromised persons).
• Measles disease: Immunity and actual disease difficult to ascertain; administer MMR or check antibody titers

PREVENTION/AVOIDANCE N/A

POSSIBLE COMPLICATIONS
Fever, malaise, local reactions (redness, pain) are the most common. Rarely, allergic reactions, febrile seizures. Encephalopathy associated with DTP is controversial.

EXPECTED COURSE AND PROGNOSIS Good, most patients develop protective antibodies

MISCELLANEOUS

ASSOCIATED CONDITIONS N/A

AGE-RELATED FACTORS
Pediatric: Most immunizations are given before entry into school. Do not delay immunization of the preterm infant unless specific contraindications exist.

Geriatric: Pneumococcal, influenza, and tetanus are needed in older age groups
Others: N/A

PREGNANCY MMR should not be routinely given to women who are pregnant or who are planning pregnancy in the next 3 months.

SYNONYMS
• Vaccinations
• Inoculations

ICD-9-CM
V05.9 Healthy person receiving prophylactic inoculation or vaccination

SEE ALSO
• Diphtheria
• Hepatitis, viral
• Influenza
• Measles, rubella
• Measles, rubeola
• Pertussis
• Pneumonia, bacterial
• Poliomyelitis
• Mumps
• Tetanus

OTHER NOTES
• PPD may be given at same time as MMR and/or TOPV or wait 4 weeks after immunization to do skin test
• Culture-proven pertussis provides immunity; use DT instead of DTP
• Haemophilus disease: Immunity not provided when child under 2 years; administer immunization as if no disease has occurred.
• Combination vaccines are available

ABBREVIATIONS
DTP = pediatric diphtheria, tetanus toxoids, and pertussis vaccine
DTaP = pediatric diphtheria, tetanus toxoids, and acellular pertussis vaccine
DT = pediatric diphtheria and tetanus toxoids
T = tetanus toxoids
Td = adult diphtheria and tetanus toxoids

HBv = hepatitis vaccine
HBIG = hepatitis B immune globulin

TOPV = trivalent oral polio vaccine
eIPV = enhanced inactivated polio vaccine

HbOC = HbCV vaccine (hibTITER)
PRP-OMP = HbCV vaccine (PedvaxHIB)

MMR = measles, mumps, and rubella vaccine
HbCV = conjugated Haemophilus influenza type b vaccine
INF = influenza vaccine
PNEU = pneumococcal vaccine
PPD = purified protein derivative
VZIG = varicella-zoster immune globulin

REFERENCES
• Immunization Practices Advisory Committee
• American Academy of Pediatrics
• American Academy of Family Physicians

Author R. Zimmerman, M.D., R. Clover, M.D.

Immunodeficiency diseases

BASICS

DESCRIPTION Disorders associated with disruption of the integrity of the immune system resulting in a wide spectrum of illnesses
• May be primary or secondary and involve any or all of the system's cells and their products (T cells, B cells, monocytes, macrophages, etc.) their receptors, metabolic pathways and products which are normally involved in health maintenance and protection
<u>Primary</u>
◊ Combined immunodeficiencies, e.g., severe combined immunodeficiency (SCID), adenosine deaminase (ADA) deficiency, and reticular dysgenesis
◊ Antibody deficiencies, e.g., X-linked agammaglobulinemia, IgA deficiency, Ig deficiency with increased IgM (hyper-IgM syndrome), common variable immunodeficiency (CVID) and transient hypogammaglobulinemia of infancy
◊ Other well-defined syndromes, e.g., Wiskott-Aldrich syndrome (eczema, thrombocytopenia and repeated infections), ataxia telangiectasia (cerebellar ataxia, oculocutaneous telangiectasia and immunodeficiency) and DiGeorge's syndrome (isolated T cell deficiency)
◊ Associated syndromes e.g., Down's syndrome, chronic mucocutaneous candidiasis, hyper-IgE syndrome, chronic granulomatous disease, partial albinism and WHIM syndrome (warts, hypogammaglobulinemia, infection, myelokathexis [retention of leukocytes in a hypercellular marrow]), phagocytic defects with early onset of periodontal disease.
<u>Secondary</u>
◊ AIDS
◊ Other infections, malignancies, malnutrition, protein-losing enteropathy, drugs, and chronic stress
System(s) affected:
Hemic/Lymphatic/Immunologic
Genetics: Included in Description
Incidence/Prevalence in USA:
• 1 in every 500 (including IgA deficiency) born with an immune system defect
• Many more will acquire a defect which may be transient or permanent
Predominant age:
• All ages. Children most likely to present with primary and/or inherited deficiencies.
• Number of newborns with AIDS increasing. In part associated with: 1) increased premature infant survival, 2) improved treatment and care of other primary diseases, 3) use of immunosuppressive agents.
Predominant sex: Male > Female

SIGNS AND SYMPTOMS
<u>Common features</u>
◊ Unusual susceptibility to infection. Frequency and severity vary with type of defect.
◊ Malignancies, especially lymphoreticular
◊ Increased tendency toward autoimmune disorders

◊ Weight loss
◊ Fever
<u>More specific features</u>
◊ Combined T and B cell deficiencies associated with severe fungal, bacterial and viral infections. Enzyme deficiencies may be involved.
◊ T cell deficiencies may be acquired (as with the human immunodeficiency virus) or congenital with wide spectrum manifestations. Children with DiGeorge's syndrome show cardiac defects, micrognathia, hypertelorism and hypocalcemic tetany.
◊ B cell or immunoglobulin deficiency syndromes may be associated with chronic sinusitis, recurrent respiratory infection, chronic diarrheal disease, rheumatoid arthritis, systemic lupus erythematosus (SLE), atopy, splenomegaly, anemia, recurrent pneumococcal pneumonia and meningococcal meningitis
◊ Chronic giardiasis, fever of unknown origin and malabsorption should cause suspicion of immunodeficiency
◊ Miscellaneous syndromes include chronic mucocutaneous candidiasis, fatal Epstein-Barr virus infection, and complement component deficiencies

CAUSES
<u>Primary immunodeficiency diseases</u>
◊ Faulty genes and gene products resulting in inherited defects of the immune system including: antibody, cellular, phagocytic and complement deficiencies
◊ Manifested by infections soon after birth but may not be expressed clinically until later in life
<u>Secondary immunodeficiency diseases</u>
◊ Treatment with immunosuppressive agents
◊ Nutritional deficiencies
◊ Use of drugs and exposure to chemicals should be considered
◊ X-ray treatment
◊ IgA deficiency associated with phenytoin or penicillamine
◊ Thymoma associated with hypogammaglobulinemia
◊ Viruses e.g., HIV-1 and HIV-2

RISK FACTORS
• Family history
• Almost anything less than good health practices
• Drug abuse and parenteral blood exposure
• Sexual lifestyle
• Aging

DIAGNOSIS

DIFFERENTIAL DIAGNOSIS
• Must consider all immunodeficiency disorders
• Careful history and physical will direct proper search

LABORATORY
• High percentage of immunodeficiencies will be discovered by a CBC with a differential smear and immunoglobulin levels including: IgG, IgA, IgM and IgE. IgG subclasses should be included.
• Further assays include mononuclear cell populations which may be quantified
• Total lymphocyte a good screen
• Functional evaluation by skin testing (anergy battery) and antibody levels to common viruses and bacterial toxins
• Complement levels
• Phagocyte function
• Specific cytokine function
• Additional specific tests for suspected acquired causes for immunodeficiencies (AIDS, chronic diarrhea, malignancy, drugs, etc.)
Drugs that may alter lab results: N/A
Disorders that may alter lab results: N/A

PATHOLOGICAL FINDINGS Vary with type of deficiency and resultant disease(s)

SPECIAL TESTS N/A

IMAGING
• MRI helpful in evaluation of CNS lesions associated with toxoplasmosis
• Techniques and technology continue to improve dramatically

DIAGNOSTIC PROCEDURES
• Careful history and physical
• Try to deduce whether infections associated with T cell response inadequacies (fungal and other opportunistic infections) or lack of B cell (antibodies) response or both

TREATMENT

APPROPRIATE HEALTH CARE
• Outpatient or inpatient management appropriate to clinical problem

GENERAL MEASURES
• Depends mainly on complexity of the immune deficiency
• Bone marrow transplant with donor T cell engraftment in severe abnormalities of T cell function. Best done at referral research centers.
• Intravenous immunoglobulin - for patients deficient in IgG. Not appropriate for treatment for Ig deficiency other than IgG, but may be helpful in the hyper-IgM syndrome.

ACTIVITY As appropriate

DIET Severe immunodeficiencies require sterile conditions

PATIENT EDUCATION Printed patient information available from: Immune Deficiency Foundation, P.O. Box 586, Columbia, MD 21045, (301)461-3127

MEDICATIONS

DRUG(S) OF CHOICE
• Antibiotics with appropriate spectra for infecting organism(s). Ketoconazole reported to be effective in some chronic fungal infections.
• Enzyme replacement therapy for ADA deficiency
• Autologous genetically corrected T cells with normal ADA gene
Contraindications: Refer to manufacturer's literature
Precautions:
• Multidisciplinary input in order
• Refer to manufacturer's literature
Significant possible interactions: Refer to manufacturer's literature

ALTERNATIVE DRUGS N/A

FOLLOWUP

PATIENT MONITORING
• Children with SCID must remain in controlled environment, exposure to any pathogen may result in death
• IgG levels monitored and maintained in common variable hypogammaglobulinemia
• Meticulous instruction and checks for infections

PREVENTION/AVOIDANCE Genetic counseling for primary cases

POSSIBLE COMPLICATIONS
• Autoimmune disorders
• Serum sickness reactions to gamma globulin treatment
• Malignancies
• Overwhelming infection
• Fatal graft-versus-host disease following blood transfusions in SCID patients

EXPECTED COURSE AND PROGNOSIS Related closely to type and degree of immunodeficiency

MISCELLANEOUS

ASSOCIATED CONDITIONS N/A

AGE-RELATED FACTORS
Pediatric: Depends on specific immunodeficiency disorder
Geriatric: Depends on specific immunodeficiency disorder
Others: N/A

PREGNANCY AIDS transmission

SYNONYMS N/A

ICD-9-CM 279.3

SEE ALSO N/A

OTHER NOTES
Research opportunities:
◊ Continue genetic studies at the molecular level
◊ Continue to develop techniques of replacing gene and gene products where deficiencies are either inherited or acquired
◊ Expand acquired immunodeficiency research and the addressing of clinical and social problems

ABBREVIATIONS N/A

REFERENCES
• NIAID Task Force on Immunology and Allergy
• Wilson, J.D., et al. (eds.): Harrison's Principles of Internal Medicine. 12th Ed. New York, McGraw-Hill, 1991
• Lichtenstein, L. & Fauci, A.: Current Therapy in Allergy, Immunology and Rheumatology. Toronto, B.C. Decker, Inc., 1988
• Stiehm, E.R. & Blaese, R.M.: Pediatric Research. Vol. 33, No. 1 (suppl)/Jan, 1993

Author H. Dix, M.D.

Impetigo

BASICS

DESCRIPTION   A superficial, intraepidermal, unilocular, vesiculopustular infection. Typically begins as erythematous tender papule that rapidly progresses through a vesicular to a honey-crusted stage. Still debated as to relative importance of staphylococci versus streptococci. Cultures give 60% mixed, 30% beta-hemolytic streptococci, and 10% coagulase-positive staphylococci.
• Bullous impetigo: Staphylococci impetigo that progress rapidly to small to large flaccid bulla
• Folliculitis: Considered by some to be staphylococci aureus impetigo of the hair follicle
• Ecthyma: A deeper, ulcerated, impetigo infection often with lymphadenitis
System(s) affected: Skin/Exocrine
Genetics: N/A
Incidence/Prevalence in USA: Unreported
Predominant age: 2-5 years
Predominant sex: Male = Female

SIGNS AND SYMPTOMS
• May be slow and indolent or rapidly spreading
• Tender red macule or papule as early lesion
• Thin roofed vesicle to bullae
• Pustules
• Weeping shallow red ulcer
• Honey-colored crusts
• Most frequent on face around mouth and nose, or at site of trauma
• Satellite lesions
• Often multiple sites

CAUSES
• Beta-hemolytic streptococci - felt to be primary cause most of time and found in pure culture 30% of the time
• Coagulase positive staphylococci - pure culture about 10%. More contagious via contact.
• Mixed infections of streptococci and staphhylococci found 60%. Streptococci usually believed to be the primary organism. Data suggest increasing importance of staphylococci.
• Direct contact or insect vector
• Can be contamination at trauma site

RISK FACTORS
• Warm, humid environment
• Tropical or subtropical climate
• Summer or fall season
• Minor trauma, insect bites, etc.
• Poor hygiene, epidemics, during war, etc.
• Familial spread
• Poor health with anemia and malnutrition
• Complication to pediculosis, scabies, chickenpox, eczema
• Contact dermatitis (Rhus)

DIAGNOSIS

DIFFERENTIAL DIAGNOSIS
• Chickenpox
• Herpes
• Folliculitis
• Erysipelas
• Insect bites
• Severe eczematous dermatitis

LABORATORY
• Culture - taken from the base of lesion after removal of crust. Blood agar grows both staphylococci and group A streptococci
• ASO titer - can be weak positive for streptococci (not usually done)
• Streptozyme - positive for streptococci (not usually done)
Drugs that may alter lab results: N/A
Disorders that may alter lab results:
Streptococci pharyngitis will alter streptococci enzyme tests

PATHOLOGICAL FINDINGS   N/A

SPECIAL TESTS   Cultures as listed under Laboratory

IMAGING   N/A

DIAGNOSTIC PROCEDURES   N/A

TREATMENT

APPROPRIATE HEALTH CARE
Outpatient

GENERAL MEASURES   Removal of crusts, cleanliness with gentle washing 2-3 times daily

ACTIVITY   No restrictions

DIET   No special diet

PATIENT EDUCATION   Good hygiene important to prevent possible spread

MEDICATIONS

DRUG(S) OF CHOICE
(Note: Increasing incidence of Staphylococcus resistant to erythromycin and penicillin may make the following suggestions inaccurate in your community). If any question of mixed etiology, would use drug with staphylococcus coverage and not start with penicillin VK.
Non-bullous (minor spread, treat 7 days; widespread, treat 10 days)
◊ Penicillin VK - adults 250-500 mg qid (or injectable penicillin G). Pediatric 25-50 mg/kg/d divided every 6 hours.
◊ Erythromycin - adults 1 gm/day divided doses q6h in adults. Pediatric 30-40 mg/kg/d divided 6 hours.
◊ Mupirocin topical ointment (Bactroban) apply tid, 7-10 days
Bullous (treat 10 days)
◊ Dicloxacillin - adult 250 mg qid. Pediatric 12-25 mg/kg/d divided q6h
◊ Erythromycin 1 gm/day divided doses q6h
Contraindications: Drug allergy
Precautions: Refer to manufacturer's profile of each drug
Significant possible interactions:
• Erythromycin with theophyllines
• Refer to manufacturer's profile of each drug

ALTERNATIVE DRUGS
Oral 1st generation cephalosporins - pediatric doses:
◊ Cephalexin - 25-50 mg/kg/24 h divide q6h
◊ Cefaclor - 40 mg/kg/24 h divide q 8 h
◊ Cephradine - 25-50 mg/kg/24 h divide q 6-12 h
◊ Cefadroxil - 30 mg/kg/24 h divide bid
Oral 1st generation cephalosporins - adult doses:
◊ Cephalexin - 250 mg qid
◊ Cefaclor - 250 mg tid
◊ Cephradine - 250 mg bid
◊ Cefadroxil - 1 gm/day

FOLLOWUP

PATIENT MONITORING
If not clear within 7-10 days, culture the lesions

PREVENTION/AVOIDANCE
Close attention to family hygiene, particularly hand washing

POSSIBLE COMPLICATIONS
• Ecthyma
• Erysipelas
• Post-streptococcal acute glomerulonephritis
• Deep cellulitis
• Bacteremia

EXPECTED COURSE AND PROGNOSIS
• Complete resolution in 7-10 days with treatment
• Antibiotic treatment will not prevent or halt glomerulonephritis as it will with rheumatic fever

MISCELLANEOUS

ASSOCIATED CONDITIONS
• Malnutrition and anemia
• Crowded living conditions
• Poor hygiene
• Neglected minor trauma

AGE-RELATED FACTORS
Pediatric: Impetigo neonatorum may occur by nursery contamination
Geriatric: N/A
Others: N/A

PREGNANCY   N/A

SYNONYMS
• Pyoderma
• Impetigo contagiosa
• Impetigo vulgaris
• Fox impetigo

ICD-9-CM   684

SEE ALSO   N/A

OTHER NOTES   N/A

ABBREVIATIONS   N/A

REFERENCES
• Braunwald E., et al. (eds.): Harrison's Principles of Internal Medicine. 12th Ed. New York, McGraw-Hill, 1991
• Moschella, S.L., and Hurley, H.J.: Dermatology. 2nd Ed. Philadelphia, W.B. Saunders Co., 1985

Author   W. Billica, M.D.

Inappropriate secretion of antidiuretic hormone

BASICS

DESCRIPTION A form of hyponatremia with inappropriately elevated urine osmolality and no discernible stimulus for ADH release. Total body sodium levels may be normal or near normal. Associated with an underlying disorder, e.g., neoplasm, pulmonary disorder, or central nervous system disease.
System(s) affected: Endocrine/Metabolic
Genetics: No known genetic pattern
Incidence/Prevalence in USA: Rare
Predominant age: Common in the elderly
Predominant sex: N/A

SIGNS AND SYMPTOMS
- Usually neurological
- Lethargy
- Restlessness
- Confusion
- Edema (rare)
- Anorexia
- Nausea/vomiting
- Headache
- Irritability
- Decreasing reflexes
- Seizures
- Coma
- Asymptomatic

CAUSES
- Oat cell carcinoma of the lung
- Drugs (vincristine, narcotics, thiazide diuretics, cyclophosphamide, carbamazepine, barbiturates, morphine, chlorpropamide, nicotine, beta-adrenergic agents, general anesthetics, oxytocin)
- Ectopic ADH production
- Hodgkin's disease
- Hypothyroidism
- Idiopathic
- Infectious diseases
- Lupus erythematosus
- Meningitis
- Myocardial infarction
- Myxedema
- Pancreatic carcinoma
- Pneumonia
- Porphyria
- Positive-pressure breathing
- Pulmonary tuberculosis
- Rocky Mountain spotted fever
- Tumor - bronchogenic carcinoma
- Vascular diseases

RISK FACTORS
- Patient with causative disorder
- Use of predisposing drugs
- Elderly patient
- Postoperative
- Institutionalized patient

DIAGNOSIS

DIFFERENTIAL DIAGNOSIS
- Postoperative: 1) caused by non-osmotic release of ADH 2) affects women more than men 3) ADH increased by pain and narcotics.
- Postprostatectomy syndrome: 1) irrigating solution must be non-conducting (i.e., electrolyte free) 2) D5W absorbed
- Psychotic polydipsia: 1) active therapy rarely needed 2) diuresis occurs when intake stopped 3) intake usually over 10 L/day 4) interaction with other psychotropic drugs.
- Acute (usually in children): 1) swallowing water during swimming 2) diluted formula 3) tap water enemas.
- Drug induced: 1) oxytocin infusion - given in D5W during labor (oxytocin has antidiuretic effect) 2) cyclophosphamide - usually with IV administration 3) chlorpropamide (oral hypoglycemic agent) 4) carbamazepine - central ADH release 5) vincristine - central SIADH 6) nonsteroidal anti-inflammatory drugs (NSAID's) - decreased renal prostaglandins
- Diuretic drug induced:- 1) usually thiazide 2) vasopressin increased by decreasing EABV 3) usually elderly patients or in bulimia 4) correct slowly
- Tumor Induced - bronchogenic carcinoma (secretes ADH-like substance)
- Unexplained persistent hyponatremia may indicate a tumor
- Pulmonary: 1) tuberculosis - secretes ADH 2) mechanical ventilation - increased intrathoracic pressure, decreased cardiac output, causes decreased EABV, causes increased ADH 3) asthma, acute respiratory failure, pneumonia
- CNS/hypothalamic irritation 1) meningitis 2) Rocky Mountain spotted fever 3) encephalitis 4) trauma - especially after CNS surgery
- Endocrine 1) Addison's Disease 2) hypothyroid

LABORATORY
- BUN low or normal
- Creatinine low or normal
- Urine osmolality 200+ milliosmols
- Urinary Na concentration > 20 mEq/L
- Elevated serum concentration ADH
- Normal adrenal and renal function
- Uric acid low
Drugs that may alter lab results: N/A
Disorders that may alter lab results: N/A

PATHOLOGICAL FINDINGS N/A

SPECIAL TESTS Oral water-loading test may be helpful in diagnosis in some patients. Response to water-load will be impaired in SIADH.

IMAGING N/A

DIAGNOSTIC PROCEDURES N/A

TREATMENT

APPROPRIATE HEALTH CARE
Outpatient or inpatient depending on severity of symptoms or underlying cause

GENERAL MEASURES
Mildly symptomatic
◊ Patient has serum Na > 125 mEq/L
◊ Restrict fluid to 800-1000 mL/day
Acute (less than 48 hours duration)
◊ Hypertonic saline
◊ Water diuresis
Symptomatic (seizure, coma)
◊ High mortality due to cerebral edema if serum Na < 120 mEq/L
◊ Decrease oral free water to 2/3 maintenance
◊ Increase oral salt
◊ Correct serum Na deficit. (mEq sodium deficit = desired sodium minus actual sodium times 0.5 times weight [kg])
◊ Increase serum sodium slowly with hypertonic saline by 0.5 mEq/L /hour until it reaches 120 mEq/L

ACTIVITY As tolerated

DIET May need increased salt or decreased water intake depending on cause

PATIENT EDUCATION Diet and fluid restrictions

MEDICATIONS

DRUG(S) OF CHOICE
• Water diuresis - furosemide (Lasix) plus hourly sodium chloride and potassium chloride replacement - requires frequent monitoring. Treatment of choice for acute management.
• Demeclocycline - blocks ADH at renal tubule - produces nephrogenic diabetes insipidus. (Dosage for long term management: 600-1200 mg/day. Onset of action is within one week, therefore not best for acute management).
• Lithium - blocks ADH at renal tubule - has the problem of lithium toxicity, antianabolic effects especially in cirrhosis and congestive heart failure

Hypertonic (3%) saline
◊ Increase serum Na by 10-12 mEq/L every 24 hrs
◊ Increase serum Na ± 5% over first few hours
◊ Increase serum Na to only 120 mEq/L, acutely
◊ Increase serum Na by 0.5 mEq/hr

Contraindications: Avoid fluids in congestive heart failure, nephrotic syndrome or cirrhosis

Precautions:

Too rapid correction can cause:
◊ Congestive heart failure
◊ Subdural and intracerebral hemorrhage
◊ Permanent CNS damage, especially with serum Na < 120 mEq/L

Significant possible interactions: Refer to manufacturer's literature

ALTERNATIVE DRUGS   N/A

FOLLOWUP

PATIENT MONITORING
• Careful, continuous, clinical and laboratory monitoring of the hyponatremic state during acute phase
• For chronic management, monitor underlying cause as needed

PREVENTION/AVOIDANCE
• Search for cause of SIADH, if unknown
• Monitor electrolytes in postoperative patients to determine if fluid intake needs restriction
• Reducing or changing medications, if a drug is the cause
• Life-long restriction of fluid intake

POSSIBLE COMPLICATIONS   Central pontine myelinolysis: Chronic hyponatremia (usually < 120 mEq/L); too rapid correction (> 12 mEq/L/day)

EXPECTED COURSE AND PROGNOSIS   Dependent on underlying cause

MISCELLANEOUS

ASSOCIATED CONDITIONS   Listed with Causes

AGE-RELATED FACTORS
Pediatric: N/A
Geriatric: Most common in this age group
Others: N/A

PREGNANCY   N/A

SYNONYMS
• SIADH
• Syndrome of inappropriate secretion of ADH

ICD-9-CM   276.9

SEE ALSO   Hyponatremia

OTHER NOTES   N/A

ABBREVIATIONS   N/A

REFERENCES
• Brenner, B.M. & Rector, F.C., Jr.: The Kidney. 3rd Ed., Philadelphia, W.B. Saunders Co., 1986
• Kokko, J.M.: Fluid and Electrolytes. Philadelphia, W.B. Saunders Co., 1989

Author   W. Arnold, M.D.

Influenza

 BASICS

DESCRIPTION An acute, usually self-limited, viral, febrile, infection caused by influenza virus types A, B, and C. It is marked by inflammation of the nasal mucosa, pharynx, conjunctiva, and respiratory tract. Outbreaks occur almost every winter with varying degrees of severity.
• The influenza virus displays antigenic drift (variation) which leads to strains of the virus to which there is little immunologic resistance in the population and may result in pandemics.
System(s) affected: Pulmonary
Genetics: N/A
Incidence in USA: 250,000-500,000 new cases each year. Attack rates in healthy children are 10-40% each year.
Prevalence in USA: N/A
Predominant age: School-aged children (3 months - 16 years); young adult (16-40 years); elderly (> 75 years)
Predominant sex: Male = Female

SIGNS AND SYMPTOMS
Sudden onset of:
• High fever
• Myalgia (sometimes severe and lasting for days)
• Sore throat/pharyngitis
• Nonproductive cough
• Abdominal pain
• Headache
• Cervical lymphadenopathy
• Chills
• Gastrointestinal pain in young children
• Nasal congestion
• Malaise
• Rales
• Rhinorrhea
• Rhonchi
• Sinusitis
• Sneezing
• Wheezes

CAUSES Orthomyxovirus (influenza antigenic types A, B, and C) that are transmitted person-to-person, or by indirect contact (e.g., use of contaminated drinking glass)

RISK FACTORS
For contracting disease:
◊ Patients in semi-closed environments such as nursing homes
◊ Students, prisoners
◊ Crowded, close environments during times of epidemics
For complications
◊ Chronic pulmonary diseases
◊ Cardiovascular diseases including valvular problems and congestive heart failure
◊ Metabolic diseases
◊ Hemoglobinopathies
◊ Malignancies
◊ Pregnancy in the 3rd trimester
◊ Neonates, elderly
◊ Immunosuppression

 DIAGNOSIS

DIFFERENTIAL DIAGNOSIS
• Febrile or afebrile common cold
• Bronchitis
• Atypical pneumonia
• Viral tonsillitis
• Infectious mononucleosis
• Coxsackie virus infections

LABORATORY
• Egg or tissue culture of nasopharyngeal swab or aspirate
Hospital tests:
• Complement fixation antibody
• Immunofluorescence or ELISA
• Hemagglutination inhibition assay
• Convalescent rise in viral titers - but not very useful clinically
• Leukopenia
• Leukocytosis may signal complications
Drugs that may alter lab results: N/A
Disorders that may alter lab results: N/A

PATHOLOGICAL FINDINGS
Inflammation of respiratory tract

IMAGING
Chest x-ray
◊ Normal (50-90%)
◊ Increased vascular markings
◊ Basilar streaking
◊ Patchy infiltrate - mild disease
◊ Diffuse alveolar infiltrates of adult respiratory distress syndrome.

SPECIAL TESTS N/A

DIAGNOSTIC PROCEDURES
• Tissue culture of nasopharyngeal swab or aspirate
• History and physical examination - close attention to epidemiology (e.g., current outbreak in community)

 TREATMENT

APPROPRIATE HEALTH CARE
Outpatient except for treatment of severe complications or treatment of those in high risk groups

GENERAL MEASURES
• Symptomatic treatment (saline nasal spray, analgesic gargle or gargle with double-strength tea for throat discomfort
• Cool-mist humidifier to increase moisture of inspired air
• Modified respiratory isolation techniques
• Hospitalized patients may require oxygen or ventilatory support
• Avoid smoking

DIET Increase fluid intake

ACTIVITY Bedrest during acute phase and for 24-48 hours after temperature returns to normal. Hospitalized individuals should have contact isolation with strict hand washing procedures.

PATIENT EDUCATION
• For patient education materials favorably reviewed on this topic, contact: American Academy of Family Physicians Foundation, PO Box 8418, Kansas City, MO 64114 (800)274-2237, ext. 440
• Educate high-risk patients about prevention

MEDICATIONS

DRUG(S) OF CHOICE
• Amantadine (only effective for influenza A) - recommended for patients with pneumonia, severe disease or at high risk for complications. 100-200 mg daily orally for 2-7 days. It shortens duration of fever, systemic and respiratory symptoms by about 50%. Effective if administered within the first 48 hours. Dose for children less than 45 kg or less than 10 years old is 4.4 mg/kg/day divided into two doses.
• Antipyretics: Acetaminophen. Important to control fever in children to avoid febrile convulsions. Aspirin should not be used in children < 16 years old due to risk of Reye's syndrome.
• Cough suppressants
• Appropriate antibiotics if complicating bacterial infection

Contraindications: Pregnancy, nursing mothers

Precautions:

Amantidine
• May cause mild CNS symptoms (e.g., lightheadedness, insomnia, anxiety) which are dose related and clear with discontinuation. It may impair ability to perform hazardous activities or to drive a motor vehicle.
• May potentiate underlying seizure disorders and exacerbate epilepsy; EEG abnormalities are increased
• May exacerbate liver disease
• Uncontrolled psychosis or severe psychoneurosis
• Observe patients with congestive heart failure for deterioration.
• Patients > 65 years old or with renal impairment should receive a reduced dose.

Significant possible interactions:
Increased atropine-like effects may occur if amantadine is given concurrently with anticholinergic drugs (e.g., antihistamines). May interact with CNS stimulants as well.

ALTERNATIVE DRUGS N/A

FOLLOWUP

PATIENT MONITORING
In mild cases, usually no follow-up required. Follow moderate or severe cases until symptoms resolved and any complications are treated effectively.

PREVENTION/AVOIDANCE
• Most infections in 24 hours before onset of symptoms and during period of peak symptoms. Incubation period is 1 to 5 days

Polyvalent influenza vaccine:
◊ Vaccine recommended for high risk individuals: chronic pulmonary disease, cardiovascular disease, immunosuppression, hemoglobinopathies, renal diseases, metabolic disease, including diabetes, HIV,

long term aspirin therapy, adults aged 65 and over
◊ Vaccine recommended for health care providers, home care providers, residents of nursing homes and other chronic care facilities, and close contacts of high risk individuals
◊ Should be administered in the fall prior to influenza season
◊ Some side effects possible, e.g., fever and mild, local reaction at vaccination site.
◊ Two vaccines: Whole and split virus
◊ Split vaccine for children < 12 years old; adults may receive either vaccine.
◊ Dose is 0.5 IM except for children < 3 years old. Children 6 through 35 months old should receive 0.25 ml.
◊ Single dose/year except for children < 9 years old who should receive 2 doses the first year that they receive influenza vaccine (1 month apart)
◊ Vaccine contraindications: Anaphylaxis to eggs (do skin testing first).
◊ 2 weeks after immunization before protection occurs
◊ Do not administer within 3 days of DTP vaccine

Amantadine:
◊ May be used prophylactically in high risk groups (that have not been vaccinated or need additional control measures) during epidemics of influenza A (ineffective against influenza B). It should not be considered as a substitute for vaccination unless vaccine contraindicated.
◊ 100 mg orally daily (for adults and children > 20 kg) for duration of outbreak, if no vaccine given. Discontinue after 14 days if used in addition to vaccine.
◊ Protective efficacy about 80% for type A influenza virus only

EXPECTED COURSE AND PROGNOSIS Favorable

POSSIBLE COMPLICATIONS
• Myocarditis (rare)
• Myoglobinuria
• Myositis (rare)
• Otitis media
• Pericarditis (rare)
• Pneumonia
• Reye's syndrome
• Rhabdomyolysis
• Post-influenza asthenia
• Acute sinusitis
• Encephalitis (rare)
• Guillain-Barré syndrome (rare)
• Transverse myelitis (rare)
• Croup
• Apnea in neonates
• Death

MISCELLANEOUS

ASSOCIATED CONDITIONS Bacterial pneumonia

AGE-RELATED FACTORS
Pediatric: Reye's syndrome is a rare and severe complication associated with Aspirin use. Do not give aspirin to children with influenza; use acetaminophen.

Geriatric:
• More susceptible to influenza infections and have increased morbidity (due to frequent and numerous complications)
• Immunization recommended for all individuals over age 65

Others: N/A

PREGNANCY
• Women with medical problems that place them at risk from complications of influenza should receive influenza vaccine. Administration after the first trimester is reasonable unless pregnant women at high risk for influenza complications would be unprotected when the influenza season begins. In such circumstances, it is undesirable to delay immunization even though it is during the first trimester.
• Amantadine is contraindicated in pregnant women.

SYNONYMS
• Flu
• Grip
• Acute catarrhal fever

ICD-9-CM
487 Influenza

OTHER NOTES
Persons with HIV infection should get annual influenza vaccination, however the antibody response to the vaccine may be low in persons with advanced HIV-related illnesses.

SEE ALSO N/A

ABBREVIATIONS N/A

REFERENCES
• Report of the Committee on Infectious Diseases, 1991. Elk Grove Village, American Academy of Pediatrics, 1991.
• Prevention and control of influenza. Recommendations of the Immunization Practices Advisory Committee (ACIP). MMWR 1991;40(RR-6):1-15.
• Mandell, G.L. (ed.): Principles and Practice of Infectious Diseases. 3rd Ed. New York, Churchill Livingstone, 1990

Author R. Zimmerman, M.D., M.P.H.

Insect bites & stings

BASICS

DESCRIPTION Arthropods affect man by being pests, inoculating poison, invading tissue, or transmitting disease. Inoculation of poison may occur as either a bite or a sting. This discussion is limited to the irritative, poisonous, allergic effects of these pests.
<u>Harmful arthropods of the U.S. include:</u>
◊ Bees: Bumblebees, sweat bees, honeybees
◊ Wasps: Hornets, wasps
◊ Ants: Fire ants, harvester ants
◊ Brown recluse spider
◊ Black widow spider
◊ Scorpions
◊ Mosquitoes
◊ Flies: Deer, horse, black, stable, and biting midges
◊ Lice: Body, head, pubic
◊ Bugs: Kissing, bed, wheel
◊ Fleas: Human, cat, dog
◊ Mites: Itch mite (scabies), red bugs (chiggers)
◊ Ticks
◊ Caterpillars: Puss, browntail, buck
◊ Centipedes
<u>Characteristic reactions include:</u>
◊ Local tissue irritation, inflammation and destruction
◊ Systemic effects related to inoculated poisons
◊ Allergic reactions: Immediate or delayed
System(s) affected: Skin/Exocrine
Genetics: N/A
Incidence/Prevalence in USA: Widespread (seasonal and regional variance)
Predominant age: All ages
Predominant sex: Male = Female

SIGNS AND SYMPTOMS
<u>Local reactions:</u>
◊ Erythema
◊ Pain
◊ Heat
◊ Swelling
◊ Itching
◊ Blisters
◊ Secondary infection - cellulitis, abscess
◊ Necrosis
◊ Ulceration
◊ Drainage
<u>Toxic reactions:</u> Non-antigenic
◊ Nausea
◊ Vomiting
◊ Headache
◊ Fever
◊ Diarrhea
◊ Lightheadedness
◊ Syncope
◊ Drowsiness
◊ Muscles spasms
◊ Edema
◊ Convulsions
<u>Systemic reactions:</u> Allergic
◊ Itching eyes
◊ Facial flushing
◊ Generalized urticaria
◊ Dry cough
◊ Chest/throat constriction

◊ Wheezing
◊ Dyspnea
◊ Cyanosis
◊ Abdominal cramps
◊ Diarrhea
◊ Nausea
◊ Vomiting
◊ Vertigo
◊ Chills/fever
◊ Stridor
◊ Shock
◊ Loss of consciousness
◊ Involuntary bowel/bladder action
◊ Frothy sputum
◊ Respiratory failure
◊ Cardiovascular collapse
◊ Death
<u>Delayed reaction:</u>
◊ Serum-sickness-like reactions
◊ Fever
◊ Malaise
◊ Headache
◊ Urticaria
◊ Lymphadenopathy
◊ Polyarthritis
<u>Unusual reactions:</u>
◊ Encephalopathy
◊ Neuritis
◊ Vasculitis
◊ Nephrosis
◊ Extreme fear/anxiety

CAUSES
• Local tissue inflammation and destruction from poison
• Allergic reaction from previous sensitization
• Toxic reaction from large inoculation of poison

RISK FACTORS
• Living environment
• Climate
• Season
• Clothing
• Lack of protective measures
• Perfumes, colognes
• Previous sensitization
• Young or elderly at more risk

DIAGNOSIS

DIFFERENTIAL DIAGNOSIS
• Local reaction: Infection, cellulitis, dermatoses, punctures, foreign bodies
• Toxic reaction: Chemical exposure/ingestion, medications, IV drug abuse, environmental, plants
• Allergic reaction: Medications, illicit drugs, foods, topical products, environmental, plants, chemicals

LABORATORY Leukocytosis, thrombocytopenia, hypofibrinogenemia, abnormal coagulation, DIC, proteinuria, hemoglobinemia, hemoglobinuria, myoglobinemia, myoglobinuria, and azotemia are uncommon but possible manifestations in severe reactions
Drugs that may alter lab results: N/A
Disorders that may alter lab results: N/A

PATHOLOGICAL FINDINGS
Inflammation, ulceration, vesiculation, pustulation, rupture, eschar, swelling

SPECIAL TESTS N/A

IMAGING N/A

DIAGNOSTIC PROCEDURES N/A

TREATMENT

APPROPRIATE HEALTH CARE
• Outpatient or inpatient, depending on individual response to injury
• Hospitalize for severe systemic reactions with threatened airway obstruction, bronchospasm, hypotension, severe angiodermatitis or pain

GENERAL MEASURES
• First aid measures, local treatment, activate emergency services in severe reactions. If history of allergy or large envenomations, don't wait to seek emergency care.
• Use ANA kit and over-the-counter antihistamines, if available and required
<u>Local (depending on severity)</u>
◊ Remove stinger (scrape it out - don't squeeze with tweezer)
◊ Cleanse wound
◊ Ice packs to bite or sting site (alternate 10 minutes on/10 minutes off)
◊ Elevation of affected part
◊ Rest the affected area
◊ Debride ulcers
◊ Drain abscesses
<u>Systemic (depending on severity, and type of reaction)</u>
◊ Adequate airway (intubation, tracheostomy) - if needed to by-pass obstruction
◊ Oxygen (4-6 L/min) - if needed for respiratory distress
◊ Hospitalize and observe 24-48 hours

ACTIVITY Rest to limit spread of poison

DIET No special diet; nothing by mouth if severe systemic reaction

PATIENT EDUCATION
• Protective measures, ANA kit use, risks
• Individuals with known sensitivity should wear medical identification (bracelet, tag) or carry a card

MEDICATIONS

DRUG(S) OF CHOICE
Local (depending on severity)
- ◊ Analgesics
- ◊ Antihistamines - Benadryl 25-50 mg qid
- ◊ Steroids topical or oral - prednisone 20-40 mg/day
- ◊ Antibiotics

Systemic (depending on severity and type of reaction)
- ◊ Epinephrine (1:1000) subcutaneous - to combat urticaria, wheezing, angioedema - child 0.01 mL/kg, adult 0.3-0.5 mL
- ◊ Benadryl - 25-50 mg IV or IM, to combat urticaria, wheezing, angioedema
- ◊ Aminophylline - adult 500 mg IV over 20-30 minutes, child 7.5 mg/kg, if needed for bronchospasm
- ◊ IV fluids (Ringer's lactate) - if needed for hypotension, hypovolemia
- ◊ Dopamine - 200 mg in 250 mL, 5 mcg/kg/min - to correct vascular collapse. Titrate to maintain systemic blood pressure > 90mm Hg.
- ◊ Hydrocortisone - 100-250 mg IV, if needed for severe urticaria
- ◊ Tetanus prophylaxis and antibiotics - if indicated
- ◊ Valium - 5-10 mg, if needed for severe muscle spasms
- ◊ Morphine or Demerol - if needed for severe pain

Contraindications: Refer to manufacturer's literature

Precautions:
- Dosing appropriate to age
- If severe reaction, don't delay treatment
- Severe vascular collapse may require central pressure monitor

Significant possible interactions: Refer to manufacturer's literature

ALTERNATIVE DRUGS N/A

FOLLOWUP

PATIENT MONITORING Followup wound care

PREVENTION/AVOIDANCE
- Avoid re-exposure in known hypersensitive individuals
- Prescribe anaphylactic (ANA Kit), if indicated
- Educate on risks of increasing anamnestic responses in future
- Consider desensitization with immunotherapy in severe cases

POSSIBLE COMPLICATIONS
- Infection
- Scarring
- Drug reactions
- Multisystem failure
- Death

EXPECTED COURSE AND PROGNOSIS
- Minor reactions - excellent
- Severe reactions - excellent with early, appropriate treatment

MISCELLANEOUS

ASSOCIATED CONDITIONS N/A

AGE-RELATED FACTORS
Pediatric: More at risk
Geriatric: More at risk
Others: N/A

PREGNANCY Not a contraindication to appropriate management

SYNONYMS N/A

ICD-9-CM
- 989.5 insect sting
- 910. - 919. (injury superficial by site, plus 4th digit 0-9 for subdivision)

SEE ALSO N/A

OTHER NOTES N/A

ABBREVIATIONS N/A

REFERENCES
- Tintinalli, J.E. & Krome, R.L. (eds.): Emergency Medicine. New York, McGraw-Hill, 1988
- Schroeder, S.A., Krupp, M.A., Tierney, L.M. & McPhee, S.J. (eds.): Current Medical Diagnosis and Treatment. Norwalk, CT, Appleton & Lange, 1989

Author R. Weston, M.D.

Insomnia

 BASICS

DESCRIPTION
Difficulty in falling asleep or maintaining sleep, intermittent wakefulness, early morning awakening or a combination of these. Can be:
• Transient - due to a life crisis, bereavement, change in environment
• Chronic - associated with medical and psychiatric conditions or drug intake.
System(s) affected: Nervous
Genetics: N/A
Incidence/Prevalence in USA: Affects an estimated 30% of the adult population. One of the most frequent complaints in primary care practice.
Predominant age: Elderly
Predominant sex: Male = Female

SIGNS AND SYMPTOMS
• Perceived reduction in sleeping time
• Initial insomnia - difficulty initiating sleep at usual time
• Middle insomnia - wakefulness during the usual sleep cycle, "tossing and turning"
• Terminal insomnia - early awakening
• Daytime sleepiness and napping
• Tiredness
• Anticipatory anxiety

CAUSES
• Medical illnesses - arthritis, primary fibromyalgia, hyperthyroidism, gastro-esophageal reflux disease, duodenal ulcer, Alzheimer's disease and other dementias, restless leg syndrome, sleep apnea, respiratory diseases, and all painful conditions (e.g., muscle cramps)
• Psychiatric illnesses - mostly depression, classically associated with early morning awakening, but can also be manifested by initial or middle insomnia
• Anxiety
• Schizophrenia
• Manic disorders
• Drug induced insomnia - alcohol, caffeine, nicotine
• Non-prescription drugs - diet aids, decongestants, cough preparations
• Prescribed drugs - steroids, theophylline, phenytoin (Dilantin), levodopa (Sinemet, Dopar)
• Obstructive sleep apnea
• Jet lag (transient)
• Heavy smoking

RISK FACTORS
• Chronic illnesses
• Age over 50
• Multiple drug intake
• Obesity

 DIAGNOSIS

DIFFERENTIAL DIAGNOSIS N/A

LABORATORY N/A
Drugs that may alter lab results: N/A
Disorders that may alter lab results: N/A

PATHOLOGICAL FINDINGS N/A

SPECIAL TESTS
Diagnosis can be confirmed by the use of polysomnography, particularly if sleep apnea is suspected. This is generally not necessary or practical.

IMAGING N/A

DIAGNOSTIC PROCEDURES
Insomnia is a self-reported condition

 TREATMENT

APPROPRIATE HEALTH CARE
Outpatient

GENERAL MEASURES
Transient insomnia
◊ Lasts less than three to four weeks
◊ Reassurance and supportive counseling are appropriate treatment modalities
Chronic insomnia
◊ Address the underlying cause: Pain, drugs, depression
◊ Avoid alcohol after 5 PM or within 6 hours of retiring because of secondary rebound stimulation
◊ Patient should be encouraged to avoid daytime napping and to develop bedtime rituals conducive to sleep
◊ A thorough review of the patient's habits, drug intake, diet, and exercise pattern may uncover correctable causes of insomnia
◊ Prescribe hypnotics only if the above strategies fail

ACTIVITY
• No restriction
• A daily exercise routine is helpful. Avoid exercise close to bedtime.

DIET
• Avoid caffeine
• Avoid heavy, late night snacks (sometimes a light snack before bedtime may help)
• Avoid alcohol after 5 PM or within 6 hours of retiring, because of secondary rebound stimulation

PATIENT EDUCATION
• Explain sleep patterns and sleep hygiene
• Show limitations and noxious effects of drugs used for insomnia

MEDICATIONS

DRUG(S) OF CHOICE
• Analgesics as indicated for pain
<u>Benzodiazepines for insomnia (3 currently used in the US)</u>
◊ Flurazepam (Dalmane), 15-30 mg, long half life, elderly might benefit from smaller dose
◊ Temazepam (Restoril), 15 mg one to two hours before bedtime
◊ Triazolam (Halcion), shortest half life, 0.125 mg to 0.25 mg, smaller dose recommended for the elderly. Useful as part of treatment regimen for jet lag.

Contraindications:
• Pregnancy and lactation
• Psychoses
• Acute narrow angle glaucoma
• Significant liver disease
• Depressed patient who may be suicide risk

Precautions:
• All benzodiazepines may cause paradoxical agitated states
• Flurazepam may cause incoordination ataxia and impairment of intellectual functions
• Triazolam has been associated with anterograde amnesia
• Withdrawal psychosis and seizures in some patients, after abrupt cessation
• Rebound insomnia
• Psychologic and, rarely, physical dependence

Significant possible interactions:
• Alcohol may potentiate the CNS effects of the benzodiazepines
• Digoxin serum concentrations may be increased
• Levodopa efficacy may be reduced

ALTERNATIVE DRUGS
• Diphenhydramine hydrochloride (Benadryl) has been used to induce sleep in the elderly, but it may also cause confusion and "hangover"
• Chloral hydrate (Noctec) is favored by some clinicians since it does not cause tolerance or withdrawal. The nightly dose is 250-500 mg.

FOLLOWUP

PATIENT MONITORING
• Need for benzodiazepines to be reassessed periodically. Avoid standing prescriptions.
• Followup as needed depending on individual patient. Refer for psychosocial counseling, if appropriate.

PREVENTION/AVOIDANCE
Avoidance, when possible, of all possible causes

POSSIBLE COMPLICATIONS
• Transient insomnia becomes chronic
• Increased daytime sleepiness

EXPECTED COURSE AND PROGNOSIS
Should resolve with time. Treatment of underlying symptoms helpful.

MISCELLANEOUS

ASSOCIATED CONDITIONS
• Obstructive sleep apnea
• Drug addiction and dependence

AGE-RELATED FACTORS
Pediatric: N/A
Geriatric:
• Exert caution when prescribing benzodiazepines or other sedative-hypnotics to the elderly
• Educate older patients about age-related sleep changes
Others: N/A

PREGNANCY
Transient insomnia occurs due to discomfort in sleeping positions

SYNONYMS
Sleeplessness

ICD-9-CM
780-52

SEE ALSO
• Sleep apnea
• Depression
• Anxiety

OTHER NOTES
L-Tryptophan - formerly widely used, - no longer available as a single ingredient

ABBREVIATIONS
N/A

REFERENCES
• Rakel, R.: Textbook of Family Practice. Philadelphia, W.B. Saunders Co., 1990
• Goldman, H.H.: Review of General Psychiatry. Norwalk, CT, Appleton & Lange, 1988
• Bahrat, R.S., Nakra, M.D., et al.: Insomnia in the Elderly. In American Family Physician, Feb, 1991, pp. 477-483

Author
M. Dodard, M.D.

Intestinal obstruction

BASICS

DESCRIPTION Intestinal obstruction exists where there is a failure, reversal or impairment of the normal transit of intestinal contents. Obstructions may be partial or complete and are manifested by abdominal pain, emesis and obstipation
System(s) affected: Gastrointestinal
Genetics: Unknown
Incidence/Prevalence in USA: Accounts, for approximately 20% of all admissions for acute abdominal conditions
Predominant age: N/A
Predominant sex: Male = Female

SIGNS AND SYMPTOMS
• Abdominal pain - diffuse, poorly localized abdominal cramping at intervals of 5 to 15 minutes
• Emesis - usually occurs immediately after obstruction of bowel. More frequent in proximal obstruction. Unusual in colon obstruction until small bowel distention occurs.
• Obstipation - common symptom. May pass contents distal to obstruction especially in high intestinal obstruction. Pain followed by explosive diarrhea often seen in partial obstruction.
• Inspection - with or without distention (a late finding), less likely in proximal obstructions
• Auscultation - high pitched bowel sounds, peristaltic rushes
• Palpation - (these 3 suggest strangulation) tenderness, mass, presence of peritoneal signs
• Rectal examination - may reveal fecal impaction. Occult blood may suggest colon malignancy

CAUSES
Luminal lesions
  ◊ Impactions
  ◊ Gallstones
  ◊ Meconium in newborns
  ◊ Intussusception in infants
Intrinsic lesions
  ◊ Congenital (e.g., atresia and stenosis, imperforate anus, duplications, Meckel's diverticulum)
  ◊ Trauma
  ◊ Inflammatory (e.g., Crohn's disease, diverticulitis, ulcerative colitis, radiation, toxic [ingestions]
  ◊ Neoplastic (most common etiology of colon obstruction)
  ◊ Miscellaneous (e.g., endometriosis)
Extrinsic lesions
  ◊ Adhesions (most common etiology of small bowel obstruction)
  ◊ Hernia and wound dehiscence
  ◊ Masses (e.g., annular pancreas, anomalous vasculature, abscess and hematoma, neoplasms)
  ◊ Volvulus
  ◊ Neuromuscular defect (e.g., megacolon, neuro/myopathic motility disorders)

RISK FACTORS
• Previous abdominal and/or pelvic surgery
• Hernia
• Chronic constipation
• Cholelithiasis
• Inflammatory bowel disease
• Ingested foreign bodies - pica, enteric potassium tablets, etc.
• Diverticular disease

DIAGNOSIS

DIFFERENTIAL DIAGNOSIS Adynamic ileus

LABORATORY
• WBC: Slight rise (15,000/mm3). Significant increases associated with strangulation.
• Hematocrit: Moderate rise associated with extracellular fluid loss
• Renal: Urine specific gravity 1.025-1.030 and rise in BUN and creatinine due to extracellular volume loss
• Amylase: May be elevated. Unreliable as an indicator of obstruction or strangulation.
• Blood gases: May be normal. Late changes are those of acidosis.
• No single or series of laboratory studies are useful in diagnosis of intestinal strangulation
Drugs that may alter lab results: N/A
Disorders that may alter lab results: N/A

PATHOLOGICAL FINDINGS
• Edema of mucosa
• Hypersecretion
• Necrosis

SPECIAL TESTS N/A

IMAGING
Abdominal and chest radiographs
  ◊ Distention of small bowel or colon
  ◊ Air-fluid levels (may be seen in ileus, gastroenteritis, constipation)
  ◊ Lack of colon gas
  ◊ Free intraperitoneal air (strangulation with perforation)
  ◊ "Bird beak" lesion in colonic volvulus
  ◊ Foreign body visualization
Contrast studies
  ◊ Barium enema useful for diagnosis of colonic obstruction and may be therapeutic in intussusception
  ◊ Barium or Gastrografin orally may differentiate obstruction from ileus
  ◊ Enteroclysis may identify site of small bowel obstruction

DIAGNOSTIC PROCEDURES
• Rigid proctoscopy. May be therapeutic in sigmoid volvulus
• Flexible sigmoidoscopy

TREATMENT

APPROPRIATE HEALTH CARE
• Inpatient
• Treatment directed at early gastrointestinal decompression, correction of fluid and electrolyte abnormalities, timely operative intervention, surgical/GI consultation required

GENERAL MEASURES
• Nasogastric suction
• Foley catheter
• Swan-Ganz catheter or other central monitor, if required
• Intravenous fluids: Normal saline/Ringer's solution with potassium supplementation as required
• Antibiotic use controversial in absence of sepsis, but prophylactic antibiotics probably appropriate
• Timing of operative intervention critical, must correct electrolytes, volume quickly prior to surgery
Surgical procedures:
  ◊ Closed bowel procedures: lysis of adhesions, reduction of intussusception, reduction of volvulus, reduction of incarcerated hernia
  ◊ Enterotomy for removal of bezoars, foreign bodies, gallstones
  ◊ Resection of bowel for obstructing lesions, strangulated bowel
  ◊ Bypasses of intestine around obstruction
  ◊ Enterocutaneous fistulae proximal to obstruction: colostomy, cecostomy

ACTIVITY Bedrest

DIET NPO

PATIENT EDUCATION N/A

MEDICATIONS

DRUG(S) OF CHOICE Surgeon's choice for prophylaxis
Contraindications: N/A
Precautions: N/A
Significant possible interactions: N/A

ALTERNATIVE DRUGS N/A

FOLLOWUP

PATIENT MONITORING Follow weekly postoperatively for 2-8 weeks

PREVENTION/AVOIDANCE N/A

POSSIBLE COMPLICATIONS
• Slow return of bowel function
• Higher risk of subsequent obstruction
• Sepsis

EXPECTED COURSE AND PROGNOSIS Usually excellent prognosis. In general, mortality from intestinal obstruction ranges from < 1% to > 20% depending upon etiology, bowel viability, co-morbidities, etc.

MISCELLANEOUS

ASSOCIATED CONDITIONS

AGE-RELATED FACTORS
Pediatric:
Different etiologies of obstruction in childhood
◊ Duodenal malformations
◊ Jejunoileal atresia
◊ Malrotation and midgut volvulus
◊ Meconium ileus
◊ Necrotizing enterocolitis
◊ Hirschsprung's disease
◊ Intussusception
◊ Duplications
◊ Meckel's diverticulum
◊ Imperforate anus
Geriatric:
• Colon neoplasms more common
• Chronic constipation/impactions more common
Others: N/A

PREGNANCY N/A

SYNONYMS N/A

ICD-9-CM 569+

SEE ALSO N/A

OTHER NOTES Rectal examination showing occult blood may represent colon malignancy as etiology of the obstruction

ABBREVIATIONS N/A

REFERENCES Sleisenger, M.H. and Fordtran, J.S. (eds.): Gastrointestinal Disease: Pathophysiology, Diagnosis, Management. 4th Ed. Philadelphia, W.B. Saunders Co., 1989

Author L. Mercer, M. D. & E. Saltzstein, M. D.

Intestinal parasites

BASICS

DESCRIPTION

The class of infectious agents called parasites is divided into two parts:
◊ Protozoa are single cell animals which characteristically divide and multiply within the host, are usually direct fecal-oral in transmission, and do not cause an eosinophilia
◊ Helminths (worms) are multi-cellular animals and with rare exceptions (i.e., Strongyloides stercoralis, Hymenolepis nana) do not multiply within the host and are often associated with some degree of eosinophilia. The level of eosinophilia is associated with the degree of mucosal invasiveness. The worms have a limited life span within the host and without reinfection would eventually die on their own.
• Not all of the parasites that start out by ingestion in the bowel will remain in the bowel. Some are invasive and some do not release their infective forms into the bowel. This later group, including Toxoplasma gondii, Echinococcus, Trichinella spiralis will not be covered in this topic.
• Most worms require either a prolonged incubation period outside the host before being infectious or need a specific vector for transmission. A notable exception to this rule is Enterobius vermicularis (pinworm), the eggs of which are infectious shortly after being passed, so auto-infection occurs readily.
• Direct person-to-person transmission is uncommon
• The likelihood of acquiring an intestinal parasite depends on several factors - the presence of the specific infectious agent, an appropriate 'vector' or mode of transmission, and a host who is susceptible to the infectious agent. The world-wide distribution of parasites is determined by geographic factors, socio-economics, age, and crowding with poor food preparation and a break in the standard of water and personal sanitation being the major factors.

System(s) affected: Gastrointestinal
Genetics: Genetic factors play a minor role in the acquisition, pathogenesis and clearance of these infections
Incidence in USA: Unknown
Prevalence in USA:
• From laboratory statistics: 5-30% general population
• From day care surveys: Asymptomatic 20-30%; symptomatic 50-80%
• Intestinal protozoa account for the majority of parasitological findings in North America (most considered to be non-pathogenic)
• In a random sampling, at least one parasite would be found in the stools of 5-10% of all people. If Blastocystis hominis were included in this accounting, 20-30% of specimens examined in parasitology will be positive.
• Helminths are considerably rarer and are highly dependent on population demographics and prior geographic exposure risk factors. In general, less than 10% of all parasitology reports include a helminth.

Predominant age: Pediatric
Predominant sex: Male = Female

SIGNS AND SYMPTOMS
• Diarrhea
• Abdominal pain/tenderness
• Excessive gas - bloating, eructation, flatulence, borborygmi
• Nausea or vomiting
• Weight loss and anorexia
• Dysentery (rare, but associated with Entamoeba histolytica, Balantidium coli)
• Pruritus ani (E. vermicularis, Trichuris trichiura, S. stercoralis, tapeworms)
• Passing a worm or a worm segment
• Increased bowel sounds
• Peri-rectal or vulvar rash

CAUSES
Protozoan pathogens:
◊ Giardia lamblia
◊ Entamoeba histolytica
◊ Cryptosporidium
◊ Isospora belli
◊ Balantidium coli
◊ Cyclospora
◊ Microsporida
Possible protozoan pathogens:
◊ Dientamoeba fragilis
Probable non-pathogenic protozoa
◊ All other Entamoeba
◊ Endolimax nana
◊ All other intestinal flagellates
Helminthic pathogens - nematodes (roundworms):
◊ Enterobius vermicularis
◊ Trichuris trichiura
◊ Ascaris lumbricoides
◊ Hookworm (Necator americanus, Ancylostoma duodenale)
◊ Strongyloides stercoralis
◊ Capillaria philippinensis
◊ Trichostrongylus
Helminthic pathogens - trematodes (flukes)
◊ Fasciolopsis buski
◊ Clonorchis sinensis
◊ Opisthorchis viverrini
◊ Heterophyes heterophyes
◊ Fasciola hepatica
◊ Paragonimus westermani
◊ Schistosoma mansoni
◊ S. japonicum
◊ S. hematobium
◊ S. mekongi
Helminthic pathogens - cestodes (tapeworms)
◊ Taenia saginata
◊ Taenia solium
◊ Diphyllobothrium latum
◊ Hymenolepis nana
◊ Hymenolepis diminuta
◊ Dipylidium caninum

RISK FACTORS
• Age (children)
• Low socioeconomic status
• Poor sanitation - personal, food, water
• International travel
• Crowding - day care centers, mental institutions
• Intercurrent medical conditions, pregnancy, gastric hypoacidity, immunosuppression (AIDS)

DIAGNOSIS

DIFFERENTIAL DIAGNOSIS
• Other intestinal infections
• Food poisoning
• Malabsorption
• Inflammatory bowel disease
• Hemorrhoids
• Rectal fissures

LABORATORY
• Examination of a single stool specimen collected into a preservative (i.e., sodium acetate formalin [SAF]), well mixed to fix and preserve all elements, will provide an accurate diagnosis in 90% of patients. Additional specimens will need to be examined for greater diagnostic accuracy.
• Newer techniques of lab exam of stool specimens (such as monoclonal antibodies, other antigen detection techniques, DNA detection) are exciting developments but currently provide little practical advantage over routine techniques
• Serology - for specific infections, especially if they do not produce a patent infection in the bowel (i.e., no eggs or parasites released into the stool), or if low numbers of parasites makes the diagnosis difficult. These tests are rarely indicated and are usually available only through referral centers.
Drugs that may alter lab results: Use of antibiotics, oil based laxatives, and the presence of barium in the stool may make a parasitological diagnosis difficult or impossible
Disorders that may alter lab results: N/A

PATHOLOGICAL FINDINGS
• Majority of intestinal parasites are not invasive and produce no or non-specific changes in the histology of the bowel
• Invasive amebiasis of the bowel produces a classical histological picture of ulceration and inflammation
• Protozoa and helminths may be seen in bowel biopsies

SPECIAL TESTS
• Special techniques for the detection of Cryptosporidium, Isospora belli, Cyclospora, and microsporidia often require that the laboratory be informed of the "risk" profile of the patient before these tests will be done
• Pinworm paddles provide a greater diagnostic yield when Enterobius vermicularis is being considered. Multiple tests (5) may be needed to exclude the diagnosis of pinworms.
• Parasite culture is possible for a few organisms - Giardia lamblia, Entamoeba histolytica, Strongyloides stercoralis, but are rarely indicated and are usually available only in referral laboratories
• String tests and upper bowel intubations are rarely needed to diagnose the upper intestinal parasites

• Rarely, a biopsy will demonstrate the presence of an invasive helminth on tissue section. Worms can be extremely difficult to diagnose in this manner, usually needing the expertise of a tissue parasite pathologist. The other parasites may be visualized on the mucosa or in the mucus layer.

IMAGING Diagnostic radiology rarely needed. Exception is for invasive infections such as amebiasis where colitis, amebomas and liver abscesses may be demonstrated by the appropriate techniques.

DIAGNOSTIC PROCEDURES
• Invasive diagnostic procedures are rarely needed or indicated
• With hemorrhagic colitis and a possible diagnosis of invasive amoebiasis, sigmoidoscopy will reveal a muco-purulent colitis with ulceration. A scraping from an ulcer, promptly examined by microscopy, will reveal the motile hematophagous trophozoites of E. histolytica.
• Upper intestinal endoscopy can yield fluid to be examined for Giardia lamblia and Strongyloides stercoralis, as can impression smears and biopsies obtained with the endoscope

TREATMENT

APPROPRIATE HEALTH CARE
Outpatient except for rare surgery

GENERAL MEASURES
• Therapy must be assessed in the best interest of the patient. Not all patients need to be treated with drugs.
• Symptomatic treatment is indicated for patient comfort once specific therapy has been initiated
• Bowel paralyzing drugs, for diarrhea caused by invasive organisms, are relatively contraindicated
• Surgical procedures play little role in treatment except when amebic liver abscesses need to be drained, e.g., multiple or large abscesses not responding to medical management, or threatened rupture, especially left lobe abscesses. Drainage of such abscesses is often accomplished by directed catheter placement in radiology, with surgical back-up as required.
• Surgery may be required if bowel or other organ obstruction occurs, as can be seen with Ascaris lumbricoides migration

ACTIVITY As tolerated

DIET
• Nutritional support may be required
• Many patients during and following bowel infections, especially when infected with Giardia lamblia, will experience irritable bowel syndrome and/or lactose intolerance. The majority of these patients will respond to a lactose free diet, reduction of caffeine intake, and an increase in dietary fiber.

PATIENT EDUCATION
• Educating the patient is important to reduce the risk of reinfection or transmission
• Education will depend on the parasite, host characteristics and the environment that the two interact in

MEDICATIONS

DRUG(S) OF CHOICE
Protozoa
 ◊ Entamoeba histolytica asymptomatic needs individual assessment
 ◊ Entamoeba histolytica symptomatic intestinal - iodoquinol or diloxanide furoate
 ◊ Entamoeba histolytica invasive disease - iodoquinol or diloxanide furoate. Plus metronidazole, alone or dehydroemetine or emetine plus chloroquine phosphate.
 ◊ Giardia lamblia - metronidazole or tinidazole or furazolidone or quinacrine. Note: albendazole (available in US only from manufacturer) may have activity against G. lamblia.
 ◊ Cryptosporidium - none proven effective
 ◊ Isospora belli protozoa - trimethoprim-sulfamethoxazole
 ◊ Balantidium coli - tetracycline or iodoquinol or metronidazole
 ◊ Cyclospora - unknown
 ◊ Microsporidia - unknown
Helminths
 ◊ Nematodes (except Strongyloides and Trichostrongylus) - mebendazole or pyrantel pamoate or piperazine citrate or albendazole (available in US only from manufacturer)
 ◊ Strongyloides and Trichostrongylus - thiabendazole or albendazole (available in US only from manufacturer)
 ◊ Cestodes - praziquantel or niclosamide
 ◊ Trematodes - niclosamide or praziquantel
Contraindications: Refer to manufacturer's profile of each drug
Precautions: Refer to manufacturer's profile of each drug
Significant possible interactions: Refer to manufacturer's profile of each drug

ALTERNATIVE DRUGS N/A

FOLLOWUP

PATIENT MONITORING Repeat examination, to ensure clearance, should be timed taking into account: The life cycle of the parasite (how long would it take to regenerate and become patent) and the risk of reinfection, as well as the specific test likely to find the parasite (stool, pinworm paddle, culture, serology)

PREVENTION/AVOIDANCE The specific nature of the infection often dictates the specific methods needed to avoid reinfection. This usually involves matters of personal, food and/or water sanitation.

POSSIBLE COMPLICATIONS See specific text on individual parasite

EXPECTED COURSE AND PROGNOSIS See specific text on individual parasite

MISCELLANEOUS

ASSOCIATED CONDITIONS N/A

AGE-RELATED FACTORS
Pediatric: Most common age group affected
Geriatric: Illness may cause more severe debilitation
Others: N/A

PREGNANCY Some of these infections can be particularly serious in pregnancy. Many of the drugs are contraindicated in pregnancy.

SYNONYMS N/A

ICD-9-CM 129 Intestinal parasitism, unspecified

SEE ALSO N/A

OTHER NOTES N/A

ABBREVIATIONS N/A

REFERENCES
• MacPherson, D.W.: Intestinal Parasites. In Conn's Current Therapy. Edited by R.E. Rakel. Philadelphia, W.B. Saunders Co., 1990:pp486-92
• Abramowicz, M. (ed.): Drugs for parasitic infections. In The Medical Letter. New York, The Medical Letter Inc.1988, Vol. 30 (issue 759)
• Mandell, G.L. (ed.): Principles and Practice of Infectious Diseases. 3rd Ed. New York, Churchill Livingstone, 1990

Author D. MacPherson, M.D. & T. Yang, M.D.

Intussusception

BASICS

DESCRIPTION   Invagination of a portion of intestine into itself (may involve any part of small intestine, ileocolic [95%], or colo-colic)
Genetics: N/A
Incidence in USA: 1.5-4/1000 live births
Prevalence in USA: N/A
Predominant age: 5-10 months (65% are less than one year of age)
Predominant sex: Male > Female (3:2) - male preponderance is more notable in older infants

SIGNS AND SYMPTOMS
• Vomiting (80-100%)
• Blood per rectum - currant-jelly stools (65%-95%) highest percent in infants
• Intermittent, colicky abdominal pain (almost all children)
• Lethargy (22%) (more pronounced with longer duration of illness)
• Palpable mass (16-41%)
• Diarrhea (7%)
• Prolapse of intussusception through anus (3%)
• Fever
• Extreme pallor in some

CAUSES
Children
   ◊ Marked hypertrophy of Peyers patches (92-98%)
   ◊ Lead point in 2%-8% (polyp, Meckel's diverticulum, duplication cyst, ectopic pancreas, lymphoma, Henoch-Schönlein purpura, lipoma, carcinoma)
   ◊ Allergic reactions, diet changes, changes in intestinal activity may be other causes
   ◊ Possible adenovirus or rotavirus infection
Adults
   ◊ Virtually always associated with lead point

RISK FACTORS
• Henoch-Schönlein purpura
• Leukemia
• Lymphoma
• Cystic fibrosis
• Recent upper respiratory infection (21%)
• Recent operation (1-24 days previously)

DIAGNOSIS

DIFFERENTIAL DIAGNOSIS
• Adhesive band small bowel obstruction
• Appendicitis
• Gastroenteritis

LABORATORY
• Electrolytes
• CBC
• Urinalysis
• Stool guaiac
Drugs that may alter lab results: N/A
Disorders that may alter lab results: N/A

PATHOLOGICAL FINDINGS
• Hyperplasia of Peyer's lymphatic patches of terminal ileum (92%) with or without mesenteric lymphadenopathy
• Recognizable lead point (see list in Causes) (2-8%)

SPECIAL TESTS   N/A

IMAGING
• Ultrasound
• Plain film - flat and upright abdominal films may suggest the diagnosis

DIAGNOSTIC PROCEDURES
• Contrast enema (barium, water soluble contrast or air)
• Abdominal ultrasound

TREATMENT

APPROPRIATE HEALTH CARE
Inpatient until problem resolved

GENERAL MEASURES
• IV fluid resuscitation
• Foley catheter (if child severely dehydrated)
• Nasogastric tube
• Antibiotics useful only if necrotic bowel present
Non-operative care:
   ◊ Hydrostatic/pneumatic reduction of intussusception (50% - 80% success)
   ◊ Barium column should be 40-42 inches high
   ◊ Enema continued as long as progress is made. Bowel may be drained and the enema repeated.
   ◊ Pneumatic reduction pressure should not exceed 120-140 mm Hg
Operative care:
   ◊ Right lower quadrant incision
   ◊ Gentle manipulation by pushing intussusception (not pulling)
   ◊ If unable to reduce or non-viable bowel, segmental resection with re-anastomosis
   ◊ Enterotomy if lead point suspected
   ◊ Incidental appendectomy commonly done

ACTIVITY   As tolerated after reduction

DIET   Liquids started after abdominal distension resolves and bowel function returns

PATIENT EDUCATION   Instruct family on possibility of recurrence (5-13%)

MEDICATIONS

DRUG(S) OF CHOICE N/A
Contraindications: N/A
Precautions: N/A
Significant possible interactions: N/A

ALTERNATIVE DRUGS N/A

FOLLOWUP

PATIENT MONITORING Office visit one week after discharge

PREVENTION/AVOIDANCE N/A

POSSIBLE COMPLICATIONS
• Bowel perforation during attempted reduction
• Prolonged ileus
• Adhesions with intestinal obstruction
• Incisional hernia
• Ischemic intestine requiring second operation
• Electrolyte abnormality
• Anemia
• Pleural effusion
• Sepsis
• Recurrence

EXPECTED COURSE AND PROGNOSIS
• Mortality should not exceed 1-2%
• Possible recurrence (5-13%) after hydrostatic reduction
• Possible recurrence (3%) after manual reduction

MISCELLANEOUS

ASSOCIATED CONDITIONS
• Henoch-Schönlein purpura
• Cystic fibrosis

AGE-RELATED FACTORS
Pediatric:
• Usually no lead point
• Postoperative intussusception (1-24 days postoperatively) is virtually always in small bowel and only rarely can be reduced hydrostatically
Geriatric: 90% have lead point
Others: N/A

PREGNANCY N/A

SYNONYMS N/A

ICD-9-CM 560.0

SEE ALSO N/A

OTHER NOTES N/A

ABBREVIATIONS N/A

REFERENCES
• Pang, L.C.: Intussusception Revisited: Clinicopathologic Analysis of 261 Cases, with Emphasis on Pathogenesis. Southern Medical J., 82(2):215-228, 1989
• Skipper, R.P., Boeckman, C.R. & Klein, R.L.: Childhood Intussusception. SGO 171:151-153, 1990
• Welch, K.J., Randolph, J.G. Ravitch, M.M., et al. (eds.): Pediatric Surgery, 4th Ed. Chicago, Year Book Medical Publishers, 1986
• West, K.W., Stephens, B., Rescorla, F.J., et al. Postoperative Intussusception: Experience with 36 Cases in Children. Surgery 104:781-787, 1988

Author T. Black, M.D., & J. Miller, M.D.

Iron deficiency anemia

 BASICS

DESCRIPTION Chronic anemia characterized by small, pale, red blood cells and depletion of iron stores. This is the most common cause of anemia in the U.S. and may be due to chronic bleed, diminished iron absorption, or both. Onset is insidious and symptoms progress slowly.
System(s) affected:
Hemic/Lymphatic/Immunologic
Genetics: No known genetic pattern
Incidence/Prevalence: It affects 10-30% of the adult population
Predominant age: All ages
Predominant sex: Female > Male

SIGNS AND SYMPTOMS
- Asymptomatic, initially
- Cheilosis
- Dyspnea on exertion
- Fatigue
- Underlying GI ulceration, neoplasm, uterine disorders, bleeding varices
- Headache
- Inability to concentrate
- Irritability
- Listlessness
- Neuralgic pain
- Pallor
- Peripheral paresthesias
- Pica (dirt, paint, ice)
- Spoon-shaped, brittle nails
- Susceptibility to infection
- Vasomotor disturbances

CAUSES
- Blood loss (e.g., GI tract, neoplasia, menorrhagia, bleeding hemorrhoids)
- Chronic occult bleeding
- Hypothyroidism
- Inadequate iron intake
- Increased demand for iron (e.g., pregnancy)
- Malabsorption of iron (such as with pica or post-gastrectomy)
- Malnutrition

RISK FACTORS
- Adolescence - increased need of iron for rapid growth and/or loss from menstruation
- Eating disorders

 DIAGNOSIS

DIFFERENTIAL DIAGNOSIS
- Chronic intravascular hemolysis
- Defects in iron metabolism
- Defects in iron utilization
- Transferrin defect

LABORATORY
- Low serum ferritin concentration (< 12 ng/mL) - the best non-invasive test
- Smear - hypochromic, microcytic (thin, pale red corpuscles)
- Hemoglobin: < 12g/100mL (males)
- Hemoglobin: < 10g/100mL (females)
- Hematocrit: < 47 mL/100mL (males)
- Hematocrit: < 42 mL/100mL (females)
- Low serum iron
- High total iron-binding capacity
- Low RBC count
- Decreased MCHC
- Decreased MCV
- Decreased hemoglobin A2
- Increased free erythrocytic protoporphyrin
Drugs that may alter lab results: Iron supplements or multivitamin-mineral preparations that contain iron
Disorders that may alter lab results:
- Occult bleeding
- Liver injury (ferritin values may be elevated)
- Some neoplasms (ferritin values may be elevated)

PATHOLOGICAL FINDINGS
- Absent marrow iron stores
- Marrow - hyperplastic, normoblastic

SPECIAL TESTS Stool examinations for blood or parasites

IMAGING GI contrast studies to discover occult bleeding sites

DIAGNOSTIC PROCEDURES
- Bone marrow aspiration
- Sigmoidoscopy
- Gastroscopy

 TREATMENT

APPROPRIATE HEALTH CARE
Outpatient

GENERAL MEASURES
- Search for cause and correct it. There can be no excuse for not searching for a bleeding site.
- Avoid transfusions except in rare instances

ACTIVITY No restrictions

DIET
- Limit milk to 1 pint a day (adults)
- Emphasize protein- and iron-containing foods (meat, beans, leafy green vegetables)
- Increase dietary fiber to decrease likelihood of constipation during iron replacement therapy
- No milk, other dairy product, antacid, or tetracycline within two hours of drug dosage

PATIENT EDUCATION For patient education materials contact: National Heart, Lung & Blood Institute, Communications & Public Information Branch, National Institutes of Health, Building 31, Room 41-21, 9000 Rockville Pike, Bethesda, MD 20892, (301)496-4236

MEDICATIONS

DRUG(S) OF CHOICE Ferrous sulfate or ferrous gluconate - administer for six months after the anemia has been corrected. A daily dose of 200 mg is usually sufficient for favorable response, but dosage varies according to tolerance of the patient.

Contraindications:
• Antacids concomitantly
• Tetracycline concomitantly

Precautions:
• Iron preparations cause black bowel movements
• Iron overdose is highly toxic. Patients should be instructed to keep tablets out of the reach of small children.

Significant possible interactions:
• Allopurinol
• Antacids
• Penicillamine
• Tetracyclines
• Vitamin E

ALTERNATIVE DRUGS
• Liquid iron preparations for individuals who cannot take tablets
• Parenteral iron - for those who do not tolerate or refuse oral iron or for those who lose blood steadily due to vascular or capillary disorders

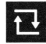
FOLLOWUP

PATIENT MONITORING Regularly after return to normal (in order to detect recurrences)

PREVENTION/AVOIDANCE
• Good nutrition with adequate iron intake
• Correction of gynecologic or other problems causing excess blood loss

POSSIBLE COMPLICATIONS
• Neglecting to identify hidden bleeding points, particularly a bleeding malignancy
• Angina pectoris
• Esophageal web
• Hypovolemic shock
• Recurrence
• Lack of patient compliance with therapy

EXPECTED COURSE AND
PROGNOSIS Curable with iron therapy if the underlying cause can be discovered and cured

MISCELLANEOUS

ASSOCIATED CONDITIONS N/A

AGE-RELATED FACTORS
Pediatric: Frequent problem in infants whose major source of nutrition is cow's milk
Geriatric: Accounts for 60% of anemias in people over 65
Others: N/A

PREGNANCY Common during pregnancy unless iron supplements are included in the diet

SYNONYMS
• Anemia of chronic blood loss
• Hypochromic, microcytic anemia
• Chlorosis

ICD-9-CM 280.9 iron deficiency anemia, unspecified

SEE ALSO N/A

OTHER NOTES N/A

ABBREVIATIONS
• MCV = mean corpuscular volume
• RBC = red blood cells
• MCHC = mean corpuscular hemoglobin concentration

REFERENCES
• Wintrobe, M.M., Lee, G.R., Boggs,D.R., et al. (eds.): Clinical Hematology. 8th Ed. Philadelphia, Lea & Febiger, 1981
• Williams, W.J., Beutler, E., Erslev, A.J., et al. (eds.): Hematology. 4th Ed. New York, McGraw-Hill, 1983

Author M. Dambro, M.D. & H. Griffith, M.D.

Irritable bowel syndrome

 BASICS

DESCRIPTION Altered bowel habits, abdominal pain, gaseousness, in the absence of organic pathology (divided into four types):
• Alternating diarrhea with constipation
• Nervous diarrhea
• Constipation predominant
• Upper abdominal bloating and discomfort
System(s) affected: Gastrointestinal
Genetics: Unknown, but more common in families of patients
Incidence in USA: Unknown, but 50% of gastrointestinal visits, and second to upper respiratory infection as cause for lost work-days
Prevalence in USA:
• At least 15% of population (uncommon in children and early teens)
Predominant age:
• Late 20's, rarely in late teens
• If over age 40, other disease more likely
Predominant sex:
• Female > Male (2:1) in the U.S.
• In other parts of the world - Male > Female

SIGNS AND SYMPTOMS
• All present in most patients but not with every episode
• Abdominal pain, usually lower quadrant, relieved by defecation
• Mucus in stools
• Globus
• Constipation
• Diarrhea
• Distention
• Upper abdominal discomfort after eating
• Straining for normal consistency stools
• Urgency of defecation
• Feelings of incomplete evacuation
• Scybalous stools
• Nausea, vomiting

CAUSES Unknown but patients show some gut motility abnormalities with increased response to stress and stimulants, and increase in the 3 cycles/minute smooth muscle contractions

RISK FACTORS Other members of the family with the same or similar gastrointestinal disorder

 DIAGNOSIS

DIFFERENTIAL DIAGNOSIS
• Inflammatory bowel syndromes
• Lactose intolerance
• Infections (Giardia lamblia, Entamoeba histolytica, Salmonella, Campylobacter, Yersinia, Clostridium difficile)
• Diverticula
• Cathartic use
• Magnesium containing antacids
• Celiac sprue
• Pancreatic insufficiency
• Depression
• Somatization
• Adenocarcinoma of the colon
• Villous adenoma
• Endocrine tumors
• Hypo/hyperthyroidism
• Diabetes mellitus

LABORATORY
As needed to rule out other pathology
◊ ESR
◊ CBC
◊ Stool for ova, parasites and culture
◊ Liver function tests
Drugs that may alter lab results: N/A
Disorders that may alter lab results: N/A

PATHOLOGICAL FINDINGS All labs normal except for sigmoidoscopy

SPECIAL TESTS Not needed for diagnosis

IMAGING Barium enema, if indicated, shows excessive muscular activity

DIAGNOSTIC PROCEDURES
Sigmoidoscopy (often normal) may show excess mucus, mucosal folds that are similar to small bowel in appearance, insufflation of air reproduces the symptoms, "winking" of mucosa or spasm seen, occasional proctitis

 TREATMENT

APPROPRIATE HEALTH CARE
Outpatient

GENERAL MEASURES
• Heat to abdomen can help
• Biofeedback may help
• Reduce stress

ACTIVITY As normal

DIET
• Increase fiber
• Avoid - large meals; spicy, fried, fatty foods; milk products

PATIENT EDUCATION
• Many materials available nationally and locally
• Stress the organicity of the disease versus any psycho-social interpretation
• Teach patient to avoid problem stimulants

MEDICATIONS

DRUG(S) OF CHOICE
Use from among this list according to need or response
◊ Bulk producing agents - psyllium containing products (Metamucil) 1 tbsp tid
◊ Constipating agents - loperamide (Imodium) 4 mg initial dose, then 2 mg after each unformed stool or diphenoxylate HCL (Lomotil) 2.5-5.0 mg (1 -2 tablets) after each unformed stool
◊ Antispasmodics - dicyclomine (Bentyl) 10-20 mg bid to qid or Lactaid 1-3 caplets ac for lactose intolerance
◊ Anticholinergics/sedatives - chlordiazepoxide HCL/clidinium bromide (Librax) 1 or 2 ac and q hs; phenobarbital/hyoscyamine sulfate/atropine sulfate/hyoscine hydrobromide (Donnatal) 1 or 2 tablets ac and hs; amitriptyline HCL (Elavil) 25-50 mg q hs
◊ Antiflatulents - simethicone (Mylicon) 2 or 4 tablets pc and hs
◊ For milk intolerance - Lactase capsules or tablets: 1 - 2 tablets prior to ingesting milk products
Contraindications: Refer to manufacturer's profile of each drug
Precautions: Refer to manufacturer's profile of each drug
Significant possible interactions: Refer to manufacturer's profile of each drug

ALTERNATIVE DRUGS N/A

FOLLOWUP

PATIENT MONITORING As needed for symptoms

PREVENTION/AVOIDANCE See Diet

POSSIBLE COMPLICATIONS N/A

EXPECTED COURSE AND PROGNOSIS
• No progression to cancer or Inflammatory disease
• Expect recurrences, when under stress, throughout life. Frequency lessens as age increases.

MISCELLANEOUS

ASSOCIATED CONDITIONS
• Migraine
• Bladder frequency
• Nocturia
• Urgency
• Radiation damage to colon
• Myalgia
• Dyspareunia
• Depression

AGE-RELATED FACTORS N/A
Pediatric: N/A
Geriatric: N/A
Others: N/A

PREGNANCY Anecdotal information implies that irritable bowel syndrome gets worse in pregnancy. But there are no increased risks to fetus or mother.

SYNONYMS
• Mucous colitis
• Spastic colon
• Irritable colon

ICD-9-CM 564.1 Irritable colon

SEE ALSO N/A

OTHER NOTES Must not give patients the impression that this is a psychiatric illness

ABBREVIATIONS N/A

REFERENCES
• Read, N.W., (ed.): Irritable Bowel Syndrome. London, Grune and Stratton, 1985
• Rakel, R., (ed.): Textbook of Family Practice. Philadelphia, W.B. Saunders Co., 1990

Author S. Duiker, M.D.

Kaposi's sarcoma

BASICS

DESCRIPTION A neoplasm characterized by vascular tumors of skin and viscera in several different forms: Indolent (classic) KS, African (endemic) KS, AIDS-related (epidemic) KS, and a form associated with immunosuppressive medications
System(s) affected: Indolent - Skin; AIDS-related - Skin and Viscera except brain
Genetics: Unknown
Incidence/Prevalence in USA:
• Indolent/lymphadenopathic - rare
• In AIDS patients - common
Predominant age: 16-75
Predominant sex: Male > Female

SIGNS AND SYMPTOMS
Indolent Kaposi's
  ◊ Multicentric red-blue violaceous tumors on the skin
  ◊ Tender skin tumors
  ◊ Pruritic skin tumors
African (endemic) Kaposi's
  ◊ Usually involves skin, viscera or lymph nodes
In Kaposi's associated with HIV infection (epidemic)
  ◊ Skin lesions widely disseminated, on the face, arms, trunk
  ◊ Lesions on mucous membranes
  ◊ Lesions in lymph nodes
  ◊ Lesions in viscera
  ◊ In older men, lesions appear first on toes or legs

CAUSES Unknown transmissible agent that leads to neoplasia

RISK FACTORS
• HIV infection
• Living in endemic area (especially Zaire or Uganda)
• Immunosuppressant medications
• Transplantation and chemotherapy

DIAGNOSIS

DIFFERENTIAL DIAGNOSIS Bacillary angiomatosis

LABORATORY Nothing specific
Drugs that may alter lab results: N/A
Disorders that may alter lab results: N/A

PATHOLOGICAL FINDINGS
• Micro - proliferation of atypical spindle cells
• Micro - proliferation of vascular channels
• Micro - large hyperchromic nuclei
• Micro - spindle-shaped perivascular cells
• Micro - hemosiderin laden macrophages

SPECIAL TESTS Tissue examination

IMAGING CT scan (chest, abdomen) may assess visceral involvement

DIAGNOSTIC PROCEDURES
• Biopsy of skin or lymph node
• Bronchoscopy with biopsy
• Liver biopsy

TREATMENT

APPROPRIATE HEALTH CARE
• Outpatient
• Outpatient surgery

GENERAL MEASURES
• If KS due to immunosuppressant medications, eliminate or reduce medication dosage
• Treatment is otherwise determined by extent of the disease
• Observation
• Cryotherapy
• Intralesional chemotherapy
• Surgical excision
• Radiotherapy (electron beam) or x-ray therapy 1000 to 2000 rads
• Systemic chemotherapy

ACTIVITY Remain active as long as possible

DIET No special diet

PATIENT EDUCATION N/A

Kaposi's sarcoma

 MEDICATIONS

DRUG(S) OF CHOICE
• Chemotherapy
• Doxorubicin
or
• Bleomycin
or
• Vinblastine
or
• Vincristine
or
• Interferon - parenteral or intralesional
• Note: Chemotherapy should be given only by those with experience in this area
Contraindications: Refer to manufacturer's literature
Precautions: Refer to manufacturer's literature. Myelosuppression with chemotherapy.
Significant possible interactions: Refer to manufacturer's literature

ALTERNATIVE DRUGS   N/A

 FOLLOWUP

PATIENT MONITORING   In HIV patients with KS, other opportunistic infections must be aggressively treated

PREVENTION/AVOIDANCE   Safe sex practices

POSSIBLE COMPLICATIONS
Aggressive form affects at least 1/3 of HIV infected patients

EXPECTED COURSE AND PROGNOSIS
• Generally poor for AIDS related disease
• Indolent form - 10 year survival

 MISCELLANEOUS

ASSOCIATED CONDITIONS
• AIDS
• HIV infection

AGE-RELATED FACTORS
Pediatric: N/A
Geriatric: Indolent form most likely to occur in men in this age group
Others: N/A

PREGNANCY   N/A

SYNONYMS
• Endotheliosarcoma
• Multiple, idiopathic hemorrhagic sarcoma

ICD-9-CM
173.9 malignant neoplasm of the skin

SEE ALSO
• HIV infection and AIDS

OTHER NOTES   N/A

ABBREVIATIONS
KS = Kaposi's sarcoma

REFERENCES
• Groopman, J.E. & Scadden, D.T.: Interferon therapy for Kaposi's sarcoma associated with the acquired immunodeficiency syndrome: A proposal for uniform evaluation, response, and staging criteria. J Clin Oncol 7:1201, 1989
• Abrams, D. Grieco, M. & McMeeking, A.: AIDS/HIV Treatment Directory. New York, American Foundation for AIDS Research (updated 4 times yearly)

Author R. Gorman, M.D.

Keloids

DESCRIPTION Abnormally large overgrowth of fibrous tissue (scar) occurring as a result of trauma or irritation that does not subside with time
System(s) affected: Skin/Exocrine
Genetics:
• 5-15 time more common in Blacks and Asians than Caucasians. In all races, more darkly pigmented individuals are at higher risk.
• Both autosomal dominant and autosomal recessive familial inheritance have been reported
Incidence/Prevalence in USA: Largely unknown, but does affect 4-16% of the Black and Hispanic population
Predominant age: N/A
Predominant sex: Male = Female

SIGNS AND SYMPTOMS
• Pain
• Tenderness
• Hyperesthesia
• Pruritis
• Firm, smooth, elevated scar with sharply demarcated borders
• Initially may be pale or mildly erythematous
• Older lesion hypo- or hyperpigmented
• Scar extends beyond margins of the initial wound
• Over period of years, keloids continue to grow and may develop claw-like projections

CAUSES
• Surgical wound
• Burn injury
• Acne scar
• Insect bite
• Folliculitis barbae

RISK FACTORS
• Family history of keloids
• Dark skin pigment
• Certain locations on the body, e.g., deltoids, chest, earlobes
• Pregnancy
• Adolescence

DIFFERENTIAL DIAGNOSIS
• Hypertrophic scar (usually spontaneously regress; do not cross wound margins)
• Dermatofibroma
• Infiltrating basal cell carcinoma (consider small punch biopsy)

LABORATORY N/A
Drugs that may alter lab results: N/A
Disorders that may alter lab results: N/A

PATHOLOGICAL FINDINGS Histology shows whorl-like arrangements of hyalinized collagen bundles with pressure thinning of papillary dermis and minimal elastic tissue

SPECIAL TESTS N/A

IMAGING N/A

DIAGNOSTIC PROCEDURES Biopsy, if unable to differentiate

APPROPRIATE HEALTH CARE
Outpatient

GENERAL MEASURES
• Intralesional corticosteroid injections - cause atrophy and are most successful therapy
• Pressure helpful for prevention. Pressure bandages must maintain 24 mm Hg, and should be worn for 6-12 months. Bandages should not be removed for more than 30 minutes/day.
• Surgery - high recurrence rate, therefore used only for debulking of large keloids or if a lesion is unresponsive to steroid injections alone
• Radiation - no advantage over other methods, therefore use only if all other methods fail, and then use in conjunction with steroids
• Laser surgery - no evidence of efficacy
• Topical agents - (e.g., retinoic acid, vitamin E, antineoplastic agents, silicone gel) no evidence to support efficacy

ACTIVITY Full activity

DIET No special diet

PATIENT EDUCATION Stress possibility of recurrence despite adequate treatment

MEDICATIONS

DRUG(S) OF CHOICE
Triamcinolone suspension 10 mg/mL (Kenalog)
◊ Using 27-30 gauge needle and a TB syringe (total dose 20-30 mg of triamcinolone). May inject 3 lesions at a time, using 10 mg/lesion.
◊ Advance needle while injecting in order to evenly distribute medication
◊ Early keloids are more responsive to this therapy than older lesions
◊ Reinject every 4 weeks until keloid shrinks to near skin surface
◊ If no response to 10 mg/mL triacinolone suspension, may try 40 mg/mL suspension
◊ May mix dilute triamcinolone (5-10 mg/mL) with local anaesthetic for excision of keloids. Postoperative steroid injections at 2-4 weeks and then monthly for 6 months helps prevent recurrences.
Contraindications: None absolute
Precautions:
• Systemic absorption with adrenal suppression (reversible)
• Local affects - skin atrophy, ulceration, depigmentation, telangiectasias
• Both types of side effects more common with 40 mg/mL triamcinolone suspension
Significant possible interactions: Rare interactions with very large doses of corticosteroids and systemic absorption

ALTERNATIVE DRUGS   None

FOLLOWUP

PATIENT MONITORING   Monthly visits for evaluation and possible steroid re-injections

PREVENTION/AVOIDANCE
Compressive pressure dressings may be useful in high risk (e.g., burn) patients. Local steroid injection postoperative in high risk patients is also effective.

POSSIBLE COMPLICATIONS   Skin atrophy, ulceration, depigmentation, telangiectasias can occur as a result of triamcinolone treatment

EXPECTED COURSE AND PROGNOSIS   Lesions gradually diminish with therapy over a 6-12 month period, leaving a flat, shiny scar

MISCELLANEOUS

ASSOCIATED CONDITIONS   None

AGE-RELATED FACTORS   Keloid formation more common during adolescence
Pediatric: None
Geriatric: None
Others: N/A

PREGNANCY   Keloid formation more likely during pregnancy

SYNONYMS   Razor bumps

ICD-9-CM   701.4

SEE ALSO   N/A

OTHER NOTES   N/A

ABBREVIATIONS   N/A

REFERENCES   Rook, A., Wilkinson, D.S., Ebling, F.J.G., et al.: Textbook of Dermatology. Oxford. Blackwell Scientific Publishing, 1986

Author   E. Lackermann, M.D.

Keratosis, actinic

BASICS

DESCRIPTION Common, usually multiple premalignant skin lesions of sun-exposed areas. They are the most common indicator of excessive cumulative ultra-violet light exposure. The risk of transformation to squamous carcinoma is quite low: 1/4% risk of malignant transformation per lesion per year.
Genetics: Relates to complexion
System(s) affected: Skin/Exocrine
Incidence/Prevalence in USA: Common in blondes and redheads; rare in blacks
Predominant age: 40+; progressive with age
Predominant sex: Male > Female (from occupational sun exposure)

SIGNS AND SYMPTOMS
• Lesions usually fairly flat, red, and rough to palpitation
• Mild hyperesthesia common over lesions
• Hypertrophic verrucous lesions (called "cutaneous horns" if extreme) may be impossible to differentiate from squamous cell carcinoma clinically
• A pigmented variant also exists
• Acute cheilitis usually involves lower lip only
• Only photo-exposed areas involved, often with other stigmata of chronic actinic damage: lentigines, actinic elastosis, atrophy

CAUSES
• Almost exclusively short-wave ultraviolet light (UVB)
• Role of long-wave ultraviolet (UVA) is questionable
• Bowen's disease can be caused by the carcinogenic types of human papilloma virus

RISK FACTORS
• Equatorial latitudes
• High elevations
• Outdoor occupation (farmers, sailors, ranchers)
• Outdoor athletics
• Sun worshippers
• Accompanying heat, wind, humidity augment carcinogenic effect
• Organ transplantation, due to immunosuppression

DIAGNOSIS

DIFFERENTIAL DIAGNOSIS
• Squamous cell carcinoma (hypertrophic type)
• Verruca vulgaris (hypertrophic type)
• Seborrheic dermatitis or psoriasis (near hairline)
• Lentigo maligna (pigmented type)
• Lupus erythematosis

LABORATORY N/A
Drugs that may alter lab results: N/A
Disorders that may alter lab results: N/A

PATHOLOGICAL FINDINGS
• (Diagnosis usually made clinically except where there is a suspicion of carcinoma)
• Hyperkeratosis
• Hypertrophic, atrophic, Bowenoid, acantholytic, and pigmented varieties show the corresponding epidermal findings
• Malignant cells sparse except in Bowenoid variety
• Usually a sparse lymphocytic and plasma cell infiltrate

SPECIAL TESTS Shave biopsy for a definitive diagnosis

IMAGING N/A

DIAGNOSTIC PROCEDURES Biopsy (shave)

TREATMENT

APPROPRIATE HEALTH CARE
Outpatient

GENERAL MEASURES
• Cryotherapy (rapid and non-scarring)
• Sun-protective techniques (See Patient Education)
• Other therapies: Dermabrasion, other destructive surgical modalities
• Photo-dynamic therapy

ACTIVITY No restrictions

DIET No special diet

PATIENT EDUCATION
• Teach sun-protective techniques
• Transfer hobbies and other outdoor activities to early morning or late afternoon
• Wear protective clothing and hats
• Daily use of topically applied sunscreens with SPF greater than 15
• Teach self-examination for cutaneous carcinoma (melanoma, squamous cell, basal cell)

MEDICATIONS

DRUG(S) OF CHOICE
- Topical 5-fluorouracil (destroys even subclinical lesions, also non-scarring)
- Topical Mesoprocol

Contraindications: N/A

Precautions: Continue treatment to involved skin

Significant possible interactions: N/A

ALTERNATIVE DRUGS   Topical tretinoin

 FOLLOWUP

PATIENT MONITORING Dependent on associated malignancy and frequency with which new actinic keratoses appear

PREVENTION/AVOIDANCE Sun protective techniques (See Patient Education)

POSSIBLE COMPLICATIONS Actinic keratosis is a premalignant lesion and may undergo carcinomatous proliferation to become squamous cell carcinoma

EXPECTED COURSE AND PROGNOSIS Excellent , if prevention taken by patient

 MISCELLANEOUS

ASSOCIATED CONDITIONS Squamous cell carcinoma

AGE-RELATED FACTORS
Pediatric: Rare
Geriatric: Frequent problem
Others: N/A

PREGNANCY N/A

SYNONYMS N/A

ICD-9-CM 701.1

SEE ALSO
- Squamous cell carcinoma
- Seborrheic dermatitis

OTHER NOTES N/A

ABBREVIATIONS N/A

REFERENCES
- Dodson, J.M., et al: Malignant potential of actinic keratoses and controversy over treatment, Archives of Dermatology:127:1029, 1991
- Lever, W.F. & Schaumburg-Lever, G.: Histopathology of the Skin. Philadelphia, J.P. Lippincott, 1983

Author J. Person, M.D.

Labyrinthitis

 BASICS

DESCRIPTION
Inflammation of the vestibular labyrinth (a system of intercommunicating cavities and canals in the inner ear). There are many possible causes (see Differential Diagnosis). The most constant and pervasive symptom is vertigo.

System(s) affected: Nervous
Genetics: No known genetic pattern
Incidence/Prevalence: Unknown
Predominant age: All ages beyond infancy
Predominant sex: Male = Female

SIGNS AND SYMPTOMS
- Vertigo
- Dizziness
- Hearing loss, fluctuating
- Nausea and vomiting
- Tinnitus
- Perspiration
- Increased salivation
- Generalized malaise
- Hypercapnia
- Nystagmus

CAUSES
- Physiologic - mismatch of vestibular, visual and somatosensory systems triggered by an external stimulus, such as a stop after whirling turns, heights, motion sickness
- Pathologic - imbalance in the vestibular system caused by a lesion within vestibular pathways (inner ear to cerebral cortex)
- Infections (especially viral)
- Tumors
- Vasculitis
- Infarction
- Ototoxic drugs, especially aminoglycosides
- Head injury
- Neuronitis

RISK FACTORS
- Trauma
- Stress
- Drug ingestion
- Predisposing virus infection
- Cardiovascular disease
- Cerebrovascular disease

 DIAGNOSIS

DIFFERENTIAL DIAGNOSIS
- Acute viral labyrinthitis
- Benign positional vertigo
- Ménierè's syndrome
- Postconcussion syndrome
- Chronic bacterial otomastoiditis
- Drug-induced damage to vestibular labyrinth
- Vascular insufficiency
- Cerebellopontine-angle tumors, such as acoustic neuroma
- Multiple sclerosis
- Para-infectious encephalomyelitis
- Para-infectious cranial polyneuritis
- Ramsay Hunt syndrome
- Cerebral or systemic vasculitis
- Temporal lobe epilepsy
- Benign positional vertigo

LABORATORY
Routine laboratory studies not helpful
Drugs that may alter lab results: All drugs with potential ototoxicity
Disorders that may alter lab results: N/A

PATHOLOGICAL FINDINGS
N/A

SPECIAL TESTS
- Electronystagmography
- Caloric test
- Doll's eye test
- Forced voluntary hyperventilation for 1 to 3 minutes to mimic symptoms if cause is physiologic or emotional

IMAGING
CT or MRI for suspected lesions

DIAGNOSTIC PROCEDURES
History and physical

 TREATMENT

APPROPRIATE HEALTH CARE
Outpatient

GENERAL MEASURES
- Treat underlying disorder when possible
- Symptomatic treatment to accompany specific treatment

ACTIVITY
Lie still with eyes closed in darkened room during acute attacks. Otherwise, activity as tolerated.

DIET
Reduced sodium

PATIENT EDUCATION
Griffith, H.W.: Instructions for Patients, page 212. Philadelphia, W.B. Saunders Company, 4th edition, 1989

MEDICATIONS

DRUG(S) OF CHOICE
• Phenergan, 25 mg qid
or
• Diazepam, 5 mg qid
or
• Prochlorperazine suppositories (25 mg) for vomiting
or
• Meclizine 25 mg qid
or
• Scopolamine transdermal

Contraindications: Refer to manufacturer's literature

Precautions: All the listed medications have significant adverse reactions. Use with caution. Avoid scopolamine in the elderly.

Significant possible interactions: Refer to manufacturer's literature

ALTERNATIVE DRUGS N/A

FOLLOWUP

PATIENT MONITORING As needed

PREVENTION/AVOIDANCE No preventive measures

POSSIBLE COMPLICATIONS
Permanent hearing loss

EXPECTED COURSE AND PROGNOSIS Depends on cause. Physiologic labyrinthitis usually clears completely.

MISCELLANEOUS

ASSOCIATED CONDITIONS
• Ménière's syndrome
• Head injury

AGE-RELATED FACTORS
Pediatric: Unusual in this age group
Geriatric:
• Very common in this age group, especially benign positional vertigo
• Avoid scopolamine or use with extreme caution in this age group
Others: N/A

PREGNANCY Avoid medications

SYNONYMS
• Acute peripheral vestibulopathy
• Vestibular neuronitis

ICD-9-CM 386.30

SEE ALSO N/A

OTHER NOTES N/A

ABBREVIATIONS N/A

REFERENCES
Baloh, R.W. & Honrobia, V.: Clinical Neurology of the Vestibular System. 2nd Ed. Philadelphia, F.A. Davis Co, 1990

Author V. Morell, MD

Lacrimal disorders

 BASICS

DESCRIPTION Lacrimal disorders refer to diseases and abnormalities of tear production and tear film. The most common lacrimal disorder is "dry eye". Lacrimal duct disorders, seen in the pediatric age group, often result in "overflow" tearing.
System(s) affected: Skin/Exocrine
Genetics: None
Incidence/Prevalence in USA: Very common and more often seen in arid climates of the desert Southwest
Predominant age: Dry eye symptoms increase with age. Most common in the elderly.
Predominant sex: Female > Male
Signs and symptoms:
• Gritty sensation to the eyes
• Visual blurring
• Redness
• Excessive tearing and mucus production
• Inadequate tear on the ocular surface

CAUSES Poor tear production and/or rapid evaporation of the tear

RISK FACTORS Individuals who live in arid regions are on diuretics and have a history of collagen vascular diseases such as rheumatoid arthritis, Sjögren's syndrome, Bell's palsy, eyelid abnormalities and thyroid disease, are most at risk.

 DIAGNOSIS

DIFFERENTIAL DIAGNOSIS Lacrimal disorders need to be differentiated from ocular infections and allergy. Another important consideration is the variety of anticholinergic affecting drugs that decrease tear production.

LABORATORY Tear production can be measured using a Schirmer's filter strip after instillation of topical anesthetic. Wetting of less than 10 mm of the slip after 5 minutes is indicative of insufficient tear production..
Drugs that may alter lab results: N/A
Disorders that may alter lab results: N/A

PATHOLOGICAL FINDINGS In Sjögren's syndrome infiltration of the lacrimal gland with inflammatory cells may be evident

SPECIAL TESTS N/A

IMAGING None

DIAGNOSTIC PROCEDURES Staining of the ocular surface with fluorescein will show areas of abnormal uptake and patches of drying. Rose bengal will be taken up by dead or dying epithelial cells and may be a more sensitive test.

 TREATMENT

APPROPRIATE HEALTH CARE
Outpatient

GENERAL MEASURES
• Those with systemic illnesses predisposed to dry eye should be informed and instructed in the appropriate use of artificial tear supplements
• Cool mist vaporizer and home humidification is helpful

ACTIVITY No restrictions

DIET No special diet

PATIENT EDUCATION All individuals with systemic illnesses predisposed to dry eye, menopausal women, and those residing in arid climates or over the age of 60 should be instructed in the use of artificial tear supplements to combat dry eye symptoms

MEDICATIONS

DRUG(S) OF CHOICE
• Artificial tear drops excluding those that have preservatives. The dosage of the drop varies depending on the severity of the symptoms. Usually one drop in each eye several times throughout the day can prevent ocular discomfort.
• The use of a bland ophthalmic ointment at bedtime between the eyelid and the eye can help prevent drying of the eye at night
Contraindications: N/A
Precautions: N/A
Significant possible interactions: N/A
Alternative drugs: N/A

 FOLLOWUP

PATIENT MONITORING Monitor early to determine the effectiveness of treatment. Occasionally the use of more viscous drops or increased frequency of tear supplements may be required.

PREVENTION/AVOIDANCE Prevent exposure to eye irritants from pollution, cigarette smoke, and sun exposure

POSSIBLE COMPLICATIONS Severe dry eye can lead to corneal break-down, secondary invasion by bacteria and eye infections

EXPECTED COURSE AND PROGNOSIS Lacrimal disorders can be adequately managed with artificial tear supplements. Blocked tear ducts can be managed with probing and punctal dilation and/or dacryocysto-rhinostomy procedures in more severe cases.

 MISCELLANEOUS

ASSOCIATED CONDITIONS Sjögren's syndrome and age-related factors more commonly seen in the elderly population

AGE-RELATED FACTORS N/A
Pediatric: May find lacrimal duct blockage in infants
Geriatric: Most common in this age group
Others: N/A

PREGNANCY Dry eyes can frequently be associated with pregnancy in an otherwise healthy individual

SYNONYMS Epiphoria (excessive tearing)

ICD-9-CM 375.15

SEE ALSO N/A

OTHER NOTES Symptoms of dry eye are most often overlooked by practitioners when considering conjunctivitis (pink eye) and allergic disorders

ABBREVIATIONS N/A

REFERENCES Orbit Eyelids And Lacrimal System, Basic and Clinical Course. San Francisco, American Academy of Ophthalmology

Author R. Kershner, M.D., F.A.C.S.

Lactose intolerance

BASICS

DESCRIPTION Inability to digest lactose (the primary sugar in milk) into its constituents, glucose and galactose, due to low levels of lactase enzyme in the brush border of the duodenum
• Congenital lactose intolerance - very rare
• Primary lactose intolerance - common in adults in whom a low level of lactase has developed after childhood. Symptoms are experienced after consumption of milk. Intolerance varies with amount of lactose consumed.
• Secondary lactose intolerance - inability to digest lactose caused by any condition injuring the intestinal mucosa (e.g., diarrhea) or a reduction of available mucosal surface (e.g., resection). This is usually transient, with the duration of the intolerance determined by the nature and course of the primary condition.
• Lactose malabsorption - inability to absorb lactose. This does not necessarily parallel lactose intolerance.
System(s) affected: Gastrointestinal, Endocrine/Metabolic
Genetics: Unknown
Incidence in USA: Unknown
Prevalence in USA:
• Primary lactose intolerance - varies according to race. 100% of American Indians, 80-90% of Blacks, Asians, Mediterraneans and Jews, less than 5% of descendants of Northern and Central Europeans.
• Secondary lactose intolerance - 50% or more of infants with acute or chronic diarrheal disease have lactose intolerance, especially with rotavirus disease. Also fairly common with giardiasis and ascariasis, inflammatory bowel disease and the AIDS malabsorptive syndrome.
Predominant age:
• Primary - teenage and adult
• Secondary - depends on the underlying condition
Predominant sex: Male = Female. However, 44% of lactose intolerant women will regain the ability to digest lactose during pregnancy.

SIGNS AND SYMPTOMS
• Bloating
• Cramping
• Abdominal discomfort
• Diarrhea or loose stools
• Flatulence
• Rumbling (borborygmi)
• Only one-third to one-fifth of people with lactose malabsorption will develop symptoms. Degree of symptoms varies with lactose load and with other foods consumed at the same time.
• In children - vomiting is common; frothy, acid stools; malnutrition can occur

CAUSES
• Primary lactose intolerance - normal decline in the lactase activity in the intestinal mucosa after weaning which is genetically controlled and permanent
• Secondary lactose intolerance - associated with gastroenteritis in children
• Also non tropical and tropical sprue, regional enteritis, abetalipoproteinemia, cystic fibrosis, ulcerative colitis, immunoglobulin deficiencies in both adults and children

RISK FACTORS
• Race
• Age

DIAGNOSIS

DIFFERENTIAL DIAGNOSIS Sucrase deficiency, diseases listed under secondary lactose intolerance

LABORATORY Low fecal pH and reducing substances only valid when stools are collected fresh and assayed immediately. Fairly insensitive.
Drugs that may alter lab results: None
Disorders that may alter lab results: None

PATHOLOGICAL FINDINGS Lactase deficiency in intestinal mucosa - may be patchy or focal. Rarely used in clinical practice.

SPECIAL TESTS
• Lactose breath hydrogen test - especially in children
• Lactose absorption test - alternative to lactose breath hydrogen test in adults

IMAGING None

DIAGNOSTIC PROCEDURES Small bowel biopsy for assay of lactase activity - may be normal if deficiency is focal or patchy (not readily available and usually not necessary)

TREATMENT

APPROPRIATE HEALTH CARE
Outpatient except severe cases of malnutrition

GENERAL MEASURES No disease specific measures

ACTIVITY Full activity

DIET
• Reduce or restrict dietary lactose to control symptoms
• Yogurt and fermented products such as hard cheeses are tolerated better than milk
• Supplement calcium in the form of calcium carbonate
• Commercially available "lactase" preparations (Lactaid or Lactrase) are effective in reducing symptoms in many people
• Prehydrolyzed milk (Lactaid) is available and effective

PATIENT EDUCATION
• Patients must read labels on commercial products since milk-sugar is used in many products and may cause symptoms
• Lactose intolerant patients may tolerate whole milk or chocolate milk better than skim
• Lactose consumed with other food products is better tolerated than when it is consumed alone
• Primary lactase deficiency is permanent; secondary lactose intolerance is usually temporary, though it may persist for several months after the inciting disease has been cured.

MEDICATIONS

DRUG(S) OF CHOICE
Lactase tablets (Lactaid or Lactrase)
◊ 1 to 2 capsules or tablets prior to ingesting milk products. These vary in effectiveness at preventing symptoms.
◊ Can add tablets or contents of capsules to milk before drinking
◊ Also available in milk in some areas
Contraindications: None
Precautions: Not effective for all people with lactose intolerance
Significant possible interactions: None

ALTERNATIVE DRUGS   None

FOLLOWUP

PATIENT MONITORING   N/A

PREVENTION/AVOIDANCE   Avoidance of lactose in large quantities will relieve symptoms. Patients can learn what level of lactose is tolerable in their diet.

POSSIBLE COMPLICATIONS   Calcium deficiency

EXPECTED COURSE AND PROGNOSIS
• Normal life expectancy
• Symptoms can be controlled

MISCELLANEOUS

ASSOCIATED CONDITIONS
• Tropical or non-tropical sprue
• Giardiasis
• Immunoglobulin deficiencies
• Crohn's disease
• Cystic fibrosis

AGE-RELATED FACTORS
Pediatric:
• Primary lactose intolerance occurs after weaning - usually beginning in late childhood
• Breast milk contains a large quantity of lactose but does not seem to worsen diarrhea associated with viral or bacterial diseases
• Lactose free formulas are available
Geriatric: No increase in lactose intolerance in this age group
Others: Secondary lactose intolerance can begin at any age

PREGNANCY   44% of lactose intolerant women will be able to tolerate lactose while pregnant

SYNONYMS   Lactase deficiency

ICD-9-CM   271.3 intolerance or malabsorption (congenital) of lactose

OTHER NOTES   N/A

SEE ALSO   N/A

ABBREVIATIONS   N/A

REFERENCES
• Saavedra, J. M., & Perman, J.A.: Current Concepts in Lactose Malabsorption and Intolerance. Annu Rev Nutr. (9)475-502, 1989
• Hurst, J.W., (ed.): Medicine for the Practicing Physician. 2nd Ed. Boston, Butterworth, 1988

Author   K. Reilly, M.D.

Laryngeal cancer

 BASICS

DESCRIPTION Most common cancer representing less than 1% of all malignant lesions. Squamous cell carcinomas comprise 5-98% of all malignant neoplasms of the larynx.
- Less than 2% of all carcinomas
- At the time of diagnosis, 62% will have local disease, 26% regional disease and 8% distant disease in the lungs, liver and/or bone
- No racial predilection

System(s) affected: Pulmonary
Genetics: Unknown
Incidence in USA: 5/100,00 (12,500 new cases per year)
Prevalence in USA: Unknown
Predominant age:
- Median age of occurrence in the 6th and 7th decades
- Less than 1% of laryngeal cancers arise in patients under 30 years of age

Predominant sex: Male > Female (5:1). However, increasing incidence in women who smoke.

SIGNS AND SYMPTOMS
- Persistent hoarseness in an elderly or middle aged cigarette smoker
- Dyspnea and stridor
- Ipsilateral otalgia
- Dysphagia
- Odynophagia
- Chronic cough
- Hemoptysis
- Weight loss due to poor nutrition
- Halitosis due to tumor necrosis
- Mass in the neck from metastatic lymph node
- Laryngeal tenderness due to tumor necrosis or suppuration
- Lump in the neck
- Broadening of the larynx on palpation with loss of crepitation
- Tenderness of the larynx
- Fullness of the cricothyroid membrane

CAUSES
- Smoking
- Alcohol abuse

RISK FACTORS Included in Causes

 DIAGNOSIS

DIFFERENTIAL DIAGNOSIS
- Acute or chronic laryngitis
- Benign vocal cord lesions such as polyps, nodules, and papillomas
- Tuberculosis or fungal infection of the larynx

LABORATORY Liver function studies to rule out metastatic disease
Drugs that may alter lab results: N/A
Disorders that may alter lab results: N/A

PATHOLOGICAL FINDINGS N/A

SPECIAL TESTS
- Laryngoscopy - fungating, friable tumor with heaped up edges and granular appearance with multiple areas of central necrosis and exudate surrounding areas of hyperemia
- CT or MRI if chest and liver or brain metastasis suspected

IMAGING
- Bone scan if bone metastasis suspected
- Screening chest x-ray to rule out metastatic disease

DIAGNOSTIC PROCEDURES Indirect and/or direct laryngoscopy and biopsy to determine stage of disease as well as histologic confirmation

 TREATMENT

APPROPRIATE HEALTH CARE
- Tracheotomy may be necessary if tumor is large enough to cause upper airway obstruction
- Early disease may be treatable by either radiation therapy or laser cordectomy on an outpatient basis
- More advanced disease needs inpatient care necessitating partial or total laryngectomy, and post-operative radiation therapy 4-5 weeks after surgery depending on the stage of disease

GENERAL MEASURES Tracheotomy care, when applicable

ACTIVITY Fully active unless the patient is debilitated from more advanced disease and/or greater degree of surgery

DIET
- Nasogastric or gastrostomy feeding may be necessary if tumor involves esophageal inlet
- No special diet otherwise

PATIENT EDUCATION Material is available from local cancer society

MEDICATIONS

DRUG(S) OF CHOICE
• Narcotics may be necessary for pain control during treatment for mucositis secondary to radiation therapy
• Nystatin mouth rinses for oral thrush
Contraindications: N/A
Precautions: N/A
Significant possible interactions: N/A

ALTERNATIVE DRUGS   N/A

FOLLOWUP

PATIENT MONITORING
• Repeat indirect laryngoscopy and complete head and neck examinations for at least five years after treatment to detect early recurrence or second primary
• Yearly chest x-ray and liver function tests
• Patients with dysphagia should undergo barium swallow and/or esophageal endoscopy to rule out second tumor in the esophagus
• Patients with unexplained pain should have appropriate radiological or nuclear medicine, bone scans
• Mental status change indicates CT scan of the brain to rule out brain metastases

PREVENTION/AVOIDANCE
• Indirect laryngoscopy for patients with persistent hoarseness lasting beyond one to two weeks
• Cessation of smoking and/or alcohol abuse

POSSIBLE COMPLICATIONS
• Temporary odynophagia or dysphagia secondary to mucositis and/or thrush during radiation therapy
• Persistent hoarseness despite adequate treatment necessitating further adjunctive procedures and/or speech therapy
• Tracheostomal stenosis requiring stenting with laryngectomy tubes or further surgery
• Dysphagia, secondary to upper esophageal stricture after total laryngectomy necessitating dilatation
• Aspiration, after partial laryngectomy necessitating completion laryngectomy or tracheotomy
• Inability to decannulate after partial laryngectomy due to laryngeal stenosis and/or aspiration
• Radiation induced chondronecrosis which mimics tumor recurrence
• Radiation edema necessitating emergent tracheotomy

EXPECTED COURSE AND PROGNOSIS
• Early disease is expected to have greater than 90% cure

MISCELLANEOUS

ASSOCIATED CONDITIONS
• Less than 10% of patients may have a synchronous squamous cell carcinoma in the lower or upper aero-digestive tract; most notably in the esophagus or lungs

AGE-RELATED FACTORS
Pediatric: N/A
Geriatric: N/A
Others: N/A

PREGNANCY
• Very rare in young patients in general
• Natural history of disease and treatment side effects have to be weighed against the possibilities of continuing on to delivery

SYNONYMS   Cancer of larynx

ICD-9-CM   161.0 malignant neoplasm of larynx

SEE ALSO   N/A

OTHER NOTES   N/A

ABBREVIATIONS   N/A

REFERENCES
• Suen, J.Y. & Myers, E.N.: Cancer of the Head and Neck. New York, Churchill Livingstone, 1981
• Ariyan, S.: Cancer of the Head and Neck. St. Louis, C.V. Mosby, 1987

Author   R. Casiano, M.D

Laryngitis

 BASICS

DESCRIPTION Inflammation of the mucosa of the larynx. Most common during peaks paralleling epidemics of individual viruses, late fall, winter, early spring. Course may be acute or chronic. Includes atrophic, hypertrophic, reflux, catarrhal, sicca, acute infectious, membranous.
System(s) affected: Pulmonary
Genetics: No known genetic pattern
Incidence/Prevalence in USA: Common
Predominant age: All ages
Predominant sex: Male = Female

SIGNS AND SYMPTOMS
- Hoarseness
- Abnormal sounding voice
- Aphonia
- Throat tickling
- Feeling of throat rawness
- Constant urge to clear the throat
- Fever
- Malaise
- Dysphagia
- Throat pain
- Cough
- Regional lymphadenopathy

CAUSES
- Virus infections - influenza A, B, parainfluenza, adenovirus, coronavirus, rhinovirus
- Bacterial infections (beta-hemolytic streptococcus or Streptococcus pneumoniae)
- Excessive use of voice
- Inhaling irritating substances
- Aspiration of caustic chemical
- Aging changes - muscle atrophy, loss of moisture in larynx, bowing of vocal cords
- Damage during surgery

RISK FACTORS
Acute
  ◊ Upper respiratory tract infection
  ◊ Bronchitis
  ◊ Pneumonia
  ◊ Influenza
  ◊ Pertussis
  ◊ Measles
  ◊ Diphtheria
Chronic
  ◊ Allergy
  ◊ Chronic rhinitis
  ◊ Chronic sinusitis
  ◊ Voice abuse
  ◊ Reflux of gastric contents
  ◊ Smoking
  ◊ Alcohol abuse
  ◊ Constant exposure to dust or other irritants

 DIAGNOSIS

DIFFERENTIAL DIAGNOSIS
- Croup
- Measles
- Diphtheria
- Vocal nodules
- Laryngeal malignancy

LABORATORY WBC elevated in bacterial laryngitis
Drugs that may alter lab results: N/A
Disorders that may alter lab results: N/A

PATHOLOGICAL FINDINGS N/A

SPECIAL TESTS Virus culture (seldom necessary)

IMAGING Only if needed for differential diagnosis

DIAGNOSTIC PROCEDURES
- Fiberoptic or indirect laryngoscopy - red, inflamed and occasionally hemorrhagic vocal cords, with rounded edges, and exudate
- Consider biopsy - chronic laryngitis in adults with history of smoking or alcohol abuse

 TREATMENT

APPROPRIATE HEALTH CARE
Outpatient

GENERAL MEASURES
Acute
  ◊ Usually a self-limited illness and not severe
    ◊ Voice rest
    ◊ Steam inhalations or cool-mist humidifier
    ◊ Increase fluid intake
    ◊ Analgesics
    ◊ Avoid smoking (or cigarette smoke from others) during acute phase
Chronic
    ◊ Symptomatic treatment as above
    ◊ Voice therapy
    ◊ Stop smoking
    ◊ Reduce alcohol intake
    ◊ Occupational change or modification, if exposure
    ◊ Vocal cord stripping of hyperplastic mucosa and areas of leukoplakia (can be used for biopsy, may produce a more normal sounding voice)
    ◊ For reflux laryngitis - elevate head of bed, other antireflux management

ACTIVITY Rest until fever subsides then, no restrictions

DIET No special diet

PATIENT EDUCATION
- Provide assistance with smoking cessation
- Help patient with modification of other predisposing habits or occupational hazards

MEDICATIONS

DRUG(S) OF CHOICE
- Usually none
- Analgesics
- Antipyretics to reduce fever
- Cough suppressants
- Penicillin G, 250 mg orally q6h for 10-12 days (for streptococcal or pneumococcal infections)

Contraindications: Refer to manufacturer's literature

Precautions: Refer to manufacturer's literature

Significant possible interactions: Refer to manufacturer's literature

ALTERNATIVE DRUGS N/A

FOLLOWUP

PATIENT MONITORING None needed (usually)

PREVENTION/AVOIDANCE
- Avoid overuse of voice
- Prompt treatment of respiratory infections
- Influenza virus vaccine for high-risk individuals

POSSIBLE COMPLICATIONS Chronic hoarseness

EXPECTED COURSE AND PROGNOSIS Complete clearing of the inflammation without sequelae

MISCELLANEOUS

ASSOCIATED CONDITIONS
- Viral pharyngitis
- Croup
- Bronchitis
- Pneumonitis

AGE-RELATED FACTORS
Pediatric: Common in this age group
Geriatric: May be sicker and slower to heal
Others: N/A

PREGNANCY Use only safe antibiotics, if antibiotics are essential

SYNONYMS
- Acute laryngitis
- Chronic laryngitis

ICD-9-CM
- 464.0 acute
- 476.0 chronic

SEE ALSO N/A

OTHER NOTES N/A

ABBREVIATIONS N/A

REFERENCES
- Avila, M.M., Carballal, G., Rovaletti, H., et al.: Viral Etiology in Acute Respiratory Infections. Am Rev Respir Dis 140:634, 1989
- Adams, G.L., et al.: Fundamentals of Otolaryngology. 6th Ed. Philadelphia, W.B. Saunders Co., 1989
- Alberti, P.W. & Ruben, R.J. (eds.); Otologic Medicine and Surgery. New York, Churchill Livingstone, 1988

Author KH Mosser, MD

Laryngotracheobronchitis

BASICS

DESCRIPTION Subacute viral illness, characterized by barking cough, stridor and fever, often causing upper airway obstruction in children.
System(s) affected: Pulmonary
Genetics: Unknown, though 15% have family history
Incidence in USA: 15,000-40,000/100,000
Prevalence in USA: Unknown
Predominant age: Childhood
Predominant sex: Male = Female

SIGNS AND SYMPTOMS
- Barking, spasmodic cough
- Biphasic stridor
- Low-grade to moderate fever
- Upper respiratory infection prodrome lasting 1-7 days
- Hypoxia/cyanosis
- Fatigue
- Non-toxic appearing child
- Normal voice, no drooling
- No change in stridor with positioning
- Non-tender larynx
- Inflamed subglottic region
- Normal appearing supraglottic region

CAUSES
Viral
- ◊ Parainfluenza 1
- ◊ Influenza virus type A
- ◊ Other parainfluenza and influenza viruses
- ◊ Respiratory syncytial virus
- ◊ Other viruses - adenovirus, rhinovirus, enterovirus, Coxsackievirus, ECHO virus, reovirus, measles virus

RISK FACTORS
- Past history of croup
- Recurrent upper respiratory infections

DIAGNOSIS

DIFFERENTIAL DIAGNOSIS
- Epiglottitis
- Foreign body aspiration
- Subglottic stenosis (congenital or acquired)
- Bacterial tracheitis
- Simple upper respiratory infection
- Subglottic hemangioma
- Diphtheria

LABORATORY
- Leukopenia early
- Leukocytosis in severe later stage
Drugs that may alter lab results: N/A
Disorders that may alter lab results: N/A

PATHOLOGICAL FINDINGS
- Inflammatory reaction of respiratory mucosa
- Loss of epithelial cells
- Thick mucoid secretions

SPECIAL TESTS N/A

IMAGING
- PA and lateral neck films show funnel-shaped subglottic region with normal epiglottis - "steeple sign" or "pencil-point sign"
- Patient should be monitored during imaging - progression of airway obstruction may be rapid

DIAGNOSTIC PROCEDURES
- Direct laryngoscopy - if child is not in acute distress
- Fiberoptic laryngoscopy - procedure of choice where available
- Bronchoscopy

TREATMENT

APPROPRIATE HEALTH CARE
- Outpatient in mild cases only
- Inpatient in Intensive Care Unit for patients with tachypnea, tachycardia, hypoxia, cyanosis, reactions, pneumonia, or congestive heart failure

GENERAL MEASURES
- Humidification - "croup tent"
- Oxygen
- Intravenous fluids
- Electrocardiographic monitoring and pulse oximetry
- Steroids, racemic epinephrine, antibiotics (see Medications)
- Intubation required in 6-10% for 3-5 days; use smallest tube possible
- Tracheotomy - rarely

ACTIVITY Must keep patient quiet, crying may exacerbate symptoms

DIET
- NPO with IV fluids for severe cases
- Frequent small feedings with increased fluids for mild cases

PATIENT EDUCATION
- Educate parents about when to seek emergency care if mild cases progress
- Emotional support and reassurance for the patient

MEDICATIONS

DRUG(S) OF CHOICE
• Dexamethasone: 1-1.5 mg/kg up to 20 mg every 8-12 hours for 8 doses
• Racemic epinephrine: 0.2-0.5 ml of 2.25 percent racemic epinephrine delivered in 2-3 ml of normal saline - one dose per 30 minutes, monitoring for side effects and rebound
• Antibiotics - controversial in this viral illness
Precautions: Refer to manufacturer's literature
Contraindications: Refer to manufacturer's literature
Significant possible interactions: Refer to manufacturer's literature

ALTERNATIVE DRUGS   N/A

FOLLOWUP

PATIENT MONITORING   Severe cases in ICU with respiratory monitoring for hypoxemia and hypercapnia

PREVENTION/AVOIDANCE   N/A

POSSIBLE COMPLICATIONS   Subglottic stenosis in intubated patients

EXPECTED COURSE AND PROGNOSIS
• Upper respiratory infection prodrome of 1-7 days
• If required, intubation is maintained for 3-5 days
• If required, tracheotomy is maintained for 3-7 days
• Recovery is usually full, without lasting effects

MISCELLANEOUS

ASSOCIATED CONDITIONS   If recurrent, search for underlying anatomic abnormality such as subglottic stenosis or consider foreign body

AGE-RELATED FACTORS
Pediatric: Common in children under the age of three
Geriatric: N/A
Others: N/A

PREGNANCY   N/A

SYNONYMS
• Croup
• Infectious croup
• Viral croup
• LTB

ICD-9-CM

SEE ALSO   N/A

OTHER NOTES
• Less severe " variant" form, spasmodic croup, consists of croupy cough which becomes worse at night, but has no fever or x-ray changes. Usually resolves with mist therapy at home.
• Most common cause of stridor in children

ABBREVIATIONS   N/A

REFERENCES
• Ballenger, J.J.: Diseases of the Nose, Throat and Ear. Philadelphia, Lea & Febiger,
• Gates, G.A.: Current Therapy in Otolaryngology - Head and Neck Surgery. 4th Ed. Philadelphia, B.C. Decker, Inc., 1990

Author   G. Suits, M.D. & L. Howell, M.D.

Lead poisoning

BASICS

DESCRIPTION Consequence of a high body burden of lead, an element with no known physiologic value
System(s) affected: Endocrine/Metabolic, Nervous, Gastrointestinal
Genetics: N/A
Incidence in USA:
Prevalence in USA:
• 17% of preschoolers in the US have a blood lead greater than 15 mcg/dL. Sporadic cases in adults.
• Estimated (1990's) in children 6 months to age 5 years (≥15 mcg/dL): 17,000/100,000
Predominant age: 1-5 years old; adult worker
Predominant sex: Male = Female

SIGNS AND SYMPTOMS
• Often asymptomatic
Mild to moderate toxicity
◊ May cause myalgia or paresthesia, fatigue, irritability, lethargy
◊ Abdominal discomfort, arthralgia, difficulty concentrating, headache, tremor, vomiting, weight loss, muscular exhaustibility
Severe toxicity - leads to 3 major clinical syndromes
◊ Alimentary type - anorexia, metallic taste, constipation, severe abdominal cramps due to intestinal spasm and sometimes associated with rigidity of the abdominal wall
◊ Neuromuscular type (characteristic of adult plumbism) - peripheral neuritis usually painless and limited to extensor muscles
◊ Cerebral type or lead encephalopathy (more common in children) - seizures, coma, long-term sequelae including neurologic defects, retarded mental development, chronic hyperactivity

CAUSES Inhalation of lead dust or fumes, or ingestion of lead

RISK FACTORS
• Children with pica
• Children with iron deficiency anemia
• Residence or frequent visitor in deteriorating, pre-1970 housing with leaded-paint surfaces
• Children with seizures
• Children with hyperkinetic or autistic behavior
• Dust from clothing of lead worker
• Lead dissolved in water from lead or lead-soldered plumbing
• Lead glazed ceramics, especially with acidic food or drink
• Food stored in inverted plastic bread bags printed with colored ink
• Colored comics
• Soil/dust near lead industries and roads
• Folk remedies (Mexican - azarcon, greta; Asian - chuifong tokuwan, pay-loo-ah, ghasard, bali goli, kandu; Middle Eastern - alkohl, surma, saoott, cebagin)
• Hobbies - glazed pottery making; target shooting at firing ranges; lead soldering; painting; preparing lead shot, fishing sinkers; stained-glass making; car or boat repair; home remodeling
• Occupational exposure - plumbers, pipe fitters, lead miners, auto repairers, glass manufacturers, shipbuilders, printers, plastic manufacturers, lead smelters and refiners, policemen, steel welders or cutters, construction workers, rubber product manufacturers, gas station attendants, battery manufacturers, bridge reconstruction workers
• Dietary - zinc or calcium deficiency

DIAGNOSIS

DIFFERENTIAL DIAGNOSIS
• Elevated erythrocyte protoporphyrin may be due to iron deficiency anemia, less commonly hemolytic anemia. Erythropoietic protoporphyria produces a very high erythrocyte protoporphyrin.
• Alimentary type may be confused with acute abdomen
• Neuromuscular type may be confused with other polyneuropathies
• Cerebral type may be confused with attention deficit disorder, mental retardation, autism, dementia, other causes of seizures

LABORATORY
• Blood lead (Pb) greater than 10 mcg/dL, collected with lead-free container
• Asymptomatic patient screening with erythrocyte protoporphyrin level (EP) greater than 35 mcg/dL indicates need for testing blood Pb
• Hgb and Hct slightly low. Eosinophilia or basophilic stippling on peripheral smear may be seen, but are not diagnostic of lead toxicity.
• Renal function decreased in late stages
CDC classification:

Class	Lead
I	< 10
II	10-19
III	20-44
IV	45-69
V	> 70

(mcg/dL whole blood)
Drugs that may alter lab results: None
Disorders that may alter lab results: None

PATHOLOGICAL FINDINGS N/A

SPECIAL TESTS Calcium ethylenediaminetetraacetic acid (Ca EDTA) mobilization test if blood Pb 25-44. This test is not widely used because it is technically difficult to perform and may delay diagnosis and treatment.

IMAGING Abdominal radiograph for lead particles in gut. X-ray of long bones for lines of increased density in the metaphyseal plate resulting from growth arrest.

DIAGNOSTIC PROCEDURES N/A

TREATMENT

APPROPRIATE HEALTH CARE
Outpatient unless parenteral chelation required

GENERAL MEASURES
• Case report to local health department. Complete inspection of home or work-place to determine source of lead. Screen all family members.
• Consider oral chelation for Class III or IV. Chelation (preferably parenteral) for Class V or symptomatic Class III or IV.

ACTIVITY No restrictions

DIET
• If symptomatic, avoid excessive fluids
• Avoidance of pica
• Consume adequate calcium and iron
• Eat a low fat diet to reduce absorption and retention of lead

PATIENT EDUCATION The Inside Story: A Guide to Indoor Air Quality, EPA/400/1-88/004. EPA and Consumer Product Safety Commission, 1988. Lead and Your Drinking Water. EPA, 1988, OPA-87-006

Lead poisoning

MEDICATIONS

DRUG(S) OF CHOICE
Oral chelation:
◊ Succimer (Chemet;
2,3-Dimercaptosuccinic acid; DMSA)10 mg/kg
q8h x 5 days, then 10 mg/kg q12h x 2 weeks.
May be repeated after 2 weeks off if lead
levels are not stabilized below < 15 mcg/dL.
Parenteral chelation (begin after establishment
of adequate urine output):
◊ Class V or symptomatic: BAL (British
anti-Lewisite, dimercaprol) 75 mg/m2 given
deep IM, then BAL 450 mg/m2/d divided q4h x
5 days + Ca EDTA (edetate calcium disodium)
1500 mg/m2/d continuous IV infusion x 5
days. If rebound lead level ≥ 45 mcg/dL,
chelation may be repeated after 2 day interval
if symptomatic, after 5 day interval if
symptomatic.
◊ Class IV asymptomatic: Ca EDTA 1000
mg/m2/d x 5 days. May be repeated after 5-7
days.
• Diazepam for initial control of seizures,
further control maintained with paraldehyde
Contraindications:
• BAL should not be given to persons allergic
to peanuts (the drug solution contains peanut
oil)
Precautions:
• Succimer: Gastrointestinal upset, rash,
nasal congestion, muscle pains, elevated liver
function tests
• Ca EDTA: Renal failure, increased excretion
of zinc, copper and iron
• BAL: Nausea, vomiting, fever, headache,
transient hypertension, hepatocellular damage
Significant possible interactions:
• Vitamins should not be given concurrently
with oral chelation
• BAL may precipitate hemolytic crisis in a
patient with G-6-PD deficiency

ALTERNATIVE DRUGS
Oral chelation with D-penicillamine: (Depen;
Cuprimine)
◊ Penicillin allergic patient should not
receive D-penicillamine (cross-sensitivity is
common)
◊ 10-20 mg/kg bid mixed in apple
juice/sauce on empty stomach (not FDA
approved)
◊ D-penicillamine may cause
gastrointestinal upset, renal failure,
granulocytopenia, liver dysfunction, iron
deficiency, drug induced lupus-like syndrome

FOLLOWUP

PATIENT MONITORING
• After chelation, check for rebound Pb level in
7-10 days. Follow with regular monitoring,
initially biweekly or monthly.
• Correct iron deficiency or any other
nutritional deficiencies present

PREVENTION/AVOIDANCE
• Family should receive counseling on
potential sources of lead and methods to
decrease lead exposure. Wet mopping and
dusting with a high phosphate solution will
help control lead-bearing dust.
• If the source is in the home, the patient must
reside elsewhere until the abatement process
is completed

POSSIBLE COMPLICATIONS
• CNS toxicity may be long lasting or
permanent
• Long-term lead exposure may cause chronic
renal failure (Fanconi-like syndrome); gout;
lead line (blue-black) on gingival tissue

EXPECTED COURSE AND PROGNOSIS
• Symptomatic lead poisoning without
encephalopathy generally improves with
chelation, but subtle CNS toxicity may be long
lasting or permanent
• If encephalopathy occurs, permanent
sequelae (mental retardation, seizure disorder,
blindness, hemiparesis) in 25-50%

MISCELLANEOUS

ASSOCIATED CONDITIONS Iron
deficiency anemia

AGE-RELATED FACTORS
Pediatric:
• Increasing evidence that low lead level
exposure (as low as 10 mcg/dL) may produce
neurotoxicity in children
• Children are at increased risk because of
incomplete development of the blood-brain
barrier before age 3 years allowing more lead
into the central nervous system; ingested lead
has 40% bioavailability in children compared
with 10% in adults
• Common childhood behaviors such as
frequent hand-to-mouth activity and pica
(repeated ingestion of nonfood products) greatly
increase the risk of ingesting lead
Geriatric: N/A
Others: N/A

PREGNANCY
• Lead exposure in pregnancy is associated
with reduced birth weight and premature birth
• Lead is an animal teratogen

SYNONYMS Lead poisoning, inorganic

ICD-9-CM 984.9; when symptomatic, or a
specific lead compound is the source, other
codes may apply

SEE ALSO N/A

OTHER NOTES Screening of all
asymptomatic children during their first 6 years
of life has been recommended. Screening EP is
not sensitive for blood Pb less than 25 mcg/dL.

ABBREVIATIONS
• Pb = lead
• EP = erythrocyte protoporphyrin
• BAL = British anti-Lewisite

REFERENCES
• Royce, S.E.: Case studies in environmental
medicine: lead toxicity. US Dept. HHS, PHS,
TSDR, 1990
• Centers for Disease Control: Preventing lead
poisoning in young children. US Dept. HHS,
PHS, CDC, Atlanta, 1991

Author J. Chao, M.D., M.S.

Légg-Calvé-Pérthes disease

BASICS

DESCRIPTION Idiopathic osteonecrosis of capital femoral epiphysis of the femoral head. 10-20% of cases are bilateral.
System(s) affected: Musculoskeletal
Genetics: No known genetic pattern
Incidence/Prevalence in USA: Incidence 15/100,000; prevalence 75/100,000
Predominant age: Susceptible age 4-12 years. However, 80% occur between 4-9 years
Predominant sex: Males > Females (4:1)

SIGNS AND SYMPTOMS
• Pain in the hip with pain referred to knee or thigh
• Hip held in flexed, abduction, and externally rotated position
• Range of motion limited, especially in internal rotation and abduction
• Atrophy of thigh musculature
• Leg length inequality

CAUSES
• Etiology remains unclear
• Felt to be related to interruption of blood flow to femoral epiphysis
• Role of trauma, hormonal and metabolic factors remains to be established

RISK FACTORS
• No genetic factors
• Increased incidence in children with low birth weight and delayed physical maturation

DIAGNOSIS

DIFFERENTIAL DIAGNOSIS
• Unilateral case - septic hip, toxic synovitis, juvenile rheumatoid arthritis, tuberculosis, lymphoma
• Bilateral cases - hypothyroidism, spondyloepiphyseal dysplasia

LABORATORY
• CBC
• Sedimentation rate
Drugs that may alter lab results: N/A
Disorders that may alter lab results: N/A

PATHOLOGICAL FINDINGS
• Early (necrotic) stage - necrosis of bone with subchondral bone fracture and subsequent collapse of subchondral bone
• Late (resorption, healing) stage - revascularization by creeping substitution of necrotic bone

SPECIAL TESTS
• Technetium 99 bone scan - helpful in delineating extent of avascular changes before they are evident on plain radiographs (sensitivity 98%, specificity 95%)
• MRI - very sensitive test, however, clinical experience is still limited
• Arthrography

IMAGING
• Serial radiographs, AP and frog lateral, are crucial determinant of extent of involvement and progression of healing. Initial findings.
• Full extent of involvement may not be evident for several months
• Classification and prognosis based on radiographic extent of involvement

DIAGNOSTIC PROCEDURES Hip
aspiration when septic joint is suspected

TREATMENT

APPROPRIATE HEALTH CARE
• Ambulatory treatment is the norm
• On occasion, inpatient traction or surgical procedure may be necessary
• When available, a pediatric orthopedic surgeon should be consulted

GENERAL MEASURES
Goals of treatment are:
• Obtain and maintain range-of-motion
• Relieve weight bearing on affected hip as necessary
• Containment of femoral epiphysis within the confines of the acetabulum in order to encourage maximal normal growth and development of the femoral head

ACTIVITY
• Bedrest and traction as necessary to relieve irritation of joint
• Ambulatory status depends on extent/stage of disease

DIET No special diet

PATIENT EDUCATION
• Patient and family should realize that LCP is a self-limited disease with revascularization occurring within 2-3 years
• Treatment is directed at maintaining an appropriate range-of-motion and maximizing the containment of the femoral head

MEDICATIONS

DRUG(S) OF CHOICE Ibuprofen
20-30 mg/kg/24 hours
Contraindications: Allergy to ibuprofen
Precautions: GI irritation
Significant possible interactions: N/A

ALTERNATIVE DRUGS N/A

FOLLOWUP

PATIENT MONITORING
• Initially, close followup needed to determine extent of necrosis and monitor clinical course
• Once healing phase entered, followup can be every 3-6 months
• Long-term followup necessary to determine final outcome

POSSIBLE COMPLICATIONS
• Permanent distortion of the femoral head
• Degenerative joint disease

PREVENTION/AVOIDANCE Since
etiology is not clearly understood, prevention is not possible

EXPECTED COURSE AND PROGNOSIS
• Most patients (60%) have a favorable outcome
• Outcome is dependent on the age at the time of the diagnosis (the younger the better)
• Prognosis is also proportional to the degree of radiologic involvement

MISCELLANEOUS

ASSOCIATED CONDITIONS
• Inguinal hernias
• Undescended testicles

AGE-RELATED FACTORS
Pediatric:
• Physical maturation is delayed
• The younger the patient at the time of diagnosis, the greater the chance for remodelling
Geriatric: N/A
Others: N/A

PREGNANCY N/A

SYNONYMS N/A

ICD-9-CM 732.1

SEE ALSO N/A

OTHER NOTES N/A

ABBREVIATIONS N/A

REFERENCES
• Catterall, A. & Chir, M.: Perthes Disease. In The Hip and its Disorders. Edited by Marvin E. Steinberg. Philadelphia, W.B. Saunders Co., 1991, pp. 419-439
• Tachdjian, M.: Pediatric Orthopedics. 2nd Ed. Philadelphia, W.B. Saunders Co., 1990, pp. 933-1003
• Wenger, D.R., Ward, T.W. & Herring, J.A.: Légg Pérthes Disease: Current Concepts Review. Journal of Bone and Joint Surgery 73A:778-788, 1991

Author F. Valencia, M.D.

Legionnaire's disease

 BASICS

DESCRIPTION Legionnaire's disease was coined for an epidemic of lower respiratory tract disease occurring in Philadelphia in 1976 in war veterans. The causative bacterium was identified and named Legionella pneumophila and may cause pneumonia or flu-like illness.
Genetics: None known
Incidence in USA: 2-4/100,000/year; 1-4% of commonly acquired pneumonias; up to 20% of nosocomial pneumonias
Prevalence in USA: N/A
Predominant Age: 15 months-84 years, increased after age 50
Predominant sex: Male > Female

SIGNS AND SYMPTOMS
• Range of illness from asymptomatic seroconversion, mild febrile illness, to severe pneumonia
• Incubation 2-10 days
• Fever, chills
• Malaise, weakness, lethargy
• Anorexia
• Myalgia
• Headache
• Watery diarrhea in up to 50%
• Nausea and vomiting in 10-20%
• Dry cough which may become productive
• Pleuritic chest pain in up to 33%
• Relative bradycardia in up to 67% of patients
• Neuropsychiatric symptoms of confusion, disorientation, obtundation, depression, hallucinations, insomnia, seizures in up to 25%
• Hyponatremia

CAUSES
• Legionella pneumophila, a weakly gram negative organism widely distributed in soil and water, acquired by inhalation of infected aerosols

RISK FACTORS
• Smoking
• Alcohol abuse
• Immunosuppression
• Chronic cardiopulmonary disease

 DIAGNOSIS

DIFFERENTIAL DIAGNOSIS Other bacterial pneumonias, atypical pneumonias with mycoplasma and chlamydia, viral pneumonias

LABORATORY
Sputum:
◊ Direct immunofluorescence 25-80% sensitive
◊ DNA probe 70% sensitive
◊ Cultures 50-90% sensitive
Blood:
◊ Indirect immunofluorescence 56% sensitive in three weeks and 90% sensitive after 6 weeks (acute and convalescent titers/seroconversion)
◊ Cultures 20% sensitive
Drugs that may alter lab results: N/A
Disorders that may alter lab results: Direct immunofluorescence can cross react with Pseudomonas and Bacteroides species

PATHOLOGICAL FINDINGS Multifocal pneumonia with alveolitis and bronchiolitis, with fibrinous pleuritis, and may have serous or serosanguinous pleural effusion

SPECIAL TESTS Silver and Gimenez stains for lung tissue/specimens

IMAGING
Chest x-ray
◊ Not specific for Legionella
◊ Commonly with lower lobe patchy alveolar infiltrate with consolidation
◊ Pleural effusion in up to 50%
◊ May take from 1-4 months for the x-ray to return to normal

DIAGNOSTIC PROCEDURES
Transtracheal aspiration or bronchoscopy for sputum/lung samples

 TREATMENT

APPROPRIATE HEALTH CARE Severity of illness and support available in the outpatient setting will dictate the appropriate site for care

GENERAL MEASURES
• Supportive care
• Maintaining oxygenation, hydration, and electrolyte balance while providing antibiotic therapy

ACTIVITY As tolerated

DIET As tolerated

PATIENT EDUCATION Can educate patients regarding prevention/avoidance measures, lowering their risk status, and if infected already, about the expected course of the disease

MEDICATIONS

DRUG(S) OF CHOICE
• Erythromycin 30-60 mg/kg/day po or IV divided into four doses for 10-21 days
• Addition of rifampin 600 mg q 12 hours po or IV should be provided along with erythromycin in very ill patients
Contraindications: Hypersensitivity reactions
Precautions: Liver disease
Significant possible Interactions:
• Erythromycin can increase theophylline, carbamazepine, and digoxin levels and can increase activity of oral anticoagulants
• Rifampin may decrease the effectiveness of oral anticoagulants, steroids, digoxin, quinidine, oral contraceptives and hypoglycemic agents

ALTERNATIVE DRUGS
• Tetracyclines may be used along with rifampin
• Trimethoprim/sulfamethoxazole, imipenem, and quinolones may also be effective
• Other macrolides (clarithromycin) or azalides (azithromycin)

 FOLLOWUP

PATIENT MONITORING Respiratory status, hydration and electrolyte status should be monitored closely

PREVENTION/AVOIDANCE
Hyperchlorination and heating water to 60-70 degrees centigrade may help prevent water contamination

POSSIBLE COMPLICATIONS
• Dehydration
• Hyponatremia
• Respiratory insufficiency requiring ventilator support
• Endocarditis
• Disseminated intravascular coagulation
• Renal failure
• Multiple organ dysfunction syndrome (MODS)
• Coma
• Death in 10% of treated non-immunocompromised patients, and in up to 80% of untreated immunocompromised patients

EXPECTED COURSE AND
PROGNOSIS Recovery is variable, some patients experience rapid improvement with defervescence in 3-5 days and recovery in 6-10 days, while others may have a much more protracted course despite treatment

 MISCELLANEOUS

ASSOCIATED CONDITIONS N/A

AGE-RELATED FACTORS
Pediatric: Less common
Geriatric: Increased over age 50
Others: N/A

PREGNANCY N/A

SYNONYMS
• Legionella pneumonia
• Pontiac fever

ICD-9-CM 482

SEE ALSO Pneumonia

OTHER NOTES N/A

ABBREVIATIONS N/A

REFERENCES
• Hoeprich, P. & Jordan, M.C.: Infectious Diseases 4th Ed. J.B. Lippincott, 1989
• Mandell, G.L. (ed.): Principles and Practice of Infectious Diseases. 3rd Ed. New York, Churchill Livingstone, 1990
• Rubenstein, E. & Federman, D.D.: Scientific American Medicine, 1988

Author M. King, M.D. & M. LeDuc, M.D.

Leukemia

BASICS

DESCRIPTION Proliferation and accumulation of abnormal immature blood cell progenitors (blasts) in the bone marrow and other tissues. The outstanding characteristic is the development of marrow failure. Intracerebral leukostasis may develop if the blood blast count becomes greatly elevated. Leukemia is classifed according to the type of blast and according to the course, if untreated:
• Acute lymphoblastic leukemia (ALL)
• Acute nonlymphoblastic leukemia (ANLL)
• Chronic myelocytic leukemia (CML)
• Chronic lymphocytic leukemia (CLL)

System(s) affected:
Hemic/Lymphatic/Immunologic
Genetics: Unknown, some are familial
Incidence/Prevalence in USA: The yearly incidence is 13.2:100,000 in males and 7.7:100,000 in females
Predominant age:
• 70% occurs in adults, mostly CLL and ANLL. 30% in children, mostly ALL.
• With the current cure rate especially good for childhood ALL, it is estimated that by the year 2010, one in 1,000 young adults (15-45 years of age) in the USA will be a childhood ALL survivor
Predominant sex: Males > Females

SIGNS AND SYMPTOMS
• Mostly nonspecific and related to marrow failure or infiltration
• Fever
• Bleeding (e.g., petechiae, purpura, easy bruising, or oozing)
• Bone pain, pallor, fatigue
• Splenomegaly
• Hepatosplenomegaly
• Lymphadenopathy
• If CNS is involved, symptoms of increased intracranial pressure can be present
• Gingival swelling

CAUSES Precise causes unknown

RISK FACTORS
• Genetic and chromosomal abnormalities (e.g., trisomy 21, breakage and translocation)
• Radiation exposure
• Immunodeficiency states
• Chemical and drug exposure (nitrogen mustard and benzene)
• Preleukemia
• Cigarette smoking

DIAGNOSIS

DIFFERENTIAL DIAGNOSIS
• Viral induced cytopenia, lymphadenopathy and organomegaly
• Immune cytopenias
• Drug induced cytopenias
• Other marrow failure and infiltrative diseases: aplastic, hypoblastic and refractory anemias; paroxysmal nocturnal hemoglobinuria; myelodysplastic syndromes, Gaucher's disease, etc.

LABORATORY
• CBC, differential, platelets show subnormal RBC, neutrophils, and possibly subnormal platelets
• In some types, no circulating leukemic blasts are necessary to be present to establish the diagnosis. If 2 of the 3 above parameters are affected, or only one profoundly decreased, bone marrow failure should be ruled out.
• Reticulocyte count < 0.5
• Sedimentation rate usually elevated
• Chemistries LDH, and URIC acid can be elevated
• Immunoglobulins IgG can be low or rarely elevated
• Coagulation profile can be normal or prolonged especially in promyelocytic leukemia (ANLL subtype)
Drugs that may alter lab results:
Chemotherapy agents, especially corticosteroids. Don't prescribe these before finalizing the bone marrow studies. Some leukemic blasts are very sensitive and can have massive cell kill from as a little as one dose of corticosteroids.
Disorders that may alter lab results: N/A

PATHOLOGICAL FINDINGS
• The marrow will be hypercellular and the normal architecture effaced
• The percentage of leukemic cells compared to the remainder of the cell population is usually more than 30%
• Liver, spleen, and kidneys can be enlarged and infiltrated with leukemic cells

SPECIAL TESTS
Spinal tap may reveal fluid with leukemic cells

IMAGING
• Chest x-ray may reveal a large mediastinal mass
• Ultrasonography or CT scan of the abdomen may discover organomegaly

DIAGNOSTIC PROCEDURES
• Bone marrow studies are necessary to make the final diagnosis
• Aspirates are stained with a buffered Wright's stain and provide good resolution for cell morphology
• Biopsies are demineralized, sectioned and stained with hematoxylin-eosin (H&E) stain. They provide valuable information for cellularity, architecture, and megakaryocytic series.
Marrow cell suspension used for:
◊ Cytochemistries (e.g., myeloperoxidase and Sudan black are positive in myeloblasts)
◊ Immunophenotyping especially useful for lymphoid leukemia and can indicate whether it is monoclonal or polyclonal, B lymphocytes or T lymphocytes, early or late, etc.
◊ Chromosome studies will show the ploidy and/or the presence of a translocation which is of prognostic value
◊ Immunofluorescent stain for terminal deoxyribonucleotidyl transferase (TdT), another marker that differentiates between myeloid and lymphoid blasts

TREATMENT

APPROPRIATE HEALTH CARE
• Consult with a chemotherapist
• Induction for acute leukemia treatment requires inpatient care

GENERAL MEASURES
• Assessment of liver, heart, and kidney functions and performance status
• In acute leukemia induction, establish good hydration and urine flow (especially in ALL patients)
• Give platelet transfusion if platelet count is < 20,000 or if patient is having bleeding symptoms
• Avoid aspirin products
• Give packed red blood cells transfusion if patient is symptomatic from the anemia (e.g., orthostatic hypotension, dizziness, fatigue, hyperactive precordium) or if a cerebral or a cardiopulmonary problem is present
• If the absolute neutrophil count (ANC) is < 1000, exert close temperature monitoring. (Formula: ANC = [WBC x Percentage of Polys + Bands] divided by 100]). If patient becomes febrile (even low grade fever), appropriate cultures should be taken and patient placed on broad spectrum IV antibiotics covering pseudomonas and gram positive bacteria.
• Isolation (when the ANC is low) has no value because majority of the infecting agents in this situation are the patient's own normal flora of the skin, mouth, or gut
• In promyelocytic leukemia (ANLL subtype), patients are especially at risk for DIC when treatment is started. Heparinization is indicated with close followup of coagulation parameters.
Bone Marrow transplant
◊ Allogenic bone marrow transplantation in first remission for ANLL is advocated if a matched sibling is available. Autologous bone marrow transplant is also acceptable in first remission.
◊ Allogenic or autologous bone marrow transplant is acceptable in first remission in high risk ALL, especially in adults. They are acceptable in second remission for childhood ALL.
◊ Early studies using an allogenic non-related match donor seem to be promising and might replace the autologous route when a full sibling match is not available

ACTIVITY
Ambulatory as tolerated

DIET
• Special attention should be given to ensure adequately balanced calorie and vitamin intake
• Weight should be followed closely because patients usually have decreased appetite.

PATIENT EDUCATION
• Extremely important, particularly regarding the chances of survival and the toxicity of the treatment.
• Leukemia Society of America has pamphlets about each of the subtypes of leukemia for patient education. Also coloring books for children and a pamphlet explaining chemotherapy. (National Headquarters: 33 Third Ave. New York, NY 10017 Telephone: (212)573-8484.)
• NCI (Bethesda, Maryland) has pamphlets: "Chemotherapy and You", "Young People with Cancer" and about "ALL" and "ANLL". NCI has a telephone number for over-the-telephone education and recent updates of treatment options.
• "You and Leukemia, A Day At A Time" by Dr. Lynn S. Baker, W. B. Saunders Co., Philadelphia

 MEDICATIONS

DRUG(S) OF CHOICE
• Change frequently as result of major cooperative research studies
For ALL
◊ Induction - vincristine plus prednisone plus asparaginase with or without doxorubicin or daunorubicin. CNS prophylaxis, intrathecal methotrexate with or without cranial irradiation.
◊ Maintenance - 6-mercaptopurine daily and methotrexate weekly for 2 years to 3 years
For ANLL
◊ Induction - cytarabine plus daunorubicin (in children and adults) or cytarabine plus idarubicin (in adults only)
◊ Continuation of therapy with combined agents and high dose cytarabine is widely applied
For promyelocytic leukemia:
◊ Retinoic acid seems to promote maturation to normal granulocyte and provide remissions with lower toxicity comparing to standard ANLL therapy
For CLL
◊ Chlorambucil with or without prednisone used only if symptomatic or cytopenic. (Fludarabine shortly to be FDA approved, is showing great promise).
For hairy cell leukemia (a lymphoid sub type seen in adults):
◊ Interferon
For CML
◊ Chronic phase CML, allogenic bone marrow transplantation. If not possible, busulfan, hydroxyurea, or interferon alfa can prolong survival.
◊ Acute phase CML - daunorubicin plus cytarabine plus vincristine plus prednisone with or without thioguanine, or
• High dose cytarabine with or without daunorubicin

Contraindications:
No absolute contraindication is present due to the variety of protocol options
Precautions:
• Administration of chemotherapy agents should be by skilled and specifically trained individuals. IV vincristine, daunorubicin, and doxorubicin may lead to chemical burns in the event of extravasation.
• If liver injury is present, the toxicity of vincristine, anthracyclines and antimetabolites can be pronounced. If liver injury is advanced and hyperbilirubinemia is present, avoid those medications or reduce dosage.
• Anthracyclines can cause cardiomyopathy. Avoid them if patient has a pre-existing cardiac problem.
• Close monitoring of the WBC's, polys, RBC and platelets is required especially in CML (chronic phase or ALL maintenance in order not to induce profound myelotoxicity
• Patients will be immunosuppressed during treatment. Avoid live vaccines. Administer varicella - zoster, or measles immunoglobulin as soon as exposure of a patient at risk becomes known.
Significant possible interactions:
Allopurinol accentuates the toxicity of 6-mercaptopurine

ALTERNATIVE DRUGS N/A

 FOLLOWUP

PATIENT MONITORING
• Repeat bone marrow studies every week or every other week during induction of acute leukemia. Less frequently later. Also perform if a relapse is suspected.
• Follow uric acid level and urinary function closely
• Physical evaluation, including weight and blood pressure, should be done with every treatment and as frequently as once a week

PREVENTION/AVOIDANCE
No intense or contact sports and no aspirin or aspirin products due to low platelets and RBC

POSSIBLE COMPLICATIONS
• Side effects of chemotherapy
• Rarely in lymphoid leukemia, acute tumor lysis syndrome may develop leading to hyperuricemia, hyperkalemia, hyperphosphatemia, hypocalcemia, and/or uric acid nephropathy

EXPECTED COURSE AND PROGNOSIS
• ALL remission rate is very good. In children, long term survival is the rule.
• AML remission rate is 60-80%, with only 20-40% long term survival
• CML invariably transforms into the acute phase within 2 years (median of 45 months). Afterward, survival rate is poor.

• CLL usually is asymptomatic for several years especially Rai, stages 0-II. In Rai's series the mean interval (in stages 0-II) is 5.3 years from diagnosis until therapy was needed. Median overall survival in CLL is thought to be 9 years.

 MISCELLANEOUS

ASSOCIATED CONDITIONS
No specific condition is associated with leukemia. Leukemia can be the first manifestation of chromosomal abnormalities or an immunodeficiency.

AGE-RELATED FACTORS
Pediatric: Tolerate intense treatments better
Geriatric:
• Do not tolerate allogenic bone marrow transplant. Cut off age for transplant is usually 50 years.
• Autologous transplant may be tried in patients above 50 years, provided no organ failure is present and performance status is good
Others: N/A

PREGNANCY
Chemotherapy is a viable option in the 2nd and 3rd trimesters. Refer patient to an oncologist.

SYNONYMS

ICD-9-CM
204.0 ALL
202.4 Hairy cell Leukemia
205.0 ANLL, AML or AGL
206.0 AMoL
204.1 CLL
205.1 CML or chronic granulocytic leukemia

SEE ALSO N/A

OTHER NOTES

ABBREVIATIONS
• ALL = acute lymphoblastic leukemia
• ANLL = acute nonlymphoblastic leukemia
• CML = chronic myelocytic leukemia
• CLL = chronic lymphocytic leukemia

REFERENCES
• Devita, V.T., Jr., Helman, S. & Rosenberg, S.A. (eds.): Cancer: Principles & Practice of Oncology. 3rd Ed. Philadelphia, J.B. Lippincott, 1989
• The Medical Letter on Drugs and Therapeutics: Drugs of Choice for Cancer Chemotherapy. Vol. (33) (issue 840), March 22, 1991

Author M. Barudi, M.D.

Leukemia, acute lymphoblastic in adults (ALL)

 BASICS

DESCRIPTION A malignant proliferation and accumulation of immature lymphocytes
System(s) affected:
Hemic/Lymphatic/Immunologic
Genetics: Increased incidence in children with Down's syndrome or in rare familial diseases such as ataxia-telangiectasia, Bloom's syndrome, Fanconi's anemia, Klinefelter's syndrome, and neurofibromatosis. Can rarely occur in adult identical twins.
Incidence/Prevalence in USA: 1000 adult cases/year
Predominant age: Median age is 30 years but incidence increases with age
Predominant sex: Male > Female (slightly)

SIGNS AND SYMPTOMS
• Anemia - fatigue, shortness of breath, lightheadedness, angina, headache
• Thrombocytopenia - petechiae, ecchymoses, epistaxis, retinal hemorrhages
• Granulocytopenia - fever, infection
• Lymphocytosis - lymphadenopathy, hepato/splenomegaly, bone pain
• Immunosuppression
• Metabolic abnormalities - hyperuricemia, renal failure, increased lactic acid dehydrogenase (LDH)
• Central nervous system - cranial nerve palsies, confusion

CAUSES Unknown. Epstein-Barr virus is implicated in Burkitt's leukemia/lymphoma.

RISK FACTORS
• Age over 60
• Incidence appears increased following exposure to chemical agents such as benzene or to radiation (but acute myeloid leukemia [AML] is more common)
• May follow aplastic anemia

 DIAGNOSIS

DIFFERENTIAL DIAGNOSIS
• Malignant disorders - other leukemias, especially AML; prolymphocytic leukemia; malignant lymphomas; multiple myeloma; bone marrow metastases from solid tumors (breast, prostate, lung, renal); myelodysplastic syndromes
• Nonmalignant disorders - aplastic anemia; myelofibrosis; autoimmune diseases (Felty's syndrome, lupus); infectious mononucleosis; autoimmune thrombocytopenic purpura; leukemoid reaction to infection

LABORATORY
• Anemia - normochromic, normocytic
• Thrombocytopenia
• Peripheral blood lymphoblasts
• Elevated LDH
• Elevated uric acid
Drugs that may alter lab results: N/A
Disorders that may alter lab results: N/A

PATHOLOGICAL FINDINGS Diffuse replacement of marrow and lymph node architecture by sheets of malignant lymphoblasts

SPECIAL TESTS
• Immunophenotyping of marrow/blood lymphoblasts: B-lineage (CD19, CD20, CD24); T-lineage (CD2, CD5, CD7); CALLA ([common ALL antigen], CD10); human leukocytic antigen (HLA)-DR; terminal deoxynucleotidyl transferase (TdT); aberrant myeloid antigens
• Cytochemical stains: Myeloperoxidase negative; Sudan black B usually negative; TdT positive; nonspecific esterase +/-; periodic acid Schiff (PAS) +/-
• Cytogenetics: Specific recurring chromosomal abnormalities have independent diagnostic and prognostic significance (hyperdiploidy > 50 chromosomes is favorable; the Philadelphia chromosome, t[9;22], the t[4;11], and the t[8;14] are unfavorable)
• Human leukocytic antigen (HLA) typing of patient and siblings for marrow transplantation

IMAGING
• Chest radiograph to evaluate for mediastinal mass or hilar adenopathy and for pulmonary infiltrates suggestive of infection
• Ultrasound exam to assess splenomegaly or renal enlargement suggestive of leukemic infiltration

DIAGNOSTIC PROCEDURES
• Bone marrow examination with aspiration, biopsy, immunophenotyping, cytochemistry, and cytogenetics
• Lymph node biopsy is rarely necessary but can be diagnostic
• Lumbar puncture should be done if neurological symptoms or signs are present. Repeat lumbar puncture after bone marrow remission is achieved to evaluate occult CNS involvement.

 TREATMENT

APPROPRIATE HEALTH CARE
• Inpatient care during remission induction chemotherapy
• Post-remission therapy is usually outpatient
• Access to the resources and expertise of a major oncology center is important for appropriate support

GENERAL MEASURES
• Surgical placement of a percutaneous silastic double-lumen central venous catheter
• Protective isolation from infection

ACTIVITY Ambulatory as tolerated

DIET
• Nutritional support including intravenous hyperalimentation, if necessary
• Avoid alcohol

PATIENT EDUCATION
• Risks of infection, transfusion, chemotherapy
• Stop smoking

Leukemia, acute lymphoblastic in adults (ALL)

MEDICATIONS

DRUG(S) OF CHOICE
• Optimal therapy is not yet known. All treatment regimens are still investigational, although clearly effective for some fraction of patients.

CALGB protocol 8811 is an example of therapy:

◊ Remission induction - cyclophosphamide 1200 mg/square meter on day 1 (800 mg/m2 if > 60 years old); daunorubicin 45 mg/m2 on days 1, 2, and 3 (30 mg/m2 if > 60 years old); vincristine 2 mg on days 1, 8, 15, and 22; l-asparaginase 6000 units/m2 on days 5, 8, 11, 15, 18, and 22; prednisone 60 mg/m2 on days 1-21 (days 1-7 if > 60 years old)

◊ Consolidation (repeat twice in 8 weeks) - cyclophosphamide 1000 mg/m2 on day 1; intrathecal (IT) methotrexate 15 mg with hydrocortisone 50 mg on day 1; 6-mercaptopurine 60 mg/m2 on days 1-14; cytarabine 75 mg/m2 SC on days 1-4 and 8-11; vincristine 2 mg on days 15 and 22; l-asparaginase 6000 units/m2 on days 15, 18, 22, and 25

◊ CNS prophylaxis and interim maintenance - 2400 cGy cranial irradiation; IT-methotrexate 15 mg with hydrocortisone 50 mg on days 1, 8, 15, 22, and 29; 6-mercaptopurine 60 mg/m2 on days 1-70; oral methotrexate 20 mg/m2 on days 36, 43, 50, 57, and 64

◊ Late intensification - doxorubicin 30 mg/m2 on days 1, 8, and 15; vincristine 2 mg on days 1, 8, and 15; dexamethasone 10 mg/m2 on days 1-14; cyclophosphamide 1000 mg/m2 on day 29; 6-thioguanine 60 mg/m2 on days 29-42; cytarabine 75 mg/m2 SC on days 29-32 and 36-39

◊ Prolonged maintenance - vincristine 2 mg/month for 16 months; prednisone 60 mg/m2 for 5 days with the vincristine; 6-mercaptopurine 60 mg/m2/day for 16 months; oral methotrexate 20 mg/m2/week for 16 months

Contraindications: Doses and schedule may need to be altered for older patients and for concurrent infection and organ toxicity

Precautions:
• Tumor lysis syndrome (elevated uric acid, potassium, and phosphate with decreased calcium leading to renal failure, disseminated intravascular coagulation, and cardiac arrhythmias) may be prevented by administering allopurinol 300-600mg/day. Begin 2 days before chemotherapy begins. Reduce doses if used with mercaptopurine or azathioprine.
• Oral sulfa-trimethoprim or aerosolized pentamidine is given for pneumocystis carinii prophylaxis
• Profound immunosuppression. Take appropriate precautions when patient is neutropenic

• High dose cyclophosphamide causes severe nausea and vomiting. Use appropriate antiemetic regimen to prevent.
• Neurotoxicity, ileus with vincristine
• Asparaginase may cause severe allergic reactions as well as impaired pancreatic and liver function. Monitor serum glucose concentrations frequently and carefully. Pancreatitis or thrombosis may occur.
Significant possible interactions: N/A

ALTERNATIVE DRUGS
Other anthracyclines, investigational chemotherapy agents

FOLLOWUP

PATIENT MONITORING
Daily during induction chemotherapy for metabolic and infectious complications. Weekly during remission consolidation chemotherapy. Monthly during maintenance therapy. Every 3 months thereafter.

PREVENTION/AVOIDANCE   N/A

POSSIBLE COMPLICATIONS
• Infections (pneumocystis carinii pneumonia; bacterial pneumonia or sepsis; fungal pneumonia)
• Bleeding
• Need for transfusions
• Sterility from treatment
• Arachnoiditis and CNS effects from intrathecal chemotherapy and irradiation
• Pancreatitis and liver dysfunction from chemotherapy
• Relapse of ALL in marrow or extramedullary sites (CNS, testis)

EXPECTED COURSE AND PROGNOSIS
• 80-95% of patients < 60 years old will achieve a complete remission, and 35-60% will remain free of disease at 5 years
• Patients with unfavorable cytogenetic subtypes should probably undergo allogeneic bone marrow transplantation in first remission if an HLA-identical donor is available

MISCELLANEOUS

ASSOCIATED CONDITIONS   N/A

AGE-RELATED FACTORS   N/A
Pediatric: Bone growth and IQ development may be affected by treatment
Geriatric: N/A
Others: N/A

PREGNANCY   Many chemotherapy drugs are teratogenic

SYNONYMS   Acute lymphocytic leukemia

ICD-9-CM   204.0

SEE ALSO   N/A

OTHER NOTES   N/A

ABBREVIATIONS   HLA = human leukocytic antigen

REFERENCES   Hoffman, R., Benz, E.J., Jr., Cohen, H., et al. (eds.): Hematology: Basic Principles and Practice. New York, Churchill Livingstone, 1991

Author   R. A. Larson, M.D.

Leukoplakia, oral

 BASICS

DESCRIPTION
A nonspecific clinical term used to describe a white patch in the oral mucosa which remains despite attempts to rub it off. It does not correlate with any specific microscopic findings and may be related to a variety of lesions, from benign hyperkeratosis to carcinoma.

System(s) affected: Gastrointestinal

Genetics: N/A

Incidence/Prevalence in USA: N/A

Predominant age: 90% of lesions found in patients over 40 years of age

Predominant sex:
• Males > Female
• Some studies show no preference

SIGNS AND SYMPTOMS
Location
  ◊ 50% on tongue, mandibular alveolar ridge, and buccal mucosa
  ◊ Also seen on maxillary alveolar ridge, palate and lower lip
  ◊ Infrequently - floor of the mouth and retromolar areas
Appearance
  ◊ Varies from nonpalpable, faintly translucent white areas to thick, fissured, papillomatous, indurated lesions
  ◊ May feel rough or leathery
  ◊ Color may be white, gray, yellowish-white, or brownish-gray
  ◊ Cannot be wiped off
  ◊ Macular or plaque-like

CAUSES
• Tobacco use
• Alcohol consumption
• Oral sepsis
• Oral snuff(smokeless tobacco)
• Human papilloma virus, types 11 and 15
• Actinic radiation
• Vitamin deficiency
• Syphilis
• Dental restorations
• Prosthetic dental appliances
• Alcoholism
• Estrogen therapy

RISK FACTORS
• Age over 40
• Tobacco or alcohol use
• Repeated or chronic trauma to oral regions

 DIAGNOSIS

DIFFERENTIAL DIAGNOSIS
White oral lesions that can be wiped away:
  ◊ Candida
  ◊ Aspirin burn
White oral lesions that cannot be rubbed off:
  ◊ Traumatic or frictional keratosis
  ◊ Leukoedema
  ◊ Galvanic keratosis
  ◊ Lichen planus
  ◊ Verrucous carcinoma
  ◊ Lupus
  ◊ Squamous cell carcinoma
  ◊ Oral hairy leukoplakia
  ◊ Leukokeratosis nicotina palati

LABORATORY N/A
Drugs that may alter lab results: N/A
Disorders that may alter lab results: N/A

PATHOLOGICAL FINDINGS
• Biopsy specimens range from hyperkeratosis to invasive carcinoma
• 6% at initial biopsy are invasive carcinoma
• 4% subsequently undergo malignant transformation
• Location is important: 60% on floor of mouth are cancerous; rarely so on buccal mucosa

SPECIAL TESTS N/A

IMAGING N/A

DIAGNOSTIC PROCEDURES Biopsy necessary to rule out carcinoma

 TREATMENT

APPROPRIATE HEALTH CARE
Outpatient biopsy, only if lesion persists despite elimination of possible etiologic factors

GENERAL MEASURES
• Eliminate habitual lip biting
• Correct ill fitting dental appliances
• Stop smoking and alcohol
• If dysplasia evident, remove lesion. Consider otolaryngologist referral.
• Some small lesions may respond to cryosurgery
• Beta-carotene may cause partial regression (experimental)

ACTIVITY Full

DIET Regular

PATIENT EDUCATION
• If biopsy negative, stress importance of periodic and careful followup
• Aid the patient in discontinuing tobacco and/or alcohol use. Referral to support groups, recommendations for stop smoking programs, etc.

MEDICATIONS

DRUG(S) OF CHOICE N/A
Contraindications: N/A
Precautions: N/A
Significant possible interactions: N/A

ALTERNATIVE DRUGS N/A

FOLLOWUP

PATIENT MONITORING Regular, close followup, even after successful treatment. Biopsy as needed.

PREVENTION/AVOIDANCE
• Avoid tobacco, alcohol, habitual biting
• Provide well-fitting dentures

POSSIBLE COMPLICATIONS
• Carcinoma
• New lesions may develop after treatment

EXPECTED COURSE AND PROGNOSIS
• Curable if detected early
• 4% of initially benign lesions subsequently develop cancer
• More likely cancerous if on floor of mouth

MISCELLANEOUS

ASSOCIATED CONDITIONS
Leukokeratosis nicotina palati is rarely malignant

AGE-RELATED FACTORS
Pediatric: N/A
Geriatric: More common in elderly
Others: Rare before age 40

PREGNANCY N/A

SYNONYMS N/A

ICD-9-CM 528.6

SEE ALSO N/A

OTHER NOTES Uncommonly - other mucosal surfaces (vaginal, anal, etc.)

ABBREVIATIONS N/A

REFERENCES
• Yeats, D. & Burns, J.: Common Oral Mucosal Lesions in Adults. American Family Physician. Dec. 91, Vol. 44, p 2043-50
• Fitzpatrick, T., et al.: Color Atlas and Synopsis of Clinical Dermatology. 2nd Ed. New York, McGraw-Hill, 1992

Author P. Johnson, M.D. & M. Sexton, M.D.

Lichen planus

 BASICS

DESCRIPTION A unique inflammatory disorder of the skin and mucous membranes. The disease is characterized by small flat, angular, violaceous, shiny, pruritic papules on the skin and white papules in the mouth. Onset abrupt or gradual. May be intermittent for years.
Genetics: N/A
System(s) affected: Skin/Exocrine
Incidence in USA: Unknown
Prevalence in USA: 450/100,000
Predominant age: 30-60 years, rare in children and the elderly
Predominant sex: Female > Male

SIGNS AND SYMPTOMS
Skin
◊ Pruritis - often severe
◊ Papules - 1-10 mm, shiny, flat
◊ Color - violaceous, with white lace-like pattern (Wickham's striae) on papules. Wickham's striae best seen after topical application of mineral oil and if present, are almost pathognomic for lichen planus.
◊ Shape - polygonal or oval shaped
◊ Arrangement - may be grouped, linear, annular, or scattered individual lesions. Koebner's phenomenon is often seen.
◊ Distribution - ventral surface of wrists, glans penis, dorsa feet, groin, sacrum, shins, eyelids, and hair of scalp
Mucous membranes
◊ Mucous membrane involvement is seen in 40-60% of patients with skin lesions. 20% of patients have mucous membrane lesions only.
◊ Milky-white papules with white lace-like pattern
◊ Usually seen on buccal mucosa, but may appear on tongue, gingiva, palate, and lips
◊ May be bullous or erosive
◊ Painful, especially if ulcers present
◊ Oral lesions may be precancerous (squamous cell carcinoma)
Hair and nails
◊ Scalp - atrophic scalp skin and destruction of hair follicles. May result in permanent and total alopecia.
◊ Nails - (10%) may cause proximal to distal linear grooves and partial or complete destruction of nail bed with pterygium formation. Large toes most commonly affected.

CAUSES Etiology unknown. Possibly a disease of keratinization or an autoimmune disease. Emotional stress can precipitate an attack.

RISK FACTORS Exposure to drugs or chemicals, graft versus host disease, or lupus erythematosus (LE-LP overlap syndrome)

 DIAGNOSIS

DIFFERENTIAL DIAGNOSIS
• Chemical exposure (chemicals used in color developing)
• Drug eruption (chloroquine, quinacrine, gold salts, methyldopa, penicillamine, arsenic, bismuth)
• Bacterial infection
• Leukoplakia
• Candidiasis
• Squamous cell carcinoma
• Aphthous ulcers
• Herpetic stomatitis
• Erythema multiforme
• Secondary syphilis
• Scabies

LABORATORY N/A
Drugs that may alter lab results: N/A
Disorders that may alter lab results: N/A

PATHOLOGICAL FINDINGS
Inflammation with hyperkeratosis, increased granular layer, irregular acanthosis, basement-membrane thinning, band-like lymphocytic infiltrate of the upper dermis

SPECIAL TESTS N/A

IMAGING N/A

DIAGNOSTIC PROCEDURES Skin biopsy

 TREATMENT

APPROPRIATE HEALTH CARE
Outpatient

GENERAL MEASURES
• Goal is to relieve itching with medications, occlusive dressings, oatmeal baths
• Psoralens and ultraviolet A (PUVA) photochemotherapy may be helpful for generalized or resistant cases
• Behavior modification for stress reduction may prevent recurrence

ACTIVITY Fully active

DIET No special diet

PATIENT EDUCATION Help with stress reduction if appropriate

Lichen planus

MEDICATIONS

DRUG(S) OF CHOICE
Skin
• Topical steroids (e.g., 0.1% triamcinolone acetonide) with occlusion
• Intralesional corticosteroids (e.g., Kenalog 5-10 mg/ml) for hypertrophic lesions
• Antihistamine (e.g., hydroxyzine, dosage - 25 mg/q6h) if needed for itching
Mucous membranes
• Topical oral retinoids (e.g., 0.05% retinoic acid in Orabase) or topical oral corticosteroids (0.1% Kenalog in Orabase) bid
• Intralesional corticosteroids for erosive, painful lichen planus (e.g., 0.5-1.0 ml Depo-Medrol 40 mg/ml)
• Oral retinoids (accutane or Tegison)
Contraindications: Patients with history of hypersensitivity to corticosteroids or retinoids
Precautions:
• Systemic absorption of steroids may result in hypothalamic-pituitary-adrenal axis suppression, Cushing's syndrome, hyperglycemia, and glucosuria
• Increased risk with high potency - i.e., use over large surface area, prolonged use, occlusive dressings
• These medications are Category C teratogens. Avoid in pregnancy.
• Children may absorb a proportionally larger amount of topical steroid due to larger skin surface to weight ratio
Significant possible interactions: See manufacturer's profile of each drug

ALTERNATIVE DRUGS
Oral prednisone - rarely used and only for a short course (e.g., prednisone 20 mg bid x 2-4 weeks)

FOLLOWUP

PATIENT MONITORING
Serial skin exams

PREVENTION/AVOIDANCE
Reduce stress

POSSIBLE COMPLICATIONS
• Alopecia
• Nail destruction
• Squamous cell carcinoma of the mouth

EXPECTED COURSE AND PROGNOSIS
• Spontaneous resolution in weeks is possible, but disease may persist for years - especially in the mouth and on shins
• There is a tendency toward relapse, especially with emotional stress
• Recurrence 12-20% especially in those with generalized involvement

MISCELLANEOUS

ASSOCIATED CONDITIONS
• Bullous pemphigoid
• Alopecia
• Vitiligo
• Chronic ulcerative colitis
• Hypogammaglobulinemia
• Graft-versus host reaction

AGE-RELATED FACTORS
Pediatric: N/A
Geriatric: N/A
Others: N/A

PREGNANCY
Avoid corticosteroids

SYNONYMS
N/A

ICD-9-CM
697.0

SEE ALSO
N/A

OTHER NOTES
Remember the 5 p's of lichen planus - purple, planar, polygonal, pruritic papules

ABBREVIATIONS
N/A

REFERENCES
• Habif, T.P.: Clinical Dermatology: A Color Guide to Diagnosis and Therapy. St. Louis, C.V. Mosby and Co., 1985
• Lazarus, G.S., et al.: Diagnosis of Skin Disease. Philadelphia, F.A. Davis and Co., 1980
• Fitzpatrick, T.B., et al.: Color Atlas and Synopsis of Clinical Dermatology. New York, McGraw-Hill, 1983
• Fitzpatrick, T.B., et al.: Dermatology in General Medicine text and Atlas. 3rd Ed. New York, McGraw-Hill, 1987

Author M. Darr, M.D.

Listeriosis

BASICS

DESCRIPTION Infection caused by the ubiquitous, weakly hemolytic, gram positive bacillus, Listeria monocytogenes, which is pathogenic to many animal species. Occurs most often in fetuses (disseminated infantile listeriosis), in neonates, and in immunosuppressed patients. 25% of patients have pre-existing disease (cirrhosis, lymphomas, solid tumors, AIDS, cancer therapy). Usual course - acute.
• In 1985 there was an epidemic affecting 142 persons in Southern California that resulted from eating contaminated Mexican cheese
System(s) affected: Pulmonary, Endocrine/Metabolic, Gastrointestinal, Renal/Urologic, Hemic/Lymphatic/Immunologic, Nervous
Genetics: No known genetic pattern
Incidence/Prevalence in USA: 1,850 cases a year (425 deaths). Rising incidence (due to AIDS) now estimated at 7.6/million.
Predominant age: Neonates, elderly
Predominant sex: Male > Female

SIGNS AND SYMPTOMS
• Asymptomatic
• Abdominal pain
• Adult respiratory distress syndrome
• Cervical lymphadenopathy
• Chills
• Conjunctivitis
• Decreased fetal movement
• Diarrhea
• Dysuria
• Fatigue
• Fever
• Hepatosplenomegaly
• Malaise
• Myalgia
• Nausea
• Pharyngitis
• Urinary frequency
• Vomiting
• Findings suggestive of meningitis - fever, headache, nausea & vomiting, stiff neck, delirium, coma
• Findings suggestive of sepsis - high fever and generalized severe illness without evidence of localized infection (in patients with alcoholism, malignancies, immunosuppression, AIDS)

CAUSES Listeria monocytogenes, a small gram-positive bacillus; infection with other species of Listeria are rare.

RISK FACTORS
• Age - fetus, neonates, elderly
• Metastatic malignant disease
• HIV infection
• Alcoholism
• Renal hemodialysis
• Pregnancy
• Immunosuppressed
• Exposure to infected animals (veterinarians, butchers, etc.). Animal-to-human transmission is rare.
• Ingesting contaminated food or drink (e.g., soft Mexican style cheese or feta cheese)

DIAGNOSIS

DIFFERENTIAL DIAGNOSIS
• Other infections - Staphylococcal, Gram negative Klebsiella, Candida, cryptococcosis,viral
• Infantile listeriosis, E. Coli, Group B streptococci
• Infectious mononucleosis

LABORATORY
CSF
◊ Gram stain - may reveal small, gram-positive rods or coccobacillary forms with "tumbling" motility. (Sometimes difficult to identify since organisms are not present in large numbers and may be confused with diphtheroids and other bacteria.)
◊ Cell count - in most cases, the predominant cell type is the neutrophil; however, mononuclear cells may predominate. Counts range from 0-1200/mm3. RBC's frequently seen.
◊ Protein concentration - within normal limits to 735 mg/dL
◊ Glucose - within normal limits to undetectable
◊ CSF cultures - demonstrates beta-hemolysis (L. monocytogenes grows well on 5% sheep's blood or chocolate agar)
◊ Counterimmunoelectrophor (CIE) latex agglutination (LA) - possibly useful for differential diagnosis
Other tests
◊ Blood cultures should be done
◊ CBC - peripheral WBC may show an elevated neutrophil count and/or left shift
◊ Other cultures in newborn - cervical vaginal secretions and lochia from the mother; cord blood; grossly abnormal portions of the placenta, meconium, and exudate expressed from an incised skin papule of the neonate
Drugs that may alter lab results:
Antibiotics
Disorders that may alter lab results:
Cultures may be confusing in patients with mixed infections

PATHOLOGICAL FINDINGS
• Gross - multi-organ miliary granulomatosis
• Micro - nodular focal abscess
• Micro - necrotic amorphous basophilic debris
• Micro - increased tissue macrophages
• Micro - gram-positive bacilli
• Motile bacilli
• Chinese-letter aggregates

SPECIAL TESTS Specimens for serologic testing should be submitted to the local public health laboratory. In outbreaks, serotyping may be desirable.

IMAGING MRI with any patient having central nervous system symptoms

DIAGNOSTIC PROCEDURES Lumbar puncture

TREATMENT

APPROPRIATE HEALTH CARE
Inpatient during acute phase

GENERAL MEASURES
• Bedrest
• Isolation if immunosuppressed
• Secretion precautions
• Respiratory assistance (if apneic, or CNS depressed)

ACTIVITY Bedrest

DIET
• Acute case, total parenteral nutrition, nasogastric tube, or softer diet if tolerated
• As a preventive, avoid eating raw or partially cooked foods and soft cheeses. Warm leftovers thoroughly and wash raw vegetables before cooking.

PATIENT EDUCATION Dietary guidelines for avoidance in high risk patients

MEDICATIONS

DRUG(S) OF CHOICE

Neonates:

◊ Meningitis - for infants older than one month: ampicillin 300-400 mg/kg/day IV

◊ Meningitis - neonate doses: < 2000 grams, less than 1 week old: ampicillin 50 mg/kg/ every 12 hours. Older than 1 week: ampicillin 50 mg/kg every 8 hours.PLUS gentamicin 7.5 mg/kg/day IV for 14 days. Discontinue gentamicin when cerebro- spinal fluid is sterile.

• Alternate therapy - penicillin G 100,000 - 200,000 u/kg/d IV x 14-21 days plus gentamicin as above

◊ Bacteremia or pneumonia - ampicillin 100-150 mg/kg/day IV x 10 days (or penicillin G 200,000 u/kg/d IV x 10 days) plus gentamicin 5.0 mg/kg/day. Discontinue gentamicin when blood cultures become negative.

Pregnant women:

◊ Ampicillin 2 gm IV q4h for 14 days plus gentamicin 120 mg IV q8h. Adjust for peak 5-6 mcg/mL.

Immunocompromised/elderly patients:

◊ Ampicillin 200 mg/kg IV x 14 days. Note: Some experts recommend addition of gentamicin 3-5 mg/kg/d IV plus intrathecal doses of 4 mg Q12h.

For endocarditis and typhoidal listeriosis:

◊ Penicillin G 75,000-100,000 u/kg IV q4h and continue for 14 days after defervescence. PLUS tobramycin 2 mg/kg load, then adjust based on levels. Aim for peak at 5-6. Continue for 4 weeks after defervescence.

For oculoglandular:

◊ Erythromycin 30 mg/kg/day as 4 equal doses q6h and continue for 1 week after defervescence

Contraindications: Allergy to penicillins

Precautions: Refer to manufacturer's literature

Significant possible interactions: Refer to manufacturer's literature

ALTERNATIVE DRUGS
In adult patients - trimethoprim-sulfamethoxazole (base on trimethoprim component) 5 mg/kg IV q6h or erythromycin 10 mg/kg IV q6h

FOLLOWUP

PATIENT MONITORING

• Frequent arterial blood gases during acute phase

• Repeat lumbar puncture at 24-48 hours and at the end of treatment

PREVENTION/AVOIDANCE

• Avoid handling livestock during pregnancy
• Avoid contaminated silage
• Avoid contaminated sewage
• Avoid raw or contaminated milk products
• Avoid soft cheeses (Mexican and feta)
• Wash carefully all raw vegetables

EXPECTED COURSE AND PROGNOSIS
High mortality if symptomatic

POSSIBLE COMPLICATIONS

• Premature delivery
• Amnionitis
• Meningitis
• Septicemia
• Pulmonary abscess
• Hepatic abscess
• Placental abscess
• Splenic abscess
• Lymph node abscess
• Endocarditis
• Peritonitis
• Abortion
• Stillbirth
• Neonatal death

MISCELLANEOUS

ASSOCIATED CONDITIONS

• Cirrhosis
• Lymphomas
• Solid tumors
• Immunodeficiencies
• Pregnancy

AGE-RELATED FACTORS

Pediatric:

• Infected fetuses are usually stillborn or premature. More than half are infected with lethal listeriosis.

• 50% mortality in treated neonates

Geriatric: Greater morbidity and mortality

Others: N/A

PREGNANCY

• Pregnant women are more susceptible to infection with Listeria monocytogenes; transmission to the fetus and neonates occurs with high mortality.

• Requires prompt and vigorous treatment to prevent transfer of disease to fetus (pregnant patient's symptoms may begin as a flu-like illness or be absent)

SYNONYMS

• Listeria monocytogenes
• Listerial disease

ICD-9-CM 027.0 listeriosis

SEE ALSO N/A

OTHER NOTES

• Notify laboratory at time of sending any specimen that listeriosis is a possibility
• Laboratory specimens must be sent to laboratory promptly (few organisms more difficult to culture)
• Need at least 10 cc of spinal fluid for culture

ABBREVIATIONS N/A

REFERENCES

• Linnan, M.J., Mascola, L., Lou, X., May, S., Salimen, C., et al.: Epidemic listeriosis associated with Mexican-style cheese. N Engl J Med. 319:823:828, 1988
• Von Lichtenberg, F.: Pathology of Infectious Diseases. New York, Raven Press, 1988
• Haft, R.F. & Kasper, D.L.: Group B Streptococcus Infection in Mother and Child. Hospital Practice, Vol. 26, Dec, 1991

Author S. May, M.D.

Low back pain

BASICS

DESCRIPTION Pain in the lower back, often accompanied by sciatica (pain radiating from the back into the buttock and into the lower extremity)
System(s) affected: Musculoskeletal, Nervous
Genetics: N/A
Incidence/Prevalence in USA: 60-90% individuals affected at some point in their life
Predominant Age: Occurs more often between ages 20-40
Predominant Sex: Male = Female

SIGNS AND SYMPTOMS Pain in varying degrees

CAUSES See Differential Diagnosis

RISK FACTORS
• Occupational risk factors
• Sedentary occupations
• Vibration
• Recreational activities such as sports (football, gymnastics, etc.)

DIAGNOSIS

DIFFERENTIAL DIAGNOSIS
• Congenital anomalies
• Peripheral nerve dysfunction
• Ruptured lumbar disk
• Nerve root entrapment
• Spondylolysis and spondylolisthesis
• Acute and chronic lumbar strain
• Degenerative back disorders
• Compression fractures
• Unstable vertebra
• Hyperlordosis
• Idiopathic lumbar scoliosis
• Tumors
• Osteoporosis
• Ankylosing spondylitis
• Infections
• Extrinsic causes
• Malingering and compensatory patients

LABORATORY
• BUN
• Creatinine
• Calcium
• Phosphorus
• Alkaline phosphate
• Liver function tests
• LDH
• Glucose
• CBC with differential
• Sedimentation rate
• Urinalysis
Drugs that may alter lab results: N/A
Disorders that may alter lab results: N/A

PATHOLOGICAL FINDINGS N/A

SPECIAL TESTS
• Rheumatoid factor
• Antinuclear antibody
• Serum protein electrophoresis
• Urine protein electrophoresis
• Thyroid tests
• Platelet thromboplastin antecedent; plasma thromboplastin
• Growth hormone
• Acid phosphatase

IMAGING
• Lumbosacral spine series in patients resistant to therapy
• CT or MRI may also be indicated

DIAGNOSTIC PROCEDURES
Myelography - reserved for patients likely to need surgery

TREATMENT

APPROPRIATE HEALTH CARE
Outpatient usually

GENERAL MEASURES
• Physiotherapy
• Traction
• Bedrest
• Exercise
• Transcutaneous electrical nerve stimulation (TENS)
• Injection therapy
• Acupuncture
• Orthotics
• Surgery
• Psychosocial issues

ACTIVITY As tolerated

DIET No restrictions

PATIENT EDUCATION
• Encourage remaining in school and work
• Physical therapy

MEDICATIONS

DRUG(S) OF CHOICE
• Non-narcotics - acetaminophen, NSAID's, aspirin
• Use narcotic analgesics sparingly and only for acute phase
• Muscle relaxants
Contraindications: Refer to manufacturer's literature
Precautions: Dependence and addiction
Significant possible interactions: Refer to manufacturer's literature

ALTERNATIVE DRUGS N/A

 FOLLOWUP

PATIENT MONITORING As needed for treatment of underlying cause

PREVENTION/AVOIDANCE
• Exercise, physiotherapy
• Weight reduction, if obese

POSSIBLE COMPLICATIONS
• Chronic low back pain
• Addiction to medication

EXPECTED COURSE AND PROGNOSIS Good if source can be identified and treated

 MISCELLANEOUS

ASSOCIATED CONDITIONS See Differential diagnosis

AGE-RELATED FACTORS
Pediatric: Relatively uncommon
Geriatric: Increased occurrence
Others: N/A

PREGNANCY Increases low back pain

SYNONYMS N/A

ICD-9-CM 724.2

SEE ALSO
• Lumbar (intervertebral) disk disorders

OTHER NOTES N/A

ABBREVIATIONS N/A

REFERENCES AAFP Home Study Self-Assessment Monograph 117, February, 1989

Author S. Jackson, M.D.

Lumbar (intervertebral) disk disorders

BASICS

DESCRIPTION
Many patients with low back pain have lumbar disc disease and involvement of surrounding spinal ligaments, muscles and skeleton. Over time may include disc degeneration, disc herniation, spinal narrowing and arthritic proliferation of the facet joint. Management is based on symptoms and disability, because the distinction between the normal aging of the spine and pathological findings are hard to distinguish.
- Non-radicular low back pain (acute and chronic) - low back pain remaining near belt-line caused by soft tissue or disc injury
- Radicular low back pain (acute and chronic) - neuropathic pain is to a greater degree in the buttocks, hips or legs rather than the back. There may or may not be signs of weakness, numbness, or loss of reflex. In younger patients, the source of the pain is likely to be mechanical compression or chemical irritation of a nerve root.
- Spinal stenosis is more likely to be the etiology of radicular pain in patients over 55 years

System(s) affected: Musculoskeletal, Nervous
Genetics: N/A
Incidence/Prevalence in USA:
- One of the most frequent complaints for which adults seek medical attention and second to the common cold for most time off work
- Lifetime prevalence of low back pain is 60-90%. The annual incidence is 5%. Among patients with acute back pain, 1% have nerve root symptoms.
- 95% of diseased disks are localized to L4-5 and L5-S1
- Less than 2% of patients with low back pain have infections, neoplasms, or inflammatory spondyloarthropathies

Predominant age: 25-45 years, first episode in 20's and 30's, infrequent before 20 years or after age 65
Predominant sex: Male = Female

SIGNS AND SYMPTOMS
- Variable pain; usually dull, originating in back, extending below knee
- Pain may or may not be followed by radiation (usually unilaterally) in nerve root distribution
- Back pain decreases at night. Bedrest usually improves symptoms at least temporarily.
- Pain increases with walking
- Constitutional symptoms absent
- Sciatica can occur without back pain
- Often sensory aberrations in extremities, paresthesia and numbness
- Occasionally muscle group weakness
- Most disc ruptures are postero-lateral and press upon lumbar nerve root with radiating pain
- Lumbar scoliosis possible, trunk tilted toward or away from affected side, depending on location of extrusion
- Paraspinal muscle spasm

CAUSES
- Trauma, major or minor
- Frequent lifting of objects weighing 25 pounds or more, especially if lifted with arms extended and knees straight, and body twisted
- Vibration; e.g., driving motor vehicles

RISK FACTORS
- Normal aging process after age 20 years
- Cigarette smoking
- Narrow lumbar vertebral canal (for prolapsed disk)
- Stress, muscle tension
- Obesity
- Osteoporosis

DIAGNOSIS

DIFFERENTIAL DIAGNOSIS
Acute lumbosacral strain, chronic lumbosacral strain, spondylosis, spondylolisthesis, spinal arthritis, fibrositis, cauda equina syndrome, compression fracture, poor posture, bursitis, metastatic and primary tumors, vertebral infection, referred pain from hip, retroperitoneum, aneurysms, or pelvis, (geriatrics) neurogenic claudication

LABORATORY
ESR - usually normal
Drugs that may alter lab results: N/A
Disorders that may alter lab results: N/A

PATHOLOGICAL FINDINGS
Difficult to distinguish normal aging process of disc degeneration from specific lesions causing low back pain and sciatica

SPECIAL TESTS
Electromyography - useful to exclude peripheral neuritis

IMAGING
- Lumbosacral plain films - rarely indicated just to initiate a conservative management program - indicated to rule out tumor or structural abnormality although presence of latter may not confirm source of pain
- Lumbosacral oblique views - controversial
- Myelography, CT scan, nuclear magnetic resonance - similar usefulness for particular surgical candidate evaluation

DIAGNOSTIC PROCEDURES
- Sciatic stretch test - in supine position, elevation of affected leg (to 15-30% for severe, 30-60%, milder) elicits pain
- Laségue's sign - dorsi flexion of foot of affected elevated leg accentuates sciatic pain
- Cross straight-leg-raising - elevating normal leg produces sciatica down other leg
- Jugular compression test - (insensitive) jugular neck veins compressed which elevates CSF pressure producing sciatica

- Doorbell sign - (insensitive) deep palpation of the spinous process over protruded disc reproduces sciatica
- Femoral stretch (for L2-3) in prone position, affected leg is extended reproducing pain along femoral nerve
- Faber's test - (positive only for hip pain) in supine position, flexion, abduction and external rotation produces pain
- Neurologic defects of lower extremities and perineum will usually locate level of lesion. Test gait, reflexes, motor strength, muscle atrophy; pulses and abdominal bruits; rectal sphincter.

TREATMENT

APPROPRIATE HEALTH CARE
Outpatient for majority. Inpatient for severe disability and/or surgery.

GENERAL MEASURES
Non-surgical
◊ Initial: 2-7 days bedrest (with bathroom privileges), local heat, pelvic traction, sedation, physical therapy (90% response)
◊ Following bedrest: up and about with midline support. Wean from support over next several weeks.
◊ For chronic non-radicular pain: improve physical fitness with low impact aerobic exercise. Manipulation and physical therapy have shown benefit.
◊ Transcutaneous electrical nerve stimulation (TENS): very short term benefit
Surgical procedures available
◊ Standard discectomy - discectomy techniques all have comparable results
◊ Microsurgical discectomy
◊ Percutaneous discectomy - relatively new, contraindicated in spinal stenosis and sequestered disc fragments
◊ Chemonucleolysis - lower rate of benefit and occasional severe complications
◊ Spinal fusion (arthrodesis) - indicated for spinal instability
Absolute indications for discectomy
◊ Cauda equina syndrome
◊ Progressive neurological deficit despite conservative treatment
Relative indications for discectomy
◊ Intolerable pain
◊ Multiple episodes of radiculopathy
◊ Severe postural list
◊ Persistent dysfunctional pain - these patients have been reported to improve more rapidly postoperatively but long term results show no difference from nonoperative treatment
◊ Static neurological deficit - no reported difference between operative or nonoperative treatment for improvement in weakness or sensory disturbance

Lumbar (intervertebral) disk disorders

ACTIVITY After pain is controlled (7-10 days) begin progressive walking program. Short walks initially 4 times a day and lengthen as tolerated. Return to work after 4-6 weeks with avoidance of high risk activities, e.g., heavy lifting, vibration, smoking.

DIET Weight reduction if appropriate

PATIENT EDUCATION
• Good posture, proper body mechanics, physical fitness, physical therapy if appropriate

MEDICATIONS

DRUG(S) OF CHOICE
• Analgesics
• Nonsteroidal anti-inflammatory medication
• Muscle relaxants (controversial)
• Mild sedatives
Contraindications: Refer to manufacturer's profile of each drug
Precautions: Elderly, prior peptic ulcer disease or bleeding, renal disease, liver disease, cardiac dysfunction
Significant possible interactions: Refer to manufacturer's profile of each drug

ALTERNATIVE DRUGS N/A

FOLLOWUP

PATIENT MONITORING Outpatient - return visit about 10 days following initial visit, should be improved. Follow pain history and neurological status. Thereafter monitor every 2 weeks until fully functional. Monitor exercise program.

PREVENTION/AVOIDANCE
• Modification of jobs to reduce exposure to known risk factors
• Selection of workers by such means as strength testing for certain jobs

POSSIBLE COMPLICATIONS
• Foot drop with weakness of anterior tibial, posterior tibial and peroneal muscles
• Loss of ankle jerk
• Bladder and rectal sphincter weakness with retention or incontinence
• Limitation of movement and restricted activity
• Narcotic addiction

EXPECTED COURSE AND PROGNOSIS
• Acute low back pain (90%) and/or radiculopathy (60-80%) can be expected to recover spontaneously with conservative therapy
• Chronic nonradicular low back pain - most patients respond to conservative management such as fitness, weight reduction, and education regarding back care
• Chronic radicular pain - good selection of surgical candidates have found satisfactory results (80% in long-term studies)

MISCELLANEOUS

ASSOCIATED CONDITIONS
• Poor physical conditioning/posture
• Obesity
• Osteoarthritis
• Osteoporosis
• Depression, other psychiatric disorders

AGE-RELATED FACTORS
Pediatric: Scoliosis, onset age 10 years, rarely symptomatic until adulthood. Detect difference in leg length.
Geriatric: Usually multifactorial lesions of spine. Degenerative spondylolisthesis (especially in women), spinal stenosis, and neurogenic claudication are more likely.
Others: N/A

PREGNANCY Commonly associated with low back pain and/or sciatica. Treatment is conservative.

SYNONYMS
• Degenerative disk disease
• Intervertebral disk dislocation

ICD-9-CM 722 intervertebral disc disorders

SEE ALSO
• Low back pain

OTHER NOTES
Features which predict best surgical outcome (90-95% improvement when all three exist)
◊ Definable neurological deficit
◊ Pathology in imaging which correlates with deficit
◊ Positive nerve root tension signs
Adverse psychosocial factors to resolving back pain
◊ Sciatica with predominant back symptoms
◊ Pending litigation or compensation
◊ Depressed or hostile patient
◊ Low IQ or poorly educated may not be able to participate in assessment or decision
◊ Prolonged use of narcotics or alcohol

ABBREVIATIONS N/A

REFERENCES
• Katz, W.A. (ed.): Diagnosis and Management of Rheumatic Diseases. 2nd Ed. Philadelphia, Lippincott Co, 1988
• Eismont, F.J. & Currier, B.: Surgical Management of Lumbar Intervertebral-Disc Disease. J Bone & Joint Surg 1989:1266-1271

Author CA Peters, M.D.

Lung abscess

 BASICS

DESCRIPTION
A localized cavity in the lung with pus resulting from necrosis of lung tissue surrounded by lung infection. May be caused by aerobic or anaerobic infection. Usual course is acute; progressive.

System(s) affected: Pulmonary

Genetics: No known genetic pattern

Incidence/Prevalence in USA: Unknown, relatively rare

Predominant age: Young adults (16-40 years); middle age (40-75 years)

Predominant sex: Male > Female

SIGNS AND SYMPTOMS
- Cough
- Sputum
- Purulent, foul-smelling
- Fever
- Chest pain
- Dyspnea
- Chills, rigors
- Fatigue
- Malaise
- Weakness
- Weight loss
- Anorexia
- Night sweats
- Hemoptysis
- Decreased breath sounds
- Rales
- Wheezing
- Tachypnea
- Tachycardia
- Diaphoresis
- Dullness to percussion
- Consolidation by auscultation
- Cavernous breath sounds
- Asymmetric chest movement
- Clubbing

CAUSES
- Aspiration pneumonia
- Necrotizing pneumonia
- Cavitary infarction
- Septic embolism
- Bacteremia
- Bronchial stenosis or obstruction
- Tumors

RISK FACTORS
- Periodontal disease
- Alcoholism
- Drug abuse
- Epilepsy
- Unconsciousness
- Lung neoplasia
- Immunosuppression
- Diabetes mellitus
- Airway foreign body
- Gastroesophageal reflux with aspiration
- Sinusitis

 DIAGNOSIS

DIFFERENTIAL DIAGNOSIS
- Bronchogenic carcinoma
- Bronchiectasis
- Empyema with bronchopulmonary fistula
- Tuberculosis
- Mycotic lung infections
- Actinomycosis
- Nocardiosis
- Infected pulmonary bulla
- Wegener's granulomatosis
- Pulmonary sequestration
- Silicotic nodule
- Subphrenic or hepatic abscess with perforation into a bronchus

LABORATORY
- Leukocytosis
- Anemia
- Hypoalbuminemia
- Sputum smear - mixed bacteria and neutrophils
- Sputum culture - mixed flora, anaerobes
- Gram-negative rods and cocci
- Transtracheal aspirate culture - anaerobes
- Pleural fluid - neutrophilia

Drugs that may alter lab results: N/A

Disorders that may alter lab results: N/A

PATHOLOGICAL FINDINGS
- Gross - solitary abscess
- Multiple abscesses
- Micro - suppuration
- Cavitation

SPECIAL TESTS
ECG - sinus tachycardia

IMAGING
- Chest x-ray - consolidation with radiolucency
- Air-fluid level
- Pleural effusion
- CT - define location and extent

DIAGNOSTIC PROCEDURES
- Bronchoscopy if obstruction suspected
- Bronchoscopic protected brushing
- Bronchoalveolar lavage
- Transthoracic needle aspiration

 TREATMENT

APPROPRIATE HEALTH CARE
- Inpatient if ill, otherwise outpatient
- Inpatient surgery

GENERAL MEASURES
- Postural drainage
- Pulmonary physiotherapy
- Treat underlying etiology (e.g. antibiotics)
- Surgery for complications (pulmonary resection)
- Tracheostomy, if imperative
- Bronchoscopy with selective therapeutic lavage

ACTIVITY
Reduced activity until x-ray evidence of clearing

DIET
No restrictions

PATIENT EDUCATION
Pulmonary physiotherapy techniques

MEDICATIONS

DRUG(S) OF CHOICE Antibiotics according to culture and sensitivity results. Most often, penicillin G 6-12 million units/day intravenously until improved, followed by 1.2 million units (750 mg) orally qid for several weeks.
Contraindications: Refer to manufacturer's literature
Precautions: Refer to manufacturer's literature
Significant possible interactions: Refer to manufacturer's literature

ALTERNATIVE DRUGS Clindamycin (except for Klebsiella or Staphylococcus infections) has been shown to be superior to penicillin in prospective trials

FOLLOWUP

PATIENT MONITORING Continue treatment until cavity has disappeared or stabilized on serial x-rays (several weeks or months)

PREVENTION/AVOIDANCE Treat predisposing diseases

POSSIBLE COMPLICATIONS
- Extension
- Brain abscess
- Meningitis
- Empyema
- Pneumothorax
- Massive hemoptysis

EXPECTED COURSE AND PROGNOSIS Guardedly favorable. 25% sequelae. Increased sequelae with concomitant disease.

MISCELLANEOUS

ASSOCIATED CONDITIONS
- Pneumonia
- Alcoholism
- Epilepsy
- Empyema
- Periodontal disease
- Unconsciousness
- Neoplasia
- Bronchogenic carcinoma
- Tuberculosis
- Fungal diseases

AGE-RELATED FACTORS
Pediatric: Occurs in children, Staphylococcus most common organism
Geriatric: More common in this age group and more grave
Others: N/A

PREGNANCY N/A

SYNONYMS Pulmonary abscess

ICD-9-CM
513.0 abscess of lung

SEE ALSO N/A

OTHER NOTES N/A

ABBREVIATIONS N/A

REFERENCES
• Barlett, J.G.: Anaerobic Bacterial Infections of the Lung. In Chest. 1987;91:901
• Murray, J.F. & Nadel, J.A. (eds.): Textbook of Respiratory Medicine. Philadelphia, W.B. Saunders Co., 1988

Author J. Cunnington, M.D., FRCP(c)

Lung, primary malignancies

 BASICS

DESCRIPTION The common lung cancers may be divided into two broad categories:
1. Non-small cell cancer: includes squamous cell cancer, (most common); adenocarcinoma and large cell carcinoma
2. Small cell cancer
Other malignancies from the lung are numerous but uncommon (lymphoma, blastoma, sarcoma, etc.)
System(s) affected: Pulmonary
Genetics: N/A
Incidence in USA: 175,000 new cases per year
Prevalence in USA: 70/100,000 population
Predominant age: 50-70 years
Predominant sex: Male > Female

SIGNS AND SYMPTOMS
May be asymptomatic.
- Hypertrophic pulmonary osteoarthropathy
- Cough
- Shortness of breath
- Hemoptysis
- Exercise limitation
- Chest pain
- Hoarseness
- Wheezing
- Excess fatigue
- Dyspnea
- Shoulder/arm pain
- Dysphagia
- Bone pain
- Weight loss
- Superior vena cava syndrome
- Anemia

CAUSES
- Smoking (greater than 90%)
- Asbestos exposure
- Chronic interstitial pneumonitis
- Halogen ethers
- Inorganic arsenic
- Radioisotopes
- Atmospheric pollution
- Other metals

RISK FACTORS Listed under Causes

 DIAGNOSIS

DIFFERENTIAL DIAGNOSIS
- Metastatic cancer
- Granuloma
- Hamartoma

LABORATORY
- CBC (look for anemia)
- SMA-18 (look for abnormalities of Na, K+, CA ++ and liver enzymes)
- PT, PTT, platelet count
Drugs that may alter lab results: None likely
Disorders that may alter lab results: None likely

PATHOLOGICAL FINDINGS Cancer cell type from positive histology or cytology (see Description)

SPECIAL TESTS
- Electrocardiogram
- Pulmonary function studies
- Exercise treadmill
- Stress thallium or Persantine scans when applicable

IMAGING
Chest x-ray, CT scan of chest, split perfusion lung scan:
  ◊ Pulmonary nodule, mass, or infiltrate
  ◊ Mediastinal widening
  ◊ Atelectasis
  ◊ Hilar enlargement
  ◊ Pleural effusion
Other CT scans:
  ◊ Of brain - when applicable
  ◊ Of abdomen (may not be necessary if CT of chest includes screen for hepatic or adrenal metastasis)
Bone scan:
  ◊ When applicable

DIAGNOSTIC PROCEDURES
- Fiberoptic bronchoscopy
- Mediastinoscopy, when applicable
- Fine needle aspiration biopsy
- Scalene node biopsy, when applicable

 TREATMENT

APPROPRIATE HEALTH CARE
- Inpatient surgical resection for non-small cell cancer, when possible
- Outpatient chemotherapy or radiation therapy for small cell cancer

GENERAL MEASURES
- Radiotherapy
- Immunotherapy
- Pain relief when applicable

ACTIVITY Fully active

DIET No special diet

PATIENT EDUCATION
- General verbal information on lung cancer
- American Cancer Society for support groups and other information

MEDICATIONS

DRUG(S) OF CHOICE Pain medication
Contraindications: Refer to manufacturer's instructions
Precautions: Refer to manufacturer's instructions
Significant possible interactions: Refer to manufacturer's instructions

ALTERNATIVE DRUGS N/A

 FOLLOWUP

PATIENT MONITORING
Surgically resectable
 ◊ First year each 3 months
 ◊ Second year each 6 months
 ◊ Third though fifth year once a year
Surgically unresectable
 ◊ As necessary for palliation

PREVENTION/AVOIDANCE
• Stop smoking
• Avoid asbestos
• Avoid occupational exposure to metals
• Consider prophylaxis with retinoid, such as beta-carotene

POSSIBLE COMPLICATIONS
• Development of metastatic disease
• Local recurrence

EXPECTED COURSE AND PROGNOSIS
• Stage I, post-surgical resection of squamous/adeno/large cell is 50% survival
• Stage II, post-surgical is 33% for squamous (stage IIIa, post-surgical survival is 15% for squamous), and 20% for adeno/large cell
• Note: Pre-surgical staging is less accurate so survival figures are lower
• If nonresectable, prognosis is poor with mean survival rate of 8 to 14 months

 MISCELLANEOUS

ASSOCIATED CONDITIONS N/A

AGE-RELATED FACTORS
Pediatric: N/A
Geriatric: More common in elderly (> 75 years)
Others: N/A

PREGNANCY N/A

SYNONYMS
• Lung cancer

ICD-9-CM
162.9

SEE ALSO N/A

OTHER NOTES N/A

ABBREVIATIONS N/A

REFERENCES
• Shields, T.W. (ed.): General Thoracic Surgery. 3rd Ed. Philadelphia, Lea and Febiger, 1989
• Baue, A.E. (ed.): Glenn's Thoracic and Cardiovascular Surgery. 5th Ed. East Norwich, Appleton and Lange, 1990
• Sabiston, D.C. (ed.): Surgery of the Chest. 4th Ed. Philadelphia, W.B. Saunders Co., 1983

Author J. Miller, M.D

Lupus erythematosus, discoid

BASICS

DESCRIPTION Discoid lupus erythematosus (DLE) is a chronic skin disease characterized by sharply marginated dull, red macules with adherent scales extending into areas of atrophy, telangiectasias, or follicular plugging
• Localized DLE - more common form with lesions occurring on the face especially the malar areas, bridge of nose, lower lip and ears
• Generalized DLE - lesions seen on upper extremities and thorax
System(s) affected: Skin
Genetics: N/A
Incidence in USA: 3/100,000 Caucasian females; 8/100,000 Black females
Prevalence in USA: 100/100,000
Predominant age: 20 to 40
Predominant sex:
• Localized DLE - Female > Male (3:1)
• Generalized DLE - Female > Male (9:1)

SIGNS AND SYMPTOMS
• Red plaque-like lesions on face, thorax, or upper extremities
• Older lesions atrophy and appear as smooth white or hyperpigmented scars with telangiectasias
• Alopecia with scalp lesions
• "Carpet tack" appearance of skin when scale removed
• Lesions occasionally pruritic
• Oral ulceration in 15 percent of patients

CAUSES Unknown

RISK FACTORS Systemic lupus erythematosus (SLE)

DIAGNOSIS

DIFFERENTIAL DIAGNOSIS
• Actinic keratoses
• Polymorphous light eruption
• Drug eruptions
• Sarcoid
• Seborrheic dermatitis
• Lichen planus
• Plaque psoriasis
• Rosacea
• Pemphigus erythematoides
• Tinea faciei
• Jessner's disease

LABORATORY
• Localized DLE - usually no lab abnormalities
• Generalized DLE (may occasionally find) - increased sedimentation rate, positive ANA, leukopenia, hematuria and albuminuria if concomitant SLE
Drugs that may alter lab results: N/A
Disorders that may alter lab results: Concomitant SLE

PATHOLOGICAL FINDINGS
• Hyperkeratosis
• Epidermal atrophy
• Liquefactive degeneration of basal cell layer
• Edema mucin, and inflammation of dermis
• Basement zone thickened with strong periodic acid-Schiff reaction staining

SPECIAL TESTS Immunofluorescent staining of skin biopsies

IMAGING N/A

DIAGNOSTIC PROCEDURES Skin biopsy

TREATMENT

APPROPRIATE HEALTH CARE
Outpatient

GENERAL MEASURES Avoid sun exposure, avoid excessive heat, cold, or trauma

ACTIVITY Full activity

DIET Regular

PATIENT EDUCATION
• Teach patients proper use of sunscreens
• Advise on symptoms of SLE that should be watched for

MEDICATIONS

DRUG(S) OF CHOICE
• Localized DLE: Higher potency topical corticosteroids applied tid (e.g., betamethasone, triamcinolone)
• Generalized DLE: Hydroxychloroquine 200 mg qid or bid and/or quinacrine 100 mg daily
Contraindications: Antimalarials such as hydroxychloroquine may have to be avoided in patients with preexisting retinal or hepatic disease. Do not give to individuals with G-6-PD deficiency.
Precautions:
• Observe for skin atrophy with topical steroids especially with use on the face
• Patients on antimalarials should have an eye examination by an ophthalmologist at start of treatment and at 3-6 month intervals to monitor signs of retinal damage
Significant possible Interactions: N/A

ALTERNATIVE DRUGS
• Localized DLE: Intralesional triamcinolone 2.5 mg/cc injected at monthly intervals. Prednisone 15 mg bid, then tapered after response.
• Generalized DLE: Chloroquine 250 mg qd, dapsone 100 mg qd, azathioprine 100 mg qd or systemic retinoids

FOLLOWUP

PATIENT MONITORING
• Recheck patients once or twice per month
• Ophthalmology followup at 6 month intervals if patient on antimalarial
• If lesions subside, reduce dosage of chloroquine over 2-3 months, then discontinue

PREVENTION/AVOIDANCE   Avoid sun exposure or excessive heat, cold, or skin trauma

POSSIBLE COMPLICATIONS
Hypertrophic scarring, hypopigmentation (especially in blacks)

EXPECTED COURSE AND PROGNOSIS
• 40% remit completely; 1-5% may develop systemic lupus (these patients usually have generalized DLE)
• Not life-threatening unless it turns into disseminated type

MISCELLANEOUS

ASSOCIATED CONDITIONS
• Systemic lupus erythematosis
• Mixed connective tissue disease (MCTD)
• Antiphospholipid syndrome

AGE-RELATED FACTORS
Pediatric: N/A
Geriatric: N/A
Others: N/A

PREGNANCY   N/A

SYNONYMS   Chronic cutaneous LE

ICD-9-CM   695.4

SEE ALSO   N/A

OTHER NOTES   N/A

ABBREVIATIONS   N/A

REFERENCES
• Habif, T.: Clinical Dermatology. 2nd Ed. St. Louis, C.V. Mosby, 1990
• Domonkos, A.N., Arnold, H.L. & Odom, R.B.: Andrews' Diseases of the Skin. 8th Ed. Philadelphia, W.B. Saunders Co., 1990

Author   G. Silko, M.D.

Lyme disease

BASICS

DESCRIPTION A multisystem infection caused by the spirochete Borrelia burgdorferi, which is transmitted primarily by Ixodid ticks
• Stage 1, early localized Lyme disease, includes a characteristic expanding skin rash (erythema migrans) and constitutional flu-like symptoms
• Stage 2, early disseminated Lyme disease, may present with involvement of one or more organ systems. Neurologic (15%) and cardiac (8%) disease are most common
• Stage 3, chronic Lyme disease, involves arthritis (50%) and chronic neurological syndromes
System(s) affected: Skin, Musculoskeletal, Hemic/Lymphatic/Immunologic
Genetics: N/A
Incidence/Prevalence in USA: Varies by region. 6.1 cases/100,000 in the Mid Atlantic region, 3.7 in New England, 0.7 in the North Central states, 0.6 in the Pacific States, 0.6 in the Southeast and southwest, and less than 0.1 in the Mountain region
Predominant age: Can occur in all ages, but most common in children under 15 and in the 25-44 year age group
Predominant sex: Male = Female

SIGNS AND SYMPTOMS
Stage 1:
◊ Erythema migrans (60-80%)
◊ Fever
◊ Headache
◊ Myalgias
◊ Arthralgias
◊ Some patients may be asymptomatic
Stage 2: (involvement of one or more organ systems)
◊ Multiple erythema migrans
◊ Facial palsies, or other cranial neuropathies
◊ Aseptic meningitis
◊ Heart block
◊ Pericarditis
◊ Orchitis, hepatitis, or iritis
◊ Arthritis (usually large joint monoarthritis)
Stage 3:
◊ Recurrent synovitis
◊ Recurrent tendinitis and bursitis
◊ Neuropsychiatric symptoms, may include: Psychotic behavior, memory loss, dementia, depression, sleep disorders
◊ Encephalopathic symptoms: Headache, decreased memory, difficulty concentrating, confusion, fatigue
◊ Symptoms mimicking other CNS diseases: Multiple sclerosis-like syndromes, stroke-like symptoms, vestibular neuronitis, transverse myelitis, parkinsonian symptoms
◊ Peripheral neuropathic symptoms: Carpal tunnel syndrome, motor, sensory, or autonomic neuropathies
◊ Ophthalmic manifestations: Iritis, keratitis, retinal vasculitis, optic neuritis

CAUSES Infection with spirochete Borrelia burgdorferi, transmitted by the bite of Ixodid ticks

RISK FACTORS Exposure to tick infested area, most common from May to September

DIAGNOSIS

DIFFERENTIAL DIAGNOSIS
• Juvenile rheumatoid arthritis
• Viral syndromes
• Later stages may mimic many other diseases (see Signs and Symptoms)

LABORATORY
• ELISA for IgM and IgG B burgdorferi antibodies (frequently negative in stage 1 disease)
• Culture of CSF for B burgdorferi
Drugs that may alter lab results: Late stage disease with negative serology may be seen in patients who received early antibiotic treatment
Disorders that may alter lab results: False positive response has been seen with Rocky Mountain spotted fever, syphilis, systemic lupus erythematosus, and rheumatoid arthritis

PATHOLOGICAL FINDINGS Culture of B burgdorferi from blood or skin biopsy specimens has a very low yield

SPECIAL TESTS N/A

IMAGING N/A

DIAGNOSTIC PROCEDURES Lumbar puncture when neurologic findings are present, with ELISA of CSF for B burgdorferi antibodies

TREATMENT

APPROPRIATE HEALTH CARE
• Stage 1, clinical diagnosis, can be treated as an outpatient
• Stage 2 and 3 may require more intensive treatment, based on symptoms

GENERAL MEASURES Prevention of infection is possible by careful examination of skin for ticks after outdoor activities. Prompt removal of ticks may limit transmission. Clothing that covers the ankles should be worn in endemic areas, and the use of insect repellants is recommended.

ACTIVITY No restriction

DIET No special diet

PATIENT EDUCATION
• In endemic areas, patients should be advised to protect themselves against tick exposure
• Information available from:
Lyme Borreliosis Foundation
P.O. Box 462
Tolland, CT 06084
(203)871-2900

MEDICATIONS

DRUG(S) OF CHOICE
Stage 1:
◊ Doxycycline (Vibramycin and others) 100 mg po bid for 14-21 days (Do not use in children under 12 or in pregnancy); or
◊ Amoxicillin 500 mg po tid for 14-21 days, (pediatric dose 25-100 mg/kg/day)
Stage 2:
◊ Normal CSF, treat for 28 days - doxycycline 100 mg po bid; or
◊ Amoxicillin 500 mg po tid with probenicid 500 mg po tid
◊ Short course of corticosteroids (5-7 days) may be helpful
◊ With abnormal CSF, treat for 3-4 weeks - ceftriaxone (Rocephin) 2 g IV qd; or cefotaxime (Claforan) 2 g IV q 8 h; or penicillin G 20-24 million units/day IV. Short course of corticosteroids (5-7 days) po.
Stage 3:
◊ Oral treatment for 28 days with doxycycline 100 mg bid; or
◊ Amoxicillin 500 mg tid plus probenecid 500 mg tid
◊ If oral treatment fails, IV treatment for 2-3 weeks with ceftriaxone 2 g qd; or cefotaxime 2 g q 8 hr

Contraindications:
• Allergy to agent
• Doxycycline contraindicated in children and in women who are pregnant or breast feeding

Precautions: Refer to manufacturer's profile of each drug

Significant possible interactions:
• Doxycycline is a tetracycline. Drug absorption may be significantly reduced if taken with milk or antacids. Oral anticoagulants may need reduced dose. Oral contraceptives may be less effective. Possible photosensitivity requires sunscreen.
• For others, refer to manufacturer's profile of each drug

ALTERNATIVE DRUGS
Erythromycin 250 mg po qid x 28 days for stage 1 disease (may be less effective)

FOLLOWUP

PATIENT MONITORING
Stage 2 and 3 disease requires careful monitoring over a period of months to years, based on severity of symptoms

PREVENTION/AVOIDANCE
Awareness of the disease, protective clothing, and careful skin inspection with timely removal of ticks may reduce the incidence of disease

POSSIBLE COMPLICATIONS
• Recurrent synovitis, tendinitis, bursitis
• Chronic neurological symptoms
• Peripheral neuropathies
• See Signs and symptoms of Stage 3 disease

EXPECTED COURSE AND PROGNOSIS
• Early treatment with antibiotics can shorten the duration of symptoms and prevent later disease
• Response of late stage disease is variable

MISCELLANEOUS

ASSOCIATED CONDITIONS
N/A

AGE-RELATED FACTORS
Pediatric: Drug of choice in pediatrics is amoxicillin. Tetracyclines are contraindicated.
Geriatric: N/A
Others: Ixodid ticks are commonly found on deer. Hunters may be at increased risk.

PREGNANCY
Because B burgdorferi can cross the placenta, pregnant patients with active disease should receive parenteral antibiotics. Doxycycline should not be used in pregnancy.

SYNONYMS
Lyme arthritis

ICD-9-CM
088.8 Other specified arthropod-borne diseases

SEE ALSO
N/A

OTHER NOTES
Ixodid ticks require white footed mice to complete their life cycle. Investigators have had some success in eradicating the ticks by providing permethrin laced cotton in areas where the mice forage for bedding material.

ABBREVIATIONS
N/A

REFERENCES
• Luger, S.W.: Questions Frequently Asked About Lyme Disease, Fam Pract Recert, 1990; 12 (10):19-39
• The Medical Letter 1989; 31 (794);57-59
• MMWR, 1989; 38:668-672

Author B. Majeroni, M.D.

Lymphogranuloma venereum

BASICS

DESCRIPTION
Lymphogranuloma venereum (LGV) is a rare, systemic, sexually transmitted disease caused by the three most virulent strains or serovars of Chlamydia trachomatis, the same organism responsible for chlamydial urethritis
• Inguinal lymphadenopathy is the most common clinical manifestation. Painless vesicular or ulcerative lesions on the external genitalia may be seen in early disease and severe anogenital inflammation and scarring may result from untreated disease.
• Usually a disease of the tropics; especially common in Africa with foci of endemicity also in the Caribbean (Haiti and Jamaica), South America, East Asia and Indonesia. In 1989, chlamydial infections required reporting in thirty states.
System(s) affected: Reproductive, Hemic/Lymphatic/Immunologic
Genetics: N/A
Incidence in USA: 277 cases reported to CDC in 1990
Prevalence in USA: The prevalence of anorectal LGV is increasing in the USA in male homosexuals
Predominant age: Third decade corresponding to the age of peak sexual activity
Predominant sex: Male > Female (5:1)

SIGNS AND SYMPTOMS
Three stages:
Primary:
• Superficial lesions such as papules, vesicles, ulcers or erosions appear on the external genitalia 3 days to 3 weeks after exposure. Lesions are painless and disappear in a few days leaving no scar. This stage frequently escapes notice.
Secondary: the inguinal syndrome or bubonic stage
• Predominantly in men (Male:Female > 10:1)
• Fever, chills
• Regional lymphadenopathy occurring a week to months after the primary stage.
• Enlarged lymph nodes (buboes) begin as a mass of firm, tender, matted lymph nodes, often unilateral and eventually involve the overlying skin with erythema and adhesions.
• As the buboes enlarge:
◊ the patient often walks with a limp
◊ Severe groin pain
◊ Within one to two weeks, the buboes may become fluctuant and rupture relieving the pain and leaving fistulas to drain, heal and scar. Other buboes slowly involute and form firm inguinal masses.
Tertiary: the anogenital stage
• Lymphatic obstruction or scarring
• Genitalia or anorectal canal inflammation
• Predominantly women and homosexual men. The rectal mucosa can be directly inoculated by receptive intercourse or may become involved through posterior lymphatic spread.
• Proctitis can present with fever, tenesmus, anal pruritis and mucous rectal discharge
• Lymphatic obstruction with perianal growths of lymphoid tissue resembling hemorrhoids or genital elephantiasis
• Perirectal abscesses, ischiorectal and rectovaginal fistulas, anal fistulas, and rectal strictures or stenosis

CAUSES
Three of fifteen known strains of C. trachomatis also described as serovars L1, L2, and L3. These serovars are more invasive and virulent and selectively infect lymphoid tissue rather than columnar epithelial cells.

RISK FACTORS
• Unprotected intercourse, especially outside of a mutually monogamous and disease-free relationship
• Anal intercourse
• Residing in or visiting tropical or developing countries
• With the increasing incidence of anorectal LGV in male homosexuals in the USA, it should be kept in mind when a patient presents with symptoms of proctocolitis

DIAGNOSIS

DIFFERENTIAL DIAGNOSIS
• Inguinal adenitis - chancroid, genital herpes or syphilis. In the USA, one or more of these is more likely than not if the adenitis is associated with a prominent genital ulceration. Other causes of inguinal adenitis include cat-scratch disease or reactive adenopathy due to skin lesions on the lower extremities. Less common: Hodgkin's disease.
• Suppurative adenitis - chancroid, donovanosis, plague, tularemia, sporotrichosis, actinomycosis and tuberculosis
• Retroperitoneal adenitis - may present as lower abdominal pain with subsequent extensive differential diagnosis
• Proctitis - gonococcal and non-LGV chlamydial proctitis as well as antibiotic-induced, infectious, and inflammatory bowel disease
• Schistosomiasis - consider if lymphatic obstruction is present

LABORATORY
• Mild leukocytosis with relative lymphocytosis or monocytosis
• Elevated erythrocyte sedimentation rate
• VDRL/RPR and HIV antibodies should be considered
Drugs that may alter lab results: Antibiotics
Disorders that may alter lab results: Chlamydial urethritis

PATHOLOGICAL FINDINGS   N/A

SPECIAL TESTS
• Bubo pus or saline injected into a bubo and re-aspirated, infected tissue or primary lesion scrapings, preserved in proper transport media, can be studied with Giemsa stain or by immunofluorescence for inclusion bodies. They can also be cultured on McCoy cells. Yield is about 30% for all of these methods.
• Antibody levels to L1, L2, and L3 serovars of C. trachomatis can be measured with complement fixation although cross-reactivity with other Chlamydial organisms is possible. Levels above 1:64, with the proper clinical scenario, are probably LGV. Levels above 1:128 minimize the cross-reactivity of this method and are likely to be true cases of LGV. Higher titers are more confirmatory for LGV. These levels are reached early in the disease course and usually do not vary much between acute and convalescent titers at six weeks.
• Microimmunofluorescent (micro-IF) titers are more sensitive and specific than the complement fixation test but are not generally available. The titers of micro-IF in LGV are usually 1:512 or higher.
• Frei's intradermal test is obsolete

IMAGING
• Computerized tomography for retroperitoneal adenitis. Lymphography does not outline buboes, but may demonstrate the extent of lymph node involvement
• Barium enema may reveal the characteristic elongated stricture of LGV

DIAGNOSTIC PROCEDURES   Incision and drainage of bubo for culture

TREATMENT

APPROPRIATE HEALTH CARE
Outpatient except for rare complications such as severe pain or for surgical repair of complications after antibiotic therapy

GENERAL MEASURES
• In the acute bubonic stage, fluctuant nodes should be aspirated before they burst and the occasional abscess should be incised and drained. Otherwise surgery should be avoided until antibiotics have been administered. Fever abates rapidly and bubo pain usually responds within a few days of starting antibiotics.
• Symptomatic treatment with nonsteroidal anti-inflammatories should be suggested in those not contraindicated. Local heat may provide some analgesia.

ACTIVITY   Sexual abstention pending treatment, otherwise limited only by symptoms

DIET Avoid milk and milk products as well as agents that chelate tetracycline, such as iron supplements and antacids. Can be taken, but not at the same time. Allow 2 hours for gastric emptying.

PATIENT EDUCATION
• LGV is a sexually transmitted disease and the patient should be counseled for other sexually transmitted diseases and toward safe sex practices
• Sexual partners should be treated
• Offer HIV counseling and testing

MEDICATIONS

DRUG(S) OF CHOICE
• For acute cases: Doxycycline 100 mg po bid for 21 days
• For chronic or relapsing cases: Consider longer course of therapy
Contraindications: Tetracycline allergy or sensitivity
Precautions:
• For patients on courses of tetracyclines longer than 21 days, changes such as leukocytosis, atypical lymphocytes, may be observed in the peripheral blood, toxic granulation of granulocytes, and thrombopenic purpura (rare)
• Suprainfections such as antibiotic-induced diarrhea may ensue
• Tetracyclines may cause photosensitization. Advise patients to use sunscreen.
• Avoid tetracyclines in pregnancy and children under 8
Significant possible interactions:
• Avoid, when taking tetracyclines: milk and milk products, sodium bicarbonate, calcium and magnesium salts, silicate, iron preparations, and bismuth subsalicylate
• As opposed to the other tetracyclines, food does not otherwise interfere with absorption of doxycycline nor does doxycycline seem to have prolonged clearance in patients with impaired renal function
• Doxycycline's half-life is shortened from 20 to 7 hours in patients who are receiving chronic treatment with barbiturates and phenytoin and hence should be administered in the same dose three to four times a day in this group of patients

ALTERNATIVE DRUGS
• Tetracycline 500 mg po qid for 21 days or
• Sulfisoxazole 500 mg po qid for 21 days or equivalent sulfonamide course
• For pregnant women or patients allergic to tetracyclines and sulfas, erythromycin 500 mg po qid for 21 days

FOLLOWUP

PATIENT MONITORING
• Fever and bubo pain usually abates within 1 to 2 days after starting antibiotics. For persistent fever or malaise, patients should be monitored closely for complications such as abscesses or superinfections.
• Treatment has no effect on preexisting scar tissue, hence patients should be monitored for surgical complications
• Dual infections with other sexually transmitted diseases are common and appropriate monitoring should also be made, especially for syphilis and HIV

PREVENTION/AVOIDANCE
• Treat sexual contacts
• Abstinence or mutual monogamy in a proven disease-free sexual relationship is the only true prevention. Condoms should be worn with sexual activity outside of such relationships.
• Condoms provide protection against genital-anogenital transmission but have no impact on transmission between other sites

POSSIBLE COMPLICATIONS
• Scarring - includes renal or bowel obstruction, persistent rectovaginal fistula or gross destruction of the anal canal, anal sphincter, or perineum. Repair of such complications as well as plastic repair of some of the complications of lymphatic obstruction such as genital elephantiasis are the more common surgical indications. Surgery should be performed only after antibiotic treatment.
• Mild rectal strictures can occasionally be dilated as an outpatient

EXPECTED COURSE AND PROGNOSIS
• Early treatment improves the prognosis
• Resolution of symptoms is usual if treatment is undertaken before scarring
• Reinfection and/or inadequate treatment may result in relapse

MISCELLANEOUS

ASSOCIATED CONDITIONS Any of the sexually transmitted diseases. Screening should be done for syphilis and HIV.

AGE-RELATED FACTORS
Pediatric: N/A
Geriatric: N/A
Others: N/A

PREGNANCY Congenital transmission does not occur, but infection may be acquired during passage through an infected birth canal

SYNONYMS
• Tropical bubo
• Climatic bubo
• Strumous bubo
• Poradenitis inguinalis
• Durand-Nicolas-Favre disease
• Lymphogranuloma inguinale
• Fourth and fifth and sixth venereal disease
• LGV

ICD-9-CM 099.1 lymphogranuloma venereum

SEE ALSO
• Chlamydia sexually transmitted disease
• Chancroid
• Syphilis
• Herpes, genital

OTHER NOTES N/A

ABBREVIATIONS N/A

REFERENCES
• Holmes, K.K., et al. (eds.): Sexually Transmitted Diseases. New York, McGraw-Hill, 1989
• Centers for Disease Control: 1989 sexually transmitted diseases treatment guidelines. MMWR 38(S-8), 1989

Author G. Fowler, M.D.

Lymphoma, Burkitt's

 BASICS

DESCRIPTION Highly undifferentiated B cell lymphoma. It may involve sites other than lymph nodes or reticuloendothelial system, particularly bone marrow and central nervous system. Endemic areas - Central Africa; New Guinea. Rare in USA.
System(s) affected:
Hemic/Lymphatic/Immunologic
Genetics: Translocation of chromosome 8 onto chromosome 14 (70%); C–MYC activation
Incidence/Prevalence in USA: Rare
Predominant age: 3 months to 16 years
Predominant sex: Male > female

SIGNS AND SYMPTOMS
African:
  ◊ Mouth pain
  ◊ Loose teeth
  ◊ Loose deciduous molars
  ◊ Jaw mass
  ◊ Anemia
North American:
  ◊ Abdominal mass

CAUSES Unknown; high association with Epstein-Barr virus

RISK FACTORS Living in endemic areas

 DIAGNOSIS

DIFFERENTIAL DIAGNOSIS N/A

LABORATORY
• Anemia
• Serum uric acid often elevated
Drugs that may alter lab results: N/A
Disorders that may alter lab results: N/A

PATHOLOGICAL FINDINGS
• Stage AR - completely resected intra-abdominal tumor
• Stages A and B - indicate single or multiple extra-abdominal sites
• Stage C - intra-abdominal disease, including kidneys and/or gonads
• Stage D - Stage C findings plus extra-abdominal sites including bone marrow, pleura and/or central nervous system
• High mitotic rate
• Starry sky pattern
• A sea of monotonous cells
• Round to oval nuclei
• 2-5 prominent nucleoli
• Pyroninophilic cytoplasm

SPECIAL TESTS
• Cytogenic studies - translocation between chromosomes 8 and 14
• Immunologic studies - presence of B cell markers (usually IgM) on cell surface

IMAGING CT scan

DIAGNOSTIC PROCEDURES
• Bone marrow aspiration
• Lumbar puncture
• Lymph node biopsy

 TREATMENT

APPROPRIATE HEALTH CARE
• Inpatient - for staging surgery and chemotherapy
• Outpatient - after definitive treatment

GENERAL MEASURES
• Symptomatic treatment for respiratory, gastrointestinal, or psychosocial problems that may follow chemotherapy
• Surgery to excise the abdominal mass if present
• Be alert to increased risk for renal failure due to tumor lysis

ACTIVITY As tolerated

DIET
• May have difficulty in swallowing or chewing. Suggest small meals of a soft diet (protein milk shakes) to help prevent malnutrition.
• Adequate fluid intake

PATIENT EDUCATION
Leukemia Society of America
733 3rd Avenue
New York, NY 10017
(212)573-8424

MEDICATIONS

DRUG(S) OF CHOICE Combination chemotherapy according to most recent protocols, e.g., cyclophosphamide alone or combined with methotrexate, vincristine and ARA-C
Contraindications: Refer to manufacturer's literature
Precautions: Myelosuppression, alopecia, mucositis, neurotoxicity with chemotherapy
Significant possible interactions: Refer to manufacturer's literature

ALTERNATIVE DRUGS N/A

FOLLOWUP

PATIENT MONITORING
• For effects of chemotherapy
• Follow for detection of recurrence

PREVENTION/AVOIDANCE Avoid endemic areas

POSSIBLE COMPLICATIONS
Tumor lysis syndrome with:
  ◊ Hyperkalemia
  ◊ Hyperphosphatemia
  ◊ Hypocalcemia
  ◊ Tetany

EXPECTED COURSE AND PROGNOSIS
• 70-80% of patients with stages A, B, and C experience long-term remission
• Without treatment, prognosis is grave

MISCELLANEOUS

ASSOCIATED CONDITIONS N/A

AGE-RELATED FACTORS
Pediatric: Common age group for this disorder
Geriatric: Unusual in this age group
Others: N/A

PREGNANCY N/A

SYNONYMS
• Monomorphic undifferentiated lymphoma
• African lymphoma
• Maxillary lymphosarcoma

ICD-9-CM 200.2

SEE ALSO N/A

OTHER NOTES N/A

ABBREVIATIONS N/A

REFERENCES
• Vietti, T. & Fernbach, D. (eds): Clinical Pediatric Oncology. 4th Ed. St. Louis, C.V. Mosby, 1992
• Williams, W.J., et al.: Hematology. 4th Ed. New York, McGraw-Hill, 1990
• Wyngaarden, J.B., Smith, L.H. (eds): Cecil Textbook of Medicine. 19th Ed. Philadelphia, W.B. Saunders Co., 1992

Author J. J. Hutter, MD

Malaria

 BASICS

DESCRIPTION Malaria is an acute and chronic protozoan infection transmitted by Anopheles mosquitoes to humans. There are four species that cause human infection: Plasmodium falciparum, P. malariae, P. vivax, P. ovale.

System(s) affected:
Hemic/Lymphatic/Immunologic
Genetics: No known genetic pattern
Incidence/Prevalence in USA: Not endemic. Cases in the U.S. are imported.
Predominant age: All ages
Predominant sex: Male = Female

SIGNS AND SYMPTOMS
- Chills
- Fever
- Hemolysis
- P. falciparum (also known as malignant tertian malaria) - does not have a specific periodicity in a non-immune individual. The patient may have persistent fever and in massive parasitemia may have serious complications including renal failure, central nervous system involvement, pulmonary edema, gastroenteritis, anemia, and thrombocytopenia. This is the only infection that is associated with fatal outcome.
- P. malariae (also known as quartan malaria) - patient will have attacks every 72 hours. This disease can become chronic. Nephrotic syndrome may be found in patients with chronic P. malariae infection.
- P. vivax (benign tertian) and P. ovale - patient will have attacks every 48 hours
- Splenomegaly is found in those with chronic infection

CAUSES Bites from infected Anopheles mosquitoes, or transfusion of infected blood

RISK FACTORS Traveling and/or living in endemic area

 DIAGNOSIS

DIFFERENTIAL DIAGNOSIS
- Severe P. falciparum infection may present with signs and symptoms suggestive of acute hepatitis, acute hemolytic anemia, acute diarrheal illness, stroke, pneumonia, and acute viral infection
- Chronic infection may have to be differentiated from other causes of tropical splenomegaly and blood dyscrasias

LABORATORY
- Anemia
- Leukopenia
- Thrombocytopenia
- Elevated alanine aminotransferase (ALT), aspartate aminotransferase (AST)
- Direct and indirect bilirubin
- Depressed albumin
Drugs that may alter lab results:
Antimalarial agents may reduce parasitemia
Disorders that may alter lab results: N/A

PATHOLOGICAL FINDINGS
- Malaria causes hemolysis
- In the case of falciparum infection, the increased stickiness of the parasitized cells results in blocking of arterioles and capillaries
- Edema, localized hemorrhage, and the presence of malarial pigments are frequent findings

SPECIAL TESTS Malarial smear; Indirect fluorescent antibody (IFA), ELISA, DNA probe

IMAGING Not contributory

DIAGNOSTIC PROCEDURES Malarial smear

 TREATMENT

APPROPRIATE HEALTH CARE
Inpatient for most cases of falciparum malaria in nonimmune patients. Outpatient for others, except during acute phase.

GENERAL MEASURES In severe cases watch for complications, such as severe anemia, and renal failure

ACTIVITY May resume activity as soon as the fever is under control

DIET No restrictions in mild cases. In severe cases, give whatever the patient can tolerate.

PATIENT EDUCATION Prevention of future exposures. These measures include prevention of mosquito bites and malarial chemoprophylaxis.

Malaria

MEDICATIONS

DRUG(S) OF CHOICE
For malarial infection except chloroquine resistant P. falciparum
◊ Oral therapy - chloroquine phosphate:
Adult dose - 600 mg base (1 gm) followed by 300 mg in 6 h then 300 mg daily for 2 days
Pediatric dose - 10 mg/kg base (maximum of 600 mg) followed by half the dose in 6 h, then daily for 2 days
◊ Parenteral therapy - quinidine or quinine IV (parenteral quinine is no longer available in the USA):
Adult dose - 10 mg/kg in 300 ml of normal saline IV over 2-4 h; repeat every 8 h until oral therapy can be started (maximum 1.8 g/d)
Pediatric dose - 25 mg/kg/d in normal saline in 3 divided doses IV over 2-4 h; repeat every 8 h until oral therapy can be started (maximum 1.8 g/d)
For chloroquine resistant P. Falciparum malaria
◊ Oral therapy - quinine sulfate plus pyrimethamine-sulfadiazine:
Adult dosages - quinine sulfate 650 mg tid for 3-7 d. Pyrimethamine-sulfadiazine available as a fixed dose combination (Fansidar - 25 mg p/500 mg s) 2-3 tablets as a single dose.
Pediatric dosages - quinine sulfate 25 mg/kg/d in 3 divided dose for 3 d.
Pyrimethamine-sulfadiazine, < 4 years 1/2 tablet, 4-8 years 1 tablet, 8-12 years 2 tablets.
◊ Parenteral therapy - quinidine or quinine IV (parenteral quinine is no longer available in the USA):
Adult dose - 10 mg/kg in 300 ml of normal saline IV over 2-4 h; repeat every 8 h until oral therapy can be started (maximum 1.8 g/d)
Pediatric dose - 25 mg/kg/d in normal saline in 3 divided doses IV over 2-4 h; repeat every 8 h until oral therapy can be started (maximum 1.8 g/d)
For P. vivax or P. ovale infection - to prevent relapse
◊ Primaquine phosphate (to be given during or after the above antimalarial therapy):
Adult dose - 15 mg base po daily times 14 d or 45 mg base weekly for 8 weeks
Pediatric dose - 0.3 mg base/kg/d for 14 days or 0.9 mg base once weekly for 8 weeks
◊ Caution - patients who have glucose-6-phosphate dehydrogenase deficiency may develop hemolysis after given primaquine
Contraindications: Refer to manufacturer's literature
Precautions: Refer to manufacturer's literature
Significant possible interactions: Refer to manufacturer's literature

ALTERNATIVE DRUGS Chloroquine resistant P. Falciparum - quinidine plus tetracycline; mefloquine

FOLLOWUP

PATIENT MONITORING Watch for relapse of clinical symptoms

PREVENTION/AVOIDANCE
• Use of malarial prophylactic agents when visiting an endemic area
Chloroquine phosphate po (chemoprophylaxis of all species except chloroquine resistant P. falciparum)
◊ Adult dose - 300 mg base once weekly. Start 2 weeks before arrival (endemic area) and continue until 4-6 weeks after leaving the area.
◊ Pediatric dose - 5 mg/kg weekly; same as for adults. Maximum 300 mg dose.
Mefloquine po (chemoprophylaxis for chloroquine resistant P. falciparum)
◊ Adult dose - 250 mg (1 tablet) weekly. Begin 1 week before arrival and continue for 4 weeks after leaving the area
◊ Pediatric dose - 15-19 kg 1/4 tablet; 20-30 kg 1/2 tablet; 31-45 kg 3/4 tablet; over 45 kg 1 tablet. Follow schedule as for adult.
• Patients with sickle cell disease, or trait, glucose-6-phosphate dehydrogenase deficiency, and hereditary ovalocytosis may have some protection against severe P. falciparum infection. Patients with Duffy-negative blood type are resistant to P. vivax infection.

POSSIBLE COMPLICATIONS
• P. falciparum - if not treated early, the patients may develop cerebral malaria, acute renal failure, acute gastroenteritis, pulmonary edema, massive hemolysis, and splenic rupture. Death from malaria is virtually limited to P. falciparum infection.
• P. malariae - nephrotic syndrome may develop in those with chronic infection
• Other complications - seizures, anuria, delirium, coma, dysentery, algid malaria, blackwater fever, hyperpyrexia

EXPECTED COURSE AND PROGNOSIS Only falciparum infection carries a poor prognosis with high mortality if untreated. However, if diagnosed early and treated appropriately the prognosis is excellent.

MISCELLANEOUS

ASSOCIATED CONDITIONS N/A

AGE-RELATED FACTORS
Pediatric: N/A
Geriatric: More serious outcome in this age group
Others: N/A

PREGNANCY Most antimalarial drugs contraindicated in pregnancy

SYNONYMS N/A

ICD-9-CM
• Blackwater fever 084.8
• Cerebral malaria 084.9
• Congenital malaria 771.2
• Hepatitis 573.2
• Mixed malarial infection 084.5
• P. falciparum infection 084.0
• P. malariae infection 084.2
• P. ovale infection 084.3
• P. vivax infection 084.1
• Recurrent malaria 084.6
• Unspecified malaria 084.6

SEE ALSO N/A

OTHER NOTES
• Most areas of the world now have chloroquine-resistant P. falciparum (the form of malaria most prevalent world-wide)
• Current information regarding malaria treatment and prophylaxis is always available from CDC, Atlanta, GA

ABBREVIATIONS N/A

REFERENCES Wyler, D.J.: Plasmodium Species (Malaria). In Principles and Practice of Infectious Diseases. Edited by G.L. Mandell, R.G. Douglas & J.E Bennett. New York, Churchill Livingstone, 1990. pp 2056-2066

Author J. Tan, M.D.

Male erectile dysfunction

BASICS

DESCRIPTION Dissatisfaction with size, rigidity, or duration of erection. Male sexual dysfunction encompasses an even larger group of complaints and disorders of arousal, desire, orgasm, sensation, and relationship. Transient periods of impotence occurs in about half of the adult males and are not considered dysfunctional.
System(s) affected: Reproductive, Nervous, Cardiovascular
Genetics: Rarely related to chromosomal disorders
Incidence/Prevalence in USA: Erectile failure involves about 10% of men, but is underreported by patients
Predominant Age:
• Patients with psychologic, gender, and primary organic problems often present themselves for help between adolescence and the third decade
• Patients with relationship problems, but concerned mainly about physical problems, tend to seek care in the sixth decade
• Most patients with physical problems are in the seventh and eighth decade, but rarely seek help
Predominant Sex: Male

SIGNS AND SYMPTOMS
• Reduction of erectile size and rigidity
• Inability to maintain erection
• Inability to achieve erection
• Reduced body hair
• Thyromegaly
• Gynecomastia
• Testicular atrophy or absence
• Deformed penis
• Peripheral vascular disease
• Neuropathy

CAUSES
• Endocrine
• Neurologic
• Vascular
• Medication
• Psychologic
• Structural

RISK FACTORS
• Prior pelvic surgery
• Medication use
• Risk factors for disorders listed in Causes

DIAGNOSIS

DIFFERENTIAL DIAGNOSIS
Endocrine
◊ Low or high thyroxine
◊ Low testosterone
◊ High prolactin
◊ Diabetes
◊ High estrogen effect
◊ Renal failure
◊ Zinc deficiency
Neurologic
◊ Central
◊ Spinal
◊ Peripheral
Vascular
◊ Arterial insufficiency
◊ Cavernosal insufficiency
◊ Venous insufficiency
Medication
◊ Many types, e.g., beta-blockers, thiazides
Psychologic
◊ Depression
◊ Schizophrenia
◊ Relationship disorders
◊ Personality disorders
◊ Anxiety
Structural
◊ Microphallus
◊ Chordee and Peyronie's disease
◊ Cavernosal scarring
◊ Phimosis
◊ Hypospadias
◊ Postsurgical sequelae

LABORATORY
• CBC
• Glucose
• K+
• Na+
• Albumin
• BUN/creatinine
• TSH
• Prolactin
• Testosterone
Drugs that may alter lab results: N/A
Disorders that may alter lab results: N/A

PATHOLOGICAL FINDINGS Most men over age 55 will have some test abnormality or risk factor, but it is not necessarily the cause of the patient's impotence

SPECIAL TESTS
• 24 hour urine zinc
• Dorsal nerve somatosensory evoked potentials
• Sacral evoked response
• Penile-brachial blood pressures
• Aortogram
• Selective pudendal angiogram
• Dynamic cavernosography
• Nocturnal penile tumescence (NPT) testing
• Penile blood pressure

IMAGING Doppler, angiogram, cavernosogram

DIAGNOSTIC PROCEDURES Response to papaverine injection

TREATMENT

APPROPRIATE HEALTH CARE Since erectile dysfunction is multifactorial, evaluation by a generalist in an outpatient setting

GENERAL MEASURES
• Early use of penile implants is now discouraged because of success with vacuum erectile devices, sensate focus therapy and injection therapy
• Improve partner communication
• Reduce performance pressure
• Use sensate focus therapy
• Try vacuum erectile device
• Use of psychiatrists, psychologists, sex therapists, vascular surgeons, urologists, endocrinologists, neurologists, plastic surgeons, etc., often necessary for refractory cases

ACTIVITY No restrictions

DIET Control diabetes if present

PATIENT EDUCATION Male Sexuality by Bernie Zilbergeld, Ph.D. and problem-specific handouts

MEDICATIONS

DRUG(S) OF CHOICE
• If hypogonadism present, testosterone cypionate 200 mg IM every two weeks
• If hyperprolactinemia present, bromocriptine 2.5 mg bid up to 40 mg/day
To induce erection
◊ Intracavernous injection of a solution containing phentolamine(0.5-1.0 mg) and papaverine (30 mg per mL, starting with 0.1 mlL) or
◊ Alprostadil 10-20 mcg/ml

Contraindications:
• Injections should be avoided in patients with bleeding disorders
• Avoid use in patients with known allergies to constituents

Precautions:
• With testosterone, watch for urinary retention, acne, sodium retention and gynecomastia
• With bromocriptine, watch for self-limiting nausea, vomiting
• With injection therapy, watch for priapism, fibrosis, hypotension and nausea

Significant possible interactions: N/A

ALTERNATIVE DRUGS
Use vacuum erection device before injections

FOLLOWUP

PATIENT MONITORING Meet with patient and, if possible, his partner, as required by cause, therapy, and response

PREVENTION/AVOIDANCE Since erectile dysfunction is multifactorial, referral to a sex therapist or couples therapist may help to speed recovery and prevent future problems

POSSIBLE COMPLICATIONS Specific to therapy

EXPECTED COURSE AND PROGNOSIS
• Given that the majority of patients have unspecified causes of their erectile disorders, vacuum erection device, injection therapy and penile implant have improved the outlook greatly
• Expect 20% failure rate of vacuum erection device, high drop-out rate from injection therapy, and a 10-30% non-use rate for penile implants
• Spontaneous cure rate is about 15%

MISCELLANEOUS

ASSOCIATED CONDITIONS see above

AGE-RELATED FACTORS
Pediatric: N/A
Geriatric: Aging alone is not a cause of impotence
Others: N/A

PREGNANCY N/A

SYNONYMS Impotence

ICD-9-CM
• 302 Sexual disorders
• 302.7 Psychosocial dysfunction
• 302.70 Psychosocial dysfunc nos
• 302.71 Inhibited sexual desire
• 302.72 Inhibited sex excitement
• 302.79 Psychosocial dysfunc nec
• 302.8 Psychosocial dis nec
• 302.89 Psychosexual dis nec
• 302.9 Psychosexual dis nos
• V41.7 Sexual function problem
• 607.84 Impotence, organic origin

SEE ALSO N/A

OTHER NOTES N/A

ABBREVIATIONS N/A

REFERENCES
• Montague, D.K.: Disorders of Male Sexual Dysfunction. Boca Raton, Year Book Medical Publishers, 1988
• Wagner, G. & Green, R.: Impotence. New York, Plenum Press, 1981
• Segraves, R.T. & Schoenberg, H.W.: Diagnosis and Treatment of Erectile Disturbances. New York, Plenum Medical Book Company, 1985

Author B. Block, M.D.

Marfan's syndrome

 BASICS

DESCRIPTION A dominantly inherited disorder of connective tissue affecting primarily the musculoskeletal system, the cardiovascular system and the eye
System(s) affected: Musculoskeletal, Endocrine/Metabolic
Genetics: Autosomal dominant with variable penetrance; 15% spontaneous mutation
Incidence/Prevalence in USA: 1 in 10,000 - 20,000 (estimated 1 in 15,000)
Predominant age: Congenital, so disorder is present from birth. However clinical manifestations do not usually become apparent until adolescence or young adulthood.
Predominant sex: No gender, ethnic or racial predilection

SIGNS AND SYMPTOMS
Musculoskeletal
◊ Tall stature
◊ Thin, gangly body habitus (limb length out of proportion to trunk)
◊ Arachnodactyly i.e. long, thin fingers
◊ Pectus deformity
◊ High arched palate
◊ Hyperextensible joints
◊ Kyphoscoliosis
◊ Joint laxity
Cardiovascular
◊ Aortic root dilatation
◊ Aortic regurgitation
◊ Aortic dissection
◊ Mitral valve prolapse
◊ Mitral regurgitation
Ocular
◊ Subluxation of lens, usually upward
◊ Myopia
◊ Retinal detachment (uncommon)
Other
◊ Easy bruising (uncommon)
◊ Excessive bleeding (uncommon)

CAUSES Genetic; at least 5% are obviously familial, the remainder arise from apparent spontaneous mutations

RISK FACTORS Advanced paternal age gives rise to a slightly increased risk only in those cases which are not clearly familial

 DIAGNOSIS

DIFFERENTIAL DIAGNOSIS
Homocystinuria, contractural arachnodactyly, Ehlers-Danlos syndrome, trisomy, all of which are rare conditions and all of which have clear cut distinguishing clinical features from the Marfan's syndrome

LABORATORY
• There are no specific laboratory abnormalities in the Marfan syndrome
• It is recommended that suspected patients have urinary homocystine measured to rule out homocystinuria
Drugs that may alter lab results: N/A
Disorders that may alter lab results: N/A

PATHOLOGICAL FINDINGS
• Cystic medial necrosis of the aorta
• Myxomatous degeneration of the cardiac valves
• Defective gene is believed to reside on chromosome 15 but specific locus is not known
• Molecular defect responsible for the syndrome is also not known but candidates include abnormal fibrillin, a large glycoprotein constituent of microfibrils; abnormal cross-linking of type I collagen; and abnormal synthesis of hyaluronic acid

SPECIAL TESTS Slit lamp examination is necessary to detect lens subluxation

IMAGING
• Plain x-rays of spine are necessary during growth years to detect and quantify scoliosis
• Annual screening echocardiograms are recommended beginning in adolescence in order to detect presymptomatic aortic root dilatation or valvular degeneration

DIAGNOSTIC PROCEDURES N/A

 TREATMENT

APPROPRIATE HEALTH CARE
Outpatient

GENERAL MEASURES
• Multidisciplinary approach including primary care physician, cardiologist, ophthalmologist and possibly orthopedic surgeon. A clinical geneticist if available, would be ideal as primary care physician.
• Many if not most of these patients will ultimately require reconstructive cardiovascular surgery

ACTIVITY
• Fully active unless limited by symptoms
• Several highly-trained athletes with the Marfan syndrome have suffered sudden death during competition leading to some concern that people with Marfan syndrome should be discouraged from participating in aerobically demanding sports

DIET No special diet

PATIENT EDUCATION N/A

MEDICATIONS

DRUG(S) OF CHOICE
• No specific medical therapy is available, however drugs are used to try to prevent certain complications
• Propranolol or other beta-adrenergic blocking drugs are used to decrease the force of cardiac contraction, in the hope of delaying the development or progression of aortic root dilatation. The dosage of these drugs are adjusted to target heart rate, i.e., resting rate of 60 per minute, with a rise to no more than 80 per minute after moderate exertion.
• Estrogen combined with progestogen has been used to induce puberty in pre-adolescent girls in an attempt to shorten the growth spurt thereby ameliorating scoliosis and preventing excessively tall stature. Do this only under the supervision of an endocrinologist.
Contraindications:
• Congestive heart failure, asthma, diabetes for the beta-adrenergic blocking drugs
• Thromboembolic disease for the estrogen/progestogen
Precautions: Refer to manufacturer's profile of each drug.
Significant possible interactions:
Amphetamines, antihistamines, anti-diabetics, oral contraceptives
Alternative drugs: N/A

FOLLOWUP

PATIENT MONITORING
• Frequent examinations (at least twice a year) while growing, with particular attention to cardiovascular system and scoliosis
• When cardiac symptoms develop or aortic root diameter becomes > 50 mm, surgical intervention must be considered
• When lens subluxation is detected, surgical correction is possible. However a high incidence of glaucoma results, so surgery should be offered only to those who cannot be treated with corrective lenses.

POSSIBLE COMPLICATIONS
• Bacterial endocarditis
• Aortic dissection
• Aortic or mitral valve insufficiency
• Dilated cardiomyopathy
• Retinal detachment

PREVENTION/AVOIDANCE
• No prenatal diagnosis yet available
• Each child has a 50% chance of inheriting the disorder from an affected parent. Clinical manifestations are variable, however, so children may be more or less severely affected.
• Antibiotic prophylaxis for endocarditis should be prescribed for all Marfan syndrome patients with either a heart murmur or echocardiographic evidence of valvular or aortic root abnormalities

EXPECTED COURSE AND PROGNOSIS
• Life-threatening complications are cardiovascular. Before routine corrective surgery was available most Marfan syndrome patients died before reaching the age of 35.
• With appropriate surgical intervention most patients can live a normal life span

MISCELLANEOUS

ASSOCIATED CONDITIONS N/A

AGE-RELATED FACTORS
Pediatric: Early medical or surgical intervention may reduce the degree of scoliosis
Geriatric: N/A
Others: N/A

PREGNANCY Pregnant women with the Marfan syndrome need to be managed as high-risk patients, preferably with involvement of a cardiologist. The outcome is usually excellent.

SYNONYMS N/A

ICD-9-CM 759.82

SEE ALSO N/A

OTHER NOTES N/A

ABBREVIATIONS

REFERENCES
• Pyeritz, R.E., McKusick,V.A.: The Marfan Syndrome: Diagnosis and Management. N Enl J Med 300:772-777, 1979
• Scriver, R.C., et. al., (eds.): The Metabolic Basis of Inherited Disease, 6th Ed. New York, McGraw Hill, 1989

Author R. Sliman, M.D.

Mastalgia

BASICS

DESCRIPTION Chronic breast pain often occurring prior to menses. Breast pain could also be acute and caused by other problems such as breast abscess.
System(s) affected: Skin/Exocrine
Genetics: Familial tendency
Incidence/Prevalence in USA: Mild form is common; severe form is uncommon
Predominant Age: Child-bearing years
Predominant Sex: Female only

SIGNS AND SYMPTOMS
• Breasts aching, heavy, or tender
• Enlarged breasts

CAUSES
• Associated with fibrocystic breast disease and premenstrual syndrome
• Hormonal influences
• Possibly related to fatty acid metabolism or prolactin

RISK FACTORS
• Caffeine consumption
• High fat diet

DIAGNOSIS

DIFFERENTIAL DIAGNOSIS
• The major alternate disease to consider is breast cancer
• Consider investigating for hypothyroidism
• Manipulation or trauma can also make symptoms worse
• Chest-wall pain must also be differentiated from mastalgia
• Often concurrent with premenstrual syndrome

LABORATORY No relevant findings
Drugs that may alter lab results: N/A
Disorders that may alter lab results: N/A

PATHOLOGICAL FINDINGS Fibrocystic changes

SPECIAL TESTS
• Possibly TSH
• Prolactin if galactorrhea

IMAGING Mammography to differentiate from breast cancer

DIAGNOSTIC PROCEDURES
• Cysts may need to be aspirated for symptom relief and diagnostic verification
• Biopsies may be indicated based on exam or mammography

TREATMENT

APPROPRIATE HEALTH CARE
Outpatient

GENERAL MEASURES
• Repeat examination within 30 days will help establish any cyclic nodularity pattern
• Good support bra
• Reassurance (this is sufficient for most women)
• Weight reduction, if obese

ACTIVITY No restrictions

DIET
• Decreased caffeine
• Decreased fat intake to 20% of total calories

PATIENT EDUCATION
• Explain that breast pain does not mean the patient has cancer
• Explain relationship to menses

MEDICATIONS

DRUG(S) OF CHOICE
• No drugs are needed unless required by severely painful symptoms. Reassurance, acetaminophen or ibuprofen may be all that is needed. (Future drugs - gonadotropin releasing hormone agonist.)
Agents often used, whose value has been questioned:
◊ Diuretics (usually spironolactone) prior to menses
◊ Vitamin B6 50 mg bid
◊ Vitamin E 600 IU/day
◊ Evening primrose oil (includes high content of fatty acids)
◊ Oral contraceptives may help some patients
Other possibilities for refractory patients, used infrequently because of potential side effects:
◊ Danazol 100 mg bid (possibly lower doses) - this may be the most effective. Major side effects - menstrual irregularities, weight gain, acne, hirsutism and voice change.
◊ Bromocriptine 2.5-5.0 mg/day. Major side effects - nausea, dizziness, orthostatic hypotension.
◊ Tamoxifen 10 mg/day. Major side effects - cataracts, hepatocellular carcinoma.
Contraindications: Refer to manufacturer's profile of each drug
Precautions: Refer to manufacturer's profile of each drug
Significant possible interactions: Refer to manufacturer's profile of each drug

ALTERNATIVE DRUGS   N/A

FOLLOWUP

PATIENT MONITORING
• As needed for patients not on prescription medications
• Time of followup will vary by type of prescription medication and patient problems

PREVENTION/AVOIDANCE   See Risk factors

POSSIBLE COMPLICATIONS   N/A

EXPECTED COURSE AND PROGNOSIS
• Premenstrual mastalgia increases with age, then generally stops at menopause
• Most patients will have control of symptoms without hormonal treatment
• Patients of hormonal treatment are likely to continue to need it for years

MISCELLANEOUS

ASSOCIATED CONDITIONS
Premenstrual syndrome

AGE-RELATED FACTORS
Pediatric: N/A
Geriatric: N/A
Others: N/A

PREGNANCY   N/A

SYNONYMS
• Mastodynia
• Breast pain

ICD-9-CM   611.71 mastalgia

SEE ALSO   N/A

OTHER NOTES
• Effects of long-term hormonal treatment are unknown
• If other treatment fails, a final possibility is subcutaneous mastectomy (used rarely)
• Oophorectomy also provides relief and may be drastic treatment for some patients

ABBREVIATIONS   N/A

REFERENCES
• Maddox, P.R. & Mansel, R.E.: Management of breast pain and nodularity. World J. Surg., 13:699-705, 1989
• Goodwin, P.J., Neelam, M. & Boyd, N.F.: Cyclical mastopathy: a critical review of therapy. Br J Surg., 75:837-844, 1988
• Nonmalignant conditions of the breast. ACOG Technical Bulletin, Number 156, June, 1991
• Gateley, C.A., Miers, M., Marisel, R.B. & Hughes, L.E.: Drug treatment for mastalgia: 17 years experience in the Cardiff Mastalgia Clinic. J Royal Soc Med. 85:12-15, 1992

Author M. Bowman, M.D.

Mastoiditis

BASICS

DESCRIPTION Inflammatory process in the mastoid air cells
• Acute mastoiditis - acute suppurative inflammatory process, typically after acute otitis media
• Chronic mastoiditis - usually associated with cholesteatoma and chronic ear disease
System(s) affected: Musculoskeletal
Genetics: No known genetic pattern
Incidence/Prevalence in USA: Unknown
Predominant age: Children, middle age
Predominant sex: Male = Female

SIGNS AND SYMPTOMS
• Otalgia
• Bulging erythematous tympanic membrane
• Post-auricular edema/mass
• Post-auricular erythema
• Post-auricular tenderness
• Protrusion of auricle
• Fever
• Increased WBC
• Clouding of mastoid air cells on plain films
• Fluid density in middle ear/mastoid air cells with or without loss of bony architecture
• Possible otorrhea if perforated tympanic membrane
• Subperiostial abscess

CAUSES
• Acute otitis media
• Inadequately treated suppurative otitis media
• Cholesteatoma
• Blockage of outflow tract of mastoid air cells (additus ad antrum)

RISK FACTORS
• Cholesteatoma
• Recurrent acute otitis media
• Immunocompromised host

DIAGNOSIS

DIFFERENTIAL DIAGNOSIS
• Post-auricular inflammatory adenopathy
• Severe external otitis
• Post auricular cellulitis
• Benign neoplasm - aneurysmal bone cyst, fibrous dysplasia
• Malignant neoplasm - rhabdomyosarcoma

LABORATORY CBC with differential - increased WBC
Drugs that may alter lab results: N/A
Disorders that may alter lab results: N/A

PATHOLOGICAL FINDINGS
• Inflammatory tissue in air cell system
• Granulation tissue
• Osteitis

SPECIAL TESTS Consider audiogram

IMAGING
• Plain mastoid films - clouding of mastoid air cells
• CT scan if complication suspected. Clouding air cells - loss of bony septation of the air cell system.

DIAGNOSTIC PROCEDURES N/A

TREATMENT

APPROPRIATE HEALTH CARE
Hospitalized during acute phase

GENERAL MEASURES
• Keep ear dry
• Frequent cleaning of ear canal under microscope to assure pressure equalization (PE) tube patency and adequate drainage of middle ear
• Myringotomy, placement of PE tube
• Culture material obtained at myringotomy
• IV antibiotics to cover the most common organisms
• If subperiosteal abscess present, it should be aspirated. If aspiration is not sufficient, incision and drainage should be performed.
• Mastoidectomy is reserved for those patients failing to respond to above measures within 18-72 hours or those with meningeal or intracranial complications
• Topical antibiotic drops are also usually used after insertion of PE tube

ACTIVITY Fully active, water precautions

DIET No special diet

PATIENT EDUCATION Griffith: Instructions for Patients; Philadelphia, W.B. Saunders Co.

MEDICATIONS

DRUG(S) OF CHOICE
IV antibiotics:
◊ Directed against most common organisms - group A beta-hemolytic strep, S. pneumonia, Hemophilus influenza
◊ In patients with cholesteatoma, consider Proteus, Bacteroides and occasional S. aureus and Pseudomonas organisms
◊ IV antibiotics for adult - ampicillin (dose: 1-2 gm q6h) or ampicillin/sulbactam (Unasyn) or cefuroxime (dose: 750 mg q 8 h) to ensure coverage of beta-lactamase producing organisms
◊ IV antibiotics for children - ampicillin (100-200 mg/kg/day divided every 6 hours) or cefuroxime (750 mg q 8 hours)
Other drugs:
◊ Topical drops - Cortisporin otic drops, gentamicin ophthalmic solution
◊ Oral antibiotic - amoxicillin/clavulanic (Augmentin)
Contraindications: Refer to manufacturer's literature
Precautions: Refer to manufacturer's literature
Significant possible interactions: Refer to manufacturer's literature

ALTERNATIVE DRUGS   N/A

FOLLOWUP

PATIENT MONITORING
• Postoperative - audiogram after acute process subsided
• Frequent cleansing of ear canal to keep PE tube patent

PREVENTION/AVOIDANCE
• Adequate antibiotic treatment for acute otitis media
• Treatment of chronic eustachian tube dysfunction (PE tubes)
• Early identification of cholesteatoma

POSSIBLE COMPLICATIONS
• Subperiosteal abscess
• Gradenigo's syndrome (sixth nerve palsy, draining ear and retro- orbital pain)
• Bezold's abscess
• Sigmoid sinus thrombosis
• Meningitis
• Intracranial abscess epidural/subdural/intraparenchymal

EXPECTED COURSE AND PROGNOSIS
• Dependent on severity of disease
• Conductive hearing loss may require reconstructive surgery
• Expect to avoid complications with early treatment

MISCELLANEOUS

ASSOCIATED CONDITIONS   N/A

AGE-RELATED FACTORS
Pediatric: N/A
Geriatric: N/A
Others: N/A

PREGNANCY   N/A

SYNONYMS   N/A

ICD-9-CM
• 383.9 coalescent mastoiditis
• 383.00 acute or subacute mastoiditis
• 383.02 acute with Gradenigo's syndrome
• 383.02 acute with petrositis
• 383.01 acute with subperiosteal abscess

SEE ALSO   N/A

OTHER NOTES   N/A

ABBREVIATIONS   PE = pressure equalization

REFERENCES Paparella, M.M., Shumrick, D.A., et al. (eds.): Otolaryngology. 4th Ed. Philadelphia, W.B. Saunders Co., 1991

Author S. McMenomey, M.D. & L. Howell, M.D.

Measles, rubella

BASICS

DESCRIPTION An endemic and epidemic viral exanthematous infection of children and adults, worldwide in distribution. Many infections are subclinical, but this virus can potentially cause fetal infection with resultant birth defects.

System(s) affected: Nervous, Skin/Exocrine

Genetics: Children with congenital rubella syndrome and children with insulin dependent diabetes mellitus share a high frequency of HLA-DR3 histocompatibility antigen and a high prevalence of islet cell antibodies

Incidence/Prevalence in USA:
• Before rubella vaccine was introduced in 1969, epidemics occurred at 6-9 year intervals. Sporadic outbreaks continue to occur in hospitals, colleges, prisons, prenatal clinics and isolated religious communities.
• In 1992, the incidence of postnatal rubella was 0.06 cases per 100,000 population.

Predominant age: Children 5-9 years of age

Predominant sex: Male = Female

SIGNS AND SYMPTOMS

Postnatal rubella
◊ Adenopathy - posterior auricular, posterior cervical, suboccipital
◊ Low-grade fever
◊ Exanthem - descending, maculopapular, may desquamate
◊ Enanthem - soft palate petechiae (Forschheimer's sign)
◊ Conjunctivitis
◊ Splenomegaly, rarely
◊ Coryza
◊ Malaise
◊ Headache
◊ Polyarthralgia/polyarthritis, especially in young women
◊ Asymptomatic (25%-50%)
Congenital rubella: (T=Transient, P=Permanent, D=Developmental)
◊ Cataracts (P)
◊ Microphthalmia (P)
◊ Chorioretinitis (P)
◊ Patent ductus arteriosis (P)
◊ Pulmonic stenosis (P,D)
◊ Atrial and ventricular septal defects (P)
◊ Sensorineural deafness (P,D)
◊ Microcephaly (P)
◊ Meningoencephalitis (T)
◊ Mental retardation (P,D)
◊ Low birth weight (T)
◊ Purpuric ("blueberry muffin") skin lesions (T)
◊ Radiolucent bone disease (T)
◊ Hepatosplenomegaly (T)
◊ Large anterior fontanelle (T)
◊ Language and behavior disorders (P,D)
◊ Cryptorchidism (P)
◊ Inguinal hernia (P)

CAUSES Rubella virus is a single-stranded RNA virus in the togavirus family. Travelling via airborne droplets of nasopharyngeal secretions, the virus replicates in the nasopharynx and regional lymph nodes during a 16-18 day incubation period. After invading the bloodstream, it may spread to skin and other distal organs or, transplacentally, to the developing fetus. Fetal viremia may then produce disseminated fetal infection. Organogenesis occurs 2 to 6 weeks postconception, so that infection is a maximum hazard (40-80% risk) to heart and eyes at that time. During the second trimester, the fetus develops increasing immunologic competence, making it less susceptible (10% risk) to the effects of intrauterine infection.

RISK FACTORS
• Inadequate immunization
• Immunodeficiency states
• Immunosuppressive therapy
• Pregnancy
• Crowded living conditions
• School, day care
• Late winter, spring seasons

DIAGNOSIS

DIFFERENTIAL DIAGNOSIS
Postnatal rubella
◊ Measles virus (rubeola)
◊ Scarlet fever
◊ Infectious mononucleosis
◊ Toxoplasmosis
◊ Roseola infantum (exanthem subitum)
◊ Erythema infectiosum (fifth disease)
◊ Drug eruptions
◊ Other exanthematous enteroviral infections
Congenital rubella
◊ Cytomegalovirus
◊ Varicella-zoster virus
◊ Picornaviruses (Coxsackie virus, echovirus)
◊ Poliovirus
◊ Herpes simplex virus
◊ Western equine virus
◊ Measles virus (rubeola)
◊ Hepatitis B virus
◊ Mumps virus
◊ Influenza virus
◊ Toxoplasmosis
◊ Congenital syphilis
◊ Malaria

LABORATORY
Postnatal rubella
◊ Mild leukopenia with relative lymphocytosis
◊ Fourfold rise in serum levels of antibody to rubella virus
◊ Pharynx, nose and blood culture positivity to rubella virus
Congenital rubella
◊ Presence of rubella-specific IgM antibody in serum up to one year of age, at which time, IgG becomes the dominant antibody
◊ Isolation of rubella virus from pharynx, blood, urine, cerebrospinal fluid

Drugs that may alter lab results: N/A

Disorders that may alter lab results: After re-exposure to rubella, a person with a low level of antibody from past infection or vaccination may experience an acute rise in antibody. This is not associated with a high incidence of contagion to others nor of fetal risk.

PATHOLOGICAL FINDINGS
• Inhibition of cellular growth after infection
• Fetal vasculitis
• Placental angiopathy
• Tissue necrosis

SPECIAL TESTS Cell-mediated immune responses (CMI) are impaired selectively in children with congenital rubella

IMAGING N/A

DIAGNOSTIC PROCEDURES Congenital rubella has been diagnosed by placental biopsy at 12 weeks

TREATMENT

APPROPRIATE HEALTH CARE
Outpatient usually

GENERAL MEASURES
• Postnatal rubella - mild and self-limited. Treat for symptomatic relief.
• Congenital rubella - supportive, unless neurologic or hemorrhagic complications develop

ACTIVITY
• For postnatal rubella - contact isolation for 7 days after onset of rash, bedrest is not necessary
• Contact isolation of congenitally infected infants for one year, unless nasopharyngeal and urine cultures after 3 months of age are negative for rubella virus

DIET No special diet

PATIENT EDUCATION Make every effort to avoid exposing infected patient to pregnant women

MEDICATIONS

DRUG(S) OF CHOICE Acetaminophen for fever every 4 hours if needed - 10-15 mg/kg/dose
Contraindications: N/A
Precautions: N/A
Significant possible interactions: N/A

ALTERNATIVE DRUGS None

FOLLOWUP

PATIENT MONITORING
• Persons immune to rubella via natural infection or vaccine may be reinfected when re-exposed. This infection is usually asymptomatic and detectable only by serologic means.
• In congenital rubella, it is extremely important to detect auditory and visual impairment early, so that adequate education and counselling can begin

PREVENTION/AVOIDANCE
Rubella vaccine
  ◊ Alone, can be given at ≥ 12 months. In combination with measles and mumps vaccine (MMR), administer at ≥ 15 months. Second dose of MMR recommended at age 6-12 years.
  ◊ Recommended for susceptible individuals in the following groups: Prepubertal boys and girls, premarital or postpartum women, college students, day care personnel, health care workers, military personnel
  ◊ It is contraindicated in: Pregnancy, immunodeficiency or immunocompromised state (except HIV), receipt within the last 3 months of immunoglobulin (IG) or blood, severe febrile illness, or hypersensitivity to vaccine components
  ◊ Persons who receive rubella vaccine do not transmit rubella to others, although the virus can be isolated from the pharynx

POSSIBLE COMPLICATIONS
Postnatal rubella
  ◊ Postinfectious encephalitis (1/5,000 cases)
  ◊ Thrombocytopenic purpura (1/3,000 cases)
  ◊ Testicular pain
  ◊ Mild hepatitis
Congenital rubella
  ◊ Spontaneous abortion
  ◊ Stillbirth
  ◊ Premature delivery
  ◊ Progressive rubella panencephalitis
  ◊ Endocrine disturbances (diabetes, thyrotoxicosis, hypothyroidism)
Rubella vaccine
  ◊ Lymphadenopathy
  ◊ Fever
  ◊ Rash
  ◊ Arthritis/arthralgia (older girls, women)
  ◊ Polyneuropathy

EXPECTED COURSE AND PROGNOSIS
Postnatal rubella
  ◊ Fever, 1-2 days
  ◊ Rash, 3 days
  ◊ Coryza, 5 days
  ◊ Lymphadenopathy, 1 week
  ◊ Arthralgia (when present), 2 weeks
  ◊ Complete and full recovery without sequelae is the rule
Congenital rubella
  ◊ Varied and unpredictable spectrum of consequences, ranging from stillbirth to completely normal infancy and childhood
  ◊ Disease characterized by chronic infection; infants may remain contagious for months after birth
  ◊ Detectable levels of hemagglutination-inhibiting antibody (IgG) persist for years, then may decline. By age 5, 20% have no detectable antibody.
  ◊ Overall mortality 10%; greatest during first 6 months
  ◊ 70% of those with encephalitis develop residual neuromotor defects, including an autistic syndrome
  ◊ Prognosis is excellent when only minor defects are present

MISCELLANEOUS

ASSOCIATED CONDITIONS N/A

AGE-RELATED FACTORS
Pediatric:
• Postnatal rubella is a milder disease in children than it is in adults
• Adolescents and young adults currently account for about 60% of all new cases
Geriatric: N/A
Others: N/A

PREGNANCY
• Women vaccinated against rubella are advised not to become pregnant for at least 3 months after receiving the vaccine
• The vaccine-type virus can cross the placenta. However, no case of congenital rubella has ever occurred in newborns of women who were inadvertently vaccinated while pregnant.
• The minimal fetal risk in women "accidentally" vaccinated while pregnant does not mandate automatic termination of a pregnancy
• If a pregnant woman is exposed to rubella (native disease, not vaccine associated), an immediate antibody titer should be obtained. Presence of antibody means that the woman is immune and not at risk. If antibody is not detectable, a second titer should be obtained 3 weeks later. If antibody is present in the second specimen, infection has occurred. If antibody is again negative, a third titer should be obtained in 3 more weeks (6 weeks after exposure). At this time, a negative test means that infection has not occurred; a positive test means that infection did occur, and that the fetus is at risk for congenital rubella.
• The use of commercially available human immunoglobulin (gamma globulin) in prophylaxis of rubella during pregnancy does not prevent rubella or the congenital rubella syndrome in a predictable or reliable fashion

SYNONYMS
• German measles
• Three-day measles

ICD-9-CM
• Uncomplicated postnatal rubella, 056.9
• Postnatal rubella with specific complications, 056.XX
• Congenital rubella syndrome, 771.0

SEE ALSO
• Measles, rubeola

OTHER NOTES   N/A

ABBREVIATIONS   N/A

REFERENCES
• Committee on Infectious Diseases, Elk Grove, Illinois, AAP Red Book, ed. 22, 1991
• Mandell, G.L. (ed.): Principles and Practice of Infectious Diseases. 3rd Ed. New York, Churchill Livingstone, 1990
• Rudolph, A.M. (ed): Rudolph's Pediatrics 19th Ed. Norwalk, CT, Appleton & Lange 1991

Author   R. Viken, M.D.

Measles, rubeola

BASICS

DESCRIPTION An acute epidemic viral exanthem which classically presents as a confluent erythematous maculopapular rash which begins over the head and spreads inferiorly to involve the trunk and extremities. The rash is preceded by the triad of cough, coryza, and conjunctivitis plus a pathognomonic enanthem (Koplik's spots).
System(s) affected: Skin/Exocrine
Genetics: N/A
Incidence in USA: Number of cases has recently increased - 1990: 27,786 cases; 1991: 9643 cases
Prevalence in USA:
• 1990 - 11/100,000
• 1991 - 3.82/100,000
Predominant Age: Recent outbreaks have primarily involved unvaccinated preschool-age children in large urban areas (including children less than 15 months) and adolescents and young adults (most of whom were previously vaccinated) in secondary schools and college
Predominant sex: Male = Female

SIGNS AND SYMPTOMS
Incubation period:
  ◊ 9-11 days from exposure to symptoms
  ◊ 14 days average to onset of rash
Prodromal period:
  ◊ Lasts 2-4 days
  ◊ Classic triad (brassy cough, coryza, and conjunctivitis)
  ◊ Fever
  ◊ Malaise
  ◊ Photophobia
  ◊ Enanthem (Koplik's spots) - minute, whitish spots over buccal/labial mucosa; number rapidly increases and these coalesce. Underlying mucosa bright red and granular, spots appear 2 days before rash and resolve within 3 days after onset of rash.
Exanthem period:
  ◊ Begins behind ears and at hairline
  ◊ Spreads centrifugally from head to feet
  ◊ Red, morbilliform, blanching rash
  ◊ Discrete lesions become confluent
  ◊ Confluence more prominent over upper body
  ◊ Clearing begins after 3-4 days
  ◊ Rash becomes coppery and nonblanching
  ◊ Fever resolves 2-3 days after onset of rash
  ◊ Pharyngitis
  ◊ Lymphadenopathy
  ◊ Croup, vomiting, and diarrhea (in young children)
  ◊ Patients contagious from 2 days before symptoms to 4 days after onset of rash
Modified illness:
  ◊ Attenuated measles in partially immune patient
  ◊ Secondary prior immune globulin, transplacental measles antibody, live vaccine failure

Atypical measles:
  ◊ Most cases secondary to natural infection following vaccination with killed vaccine (available in U.S. 1963-68 and in Canada until 1975)
  ◊ Maculopapular rash begins distally and spreads centrally
  ◊ Rash frequently is petechial, purpuric, or urticarial
  ◊ Pulmonary involvement in all cases

CAUSES Single antigenic type of a RNA morbillivirus in the paramyxovirus family

RISK FACTORS
• Not being vaccinated
• Exposure to infected person

DIAGNOSIS

DIFFERENTIAL DIAGNOSIS
Typical measles:
  ◊ Any erythematous maculopapular rash
Exanthems secondary to:
  ◊ Drug eruptions
  ◊ Infectious mononucleosis
  ◊ Mycoplasma pneumoniae
  ◊ Rubella
  ◊ Erythema infectiosum
  ◊ Roseola
  ◊ Enteroviruses
Atypical measles:
  ◊ Rocky mountain spotted fever
  ◊ Drug eruptions
  ◊ Anaphylactoid purpura
  ◊ Mycoplasma pneumoniae infection

LABORATORY
• Viral isolation in tissue culture
• Detection of measles antigen in exfoliative cells by immunofluorescence
• Demonstration of measles specific IgM or substantial rise in IgG tilers between acute and convalescent sera
Drugs that may alter lab results:
Immunosuppressive agents which may impair rise in specific antibody titers
Disorders that may alter lab results:
• Primary (severe combined immunodeficiency [SCID], etc.)
• Acquired immune deficiencies (HIV-I infection, cancer chemotherapy)

PATHOLOGICAL FINDINGS
Multinucleated giant cells
  ◊ Reticuloendothelial types (Warthin-Finkeldey) in lymphoid tissues
  ◊ Epithelial syncytial giant cells in skin, and respiratory mucosa
  ◊ Damaged respiratory ciliated epithelium

SPECIAL TESTS N/A

IMAGING Pneumonia frequent; detected on radiologic exam

DIAGNOSTIC PROCEDURES N/A

TREATMENT

APPROPRIATE HEALTH CARE
Outpatient except when complications develop (encephalitis, pneumonitis)

GENERAL MEASURES Symptomatic therapy (i.e., antipyretics, antitussives, humidification, encourage oral fluids)

ACTIVITY Restricted during febrile phase

DIET No special diet

PATIENT EDUCATION Avoid exposure to other children and potential secondary bacterial pathogens until respiratory symptoms resolve

MEDICATIONS

DRUG(S) OF CHOICE
• No proven specific antiviral agent is available
• Antipyretics, if necessary
• Antibiotics if there are secondary bacterial infections
• Antitussives
Contraindications: N/A
Precautions: N/A
Significant possible interactions: N/A

ALTERNATIVE DRUGS N/A

FOLLOWUP

PATIENT MONITORING Not required unless complications develop

PREVENTION/AVOIDANCE
• For a comprehensive discussion of the complete indications and contraindications for measles vaccine use and control of measles outbreaks, see first listing in References
<u>Postexposure prophylaxis</u>
◊ Vaccine use - protective if given within 72 hours postexposure
◊ Immune globulin (IG) - prevents/modifies illness if given within 6 days postexposure. Dose - usually 0.25 mL/kg IM (for immunocompromised children 0.5 mL/kg IM) not to exceed 15 mL.
<u>Active immunization:</u>
◊ Moraten Strain Vaccine - only currently licensed vaccine available as monovalent vaccine or in combination with mumps and rubella i.e., measles and rubella (MR); measles, mumps and rubella (MMR)
◊ Primary vaccination: Two doses of vaccine; 1st MMR at 15 months, 2nd at 6-12 years. Need for 2nd dose necessitated by recent outbreaks among adolescents and young adults.
<u>Adverse events associated with vaccination (occur in < 5%):</u>
◊ Fever
◊ Transient rashes
◊ Convulsions (most likely febrile)
◊ Encephalitis (incidence post-measles vaccination [<1/106 vaccine doses] is lower than the incidence of idiopathic encephalitis in the United States, hence post-vaccination encephalitis may be temporally and not casually related).

POSSIBLE COMPLICATIONS
<u>Measles infection (not associated with vaccination):</u>
◊ Otitis media (most common)
◊ Laryngotracheitis
◊ Broncopneumonia, viral (Hecht's or giant cell pneumonitis) or bacterial in origin
◊ Encephalitis (incidence - 1 per 1000)
◊ Hemorrhagic lesions ("Black measles") of skin and bowel
◊ Thrombocytopenic purpura
◊ Mesenteric adenitis
◊ Myocarditis and pericarditis
◊ Subacute sclerosing panencephalitis - secondary to persistent infection following natural disease (disappearing as a result of mass vaccination)

EXPECTED COURSE AND PROGNOSIS Self-limited, prognosis good

MISCELLANEOUS

ASSOCIATED CONDITIONS
• Primary measles in an immunosuppressed patient with leukemia or symptomatic HIV-1 infection may present with or without a rash and giant cell pneumonitis
• Increased mortality with malnutrition
• Possible reactivation of latent tuberculosis secondary to measles

AGE-RELATED FACTORS
Pediatric: Infants have higher rate of complications than older children
Geriatric: N/A
Others: N/A

PREGNANCY Increased fetal morbidity and mortality with infection during pregnancy

SYNONYMS
• Rubeola
• Red measles
• Hard measles
• Ten-day measles

ICD-9-CM 055.9

SEE ALSO Rubella

OTHER NOTES N/A

ABBREVIATIONS N/A

REFERENCES
• Measles. In Report of the Committee on Infectious Diseases, 277-289, American Academy of Pediatrics, 1991
• Measles Prevention: Recommendations of the Immunization Practices Advisory Committee (ACIP). Morbidity and Mortality Weekly Report, Recommendations and Reports. 1989, 38 (S-9):1-13
• Cherry, J.: Measles. In Textbook of Pediatric Infectious Diseases. Edited by R. Feigin & J. Cherry. Philadelphia, W.B. Saunders Co., 1987

Author C. Mitchell, M.D.

Melanoma

 BASICS

DESCRIPTION Malignant degeneration of cells from the melanocytic system. The overwhelming majority of melanoma arises in the skin, but it may also present as a primary lesion in any tissue pigmentation. Metastatic spread may be to any region in the body.

System(s) affected: Skin/Exocrine

Genetics:
• The only genetic predisposition is in the familial dysplastic nevus syndrome. If the family history of a person with dysplastic nevus syndrome includes one relative with melanoma, then the risk of developing melanoma is 100%.
• Skin pigmentation is the only other risk factor transmitted genetically

Incidence/Prevalence in USA:
• 4.5/100,000 people in the USA
• Estimated year 1992, 32,000 cases, 6,700 deaths
• Estimated year 2000, 1 in 75 persons then living will eventually die of malignant melanoma

Predominant age: A median age is 53 with the highest annual incidence rate of any cancer in whites between the ages of 25-29 and in white males between 35-39

Predominant sex: Male = Female

SIGNS AND SYMPTOMS Any change in a pigmented lesion including hypo- or hyperpigmentation, bleeding, scaling, size change, texture change

CAUSES Under investigation. Probably radiation in the ultraviolet B range.

RISK FACTORS
• Adulthood
• Previous pigmented lesions (especially dysplastic nevi)
• Fair complexioned, freckling, blue eyes and blond hair
• Twice the risk in persons with adolescent blistering sunburn, family history of previous melanoma, congenital nevi

 DIAGNOSIS

DIFFERENTIAL DIAGNOSIS
• Dysplastic nevi
• Vascular skin tumors
• Pigmented squamous cell and basal cell carcinomas, seborrheic keratoses, other changing nevi. It follows the ABCDE mnemonic which stands for 1) asymmetry, 2) border irregularity, 3) color variegation, and 4) diameter great than 6 millimeters with the location on whites being primarily back and lower leg, and on African Americans being hands, feet, and nails, 5) elevation above skin surface.

LABORATORY N/A
Drugs that may alter lab results: N/A
Disorders that may alter lab results: N/A

PATHOLOGICAL FINDINGS
Gross pathologic features include four clinical types:
◊ Superficial spreading melanoma - 70% of all cases
◊ Nodular - 15% of all cases
◊ Acral lentiginous - 2-8% of all cases
◊ Lentigo-maligna - 4-10% of all cases
◊ Note: Nodular melanoma is primarily vertical growth while the other three types are horizontal

SPECIAL TESTS The only special tests that exist for melanoma are those designed to follow metastatic disease

IMAGING Imaging studies are of benefit only in detecting metastatic disease which is usually to the brain, lymph nodes and lungs

DIAGNOSTIC PROCEDURES Surgical biopsy is the only form of appropriate diagnostic procedure

 TREATMENT

APPROPRIATE HEALTH CARE
Outpatient or inpatient surgery

GENERAL MEASURES
• The appropriate health care for melanoma is surgical excision. Much debate exists as to the extent of the margins of excision once diagnosis has been made. The tendency now is toward margins of 1 cm if the lesion is less than 2 mm thick. If thicker, then margins can be extended to 3 cm. Regional lymph node dissection is of questionable benefit.
• The key to the cure of melanoma is prevention: Avoidance of blistering solar radiation and the use of a sunscreen when exposure is unavoidable

ACTIVITY Avoid sun exposure

DIET No restrictions

PATIENT EDUCATION
• It is critical that a patient with melanoma or dysplastic nevi syndrome has frequent total body examinations for any abnormal appearing or changing nevi
• National Cancer Institute, Dept. of Health And Human Services, Public Inquiries Section, Office of Cancer Communications, Building 31, Room 101-18, 9000 Rockville Pike, Bethesda, MD 20892, (301)496-5583

MEDICATIONS

DRUG(S) OF CHOICE
• There is no clear choice in the chemotherapy of malignant melanoma
• Adjuvant chemotherapy has included bacillus Calmette-Guérin (BCG) and levamisole
• Standard chemotherapy includes dacarbazine and cisplatin
• Adoptive immunotherapy with leukapheresis and IL-2 with LAK's (under investigation)
Contraindications: Refer to manufacturer's literature
Precautions:
• Dacarbazine - myelosuppression, alopecia
• Cisplatin - severe nausea/vomiting, renal tubular damage, ototoxicity, peripheral neuropathies, hypokalemia, and hypomagnesemia
Significant possible interactions: Refer to manufacturer's literature

ALTERNATIVE DRUGS
Many have been tried, none successfully

FOLLOWUP

PATIENT MONITORING
• Current recommendations after diagnosis of malignant melanoma are skin exams every 3-6 months
• Chemical screens, liver function tests, and CT scans of the brain should be followed regularly (debated)
• The patient should conduct his/her own skin examinations on a weekly basis. They must be thorough.

PREVENTION/AVOIDANCE
Avoidance of burning solar exposures and the use of sunscreens is critical. Those at high risk should do all they can to avoid sunburn especially during the adolescent years.

POSSIBLE COMPLICATIONS
• Metastatic spread
• Unsatisfactory cosmetic results following the primary surgery

EXPECTED COURSE AND PROGNOSIS
• Prognosis is entirely based on staging of the initial lesion
Staging (falls into two categories)
◊ Breslow: This shows a 70% five-year survival of all patients who have no local or distant lymphatic spread.
◊ Clark's staging depends on depth of invasion by skin layer. The best prognosis is for those lesions which are less than .85 mm which carry 95-100% five-year survival. Spread to lymphatics or regional lymph nodes carries less than a 5% five-year survival.

MISCELLANEOUS

ASSOCIATED CONDITIONS
As above

AGE-RELATED FACTORS
Pediatric: Rarely seen in pediatric age group
Geriatric: Lentigo maligna is most commonly seen in elderly patients who have had a slowly enlarging pigmented lesion, usually found on the face
Others: The most recent data on melanoma indicates that its highest incidence is between ages 30-50. However, it can occur at any age.

PREGNANCY
• Due to the facts that melanocyte-stimulating hormone (MSH) levels are markedly increased during pregnancy and that melanoma is one of the few carcinomas that can spread to the placenta, concern has been that pregnancy exacerbates melanoma. This has been neither proven nor disproven.
• If a person has had recent melanoma, many authors suggest waiting at least two years if further pregnancy is desired
• If invasion extends into the lymphatic structures, then further pregnancy is probably contraindicated
• If pregnancy occurs during metastatic melanoma, then there is clear risk to the fetus

SYNONYMS
N/A

ICD-9-CM
172.9

SEE ALSO
N/A

OTHER NOTES
It is imperative for the physician to realize that any nevus or pigmented lesion that is in any way suspect should be excised. A full thickness total excisional biopsy must be sent for pathologic specimen and never to be curetted, electrodesiccated, or shaved.

ABBREVIATIONS
N/A

REFERENCES
• Koh, H.K.: Cutaneous Melanoma. N Engl J Med 1991; 325:171-182
• NIH Consensus Conference. Diagnosis and Therapy of Early Melanoma: NIH consensus development panel on early melanoma. JAMA 1992; 268:1314-19
• Cancer Facts & Figures-1992-Atlanta, GA: ACS 1991. American Cancer Society publication 92-425M-No. 5008.92-LE

Author D. Sealy, M.D.

Ménière's disease

 BASICS

DESCRIPTION An inner ear (labyrinthine) disorder in which there is an increase in volume and pressure of the inner-most fluid of the inner ear (endolymph), resulting in recurrent attacks of hearing loss, tinnitus, vertigo, and fullness
• Usually unilateral, but in 10-50% may later involve the second ear
• Severity and frequency may diminish over the years, but with increasing loss of hearing. It is not a synonym for dizziness.
System(s) affected: Nervous
Genetics: N/A
Incidence in USA: No reliable figures are available to provide comprehensive numbers for incidence and prevalence by age and sex, but using incidence figures from a Swedish study conducted in 1973, it is estimated that the incidence of Ménière's disease in the US is 46 (new cases/100,000/year). No figures for sex and age are available, but the disease is relatively equal in males and females, and is extremely rare in children.
Prevalence in USA: Using extrapolation, the estimated prevalence is 1,150 (cases/100,000 population).
Predominant age: Usual age of onset 20-60
Predominant sex: Male = Female

SIGNS AND SYMPTOMS
• Hearing loss - low frequency, fluctuating
• Vertigo - spontaneous attacks, duration 20 minutes to several hours
• Ear fullness
• Occurs as attacks, with intervening remission
During severe attacks
  ◊ Pallor
  ◊ Sweating
  ◊ Nausea and vomiting
  ◊ Falling
  ◊ Prostration
  ◊ All symptoms aggravated by motion
  ◊ Between attacks may experience motion-related imbalance without vertigo

CAUSES
• Unknown. Best theory is inner ear response to variety of injuries (reduced middle ear pressure, allergy, endocrine disease, lipid disorders, vascular, viral, luetic).
• Recent theory is intracranial compression of balance nerve by blood vessel

RISK FACTORS
• Caucasian
• Stress
• Allergy
• Increased salt intake
• Noise

 DIAGNOSIS

DIFFERENTIAL DIAGNOSIS
• Acoustic tumor
• Syphilis
• Perilymph fistula
• Multiple sclerosis
• Viral labyrinthitis
• Vertebro-basilar disease
• Other labyrinthine disorders producing same symptoms (Cogan's syndrome, benign positional vertigo, temporal bone trauma)

LABORATORY
• Lab studies done to rule out other conditions
• Serologic tests specific for Treponema pallidum - microhemagglutination (MHA), fluorescent treponemal antibody (FTA), Treponema immobilization test (TPI)
• Thyroid studies
• Lipid studies
Drugs that may alter lab results: Any medication that produces a significant degree of sedation is likely to affect vestibular testing and invalidate it
Disorders that may alter lab results: Many conditions may produce auditory and vestibular findings identical to those associated with Ménière's disease, making it a diagnosis of exclusion. A low frequency sensorineural hearing loss (nerve loss as opposed to conductive loss) is seen on audiometry, and a reduced caloric response on caloric testing is usual.

PATHOLOGICAL FINDINGS
Autopsy only. Shows dilation of inner ear fluid system (endolymph).

SPECIAL TESTS
• Otoscopy with air pressure applied to the tympanic membrane
Auditory
  ◊ Hearing test (audiometry using pure tone and speech) to show low frequency sensorineural [nerve] loss and impaired speech discrimination
  ◊ Tuning fork test (Weber and Rinne) to confirm validity of audiometry
  ◊ Auditory Brainstem Response audiometry (ABR) to rule out acoustic neuroma
Vestibular
  ◊ Spontaneous nystagmus (rapid rhythmic eye motion) seen visually. Must avoid eye fixation by having patient use 40 diopter glasses for test.
  ◊ Caloric testing - electronystagmography (ENG) may show reduced caloric response. Can obtain reasonably comparable information with use of 0.8 cc ice water instilled in ear canal, then noting duration and frequency of resulting nystagmus with 40 diopter lenses in place. Reduced activity on either side is consistent with Ménière's diagnosis, but is not diagnostic.

IMAGING MRI to rule out acoustic tumor, which can produce identical symptoms and findings

DIAGNOSTIC PROCEDURES N/A

 TREATMENT

APPROPRIATE HEALTH CARE Can usually be managed in outpatient setting. Inpatient for surgery.

GENERAL MEASURES
• Medications are given primarily for symptomatic relief of vertigo and nausea. There is no medication available that influences the disease process.
• For attacks, bedrest with eyes closed and protection from falling. Attacks rarely last longer than four hours.
• Streptomycin therapy for bilateral Ménière's disease, when conventional management has failed. Streptomycin may be administered over a period of several days or weeks intentionally to damage the neuro-epithelium of the balance centers and reduce their function. Hearing must be carefully monitored during this time so that the treatment does not proceed to the point of damaging the hearing structures. This form of treatment should be administered only by an otolaryngologist and after careful patient education.
Surgery:
  ◊ Hearing good: Endolymphatic sac surgery, either (1) decompression or (2) drainage of endolymph into mastoid or subarachnoid space. Alternative procedure is to cut the vestibular nerve (intracranial procedure).
  ◊ Hearing poor, but usable: Can do sac procedure or nerve section depending on quality of hearing. For poor hearing, can decompress cochlea (cochleocentesis), or perfuse cochlea with streptomycin.
  ◊ Hearing not useful: Destruction of inner ear (labyrinthectomy)

ACTIVITY
• Limit activity during attacks
• Between attacks patient may be fully active, but this may be limited by (1) fear of impending attack, (2) unsteadiness following attacks, (3) ear fullness or tinnitus, or (4) hearing loss in involved ear that may severely limit the patient's ability to perform work duties or to participate in social life

DIET Limit total intake during attacks because of nausea. Otherwise diet is usually not a factor unless attacks are brought on by certain foods. A restricted salt diet may be useful in some cases.

PATIENT EDUCATION Many otolaryngologists keep booklets on Ménière's disease as handouts. Ask your otolaryngology consultant for a supply.

MEDICATIONS

DRUG(S) OF CHOICE
<u>Acute attack. For severe episode, one of the following may be used. Adult doses are indicated</u>
◊ Atropine 0.2-0.4 mg IV
◊ Diazepam (Valium) 5-10 mg IV slowly
◊ Transderm scopolamine, 1 patch, or smaller segment of patch, applied to skin surface and not replaced sooner than 3 days
<u>Maintenance. Adult doses are indicated (frequently must be reduced to avoid sedating effects)</u>
◊ Meclizine (Antivert, Bonine) 25-100 mg orally, either at bedtime or in divided doses
◊ Bellergal Spacetabs, one q 12 hr
◊ Diazepam (Valium), 2 mg (or less) tid
Contraindications:
• Atropine - cardiac disease, especially supraventricular tachycardia and other arrhythmias
• Scopolamine - children and elderly
Precautions:
• Sedating drugs should be used with caution, particularly in elderly people. The need to reduce the dosage is common. Patients should be cautioned not to operate motor vehicles when they are sedated.
• Atropine, scopolamine, and Bellergal should be used with particular caution. If not prescribed frequently, refer to manufacturer's literature.
Significant possible interactions:
• Bellergal - oral anticoagulants, tricyclic antidepressants, phenothiazines, narcotics, beta blockers, estrogens, and others
• Transderm scopolamine - anticholinergics, belladonna products, antihistamines, tricyclic antidepressants, and others

ALTERNATIVE DRUGS
<u>Acute attack</u>
◊ Droperidol, 1.5-2.5 mg IV slowly (in hospital setting)
◊ Promethazine (Phenergan) 12.5-25 mg IV slowly
◊ Diphenhydramine HCl (Benadryl) 50 mg IV slowly
◊ Carbogen (5% carbon dioxide and 95% oxygen) by mask from tank
<u>Maintenance</u>
◊ Dimenhydrinate (Dramamine) 50 mg q 4-6 hr po
◊ Promethazine (Phenergan) 12.5-25 mg q 4-6 hr po
◊ Diphenidol (Vontrol) 25-50 mg tid po
◊ Diphenhydramine HCl (Benadryl), 25-50 mg q 6-8 hr po. Maximum, 100 mg/24 hours
◊ Chlorothiazide (Diuril) 500 mg daily po with potassium supplement

FOLLOWUP

PATIENT MONITORING
The most common complaint by Ménière's patients regarding prior treatment is that the primary care physician did not take the condition seriously and that he or she didn't seem interested in providing ongoing care. Because of the emotional impact alone, these patients need close followup care. It is important to monitor the status of their hearing, since it is at risk, and to continue to consider the possibility of a more serious underlying problem such as an acoustic tumor.

PREVENTION/AVOIDANCE
• Reduce stress
• Reduce salt intake
• Don't smoke
• Avoid significant noise exposure, or use ear protectors
• Avoid use of ototoxic medications (aspirin, quinine, kanamycin, and many others)

POSSIBLE COMPLICATIONS
• Failure to diagnose acoustic neuroma
• Loss of hearing
• Injury during attack
• Inability to work

EXPECTED COURSE AND PROGNOSIS
• Alternating attacks and remission
• Over time the balance problem tends to resolve, but the hearing worsens
• The great majority of patients can be managed successfully with medication. About 5-10% of patients require surgery for incapacitating vertigo.
• Very important not to overlook acoustic tumor, which produces an identical clinical picture

MISCELLANEOUS

ASSOCIATED CONDITIONS
• Cochlear hydrops (hearing problem only)
• Vestibular hydrops (balance problem only)
• Drop attacks

AGE-RELATED FACTORS
Pediatric: Unusual, but occasional. Dizziness in children likely to be on basis of significant central nervous system disease.
Geriatric: Less likely to occur in elderly. Patients exposed to loud noise levels over many years are more susceptible.
Others: Usual onset age 20-60

PREGNANCY Not a common problem, but difficult to treat because of risk of producing fetal abnormalities with medication

SYNONYMS
• Ménière's syndrome
• Endolymphatic hydrops

ICD-9-CM 386.01

SEE ALSO N/A

OTHER NOTES N/A

ABBREVIATIONS N/A

REFERENCES
• Paparella, M.M. & Shumrick, D.A. (eds.): Otolaryngology. 2nd Ed. Philadelphia, W.B. Saunders Co., 1980. pp 1878-1889
• Schuknecht, H.F.: Ménière's Disease. In Common Problems in Otology. Edited by B.H. Britton. St. Louis, Mosby Year Book, 1991. pp 180-185

Author G. Gardner, M.D.

Meningitis, bacterial

 BASICS

DESCRIPTION Inflammation in response to bacterial infection of the pia-arachnoid and its fluid and the fluid of the ventricles. Meningitis is always cerebrospinal.
System(s) affected: Nervous
Genetics: Navajo Indian and American Eskimo may have genetic or acquired vulnerability to invasive disease
Incidence/Prevalence in USA: 3-10 cases per 100,000 population
Predominant age: Neonates, infants and geriatric aged
Predominant sex: Male = Female

SIGNS AND SYMPTOMS
• Antecedent URI
• Fever
• Headache
• Meningismus
• Signs of cerebral dysfunction
• Vomiting
• Photophobia
• Seizures
• Nausea
• Rigors
• Profuse sweats
• Weakness
• Altered mental status
• Focal neurologic deficits
• Elderly have subtle findings commonly including confusion
• Meningococcemia has rash - macular and erythematous at first, then petechial or purpuric

CAUSES
• Neonates: Escherichia coli, group B Streptococcus, Listeria monocytogenes and non-group B Streptococcus
• Infants/children: H. influenza (48%), Streptococcus pneumoniae (13%), and Neisseria meningitidis
• Adults: Streptococcus pneumoniae (30-50%), Haemophilus influenza (1-3%), Neisseria meningitidis (10-35%), Gram-negative bacilli (1-10%), Staphylococci (5-15%), Streptococci (5%) and Listeria species(5%)

RISK FACTORS
• Immunocompromised host
• Alcoholism
• Neurosurgical procedure or head injury

 DIAGNOSIS

DIFFERENTIAL DIAGNOSIS
• Bacteremia
• Sepsis
• Brain abscess
• Seizures
• Other non-bacterial meningitides

LABORATORY
• Turbid CSF
<u>Neonates</u>
◊ > 10 WBC's in CSF
◊ CSF: blood glucose ratio < 0.6
◊ CSF protein >150 mg/dL
<u>Infants/children</u>
◊ > 5 WBC's in CSF
◊ CSF: blood glucose ratio < 0.6
◊ CSF protein > 50 mg/dL
<u>Adults</u>
◊ 1000-100,000 WBC's in CSF (average 5000-20,000)
◊ CSF: blood glucose ratio < 0.4
◊ CSF protein >45 mg/dL (usually 150-400 mg/dL)
<u>In all age groups:</u>
◊ CSF opening pressure > 180 mm H20
◊ CSF gram stain + in 75% of untreated patients
◊ CSF culture + 70-80% of the time
◊ Blood culture + 40-60% of the time
◊ CSF bacterial antigen test (sensitivity varies)
Drugs that may alter lab results: N/A
Disorders that may alter lab results: N/A

PATHOLOGICAL FINDINGS N/A

SPECIAL TESTS N/A

IMAGING
• CT scan of head if concern for increased ICP
• Chest x-ray may reveal silent area of pneumonitis or abscess
• Sinus/skull x-rays may reveal cranial osteomyelitis, paranasal sinusitis or skull fracture
• Later in course, head CT scan, if hydrocephalus, brain abscess, subdural effusions or subdural empyema are considered

DIAGNOSTIC PROCEDURES Lumbar puncture

 TREATMENT

APPROPRIATE HEALTH CARE
Inpatient often with ICU. If diagnosis is suspected, lumbar puncture should be done in office with antimicrobial therapy begun before transfer to hospital.

GENERAL MEASURES
• Appropriate antibiotic therapy
• Vigorous supportive care with constant nursing to ensure prompt recognition of seizures and prevention of aspiration
• Therapy for any coexisting conditions
• Measures to prevent hypothermia and dehydration

ACTIVITY As tolerated in hospital and on discharge

DIET Regular as tolerated, except when SIADH complicates course

PATIENT EDUCATION For patient education materials on this topic, contact: American Academy of Pediatrics, 141 Northwest Point Blvd., P.O. Box 927, Elk Grove Village, IL 60009-0927, (800)433-9016

Meningitis, bacterial

 MEDICATIONS

DRUG(S) OF CHOICE Empiric therapy until culture results available (need to consider local patterns of bacterial sensitivity)
• 0 to 4 weeks - ampicillin (300–400 mg/kg/d) plus a third-generation cephalosporin (cefotaxime [200 mg/kg/d q4-6h], or ceftriaxone [100 mg/kg/d q12-24h]); or ampicillin plus an aminoglycoside (tobramycin 7.5 mg/kg/d q6-8 h prematures or infants < 1 week, 2.5 mg/kg q 12 h). 14-21 days treatment
• 4 to 12 weeks - ampicillin plus a third-generation cephalosporin. 10 days treatment (same doses as above).
• 3 months to 18 years - third generation cephalosporin; or ampicillin plus chloramphenicol(75-100mg/kg/d). 10 days treatment.
• 18 to 50 years: penicillin G(18-24 million units q4-6h) or ampicillin(12-18gm/d divided doses). 10 days treatment.
• Older than 50 years - ampicillin plus a third-generation cephalosporin (cefotaxime 2gm q4h or ceftriaxone 2gm/d). 14-21 days treatment.
Contraindications: Allergies to antibiotics
Precautions:
• Ototoxicity from aminoglycoside
• Hearing loss
• Developmental abnormalities related to meningitis
Significant Possible Interactions: Refer to manufacturer's literature

ALTERNATIVE DRUGS
• Vancomycin
• Antipseudomonal penicillins
• Aztreonam
• Quinolones

 FOLLOWUP

PATIENT MONITORING Brainstem Auditory Evoked Response (BAER) test should be done with infants prior to hospital discharge. Further followup will depend on its results and course of meningitis while in hospital.

PREVENTION/AVOIDANCE
• Prompt medical treatment for infections
• Strict aseptic techniques when treating patients with head wounds or skull fractures

POSSIBLE COMPLICATIONS
• Seizures (20-30% during course of illness)
• Focal neurologic deficit
• Cranial nerve palsies (III, VI, VII, VIII) 10-20% of cases, usually disappear within a few weeks
• Sensorineural hearing loss (10% in children)
• Neurodevelopmental sequelae (subtle learning deficits 30%)
• Obstructive hydrocephalus
• Subdural effusions

EXPECTED COURSE AND PROGNOSIS
• Overall case fatality 14%
• H. influenza 6%
• Neisseria meningitidis 10.3%
• Streptococcus pneumoniae 26.3%

 MISCELLANEOUS

ASSOCIATED CONDITIONS
Which worsen prognosis:
• Coma
• Seizures
• Alcoholism
• Old age
• Infancy
• Diabetes mellitus
• Multiple myeloma
• Head trauma

AGE-RELATED FACTORS
Pediatric: N/A
Geriatric: Several signs and symptoms may be less evident in elderly patients with other disorders (congestive heart failure, pneumonia)
Others: Different etiologic agents, antimicrobials and dosing, and CSF findings as listed above

PREGNANCY N/A

SYNONYMS N/A

ICD-9-CM 320 bacterial meningitis

SEE ALSO N/A

OTHER NOTES Adrenocortical steroids (dexamethasone) use as adjunct therapy - beneficial in decreasing overall neurologic sequelae and decrease in mortality for pneumococcal meningitis. Clinical trials still pending regarding dosage and timing of steroids.

ABBREVIATIONS N/A

REFERENCES
• Tunkel, A.R., Wispelwey, B. & Scheld, W.M.: Bacterial meningitis: Recent advances in pathophysiology and treatment. Annals of Int Med 1990;112:610-623
• Shelton, M.M. & Marks, W.A.: Bacterial meningitis: An update. Neurologic Clinics of North America 1990;8:3:605-617
• Braunwald E., et al. (eds.): Harrison's Principles of Internal Medicine. 12th Ed. New York, McGraw-Hill, 1991

Author P. Gordon, M.D.

Meningitis, viral

 BASICS

DESCRIPTION Viral infection of the meninges and spinal fluid. The usual cause is acute and may be relapsing. Peak incidence occurs in summertime.

System(s) affected: Nervous

Genetics: N/A

Incidence/Prevalence in USA: Average of 10,000 reported cases per year. Probably many more unreported.

Predominant age: May affect all ages, but most common in young adults

Predominant sex: Male = Female

SIGNS AND SYMPTOMS
- Fever
- Headache, often severe
- Stiff neck
- Nausea and vomiting
- Photophobia
- Generalized aches and pains
- Occasional rash

CAUSES
- Coxsackie A, B
- ECHO virus (enteroviruses 70-75% of all cases)
- Poliovirus
- Lymphocytic choriomeningitis (LCM)
- Mumps
- Herpes (simplex and zoster)
- Epstein-Barr virus (EBV)
- Arthropod borne viruses
- Cytomegalovirus (CMV)
- Adenovirus

RISK FACTORS
- No specifics known
- Immunocompromised hosts may be more susceptible to CMV and adenovirus

 DIAGNOSIS

DIFFERENTIAL DIAGNOSIS
- Bacterial meningitis
- Encephalitis
- Acute encephalopathy
- Postinfectious encephalomyelitis
- Parameningeal infections (e.g., subdural empyema)
- Carcinomatous meningitis
- Meningeal leukemia
- Migraine headache
- Viral syndrome (e.g., influenza)
- Chemical meningitis
- Brain abscess
- Other infectious agents (TB, syphilis, ameba, leptospirosis)

LABORATORY
- CSF pleocytosis - usually predominantly mononuclear but may show more polys early on
- CSF cell count up to 3000-4000, but usually 50-200
- CSF - increased pressure
- CSF - serum antiviral antibody
- Elevated CSF protein, but usually < 150 mg/dL
- CSF sugar usually normal
- Negative CSF gram stain and culture for bacteria
- Negative CSF latex agglutination or CIEP for bacterial antigens
- Normal or mildly elevated WBC (blood)
- Viral cultures and/or antibody titers are seldom helpful

Drugs that may alter lab results: Pretreatment with antibiotics may result in a "partially treated" bacterial meningitis, mimicking viral meningitis

Disorders that may alter lab results:
- Diabetes (alteration in spinal fluid sugar)
- Pre-existing neurologic diseases (e.g., brain tumor, demyelinating disease) could affect CSF findings

PATHOLOGICAL FINDINGS Lymphocyte infiltration of meninges and ventricles

SPECIAL TESTS EEG in some cases, especially if encephalitis is a consideration

IMAGING
- CT scan or MRI scan of the brain
- Usually CT or MRI performed prior to lumbar puncture

DIAGNOSTIC PROCEDURES Lumbar puncture

 TREATMENT

APPROPRIATE HEALTH CARE
- Usually inpatient, depending on severity of symptoms
- Private room indicated with moderate sterile precautions. Stress hand washing.

GENERAL MEASURES
- Fever control
- IV fluids if oral intake is poor or vomiting is present

ACTIVITY Bedrest initially, then activity as tolerated

DIET Determined by symptoms; may need to NPO due to nausea or vomiting, advance to clear fluids and regular diet as tolerated

PATIENT EDUCATION
- Discuss possibility, but low probability, of transmission to contacts
- Expected duration of illness (2-7 days)
- For patient education materials favorably reviewed on this topic, contact: American Academy of Pediatrics, 141 Northwest Point Blvd., P.O. Box 927, Elk Grove Village, IL 60009-0927, (800)433-9016

MEDICATIONS

DRUG(S) OF CHOICE
• May require parenteral narcotic analgesics for pain (e.g., meperidine (Demerol) 25-50 mg IM q 3-4h or nalbuphine (Nubain) 10 mg IM q 3-4h (adult doses) or morphine 2-5 mg IM or IV q 3-4h)
• May require anti-emetics (e.g., promethazine (Phenergan) 25 mg IM q 3-4h or prochlorperazine (Compazine) 10 mg IM q 3-4h (adult doses)
• Use oral pain medications when nausea and vomiting subside, e.g., Tylenol with codeine or Percocet, 1 or 2 q 3-4h prn for adults
• Specific antiviral agents are not indicated in the usual care of viral meningitis
• Antipyretics are indicated for fever, preferably acetaminophen (Tylenol) 650 mg po or suppository q4h for adults. Approximately 60 mg per year of age in children or 10-15 mg/kg/dose.
• Antibiotics are not indicated for treatment of viral meningitis, but are often initiated until a diagnosis is firmly established. If all parameters suggest a viral etiology, it is usually prudent to treat symptomatically and follow the patient closely in the hospital setting. If in doubt, a broad spectrum antibiotic with good CSF penetration should be started intravenously. The choice may be dictated by local custom and sensitivities, as well as a consideration of age related pathogens. (See section on Bacterial meningitis.)
Contraindications: Refer to manufacturer's profile of each drug
Precautions:
• Aspirin should be avoided in children and adolescents due to a possible association with Reye's syndrome
• Phenothiazines may produce a dystonic reaction, especially in adolescents
Significant possible interactions: Refer to manufacturer's profile of each drug

ALTERNATIVE DRUGS
Symptomatic relief may be provided by a variety of anti-emetics and analgesics (e.g., nonsteroidal anti-inflammatory drugs)

 FOLLOWUP

PATIENT MONITORING
• Once the acute illness begins resolving, follow at least once within 7-10 days
• Repeat of lumbar puncture is not necessary unless the clinical course is atypical

PREVENTION/AVOIDANCE   N/A

POSSIBLE COMPLICATIONS
• Deafness
• Fatigue
• Irritability
• Muscle weakness
• Seizures (rare)

EXPECTED COURSE AND PROGNOSIS
Complete recovery in 2-7 days; headaches and other uncomfortable symptoms may sometimes persist intermittently for 1-2 weeks

 MISCELLANEOUS

ASSOCIATED CONDITIONS
Encephalitis

AGE-RELATED FACTORS
Pediatric: N/A
Geriatric: Viral meningitis is rarely seen in the elderly, and suspicions should be raised about an alternative diagnosis, e.g., carcinomatous meningitis
Others: N/A

PREGNANCY   N/A

SYNONYMS
• Abacterial meningitis
• Aseptic meningitis

ICD-9-CM   047.9

SEE ALSO   Bacterial meningitis

OTHER NOTES
Enteroviruses and arthropod-borne viruses predominate in warm months; mumps usually occurs in the winter and spring, often in epidemics

ABBREVIATIONS
• CIEP - counterimmunoelectrophoresis
• CSF - cerebrospinal fluid

REFERENCES
• Mandell, G., Douglas, R.G., Jr., Bennett, J.E.: Principles and Practice of Infectious Diseases, 3rd Ed. New York, Churchill Livingstone, 1990
• Krugman, S., Katz, S., Gershon, A., Wilfert, C.: Infectious Diseases of Children. 9th Ed. New York, C.V. Mosby, 1990

Author   G. Miller, M.D.

Meningomyelocele

BASICS

DESCRIPTION
A defective closure of the vertebral column, in which the protruding sac contains meninges and spinal cord
- Meningomyelocele, anencephaly, and encephalocele belong to a group of disorders known as spina bifida, neural tube defects, or spinal dysraphism
- Meningomyelocele, anencephaly and encephalocele are serious congenital abnormalities of the nervous system, which develop in the first 4 weeks of gestation and represent faulty formation of the neural tube.

Postneurulation defects:
◊ By 25 days of intrauterine life, neurulation is complete
◊ At this stage postneurulation defects of dysraphism develop
◊ Characterized by intact skin over the underlying lesion
◊ Lesions include simple meningocele, lipomyelomeningocele, diastematomyelia, myelocystocele, neurenteric cyst, intraspinal and pelvic meningoceles

System(s) affected:
Nervous, Musculoskeletal, Skin/Exocrine

Genetics:
- Meningomyelocele, as well as the other forms of spina bifida (anencephaly and encephalocele) are a common example of multifactorial inheritance, i.e., they result from a number of genes and environmental factors acting together to determine the final result
- The parents of an affected infant have about a 1:30 chance of producing a 2nd affected offspring (this 3% risk has been calculated mathematically and confirmed by empiric data from population studies). Similarly, the patient with a neural tube defect, if able to have children, has a 3-4% chance of having an affected child. In the relatively rare instance where a couple has had 2 affected children, the risk for a 3rd rises further (7-8%). 2nd degree relatives of an affected individual (nieces, nephews) have about a 1:100 risk; for 1st cousins, the risk is about 1:200. There is little if any increased risk for other family members.
- Recent data have implicated vitamin deficiency as an environmental factor that plays a role in neural tube defects

Incidence/Prevalence in USA:
Neural tube defects (also called spina bifida) incidence in Caucasians is about 1:700 live births. The incidence among Blacks is < 1:3000.

Predominant age:
Congenital abnormality which is usually apparent at birth

Predominant sex:
Male = Female

SIGNS AND SYMPTOMS
- 75% of the lesions are situated in the lumbosacral spine
- The bony defect extends to the bottom of the vertebral column. Most are flat at birth but become cystic as time progresses.
- Infants are usually born with a single myelomeningocele
- Hydrocephalus - occurs in > 80% of infants with spina bifida and tends to arrest spontaneously over time
- Eventually only 1/2 of spina bifida patients are shunt-dependent

Arnold-Chiari malformation (ACM)
◊ All spina bifida patients have an Arnold-Chiari malformation - overgrowth of cerebellar tissue into the spinal canal, elongated 4th ventricle and buckled medulla in the spinal canal
◊ ACM is symptomatic in only 20% of affected children
◊ If symptomatic - can impair nerve control of swallowing/breathing, can also lead to weakness of arms and legs
◊ In older children, ACM can lead to syringomyelia - cystic expansion of central spinal canal
◊ Syringomyelia causes weak legs/arms, cranial nerve dysfunction
◊ Decompression may reverse or arrest these problems

CAUSES
- Cause of spinal dysraphism is unclear
- General belief is that dysraphic malformations occur when environmental factors trigger an underlying hereditary predisposition that manifests itself in some form of spinal dysraphism

RISK FACTORS
- 1st trimester valproic acid and derivatives (Valproate Sodium) use
- High risk pregnancy - mother with one child with spina bifida
- High risk pregnancy - mother with close relative with spina bifida
- > 90% of spina bifida infants are from low-risk pregnancies

DIAGNOSIS

DIFFERENTIAL DIAGNOSIS N/A

LABORATORY
- Prenatal: Maternal serum alpha-fetoprotein (AFP) levels - if AFP level at 16-18 weeks is high, may suggest fetal neural defects. Amniocentesis is indicated.
- Newborn: No specific lab tests indicated

Drugs that may alter lab results: N/A
Disorders that may alter lab results: N/A

PATHOLOGICAL FINDINGS N/A

SPECIAL TESTS
Prenatal
◊ Amniocentesis: Increased alpha-fetoprotein in amniotic fluid (by 14 weeks) indicates neural tube defects
◊ Ultrasound: Hydrocephalus usually easily diagnosable by ultrasonography. > 80% of open neural tube defects have hydrocephalus. Banana sign - compression/anterior alignment of cerebellum. Banana sign on ultrasound may be sign of open spina bifida.
Newborn
◊ Neurological testing to determine severity of functional defect
◊ Pinprick examination of trunk and legs shows level of sensory and motor involvement. Functional integrity is present if stimulus leads to limb movements, arousal, and crying.

IMAGING
Newborn: MRI or CT scan of the brain may reveal an Arnold-Chiari malformation

DIAGNOSTIC PROCEDURES
Newborn
◊ Usually, meningomyelocele is obvious on examination
◊ Defective innervation of the bladder is indicated by urinary dribbling

TREATMENT

APPROPRIATE HEALTH CARE
Inpatient

GENERAL MEASURES
• A team approach is necessary for effective care (neurosurgeon, orthopedist, urologist, nurse, social worker, occupational and physical therapist)
• Most patients with myelomeningocele have neurogenic bladder. Intermittent catheterization prevents severe urologic disorders.
Surgical procedures:
◊ Myelomeningocele repair - should be within 24-48 hours of birth. Orthopedist must address deformities of lower limbs and spine.
◊ ACM decompression - bony removal below level of herniated cerebellar tissue; dura opened and dural sac enlarged by sewing in a dural graft

ACTIVITY
• Guided by level of the lesion
• Activity assisted by physical therapy, braces, and wheelchair

DIET
Liquid and food intake may need to be modified depending on bladder and bowel involvement

PATIENT EDUCATION
• Urologist instructs parents for protocol and techniques of catheterization
• Urologist instructs parents for prevention of urinary tract infections
• Neurosurgeon instructs parents about signs of shunt obstruction
• Genetic counseling
• Printed patient information available from: Spina Bifida Association of America, 1700 Rockville Pike, Suite 540, Rockville, MD, (800)621-3141

MEDICATIONS

DRUG(S) OF CHOICE N/A
Contraindications: N/A
Precautions: N/A
Significant possible interactions: N/A

ALTERNATIVE DRUGS N/A

FOLLOWUP

PATIENT MONITORING
• Physiotherapist looks for any deterioration in function
• Neurosurgeon follows patient's shunt function
• Urologist assesses urologic function
• Family physician provides general medical care/coordination

PREVENTION/AVOIDANCE
Early recognition/decompression of ACM may reverse symptoms

POSSIBLE COMPLICATIONS
• Causes of late deterioration secondary to myelomeningocele repair
• Shunt obstruction - back pain and increasing neurologic deficit
• Shunt obstruction - can lead to hydrosyringomyelia
• Hydronephrosis - most occurs in 1st 5 years of life
• If operative procedures are not carried out, infants usually die within one year.

EXPECTED COURSE AND PROGNOSIS
• > 80% of treated open neural tube defects have normal IQ
• Since 1970's, management techniques have improved tremendously
• Shunt infection and malfunction are now uncommon
• Early assessment in spina bifida may give misleading prognosis, i.e., a child with hydrocephalus and paraplegia may have normal IQ
• Small sacral lesion may result in severe physical/intellectual impairment from hydrocephalus or Arnold-Chiari malformation

MISCELLANEOUS

ASSOCIATED CONDITIONS
Infants with a simple meningocele may have an associated intraspinal abnormality that also requires treatment

AGE-RELATED FACTORS
Pediatric: Congenital defect
Geriatric: N/A
Others: N/A

PREGNANCY
Diagnosable during pregnancy

SYNONYMS
Myelomeningocele

ICD-9-CM
741.0 Spina bifida with hydrocephalus
741.9 Spina bifida without mention of hydrocephalus

SEE ALSO N/A

OTHER NOTES
When an infant is severely affected, a decision about performing operative procedures or letting the disorder take its natural course presents serious ethical problems.

ABBREVIATIONS
ACM = Arnold Chiari malformation

REFERENCES
• Berklow, R., et al. (eds.): Merck Manual. 14th Ed. Rahway, NJ, Merck Sharp & Dohme, 1986
• Hoffman, H.J.: Spinal Dysraphism. American Family Physician December, 1987 Volume 36 Number 6

Author S. Owen, M.D.

Menopause

 BASICS

DESCRIPTION
The cessation of spontaneous menstrual cycles
• Climacteric: That period of time during which there is a decline in ovarian function. Although a woman may continue to have periodic uterine bleeding, such cycles may be anovulatory. During this time estrogen production diminishes and a woman may experience early signs of estrogen deficiency, such as vasomotor symptoms, even though she still has periodic bleeding.
• Postmenopause: The period after menopause usually accounting for more than a third of a women's total life.
System(s) affected: Reproductive, Endocrine/Metabolic, Skeletal
Genetics: N/A
Incidence/Prevalence in USA: Increasingly common as life span increases - currently affects more than 30 million women
Predominant age:
• Average age is 51 and is unrelated to the age of the menarche. Virtually all women will be postmenopausal by age 58.
• If the menopause occurs before age 30, it is defined as premature menopause and may be associated with abnormalities of the sex chromosomes. A karyotype is indicated in such young women to rule out the presence of a Y chromosome.
Predominant sex: Female only

SIGNS AND SYMPTOMS
• Cessation of menses - either abruptly or preceded by a period of irregular cycles and/or diminished bleeding
• Vasomotor symptoms - hot flashes, sweating (85%)
• Psychologic symptoms - depression, nervousness, insomnia
• Vaginal atrophy - dyspareunia
• Urinary tract atrophy - stress or urge urinary incontinence
• Skin atrophy - wrinkles
• Osteoporosis - fractures (20% by age 85)
• Arteriosclerosis - coronary artery disease

CAUSES
• Physiologic - when due to depletion of oocytes
• Surgical - when due to removal of functioning ovaries because of disease or incidental to hysterectomy
• Medical - as a result of treatment of endometriosis (Danocrine or GnRH analogues) or of breast cancer (antiestrogens). This etiology is reversible.

RISK FACTORS
• Increasing age
• Pelvic surgery
• Sex chromosome abnormalities

 DIAGNOSIS

DIFFERENTIAL DIAGNOSIS
• Pregnancy
• Polycystic ovarian disease
• Microadenoma of pituitary
• Hypothalamic dysfunction
• Asherman's syndrome
• Obstruction of uterine outflow tract

LABORATORY
• Usually none is required because patient's age and symptoms readily establish the diagnosis
• If the diagnosis is questionable in a young patient, an elevated serum FSH indicates ovarian failure (FSH greater than 100 mIU/mL). Measurement of LH is not necessary.
Drugs that may alter lab results:
• Estrogens
• Androgens
Disorders that may alter lab results:
Temporary, reversible cessation of ovarian function, e.g., during chemotherapy

PATHOLOGICAL FINDINGS
• Atrophy of endometrium - virtually 100% if untreated. The uterus may seem smaller on bimanual examination.
• Atrophy of vagina - loss of rugae, appearance of petechiae - virtually 100% after several years if untreated
• Atrophy of urinary tract
• Osteoporosis - approximately 2% loss of bone mass per year. This is most common in Caucasians and Orientals and least common in African-Americans.
• Arteriosclerosis
• Ovarian stroma only - or only a few inactive oocytes

SPECIAL TESTS
Endometrial biopsy and/or D and C in patients who have intermenstrual or postmenopausal bleeding - may be accompanied by hysteroscopic examination of uterine cavity if available. Investigation for endometrial cancer is necessary even in the presence of an atrophic vagina (usually the cause of the bleeding).

IMAGING
• None for physiologic menopause
• CT scan of head if pituitary tumor is suspected
• Some physicians monitor bone density with photon beam absorptiometry - abnormal only after bone loss has occurred

DIAGNOSTIC PROCEDURES
• Serum FSH if diagnosis is questionable
• Peripheral blood karyotype if under age 30
• Endometrial sampling if intermenstrual or post menopausal bleeding occurs
• Pap smear
• Bimanual pelvic examination
• Mammography annually

 TREATMENT

APPROPRIATE HEALTH CARE
Periodic office visits

GENERAL MEASURES
• To retard development of osteoporosis - adequate calcium intake - at least 1500 mg elemental calcium per day obtained by diet or possibly by supplemental calcium; exercise; avoid smoking, excessive alcohol or caffeine intake
• Estrogen replacement therapy is indicated for long-term prophylaxis against osteoporosis and coronary artery disease as well as relief of vasomotor symptoms and urogenital atrophy. Exceptions are women with contraindications to therapy and obese women (who usually have sufficient endogenous estrogens produced by peripheral conversion of androgens by adipose tissue).
• Estrogen replacement has a favorable effect on lipoproteins, elevating the HDL levels, as well as retarding the development of osteoporosis, thereby reducing the incidence of fractures

ACTIVITY
Active exercise to the extent possible. Some type of weight-bearing exercise is recommended.

DIET
Increased calcium intake

PATIENT EDUCATION
Printed material available from:
• American College of Obstetricians and Gynecologists (ACOG), 409 12th St. S.W., Washington, D.C. 20024, (800)673-8444
• American Academy of Family Physicians Foundation, P.O. Box 8418, Kansas City, MO, 64114,(800)274-2237, ext. 4400

MEDICATIONS

DRUG(S) OF CHOICE
• Oral estrogens - most commonly used are conjugated estrogens (Premarin). Daily dose effective in retarding osteoporosis is 0.625 mg. Lesser doses are not effective. If vasomotor symptoms persist at 0.625 mg, a dose of 0.9 mg or 1.25 mg may be utilized.
• Because estrogens are carcinogenic to the endometrium, a progestogen should be added for its protective effect against endometrial cancer. (If the uterus has been removed, a progestogen is not needed). Most often, medroxyprogesterone acetate (Provera) is used in a daily dose of 2.5 mg (for continuous use) or 5 mg (for cyclic use).
• Estrogens and progestogens may be administered continuously or cyclically. The advantage of continuous use is that withdrawal uterine bleeding is not expected. With cyclic therapy, withdrawal bleeding may occur during the time that the patient is not on medication. The most frequently used formulations are: Premarin 0.625 mg plus Provera 2.5 mg daily or Premarin 0.625 mg for 25 days per month - add Provera 5 mg during the last 10-14 days of estrogen therapy.
Contraindications:
• Estrogen dependent malignancies
• Unexplained abnormal uterine bleeding
• History of thrombophlebitis
• Active liver disease
Precautions:
• Continuous therapy should not result in uterine bleeding
• Women on cyclic therapy may bleed normally only during those days when no therapy is given. Any bleeding other than that normally expected must be evaluated for the possibility of endometrial cancer.
Significant possible interactions: The estrogen dosage recommended is very low. It is unlikely that it will result in some of the complications that are associated with higher doses of estrogen, including hypercoagulability, breast tenderness, gall bladder disease and hypertension. The possible relationship to breast cancer is still controversial.

ALTERNATIVE DRUGS
• Oral - estropipate (Ogen) 0.625 mg, estradiol (Estrace) 1-2 mg
• Transdermal (patch) - estradiol (Estraderm) 0.05-0.1 mg applied twice weekly
• Vaginal - conjugated estrogens (Premarin cream) - best for local therapy of atrophic vaginitis only. Systemic absorption occurs, but blood levels are unpredictable.
• Intramuscular - not recommended - may not be protective against coronary artery disease without first passing through the liver
• For women who cannot take estrogens - using progestogens (Depo-Provera) 150 mg IM every month is helpful in alleviating hot flashes. This may also retard the development of osteoporosis but is not helpful in preventing coronary artery disease or urogenital atrophy.

• Vitamin D is not helpful as the sole treatment for preventing osteoporosis
• Calcitonin produces only a temporary increase in body calcium
• Sodium fluoride increases bone volume but has toxic side effects
• Etidronate may increase bone volume. Still an investigational drug

FOLLOWUP

PATIENT MONITORING
• Annual Pap smear and pelvic and breast examinations
• Annual mammography
• Endometrial sampling only in patients with abnormal bleeding

PREVENTION/AVOIDANCE
Menopause is a physiological process. It cannot be avoided, but the untoward effects can be moderated or eliminated by estrogen replacement therapy.

POSSIBLE COMPLICATIONS
• Vasomotor symptoms
• Uncomfortable psychologic symptoms
• Vaginal atrophy
• Skin wrinkles
• Osteoporosis
• Arteriosclerosis

EXPECTED COURSE AND PROGNOSIS
If untreated
◊ Ultimate disappearance of vasomotor symptoms - usually takes several years
◊ Urogenital atrophy
◊ Osteoporosis - possible fractures especially of the hip, vertebrae and wrists. Mortality associated with hip fractures is 15%.
◊ Coronary artery disease
If treated
◊ Minimal effects of estrogen deprivation
◊ Slower development of significant bone loss and reduced incidence of coronary artery disease
◊ Therapy may be continued indefinitely if no contraindications appear since osteoporosis will rapidly occur after stopping therapy

MISCELLANEOUS

ASSOCIATED CONDITIONS
Any medical problems that may occur with increasing age, especially osteoporosis

AGE-RELATED FACTORS
Pediatric: N/A
Geriatric: N/A
Others: N/A

PREGNANCY
Mutually exclusive

SYNONYMS
• Climacteric
• Ovarian failure

ICD-9-CM
• 627.0 Premenopausal menorrhagia
• 627.2 Menopausal or female climacteric states
• 627.4 States associated with artificial menopause
• 716.3 Climacteric arthritis

SEE ALSO
N/A

OTHER NOTES
• Estrogen replacement therapy is especially important in women having an early menopause, either spontaneous or surgical because of their long expected life without endogenous estrogens. Without such therapy, they may be at a significantly increased risk for osteoporosis and its life threatening or debilitating effects.
• Following surgical menopause, vasomotor symptoms often appear very rapidly. Estrogen replacement therapy may be started in the early postoperative period.
• In perimenopausal women bothered by severe vasomotor symptoms, cyclic estrogen and progestogen therapy may be started even though the patient is still having periodic uterine bleeding

ABBREVIATIONS
N/A

REFERENCES
Mishell, D.R., Jr.: Menopause. Physiology and Pharmacology. Chicago, Year Book Medical Publishers, 1987

Author A. Langer, M.D.

Menorrhagia

BASICS

DESCRIPTION
Excessive amount or duration of menstrual flow, at more or less regular intervals

Distinguish from, but may overlap with:
◊ Metrorrhagia - irregular or frequent flow, noncyclic
◊ Menometrorrhagia - frequent, excessive, irregular flow (menorrhagia plus metrorrhagia
◊ Polymenorrhea - frequent flow, cycles of 21 days or less
◊ Intermenstrual bleeding - bleeding between regular menses
◊ Dysfunctional uterine bleeding (DUB) - abnormal endometrial bleeding of hormonal cause and related to anovulation

System(s) affected: Reproductive
Genetics: N/A
Incidence/Prevalence in USA: Abnormal bleeding is common; prevalence varies with definition (endometrial carcinoma: about 40,000 new cases per year)
Predominant age:
• Menarche to menopause; about 50% of cases occur after 40 years of age
• Dysfunctional bleeding is fairly common in adolescence and near menopause
Predominant sex: Female only

SIGNS AND SYMPTOMS
• "Excessive" menstrual flow defined subjectively varies greatly from woman to woman (average normal menstrual flow is about 30 mL per cycle)

Useful historical features include:
◊ Bleeding substantially heavier than the patient's usual flow
◊ Bleeding lasting more than 7 days
◊ Flow associated with passage of significant clots
◊ Anemia

The following symptoms tend to suggest that cycles are ovulatory:
◊ Regular menstrual interval
◊ Mid-cycle pain (mittelschmerz)
◊ Dysmenorrhea
◊ Premenstrual symptoms - breast soreness, mood changes, etc.

Abdominal pain or cramps at other times of the cycle may be associated with structural causes:
◊ Myomas
◊ Polyps
◊ Ovarian tumors

Hirsutism or acne
◊ May accompany Stein-Leventhal syndrome

CAUSES
• Hypothyroidism

Endometrial proliferation/ excess/hyperplasia:
◊ Anovulation, oligo-ovulation
◊ Polycystic ovarian disease (PCOD), Stein-Leventhal syndrome
◊ Ovarian tumor
◊ Obesity
◊ Hormone (estrogen) therapy

Endometrial atrophy:
◊ Postmenopause
◊ Prolonged progestin or oral contraceptive administration

Local factors:
◊ Endometrial polyps
◊ Endometrial neoplasia
◊ Adenomyosis/endometriosis
◊ Uterine myomata (fibroids)
◊ Intrauterine device (IUD)
◊ Uterine sarcoma

Coagulation disorders:
◊ Thrombocytopenia, platelet disorders
◊ von Willebrand's disease
◊ Leukemia
◊ Ingestion of aspirin or anticoagulants
◊ Renal failure/dialysis

RISK FACTORS
• Obesity
• Anovulation
• Estrogen administration (without progestin)
• Prior treatment with progestational agents or oral contraceptives increases the risk of endometrial atrophy, but decreases the risk of endometrial hyperplasia or neoplasia

DIAGNOSIS

DIFFERENTIAL DIAGNOSIS
Pregnancy complications:
◊ Threatened abortion
◊ Incomplete abortion
◊ Ectopic pregnancy

Nonuterine bleeding:
◊ Cervical ectropion/erosion
◊ Cervical neoplasia/polyp
◊ Cervical or vaginal trauma
◊ Condylomata
◊ Atrophic vaginitis
◊ Foreign bodies

Pelvic inflammatory disease (PID):
◊ Endometritis
◊ Tuberculosis

LABORATORY
• Pregnancy test
• CBC to assess severity of blood loss, exclude thrombocytopenia and leukemia

In selected cases:
◊ TSH - elevated in hypothyroidism
◊ Platelet count, bleeding time, prothrombin time (PT), partial thromboplastin time (PTT) for coagulation screen
◊ Creatinine, BUN
◊ Serum progesterone - 5-20 ng/mL in luteal phase, < 1 ng/mL in follicular phase or anovulatory cycle

Drugs that may alter lab results:
Progestins used prior to endometrial biopsy may cause decidualization and obscure true diagnosis
Disorders that may alter lab results: N/A

PATHOLOGICAL FINDINGS
Vary with cause: see Causes

SPECIAL TESTS
Endometrial biopsy detects hyperplasia, dysplasia, or atrophy. If done prior to expected menses, may also help make the diagnosis of anovulation or luteal phase defect.

IMAGING
• Ultrasonography to evaluate adnexal masses or fibroids suspected from pelvic exam
• Computerized tomography used in investigation of potentially malignant pelvic masses

DIAGNOSTIC PROCEDURES
• Pelvic and rectal examination
• Pap smear
• Endometrial biopsy
• Diagnostic D&C
• Hysteroscopy

TREATMENT

APPROPRIATE HEALTH CARE
• Most cases can be managed as outpatients in office or emergency department
• Hospitalize for bleeding accompanied by orthostatic hypotension or hematocrit < 25%

GENERAL MEASURES
• Rule out pregnancy complications and non-uterine bleeding

Treat severe or life-threatening bleeding acutely:
◊ Intravenous estrogen
◊ Curettage if necessary
◊ Hysterectomy in extreme case

Proceed to identify underlying cause of bleeding and treat to prevent recurrence
◊ Hormonal therapy
◊ Dilatation and curettage for hormone-unresponsive cases
◊ Consider endometrial ablation or hysterectomy in persistent cases where fertility is not desired
◊ Specific treatment for neoplasia, polyps, systemic disease, etc.
◊ Patients who desire fertility may also need appropriate treatment for anovulation, endometriosis, myomata, etc.

ACTIVITY
As tolerated. Resting with feet elevated may be helpful.

DIET
Iron supplementation may help correct for increased blood loss

PATIENT EDUCATION
Information about side effects of medications

MEDICATIONS

DRUG(S) OF CHOICE
For acute control of severe bleeding:
◊ Conjugated estrogen (Premarin) 25 mg IV every 4 hours up to 6 doses until bleeding abates
For less severe bleeding or after control of acute bleeding:
◊ Medroxyprogesterone acetate (Provera) 10-30 mg daily for 5-10 days
◊ Any combination oral contraceptive, (usually one of the "high dose" oral contraceptives) one tablet 4 times a day for 5-7 days
To prevent heavy bleeding in subsequent cycles:
◊ Medroxyprogesterone acetate 10-20 mg daily for 10 days per month
◊ Usual cyclic dose of a combination oral contraceptive
For endometrial atrophy in postmenopausal woman:
◊ Estrogen plus progesterone replacement therapy

Contraindications:
To estrogen, oral contraceptives, or progestins:
◊ Pregnancy
◊ Breast or endometrial cancer
◊ Thromboembolic disease, past or present
◊ Impaired liver function

Precautions:
• Nausea and vomiting are common from IV estrogen; antiemetics are helpful
• Estrogen may precipitate acute intermittent porphyria or cholestatic jaundice in susceptible individuals

Significant possible Interactions: Refer to manufacturer's profile of each drug

ALTERNATIVE DRUGS
• Norethindrone acetate (Norlutin, Norlutate) 2.5-10 mg daily for 10 days per month, during the assumed latter half of menstrual cycle
• Megestrol acetate (Megace) 40 mg daily for 10 days per month
• Megestrol acetate (Megace) 40 mg daily continuously to treat atypical hyperplasia
• Nonsteroidal prostaglandin-synthetase inhibitors (naproxen, mefenamic acid, ibuprofen, and others) can reduce blood loss with ovulatory cycles and reduce dysmenorrhea

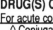

FOLLOWUP

PATIENT MONITORING
• Varies with cause of bleeding
• Medical treatment of hyperplastic/dysplastic endometrium should be followed by repeat biopsy to confirm that histologic structure has returned to normal

PREVENTION/AVOIDANCE   Pap smear and pelvic examination annually

POSSIBLE COMPLICATIONS   Anemia

EXPECTED COURSE AND PROGNOSIS
• Varies with cause of bleeding
• Most patients with hormonal causes will respond to hormonal manipulation

MISCELLANEOUS

ASSOCIATED CONDITIONS
Metrorrhagia, menometrorrhagia, androgenic disorders

AGE-RELATED FACTORS
Pediatric: Genital bleeding prior to puberty can result from trauma, foreign bodies, vaginal infection, or exogenous hormone administration
Geriatric: Genital atrophy may predispose to bleeding with minimal trauma. Neoplasm of ovary or endometrium must be ruled out.
Others:
• In adolescence, irregular bleeding due to anovulation and immaturity of the hypothalamic-pituitary-ovarian axis is common
• Beyond age 35-40, endometrial dysplasia and endometrial carcinoma are significant causes of bleeding. Obtain endometrial sampling before attempting hormonal treatment.

PREGNANCY   Bleeding in pregnancy is not menorrhagia. Complications of pregnancy or cervical/vaginal lesions should be considered.

SYNONYMS   N/A

ICD-9-CM
• Endometrial polyp 621.0
• Endometrial hyperplasia 621.3
• Endometrial atrophy 621.8
• Menorrhagia, menometrorrhagia, polymenorrhea 626.2
• Pubertal menorrhagia 626.3
• Irregular menses 626.4
• Metrorrhagia 626.6
• Dysfunctional uterine bleeding 626.8
• Postmenopausal bleeding 627.1

SEE ALSO   Amenorrhea, cervical disorders, dysmenorrhea, fibroid tumors, menopause, Stein-Leventhal syndrome

OTHER NOTES   N/A

ABBREVIATIONS   N/A

REFERENCES
• Wentz, A.C.: Abnormal Uterine Bleeding. In Novak's Textbook of Gynecology. 11th Ed. Edited by H.W. Jones. Baltimore, Williams & Wilkins, 1988
• Cowan, B.D. & Morrison, J.C.: Management of Abnormal Genital Bleeding in Girls and Women. N Engl J Med. 324(24):1710-15, June 13, 1991
• Speroff, L.: Clinical Gynecologic Endocrinology and Infertility. 4th Ed. Baltimore, Williams & Wilkins, 1989
• Carlson, J.M.: Menorrhagia and Metrorrhagia. In Gynecologic Decision Making. 2nd Ed. Edited by E.A. Friedman. Philadelphia, B.C. Decker, 1988

Author   D. Nelson, M.D.

Mental retardation

BASICS

DESCRIPTION Mental retardation (MR) is a symptom with multiple etiologies including chromosomal abnormalities, genetic defects, intrauterine, perinatal, neonatal, and postnatal causes. Mental retardation refers to substantial limitations in present functioning. It is characterized by significantly subaverage intellectual functioning, existing concurrently with related limitations in two or more of the following applicable adaptive skills areas: communication, self-care, home living, social skills, community use, self-direction, health and safety, functional academics, leisure and work. Mental manifestations manifest before age 18.
Subgroups:
◊ Mild mental retardation IQ 55-69 (approximately 85% of mentally retarded)
◊ Moderate mental retardation IQ 40-54 (12% of mentally retarded)
◊ Severe mental retardation IQ 25-39 (7% of mentally retarded)
◊ Profound mental retardation IQ 0-24 (1% of mentally retarded)
System(s) affected: Nervous
Genetics:
• Autosomes: Trisomies and rearrangements - approximately 1500 variations are all associated with MR
• Sex chromosomes: 80 of 336 disorders cause MR
• Autosomal dominant: 180 of 3,000 disorders cause MR
• Autosomal recessive: 400 of 1,550 disorders cause MR
Incidence/Prevalence in USA: Incidence and prevalence are closely related to social, economic, and health conditions of the society. The general incidence of mental retardation in the United States has been estimated at 125,000 births per year by the American Association on Mental Retardation. This would correspond to approximately 3% of the population. The research on both incidence and prevalence of mental retardation in the U.S. is exceedingly scant. A comprehensive Canadian study of the maritime Provinces found prevalences of 3.65 per 1000. Most professionals associated with the American Association on Mental Retardation accept a prevalence of 2.5% and they recognize that the prevalence varies with chronological age. Specifically, mildly retarded preschoolers are able to meet societies demands but are identified by the school system due to demands for cognitive processing. Conversely, once they leave the requirements of the educational system they may adapt to societies demands and the diagnosis need not apply.
Predominant age: By definition mental retardation occurs during the developmental period. Older adults who lose mental faculties are usually diagnosed as demented.
Predominant sex: Male > Female (1.5:1)

SIGNS AND SYMPTOMS
• Profoundly and severely retarded children are frequently diagnosed at the time of birth or during the newborn period. Children with dysmorphic features are more likely to be retarded
• Moderately retarded children may go undiagnosed until they fail to meet normal developmental milestones
• Mildly retarded children may go undiagnosed until well into the school years

CAUSES
Chromosomal abnormalities
◊ Autosomal abnormalities
◊ Trisomy (Down's syndrome)
◊ Translocations
◊ Inversions
◊ Duplications
◊ Deletions (Prader-Willi)
Sex chromosome abnormalities
◊ Fragile X syndrome
◊ Turner syndrome
◊ Klinefelter's syndrome
◊ Various multiple X and/or Y conditions
Autosomal dominant conditions
◊ Neurocutaneous syndromes (neurofibromatosis, tuberous sclerosis)
Autosomal recessive conditions
◊ Amino acid metabolism (phenylketonuria, Maple syrup urine disease)
◊ Carbohydrate metabolism (galactosemia, fructosuria)
◊ Lipid metabolism
◊ Tay-Sachs
◊ Gaucher's
◊ Niemann-Pick (mucopolysaccharidosis)
◊ Purine metabolism (Lesch-Nyhan)
◊ Other (Wilson's)
Multifactorial and sporadic conditions
◊ Cornelia de Lange's Syndrome
◊ Spinal cord disorders (spina bifida, Arnold-Chiari malformation)
◊ Disorders of brain and skull
◊ Prenatal factors
◊ Rh incompatibility
◊ Maternal infections - all the TORCH viruses -rubella, toxoplasmosis, cytomegalic virus, and herpes simplex)
◊ Maternal diseases (diabetes mellitus, toxemia)
◊ Maternal substance abuse (alcohol use/abuse, cocaine). Fetal alcohol syndrome felt to be one of the leading causes of mental retardation.
◊ Prescription medications, such as Accutane or Dilantin
Perinatal factors
◊ Prematurity
◊ Postmaturity
◊ Birth injuries
◊ High risk mothers
Postnatal factors
◊ Childhood diseases (meningitis, encephalitis, general inflammatory disease with high fever, hypothyroidism)
◊ Trauma (accidents, physical abuse, marked deprivation)
◊ Poisoning (lead, carbon monoxide, household products)

RISK FACTORS Risk factors for future offspring of the parent couple must be calculated based upon the specific etiology of related retarded individuals

DIAGNOSIS

DIFFERENTIAL DIAGNOSIS
• Brain tumors
• Hearing impairment
• Infantile autism
• Cerebral palsy
• Emotional disturbance
• Environmental opportunities for appropriate development

LABORATORY
• Specific studies are available for those patients with identifiable genetic disease entities
• Chromosome studies
• Metabolic screens
• Amino acid
• Sugar substrates
• Molecular studies (e.g., DNA)
Drugs that may alter lab results: N/A
Disorders that may alter lab results: N/A

PATHOLOGICAL FINDINGS   N/A

SPECIAL TESTS
Individually administered measure of intellectual abilities
◊ Measure utilized depends upon the age of the patient
◊ Birth through 2 years - Bayley's Scales of Infant Development
◊ 2 years of age through adulthood - Stanford Binet (form LM), Stanford Binet (4th edition), Wechsler Scales
◊ Preschool children - WIPPSI
◊ School age - WISC-III
◊ Adults- WAIS-R, and an adaptive behavior scale (Vineland Adaptive Scales)
◊ Other measures are available; however, these are the most widely recognized and utilized measures of individual ability and adaptive behavior

IMAGING   N/A

DIAGNOSTIC PROCEDURES   See Special tests

TREATMENT

APPROPRIATE HEALTH CARE
• Some specialized care may be necessary based upon the etiology of the retardation
• Care for the retarded is educational, not medical

GENERAL MEASURES N/A

ACTIVITY Full activity

DIET No research evidence supports the use of specific diets for mental retardation and/or Attention Deficit Hyperactivity Disorder (ADHD). Exception: Some metabolic and storage disorders, i.e., PKU.

PATIENT EDUCATION Parental education and consultation as to the development of appropriate behavioral and educational expectations are strongly advised. Families should be referred to the local Association for Retarded Citizens.

MEDICATIONS

DRUG(S) OF CHOICE None
Contraindications: N/A
Precautions: N/A
Significant possible interactions: N/A

ALTERNATIVE DRUGS N/A

FOLLOWUP

PATIENT MONITORING Regular pediatric care

PREVENTION/AVOIDANCE N/A

POSSIBLE COMPLICATIONS Learning inappropriate behaviors

EXPECTED COURSE AND PROGNOSIS
• Mild retardation: Social and communication skills appropriate for community functioning, basic job skills, and functional literacy
• Moderate mental retardation: Speech deficits, social awareness, personal care skills, i.e., dressing, feeding, washing, sheltered employment, group home living
• Severe mental retardation: Limited speech and language, poor motor development, in need of supervision
• Profound mental retardation: Neurological defect, poor cognitive social ability, absent speech, possible self harm, extended care

MISCELLANEOUS

ASSOCIATED CONDITIONS
• Speech problems
• Seizures
• Maladaptive behaviors
• Attention deficit hyperactivity disorder (ADHD) (found with greater frequency among individuals with neuropsychological dysfunction. Treatment for ADHD among the mentally retarded is not unlike that for the "normal" population. Data indicates overuse of psychoactive substances to aid caretakers).

AGE-RELATED FACTORS
Pediatric: N/A
Geriatric: N/A
Others: N/A

PREGNANCY Parents and first degree relatives could benefit from consultation with a genetic associate or counselor

SYNONYMS Mental deficiency

ICD-9-CM
• 317.00 - Mild mental retardation
• 318.00 - Moderate mental retardation
• 318.10 - Severe mental retardation
• 318.20 - Profound mental retardation
• 319.00 - Unspecified mental retardation

SEE ALSO
• Cerebral palsy
• Down syndrome
• Fragile X syndrome
• Lead poisoning

OTHER NOTES Extensive family history to aid in diagnosis is mandatory. Genetic referral in cases without known etiology is appropriate.

ABBREVIATIONS MR = mental retardation

REFERENCES Holmes, L.B., et al.: Mental Retardation: An Atlas of Diseases with Associated Physical Abnormalities. New York, The Macmillan Company, 1972

Author R. Simensen, Ph.D.

Metatarsalgia

BASICS

DESCRIPTION A catch-all term for pain in the forefoot, usually in the plantar aspect
• Pain and inflammation along the medial and transverse arches of the mid - and forefoot, involving the muscles, tendons and ligaments
System(s) affected: Musculoskeletal
Genetics: N/A
Incidence/Prevalence in USA: Common
Predominant age: 30's-80's
Predominant sex: Female > Male

SIGNS AND SYMPTOMS
• Predominantly located in the dorsal and plantar forefoot, especially distal half of metatarsal shaft
• Pain
• Swelling
• Tenderness
• Occasionally erythema

CAUSES
<u>Excess strain (anatomical variations)</u>
◊ Hallux valgus and rigidus
◊ Plantar flexed metatarsals
◊ Hammer toe
◊ Obesity
<u>Repetitive and/or excessive and/or unaccustomed walking and running</u>
◊ Long distance
◊ Hard surfaces
◊ Poor shoe construction
◊ Skeletal abnormalities
<u>Systemic disorder</u>
◊ Gout
◊ Rheumatoid arthritis

RISK FACTORS
• Pes planus (flat foot)
• Old or poorly constructed shoes
• Poor physical condition

DIAGNOSIS

DIFFERENTIAL DIAGNOSIS
• Stress fracture
• Cellulitis or infection
• Neuroma (plantar or Morton's)
• Inflammatory arthritis
• Traumatic arthritis
• Foreign body
• Tumor (rare)

LABORATORY
• WBC - normal (elevated in infection)
• Sedimentation rate - normal (elevated in infection and inflammatory arthritis)
• Tests for gout, rheumatoid arthritis, or other systemic disorders if strongly suspect
Drugs that may alter lab results: N/A
Disorders that may alter lab results: N/A

PATHOLOGICAL FINDINGS N/A

SPECIAL TESTS N/A

IMAGING
• Routine anteroposterior and lateral foot x-ray - normal
• Bone scan if high index of suspicion of stress fracture
• MRI if suspect mass lesion

DIAGNOSTIC PROCEDURES N/A

TREATMENT

APPROPRIATE HEALTH CARE
Outpatient

GENERAL MEASURES
• Ice initially
• Moist heat later
• Taping or Gelcast
• Walking cast - rarely
• Physical therapy - rarely
• Cane or crutch - temporary
• Arch support in a well-fitted, low-heel shoe
• Energy-absorbing sole on shoe

ACTIVITY
• Rest during active, symptomatic phase
• Weight bearing as tolerated
• Progressive return to previous level of activities and sports - bike riding to jogging to running (with an arch support in running shoes)

DIET No special diet

PATIENT EDUCATION Instruct about proper shoes for specific activity and gradual return to usual activities

MEDICATIONS

DRUG(S) OF CHOICE
Nonsteroidal anti-inflammatories such as:
◊ Piroxicam (Feldene) 20 mg daily 7-14 days
◊ Naproxen (Naprosyn) 500 mg bid 7-14 days
◊ Flurbiprofen (Ansaid) 100 mg bid 7-14 days
◊ Ibuprofen (Motrin) 800 mg tid 7-14 days

Contraindications:
- GI bleeding or ulcer history
- Liver diseases

Precautions:
- Renal disease
- Hepatic disease
- Fluid retention
- GI disorders, especially ulcers
- Coagulation disorders
- Anemia

Significant possible interactions:
- Anticoagulants
- Digoxin
- Lithium
- Methotrexate
- Cyclosporine

ALTERNATIVE DRUGS N/A

FOLLOWUP

PATIENT MONITORING Weekly for 2-4 weeks

PREVENTION/AVOIDANCE
- Appropriate shoes for appropriate activity
- Avoid overuse
- Treat systemic disorders

POSSIBLE COMPLICATIONS Back and knee problems due to change in weight bearing dynamics

EXPECTED COURSE AND PROGNOSIS Expect complete healing with appropriate treatment

MISCELLANEOUS

ASSOCIATED CONDITIONS See Causes

AGE-RELATED FACTORS
Pediatric: N/A
Geriatric:
- More frequent in older athletes and the aging
- Symptoms more pronounced

Others: N/A

PREGNANCY N/A

SYNONYMS N/A

ICD-9-CM 726.70

SEE ALSO N/A

OTHER NOTES N/A

ABBREVIATIONS N/A

REFERENCES Sullivan, J.A. & Finberg, L.: The Pediatric Athlete. Park Ridge, Ill, American Academy of Orthopedic Surgeons, 1990

Author R. Cohen, M.D.

Migraine

BASICS

DESCRIPTION Paroxysmal, usually unilateral, severe headache lasting 2-72 hours, accompanied by gastrointestinal, visual, or other neurological signs, and with complete freedom from symptoms between episodes. Episodes vary in frequency from weekly to less than one per year. International Classification of Headaches (1988) has seven sub-types based on symptom complex. There is wide variety of alternative subtypes and taxonomies.
• Without aura - common migraine affects 80% of patients
• With aura - classic migraine affects less than 20% of patients. Patients experience some consistent warning symptoms before headache. Wide variety of aura reported from a specific neurologic sign or symptom, e.g., scotoma, to non-specific mood change. Rare forms include "hemiplegic migraine" with aura of transient hemiparesis and/or paraesthesia; basilar migraine (Bickerstaff's migraine) has aura of mixed symptoms suggesting ischemia in hind brain.
• Ophthalmoplegic (rare) - palsy of third cranial nerve ipsilateral to migraine pain during headache
• Retinal (rare) - symptoms of retinal vascular lesions during headache
• Childhood periodic syndromes - migraine equivalents in children. Recurrent episodes with symptoms such as vomiting, abdominal pain, vertigo predominating over headache.
• Complication of migraine (very rare) - status migrainous occurs if attack does not resolve spontaneously. Also reported cases of cerebral infarction during migraine episode.
• Other migraine patterns are less common
System(s) affected: Nervous, Musculoskeletal, Cardiovascular, Gastrointestinal
Genetics: Over 70% of patients give a family history. Clearly some genetic component but mechanism unclear. A recessive gene of approximately 70% penetration or a dominant gene with greater penetration in females are suggested.
Incidence in USA:
• Number of new cases cannot be measured due to problems of diagnosis and reporting. Up to 75% of patients do not consult physician.
• Proportion of population reporting a migraine attack in any previous year (period prevalence) ranges from 1-25% in different studies
Prevalence in USA:
• Difficult to measure because of problems of definition and reporting. Estimates of lifetime prevalence (percentage of population reporting at least one attack during life) approximately 10%; 6% of men (age 12-80) and 18% females (age12-80)
Predominant age: Young adults < 50 years. Onset teens-30 years.
Predominant sex: Female > Male

SIGNS AND SYMPTOMS
• Aura preceding headache by less than one hour in classical migraine
• Visual disturbances (photopsia, hemianopia, scotoma, fortification spectra, "zig-zag" lines, hallucinations)
• CNS signs (paresthesia, aphasia, hemiparesis of face and/or upper limb, ophthalmic and other CNS signs)
• Sensory disturbances of vision (photophobia), taste, smell, hearing
• Psychological symptoms (déjà vu, euphoria, anxiety, fatigue, mood changes)
• Headache: unilateral (< 30% bilateral), severe, throbbing, aggravated by movement
• Nausea (87%), vomiting (56%), diarrhea (16%)
• Photophobia (82%)
• Scalp tenderness (65%)
• Lightheadedness (72%), vertigo (33%), syncope (10%)
• Perioral paresthesia
• Other (pallor, fever, facial flushing, polyuria)

CAUSES
• Exact etiology unknown
• Abnormality of serotonin metabolism
• Disturbance of regional cerebral blood flow
• Dilatation of scalp arteries
Individual attacks may be precipitated by
◊ Specific foods or alcohol (chocolate, cheese, smoked meats, red wine)
◊ Missing meals
◊ Menstrual cycle
◊ Oral contraceptives
◊ Fatigue or excessive sleep
◊ Excessive or flickering light
◊ Stress or relief of stress ("weekend migraine")

RISK FACTORS
• Family history of migraine
• Female sex
• Young age
• Personal history of childhood recurrent abdominal pain, cyclical vomiting, or motion sickness
• No association with intelligence, social class, or specific psychological profiles

DIAGNOSIS

DIFFERENTIAL DIAGNOSIS
• Cluster, tension or headache secondary to any cause
• Drug-seeking behavior, psychogenic headache
• Rarely, migraine symptoms similar to certain forms of epilepsy

LABORATORY Only useful to rule out alternative causes of headache, e.g., sedimentation rate for temporal arteritis, complete blood count if meningitis/encephalitis is suspected
Drugs that may alter lab results: N/A
Disorders that may alter lab results: N/A

PATHOLOGICAL FINDINGS
• Changes in serotonin levels in blood and metabolites in urine immediately before and during attacks
• Changes in regional intracranial blood flow

SPECIAL TESTS Only to rule out alternative diagnoses

IMAGING Used in research or to rule out alternative diagnoses especially cerebral tumor or vascular malformation

DIAGNOSTIC PROCEDURES Based on history

TREATMENT

APPROPRIATE HEALTH CARE
Outpatient except for status migrainous

GENERAL MEASURES
• Compression of ipsilateral temporal artery
• Cold compress to ipsilateral temple/eye/occiput
• Lie completely still. Wedge pillows to support head and neck.
• Minimize light, noise, odors (especially from cooking, tobacco smoke)

ACTIVITY Usually most comfortable in bed in a dark room

DIET Avoid precipitants if known

PATIENT EDUCATION
• Multiple resources available
• Emphasize to patient migraine is inherited recurrent biochemical abnormality which cannot be cured. Address and correct myths about condition.
• Negotiate with patient and family a treatment plan to minimize number and severity of attacks
• Advise patient to anticipate changes over time in pattern of symptoms and frequency of attacks
• Emphasize that narcotics have little, if any, role in treatment

MEDICATIONS

DRUG(S) OF CHOICE
• No single drug of choice. Wide variety of vasoconstrictors, analgesics, antiemetics, sedatives used alone or in combination depending on patient's symptom and other factors. All medications need to be given early in attacks.

Ergotamines (in order of speed of onset)

◊ Dihydroergotamine mesylate (DHE 45) 1 mg/mL. One mg IM or IV promptly followed by 1 mg every hour prn up to 3 mg IM or 2 mg IV. Maximum in one week 6 mg. Many protocols add anti-emetic e.g., 10 mg prochlorperazine IM or 5 mg IV before DHE.

◊ Ergotamine suppositories 2 mg (Wigraine, Cafergot, Cafergot PB). Start with half and increase up to 2 suppositories per attack. Maximum ergotamine is 6 mg in 24 hours and no greater than 10 mg in 1 week. All suppositories contain 100 mg caffeine. Cafergot PB also contains 60 mg pentobarbital and 0.25 mg belladonna.

◊ Medihaler-ergotamine. Metered-dose oral inhaler 0.36 mg/inhalation. One inhalation promptly repeated prn after 5 minutes. Maximum daily dose 6 inhalations/24 hours or 15/week.

◊ Ergotamine 2 mg sublingual (Ergostat, Ergomar). One dissolved under tongue at onset of symptoms. Repeat after 30 minutes to maximum of 3/day or 5/week.

◊ Ergotamine 1 mg plus caffeine 100 mg (Wigraine, Cafergot, Cafergot PB). Two tablets po at onset of symptoms. Then one after 30 minutes. Then prn to maximum of 6/day, 10/week. Cafergot PB also contains 30 mg pentobarbital and 0.125 mg belladonna.

◊ Ergotamine 0.6 mg plus belladonna 0.2 mg plus phenobarbital 40 mg (Bellergal-S). One at onset of symptoms. Maximum weekly dose 16 tablets.

Analgesics

◊ Aspirin 650-1,000 mg po every 4 hours

◊ Acetaminophen 650 mg po every 4 hours

◊ Ibuprofen (Nuprin, Motrin) 800 mg po, followed by 400 mg after 30-60 minutes prn

◊ Naproxen 500 mg (Naprosyn) or naproxen sodium 550 (Anaprox DS), one tablet po. Maximum daily dose 1,375 mg.

◊ Ketorolac (Toradol) IM 15 or 30 mg/mL. One IM injection of 30 or 60 mg for severe migraine pain.

Combination drugs

◊ Acetaminophen 325 mg, isometheptene 65 mg, dichloralphenazone 100 mg (Midrin, Isocom). Two capsules at onset of symptoms followed by one per hour if needed up to five capsules in 12 hours.

◊ Acetaminophen 325, butalbital 50 mg (Phrenilin). One or two tablets every four hours. Maximum of six tablets per day. (Phrenilin Forte contains 650 mg of acetaminophen.)

◊ Acetaminophen 325 mg, butalbital 50 mg caffeine 40 mg (Fioricet). Brand name Fiorinal substitutes 325 mg aspirin for acetaminophen and is also available with additional 30 mg of codeine (Fiorinal #3).

Sumatriptan (Imitrex)

◊ 6 mg subcutaneous self-administered injection, or 100 mg oral tablet

Contraindications:

• Avoid ergotamines in pregnancy, peripheral vascular disease, myocardial ischemia
• Avoid aspirin and NSAID's containing drugs if danger of gastric erosion
• Combination drugs including barbiturates and codeine have the potential for addiction

Precautions:

• Match choice of treatment to patient
• Ergotamines must be administered early and may increase vomiting in susceptible patients

• Monitor use of analgesics for symptoms of gastric erosion
• Monitor use of potentially-addictive medications (codeine, butalbital)
• Combination drugs with vasoconstrictors (ergotamines, Midrin, Isocom) may increase blood pressure

Significant possible interactions: Other sedatives, analgesics, alcohol, vasoconstrictors

ALTERNATIVE DRUGS

• Any analgesic, anti-emetic, sedative, oxygen

In Emergency-room situation

◊ Try adequate analgesia plus anti-emetic as above

◊ Oxygen 8-10 L/minute for ten minutes

◊ Prochlorperazine (Compazine) 10 mg IV or IM

◊ Ketorolac (Toradol) 30-60 mg IM

◊ Dihydroergotamine mesylate (DHE 45) 1 mg IM at presentation. May repeat after one hour to maximum of three doses. Or 0.75-1 mg IV slowly over 2-3 minutes with or without 5 mg prochlorperazine. Additional 0.5 mg IV after 30 minutes prn.

◊ Avoid narcotic use in migraine. If above protocols unsuccessful, consider alternative diagnosis, especially intracranial lesion or drug-addiction.

FOLLOWUP

PATIENT MONITORING

• Frequency of attacks
• Management of medications, monitor side-effects
• Continue patient education

PREVENTION/AVOIDANCE

• Avoid precipitants of attacks
• Prophylactic therapy: If attacks significantly interfere with lifestyle in timing or severity, daily prophylactic medication may be appropriate. Regular follow-up mandatory to monitor effect on migraine and side-effects of individual drugs. Only propranolol indicated by FDA for migraine prophylaxis.
- Propranolol (Inderal) 80-320 mg daily
- Atenolol (Tenormin) 50-100 mg daily
- Nadolol (Corgard) 40-80 mg daily
- Metoprolol (Lopressor) 100-450 mg daily
- Amitriptyline (Elavil) 50-150 mg daily
- Methysergide (Sansert) 5-8 mg daily
- Cyproheptadine (Periactin) 4-16 mg daily
- Ergonovine (Ergotrate) 0.4 - 2 mg mg daily
- Verapamil (Isoptin, Calan) 80-120 mg tid

POSSIBLE COMPLICATIONS

• Rare status migrainous. Attack lasting longer than 72 hours leading to dehydration, sterile meningeal inflammation, exhaustion.
• Rare cerebral ischemic episodes during attack
• Iatrogenic effects of treatment, including drug addiction if narcotics are given for acute attacks. Side-effects of prophylaxis must be balanced against effectiveness.

EXPECTED COURSE AND PROGNOSIS

• Reduction in severity and frequency of attacks with age
• Change in nature of attacks with age
• Most migraine attacks should subside within 72 hours

MISCELLANEOUS

ASSOCIATED CONDITIONS Motion
sickness

AGE-RELATED FACTORS

Pediatric: May present with abdominal pain and cyclical vomiting as dominant symptoms rather than headache

Geriatric:

• Very rare onset after 40 years of migraine equivalent - episodic neurological dysfunction with or without headache. Possible relationship to transient global amnesia
• Late onset of migraine or equivalent requires investigation for intra-cranial lesion

Others:

• No racial or social class predominance in migraine. No relationship to intelligence or psychological profile.
• Majority of migraine patients do not consult physicians but manage attacks in family context

PREGNANCY Attacks appear to diminish or
abate during pregnancy. Use of ergotamines contraindicated.

SYNONYMS

• Hemicrania
• Sick headache

ICD-9-CM 346.9

SEE ALSO N/A

OTHER NOTES

New drugs in development (some in use outside USA)

◊ Pizotyline - 5HT antagonist. Prophylaxis 1.5-3 mg daily.

◊ Nimodipine - calcium channel blocker

◊ Flunarizine - calcium channel blocker 20 mg IV for acute attacks. Oral for prophylaxis.

◊ Pirprofen - NSAID 600 mg suppositories for acute attack

ABBREVIATIONS N/A

REFERENCES

• Sandler, M. & Collins, G.M., (eds.): Migraine: A Spectrum of Ideas. New York, Oxford University Press, 1990
• Raskin, N.H.: Headache. 2nd Ed. New York, Churchill Livingstone, 1986
• Dalessio, D.J. (ed.): Wolff's Headache. 5th Ed. New York, Oxford University Press, 1987

Author A. Walling, M.D.

Miliaria rubra

BASICS

DESCRIPTION Miliaria rubra or prickly heat is a papulovesicular eruption
System(s) affected: Skin/Exocrine
Genetics: N/A
Incidence/Prevalence in USA: N/A
Predominant age: Common in infants, less common in adults
Predominant sex: Male = Female

SIGNS AND SYMPTOMS
• Fine papules and vesicles on an erythematous base
• May become inflamed pustules (miliaria pustulosa)
• Prevalent in areas of friction caused by clothing and in areas of flexure
• In infants - trunk, diaper area, neck, groin, axilla, face
• Pilosebaceous follicles, palms, soles spared
• Lesions appear after individual has been in a hot humid environment, resulting in sweating
• Pruritus or prickly, mildly stinging sensation in affected areas

CAUSES
• Keratinous plugging of the sweat ducts as a result of toxins produced by resident bacteria
• This leads to rupture of sweat duct producing sweat retention vesicle

RISK FACTORS
• Hot humid environment
• Occlusive bandages
• Plastic undersheets
• High fever

DIAGNOSIS

DIFFERENTIAL DIAGNOSIS
• Acne
• Folliculitis
• Viral exanthems
• Drug eruptions
• Erythema toxicum
• Yeast infections
• Pyogenic infections

LABORATORY N/A
Drugs that may alter lab results: N/A
Disorders that may alter lab results: N/A

PATHOLOGICAL FINDINGS
• Keratinous plugging of sweat ducts
• Sweat retention vesicle

SPECIAL TESTS N/A

IMAGING N/A

DIAGNOSTIC PROCEDURES N/A

TREATMENT

APPROPRIATE HEALTH CARE
Outpatient

GENERAL MEASURES
• Avoid wearing heavy, tight clothing or garments causing friction
• Avoid plastic or occlusive dressings/garments in hot environments
• Avoid excessive use of soap and contact with irritants
• Frequent cool baths with Aveeno colloidal, oatmeal or cornstarch
• Provide cool, dry environment for 8-10 hours a day

ACTIVITY Avoid vigorous activity leading to sweating

DIET No special diet

PATIENT EDUCATION
• Cause of eruption/avoidance
• General measures for home care

MEDICATIONS

DRUG(S) OF CHOICE
• Topical steroids to relieve pruritus - 0.1% Valisone bid for 3 days
• Systemic antibiotics in cases of bacterial secondary infection - Staphylococcicidal antibiotic, e.g., dicloxacillin 250 mg qid for 10 days (unless resistance)
• If sweating due to fever, antipyretic drugs may be useful

Contraindications: N/A

Precautions: Care with fluorinated steroid application in children. They may cause systemic effects.

Significant possible Interactions: N/A

ALTERNATIVE DRUGS   N/A

FOLLOWUP

PATIENT MONITORING   As needed for persistence of symptoms

PREVENTION/AVOIDANCE
• See General measures
• Acclimatize slowly to hot weather

POSSIBLE COMPLICATIONS
Secondary bacterial infections

EXPECTED COURSE AND PROGNOSIS
• Benign - responds to cooling
• Avoidance of causative agents is key

MISCELLANEOUS

ASSOCIATED CONDITIONS   N/A

AGE-RELATED FACTORS
Pediatric: More common
Geriatric:
• Less common
• Backs of hospitalized patients
Others: N/A

PREGNANCY   N/A

SYNONYMS   Prickly heat

ICD-9-CM
705.1 Prickly heat

SEE ALSO   N/A

OTHER NOTES   N/A

ABBREVIATIONS   N/A

REFERENCES   Bondi, E., Jegasothy, B. & Lazarus, G.: Dermatology, Diagnosis and Therapy, 1991

Author   J. Stearns, M.D.

Milk-alkali syndrome

 BASICS

DESCRIPTION A condition resulting from ingestion of excessive amounts of calcium and absorbable alkali (e.g., sodium bicarbonate and calcium carbonate) usually during self-treatment for peptic ulcer or gastro-esophageal reflux
System(s) affected: Gastrointestinal, Renal/Urologic, Endocrine/Metabolic
Genetics: Unknown
Incidence/Prevalence in USA: Infrequent
Predominant age: 40-75 years
Predominant sex: Male = Female

SIGNS AND SYMPTOMS
• Anorexia
• Band keratopathy
• Constipation
• Dehydration
• Depression
• Dizziness
• Food distaste
• Headache
• Irritability
• Mental status changes
• Myalgias
• Nausea
• Periarticular calcinosis
• Polydipsia
• Polyuria
• Vomiting
• Weakness

CAUSES Excess intake of milk and alkali as therapy for gastrointestinal problems accompanied with gastric hyperacidity (e.g., peptic ulcer, esophageal reflux)

RISK FACTORS
• Peptic ulcer
• Hiatal hernia
• Malignancies

 DIAGNOSIS

DIFFERENTIAL DIAGNOSIS Other causes of hypercalcemia, such as excessive osteolysis with malignant disease, vitamin intoxication, thyroid disease, sarcoidosis, thiazide diuretic treatment, hyperparathyroidism

LABORATORY
• Mild alkalosis
• Hypercalcemia
• Normocalciuria
• Decreased urine phosphate
• Increased BUN and serum creatinine
• Normal alkaline phosphatase
Drugs that may alter lab results: N/A
Disorders that may alter lab results: N/A

PATHOLOGICAL FINDINGS
Nephrocalcinosis, ectopic calcification

SPECIAL TESTS N/A

IMAGING N/A

DIAGNOSTIC PROCEDURES N/A

 TREATMENT

APPROPRIATE HEALTH CARE
Inpatient

GENERAL MEASURES
• Withdraw milk and alkali
• Treat the hypercalcemia
• Intravenous treatment to cause calcinosis (usually with sodium chloride solution)
• Goal of treatment: Maintain urine volume of 3 liters per day
• With significant renal insufficiency, employ renal dialysis

ACTIVITY Bedrest during active treatment

DIET Increased fluid intake

PATIENT EDUCATION N/A

MEDICATIONS

DRUG(S) OF CHOICE
• To treat hypercalcemia: Isotonic sodium chloride 0.9% intravenously when serum calcium exceeds 15 mg/dL (see Hypercalcemia), plus
• Furosemide 80 to 100 mgm IV q 2h for 24 hours after volume depletion has been corrected
Contraindications: Refer to manufacturer's literature
Precautions: Replace sodium and potassium losses associated with furosemide use
Significant possible interactions: Refer to manufacturer's literature

ALTERNATIVE DRUGS
Disodium and monopotassium phosphate. (HAZARDOUS - should be used only by experienced nephrologist and only if dialysis is unavailable.)

FOLLOWUP

PATIENT MONITORING
• Kidney function
• Fluid intake and output
• Urine electrolytes

PREVENTION/AVOIDANCE
Avoid excess milk and/or absorbable antacids

POSSIBLE COMPLICATIONS
• Renal failure
• Nephrocalcinosis

EXPECTED COURSE AND PROGNOSIS
Favorable with appropriate therapy

MISCELLANEOUS

ASSOCIATED CONDITIONS
• Peptic ulcer disease
• Hiatal hernia
• Gastro-esophageal reflux
• Hyperparathyroidism
• Hypercalcemia of malignancy

AGE-RELATED FACTORS
Pediatric: N/A
Geriatric: Occurs predominately in this age group
Others: N/A

PREGNANCY   N/A

SYNONYMS   N/A
• Burnett's syndrome
• Milk poisoning
• Milk drinker syndrome

ICD-9-CM
999.9

SEE ALSO   N/A

OTHER NOTES   N/A

ABBREVIATIONS   N/A

REFERENCES
• Wilson, J.D. & Foster, D.W. (eds): Williams' Textbook of Endocrinology. 7th ed. Philadelphia, Saunders, 1985
• Labhart, A.: Clinical Endocrinology: Theory & Practice. 2nd Ed. Springhouse, PA, Springer-Verlag, 1987

Author S. Smith

Mitral stenosis

BASICS

DESCRIPTION Resistance to diastolic filling of the left ventricle due to valvular narrowing. In the adult, the most common etiology is rheumatic heart disease.
System(s) affected: Cardiovascular
Genetics: Congenital mitral stenosis is a rare congenital malformation, manifested in only 0.42% of children with congenital heart disease
Incidence/Prevalence in USA: The overall incidence of rheumatic heart disease is decreasing. The mitral valve is the valve most commonly affected with rheumatic heart disease.
Predominant age: Symptoms primarily occur in middle age (40-70 years)
Predominant sex: Female > Male

SIGNS AND SYMPTOMS
History:
◊ History of murmur
◊ History of rheumatic fever
◊ History of pulmonary edema with pregnancy, exercise, infection or arrhythmia (commonly atrial fibrillation)
Most common signs and symptoms:
◊ Effort induced dyspnea
◊ Palpitations
◊ Effort fatigue
◊ Hemoptysis (late)
◊ Apical early diastolic low-pitched rumble often with presystolic accentuation (listen with bell of stethoscope in left lateral decubitus position)
◊ Loud S1 (early in disease - as the valve becomes more stenotic and less mobile, this is less common)
◊ Opening snap after S2 (may also diminish in intensity with increasing stenosis)
◊ Right ventricle enlargement
Other signs and symptoms:
◊ Paroxysmal nocturnal dyspnea
◊ Orthopnea
◊ Recumbent cough
◊ Hoarseness
◊ Digital clubbing
◊ Chest pain
◊ Peripheral edema
◊ Systemic embolization
◊ Rales, atrial fibrillation, malar rash (rare)
◊ Holosystolic murmur of mitral regurgitation may accompany the valvular deformity of mitral stenosis
◊ If pulmonary hypertension is present: right ventricular lift, increased pulmonic second sound, a high pitched decrescendo diastolic murmur of pulmonic insufficiency (Graham Steell's murmur)
◊ If right ventricular failure has developed: increased jugular venous distention, holosystolic murmur of tricuspid regurgitation at left sternal border, hepatomegaly and peripheral edema are often found
◊ May also find associated aortic, or less commonly, tricuspid murmurs (due to aortic or tricuspid valve involvement with rheumatic heart disease)

CAUSES In the adult, mitral stenosis is almost always secondary to rheumatic heart disease. Rarely, congenital in etiology.

RISK FACTORS History of rheumatic fever

DIAGNOSIS

DIFFERENTIAL DIAGNOSIS The major differential diagnosis to be considered in a patient with the relatively characteristic findings of mitral stenosis is the uncommon atrial myxoma or vegetation due to endocarditis obstructing left ventricle (LV) inflow. Diastolic flow murmurs can be also heard in the absence of true stenosis due to increased flow across a normal valve. These murmurs are generally limited to early diastole and may be associated with anemia, thyrotoxicosis, shunts as well as with significant mitral regurgitation.

LABORATORY N/A
Drugs that may alter lab results: N/A
Disorders that may alter lab results: N/A

PATHOLOGICAL FINDINGS
• Scarring of the leaflets with fibrosis restricting valve mobility
• Retraction then leads to further valvular narrowing, often with a funnel shaped deformity
• Chordal involvement leads to fusion of the chords and obliteration of the interchordal spaces, further limiting LV inflow
• Left atrial dilatation
• Left atrial thrombi may be found
• Right ventricular hypertrophy
• Pulmonary arterial thickening

SPECIAL TESTS
ECG:
◊ Left atrial enlargement (manifested by broad, notched P waves in lead II with a negative terminal deflection of the P wave in lead V1)
◊ Atrial fibrillation is commonly noted
◊ With right ventricular hypertrophy, right axis deviation may be noted

IMAGING
Chest x-ray:
◊ Left atrial enlargement with straightening of the left heart border, a "double density", and elevation of the left main stem bronchus
◊ Pulmonary venous patterns changes with redistribution of flow toward the apices
◊ Prominent pulmonary arteries at the hilum with rapid tapering
◊ Right ventricular enlargement
◊ Kerley's B lines
◊ Pulmonary edema pattern (late)

DIAGNOSTIC PROCEDURES
Echocardiography: (2-D):
◊ Mitral valve thickening with decreased diastolic excursion and "doming" of the anterior leaflet in diastole
◊ Valvular calcification
◊ Decreased mitral orifice as directly measured by planimetry
◊ Enlarged left atrium
◊ Right ventricular enlargement
◊ Atrial thrombi
Doppler:
◊ Transvalvular pressure gradients
◊ Calculated valve area
◊ Concomitant mitral regurgitation (MR), pulmonary insufficiency (PI), tricuspid regurgitation (TR)
Cardiac catheterization:
◊ Increased left atrial or pulmonary capillary wedge pressure (PCWP)
◊ Increased left atrial or PCWP to left ventricular pressure gradient
◊ Calculated mitral valve orifice area
◊ Calcified mitral valve
◊ Concomitant mitral regurgitation
◊ Presence of coronary artery disease

TREATMENT

APPROPRIATE HEALTH CARE
Outpatient except for complications or surgery

GENERAL MEASURES
• Mitral stenosis is generally a progressive disease. The asymptomatic patient with non-critical mitral stenosis can be followed with appropriate evaluation.
• The patient should avoid unusual stresses (emotional and physical)
• All patients should receive endocarditis prophylaxis, prior to dental work or invasive procedures, regardless of age, etiology or severity of the stenosis (as recommended by the American Heart Association in Circulation, Vol 83, No 3, March, 1991)
• Patients who have mitral stenosis on the basis of rheumatic fever should also receive rheumatic fever prophylaxis (in addition to endocarditis prophylaxis) if under 35 years of age or continues to be in contact with young children
• If atrial fibrillation develops, it is important to slow the heart rate to allow more time for diastolic filling through the stenotic valve
• The development of pulmonary edema is often associated with atrial fibrillation and a rapid ventricular response. It is important to slow the heart rate. Cardioversion could be considered, particularly if the patient is chronically anticoagulated.

• Surgical intervention: If the patient is eligible for a commissurotomy or balloon valvuloplasty, the onset of symptoms clearly referable to the mitral stenosis is generally considered an indication for early surgical intervention. If, however, the patient requires placement of a prosthetic mitral valve prosthesis, often the timing of the surgical intervention is delayed until the symptoms are more severe.

• Consider anticoagulation with warfarin (coumadin) in all patients with mitral stenosis, particularly if a history of systemic embolism, or have atrial fibrillation or a large left atrium

ACTIVITY Adequate rest and reasonable physical activity

DIET Low salt

PATIENT EDUCATION Educate the patient about symptoms of mitral stenosis and report them should they occur

MEDICATIONS

DRUG(S) OF CHOICE

• Judicious addition of diuretics if symptoms indicate

• Atrial fibrillation - consider digoxin plus anticoagulation with coumadin. Beta or calcium channel blockers have been used in place of digoxin. Digoxin is used for rate control, not to convert to normal sinus rhythm. May require high levels (1.5-2.0 nanograms/mL) to be effective. Monitor serum levels.The use of anti-arrhythmic therapy should be considered to maintain normal sinus rhythm.

• Rheumatic fever prophylaxis - preferably penicillin G benzathine, 1.2 million units IM every four weeks or penicillin V 250 mg twice daily

• Bacterial endocarditis prophylaxis - depends on procedure. For dental procedures - amoxicillin 3.0 g 1 hour prior to procedure and 1.5 g 6 hours after initial dose.

Contraindications: Penicillin allergy

Precautions: Refer to manufacturer's profile of each drug

Significant possible interactions: There are many when using the combination of warfarin and digoxin. Use caution when adding new medications. Refer to manufacturer's profile of each drug.

ALTERNATIVE DRUGS Erythromycin for prophylaxis

FOLLOWUP

PATIENT MONITORING Close regular visits for assessment of the gradually progressive symptoms

PREVENTION/AVOIDANCE

• Bacterial endocarditis prophylaxis for dental and invasive procedures continued for life

• Strep throat - treat appropriately when it occurs

• Rheumatic fever prophylaxis when indicated (See GENERAL MEASURES)

POSSIBLE COMPLICATIONS

• Thromboembolism from mitral stenosis is a major potential complication (anticoagulation therapy has lessened this risk substantially)

• Recurrent rheumatic fever

• Bacterial endocarditis

• Pulmonary hypertension

• Pulmonary edema

EXPECTED COURSE AND PROGNOSIS

• Although a milder course is now seen in North America, the classic mitral stenosis history is 10 years from the episode of rheumatic fever to the development of a murmur, another 10 years until symptomatic and another 10 years for the patient to develop serious disability

• Operative mortality 1-2% for mitral commissurotomy; 2-5% for mitral valve replacement

MISCELLANEOUS

ASSOCIATED CONDITIONS Congestive heart failure

AGE-RELATED FACTORS

Pediatric: N/A

Geriatric:

• Atrial fibrillation and complicating arterial embolism more common

• Though there is an increased risk for bleeding, anticoagulation therapy recommended (unless specifically contraindicated) due to high risk of embolism and valve thrombosis (especially if atrial fibrillation present)

Others: N/A

PREGNANCY

• Can cause marked deterioration in cardiac function due to hemodynamic changes associated with increased intravascular volume and heart rate, with decreased diastolic filling time

• The associated pulmonary hypertension also poorly tolerated in pregnancy

SYNONYMS N/A

ICD-9-CM 394.0

SEE ALSO N/A

OTHER NOTES N/A

ABBREVIATIONS N/A

REFERENCES

• Brandenburg, R.O., et al.: Cardiology: Fundamentals and Practice, Chicago, Year Book Medical Publishers, 1987

• Dalen, J.E. & Alpert, J.S.: Valvular Heart Disease. 2nd Ed. New York, Little Brown, 1987

• Cotran, R.S. et al.(eds.): Robbins Pathological Basis of Disease, 4th Ed. Philadelphia, W.B. Saunders Co., 1989

• Hurst, J.W, et al.: The Heart. 7th Ed. New York, McGraw-Hill, 1990

Author J. Galloway, M.D., F.A.C.P.

Mitral valve prolapse

BASICS

DESCRIPTION Systolic bulging of the mitral valve leaflets into the left atrium during systole. This anatomic abnormality frequently is associated with vague symptoms. The prolapse causes a crisp systolic sound or click and a late systolic murmur of mitral regurgitation.
System(s) affected: Cardiovascular
Genetics: Occasionally runs in families
Incidence/Prevalence in USA: Unknown
Predominant age: Early adulthood
Predominant sex: Female > Male

SIGNS AND SYMPTOMS
• Early to midsystolic click and a midsystolic or late systolic murmur
• May be asymptomatic
• Orthostatic hypotension
• Chest pain - recurrent, located in left precordial and substernal areas
• Fatigue
• Narrow chest in the A-P diameter
• Psychological changes
• Shortness of breath
• Thin body habitus

CAUSES
• May have familial tendency
• Possible fibromyxomatous degeneration of connective tissue of the mitral valve
• Dysautonomia
• May be associated with congenital heart disease

RISK FACTORS
• Mitral commissurotomy
• Cardiomyopathy

DIAGNOSIS

DIFFERENTIAL DIAGNOSIS
• Hypertrophic cardiomyopathy
• Papillary muscle dysfunction

LABORATORY N/A
Drugs that may alter lab results: N/A
Disorders that may alter lab results: N/A

PATHOLOGICAL FINDINGS
• Myxomatous degeneration of the mitral valve
• Redundancy of mitral valve leaflets

SPECIAL TESTS
ECG:
◊ T-wave and ST-segment changes
◊ Atrial or ventricular ectopic beats
◊ Runs of premature beats

IMAGING Chest x-ray - asthenic habitus, narrow anteroposterior diameter, elongated cardiac silhouette

DIAGNOSTIC PROCEDURES
• 2 dimension echocardiography - the diagnostic technique of choice to demonstrate mitral valve prolapse
• Color Doppler displays the amount of mitral regurgitation
• Exercise testing - documents patient's fatigue and musculoskeletal symptoms
• Cardiac catheterization - confirms the diagnosis, but seldom necessary because of precision of echocardiography. May need to proceed to coronary angiography if coronary heart disease cannot be ruled out.

TREATMENT

APPROPRIATE HEALTH CARE
Outpatient

GENERAL MEASURES
• The majority require no treatment
• Rarely - mitral valve replacement if mitral regurgitation becomes progressive with enlarged ventricle or ruptured chordae. Instead of valvular replacement, some authorities prefer mitral valve reconstruction or mitral valve annuloplasty.

ACTIVITY No restrictions

DIET No limitations unless there are complications

PATIENT EDUCATION
• Assurance of usual benign course
• Approved printed material for patient information can be obtained from: American Heart Association, 7320 Greenville Avenue, Dallas, TX 75231, (214)373-6300

Mitral valve prolapse

MEDICATIONS

DRUG(S) OF CHOICE
• Usually none
• Beta-blockers if palpitations and/or ventricular atopy become disabling
Contraindications: Refer to manufacturer's literature
Precautions: Beta-blockers will increase fatigue - already a problem for many patients with this syndrome
Significant possible interactions: Refer to manufacturer's literature

ALTERNATIVE DRUGS   None

FOLLOWUP

PATIENT MONITORING   Conservative followup. Evaluate every 2-3 years for development of mitral regurgitation or other complications.

PREVENTION/AVOIDANCE   Antibiotic prophylaxis to prevent infective endocarditis

POSSIBLE COMPLICATIONS
• Note - incidence of complications is low
• Infective endocarditis
• Stroke
• Congestive heart failure
• Cardiac dysrhythmias
• Sudden death
• Mitral regurgitation

EXPECTED COURSE AND PROGNOSIS   Uncertain, but usually benign

MISCELLANEOUS

ASSOCIATED CONDITIONS
• Marfan's syndrome
• Osteogenesis imperfecta
• Coronary artery disease
• Rheumatic endocarditis
• Autoimmune thyroid disorders
• Anorexia nervosa
• Bulimia
• Ehlers-Danlos syndrome

AGE-RELATED FACTORS
Pediatric: Not a problem in this age group
Geriatric: Usually discovered before age 50
Others: N/A

PREGNANCY   N/A

SYNONYMS
• Systolic murmur-click syndrome
• Mitral click murmur syndrome

ICD-9-CM
424.0 Mitral valve disorders
394.0 Mitral stenosis
394.1 Rheumatic mitral insufficiency
394.2 Mitral stenosis with insufficiency
394.9 Other and unspecified mitral value diseases

SEE ALSO   N/A

OTHER NOTES   N/A

ABBREVIATIONS   N/A

REFERENCES
• Hurst, J.W., et al.: The Heart. 7th Ed. New York, McGraw-Hill, 1990
• Wyngaarden, J.B. & Smith, L.H. (eds): Cecil Textbook of Medicine. 18th Ed. Philadelphia, W.B. Saunders Co., 1992

Author   H. Griffith, M.D. & M. Dambro, M.D.

Molluscum contagiosum

 BASICS

DESCRIPTION
Common, benign viral skin disorder consisting of small umbilicated papules which tend to occur on the face, trunk and extremities in children and on the groin and genitalia in adults. Incubation period is 2 weeks to 2 months.
Genetics: No known genetic pattern
Systems(s)affected: Skin/Exocrine
Incidence in USA: Common
Prevalence in USA: Common
Predominant age: Children and young adults
Predominant sex: Male = Female

SIGNS AND SYMPTOMS
• Discrete pearly to flesh colored firm papules
• Diameter 2 to 6 mm (rarely giant nodules up to 3 cm occur)
• Usually grouped in one or two areas
• Centrally umbilicated with erythematous base
• Beneath umbilicated center is white curdlike core
• Distribution: Anywhere. Predilection for face, trunk and extremities in children and groin and genitalia in adults.

CAUSES
DNA virus of the poxvirus group. The virus cannot be grown in cell cultures. Incubation period is 2 weeks to 2 months after contact.

RISK FACTORS
Close personal contact with infected persons. In children, transmission can occur from swimming pools. In adults, sexual transmission is common. In immune compromised patients, infections may be extensive.

 DIAGNOSIS

DIFFERENTIAL DIAGNOSIS
• Furunculosis
• Keratoacanthomas
• Warts
• Pyodermas
• Vesicular skin disorders
• Disseminated mycosis in AIDS patients

LABORATORY
Virus particles cannot be cultured
Drugs that may alter lab results: N/A
Disorders that may alter lab results: N/A

PATHOLOGICAL FINDINGS
• Intracytoplasmic inclusion bodies in histological or cytological specimens
• Hypertrophied and hyperplastic epidermis

SPECIAL TESTS
N/A

IMAGING
N/A

DIAGNOSTIC PROCEDURES
• White, curdlike core easily expressed from beneath umbilication
• Biopsy

 TREATMENT

APPROPRIATE HEALTH CARE
Outpatient

GENERAL MEASURES
• Spontaneous resolution common in 6 to 12 months
• Topical applications including cantharidin (may be too irritating for genital lesions), trichloroacetic acid and liquid nitrogen. Podophyllin is ineffective.
• Removal by curettage

ACTIVITY
No restrictions

DIET
No special diet

PATIENT EDUCATION
Instructions for Patients, W.B. Saunders Co., Philadelphia

MEDICATIONS

DRUG(S) OF CHOICE Topical cantharidin (sloughing of tissue in 7 to 10 days, scarring is none or minimal, pain on application is minimal, but may be too irritating for some genital lesions)
Contraindications: Refer to manufacturer's literature. For external use only. Do not allow exposure to normal skin or mucous membranes.
Precautions: Refer to manufacturer's literature
Significant possible interactions: None expected

ALTERNATIVE DRUGS
• Liquid nitrogen
• Trichloroacetic acid applied by cotton tipped applicator, Calgiswab or toothpick like applicator.

FOLLOWUP

PATIENT MONITORING
Recheck in 2 to 4 weeks after treatment for development of new lesions. Two to 4 visits are often required for complete course of treatment.

PREVENTION/AVOIDANCE In adults, avoid sexual contact with infected individuals

POSSIBLE COMPLICATIONS
• Autoinoculation is common
• Contagious to others
• Immunocompromised individuals may have extensive infections

EXPECTED COURSE AND PROGNOSIS
• Untreated, the condition is usually self limited. Individual lesions spontaneously involute in 2 months. Total resolution usually takes 6 to 12 months.
• Recurrences are uncommon.

MISCELLANEOUS

ASSOCIATED CONDITIONS N/A

AGE-RELATED FACTORS
Pediatric: Commonly seen on face, trunk and extremities. May be spread through swimming pools.
Geriatric: N/A
Others: In adults, is often a sexually transmitted disease.

PREGNANCY N/A

SYNONYMS N/A

ICD-9-CM 078.0 Molluscum contagiosum

SEE ALSO N/A

OTHER NOTES Spontaneous healing depends on triggering of a cell mediated immune response

ABBREVIATIONS N/A

REFERENCES
• Billstein, S.A., & Mattaliano, V.J.: The "nuisance" sexually transmitted diseases: Molluscum contagiosum, scabies, and crab lice. Med Clin North America 1990;74(6):1487-1491
• Buntin, D.M, et al.: Sexually transmitted diseases: Viruses and ectoparasites. J Am Acad Dermatol, 1991;25:527-34
• Lowy, D.R.: Milker's nodules, Molluscum Contagiosum. In Dermatology in General Medicine. 3rd Ed. Edited by T.B. Fitzpatrick, et al. New York, McGraw-Hill, 1987

Author N. Elder, M.D., MSPH

Mononucleosis

 BASICS

DESCRIPTION Mononucleosis is a viral illness caused by the Epstein-Barr virus (EBV) of the herpes family. It causes 90% of the mono-like syndromes. EBV infection causes general involvement of the lymphoreticular system. The "mono" syndrome is characterized by fatigue, fever, splenomegaly, adenopathy and pharyngitis. Transmission is fecal-oral, often attributed to kissing. Incubation period is 20-50 days.

System(s) affected:
Hemic/Lymphatic/Immunologic

Genetics: N/A

Incidence/Prevalence in USA:
• Lower socioeconomic status: 50-85% seropositive by age 4
• Middle-upper socioeconomic status: 14-50% seropositive by college age
• By young adult life, 60-90% of persons are antibody positive
• Incidence is about 50/100,000 in general population to 5,000/100,000 in susceptible college students

Predominant age: High school and college predominate

Predominant sex: Male = Female

SIGNS AND SYMPTOMS
• Malaises (100%)
• Fatigue (100%)
• Headache (50%)
• Fever (85%)
• Adenopathy (85%)
• Tonsillitis (60%)
• Headache (50%)
• Splenomegaly (45%)
• Hepatomegaly (35%)
• Petechiae (palate) (35%)
• Edema (periorbital) (35%)
• Rash (3-15%)

CAUSES Epstein-Barr virus - double-stranded DNA virus (herpes family)

RISK FACTORS
• College and high school students
• Kissing
• 70-90% shed virus 2-6 months after initial infection
• 20-30% individuals shed virus at any one time after 6 months

 DIAGNOSIS

DIFFERENTIAL DIAGNOSIS
• Cytomegalovirus (CMV)
• Toxoplasmosis
• Rubella
• Adenovirus
• Herpes simplex
• Drug side effects
• Streptococcal pharyngitis
• Viral tonsillitis
• Vincent's angina
• Diphtheria
• Viral hepatitis A and B
• Lymphoma or leukemia

LABORATORY
• Positive EBV titers (IgG or IgM) (100%)
• Lymphocytosis (95%)
• Atypical monocytosis (95%)
• Elevated liver function tests (80%)
• Hypergammaglobulinemia (80%)
• Positive heterophil antibodies (70%)
• Thrombocytopenia (50%)
• Elevated bilirubin (40%)
• Cold agglutinins (30-80%)
• Monospot test useful as screen

Drugs that may alter lab results: N/A

Disorders that may alter lab results:
• CMV most frequently confused with EBV-induced mononucleosis
• Group A beta streptococcus often present (30%); does not rule out mononucleosis

PATHOLOGICAL FINDINGS
• B-Cell lymphocytes infected
• Polyclonal proliferation of B-Cells
• Strong T-Cell response

SPECIAL TESTS
• Positive results most likely during 2nd to 3rd week of clinical illness
• Heterophil antibody tests (Monospot or differential absorption) . Tends to be negative in young children
Specific EBV titers (use in heterophil negative or complications)
◊ Viral capsid antigen (VCA): IgG and IgM - peak at 3-4 weeks. IgG then declines, but persists for life. IgM declines rapidly and is undetectable by 3 months. High persisting IgG suggests remote infection, systemic lupus, chronic renal failure, Burkitt's lymphoma, nasopharyngeal cancer, leukemia, sarcoidosis, cancer, AIDS, Hodgkin's lymphoma, rheumatoid arthritis, and immunodeficiency state.
◊ Early antigen (EA): Occur in 70-90%, persist 2-3 months. May persist in up to 20% of remote infections. High persisting titers might suggest: Pregnancy, immunodeficiency states, Hodgkin's lymphoma, lymphoma, leukemia, AIDS, Burkitt's, nasopharyngeal carcinoma.
◊ Epstein-Barr nuclear antigen (EBNA): Develop after 2 months and persist indefinitely. E antigen in mononucleosis primarily. K antigen in nasopharyngeal carcinoma primarily. Absent suggests immunodeficiency.

IMAGING Possible splenomegaly and/or hepatomegaly

DIAGNOSTIC PROCEDURES
• History and physical - fatigue, fever, splenomegaly, adenopathy, pharyngitis
• Heterophil antibodies - positive serology
CBC/differential - abnormal white count
◊ Absolute lymphocytosis (> 4,000 cells/cc)
◊ Relative lymphocytosis (> 50%)
◊ Atypical lymphocytosis (10-20% or more)

 TREATMENT

APPROPRIATE HEALTH CARE
Outpatient usually

GENERAL MEASURES
• No specific treatment
• Quarantine not indicated
• General supportive measures
• Gargles
• If splenic rupture, splenectomy
• Avoid vigorous splenic palpation

ACTIVITY
• Rest (bed rest possibly during acute phase)
• Avoid contact sports, heavy lifting, strenuous athletics

DIET
• Healthy diet important
• To ease throat discomfort, patient may want to drink milk shakes, fruit juices and consume soft foods

PATIENT EDUCATION
• Convalescence may take several weeks
• Avoid stress
• Discuss feasibility of continuing with school or work
• Emphasize risk of splenic rupture from contact sports

MEDICATIONS

DRUG(S) OF CHOICE
• Antibiotics for secondary infections only
• Analgesics (Tylenol or Tylenol with codeine)
• Steroids may be indicated in certain complications only - prednisone (40-80 mg/d then less over 5-7 days). Consider in threatened airway obstruction, hemolytic anemia, and thrombocytopenic purpura.
Contraindications: Aspirin (associated with Reye's Syndrome)
Precautions: Refer to manufacturer's profile of each drug
Significant possible Interactions: Refer to manufacturer's profile of each drug

ALTERNATIVE DRUGS N/A

FOLLOWUP

PATIENT MONITORING
• Re-evaluate as needed based on clinical findings
• Preferable documentation of resolution of splenomegaly before resuming contact sports

PREVENTION/AVOIDANCE Most likely spread by saliva

POSSIBLE COMPLICATIONS
• Chronic EBV Infections (chronic fatigue syndrome- very controversial)
• Splenic rupture (rare, 0.1-0.5%of patients with proven monoucleosis)
• Hemolytic anemia (mild)
• Thrombocytopenia purpura
• Coagulopathy
• Aplastic anemia
• Hemolytic-uremic syndrome
• Seizures
• Cerebellar syndrome
• Nerve palsies
• Meningoencephalitis
• Optic neuritis
• Reye's syndrome
• Coma
• Transverse myelitis
• Guillain-Barré syndrome
• Psychosis
• Pericarditis
• Myocarditis
• ECG changes
• Airway obstruction
• Pneumonitis
• Pleural effusion
• Pulmonary hemorrhage
• Hepatitis/liver necrosis
• Malabsorption
• Dermatitis
• Urticaria
• Erythema multiforme
• Glomerulonephritis
• Nephrotic syndrome
• Mild hematuria/proteinuria
• Conjunctivitis
• Episcleritis
• Uveitis
• B-hemolytic streptococcal infections
• Staphylococcal infection
• Mycoplasma infection
• Bullous myringitis
• Orchitis
• Parotitis
• Monoarticular arthritis

EXPECTED COURSE AND PROGNOSIS
• Fever subsides in about 10 days
• Adenopathy and splenomegaly subside in about 4 weeks
• Children should be able to return to school when signs of infection have decreased, appetite returns, and alertness, strength, and sense of well-being allow.
• Death is uncommon (splenic rupture, blood dyscrasias, hypersplenism, or encephalitis)

MISCELLANEOUS

ASSOCIATED CONDITIONS
Streptococcal pharyngitis

AGE-RELATED FACTORS
Pediatric:
• Children have subclinical or mild infections
• Most adolescents have clinically apparent infections
Geriatric: N/A
Others: N/A

PREGNANCY No other specific recommendations

SYNONYMS
• Mono
• Infectious mononucleosis (IM)

ICD-9-CM 075 infectious mononucleosis

SEE ALSO Epstein-Barr virus infections

OTHER NOTES N/A

ABBREVIATIONS N/A

REFERENCES
• Neinstein, L.S.: Adolescent Health Care: A Practical Guide. 2nd Ed. Baltimore, Urban & Schwarzenberg, Inc., 1991
• Schroeder, S.A., Krupp, M.A., Tierney, L.M. & McPhee, S.J. (eds.): Current Medical Diagnosis and Treatment. Norwalk, CT, Appleton & Lange, 1989
• Braunwald, E., et al. (eds.): Harrison's Principles of Internal Medicine. 12th Ed. New York, McGraw-Hill, 1991
• Safran, D. & Bloom, G.P.: Spontaneous Splenic Following Mononucleosis. American Surgeon, 56(10):601-5 (VI:91093752) Oct, 1990

Author R. Weston, M.D.

Motion sickness

 BASICS

 DIAGNOSIS

 TREATMENT

DESCRIPTION Not a true sickness but a normal response to an abnormal situation in which there is a sensory conflict about body motion between the visual receptors, vestibular receptors and body proprioceptors. It can also be induced when patterns of motion differ from those previously experienced.
System(s) affected: Nervous
Genetics: N/A
Incidence/Prevalence in USA: N/A
Predominant age: N/A
Predominant sex: N/A

SIGNS AND SYMPTOMS
• Nausea
• Vomiting
• Diaphoresis
• Pallor
• Hypersalivation
• Yawning
• Hyperventilation
• Anxiety
• Panic
• Malaise
• Fatigue
• Weakness
• Confusion

CAUSES Motion (auto, plane, boat, amusement rides)

RISK FACTORS
• Travel
• Visual stimuli (i.e. moving horizon)
• Poor ventilation (fumes, smoke, carbon monoxide)
• Emotions (fear, anxiety)
• Zero gravity
• Other illness or poor health

DIFFERENTIAL DIAGNOSIS
• Mountain sickness
• Vestibular disease
• Gastroenteritis
• Metabolic disorders
• Toxin exposure

LABORATORY N/A
Drugs that may alter lab results: N/A
Disorders that may alter lab results: N/A

PATHOLOGICAL FINDINGS N/A

SPECIAL TESTS N/A

IMAGING N/A

DIAGNOSTIC PROCEDURES N/A

APPROPRIATE HEALTH CARE
Remove triggers or noxious stimuli

GENERAL MEASURES
• Minimize exposure (seat in middle of plane or boat)
• Improve ventilation

ACTIVITY
• Semi-recumbant seating
• Fix vision at 45 degree angle above horizon
• Avoid fixation of vision on moving objects (i.e. waves)
• Avoid reading

DIET
• Decrease oral intake or take frequent small feedings
• Avoid alcohol

PATIENT EDUCATION N/A

MEDICATIONS

DRUG(S) OF CHOICE Scopolamine (Transdermal) patch every 3 days
Contraindications: Glaucoma
Precautions:
• Young children
• Elderly
• Pregnancy
• Urinary obstruction
• Pyloric obstruction
Significant possible interactions:
• Sedatives (antihistamines, alcohol, antidepressants)
• Anticholinergics (belladonna alkaloids)

ALTERNATIVE DRUGS Antihistamines (dimenhydrinate/Dramamine, meclizine/Antivert)

FOLLOWUP

PATIENT MONITORING N/A

PREVENTION/AVOIDANCE
• Minimize exposure (seat in middle of plane or boat)
• Improve ventilation
• Semi-recumbant seating
• Fix vision at 45 degree angle above horizon
• Avoid fixation of vision on moving objects (i.e. waves)
• Avoid reading

POSSIBLE COMPLICATIONS
• Hypotension
• Dehydration
• Depression
• Panic

EXPECTED COURSE AND PROGNOSIS Symptoms should resolve when motion exposure ends

MISCELLANEOUS

ASSOCIATED CONDITIONS N/A

AGE-RELATED FACTORS
Pediatric: All ages
Geriatric: All ages
Others: N/A

PREGNANCY N/A

SYNONYMS
• Car sickness
• Sea sickness
• Air sickness
• Space sickness

ICD-9-CM
994.6 Motion sickness

SEE ALSO N/A

OTHER NOTES N/A

ABBREVIATIONS N/A

REFERENCES
• Postgraduate Medicine. May, 1991
• Wyngaarden, J.B., Smith, L.H. (eds): Cecil Textbook of Medicine. 18th Ed., Philadelphia, W.B. Saunders Co., 1988

Author R. Oates, M.D.

Multiple myeloma

 BASICS

DESCRIPTION
Multiple myeloma (malignant tumor of plasma cells) is the most common primary malignancy of bone. It is the prototype of a monoclonal tumor cell proliferation that usually reveals monoclonal protein in the serum or urine of more than 90% of patients.
• The disease process encompasses a spectrum of localized and disseminated disease forms
System(s) affected:
Hemic/Lymphatic/Immunologic, Nervous, Musculoskeletal
Genetics: Occasional familial occurrence, indicating recessive heredity
Incidence/Prevalence in USA: Multiple myeloma accounts for approximately 1% of all types of malignant disease and slightly more than 10% of hematologic malignancies
Predominant age: Ages 40 to 80 (with a peak incidence in the 70's)
Predominant sex: Male = Female

SIGNS AND SYMPTOMS
• The majority of patients (65%) present with bone pain
• Pathologic fracture occurs in approximately one-third of these patients
• Weakness and fatigue are common
• Bleeding (nose, gums), often evidenced by purpura or epistaxis, may occur in the presence of thrombocytopenia or secondary amyloidosis
• Recurrent infections may occur
• Patients may also present with renal insufficiency or renal failure
• Swelling on ribs, skull, sternum, vertebrae, clavicles, shoulder, pelvis
• Weight loss
• Hyperviscosity syndrome

CAUSES
Unknown. There are tumor cells characteristic of plasma cells arising from bone marrow.

RISK FACTORS
Family history of myeloma

 DIAGNOSIS

DIFFERENTIAL DIAGNOSIS
Metastatic carcinoma, primary malignancy of bone (sarcoma, lymphoma), metabolic bone disease, monoclonal gammopathy of undetermined significance (MGUS)

LABORATORY
• Anemia is present in 70% of the patients at the time of diagnosis. Nearly all patients will develop anemia as the disease progresses.
• Peripheral blood smear - Rouleaux's formation
• Serum protein electrophoresis - usually shows a spike or a localized band (M spike in approximately 80% of patients). Of these, 50% are IgG protein, 20% IgA, and 17% free monoclonal light chains (Bence Jones protein).
• Urine electrophoresis - positive about 70% of the time for light chains, but inconsistencies hinder diagnosis
• Hypercalcemia
• Decreased platelets
• Elevated sedimentation rate
• Elevated creatinine and BUN
Drugs that may alter lab results: N/A
Disorders that may alter lab results: N/A

PATHOLOGICAL FINDINGS
• Secondary amyloidosis
• Myeloma kidney

SPECIAL TESTS N/A

IMAGING
• Skeletal x-rays often show a radiolucent or a lytic lesion when the long bones are involved. The skull often shows punched-out lytic lesions with no sclerotic or reactive border. Periosteal reaction is uncommon. Vertebral compression fractures, with occasional extraosseous or extradural cord compression, are commonly seen.
• Although Technetium 99 bone scans have often been described as cold, they will actually show some slight uptake increase in involved skeletal regions, particularly in the presence of fracture; however, the amount of uptake is far less than that demonstrated in other malignancies of bone
• MRI scans can be extremely valuable in determining the extent of marrow involvement as well as the difference between benign compression fractures and multiple myeloma lesions

DIAGNOSTIC PROCEDURES
The laboratory test most likely to yield a definitive diagnosis is a bone marrow biopsy. The bone marrow will contain increased numbers of plasma cells at various stages of maturation.

 TREATMENT

APPROPRIATE HEALTH CARE
Outpatient, except during intensive chemotherapy periods

GENERAL MEASURES
• Radiation therapy is limited to patients with intractable bone pain (failing chemotherapy)
• Patients with impending or pathologic fractures should have those fractures rigidly stabilized along with removal of the tumor, if possible. Patients with impending paraplegia secondary to spinal cord involvement should undergo immediate radiation therapy and bracing and/or surgical decompression and stabilization.

ACTIVITY As tolerated

DIET No special diet

PATIENT EDUCATION
American Cancer Society has literature available

MEDICATIONS

DRUG(S) OF CHOICE
• Chemotherapy is the primary treatment for symptomatic multiple myeloma, but the ideal chemotherapy is unknown. The most common initial protocol management includes the oral administration of melphalan (Alkeran) and prednisone. This protocol produces an objective response in 50-60% of the patients. This is usually given in oral doses of 0.25 mg/kg/day for four days, along with 50 mg of prednisone bid for the same period of time. The dosage should be repeated every six weeks with leukocyte and platelet counts evaluated at three-week intervals.

Contraindications: Refer to manufacturer's profile of each drug

Precautions:
• Melphalan - myelosuppression is the major dose-limiting toxicity of this drug (mainly leukopenia, thrombocytopenia). Monitor CBC, platelets every 3 weeks.
• Prednisone - usual hazards of long-term corticosteroid administration. Refer to manufacturer's literature.

Significant possible interactions: Refer to manufacturer's profile of each drug

ALTERNATIVE DRUGS
In the event of failure of the above-mentioned regimen, alternate protocols include
◊ Cyclophosphamide, carmustine (BCNU), vincristine, and prednisone
◊ VAD - combination of Vincristine, doxorubicin (Adriamycin), and dexamethasone

FOLLOWUP

PATIENT MONITORING
CBC, platelets q 6 weeks

PREVENTION/AVOIDANCE N/A

POSSIBLE COMPLICATIONS
• Skeletal destruction
• Spontaneous fractures
• Secondary amyloidosis
• Renal insufficiency
• Recurrent infections (e.g., Streptococcus pneumoniae, Haemophilus influenza)
• Hyperviscosity syndrome

EXPECTED COURSE AND PROGNOSIS
• Average survival time varies considerably. The median survival of all patients is approximately 24 months. A significantly large number of patients survive for much longer periods of time with evidence of disease present.
• There are occasional temporary remissions with therapy
• Bone marrow transplant should be considered in younger patients

MISCELLANEOUS

ASSOCIATED CONDITIONS
Multiple myeloma has an association with systemic amyloidosis in which the amyloid is derived from immunoglobulin light chains. In one autopsy series, 15% of the patients had generalized amyloidosis with deposits in the kidneys, spleen, adrenal bodies, and liver. Kidney involvement often leads to azotemia and secondary renal failure.

AGE-RELATED FACTORS
Pediatric: N/A
Geriatric: More common in older adults
Others: N/A

PREGNANCY N/A

SYNONYMS Myeloma, plasma cell

ICD-9-CM 203.0 multiple myeloma

SEE ALSO N/A

OTHER NOTES N/A

ABBREVIATIONS N/A

REFERENCES
DeVita, V.T., Hellman, S. & Rosenberg, S.A.: The Principles and Practices of Oncology. Philadelphia, J.B. Lippincott, 1985

Author M. Leeson, M.D.

Multiple sclerosis

 BASICS

DESCRIPTION
Multiple sclerosis (MS) is an inflammatory progressive demyelinization of the white matter of the brain and spinal cord resulting in multiple and varied neurologic symptoms and signs. Usual course - intermittent, progressive and relapsing. It may pursue an acute course. It is a major cause of disability in young adults.
System(s) affected: Nervous
Genetics: Appears to be a strong genetic component in determining susceptibility to the disease.
Incidence/Prevalence in USA: 25,000 new cases each year
Predominant age: Young adult (16-40 years)
Predominant sex: Female > Male

SIGNS AND SYMPTOMS
- Ataxia
- Babinski sign
- Blurred, double or loss of vision in a single eye; often triggered by retro-bulbar neuritis and its visual sequelae
- Clonus
- Clumsiness
- Dysarthria
- Emotional
- Lability
- Fatigue
- Genital anesthesia in women
- Hand paralysis
- Hemiparesis
- Hyperactive deep tendon reflexes
- Hyperesthesia
- Incoordination
- Loss of position sense
- Loss of vibration sense
- Monoparesis
- Ocular paralysis
- Paresthesias
- Sexual impotence in men
- Urinary frequency, hesitancy, incontinence
- Trigeminal neuralgia

CAUSES
- Unknown
- Autoimmune theory - supported by HLA linkage, hereditary pattern, immunocytes in plaques, changes in peripheral blood immunocytes
- Viral theory - supported by increasing incidence of disease at higher latitudes, clusters of cases with families, geographical clusters of cases, animal studies of infectious diseases of myelin
- Combined theory - autoimmune disorder triggered by environmental exposure to toxin or virus early in life

RISK FACTORS
- Living in temperate zone
- Northern European descent
- Family history of the disease

 DIAGNOSIS

DIFFERENTIAL DIAGNOSIS
- Amyotrophic lateral sclerosis
- Behcet's disease
- Brain stem tumors
- Central nervous system infections
- Cerebellar tumors
- Friedreich's ataxia
- Hereditary ataxias
- Leukodystrophies
- Neurofibromatosis
- Pernicious anemia
- Ruptured intervertebral disk
- Small cerebral infarcts
- Sarcoidosis
- Spinal cord tumors
- Syphilis
- Syringomyelia
- Systemic lupus erythematosus

LABORATORY
Cerebrospinal fluid
- ◊ Abnormal colloidal gold curve
- ◊ Gamma globulin IgG elevated
- ◊ Mild mononuclear pleocytosis (less than 40 ceils/mL)
- ◊ Myelin debris
- ◊ Negative serology for syphilis
- ◊ Protein normal or slightly elevated (50◊ 100 mg/100 mL)
Tests to exclude other disorders
- ◊ FTA-ABS
- ◊ Sedimentation rate
- ◊ Screens for clinically suspected vasculitic disorders
- ◊ HTLV-I serology
Drugs that may alter lab results: N/A
Disorders that may alter lab results: N/A.

PATHOLOGICAL FINDINGS
- Destruction of myelin sheaths of nerve fibers and axis cylinders, sparing axons, glia and other structures
- Atrophy of optic nerves and cerebral hemispheres
- T-cell lymphocytes about venules

SPECIAL TESTS
- Visual evoked response (VER) - abnormal in 75-97% of definite MS cases
- Somatosensory evoked potentials - abnormal in 72-96% of cases
- Brain stem auditory evoked responses - abnormal in 57-65% of cases

IMAGING N/A
- MRI -(more sensitive than CT) may show many plaques
- CT scan (double-dose, delayed) - plaques

DIAGNOSTIC PROCEDURES
- No test specific to diagnose MS
- History, physical, CSF analysis, MRI, evoked potential studies, repeated observations over a period of time

 TREATMENT

APPROPRIATE HEALTH CARE
- Outpatient as long as possible
- Long-term care facility for physical therapy or complications such as pyelonephritis

GENERAL MEASURES
- No specific therapy. Remissions occur spontaneously and make treatment evaluations difficult
- Emotional support, encouragement, and reassurances are necessary to help avoid a hopeless outlook
- Occupational therapy
- Urologic evaluation including any sexual dysfunction problems (impotence common in male patients)
- Self-catheterizations for inadequate bladder emptying (indwelling catheter may be necessary in a few patients)
- Custodial care, if patient cognitively impaired
- Physiotherapy to maintain range of movement and strength and to avoid contractures

ACTIVITY
- Maintain activity, avoid overwork and fatigue
- Rest during periods of acute relapse

DIET If constipation a problem, high fluid intake, plus a high fiber diet

PATIENT EDUCATION For patient education materials favorably reviewed on this topic, contact: National Multiple Sclerosis Society, 205E-42nd Street, New York, NY, 10017; 1-800-624-8236

MEDICATIONS

DRUG(S) OF CHOICE
• Drug therapy directed toward relieving symptoms
• Prednisone 60 mg/day or methylprednisolone IV 500 mg for 5-7 days for acute attacks, especially retrobulbar neuritis (recommended by some clinicians)
• Chronic fatigue: amantadine 200-300 mg/day (no specific evidence that this works)
• Spasticity: baclofen (low dosage to start, 5 mg 1-3 times a day, increase as needed) or diazepam 2-5 mg at night
• Constipation: stool softeners, bulk producing agents, laxative suppositories
• Urinary problems: propantheline 7.5 mg every 3-4 hours to start, increase to 15 mg 3-4 times a day plus 15-30 mg at bedtime; or oxybutynin chloride 5 mg 3-4 times a day
• Prophylactic antibiotic therapy for urinary infections may be indicated
• Incoordination or tremors: no ideal therapy. May try beta-blockers (if not contraindicated), primidone, or clonazepam
• Depression and emotional lability: amitriptyline 10-25 mg at bedtime to start, increase as tolerated
• Paranoia or mania: haloperidol or lithium
• Musculoskeletal pain or discomfort: nonsteroidal anti-inflammatories
• Hemifacial and dysesthesias: carbamazepine 100-200 once or twice a day to start, increase to total daily dosage of 600-1600 mg 3-4 times a day. Must monitor serum levels.
• Immunosuppressive agents (e.g., azathioprine, adrenocorticotropic hormone (ACTH), methylprednisolone, cyclophosphamide, interferons, cyclosporine) still investigational
Contraindications: Refer to manufacturer's literature
Precautions: Refer to manufacturer's literature
Significant possible interactions: Refer to manufacture

ALTERNATIVE DRUGS
• Baclofen 40-80 mg/day in divided doses for reduction of spasticity
• Interferon (investigational)

FOLLOWUP

PATIENT MONITORING Requires FOLLOWUP

PREVENTION/AVOIDANCE No known preventive measures. Avoid factors that may precipitate an attack, particularly stress from hot weather.

POSSIBLE COMPLICATIONS
• Coma
• Delirium
• Emotional lability
• Nystagmus
• Optic nerve atrophy
• Paraplegia
• Sexual impotence (men)
• Urinary tract infections

EXPECTED COURSE AND PROGNOSIS
• Highly variable and unpredictable. Approximately 70% of patients lead active, productive lives with prolonged remissions.
• May disable the patient by early adulthood or cause death within months of onset
• Average duration exceeds 25 years
• 30% relapse in one year, 20% in 5-9 years, 10% in 10-30 years

MISCELLANEOUS

ASSOCIATED CONDITIONS N/A

AGE-RELATED FACTORS
Pediatric: Unlikely before puberty.
Geriatric: Remissions less frequent in this age group
Others: N/A

PREGNANCY A triggering factor for multiple sclerosis in some cases

SYNONYMS
• Disseminated sclerosis
• Insular sclerosis

ICD-9-CM
340 multiple sclerosis

SEE ALSO N/A

OTHER NOTES
• Since the course is highly variable and unpredictable, avoid a hopeless outlook
• 30-40% of patients with optic neuritis alone eventually develop other signs

ABBREVIATIONS
MS = multiple sclerosis

REFERENCES
• Sibley, W.A.: Therapeutic claims in multiple sclerosis. 2nd Ed. New York, Demos, 1988
• Matthews, W.B., et al.: McAlpine's Multiple Sclerosis. New York, Churchill Livingstone, 1985
• Adams, R.D. & Victor, M.: Principles of Neurology. New York, McGraw-Hill, 1986
• Rowland, L.P. (ed.): Merritt's Textbook of Neurology. 8th Ed. Philadelphia, Lea & Febiger, 1989

AUTHOR S. Smith, M.D.

Mumps

BASICS

DESCRIPTION Acute generalized paramyxovirus infection usually presenting with unilateral or bilateral parotitis. Epidemics occur in late winter and spring with transmission by respiratory secretions. Incubation is approximately 14 to 24 days.
System(s) affected: Reproductive, Hemic/Lymphatic/Immunologic, Skin/Exocrine
Genetics: N/A
Incidence in USA: 0.96/100,000 (2400 per year)
Prevalence in USA:
• 0 .0064/100,000
• 90% of adults are sero-positive even without history
Predominant age: 85% occur before age 15 years, but more severe in adults
Predominant sex: Male = Female

SIGNS AND SYMPTOMS
• Parotid pain and swelling in one or both glands
• Rare prodrome of fever, neck muscle ache, malaise
• Initial parotid swelling just behind jaw
• Swelling peaks in 1-3 days, lasts 3-7 days
• Obscures angle of mandible
• Elevates earlobe
• Redness at opening of Stensen's duct
• Sour foods cause pain in the parotid gland region
• Moderate fever, usually not above 104° F. High fever is frequently associated with complications.
• Meningeal signs in 15%, encephalitis in 0.5%
• Rarely arthritis, orchitis, thyroiditis, mastitis, pancreatitis
• Rare maculopapular erythematous rash
• Up to 50% of cases may be asymptomatic
• Swelling in the sternal area, rare, but pathognomonic of mumps

CAUSES
• Mumps Paramyxovirus
• Other viruses, such as Coxsackie (rare)

RISK FACTORS
• Urban epidemics, non-vaccinated population
• Usual communicable period is 2 days before to 6-10 days after onset of parotitis

DIAGNOSIS

DIFFERENTIAL DIAGNOSIS
• Parainfluenza parotitis, other viruses
• Suppurative parotitis with pus - often associated with Staphylococcus aureus (presence of Wharton's duct pus nearly excludes diagnosis of mumps).
• Recurrent allergic parotitis
• Salivary calculus with intermittent swelling
• Lymphadenitis from any cause
• Cytomegalovirus parotitis in immunocompromised patients
• Mikulicz's syndrome (chronic, painless parotid and lacrimal gland swelling of unknown cause that occurs in tuberculosis, sarcoidosis, lupus, leukemia, and lymphosarcoma patients)
• Malignant or benign salivary gland tumors
• Drug-related parotid enlargement (iodides, guanethidine)
• Other causes of the complications of mumps (meningoencephalitis, orchitis, oophoritis, pancreatitis, polyarthritis, nephritis, myocarditis, prostatitis)
• Mumps orchitis must be differentiated from testicular torsion. (Testicular scan can be useful.)

LABORATORY
• Viral isolation from throat washings, urine, blood, or spinal fluid
• Serum amylase elevated
• Rise in paired antibodies: Anti-"S" antibodies peak early and may be seen at the time of presentation
• Cerebrospinal fluid (CSF) - leucocytosis
• Leukopenia
Drugs that may alter lab results: N/A
Disorders that may alter lab results: N/A

PATHOLOGICAL FINDINGS Periductal edema and lymphocytic infiltration

SPECIAL TESTS Rarely necessary

IMAGING Useful to differentiate mumps orchitis from testicular torsion

DIAGNOSTIC PROCEDURES N/A

TREATMENT

APPROPRIATE HEALTH CARE
Outpatient, if no complications

GENERAL MEASURES
• Supportive and symptomatic
• For patients with orchitis, ice packs to scrotum can help relieve pain
• Scrotal support with adhesive bridge while recumbent and/or athletic supporter while ambulatory
• Use IV fluids if severe nausea or vomiting accompanies pancreatitis

ACTIVITY Mumps Orchitis - bedrest and local supportive clothing, such as wearing 2 pairs of briefs, or adhesive-tape bridge

DIET Liquids if cannot chew

PATIENT EDUCATION
• Must be out of school until no longer contagious - about 9 days after onset of pain
• Orchitis is common in older children but rarely results in sterility
• Immunization of family may protect against later exposures but not the present one

MEDICATIONS

DRUG(S) OF CHOICE Corticosteroids or a nonsteroidal anti-inflammatory may diminish pain and swelling in acute orchitis and arthritis mumps, but usually not necessary. May use acetaminophen for fever and/or pain.
Contraindications: Refer to manufacturer's profile of each drug
Precautions: Avoid aspirin for pain in children. There may be an association of aspirin, virus infection, and Reye's syndrome in children.
Significant possible interactions: Refer to manufacturer's profile of each drug

ALTERNATIVE DRUGS Mumps arthritis may improve with corticosteroids or a nonsteroidal anti-inflammatory

FOLLOWUP

PATIENT MONITORING Most cases will be mild. Monitor hydration status.

PREVENTION/AVOIDANCE
• 2 doses of live mumps vaccine recommended for active immunization: At 15 months and at entry to middle school. (Postexposure vaccination does not protect from recent exposure).
• Isolate hospitalized patients until 9 days past onset

POSSIBLE COMPLICATIONS
• May precede, accompany, or follow salivary gland involvement and may occur (rarely) without primary involvement of the parotid gland
• Meningoencephalitis occurs clinically in approximately 10%. These symptoms may begin as late as 10 days following symptoms that signal onset of the illness.
• Cerebrospinal fluid (CSF) pleocytosis found in 65% of cases with parotitis
• Orchitis common (30%) in postpubertal boys, starts within 8 days after parotitis, fever, swollen testis of 4 day duration, fertility impaired in 13% but absolute sterility is rare
• Oophoritis in 7% of postpubertal females, no decreased fertility
• Pancreatitis, usually mild
• Nephritis thyroiditis, or arthralgias are rare
• Myocarditis - usually mild, but may depress ST segment
• Deafness - 1/15,000 unilateral nerve deafness, may not be permanent
• Inflammation about the eye (rare)

EXPECTED COURSE AND PROGNOSIS
• Complete recovery is usual, immunity is permanent
• Sensorineural hearing loss in 4% of adults - transient
• Rare recurrence after 2 weeks may be recurrent nonepidemic parotitis

MISCELLANEOUS

ASSOCIATED CONDITIONS N/A

AGE-RELATED FACTORS
Pediatric:
• In adolescents - orchitis more common
• Most cases of acute epidemic mumps occur in children aged 5 to 15. Unusual in children less than 2 years. Most infants less than 1 year are immune.
• Less likely to develop complications
Geriatric: Most are immune
Others: Most complications occur in post-pubertal group

PREGNANCY No proven complications of vaccine or virus but theoretically should not vaccinate in pregnancy

SYNONYMS
• Epidemic parotitis
• Infectious parotitis

ICD-9-CM 072.9

SEE ALSO N/A

OTHER NOTES A portion of people infected with mumps virus have no parotid swelling and a clinically inapparent infection

ABBREVIATIONS N/A

REFERENCES
• Behrman, R.E. (ed.): Nelson's Textbook of Pediatrics. Philadelphia, W.B. Saunders, 1991
• Report of the Committee on Infectious Diseases (Red Book). Elk Grove Village, Ill, American Academy of Pediatrics, 1991

Author F. Wu, M.D.

Muscular dystrophy

BASICS

DESCRIPTION Inherited, progressive diseases of muscle with wide ranges of clinical expression. Included: Congenital muscular dystrophy, congenital myotonic dystrophy, Duchenne's muscular dystrophy (DMD), Becker's muscular dystrophy (BMD), myotonic dystrophy, fascioscapulohumeral dystrophy (FHS).
System(s) affected: Musculoskeletal, Nervous
Genetics: See Causes and Risk factors
Incidence/Prevalence in USA:
• Duchenne's muscular dystrophy (DMD) -1 per 3000 male births
• Myotonic dystrophy - 1 per 10,000 births
Predominant age:
• Birth to infancy: Congenital muscular dystrophy with or without cerebral involvement, congenital myotonic dystrophy
• Infancy to early childhood: Duchenne's muscular dystrophy (DMD), Becker's muscular dystrophy (BMD), fascioscapulohumeral dystrophy (FHS)
• Late childhood to adolescence: BMD, FSH, myotonic dystrophy
Predominant sex: Male > Female (DMD and BMD caused by defect in same gene)

SIGNS AND SYMPTOMS
DMD and BMD:
◊ Normal motor milestones until child begins to walk
◊ Clumsiness - frequent falls, toe-walking, waddling gait
◊ Weakness - inability to jump or climb stairs, weak neck flexors, Gower's sign, lumbar lordosis
◊ Pseudohypertrophy of calf muscles and contractures of heel cords
◊ Kyphosis and scoliosis
Myotonic dystrophy:
◊ Facial weakness - open, triangular mouth and droopy eyelids
◊ Sustained muscle contraction with percussion of thenar eminence
◊ High forehead with receding hairline
◊ Neonatal form - hypotonia, respiratory distress, hip dislocations
FSH:
◊ Facial weakness - inability to completely close eyes or whistle, pouting expression with transverse smile
◊ Shoulder and proximal arm weakness - inability to do push-ups, horizontal clavicles, "Popeye" arms, winging of the scapula

CAUSES
• X-linked: DMD and milder allelic form BMD have abnormal gene for production of "dystrophin" on short arm of X chromosome
• Autosomal dominant: Myotonic dystrophy gene mapped to short arm of chromosome 19. FSH gene mapped to long arm of chromosome 4.

RISK FACTORS
• X-linked - affected male on maternal side of family
• Autosomal dominant - affected parent. Myotonic dystrophy more severe if mother is affected parent.

DIAGNOSIS

DIFFERENTIAL DIAGNOSIS
• Onset from birth to early infancy: Encephalopathy, spinal muscular atrophy, infantile botulism, myasthenia gravis, congenital myopathies, metabolic myopathies, chromosomal disorders, paroxysmal disorders, neonatal spinal cord injury
• Onset from infancy to early childhood: Carnitine deficiency, acid maltase deficiency, spinal muscular atrophy, myotonia congenita
• Onset from childhood to adolescence: Other muscular dystrophies, spinal muscular atrophy, congenital myopathies, metabolic or inflammatory myopathies, myasthenia gravis, periodic paralysis

LABORATORY
Creatine kinase:
◊ Marked elevation in DMD
◊ Moderate elevation in BMD, FSH
◊ Normal in congenital muscular dystrophy, late DMD
Drugs that may alter lab results:
• Opiates including codeine, heroin, meperidine, and morphine
• Dexamethasone
• Ethanol
• Digoxin
• Furosemide
• Aminocaproic acid
• Halothane anesthetic
• Imipramine
• Phenobarbital
• Lithium
• Clofibrate
Disorders that may alter lab results:
• Polymyositis/dermatomyositis
• Muscle trauma - exercise, seizures, IM injections, needle EMG
• Hypothyroidism, hyperthyroidism
• Myocardial infarction, stroke, sepsis, shock

PATHOLOGICAL FINDINGS Muscle biopsy in DMD - fiber splitting, necrosis, regeneration with interspersed fibrosis

SPECIAL TESTS EMG in myotonic dystrophy - high frequency repetitive discharges ("dive-bomber" effect)

IMAGING N/A

DIAGNOSTIC PROCEDURES
• Muscle biopsy of moderately weak muscle (vastus lateralis, triceps) not studied by needle electromyography
• Dystrophin level from frozen muscle (Genica, 373 Plantation St., Worcester, MA 01605, telephone (508)756-2886)

TREATMENT

APPROPRIATE HEALTH CARE
Outpatient with team approach - neurologist, orthopedic surgeon, physical and occupational therapists, social worker, and orthotist

GENERAL MEASURES
• Physical therapy to maintain neuromuscular function
• Orthoses to sustain walking and delay development of scoliosis
• Surgical release of contractures or fixation of joints
• Respiratory care, ventilation during sleep for nocturnal hypoventilation syndrome

ACTIVITY Exercise as desired, but stop short of muscle pain or exhaustion

DIET Monitor nutrition and fat stores because of increased caloric requirements

PATIENT EDUCATION
• Family and individual counseling
• Genetic counseling
• Printed material and clinical services available through the Muscular Dystrophy Association, 3561 E. Sunrise Dr., Tucson, AZ 85718. Telephone (800)221-1142

MEDICATIONS

DRUG(S) OF CHOICE
• No drug treatment recommended at present
• Prednisone 0.15-0.75 mg/kg/day improves muscle strength in boys with DMD
Contraindications: N/A
Precautions: Careful monitoring for side effects of long-term steroid therapy is required; these include weight gain, hypertension, GI bleeding, immunosuppression
Significant possible interactions: N/A

ALTERNATIVE DRUGS   N/A

FOLLOWUP

PATIENT MONITORING   Determined by interdisciplinary health care team

PREVENTION/AVOIDANCE
• Maternal carrier status evaluation in DMD (80% sensitive) and BMD (60% sensitive) by creatine kinase levels
• DNA probes for carrier status determination and antenatal diagnosis in DMD and BMD
• DNA linkage techniques in selected families for antenatal diagnosis of myotonic dystrophy

POSSIBLE COMPLICATIONS
• Cardiac arrhythmias or myopathy, in DMD (< 80%); in BMD (< 40%)
• Hypertension - FSH
• Dysphagia or acute gastric dilation - DMD, myotonic dystrophy
• Malignant hyperthermia - DMD
• Respiratory failure and early death - congenital muscular dystrophy (15%), neonatal-onset myotonic dystrophy (> 50%)
• Endocrinopathies - myotonic dystrophy
• Cataracts - myotonic dystrophy
• Sensorineural hearing loss - FSH
• Seizures and cerebral dysplasia - congenital muscular dystrophy with cerebral involvement (> 50%)

EXPECTED COURSE AND PROGNOSIS
DMD and BMD:
◊ Progressive weakness, contractures, inability to walk
◊ Kyphoscoliosis and respiratory compromise
◊ Early death (Duchenne's 16 +/- 4 years; Becker's 42 +/- 16 years)
Myotonic dystrophy (neonatal onset) and congenital muscular dystrophy with cerebral involvement:
◊ Progressive hypotonia and weakness
◊ Respiratory failure and early death
Other types
◊ Slow progression and near normal life span

MISCELLANEOUS

ASSOCIATED CONDITIONS   Mental retardation - DMD (25%), myotonic dystrophy with early onset

AGE-RELATED FACTORS
Pediatric: N/A
Geriatric: N/A
Others: N/A

PREGNANCY   Refer mother with myotonic dystrophy to perinatologist

SYNONYMS
• Pseudohypertrophic muscular dystrophy; DMD
• Steinert's disease; Myotonic dystrophy
• Landouzy-Déjèrine dystrophy; FSH
• Fukuyama syndrome; congenital muscular dystrophy with cerebral involvement

ICD-9-CM
• 359.0 Congenital muscular dystrophy
• 359.1 DMD, BMD, FSH and others
• 359.2 Myotonic dystrophy

SEE ALSO   N/A

OTHER NOTES   N/A

ABBREVIATIONS
• DMD = Duchenne's muscular dystrophy
• BMD = Becker's muscular dystrophy
• FSH = fascioscapulohumeral dystrophy

REFERENCES   Brooke, M.H.: Clinician's View of Neuromuscular Diseases. 2nd Ed. Baltimore, Williams & Wilkins, 1986

Author   D. Griesemer, M.D. & E. Bailey, M.D.

Myasthenia gravis

BASICS

DESCRIPTION
Myasthenia gravis - a disorder of the neuromuscular junction which results in a pure motor syndrome characterized by weakness and fatigue particularly of the extraocular, pharyngeal, facial, cervical, proximal limb and respiratory musculature. Typical and neonatal forms are immunologically mediated. A number of congenital forms of obscure pathogenesis exist. Onset may be sudden and severe (myasthenic crisis) but, more typically, is mild and intermittent over many years.

System(s) affected: Musculoskeletal, Hemic/Lymphatic/Immunologic

Genetics:
• 15% of infants born to myasthenic mothers have neonatal myasthenia gravis, due to the transplacental passage of anti-acetylcholine receptor antibodies. The condition completely resolves in weeks to months. Neonatal myasthenia gravis is not a genetic disorder.
• Infants with congenital myasthenia gravis syndromes are born to normal mothers. The onset is at birth or in early childhood. Inheritance is typically autosomal recessive. The condition is persistent.
• Typical adult and juvenile myasthenia gravis does have a familial predisposition (5% of cases) and an increased frequency of HLA-B8 and DR3.

Incidence/Prevalence in USA:
2-5/year/million; 3/100,000

Predominant age: Ages 20-40, but occurs at any age (1-80). Incidence in females peaks in the 3rd decade, in males in the 5th and 6th decades.

Predominant sex:
• Adults - Female > Male (3:2)
• Children - Female > Male (3:2)
• Children with myasthenia plus associated disease - Female > Male (5:1)

SIGNS AND SYMPTOMS
• Ptosis
• Diplopia
• Facial weakness
• Fatigue on chewing
• Dysphagia
• Dysarthria
• Dysphonia
• Neck weakness
• Proximal limb weakness
• Respiratory weakness
• Generalized weakness

CAUSES Humoral and cellular immune-mediated injury of the post-synaptic neuromuscular junction acetylcholine receptors

RISK FACTORS
• Female
• Age 20-40
• Familial myasthenia gravis
• D-penicillamine ingestion
• Other autoimmune diseases

DIAGNOSIS

DIFFERENTIAL DIAGNOSIS
• Chronic fatigue syndrome
• Neurasthenia
• Oculopharyngeal muscular dystrophy
• Thyrotoxic ophthalmopathy
• Other disorders of neuromuscular transmission (myasthenic syndrome, botulism)
• Polymyositis
• Other myopathies
• Intracranial focal lesions involving cranial nerves
• Multiple sclerosis

LABORATORY
• Acetylcholine receptor antibody - generalized myasthenia 80% positive; ocular myasthenia 50% positive; myasthenia + thymoma 100% positive; congenital myasthenia 0% positive; no clear correlation between antibody titer and disease severity
• Check thyroid function tests

Drugs that may alter lab results: N/A
Disorders that may alter lab results: N/A

PATHOLOGICAL FINDINGS
• Muscle electron microscopy - receptor infolding and the tips of the folds are lost, synaptic clefts are widened
• Immunofluorescence - IgG antibodies and complement on receptor membranes

SPECIAL TESTS
• Motor nerve conduction velocity - normal
• Sensory nerve conduction velocity - normal
• Concentric needle (conventional) electromyography- normal in mild cases; low amplitude, short duration, polyphasic motor unit potentials with a varying morphology (may be called "myopathic")
• Repetitive nerve stimulation - shows a decremental response at 3Hz which is seen more frequently in the proximal, cervical or facial muscles. The decrement is less pronounced 30 seconds after a 30 second maximal voluntary contraction (post-tetanic facilitation) and most pronounced 120 seconds after the contraction (post-tetanic depression).
• Single fiber EMG (SFEMG) - highly sensitive but less specific, technically difficult to perform, limited availability. SFEMG assesses the temporal variability between two muscle fibers within the same motor unit (jitter). Myasthenia is one condition that increases jitter.
• Edrophonium (Tensilon) test - initial dose is 2 mg IV, followed in 30 seconds by 3 mg, followed in 30 seconds by 5 mg to a maximum dose of 10 mg. A positive test is characterized by improvement of strength (of striated muscle) within 30 seconds of administration. False positives make a saline placebo control desirable. Atropine .4 mg IV may rarely be required as an antidote for severe bradycardia, but should always be available.

IMAGING Chest CT scan - thymoma

DIAGNOSTIC PROCEDURES
• History and physical
• Electrodiagnostic studies; repetitive nerve stimulation (RNS)
• Edrophonium (Tensilon) test

TREATMENT

APPROPRIATE HEALTH CARE
• Typically outpatient
• Inpatient care for plasmapheresis, intravenous gamma globulin, management of pulmonary infections, myasthenic or cholinergic crises

GENERAL MEASURES
• Management of myasthenia gravis is difficult and should be carried out by a neurologist with experience in the field.
• There are three basic approaches to treatment, the first being symptomatic, the second being immunosuppressive and the third being supportive. No or few patients should be receiving a single therapeutic modality.
• Symptomatic therapy consists of reversal of weakness with an acetylcholinesterase inhibitor such as pyridostigmine bromide which is also available in a slow release oral preparation, or neostigmine methylsulfate which can be administered parenterally. Symptomatic therapy does nothing to stop the ongoing immunologically mediated damage to the muscle receptor. An overdose of these agents may induce severe weakness known as a cholinergic crisis. A cholinergic crisis should be suspected if there are other signs of cholinergic overactivity (excessive secretions, diarrhea, bradycardia).
• Immunosuppressive therapy in some form is necessary for all patients with myasthenia gravis. This includes thymectomy, corticosteroids, plasmapheresis, immunosuppressive drugs (azathioprine, cyclophosphamide, cyclosporine) and/or intravenous human gammaglobulin.
• Supportive therapy may be intermittently or occasionally eventually continually required and may include intubation, tracheostomy, artificial ventilation, respiratory therapy, administration of antibiotics, nasogastric tube and/or gastrostomy

ACTIVITY As tolerated. Heat and exercise both temporarily exacerbate symptoms.

DIET As tolerated

PATIENT EDUCATION Printed materials, reference lists and other forms of patient and family support available from: 1. Myasthenia Gravis Foundation, 53 W. Jackson, Suite 660, Chicago, IL 60604, (312)427-6252. 2. Muscular Dystrophy Association, 3300 E. Sunrise Drive, Tucson, AZ 85718-3208, (800)221-1142.

MEDICATIONS

DRUG(S) OF CHOICE
• Pyridostigmine bromide (Mestinon), 60 mg tablets and 180 mg sustained release tablets. Titrate dosage to clinical need. An average requirement would be 600 mg per day.
• Neostigmine methylsulfate (Prostigmin), 0.25, 0.5 and 1 mg/mL concentrations. Titrate dosage to clinical need. Starting dosages would be 0.5 mg SC or IM every 3 hours.
• Prednisone should be initiated with a daily, followed by a switch to an alternate day, regimen. Start with a 60-80 mg/day, taper the dosage every 3 days. Switch to an alternate day regimen within 2 weeks, continue to taper very slowly attempting to establish the minimum dosage necessary to maintain remission. A typical maintenance dosage would be 35 mg every other day.
• Azathioprine or cyclophosphamide 150-200 mg per day.
• Immune globulin

Contraindications: Refer to manufacturer's literature

Precautions: Numerous. Avoid aminoglycosides which may precipitate weakness. Refer to manufacturer's literature.

Significant possible interactions: Numerous. Refer to manufacturer's literature.

ALTERNATIVE DRUGS
• Cyclosporine

FOLLOWUP

PATIENT MONITORING
Constant in an intensive care unit setting during myasthenic or cholinergic crises

PREVENTION/AVOIDANCE
Not possible

POSSIBLE COMPLICATIONS
• Acute respiratory arrest
• Chronic respiratory insufficiency
• Atelectasis, aspiration, pneumonia

EXPECTED COURSE AND PROGNOSIS
Highly variable, ranging from remission to death. Mortality is probably less than 10%

MISCELLANEOUS

ASSOCIATED CONDITIONS
• Thymoma
• Thymic hyperplasia
• Thyrotoxicosis
• Other autoimmune diseases

AGE-RELATED FACTORS
Pediatric: N/A
Geriatric: N/A
Others: Occurs in patients of all ages

PREGNANCY   N/A

SYNONYMS   N/A

ICD-9-CM   358.0 myasthenia gravis

SEE ALSO   N/A

OTHER NOTES   N/A

ABBREVIATIONS
MG = myasthenia gravis

REFERENCES
• Rowland, L.P. (ed.): Merritt's textbook of Neurology. 8th ED. Philadelphia, Lea & Febiger, 1989
• Kimura, J.: Electrodiagnosis in diseases of nerve and muscle: principles and practice. 2nd Ed. Philadelphia, F.A. Davis, 1989
• Snead, O.C., Benton, J.W., Dwyer, D. et al.: Juvenile myasthenia gravis. Neurology 30:732-739, 1980
• Soliven, B.C., Lang, D.J., Penn, A.S., et al.: Seronegative myasthenia gravis. Neurology 38:514-517, 1988

Author   C. Bamford, M.D.

Myelodysplastic syndromes (MDS)

BASICS

DESCRIPTION A heterogeneous group of acquired hematopoietic stem cell disorders, characterized by cytologic dysplasia in the bone marrow and blood and by various combinations of anemia, neutropenia, and thrombocytopenia
• There is a natural progression of disease between categories as cellular maturation becomes more arrested and blast cells accumulate. There is a great deal of overlap between arbitrary diagnostic subgroups.
• Refractory anemia (RA) - < 5% blasts in marrow; < 1% blasts in blood
• Refractory anemia with ringed sideroblasts (RARS) - < 5% blasts in marrow; > 15% ringed sideroblasts; < 1% blasts in blood. Also known as acquired idiopathic sideroblastic anemia (AISA).
• Refractory anemia with excess of blasts (RAEB) - 5-20% blasts in marrow; < 5% blasts in blood
• Refractory anemia with excess of blasts in transformation (RAEBT) - 20-30% blasts in marrow; or > 5% blasts in blood; or Auer rods present
• Chronic myelomonocytic anemia (CMMOL) - 1-20% blasts in marrow; < 5% blasts in blood with > 1000 monocytes/µl
• Refractory cytopenia - same as RA but with leukopenia or thrombocytopenia without anemia
• Unclassifiable MDS - marked trilineage dysplasia but without excess of blasts
• Acute MDS with sclerosis - RAEB with marked myelosclerosis
• Refractory anemia with 5q minus syndrome - RA or RAEB with erythroid hyperplasia, mono- or bilobulated megakaryocyte nuclei and normal or increased platelets. Incidence is 2:1 female > male. Characteristic interstitial deletion on the long arm of chromosome 5.
• Therapy-related (t-MDS) - seen 3-7 years after treatment with alkylating agents and/or radiation therapy. Evolves to acute myeloid leukemia (AML) over about 6 months.
System(s) affected:
Hemic/Lymphatic/Immunologic
Genetics: Most are clearly clonal neoplasms by cytogenetics, G6PD isoenzyme analysis, or RFLP analysis. Mutations in RAS oncogene have been reported.
Incidence/Prevalence in USA: Apparent increased incidence (1-2/100,000/year) in recent years may be due to more accurate diagnosis
Predominant age: Median age is > 65 years; uncommon in children and young adults
Predominant sex: Male = Female

SIGNS AND SYMPTOMS
• Anemia - fatigue, shortness of breath, lightheadedness, angina
• Leukopenia - fever, infection
• Thrombocytopenia - ecchymoses, petechiae, epistaxis, purpura
• Splenomegaly - uncommon; mild to moderate enlargement may be encountered, particularly in CMMOL
• Skin infiltrates

CAUSES Unknown

RISK FACTORS
• Primary MDS is associated with occupational exposure to petroleum solvents (benzene, toluene, gasoline)
• Secondary (therapy-related) MDS is associated with prior treatment with alkylating agents or radiation therapy

DIAGNOSIS

DIFFERENTIAL DIAGNOSIS
• Other malignant disorders - evolving acute myeloid leukemia (AML) or erythroleukemia; chronic myeloproliferative disorders (chronic myelogenous leukemia (CML), polycythemia vera, myeloid metaplasia with myelofibrosis); malignant lymphoma; metastatic carcinoma
• Nonmalignant disorders - aplastic anemia; autoimmune disorders (Felty's syndrome, lupus); nutritional deficiencies (pyridoxine, vitamin B12, protein malnutrition); heavy metal intoxication; alcoholism; chronic liver disease; hypersplenism; chronic inflammation; recent cytotoxic therapy or irradiation

LABORATORY
• Anemia - often macrocytic; occasional poikilocytosis, anisocytosis; variable reticulocytosis
• Granulocytopenia - hypogranular or agranular neutrophils with poorly condensed chromatin. Pelger-Huet anomaly with hyposegmented nuclei.
• Thrombocytopenia - occasionally giant platelets or hypogranular platelets
• Fetal hemoglobin - increased in 70%
• Sugar water (Ham's) test - increased RBC membrane sensitivity to complement lysis in some
• Direct antiglobulin (Coombs) test - positive in some
• Paraprotein - present in some
• Erythropoietin - usually normal or physiologically compensated levels unless renal failure is present
Drugs that may alter lab results: N/A
Disorders that may alter lab results: N/A

PATHOLOGICAL FINDINGS
• Ineffective hematopoiesis with dysplasia in one or more cell lineages dominates the bone marrow picture in MDS. Marrow cellularity is usually normal or increased for the patient's age but may be hypoplastic in about 10%.

• Reticulin fibrosis is usually minimal except in therapy-related MDS
• Myeloblasts may be clustered in the intertrabecular spaces, abnormal localization of immature precursors (ALIP)

SPECIAL TESTS
• Cytogenetics - at least half of patients with primary MDS and nearly all with therapy-related MDS have clonal chromosomal abnormalities (+8,-7,-5, del(5q), del(7q), del(20q), iso(17), and complex karyotypes). Detection of such a clonal abnormality establishes a diagnosis of neoplasm and rules out a nutritional, toxic, or autoimmune etiology.
• Granulocyte function tests - abnormal in half (decreased myeloperoxidase activity, phagocytosis, chemotaxis, and adhesion)
• Platelet function tests - impaired aggregation
• Marrow colony assays in vitro - results variable and correlate poorly with clinical course. Poor clonal growth may suggest more rapid evolution to AML.
• Immunophenotyping - nonspecific myeloid markers present. Occasionally evidence can be found for concomitant lymphoproliferative disorder.

IMAGING Liver/spleen scan or CT although rarely necessary may disclose occult splenomegaly or lymphadenopathy

DIAGNOSTIC PROCEDURES
• Bone marrow aspiration, biopsy, and cytogenetics
• Review peripheral blood smear

TREATMENT

APPROPRIATE HEALTH CARE Usually outpatient except when necessary to hospitalize for treatment of infection, blood transfusions, or intensive chemotherapy

GENERAL MEASURES
• Immunize for pneumococcal pneumonia and influenza
• RBC transfusions to alleviate symptoms
• Platelet transfusions only for bleeding or prior to surgery in order to avoid alloimmunization
• Early use of antibiotics for fever, even while culture results are pending, due to quantitative and qualitative granulocyte disorder
• Iron chelation therapy to avoid iron overload from chronic transfusions

ACTIVITY As tolerated

DIET Reduce alcohol use. Reduce iron intake.

PATIENT EDUCATION
• Stop smoking
• Seek early medical attention for fever, bleeding, or symptoms of anemia
• Advise about the risks of chronic transfusion therapy

MEDICATIONS

DRUG(S) OF CHOICE
• No medication has been proven more effective for these heterogeneous disorders than supportive care with antibiotics and transfusions as needed. Vitamins, iron, corticosteroids, androgens, or thyroid hormone are rarely helpful unless evidence of a specific deficiency exists.
• Investigational agents - low doses of cytarabine or 5-azacytidine, 13-cis- retinoic acid, interferon, granulocyte-macrophage (GM-CSF) or granulocyte colony stimulating factor (G-CSF), interleukin 3 (IL-3)
• Intensive chemotherapy - younger patients with MDS may benefit from AML chemotherapy, especially if Auer rods are present, but toxicity may be severe for older patients. Remission durations are variable (median, about 1 year).
• Allogeneic bone marrow transplantation - recommended for younger patients with HLA-matched donors to eradicate the malignant clone and re-supply normal hematopoietic stem cells
• Epsilon-aminocaproic acid or tranexamic acid may benefit patients with chronic, severe thrombocytopenia and bleeding.
Contraindications: Cytotoxicity of chemotherapy may increase the risk of bleeding and infection and the need for transfusion support
Precautions: Aspirin, salicylates, and NSAID's should be avoided
Significant possible interactions: N/A

ALTERNATIVE DRUGS
• Possible differentiating agents such as all-trans-retinoic acid or homoharringtonine and other hematopoietic growth factors are under investigation
• Danazol or prednisone may benefit concomitant autoimmune thrombocytopenia

FOLLOWUP

PATIENT MONITORING
At least monthly during supportive care. More frequently if receiving treatment.

PREVENTION/AVOIDANCE N/A

POSSIBLE COMPLICATIONS
Infection, bleeding, complications of anemia and transfusions

EXPECTED COURSE AND PROGNOSIS
• Median survival for RA and RARS is 5 years but may extend much longer. Refractory anemia with 5q minus syndrome is quite favorable.
• Median survival for RAEB, RAEBT, and CMMOL is about 1 year with half of patients evolving to AML and the other half dying of infection or bleeding

MISCELLANEOUS

ASSOCIATED CONDITIONS N/A

AGE-RELATED FACTORS
Pediatric: Monosomy 7 syndrome; juvenile chronic myelogenous leukemia
Geriatric: N/A
Others: N/A

PREGNANCY N/A

SYNONYMS
• Dysmyelopoietic syndrome
• Hemopoietic dysplasia
• Preleukemia
• Smoldering or subacute myeloid leukemia
• CMMOL; Chronic myelomonocytic anemia
• CMML; Chronic myelomonocytic anemia

ICD-9-CM N/A

SEE ALSO N/A

OTHER NOTES N/A

ABBREVIATIONS N/A

REFERENCES
Hoffman, R., Benz, E.J., Jr., Cohen, H., et al. (eds.): Hematology: Basic Principles and Practice. New York, Churchill Livingstone, 1991

Author R. A. Larson, M.D.

Myeloproliferative disorders

BASICS

DESCRIPTION The myeloproliferative disorders are neoplasms of the pluripotent hematopoietic stem cell. They include chronic myelogenous leukemia (CML), polycythemia vera (PV), agnogenic myeloid metaplasia with myelofibrosis (AMM/MF), and essential thrombocytosis (ET). PV is discussed in another chapter.
• With each disorder, the proliferation of one particular cell line tends to dominate. There is a variable tendency for reactive proliferation of the bone marrow fibroblast, which is not a part of the malignant clone, resulting in myelofibrosis, and for termination in an acute blastic leukemia.
CML
◊ Characterized by marked splenomegaly and increased granulocytes, particularly neutrophils
◊ Runs a generally mild course until it transforms to a frankly leukemic (blastic) phase
AMM/MF
◊ Characterized by the tendency of the neoplastic cells to lodge and grow in multiple sites outside the marrow. There is no evidence that this arises in compensation for replacement of the marrow by fibrosis.
◊ Myelofibrosis appears to be a reaction to the presence of the abnormal, proliferating hematopoietic clone
ET
◊ Dominated clinically by a markedly elevated platelet count
System(s) affected:
Hemic/Lymphatic/Immunologic
Genetics:
• CML - no genetic predisposition known
• AMM/MF - rare familial occurrence
• ET - may be familial
Incidence in USA:
• CML - one-fifth of all leukemia cases in the United States. Incidence of 1-2 cases per 100,000 persons per year. Incidence increases with age.
• AMM/MF - unknown
Prevalence in USA:
• CML - 1/5 of all leukemia cases
• ET - the least common of the myeloproliferative disorders
Predominant age:
• CML - median age at diagnosis is 45-50
• AMM/MF - generally begins in late middle life
• ET - generally begins in late middle life. Distinct second peak of incidence occurs in younger patients.
Predominant sex: Male = Female

SIGNS AND SYMPTOMS
General
◊ Most are asymptomatic at the time of diagnosis
◊ Vague constitutional symptoms
◊ Hypermetabolic state (fever, sweating)
◊ Acute gouty arthritis
◊ Left-upper-quadrant abdominal pain or fullness from splenomegaly

CML
◊ Marked splenomegaly (palpable in 90% of patients)
AMM/MF
◊ Splenomegaly in virtually all patients, and can be massive
◊ Hepatomegaly in 50%
◊ Lymph node enlargement in 10%
◊ Jaundice, edema, and ascites in 10-20%
◊ Petechiae in up to 25%
ET
◊ Easy bruisability, unusual bleeding after minor dental procedures, large-vessel bleeding in the absence of trauma
◊ Transient ischemic attacks, or even frank strokes, may occur in patients with markedly elevated platelet counts

CAUSES Unknown. May be familial for some types

RISK FACTORS
• Family history of myeloproliferative disorder (rare)
• CML - increased incidence in atomic bomb survivors and following radiation treatment of ankylosing spondylitis and cervical cancer

DIAGNOSIS

DIFFERENTIAL DIAGNOSIS
CML
◊ Low or absent leukocyte alkaline phosphatase (LAP) also seen in paroxysmal nocturnal hemoglobinuria, and occasional cases of myelodysplasia and AMM/MF
◊ Leukemoid reaction
AMM/MF
◊ Hepatomegaly in the absence of splenomegaly is extremely rare in AMM/MF, and suggests secondary myeloid metaplasia
◊ Spent PV (late stage of PV)
◊ Secondary myelofibrosis
ET
◊ Secondary thrombocytosis

LABORATORY
• Basophilia
• Elevated serum vitamin B12 level
• Hyperuricemia
CML
◊ Marked leukocytosis consisting of mature polymorphonuclear neutrophils and myelocytes or metamyelocytes
◊ Chronic phase typically with less than 5% myeloblasts in peripheral blood
◊ Blast crisis is defined when 30% or more blast cells are present in the bone marrow and/or peripheral blood
◊ Markedly decreased leukocyte alkaline phosphatase (absent in 5-10% of patients)
AMM/MF
◊ Mild anemia - in more than 50% of patients at time of diagnosis, eventually in almost all patients, and is progressive
◊ Leukocytosis in 50% of patients (up to 50,000 leukocytes per mL, up to 10% blasts)
◊ Leukoerythroblastic blood picture
◊ Occasional RBC autoantibodies

ET - the Polycythemia Vera Study group diagnostic criteria are:
◊ Thrombocytosis persistently greater than 1,000,000 per mL in the absence of an identifiable cause
◊ Normal total RBC volume
◊ Presence of iron in the bone marrow
◊ Absence of fibrosis in bone marrow biopsy
◊ Absence of the Philadelphia chromosome
Drugs that may alter lab results: N/A
Disorders that may alter lab results: In CML, LAP rises during infection, glucocorticoid use, or successful therapy

PATHOLOGICAL FINDINGS
AMM/MF
◊ Foci of extramedullary hematopoiesis seen in kidneys, lymph nodes, adrenal glands, and lungs
◊ Special stains of the bone marrow reveal increased reticulin deposition, even in hypercellular areas

SPECIAL TESTS CML - 95% of patients are Philadelphia chromosome positive (shortened chromosome 22 due to a reciprocal translocation between chromosomes 22 and 9)

IMAGING AMM/MF - radiographic osteosclerosis in 70% of patients, particularly in the axial skeleton and proximal long bones

DIAGNOSTIC PROCEDURES Bone marrow aspiration

TREATMENT

APPROPRIATE HEALTH CARE
Outpatient therapy. Inpatient for surgery when required.

GENERAL MEASURES
• Treatment to relieve symptoms and prevent infections
• Splenectomy has no impact on mortality, but is occasionally done for symptomatic relief. Extreme thrombocytosis, progressive and massive liver enlargement may ensue.
CML
◊ Benign phase typically treated with hydroxyurea or an alkylating agent, reducing the dose as the blood counts return to normal. Interferons, aggressive chemotherapy, and allogeneic transplantation have resulted in loss of the Philadelphia chromosome and cures.
◊ Aggressive chemotherapy generally only leads to transient remissions
◊ Allogeneic bone marrow transplantation has a 30% treatment-related early mortality, but 50-60% of patients will be in hematologic or cytogenetic remission 3-5 years after transplantation
◊ Interferon-alpha produces hematologic remissions in 70-80% of patients, while 10% will have a complete or partial suppression in the Philadelphia chromosome
◊ Accelerated phase and blast crisis usually treated with regimens designed for the treatment of acute leukemia

AMM/MF
◊ No definitive therapy
◊ Anemia is treated with transfusions as required
◊ Radiotherapy for localized bone pain, or symptomatic extramedullary hematopoietic tumors
◊ Successful bone marrow transplantation leads to the reversal of established fibrosis

ET
◊ Young, asymptomatic patients generally not treated
◊ Patients with symptomatic thrombocytosis who have had bleeding or thrombotic episodes should be treated

ACTIVITY
Restrictions will be dependent on symptoms and progression of the disorder

DIET
• No special diet, but important to maintain nutrition
• Small frequent meals, high-protein drinks may help
• May need to relieve symptoms of GI hyperacidity with antacids

PATIENT EDUCATION
• Explanations about the disorder, treatment protocols, and prognosis
• Symptoms of recurrence to watch for
• Importance of followup examinations and lab studies

MEDICATIONS

DRUG(S) OF CHOICE
• Hydroxyurea 20-30 mg/kg/day as a single daily dose, generally favored over alkylating agents in the control of leukocytosis or thrombocytosis, as it has no known leukemogenic potential
• Allopurinol to control hyperuricemia - begin prior to hydroxyurea therapy
Contraindications: ET - because platelet function is often defective, drugs such as salicylates that impair platelet function are generally avoided
Precautions: ET - prolonged administration of platelet-antiaggregating agents may increase the risk of gastrointestinal hemorrhage
Significant possible interactions: Toxicity (bone marrow depression) of cyclophosphamide (Cytoxan) may be increased by allopurinol

ALTERNATIVE DRUGS
AMM/MF
◊ Androgens and glucocorticoids may improve the anemia
◊ Corticosteroids if autoimmune hemolysis is present

ET
◊ Aspirin with or without dipyridamole may prove useful in preventing thrombotic or ischemic symptoms in some patients
◊ Erythromelalgia (described below) responds to rapid reduction of the platelet count or to administration of nonsteroidal anti-inflammatory agents

FOLLOWUP

PATIENT MONITORING
Individualized and dependent on therapy prescribed, ongoing studies, and stage of the illness

PREVENTION/AVOIDANCE N/A

POSSIBLE COMPLICATIONS
• Transformation to acute leukemia
• Gout due to the hyperuricemia, or uric acid nephropathy
AMM/MF
◊ Portal hypertension
◊ Splenic infarcts
◊ Budd-Chiari syndrome
ET
◊ Hemorrhage, fatal thrombosis
◊ Erythromelalgia (a vaso-occlusive syndrome characterized by localized pain, burning, warmth of distal extremities, which may progress to gangrene)

EXPECTED COURSE AND PROGNOSIS
CML
◊ In the first 2 years following diagnosis, 10% of patients per year will develop into the accelerated phase or blast crisis. This rate then increases to 15-20% per year.
◊ Median survival is greater than 5 years from the time of diagnosis, approximately 12-18 months after development of the accelerated phase, and 3 months after developing blast crisis
◊ Adverse prognostic factors include advanced age, large liver size, degree of splenomegaly, elevated platelet count, degree of leukocytosis, presence of large numbers of eosinophils or basophils, percent of immature cells in the marrow, and clonal evolution
◊ 85% will die in blast crisis
AMM/MF
◊ Progressive splenomegaly, anemia and thrombocytopenia
◊ Median survival is 5 years from the time of diagnosis, and 10 years from disease onset
◊ Adverse prognostic factors include platelet count less than 100,000 per mL, hemoglobin of less than 10 gm/dl, and hepatomegaly
ET
◊ Median survival not well defined, but approximates 10-12 years

MISCELLANEOUS

ASSOCIATED CONDITIONS
AMM/MF - associations with systemic lupus erythematosus, periarteritis nodosa, scleroderma, and vasculitis have been reported

AGE-RELATED FACTORS
Pediatric: Rare in the young
Geriatric: These disorders more often found in middle and later years
Others: N/A

PREGNANCY
CML
◊ Pregnancy does not affect the course of the disease
◊ Greater than 95% of mothers survive to delivery, with greater than 80% fetal survival rate through gestation
◊ Severe congenital defects have been reported with busulfan

SYNONYMS N/A

ICD-9-CM
• CML - 205.1
• AMM/MF - 289.8
• ET - 238.7

SEE ALSO N/A

OTHER NOTES N/A

ABBREVIATIONS
• CML = chronic myelogenous leukemia, chronic myelocytic leukemia, chronic granulocytic leukemia
• PV = polycythemia vera
• AMM/MF = agnogenic myeloid metaplasia with myelofibrosis
• ET - essential (primary) thrombocythemia, hemorrhagic thrombocythemia

REFERENCES
Williams, W.J., et al.: Hematology. 4th Ed. New York, McGraw-Hill, 1990

Author R. Dolin, M.D.

Myocardial infarction

BASICS

DESCRIPTION Acute myocardial infarction (AMI) is the rapid development of myocardial necrosis resulting from a sustained and complete reduction of blood flow to a portion of the myocardium, produced by a superimposed thrombosis, engrafted upon a coronary atherosclerotic plaque
• Clinical consequences - dependent on the size and location of the infarction and the rapidity with which blood flow can be re-established by either pharmacologic or mechanical modalities
• Experimental data suggest that myocardial necrosis secondary to total occlusion is complete within 4-6 hours. Data suggests that flow to ischemic area must remain above 40% of pre-occlusion levels for that area to survive.
• Infarctions can be divided into Q-wave and non Q-wave infarctions with the former being transmural and associated with totally obstructed infarct-related artery and the latter being non-transmural and associated with patent, but highly narrowed infarct-related artery
• Total occlusion of the left main coronary artery which supplies 70% of the LV mass is catastrophic and results in death in minutes to hours
System(s) affected: Cardiovascular
Genetics: N/A
Incidence/Prevalence in USA: 600/100,000
Predominant age: Over 40
Predominant sex:
• Age 40-70 - Male > Female
• Over age 70 - Male = Female

SIGNS AND SYMPTOMS
• Pain - abdomin, arm, back, jaw, neck, chest
• Anxiety
• Cannon jugular venous A waves (in presence of heart block or right ventricular failure)
• Chest heaviness, tightness
• Cough, diaphoresis, dyspnea, rales, wheezing
• Fever
• Gallop rhythm, murmur, tachycardia, bradycardia, pulsus alternans, pericardial friction rub
• Hypertension, hypotension
• Jugular venous distention
• Lightheadedness, pallor, weakness, syncope
• Nausea, vomiting
• Orthopnea

CAUSES
• Coronary thrombosis - most common cause
• Coronary artery spasm
• Arteritis
• Trauma (e.g., chest contusion)
• Metabolic disease (rare, e.g., amyloidosis)
• Embolic infarction
• Congenital coronary anomalies
• Oxygen supply - demand imbalance; carbon monoxide poisoning
• In situ thrombosis - hematologic in origin (e.g., polycythemia rubra vera)
• Cocaine

RISK FACTORS
• Hypercholesterolemia (increased LDL; decreased HDL)
• Hypertriglyceridemia
• Premature familial onset of coronary disease (before the age of 55)
• Smoking
• Hypertension
• Obesity
• Sedentary life style
• Diabetes mellitus
• Aging
• Stress
• Hostile, frustrated personality as opposed to simply hard-driving

Diagnosis

DIFFERENTIAL DIAGNOSIS
• Unstable angina pectoris - serial ECG and enzymes to differentiate
• Aortic dissection
• Pulmonary embolism
• Pericarditis - differentiated by history of postural improvement of pain and pleuritic component, plus presence of a pericardial friction rub and upward concave diffuse ST segment elevation on ECG
• Esophageal spasm - no ECG or enzyme elevations
• Pancreatitis and biliary tract disease

LABORATORY
• Creatine kinase (CK) and its isoenzymes are earliest to rise following infarction; CK begins to rise within 4-8 hours post infarction; average peak within 24 hours and subsides within 3-4 days. Most sensitive indicator for myocardial necrosis. Has 15% false positive rate.
• CK isoenzyme analysis - MM, MB, and BB forms identified with skeletal muscle, BB in brain and kidney, and MB and MM in cardiac. Elevation of CK-MB in serum can be considered diagnostic of myocardial infarction with the exception of a recent history of trauma or surgery involving brain, kidney or muscle.

• LDH rises above normal values within 24 hours of MI and reaches a peak within 3-6 days and returns to baseline within 8-12 days. Can be used to date recent episode of acute MI well past the acute episode.
• ESR - rises above normal level within 3 days and may remain elevated for several weeks
• Leukocytosis - rises within several hours after onset of MI, peaks in 2-4 days, and is normal within 1 week
Drugs that may alter lab results: Refer to standard cardiology texts
Disorders that may alter lab results: Refer to standard cardiology texts

PATHOLOGICAL FINDINGS Necrosis of myocardium in areas deprived of blood supply

SPECIAL TESTS
Electrocardiography
◊ ST segment elevation in a regional pattern - typical of acute transmural myocardial ischemia
◊ ST segment depression with T-wave inversions - typical of subendocardial ischemia
◊ ST segment elevation and depression are early findings of myocardial ischemia and injury. A significant percent of patients will have non-specific findings on presentation, such as peaking of the T-waves and ST-segment elevation less than 0.1 mv. Very small percentage of patients with transmural infarction present with normal electrocardiograms.
◊ Q-waves representing transmural myocardial necrosis appear with 24-48 hours
Echocardiography
◊ 2D and M-mode echocardiography useful in evaluating wall motion abnormalities in MI and overall left ventricular function
◊ Useful in delineating and assessing mechanical complications

IMAGING
Chest x-ray
◊ Findings dependent on severity and evolution of myocardial infarction
Radionuclide studies
◊ Pyrophosphate scanning
◊ Thallium scanning
◊ Technetium-99 gated blood pool scanning-noninvasive means of measuring ventricular function

DIAGNOSTIC PROCEDURES
Angiography prior to procedures to re-establish coronary perfusion

TREATMENT

APPROPRIATE HEALTH CARE
Inpatient coronary care unit

GENERAL MEASURES
• Based on several guiding principles: Analgesia, prevention and treatment of complications both electrical and mechanical, limitation of infarct size, and salvage of myocardium
• Routine administration of O2 for first 24-48 hours in an attempt to prevent CHF, bradyrrhythmia, and A-V block
• Intra-aortic balloon counter pulsation
• Ventricular tachycardia - treated with DC counganshock, lidocaine, and/or procainamide (Pronestyl)
• Ventricular fibrillation - treated with prompt countershock and repeated countershocks; if unsuccessful, then cardiopulmonary resuscitation with pharmacologic therapy, assisted ventilation, and repeated countershock
• Atrial flutter and fibrillation - digitalis or IV verapamil. If hemodynamic compromise - DC countershock or rapid atrial pacing.
• Sinus bradycardia - no treatment unless accompanied by hypotension or hemodynamic compromise. Then treat with atropine and if ineffective, electrical pacing.
• Atrioventricular block - complete heart block in inferior infarction requires transvenous pacing if patient hemodynamically compromised. In anterior infarction, pacing usually required as escape rhythm is unstable with ventricular asystole occurring quite suddenly.
Coronary reperfusion
◊ A relatively recent treatment modality to establish reperfusion of ischemic muscle. Involves intravenous thrombolysis with the following agents (none is superior to others):
◊ Streptokinase - produces systemic lytic effect in addition to local thrombolysis
◊ Tissue plasminogen activator (TPA) - more effective lytic agent with higher rate of patency 90 minutes after administration than streptokinase. Has a lesser systemic lytic effect and higher rate of re-occlusion.
◊ Emergency percutaneous transluminal angioplasty (PTCA) - mechanical form of coronary reperfusion. There are no controlled studies to show that this technique is superior to intravenous thrombolysis.
◊ Emergency surgical reperfusion - can be accomplished with low mortality. Must be carried out within 4 hours of beginning of the event. Many consider this treatment to be rarely indicated.

ACTIVITY
• Strict bedrest for first 24 hours
• Medically supervised rehabilitation plan

DIET
Nothing by mouth until stable; later, low-fat, low salt diet

PATIENT EDUCATION
Printed patient information available from: American Heart Association, 7320 Greenville Avenue, Dallas, TX 75231, (214)373-6300

MEDICATIONS

DRUG(S) OF CHOICE
• Intravenous nitrates 5 mcg/min, increase slowly. Do not lower arterial blood pressure beyond 20 mm Hg.
• Lidocaine 1-2 mg/kg once, then 1-4 mg/min. Use for arrhythmias only. Do not expect arrhythmia prophylaxis.
• Minidose heparin
• Nasal O2 (2-4 L per minute)
• Oxazepam 10 mg po q 6 hr if needed for sedation
• Opiates for analgesia - specifically morphine 2 mg IV in 25 minutes for severe pain
B-blockades (choose 1) - contraindicated in setting of incipient congestive heart failure:
◊ Metoprolol 5 mg IV x 3, approximately 2 minutes apart, then 50 mg q6h x 48 hours. Then 100 mg bid. If IV not tolerated well, use lower dosage po.
◊ Atenolol 5 mg IV over 5 minutes. Follow with a second dose 10 minutes later. Follow with 50 mg po in 10 minutes after the 2nd IV dose. Then q12h for at least 7 days.
Contraindications: Refer to manufacturer's literature
Precautions: Refer to manufacturer's literature
Significant possible interactions: Refer to manufacturer's literature

ALTERNATIVE DRUGS   N/A

FOLLOWUP

PATIENT MONITORING   Determined by needs of patient

PREVENTION/AVOIDANCE   Avoid risk factors for coronary artery disease

POSSIBLE COMPLICATIONS
• Congestive heart failure
• Cardiogenic shock
• Myocardial rupture
• Left ventricular aneurysm
• Left ventricular thrombus and peripheral embolism
• Deep venous thrombosis and pulmonary embolism
• Pericarditis
• Dysrhythmias
• Mitral regurgitation
• Ventricular septal defect
• Dressler's syndrome
• Cardiac arrest
• Death

EXPECTED COURSE AND PROGNOSIS
• Overall mortality rate is 10% during the hospital phase with an additional 10% mortality rate during the year after. More than 60% of the deaths occur within one hour of the onset of the event.
Killip classification
◊ Class I - no evidence of CHF; mortality rate < 5%
◊ Class II - mild to moderate CHF, bibasilar rales and/or S3 gallop; mortality rate 10%
◊ Class III - severe CHF, rales over greater than 50% lung fields, S3 gallop, pulmonary edema; mortality rate 30%
◊ Class IV - cardiogenic shock, BP < 90 and signs of systemic hypoperfusion, i.e., oliguria, confusion, clammy skin; mortality rate 80-100%

MISCELLANEOUS

ASSOCIATED CONDITIONS
• Abdominal aortic aneurysm
• Extracranial cerebrovascular disease
• Atherosclerotic peripheral vascular disease

AGE-RELATED FACTORS
Pediatric: N/A
Geriatric: All incidences of complications are higher
Others: N/A

PREGNANCY   N/A

SYNONYMS
• Coronary thrombosis
• Coronary occlusion
• Heart attack

ICD-9-CM   410.9

SEE ALSO   N/A

OTHER NOTES   N/A

ABBREVIATIONS   N/A

REFERENCES
• Braunwald, E.: Heart Disease. 3rd Ed. Philadelphia, W. B. Saunders Co., 1988
• Harvey, A.M.:The Principles and Practice of Medicine. 22nd Ed. Norwalk, CT, Appleton & Lange, 1988

Author F. Griff, M.D.

Narcolepsy

BASICS

DESCRIPTION Narcolepsy is characterized by a tetrad consisting of irresistible attacks of sleepiness and a series of auxiliary symptoms - cataplexy, sleep paralysis, and hypnagogic hallucinations, which appear during rapid-eye-movement (REM) sleep. Commonly misconceived as representing low intelligence and/or poor motivation. The syndrome is frequently overlooked with an average of 15 years of symptoms prior to diagnosis.
System(s) affected: Nervous
Genetics:
• Inherited dominant with incomplete penetrance
• 60 fold increased incidence in families with positive history
• Incidence in first degree relative of index case is 30%
• Biologic marker HLA-DR2 allele on short arm of chromosome 6 in 100% of Caucasian patients; 1/3 normal patients are also positive. 30% of Black narcoleptic patients are non DR 2, but all with HLA-DW1.
Incidence in USA: 1 in 1000
Prevalence in USA: 100,000-200,000
Predominant age: Mean age onset 18
Predominant sex: Male = Female

SIGNS AND SYMPTOMS
• Tetrad: 10-20% with all symptoms
• 10% with excessive daytime sleepiness (EDS) alone
• 25% with EDS plus one auxiliary symptom
• 50% with EDS plus all 3 auxiliary
Sleep attacks (100%) - primary symptom
◊ Instantaneous, irresistible REM sleep
◊ First and most disabling symptom
◊ Satisfied by naps lasting 5-10 minutes
◊ Lasts minutes to hours
◊ 1-8 naps per day
◊ Increased in monotonous environment, warm environment, after a large meal, or with strong emotions
Cataplexy (80%) auxiliary symptom
◊ Momentary paralysis of voluntary muscles in association with sudden emotional reaction
◊ Can be limited to a particular muscle group, e.g., jaw droop with inability to speak; arm, neck or leg weakness
◊ Can be generalized causing patient to slump to floor while remaining fully conscious
◊ Can last seconds or minutes
Sleep paralysis - auxiliary symptom
◊ When falling asleep or on awakening the patient wants to move but cannot
◊ The brain wakes from sleep while the body remains in REM sleep
◊ Lasts seconds to minutes
◊ Patients are aware of events around them, but cannot open eyes or move
◊ Can be preceded by hallucinatory phenomena
Hypnagogic hallucinations - auxiliary symptom
◊ Vivid, frightening auditory or visual illusions or hallucinations at onset of sleep
◊ Dream-like experiences that occur during

wakefulness or suddenly at sleep onset
◊ Characteristic hallucinations include seeing human or animal faces or feeling that someone else is in the room
Disturbed nocturnal sleep
◊ Normal total sleep with decreased sleep efficiency
◊ More frequent transitions from wakefulness to sleep
◊ Retrograde amnesic and automatic behavior lasting minutes to hours
◊ Increased periodic leg movements

CAUSES
• Unknown
• Possible involvement of the immune system
• Widespread under-release of dopamine and a brainstem-specific proliferation of acetylcholine receptors and hypersensitivity to acetylcholine

RISK FACTORS
• Head trauma
• CNS infectious disease
• Anesthesia
• Family history

DIAGNOSIS

DIFFERENTIAL DIAGNOSIS
• Sleep apnea syndromes
• Epileptic seizures and syncope
• Idiopathic CNS hypersomnolence
• Nocturnal myoclonus
• Psychomotor seizures
• Abuse of sedative drugs

LABORATORY HLA-DR2
Drugs that may alter lab results: N/A
Disorders that may alter lab results: N/A

PATHOLOGICAL FINDINGS N/A

SPECIAL TESTS
• Nighttime polysomnography - monitoring of patients in a sleep laboratory will usually document fragmented sleep with a normal amount of REM sleep but a pattern of sleep onset REM. Polysomnography rules out other causes of excessive daytime sleepiness including sleep apnea syndromes and nocturnal myoclonus.
• Multiple sleep latency test (MSLT) - begins at least 90 minutes after nighttime test. Patient is monitored during 4-5 naps taken at two-hour intervals. The rapidity of sleep onset and type of sleep pattern are documented. A supportive test includes a mean sleep latency (time to fall asleep) of five minutes or less and at least two sleep-onset REM periods.
• HLA typing in ambiguous cases

IMAGING N/A

DIAGNOSTIC PROCEDURES
• Presence of excessive daytime sleepiness
• Documentation of at least two sleep-onset REM periods during MSLT

TREATMENT

APPROPRIATE HEALTH CARE
Inpatient for sleep laboratory analysis, outpatient for followup

GENERAL MEASURES
• Usually managed with medication
• Regularly scheduled time for naps may help in mild cases

ACTIVITY
Exercise can sometimes decrease the number of sleep attacks. Seek to achieve optimal physical fitness.

DIET
No special diet, avoid alcohol

PATIENT EDUCATION
• Symptoms can spontaneously improve or worsen
• The American Narcolepsy Association, P.O. Box 1187, San Carlos, CA 94070, (800)327-6085

MEDICATIONS

DRUG(S) OF CHOICE
• Recommended drugs either block norepinephrine uptake or cause central anticholinergic effects
• For excessive daytime sleepiness - stimulants that increase levels of daytime alertness, such as non-amphetamine stimulants. Methylphenidate (Ritalin) 30-60 mg/day) or pemoline (Cylert)18.75-150 mg/day.
• For auxiliary symptoms (cataplexy, hypnagogic hallucination, sleep paralysis) - tricyclic antidepressants suppress REM sleep. Imipramine 75-150 mg/day, protriptyline 10-40 mg/day, fluoxetine 20-60 mg/day.

Contraindications: Stimulants in hypertensive patients

Precautions:
• If patient develops tolerance to stimulants, switch drugs rather than increasing the dose - there is little cross-tolerance
• Patient may develop tolerance to the anticataplectic effect of tricyclic antidepressants and can get a rebound in cataplexy when withdrawn
• Stimulants - headaches, irritability, hypertension, psychosis, anorexia, habituation
• Pemoline - less cardiovascular side effects, longer acting, liver toxicity
• Imipramine - dry mouth, sedation, urinary retention, impotence

Significant possible interactions:
Combination of tricyclic antidepressants and stimulants can lead to significant hypertension

ALTERNATIVE DRUGS
Excessive daytime sleepiness:
◊ Propranolol - 280-480 mg/day, good for patients during withdrawal from stimulants or patients with hypertension
◊ Dextroamphetamines 5-60 mg/day
◊ L-Tyrosine 64-120 mg/day
Ancillary symptoms
◊ Gamma-hydroxybutyrate - 5.25-6.75 g during sleep, has little effect on sleep architecture of REM sleep but increases slow-wave sleep. Also has mild effect on excessive daytime sleepiness without tolerance development.
Gamma-hydroxybutyrate can increase sleep walking by increasing slow-wave sleep.
◊ Codeine 150 mg/day
◊ Triazolam 0.25 mg improves nocturnal sleep quality

FOLLOWUP

PATIENT MONITORING Frequent blood pressure checks

PREVENTION/AVOIDANCE N/A

POSSIBLE COMPLICATIONS N/A

EXPECTED COURSE AND PROGNOSIS
• Life-long disease
• Symptoms can worsen with aging
• In women, symptoms can improve after menopause

MISCELLANEOUS

ASSOCIATED CONDITIONS Obstructive sleep apnea

AGE-RELATED FACTORS
Pediatric: Uncommon syndrome of childhood
Geriatric: Symptoms worsen with aging
Others: N/A

PREGNANCY N/A

SYNONYMS N/A

ICD-9-CM 347

SEE ALSO Obstructive sleep apnea

OTHER NOTES N/A

ABBREVIATIONS
• REM = rapid eye movement
• MSLT = multiple sleep latency test

REFERENCES
• Mitler, M., Hajdukovic, R., et al.: Narcolepsy. Journal of Clinical Neurophysiology. 7(1):93-118, 1990
• Scharf, M., Fletcher, K., et al.: Current Pharmacologic Management of Narcolepsy. AFP 38(1):143-148, 1988
• Nahmias, J. & Karetzky, M.: Current Concepts in Narcolepsy. New Jersey Medicine. 86:617-622,1989
• Chaudhary, B. & Husain, I.: Narcolepsy. Jour Fam Prac. 36(2);207-213, 1993

Author J. Minteer, M.D.

Near drowning

BASICS

DESCRIPTION Multisystem, potentially fatal disease, resulting from near suffocation secondary to submersion of a person's face or head. Approximately 10% of drowned patients die without actually aspirating. Most near drowning victims do not aspirate large volumes of fluid

Genetics: N/A

Incidence in USA:
• 7,000 deaths yearly
• Drowning is the third leading cause of accidental death in the United States

Prevalence in USA: N/A

Predominant age: Teenagers

Predominant sex: Male > Female

SIGNS AND SYMPTOMS
• Altered level of consciousness or comatose
• Absent or thready pulse
• Tachypnea or agonal respirations
• Cyanosis
• Wheezing
• Hypothermia
• Poorly reactive, dilated and fixed pupils

CAUSES
• Swimming accidents
• Hyperventilation before underwater swimming
• Boating mishaps
• Motor vehicle accidents (i.e., auto submerged in water)
• Suicide
• Drug overdose (including alcohol)

RISK FACTORS
• Low socioeconomic class
• Alcohol
• Seizure disorder
• Inability to swim
• Improper pool fencing
• Inadequate adult supervision of children

DIAGNOSIS

DIFFERENTIAL DIAGNOSIS The submersion may have resulted from loss of consciousness and accidently falling into water because of another medical condition (i.e. trauma, arrhythmia, seizure, etc.)

LABORATORY
Salt water
◊ Hypoxemia
◊ Hypercarbia
◊ Mixed acidosis
◊ Slight increase in serum sodium
◊ Normal or minimally increased Hb
◊ Rare albuminuria
◊ Rare oliguria
◊ Rare hemoglobinuria
◊ Hypovolemia possibly, or hypervolemia
Fresh water
◊ Hypoxemia
◊ Hypercarbia
◊ Mixed acidosis
◊ Slight decrease in serum sodium
◊ Normal or slightly decreased Hb
◊ Albuminuria rarely
◊ Oliguria rarely
◊ Rare hemoglobinuria
◊ Evidence of hemolysis

Drugs that may alter lab results: N/A

Disorders that may alter lab results: Any underlying condition that may alter normal fluid and electrolyte balance (i.e., congestive heart failure) or alter normal pulmonary function (i.e., emphysema)

PATHOLOGICAL FINDINGS
• "Dry lungs" 10% of time
• Loss of normal pulmonary architecture (fresh water). Alveolar consolidations, collapse, hyaline membrane formation.
• Increased lung weight and intra-alveolar hemorrhages (salt water)
• Lung hyperexpansion
• Pneumonia, abscess and adult respiratory distress (ARDS) in those who survive only a few hours or days

SPECIAL TESTS
• Lung compliance (reduced)
• Central venous pressure monitoring
• ECG
• EEG
• Calculation of V/Q mismatch, shunt, AaDO2

IMAGING Chest x-ray may show pulmonary edema or consolidation from aspiration

DIAGNOSTIC PROCEDURES N/A

TREATMENT

APPROPRIATE HEALTH CARE
Hospitalize all patients initially. Monitor patients in an Intensive Care setting except for those few who present to the Emergency Room in an alert condition without evidence of respiratory compromise. The incidence of delayed drowning is 5%. Therefore all patients who have had a significant submersion accident should be hospitalized for 24-48 hours.

GENERAL MEASURES
• Begin resuscitation at the scene while the victim is still in the water, if possible. Remove from water quickly and place in normal CPR position.
• Supplemental oxygen
• Positive airway pressure - positive end-expiratory pressure (PEEP) or continuous positive airway pressure (CPAP) for persistent hypoxia
• Avoid abdominal thrust unless airway obstruction is present
• Monitor pH and adjust bicarbonate administration accordingly
• Monitor arterial oxygenation
• Avoid steroids
• Avoid prophylactic antibiotics

ACTIVITY Bedrest for at least the initial 24 hours

DIET N/A

PATIENT EDUCATION Proper water safety techniques may help to avoid this problem

MEDICATIONS

DRUG(S) OF CHOICE
• All patients: Oxygen
• Unconscious patient without known pH: Sodium bicarbonate - 1.0 mEq/kg
• Bronchospastic patient: Aerosolized bronchodilator such as metproterenol (Alupent) 0.3 cc in 2.7 cc normal saline solution or albuterol (Proventil or Ventolin) 0.5 cc in 2.5 cc normal saline solution
• Patients who develop pneumonia: Appropriate antibiotic based on sputum or endotracheal lavage culture
• Fresh water drowning patients with hemolysis: Transfusion may be necessary
Contraindications: Refer to manufacturer's profile of each drug
Precautions: Refer to manufacturer's profile of each drug
Significant possible interactions: Refer to manufacturer's profile of each drug

ALTERNATIVE DRUGS
Aminophylline for bronchospasm

FOLLOWUP

PATIENT MONITORING
• Frequent check of vital signs
• Arterial blood gas monitoring
• Pulmonary artery catheter may be needed for hemodynamic monitoring
• Pulse oximeter for oxygen saturation trending
• Intracranial pressure monitoring in selected patients
• Serial chest x-rays
• Serum electrolyte determinations

PREVENTION/AVOIDANCE
• Proper adult supervision of children
• Knowledge of water safety guidelines
• Mandatory pool fencing
• Avoidance of alcohol or recreational drugs around water
• Swimming instruction at an early age

POSSIBLE COMPLICATIONS
• Prolonged neurologic sequelae
• Fear of water
• Pneumonitis/lung abscess
• Secondary drowning

EXPECTED COURSE AND PROGNOSIS
• Patients who are alert or somewhat obtunded at the time they present to the hospital have an excellent chance for a full recovery
• Patients who are comatose or receiving CPR at the time of presentation have a more guarded and often poor prognosis

MISCELLANEOUS

ASSOCIATED CONDITIONS
• Cardiopulmonary arrest before the submersion
• Trauma, especially to the head causing altered mental status
• Seizure disorder
• Alcohol or drug overdose

AGE-RELATED FACTORS
Pediatric: Children frequently don't swim well
Geriatric: N/A
Others:
• Adolescents - may be intoxicated or using drugs
• Adults - most near-drownings are associated with boating accidents with or without alcohol

PREGNANCY N/A

SYNONYMS N/A

ICD-9-CM 994.1 or 518.5

SEE ALSO
• Aspiration pneumonia
• Pneumonia

OTHER NOTES
Accomplished swimmers may drown by hyperventilation before prolonged underwater swimming or by becoming fatigued following a particularly strenuous or long swim. Approximately 10% of victims drown without aspiration.

ABBREVIATIONS N/A

REFERENCES
• Wintemute, G.: Childhood Drowning and Near-Drowning in the United States. AJDC 144:663, 1990
• Modell, J., Graves, S. & Ketover, A.: Clinical Course of 91 Consecutive Near-Drowning Victims. Chest 70:231, 1976

Author A. Cropp, M.D., F.C.C.P.

Nephropathy, urate

BASICS

DESCRIPTION Renal parenchymal damage and dysfunction associated with disordered uric acid metabolism. Several syndromes can present.

Gout: Acute urate crystal-induced arthritis related to chronic hyperuricemia due to uric acid renal underexcretion in 80-90% and uric acid overproduction in 10-20%.

Hyperuricemic acute renal failure: Precipitated by distal tubular obstruction resulting from acute massive overproduction of uric acid due to cell lysis. Serum uric acid usually greater than 15-20 mg/dl.

Uric acid nephrolithiasis: Most commonly seen in gouty patients who are uric acid overproducers and have hyperuricosuria. Frequency of stone formation increases with increasing serum uric acid levels and urinary uric acid excretion rates. About 22% of gouty patients will form uric acid stones.

Hyperuricemia of chronic renal failure: Occurs when creatinine clearance less than 15. Serum uric acid usually greater than 10 mg/dl. Secondary gout rare. Acute deterioration of renal function can be precipitated by an abrupt rise in serum uric acid.

Chronic urate nephropathy: Renal insufficiency attributed to parenchymal damage secondary to medullary urate deposition. Bulk of evidence supports conclusion that typical gout or asymptomatic hyperuricemia are unlikely to lead to serious renal insufficiency. In patients with gout, renal insufficiency can usually be attributed to a complicating medical condition, most often hypertension, diabetes, renal vascular disease, obstructive uropathy, urinary tract infection or lead intoxication.

Incidence/Prevalence in USA: Gout 0.3%, Hyperuricemia 5-10%

System(s) affected: Renal/Urologic

Genetics: N/A

Predominant age: Adults

Predominant sex: Male > Female

SIGNS AND SYMPTOMS

Hyperuricemic acute renal failure
◊ Precipitated by chemotherapy for leukemia or lymphoma
◊ Precipitated by heat stress and exercise
◊ Oliguria
◊ Anuria
◊ Anorexia, nausea, vomiting, encephalopathy and other manifestations of uremia
◊ Hypertension
◊ Anemia
◊ Dehydration
Uric acid nephrolithiasis
◊ Flank pain
◊ Groin pain
◊ Micro or gross hematuria
◊ Anorexia
◊ Nausea
◊ Vomiting
◊ Dehydration

Hyperuricemia of chronic renal failure
◊ Established chronic renal failure with GFR less than 15-20
◊ Serum uric acid greater than 10 mg/dL chronically
◊ Intercurrent cause of abrupt increase in serum uric acid
◊ Acute decrease in GFR
◊ Acute onset of uremic symptoms

CAUSES

Primary
◊ Congenital gout and hyperuricemia
◊ Congenital HGPRT deficiency (X-linked recessive)
◊ Congenital PRPP overactivity (X-linked recessive)
◊ Congenital glycogen storage disease, type I
Secondary
◊ Lead intoxication
◊ Diuretics
◊ Cytotoxic chemotherapy in leukemia or lymphoma
◊ Heat stress and exercise
◊ Diabetic ketoacidosis
◊ Starvation ketosis
◊ Chronic myeloproliferative disease
◊ Psoriasis

RISK FACTORS
• Sudden increase in uric acid load
• Dehydration
• Urine pH less than 5
• Hypertension
• Diabetes mellitus
• Renal insufficiency
• Renal vascular disease

DIAGNOSIS

DIFFERENTIAL DIAGNOSIS Other causes of acute renal failure, other causes of nephrolithiasis, other causes of chronic renal failure

LABORATORY

Gout and hyperuricemia
◊ Hyperuricemia
◊ Hyperuricosuria in 10-20%
◊ Decreased urinary ammonia production
Hyperuricemic acute renal failure
◊ Serum uric acid greater than 15-20 mg/dL
◊ Rising BUN and creatinine
◊ Urinary uric acid to creatinine ratio > 1
◊ Uric acid crystals in urine
Uric acid nephrolithiasis
◊ Uric acid crystals in urine
◊ Urinary uric acid greater than 600-700 mg per 24 hours (hyperuricosuria) on purine-free diet
◊ Hyperuricemia
◊ Microhematuria
◊ Pyuria
◊ Positive urine culture
◊ Stone composition uric acid or mixed uric acid and calcium oxalate or calcium phosphate

Hyperuricemia of chronic renal failure
◊ Acute exacerbation of hyperuricemia with serum uric acid greater than 10 mg/dL
◊ Acute on chronic BUN and creatinine elevations
Drugs that may alter lab results: N/A
Disorders that may alter lab results: N/A

PATHOLOGICAL FINDINGS
• Renal tophi-medullary monosodium urate deposits with inflammatory reaction and interstitial fibrosis
• Poor correlation between severity of renal pathology and severity of gout
• Tubulointerstitial nephritis with obstruction, recurrent infection or lead intoxication

SPECIAL TESTS Stone analysis

IMAGING
• IVP
• Renal ultrasound

DIAGNOSTIC PROCEDURES
• Cystoscopy and retrograde pyelography
• Renal biopsy

TREATMENT

APPROPRIATE HEALTH CARE
Outpatient except for complicated nephrolithiasis and hyperuricemic acute renal failure

GENERAL MEASURES
• Hydration to increase urine output
• Normalize serum uric acid
• Normalize renal uric acid excretion
• Decrease uric acid production
• Maintain urine pH greater than 6
• Antibiotic treatment of urinary tract infection
Hyperuricemic acute renal failure:
◊ IV hydration
◊ hemodialysis
Uric acid nephrolithiasis:
◊ Cystoscopic or surgical stone removal for persistent ureteral obstruction

ACTIVITY Limited during attacks of acute gouty arthritis

DIET
• Purine restriction
• Protein restriction
• For nephrolithiasis, fluid intake adequate to produce urine output at least 2 L per day unless urine output is limited by acute or chronic renal failure
• In acute renal failure restrict sodium for hypertension and potassium for hyperkalemia

PATIENT EDUCATION Griffith, H.W.: Instructions for Patients. Philadephia, W.B. Saunders Co., 1988, p166-167

MEDICATIONS

 FOLLOWUP

 MISCELLANEOUS

DRUG(S) OF CHOICE

Gout and hyperuricemia

◊ Uricosuric agent - probenicid (Benemid) starting with 250 mg bid and doubling 7-10 day intervals up to 500-1000 mg bid (max. 3 gms/day)

◊ Xanthine oxidase inhibitor preferred for hyperuricosuria (Zyloprim) 200-300 mg/day.

◊ Treatment of symptomatic or asymptomatic hyperuricemia with uric acid-lowering drugs has no apparent favorable or adverse effect with respect to development of renal insufficiency.

Hyperuricemic acute renal failure

◊ Prevent by pretreating with allopurinol and hydrating patient prior to administration of chemotherapeutic agents for leukemia or lymphoma

◊ Loop diuretic

◊ IV alkalinizing solution

Uric acid nephrolithiasis

◊ Allopurinol 200-300 mg/day

◊ Alkali to maintain urine pH 6.0-6.5 - sodium bicarbonate or potassium citrate/citric acid 0.5-1.5 meq/kg in 5 or 6 divided doses.

Hyperuricemia of chronic renal failure

◊ Allopurinol in patients with prior history of gout

Contraindications: Avoid uricosuric agents in patients with hyperuricosuria, uric acid nephrolithiasis or chronic renal failure

Precautions:

• Avoid abrupt decreases or increases in serum uric acid, which may precipitate acute gouty arthritis

• Administer colchicine 0.5-0.65 mg/day 1-4 times/week concomitantly with allopurinol first 2-3 months to prevent precipitation of acute gouty arthritis

Significant possible interactions:

Phenylbutazone, diflunisal, aspirin (1-2 gm/day), radio-contrast agents, glyceryl guaiacolate, pyrazinamide, ethambutol, ethanol, diuretics, ascorbic acid(high dose), nicotinic acid

ALTERNATE DRUGS Sulfinpyrazone (Anturane)

PATIENT MONITORING

• Serum uric acid, urinary uric acid excretion, BUN and/or serum creatinine at least twice a year

• Blood pressure screening at least once a year

PREVENTION/AVOIDANCE

• Appropriate pretreatment prior to chemotherapy of leukemia or lymphoma

• Avoid factors that can cause abrupt or persistent increases of serum uric acid or urinary uric acid excretion

• Prompt treatment of urinary obstruction or infection

• Control blood pressure in hypertensives

POSSIBLE COMPLICATIONS

Gout and hyperuricemia

◊ No apparent renal complications

Hyperuricemic acute renal failure

◊ Irreversible renal failure (end-stage renal disease)

◊ Residual renal insufficiency

◊ Persistent renal tubular functional defects

Uric acid nephrolithiasis

◊ Urinary obstruction

◊ Urinary infection

◊ Renal insufficiency

Hyperuricemia of chronic renal failure

◊ Progression to end-stage renal failure

EXPECTED COURSE AND PROGNOSIS

• With effective drug therapy and general management prognosis is excellent in patients with gout, hyperuricemia, or nephrolithiasis

• Development or progression of renal insufficiency should not occur unless due to underlying renal disease or associated medical conditions with adverse renal effects

ASSOCIATED CONDITIONS

• Hypertension

• Diabetes mellitus

AGE-RELATED FACTORS

Pediatric:

• Gout and uric acid nephrolithiasis may have onset in infancy or childhood with HGPRT deficiency, PRPP overactivity or glycogen storage disease, type I

Geriatric: Renal insufficiency more likely due to age and associated medical conditions

Others: N/A

PREGNANCY Women with nephrolithiasis have a slightly higher incidence of urinary tract infection, but no increase in stone formation rate

SYNONYMS N/A

ICD-9-CM

• Gouty nephropathy 274.10

• Uric acid nephrolithiasis 274.11

OTHER NOTES N/A

REFERENCES

• Jacobson, H.R., Striker, G.E. & Klahr, S. (eds.): The Principles and Practice of Nephrology. Philadelphia, B.C. Decker, Inc., 1991

• Brenner, B.M. & Rector, F.C., Jr., (eds.): The Kidney. 4th Ed. Philadelphia, W.B. Saunders Co., 1991

Author D. Eipper, M.D.

Nephrotic syndrome

BASICS

DESCRIPTION
A syndrome comprising glomerular proteinuria (> 3 gm/day), hypoalbuminemia, lipiduria, hypercholesterolemia and edema.
Classification - primary or idiopathic; secondary.
Primary renal disease:
◊ Focal glomerulonephritis
◊ Focal glomerulosclerosis (FGS)
◊ IgA nephropathy
◊ Membranoproliferative glomerulonephritis (MPGN)
◊ Membranous glomerulopathy (MGN)
◊ Mesangial proliferative glomerulonephritis
◊ Minimal change disease (MCD)
◊ Rapidly progressive glomerulonephritis (RPGN)
◊ Congenital nephrotic syndrome
Secondary renal disease
◊ Allergens (Snake venoms, antitoxins, poison ivy, insect stings)
◊ Amyloidosis
◊ Carcinoma (bronchogenic, breast, colon, stomach, kidney) MGN
◊ Diabetes mellitus
◊ Erythema multiforme
◊ Henoch-Schonlein purpura
◊ Heredofamilial (Alport's syndrome, Fabry's disease)
◊ HIV infection
◊ Hodgkin's lymphoma (MCD)
◊ Infections: ventriculo atrial shunt infection, bacterial endocarditis (MPGN), viral (Hepatitis B MPGN, mesangial, MGN) other viral (hepatitis C), protozoal and helminthic
◊ Leukemias
◊ Lymphomas-MGN
◊ Non-Hodgkin's
◊ Focal glomerulosclerosis (reflux nephropathy, heroin abuse, nephron ablation, extensive glomerular scarring in acute glomerulonephritis, chronic renal allograft rejection, end stage kidney, morbid obesity)
◊ Malignant hypertension
◊ Melanoma
◊ Multiple myeloma - amyloid
◊ Nephrotoxins and drugs (gold penicillamine, mercury, MGN)
◊ Nonsteroidal antiinflammatory drug induced nephrotic syndrome (MCD) and interstitial nephritis.
◊ Polyarteritis nodosa
◊ Post strep glomerulonephritis (PSGN) 20% are nephrotic
◊ Sarcoid
◊ Serum sickness
◊ Sjogren's syndrome
◊ Systemic lupus erythematosus (SLE) MGN, FGS, focal, mesangial, diffuse, proliferative
◊ Toxemia of pregnancy
Incidence/Prevalence in USA:
• Children - 2:100,000 new cases/year
• Adults - 3:100,000 new cases/year
System(s) affected: Renal/Urologic - primarily, edema generalized

Genetics: N/A
Predominant age:
• Children - 1.5 - 6 years (MCD)
• Adults - all ages (FGS, MGN more common U.S.A., IgG-IgA worldwide)
Predominant sex: Male = Female

SIGNS AND SYMPTOMS
• Abdominal distention
• Anorexia
• Ascites
• Edema
• Hypertension
• Oliguria
• Orthostatic hypotension
• Puffy eyelids
• Retinal sheen
• Scrotal swelling
• Shortness of breath
• Skin striae
• Weight gain

CAUSES
See classifications listed in description

RISK FACTORS
• Drug addiction, HIV, hepatitis B, C, heroin (FGS)
• Immunosuppression
• Nephrotoxic drugs
• Infections
• Homosexuality and HIV
• Vesicoureteral reflux (FGS)
• Cancer (MGN)

DIAGNOSIS

DIFFERENTIAL DIAGNOSIS
See secondary renal disease in description

LABORATORY
• Proteinuria (> 3 gm/24 hr)
• Hypoalbuminemia
• Hyperlipidemia
• Lipiduria
• Some diseases - low complement (MPGN, SLE, infectious, PSGN)
• Azotemia
• Hypercholesterolemia
• Glycosuria
• Hematuria
• Aminoaciduria
• Increased serum beta-globulin
• Increased serum IgG
Urine
◊ RBC casts
◊ Granular casts
◊ Proteinuria
◊ Hyaline casts
◊ Fatty casts
◊ Foamy appearance
Drugs that may alter lab results: See description
Disorders that may alter lab results: Many

PATHOLOGICAL FINDINGS
• Light microscopy
• Nothing (MCD)
• Other specific for disease: sclerosis (FGS, diabetes), etc.
• Immunofluorescence: Mesangial IgA, (Henoch Schonlein, IgG-IgA nephropathy). Other specific for disease
• Electron microscopy (specific for disease, e.g., sub-epithelial deposits of IgG:MGN)

SPECIAL TESTS
• Complement levels
• Antinuclear antibody
• Serum protein electrophoresis
• Urine immune electrophoresis
• Blood cultures
• Renal venogram for thrombosis

IMAGING
• X-ray
• Ultrasound
• CT
• MRI or venography for renal vein thrombosis

DIAGNOSTIC PROCEDURES
History, physical, basic laboratory including electrolytes, renal biopsy with light, immunofluorescence, electronic microscopy for definitive diagnosis

TREATMENT

APPROPRIATE HEALTH CARE
Outpatient

GENERAL MEASURES
• Salt restriction
• Fluid restriction if hyponatremic
• Treat infections vigorously (especially bacteriuria, endocarditis, peritonitis)
• Anticoagulant (heparin and warfarin) if thromboses occur
• Vaccines: Pneumovax, flu vaccine
• Avoid excess sunlight
• Avoid nephrotoxic drugs
• Judicious use of diuretics

ACTIVITY
Bedrest as tolerated

DIET
• Normal protein (1 g/kg/day)
• Low fat
• Reduced sodium
• Liberal potassium (unless hyperkalemic)
• Supplemental multivitamins and minerals, especially D and iron
• Fluid restriction if hyponatremic
• Caloric restriction if obese or diabetic

PATIENT EDUCATION
Printed material for patients: National Kidney Foundation, 30 E. 33rd Street, Suite 1100, NY, NY 10016 (800)622-9010
• "Childhood Nephrotic Syndrome" (Order #02-23NN)
• "Diabetes and Kidney Disease" (Order #02-09CP) and "Focal Glomerulosclerosis" (Order #02-28NN)

MEDICATIONS

DRUG(S) OF CHOICE
Treat underlying disorder
For steroid-responsive disease: MCD, MGN (sometimes), FGS (rarely)
◊ Adults - prednisone 1.0-1.5 mg/kg/day for 4-6 weeks. After response, continue steroid for 2 additional weeks, then shift to maintenance dose of 2-3 mg/kg on alternate days for 4 weeks. Taper to zero during the next 4-6 months, or 120 mg po qod daily same duration, same period of taper.
◊ Children - prednisone 60 mg/sq m or 2 mg/kg/day orally for 4 weeks. After response - continue steroid for 2 additional weeks, then shift to maintenance dose of 2-3 mg/kg on alternate days for 4 weeks. Taper to zero during the next four months.
For edema
◊ Most importantly salt restriction; then judicious thiazide, loop diuretics
◊ If resistant, a combination of loop and distal diluting segment diuretics [e.g., metolazone (Zaroxolyn)] are synergistic
◊ It is possible that furosemide (Lasix) and albumin mixed and given IV may potentiate diuresis. Be wary of possible thromboses (especially renal vein thrombosis).
Other nephrotic renal diseases: frequently relapsing MCD, RPGN, ?MGN, SLE
◊ Are treated with bolus steroids and/or immune suppression (cyclophosphamide, chlorambucil, cyclosporine)
◊ Consultation often required
Hypercholesterolemia
◊ Should be treated with diet and cholesterol lowering drugs
Contraindications: See manufacturer's information
Precautions: See manufacturer's information
Significant possible interactions: See manufacturer's information

ALTERNATIVE DRUGS N/A

FOLLOWUP

PATIENT MONITORING Frequent monitoring for azotemia, hypertension, edema, nephrotoxicity, serum cholesterol, weight

PREVENTION/AVOIDANCE
• Avoid causative factors whenever possible
• Detect and treat infections vigorously. Infections may involve the common (pneumococcus) to the unusual (strongyloides) especially with immune suppression.

POSSIBLE COMPLICATIONS
• Low levels of: 25-hydroxycholecalciferol, serum calcium, adrenocortical hormones, thyroid hormones
• Hypercoagulability, thrombosis
• Pulmonary emboli
• Hyperlipidemia/accelerated cardiovascular disease
• Acute renal failure
• Progressive renal failure
• Renal vein thrombosis
• Protein malnutrition
• Infection
• Pleural effusion
• Ascites

EXPECTED COURSE AND PROGNOSIS Varies with specific causes. Complete remission expected if basic disease is treatable (infection, malignancy, drug-induced)

MISCELLANEOUS

ASSOCIATED CONDITIONS
• Cancer (see classification)
• Drugs
• Diabetes mellitus
• Connective tissue disease (SLE)
• Multiple myeloma
• Congenital

AGE-RELATED FACTORS
Pediatric: Relatively common in children aged 1.5 - 4 years (MCD)
Geriatric: Occurs in this age group. Prognosis is worse.
Others: N/A

PREGNANCY Toxemia of pregnancy may be nephrotic

SYNONYMS N/A

ICD-9-CM 581.9 nephrotic syndrome with unspecified lesion in kidney

SEE ALSO
• Chronic renal failure
• Acute renal failure
• Diabetes mellitus
• Multiple myeloma
• Systemic lupus erythematosis
• Endocarditis

OTHER NOTES N/A

ABBREVIATIONS
• FGS - Focal segmental glomerulosclerosis
• MGN - Membranous nephropathy
• MPGN - Chronic hypocomplementemic glomerulonephritis, chronic mesangiocapillary glomerulonephritis
• MCD - lipid nephrosis, four process disease, nil disease
• RPGN - Crescentic glomerulonephritis

REFERENCES
• The nephrotic syndrome and its complications. Am J Kidney Dis 10:157, 1987
• Glomerular Disorders. In Cecil Textbook of Medicine. Edited by J.B. Wyngaarden & L.H. Smith. Philadelphia, W.B. Saunders Co., 1992
• Schena, F.P. & Cameron, J.S.: Treatment of Proteinuric Idiopathic Glomerulonephritides in Adults: A Retrospective Survey. Amer J Med 1988;85:315-326

Author G. Rutecki, M.D.

Neuroblastoma

 BASICS

DESCRIPTION
A neoplasm of neural crest origin which may arise anywhere along the sympathetic ganglion chain or in the adrenal medulla. The most common tumor in children less than 1 year of age in the USA.

Genetics:
- Familial cases reported
- Genetic abnormalities in 80%
- Deletions in short arm of chromosome 1(1P)
- Amplification of n-myc oncogene occurs on chromosome 2 (poor prognostic sign)

System(s) affected: Nervous, Endocrine

Incidence in USA: N/A

Prevalence in USA: 27.8 cases/million children/year for 1st five years of life in USA; Denmark: 1/12,000 - 14,000 live births; Japan: 1/15,000-18,749 infants

Predominant age:
- 90% occur in 1st 8 years of life
- More than 1/2 are under 2 years of age
- Most common intra-abdominal malignancy in the newborn

Predominant sex: Slightly more common in boys than girls(1.2:1)

SIGNS AND SYMPTOMS
- 50% present with metastatic disease
- Abdominal mass (50-75%)
- Weight loss
- Anemia
- Failure to thrive
- Abdominal pain and distension
- Bone pain
- Fever
- Diarrhea
- Hypertension (25%)
- Horner's syndrome (ptosis, miosis, enophthalmos, heterochromia of iris)
- Orbital ecchymosis (panda eyes)
- Respiratory distress
- Dysphagia
- Paraplegia
- Cauda equina syndrome
- Flushing, sweating, irritability
- Cerebellar ataxia (chaotic nystagmus): dancing eye syndrome

CAUSES
- Genetic abnormalities in 80% of cases

RISK FACTORS
- Beckwith-Weidemann syndrome
- Pancreatic islet cell dysplasia
- Maternal phenytoin treatment
- Fetal alcohol syndrome
- Hirschsprung's disease

 DIAGNOSIS

DIFFERENTIAL DIAGNOSIS
- Rhabdomyosarcoma
- Wilms' tumors
- Other tumors of neck, chest, abdomen and pelvis

LABORATORY
- CBC, platelet count
- Liver function studies
- Renal function studies
- Urinary catecholamines
- Uric acid
- Creatinine
- Magnesium, calcium
- LDH
- Electrolytes
- Bilirubin, SGOT, SGPT
- Gd2 monoclonal antibody levels
- Serum neuron-specific enolase
- Serum ferritin
- Bone marrow aspiration
- Assay for V.I.P.

Drugs that may alter lab results: N/A
Disorders that may alter lab results: N/A

PATHOLOGICAL FINDINGS
- Small, dark, round cells
- Immature tumors tend to be large, red, lobular soft, friable
- Mature tumors are fibrous, contain calcification, hemorrhage, necrosis, cysts, rosettes, nerve filaments
- May be neuroblastoma, ganglioneuroblastoma, or benign neuroblastoma (depends on cell maturity)
- Favorable histology(Shimada): Stroma-rich, well-differentiated and intermixed tumors
- Unfavorable histology (Shimada): Stroma-rich nodular and stroma-poor, undifferentiated tumors

Staging (Evans)
- ◊ I - confined to single organ, completely resected
- ◊ II - Extends beyond organ of origin but does not cross midline
  - ◊ III - Extends across midline
  - ◊ IV -Distant metastases
  - ◊ IVS - Infants under I year with metastases to liver, skin or bone marrow, sparing cortical bone
- Amplification of n-myc oncogene (poor prognosis)
- Normal DNA ploidy - worse prognosis than hyperploidy

SPECIAL TESTS N/A

IMAGING
- Chest x-ray
- Skeletal survey (including orbital views)
- Bone scan
- CT or MRI of neck, chest, abdomen or pelvis (depending on location of tumor)
- Myelogram for neurologic symptoms

DIAGNOSTIC PROCEDURES
- Myelogram if needed
- Bone marrow aspiration

 TREATMENT

APPROPRIATE HEALTH CARE
Inpatient workup and treatment until stable and induction chemotherapy completed

GENERAL MEASURES
- Surgical resection may be complete, incomplete or biopsy only (for Stage I, excision only)
- If resection incomplete or biopsy, chemotherapy followed by 2nd look operation
- Dumbbell extension through vertebral foramina, chemotherapy alone vs. laminectomy and decompression
- Stage IVS: resection of primary tumor and chemotherapy
- Radiation therapy in Stage III over 1 year of age
- Bone marrow transplantation considered in stages III & IV

ACTIVITY As tolerated

DIET No special diet

PATIENT EDUCATION
- Patient and family teaching regarding long term outlook
- Possibility of second malignancy
- Side effects of treatment

MEDICATIONS

DRUG(S) OF CHOICE
- Cyclophosphamide
- Melphalan
- Vincristine
- Dacarbazine (DTIC)
- Teniposide (VM-26)
- Etoposide (VP16)
- Adriamycin
- Cisplatin
- Peptichemio
- Carboplatin
- Ifosfamide

Contraindications: See manufacturer's information
Precautions: See manufacturer's information
Significant possible interactions: See manufacturers information

ALTERNATIVE DRUGS By protocol

FOLLOWUP

PATIENT MONITORING
- Multi-agent chemotherapy every 3-4 weeks for 4 courses then re-evaluate with bone marrow or second look operation
- Follow every 3 months for 1st year, every 4 months for 2nd year, every 6 months for 3rd year, then at least yearly
- Follow with CT or MRI every 3-6 months initially, then yearly

PREVENTION/AVOIDANCE N/A

POSSIBLE COMPLICATIONS
- Nausea, vomiting
- Alopecia
- Bone marrow depression
- Immunosuppression
- Hemorrhagic cystitis
- Azotemia
- Diarrhea
- ADH secretion
- Local tissue necrosis
- Myocardiopathy
- Renal toxicity
- Hearing loss
- Hypocalcemia, hypomagnesemia

EXPECTED COURSE AND PROGNOSIS
- Overall survival 55%
- Stage I - expected survival approximates 100%
- Stage II - Survival 75%
- Stage III - Survival 43%
- Stage IV - Survival 15%
- Stage IVS - Survival 70'80%
- Normal DNA ploidy, n-myc amplifications, unfavorable histology indicates worse than usual prognosis for same tumor
- Infants under 1 year of age have better outcome
- Patients with cervical, pelvic, and mediastinal tumors have better prognosis than those with retroperitoneal, paraspinal or adrenal tumors
- Survival for those presenting with opsoclonus and nystagmus is nearly 90% (seen especially in mediastinal tumors in infants under 1 year of age)

MISCELLANEOUS

ASSOCIATED CONDITIONS See Risk factors

AGE-RELATED FACTORS
Pediatric: Occurs only in children
Geriatric: N/A
Others: N/A

PREGNANCY N/A

SYNONYMS N/A

ICD-9-CM
194.0 malignant neoplasm of adrenal medulla
171.8 malignant pelvo-abdominal neoplasm
195.1 thoracic neoplasm
173.4 cervical neoplasm

SEE ALSO N/A

OTHER NOTES N/A

ABBREVIATIONS N/A

REFERENCES
- Ashcraft, K.W. & Holder, T.M.: Pediatric Surgery. 2nd Ed. Philadelphia, W.B. Saunders Co., 1993.
- Grosfeld, J.L., Rscorla, F., West, K.W., & Goldman J: Neuroblastoma in the First Year of Life: Clinical and Biologic Factors Influencing Outcome. Seminars in Pediatric Surgery. 2 (1): 37-46, 1993.
- Welch, K.J., Randolph, J.G., Ravitch, M.M., O'Neill, S.A. & Rowe, M.I.: Pediatric Surgery. 4th Ed. Chicago, Year Book Medical Publishers, 1986.

Author T. Black, M.D.

Neurodermatitis

 BASIC INFORMATION

DESCRIPTION
A chronic dermatitis resulting from continued, repeated rubbing or scratching part of the skin
System(s) affected: Skin/Exocrine
Genetics: None known
Incidence/Prevalence in USA: Common
Predominant Age: May occur in any age
Predominant sex: Female > Male

SIGNS AND SYMPTOMS
• Lichenified, pruritic, scaly patch on any part of the body
• Accentuation of normal skin lines
• Surface often excoriated
• Vesicles or weeping are rare
• Non-erythematous
• Postinflammatory hypopigmentation or hyperpigmentation may be present
• Scarring is rare except after serious secondary infections
• Most commonly involves nape of neck, lower legs, ankles, wrist, extensor surface of forearms, scalp, external ear or anogenital region
• Nuchal and suboccipital regions more commonly affected in women
• Perineal region more commonly affected in men
• Social stress or obsessive-compulsive personality trait may play a role in development of this disease

CAUSES
• Idiopathic in many instances
• Some causes of apparent idiopathic disease may be secondary to a previously unrecognized dermatosis
• Secondary forms may begin as another pruritic skin disease which evolves into neurodermatitis after resolution of the primary dermatitis
• Primary dermatoses from which neurodermatitis may develop include lichen planus, stasis dermatitis, atopic dermatitis, tinea corporis, seborrheic dermatitis, xerosis and eczema

RISK FACTORS
• Any pre-existing pruritic dermatosis as noted above
• Obsessive-compulsive personality

 DIAGNOSIS

DIFFERENTIAL DIAGNOSIS
• Atopic dermatitis
• Contact dermatitis
• Lichen planus
• Lichenified psoriasis
• Stasis dermatitis
• Fungal infections
• Seborrheic dermatitis

LABORATORY
None diagnostic
Drugs that may alter lab results: N/A
Disorders that may alter lab results: N/A

PATHOLOGICAL FINDINGS
Thickening of all skin layers with minimal cellular infiltration is noted on skin biopsy

SPECIAL TESTS
None

IMAGING
N/A

DIAGNOSTIC PROCEDURES
Skin biopsy

 TREATMENT

APPROPRIATE HEALTH CARE
Outpatient management

GENERAL MEASURES
• Primary goal in treatment is to interrupt the scratch-itch cycle
• In addition to the medications listed below, occlusive dressings to prevent rubbing/scratching may be beneficial

ACTIVITY
As tolerated. May want to encourage exercise in those cases where stress may play a role.

DIET
Regular

PATIENT EDUCATION
Patients should understand the cause of this disease and their role in helping resolve the condition. Various stress reduction techniques can also be used in those patients in whom stress plays a significant role.

MEDICATIONS

DRUG(S) OF CHOICE
Topical steroids
  ◊ Especially high potency ointments, can break the scratch-itch cycle
  ◊ If necessary these can be used under occlusion initially
  ◊ They should be used for no longer than two weeks, after which low potency topical steroids can be used if needed
Steroid tape (Cordran)
  ◊ Optimized penetration
  ◊ Provides some barrier to further trauma
Contraindications: High potency topical steroids are contraindicated for use on the face and intertriginous areas
Precautions: Topical and intralesional steroid therapy can cause epidermal and dermal atrophy as well as hypopigmentation
Significant possible interactions: N/A

ALTERNATIVE DRUGS
 • Tar preparations are useful but cosmetically less appealing
 • Oral antihistamines can be used for both their antipruritic and sedative effects
 • In extreme cases, a short tapering course of oral prednisone could be considered

FOLLOWUP

PATIENT MONITORING Patients should be followed closely and regularly for response to therapy and for development of complications from therapy

PREVENTION/AVOIDANCE Avoid known pruritic substances/exposure

POSSIBLE COMPLICATIONS
 • Secondary infection
 • Complications related to therapy, as mentioned

EXPECTED COURSE AND
PROGNOSIS Often runs a very chronic course, however, the prognosis is good for those patients in whom the scratch-itch cycle can be broken

MISCELLANEOUS

ASSOCIATED CONDITIONS Prurigo nodularis is a nodular variety of the same disease process

AGE-RELATED FACTORS
Pediatric: Rare in pre-adolescents
Geriatric: N/A
Others: N/A

PREGNANCY N/A

SYNONYMS Lichen simplex (chronicus)

ICD-9-CM 698.3

SEE ALSO
 • Pruritis ani
 • Pruritis vulvae
 • Dermatitis, contact
 • Dermatitis, stasis
 • Dermatitis, seborrheic

OTHER NOTES N/A

ABBREVIATIONS N/A

REFERENCES
 • Orkin, M. & Maibach, H.I.: 1st Ed. Dermatology. San Nateo, CA, Appleton & Lange, 1991
 • Moschella, S.L., Hurley, H.J.: Dermatology, 2nd ed. Philadelphia, W.B. Saunders, 1985
 • Arnold, H.L., Odom, R.B. & Jamos, W.D.: Andrews' Diseases of the Skin. 8th Ed. Philadelphia, W.B. Saunders Co., 1990
 • Sauter, G.C.: Manual of Skin Disease, 6th Ed. Philadelphia, J.B. Lippincott, 1991
 • Sams, W.M. & Lynch, P.J.: Principles and Practice of Dermatology. 1st Ed. New York, Churchill Livingstone, 1990

Author M. King, M.D. & M. LeDuc, M.D.

Nocardiosis

BASICS

DESCRIPTION Nocardiosis is an acute, subacute, or chronic infection occurring in cutaneous, pulmonary, and disseminated forms. Nocardiosis produces suppurative necrosis and abscess formation at sites of infection.
• Primary cutaneous nocardiosis presents as cutaneous infection (cellulitis or abscess), lymphocutaneous infection (similar to sporotrichosis), or subcutaneous infection (actinomycetoma)
• Pulmonary infection presents as an acute, subacute, or chronic pneumonitis
• Disseminated nocardiosis may involve any organ (lesions in the brain or meninges most frequent)
System(s) affected:
Pulmonary/Nervous/Skin, Renal/Urologic
Genetics: N/A
Incidence in USA: 0.4/100,000 (it is estimated that 500-1000 new cases occur per year)
Prevalence in USA: N/A
Predominant age: All ages are susceptible, mean age at diagnosis is the fourth decade of life
Predominant sex: Males > Female (3:1)

SIGNS AND SYMPTOMS
Pulmonary nocardiosis:
◊ Fever (66%)
◊ Cough (52%)
◊ Pleuritic chest pain (32%)
◊ Dyspnea (16%)
◊ Anorexia
◊ Weight loss
◊ Hemoptysis
◊ Fever (70%)
◊ Tachypnea
◊ Rales
◊ Central nervous system dysfunction in those with CNS involvement
◊ Other focal infections in those with disseminated infection
Cutaneous nocardiosis
◊ Abscesses
◊ Lymphadenopathy
Disseminated nocardiosis
◊ Confusion
◊ Disorientation
◊ Dizziness
◊ Headache
◊ Nausea and/or vomiting
◊ Seizures

CAUSES Nocardiosis is caused by traumatic or inhalation inoculation Nocardia species bacteria (predominantly Nocardia asteroides, but also Nocardia brasiliensis and Nocardia caviae) from soil

RISK FACTORS
• Most cases occur as opportunistic infection of immunocompromised hosts or hosts with predisposing pulmonary abnormalities
• Solid organ transplantation, chronic granulomatous disease of childhood, dysgammaglobulinemias, pemphigus, Cushing's disease, hemochromatosis, cirrhosis, bronchiectasis, tuberculosis, sarcoidosis, anthrosilicosis, pulmonary alveolar proteinosis, lymphoma, leukemia, glucocorticoid and cytotoxic therapy, solid malignancies, and AIDS.

DIAGNOSIS

DIFFERENTIAL DIAGNOSIS Includes other causes of acute, subacute, or chronic pneumonitis, particularly those occurring principally in immunocompromised hosts; tuberculosis, histoplasmosis, mixed bacterial lung abscess, and carcinoma

LABORATORY The diagnosis is established by observing the characteristic microscopical appearance of the organism in Gram stained and modified acid-fast stained preparations of sputum or pus or histopathologic samples. Confirmation is by culture of these same specimens.
Drugs that may alter lab results: N/A
Disorders that may alter lab results: N/A

PATHOLOGICAL FINDINGS
Histopathology reveals a suppurative lesion with acute necrosis and abscess formation and the microorganism

SPECIAL TESTS N/A

IMAGING
• X-ray - confluent bronchopneumonia with or without cavitation. Pleural effusion is common (up to 50%). Other chest x-ray presentations include masses, nodules, cavities, interstitial infiltrates.
• Imaging of the brain (brain scan, CT, or MRI) may reveal single or multiple intracranial abscesses, and is indicated in all patients with pulmonary nocardiosis. Other sites of focal infection may be identified by imaging in disseminated disease.

DIAGNOSTIC PROCEDURES If
evaluation of sputum is nondiagnostic, bronchoscopy for bronchoalveolar lavage and transbronchial lung biopsy may prove valuable for diagnosis

TREATMENT

APPROPRIATE HEALTH CARE
Patients with moderate or severe illness generally require hospitalization

GENERAL MEASURES
• Respiratory support is often necessary in such hospitalized patients
• Surgical drainage of abscesses other than intrapulmonary abscesses is generally indicated if technically feasible

ACTIVITY Acute phase usually requires bedrest. Increase activity as condition improves.

DIET No special diet

PATIENT EDUCATION
• Not a contagious disease
• Advise patients of the need for long-term antimicrobial therapy to reduce the likelihood of relapse

MEDICATIONS

DRUG(S) OF CHOICE
• Sulfonamides are the traditional mainstay of treatment for all forms of nocardiosis. Some prefer sulfadiazine because of possibly better CNS activity. Sulfadiazine should be given as 4-8 gm po per day in 4 divided doses. Dosage should be adjusted to maintain sulfonamide serum levels in the range of 8-16 mg/dL.
• Some prefer to use trimethoprim/sulfamethoxazole. This agent must be used if parenteral sulfonamide therapy is required. Initial dose based on trimethoprim component. 640 mg trimethoprim daily. Base subsequent doses on sulfamethoxazole level. Dosage should provide equivalent sulfonamide dosing and levels as when a sulfonamide is used alone.

Contraindications:
• Sulfonamides - in the last month of pregnancy (should only be used when the potential benefits outweigh the risks)
• All antimicrobial agents above are contraindicated in the presence of known hypersensitivity to the agent

Precautions: With the use of high dose sulfadiazine, high urine flow should be maintained to minimize risk of crystalluria. Generally, patient should be advised to drink 2-3 L/day.

Significant possible interactions:
• Sulfonamides can increase the therapeutic effects of oral anticoagulants, phenytoin, sulfonylurea hypoglycemic agents, methotrexate, and thiopental
• Decreased absorption of digoxin may be encountered

ALTERNATIVE DRUGS
Alternatives for sulfonamide allergic patients include doxycycline or minocycline, ampicillin plus erythromycin, amikacin, imipenem, b-lactam/b-lactamase inhibitor combinations, and cefotaxime or ceftriaxone. Clinical experience with these alternative regimens is limited.

FOLLOWUP

PATIENT MONITORING
Patients on high dose sulfonamide therapy should have a complete blood count and assessment of hepatic and renal function performed at least every other week

PREVENTION/AVOIDANCE   N/A

POSSIBLE COMPLICATIONS
• Central nervous system infection (brain abscess or meningitis) (16%)
• Secondary cutaneous nocardiosis (13%)
• Septic arthritis (2%)
• Hematogenous osteomyelitis (1%)
• Other focal manifestations of disseminated infection (13%)

EXPECTED COURSE AND PROGNOSIS
Overall modern mortality is 7-44%. In renal transplant recipients: overall mortality 25%, 0% mortality with isolated cutaneous involvement, 29% mortality with localized pleuropulmonary disease, 42% mortality with central nervous system involvement. In patients with the acquired immunodeficiency syndrome, mortality is 30%.

MISCELLANEOUS

ASSOCIATED CONDITIONS   See Risk factors

AGE-RELATED FACTORS
Pediatric: Reported association between chronic granulomatous disease of childhood and nocardiosis
Geriatric: N/A
Others: N/A

PREGNANCY
Sulfonamides - in the last month of pregnancy (should only be used when the potential benefits outweigh the risks)

SYNONYMS   N/A

ICD-9-CM   039.9

SEE ALSO   N/A

OTHER NOTES
Unusual nocardial infections: Keratoconjunctivitis associated with contact lenses, peritonitis in patients on continuous ambulatory peritoneal dialysis, upper aerodigestive tract infections, pericarditis, hematogenous endophthalmitis, prosthetic joint infections, natural or prosthetic valve endocarditis

ABBREVIATIONS   N/A

REFERENCES
• Kalb, R.E., Kaplan, M.H. & Grossman, M.E.: Cutaneous nocardiosis. J Am Acad Derm 13:125-133, 1985
• Wilson, J.P., Turner, H.R., Kirchner, K.A. & Chapman, S.W.: Nocardial infection in renal transplant recipients. Medicine 68:38-57, 1989
• Kim, J., Minamoto, G.Y. & Grieco, M.H.: Nocardial infection as a complication of AIDS: Report of six cases & review. Rev Infect Dis 13:624-629, 1991

Author R. Greenfield, M.D. & D. Fine, M.D.

Obesity

 BASICS

DESCRIPTION
A condition of increased body weight (consisting of both lean and fat tissue) that leads to increased morbidity and mortality. Also defined as weight 20% greater than an individual's desirable weight as defined by the Metropolitan Life Insurance Company.
• Android obesity (male pattern or abdominal obesity) is higher risk and gynoid obesity (female pattern or gluteal obesity) is lower risk for long-term health problems.

System(s) affected: Gastrointestinal, Endocrine/Metabolic

Genetics: 25-30% of the variance in body fat is genetically transmitted

Incidence in USA: N/A

Prevalence in USA:
• 20-30% of adult men and 30-40% of adult women (according to an NIH panel)
• Ages 35-44 - 1600/100,000 males; 1400/100,000 females
• Ages 65-74 - 500/100,000 males; 400/100,000 females

Predominant age: All ages

Predominant sex: Female > Male

SIGNS AND SYMPTOMS
Increased body weight and adipose tissue

CAUSES
• Multifactorial
• Rare genetic syndromes have been described
• Idiopathic obesity is assumed to be due to an imbalance between food intake and energy expenditure (physical activity and metabolic rate)
• Insulinoma
• Hypothalamic disorders
• Cushing's syndrome
• Corticosteroid drugs

RISK FACTORS
• Parental obesity
• Pregnancy
• Sedentary lifestyle
• High fat diet
• Low socioeconomic status

 DIAGNOSIS

DIFFERENTIAL DIAGNOSIS N/A

LABORATORY
• Not needed for diagnosis
• Consider thyroid function tests
• Cardiac risk factors: serum cholesterol, triglycerides, glucose

Drugs that may alter lab results: N/A

Disorders that may alter lab results: Hypothyroidism

PATHOLOGICAL FINDINGS
• Hypertrophy and/or hyperplasia of adipocytes
• Cardiomegaly
• Hepatomegaly

SPECIAL TESTS
• Body mass index (BMI) = body weight (kg) divided by the square of body height (m). Obesity is BMI > 30 kg/m2
• Determine fat distribution pattern by measuring waist and hips circumferences and calculating the waist to hips ratio (WHR)
• Android (male pattern, or abdominal obesity) has WHR greater than 0.85 for females; 0.95 for males
• Gynoid (female pattern, or gluteal obesity) has WHR less than 0.85 for females; 0.95 for males

IMAGING N/A

DIAGNOSTIC PROCEDURES N/A

 TREATMENT

APPROPRIATE HEALTH CARE
Outpatient

GENERAL MEASURES
• Appropriate functions for the primary care physician include: assessment of degree of health risk from BMI and WHR (see Diagnosis); assessment of motivation to lose weight; helping patients to set goals of therapy; office counselling or referral to a registered dietician or weight loss program for in depth counselling on diet, exercise, and behavior modification; and long term follow-up
• Occasionally, patients with severe obesity (BMI > 40 kg/m2) are treated with a gastric stapling procedure. This involves complex pre-surgical evaluation, surgery and followup and should only be done in a center skilled in this treatment. Surgical treatment is the most effective long term weight loss treatment available for morbid obesity.
• Many reputable commercial and community programs exist for obesity treatment. Desirable programs should include diets which meet the RDA for nutrients, exercise counselling, behavior modification, and provision for long term maintenance. Physicians can provide valuable additional monitoring and long term followup.

ACTIVITY
Exercise alone rarely causes significant weight loss. It may improve long term results of weight loss treatment and should be an integral part of any weight loss program.

DIET
• Diet restriction is the cornerstone of obesity management (low-fat, high-complex carbohydrate and high-fiber)
• A 500 kcal reduction in calorie intake will result in approximately 1 pound weight loss per week

Very low calorie diets (VLCD)
◊ (400-800 kcal per day) are usually based on liquid formulas and cause more rapid weight loss
◊ Complications of VLCD include: dehydration, orthostatic hypotension, fatigue, muscle cramps, constipation, headache, cold intolerance, and relapse after discontinuation
◊ Contraindications of VLCD include: recent myocardial infarction or cerebrovascular accident, renal or hepatic disease, cancer, pregnancy, insulin-dependent diabetes mellitus, some psychiatric disturbances
◊ Physician supervision is important for VLCD

PATIENT EDUCATION
• Educating the patient about the value of weight reduction is important
• Behavior modification can improve dietary adherence and long term results of weight loss and should be included in any weight loss program

MEDICATIONS

DRUG(S) OF CHOICE
• Drug treatment is not usually recommended
• Appetite suppressants - diethylpropion, phentermine, fenfluramine, mazindol (Schedule IV drugs) or phendimetrazine, benzphetamine (Schedule III drugs) may be indicated for short-term use (few weeks) in conjunction with a weight loss regimen
Contraindications: Advanced atherosclerosis, symptomatic cardiovascular disease, hypertension, hyperthyroidism, glaucoma, history of drug abuse, agitated states, use of MAO inhibitors
Precautions:
• Abuse potential, especially for Schedule III
• Relapse after discontinuation of drug
Significant possible interactions:
Concurrent use with general anesthetics may cause arrhythmias

ALTERNATIVE DRUGS
Phenylpropanolamine is used in over the counter weight loss preparations

FOLLOWUP

PATIENT MONITORING
Long term followup is crucial to prevent further weight gain or regain after weight loss

PREVENTION/AVOIDANCE
Counselling in regular exercise and prudent diet with regular follow-up, especially in children and young adults and those with family history of obesity or diabetes mellitus

POSSIBLE COMPLICATIONS
• Increased mortality due largely to cardiovascular disease
• Diabetes mellitus
• Hypertension
• Hyperlipidemia
• Gall bladder disease with cholelithiasis
• Osteoarthritis
• Gout
• Thromboembolism
• Hypoventilation and sleep apnea syndromes
• Poor self-esteem
• Occupational discrimination

EXPECTED COURSE AND PROGNOSIS
• Long term maintenance of weight loss is extremely difficult
• If patient is not motivated, successful weight loss is unlikely

MISCELLANEOUS

ASSOCIATED CONDITIONS
See Possible complications

AGE-RELATED FACTORS
Pre-puberty and young adulthood appear to be sensitive periods for development of obesity
Pediatric: Prevalence of obesity is increasing. Among other factors, decreased physical activity and increased television viewing have been implicated.
Geriatric: Desirable weights (those associated with the lowest risk of mortality) increase with age
Others: N/A

PREGNANCY
Pregnancy is a common time for onset or increase in obesity

SYNONYMS
• Overweight
• Adiposis
• Adiposity

ICD-9-CM
278.0

SEE ALSO
N/A

OTHER NOTES
N/A

ABBREVIATIONS
N/A

REFERENCES
• Bray, G.A.: West J Med. 149:429-441 and 555-571, 1988
• Bray, G.A.: Obesity: Basic aspects and clinical applications. Med Clin North Am, January 1989
• Harrison's Textbook of Medicine, 19th edition, p. 411.

Author D. Gray, M.D.

Obsessive compulsive disorder

BASICS

DESCRIPTION Psychiatric condition classified as an anxiety disorder in Diagnostic and Statistical Manual of Mental Disorders (DSM-III-R) and characterized by recurrent, intrusive thoughts (obsessions) and ritualistic behaviors (compulsions)
• Obsessions and compulsions consume more than an hour per day and cause occupational/social impairment
• Patients know thoughts (obsessions) come from their own minds and are not imposed from outside (as in thought insertion). Thoughts are not associated with another disorder (for example, thought of food if an eating disorder is present).
• Compulsions are ritualistic behaviors designed to relieve the anxiety of obsessions
Common obsessive themes:
◊ Violence, such as harming a beloved child
◊ Doubt, such as whether doors or windows locked or iron turned off
◊ Blasphemous thoughts, such as in a devoutly religious person
◊ Contamination, dirt or disease
◊ Symmetry or orderliness
Common rituals or compulsions:
◊ Hand washing
◊ Checking
◊ Counting
◊ Hoarding
◊ Repeaters - such as dressing rituals
System(s) affected: Nervous
Genetics: Positive family history in about 20% of cases, no mode of transmission identified
Incidence/Prevalence in USA: 2.5% lifetime prevalence
Predominant age: Mean age 20. 1/3 cases present by age 15, new cases after age 50 rare.
Predominant sex: Male = Female (males tend to present at a younger age)

SIGNS AND SYMPTOMS
• Obsessions and/or compulsions that consume more than an hour a day and cause significant distress or impairment
• Obsessions (thoughts) are recurrent; patient attempts to ignore or neutralize thoughts with another thought or action
• Neither obsessions nor compulsions are related to another mental disorder
• Compulsions (actions) are repetitive, purposeful behaviors in response to thoughts in attempt to neutralize the thought - such as checking in response to doubt (locks, doors, windows or driving back over route to check for any possible damage inadvertently done while driving one's car)

• Repeated handwashing or ritualistic handwashing in response to fear of contamination
• 80-90% of patients have obsessions and compulsions
• 10-19% are pure obsessional
• 5% perform rituals until they "feel right" and may not have an identifiable obsession
• Hoarding and obsessional slowness comprise two other categories

CAUSES Dysregulation of neurotransmitter, serotonin

RISK FACTORS Greater concordance in monozygotic twins family history as above

DIAGNOSIS

DIFFERENTIAL DIAGNOSIS
• Impulse control disorders: Compulsive gambling, sex or substance abuse - the "compulsive" behavior is not in response to obsessive thought and patient derives pleasure from the activity, unlike OCD where obsessions and compulsions are ego dystonic
• Depression: Can see brooding, but ideas not perceived as senseless as in OCD
• Schizophrenia: Patient perceives thought to be true and from an external source
• Compulsive personality disorder: Not to be confused with OCD. In personality disorder, traits are ego-syntonic. Traits include perfectionism, preoccupation with detail, trivia or procedure and regulation. Patient tends to be rigid, moralistic and stingy. Often traits are rewarded in patient's job as desirable traits.

LABORATORY N/A
Drugs that may alter lab results: N/A
Disorders that may alter lab results: N/A

PATHOLOGICAL FINDINGS N/A

SPECIAL TESTS Yale Brown OCD checklist (Y-BOCS)

IMAGING PET scan - abnormal metabolism in frontal cortex and caudate nuclei (not generally available other than in research centers)

DIAGNOSTIC PROCEDURES
Psychiatric interview

TREATMENT

APPROPRIATE HEALTH CARE
Psychiatric referral for therapy (in vivo exposure)

GENERAL MEASURES In vivo exposure with response prevention (prevention or delay of ritual)

ACTIVITY No restriction

DIET With use of phenelzine must have tyramine free diet to prevent precipitation of hypertensive crisis

PATIENT EDUCATION
• OCD Foundation, P.O. Box 9573, New Haven, CT 06535, (203) 772-0565
• Printed patient information available from: Obsessive-Compulsive Anonymous, P.O. Box 215, New Hyde Park, NY 11040, (516)741-4901

Obsessive compulsive disorder

MEDICATIONS

DRUG(S) OF CHOICE
Clomipramine
◊ Adults - beginning at 25 mg/day and increased gradually to 100 mg over first 2 weeks. Then to 250 mg over next several weeks, as tolerated.
◊ Children - beginning at 25 mg /day over first two weeks as in adults. Then titrated up to 3 mg/kg or 200 mg/day (which ever is smaller) over the next several weeks.

Contraindications:
• Clomipramine is of the tricyclic antidepressant class, so carries same contraindications as drugs in that class
Absolute clomipramine contraindications:
◊ Within 6 months of myocardial infarction
◊ Narrow angle glaucoma
◊ 3rd degree AV block
◊ Within 14 days of MAO inhibitor
Relative clomipramine contraindications:
◊ Prostatic hypertrophy (urinary retention)
◊ Seizure disorder (lower seizure threshold)
◊ 1st, 2nd degree AV block, bundle branch block and CHF (pro-arrhythmic effect)

Precautions:
• Drug needs to be continued for a minimum of 8 weeks before considering it a treatment failure (as in depression)
• Because patients with OCD may have concomitant depression, suicide potential must be ascertained as well
• Tricyclic class of antidepressants dangerous in overdose

Significant possible interactions:
• Not yet fully elucidated
• May interfere with guanethidine, clonidine
• Serum level increased if used concomitantly with haloperidol
• Probable plasma increase if used with cimetidine, fluoxetine, methylphenidate
• Increases serum level of phenobarbital

ALTERNATIVE DRUGS
• Fluoxetine (serotonin reuptake inhibitor)
• Psychosurgery (last resort)

FOLLOWUP

PATIENT MONITORING Y-BOCS

PREVENTION/AVOIDANCE N/A

POSSIBLE COMPLICATIONS
• Depression
• Avoidant behavior (phobic avoidance)
• Anxiety and panic-like episodes associated with obsessions

EXPECTED COURSE AND PROGNOSIS
• Chronic waxing and waning course in majority
• 24-33% fluctuating course
• 11-14% phasic with periods of remission
• 54-61% chronic progressive course

MISCELLANEOUS

ASSOCIATED CONDITIONS
• Depression
• Panic disorder
• Social phobia
• Phobia
• Tourette's
• Alcoholism
• Substance abuse

AGE-RELATED FACTORS
Pediatric: Adolescent onset in 15%. At this age males outnumber females 3:1.
Geriatric: Diagnosis not generally made after age 50
Others: N/A

PREGNANCY
• Onset of OCD has been noted after delivery
• Safety of clomipramine has not been established in pregnancy nor lactation

SYNONYMS Obsessive compulsive neurosis

ICD-9-CM 300.3 (same as DSM-III-R code)

SEE ALSO N/A

OTHER NOTES Not to be confused with obsessive compulsive personality disorder (see differential diagnosis, above)

ABBREVIATIONS
Y-BOCS = Yale Brown OCD checklist

REFERENCES
• American Psychiatric Association: Diagnostic and Statistical Manual of Mental Disorders (DSM-III-R). 3rd Ed. Washington, D.C., 1987
• Talbot
• Hales and Yudofsky 88

Author K. Hall, M.D.

Ocular chemical burns

BASICS

DESCRIPTION Chemical exposure to the eye can result in rapid, devastating, and permanent damage and is one of the true emergencies in ophthalmology
<u>Separate alkaline from acid chemical exposure:</u>
◊ Alkaline burns - more severe, alkali penetrates and saponifies tissues easily, may produce injury to lids, conjunctiva, cornea, sclera, iris, lens, and retina
◊ Acid burns - usually acid does not damage internal structures since protein coagulation limits acid penetration. Injury often limited to lids, conjunctiva, and cornea.
System(s) affected: Nervous, Skin/Exocrine
Genetics: N/A
Incidence in USA: Estimated 300/100,000/year
Prevalence in USA: Unknown
Predominant age: 18-65
Predominant sex: Male > Female

SIGNS AND SYMPTOMS
<u>Mild burns:</u>
◊ Pain and blurred vision
◊ Eyelid skin erythema and edema
◊ Corneal epithelial defects
◊ Conjunctival chemosis, hyperemia, and hemorrhages without perilimbal ischemia
◊ Mild anterior chamber reaction
<u>Moderate to severe burns:</u>
◊ Symptoms of severe pain and markedly reduced vision
◊ Second and third degree burns of eyelid skin
◊ Corneal edema and opacification
◊ Corneal epithelial defects
◊ Marked conjunctival chemosis and perilimbal blanching
◊ Moderate anterior chamber reaction
◊ Increased intraocular pressure
◊ Local necrotic retinopathy
◊ In alkaline burns, can have initial pain which later diminishes

CAUSES
• Alkali: Ammonia (NH3), lye (NaOH), magnesium hydroxide [Mg(OH)2], potassium hydroxide (KOH), and lime [Ca(OH)2]
• Acids: Hydrochloric (HCl), hydrofluoric (HF), acetic (CH3COOH), nitrous (HNO2), and sulfuric (H2SO4)

RISK FACTORS
• Construction work (plaster, cement, whitewash)
• Use of cleaning agents (drain cleaners, ammonia)
• Automobile battery explosions (sulfuric acid)
• Industrial work (many possible agents)
• Alcoholism

DIAGNOSIS

DIFFERENTIAL DIAGNOSIS
• Thermal burns
• Ocular cicatricial pemphigoid
• Other causes of corneal opacification

LABORATORY None
Drugs that may alter lab results: N/A
Disorders that may alter lab results: None

PATHOLOGICAL FINDINGS
• Precipitation of glycosaminoglycans causes corneal opacification
• Saponification of cell membranes causes cell death
• Cation binding to collagen results in hydration, thickening, and shortening of collagen fibrils

SPECIAL TESTS Measure pH of tear film with litmus paper or electronic probe (irrigating fluid with non-neutral pH [e.g., normal saline has pH of 4.5] may alter results)

IMAGING Not necessary unless suspicion of intraocular or orbital foreign body is present

DIAGNOSTIC PROCEDURES
• Careful slit lamp examination, fundus ophthalmoscopy, tonometry, and measurement of visual acuity
• Full extent of damage from alkaline burns may not be apparent until 48-72 hours after exposure

TREATMENT

APPROPRIATE HEALTH CARE
Emergency room with inpatient admission depending on severity

GENERAL MEASURES
• Copious irrigation and removal of corneal or conjunctival foreign bodies are always the initial treatment. Continue irrigation until the tear film is of neutral pH and pH is stable. Sweep the conjunctival fornices every 12-24 hours to prevent adhesions.
<u>Surgical procedures:</u>
◊ Punctal occlusion for tear film preservation and corneal epitheliopathy
◊ Tarsorrhaphy for persistent epithelial defects
◊ Tissue adhesive (e.g., isobutyl cyanoacrylate) for impending or actual corneal perforation
◊ Conjunctival or limbal autograft transplantation for epithelial stem cell restoration
◊ Lamellar or penetrating keratoplasty for tectonic stabilization or visual rehabilitation

ACTIVITY Ambulatory

DIET Usual for patient

PATIENT EDUCATION Safety glasses

Ocular chemical burns

MEDICATIONS

DRUG(S) OF CHOICE
Immediate treatment (any non-toxic irrigant):
◊ In hospital setting, sterile water, normal saline, lactated Ringer's solution are effective
◊ In the field, use what is available (tap water). Rapidity of irrigation is critical.
◊ Irrigation is continued until pH of superior/inferior cul-de-sac is neutral
◊ It is impossible to over-irrigate
Further treatment
◊ Topical prophylactic antibiotics: Any broad spectrum agent, e.g., bacitracin/polymyxin ointment (Polysporin) q 2-4 h, ciprofloxacin drops (Ciloxan) q 2-4 h, chloramphenicol ointment (Chloroptic) q 2-4 h
◊ Tear substitutes: Hypotears PF or Cellufresh drops q 4 h, Refresh P.M. ointment q hs
◊ Cycloplegics: Cyclopentolate 1% tid, or scopolamine 1/4% bid
◊ Anti-glaucoma for elevated intraocular pressure (IOP): Timolol (Timoptic 0.5%) bid or levobunolol (Betagan 0.5%) bid and/or acetazolamide (Diamox) 125-250 mg po q6h or methazolamide (Neptazane) 25-50 mg po bid and/or mannitol 20% 1-2 g/kg IV prn
◊ Corticosteroids: Prednisolone acetate 1% or equivalent (Pred Forte) q 1-4 h for 10-14 days; if severe, prednisone 20-60 mg po qd for 5-7 days. Taper rapidly if epithelium intact by this time.
◊ Consider collagen shield to help absorb collagenases and re-epithelialize cornea
◊ Consider ascorbic acid 500 mg po qid and/or acetylcysteine (Mucomyst) 10-20% top q 4 h if corneal melting occurs

Contraindications: None
Precautions:
• For timolol and levobunolol - history of congestive heart failure or chronic obstructive pulmonary disease
• For acetazolamide and methazolamide - history of nephrolithiasis or metabolic acidosis
• For mannitol - history of congestive heart failure or renal failure
• For scopolamine - history of urinary retention
Significant possible interactions: Refer to manufacturer's literature

ALTERNATIVE DRUGS   Already listed

FOLLOWUP

PATIENT MONITORING
• Depending on severity of ocular injury, from daily to weekly visits initially
• May be inpatient
• If on mannitol or prednisone, consider frequent serum electrolytes

PREVENTION/AVOIDANCE   Safety glasses to safeguard uninvolved eye

POSSIBLE COMPLICATIONS
• Persistent epitheliopathy
• Fibrovascular pannus
• Corneal ulcer/perforation
• Progressive symblepharon and entropion
• Neurotrophic keratitis
• Glaucoma
• Cataract
• Hypotony
• Phthisis bulbi

EXPECTED COURSE AND PROGNOSIS
• Depends on severity of initial injury
• Increasing amounts of limbal ischemia and corneal opacification correlate with poorer prognosis
• For severely injured eyes, permanent loss of vision is not uncommon

MISCELLANEOUS

ASSOCIATED CONDITIONS   Facial cutaneous chemical or thermal burns

AGE-RELATED FACTORS
Pediatric: N/A
Geriatric:
• Compromised ocular surface from keratitis sicca or other disease associated with poorer prognosis
• Compromised corneal endothelium or pre-existing glaucoma may also complicate clinical management
Others: N/A

PREGNANCY   N/A

SYNONYMS   Chemical ocular injuries

ICD-9-CM
• Alkali burn: 940.2
• Acid burn: 940.3

SEE ALSO   Burns

OTHER NOTES   N/A

ABBREVIATIONS   N/A

REFERENCES
• Fraunfelder, F.T. & Roy, F.H.: Current Ocular Therapy, 3rd ed, Philadelphia, W.B. Saunders Co., 1990
• McCulley, J.P.: Chemical Injuries. In The Cornea: Scientific Foundations and Clinical Practice. Edited by G. Smolin & R.A. Thoft. New York, Little, Brown, 1987
• Shingleton, B.J., Hersh, P.S. & Kenyon, K.R.: Eye Trauma. St. Louis, Mosby Year Book, 1991
• Ralph, R.A.: Chemical Burns of the Eye. In Clinical Ophthalmology. Edited by W. Tasman. Philadelphia, J.B. Lippincott, 1992

Author   R. Fante, M.D.

Onychomycosis

BASICS

DESCRIPTION Infection of the nail by fungi
System(s) affected: Skin/Exocrine
Genetics: N/A
Incidence/Prevalence in USA: 22-130 cases/1000 population
Predominant age: Varies with type. Rare before puberty.
Predominant sex: Varies with type

SIGNS AND SYMPTOMS
• Dermatophyte onychomycosis (four distinct clinical forms occur)
◊ Commonly preceded by dermatophyte infection at another site
◊ Most frequent form in adults
◊ 80% involve toenails - especially hallux
◊ Simultaneous infection of finger and toe nails rare
Distal subungual onychomycosis
◊ Spreads from hyponychium to nailbed to nailplate, involving one or more digits of hands or feet
◊ Subungual hyperkeratosis - yellowish-gray mass which lifts off free border of nail
◊ Subungual paronychia - thickening of subungual region which lifts off nailplate
◊ Onycholysis (detachment of nailplate from nailbed)
◊ Dystrophic changes - thickening, deformation, crumbling
◊ Discoloration - yellow-brown
◊ Bois vermoulu - end stage nail, looks like worm-eaten wood
◊ Onychomadesis (shedding of nail) or traumatic avulsion may occur
◊ Subjective symptoms minimal except from secondary infection or deformity
◊ Rate of spread depends on pathogen
Lateral onychomycosis (common)
◊ Yellowish discoloration lateral nail groove
◊ Progressive onycholysis, proximal or distal
◊ Very rarely will invade nailplate and spread to opposite lateral fold
Proximal onychomycosis (rare)
◊ Hands or feet
◊ Leukonychia - yellowish-white spots begin under posterior nail groove, spreading to nail plate and lunula
White superficial onychomycosis (rare)
◊ Hallux preferentially affected
◊ Infection of upper part of nailplate
◊ Opaque white spots on nail plate eventually merge to involve entire surface of the nail
◊ Trichophyton mentagrophytes most common pathogen
Candidal onychomycosis
◊ Predominantly adult women
◊ Hands 70% - especially dominant hand
◊ Middle finger most common
◊ Pain mild, unless secondarily infected
◊ Pain increases with frequent or prolonged contact with water
◊ Attacks the soft tissue surrounding the nail - penetrates keratin only secondarily
◊ Begins with detachment of cuticle from nailplate
◊ Dark yellowish to blackish-brown zone along lateral border of nail
◊ Secondary ungual changes - convex, irregular, striated nailplate with dull rough surface
◊ Onycholysis - frequent, especially on hands
◊ Distal subungual onychomycosis may occur
◊ Primary involvement of the nailplate uncommon (thin, crumbly, opaque, brownish nailplate deformed by transverse grooves)
◊ Periungual edema/erythema may occur (club-shaped, bulbous fingertips)
◊ Superficial white onychomycosis - young children
Mold onychomycosis
◊ More common over 60 years old
◊ More common in nails of hallux
◊ Resembles distal and lateral onychomycosis

CAUSES
Dermatophytes
◊ Invade normal keratin
◊ Trichophyton rubrum - most common
◊ Trichophyton mentagrophytes var. interdigitale - 25% as common as T. rubrum
◊ Epidermophyton floccosum, T. violaceum and Microsporum less common
Candida
◊ 70% Candida albicans
◊ C. parapsilosis, C. tropicalis, C. krusei (less common)
Molds
◊ Invade altered keratin
◊ Found in following order of frequency: Scopulariopsis brevicaulis, Hendersonula toruloidea, Aspergillus species, Alternaria tenuis, Cephalosporium, Scytalidium hyalinium

RISK FACTORS
Dermatophyte onychomycosis
◊ Warmth
◊ Moisture - hyperhidrosis, rubber shoes
◊ Cramped or tight fitting foot wear
◊ Peripheral vascular disease
◊ Depressed cell-mediated immunity
◊ Indirect contamination
Candidal onychomycosis
◊ Direct contamination - ano-vulvar, perirectal pruritus
◊ Chemical or mechanical damage to cuticle
◊ Maceration
◊ Occlusion
◊ Contact with substances containing sugar
◊ Hyperhidrosis
◊ Chilblain
◊ Cold hands (Raynaud's phenomenon)
◊ Psoriatic onycholysis
◊ Diabetes mellitus
◊ Hyperparathyroidism
◊ Addison's disease
◊ Malnutrition
◊ Malabsorption
◊ Dyscrasias
◊ Malignant tumors
◊ Postoperative conditions
◊ Altered immune function

Mold onychomycosis
◊ Soil contamination
◊ Peripheral vascular disease
◊ Overlapping toes
◊ Onychogryposis - deforming overgrowth of nails resulting in hooked or curved state

DIAGNOSIS

DIFFERENTIAL DIAGNOSIS Bacterial paronychia, herpetic whitlow, eczema, pustular psoriasis, tumor, Darier's disease, pityriasis rubra pilaris, trophic changes, endocrine disease, drugs, peripheral vascular disease, trauma, chemicals, alopecia areata, lichen planus, yellow nail syndromes (icterus, carotenemia, amyloidosis), white acquired nail discoloration (trauma, acute infections, chronic disease, thallium or arsenic poisoning, hepatic cirrhosis, chronic hypoalbuminemia), brown-black pigment (melanotic, hematoma), or green dyschromia (Pseudomonas aeruginosa)

LABORATORY
• Direct microscopy (KOH preparation) - clip or file away some of nailplate as needed, collect scales from stratum corneum of most proximal area (beneath nail or crumbling nail itself), 5% KOH + gentle heat, 100% sensitive if > 2 preps examined
• Cultures - negative in 30% (secondary to loss of dermatophyte viability)
• Histologic examination of keratin
• All are influenced by quality of sampling
Drugs that may alter lab results: Discontinue all topical medication several days before obtaining sample
Disorders that may alter lab results: N/A

PATHOLOGICAL FINDINGS Pathogens within the nail keratin

SPECIAL TESTS N/A

IMAGING N/A

DIAGNOSTIC PROCEDURES
• Punch or scalpel biopsy - proximal lesions with PAS stain
• Nail scraping - KOH prep

TREATMENT

APPROPRIATE HEALTH CARE
Outpatient - unless secondary cellulitis/osteomyelitis

GENERAL MEASURES
• Avoid factors that promote fungal growth (heat, darkness, moisture)
• Treat underlying disease risk factors
• Treat associated fungal infections in other locations (40%)
• Treat secondary infection, if present
Nail removal to remove infected keratin
◊ Mechanical - soften with occlusive dressing, detach from nailbed with tweezers or file with abrasive paper/grinding stone
◊ Chemical - protect peripheral tissue with adhesive strips, apply ointment of 30% salicylic acid, 40% urea or 50% potassium iodide under occlusive dressing
◊ Surgical avulsion - for involvement of just one or only a few nails

ACTIVITY
Restrictions are based solely on local promoting factors, underlying disease or secondary infection

DIET
No special diet

PATIENT EDUCATION
• Keep affected area clean and dry
• Avoid rubber or other occlusive footwear
• Avoid tight or ill-fitting footwear
• Wear absorbent cotton socks - avoid wool or synthetic fibers
• Change clothing and towels frequently and launder in hot water

MEDICATIONS

DRUG(S) OF CHOICE
• Dermatophyte onychomycosis
Local treatments
◊ Less effective than oral
◊ Apply under occlusive dressing
◊ May mix with keratolytic chemicals
◊ Most common agents: Imidazoles - clotrimazole (Lotrimin, Mycelex), miconazole (Monistat), butoconazole, tioconazole, econazole (Spectazole), ketoconazole (Nizoral), sulconazole (Exelderm), oxiconazole (Oxistat); unsaturated fatty acid derivatives - propionic acid, undecylenic acid; haloprogin (Halotex); tolnaftate (Tinactin)
◊ Other available agents: Ciclopirox (Loprox), naftifine (Naftin), cationic surfactants - benzalkonium chloride (Cetylcide, Fungoid), cetrimide, cetylpyridinium chloride, halogenated/chlorinated/iodinated derivatives - chloramine, tincture of iodine; dyes - malachite green, crystal violet; mercury derivatives - thimerosal; phenols; glutaraldehyde

• Dermatophyte onychomycosis
Systemic therapy
◊ Griseofulvin ultramicrosize (Fulvicin, Gris-PEG, Grisactin) usual adult dose 250-500mg bid with meals
◊ Fluconazole 50-100mg/d, overall better tolerated than ketoconazole; expensive; reserve for extreme cases (disseminated disease, immunocompromised)
◊ Itraconazole: 200mg po qd 3 months for fingernails and 6 months for toenails.
◊ New drugs: oral terbinafine, topical 5% amorolfine lacquer (Loceryl)
• Candidal onychomycosis
◊ Treat with preparation effective against both Candida and bacteria - imidazole derivatives
◊ If bacterial infection present, treat with antibacterial plus agent effective against Candida e.g., nystatin (Mycostatin), topical amphotericin B (Fungizone), itraconazole (Sporinox) 200mg po qd, or fluconazole 100mg po qd.
• Mold onychomycosis
◊ 1% iodinated alcohol, Whitfield's ointment, silver nitrate, glutaraldehyde, imidazole derivatives, itraconazole
Contraindications:
• Griseofulvin: porphyria, hepatocellular failure, serious side effects (leukopenia, persistent anemia), pregnancy
• Ketoconazole: prior sensitivity to drug, hepatocellular disease, pregnancy
• Fluconazole: hepatocellular failure, pregnancy
Precautions:
• Topical agents: use caution on broken skin, vascular compromise, decreased sensation
• Griseofulvin: monitor periodically for hepatic, renal, hematopoietic side effects; photo-sensitivity; lupus-like symptoms or exacerbation. Best taken with meals to enhance absorption.
• Ketoconazole: hepatotoxicity (may be severe or fatal), anaphylaxis may (rarely) occur with first dose, decreased testosterone levels
• Fluconazole: decrease dose in renal failure, hepatotoxicity
Significant possible interactions:
• Griseofulvin: warfarin, barbiturates, alcohol, oral contraceptives
• Ketoconazole: H2-blockers, antacids, warfarin, omeprazole, rifampin, cyclosporine, phenytoin, terfenadine
• Fluconazole: phenytoin (Dilantin), cyclosporine, oral hypoglycemics, oral anticoagulants, rifampin, hydrochlorothiazide

ALTERNATIVE DRUGS N/A

FOLLOWUP

PATIENT MONITORING
• Topical agents: slow response expected; visits can be every 6-12 weeks, after initial followup to assess compliance
• Griseofulvin: periodic monitoring of CBC and liver function tests initially and every 3 months

• Ketoconazole: liver function tests every 3 weeks for the first 3 months, then monthly
• Treatment duration: fingernails 6-9 months, toenails 9-12 months, great toe nail 12-24 months

PREVENTION/AVOIDANCE See Patient education

POSSIBLE COMPLICATIONS
Secondary infections with progression to cellulitis/osteomyelitis in compromised individuals

EXPECTED COURSE AND PROGNOSIS
• Relapse common; prognosis especially poor if one hand and 2 feet or multiple nails involved
• 20-40% of nails fail to respond
• 40-70% of patients show long term relapse

MISCELLANEOUS

ASSOCIATED CONDITIONS Consider underlying immunodeficiency or chronic metabolic disease in cases which present with rapid spread

AGE-RELATED FACTORS
Pediatric: Dermatophyte onychomycosis rare before puberty, candidal infection presents more commonly as superficial white onychomycosis, drug dosing based on body mass and approved drugs more limited
Geriatric: Mold onychomycosis more common, predisposing medical conditions more common and hepatic renal reserve may be more limited; decreased ability to do adequate topical self-treatment
Others: N/A

PREGNANCY Drug choices limited

SYNONYMS
• Tinea unguium
• Ringworm of the nail

ICD-9-CM 1101

SEE ALSO HIV infection

OTHER NOTES N/A

ABBREVIATIONS N/A

REFERENCES
• Pariser, D.M.: Superficial fungal infections. Postgraduate medicine. Vol 87 No 5, April 1990;205-214
• Baden, H.P.: Diseases of the Hair and Nails. Chicago, Year Book Medical Publishers, 1987

Author D. Phillips, M.D.

Optic atrophy

BASICS

DESCRIPTION End result of loss of ganglion cells or axons of the optic nerve
System(s) affected: Nervous
Genetics: Inherited forms may be autosomally recessive, autosomally dominant or X-linked recessive
Incidence/Prevalence in USA: Unknown
Predominant age:
• Inherited forms occur shortly after birth to the third decade
• Acquired forms tend to occur later
Predominant sex: Male > Female (inherited forms)

SIGNS AND SYMPTOMS
• Loss of visual acuity
• Pallor of the optic disk
• Loss of pupillary reactions
• Visual field defects

CAUSES
• Glaucoma
• Status post central retinal artery or vein occlusion
• Ischemic optic neuropathy
• Chronic optic neuritis
• Chronic papilledema
• Compression of the optic nerve or chiasm or tract by tumor or by aneurysm
• Trauma
• Syphilis
• Retinal degeneration (i.e., retinitis pigmentosa)
• Congenital optic atrophy
• Radiation neuropathy
• Drugs (amiodarone, chloroquine, ethambutol, oral contraceptives, streptomycin, vincristine)
• Thiamine deficiency

RISK FACTORS
Hereditary
◊ Family history
Acquired
◊ Diabetes mellitus
◊ Hypertension
◊ Radiation exposure
◊ Alcoholism
◊ Renal failure
◊ Arteriosclerosis

DIAGNOSIS

DIFFERENTIAL DIAGNOSIS
• Myopia
• S/p cataract extraction (no natural yellow color from the human lens)

LABORATORY
• CBC
• Antinuclear antibody (ANA)
• ESR
• Rapid plasma reagin (RPR)
• Fluorescent treponemal antibody absorption (FTA-ABS)
• Serological test for syphilis
• Heavy metal screen

SPECIAL TESTS Automated visual field test (i.e., Humphrey)
Drugs that may alter lab results: N/A
Disorders that may alter lab results: N/A

PATHOLOGICAL FINDINGS N/A

IMAGING CT or MRI of head

DIAGNOSTIC PROCEDURES
• Carotid Doppler (adult acquired optic atrophy)
• Complete ophthalmologic exam including dilated evaluation of retina

TREATMENT

APPROPRIATE HEALTH CARE
Outpatient

GENERAL MEASURES
• Treat underlying cause (rarely possible)
• Discontinue causative drug if possible
• If pressure against optic nerve is cause, neurosurgery to relieve it may help if done early

ACTIVITY Fully active

DIET No special diet

PATIENT EDUCATION
• Low vision counseling if bilateral
• Genetic counseling if inherited
• For patient education materials favorably reviewed on this topic, contact: National Eye Institute, Information Officer, Dept. of Health and Human Services, 9000 Rockville Pike, Bethesda, MD 20892, (301)496-5248

MEDICATIONS

DRUG(S) OF CHOICE None
Contraindications: N/A
Precautions: N/A
Significant possible interactions: N/A

ALTERNATIVE DRUGS N/A

 FOLLOWUP

PATIENT MONITORING Annual evaluations if stable

PREVENTION/AVOIDANCE N/A

POSSIBLE COMPLICATIONS N/A

EXPECTED COURSE AND PROGNOSIS
• Rarely possible to treat the underlying cause effectively
• Visual loss occurs over weeks to months
• Optic atrophy secondary to vascular, trauma, degenerative changes and some toxic causes has a very bad prognosis

 MISCELLANEOUS

ASSOCIATED CONDITIONS
Inherited neurodegenerative conditions
◊ Hereditary ataxia
◊ Charcot-Marie-Tooth disease
◊ Storage diseases
◊ Leukodystrophies

AGE-RELATED FACTORS
Pediatric: Optic atrophy in small children is difficult to recognize because disks normally have a pale appearance
Geriatric: None
Others: None

PREGNANCY None

SYNONYMS N/A

ICD-9-CM 377.10

SEE ALSO N/A

OTHER NOTES American Council of the Blind (800)424-8666

ABBREVIATIONS N/A

REFERENCES
• Miller, N.R.: Walsh and Hoyt's Clinical Neuro-Ophthalmology. 4th Ed. Baltimore, Williams & Wilkins, 1982
• Fraunfelder, F.T. & Roy, F.H.: Current Ocular Therapy. 3rd Ed. Philadelphia, W.B. Saunders Co., 1990

Author R. Noecker, M.D.

Optic neuritis

 BASICS

DESCRIPTION
Inflammation of the optic nerve

System(s) affected: Nervous
Genetics: N/A
Incidence/Prevalence in USA: N/A
Predominant age: Typically 18-50 years
Predominant sex: Female > Male

SIGNS AND SYMPTOMS
• Loss of vision, deteriorating from hours to days, usually reaching lowest level in one week
• Usually unilateral in adults, bilateral disease more common in children
• Tenderness of the globe, deep orbital pain or brow ache, especially with eye movement
• Central, cecocentral or arcuate visual field deficits
• Decreased color vision
• Apparent dimness of light intensities
• Impairment of depth perception
• Increase in visual symptoms with increased body temperature (Uhthoff's sign)
• May be either swollen optic disk (most commonly seen in children) or normal optic disc
• Relative afferent pupillary defect (Marcus Gunn's pupil)

CAUSES
• Idiopathic
• Multiple sclerosis
• Viral infections of childhood (measles, mumps, chickenpox)
• Other viral infections (mononucleosis, herpes zoster, encephalitis)
• Contiguous inflammation of the meninges, orbit, or sinuses
• Granulomatous inflammations (syphilis, tuberculosis, cryptococcus, sarcoidosis)
• Intraocular inflammations
• Lead toxicity
• Chronic high doses chloramphenicol

RISK FACTORS N/A

 DIAGNOSIS

DIFFERENTIAL DIAGNOSIS
• Acute papilledema
• Anterior ischemic optic neuropathy
• Severe systemic hypertension
• Toxic/nutritional optic neuropathy
• Orbital tumor compressing the optic nerve
• Intracranial tumor pressing on the afferent visual pathway
• Leber's congenital optic neuropathy

LABORATORY
• CBC
• Antinuclear antibody (ANA)
• ESR
• Rapid plasma reagin (RPR)
• Fluorescent treponemal antibody absorption (FTA-ABS)
• Serological test for syphilis
Drugs that may alter lab results: N/A
Disorders that may alter lab results: N/A

PATHOLOGICAL FINDINGS N/A

SPECIAL TESTS   Visual field test
(preferably automated Humphrey or Octopus)

IMAGING
• Chest x-ray
• MRI head or CT head/orbits in atypical cases or when patient is not improving after 10-14 days and other tests are negative

DIAGNOSTIC PROCEDURES
• Check blood pressure
• Complete ophthalmologic exam including pupillary assessment, color vision evaluation with color plates, dilated retinal examination with optic nerve assessment
• Neurologic work-up

 TREATMENT

APPROPRIATE HEALTH CARE
Outpatient observation

GENERAL MEASURES   No disease specific measures

ACTIVITY   Fully active

DIET   No special diet

PATIENT EDUCATION
• Reassurance about recovery of vision
• If felt to be secondary to demyelinating disease, patient should be informed of the risk of developing multiple sclerosis
• For patient education materials favorably reviewed on this topic, contact: National Eye Institute, Information Officer, Dept. of Health and Human Services, 9000 Rockville Pike, Bethesda, MD 20892, (301)496-5248

MEDICATIONS

DRUG(S) OF CHOICE None
Contraindications: N/A
Precautions: N/A
Significant possible interactions: N/A

ALTERNATIVE DRUGS
• Prednisone (controversial) 1 mg/kg/day po for 2 weeks, then taper over 1-2 weeks
• Pulse steroids - methylprednisolone 250 mg IV q 6 hours x 12 doses in the hospital followed by prednisone 1 mg/kg/day po for 11 days, taper over 1-2 weeks
• Anti-ulcer medication is given with steroids

FOLLOWUP

PATIENT MONITORING Monthly followup to monitor visual changes

PREVENTION/AVOIDANCE N/A

POSSIBLE COMPLICATIONS
Permanent loss of vision

EXPECTED COURSE AND PROGNOSIS
• Visual acuity begins to improve 2-3 weeks after onset
• Improvement continues over several months and vision often returns to normal or near normal levels

MISCELLANEOUS

ASSOCIATED CONDITIONS Over 50% of adult optic neuritis patients will develop multiple sclerosis

AGE-RELATED FACTORS
Pediatric: N/A
Geriatric: N/A
Others: N/A

PREGNANCY N/A

SYNONYMS
• Papillitis
• Retrobulbar neuritis

ICD-9-CM 377.30

SEE ALSO Multiple sclerosis

OTHER NOTES N/A

ABBREVIATIONS N/A

REFERENCES
• Sergott, R. & Brown, M.: Current concepts of the pathogenesis of optic neuritis associated with multiple sclerosis. Surv Ophthalmol. 1988;33:108-116
• Miller, N.: Walsh and Hoyt's Clinical Neuro-Ophthalmology. 4th Ed. Baltimore, Williams & Wilkins, 1982
• Fraunfelder, F.T. & Roy, F.H.: Current Ocular Therapy. 3rd Ed. Philadelphia, W.B. Saunders Co., 1990

Author R. Noecker, M.D.

Oral cavity neoplasms

 BASICS

DESCRIPTION Malignant tumors affecting the lip, tongue, floor of the mouth, salivary glands, inside of cheeks, gums, and palate. 90% of the neoplasms are squamous cell carcinomas and the remainder are lymphomas, melanomas, adenocarcinomas from minor salivary gland origin and sarcomas.
System(s) affected: Gastrointestinal
Genetics: N/A
Incidence in USA:
• 12/100,000 (30,300 new cases a year). 5000 persons die of this disease annually.
• Oral cavity neoplasms account for 4% of all cancers occurring in men and 2% in women
• High incidence in Asia, related to the habit of chewing betelnut, fresh betel leaf, and habitual reverse smoking in which the lighted end of the cigarette is held within the oral cavity
Prevalence in USA: Unknown
Predominant sex: Male > Female
Predominant age: 50 and over. However, increasingly being seen in younger age group with the use of smokeless tobacco.

SIGNS AND SYMPTOMS
• Dysphagia
• Odynophagia
• Problems articulating
• Regurgitation of liquids secondary to nasopharyngeal incompetence from the tumor
• Ipsilateral otalgia from referred pain
• Friable granular exophytic and/or infiltrative mass or ulcer which frequently is tender and confused for infection. Usually has hard indurated margins by palpation which extend beyond the confines of the ulcer itself.
• Hard neck mass suggesting metastatic disease in the nodal chain along the internal jugular vein

CAUSES
• Tobacco use (smokeless or smoked)
• Use of snuff (common in the Southwestern United States)
• Excess alcohol consumption
• Exposure to ultra violet light in the instances of lip carcinoma
• Riboflavin or iron deficiency anemia, and Plummer-Vinson syndrome associated with oral cancers

RISK FACTORS   See Causes

 DIAGNOSIS

DIFFERENTIAL DIAGNOSIS
• Exudative tonsillitis (usually bilateral involvement)
• Stomatitis or glossitis secondary to infectious etiology, most commonly candidiasis
• Benign tumors of the oral cavity (slow growing and usually not erosive or ulcerative)
• Kaposi's sarcoma
• Mycosis fungoides
• Premalignant lesions such as leukoplakia or erythroplasia
• Lichen planus

LABORATORY   Liver function test to rule out metastasis to the liver
Drugs that may alter lab results: N/A
Disorders that may alter lab results:
• Alcoholism
• Hepatitis

PATHOLOGICAL FINDINGS   Malignant changes characteristic of cell types

SPECIAL TESTS   N/A

IMAGING
• Chest x-ray to rule out metastasis to the lungs
• Imaging bone scans if there is pain in the bones suggesting bone metastasis
• CT or MRI scan if clinical suggestion of intracranial or liver metastasis

DIAGNOSTIC PROCEDURES   Transoral biopsy as an outpatient makes the definitive diagnosis

 TREATMENT

APPROPRIATE HEALTH CARE
• Inpatient for surgery
• The treatment varies depending on location, i.e., tongue, buccal wall, pharynx, palate, lip

GENERAL MEASURES
• Wide resection with or without radiation therapy and/or chemotherapy is the treatment of choice
• Unresectable lesions usually are treated with radiation therapy and/or chemotherapy for palliation
• Nutrition is of prime importance for normal wound healing should patient require surgery. Patients may necessitate naso-gastric and/or gastrostomy feedings if orally disabled.
• Tracheotomy may be necessary if the patient has problems handling secretions or difficulty breathing

ACTIVITY   As tolerated by patient's nutritional and physical status

DIET
• Depends on the extent of disease and whether the patient is able to chew or swallow
• Usually early lesions can be managed with a regular diet. As disease progresses, a soft diet is necessary.

PATIENT EDUCATION   Literature is available from American Cancer Society

MEDICATIONS

DRUG(S) OF CHOICE Narcotics for pain relief
Contraindications: N/A
Precautions: N/A
Significant possible interactions: N/A

ALTERNATIVE DRUGS N/A

FOLLOWUP

PATIENT MONITORING Routine periodic head and neck exams to detect possible second primary or recurrence in the upper aerodigestive tract

PREVENTION/AVOIDANCE
• Avoidance of smoking or the use of smokeless tobacco
• Avoid alcohol use

POSSIBLE COMPLICATIONS
• Functional and/or cosmetic disabilities proportional to the degree of surgery and stage of tumor
• Stomatitis with or without candidiasis secondary to radiation therapy or chemotherapy
• Persistent dysphagia secondary to surgery or radiation therapy
• Persistent problems with articulation or deglutition depending on the amount of tongue resection

EXPECTED COURSE AND PROGNOSIS
Early lesions with adequate treatment leads to a greater than 80% cure

MISCELLANEOUS

ASSOCIATED CONDITIONS Leukoplakia or erythroplasia should be biopsied, since they are considered premalignant and associated with carcinoma at least 10% of the time

AGE-RELATED FACTORS None
Pediatric: N/A
Geriatric: Greater incidence after 50
Others: N/A

PREGNANCY N/A

SYNONYMS N/A

ICD-9-CM
• 145.9 Malignant neoplasm of mouth, unspecified
• 198.89 Secondary malignant neoplasm, other specified sites, other
• 230.0 Carcinoma in situ lip, oral cavity and pharynx
• 210.4 Benign neoplasm other and unspecified parts of mouth
• 235.1 Neoplasm of uncertain behavior of lip, oral cavity and pharynx

SEE ALSO N/A

OTHER NOTES N/A

ABBREVIATIONS N/A

REFERENCES Cummings, C.W., Fredrickson, J.M., Harker, L.A., Crause, C.J., & Schuller, D.E.: Otolaryngology: Head and Neck Surgery. Volume 2. New York, C.V. Mosby Company, 1986

Author R. Casiano, M.D.

Oral rehydration

BASICS

DESCRIPTION
• Dehydration and ongoing fluid losses from infectious gastroenteritis (GE) can be effectively treated with oral rehydration solutions (ORS), except in the most severe cases where initial parenteral fluid resuscitation is required. This therapy takes advantage of the coupled transport of sodium and glucose in the small intestine even during cases of GE. Water follows osmotically after sodium entry. Potassium is passively absorbed via solvent drag. A glucose concentration of 2% allows maximal sodium absorption.
• ORS for rehydration and the ORS to be used when ongoing losses from GE have a high sodium content (e.g., cholera) generally contain 75-90 meq/L of sodium. Maintenance ORS with sodium content of 40-50 meq/L are useful for mild dehydration and treatment of ongoing losses with a lower sodium content (e.g., rotavirus).

System(s) affected: Gastrointestinal, Endocrine/Metabolic

Genetics: N/A

Incidence/Prevalence in USA: N/A

Predominant age: Primarily aimed at infants and children but effective for all ages

Predominant sex: Male = Female

SIGNS AND SYMPTOMS N/A

CAUSES N/A

RISK FACTORS N/A

DIAGNOSIS

DIFFERENTIAL DIAGNOSIS N/A

LABORATORY N/A

SPECIAL TESTS N/A
Drugs that may alter lab results: N/A
Disorders that may alter lab results: N/A

PATHOLOGICAL FINDINGS N/A

IMAGING N/A

DIAGNOSTIC PROCEDURES N/A

TREATMENT

APPROPRIATE HEALTH CARE
Primarily outpatient. Designed to be administered by family members.

GENERAL MEASURES
• Sufficient ORS to replace the fluid deficit and any ongoing losses should be offered in the first 4-12 hours. Estimate replacement at 60 cc/μg for mild and 80 cc/μg for moderate dehydration.
• If the patient has hypertonic dehydration, oral rehydration should be planned for 12-24 hours
• If vomiting occurs, small amounts of ORS given frequently is usually effective
• Replace ongoing stool losses with ORS. Estimate 5-10 cc/μg per stool.
• Traditional clear fluids are inappropriate for oral rehydration therapy
• ORS is not to be diluted
• Maintenance oral rehydration therapy begins when the deficit is replaced and provides for ongoing losses. Maintenance ORS or a combination of ORS and water or other clear liquids can be used.

ACTIVITY As tolerated

DIET
• For breast feeding infants - mother should continue nursing
• For bottle fed babies - early institution of lactose-free formulas. Delay using milk-based formula for several days.
• For older infants, children and adults - easily digestible, carbohydrate rich, low lactose foods should be offered as soon as the dehydration deficit is replaced. Cow's milk can be added to diet after several days.

PATIENT EDUCATION
• Awareness and availability of ORS markedly diminishes morbidity from gastroenteritis
• Travelers concerned with severe diarrhea should carry ORS packets on trips

MEDICATIONS

DRUG(S) OF CHOICE
The prototype ORS is the World Health Organization solution
WHO ORS:
 ◊ 1 liter of clean water
 ◊ 1/2 tsp sodium chloride (salt)
 ◊ 1/2 tsp trisodium citrate
 ◊ 1/4 tsp potassium chloride (salt substitute)
 ◊ 2 tbsp glucose (table sugar)
Note:
 ◊ Glucose can be replaced by either sucrose or rice powder which are less expensive.
 ◊ Trisodium citrate can be replaced by sodium bicarbonate (baking soda). (Sodium bicarbonate was used in previous formulation).
 ◊ In developed countries, when GE is unlikely to be caused by cholera, a lower sodium solution such as Rehydralyte is advisable.
Comparison of ORS's

Solution	Type†	Sodium Meq/L
WHO ORS	R	90
Rehydralyte	R	75
Ricelyte	M	50
Pedialyte	M	45

† R=rehydration
  M=maintenance

Solution	Storage form
WHO ORS	Powder
Rehydralyte	Liquid
Ricelyte	Liquid
Pedialyte	Liquid

Contraindications:
• Conditions predisposing to risk of aspiration: Altered consciousness, seizure activity, severe hypotension, shock
• Persistent vomiting (as in pyloric stenosis)
• Absent bowel sounds
Precautions:
• The ingredients should be provided in pre-mixed packets in order to avoid iatrogenic errors in mixing
• If water safety is questionable, it should be boiled or treated for purification
• Discard the solution after 12 hours if held at room temperature, or 24 hours if refrigerated
• After rehydration is complete, ORS's should not be used as the only fluid intake because the high sodium content may lead to hypernatremia
Significant possible interactions: N/A

ALTERNATIVE DRUGS   N/A

FOLLOWUP

PATIENT MONITORING   The patient needs to be frequently evaluated to ensure establishment of an improving clinical status and an adequate urine output

PREVENTION/AVOIDANCE   N/A

POSSIBLE COMPLICATIONS   If in increasing weight loss (fluid deficit), clinical deterioration, or intractable vomiting, switch to IV hydration.

EXPECTED COURSE AND PROGNOSIS
• Rapid clinical improvement despite continuing diarrhea is the usual course
• The overall complication rate for oral rehydration is the same as that for parenteral rehydration in cases of mild and moderate dehydration.

MISCELLANEOUS

ASSOCIATED CONDITIONS   N/A

AGE-RELATED FACTORS   N/A
Pediatric: See Diet
Geriatric: N/A
Others: N/A

PREGNANCY   N/A

SYNONYMS   N/A

ICD-9-CM   N/A

SEE ALSO   Dehydration

OTHER NOTES   Advantages of oral rehydration include a much lower cost, minimal storage requirements (for powder forms) and no need for sterile conditions

ABBREVIATIONS
• GE = gastroenteritis
• ORS = oral rehydration solutions

REFERENCES
• Primack, W.A.: Parenteral fluid therapy in infants and children. In Conn's Current Therapy. Edited by R. A. Rakel. Philadelphia, W.B. Saunders Co., 1991
• The management of acute diarrhea in children: Oral rehydration, maintenance and nutritional therapy. MMWR 41:RR16:10/16/92
• Goepp, J. & Santosham, M.: Oral rehydration therapy. In Principles and Practice of Pediatrics. Edited by F. Oski. Philadelphia, J.B. Lippincott, 1992

Author   W. Primack, M.D. & C. Jacobs, M.D.

Osgood-Schlatter disease

BASICS

DESCRIPTION The syndrome associated with traction apophysitis in adolescent boys and girls consisting of pain of the tibial tubercle with swelling
System(s) affected: Musculoskeletal
Genetics: Unknown
Incidence in USA: Not known, but common
Prevalence in USA: Not known, but common (13% of atheletes in one Finnish study)
Predominant age:
• Females 10-16
• Males 11-18
Predominant sex: Male > Female

SIGNS AND SYMPTOMS
• Unilateral or bilateral (30%) tibial tuberosity pain
• Pain exacerbated by exercise
• Tibial tuberosity swelling
• Pain increased with knee extension against resistance or kneeling
• Knee pain with squatting or crouching
• Absence of effusion or condyle tenderness
• Erythema of tibial tuberosity

CAUSES Basic etiology unknown, but clearly exacerbated by exercise - jumping and pivoting sports are the worst

RISK FACTORS
• Age between 11 and 18
• Male sex
• Rapid skeletal growth
• Involvement in repetitive jumping sports

DIAGNOSIS

DIFFERENTIAL DIAGNOSIS
• Stress fracture of the proximal tibia
• Pes anserinus bursitis
• Quadriceps tendon avulsion
• Patellofemoral stress syndrome
• Villonodular synovitis
• Chondromalacia patellae
• Proximal tibial neoplasm
• Osteomyelitis of the proximal tibia
• Tibial plateau fracture
• Patellar tendon rupture

LABORATORY No blood tests indicated unless other diagnostic considerations are entertained
Drugs that may alter lab results: N/A
Disorders that may alter lab results: N/A

PATHOLOGICAL FINDINGS
• Osteochondritis of the tibial tubercle
• Heterotopic bone formation of the patellar tendon
• Bony fusion of the tibial metaphysis
• Inflammatory infiltrate of the epiphysis in severe cases
• Complete avulsion of the tibial tubercle with nonunion of the tubercle with the tibia

SPECIAL TESTS N/A

IMAGING
• X-ray imaging of the proximal tibia and knee may show heterotopic calcification in the patellar tendon
• Calcific thickening of the tibial tuberosity with irregular ossification in the tibial tuberosity
• Bone scan may show increased uptake in the area of the tibial tuberosity

DIAGNOSTIC PROCEDURES N/A

TREATMENT

APPROPRIATE HEALTH CARE
Outpatient

GENERAL MEASURES
• Frequent ice applications (20 minutes every two hours)
• Rest
• Knee immobilization in extension
• In more severe cases, avoidance of activities that increase pain or swelling
• Quadriceps isometric strengthening, hip extensions, adductor strengthening, hamstring and quadriceps stretching exercises
• Intercurrent upper body strengthening may continue unhindered
• Cushioned knee pad
• A cylinder walking cast for severe symptoms, unless symptoms are bilateral
• Surgical treatment for fixation of an avulsed tibial tuberosity
• Débridement of a thickened cosmetically unsatisfactory tibial tubercle

ACTIVITY Activity to be restricted to those activities not causing pain

DIET N/A

PATIENT EDUCATION Stress avoidance of jumping sports. Assure family that symptoms and findings will diminish with time and rest.

MEDICATIONS

DRUG(S) OF CHOICE None in particular, but all analgesics may be considered. NSAID's are of minimal benefit.
Contraindications: N/A
Precautions: N/A
Significant possible interactions: N/A

ALTERNATIVE DRUGS More potent analgesics such as narcotics may be considered for short term use or in extreme situations

FOLLOWUP

PATIENT MONITORING Follow up on a prn basis for management of pain and disability

PREVENTION/AVOIDANCE
• Avoidance of those sports involving heavy quadriceps loading
• Patients may compete if the pain is minimal
• Increase hamstring and quadriceps flexibility

POSSIBLE COMPLICATIONS
• Nonunion of the tubercle to the tibia
• Upriding of the patella
• Patellar tendon avulsion
• Genu recurvatum
• Patellofemoral degenerative arthritis
• Subluxation of the patella
• Patella alta
• Chondromalacia

EXPECTED COURSE AND PROGNOSIS
Except in rare complicated cases, this is a self-limiting illness resolved within two years after full skeletal maturation

MISCELLANEOUS

ASSOCIATED CONDITIONS N/A

AGE-RELATED FACTORS
Pediatric: In skeletally mature boys and girls, with boys more frequent than girls
Geriatric: N/A
Others: Participants in sports involving heavy quadriceps activity

PREGNANCY N/A

SYNONYMS Osteochondritis of the tibial tubercle

ICD-9-CM 732.4

SEE ALSO Tendinitis

OTHER NOTES N/A

ABBREVIATIONS N/A

REFERENCES
• Kujala, U.M., Koist, M. & Heiwomen, O.: Osgood-Schlatter's disease in adolescent athletes. Retrospective Study of Incidence and Duration. Am J Sports Med. 13:236-241, 1985
• Micheli, L.J.: The Traction Apophysitises, Clinics in Sports Medicine. 6:389, 1987

Author D. Sealy, M.D.

Osteitis deformans

BASICS

DESCRIPTION Inflammatory focal (sometimes generalized) condition of the skeleton characterized by rapid, chaotic bone resorption followed by equally chaotic and excessive bone formation. Leads to enlarged but weakened and highly vascularized bone which is painful, easily deformed and subject to fractures with minimal trauma. Cranial and vertebral involvement can also cause neurologic deficits.

System(s) affected: Musculoskeletal

Genetics: 15-50% of patients have one or more involved first order relatives with osteitis deformans

Incidence/Prevalence in USA: 3% of Caucasian individuals above age 50 have at least one focus. Rare in African Americans and Asians.

Predominant age: Above age 50, occasional cases ages 20-50

Predominant sex: Male = Female

SIGNS AND SYMPTOMS
- Asymptomatic frequently
- Bone pain
- Skeletal deformities
- Bowing of extremities
- Acetabular protrusion
- Headaches
- Head enlargement
- Frequent fractures
- Secondary osteoarthritis
- Vertebral compression
- Neurologic deficits
- High output congestive heart failure (rare)
- Hypercalcemia (rare)
- Renal calculi (calcium, uric acid)
- Angioid streaks (rare)
- Mottled retinal degeneration (rare)
- Increased skin temperature over affected areas
- Bone sarcomas (rare)
- Peripheral neuropathies
- Carpal/tarsal tunnel syndromes
- Valvular/endocardial calcification
- Accelerated atherosclerosis
- Gouty diathesis
- Hyperparathyroidism
- Sensorineural hearing loss
- Conductive hearing loss

CAUSES Unknown; best evidence to date is for slow virus infection

RISK FACTORS None known

DIAGNOSIS

DIFFERENTIAL DIAGNOSIS
- Polyostotic fibrous dysplasia
- Osteitis fibrosis cystica (skeletal hyperparathyroidism)
- Primary bone neoplasms
- Osteolytic, osteoblastic metastases

LABORATORY
- Serum calcium - usually normal, occasionally increased
- Serum alkaline phosphatase - usually increased
- Serum GGT - normal
- Serum osteocalcin (BGP) - usually increased
- Urine total hydroxyproline - usually increased

Drugs that may alter lab results:
- Vitamin D and its metabolites
- Hepatotoxic drugs

Disorders that may alter lab results:
- See Differential diagnosis
- Osteomalacia
- Liver disorders
- Traumatic fractures

PATHOLOGICAL FINDINGS
- Chaotic bone resorption at advancing edge of disease. Osteoclasts are large, contain 10-100 nuclei and have abnormal configuration.
- Electrophotomicroscopically, the nuclei and cytoplasm contain myriad inclusion bodies resembling viral nucleocapsids
- Later, excessive osteoblastic bone formation predominates with sclerotic bone containing cement lines forming mosaic pattern

SPECIAL TESTS
- Neurologic examination
- Audiogram, if skull involvement
- Visual field study, if skull involvement

IMAGING
- X-rays show irregular pattern of alternating bone formation and resorption in enlarged deformed bones. Resorptive fronts at advancing edge.
- Bone scans show intense uptake in focal pattern
- CT/MRI show extra-bony extension if sarcomatous degeneration occurs

DIAGNOSTIC PROCEDURES Bone biopsy needed only in confusing cases (rare)

TREATMENT

APPROPRIATE HEALTH CARE
Outpatient, except when intravenous treatment is used

GENERAL MEASURES
- Rarely, splints for severely resorbed areas causing high risk of fracture
- Hearing aids for severe deafness; of some (but not great) value in sensorineural deafness

ACTIVITY
- Full activity to maintain function
- Avoid excessive mechanical stress on involved bones

DIET No special diet

PATIENT EDUCATION Paget's Disease Foundation, 200 Varick St., Suite 1004, New York, NY 10014-4810, (718)596-1043

MEDICATIONS

DRUG(S) OF CHOICE
• Synthetic salmon calcitonin (Calcimar, Miacalcin), 50 IU three times weekly to 100 IU qd, courses 1.5 to 3 years
or
• Synthetic human calcitonin (Cibacalcin), 0.5 mg, three times a week or up to once a day, courses 1.5 to 3 years
or
• Etidronate disodium (Didronel), 5 mg/kg/day (approximately 400 mg) x 6 mos. Rarely, 20 mg/kg/day x 1 month. Courses may be repeated after a 3-6 month rest period
or
• Pamidronate disodium (Aredia) 60 mg/day by 4-6 hour infusions times 3 days. Alternately, 30 mg/day by 4-6 hour infusions once a week for 6 weeks. May be repeated several months later when effect wears off.
or
• Plicamycin (Mithracin), 25 mcg/kg/day or qod by 4-6 hr infusions x 9-10 infusions
• Add nonsteroidal anti-inflammatories (NSAID's) to above drugs for secondary osteoarthritis

Contraindications:
• Prior history of allergy or hypersensitivity
• For plicamycin, manifest hepatic or renal impairment or bone marrow depression

Precautions:
• Adverse side effects may require ameliorative measures or temporary dose reduction
• Salmon and human calcitonin - nausea, vomiting, anorexia, flushing, rash, including urticaria (rare)
• Etidronate disodium - nausea, vomiting, diarrhea, increased bone pain
• Pamidronate disodium - transient fever, leukopenia, hypocalcemia, headache, malaise, loss of appetite
• Plicamycin - vomiting, anorexia, malaise, abnormal liver/renal function, thrombocytopenia with bleeding

Significant possible Interactions: None

ALTERNATIVE DRUGS
NSAID's for mildly symptomatic disease in nonstrategic areas

FOLLOWUP

PATIENT MONITORING
• Followup visits every 2 months during drug therapy; yearly if drugs not being used. Alkaline phosphatase before each visit.
• Repeat x-rays and bone scan every 3-5 years

PREVENTION/AVOIDANCE
Avoid excessive mechanical stress on afflicted bones to reduce chance of fractures and other complications

POSSIBLE COMPLICATIONS
Fractures, severe deformities, head enlargement, acetabular protrusion, carpal/tarsal tunnel syndromes, neurologic deficits, deafness, visual impairment, congestive heart failure (high output), renal calculi, sarcomatous degeneration

EXPECTED COURSE AND PROGNOSIS
• Depends on severity
• Slow progression if untreated
• Significant amelioration with treatment (85%)
• Poor prognosis if bone sarcoma develops

MISCELLANEOUS

ASSOCIATED CONDITIONS
Hyperparathyroidism, gouty diathesis, secondary osteoarthritis, angioid streaks, mottled retinal degeneration, bone sarcoma (rare)

AGE-RELATED FACTORS
Pediatric: N/A
Geriatric: Common
Others: More prevalent if ancestry Caucasian, especially United Kingdom, Northern Europe (excluding Scandinavia), Italy, Australia and New Zealand. Rare in African Americans and Asians.

PREGNANCY N/A

SYNONYMS Paget's disease of bone

ICD-9-CM 731.0

SEE ALSO N/A

OTHER NOTES N/A

ABBREVIATIONS N/A

REFERENCES
• Singer, F.R. & Wallach, S. (eds.): Paget's Disease of Bone. Clinical Assessment, Present and Future Therapy. New York, Elsevier, 1991
• Calkins, E., Ford, A.B., & Katz, P.R. (eds.): The Practice of Geriatrics. 2nd Ed. Philadelphia, W.B. Saunders Co., 1992
• Rakel, R.E. (ed.): Paget's Disease of Bone. In Conn's Current Therapy. Philadelphia, W.B. Saunders, 1990
• Bone, H.G. & Kleerekoper, M.: Paget's Disease of Bone. J Clin Endocrinol Metab. 75:1179-1182, 1992

Author S. Wallach, M.D.

Osteoarthritis

BASICS

DESCRIPTION Osteoarthritis (OA) is the most common form of joint disease. Involves progressive loss of articular cartilage and reactive changes at joint margins and in subchondral bone.
<u>Primary</u>
◊ Idiopathic
◊ Divided into subsets depending on clinical features
<u>Secondary</u>
◊ Childhood anatomic abnormalities (e.g., congenital hip dysplasia, slipped femoral epiphyses)
◊ Inheritable metabolic disorders (e.g., alkaptonuria, Wilson's disease, hemochromatosis)
◊ Neuropathic arthropathy (Charcot's joints)
◊ Hemophiliac arthropathy
◊ Acromegalic arthropathy
◊ Paget's disease
◊ Rheumatoid arthritis
◊ Gout, calcium pyrophosphate deposition disease (pseudogout)
◊ Septic or tuberculous arthritis
◊ Spondyloarthropathies
◊ Post-traumatic
System(s) affected: Musculoskeletal
Genetics: Unknown
Incidence in USA: Unknown
Prevalence in USA:
• Estimates of radiographic evidence of OA - range from 33% to almost 90% in those people over the age of 65
• Approximately 60 million patients at any one time
Predominant age:
• Over age 40 (for symptomatic disease)
• Leading cause of disability in those over age 65
Predominant sex: Male = Female

SIGNS AND SYMPTOMS
• Slowly developing joint pain
• Pain that follows use of a joint
• Stiffness (especially morning and after sitting) of less than 15 minutes duration
• Joint enlargement (e.g., Heberden's nodes of distal interphalangeal joints)
• Decreased range of motion
• Tenderness usually absent; may be associated with synovitis, with tenderness along joint margin
• Crepitation as late sign
• Local pain and stiffness with osteoarthritis of spine, with radicular pain (if there is compression of nerve roots)

CAUSES Biomechanical, biochemical, inflammatory, and immunological factors are all implicated in pathogenesis of osteoarthritis

RISK FACTORS
• Age over 50
• Obesity (weight bearing joints)
• Prolonged occupational or sports stress
• Injury to a joint

DIAGNOSIS

DIFFERENTIAL DIAGNOSIS
• Distinguish from other types of arthritis by absent systemic findings, minimal articular inflammation, and distribution of involved joints (e.g., distal and proximal interphalangeal joints, not wrist and metacarpophalangeal joints)
• In spine, distinguish from osteoporosis, metastatic disease, multiple myeloma, other bone disease

LABORATORY Not helpful (sedimentation rate not increased)
Drugs that may alter lab results: N/A
Disorders that may alter lab results: N/A

PATHOLOGICAL FINDINGS
• Synovial fluid may have a slightly increased white blood cell count, especially mononuclear
• Calcium pyrophosphate dihydrate and/or apatite crystals may occasionally be seen in effusions and require polarized light microscopy or special techniques to see
• Subchondral bone trabecular microfractures
• Degradation response produced by release of proteolytic enzymes, collagenolytic enzymes, prostaglandins, and immune responses

SPECIAL TESTS N/A

IMAGING X-rays usually normal early; later often show narrowed joint space, osteophyte formation, subchondral bony sclerosis, and cyst formation. Erosions may occur on surface of distal interphalangeal (DIP) and proximal interphalangeal (PIP) joints when OA is associated with inflammation (erosive osteoarthritis).

DIAGNOSTIC PROCEDURES
<u>Joint aspiration</u>
◊ May be helpful to distinguish between OA and chronic inflammatory arthritides
◊ OA - cell count usually < 500 cells/m3, predominantly mononuclear
◊ Inflammatory - cell count usually > 2000 cells/m3, predominantly neutrophils

TREATMENT

APPROPRIATE HEALTH CARE
Outpatient

GENERAL MEASURES
• Reassurance of absence of generalized systemic disease, with recognition of potential disability from osteoarthritis
• Weight reduction if obese
• Heat (local, tub baths, etc.)
• Physical therapy to maintain or regain joint motion and muscle strength
• Protect joints from overuse (e.g., cane, crutches, walker, neck collar, elastic knee support)
• Surgery may be indicated in advanced disease (e.g., fusion, joint replacement)

ACTIVITY As active as tolerated

DIET No special diet

PATIENT EDUCATION Information concerning patient education materials is available from the AAFP/F Herb H. Huffington Memorial Library at (800)274-2237, (ext 4400). P.O. Box 8418; Kansas City, MO 64114

MEDICATIONS

DRUG(S) OF CHOICE Aspirin or other NSAID's for both analgesic and anti-inflammatory use. Acetaminophen (Tylenol) is also effective and doesn't have side effects of ASA and other NSAID's. For maintenance, tailor dosage to maximum benefit within range of tolerance of side effects.

Contraindications: NSAID's - relative contraindication if there is renal disease or cardiac disease, especially congestive failure and hypertension. See manufacturer's profile of each drug.

Precautions:
• NSAID's contraindicated if previous hypersensitivity reaction to any NSAID's, active peptic ulcer disease, nasal polyps, asthma
• Oral or parenteral adrenal corticosteroids are contraindicated
• No more than 3-4/year intra-articular corticosteroid injections up to a maximal total of 12 injections per joint
• For aspirin and other NSAID's - asthma, hemophilia, intrinsic coagulation defects, history of peptic ulcer, cardiac decompensation, hypertension, renal dysfunction
• Intra-articular corticosteroid injections, if excessive, can accelerate joint deterioration

Significant possible interactions:
• NSAID's reduce effectiveness of ACE inhibitors
• Aspirin and NSAID's may increase effects of anticoagulants
• Increased hypoglycemic effects of oral hypoglycemics with aspirin
• Avoid concomitant use of aspirin with NSAID's
• Salicylates reduce effectiveness of spironolactone (Aldactone) and uricosurics
• Corticosteroids and some antacids increase salicylate excretion, while ascorbic acid and ammonium chloride reduce salicylate excretion and may cause toxicity

ALTERNATIVE DRUGS
• Tailor drug to patient, and switch if tolerance develops
• Judicious use of intra-articular injections of corticosteroids for selected acute flare-ups of joints
• Non-acetylate salicylates - salsalates (magnesium choline salicylates) provide anti-inflammatory action without significant antiplatelet effects, also have less GI toxicity

FOLLOWUP

PATIENT MONITORING
• Follow range of motion and functional status at regular intervals
• Watch for GI blood loss and follow cardiac, renal and mental status in older patients on NSAID's or ASA
• Periodic CBC, renal function tests, stool for occult blood

PREVENTION/AVOIDANCE Followup of secondary causes

POSSIBLE COMPLICATIONS
• Decompensated CHF, GI bleeding, decreased renal function on NSAID's or ASA
• Hypoglycemic reactions in diabetic patients taking aspirin (rare)
• Infection or accelerated cartilage loss with intra-articular corticosteroids

EXPECTED COURSE AND PROGNOSIS
• Tends to be progressive
• Early in course, pain relieved by rest; later, pain may occur at rest
• Joint effusions may occur, especially in knees
• Joint enlargement occurs later in course due to bony enlargement
• Osteophyte spur formation, especially at joint margins, as disease progresses
• Advanced stage with full thickness loss of cartilage down to bone

MISCELLANEOUS

ASSOCIATED CONDITIONS N/A

AGE-RELATED FACTORS
Pediatric: N/A
Geriatric:
• Prevalence increases with age
• Almost universal over 65 (by x-ray but not clinically)
Others: N/A

PREGNANCY ASA and NSAID's with some risk to fetus during pregnancy; compatible with breast feeding

SYNONYMS
• Osteoarthrosis
• Degenerative joint disease

ICD-9-CM 715.9 Osteoarthritis, unspecified whether generalized or localized

SEE ALSO N/A

OTHER NOTES Surgery may be indicated in advanced disease (for example joint replacement, fusion)

ABBREVIATIONS N/A

REFERENCES
• Kelly, H.E., Ruddy, S. & Sledge, C.B. (eds.): Textbook of Rheumatology. 4th Ed. Philadelphia, W.B. Saunders Co., 1993
• Schroeder, S.A., Krapp, M.A., Tierney, L.M. & McPhee, S.I.: Current Medical Diagnosis and Treatment. Norwalk, CT, Appleton and Lange, 1991, 593-594
• Johnson, G.E.: Essentials of Drug Therapy. Philadelphia, W.B. Saunders Co., 1991
• Ellsworth, A.J., Bray, R.F., Bray, B.S. & Geyman, J.P.: The Family Practice Drug Handbook. Chicago, Mosby-Year Book, 1991, 180, 186-187

Author J. Geyman, M.D. & B. Gilliland, M.D.

Osteomalacia and rickets

BASICS

DESCRIPTION Osteomalacia (referred to as rickets in children) is defined as an excess organic bone matrix secondary to defective or inadequate bone mineralization
System(s) affected: Musculoskeletal
Genetics: N/A
Incidence/Prevalence in USA: N/A
Predominant age: All ages. In adults, osteomalacia is usually a disease of the older population (50-80).
Predominant sex: Female > Male (slightly)

SIGNS AND SYMPTOMS
• Bone pain, tenderness, muscle weakness
• Bone pain is dull and tends to be poorly localized, usually affecting the ribs and upper thighs
• Muscle weakness is usually proximal
• Other symptoms of malnutrition or an underlying problem such as chronic renal disease may also be clinically evident
• Weight loss
• Anorexia
• Tetany
• In young children - restlessness, poor sleep patterns, craniotabes, costochondral beading, bowlegs, kyphoscoliosis

CAUSES
• Can be caused by a wide variety of pathogenic processes, including, but not limited to, vitamin D deficiency (reduced exposure to sunlight, poor nutrition, malabsorption syndromes)
• Defective metabolism of parent vitamin D to active metabolites (drug-induced, i.e., anticonvulsants—Dilantin, chronic renal failure), hypophosphatemia (renal tubular acidosis, hypophosphatemic syndrome), miscellaneous (long-term hemodialysis, malnutrition, vitamin D-dependent rickets)

RISK FACTORS
• Poverty
• Inadequate nutrition and sunlight exposure

DIAGNOSIS

DIFFERENTIAL DIAGNOSIS
• Osteoporosis
• Metastatic bone disease
• Primary bone malignancies (lymphoma, myeloma)

LABORATORY
• Alkaline phosphatase - increased
• Serum calcium is low or normal (never high)
• Hypophosphatemia
• Aminoaciduria
• Acidosis
• Glucosuria
• Hypouricemia
Drugs that may alter lab results: N/A
Disorders that may alter lab results: N/A

PATHOLOGICAL FINDINGS
• Defective calcification of growing bone
• Hypertrophy of epiphyseal cartilages

SPECIAL TESTS N/A

IMAGING Radiographic changes are non-specific. Earliest manifestations are thinning of cortical bone. In long-term osteomalacia - bone softening (protrusio acetabuli), looser lines, stress fractures, and pathologic fractures.

DIAGNOSTIC PROCEDURES Bone biopsy and subsequent histopathologic evaluation deliver the most accurate diagnosis of osteomalacia. This is usually the iliac crest, and both calcified, and non-calcified studies, as well as special stains (including von Kossa's stain)

TREATMENT

APPROPRIATE HEALTH CARE Can be managed on an outpatient basis, except for complicating emergencies/fractures

GENERAL MEASURES
• Treatment of osteomalacia depends upon the cause. The important aspect in designing treatment is determining the underlying etiology, i.e., gastrointestinal, renal, or nutritional.
• For nutritional osteomalacia, calcium and vitamin D have been shown to correct the disease process
• Treatment can be monitored by observing simple bone biochemistry
• Ultimate treatment results depend on identifying and correcting the etiologic cause

ACTIVITY Full activity is encouraged, including a neuroconditioning program

DIET
• Ensure adequate vitamin D intake
• Provide instructions for a high calcium diet and information on calcium supplements if appropriate

PATIENT EDUCATION Educate family and patient on nutrition

Osteomalacia and rickets

MEDICATIONS

DRUG(S) OF CHOICE For adults and uncomplicated rickets, ergocalciferol (vitamin D) 2000-4800 IU once a day for one month. Then reduce dose gradually.
Contraindications: N/A
Precautions: N/A
Significant possible interactions: N/A

ALTERNATIVE DRUGS IV calcium salts if tetany complicates. Single IM dose of 100,000 IU in adolescent each fall.

FOLLOWUP

PATIENT MONITORING Office visits every 6 months

PREVENTION/AVOIDANCE
- Adequate dietary intake of vitamin D
- Adequate sunlight exposure
- Fortified cow's milk

POSSIBLE COMPLICATIONS
- Fractures
- Osteomyelitis
- Renal failure
- Renal tabular acidosis
- Seizures

EXPECTED COURSE AND PROGNOSIS Variable

MISCELLANEOUS

ASSOCIATED CONDITIONS
- Chronic renal disease
- Epilepsy
- Malnutrition
- Previous gastric surgery
- Pregnancy-nutritional factors

AGE-RELATED FACTORS
Pediatric: N/A
Geriatric: Studies have suggested that vitamin D deficiency osteomalacia is a relatively common condition in the acutely ill elderly population, with an estimated prevalence of about 3-5%; however, it often goes undiagnosed
Others: N/A

PREGNANCY N/A

SYNONYMS Rickets

ICD-9-CM 268.2

SEE ALSO N/A

OTHER NOTES N/A

ABBREVIATIONS N/A

REFERENCES Mare, G.M., McKenna, M.J. & Frame, B.: Osteomalacia. Bone Mineral Res 4:335, 1986

Author M. Leeson, M.D.

Osteomyelitis

 BASICS

DESCRIPTION Osteomyelitis is an acute or chronic inflammation of the bone and its structures caused most commonly by bacteria and rarely by other microorganisms. This infection may be acquired either by hematogenous, contiguous, or direct inoculation.
System(s) affected: Musculoskeletal
Genetics: There is no genetic predisposition known in this disease
Incidence/Prevalence in USA: Uncommon
Predominant age: This infection is commonly seen in older adults; hematogenous is bimodal, also seen in infants and children
Predominant sex: Males > Females

SIGNS AND SYMPTOMS
Hematogenous long bone infection (in children with hematogenous osteomyelitis):
◊ Abrupt onset of high fever
◊ Irritability
◊ Malaise
◊ Restriction of movement of the involved extremity
◊ Signs of localized inflammation
Hematogenous vertebral infection (in adults with vertebral osteomyelitis):
◊ Illness is insidious and behaves more like a chronic infection
◊ History of an acute bacteremic episode associated with infection of a specific organ may be found in some patients
Contiguous and vascular insufficiency associated infection:
◊ Acute constitutional manifestations are seldom seen
◊ Localized signs and symptoms of inflammation with or without drainage frequently found
Chronic osteomyelitis:
◊ Non-healing ulcer or draining sinus
◊ Constitutional symptoms, when present, indicate acute suppurative condition in the bone or surrounding tissues
Prosthetic device associated infection:
◊ Infection may be acquired either by hematogenous route, or by contiguous foci such as local infection, operative contamination, or postoperative infection
◊ Acute postoperative infection may present as fever, localized swelling, tenderness, and drainage
◊ Chronic infection is characterized by joint discomfort, swelling, erythema, and joint dysfunction

CAUSES
Acute hematogenous osteomyelitis:
◊ Staphylococcus aureus (most common)
◊ Streptococcus, coagulase negative Staphylococcus, Haemophilus influenzae, and gram negative organisms (less common)
Vertebral osteomyelitis:
◊ Staphylococcus aureus and gram negative enteric organisms (common)
◊ Other microorganisms to consider include Mycobacterium tuberculosis, and fungi
Contiguous focus osteomyelitis and vascular insufficiency osteomyelitis:
◊ Mixed aerobic/anaerobic microorganisms are frequently found
Prosthetic device infection:
◊ Coagulase negative Staphylococcus, and S. aureus (most common)
◊ Diphtheroids, and gram negative bacteria (less common)

RISK FACTORS
• Sickle cell disease
• Other conditions which predispose to bone infarcts
• IV drug use
• Hemodialysis
• Local trauma
• Open fractures
• Presence of prosthetic orthopedic implant
• Vascular insufficiency
• Neuropathy
• Diabetes mellitus

 DIAGNOSIS

DIFFERENTIAL DIAGNOSIS
• Systemic infection from other source
• Aseptic bone infarction
• Other localized inflammation of skin and soft tissues
• Neuropathic joint disease
• Fractures
• Gout

LABORATORY
• Definitive diagnosis is made by needle aspiration or bone biopsy and demonstration of the microorganism by culture or histology
• Blood culture may be positive in about 50% of younger patients with acute hematogenous disease
• Leukocyte count is usually elevated in the acute cases, but not in the chronic cases
• Sedimentation rate is usually elevated, but non-specific
• Teichoic acid antibody may be elevated in a patient who has S. aureus infection for more than 2 weeks
Drugs that may alter lab results:
Antimicrobial agents given before bone culture
Disorders that may alter lab results:
Cultures from the sinus tract are unreliable because of frequent contamination

PATHOLOGICAL FINDINGS
Inflammatory process of the bone with pyogenic bacteria

SPECIAL TESTS N/A

IMAGING
• Radiographic - routine x-ray (findings on plain x-ray often delayed for 10-14 days in acute infection), computed tomography, magnetic resonance imaging
• Radionuclide (technetium, indium, or gallium) are also useful

DIAGNOSTIC PROCEDURES Needle biopsy or open bone biopsy for bacterial culture

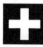 **TREATMENT**

APPROPRIATE HEALTH CARE
Hospitalize the patient with suspected acute osteomyelitis for diagnostic work-up and initial treatment

GENERAL MEASURES
• Symptomatic treatment of pain
• Surgical drainage and removal of necrotic tissues are of utmost importance to effect cure
• In patients with vascular insufficiency or severe gangrenous infection, amputation may be the only effective treatment

ACTIVITY Bedrest and immobilization of the involved bone and joint

DIET No restriction

PATIENT EDUCATION Stress need for long-term treatment and follow up

Osteomyelitis

MEDICATIONS

DRUG(S) OF CHOICE
• The antimicrobial agent/agents chosen should be based on susceptibility testing and known clinical efficacy. The duration of therapy for acute osteomyelitis should be at least 4-6 weeks. In chronic osteomyelitis, longer duration of therapy may be needed.
• Staphylococcus aureus and coagulase negative staphylococcus - nafcillin 2g IV q4-6h. Vancomycin 1g q12h for methicillin resistant Staph.
• Streptococcus spp. - penicillin G 2-4 million units q4h IV
• Enteric gram negative bacilli, and Pseudomonas aeruginosa - piperacillin 4g q4-6h IV, plus aminoglycoside
• Mixed aerobic/anaerobic infection (diabetic foot, bite wound) - beta-lactamase inhibitor combination (ticarcillin/clavulanate 3.1g q6h IV; ampicillin/sulbactam 3g q6h IV)
Contraindications: Allergy
Precautions: In patients with renal or hepatic insufficiency, antimicrobial dose may need adjustment
Significant possible Interactions: Refer to manufacturer's literature

ALTERNATIVE DRUGS
• Staphylococcus aureus and coagulase negative staphylococcus: clindamycin 600mg IV q6h, nafcillin 2g q4h, or cefazolin 1g q8h IV, or vancomycin 1g q12h
• Streptococcus spp.: penicillin 2 million units q4h, cefazolin 1g q8h IV, or clindamycin 600mg q6h IV
• Enteric gram negative bacilli and Pseudomonas aeruginosa: ceftazidime 1g q8h IV or ciprofloxacin (or other quinolone) 750mg q12h orally.
• Mixed aerobic/anaerobic infection (diabetic foot, bite wound): ampicillin/sulbactam 3g q6h IV, ticarcillin/clavulanate 3.1g q6h IV, clindamycin plus third generation cephalosporin or quinolone
• Home therapy often used - consider a simplified antibiotic regimen for outpatient use or oral therapy

FOLLOWUP

PATIENT MONITORING   Blood level of antimicrobial agents, serum antibacterial titers, sedimentation rate

PREVENTION/AVOIDANCE   Avoid further stress and weight bearing until healing

POSSIBLE COMPLICATIONS
• Abscess formation
• Bacteremia
• Fracture
• Loosening of the prosthetic implant
• Postoperative infection

EXPECTED COURSE AND PROGNOSIS
• Cure of osteomyelitis with medical treatment is notoriously unpredictable especially when not accompanied by surgical debridement
• In patients with acute hematogenous osteomyelitis, the prognosis is usually good even without surgery. Cure takes about 6 weeks.
• The prognosis is improved if all infected bone has been removed

MISCELLANEOUS

ASSOCIATED CONDITIONS   Listed with Causes

AGE-RELATED FACTORS
Pediatric: Occurs most often in 5-14 age group and more frequently in boys
Geriatric:
• Vertebral osteomyelitis more common
• Contiguous focus of infection more common
• Vascular insufficiency is most common cause of osteomyelitis in 50-70 age group (usually due to presence of associated conditions)
Others: N/A

PREGNANCY   N/A

SYNONYMS   N/A

ICD-9-CM
• Acute osteomyelitis 730.0
• Chronic osteomyelitis 730.1
• Jaw osteomyelitis 526.4
• Orbital osteomyelitis 376.03
• For specific microbial etiology, see the ICD code of the the specific organism, e.g., Salmonella - see Salmonella osteomyelitis 003.24. N.B.: 5th digit code required for site
0 - site unspecified
1 - shoulder
2 - upper arm
3 - forearm
4 - hand
5 - pelvis/thigh
6 - lower leg
7 - ankle/foot
8 - other, specified
9 - multiple sites

SEE ALSO   N/A

OTHER NOTES   N/A

ABBREVIATIONS   N/A

REFERENCES   Waldvogel, F.A.: Osteomyelitis. In Infectious Diseases. Edited by S.L. Gorbach, J.G. Bartlett & N.R. Blacklow. Philadelphia, W.B. Saunders Co., 1992, pp.1125-1129

Author   J. S. Tan, M.D.

Osteonecrosis

BASICS

DESCRIPTION Death of the cellular components of bony tissue
System(s) affected: Musculoskeletal
Genetics: The underlying condition of hemoglobinopathies, especially sickle cell disease, diabetes, and type II or IV hyperlipemia are inheritable and associated with a high incidence of osteonecrosis. Other forms have no proven genetic relationship.
Incidence/Prevalence in USA: Dependent upon the underlying condition
Predominant age: 3rd to 6th decade
Predominant sex: Male > Female

SIGNS AND SYMPTOMS
• The symptoms may be acute as in osteonecrosis of sickle cell disease or renal transplant. Usually insidious in other forms. Diagnosis may not be made for two years after onset of symptoms.
• Pain, the prominent symptom, is made worse with activity
• Loss of motion of the affected joint
• Stiffness (especially early morning)
• Swelling if the involved joint is superficial
• Locking may occur if a loose body has developed
• Proximal femur is the most common site and more prevalent in males in the 3rd-6th decade
• The distal femur, especially the medial femoral condyle, is the second most frequent site. This area is unique in that night pain is a prominent early symptom. Most common in females in the 6th-7th decade.
• Other sites in decreasing frequency are the proximal humerus, talus, carpal lunate (Kienböck's disease) and the humeral capitulum

CAUSES
• Idiopathic
• Fractures, especially the femoral neck
• Traumatic (fractures, dislocation)
• Dislocations
• Legg-Calvé-Perthes (seen in 6-12 year age group)
• Hemoglobinopathies (especially sickle cell disease)
• Metabolic (hemoglobinopathies, ETOH, steroid use, renal failure/transplantation)

RISK FACTORS
• Gaucher's disease - especially likely as a postoperative infection
• Diabetes mellitus
• Alcoholism - the most frequent cause
• Type II or IV hyperlipemia
• Cortisone therapy (may be seen with Cushing's disease)
• Obesity
• Oral contraceptives
• Organ transplant, especially kidney
• Pregnancy
• Decompression sickness ("bends")

DIAGNOSIS

DIFFERENTIAL DIAGNOSIS Rheumatoid arthritis, septic necrosis and severe secondary parathyroidism. A crescent sign (a linear subchondral lucency indicates collapse of subchondral bone. Patchy lucencies reflect resorption; patchy sclerosis indicates growth of new bone over the scaffolding of dead trabeculae) in these conditions may occur because the bone may be so soft that it collapses producing a crescent sign.

LABORATORY N/A
Drugs that may alter lab results: N/A
Disorders that may alter lab results: N/A

PATHOLOGICAL FINDINGS The subchondral fracture occurs during bone repair as necrotic bone is resorbed. Later, a collapse of the bone occurs with subsequent irregularities at the joint surface. This will eventually produce osteoarthritic changes.

SPECIAL TESTS Bone scan with radioactive materials show decreased bone uptake. Later, the uptake increases as reparative processes begin within the bone.

IMAGING MRI will show a decreased signal intensity of the involved bone and is the most sensitive diagnostic exam.

DIAGNOSTIC PROCEDURES The presence of a crescent sign is practically diagnostic (see Differential Diagnosis of osteonecrosis). It is caused by a subchondral fracture.

TREATMENT

APPROPRIATE HEALTH CARE Outpatient normally; inpatient if surgery indicated

GENERAL MEASURES
• Surgery: bone grafts, arthroplasty, allografts and arthrodesis may be used, dependent upon the joint involved
• Only four conditions can be treated to decrease the incidence of osteonecrosis
  ◊ Alcoholism - abstinence is obvious, but quite difficult to attain
  ◊ Dysbarism - new tables of decompression, if followed, will lower osteonecrosis incidence of divers
  ◊ Transplant patients - decreased doses of cortisone and regulation of calcium and phosphorous metabolism
  ◊ Sickle cell disease - treat a crisis vigorously with hydration, possible exchange transfusion and oxygenation, especially hyperbaric oxygen

ACTIVITY As tolerated

DIET No special diet

PATIENT EDUCATION The patient should be instructed in the use of crutches and/or canes when the lower extremity is involved. Proper use of a walking cane can decrease the pressure on the femoral head 20-30% when walking.

MEDICATIONS

DRUG(S) OF CHOICE
• NSAID's - consistent with the underlying disease may be used for painful episodes
• Acetaminophen - 500 mg qid can be quite helpful in alleviating symptoms
Contraindications: See manufacturer's profile of each drug
Precautions: Nonsteroidals - if history of peptic ulcer is present, the use of Zantac 150 mg bid or 300 mg hs can be given. Cytotec 100 micrograms bid will usually prevent gastritis (not needed with acetaminophen).
Significant possible interactions: See manufacturer's profile of each drug

ALTERNATIVE DRUGS N/A

FOLLOWUP

PATIENT MONITORING X-rays should be made every 12-18 months, more frequently if symptoms become more severe

PREVENTION/AVOIDANCE Early diagnosis and treatment of underlying disease

POSSIBLE COMPLICATIONS
• Progression of disease
• The pressure of osteonecrosis leads to osteoarthritis of the involved joint to a varying degree. Arthroplasty of the hip carries a much poorer prognosis than osteoarthritis alone. It should be postponed as long as possible.

EXPECTED COURSE AND PROGNOSIS Gaucher's disease is associated with a high risk of infection following surgery

MISCELLANEOUS

ASSOCIATED CONDITIONS N/A

AGE-RELATED FACTORS
Pediatric:
• Legg-Calvé-Perthes occurs in the 6-12 year age group. Prognosis is better in younger patients.
Geriatric: N/A
Others: N/A

PREGNANCY Is a risk factor

SYNONYMS
• Idiopathic osteonecrosis
• Avascular necrosis
• Kienböck's disease
• Subchondral fracture

ICD-9-CM 730.1

SEE ALSO
• Osteoarthritis
• Legg-Calvé-Perthes disease

OTHER NOTES N/A

ABBREVIATIONS N/A

REFERENCES
• Harris, W.H.: Total Hip Replacement. American Academy of Orthopedic Surgeons, Institutional Course Lectures, Vol 23. St. Louis, C.V. Mosby Company, 1974
• Eftekhaur Khaur, N.S. & Keirwam, H.: Systemic and Local Complications following low friction. Arthroplasty. In Archives of Surgery, 111:150, 1976
• Nicholson, O.R.: Total Hip Replacement. In Clinical Orthopedics, 95:217, 1973

Author F. Johnston, M.D.

Osteoporosis

 BASICS

DESCRIPTION
A multifactorial skeletal disease characterized by severe bone loss sufficient to predispose to atraumatic fractures of the vertebral column, upper femur; distal radius, proximal humerus, pubic rami and ribs
• Postmenopausal osteoporosis (Type I): The most common form in Caucasian and Asian women. Due to excessive and prolonged acceleration of bone resorption following menopausal loss of estrogen secretion.
• Involutional osteoporosis (Type II): Occurs in both sexes above age 75. Due to a subtle, prolonged imbalance between rates of bone resorption and formation.
• Idiopathic osteoporosis: A rare form of primary osteoporosis occurring in premenopausal women and in men below age 75. Not related to secondary causes or risk factors predisposing to bone loss. Causes unknown.
• Juvenile osteoporosis: A rare form of variable severity occurring in prepubertal children. Self-limited with cessation of fractures at puberty. Cause unknown. (Not covered in this topic.)
• Secondary osteoporosis: Severe bone loss sufficient to cause atraumatic fractures due to extrinsic factors such as corticosteroid excess, rheumatoid arthritis, chronic liver/kidney disease, malabsorption syndromes, systemic mastocytosis, hyperparathyroidism, hyperthyroidism, a variety of hypogonadal states, and others
System(s) affected: Musculoskeletal
Genetics: Familial predisposition to suboptimal skeletal mass during growth and development and to rapid bone loss after the menopause have been described in some patients. Also, osteoporosis more common in Caucasians and Orientals than in Black and Latino ethnic groups.
Incidence in USA: Unknown
Prevalence in USA:
• 30-40% cumulatively in women, 5-15% in men
• Prevalence of idiopathic and juvenile types unknown
• Secondary osteoporosis cumulatively 5-10%, both sexes
Predominant age: Age 8 to senescence, depending on type
Predominant sex: Female > Male

SIGNS AND SYMPTOMS
• Back ache/pain; acute/chronic
• Kyphosis/scoliosis
• Atraumatic fractures
• No peripheral bone deformities
• Sclerae not blue/green/grey
• Loss of height

CAUSES
• Postmenopausal (Type I): Hypoestrogenemia
• Involutional (Type II): Unknown
• Idiopathic: Unknown
• Juvenile: Unknown
• Secondary: Various (see Description)
• Although bone loss is an inevitable consequence of aging, osteoporosis occurs most frequently in individuals who fail to achieve optimal skeletal mass during development or lose bone rapidly thereafter due to excessive postmenopausal and/or involutional bone loss, or medical conditions/risk factors that increase bone loss

RISK FACTORS
• Dietary - inadequate calcium, excessive phosphate/protein
• Physical - immobilization, sedentary lifestyle
• Social - alcohol, cigarettes, caffeine
• Medical - chronic diseases, endocrinopathies, (see Secondary osteoporosis)
• Iatrogenic - corticosteroids, excess thyroid hormone replacement, chronic heparin, chemotherapy, loop diuretics, anticonvulsants, tetracyclines, radiation therapy
• Genetic/familial - suboptimal bone mass at maturity, "familial fast bone losers"

 DIAGNOSIS

DIFFERENTIAL DIAGNOSIS
• Multiple myeloma
• Other neoplasia
• Osteomalacia
• Osteogenesis imperfecta tarda (Type I)
• Skeletal hyperparathyroidism (primary and secondary)
• Mastocytosis (rare)

LABORATORY
• All "routine" tests usually normal
• Alkaline phosphatase may be transiently increased following fractures
• Serum and/or urine protein electrophoresis normal
• Thyroid function tests and urinary free cortisol normal in primary types
• Serum osteocalcin, if high, indicates high turnover type
• Urine calcium normal
Drugs that may alter lab results:
• Hepatotoxins cause changes in alkaline phosphatase
• Estrogens cause changes in thyroid function tests
Disorders that may alter lab results:
• Multiple myeloma or other neoplasia
• Osteomalacia
• Osteogenesis imperfecta
• Hyperparathyroidism

PATHOLOGICAL FINDINGS
• Reduced skeletal mass, trabecular bone more so than cortical bone. Loss of trabecular connections.
• Osteoclast and osteoblast number variable
• No evidence of other metabolic bone diseases and no increase in unmineralized osteoid
• Marrow normal or atrophic

SPECIAL TESTS N/A

IMAGING
• X-rays - "early" changes of increased width of intervertebral spaces, relative accentuation of cortical plates, vertical striations of vertebral bodies
• "Late" changes of cortical plate fractures, vertebral compression, wedge and crush fractures, peripheral fractures at ends of long bones
• Bone scan may show increased uptake at previous fracture sites, otherwise negative
• Bone mineral density (BMD) by dual energy x-ray absorptiometry (DXA) or quantitative CT scan (QCT)
◊ DXA: Utilizes filtered x-ray beam to quantitate BMD of lumbar spine and upper femur. Normal range is plus or minus 1 standard deviation (SD) from mean peak BMD for skeletal site and population group.
◊ QCT: Utilizes fourth generation CT scanner, special program and plastic phantom containing bone mass standards to quantitate either trabecular or cortical bone mass, or both (integral data) of lumbar spine. Normal range - plus or minus 1 SD.
◊ Quantitative bone histomorphometry: Histologic method of quantitating various elements of bone physiology utilizing iliac crest biopsy cores and special methods of handling and staining, including prior administration of tetracycline pulses to permit fluorescent measurements of bone mineralization rate. Normative data for various populations exist.

DIAGNOSTIC PROCEDURES
Bone biopsy needed rarely, to rule out other metabolic bone diseases. Sometimes used to quantitate bone loss, utilizing quantitative histomorphometric technique.

TREATMENT

APPROPRIATE HEALTH CARE
• Usually outpatient
• Inpatient care for acute back pain, especially for new vertebral fractures and for acute treatment of upper femoral and pelvic fractures
• Nursing home or home care may be needed following peripheral fractures

GENERAL MEASURES
As required by pain and disability, e.g., heat, analgesics, physical therapy

ACTIVITY
• Maintain ambulation, walking 1 mile twice a day, if possible, swimming, tricycling
• Avoid exercises and maneuvers that increase compressive forces and mechanical stress on spine and peripheral bone sites
• Rehabilitation procedures for back muscle spasm and ambulation encouragement

DIET
• Reducing diet if overweight
• Calcium intake 1500 mg/day from all sources, if not hypercalciuric or with past medical history of calcium stones
• Avoid excess phosphate or protein intake, i.e., avoid phosphoric-acid-containing beverages and excess meat intake

PATIENT EDUCATION
Teaching resources and patient literature available from National Osteoporosis Foundation, 2100 M St., Suite 602, Washington, D.C. 20037

MEDICATIONS

DRUG(S) OF CHOICE
• Synthetic salmon calcitonin (Calcimar, Miacalcin) 100 IU qd or qod preferred, 50 IU qd or 3 times a week may be effective in high turnover types. Should be used in conjunction with adequate calcium and vitamin D.
• Synthetic human calcitonin (Cibacalcin), 0.5 mg qd to 3 times a week. Not FDA approved for this indication; may be used when allergy or resistance to synthetic salmon calcitonin intervenes.
• Hormone replacement therapy (HRT) (estrogen/progesterone) - several preparations of each available, doses depend on preparation
Contraindications:
• Calcitonins - none except allergy
• HRT absolute - past medical history of endometrial or breast cancer or premalignant breast conditions
• HRT relative - past medical history hypertension, thromboembolic conditions, edematous conditions, endometriosis, migraine, stress incontinence, severe hepatic dysfunction; family history of breast cancer

Precautions:
• Calcitonins - none
• HRT - annual gynecology exam, including Pap smear or endometrial biopsy, annual breast exam and mammography. Check blood pressure twice a week during initiation of HRT.
Significant possible interactions: None

ALTERNATIVE DRUGS
• Etidronate disodium - research drug, long-term effects uncertain
• Other biphosphonates - research drugs, inhibitors of bone resorption, possible effects on bone formation
• Sodium fluoride - research drug, stimulates bone formation but may have adverse effects on cortical bone
• Tamoxifen - research drug, that may have estrogen effects on bone without potential for breast stimulation
• Progestogens - research drugs, may have effects on bone similar to estrogens or androgens
• Androgens/anabolics - research drugs, may stimulate bone formation
• Ipriflavone - research drug - inhibitor of bone resorption

FOLLOWUP

PATIENT MONITORING
• Monthly during initiation, every 2-4 months thereafter
• Annual multiphasic screening, annual gynecological exam, breast exam, and mammography
• Annual BMD using same technique and instrument as for baseline measurement
• Repeat x-rays of spine every 3 years. More often when indicated for acute pain, suspected fractures.
• Peripheral bone x-rays if acute pain

PREVENTION/AVOIDANCE
General guidelines
◊ Diet, exercise, hormone replacement at menopause
◊ Increased calcium intake
Prevention during the osteopenic phase (prolonged, usually asymptomatic phase prior to fracturing)
◊ Identification of osteopenia: BMD (regardless of method) between -1 and -2 standard deviations (SD) below mean peak bone mass for the skeletal site and population group (Z score)
◊ Correction of treatable medical conditions and other risk factors (see Risk factors); will also help achieve optimal skeletal mass during development
◊ HRT if postmenopausal and no absolute contraindications

POSSIBLE COMPLICATIONS
• Severe disabling pain
• Dorsal/lumbar neurologic deficits 2° to vertebral fracture (rare)
• Invalidism/death secondary to complications of upper femoral fractures

EXPECTED COURSE AND PROGNOSIS
• In 70% patients, treatment will lead to stabilization of skeletal manifestations
• Small increases in bone mass in some cases
• Reduced pain, increased mobility
• 20-30% of upper femoral fractures will lead to chronic care status and/or premature death from complications despite treatment

MISCELLANEOUS

ASSOCIATED CONDITIONS
• Corticosteroid excess
• Rheumatoid arthritis
• Chronic liver/kidney disease
• Malabsorption syndromes
• Systemic mastocytosis
• Hyperparathyroidism
• Hyperthyroidism
• Various hypogonadal states

AGE-RELATED FACTORS
Pediatric: Juvenile osteoporosis not discussed herein
Geriatric: Postmenopausal/involutional/mixed types
Others: Primary types rare in African Americans. Patients with British, North European, Scandinavian, and Oriental ancestry most susceptible.

PREGNANCY
Rare acute osteoporosis of pregnancy, not discussed herein

SYNONYMS N/A

ICD-9-CM 733.0

SEE ALSO N/A

OTHER NOTES N/A

ABBREVIATIONS
• BMD = bone mineral density
• SD = standard deviation
• HRT = hormone replacement therapy

REFERENCES
• Christiansen, C.: Consensus Development Conference: Prophylaxis and Treatment of Osteoporosis. Amer J.Med. 90:107-110, 1991
• Wisneski, L.A.: Choosing the Best Regimen in Postmenopausal Osteoporosis. J. Musculoskel Med. 3:33-45, 1991
• Chestnut, C.H., III, Cummings, S.R., Drinkwater, B.L., & Johnston, C.C.: New Options in Osteoporosis. Patient Care. pp 160-194, Jan. 15, 1988
• Recker, R.R.: Current Therapy for Osteoporosis. J Clin Endocrinol Metab. 76:14-16, 1993

Author S. Wallach, M.D.

Otitis externa

BASICS

DESCRIPTION Inflammation of the external auditory canal
• Acute diffuse otitis externa - the most common form, an infectious process usually bacterial, occasionally fungal
• Acute circumscribed otitis externa - synonymous with furuncle. Associated with infection of the hair follicle.
• Chronic otitis externa - same as acute diffuse, but of longer duration (greater than 6 weeks)
• Eczematous otitis externa - may accompany typical atopic eczema or other primary skin conditions
• Necrotizing "malignant" otitis externa - an infection which extends into the deeper tissues adjacent to the canal. May include osteomyelitis and cellulitis. Rare in children.
Incidence in USA: Unknown. Incidence is higher in the summer months.
Prevalence in USA:
• Acute, chronic and eczematous - common
• Necrotizing - uncommon
System(s) affected: Skin
Genetics: N/A
Predominant age: All ages
Predominant sex: Male = Female

SIGNS AND SYMPTOMS
• Itching
• Plugging of the ear
• Otalgia
• Periauricular adenitis
• Erythematous canal
• Purulent discharge
• Eczema of pinna
• Cranial nerve involvement (VII, IX-XII)

CAUSES
Acute diffuse otitis externa
◊ Traumatized external canal
◊ Bacterial infection - pseudomonas (67% cases); staphylococcus; streptococcus; gram negative rods
◊ Fungal infection - aspergillus (90% cases); Phycomycetes; Rhizopus; actinomyces; Penicillium; yeast
Chronic otitis externa
◊ Bacterial infection - pseudomonas
Eczematous otitis externa (associated with primary skin disorder):
◊ Eczema
◊ Seborrhea
◊ Neurodermatitis
◊ Contact dermatitis
◊ Purulent otitis media
◊ Sensitivity to topical medications
Necrotizing otitis externa
◊ Invasive bacterial infection - pseudomonas

RISK FACTORS
Acute and chronic otitis externa
◊ Traumatization of external canal
◊ Swimming
◊ Hot humid weather
◊ Use of a hearing aid
Eczematous
◊ Primary skin disorder
Necrotizing otitis externa in adults
◊ Elderly
◊ Diabetes
◊ Debilitating disease
Necrotizing otitis externa in children (rare)
◊ Leukopenia
◊ Malnutrition
◊ Diabetes mellitus
◊ Diabetes insipidus

DIAGNOSIS

DIFFERENTIAL DIAGNOSIS
• Ear pain
• Purulent ear discharge
• Hearing loss
• Cranial nerve palsy (VII, IX-XII) with necrotizing otitis externa

LABORATORY Gram stain and culture of canal discharge (occasionally helpful)
Drugs that may alter lab results: Antibiotic pretreatment
Disorders that may alter lab results: N/A

PATHOLOGICAL FINDINGS
• Acute and chronic otitis externa - desquamation of superficial epithelium of external canal with infection
• Eczematous otitis externa - pathologic findings consistent with primary skin disorder, secondary infection on occasion
• Necrotizing otitis externa - vasculitis, thrombosis and necrosis of involved tissues; osteomyelitis

SPECIAL TESTS N/A

IMAGING Radiologic evaluation of deep tissues in necrotizing otitis externa

DIAGNOSTIC PROCEDURES N/A

TREATMENT

APPROPRIATE HEALTH CARE
Outpatient, except for resistant cases and necrotizing otitis externa

GENERAL MEASURES
• Thorough cleansing of external canal
• Pain medications
• Antipruritic and antihistamines (eczematous form)

ACTIVITY No restrictions

DIET No restrictions

PATIENT EDUCATION Methods for prevention

MEDICATIONS

DRUG(S) OF CHOICE
Acute bacterial and chronic otitis externa
◊ Topical therapy for approximately 10 days
◊ 2% acetic acid
◊ Antibiotics
◊ Corticosteroids
Fungal otitis externa
◊ Topical therapy anti-yeast for candida or yeast - nystatin
◊ Parenteral antifungal therapy - amphotericin B
Eczematous otitis externa - topical therapy
◊ Aluminum acetate 8%
◊ Acetic acid 2% in aluminum acetate
◊ Burrow's solution
◊ Steroid cream, lotion, ointment
◊ Antibacterial, if superinfected
Necrotizing otitis externa
◊ Parenteral antibiotics - antistaphylococcus and antipseudomonal
◊ 4-6 weeks of therapy
Contraindications:
• Hypersensitivity to topical or parenteral therapy
• Renal or hepatic failure when using amphotericin B
Precautions: Dosage adjustment for amphotericin B in patients with renal or hepatic dysfunction
Significant possible interactions:
• Hypokalemia associated with amphotericin B may lead to digitalis toxicity
• Concurrent administration of nonabsorbable anions, such as carbenicillin, may exacerbate hypokalemia

ALTERNATIVE DRUGS N/A

FOLLOWUP

PATIENT MONITORING
Acute otitis externa
◊ 48 hours after therapy instituted to assess for improvement
◊ At the end of treatment
Chronic otitis externa
◊ Every 2-3 weeks for repeated cleansing of canal
◊ May require alterations in topical medication, including antibiotics and steroids
Necrotizing otitis externa
◊ Daily monitoring in hospital for extension of infection
◊ Baseline auditory and vestibular testing at beginning and end of therapy

PREVENTION/AVOIDANCE
• Avoid prolonged exposure to moisture
• Utilize preventive antiseptics
• Treat predisposing skin conditions
• Eliminate self-inflicted trauma to canal
• Diagnose and treat underlying systemic conditions

POSSIBLE COMPLICATIONS
• Mainly a problem with necrotizing otitis externa. May spread to infect contiguous bone and CNS structures.
• Acute otitis externa may spread to pinna causing a chondritis

EXPECTED COURSE AND PROGNOSIS
• Acute otitis externa - rapid response to therapy with total resolution
• Chronic otitis externa - with repeated cleansing and antibiotic therapy the majority of cases will resolve. Occasionally, surgical intervention is required for resistant cases.
• Eczematous otitis externa - resolution will occur with control of the primary skin condition
• Necrotizing otitis externa - can usually be managed with debridement and prolonged parenteral antibiotics. Recurrence rate is 100% when treatment is inadequate. Surgical intervention may be necessary in resistant cases or if there is cranial nerve involvement. Mortality rate is significant, probably secondary to the underlying disease.

MISCELLANEOUS

ASSOCIATED CONDITIONS See Risk Factors

AGE-RELATED FACTORS N/A
Pediatric: N/A
Geriatric: N/A
Others: N/A

PREGNANCY N/A

SYNONYMS Swimmer's ear

ICD-9-CM 380.10 infective otitis externa, unspecified

SEE ALSO N/A

OTHER NOTES N/A

ABBREVIATIONS N/A

REFERENCES
• Marcy, S.M.: Swimmer's Ear. Contemporary Pediatrics 1986; 3:20
• Bluestone, C. & Stool, S. (eds.): Pediatric Otolaryngology. 2nd Ed. Philadelphia, W.B. Saunders Co., 1990

Author J. Nard, M.D.

Otitis media

BASICS

DESCRIPTION
Inflammation of the middle ear
• Acute otitis media (AOM): Usually a bacterial infection accompanied by viral upper respiratory infection
• Recurrent AOM: 3 or more AOM in 6 months, or 4 or more AOM in 1 year
• Otitis media with effusion (OME): Persistent inflammation manifested as asymptomatic middle ear fluid that follows AOM or arises without prior AOM
System(s) affected: Nervous
Genetics: N/A
Incidence/Prevalence in USA: (Incidence) By age 7 years 93% of children have 1 or more AOM; 39% have 6 or more AOM; after AOM 10 to 20% still have OME 3 months later
Predominant age: Peak incidence age 6-12 months; declines after age 7 years; rare in adults
Predominant sex: Male = Female

SIGNS AND SYMPTOMS
AOM:
◊ Earache
◊ Fever, although more often afebrile
◊ Accompanying nasal discharge and cough common
◊ Decreased hearing
◊ Otorrhea if eardrum perforated
◊ Eardrum mobility decreased (as observed by pneumatic otoscopy)
◊ Eardrum bulging, opaque, often yellowish or inflamed. Redness alone is not a reliable sign.
AOM in infants:
◊ May cause no symptoms in the first few months of life
◊ Irritability is sometimes the only indication of earache
◊ Eardrum bulging, opaque, often yellowish or inflamed. Redness alone not a reliable sign.
OME:
◊ Usually asymptomatic
◊ Decreased hearing probably universal, but not always measurable, and rarely appreciated by parents
◊ Eardrum often dull, but not bulging
◊ Eardrum mobility decreased (as observed by pneumatic otoscopy)

CAUSES
AOM: A preceding viral upper respiratory infection produces eustachian tube dysfunction that is thought to promote bacterial infection via eustachian tube. Bacteriology:
◊ Pneumococci - 30-35%
◊ Haemophilus influenzae - 20-25%
◊ Moraxella (Branhamella) catarrhalis - 10-15%
◊ Group A streptococci 1-2%
◊ Staphylococcus aureus - 1-2%
◊ Sterile/non-pathogens - 25-30%
OME:
◊ 20-40% silent bacterial infection
◊ Eustachian tube dysfunction thought important
◊ Allergic causes rarely substantiated

RISK FACTORS
• Day care
• Formula feeding
• Smoking in household
• Male gender
• Family history of middle ear disease
• AOM in 1st year of life is a risk factor for recurrent AOM

DIAGNOSIS

DIFFERENTIAL DIAGNOSIS
• Should not be confusing if otoscopic exam is performed
• Earache with a normal ear exam may be caused by referred pain from the jaw or teeth

LABORATORY
WBC not helpful
Drugs that may alter lab results: N/A
Disorders that may alter lab results: N/A

PATHOLOGICAL FINDINGS
N/A

SPECIAL TESTS
• To document the presence of middle ear fluid - tympanometry, acoustic reflex measurement or acoustic reflectometry
• Hearing testing helpful to assess the need for early surgical intervention in OME

IMAGING
N/A

DIAGNOSTIC PROCEDURES
Tympanocentesis for microbiologic diagnosis in selected cases

TREATMENT

APPROPRIATE HEALTH CARE
Outpatient except when surgery is indicated

GENERAL MEASURES
• AOM: Outpatient except for febrile infants < 2 months
• OME: Referral for surgery if: > 3 months bilateral OME, and/or > 6 months unilateral OME, and/or hearing loss > 25 decibels
• Recurrent AOM: Referral for surgery if > 2 or 3 AOM while on chemoprophylaxis. Tympanostomy tubes and adenoidectomy effective surgical procedures for OME and recurrent AOM, but not in all cases.

ACTIVITY
No restrictions

DIET
No special diet

PATIENT EDUCATION
N/A

MEDICATIONS

DRUG(S) OF CHOICE
• AOM: Amoxicillin 40 mg/kg/day divided tid for 10 days
• Recurrent AOM: Amoxicillin 20 mg/kg daily dose for 3-6 months or until summer
• OME: Antihistamines and decongestants ineffective, indications for steroids not defined, amoxicillin promotes resolution in 10-15% but effect is usually transitory
Contraindications: Allergy to penicillins
Precautions: Refer to manufacturer's profile of each drug
Significant possible interactions: Refer to manufacturer's profile of each drug

ALTERNATIVE DRUGS
Alternative drugs are indicated for following AOM patients:
◊ Patients with penicillin allergy
◊ Persistent symptoms after 48-72 hrs of amoxicillin
◊ Recurrence of AOM within 3-4 weeks of a previous AOM
◊ AOM with severe earache
◊ Infants less than 6 months with high fever
◊ Immunocompromised hosts
Alternative drugs effective against amoxicillin resistant pathogens:
◊ Amoxicillin plus clavulanic (Augmentin) 40 mg/kg/day of amoxicillin component tid
◊ Cefixime (Suprax) 8 mg/kg/day bid or single daily dose
◊ Trimethoprim-sulfamethoxazole (Septra, Bactrim) 40 mg trimethoprim, 8 mg sulfamethoxazole/kg/day divided bid
◊ Erythromycin plus sulfisoxazole (Pediazole) 40 mg erythromycin component/kg/day divided qid
◊ Cefaclor (Ceclor) is less effective than other alternatives
Recurrent AOM:
◊ Sulfisoxazole 75 mg/kg single daily dose for penicillin allergic patients

FOLLOWUP

PATIENT MONITORING
• AOM: Otoscopic examination 2-4 weeks after diagnosis
• OME: Monthly otoscopic or tympanometric exams as long as OME persists

PREVENTION/AVOIDANCE
• Breast feeding decreases incidence of AOM
• Eliminate cigarette smoking in the household

POSSIBLE COMPLICATIONS
• AOM: Perforation/otorrhea, acute mastoiditis, facial nerve paralysis, otitic hydrocephalus
• OME: Hearing loss. Extent and significance of impaired speech and language is controversial.
• Recurrent AOM and OME: Atrophy and scarring of eardrum, chronic perforation and otorrhea, cholesteatoma, permanent hearing loss, chronic mastoiditis, brain abscess and other intracranial suppurative complications

EXPECTED COURSE AND PROGNOSIS
• AOM: Symptoms usually improve in 48-72 hrs; OME following AOM resolved in 90% by 3 months
• OME: Approximately 50% resolve after 8 weeks of observation
• Recurrent AOM and OME: Usually subside in school age children; only a small percentage have complications

MISCELLANEOUS

ASSOCIATED CONDITIONS
• Upper respiratory infection
• Bacteremia
• Meningitis

AGE-RELATED FACTORS
Pediatric: Primarily a pediatric disease
Geriatric: N/A
Others: N/A

PREGNANCY N/A

SYNONYMS
• Secretory otitis media
• Serous otitis media

ICD-9-CM
• 382.0 acute otitis media
• 381.0 acute suppurative otitis media

SEE ALSO N/A

OTHER NOTES
In first few months of infancy, the eardrum is normally at an angle and less mobile in older adults

ABBREVIATIONS
• AOM = acute otitis media
• OM = otitis media
• OME = otitis media with effusion

REFERENCES
Bluestone, C.D. & Klein, J.O.: Otitis Media in Infants and Children. Philadelphia, W.B. Saunders Co., 1988

Author C. Marchant, M.D.

Otosclerosis (Otospongiosis)

BASICS

DESCRIPTION A primary bone dyscrasia involving the otic capsule. It is the leading cause of conductive hearing loss in adults.
• Histologic otosclerosis: Asymptomatic form in which abnormal bone spares vital structures of the ear
• Clinical otosclerosis: Abnormal spongy bone involves ossicular chain or other structures leading to altered physiology
System(s) affected: Nervous
Genetics:
• 60% of those affected give positive family history
• Appears to be transmitted by autosomal dominant gene with variable penetrance
Incidence in USA: 4-8% among Caucasians; 1% among African-Americans (histologic form)
Prevalence in USA: Caucasians 5000/100,000; Blacks 1000/100,000 (histologic form)
Predominant age: Clinical onset usually in early 20's. Peak incidence fourth and fifth decades.
Predominant sex: Female > Male (2:1)

SIGNS AND SYMPTOMS
• Progressive conductive hearing loss, usually with well preserved speech discrimination. May have sensorineural hearing loss with cochlear involvement.
• Carhart's notch: A dip in bone conductive threshold at 2000 Hz. on audiometric testing
• Schwartze's sign: Reddish hue on promontory upon otoscopic examination
• Patients often soft spoken and aware they seem to hear better in noisy environments

CAUSES Unknown; fluoride metabolism felt by some authorities to play a role in etiology

RISK FACTORS Unknown

DIAGNOSIS

DIFFERENTIAL DIAGNOSIS
• Chronic suppurative otitis media
• Serous otitis media
• External auditory canal occlusion
• Ossicular chain disruption
• Congenital fixation of stapes
• Presbycusis

LABORATORY N/A
Drugs that may alter lab results: N/A
Disorders that may alter lab results: N/A

PATHOLOGICAL FINDINGS
• Gross: Off-white to reddish bone formation, most often located anterior to the oval window and extending to involve the stapedial footplate. Sometimes covers entire oval window (obliterative). May be found anywhere in otic capsule. Bilateral in 75% of cases.
• Micro: "Spongy" appearing bone with increased vascular spaces. Osteoblasts and osteoclasts are plentiful.

SPECIAL TESTS
Tuning fork and audiometric testing for conductive and/or sensorineural hearing loss. Will lateralize to more impaired ear with Weber's test.

IMAGING
Coaxial or computerized tomography sometimes helpful

DIAGNOSTIC PROCEDURES N/A

TREATMENT

APPROPRIATE HEALTH CARE
Inpatient for surgery. Outpatient if surgery not feasible.

GENERAL MEASURES
• Hearing aids
• Surgical correction (stapedectomy): Usually involves mobilization or removal of the stapedial foot plate with placement of a stapes prosthesis. Recent procedural innovations have involved use of lasers.
• Relative indications for surgery include: Negative Rinne's test (air-bone audiometric gap at least 20 dB); bilateral involvement

ACTIVITY No restrictions

DIET No special diet

PATIENT EDUCATION
• Because speech discrimination is usually preserved, patients should be advised of the possible benefit from hearing aids (as an alternative or adjunct to surgery)
• Mayo Foundation for Medical Education and Research, Section of Patient and Health Education, Sieber Subway, Rochester, MN 55905, (507)284-8140

MEDICATIONS

DRUG(S) OF CHOICE No specific drug therapy but sodium fluoride, vitamin D and calcium gluconate have been tried, especially in cases of predominantly sensorineural hearing loss
Contraindications: Refer to manufacturer's literature
Precautions: Refer to manufacturer's literature
Significant possible interactions: Refer to manufacturer's literature

ALTERNATIVE DRUGS N/A

FOLLOWUP

PATIENT MONITORING Interval audiometric testing

PREVENTION/AVOIDANCE N/A

POSSIBLE COMPLICATIONS Surgical risks include chorda tympani nerve injury, tympanic membrane laceration, ossicular chain disruption, otitis media and externa, labyrinthitis, granuloma formation, perilymph fistulae, and total deafness ("dead ear")

EXPECTED COURSE AND PROGNOSIS Progressive hearing loss if not treated. Surgery improves hearing by at least 15 dB in 90% of cases.

MISCELLANEOUS

ASSOCIATED CONDITIONS
• Van der Hoeve's syndrome (rare triad of osteogenesis imperfecta, blue sclera, and otospongiosis)
• Tinnitus
• Vertigo

AGE-RELATED FACTORS
Pediatric: N/A
Geriatric: Important differential diagnosis for presbycusis
Others: N/A

PREGNANCY Progression may accelerate during pregnancy. Some women first notice hearing loss at this time.

SYNONYMS N/A

ICD-9-CM 387.9

SEE ALSO N/A

OTHER NOTES N/A

ABBREVIATIONS N/A

REFERENCES
• English, G.M.: Otolaryngology: A Textbook. New York, Harper & Rowe, 1976, chap. 17
• Lee, K.J.: Essential Otolaryngology: Head & Neck Surgery. 4th Ed. New Hyde Park, NY, Medical Examination Pub. Co., 1987

Author J. Wolfrey, M.D.

Ovarian cancer

BASICS

DESCRIPTION A variety of malignancies that arise from the epithelium, stromal cells, or germ cells or are metastatic to the ovary
System(s) affected: Reproductive, Endocrine/Metabolic
Genetics: Epithelial ovarian cancer may have a subset of inherited tendencies - two documented first degree relatives with epithelial ovarian cancer may give risk of 50%
Incidence/Prevalence in USA:
• 12,000 deaths/year
• 5th leading cause of cancer death in women
Predominant age:
• Epithelial: 40-75 years
• Germ cell malignancies: 12-40 years (although epithelial still the most common malignancy in this age)
Predominant sex: Female only

SIGNS AND SYMPTOMS
• Vague gastrointestinal symptoms
• Bloating and dyspepsia
• Abdominal swelling, pain, and distention
• Occasional vaginal discharge
• Irregular vaginal bleeding
• Ascites
• Cul-de-sac and/or pelvic nodularity
• Pelvic mass
• Dyspareunia
• Weight loss

CAUSES Etiology unknown

RISK FACTORS
• Low parity
• Late pregnancies (over 30)
• Family history

DIAGNOSIS

DIFFERENTIAL DIAGNOSIS
• Gastrointestinal or other gynecologic malignancies
• Irritable bowel syndrome
• Colitis
• Hepatic failure with ascites

LABORATORY
• Cancer antigen (CA) 125 (normal < 35)
• Liver function tests (LFT) to rule out hepatic involvement
• Carcinoembryonic antigen (CEA) if gastrointestinal primary suspected
• Chorionic gonadotropin (beta-hCG); LDH isoenzymes if patient less than 40 years (for germ cell malignancies)
Drugs that may alter lab results: N/A
Disorders that may alter lab results: CA 125 may be elevated with benign disease (endometriosis, peritonitis, myomas) and with other malignancies

PATHOLOGICAL FINDINGS At surgery, most common type will be epithelial ovarian cancer and most common subtype will be serous cystadenocarcinoma

SPECIAL TESTS Pelvic ultrasound to differentiate other pelvic masses when ascites is not present, and examination not characteristic of ovarian cancer.

IMAGING If site of cancer is in question: Mammogram, barium enema (BE), upper gastrointestinal series (UGI), CT

DIAGNOSTIC PROCEDURES
• Surgery is definitive
• Occasionally paracentesis and thoracentesis for cytology may be helpful
• Guided needle aspiration of ovarian masses is not helpful

TREATMENT

APPROPRIATE HEALTH CARE
• Inpatient
• Surgical staging and primary debulking are critical. Chemotherapy and/or radiotherapy as recommended by oncologist.

GENERAL MEASURES
For epithelial malignancies:
◊ Total abdominal hysterectomy (TAH)/bilateral salpingo-oophorectomy (BSO)
◊ Omentectomy/debulking
◊ Staging biopsies including node sampling as indicated
For germ cell cancers (which are less likely to be bilateral):
◊ Salpingo-oophorectomy (unilateral if only one ovary involved)
◊ Careful staging, including lymph node dissection, may be adequate

ACTIVITY As tolerated

DIET
• High protein diet
• Follow serum protein closely with significant ascites

PATIENT EDUCATION
• "What You Need to Know About Ovarian Cancer" - National Institutes of Health pamphlet
• "Chemotherapy and You: A Guide to Self-Help During Treatment" - National Institutes of Health pamphlet

MEDICATIONS

DRUG(S) OF CHOICE
• Platinum-based regimen (cisplatin or carboplatin)
• Cyclophosphamide (Cytoxan)
• Paclitaxel (Taxol) presently released for therapy after failure of first-line or subsequent chemotherapy
• Other drugs based on current protocol
Contraindications: Cisplatin - impaired renal function, hearing loss, neuropathy
Precautions: All regimens cause bone marrow suppression. Cisplatin associated with ototoxicity, renal toxicity, and peripheral neuropathy.
Significant possible interactions: All regimens may cause clinically significant bone marrow suppression

ALTERNATIVE DRUGS
• Etoposide
• 5-Fluorouracil
• Adriamycin
• Other members of the alkylating agent family (melphalan, hexamethylmelamine, ifosfamide)

 FOLLOWUP

PATIENT MONITORING
• A logarithmic or sevenfold fall in CA 125 suggests a good response, but normal reading has only mild correlation with absence of disease
• A rise in CA 125 usually requires a change in therapy
• In germ cell cancers, markers should fall to normal range. Normal levels correlate closely with absence of disease.

PREVENTION/AVOIDANCE
• Prophylactic oophorectomy has been suggested for women with two first degree relatives with epithelial ovarian cancer
• Possible preventive role of oral contraceptive agents
• Mass screening for ovarian cancer by sonography and CA 125 still not cost-effective

POSSIBLE COMPLICATIONS
• Pleural effusion
• Pseudomyxoma
• Ascites
• Radiotherapy and chemotherapy adverse reactions
• Bowel obstruction

EXPECTED COURSE AND PROGNOSIS
• Dependent on cell type, stage and residual disease
• For stage I, 80% 5 year survival
• For stage II, 60% 5 year survival
• For stage III, (grade III epithelial cancer) 15-30% 5 year survival
• For stage IV, 10% 5 year survival

 MISCELLANEOUS

ASSOCIATED CONDITIONS
• Ascites
• Pleural effusion
• Decrease of serum albumin
• Breast carcinoma

AGE-RELATED FACTORS
Pediatric: N/A
Geriatric: N/A
Others: Patients under 60 have better prognosis

PREGNANCY N/A

SYNONYMS N/A

ICD-9-CM 183.0

SEE ALSO N/A

OTHER NOTES N/A

ABBREVIATIONS N/A

REFERENCES
• Bast, R.C., et al.: A Radioimmunoassay Using a Monoclonal Antibody to Monitor the Course of Epithelial Ovarian Cancer. New England Journal of Medicine, 1983:309:883-7
• Griffiths, T. & Parker, L.: Cancer of the Ovary. In Gynecologic Oncology. Edited by Knapp & Berkowitz. New York, Macmillan, 1986
• Classification and Staging of Gynecologic Malignancies. ACOG Technical Bulletin, 155, May 1991

Author J. Cain, M.D.

Ovarian tumor, benign

 BASICS

DESCRIPTION The ovaries are a source of more varieties of tumors (benign and malignant) than any other part of the body. Benign tumors of the ovary create difficulties in differential diagnosis because of the need to identify malignancy. The tumors are often clinically silent until well developed; may be solid, cystic or mixed; may be functional (producing sex steroids) or nonfunctional.
System(s) affected: Reproductive, Endocrine/Metabolic
Genetics: N/A
Incidence/Prevalence in USA: Unknown due to asymptomatic character
Predominant age:
• All ages
• Concern for malignancy greater in postmenopausal women
Predominant sex: Female only

SIGNS AND SYMPTOMS
• Usually asymptomatic
• Pain related to torsion, endometriosis, or rupture
• Swelling in abdomen or bladder
• Bowel pressure or bladder pressure sensations

CAUSES
• Endometriosis with localized, repeated ovarian hemorrhage
• Physiologic cysts
• Etiology unknown

RISK FACTORS None known

 DIAGNOSIS

DIFFERENTIAL DIAGNOSIS
• Malignancies
• Uterine myomas
• Appendiceal cysts
• Diverticulitis and abscesses
• Pelvic inflammatory disease with tubo-ovarian abscess
• Distended urinary bladder

LABORATORY
Serum tumor markers as indicated
  ◊ Cancer antigen (CA) 125
  ◊ Alpha fetoprotein (FP)
  ◊ Chorionic gonadotropin (beta-hCG)
Drugs that may alter lab results: N/A
Disorders that may alter lab results:
CA 125
  ◊ Endometriosis
  ◊ Peritonitis
  ◊ Pelvic inflammatory disease (PID)
  ◊ Other cancers

PATHOLOGICAL FINDINGS
Benign
  ◊ Simple cysts
  ◊ Physiologic cysts
  ◊ Endometrioma
  ◊ Epithelial cysts
  ◊ Granulosa cell/stromal tumors
  ◊ Fibroma
  ◊ Cystic teratoma

DIAGNOSTIC PROCEDURES N/A

SPECIAL TESTS
• Pelvic exam is the most important
• Careful physical exam

IMAGING May differentiate tumors from other pelvic masses and identify features at high risk for malignancy, e.g., solid component, papillations, multiple septations

 TREATMENT

APPROPRIATE HEALTH CARE
Inpatient if surgery necessary

GENERAL MEASURES
Surgical removal of tumor to establish diagnosis
  ◊ Premenopausal cysts greater than 5 cm or that persist
  ◊ Postmenopausal cysts
  ◊ Cysts with worrisome ultrasound features

ACTIVITY As tolerated

DIET No special diet

PATIENT EDUCATION Dependent on etiology, e.g., endometriosis vs. pelvic inflammatory disease vs. physiologic

MEDICATIONS

DRUG(S) OF CHOICE Oral contraceptives may be helpful in premenopausal patients to differentiate physiologic cysts. Suppression of formation of new cysts by this method and reexamination may resolve the issue.
Contraindications: Refer to manufacturer's profile of each drug
Precautions: Refer to manufacturer's profile of each drug
Significant possible interactions: Refer to manufacturer's profile of each drug

ALTERNATIVE DRUGS N/A

FOLLOWUP

PATIENT MONITORING
• Most require only yearly exams
• Varies by diagnosis

PREVENTION/AVOIDANCE Use of oral contraceptives may decrease risk

POSSIBLE COMPLICATIONS
Complications of untreated dermoid and mucinous cysts may include pseudomyxoma peritonei

EXPECTED COURSE AND PROGNOSIS Complete cure

MISCELLANEOUS

ASSOCIATED CONDITIONS N/A

AGE-RELATED FACTORS
Pediatric: N/A
Geriatric: Concern greater with postmenopausal emergence of ovarian masses
Others: N/A

PREGNANCY Rarely, tumors may be detected during pregnancy examinations

SYNONYMS N/A

ICD-9-CM 220 benign neoplasm of ovary

SEE ALSO N/A

OTHER NOTES N/A

ABBREVIATIONS N/A

REFERENCES
• Benacerrif, B.R., Finkler, N.J., et al: Sonographic Accuracy in the Diagnosis of Ovarian Masses. Journal of Reproductive Medicine 35:491-5, 1990
• Bird, C., et al.: Benign Neoplasms of the Ovary. In Clinical Gynecology. Edited by J. Sciarra and W. Droegmuller. Philadelphia, J.B. Lippincott, 1990
• Cain, J.: Pelvic Mass: Detection, Diagnosis and Management. In Office Gynecology. Edited by M. Stenchever. St. Louis, Mosby Year Book, Inc., 1991

Author J. Cain, M.D.

Paget's disease of the breast

BASICS

DESCRIPTION Rare type of carcinoma that appears unilaterally as dermatitis of the nipple, representing an extension to the epidermis of an underlying carcinoma of a mammary duct.
System(s) affected: Skin/Exocrine
Genetics: No known genetic pattern
Incidence in USA: 1000-4000 new cases each year
Prevalence in USA: Approximately 2% of all cases of breast cancer
Predominant age: 40-75
Predominant sex: Female

SIGNS AND SYMPTOMS
• Nipple skin changes that do not respond to conservative treatment
• Nipple itching
• Nipple burning
• Nipple oozing
• Nipple bleeding
• Eczematoid nipple changes
• Breast mass
• Nipple fissures
• Nipple ulceration
• Local hyperemia
• Local edema

CAUSES   Unknown

RISK FACTORS   Same as for non-heritable breast carcinoma

DIAGNOSIS

DIFFERENTIAL DIAGNOSIS
• Eczema
• Psoriasis
• Skin tumors (e.g., Bowen's disease)
• Squamous cell carcinoma
• Basal cell carcinoma

LABORATORY   N/A
Drugs that may alter lab results: N/A
Disorders that may alter lab results: N/A

PATHOLOGICAL FINDINGS
• Micro - malignant cell invasion of the epidermis with large pale staining sells
• Underlying ductal adenocarcinoma

SPECIAL TESTS   N/A

IMAGING   Mammography - useful, but cannot exclude malignancy without clinicopathological correlation

DIAGNOSTIC PROCEDURES   Any chronic or nonhealing nipple lesion should be biopsied

TREATMENT

APPROPRIATE HEALTH CARE As determined by surgical consultant

GENERAL MEASURES
• Surgery
• Radiotherapy
• Chemotherapy
• Hormonal manipulation

ACTIVITY   Full activity

DIET   No special diet

PATIENT EDUCATION   National Cancer Institute, Dept. of Health And Human Services, Public Inquiries Section, Office of Cancer Communications, Building 31, Room 101-18, 9000 Rockville Pike, Bethesda, MD 20892, (301)496-5583

MEDICATIONS

DRUG(S) OF CHOICE According to protocols supervised by an oncologist
Contraindications: Refer to manufacturer's literature
Precautions: Refer to manufacturer's literature
Significant possible interactions: Refer to manufacturer's literature

ALTERNATIVE DRUGS N/A

FOLLOWUP

PATIENT MONITORING As dictated by needs of the various therapy modalities

PREVENTION/AVOIDANCE None known

POSSIBLE COMPLICATIONS
Metastases

EXPECTED COURSE AND PROGNOSIS
• Dependent on stage of underlying breast carcinoma
Stage and 10 year disease free survival
◊ 1 - 70-95%
◊ 2 - 40-45%%
◊ 3 - 10-15%
◊ 4 - < 5%

MISCELLANEOUS

ASSOCIATED CONDITIONS Underlying carcinoma

AGE-RELATED FACTORS
Pediatric: N/A
Geriatric: N/A
Others: N/A

PREGNANCY N/A

SYNONYMS N/A

ICD-9-CM
174.0 malignant neoplasm of breast and areola

SEE ALSO N/A

OTHER NOTES Extramammary Paget's disease can also occur

ABBREVIATIONS N/A

REFERENCES
• Bland, K.I. & Copeland, E.M. (eds.): The Breast. Philadelphia, W.B. Saunders Co., 1991
• Fitzpatrick, T.B., et al. (eds.): Dermatology In General Medicine, 3rd Ed. New York, McGraw-Hill, 1987
• DeVita, V.T., Jr., Hellman, S. & Rosenberg, S.A. (eds.): Cancer: Principles and Practices of Oncology. 3rd Ed. Philadelphia, J.B. Lippincott, 1989

Author M. Horattas, M.D.

Pancreatic cancer, exocrine

BASICS

DESCRIPTION Pancreatic exocrine malignancies (including adenocarcinoma, 90%; cystadenocarcinoma; and acinar cell carcinoma) represent 3% of all cancers but the fifth most common cause of cancer deaths in the United States.
These malignancies are divided into two broad categories:
◊ Periampullary lesions - most commonly adenocarcinoma of the head of the pancreas. Of lesser frequency are malignant lesions of the ampulla, duodenum and common bile duct. Lesions in these areas are characterized by jaundice, weight loss and abdominal pain.
◊ Lesions of body and tail - account for thirty percent of adenocarcinomas of the pancreas. Due to retroperitoneal location and distance from common bile duct, lesions tend to be much larger at diagnosis. Common symptoms are those of weight loss and pain.
System(s) affected: Gastrointestinal
Genetics: More common in Blacks, diabetic patients
Incidence/Prevalence in USA:
• Approximately 28,000 new cases diagnosed per year
• Varies among ethnic groups, highest in Blacks and Hawaiians
Predominant age: Mean age in males = 63 years, females = 67 years
Predominant sex: Male > Female (1.5-2:1)

SIGNS AND SYMPTOMS
• Weight loss (90%)
• Pain (75%)
• Jaundice (65%)
• Anorexia (60%)
• Pruritis (40%)
• Diabetes mellitus (15%)
• Malnutrition (75%)
• Hepatomegaly (65%)
• Jaundice (70%)
• Palpable gallbladder (25%)
• Abdominal tenderness (20%)
• Mass (10%)
• Ascites (5%)

CAUSES
• No known etiology, though many associations
• Associations include race, diabetes mellitus, tobacco, environmental and occupational exposures, and dietary lipids
• Of interest, seemingly no association between pancreatitis, alcohol and coffee consumption when data adjusted for effect of tobacco use

RISK FACTORS
• Probable: Race, diabetes mellitus, tobacco
• Possible: Environmental/occupational exposures, dietary lipids

DIAGNOSIS

DIFFERENTIAL DIAGNOSIS
• Choledocholithiasis
• Pancreatitis
• Pancreatic pseudocyst
• Cholangiocarcinoma
• Carcinoma of the ampulla of Vater
• Duodenal neoplasms
• Miscellaneous malignancies with extrinsic bile duct compression
• Biliary tract stricture
• Choledochal cyst

LABORATORY
• Bilirubin level mean of 15 mg/dl in patients with jaundice due to pancreatic cancer; considerably higher than that in patients with benign diseases (choledocholithiasis, strictures)
• Patients with recent onset of jaundice with bilirubin greater than 10 mg/dl should be considered to have neoplastic obstruction of common bile duct until proven otherwise
• Alkaline phosphatase elevated in most patients. Mean of 550 IU/L not significantly different from level in patients with bile duct obstruction from benign disease
• Anemia present in approximately 60% of patients
• Stool occult blood present in approximately 90% of patients with periampullary tumors
• Elevated amylase found in less than 5% of patients
Tumor markers:
◊ Relatively recent developments. In general, useful for screening and assessment of extent of disease. Likely to have good specificity when multiple marker assays combined. Represent a dynamic area of research and discovery of new markers and development of sensitive and specific assays likely in the future.
◊ CA 19-9: Elevated in serum and pancreatic juice of patients with pancreatic cancer. Sensitivity/specificity in differentiating pancreatitis is undetermined.
◊ Carcinoembryonic antigen (CEA): Serum and pancreatic juice levels elevated beyond 10 ng./ml and 30 ng./ml respectively in patients with pancreatic cancer.
◊ Pancreatic-oncofetal antigen: Sensitivity of 68% when used as screening test. Combining test with CEA and alpha-fetoprotein increases specificity.
◊ Galactosyltransferase isoenzyme II: Sensitivity of 67.2% and specificity of 98.2% in pancreatic cancer. Cannot distinguish between pancreatic cancer and malignancies of other intra-abdominal organs.
Drugs that may alter lab results: N/A
Disorders that may alter lab results: N/A

PATHOLOGICAL FINDINGS
• Adenocarcinoma (90%)
• Acinar cell carcinoma (1.2%)
• Other (0.8%)
• Uncertain (9.2%)

SPECIAL TESTS Pancreatic juice - for cytology and CEA, CA 19-9 assays

IMAGING
• Upper GI series - widening of duodenal sweep in large tumors
• CT scan - most useful imaging modality
• Ultrasound - limited by overlying bowel, less accuracy in staging
• MRI
• Endoscopic retrograde cholangiopancreatography (ERCP) - particularly useful in ampullary or duodenal lesions where biopsy may be performed, pancreatic juice sampled and pancreatic duct cytology
• PTC - delineates proximal biliary tree, important data in planning reconstruction following surgical procedure
• Angiography - role in preoperative staging, not in tumor localization

DIAGNOSTIC PROCEDURES
Biopsy:
◊ CT-guided percutaneous needle aspiration has sensitivity of 85% with specificity of approximately 100% in pancreatic adenocarcinoma. Few complications and extremely low risk of tract seeding.
◊ Pseudocyst aspiration can differentiate benign pseudocysts from cystadenocarcinoma. Fluid in cystadenocarcinoma has low amylase, high CEA and lactate dehydrogenase (LDH) levels, and malignant cells are usually present.
◊ Liver biopsy may be useful in patients with hepatic metastases
◊ Laparoscopy with biopsy is becoming a popular technique and is likely to be more frequently used in the future
Esophagogastroduodenoscopy:
◊ Useful for evaluation of ampulla and duodenal regions in patients with periampullary picture and normal CT or MRI

TREATMENT

APPROPRIATE HEALTH CARE
Inpatient for testing, preliminary therapy, surgery or other protocols

GENERAL MEASURES
• Management highly variable and influenced by the overall health of the patient, presence of metastases, and location and size of tumor
• Analgesia
• Management of pruritis
• Control of diabetes (usually "brittle") if total pancreatectomy performed
Surgical procedures
◊ Pancreaticoduodenectomy (Whipple's procedure)
◊ Total pancreatectomy
◊ Regional pancreatectomy - resection pancreas, portal vein, regional nodes, subtotal gastrectomy
◊ Biliary decompression for unresectable disease - T-tube, bilio-enteric anastomoses
◊ Gastrojejunostomy for gastric outlet obstruction in unresectable disease
Non-operative procedures
◊ Biliary decompression by use of endoprostheses, transhepatic drainage catheters
◊ Celiac blockade and epidural catheter placement for analgesia
◊ Chemotherapy - multiple protocols
◊ Radiation therapy - external beam (intraoperative - largely investigational)

ACTIVITY   Ad lib

DIET   As tolerated. Serve small frequent meals.

PATIENT EDUCATION   Printed patient information available from: National Cancer Institute, Dept. of Health And Human Services, Public Inquiries Section, Office of Cancer Communications, Building 31, Room 101-18, 9000 Rockville Pike, Bethesda, MD 20892, (301)496-5583

MEDICATIONS

DRUG(S) OF CHOICE
• Analgesics
• Management of pruritis, e.g., phenothiazines or cholestyramine
• Chemotherapy - multiple protocols
• Antacids
• Pancreatic enzymes
• Diabetes control
Contraindications: N/A
Precautions: N/A
Significant possible interactions: N/A

ALTERNATIVE DRUGS   N/A

FOLLOWUP

PATIENT MONITORING   Variable

PREVENTION/AVOIDANCE   Avoid tobacco

POSSIBLE COMPLICATIONS
• Pain
• Jaundice
• Malnutrition
• Diabetes - especially in patients undergoing total pancreatectomy
• Operative mortality - varies from 10-40%

EXPECTED COURSE AND PROGNOSIS
• Three year survival - 2.5%
• Five year survival - 1%
• Following surgery for potentially curable disease, five year survival is about 4%. Reflects high likelihood of metastases at the time of diagnosis.

MISCELLANEOUS

ASSOCIATED CONDITIONS
• Diabetes
• Other findings associated with metastases, e.g., superior vena cava syndrome, Horner's syndrome

AGE-RELATED FACTORS
Pediatric: N/A
Geriatric: More common in this age group, particularly males
Others: N/A

PREGNANCY   N/A

SYNONYMS   N/A

ICD-9-CM   157.0 (site specified 157.x)

SEE ALSO   N/A

OTHER NOTES   N/A

ABBREVIATIONS
• CEA = carcinoembryonic antigen
• CA = cancer antigen

REFERENCES   Howard, J.M., Jordan, G.L. & Reber, H.A. (eds.): Surgical Diseases of the Pancreas. Philadelphia, Lea and Febiger, 1987

Author   L. Mercer, M.D. & E.C. Saltzstein, M.D.

Pancreatitis

 BASICS

DESCRIPTION An inflammatory,
auto-digestive process of the pancreas
Acute pancreatitis
◊ Inflammatory episode with symptoms related to intrapancreatic activation of enzymes with pain, nausea and vomiting, and associated intestinal ileus
◊ It varies widely in severity, complications and prognosis
Chronic pancreatitis
◊ Progressive functional destruction of the pancreas that may exist in the absence of an etiology
◊ Results in both exocrine and endocrine deficiencies
◊ Pain, maldigestion and diabetes mellitus are the major features
System(s) affected: Gastrointestinal
Genetics: Hereditary pancreatitis is a very rare condition with an autosomally dominant inheritance pattern
Incidence/Prevalence in USA: Urban - 22/100,00; rural - 10/100,000
Predominant age:
• Acute pancreatitis - none
• Chronic pancreatitis - 35-45 years (usually related to alcohol)
Predominant sex: Male = Female

SIGNS AND SYMPTOMS
• Abdominal pain - epigastric, may radiate straight through to back
• Nausea and/or vomiting
• Mild abdominal distention
• Fever (100-101° F)
• Hypotension/shock (40%)
• Mild jaundice
• Diminished or absent bowel sounds
• Flank discoloration (Grey Turner's sign)
• Umbilical discoloration (Cullen's sign)
• Pleural effusion

CAUSES
• Cholelithiasis/choledocholithiasis
• Alcoholism and acute intoxication
• Medications
• Metabolic hypercalcemia, hypertriglyceridemia
• Penetrating peptic ulcer
• Trauma/surgery
• Viral infections
• Endoscopic retrograde cholangiopancreatography (ERCP)
• Idiopathic
• Biliary tract disease
• Tumor
• Systemic lupus erythematosus
• Mumps
• Salmonella
• Streptococcus
• Cytomegalovirus
• Cystic fibrosis

RISK FACTORS Listed with Causes

 DIAGNOSIS

DIFFERENTIAL DIAGNOSIS
Acute pancreatitis
◊ Penetrating or perforated peptic ulcer
◊ Acute cholecystitis
◊ Choledocholithiasis
◊ Macroamylasemia, macrolipasemia
◊ Mesenteric vascular obstruction and/or infarction
◊ Perforation of a viscous
◊ Intestinal obstruction
Chronic pancreatitis
◊ Pancreatic cancer
◊ Other malabsorptive processes

LABORATORY
Acute pancreatitis
◊ Elevated serum amylase
◊ Elevated serum lipase
◊ Elevated (mild) alanine aminotransferase (ALT) and/or aspartate aminotransferase (AST) - when associated with alcoholic hepatitis or choledocholithiasis
◊ Elevated alkaline phosphatase (mild) - when associated with alcoholic hepatitis or choledocholithiasis
◊ Hyperbilirubinemia - when associated with alcoholic hepatitis or choledocholithiasis
◊ Glucose increased - in severe disease
◊ Calcium decreased - in severe disease
◊ WBC 10,000 - 25,000
Chronic pancreatitis
◊ Sometimes none
◊ Hyperglycemia
◊ Steatorrhea
◊ Flare-ups may mimic acute pancreatitis
Drugs that may alter lab results: Insulin and corticosteroids
Disorders that may alter lab results:
• Biliary tract disease
• Penetrating peptic ulcer
• Intestinal obstruction
• Intestinal ischemia/infarction
• Ruptured ectopic Pregnancy
• Renal insufficiency
• Burns
• Macroamylasemia

PATHOLOGICAL FINDINGS
Acute pancreatitis
◊ Autodigestion of the pancreas
◊ Interstitial edema
◊ Hemorrhage
◊ Cell and fat necrosis
Chronic pancreatitis
◊ Calcification
◊ Fibrosis

SPECIAL TESTS N/A

IMAGING
Acute pancreatitis
◊ Plain film of abdomen - signs of ileus
◊ Chest x-ray - pleural effusion
◊ Ultrasound/CT scan of abdomen
◊ Endoscopic retrograde cholangiopancreatography (ERCP)
Chronic pancreatitis
◊ X-ray of abdomen - pancreatic calcification
◊ Ultrasound and/or CT scan of abdomen - pseudocyst formation/calcification
◊ Endoscopic retrograde cholangiopancreatography (ERCP) - ductal deformity, retained common bile duct (CBD) stone
◊ Endoscopic sphincterotomy - early CBD stone removal improves outlook

DIAGNOSTIC PROCEDURES For
chronic pancreatitis - secretin stimulation test; para-aminobenzoic acid test (bentiromide [Chymex] test)

 TREATMENT

APPROPRIATE HEALTH CARE
• Acute pancreatitis - hospitalization, unless mild and able to maintain po intake
• Chronic pancreatitis - outpatient except for complications

GENERAL MEASURES
Acute pancreatitis
◊ P - pain control: meperidine
◊ A - arrest shock: IV fluids
◊ N - nasogastric tube for vomiting
◊ C - calcium monitoring
◊ R - renal evaluation
◊ E - ensure pulmonary function
◊ A - avoid oral feeding
◊ S - surgery
Chronic pancreatitis
◊ Pain - abstinence from alcohol, analgesia (avoid narcotics if possible), celiac ganglion block, surgery, pancreatic enzyme preparations
◊ Maldigestion - pancreatic enzyme supplements, H2-blockers
◊ Diabetes mellitus - insulin

ACTIVITY
• Acute pancreatitis - usually bedrest although sitting in a chair may be more comfortable. Advance as able.
• Chronic pancreatitis - not restricted

DIET
• Acute pancreatitis - begin diet after pain, tenderness and ileus have resolved; small amounts of high carbohydrate, low fat and low protein foods. Advance as tolerated.
• Chronic pancreatitis - small meals high in protein. Adjust if diabetes mellitus is present.

PATIENT EDUCATION For patient
education materials favorably reviewed on this topic, contact: National Digestive Diseases Information Clearinghouse, Box NDDIC, Bethesda, MD 20892, (301)468-6344

MEDICATIONS

DRUG(S) OF CHOICE
Acute pancreatitis
◊ Meperidine (Demerol) 50-100 mg IM/IV every 3-4 hours
Chronic pancreatitis
◊ Analgesics (acetaminophen [Tylenol], oxycodone/hydrocodone [Tylox/Vicodin])
◊ Pancreatic enzyme supplements (Pancrease MT, Creon)
◊ H2-blockers (reducing gastric acid increases availability of pancreatic enzymes)
Contraindications: Nor-meperidine, a metabolite of meperidine, may accumulate following several days of round-the-clock dosing. May cause mental status changes or seizures.
Precautions: Narcotic addiction
Significant possible interactions: Refer to manufacturer's profile of each drug

ALTERNATIVE DRUGS   N/A

FOLLOWUP

PATIENT MONITORING
• Assure alcohol abstinence
• Follow and correct any etiologic cause - hypertriglycerides, choledocholithiasis

PREVENTION/AVOIDANCE   Avoid alcohol

POSSIBLE COMPLICATIONS
• Acute pancreatitis - pseudocyst
• Chronic pancreatitis - pseudocyst, abscess, biliary/duodenal obstruction, portal/splenic vein thrombosis

EXPECTED COURSE AND PROGNOSIS
• Acute pancreatitis - 85-90% resolve spontaneously, 3-5% mortality
• Chronic pancreatitis - may have recurrent episodes of "acute pancreatitis", slow progression, may "burn out" with resolution of symptoms. Narcotic addiction frequent.
• The following factors are accompanied by poor prognosis:
On admission
◊ Age > 55 years
◊ WBC > 16,000/mm
◊ Blood glucose > 200 mg/dL
◊ Serum LDH > 2 x normal
◊ Serum SGOT > 6 x normal
Within 48 hours
◊ Hematocrit decrease > 10%
◊ Serum calcium < 8 mg/dL
◊ BUN increase > 5 mg/dL
◊ Arterial pO2 < 60 mm Hg
◊ Base deficit > 4 mEq/L
◊ Fluid retention > 61

MISCELLANEOUS

ASSOCIATED CONDITIONS   N/A

AGE-RELATED FACTORS
Pediatric: Mumps, sometimes complicated by pancreatitis
Geriatric: Vascular disease
Others: N/A

PREGNANCY   Acute fatty liver of pregnancy

SYNONYMS   N/A

ICD-9-CM
• Acute pancreatitis - 577.0
• Chronic pancreatitis - 577.1

SEE ALSO
• Choledocholithiasis
• Alcoholism
• Peptic ulcer

OTHER NOTES   N/A

ABBREVIATIONS   N/A

REFERENCES
• Silverman, A. & Roy, C.R.: Pediatric Clinical Gastroenterology. St Louis, The C.V. Mosby Co., 1983
• Sleisenger, M.H. & Fordtran, J.S. (eds.): Gastrointestinal Disease: Pathophysiology, Diagnosis, Management. 4th Ed. Philadelphia, W.B. Saunders Co., 1989

Author   D. Roe, M.D.

Parkinson's disease

 BASICS

DESCRIPTION Parkinson's disease is an adult onset neurodegenerative disorder of the extrapyramidal system characterized by a combination of tremor at rest, rigidity and bradykinesia. The diagnosis requires therapeutic response to levodopa which implies normal striatal neurons. This is the only neurodegenerative disease which is treatable long term.
Genetics: Five percent of the patients have a positive family history
System(s) affected: Neurologic and musculoskeletal
Incidence/Prevalence in USA: 50,000 per year
Predominant age: Age 60 with 5% between the ages of 21 and 39
Predominant sex: Male > female (1.4:1)

SIGNS AND SYMPTOMS
Cardinal signs
Tremor in repose
  ◊ Diagnostic but not required
  ◊ Brings most patients to treatment
  ◊ 48 cycles per second
  ◊ Relieve with activity, concentration, and sleep
  ◊ Increased with stress
  ◊ 10% present with only tremor
  ◊ 30% present without
  ◊ Most begin unilateral tremor
Bradykinesia
  ◊ Required for diagnosis
  ◊ Most disabling
  ◊ Problem with initiation with movement
  ◊ Can be overcome with will to do so
  ◊ Etiology of the gait disturbance
  ◊ Postural abnormalities
Rigidity
  ◊ Lead pipe type
  ◊ Cogwheeling with tremor
Other associated signs and symptom
 • Speech is poorly enunciated, low volume, clipped
 • Ocular abnormalities consisting of: Decreased blinking, blepharospasm, impaired conugate upward gaze
 • Seborrhea
 • Dysautonomia presenting as constipation, incontinence, sexual dysfunction
 • Depression in 2/3 of patients
 • Dementia in 20% of patients
 • Gait disturbances including:no arm swing, en mass turning, problems getting up from chair, festination, freezing
 • Leaning posture
 • Propulsion or retropulsion
 • Micrographia
 • Mask faces
 • Neglect of swallowing with drooling

CAUSES
 • Unknown
 • Lost of dopaminergic neurons in the substantia nigra with rate of loss 1% per year in patients with Parkinson's versus 0.5% in normal aging.
 • Probably not genetic rather toxic or infectious
 • Known toxic substance is MPTP exposure
 • Other non-dopaminergic neurons can also be effected.

RISK FACTORS Unknown in the idiopathic disease

 DIAGNOSIS

DIFFERENTIAL DIAGNOSIS
Parkinsonism: bradykinesia and occasionally tremor with little or no response to levodopa indicating that the striatal neurons are also degenerated
  ◊ Progressive supranuclear palsy
  ◊ Multisystem atrophy
  ◊ Alzheimer's disease with extrapyramidal features
  ◊ Side effects of neuroleptic medications
  ◊ Infectious - postencephalitic
  ◊ Vascular - lacunar state
  ◊ Toxins
  ◊ Metabolic - Wilson's disease
Benign essential tremor

LABORATORY N/A
Drugs that may alter lab results: N/A
Disorders that may alter lab results: N/A

PATHOLOGICAL FINDINGS Typical changes that allow precise pathological diagnosis. Lewy bodies

SPECIAL TESTS N/A

IMAGING
 • CT or MRI can eliminate disorders that mimic Parkinson's
 • PET scanning

DIAGNOSTIC PROCEDURES N/A

 TREATMENT

APPROPRIATE HEALTH CARE
Outpatient except for complications or elective surgery

GENERAL MEASURES
 • Investigate for a possible drug-induced cause and if found, discontinue the drug. Complete resolution of symptoms may take weeks to months.
 • No curative therapy available for primary Parkinson's. Therapy is individualized.
 • Disease involves lifelong treatment directed toward symptom control and slowing progression of the disease
 • Physical, occupational and speech therapy may be useful
 • Patient's physical limitations may require many adjustments in the home, e.g., special chairs, elevated toilet seat, eating utensils, dressing oneself
 • Surgery (sometimes)

ACTIVITY
 • Maintain activity to whatever degree possible
 • Use cane for walking

DIET
 • Small frequent meals, if patient has difficulty eating
 • High liquid intake important
 • High bulk foods
 • Reduced protein diet is unnecessary

PATIENT EDUCATION
 • Refer patient to local support groups, when available
Printed patient information available from:
  ◊ United Parkinson Foundation, 360 W. Superior St., Chicago, IL 60610, (312)664-2344
  ◊ Parkinson's Education Program - USA, 3900 Birch Street, #105, Newport Beach, CA 92660, (800)344-7872

MEDICATIONS

DRUG(S) OF CHOICE
General principles
◊ Treat disability
◊ Drugs can have added therapeutic and toxic effects
◊ Acute worsening may indicate failure to take medications or depression or a supervening illness
◊ Course is progressive with or without medication
Levodopa/carbidopa
◊ Mainstay of treatment for disability
◊ Start with 1/2 of a 25/100 mg tablet 3 times a day
◊ Dosage range is from 300-1,000/75-200 of the combination daily
◊ If using continued release form start with 50/200 2 times daily
◊ If switching to the continuous release increase the usual daily dose 110%
Agonist - bromocriptine, pergolide
◊ Low potency
◊ Works best as an adjunct to levodopa/carbidopa
◊ Titrate the Levodopa/carbidopa combination downward as these agents are added such that 1 mg of bromocriptine equals 10 mg of levodopa and 1 mg of pergolide = 10 mg of bromocriptine
◊ Usual starting dose 2.5 mg of bromocriptine or .05 mg of pergolide t.i.d
MAO inhibitors - selegiline
◊ Blocks metabolism of dopa in the brain
◊ May prevent progression
◊ Is being used early in patients without significant disability to prolong the time prior to need for levodopa/carbidopa
◊ Usual dose is 5 mg in the morning and 5 mg at noon to avoid sleep disturbance
Anticholinergic
◊ Thirty percent improvement in 50% of the patients
◊ For tremor in early stages or as an adjunct
◊ Trihexyphenidyl hydrochloride (Artane): 1 mg on may 1, increase by 2 mg every 3-5 days until dose of 6-10 mg/day is given
◊ Benztropine (Cogentin): Usual dose 1-2 mg once a day. Start with low doses, 0.5 mg/day and increase dose slowly by 0.5 mg every 5-6 days. Maximum dose 6 mg.
Dopamine release stimulator-Amantadine
◊ Useful early in the disease for bradykinesia and rigidity
◊ Synergistic with L-dopa
◊ Start with 100 mg daily then maybe increased to 100 mg bid
Contraindications: Refer to manufacturer's literature
Precautions:
L-dopa/carbidopa
◊ Time related dosage problems which occur in 50% of patients in 4-5 years
◊ Dyskinesia's (chorea, athetosis, and dystonia) probably secondary to receptor hypersensitivity. Usually occurs at peak levels of the drug or 2 hours after the immediate release form.

◊ Wear-off phenomena usually occurs 3-4 hours after the last dose.Can be improved using the sustained release form with the addition of an agonist
◊ On/off phenomena. 15-20% of patients develop severe fluctuation of response causing this syndrome. Most difficult side effect to treat.
Agonist
◊ Can induce nausea, orthostatic hypertension nightmares, hallucinations, agitation
◊ Can induce Raynaud's phenomena in doses greater than 30 mg per day, edema, hypertension, worsening CHF
MAO inhibitor:
◊ Can cause anxiety and sleep disturbance
Anticholinergics:
◊ Can induce confusion, constipation, urinary retention, dry mouth and glaucoma
Dopamine release stimulator:
◊ Can induce confusion, hallucinations, edema, livedo reticularis, and worsening CHF
Significant possible interactions: Most of the drugs have additive therapeutic and side effects

ALTERNATIVE DRUGS
• Tricyclic antidepressants for night time sedation and associated depression
• Antioxidants or vitamin-E have shown no definite benefit to this point
• Current investigation includes selective catechol-O-methyltransferase inhibitors
• New agonist to effect another of the 5 dopamine receptors
• Inhibition of the subthalamic nucleus, and neuronal growth factors
• Adrenal brain transplants
• Thalamotomy, unilateral for tremor are being studied

FOLLOWUP

PATIENT MONITORING   Lifelong for medication adjustment and physical therapy

PREVENTION/AVOIDANCE
Avoid drugs known to cause tardive dyskinesia, such as:
◊ Fluphenazine
◊ Perphenazine
◊ Prochlorperazine
◊ Thiopropazate
◊ Trifluoperazine
◊ Promazine
◊ Thioridazine
◊ Haloperidol
◊ Droperidol
◊ Benperidol
◊ Fluspirilene
◊ Pimozide
◊ Trifluperidol
◊ Chlorprothixene
◊ Clopenthixol
◊ Thiothixene

EXPECTED COURSE AND PROGNOSIS
Slowly progressive

POSSIBLE COMPLICATIONS
• Dementia
• Depression
• Aspiration pneumonia
• Falls
• Freezing
• Dyskinesias

MISCELLANEOUS

ASSOCIATED CONDITIONS
• Psychosis
• Depression

AGE-RELATED FACTORS
Pediatric: May occur as secondary parkinsonism in this age group
Geriatric: Common among elderly
Others: N/A

PREGNANCY   N/A

SYNONYMS
• Paralysis agitans
• Shaking palsy

ICD-9-CM   332.0 paralysis agitans

SEE ALSO   N/A

OTHER NOTES   New approaches in treatment of Parkinson's disease currently undergoing study (e.g., earlier diagnosis, experimental medications, surgical procedures and treatment to prevent its progression)

ABBREVIATIONS   N/A

REFERENCES
• Koller, W.C. & Zilkoski, M.: Parkinson's Disease. Amer Acad Fam Phy Monograph, Spring, 1992
• Stern, M: Parkinson's Disease: Early Diagnosis and Management. J Fam Pract. 1993: 36:439-446

Author   J. Minteer, M.D.

Paronychia

BASICS

DESCRIPTION Infectious inflammation of the folds of skin surrounding the fingernail or toenail. May be acute or chronic.
System(s) affected: Skin/Exocrine
Genetics: No known genetic pattern
Incidence/Prevalence in USA: Common
Predominant age: All ages
Predominant sex: Female > Male

SIGNS AND SYMPTOMS
• Separation of nail fold from nail plate
• Red, painful swelling of skin around nail plate
• Purulent

CAUSES
• Acute - Staphylococcus aureus. Less frequently by Streptococci and Pseudomonas.
• Chronic - Candida albicans. Less frequently by fungi.

RISK FACTORS
• Acute - trauma to skin surrounding nail, ingrown nails
• Chronic - frequent immersion of hands in water, diabetes mellitus

DIAGNOSIS

DIFFERENTIAL DIAGNOSIS Herpetic whitlow, felon

LABORATORY
• Gram stain
• KOH preparation
• Culture and sensitivity
Drugs that may alter lab results: N/A
Disorders that may alter lab results: N/A

PATHOLOGICAL FINDINGS N/A

SPECIAL TESTS None

IMAGING N/A

DIAGNOSTIC PROCEDURES N/A

TREATMENT

APPROPRIATE HEALTH CARE
Outpatient

GENERAL MEASURES
• Incision and drainage (I&D) of abscess, if present. If there is a subungual abscess or ingrown nail present, will need partial or complete removal of nail.
• Acute - warm compresses or soaks, elevation
• Chronic - keep fingers dry

ACTIVITY Full activity

DIET No special diet

PATIENT EDUCATION Chronic - keep fingers dry

MEDICATIONS

DRUG(S) OF CHOICE
• Acute (if diabetic, suppurative or more severe cases) - dicloxacillin 125-500 mg q6h, cloxacillin 250-500 mg q6h, erythromycin 500 mg q6h, cephalexin (Keflex) 250 mg q6h
• Chronic - topical antifungals - nystatin, imidazoles (e.g., clotrimazole, ketoconazole) for 2-3 months. Drying agents prn, e.g., Castellani's paint.
• Systemic ketoconazole also of help
Contraindications: Allergy to antibiotic
Precautions: Erythromycin may cause significant gastrointestinal upset
Significant possible interactions:
• Erythromycin affects levels of theophylline and effects of carbamazepine, digoxin and corticosteroids
• Ketoconazole - terfenadine

ALTERNATIVE DRUGS N/A

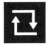
FOLLOWUP

PATIENT MONITORING Routine followup until healed

PREVENTION/AVOIDANCE
• Chronic - avoid frequent wetting of hands, wear rubber gloves
• Good diabetic control

POSSIBLE COMPLICATIONS
• Acute - subungual abscess
• Chronic - secondary ridging, thickening and discoloration of nail, nail loss

EXPECTED COURSE AND PROGNOSIS With adequate treatment and prevention, healing can be expected

MISCELLANEOUS

ASSOCIATED CONDITIONS Diabetes mellitus

AGE-RELATED FACTORS
Pediatric: Anaerobes may be involved in cases with thumb/finger sucking
Geriatric: N/A
Others: N/A

PREGNANCY N/A

SYNONYMS
• Eponychia
• Perionychia

ICD-9-CM
• Finger - 681.02
• Chronic candidal - 112.3

SEE ALSO N/A

OTHER NOTES May be considered work-related in bartenders, waitresses, nurses and others who often wet their hands

ABBREVIATIONS N/A

REFERENCES Fitzpatrick, T.B., et al. (eds.): Dermatology In General Medicine. 3rd Ed. New York, McGraw-Hill, 1987

Author M. Davidson, M.D.

Patent ductus arteriosus

BASICS

DESCRIPTION Patent ductus arteriosus (PDA) is the failure of the ductus arteriosus to close after birth. 75% of time occurs as isolated defect.
System(s) affected: Cardiovascular
Genetics: No Mendelian inheritance. 1% chance of PDA in infant if one parent affected.
Incidence/Prevalence in USA: 8/1000 live births
Predominant age: Infancy
Predominant sex: Female > Male (2-3:1)

SIGNS AND SYMPTOMS
Children
  ◊ Failure to grow
  ◊ Recurrent respiratory infections
  ◊ Easy fatigability
  ◊ Dyspnea on exertion
Adult
  ◊ Leg fatigue
  ◊ Fatigue
  ◊ Shortness of breath
  ◊ Angina
  ◊ Syncope
Signs (left-to-right shunt)
  ◊ Rough systolic murmur
  ◊ Continuous "machinery" murmur
  ◊ Thrill at left upper sternal border
  ◊ Bounding pulse with wide pulse pressure
  ◊ Prominent, displaced apical impulse
  ◊ Systolic ejection click
  ◊ Diastolic flow murmur (across mitral valve)
  ◊ Excessive sweating
  ◊ Tachypnea, tachycardia, rales if failure ensues
Signs (right-to-left shunt)
  ◊ Cyanosis, especially lower extremities
  ◊ Clubbing
  ◊ Diastolic Graham-Steele murmur (pulmonic insufficiency)
  ◊ Right ventricular heave
  ◊ Polycythemia

CAUSES
• Prematurity
• Congenital
• Hypoxia
• Prostaglandins

RISK FACTORS
• Premature birth
• High altitudes
• Maternal rubella
• Coexisting cardiac anomalies
• Any condition resulting in hypoxia (pulmonary, hematologic, etc.)

DIAGNOSIS

DIFFERENTIAL DIAGNOSIS
• Venous hum
• Total anomalous pulmonary venous return
• Ruptured sinus of Valsalva
• Arteriovenous communications
• Anomalous origin of left coronary artery from pulmonary artery
• Absence or atresia of pulmonary valve
• Aortic insufficiency with ventricular septal defect
• Peripheral pulmonary stenosis (maternal rubella)
• Truncus arteriosus
• Aortopulmonary fenestration
• Coronary artery fistula

LABORATORY Arterial blood gas
Drugs that may alter lab results: None
Disorders that may alter lab results: None

PATHOLOGICAL FINDINGS
• Left ventricular and atrial enlargement
• Patent ductus may have abnormal intima (maternal rubella)

SPECIAL TESTS
• ECG in children and adults may show left ventricle and left atrial hypertrophy
• ECG in infants usually normal

IMAGING
• Echocardiography/Doppler
• Contrast echocardiography
• Radionuclide angiography
• Magnetic resonance imaging (MRI)
• Chest x-ray usually normal in infants
• Chest x-ray in children and adults (shunt vascularity, calcifications, left ventricle and left atrial enlargement, dilated ascending aorta, dilated pulmonary arteries)

DIAGNOSTIC PROCEDURES
• Cardiac catheterization and angiography - will demonstrate the shunt and determine the amount of shunt, pulmonary pressures, and other coexisting cardiac abnormalities
• Echocardiography - left atrial enlargement
• Doppler - displays direction of shunt and size of the patent ductus

TREATMENT

APPROPRIATE HEALTH CARE
Inpatient surgery

GENERAL MEASURES
• Surgical transection and ligation for moderate/large shunts
• Transfemoral catheter technique to occlude PDA with foam plastic plug or double umbrella
• Small, asymptomatic shunts may not need closure
• Pulmonary support
• Oxygen to correct hypoxia
• Sodium and fluid restriction
• Correction of anemia (hematocrit > 45)

ACTIVITY As tolerated

DIET No special diet

PATIENT EDUCATION Discuss prematurity and explain different treatments of premature infants and full-term infants

MEDICATIONS

DRUG(S) OF CHOICE
• Indomethacin 0.2-0.25 mg/kg/dose IV preferred. Repeat every 12-24 hours x 3 doses. (Decreased efficacy in term infants; not effective in children or adults.)
• Oxygen
• Diuretics
• Antibiotic prophylaxis if not surgically repaired

Contraindications:
To treatment with indomethacin
◊ Renal dysfunction
◊ Overt bleeding
◊ Shock
◊ Necrotizing enterocolitis
◊ Myocardial ischemia

Precautions: With indomethacin treatment - oliguria, hyponatremia

Significant possible Interactions: Refer to manufacturer's profile of each drug

ALTERNATIVE DRUGS None

FOLLOWUP

PATIENT MONITORING
• Annual, routine followup after closure
• Shunts that have not been closed should be followed more closely

PREVENTION/AVOIDANCE N/A

POSSIBLE COMPLICATIONS
• Left heart failure
• Pulmonary hypertension
• Right heart hypertrophy and failure
• Eisenmenger's physiology
• Bacterial endocarditis
• Myocardial ischemia
• Necrotizing enterocolitis

EXPECTED COURSE AND PROGNOSIS
• Spontaneous closure after 3 months is rare
• Before 3 months, closure in premature infants is 75%
• Before 3 months, closure in term infants is 40%
• Best postoperative results if closed before age 3 years
• Increased pulmonary vascular resistance and pulmonary hypertension more common if closed after age 3 years
• No firm statistics but decreased survival for large shunts

MISCELLANEOUS

ASSOCIATED CONDITIONS
• Coarctation of the aorta
• Pulmonary valve stenosis or atresia
• Peripheral pulmonary stenosis (maternal rubella)
• Aortic stenosis
• Ventricular septal defect
• Necrotizing enterocolitis
• Club feet, cataracts, blindness, systemic arterial stenosis (associated with maternal rubella)

AGE-RELATED FACTORS Moderate to large shunts usually diagnosed in infancy or childhood. Small shunts occasionally diagnosed in adults.
Pediatric:
• Symptoms and signs depend largely on size of shunt
• Some infants with coexisting cardiac anomalies benefit temporarily from a patent ductus to provide shunting to the lungs (right heart obstructions) or periphery (coarctation of the aorta). This benefit is short lived, so definitive treatment should proceed as soon as feasible
Geriatric: Good results expected with repair age 50-70 years
Others: N/A

PREGNANCY
• Women with small to moderate sized ductus and left-to-right shunt can expect an uncomplicated pregnancy
• High risk in those with high pulmonary resistance and right-to-left shunt

SYNONYMS Aorticopulmonary shunt or communication

ICD-9-CM 747.0

SEE ALSO N/A

OTHER NOTES No need for antibiotic prophylaxis after surgical repair

ABBREVIATIONS N/A

REFERENCES
• Adams, F.H., Emmanouilides, G.C. & Riemenschneider, T.A.: Moss' Heart Disease in Infants, Children and Adolescents. 4th Ed. Baltimore, Williams & Wilkins, 1989
• Brandenburg, R.O., et al.: Cardiology: Fundamentals and Practice. Chicago, Year Book Medical Publishers, 1987

Author K. Bellah, M.D.

Pediculosis

BASICS

DESCRIPTION
Pediculosis is an infestation of lice
• Lice are ectoparasites that when removed from their human host die of starvation within ten days
• Lice feed solely on human blood by piercing the skin, injecting saliva, and then sucking blood
• Lice are mobile and can move quickly, thereby aiding their transmission
• A mature adult female lays 3-6 eggs, or nits, a day. Nits are 0.8 mm long, white, and appear cemented to the base of the hair. They hatch in 8-10 days and reach maturity in 8-18 days. Adults live 9-10 days.
• Nits may survive three weeks when removed from host
Two species of lice infest humans:
◊ Pediculus humanus has two subspecies, the head louse, (Pediculus humanus capitis), and the body louse, (Pediculus humanus corporis). The head and body lice are anatomically identical although the head louse is smaller. Both species are smaller than 2 mm, are flat, wingless, and have three pairs of legs that attach closely behind the head.
◊ Phthirus pubis (pubic or crab louse). The pubic louse resembles a sea crab and is shorter than the Pediculosis species with large, widespread claws on the 2nd and 3rd legs.
System(s) affected: Skin
Genetics: No genetic pattern
Incidence/Prevalence in USA: 10-40% in schools where accurate surveys have been conducted
Predominant age:
• Most common in adults - pubic lice
• Most common in children - Pediculosis capitis
Predominant sex: Female > Male

SIGNS AND SYMPTOMS
Pediculosis capitis (head louse)
◊ Found most often on the back of the head and neck and behind the ears (warmer areas of the hair)
◊ Nits are white spheres found on the hair shaft. They cannot be moved. This distinguishes them from pilar casts or dandruff scale.
◊ Nits are more prevalent than adult lice
◊ Itching common
◊ Prickling sensation of the scalp
◊ Scratching can cause inflammation and secondary bacterial infection, with pyoderma and posterior cervical lymphadenopathy
◊ Eyelashes may be involved
Pediculosis corporis (body louse)
◊ Affects individuals with poor hygiene
◊ Adult lice live, and lay their nits, in the seams of clothing
◊ Most common symptom is pruritus that leads to scratching, and in later stages, secondary infection
◊ Uninfected bites present as red papules, 2-4 mm in diameter, with an erythematous base

◊ In chronic cases - skin of axilla, groin, and truncal areas can show diffuse pigmentation with skin thickening
Phthirus pubis (pubic louse)
◊ Anogenital pruritus
◊ May have no symptoms during 30-day incubation period
◊ Small brown adults are found at base of hairs attached to two different hairs
◊ Nits are present at the base of hair shafts
◊ Delay in treatment may lead to development of widespread groin inflammation, infection, and regional adenopathy
◊ Gray-blue macules may be seen in the groin in areas adjacent to the infestation
◊ Pubic hair most common site
◊ Lice may spread to hair around anus, abdomen, axillae, chest, beard, eyebrows, and eyelashes
◊ Infested adult patients may spread lice to eyelashes of children. This may induce blepharitis with localized pruritus and/or infection.

CAUSES
Lice are transmitted by close personal contact and contact with objects such as combs, hats, clothing, and bed linen

RISK FACTORS
• Pediculosis corporis - inability to change and launder clothing, overcrowded sleeping quarters
• Phthirus pubis - sexual contact with an infected person

DIAGNOSIS

DIFFERENTIAL DIAGNOSIS
Scabies and other mite species that can cause cutaneous reactions in humans

LABORATORY N/A
Drugs that may alter lab results: N/A
Disorders that may alter lab results: N/A

PATHOLOGICAL FINDINGS N/A

SPECIAL TESTS
• Scalp and pubic lice are apparent with careful examination of individual hairs
• Lice and nits can easily be seen under a microscope
• On Wood's lamp exam, live nits fluoresce white, empty nits fluoresce gray
• Examination of the seams of clothing, particularly the crotch and armpits, reveals body lice and their eggs

IMAGING N/A

DIAGNOSTIC PROCEDURES
History and physical exam

TREATMENT

APPROPRIATE HEALTH CARE
Outpatient

GENERAL MEASURES
Nit removal:
◊ After treatment with shampoo or lotion, nits remain in scalp or pubic hair
◊ Nits are best removed with a very fine comb (nit comb). Removal may be made easier by soaking the hair in a solution of equal parts water and white vinegar and wrapping wet scalp in a towel for at least 15 minutes.
◊ Repeat treatment periodically as needed for stubborn nits
◊ All family contacts possibly infested with head lice should be treated concomitantly

ACTIVITY No restrictions

DIET No special diet

PATIENT EDUCATION
• Poor hygiene is not a risk factor in acquiring pediculosis capitis
• Printed patient information available from: Mayo Foundation for Medical Education and Research, Section of Patient and Health Education, Sieber Subway, Rochester, MN 55905, (507)284-8140

MEDICATIONS

DRUG(S) OF CHOICE
• Head lice - treatments available include lindane (Kwell), synergized pyrethrins (RID) and 1% permethrin (NIX). A single application of permethrin has been found to be as effective as two applications of synergized pyrethrins and more effective than a single application of lindane.
• Pubic lice - treatments available include lindane, synergized pyrethrins, or permethrin. These can be used either as the shampoo left on for 10 minutes or the lotion which can be left on for several hours for best results.
• Body lice - best treated with lindane or synergized pyrethrins lotion applied once and left on for several hours
• Eyelash infestation - treated by careful manual removal of lice and nits, or by application of petroleum jelly (Vaseline) three or four times a day for 8-10 days

Contraindications: Avoid lindane in infants and pregnant women

Precautions:
• Pediculicides should never be used to treat eyelash infections
• Accidental ingestion and gross overuse of lindane may be associated with CNS toxicity

Significant possible Interactions: N/A

ALTERNATIVE DRUGS
Malathion (Ovide) 0.5% lotion

FOLLOWUP

PATIENT MONITORING
As needed

PREVENTION/AVOIDANCE
• Ability to change and launder clothing eliminates risk of acquiring Pediculosis corporis
• Careful followup in schools by public health nurses may help prevent recurrence and spread of head lice
• Washing combs, brushes, hats, coats, collars, sheets, pillow cases, etc., will help to prevent reinfestation by head lice

POSSIBLE COMPLICATIONS
Persistent itching may be caused by too-frequent use of the pediculicide

EXPECTED COURSE AND PROGNOSIS
• With appropriate treatment over 90% cure rate
• Recurrence common, mainly from reinfection, failure to comply with treatment

MISCELLANEOUS

ASSOCIATED CONDITIONS
• Pubic lice are readily transmitted by sexual contact, with a 90% transmission rate. Up to 1/3 of patients have at least one concomitant sexually transmitted disease.
• Eyelash infestation on a child may be a sign of childhood sexual abuse

AGE-RELATED FACTORS N/A
Pediatric: N/A
Geriatric: N/A
Others: Typhus, relapsing fever, and trench fever are spread by body lice during wartime and in underdeveloped countries

PREGNANCY N/A

SYNONYMS
• Lice
• Crabs

ICD-9-CM 132.9

SEE ALSO N/A

OTHER NOTES N/A

ABBREVIATIONS N/A

REFERENCES
• Elgart, M.L.: Pediculosis. Dermatol Clinics 8:219-27, 1990
• Habif, T.: Clinical Dermatology. 2nd Ed. St. Louis, C.V. Mosby, 1990

Author P. Duey, M.D. & C. Zucker, M.D.

Pelvic inflammatory disease (PID)

BASICS

DESCRIPTION PID is a clinical syndrome caused by the ascent of microorganisms from the vagina and endocervix to the endometrium, fallopian tubes, ovaries, and contiguous structures. PID is a broad term that includes a variety of upper genital tract infections, unrelated to pregnancy or surgical procedures, such as salpingitis, salpingo-oophoritis, endometritis, tubo-ovarian inflammatory masses, and pelvic or diffuse peritonitis.
Pathogenesis: The precise mechanism by which microorganisms ascend from the lower genital tract is not known. One possibility is that chlamydial or gonococcal endocervicitis alters the defense mechanisms of the cervix allowing ascent of the vaginal flora with or without the original pathogen. Other possibilities suggest that polymicrobial infection can occur without N. gonorrhoeae or C. trachomatis. Factors that predispose to the ascent of bacteria include the use of an intrauterine device (IUD) and the hormonal and physical changes associated with menstruation.
System(s) affected: Reproductive
Genetics: N/A
Incidence in USA: Estimated 1 million women are treated each year
Prevalence in USA: 100-200/100,000
Predominant age: 16-40
Predominant sex: Female only

SIGNS AND SYMPTOMS
• May be asymptomatic
• Lower abdominal pain
• Fever and malaise
• Vaginal discharge
• Irregular bleeding
• Urinary discomfort, proctitis
• Nausea and vomiting
• Abdominal tenderness
• Tenderness with cervical motion
• Adnexal tenderness
• Unilateral or bilateral tender adnexal mass

CAUSES
• Bacteriology - multiple organisms act as etiologic agents in PID and most cases are polymicrobial. Chlamydia trachomatis, Neisseria gonorrhoeae, and a wide variety of aerobic and anaerobic bacteria are recognized as etiologic agents. Mycoplasmas have also been implicated but their role is less clear. The proportion of cases infected with chlamydia or gonorrhea varies widely depending on the population studied. The most common anaerobes include Bacteroides, Peptostreptococcus, and Peptococcus species. The organisms involved in bacterial vaginosis are similar to the nongonococcal, nonchlamydial bacteria often found in the upper genital tract of women with PID, however, the relationship between these conditions is unclear.

RISK FACTORS
• Sexually active, reproductive age
• Most common in adolescents
• Multiple sexual partners
• Use of an IUD, greatest risk in first few months after insertion
• Previous history of PID; 20-25% will have a recurrence
• Chlamydial or gonococcal cervicitis; 8-10% will develop PID
• Gonococcal salpingitis occurs commonly within 7 days of onset of menses
• Condoms and vaginal spermicides lessen the risks of PID
• Oral contraceptives may reduce the risk of PID

DIAGNOSIS

DIFFERENTIAL DIAGNOSIS
• Appendicitis
• Ectopic pregnancy
• Ovarian torsion
• Hemorrhagic or ruptured ovarian cyst
• Endometriosis
• Irritable bowel syndrome
• Somatization disorder

LABORATORY
• Pregnancy test
• Leukocyte count greater than 10,000 cells per mm3
• Endocervical gram stain for gram-negative intracellular diplococci
• ESR of 15 mm/hour or higher
• Endocervical culture for gonorrhea
• Endocervical culture or antigen test for chlamydia
• Plasma cell endometritis on endometrial biopsy
Drugs that may alter lab results: N/A
Disorders that may alter lab results: N/A

PATHOLOGICAL FINDINGS N/A

SPECIAL TESTS
• Culdocentesis with culture of aspirated material
• Diagnostic laparoscopy with culture of fallopian tubes

IMAGING Pelvic ultrasound

DIAGNOSTIC PROCEDURES
• PID diagnosis is elusive and even asymptomatic patients are at risk for sequelae. Diagnosis incorrect in up to a third of women diagnosed. Laparoscopic diagnosis best but impractical as routine and generally reserved for problem situations. In general, wiser to over-treat lower tract genital infection than to miss an upper tract infection.

Suggested criteria for diagnosis:
◊ Lower abdominal tenderness
◊ Cervical motion tenderness
◊ Adnexal tenderness
All of the above should be present, PLUS one of the following:
◊ Temperature greater than or equal to 38° C
◊ WBC greater than or equal to 10,500/mm3
◊ Purulent material by culdocentesis
◊ Adnexal mass
◊ ESR > 15 mm/hour
◊ Laboratory evidence of gonorrhea or chlamydia

TREATMENT

APPROPRIATE HEALTH CARE
• Outpatient, normally
Hospitalization recommended in the following situations:
◊ Uncertain diagnosis
◊ Surgical emergencies cannot be excluded, e.g., appendicitis
◊ Suspected pelvic abscess
◊ Pregnancy
◊ Adolescent patient with uncertain compliance with therapy
◊ Severe illness
◊ Cannot tolerate outpatient regimen
◊ Failed to respond to outpatient therapy
◊ Clinical follow-up within 72 hours of starting antibiotics cannot be arranged
◊ HIV-infected

GENERAL MEASURES
• Avoidance of sex until treatment is completed
• Insure that sex partners are referred for appropriate evaluation and treatment. Partners should be treated, irrespective of evaluation, with regimens effective against chlamydia and gonorrhea.
Surgical Intervention
◊ Reserved for failures of medical treatment and for suspected ruptured adnexal abscess with resulting acute surgical abdomen
◊ Conservative surgery preferred. This allows a 10-15% postoperative fertility rate
◊ Hysterectomy and adnexectomy for older patients with completed childbirth
◊ Failure of medical therapy generally associated with adnexal abscess which may be amenable to transabdominal or transvaginal drainage under guidance by ultrasonography, computed tomography, or laparoscopy

ACTIVITY According to severity of illness

DIET According to severity of illness

PATIENT EDUCATION Information on written materials for patient distribution can be obtained from local and state health departments or from Information Services, CDC, E06, Atlanta, GA 30333, (404)639-1819

MEDICATIONS

DRUG(S) OF CHOICE
• Several antibiotic regimens are highly effective with no single regimen of choice
• Coverage must extend to include chlamydia, gonorrhea, anaerobes, gram-negative rods, and streptococci. The CDC regimens that follow are recommendations and the specific antibiotics named are examples.
Inpatient treatment - recommended regimen A
  ◊ Cefoxitin 2 g IV every 6 hours or cefotetan IV 2 g every 12 hours (or other cephalosporins such as ceftizoxime, cefotaxime, and ceftriaxone) plus doxycycline 100 mg orally or IV every 12 hours
  ◊ Therapy for 48 hours after clinical improvement and doxycycline continued after discharge for a total of 10-14 days
Inpatient treatment - recommended regimen B
  ◊ Clindamycin 900 mg IV every 8 hours plus gentamicin loading dose IV or IM (2 mg/kg of body weight) followed by a maintenance dose (1.5 mg/kg) every 8 hours
  ◊ Therapy for 48 hours after clinical improvement with doxycycline after discharge as above
Outpatient treatment - recommended regimen
  ◊ Cefoxitin 2 g IM plus probenecid, 1 g orally, concurrently or ceftriaxone 250 mg IM or equivalent cephalosporin plus doxycycline 100 mg orally bid for 10-14 days or tetracycline 500 mg orally qid for 10-14 days or erythromycin 500 mg orally qid for 10-14 days in patients who do not tolerate tetracyclines
Contraindications: Refer to manufacturer's profile of each drug
Precautions: Refer to manufacturer's profile of each drug
Significant possible interactions: Refer to manufacturer's profile of each drug

ALTERNATIVE DRUGS
Many other antibiotic regimens have been proposed and used with success

FOLLOWUP

PATIENT MONITORING
• Close observation of clinical status, in particular for fever, symptoms, level of peritonism, white cell count
• Follow adnexal abscess size and position with ultrasonography

PREVENTION/AVOIDANCE
• Educational programs about safe sex practices
• Education, particularly for those who have had an episode of PID
• IUD contraindicated in women with history of PID or lifestyle associated with STD
• Oral contraceptive appears to decrease risk of PID in cases with cervicitis and the PID cases which do occur are generally less severe
• Barrier contraceptives, especially condoms, and spermicidal creams or sponges provide protection, the extent of which is not well documented
• Insure evaluation and treatment of sex partners
• Comply with management instructions
• Seek medical care early when genital lesions or discharge appear
• Seek routine check-ups for STD if in non-mutually monogamous relationship(s)

POSSIBLE COMPLICATIONS
• A tubo-ovarian abscess will develop in approximately 7-16% of patients
• Recurrent infection occurs in 20-25% of patients
• Risk of ectopic pregnancy increased by 7-10-fold to about 8% of women who have had PID
• Tubal infertility in 15, 35, and 55% of women after one, two, and three episodes of PID, respectively
• Chronic pelvic pain in 20% related to adhesion formation, chronic salpingitis, or recurrent infections

EXPECTED COURSE AND PROGNOSIS
• Wide variation with good prognosis if early, effective therapy instituted and further infection avoided
• Poor prognosis related to late therapy and continued unsafe lifestyle

MISCELLANEOUS

ASSOCIATED CONDITIONS
• In PID patients with an IUD in situ, especially if an adnexal abscess is present, the possibility of actinomyces infection requiring penicillin treatment must be kept in mind
• The IUD is contraindicated in women with a previous episode of PID
• Rupture of an adnexal abscess is rare but life-threatening. Early surgical exploration is mandatory.
• Chlamydia or gonococcal perihepatitis may occur with PID. This combination is termed the Curtis-Fitz-Hugh Syndrome.

AGE-RELATED FACTORS
Pediatric:
• PID is rare before puberty
• Adolescents are highly vulnerable to sexually transmitted diseases (STD) including PID. Early vigorous therapy to prevent infertility is especially important in this age group.
Geriatric: PID is rare after menopause, although postmenopausal adnexal abscess is a well-documented entity.
Others: N/A

PREGNANCY PID is rare during pregnancy but occurs occasionally and the possibility must be kept in mind

SYNONYMS
• Salpingitis
• Salpingo-oophoritis
• Adnexitis
• Pyosalpinx
• Tubo-ovarian abscess
• Pelvic peritonitis

ICD-9-CM 614.9

SEE ALSO
• Chlamydia sexually transmitted disease
• Gonococcal infections

OTHER NOTES N/A

ABBREVIATIONS PID

REFERENCES
• Pelvic inflammatory disease: Guidelines for prevention and management. MMWR. 40:1-25,1991

Author M. Rivlin, M.D.

Pemphigoid, bullous

BASICS

DESCRIPTION Chronic benign bullous eruption considered to be an autoimmune disease. Confined to people over 60.
System(s) affected: Skin/Exocrine, Hemic/Lymphatic/Immunologic
Genetics: HLA typing does not reveal any typical pattern
Incidence/Prevalence in USA: Uncommon
Predominant age: Greater than 60 years
Predominant sex: Male = Female

SIGNS AND SYMPTOMS
• Large bullae 2 to 5 cm in diameter. Occasional tiny peripheral vesicles.
• Bullae that arise from normal-appearing skin (usually) or erythematous skin (sometimes)
• Bullae stay intact for many days
• Located on extremities at first, trunk later
• Occasionally located on the scalp, palms, soles, mucous membranes
• Intact blisters outnumber erosions (reverse is true with pemphigus)
• Clear fluid fills bullae (usually)
• Blood tinged fluid in bullae (sometimes)
• Itching (sometimes severe)
• Some patients are asymptomatic
• 10-20% of skin surface is continuously involved

CAUSES Autoimmune disorder

RISK FACTORS Male, age over 60

DIAGNOSIS

DIFFERENTIAL DIAGNOSIS
• Pemphigus
• Bullous erythema multiforme
• Dermatitis herpetiformis
• Drug eruptions

LABORATORY Circulating autoantibodies in 70% directed at the basement membrane (by immunofluorescence). These can be demonstrated in serum or skin.
Drugs that may alter lab results: N/A
Disorders that may alter lab results: N/A

PATHOLOGICAL FINDINGS Bullae located in a subepidermal location

SPECIAL TESTS
• Light microscopy reveals subepidermal blister with perilesional inflammation containing many eosinophils
• Immunofluorescent studies

IMAGING N/A

DIAGNOSTIC PROCEDURES
• History and physical
• Biopsy - essential for precise diagnosis

TREATMENT

APPROPRIATE HEALTH CARE
Outpatient, unless significant complications

GENERAL MEASURES
• Soaks to active lesions to debride and remove crusts
• Analgesic mouth washes (see Medications)

ACTIVITY Depends on severity of disease and/or complications

DIET Liquid. Regular diet when tolerated.

PATIENT EDUCATION
• Use of oral analgesics
• Teach side effects and adverse reactions of steroids

MEDICATIONS

DRUG(S) OF CHOICE
• Prednisone 60 to 80 mg in single morning dose. Gradually taper in several weeks to maintenance level of 20 to 40 mg per day. Attempt switch to alternate day treatment.
• Consider adjunctive azathioprine if switch to alternate day treatment is not successful. Trial of cyclosporine for resistant disease.
• Topical intralesional corticosteroids may be sufficient for patients with localized disease
• Oral analgesics prn:
  ◊ Elixir of Benadryl for oral ulcers
  ◊ Xylocaine viscous
  ◊ Dyclone solution
Contraindications: Refer to manufacturer's literature
Precautions: Some patients (who have only occasional lesions) can be managed without the need for internal medication
Significant possible interactions: Refer to manufacturer's literature

ALTERNATIVE DRUGS Dapsone

FOLLOWUP

PATIENT MONITORING Blood levels mandatory if prescribing cyclosporine

PREVENTION/AVOIDANCE N/A

POSSIBLE COMPLICATIONS
• Superimposed infection (may result in death in elderly debilitated patient)
• Complications of steroid therapy
• Associated malignancy
• Untreated severe disease can be fatal

EXPECTED COURSE AND PROGNOSIS
• A chronic disease that lasts indefinitely
• Old lesions heal rapidly as new lesions appear
• Accompanying debilitation not as great as with pemphigus

MISCELLANEOUS

ASSOCIATED CONDITIONS May have an associated malignancy

AGE-RELATED FACTORS
Pediatric: Not a problem in pediatric age group
Geriatric: Older people with pemphigoid may have higher than expected rate of malignancy
Others: N/A

PREGNANCY N/A

SYNONYMS Pemphigoid

ICD-9-CM 694.5 pemphigoid

SEE ALSO N/A

OTHER NOTES N/A

ABBREVIATIONS N/A

REFERENCES
• Fitzpatrick, T.B, et al (eds.): Dermatology in General Medicine. 3rd Ed. New York, McGraw-Hill, 1987
• Habif, T.: Clinical Dermatology. 2nd Ed. St. Louis, C.V. Mosby, 1990

Author M. Dambro, M.D. & H. Griffith, M.D.

Pemphigus vulgaris

 BASICS

DESCRIPTION Uncommon, debilitating, potentially fatal skin disorder characterized by intraepidermal bullae that appear on normal appearing skin without surrounding inflammation
System(s) affected: Skin/Exocrine, Gastrointestinal
Genetics: HLA-A10 and HLA-DR4 antigens; higher incidence among persons of Jewish or Mediterranean descent
Incidence/Prevalence in USA: Rare
Predominant age: Mid to late adult life
Predominant sex: Male = Female

SIGNS AND SYMPTOMS
• Oral mucous membrane lesions (particularly in the posterior mouth) often precede the cutaneous lesions (sometimes by several weeks or months)
• Lesion distribution - upper trunk or back initially. Gradual extension to face, groin, and axillae.
• Bullae arise from normal appearing skin
• Multiple shallow erosions which heal slowly
• Blisters are fragile
• Intact bullae are found only on the first day or two of their existence
• After blister roof breaks, a bright red or crusted shallow erosion follows which requires weeks or months to heal
• Outer layer of skin can easily be rubbed off (Nikolsky's sign)

CAUSES An autoimmune disorder with specific IgG antibodies and sometimes complement which are deposited at sites of epidermal cell damage

RISK FACTORS
• Genetic factors (more common in persons of Jewish or Mediterranean descent)
• Medications (particularly penicillamine)

 DIAGNOSIS

DIFFERENTIAL DIAGNOSIS
• Eczematous disorders
• Herpes
• Tinea
• Varicella-zoster
• Erythema multiforme
• Bullous impetigo
• Pemphigoid
• Dermatitis herpetiformis
• Drug eruptions
• Transient acantholytic dermatosis

LABORATORY
• Autoantibody titers (by immunofluorescent studies)
• Titer corresponds to severity of the disease
Drugs that may alter lab results: N/A
Disorders that may alter lab results: N/A

PATHOLOGICAL FINDINGS
• Causative antigens are located on the exterior surface of the cytoplasmic membrane of epithelial cells
• Biopsy shows acantholytic intraepidermal bullae

SPECIAL TESTS N/A

IMAGING N/A

DIAGNOSTIC PROCEDURES
• Biopsy of lesions
• Light microscopy - suprabasal cleft formation and acantholysis

 TREATMENT

APPROPRIATE HEALTH CARE
Depends on severity of the disease and medical status of patient

GENERAL MEASURES
• May require reverse isolation procedures
• Topical treatment to prevent oozing skin from adhering to bed sheets
• Soaks to active lesions to debride and remove crusts
• Analgesic mouth washes (see Medications)
• Plasmapheresis, or cyclosporine, if patient fails to respond to an adequate trial of recommended regimens

ACTIVITY Severity of disease and medical status of patient dictates

DIET Liquid or soft for patient with mouth lesions. Regular diet when tolerated.

PATIENT EDUCATION
• Use of oral analgesics
• Teach side effects and adverse reactions of steroids

Pemphigus vulgaris

MEDICATIONS

DRUG(S) OF CHOICE
• Prednisone - high doses 60-100 mg, higher if necessary. Reduce to every other day dosage when possible.
• Consider concomitant immunosuppressants, such as azathioprine, or cyclophosphamide
• Oral analgesics prn, choose one:
  ◊ Diphenhydramine (Benadryl elixir)
  ◊ Lidocaine (Xylocaine Viscous)
  ◊ Dyclonine solution or lozenges
Contraindications: Refer to manufacturer's literature
Precautions: Refer to manufacturer's literature
Significant possible interactions: Refer to manufacturer's literature

ALTERNATIVE DRUGS
• Gold therapy (with or without concomitant corticosteroids)
• Dapsone controls some cases

FOLLOWUP

PATIENT MONITORING
• Frequent visits during acute phases
• If immunosuppressants prescribed, monitor blood levels frequently
• In elderly patients, chest x-ray to rule out reactivation of old tuberculosis, test urine daily for glycosuria

PREVENTION/AVOIDANCE   N/A

POSSIBLE COMPLICATIONS
• Steroid complications that can lead to morbidity and mortality
• Inadequate nutrition and debilitation due to pain of oral lesions

EXPECTED COURSE AND PROGNOSIS
• Chronic. Inevitably fatal if not treated.
• 10% fatality with vigorous treatment
• Raptured bullae require weeks to heal

MISCELLANEOUS

ASSOCIATED CONDITIONS
• Thymomas
• Other internal malignancies
• Other autoimmune diseases

AGE-RELATED FACTORS
Pediatric: Unusual in this age group
Geriatric:
• This is the age group in which pemphigus is most likely to occur
• Close followup is needed for elderly patients on high doses of steroids
Others: N/A

PREGNANCY   N/A

SYNONYMS   Pemphigus

ICD-9-CM   694.4 pemphigus

SEE ALSO   N/A

OTHER NOTES
• Atypical presentation - pemphigus foliaceus has infrequent oral lesions and is not as debilitating
• In mild disease, gold salts alone can sometimes produce remission. This has the obvious advantage of avoiding immunosuppression.

ABBREVIATIONS   N/A

REFERENCES
• Fitzpatrick, T.B., et al. (eds.): Dermatology In General Medicine. 3rd Ed. New York, McGraw-Hill, 1987
• Habif, T.: Clinical Dermatology. 2nd Ed. St. Louis, C.V. Mosby, 1990

Author   M. Dambro, M.D. & H. Griffith, M.D.

Peptic ulcer disease

BASICS

DESCRIPTION A chronic ulcer in the lining of the gastrointestinal tract.
• Duodenal ulcer (DU): Most common form; four times more common than gastric ulcers. Nearly all DU's are located in the duodenal bulb. Multiple ulcers, and ulcers located distal to the bulb raise the possibility of Zollinger-Ellison syndrome. Etiology of DU is multifactorial, but gastric acid and Helicobacter pylori gastritis are present in nearly all patients.
• Gastric ulcer (GU): Much less common than DU (in the absence NSAIDs). Most commonly located along the lesser curvature of the antrum near the incisura and in the pre-pyloric area. Etiology is multifactorial. GU is 3-4 times as common as DU among NSAID users.
• Esophageal ulcers: A peptic ulcer in the distal esophagus may be part of Barrett's epithelial change due to chronic reflux of gastroduodenal contents
• Ectopic gastric mucosal ulceration: May develop in patients with Meckel's diverticula or other sites of ectopic gastric mucosa
Genetics: Higher incidence with HLA-B12, B5, BW 35 phenotypes
Incidence/Prevalence in USA:
• DU: lifetime prevalence of about 10% for men and 5% for women (although the gender gap is closing). The incidence of uncomplicated DU and need for hospitalization has declined for the past four decades. Between 200,000 and 400,000 new cases of DU are diagnosed annually.
• GU: approximately 87,500 new cases diagnosed annually with an incidence of new GU in adults being approximately 50/100,000 persons
Predominant age:
• DU 25-75 years (rare before age 15)
• GU peak incidence age 55-65 (rare prior to age 40)
Predominant sex:
• DU: Male > Female (slightly)
• GU: Male = Female (female predominance among NSAID users)

SIGNS AND SYMPTOMS
In adults (DU)
◊ Gnawing or burning epigastric pain 1-3 hours after meals, relieved by food or antacids (or antisecretory agents)
◊ Nocturnal pain causing awakening in early morning hours in 50-90% (rarely before breakfast)
◊ Epigastric pain in 60-90% (often vague discomfort, cramping, hunger pangs). Non-specific dyspeptic complaints (belching, bloating, abdominal distention, food intolerance) occur in 40-70%.
◊ Symptomatic periods occur in clusters lasting a few weeks followed by symptom-free periods for weeks to months. Some seasonal occurrence (spring and fall).
◊ Early satiety, anorexia, nausea, vomiting suggest pyloric obstruction
◊ Heartburn (suggesting reflux disease)
◊ Sudden onset of severe diffuse abdominal pain may indicate perforation
◊ Dizziness, syncope, hematemesis or melena suggest hemorrhage
In adults (GU)
◊ Symptom complex similar to DU
◊ Ulcers related to NSAID often silent
◊ Perforation or bleeding may be the initial presentation in NSAID-related ulcers
◊ Epigastric pain following a meal an uncommon finding; early satiety, nausea, vomiting suggest gastric outlet obstruction
◊ Weight loss can occur with either benign or malignant gastric ulcers
In children (DU)
◊ Positive family history in 50% of early onset DU patients (under age 20)
◊ May account for chronic abdominal pain syndrome in young children
◊ Symptoms in older children - same as adults
◊ Gastric outlet obstruction from ulcer must be distinguished from congenital infantile hypertrophic pyloric stenosis (seen within the first month after birth along with visible peristalses and a palpable pyloric mass)

CAUSES
• Imbalance between aggressive factors (e.g., gastric acid, pepsin, bile salts, pancreatic enzymes) and defensive factors maintaining mucosal integrity (e.g., mucus, bicarbonate, blood flow, prostaglandins, growth factors, cell turnover)
• Helicobacter pylori is present in most patients and appears to be a requisite factor (the organism contains urease and other enzymes that may play a pathogenic role)
• Ulcerogenic drugs such as aspirin and other NSAIDs may cause ulcers (GU > DU) or exacerbate existing or latent ulcers

RISK FACTORS
• Strongly associated: Cigarette smoking (more than 1/2 pack/day), drugs (e.g., NSAID use), family history of ulcer, Zollinger-Ellison syndrome (gastrinoma)
• Possibly associated: Corticosteroids (high dose and/or prolonged therapy); blood group O; HLA-B12, B5, BW35 phenotypes; stress; lower socioeconomic status; manual labor
• Poorly or not associated: Dietary spices, alcohol, caffeine, acetaminophen

DIAGNOSIS

DIFFERENTIAL DIAGNOSIS
• Gastroesophageal reflux (with or without esophagitis)
• Non-ulcer dyspepsia
• Gastric carcinoma
• H. pylori-associated gastritis
• Crohn's disease (gastroduodenal)
• Pancreatitis
• Variant angina pectoris
• Cholelithiasis syndrome

LABORATORY
• Anemia uncommon in absence of hemorrhage. Fecal occult blood requires colonic evaluation before attributing positive test to ulcer alone (esp. in patients > 40yrs).
• Elevated serum gastrin (to rule out Zollinger-Ellison syndrome)
• Gastric analysis (to rule out achlorhydria, acid hypersecretion)
• Secretin stimulation test (paradoxical rise seen in ZE)
• Serum pepsinogen
Drugs that may alter lab results:
Antisecretory medications may give falsely low gastric analysis
Disorders that may alter lab results:
Malignant gastric ulcer may go unrecognized
Pathological findings:
• Helicobacter pylori present in > 90% in DU and > 75% in GU
• Ulcer crater usually > 5 mm diameter; extends through the entire thickness of the mucosa

SPECIAL TESTS N/A

IMAGING
• Endoscopy more accurate than barium meal and radiography
• Radiographic features of benign GU include ulcer projecting beyond the lumen, radiolucent band (Hampton line) paralleling ulcer base, radiating folds

DIAGNOSTIC PROCEDURES
• Endoscopy (accuracy > 95%)
• Barium meal (accuracy 70-90%)
• Mucosal biopsy, cytology (excludes malignancy in > 99%)
• Exploratory laparotomy

TREATMENT

APPROPRIATE HEALTH CARE
• Empiric treatment justified for young healthy patients with dyspepsia, otherwise elective diagnostic outpatient endoscopy or barium meal for uncomplicated cases
• Emergency endoscopy and hospitalization for suspected ulcer bleeding
• ICU care for severe hemorrhage
• Surgical consultation for suspected perforation/obstruction, uncontrolled bleeding

GENERAL MEASURES
• Reduce or avoid cigarette smoking
• Reduce use of aspirin or NSAID's
• Reduce psychic stress

ACTIVITY Fully active for uncomplicated disease; exercise to tolerance after hemorrhage

DIET 3 regular meals daily with avoidance of dietary irritants; successful therapy usually overcomes dietary indiscretions.

PATIENT EDUCATION National Digestive Diseases Information Clearinghouse, Box NDDIC, Bethesda, MD 20892, (301)468-6344

MEDICATIONS

DRUG(S) OF CHOICE
Acute DU, GU
◊ Histamine-2 receptor antagonists: cimetidine 400 mg bid or 800 mg hs; ranitidine 150 mg bid or 300 mg hs; famotidine 20 mg bid or 40 mg hs; nizatidine 150 mg bid or 300 mg hs. Expected healing 65-85% at 4 weeks and 90-95% at 8 weeks.
◊ Sucralfate 1 gm qid or 2 gm bid for 4-8 weeks. Efficacy similar to H2 blockers.
◊ Proton-pump inhibitors, e.g., omeprazole 20 mg daily. Expected healing 75-85% at 4 weeks, > 95% at 8 weeks.
◊ Antacids, e.g., magnesium hydroxide (Mylanta, Maalox), aluminum hydroxide (ALternaGEL) 1-3 hr after meals (4-7 doses/day). Healing similar to H2 blockers.
Contraindications: H2 blockers, or omeprazole - known hypersensitivity to the drug or another member of the class
Precautions:
• Renal insufficiency (GFR < 30 cc/min): reduce H2 blocker dose by 50%. Avoid magnesium - containing antacids, avoid cimetidine when potentially interacting medications are co-administered or closely monitor levels of interacting drugs.
• Symptomatic response to therapy does not preclude malignancy
• Omeprazole: short-term treatment only
• Give sucralfate distant from meals to avoid binding with food proteins
Significant possible interactions:
• Cimetidine interacts with many drugs (e.g., theophylline, warfarin, phenytoin, lidocaine) via inhibition of cytochrome P-450 isozymes, leading to reduced drug clearance
• Ranitidine and famotidine have rarely been associated with increased theophylline levels
• Nizatidine has not been associated with drug interactions (but clinical usage is significantly less than with other H2 blockers)
• Omeprazole may prolong the elimination of diazepam, warfarin and phenytoin
• Sucralfate may reduce absorption of tetracycline, norfloxacin, ciprofloxacin, and theophylline leading to subtherapeutic blood levels

ALTERNATIVE DRUGS
• Unhealed refractory ulcer - double dose of H2 blocker or proton pump inhibitor
• Therapy directed at eradication of H. pylori is becoming less controversial; several regimens proposed:
◊ Classic "triple therapy" - Pepto-Bismol 30cc qid + metronidazole 200-500mg tid + amoxicillin 250-500mg qid or tetracycline 500mg qid
◊ H2 blocker (e.g., ranitidine 150 mg bid or 300 mg hs) + 2 antibiotics (e.g., amoxicillin 250 mg tid and metronidazole 500mg tid) or combined with triple therapy
◊ Omeprazole 40mg qd + amoxicillin 500mg tid or clarithyromycin 500mg TID
• Antibiotic therapy usually given for 2-3 weeks, but is associated with possible complications, including diarrhea, Clostridium difficile colitis and antibiotic resistance
• Adjunctive use of antidepressants, anticholinergics
• Combination therapy (e.g., H2 blocker plus sucralfate). Not recommended for uncomplicated ulcers.

FOLLOWUP

PATIENT MONITORING
• Acute DU - monitor clinical response. No need to repeat endoscopy or x-ray exam to document healing unless recurrence or complication suspected.
• Acute GU - documentation of complete healing recommended (endoscopy after 6-12 weeks allows for cytology and biopsy of poorly or unhealed ulcer)

PREVENTION/AVOIDANCE
• H2 blockers or sucralfate indicated in 1/2 the acute healing dose. Take at bedtime to prevent recurrence in high-risk patients (e.g., more than 2 symptomatic recurrences per year, history of ulcer complications).
• Stop/avoid risk factors
• Intermittent use of H2 blocker for symptomatic relapses is less cost-effective than daily maintenance therapy
• H. pylori eradication regimen may become best means of prevention

POSSIBLE COMPLICATIONS
• Hemorrhage occurs in up to 25% of cases (initial presentation in 10%). Most bleeding episodes related to NSAID use. Suspect with melena, hematemesis, anemia, syncope.
• Perforation occurs in < 5%, usually related to NSAID use. Suspect with sudden, severe mid-epigastric pain radiating to right shoulder, peritoneal signs and free peritoneal air on x-ray.
• Gastric outlet obstruction occurs in up to 5% of patients with duodenal or pyloric channel ulcers. Men predominate. Suspect obstruction with symptoms of gastric stasis, vomiting, early satiety, weight loss, abnormal saline load test, succussion splash, gastric retention of barium.
• Intractability rare since H2 blockers/omeprazole available

EXPECTED COURSE AND PROGNOSIS
• Ulcer relapse rate, off therapy, after initial healing remains high (50-80% at one year)
• Long-term daily maintenance therapy with H2 blockers or sucralfate in patients with frequent symptomatic recurrences or prior complications can prevent future exacerbations of disease indefinitely
• Successful eradication of H. pylori is associated with very low relapse rates and infrequent reinfection

MISCELLANEOUS

ASSOCIATED CONDITIONS
• Zollinger-Ellison syndrome (gastrinoma)
• Systemic mastocytosis
• Multiple endocrine neoplasia syndrome (type I)
• COPD, chronic renal failure, cirrhosis, hyperparathyroidism, carcinoid syndrome, polycythemia rubra vera, basophilic leukemia, porphyria cutanea tarda

AGE-RELATED FACTORS
Pediatric:
• Uncommon prior to puberty
• Hemorrhage and perforation may be more common than in adults
Geriatric: Ulcers often silent, especially those associated with NSAIDs. Acute bleeding or perforation often initial presentation.
Others: N/A

PREGNANCY
• Unusual during gestation
• Safety of H2 blockers not established in the first 16 weeks, but considered reasonably safe later; sucralfate and antacids relatively non-systemic and preferred as initial therapy

SYNONYMS
• Duodenal ulcer
• Gastric ulcer

ICD-9-CM DU 532.9, GU 531.9

SEE ALSO
Zollinger-Ellison syndrome

OTHER NOTES N/A

ABBREVIATIONS
NSAID = nonsteroidal anti-inflammatory drug
GFR = glomerular filtration rate

REFERENCES
• Soll, A.H.: Duodenal ulcers and drug therapy. In Gastrointestinal Disease: Pathophysiology, Diagnosis, Management. 4th Ed. Edited by M.H. Sleisenger & J.S. Fordtran. Philadelphia, W.B. Saunders Co., 1989
• Richardson, C.T.: Gastric ulcer. In Gastrointestinal Disease: Pathophysiology, Diagnosis, Management. 4th Ed. Edited by M.H. Sleisenger & J.S. Fordtran. Philadelphia, W.B. Saunders Co., 1989
• Chilbu, N., Rao, B.V. & Hunt, R.H.: Meta-analysis of the efficacy of antibiotic therapy in eradicating Helicobacter pylori. Amer J of Gastro. 87:1716-1727, 1992
• Graham DY. Treatment of Peptic Ulcers caused by H. pylori, N Engl J Med. 1993; 328:349-350.

Author J. Lewis, M.D.

Pericarditis

BASICS

DESCRIPTION The clinical manifestations of disease processes involving the pericardial sac surrounding the heart
• Acute pericarditis - an inflammatory process from a wide spectrum of etiologies of the pericardium with or without associated effusion. The most common etiology is idiopathic or nonspecific pericarditis.
• Pericardial tamponade - cardiac compression from pericardial effusion causing hemodynamic compromise and disruption of compensatory mechanisms
• Constrictive pericarditis - thickening and adherence of the pericardium to the heart after chronic inflammation
System(s) affected: Cardiovascular
Genetics: Unknown
Incidence/Prevalence in USA: N/A
Predominant age: Adolescents and young adults
Predominant sex: Male > Female

SIGNS AND SYMPTOMS
Acute pericarditis
◊ Chest pain, typically sharp, retrosternal with radiation to the trapezial ridge
◊ Pain frequently sudden in onset
◊ Pain reduced by leaning forward and sitting up
◊ Splinted breathing
◊ Odynophagia
◊ Fever
◊ Myalgia
◊ Anorexia
◊ Anxiety
◊ Pericardial friction rub
◊ Cardiac arrhythmias often intermittent, supraventricular tachycardia (SVT)
◊ Tachypnea
◊ Localized rales
Pericardial tamponade
◊ Dyspnea
◊ Tachycardia
◊ Distended jugular neck veins,
◊ Cyanosis
◊ Relative or absolute hypotension
◊ Quiet precordium with little palpable cardiac activity
◊ Pericardial friction rub
◊ Lungs clear
◊ Ewart's sign - dullness and bronchial breathing between the tip of the left scapula and vertebral column
◊ Rapid thready pulse
◊ Varying degrees of consciousness
◊ Pulsus paradoxus: > 10 mm Hg decrease in systolic pressure with inspiration

Constrictive pericarditis
◊ Asymptomatic, early
◊ Dyspnea, pulmonary congestion
◊ Fatigue very common
◊ Peripheral edema
◊ Hepatomegaly
◊ Ascites
◊ Jugular venous distention - elevated, deep Y trough (not seen in tamponade)
◊ Kussmaul's sign - inspiratory increase in jugular venous pressure
◊ Pericardial "knock" - follows S2 by 0.06-0.12 sec, increases with squatting
◊ Hypovolemia may mask the signs of constriction

CAUSES
• Idiopathic
• Viral: Coxsackie, echo, adenovirus, Epstein-Barr, mumps
• Bacterial: Haemophilus (especially children), Staphylococcus, Pneumococcus, Salmonella
• Fungal: Candida, Histoplasmosis, Aspergillus, Nocardia
• Mycobacterial: Mycobacterium tuberculosis
• Neoplastic: Breast, lung, lymphoma
• Drug-induced: Procainamide, hydralazine, bleomycin, phenytoin, minoxidil and perhaps others
• Connective tissue disease: Systemic lupus erythematosis, rheumatoid arthritis, scleroderma
• Radiation
• Myocardial infarction
• Postpericardiotomy
• Chest trauma
• Uremia
• Myxedema
• Cholesterol pericarditis
• Aortic dissection
• Sarcoidosis
• Pancreatitis
• Inflammatory bowel disease
• AIDS

RISK FACTORS Dependent on etiology

DIAGNOSIS

DIFFERENTIAL DIAGNOSIS
• Acute myocardial infarction
• Pneumonia with pleurisy
• Pulmonary emboli
• Aortic dissection
• Pneumothorax
• Mediastinal emphysema
• Cholecystitis
• Pancreatitis

LABORATORY
• Leukocytosis and increased ESR
• May see elevated creatine phosphokinase (CPK), lactate dehydrogenase (LDH), serum glutamic-oxaloacetic (SGOT)
Drugs that may alter lab results: N/A
Disorders that may alter lab results: N/A

PATHOLOGICAL FINDINGS
Micro: acute inflammation

SPECIAL TESTS
• Electrocardiogram
• Echocardiogram
• Right heart catherization

IMAGING
• Chest x-ray - small pleural effusion, transient infiltrates; "water bottle" silhouette in large associated pericardial effusion
• Chest CT or MRI in suspected constrictive pericarditis may reveal calcified or thickened pericardium; delineate effusions

DIAGNOSTIC PROCEDURES
• Pericardiocentesis
• Pericardial biopsy

TREATMENT

APPROPRIATE HEALTH CARE
• Outpatient unless signs of complications
• Inpatient with complications (hemodynamic compromise or effusion present)

GENERAL MEASURES
• Pericardiectomy may be required if drugs are not effective

ACTIVITY No restrictions; limited by patients symptoms only

DIET No restriction. If patient overweight, suggest a weight loss program.

PATIENT EDUCATION Since 15% of patients have a recurrence, must educate for return of symptoms and followup

MEDICATIONS

DRUG(S) OF CHOICE Uncomplicated: aspirin 650mg q4h. If effective, continue for 2 weeks.
Contraindications: Hypersensitivity to aspirin, known coagulopathy
Precautions: Use with caution in patients with asthma, nasal polyps, severe carditis, pregnancy in the third trimester, history of GI disturbances or bleeding, bleeding disorders or diathesis, telangiectasis, anticoagulation, renal or hepatic dysfunction
Significant possible interactions:
Acetaminophen, acetazolamide, ammonium chloride, antacids, aurothioglucose, chlorpropamide, cimetidine, corticosteroids, diclofenac, dicumarol, diltiazem, dipyridamole, etodolac, flurbiprofen, ibuprofen, indomethacin, insulin, ketorolac, meclofenamate, mefenamic acid, methotrexate, metoclopramide, naproxen, nitroglycerin, nizatidine, penicillin G, phenprocoumon, phenylbutazone, phenytoin piroxicam, probenicid, protirelin, quinidine, spironolactone, sulfinpyrazone, sulfonylureas, sulindac, suprofen, tolmetin, valproic acid, warfarin

ALTERNATIVE DRUGS

• Ibuprofen 400-600mg q6h for 2 weeks
• Indomethacin 25-50mg q6-8h for 2 weeks
• Colchicine 1mg q day
• Azathioprine, phenylbutazone, prednisone 60mg q day x 2-3 days and quickly taper (last resort)

FOLLOWUP

PATIENT MONITORING

• Followup patients in office in 2 weeks and re-evaluate cardiac status and symptomatology
• Repeat chest x-ray and electrocardiogram should be considered at 4 weeks

PREVENTION/AVOIDANCE N/A

POSSIBLE COMPLICATIONS

• Pericardial tamponade
• Recurrence of pericarditis
• Non-compressive effusion
• Chronic, constrictive pericarditis

EXPECTED COURSE AND PROGNOSIS

• The majority of patients have complete resolution of pain and symptoms during the 2 weeks of therapy
• Fifteen per cent will have at least one recurrence in the first few months
• A rare patient may become refractory and require corticosteroids or pericardiectomy
• The hemodynamic effects of effusions depends on the volume and rapidity of development
• A very small percentage of patients can develop signs of right sided heart failure secondary to constriction. These patients are best treated with pericardiectomy.

MISCELLANEOUS

ASSOCIATED CONDITIONS
• Dependent on etiology
• Pericarditis, constrictive
• Pericarditis, acute suppurative

AGE-RELATED FACTORS
Pediatric: N/A
Geriatric: N/A
Others: N/A

PREGNANCY N/A

SYNONYMS Acute nonsuppurative pericarditis,

ICD-9-CM
• 420.91
• 420.99 other acute pericarditis

SEE ALSO N/A

OTHER NOTES N/A

ABBREVIATIONS N/A

REFERENCES
• Rippe, J.M.: Intensive Care Medicine. 1st ed. Boston/Toronto, Little, Brown, 1985
• Wyngaarden, J.B. & Smith, L.H. (eds.): Cecil Textbook of Medicine. 19th Ed. Philadelphia, W.B. Saunders Co., 1992
• Harvey, A.M.:The Principles and Practice of Medicine. 22nd Ed. Norwalk, CT, Appleton & Lange, 1988
• Shabetai, R.: Diseases of the Pericardium. Cardio Clinics, Nov, 1990

Author D. Heiselman, D.O.

Peritonitis, acute

 BASICS

DESCRIPTION Acute inflammation of the visceral and parietal peritoneum
System(s) affected: Gastrointestinal, Endocrine/Metabolic, Cardiovascular
Genetics: No known genetic pattern
Incidence/Prevalence in USA: Common
Predominant age: None
Predominant sex: Male > Female

SIGNS AND SYMPTOMS
- Acute abdominal pain
- Fever
- Nausea
- Vomiting
- Constipation
- Abdominal pain exacerbated by motion
- Abdominal distention
- Dyspnea
- Diffuse abdominal rebound
- Generalized abdominal rigidity
- Decreased bowel sounds
- Abdominal hyper-resonance to percussion
- Hypotension
- Tachycardia
- Hippocratic facies
- Tachypnea
- Dehydration
- Ascites

CAUSES
Primary - spontaneous bacterial peritonitis
  ◊ Ascites associated with cirrhosis, nephrotic syndrome
Secondary
  ◊ Following abdominal trauma
  ◊ Penetrating wounds
  ◊ Continuous ambulatory peritoneal dialysis
  ◊ Perforation
  ◊ Appendicitis
  ◊ Colitis - infectious, inflammatory
  ◊ Peptic ulcer perforation
  ◊ Gangrene of the bowel
  ◊ Diverticulitis
  ◊ Pancreatitis
  ◊ Postoperative
  ◊ Acute cholecystitis

RISK FACTORS
- Recent surgery
- Advanced liver disease
- Corticosteroid medication
- Nephrotic syndrome
- Continuous ambulatory peritoneal dialysis

 DIAGNOSIS

DIFFERENTIAL DIAGNOSIS
- Abscess formation (subdiaphragmatic, subhepatic, peritoneal, pelvic)
- Other causes of ileus (volvulus, intussusception)
- Mesenteric adenitis
- Appendicitis
- Pancreatitis

LABORATORY
- Positive culture of peritoneal aspirate
- Leukocytosis
- Increased BUN
- Hemoconcentration
- Positive blood culture
- Metabolic acidosis
- Respiratory acidosis
- elevated amylase
- Ascitic fluid analysis
Drugs that may alter lab results:
Antibiotics prior to blood studies
Disorders that may alter lab results: N/A

PATHOLOGICAL FINDINGS
- Peritoneum - generalized fibrinopurulent exudate
- Peritoneum - polymorphonuclear infiltration

SPECIAL TESTS   N/A

IMAGING
- Abdominal film - free air in peritoneal cavity, large bowel dilatation, small bowel dilatation, intestinal wall edema
- Chest x-ray - elevated diaphragm
- CT - intra-abdominal mass, ascites
- Sonography - intra-abdominal mass, ascites

DIAGNOSTIC PROCEDURES   N/A

 TREATMENT

APPROPRIATE HEALTH CARE
Inpatient

GENERAL MEASURES
- Treat underlying condition(s) and infection (by surgery if necessary)
- Treat paralytic ileus (naso-gastric decompression until aspirate becomes clear and scanty)
- Treat dehydration
- Antibiotics (after culture results)
- Respiratory support if needed
- IV fluids
- Blood transfusions (sometimes)

ACTIVITY   Bedrest until infection is under control

DIET
- IV fluids and electrolytes, liquid, or soft diet as tolerated
- Oral feedings only after return of bowel sounds, and passage of flatus and/or feces
- Total parenteral nutrition may be necessary

PATIENT EDUCATION   N/A

MEDICATIONS

DRUG(S) OF CHOICE
Primary
◊ Cefotaxime 1-2 g IV q4-8h
or
◊ Ceftriaxone 1-2 g IV q24h
Secondary
◊ Ampicillin 1-2g q6h plus gentamicin 1.5 mg/kg/dose plus clindamycin 600-900mg q8h
or
◊ Ampicillin plus gentamycin plus metronidazole 500mg q6-8h
or
◊ Gentamicin plus clindamycin
or
◊ Imipenem 0.5-1.0g q6-8h
Continuous abdominal peritoneal dialysis
◊ Intraperitoneal vancomycin (20mg/L dialysate + 1gm IV "load") plus gentamicin (6-8mg/L dialysate)
or
Intraperitoneal cefazolin
Other
◊ Morphine 2-10mg IV or IM q3-4h, as needed, for pain
Contraindications: Refer to manufacturer's literature
Precautions: Refer to manufacturer's literature
Significant possible interactions: Refer to manufacturer's literature

ALTERNATIVE DRUGS
• Initial therapy with a third-generation cephalosporin (e.g., cefotaxime or ceftriaxone)
• Antibiotics, other than those mentioned, if indicated by culture of blood or peritoneal fluid

FOLLOWUP

PATIENT MONITORING Inpatient and sometimes intensive care unit as indicated

PREVENTION/AVOIDANCE
Prophylactic antibiotics during abdominal surgery

POSSIBLE COMPLICATIONS
• Hypovolemic consequences
• Septicemia
• Septic shock
• Acute renal failure
• Acute respiratory insufficiency
• Liver failure
• Abscess formation

EXPECTED COURSE AND PROGNOSIS
• Fully developed paralytic ileus requires 48 hours for recovery
• Mortality dependent on - age, duration, cause, and on pre-existing conditions

MISCELLANEOUS

ASSOCIATED CONDITIONS
• Abscesses: Subdiaphragmatic, subhepatic, peritoneal, pelvic
• Ileus

AGE-RELATED FACTORS
Pediatric: Get pediatric and surgical consultation, if available
Geriatric: Mortality greater in this age group. Symptoms may be muted.
Others: N/A

PREGNANCY Ruptured ectopic pregnancy may lead to peritonitis

SYNONYMS N/A

ICD-9-CM
567.2 acute generalized peritonitis

SEE ALSO N/A

OTHER NOTES N/A

ABBREVIATIONS N/A

REFERENCES
• Braunwald E., et al. (eds.): Harrison's Principles of Internal Medicine. 12th Ed. New York, McGraw-Hill, 1991
• Sleisenger, M.H. and Fordtran, J.S. (eds.): Gastrointestinal Disease: Pathophysiology, Diagnosis, Management. 4th Ed. Philadelphia, W.B. Saunders Co., 1989
• Wyngaarden, J.B., Smith, L.H., Jr. & Bennett, J.C. (eds.): Cecil Textbook of Medicine. 19th Ed. Philadelphia,
• Sabiston, D.C., Jr. (ed.): Textbook of Surgery: The Biological Basis of Modern Surgical Practice. 14th Ed. Philadelphia, W.B. Saunders Co., 1991
• Woodley, M. & Whelan, A. (eds.): Manual of Medical Therapeutics. 27th Ed. Boston, Little-Brown & Co., 1992

Author A. Adelman, M.D.

Pertussis

 BASICS

DESCRIPTION
Pertussis or whooping cough is a highly communicable, respiratory, bacterial infection. Characteristically, it produces a paroxysmal spasmodic cough, ending in prolonged high-pitched inspiratory whoop or crow. Transmission is by direct contact and patients are contagious for 3 weeks. Incubation period averages 7 to 14 days (maximum 3 weeks). Usual course - acute (lasts 3-10 weeks after catarrhal period).

System(s) affected: Pulmonary
Genetics: N/A
Incidence/Prevalence in USA:
• 1.740 cases/100,000 people
• Annual average cases - 3,500, with 10 deaths
• Increasing as immunization rates decline.
Predominant age: 3 months-6 years (infants comprise about half of the cases)
Predominant sex: Female > Male

SIGNS AND SYMPTOMS
• Cough paroxysms
• Stacatto cough
• Mild fever
• Rhinorrhea
• Anorexia
• "Whoop" cough
• Apnea, episodic
• Posttussive inspiratory gasp

CAUSES
Bordetella pertussis. Bordetella parapertussis and Bordetella bronchiseptica produce a similar, but milder clinical illness.

RISK FACTORS
• Unimmunized children
• Contact with an infected person
• Epidemic exposure
• Pregnancy

 DIAGNOSIS

DIFFERENTIAL DIAGNOSIS
• Common cold
• Adenoviral syndromes
• Bronchiolitis
• Influenza
• Bacterial pneumonias
• Cystic fibrosis
• Tuberculosis
• Interstitial pneumonitis
• Foreign body

LABORATORY
• ELISA: IgA against Bordetella pertussis
• WBC: 15,000-20,000; 60-80% lymphocytes
• Bordetella pertussis on Bordet-Gengou culture medium
Drugs that may alter lab results: N/A
Disorders that may alter lab results: N/A

PATHOLOGICAL FINDINGS
• Focal emphysema
• Mucopurulent exudate
• Patchy ulceration of respiratory epithelium

SPECIAL TESTS N/A

IMAGING
Chest x-ray - focal atelectasis, peribronchial cuffing, emphysema

DIAGNOSTIC PROCEDURES N/A

 TREATMENT

APPROPRIATE HEALTH CARE
Hospitalization for seriously ill infants. Outpatient for milder cases.

GENERAL MEASURES
• General supportive, skilled nursing care
• Isolation and quarantine for 4 weeks; 1 week after erythromycin started
• Parenteral fluid therapy if needed
• Oxygen
• Careful observation for apnea in young infants, and, to avoid stimuli that trigger paroxysms
• Mechanical ventilation
• Nutritional support

ACTIVITY
Rest during active phase in quiet environment

DIET
Encourage extra fluids. May need to provide small frequent meals to assure adequate nutrition.

PATIENT EDUCATION
For patient education materials favorably reviewed on this topic, contact: American Academy of Pediatrics, 141 Northwest Point Blvd., P.O. Box 927, Elk Grove Village, IL 60009-0927, (800)433-9016

MEDICATIONS

DRUG(S) OF CHOICE
• Erythromycin during catarrhal stage, 30-40 mg/kg/24h divided every 6 hours
• Other antibiotics for bacterial complications such as bronchopneumonia or otitis media
• Antibiotics do not alter course of illness, but prevent spread
Contraindications: Do not use cough suppressants
Precautions: N/A
Significant possible interactions: N/A

ALTERNATIVE DRUGS
• Steroids and/or theophylline have been suggested for treatment of severely ill patients (their effectiveness and potential hazards require further controlled studies)
• Beta-2 agonists may help with cough paroxysms.

FOLLOWUP

PATIENT MONITORING
• Intensive care unit may be necessary for severely ill infants
• Older children and adults with mild cases do not need to be confined to bed

PREVENTION/AVOIDANCE
• Isolate infected persons
• Active immunization for all infants, usually combined with diptheria and tetanus toxoids (DPT). Immunization or booster not recommended after age 6 years. (New vaccine for the 4th and 5th DPT shots [Acel-Immune] available since December, 1991 may have fewer side effects.)
• Erythromycin - for susceptible children (under 2 months or unvaccinated) if they are exposed to an infected person during the contagious period

POSSIBLE COMPLICATIONS
• Can infect up to 90% of household members who are not immune
• Death in infants
• Pneumonia
• Hypoxic encephalopathy
• Coma
• Otitis media
• Tuberculosis activation
• Epistaxis
• Hernia
• Re-induction of paroxysmal coughing (for several months) especially with upper respiratory infections
• Convulsions
• Cerebral hemorrhage
• Neurologic disorders
• Weight loss
• Hemoptysis
• Atelectasis

EXPECTED COURSE AND PROGNOSIS Complete recovery

MISCELLANEOUS

ASSOCIATED CONDITIONS
• Otitis media
• Bronchopneumonia
• Failure to thrive

AGE-RELATED FACTORS
Pediatric: Most serious and highest mortality in infants less than 6 months of age (death usually due to complications)
Geriatric: May be more serious in this age group
Others: N/A

PREGNANCY N/A

SYNONYMS
Whooping cough

ICD-9-CM
033 whooping cough

SEE ALSO N/A

OTHER NOTES
• Do not use cough suppressants
• Reporting of selected adverse reactions with certain vaccines is now required by the National Childhood Vaccine Injury Act of 1986. Toll-free information number - (800)822-7967.

ABBREVIATIONS N/A

REFERENCES
• Mandell, G.L. (ed.): Principles and Practice of Infectious Diseases. 3rd Ed. New York, Churchill Livingstone, 1990
• Centers for Disease Control: National Childhood Vaccine Injury Act: Requirements for permanent vaccination records and for reporting of selected events after vaccination. MMWR 1988;37:197-200

Author N. Dambro, M.D.

Pharyngitis

BASICS

DESCRIPTION Inflammation of the pharynx most commonly caused by acute infection. Group A streptococcus is a focus of diagnosis due to its potential for preventable rheumatic sequelae.

System(s) affected: Gastrointestinal

Genetics: Individuals with a positive family history of rheumatic fever have a higher risk of rheumatic sequelae following an untreated group A beta hemolytic streptococcal infection

Incidence/Prevalence in USA:
• Estimated 30 million cases diagnosed yearly
• 11% of all school age children visit a physician annually with pharyngitis
• 12-25% of sore throats seen by physicians
• Incidence of rheumatic fever is decreasing with estimate of 64 cases per 100,000

Predominant age:
• Pharyngitis occurs in all age groups
• Streptococcal infection has greatest incidence 5 to 18 years of age

Predominant sex: Male = Female

SIGNS AND SYMPTOMS
• Sore throat
• Enlarged tonsils
• Pharyngeal erythema
• Tonsillar exudates
• Soft palate petechiae
• Cervical adenopathy
• Absence of cough hoarseness or lower respiratory symptoms
• Fever (> 102.5° F. suggests streptococcus)
• Scarlet fever rash - punctate erythematous macules with reddened flexor creases and circumoral pallor (streptococcal pharyngitis)
• Gray pseudomembrane found in diphtheria
• Characteristic erythematous based clear vesicles in herpes stomatitis
• Anorexia
• Chills
• Malaise
• Headache

CAUSES
Acute - bacterial:
◊ Group A beta-hemolytic streptococci
◊ Neisseria gonorrhoeae
◊ Corynebacterium diphtheriae
◊ Haemophilus influenzae
◊ Moraxella (Branhamella) catarrhalis
◊ Group C and G streptococcus rarely
Acute - virus:
◊ Rhinovirus
◊ Adenovirus
◊ Parainfluenza virus
◊ Coxsackie virus
◊ Coronavirus
◊ Echovirus
◊ Herpes simplex virus
◊ Epstein-Barr virus
◊ Cytomegalovirus

Chronic
◊ More likely non-infectious
◊ Irritation from post-nasal discharge of chronic allergic rhinitis
◊ Chemical irritation
◊ Neoplasms and vasculitides

RISK FACTORS
• Group A beta hemolytic streptococcal epidemics occur
• Age (young are more susceptible)
• Family history
• Close quarters, such as in new military recruits
• Immunosuppression
• Fatigue
• Smoking
• Excess alcohol consumption
• Oral sex
• Diabetes mellitus
• Recent illness

DIAGNOSIS

DIFFERENTIAL DIAGNOSIS
• See causative factors
• Sore throat can be seen with leukopenia

LABORATORY
• Blood agar throat culture from swab. Bacitracin disc sensitivity of hemolytic colonies suggest group A streptococci.
• Rapid screening for streptococci can be done from throat swab with antigen agglutination kits. 5-10% false negatives lead some to suggest routine backup of all negatives with blood agar culture.
• Leukocytosis (if bacterial)

Drugs that may alter lab results: N/A
Disorders that may alter lab results: N/A

PATHOLOGICAL FINDINGS
Culture of pathogens to identify causes

SPECIAL TESTS
• Special tests usually only done based on suggestive history
• Screening for gonococcal infection requires warm Thayer-Martin plate
• Viruses can be cultured in special media
• Mono spot test for Epstein-Barr virus
• Gram stain can be suggestive
• Streptococcal isolates can be immunologically typed

IMAGING N/A

DIAGNOSTIC PROCEDURES
History and physical probably only 50% accurate. Laboratory required unless in epidemic setting.

TREATMENT

APPROPRIATE HEALTH CARE
Outpatient

GENERAL MEASURES
• Salt water gargles
• Acetaminophen
• Dyclonine lozenges
• Cool-mist humidifier

ACTIVITY As tolerated

DIET No restrictions. Encourage extra fluids.

PATIENT EDUCATION
• Important to complete 10 day course of antibiotics regardless of symptom response
• Patients presumed to be non-infectious after 24 hours of antibiotic coverage

MEDICATIONS

DRUG(S) OF CHOICE
For streptococcal pharyngitis:
• Penicillin for 10 day course is the standard. All choices should have complete 10 day course.
• Penicillin VK 250 mg tid (25-50 mg/kg/day), or
• For penicillin allergic patients, erythromycin ethylsuccinate 300 to 400 mg tid (30 mg/kg/day), or
• Cephalexin 250 mg tid (30 mg/kg/day)
Contraindications: Allergy to specific antibiotic
Precautions: Refer to manufacturer's profile of each drug
Significant possible interactions: Refer to manufacturer's profile of each drug

ALTERNATIVE DRUGS
• Treatment of carrier state is difficult, usually requiring addition of rifampin to penicillin regimen
• Penicillin is the most documented treatment to prevent rheumatic sequelae but cephalosporins have lower rate of bacteriologic failure
• The newer macrolides, azithromycin and claithromycin, are also effective against streptococcal pharyngitis, but more expensive. The chief advantage of azithromycin is its 5 day course with 10 day effective duration.
• Other cephalosporins are generally effective for streptococcal pharyngitis, but more expensive than cephalexin

FOLLOWUP

PATIENT MONITORING
• Routine followup cultures not necessary
• Telephone consult for duration of symptoms

PREVENTION/AVOIDANCE
Avoid contact with infected people

POSSIBLE COMPLICATIONS
• Rheumatic fever
• Post-streptococcal glomerulonephritis
• Peritonsillar abscess
• Systemic infection
• Otitis media
• Septicemia
• Rhinitis
• Sinusitis
• Pneumonia

EXPECTED COURSE AND PROGNOSIS
• Streptococcal pharyngeal infection runs a 5-7 day course with peak of fever at 2-3 days
• Symptoms will resolve spontaneously without treatment, but rheumatic complications are still possible
• Suppurative complications such as peritonsillar abscess require surgical intervention

MISCELLANEOUS

ASSOCIATED CONDITIONS N/A

AGE-RELATED FACTORS
Pediatric: N/A
Geriatric: N/A
Others: N/A

PREGNANCY N/A

SYNONYMS
• Sore throat
• Tonsillitis
• Streptococcal throat

ICD-9-CM
• Acute pharyngitis - 462
• Streptococcal - 034.0

SEE ALSO
• Rheumatic fever
• Herpes simplex
• Mononucleosis

OTHER NOTES Unless clinical presentation is unusual, treatment is based on presence or absence of group A streptococci

ABBREVIATIONS N/A

REFERENCES
• Pichichero, M.E.: Controversies in the Treatment of Streptococcal Pharyngitis. American Fam Phys. December, 1990
• Wyngaarden, J.B., Smith, L.H. (eds): Cecil Textbook of Medicine. 19th Ed. Philadelphia, W.B. Saunders Co., 1992

Author D. Burtner, M.D.

Pheochromocytoma

 BASICS

DESCRIPTION Catecholamine-producing tumor. In 80% of cases, the tumors are found in the adrenal medulla, but may also be found in other tissues derived from neural crest cells.
System(s) affected: Endocrine/Metabolic
Genetics: N/A
Incidence/Prevalence in USA:
• 0.01% to 0.1% of the hypertensive population
Predominant age: Any age, peak incidence ages 30 to 60 years
Predominant sex: Male = Female

SIGNS AND SYMPTOMS
Paroxysmal spells (the "5 P's")
◊ Pressure - sudden increase in blood pressure
◊ Pain - headache, chest and abdominal pain
◊ Perspiration
◊ Palpitations
◊ Pallor
Additional symptoms
◊ Constipation
◊ Tremor
◊ Weight loss
◊ Anxiety
Signs
◊ Hypertension - paroxysmal in half of the patients
◊ Orthostatic hypotension
◊ Grade II to IV retinopathy
◊ Fever
◊ Hyperglycemia
◊ Hypercalcemia
◊ Erythrocytosis

CAUSES
Catecholamine-producing tumor - "Rule of 10:"
◊ 10% are extra-adrenal
◊ 10% are multiple or bilateral
◊ 10% are malignant
◊ 10% recur after surgical removal
◊ 10% occur in children
◊ 10% are familial

RISK FACTORS
• Familial pheochromocytoma
• Multiple endocrine neoplasia types II A and B
• Neurofibromatosis
• Von Hippel-Lindau syndrome

 DIAGNOSIS

DIFFERENTIAL DIAGNOSIS
• Labile essential hypertension
• Anxiety and panic attacks
• Paroxysmal cardiac arrhythmia
• Thyrotoxicosis
• Menopausal syndrome
• Hypoglycemia
• Mastocytosis
• Withdrawal of adrenergic-inhibiting medications
• Angina
• Hyperventilation
• Migraine headache
• Amphetamine or cocaine use
• Sympathomimetic ingestion

LABORATORY
• Elevated 24-h urine metanephrine
• Elevated 24-h urine or plasma catecholamines measured by high performance liquid chromatography (HPLC)
• If results equivocal or normal, repeat 24-h urine collection with a spell
Drugs that may alter lab results:
Increased by:
◊ Amphetamines
◊ Clonidine or other drug withdrawal
◊ Labetalol
◊ Ethanol
◊ Methyldopa
◊ Sotalol
◊ Levodopa
Decreased by:
◊ Central alpha-2 agonists
◊ Reserpine
Disorders that may alter lab results:
Major physical stress (e.g., surgery, stroke)

PATHOLOGICAL FINDINGS
Catecholamine-producing tumor in the adrenal medulla, para-aortic sympathetic chain, wall of the urinary bladder, sympathetic chain in the neck or mediastinum

SPECIAL TESTS Clonidine suppression test, suppression/provocative tests

IMAGING
• Computerized abdominal imaging (MRI preferred over CT)
• M-131-I-iodobenzylguanidine scan

DIAGNOSTIC PROCEDURES N/A

 TREATMENT

APPROPRIATE HEALTH CARE
Inpatient surgery

GENERAL MEASURES
• Combined alpha- and beta-adrenergic blockade
• High risk surgical procedure
• Experienced surgeon/anesthesiologist team required
• Cardiovascular and hemodynamic variables must be monitored closely

ACTIVITY No limitations

DIET High in salt content preoperatively

PATIENT EDUCATION N/A

MEDICATIONS

DRUG(S) OF CHOICE
• Combined alpha- and beta-adrenergic blockade required preoperatively
• Initiate alpha-blockade first - phenoxybenzamine (Dibenzyline) 10 mg daily and increase by 10-20 mg every 2 days as needed to control blood pressure and paroxysmal spells (average dose is 0.5-1.0 mg/kg daily)
• Beta-blockade after alpha-blockade is established - propranolol (Inderal) 10 mg every 6 hours initially and increase as necessary to control tachycardia
• Acute hypertensive crises should be treated with phentolamine (Regitine) administered intravenously
Contraindications: Beta-adrenergic blockade in patients with asthma, sinus bradycardia and greater than first degree block, or congestive heart failure
Precautions:
• Beta-adrenergic blockade alone may result in more severe hypertension due to the unopposed alpha-adrenergic stimulation; patients should be cautioned about postural hypotension
• Beta-adrenergic blockade is initiated at low doses of a short acting agent due to the possible side effect of pulmonary edema in the patient with catecholamine myocardiopathy
Significant possible Interactions: For beta-adrenergic blockade - verapamil, phenytoin, phenobarbitone, rifampin, chlorpromazine, cimetidine

ALTERNATIVE DRUGS
• Alpha-adrenergic blocking agents - prazosin (Minipress), terazosin (Hytrin), doxazosin (Cardura)
• Beta-adrenergic blocking agents - nadolol (Corgard), atenolol (Tenormin), metoprolol (Lopressor)
• Combined beta- and alpha-adrenergic blocker - labetalol (Normodyne, TranDate)
• Catecholamine synthesis inhibitor - metyrosine (Demser)

FOLLOWUP

PATIENT MONITORING
• Daily blood pressure monitoring prior to surgery
• Intra-operative hemodynamic monitoring
• Two weeks postoperatively - 24-h urine for measurement of catecholamines and metanephrines; if normal, re-check annually for five years

PREVENTION/AVOIDANCE   N/A

POSSIBLE COMPLICATIONS
• Postural hypotension with alpha-adrenergic blockade
• Pulmonary edema with beta-adrenergic blockade
• Intra-operative hypertensive crisis

EXPECTED COURSE AND PROGNOSIS
The survival rate after removal of a benign pheochromocytoma is nearly that of age- and sex-matched controls. For malignant pheochromocytoma the 5-year survival rate is less than 50%.

MISCELLANEOUS

ASSOCIATED CONDITIONS
• Multiple endocrine neoplasia type IIA (medullary thyroid carcinoma and primary hyperparathyroidism)
• Multiple endocrine neoplasia type IIB (medullary thyroid carcinoma and mucosal neuromas)
• Neurofibromatosis
• Von Hippel-Lindau syndrome (retinal angiomatosis and cerebellar hemangioblastoma)
• Ataxia-telangiectasia
• Tuberous sclerosis
• Sturge-Weber syndrome
• Cholelithiasis
• Renal artery stenosis

AGE-RELATED FACTORS
Pediatric: N/A
Geriatric: N/A
Others: N/A

PREGNANCY
• First and second trimester - surgical resection
• Third trimester - cesarean section and removal of the pheochromocytoma in the same operation

SYNONYMS   Paraganglioma

ICD-9-CM   194.0

SEE ALSO   Hypertension

OTHER NOTES
All patients with paroxysmal spells and hypertension or with difficult to control hypertension should be screened

ABBREVIATIONS   HPLC = high performance liquid chromatography

REFERENCES
• Sheps, S.G., Jiang, N.S. & Klee, G.G.: Diagnostic evaluation of pheochromocytoma. Endocrinol Metab Clinic North America, 1988
• Bravo, E.L. & Gifford, R.W.: Pheochromocytoma: Diagnosis, localization, and management. N Engl J Med., 1984;311:1298

Author   W. F. Young, Jr., M.D.

Phimosis and paraphimosis

 BASICS

DESCRIPTION
• Phimosis - tightness of the penile foreskin which prevents it from being drawn back from over the glans
• Paraphimosis - constriction of glans penis by proximally placed phimotic foreskin
System(s) affected: Renal/Urologic, Reproductive, Skin/Exocrine
Genetics: N/A
Incidence/Prevalence in USA: 1% of boys over 16 years of age
Predominant age: Infancy and adolescence
Predominant sex: Male only

SIGNS AND SYMPTOMS
Phimosis
◊ Unretractable foreskin
◊ Pain in erection
◊ Superimposed balanitis
Paraphimosis
◊ Penile pain
◊ Drainage
◊ Ulceration
◊ Swelling

CAUSES
Phimosis
◊ "Physiologic" - present at birth and resolves spontaneously during the first 2-3 years of life by nocturnal erections which slowly dilate the phimotic ring
◊ Congenital - unresolved physiologic phimosis
◊ Acquired - recurrent infection or irritation
Paraphimosis
◊ Foreskin not retracted back over the glans after cleaning, cystoscopy or catheter insertion

RISK FACTORS
Phimosis
◊ Poor hygiene
◊ Diabetes
◊ Frequent diaper rash in infant
Paraphimosis
◊ Presence of foreskin
◊ "Inexperienced" health care provider, i.e., leaving foreskin retracted after catheter placement

 DIAGNOSIS

DIFFERENTIAL DIAGNOSIS Penile lymphedema which can be related to insect bites, trauma or allergic reactions

LABORATORY N/A
Drugs that may alter lab results: N/A
Disorders that may alter lab results: N/A

PATHOLOGICAL FINDINGS N/A

SPECIAL TESTS N/A

IMAGING N/A

DIAGNOSTIC PROCEDURES N/A

 TREATMENT

APPROPRIATE HEALTH CARE
Outpatient except for complications

GENERAL MEASURES
• Phimosis: Circumcision
• Paraphimosis: Reduction if possible (should be done with the patient sedated). Place the middle and index fingers of both hands on the engorged skin proximal to the glans. Place both thumbs on glans and with gentle pressure pushing on the glans and pulling on foreskin, attempt reduction. If unsuccessful, a dorsal slit will be necessary with eventual circumcision after the edema resolves.

ACTIVITY No sexual activity following circumcision until healing is complete

DIET No limitations

PATIENT EDUCATION If the patient is uncircumcised, appropriate hygiene and care of the foreskin is necessary to prevent phimosis and paraphimosis

MEDICATIONS

DRUG(S) OF CHOICE N/A
Contraindications: N/A
Precautions: N/A
Significant possible interactions: N/A

ALTERNATIVE DRUGS N/A

FOLLOWUP

PATIENT MONITORING 1 week after reduction of paraphimosis and 1 to 2 weeks after a circumcision

PREVENTION/AVOIDANCE Good patient and parental education

POSSIBLE COMPLICATIONS
• Unreduced paraphimosis can lead to gangrene of the glans
• Posthitis (inflammation of the prepuce)

EXPECTED COURSE AND PROGNOSIS Complete resolution if treatment is carried out effectively

MISCELLANEOUS

ASSOCIATED CONDITIONS N/A

AGE-RELATED FACTORS
Pediatric:
• Recurrent balanitis, either chemical or infectious, can lead to an acquired phimosis
• Forced reduction of a physiologic foreskin can lead to chronic scarring and acquired phimosis
Geriatric: Recurrent infection and irritations (condom catheterizations) can lead to phimosis
Others: N/A

PREGNANCY N/A

SYNONYMS N/A

ICD-9-CM
• Phimosis 605
• Paraphimosis 605

SEE ALSO N/A

OTHER NOTES N/A

ABBREVIATIONS N/A

REFERENCES Kelalis, P.P., King, L.R. & Belman, A.B.: Clinical Pediatric Urology. 3rd Ed. Philadelphia, W. B. Saunders Co., 1991

Author J. Miller, M.D. & T. Black, M.D.

Phobias

BASICS

DESCRIPTION Psychiatric conditions classified in Diagnostic and Statistical Manual of Mental Disorders (DSM-III-R) as anxiety disorders. When confronted with the phobic stimulus, patient reacts with intense anxiety, usually realizes the fear is excessive or exaggerated. When a fear causes significant distress and interferes with normal functions of life, then it is considered a psychiatric disorder.
• Agoraphobia: Fear of being trapped in a situation where escape is impossible or difficult. Fear centers on 1) fear of being alone, 2) fear of being away from home and 3) fear of being in place where escape is difficult - seen most often in association with panic disorder.
• Simple phobia: Fear of a discrete stimulus such as animals, insects, heights, flying, claustrophobia, blood-injury phobia
• Social phobia: Fear of humiliation or embarrassment in social situations where person may be under scrutiny by others, e.g., performance anxiety, speaking in public, or fear of using public toilets

Incidence/Prevalence in USA: 1 month prevalence of all phobic conditions: 6.2%
System(s) affected: Nervous
Genetics: No consistent genetic pattern
Predominant age:
• Agoraphobia - onset 18-35 (mean 24)
• Simple phobia fear of animals - onset usually in childhood (mean 4.4 years)
• Simple phobia fear of heights, claustrophobia - 4th decade
• Other simple phobias - mean 22.7 years
• Social phobia - late childhood, adolescence (mean 19 years)
Predominant sex:
• Female > Male, overall phobias
• Male = Female, social phobia

SIGNS AND SYMPTOMS
• Extreme anxiety when exposed to phobic stimulus
• Tremors
• Palpitations
• Sweating
• Blushing
• Dyspnea
• Associated nausea

CAUSES
• Persistence or exaggeration of learned response, learned initially as a protective mechanism (such as avoidance of large dogs by small children)
• Social - learned maladaptive anxiety response to social situation

RISK FACTORS
• For all phobias - presence of another psychiatric disorder
• Separation anxiety in childhood
• Introverted or dependent personality

DIAGNOSIS

DIFFERENTIAL DIAGNOSIS
For agoraphobia:
 ◊ Paranoid and psychotic states
 ◊ PTSD (posttraumatic stress disorder)
 ◊ Depression - but do not see the other aspects of depression (anhedonia, loss of appetite and libido, sleep disturbance-early morning awakening, frequent night awakening, difficulty falling asleep)
For simple phobia:
 ◊ Schizophrenia - avoidance can be seen but usually in response to a delusion and patient does not realize that fear is excessive. Schizophrenia is intimately intertwined with delusion.
 ◊ PTSD - phobic avoidance seen and is associated with the original trauma
 ◊ Obsessive compulsive disorder (OCD) - avoidance associated with obsessions (such as dirt avoidance)
For social phobia:
 ◊ Avoidant personality disorder - central fear in avoidant personality disorder is that of rejection, not of humiliation or embarrassment as in social phobia
 ◊ Paranoid personality disorder
 ◊ Schizophrenia

LABORATORY None
Drugs that may alter lab results: N/A
Disorders that may alter lab results: N/A

PATHOLOGICAL FINDINGS N/A

SPECIAL TESTS None

IMAGING N/A

DIAGNOSTIC PROCEDURES
• Careful history and observation of the patient
• Description of the behavior by patient, family or friends
• Psychiatric examination

TREATMENT

APPROPRIATE HEALTH CARE
Outpatient

GENERAL MEASURES
Agoraphobia:
 ◊ Behavioral treatment
 ◊ Graduated exposure
 ◊ Different treatment required when agoraphobia is associated with panic disorder
Simple phobia:
 ◊ In vivo or graduated exposure
 ◊ Fear of flying specifically - benzodiazepine
Social phobia:
 ◊ Social skills training
 ◊ Graduated exposure
 ◊ Performance anxiety or situations where patient in a circumscribed setting - beta blocker

ACTIVITY No restriction

DIET Consider restriction of stimulants - such as caffeine, nicotine, xanthines, sympathomimetics, which can overdrive anxiety. Phenelzine - requires tyramine free diet.

PATIENT EDUCATION
• Cognitive therapy
• Phobia clinic or group therapy, if available

MEDICATIONS

DRUG(S) OF CHOICE
• Agoraphobia - none recommended
• Simple phobia - none recommended, except for fear of flying. A benzodiazepine, such as alprazolam, may help. Initial dose as low as 0.5 mg titrated upward as needed.
• Social phobia (acute) - beta-blocker, e.g., propranolol (Inderal) 10-40 mg, 45-60 minutes before anticipated performance, atenolol 50-100 mg/day for more generalized social phobia
• Social phobia (chronic) - phenelzine (a MAO inhibitor), up to 90 mg/day, if social phobia more generalized and requires more constant medication (as opposed to the sporadic treatment for performance anxiety)
Contraindications:
• Beta-blocker - asthma or bronchospasm, congestive heart failure, bradycardia
• Phenelzine - not with other antidepressants, tyramine in diet, decongestants, diet pills, Demerol
Precautions:
• Do not abruptly discontinue alprazolam due to potential for withdrawal seizures to develop
• Monitor blood pressure in patients on beta-blockers
Significant possible interactions:
Phenelzine - significant dietary restrictions due to potential for hypertensive crisis. Drugs to avoid include: Sympathomimetics, TCA's, fluoxetine, CNS depressants. Consult drug information sources before adding new medications in patients.

ALTERNATIVE DRUGS As above

FOLLOWUP

PATIENT MONITORING Outpatient as needed

PREVENTION/AVOIDANCE N/A

POSSIBLE COMPLICATIONS
• Avoidance behavior
• Episodic alcohol, barbiturate and anxiolytic abuse/overuse and dependence as patients try to self-medicate to ameliorate symptoms
• Development of mild depression

EXPECTED COURSE AND PROGNOSIS
• Agoraphobia - usually associated with panic disorder, chronic. Often patient becomes more and more home-bound as condition continues.
• Simple phobia - some spontaneously remit as person ages (as in some simple phobias of childhood), alternatively some become chronic. Impairment can be minimal if object can be avoided (such as snakes). Although improvement occurs with in vivo exposure, phobia can recur after successful treatment.
• Social phobia - chronic course

MISCELLANEOUS

ASSOCIATED CONDITIONS
• For all phobias - depression, substance abuse
• Social and agoraphobia - panic attacks or panic disorder

AGE-RELATED FACTORS
Pediatric: Animal phobia mean age of onset 4.4 years
Geriatric: N/A
Others: N/A

PREGNANCY No data

SYNONYMS N/A

ICD-9-CM
• Agoraphobia 300.22
• Simple phobia 300.29
• Social phobia 300. 23

SEE ALSO N/A

OTHER NOTES ICD-9-CM codes identical to DSM-III-R

ABBREVIATIONS PTSD = (posttraumatic stress disorder)

REFERENCES
• American Psychiatric Association: Diagnostic and Statistical Manual of Mental Disorders (DSM-III-R). 3rd Ed. Washington, D.C., 1987

Author K. Hall, M.D.

Photodermatitis

BASICS

DESCRIPTION Light-induced eruptions seen in a pattern of photo-distribution
• Phototoxic reactions - result of the acute toxic effect on skin of ultraviolet light alone (sunburn) or together with a photosensitizing substance (non-allergic)
• Photoallergic eruptions - a form of allergic dermatitis resulting from combined effects of a photosensitizing substance (drugs or chemical) plus ultraviolet light (immunologic/delayed hypersensitivity)
• Polymorphous light eruption (PLE) - chronic, intermittent light-induced eruption with erythematous papules, urticaria, or vesicles on areas exposed to sunlight
System(s) affected: Skin
Genetics: Predisposition occurs in inbred populations (e.g., Pima Indians)
Incidence/Prevalence in USA: Unknown
Predominant age: All ages
Predominant sex: Male = Female

SIGNS AND SYMPTOMS
Phototoxic
◊ Erythema
◊ With increasing severity - vesicles and bullae
◊ Classic example - sunburn
◊ Nails may exhibit onycholysis
◊ Chronic - epidermal thickening, elastosis, telangiectasia and pigmentary changes
◊ Sharp lines of demarcation between involved and uninvolved skin (sunlight exposure)
◊ Phototoxic eruption due to topicals - area of application
◊ Usually develops shortly after sun exposure
◊ Hyperpigmentation may follow resolution
◊ Pain
Photoallergic
◊ Papules with erythema and occasionally vesicles
◊ Area exposed to light with less distinct borders
◊ Usually delayed - 24 hours or more after exposure
◊ May spread to unexposed areas
◊ Pruritus
Polymorphous light eruption (PLE)
◊ Erythematous papules
◊ Occasionally urticaria or vesicles
◊ Scattered over sun exposed areas with normal skin in between
◊ Can spread to non-exposed areas
◊ Often flares in spring or early summer
◊ Desensitization affect (less over the course of the summer)
◊ Burning or pruritus may precede lesions

CAUSES
• Sunlight
• Phenothiazines
• Diuretics
• Tetracyclines
• Sulfonamides
• Oral contraceptives
• Topicals - psoralens, coal tars, photo-active dyes (eosin, acridine orange)

RISK FACTORS N/A

DIAGNOSIS

DIFFERENTIAL DIAGNOSIS
• Systemic lupus erythematosus

LABORATORY Antinuclear antibody (ANA) to rule out systemic lupus erythematosus
Drugs that may alter lab results: N/A
Disorders that may alter lab results: N/A

PATHOLOGICAL FINDINGS Nonspecific

SPECIAL TESTS
• Photo-testing
• Photopatch testing
• Skin biopsy - to rule out other disorders

IMAGING N/A

DIAGNOSTIC PROCEDURES Physical examination and medical history

TREATMENT

APPROPRIATE HEALTH CARE
Outpatient

GENERAL MEASURES
• Avoid sunlight/limit exposure
• Protective clothing/sunscreens
• Ice packs/cold water compresses

ACTIVITY Avoid sunlight

DIET No special diet

PATIENT EDUCATION
• Avoidance of sunlight
• Avoidance of photosensitizing drugs
• Protective clothing
• Sunscreens

Photodermatitis

MEDICATIONS

DRUG(S) OF CHOICE
• Topical corticosteroids (betamethasone valerate 0.1% cream)
• Salicylates or nonsteroidal anti-inflammatory agents (indomethacin 25 mg tid)
• Prednisone for severe reactions (0.5-1 mg/kg/d) for 3-10 days
• Antihistamines for pruritus (hydroxyzine 25-50 mg qid)
• Sunscreens for prevention. Use broad-spectrum sunscreen to block both UVA and UVB. PABA may aggravate photodermatitis in sensitized patients (due to the sulfa moiety).
Contraindications: Refer to manufacturer's profile of each drug
Precautions: Refer to manufacturer's profile of each drug
Significant possible interactions: Refer to manufacturer's profile of each drug

ALTERNATIVE DRUGS N/A

FOLLOWUP

PATIENT MONITORING As necessary for persistence or recurrence

PREVENTION/AVOIDANCE
• Sunlight avoidance/protective clothing
• Identification and avoidance of causative drugs (see under Causes)
Sunscreens - apply before exposure
  ◊ Zinc oxide - opaque, cosmetically less acceptable
  ◊ Chemical - use sun-protective factor > 15 for maximum protection; substantively resistant to sweat and swimming; cosmetically more acceptable

POSSIBLE COMPLICATIONS N/A

EXPECTED COURSE AND PROGNOSIS Good with avoidance/protection measures

MISCELLANEOUS

ASSOCIATED CONDITIONS
• Sunlight aggravation of systemic lupus
• Persistent light reactivity
• Actinic reticuloid

AGE-RELATED FACTORS N/A
Pediatric: N/A
Geriatric: More likely to experience adverse reactions to causative drugs
Others: N/A

PREGNANCY N/A

SYNONYMS
• Sun poisoning

ICD-9-CM
• 692.79 due to solar radiation, other
• 692.89 due to other specified agents, other

SEE ALSO N/A

OTHER NOTES N/A

ABBREVIATIONS N/A

REFERENCES Bondi, J., Jegasothy, B. & Lazarus, G.: Dermatology, Diagnosis and Therapy. Norwalk, CT, Appleton & Lange, 1991

Author J. Stearns, M.D.

Pinworms

 BASICS

DESCRIPTION Intestinal infection with Enterobius vermicularis. Characterized by perianal itching, usually worse at night.
System(s) affected: Gastrointestinal, Skin
Genetics: N/A
Incidence in USA: N/A
Prevalence in USA: Approximately 20% of young children (ages 5-10)
Predominant age: 5 to 14
Predominant sex: Female > Male

SIGNS AND SYMPTOMS
- Perianal itching
- Perineal itching
- Vulvovaginitis
- Enuresis
- Abdominal pain
- Insomnia

CAUSES The intestinal nematode Enterobius (Oxyuris) vermicularis

RISK FACTORS
- Institutionalization (50-90% of institutionalized children have pinworms)
- Crowded living conditions
- Poor hygiene
- Warm climate

 DIAGNOSIS

DIFFERENTIAL DIAGNOSIS
- Idiopathic pruritus ani
- Atopic dermatitis
- Contact dermatitis
- Psoriasis
- Lichen planus
- Infection with human papilloma virus
- Herpes simplex
- Fungal infections
- Erythrasma
- Scabies
- Vaginitis

LABORATORY N/A
Drugs that may alter lab results: N/A
Disorders that may alter lab results: N/A

PATHOLOGICAL FINDINGS
Identification of ova on low power microscopy or direct visualization of the female worm (10 mm in length). Ova are asymmetric, flattened on one side, and measure 30 by 60 mm.

SPECIAL TESTS
- Transparent tape test - a piece of transparent cellophane tape is adhered to the perianal skin in the early morning and then affixed to a microscope slide. This procedure must be performed at least 3 times to achieve 90% sensitivity.
- Flashlight to perianal region at night for direct observation
- Digital rectal examination with saline slide preparation of stool on gloved finger

IMAGING N/A

DIAGNOSTIC PROCEDURES N/A

 TREATMENT

APPROPRIATE HEALTH CARE
Outpatient

GENERAL MEASURES
- All symptomatic family members should be treated simultaneously
- Bedclothes and underwear of infected individuals should be washed in hot water at the time of treatment (ova can remain viable for 2-3 weeks in a moist environment)
- Strict hand washing can help prevent fecal-oral transmission
- Practice good hygiene (showers, nail cleaning)
- Topical use of antipruritic creams or ointments may help relive itching in the perianal region

ACTIVITY No restrictions

DIET No restrictions

PATIENT EDUCATION For patient education materials on this topic: Centers for Disease Control, Dept. of Health and Human Services, Office of Public Affairs, Atlanta, GA 30333, (404)329-3534

MEDICATIONS

DRUG(S) OF CHOICE
• Mebendazole (Vermox) chewable tablet 100 mg as a single dose. Repeat same dose in 2 weeks. Use with caution in children < age 2, or
• Pyrantel pamoate (Antiminth) oral suspension 11 mg/kg as a single dose. Repeat same dose in 2 weeks. Maximum dose 1 gram. Use with caution in children < age 2, or
• Pyrvinium pamoate (Povan) tablets 5 mg/kg as a single dose. Repeat same dose in 2 weeks. Maximum dose 350 mg, or
• Piperazine citrate (Vermizine) tablets or suspension 50 mg/kg/day x 7 days. Second course given after 2-4 weeks. Maximum daily dose 2.5 g.
Contraindications: Refer to manufacturer's profile of each drug
Precautions:
• All family members should be treated
• Take medicine on empty stomach
• May cause diarrhea and/or nausea
Significant possible interactions: Refer to manufacturer's profile of each drug

ALTERNATIVE DRUGS N/A

FOLLOWUP

PATIENT MONITORING Unnecessary
unless symptoms do not abate following drug therapy

PREVENTION/AVOIDANCE
• Careful hand washing, keep nails short and clean
• Wash anus and genitals at least once a day, preferably in a shower
• Don't scratch anus or put fingers near nose or mouth

POSSIBLE COMPLICATIONS
• Perianal scratching may cause impetigo or excoriation
• Young girls - vulvovaginitis, urethritis, endometritis, salpingitis
• Urinary tract infections

EXPECTED COURSE AND PROGNOSIS
• Asymptomatic carriers are common
• Symptomatic infections are cured > 90% of the time with drug therapy
• Reinfection is common

MISCELLANEOUS

ASSOCIATED CONDITIONS Pruritis ani

AGE-RELATED FACTORS
Pediatric: More common in children and more likely to get reinfected
Geriatric: N/A
Others: N/A

PREGNANCY Drug therapy is
contraindicated in pregnancy

SYNONYMS Enterobiasis

ICD-9-CM 127.4 Enterobiasis

SEE ALSO N/A

OTHER NOTES N/A

ABBREVIATIONS N/A

REFERENCES
• Wyngaarden, J.B., Smith, L.H. (eds.): Cecil Textbook of Medicine. 19th Ed. Philadelphia, W.B. Saunders Co., 1992
• Berman, R.E., et al (eds.): Nelson Textbook of Pediatrics. 14th Ed., Philadelphia, W.B. Saunders Co., 1992

Author S. Eisenstein, M.D.

Pityriasis alba

BASICS

DESCRIPTION A chronic skin disorder characterized by one or more groups of poorly marginated, white patches and plaques that appear on the cheeks and lateral arms of children and young adults

Genetics: Unknown, but is primarily seen in children with a genetic predisposition to atopic disease

System(s) affected: Skin/Exocrine

Incidence in USA: Common, exact incidence unknown

Prevalence in USA: Common, especially in darked skin individuals in sunnier climates (90% for ages 6-12)

Predominant age: 3-10 years. Rare after 25.

Predominant sex: Male = Female

SIGNS AND SYMPTOMS

- Description - small white patches
- Location - cheeks and lateral arms
- Number - 1-12 or more patches
- Palpation - smooth or slightly rough, and dry
- Appearance - pinpoint white papules (representing accentuation and keratinization of follicular orifices)
- Scale is either invisible or fine and light
- More common in dark skinned individuals
- Usually asymptomatic
- Pruritic (rare)
- More apparent in summertime in light skinned individuals
- Lesions do not tan in summer
- Even a small amount of sunlight exposure causes lesions to redden

CAUSES

- Unknown. Maybe part of an atopic diathesis.
- Possibly defects in melanin production or transfer

RISK FACTORS Children with a genetic predisposition to atopic disease

DIAGNOSIS

DIFFERENTIAL DIAGNOSIS

- Pityriasis versicolor
- Vitiligo
- Milia
- Keratosis pilaris
- Indeterminate or uncharacteristic leprosy

LABORATORY N/A

Drugs that may alter lab results: N/A

Disorders that may alter lab results: N/A

PATHOLOGICAL FINDINGS N/A

SPECIAL TESTS N/A

IMAGING N/A

DIAGNOSTIC PROCEDURES History and physical exam. Atopic diathesis is of diagnostic significance.

TREATMENT

APPROPRIATE HEALTH CARE
Outpatient

GENERAL MEASURES No truly effective therapy available. Lubricating cream application may improve roughness and/or dryness.

ACTIVITY No restrictions

DIET No special diet

PATIENT EDUCATION Stress long-term chronicity and permanent resolution in second or third decade of life

MEDICATIONS

DRUG(S) OF CHOICE
• Coal tar preparations (e.g., Alphosyl or Estar or Balnetar) applied topically once or twice a day. Treatment is not mandatory.
• Topical steroids if needed to reduce redness due to sunburn or spontaneous inflammation
• Note: Neither will change the pigmentation, but may improve pruritus, roughness and/or dryness, if the lubricating cream is not sufficient
• Phototherapy (e.g., UVB)
Contraindications: N/A
Precautions: Refer to manufacturer's literature
Significant possible interactions: N/A

ALTERNATIVE DRUGS N/A

 FOLLOWUP

PATIENT MONITORING As needed only if lesions become symptomatic

PREVENTION/AVOIDANCE No known preventive measures

POSSIBLE COMPLICATIONS None expected

EXPECTED COURSE AND PROGNOSIS Permanent resolution during second or third decade of life

 MISCELLANEOUS

ASSOCIATED CONDITIONS N/A

AGE-RELATED FACTORS
Pediatric: More common in children 3 to 10 years
Geriatric: Rare in this age group
Others: N/A

PREGNANCY N/A

SYNONYMS
• Pityriasis streptogenes
• Pityriasis simplex
• Pityriasis sicca faciei
• Erythema streptogenes
• Furfuraceous impetigo

ICD-9-CM 696.5

SEE ALSO
• Pityriasis versicolor
• Vitiligo
• Keratosis

OTHER NOTES N/A

ABBREVIATIONS N/A

REFERENCES
• Habif, T.: Clinical Dermatology. 2nd Ed. St. Louis, C.V. Mosby, 1990
• Sams, W.M. & Lynch, P.J. (eds): Principles and Practices of Dermatology. New York, Churchill Livingstone, 1990
• Fitzpatrick, T.B., et al. (eds.): Dermatology in General Medicine. 3rd Ed. New York, McGraw-Hill, 1987
• Domankos, A.N., Arnold, K.L. & Odom, R.B.:Andrews' Diseases of the Skin. 8th Ed. Philadelphia, W.B. Saunders Co., 1990

Author M. King, M.D.

Pityriasis rosea

 BASICS

DESCRIPTION An idiopathic self-limited skin eruption characterized by widespread papulosquamous lesions
System(s) affected: Skin/Exocrine
Genetics: Less than 5 percent of those affected give a positive family history
Incidence/Prevalence in USA: Relatively common but exact frequency unknown
Predominant age: 10-35, but occurs in all age groups
Predominant sex: Male = Female

SIGNS AND SYMPTOMS
• Salmon to light brown oval plaques with fine scales centrally and "collarette" of loose scales along borders
• Lesions average 1-2 cm in diameter and usually spare face, hands and feet in adults
• Lesions frequently oriented along skin cleavage lines in "Christmas tree" pattern
• Eruption often preceded by 2-6 cm "herald patch" of similar appearance days to weeks before generalized rash
• Mild pruritus, rarely severe
• Fever and malaise rare
• Variant forms include purpuric, urticarial, and vesicular lesions

CAUSES Unknown, may be a viral agent or an autoimmune disorder

RISK FACTORS Unknown

 DIAGNOSIS

DIFFERENTIAL DIAGNOSIS
• Secondary syphilis
• Viral exanthems
• Drug rashes
• Psoriasis
• Parapsoriasis
• Eczema
• Lichen planus
• Tinea corporis

LABORATORY WBC normal. No specific lab markers. Serology to rule out syphilis.
Drugs that may alter lab results: N/A
Disorders that may alter lab results: N/A

PATHOLOGICAL FINDINGS Chronic inflammation with cytolytic degeneration of keratinocytes adjacent to Langerhans cells

SPECIAL TESTS KOH preparation to distinguish from tinea corporis

IMAGING N/A

DIAGNOSTIC PROCEDURES N/A

 TREATMENT

APPROPRIATE HEALTH CARE
Outpatient

GENERAL MEASURES
• Symptomatic treatment
• Topical antipruritics as needed
• Ultraviolet therapy has been used but efficacy not proven
• Lukewarm oatmeal baths (not hot as it can intensify itching)

ACTIVITY Full activity with good skin hygiene to prevent secondary infection

DIET N/A

PATIENT EDUCATION
• Reassurance as to self-limited nature of condition
• Printed patient information available from: American Academy of Dermatology (708) 330-0230.

MEDICATIONS

DRUG(S) OF CHOICE Topical steroids to reduce itching, if needed
Contraindications: N/A
Precautions: N/A
Significant possible interactions: N/A

ALTERNATIVE DRUGS N/A

FOLLOWUP

PATIENT MONITORING
• Check syphilis serology
• Return visit for reevaluation, if lesions persist longer than 8-10 weeks

PREVENTION/AVOIDANCE N/A

POSSIBLE COMPLICATIONS
Secondary infection (e.g., impetigo)

EXPECTED COURSE AND PROGNOSIS Gradual resolution in 1-14 weeks (usually 2-6)

MISCELLANEOUS

ASSOCIATED CONDITIONS N/A

AGE-RELATED FACTORS
Pediatric: Face, distal extremities more often involved in children and lesions may be more papular
Geriatric: N/A
Others: N/A

PREGNANCY N/A

SYNONYMS N/A

ICD-9-CM 696.3

SEE ALSO N/A

OTHER NOTES N/A

ABBREVIATIONS N/A

REFERENCES
• Fitzpatrick, T.B. et al. (eds.): Dermatology In General Medicine. 3rd Ed. New York, McGraw-Hill, 1987
• Cheong, W.K. & Wong, K.S.: Pityriasis Rosea. Singapore Medical J, Feb, 1989

Author J. Wolfrey, M.D.

Placenta previa

BASICS

DESCRIPTION Placental placement near, partially, or completely over the cervical os
Marginal previa: Placement near enough to cervical os to cause risk of hemorrhage during effacement and dilation of the cervix during labor
Partial previa: Placement causing partial covering of the cervical os
Total previa: Placement that causes entire os to be covered by placenta
System(s) affected: Reproductive, Cardiovascular
Genetics: N/A
Incidence in USA: 0.5% to 0.8% of all pregnancies; low lying placenta 4-8% in early pregnancy with < 10% persisting to term
Prevalence in USA: N/A
Predominant age: Childbearing ages
Predominant sex: Female only

SIGNS AND SYMPTOMS
• Typically painless bright red bleeding 2nd or 3rd trimester
• Average time of first bleed, 27-32 weeks
• Contractions variably present
• First bleed usually self limited
• Maternal hemodynamic status consistent with clinical blood loss estimate
• Complete previas may bleed earlier and not "migrate"

CAUSES Prior uterine insult or injury or other uterine factors

RISK FACTORS
• Prior previa (4%-8%)
• First subsequent pregnancy following a cesarean section delivery
• Multiparity (5% in grand multiparous patient)
• Advanced maternal age
• Multiple gestation
• Prior induced abortions
• Smoking

DIAGNOSIS

DIFFERENTIAL DIAGNOSIS Abruptio placentae, vasa previa, vaginal and cervical causes including marked "bloody show" and infections

LABORATORY
• Maternal blood type and Rh
• Hemoglobin and hematocrit
• Platelet count
• PT, PTT, fibrinogen
• Type and cross match packed RBC (at least three units)
• Apt test: To determine fetal origin of blood (as in vasa previa). Mix vaginal blood with small amount tap water to cause hemolysis, centrifuge for several minutes, mix 1 cc of 1% NaOH with each 5 cc of the pink-hemoglobin-containing supernatant, observing pink fluid if fetal hemoglobin, and yellow-brown if adult origin.
• Wright's stain applied to a slide smear of vaginal blood looking for nucleated RBC's which are usually from cord blood and not adult blood
• L/S ratio for fetal maturity if needed
Drugs that may alter lab results: Drugs altering cell counts or clotting studies
Disorders that may alter lab results:
• Coagulopathies from other causes
• Red cell and hemoglobin disorders from other causes

PATHOLOGICAL FINDINGS
• Normocytic, normochromic anemia with acute bleed
• Coagulopathy rare, but may occur
• Positive Kleihauer-Betke if fetal/maternal transfusion

SPECIAL TESTS
• Kleihauer-Betke if concerned about fetal-maternal transfusion
• Bedside clot test: Draw red top tube from mother and observe for clot quality at 7-10 minutes. If there is no clot or if clot is friable may indicate disseminated intravascular coagulation (DIC).

IMAGING
• External sector sonography with moderately full and empty bladder
• Vaginal probe sonography may be done if not actively bleeding. Place the probe just inside os and use 5 or 6.5-mHz transducers.
• Magnetic resonance imaging (MRI) accurate, but more expensive, less available, and time consuming

DIAGNOSTIC PROCEDURES
• If placenta location unknown and sonography not available, a double setup bimanual vaginal exam may be done in operating room with complete cesarean section readiness

• Careful vaginal speculum exam is not contraindicated and allows checking for cervical or vaginal source of bleeding, fern and nitrazine testing, cultures, and fluid for determining bleeding source
• Since fibrin degradation products rise in pregnancy, these levels are less helpful

TREATMENT

APPROPRIATE HEALTH CARE
• Inpatient observation at bedrest initially; once stable, and preterm, may be followed as outpatient
• May consider transfer to high risk center based on condition and local services

GENERAL MEASURES
• Optimizing maternal stability while delaying delivery, if possible, or if preterm to improve perinatal outcome
• Cesarean section indicated for partial or complete previa if fetus is mature or if the situation is urgent and the fetus is immature
• A trial of labor may be considered with anterior marginal previa, including oxytocin (Pitocin) augmentation IV
• Amniocentesis for L/S ratio for maturity as needed
• IV fluid support, oxygen, transfusions of packed RBC's, platelets and fresh frozen plasma if needed
• External fetal and labor monitoring
• Other intervention or observation based on maternal condition
• DIC risk low unless massive bleed. Follow coagulation studies and give fresh frozen plasma (FFP), platelets as needed, or cryoprecipitate if fibrinogen < 100-150.
• Transfuse platelets at < 20,000 or < 50,000 if surgery needed
• Low lying posterior marginal previa associated with tissue dystocia and greater need for cesarean section
• Blood volume increased in pregnancy; can lose > 30% maternal blood volume before shock findings
• Central line placement only after checking coagulation studies
• May use sector probe with condom at introitus if vaginal probe unavailable

ACTIVITY
• Bedrest
• Intercourse abstinence

DIET NPO initially, then based on delivery decisions

PATIENT EDUCATION
• First bleed rarely fatal
• Rebleed risk with activity or cervical stimulation
• Greatest cause of perinatal mortality is prematurity
• Risks and conditions associated with previa

MEDICATIONS

DRUG(S) OF CHOICE
• For IV fluids: Lactated Ringer's or saline
• Oxygen for all, since O2 consumption up 20% in pregnancy and fetus is more prone to hypoxia
• Fresh frozen plasma and platelets as needed
• Cryoprecipitate and fibrinogen if above unsuccessful
• Tocolytics may have role in certain preterm patients, but tachycardia of B-agonists (terbutaline) and risk of placental hypoperfusion with calcium channel blockers may make MgSO4 the drug of choice. For MgSO4, use 4 grams IV load and 1-4 grams/hour as indicated.
Contraindications:
Avoid tocolytics with term infant or unstable mother
Precautions:
• Beta-agonists and calcium channel blockers may complicate clinical picture
• Cryoprecipitate and fibrinogen may increase infection transmission risk
Significant possible interactions: Refer to manufacturer's profile of each drug

ALTERNATIVE DRUGS
Ritodrine (Yutopar) IV may be an alternate beta-agonist, but carries same concerns as terbutaline

 FOLLOWUP

PATIENT MONITORING
• Inpatient followup
• Outpatient care with frequent visits

PREVENTION/AVOIDANCE
• Decrease activity to avoid rebleeding
• All vaginal exams, sexual intercourse, douching, or other vaginal manipulation may cause rebleeding

POSSIBLE COMPLICATIONS
• Maternal mortality is rare with cesarean section available. Greatest fetal risk is preterm delivery.
• Attempted tocolysis may compromise maternal status
• Rebleeding risk may be more risky than delivery and management
• If previa present after 30 weeks, there is greater risk of persisting previa

EXPECTED COURSE AND PROGNOSIS
• If term and complete or partial: Cesarean delivery
• If term and anterior marginal: Trial of labor may be okay
• If preterm and maternal and fetal status stable: May observe and delay delivery

 MISCELLANEOUS

ASSOCIATED CONDITIONS
• Abnormal presentations such as oblique and/or transverse lie
• Persistent high fetal station
• If previa present, then increased risk of intrauterine growth retardation (IUGR)
• Placenta accreta
• Postpartum hemorrhage
• Increased incidence of small for gestational age (SGA) babies with previas

AGE-RELATED FACTORS
Pediatric: N/A
Geriatric: N/A
Others: Advanced maternal age increases risk

PREGNANCY As above

SYNONYMS N/A

ICD-9-CM
• 641.1 hemorrage from placenta previa
• 641.0 placenta previa without hemorrhage

SEE ALSO Abruptio placenta

OTHER NOTES N/A

ABBREVIATIONS
• DIC = disseminated intravascular coagulation
• L/S ratio = lecithin/sphingomyelin ratio
• PT = prothrombin time
• PTT = partial thromboplastin time

REFERENCES
• Pritchard, J.A., McDonald, P.C., & Gant, N.F.: Williams Obstetrics. Norwalk, CT, Appleton-Century-Crofts,1985, pp. 407-411
• Lavery, J.P.: Placenta Previa. Obstetrics and Gyn, vol. 33, No 3, September 1990

Author M. Sexton, M.D.

Plague

BASICS

DESCRIPTION
• Acute infection
• Sporadic world wide, especially Third World nations
• Epidemics associated with war, famine, and disaster
• Disease of rats and other small vertebrates
• Transmitted to humans by rat flea
• Occasional transmission to humans handling infected tissues
• Occasional human to human transmission by secretions or human flea
Genetics: N/A
Incidence/Prevalence in USA: Few cases annually in Southwestern states, usually Spring, Summer, Fall
Predominant age: N/A
Predominant sex: Male = Female

SIGNS AND SYMPTOMS
Bubonic plague
◊ Acute onset after 2-8 days incubation
◊ Fever
◊ Chills
◊ Weakness
◊ Headache
◊ Bubo - painful, very tender enlargement of regional lymph node(s) draining inoculation site. Overlying edema. Typically, absence of overlying skin lesion, ascending lymphangitis.
◊ Skin lesions - pustules, vesicles, eschars in area of flea bite(s)
Purpura septicemic plague
◊ Features of bubonic plague
◊ Occasional occurrence without bubo
◊ Hypotension
◊ Hepatosplenomegaly
◊ Delirium
◊ Seizures in children
◊ Shock
Secondary pneumonic plague
◊ Features of bubonic and septicemic plague
◊ Cough
◊ Chest pain
◊ Hemoptysis
Primary pneumonic plague
◊ Acute onset within hours to one day after inhalation of bacteria
◊ Fever
◊ Chills
◊ Cough
◊ Chest pain
◊ Dyspnea
◊ Hemoptysis
◊ Lethargy
◊ Hypotension
◊ Shock

CAUSES
• Yersinia pestis, transmitted by bite of a flea from an infected rodent
• Untreated bubonic plague may progress to secondary pneumonic type which can be transmitted by contaminated respiratory droplets

RISK FACTORS
• Environmental exposure to rats and fleas
• Close contact with pneumonic plague patient
• Plague bacillus in laboratory
• Hunters who skin wild animals

DIAGNOSIS

DIFFERENTIAL DIAGNOSIS Other causes of fulminant bacteremia, pneumococcal pneumonia, lymphangitis

LABORATORY
• Elevated white cell count, predominantly mature and immature neutrophils. Leukemoid reaction sometimes.
• Stained smears of aspirate of bubo, sputum, peripheral blood reveal gram-negative coccobacilli with bipolar staining, "safety pin" appearance
• Aspirate, blood, sputum cultures (infusion broth, blood and MacConkey's agar) grow typical bacteria. Public health authorities arrange definitive identification and serological followup.
Drugs that may alter lab results:
Antibiotics
Disorders that may alter lab results: N/A

PATHOLOGICAL FINDINGS Acute inflammation dominated by neutrophils, necrosis, masses of plague bacilli, seropurulent pericarditis

SPECIAL TESTS Low platelet number; evidence of disseminated intravascular coagulation may occur

IMAGING Chest x-ray - patchy or confluent pulmonary consolidation in pneumonic plague

DIAGNOSTIC PROCEDURES N/A

TREATMENT

APPROPRIATE HEALTH CARE
Hospitalization. For suspected pneumonic plague, respiratory isolation until 48 hours after initial effective therapy or after sputum negative.

GENERAL MEASURES
• Do not create aerosol
• Handle blood and bubo aspirate with gloves
• Notify laboratory to take precautions
• Intravenous fluids as required
• Hot, moist compresses for buboes

ACTIVITY Bedrest until convalescent

DIET As tolerated during recovery

PATIENT EDUCATION
• Avoid contact with wild animals
• Reduce rat and flea population in environment

Plague

MEDICATIONS

DRUG(S) OF CHOICE
• Streptomycin - 30 mg/kg IM in two divided doses daily for 10 days. If streptomycin not available, CDC recommends gentamicin.
• If streptomycin contraindicated or condition allows oral medication - tetracycline (Achromycin) 25-50 mg per kg daily, equally divided, every 6 hours for 10 days
• For meningitis - chloramphenicol (Chloromycetin) 25 mg/kg followed by 60 mg/kg in 4 equally divided doses, daily for 10 days

Contraindications: None to antibiotic treatment of this often fatal infection

Precautions:
• Reduce dose of streptomycin for renal impairment, 20 mg/kg daily if mild and 8 mg/kg each 3 days if advanced
• Pregnant women and those with hearing disorders, shorten streptomycin to 3 days after afebrile
• Chloramphenicol associated with hematologic toxicity

Significant possible interactions: N/A

ALTERNATIVE DRUGS
None demonstrated to be as effective or less toxic

FOLLOWUP

PATIENT MONITORING Appropriate to clinical status

PREVENTION/AVOIDANCE
• Avoid contact with vectors, infected tissue or aerosol, e.g., pneumonic plague case
• Killed vaccine for people at high risk to reduce risk and/or severity; tetracycline prophylaxis. Vaccine available from C.D.C., Atlanta.

POSSIBLE COMPLICATIONS
Progression of bubonic form to septicemic and pneumonic forms
• Necrosis of bubo may require aspiration or incision and drainage
• Pericarditis
• Adult respiratory distress syndrome
• Meningitis

EXPECTED COURSE AND PROGNOSIS
• Untreated plague mortality > 50%; 100% in primary pneumonic plague
• Plague may be fulminant, e.g., exposure, first symptoms and death in one day in primary pneumonic plague. Must not delay treatment of suspected cases until laboratory-confirmed diagnosis. Delay of initial therapy beyond 24 hours after onset of primary pneumonic plague regularly followed by death.

MISCELLANEOUS

ASSOCIATED CONDITIONS N/A

AGE-RELATED FACTORS N/A
Pediatric: N/A
Geriatric: N/A
Others: N/A

PREGNANCY N/A

SYNONYMS Black death

ICD-9-CM
• Bubonic plague 020.0
• Septicemic plague 020.2
• Unspecified pneumonic plague 020.5
• Primary pneumonic plague 020.3
• Secondary pneumonic plague 020.4

SEE ALSO N/A

OTHER NOTES N/A

ABBREVIATIONS N/A

REFERENCES Mandel, G.L., Douglas, R.G., & Bennett, J.E., (eds.): Principles and Practice of Infectious Diseases. 3rd Ed. New York, Churchill Livingstone, 1990

Author W. Sawyer, M.D.

Pleural effusion

BASICS

DESCRIPTION Excessive fluid collection in the pleural space, almost always caused by an underlying disease. Effusions may be from transudates (effusions due to imbalances in hydrostatic and oncotic pressures, such as those seen in congestive heart failure or hypoalbuminuria) or exudates (effusions that may be associated with many diseases - see Causes below). Normal individuals will have a small amount of extracellular fluid that lubricates the pleural surfaces. Most patients with effusions will demonstrate symptoms relating to the underlying pathology.

Genetics: N/A
Incidence/Prevalence in USA: Not known
Predominant age: All ages
Predominant sex: Male = Female

SIGNS AND SYMPTOMS
- None in mild effusion
- Chest pain
- Cough
- Splint of chest wall
- Dyspnea
- Tachypnea
- Diminished chest wall excursion
- Reduced tactile fremitus
- Dullness to percussion
- Diminished or absent breath sounds over the effusion
- Displacement of trachea and the cardiac apex toward the contralateral side
- Friction rub in small effusion
- Weight loss
- Chills
- Hemoptysis
- Night sweats

CAUSES
- Parapneumonic effusion
- Empyema: Often associated with pneumonia exudate caused by pneumococcal or gram negative organisms in adult; pneumococcal, H. influenzae, staphylococcus aureus, and mycoplasma organisms in children. Occasionally mycobacterial or fungal organism can be responsible in all age groups.
- Malignancy: Exudates, primary pleural malignancy vs. metastatic malignancy. Frequency scale - lung > breast > lymphoma > others.
- Congestive heart failure: Transudate often bilateral
- Renal: Nephrotic syndrome, renal failure. Transudates often bilateral.
- Cirrhosis: Transudate, usually right-sided
- Rheumatic disease: Exudate (small)
- Drug induced effusion: Exudate often with eosinophilia
- Dressler's Syndrome (post cardiotomy or myocardial infarction syndrome): Exudate often associated with myocardial effusion
- Intra-abdominal abscess: Exudate, WBC, normal glucose, sterile
- Esophageal perforation: Exudate, air-fluid level, high amylase, unilateral, toxicity
- Pancreatitis: Exudate with high amylase, often left-sided

RISK FACTORS N/A

DIAGNOSIS

DIFFERENTIAL DIAGNOSIS See Causes

LABORATORY
- Leukocytosis
- Anemia

Drugs that may alter lab results: N/A
Disorders that may alter lab results: N/A

PATHOLOGICAL FINDINGS N/A

SPECIAL TESTS
Examination of pleural fluid obtained by thoracentesis
   ◊ Cell count and differential
   ◊ Glucose, usually < 60 in empyema and rheumatoid arthritis. May also be this low in tuberculosis and parapneumonia effusions.
   ◊ Protein > 3 gm/100 mL with pleural serum ratio > 0.5 in exudate
   ◊ Pleural fluid lactic dehydrogenase (LDH) > 200 IU, with pleural/serum ratio > 0.6 in exudate
   ◊ PH < 7.2 in empyema
   ◊ Amylase, elevated in effusion secondary to pancreatitis or esophageal perforation
   ◊ RBC's in malignant, traumatic, or pulmonary embolism effusions. Large amounts of RBC (> 100,000) is termed hemorrhagic effusion and may also be seen in other causes
   ◊ Cytology (tumor cells)
   ◊ Cultures, gram stain bacterial, fungal, mycobacterial.

IMAGING N/A
- Chest x-ray, anteroposterior (upright), lateral decubitus
- Chest ultrasounds: Echo-transmitting space due to encapsulated fluid
- CT scan, rarely required

DIAGNOSTIC PROCEDURES N/A
- Pleural biopsy in selective cases (useful in diagnosis of cancer or tuberculosis)
- Pleuroscopy in selective cases
- Thoracentesis

TREATMENT

APPROPRIATE HEALTH CARE
Inpatient

GENERAL MEASURES
- Supportive, oxygen, hydration, chest physiotherapy
- Treat the primary disorder
Empyema
   ◊ Antibiotics alone in selective cases (children)
   ◊ Chest tube drainage (initial therapy in adults)
   ◊ Pleurectomy (pleural stripping) in cases of "trapped lung"
Malignant pleural effusion
   ◊ Treatment of the primary malignancy
   ◊ Thoracentesis, chest tube drainage for symptomatic management
   ◊ Chemical pleurodesis in some patients
Chylothorax
   ◊ Radiation therapy in some malignant chylothorax
   ◊ Surgical ligation of thoracic duct in traumatic chylothorax
Hemothorax
   ◊ Fluid hematocrit equal to or similar to blood hematocrit - almost always caused only by trauma
   ◊ Thoracostomy tube drainage in traumatic hemothorax
Hemorrhagic effusion
   ◊ Treatment of primary disease (usually malignancy)

ACTIVITY As tolerated

DIET No special diet

PATIENT EDUCATION Patient instruction materials available from American Lung Association (local agency or 1740 Broadway, New York, NY 10038)

MEDICATIONS

DRUG(S) OF CHOICE
• Antimicrobial treatment if appropriate
• Chemical pleurodesis with doxycycline 500 mg or bleomycin 60 units in some patients
Contraindications: Refer to manufacturer's profile of each drug
Precautions: Refer to manufacturer's profile of each drug
Significant possible interactions: Refer to manufacturer s profile of each drug

ALTERNATIVE DRUGS   N/A

FOLLOWUP

PATIENT MONITORING
• Chest x-ray every three months until return to normal
• Pulmonary function tests (PFT's) every three months until return to normal

PREVENTION/AVOIDANCE   N/A

POSSIBLE COMPLICATIONS
• Chronic empyema
• Drainage through chest wall - pleurocutaneous fistula
• Bronchopleural fistula
• Toxic shock syndrome

EXPECTED COURSE AND
PROGNOSIS   Mortality rate around 20% for exudative effusions; worse for elderly patients or those with serious underlying conditions

MISCELLANEOUS

ASSOCIATED CONDITIONS   N/A

AGE-RELATED FACTORS   N/A
Pediatric: N/A
Geriatric: N/A
Others: N/A

PREGNANCY   N/A

SYNONYMS   N/A

ICD-9-CM
• 511.9 unspecified pleural effusion
• 511.1 pleurisy with effusion, with mention of a bacterial cause other than tuberculosis
• 197.2 secondary malignant neoplasm of respiratory and digestive system, pleura

SEE ALSO   N/A

OTHER NOTES   N/A

ABBREVIATIONS   N/A

REFERENCES
• Braunwald, E., et al. (eds.): Harrison's Principles of Internal Medicine. 12th Ed. New York, McGraw-Hill, 1991
• Kendig, R. & Chernick, V.: Disorders of the Respiratory Tracts in Children. 5th Ed. Philadelphia, W.B. Saunders Co., 1990

Author S. Hadeed, M.D.

Pheumonia, bacterial

BASICS

DESCRIPTION An acute, bacterial infection of the lung parenchyma. It is more common in adults and much less common in children than viral pneumonia. Infection may be community acquired or nosocomial (hospital acquired by an inpatient for at least 72 hours). Most commonly, community acquired disease is caused by Streptococcus pneumoniae or Haemophilus influenzae. Hospital acquired pneumonia is usually due to gram negative rods (60%) such as pseudomonas, or if gram positive from staphylococcus (14.5%).

System(s) affected: Pulmonary/respiratory
Genetics: No known genetic pattern
Incidence/Prevalence in USA:
• Incidence - community acquired: 1200 cases/100,000 population per year.
• Incidence - nosocomial: 800 cases/100,000 admissions per year.
• Prevalence - community acquired: 120 cases/100,000 population†
• Prevalence - nosocomial: 80 cases/100,000 admissions†
† Note: Assumes each case of pneumonia lasts 10 days or less, and that pneumonia cases are evenly spread throughout the year. These assumptions yield the approximate prevalence figures given.
Predominant age: All ages
Predominant sex: Male > Female

SIGNS AND SYMPTOMS
Cardinal signs and symptoms
◊ Cough
◊ Fever
◊ Chest pain
◊ Chill, with sudden onset
◊ Dark, thick or bloody (rusty) sputum
Others
◊ Abdominal distension
◊ Abdominal pain
◊ Anorexia
◊ Anxiety
◊ Bronchial breath sounds
◊ Chest dullness to percussion
◊ Confusion
◊ Crackles (rales)
◊ Cyanosis
◊ Decreased breath sounds
◊ Dehydration
◊ Delirium
◊ Diaphoresis
◊ Distress
◊ Dyspnea
◊ Egophony
◊ Facial flush
◊ Headache
◊ Hemoptysis
◊ Malaise
◊ Myalgia
◊ Pleural friction rub
◊ Pleurisy
◊ Pleuritic pain
◊ Prostration
◊ Restlessness
◊ Rhonchi
◊ Rigors

◊ Shoulder pain
◊ Stupor
◊ Tachycardia
◊ Tachypnea
◊ Vocal fremitus
◊ Weakness
◊ Whispered pectoriloquy

CAUSES
• Hematogenous spread of the microorganism
• Inhalation of the microorganism
• Aspiration of the infectious agent from the oropharynx
Bacterial pathogens
◊ Streptococcus pneumoniae (pneumococcus)
◊ Haemophilus influenzae
◊ Staphylococcus aureus
◊ Legionella pneumophila (see separate topic)
◊ Moraxella catarrhalis (Branhamella catarrhalis)
◊ Mycoplasma pneumoniae
◊ Klebsiella pneumoniae
◊ Pseudomonas aeruginosa
◊ Escherichia coli

RISK FACTORS
• Viral infections
• Hospitalization
• Age extremes
• Alcoholism
• AIDS or other immunosuppression
• Tobacco smoking
• Renal failure
• Cardiovascular disease
• Functional asplenia
• Chronic obstructive pulmonary disease
• Diabetes mellitus
• Malnutrition
• Malignancy
• General anesthesia
• Mechanical ventilation
• Altered level of consciousness or gag (e.g., seizures, stroke, neuromuscular disease, etc.)

DIAGNOSIS

DIFFERENTIAL DIAGNOSIS Other causes of infectious pneumonitis: Viruses (respiratory syncytial, adenovirus, parainfluenza, influenzae A and B, varicella, measles, rubella, enterovirus, Epstein-Barr); Nocardia; Fungi (Blastomyces, cryptococcus, aspergillus, histoplasma, Coccidioides, pneumocystis carinii); Protozoans (Toxoplasma); Chlamydia (pneumoniae, psittaci, trachomatis); Rickettsia (Coxiella burnetti - Q fever). Also tuberculosis, pulmonary embolism with infarction, bronchiolitis obliterans with organizing pneumonia (BOOP), pulmonary contusion, pulmonary vasculitis, acute sarcoid, hypersensitivity pneumonitis, pneumothorax, and other causes.

LABORATORY
• Leukocytosis with left shift on differential
• Hemoconcentration
• Hyponatremia (SIADH)

• Transaminase elevation
• Proteinuria
• Hypoxemia
• Hypocapnia initially, then hypercapnia
• Blood culture - positive in 20-30% of patients with community acquired pneumonia
• Serum or urine - pneumococcal antigen
• Bronchoscopic protected telescoping catheter brushing culture - significant at greater than or equal to 1000 organisms
• Bronchoscopic bronchoalveolar lavage culture - significant at greater than or equal to 10,000 organisms
Drugs that may alter lab results: Refer to lab test reference
Disorders that may alter lab results: Refer to lab test reference

PATHOLOGICAL FINDINGS
Lung:
◊ Positive gram stain for bacteria
◊ Edema fluid
◊ Red hepatization
◊ Gray hepatization
◊ Segmental, lobar, or multifocal peribronchial consolidation

SPECIAL TESTS
• Culture of transtracheal aspirate
• Culture of bronchoalveolar lavage
• Culture of protected telescoping catheter brushing
• Decubitus chest roentgenograms to investigate for parapneumonic effusion
• Culture of pleural fluid
• pH of pleural fluid (iced, airless sample sent to blood gas laboratory)

IMAGING
Chest roentgenogram
◊ Air bronchogram
◊ Lobar or segmental consolidation
◊ Bronchopneumonia
◊ Pleural effusion

DIAGNOSTIC PROCEDURES
• Induced sputum for culture (15 minutes of 3% saline by nebulizer after patient has rinsed their mouth)
• Nasal trachea suctioning for culture
• Transtracheal aspirate for culture
• Bronchoscopy with bronchoalveolar lavage or protected telescoping catheter brushing for culture
• Thoracentesis for pleural fluid studies
• Transthoracic fine needle aspiration for culture
• Blood culture

TREATMENT

APPROPRIATE HEALTH CARE
• Community acquired - outpatient for mild case, inpatient for moderate to severe case such as multilobar presentation, hypoxemia, hypotension, significant co-morbid illness, and age extremes.
• Nosocomial - patients already hospitalized

GENERAL MEASURES
• Antimicrobial therapy for most likely pathogen(s)
• Consider oxygen for patients with cyanosis, hypoxia, dyspnea, circulatory disturbances or delirium
• Mechanical ventilation for respiratory failure
• Chest physiotherapy
• Hydration
• Nasotracheal suction
• Analgesia for pain
• Electrolyte correction
• Respiratory isolation if TB is a possibility

ACTIVITY Bedrest and/or reduced activity during acute phase

DIET
• Nothing by mouth if there is incipient respiratory failure
• Consider soft, easy-to-eat foods

PATIENT EDUCATION Printed patient information available from: American Lung Association, 1740 Broadway, New York, NY 100019 (212)315-8700

MEDICATIONS

DRUG(S) OF CHOICE
Initial therapy
◊ Usually empiric for most likely pathogens (if specific etiology is identified, antimicrobial therapy can be adjusted)
◊ For otherwise healthy adult with community acquired pneumonia - erythromycin 500 mg IV every 6 hours (adequately treats Mycoplasma and Legionella)
◊ For hospital acquired pneumonia - third generation cephalosporin (cefotaxime or ceftizoxime) plus vancomycin. If Pseudomonas is a concern, use antipseudomonal penicillin (piperacillin, mezlocillin or ticarcillin) or cephalosporin (ceftazidime) plus an aminoglycoside
◊ Analgesics for pleuritic pain
Therapy for specific organism
◊ S. pneumoniae - penicillin G or oral penicillin V. If high incidence of penicillin resistant S. pneumoniae in the area consider vancomycin or fluoroquinolone (ciprofloxacin, ofloxacin)
◊ H. influenzae - ampicillin or amoxicillin. For severe infections - cefotaxime or ceftriaxone
◊ S. aureus - nafcillin; vancomycin (if there is a high incidence of methicillin resistant S. aureus)
◊ Klebsiella species - aminoglycoside plus cephalosporin
◊ E. coli - aminoglycoside plus cephalosporin
◊ Pseudomonas - aminoglycoside plus antipseudomonal penicillin or ceftazidime
◊ Moraxella catarrhalis - 2nd generation cephalosporin (cefaclor, cefuroxime axetil)
◊ Chlamydia pneumoniae - tetracycline
◊ Mycoplasma pneumoniae - erythromycin
◊ Legionella pneumophila - erythromycin

Contraindications: Allergy or likely cross-allergy to the prescribed antibiotic
Precautions: Possible significant sodium overload with antipseudomonal penicillins
Significant possible interactions: Refer to manufacturer's literature

ALTERNATIVE DRUGS
• S. pneumoniae - erythromycin; cephalosporin
• H. influenzae - cefuroxime; trimethoprim-sulfamethoxazole; tetracycline; chloramphenicol
• S. aureus - a first generation cephalosporin; vancomycin; clindamycin; ciprofloxacin
• Klebsiella - chloramphenicol; ciprofloxacin
• E. coli - ampicillin; cephalosporin; ciprofloxacin; chloramphenicol
• Pseudomonas - aminoglycoside plus ceftazidime; ciprofloxacin; imipenem
• Moraxella catarrhalis - amoxicillin clavulanate; trimethoprim sulfamethoxazole; tetracycline; clarithromycin; cefixime
• Chlamydia pneumoniae - doxycycline; clarithromycin; azithromycin; ciprofloxacin; ofloxacin
• Mycoplasma pneumoniae - clarithromycin; azithromycin; tetracycline
• Legionella pneumophila - clarithromycin; azithromycin; rifampin; ciprofloxacin; ofloxacin

FOLLOWUP

PATIENT MONITORING
• If outpatient therapy, daily assessment of the patient's progress
• Chest roentgenograms take time to clear and may not show clearing, even though patient is improving. Repeat study about 6 weeks after recovery to verify the pneumonia was not caused by an obstructing endobronchial lesion.
• Repeating the cultures after treatment has been started is unnecessary

PREVENTION/AVOIDANCE
• Polyvalent pneumococcal vaccine; pneumovax (see Other notes)
• Reduce risk factors where possible
• Avoid indiscriminate use of antibiotics during minor viral infections
• Annual influenza vaccine for high risk individuals
• Bedridden and postoperative patients - deep breathing and coughing exercises; prevent aspiration during nasogastric tube feedings

POSSIBLE COMPLICATIONS
• Empyema
• Pulmonary abscess
• Purulent pericarditis
• Pleurisy
• Pleural effusion
• Lung necrosis
• Superinfections
• Multiple organ dysfunction syndrome (MODS)
• Adult respiratory distress syndrome (ARDS)

EXPECTED COURSE AND PROGNOSIS
• Usual course - acute. In otherwise healthy individual, improvement seen and fever resolved in 1-3 days.
• Overall mortality is about 5%
• Poorest prognosis - age extremes, positive blood cultures, low WBC, presence of associated disease, immunosuppression

MISCELLANEOUS

ASSOCIATED CONDITIONS
• Alcoholism
• Tobacco smoking
• Upper respiratory infection

AGE-RELATED FACTORS
Pediatric: Morbidity and mortality high in children under age 1
Geriatric:
• Morbidity and mortality high if over 70, especially with associated disease or risk factor
• For prophylaxis - vaccinate if 65 years or older, even if healthy
Others: N/A

PREGNANCY N/A

SYNONYMS
• Lobar pneumonia
• Classic pneumococcal pneumonia

ICD-9-CM 481 pneumococcal pneumonia

SEE ALSO N/A

OTHER NOTES Vaccination recommended for children over 2 years and adults with increased risk: Chronic disease, splenic dysfunction or asplenia, Hodgkin's, multiple myeloma, cirrhosis, alcoholism, renal failure, organ transplant, immunosuppression, nephrosis, over age 65

ABBREVIATIONS N/A

REFERENCES
• Coonrod, J.D.: Pneumococcal Pneumonia. Semin Respir Infect 4:4, 1989
• Fishman, A.P.: Pulmonary Diseases and Disorders. 2nd Ed. New York, McGraw-Hill, 1988
• George, R.B., Light, R.W., Matthay, R.A., Matthay, M.A. (eds.): Chest Medicine. 2nd Ed. Baltimore, Williams & Wilkins, 1990

Author S. Knoper, M.D.

Pneumonia, Mycoplasma

 BASICS

DESCRIPTION Interstitial pneumonia caused by extensive infection of the lungs and bronchi, particularly the lower lobes of the lungs, by Mycoplasma pneumoniae. It may be distinguished from viral pneumonia by the presence of cold agglutinins. Usual course - acute. Incubation period is about 18-21 days and includes prodromal symptoms.
• Cases tend to occur in summer and peak in autumn. Epidemics in communities tend to be prolonged (over many months) and occur every 4-5 years.
System(s) affected: Pulmonary
Genetics: None
Incidence/Prevalence in USA:
• 130 cases/100,000 people
• Estimated to be most common cause of pneumonia in school children and young adults (without chronic underlying condition)
Predominant age: Ages 5-15, but occurs at any age
Predominant sex: Male > Female

SIGNS AND SYMPTOMS
• Early symptoms - mild sore throat, dry cough, low-grade fever, and malaise (increased in severity with time)
• Blood-streaked sputum
• Bullous myringitis
• Decreased breath sounds
• Fever
• Fine inspiratory rales
• Headache
• Myalgias
• Nasal congestion
• Paroxysmal cough
• Pleural effusion
• Pleural friction rub
• Sore throat

CAUSES Mycoplasma pneumoniae infection

RISK FACTORS
• Living on military base (some of largest outbreaks have been in army recruits)
• College campus exposure (e.g., fraternity house living)
• Other close community living, e.g., hospitals, prisons
• Family exposure
• Immunocompromised patients

 DIAGNOSIS

DIFFERENTIAL DIAGNOSIS
• Viral pneumonia
• Bacterial pneumonia (including plague and tularemia in severe cases)
• Fungal pneumonias
• Pneumocystis carinii pneumonia

LABORATORY
• Increased sedimentation rate
• Increased complement fixation
• Positive cold agglutinins (titer of 1:64 or greater; or rising fourfold) in 50% of infections
• False-positive VDRL
• M. pneumoniae culture (requires 7-10 days)
• Peripheral white blood cell count - normal
• Complement fixation serologic assay shows fourfold rise in titer at 2-4 weeks after symptom onset
Drugs that may alter lab results: N/A
Disorders that may alter lab results: N/A

PATHOLOGICAL FINDINGS Absence of bacterial pathogens on Gram stain and culture of sputum or transtracheal aspirate. Mycoplasma is a fastidious and slow-growing organism

SPECIAL TESTS Radiolabeled DNA probe which detects M. pneumoniae ribosomal RNA in respiratory secretions. 90% sensitive.

IMAGING Chest x-ray - diffuse interstitial infiltrates; small bilateral pleural effusion

DIAGNOSTIC PROCEDURES N/A

 TREATMENT

APPROPRIATE HEALTH CARE
Outpatient usually, inpatient if symptoms severe

GENERAL MEASURES N/A

ACTIVITY Rest during acute phase

DIET Drink plenty of fluids

PATIENT EDUCATION Printed patient information available from American Lung Association, 1740 Broadway, New York, NY 10019, (212)315-8700

MEDICATIONS

DRUG(S) OF CHOICE
• Children 9 years and over and adults: Tetracycline or erythromycin 500 mg every 6 hours for 7 days
• Children under 8 years of age: Erythromycin - 30-50 mg/kg/day for 7 days
• Antibiotics such as penicillins are ineffective against M. pneumoniae
Contraindications: Refer to manufacturer's literature
Precautions: Refer to manufacturer's literature
Significant possible interactions: Refer to manufacturer's literature

ALTERNATIVE DRUGS
In adults
These drugs are erythromycin analogues and have a diminished incidence of gastrointestinal upset compared to erythromycin; reserve use for patients who experience severe GI upset with erythromycin because these agents are very expensive.
◊ Clarithromycin 250 mg bid x 7 days
◊ Azithromycin 500 mg first day, then 250 mg on days 2 to 5

FOLLOWUP

PATIENT MONITORING
• Phone or in person followup
• Clearing of chest x-ray should be documented if patient is a nonsmoker, but older than 50. In smokers, document a clear x-ray in 6-8 weeks.

PREVENTION/AVOIDANCE   Isolation of active cases. Antibiotic prophylaxis of contacts is not indicated.

POSSIBLE COMPLICATIONS
Note: All complications are rare except reactive airway disease, hemolytic anemia, and erythma multiforme.
• Reactive airway disease
• Hemolytic anemia
• Erythma multiforme
• Meningoencephalitis
• Polyneuritis
• Polyarthritis
• Stevens-Johnson syndrome
• Pericarditis
• Myocarditis
• Respiratory distress syndrome
• Cerebral ataxia
• Thromboembolic phenomena

EXPECTED COURSE AND PROGNOSIS
• Mycoplasma infection symptoms usually resolve in about 2 weeks
• Some constitutional symptoms may persist for several weeks
• With correct therapy, even most severe cases can expect complete recovery

MISCELLANEOUS

ASSOCIATED CONDITIONS   N/A

AGE-RELATED FACTORS
Pediatric:
• Unusual in infants
• M. pneumoniae is associated with an increased incidence of asthma attacks in older children
Geriatric: Unusual in this age group
Others: N/A

PREGNANCY   Tetracycline contraindicated in pregnancy

SYNONYMS
• Primary atypical pneumonia (PAP)
• Eaton agent pneumonia
• Cold agglutinin-positive pneumonia

ICD-9-CM   483 mycoplasma pneumonia

SEE ALSO   N/A

OTHER NOTES   N/A

ABBREVIATIONS   N/A

REFERENCES
• Mandell, G.L. (ed.): Principles and Practice of Infectious Diseases. 3rd Ed. New York, Churchill Livingstone, 1990
• Luby, J.P.: Pneumonia caused by Mycoplasma pneumonia infection. Clinics in Chest Medicine. 12:237-99, 1991

Author   G. Bergus, M.D.

Pneumonia, Pneumocystis carinii (PCP)

 BASICS

DESCRIPTION
A pneumonia arising in immunosuppressed persons caused by Pneumocystis carinii (PCP). This is one of the most common opportunistic infections occurring in patients with human immunodeficiency virus (HIV) infections.
Genetics: N/A
Incidence/Prevalence in USA: Causes 43% of all opportunistic infections in AIDS patients
Predominant age:
• In HIV infected children, median age of onset is 5 months of age
• In HIV infected adults, PCP may occur at any age
Predominant sex: Male > Female

SIGNS AND SYMPTOMS
• Usually insidious but occasionally may be abrupt in onset
• Weakness, fatigue, malaise
• Fever, chills
• Dyspnea on exertion progressing to continuous dyspnea
• Cough - non-productive or productive of scant white or clear sputum
• Tachypnea

CAUSES
The ubiquitous Pneumocystis carinii may cause infection in normal hosts (65%-100% of young children have positive serology) but will rarely cause symptoms in immunocompetent individuals

RISK FACTORS
Immunodeficiency (premature infants, neoplasia, congenital or drug-induced immunodeficiency states)

 DIAGNOSIS

DIFFERENTIAL DIAGNOSIS
• Tuberculosis
• Mycobacterium avium intracellulare
• Viral pneumonias
• Fungal pneumonias
• Lymphoid interstitial pneumonitis (in children)

LABORATORY
• Serum LDH frequently elevated (mean elevation of 340 IU)
• Arterial blood gases reveal hypoxemia and increased alveolar-arterial gradient (varies with severity of disease)
• Sputum induced with inhaled 3-5% hypertonic saline may reveal pneumocystis on cytologic evaluation using Pap and Gomori methenamine-silver (GMS) stains. An IF (immunofluorescence) technique is also available. (Sensitivity may be as high as 78% in labs with experienced personnel.)
• CD4 cell count generally below 200 in HIV infected patients with PCP.
Drugs that may alter lab results: Inhaled pentamidine used to prevent PCP may change radiographic picture to infiltrates in predominantly upper-lobe distribution
Disorders that may alter lab results: N/A

PATHOLOGICAL FINDINGS
Pneumonitis caused by presence of organism and inflammatory response

SPECIAL TESTS
Gallium scanning of the lungs is highly sensitive for PCP but is not very specific. May be useful when sputum studies are inconclusive and bronchoscopy is not available.

IMAGING
Chest x-ray
◊ Shows bilateral interstitial or perihilar infiltrate in 75% of cases
◊ May also show a normal chest x-ray, unilateral disease, pleural effusions, abscesses or cavitations, pneumothorax, and lobar consolidations

DIAGNOSTIC PROCEDURES
• Fiberoptic bronchoscopy with bronchoalveolar lavage or transbronchial biopsy is the preferred method of diagnosis when sputums are negative
• Open lung biopsy is rarely required

 TREATMENT

APPROPRIATE HEALTH CARE
Outpatient in mild cases, otherwise inpatient

GENERAL MEASURES
Oxygen therapy often necessary

ACTIVITY
As tolerated

DIET
No special diet

PATIENT EDUCATION
For patient education materials on this topic, contact: American Lung Association, 1740 Broadway, New York, NY 10019, (212)315-8700

Pneumonia, Pneumocystis carinii (PCP)

MEDICATIONS

DRUG(S) OF CHOICE
• Trimethoprim/sulfamethoxazole (Bactrim, Septra) 10-20 mg/kg/day of trimethoprim component po or IV divided q6h daily for 21 days
• Reduce dose of trimethoprim/sulfamethoxazole in patients with renal failure
• Adjunctive corticosteroid (prednisone) therapy begun within 72 hours of diagnosis (found to benefit AIDS patients with moderate to severe PCP)
Contraindications: Use with care in pregnant patient and infants less than 2 months
Precautions:
• History of sulfa allergy
• A high percentage of patients with AIDS will develop intolerance to trimethoprim/ sulfamethoxazole. Especially common are dermatologic reactions, hematologic toxicity, or fever.
Significant possible interactions:
Phenytoin, oral anti-coagulants, oral sulfonylureas, digitalis

ALTERNATIVE DRUGS
• Pentamidine 4 mg/kg/day IM or IV for 21 days
• Dapsone 100 mg po daily plus trimethoprim 20 mg/kg/day po in 4 divided doses. Check G6PD level before beginning Dapsone as hemolysis may result.
• Clindamycin 450mg po QID plus primaquine 15-30mg po daily for 21 days
• Atovaquone 750mg po TID with meals for 21 days

FOLLOWUP

PATIENT MONITORING Serum LDH, pulmonary function tests and arterial blood gases generally normalize with treatment

PREVENTION/AVOIDANCE All AIDS patients with a history of PCP (or CD4 cells less than 200) require life-long prophylaxis with daily or thrice-weekly trimethoprim/sulfamethoxazole, daily dapsone or monthly aerosolized pentamidine

POSSIBLE COMPLICATIONS
• Respiratory failure
• Pneumothorax (even after successful treatment)
• Extrapulmonary pneumocystis (especially in patients on inhaled pentamidine prophylaxis)

EXPECTED COURSE AND PROGNOSIS
• Previously, mortality from first episode PCP was 30-40%. Has declined to 10-15%. With prophylactic therapy, mean survival has increased.
• Approximately 11% of patients with PCP develop respiratory failure and 86% of these die

MISCELLANEOUS

ASSOCIATED CONDITIONS
• AIDS
• HIV infection

AGE-RELATED FACTORS
Pediatric:
• Early onset (5 months of age) and high mortality (median survival 1 month)
• Important to distinguish from lymphoid interstitial pneumonitis (LIP) as treatment and prognosis differ
• PCP prophylaxis for HIV positive children is recommended
Geriatric: N/A
Others: N/A

PREGNANCY
Trimethoprim/sulfamethoxazole has been used for treatment and prophylaxis. Avoid pentamidine.

SYNONYMS
• Pneumocystosis
• Pulmonary pneumocystosis
• Interstitial plasma cell pneumonia

ICD-9-CM 136.3

SEE ALSO
• HIV infection and AIDS

OTHER NOTES N/A

ABBREVIATIONS
• LDH = lactic acid dehydrogenase
• G6PD = glucose 6-phosphate dehydrogenase

REFERENCES
• Cohen, M., Sande, M. & Volberding, P.: The AIDS Knowledge Base. Waltham, MA, The Medical Publishing Group, 1990
• Masur, H.: Consensus statement on the use of corticosteroids as adjunctive therapy for pneumocystis pneumonia in the acquired Immunodeficiency syndrome. N Engl J Med 32:1500-4, 1990, Nov 22
• Guidelines for prophylaxis against PCP for children infected with Human Immunodeficiency virus. MMWR, Recommendations and Reports, 40 RR-2 (March 15, 1991)
• Recommendations of prophylaxis against PCP for adults and adolescents with Human Immunodeficiency Virus. MMWR, Recommendations and Reports, 41 RR-4 (April 10, 1992).

Author C. Carmichael, M.D.

Pneumonia, viral

 BASICS

DESCRIPTION Inflammatory disease of the lungs. Most viral pneumonia results from exposure of a non-immune individual to infected persons who are shedding the implicated agent.
System(s) affected: Pulmonary
Genetics: No known genetic pattern
Incidence/Prevalence in USA:
• More common in children than in adults
• Approximately 90% of childhood pneumonia is viral
• 1, 3, and 5% of pneumonia in adults has been attributed to viral etiologies in different series
• Incidence is roughly 60 cases/100,000 population per year
• Prevalence is unknown and variable due to seasonal variation
Predominant age: All ages
Predominant sex: Male = Female

SIGNS AND SYMPTOMS
• Fever
• Chills
• Cough (productive of mucopurulent sputum)
• Dyspnea
• Recent history of upper respiratory tract infection
• Referred abdominal pain
• Pulmonary rales and rhonchi
• Altered breath sounds
• Pleurisy
• Friction rub
• Headache

CAUSES
• Influenza A and B
• Parainfluenza 1, 2, 3, and 4
• Respiratory syncytial virus (RSV, especially in young children)
• Adenovirus
• Cytomegalovirus (CMV), particularly in immunocompromised patients)
• Varicella (chicken pox)
• Herpes simplex
• Rubeola (hard measles)
• Hemorrhagic fever viruses (arboviruses, arenaviruses, bunyaviruses, Hantaan virus, Marburg virus, Ebola virus)

RISK FACTORS
• Immunocompromised
• Living in close quarters
• Seasonal - epidemic upper respiratory illness
• Elderly

 DIAGNOSIS

DIFFERENTIAL DIAGNOSIS
• Pulmonary edema
• Pulmonary embolus/infarction
• Bronchial carcinoma with lymphangitic spread
• Bacterial pneumonia (especially atypical etiologies - Chlamydia pneumoniae and psittaci, Mycoplasma pneumoniae, Legionella pneumophila)
• Cystic fibrosis (in infants)
• Pneumothorax
• Hypersensitivity pneumonitis
• Bronchiolitis obliterans with organizing pneumonia (BOOP)
• Pneumocystis carinii pneumonia (PCP)
• Aspiration pneumonia

LABORATORY
• Sputum gram stain and culture
• Viral culture and appropriate direct fluorescent antigen from throat swab
• Cytopathology
• Normal or near normal granulocyte count, occasionally leukopenic with increased lymphocyte percentage
• Hypoxemia with severe disease
Drugs that may alter lab results: N/A
Disorders that may alter lab results: N/A

PATHOLOGICAL FINDINGS
• Heavy lungs
• Enlarged regional lymph nodes
• Atelectasis, edema, emphysema
• Cytoplasmic inclusion bodies (CMV)
• Intranuclear inclusion bodies (adenovirus, CMV, herpes virus, varicella)
• Intense inflammatory reaction with mononuclear cells

SPECIAL TESTS   Serologic assays

IMAGING Chest roentgenogram - interstitial pneumonia, peribronchial thickening, pleural effusion

DIAGNOSTIC PROCEDURES
• Nasopharyngeal throat swab
• Transtracheal aspiration (seldom needed)
• Bronchoscopy with bronchoalveolar lavage (BAL)

 TREATMENT

APPROPRIATE HEALTH CARE
Outpatient for most cases. Inpatient for infants under 4 months of age or for any patient with diffuse, severe infection (hypoxemia, hypercarbia, hypotension or shock, adult respiratory distress syndrome)

GENERAL MEASURES
• Encourage coughing and deep breathing exercises to clear secretions
• Dispose of secretions carefully
• Hydration
• Consider respiratory isolation for Varicella which is highly contagious (i.e., negative pressure)

ACTIVITY Rest in quiet, calm environment

DIET Increase fluids (2-3 L/day), high calorie, high protein, soft diet

PATIENT EDUCATION For patient education materials on this topic, contact: American Lung Association, 1740 Broadway, New York, NY 100919, (212)315-8700

MEDICATIONS

DRUG(S) OF CHOICE

<u>Amantadine:</u> Influenza A (not effective for influenza B)

◊ Age < 10: 5-8 mg/kg/day in 2 divided doses. Not to exceed 150 mg/day.

◊ Age 10-65: 100 mg orally q 12 h (adults may be given a loading dose of 200 mg initially)

◊ Age > 65: 100 mg orally once a day

<u>Acyclovir:</u> Pulmonary infections involving herpes simplex, herpes zoster or varicella

◊ Adults 5 mg/kg IV q 8 h

◊ Children 250 mg/square meter body surface area IV q8h

<u>Ganciclovir:</u> CMV infection

◊ 5 mg/kg IV q12h

Contraindications: Refer to manufacturer's literature

Precautions: Amantadine should be used cautiously in patients with liver disease, epilepsy, and those with a history of psychotic illness

Significant possible interactions: Refer to manufacturer's literature

ALTERNATIVE DRUGS

• Rimantadine, an amantadine analog, is equally effective as amantadine and has fewer CNS adverse effects. Useful for influenza A.

• Ribavirin by small particle aerosol generator (SPAG) for select hospitalized patients (e.g., life threatening infections with RSV, possibly influenza B, adenovirus, hemorrhagic fever virus). Usually given by mask, tent, or through ventilator if patient is intubated, for 18 hours per day for 5 days. Because it is teratogenic, health care workers who are pregnant should not prepare, administer, or be in a room where it is being given. An air filtering scavenging system is frequently employed in the treatment room.

• Antibiotics for superimposed bacterial infections.

• Foscarnet for CMV infections, 60 mg/kg IV q 8 h

• IVIG may increase response in patients with CMV pneumonia. Dose and dosage regimen not well established, but 500mg/kg IV qDx3 may be beneficial.

 FOLLOWUP

PATIENT MONITORING
Physical examinations and/or chest roentgenograms until fully active

PREVENTION/AVOIDANCE

• Influenza A and B vaccine: Use for patients with chronic cardiovascular lung disease, residents of chronic care facilities, medical personnel with extensive contact with high risk patients, people over 65 years of age or those with chronic diseases

• For those patients unable to receive influenza vaccine (egg allergy or other) and are at high risk because of age, co-morbid illness, or other risk factor, amantadine can be given throughout the infectious season if tolerated

• For those who did not receive the vaccine and have been exposed to influenza, or there is an influenza A outbreak, amantadine may also be taken for 2 weeks until vaccination has produced immunity

• Health care workers who are pregnant need to take proper precautions to avoid infectious patients

POSSIBLE COMPLICATIONS

• Superimposed bacterial infections such as S. pneumoniae, S. aureus, H. influenza and others. These require antibiotics.

• Respiratory failure

• Adult respiratory distress syndrome (ARDS)

EXPECTED COURSE AND PROGNOSIS
Usually favorable prognosis with illness lasting several days to a week. Post-viral fatigue is common. However, death can occur, especially in pediatric adenovirus or elderly influenza infections.

 MISCELLANEOUS

ASSOCIATED CONDITIONS

• Bacterial pneumonias

• Fungi, pneumocystis carinii in immunosuppressed patients

AGE-RELATED FACTORS

Pediatric: Adenovirus infections in children are most serious. Also serious RSV infection is almost exclusively seen in infants.

Geriatric: Morbidity and mortality greatest in this age group

Others: N/A

PREGNANCY
Important to avoid contact with individuals who may have viral infections

SYNONYMS
N/A

ICD-9-CM
480.9

SEE ALSO
N/A

OTHER NOTES
N/A

ABBREVIATIONS

• RSV - respiratory syncytial virus

• PCP - pneumocystis carinii pneumonia

• ARDS - adult respiratory distress syndrome

• BOOP - bronchiolitis obliterans with organizing pneumonia

• CMV - cytomegalovirus

REFERENCES

• Mandell, G.L. (ed.): Principles and Practice of Infectious Diseases. 3rd Ed. New York, Churchill Livingstone, 1990

• Fields, B.N. (ed.): Virology. 2nd Ed. New York, Raven Press, 1990

Author S. Knoper, M.D.

Pneumothorax

 BASICS

DESCRIPTION
Accumulation of air or gas between the parietal and visceral pleurae. The amount trapped determines the degree of lung collapse.
• Spontaneous pneumothorax - may be primary or secondary
• Traumatic pneumothorax - may coexist with hemothorax
• Tension pneumothorax - the air in the pleural space is under higher pressure than air in adjacent lung and vascular structures
System(s) affected: Pulmonary, Cardiovascular
Genetics: No known genetic pattern, possible congenital predisposition in young men
Incidence/Prevalence in USA: 9/100,000
Predominant age: Adults 20-40 years
Predominant sex: Male > Female

SIGNS AND SYMPTOMS
• Chest pain, sudden, sharp, made worse by breathing, coughing or moving the chest
• Chest movements - asymmetrical
• Dyspnea
• Cyanosis (sometimes)
• Moderate to severe - profound respiratory distress
• Tension pneumothorax - weak, rapid pulse, pallor, neck vein distension, anxiety, tracheal deviation
• Shock
• Circulatory collapse
• Diminished breath sounds and voice sounds

CAUSES
• Perforation of the visceral pleura and entry of gas from the lung
• Gas generated by microorganisms in an empyema
• Penetration of the chest wall, diaphragm, mediastinum, or esophagus

RISK FACTORS
• Trauma (broken rib, ruptured bronchus, perforated esophagus)
• Rupture of superficial lung bulla following cough or blowing a musical instrument
• Vigorous exercise
• Stretching exercises
• Flying (high altitude)
• Pneumoconioses
• Tuberculosis
• Bronchial obstruction
• COPD (particularly emphysema)
• Diving
• Asthma
• Neoplasms
• Endometriosis
• Rare diseases (Marfan's, Ehlers-Danlos)
• Rupture of an infected abscess
• Lymphangioleiomyomatosis
• Cystic fibrosis
• Subpleural Pneumocystis carinii pneumonia (PCP) (in AIDS patients on PCP prophylaxis via pentamidine aerosol)
• Cigarette smoking

 DIAGNOSIS

DIFFERENTIAL DIAGNOSIS
• Pleurisy
• Pericarditis
• Myocardial infarction
• Pulmonary embolism
• Diaphragmatic hernia
• Stomach herniation through diaphragm
• Dissecting aneurysm

LABORATORY
Arterial blood gases in significant pneumothorax - pH < 7.35, pO2 < 80 mmHg, pCO2 > 45 mmHg
Drugs that may alter lab results: N/A
Disorders that may alter lab results: N/A

PATHOLOGICAL FINDINGS   N/A

SPECIAL TESTS   N/A

IMAGING
Chest x-ray:
◊ Air without lung markings peripherally, mediastinal shift to contralateral side
◊ Small pneumothorax may be evident only with expiratory or lateral decubitus film

DIAGNOSTIC PROCEDURES
Careful history and physical. The physical findings depend on size of pneumothorax.

 TREATMENT

APPROPRIATE HEALTH CARE
• Outpatient - lung collapse less than 30%, no dyspnea, no signs of tension pneumothorax
• Inpatient - if more than 30% collapse or tension

GENERAL MEASURES
Outpatient
◊ Bedrest
◊ Monitoring blood pressure, pulse rate, respirations
Inpatient
◊ Thoracotomy tube - inserted in second or third intercostal space in midclavicular line connected to water seal or low suction pressures
◊ Tension pneumothorax - insert 19-gauge or larger needle into the chest followed by using a 3-way stopcock attached to a large syringe to withdraw air rapidly through the needle. Follow this with tube insertion
◊ Oxygen by nasal cannula
◊ Treatment of any underlying condition
Recurrent pneumothorax
◊ Can cause severe disability
◊ Consider surgery (thoracotomy or thoracoscopy with pleurectomy) following 2 or more spontaneous pneumothoraces

ACTIVITY   Bedrest until re-expanded

DIET   No special diet

PATIENT EDUCATION   Help with smoking cessation, if appropriate

MEDICATIONS

DRUG(S) OF CHOICE Intrapleural doxycycline or bleomycin or talc pleurodesis for persistent or recurrent pneumothorax in patients who are poor risk for thoracotomy (emphysema, cystic fibrosis)
Contraindications: Talc pleurodesis can be performed via thoracoscopy, but would not be a therapy to consider in a debilitated patient because it is usually performed under general anesthesia due to pain
Precautions: Fever, mild-moderate pain are the most common adverse effects. Myelosuppression is not a problem with intrapleural bleomycin.
Significant possible interactions: Refer to manufacturer's literature

ALTERNATIVE DRUGS None

FOLLOWUP

PATIENT MONITORING Blood pressure, respiratory rate, arterial blood gases, for patients requiring hospitalization

PREVENTION/AVOIDANCE No preventive measures known, but patients may avoid some risk factors, e.g. exposure to high altitudes, flying in unpressurized aircraft, scuba diving, smoking

POSSIBLE COMPLICATIONS
• Re-expansion pulmonary edema following suction
• Bronchopleural fistulae requiring surgical repair
• Surgery indicated following 2 spontaneous pneumothoraces on the same side

EXPECTED COURSE AND PROGNOSIS
• Air reabsorbed from small spontaneous pneumothorax in a few days
• Air reabsorbed from larger air space in 2-4 weeks

MISCELLANEOUS

ASSOCIATED CONDITIONS Listed with Causes

AGE-RELATED FACTORS
Pediatric: Unusual in this age group except following trauma
Geriatric: Higher morbidity and mortality
Others: N/A

PREGNANCY N/A

SYNONYMS N/A

ICD-9-CM 512.8

SEE ALSO N/A

OTHER NOTES Chest pain may simulate an acute coronary occlusion or acute abdomen

ABBREVIATIONS N/A

REFERENCES
• O'Rourke, J.P. & Yee, E.: Civilian spontaneous pneumothorax: Treatment options and long-term results. Chest 96:1302, 1989
• Murray, J.F. & Nadel, J.A. (eds.): Textbook of Respiratory Medicine. Philadelphia, W.B. Saunders Co., 1988

Author H. Griffith, M.D. & M. Dambro, M.D.

Poliomyelitis

 BASICS

DESCRIPTION Acute, highly contagious, viral infection with wide range of manifestations including nonparalytic, aseptic meningitis, and paralytic poliomyelitis accompanied with flaccid weakness of various muscle groups. Usual course - acute. Paralysis develops within hours to 5 days; chronic. Prior to availability of vaccine, polio occurred sporadically and in epidemics. The disease is presently controlled by worldwide vaccine use.
<u>Three types</u>
   ◊ Encephalitic - coma
   ◊ Bulbar - cranial nerve paralysis
   ◊ Spinal - arm(s) and leg(s) weaknesses
Systems affected: Nervous/Mental
Genetics: N/A
Incidence/Prevalence in USA: 5-32 new cases per year
Predominant age: 3 months-16 years
Predominant sex: Male = Female

SIGNS AND SYMPTOMS
- Nuchal rigidity
- Myalgias
- Fever
- Headache
- Muscle cramps
- Malaise
- Anorexia
- Nausea
- Vomiting
- Diarrhea
- Sore throat
- Constipation
- Asymmetrical paralysis
- Sensory loss
- Meningeal irritation
- Flaccid motor paralysis
- Fasciculations
- Hyporeflexia
- Dysesthesias
- Transient urinary retention
- Muscle atrophy
- Hyperreflexia
- Ileus
- Shoulder girdle paralysis
- Intercostal paralysis
- Cyanosis
- Stridor
- Lethargy
- Coma

CAUSES Poliovirus

RISK FACTORS
- Living in areas where sanitation and hygiene are poor
- Low socioeconomic status
- Increasing age, if not immunized
- Pregnancy
- Recent tonsillectomy
- Inoculation (e.g., DPT injection)

 DIAGNOSIS

DIFFERENTIAL DIAGNOSIS
- Guillain-Barré syndrome
- Mumps, herpes, Coxsackievirus infection
- Aseptic meningitis
- Paralysis from a tick bite

LABORATORY
- Cerebrospinal fluid - pleocytosis
- Increased protein
- Normal glucose
- Complement fixation antibody - increased titer
- Leukocytosis
- Virus culture

Drugs that may alter lab results: N/A
Disorders that may alter lab results: N/A

PATHOLOGICAL FINDINGS
- Spinal cord - perivascular cuffing, abnormal motor nuclei, chromatolysis of motor neurons, intermediate column inflammation, posterior column inflammation
- Diffuse mononuclear infiltrate
- Abnormal anterior horn cells
- Hypothalamic lesion
- Thalamic lesion
- Brainstem lesion
- Vestibular nuclei lesions
- Cerebellar deep nuclei lesions
- Reticular formation lesions
- Cortical motor area lesions
- Cerebral edema
- Edematous cord

SPECIAL TESTS Spinal fluid virus isolation from throat (early in disease) and/or feces (early and late in the disease)

IMAGING N/A

DIAGNOSTIC PROCEDURES Lumbar puncture

 TREATMENT

APPROPRIATE HEALTH CARE
Inpatient for acute phase. Outpatient or rehabilitation facility for therapy.

GENERAL MEASURES
- Provide bed that has firm mattress, footboard, foam rubber pads or sandbags. Change positions frequently. Give good skin care.
- Mechanical ventilation, if required
- Tracheostomy is frequently required in respiratory failure
- Management of fecal impaction and urinary retention. Catheterization may be necessary.
- Non-narcotic analgesics
- Hot, moist packs
- Physical therapy

ACTIVITY
- Bedrest during active phase. With paralysis, may require an extended period.
- Long-term rehabilitation plan - using physical therapy, braces, special shoes, possibly orthopedic surgery. Team effort with doctors, physical and occupational therapists, and social worker or psychiatrist, if necessary.

DIET Be sure patient has adequate well-balanced diet. May require tube feedings.

PATIENT EDUCATION For patient education materials favorably reviewed on this topic, contact: International Polio Network, 4502 Maryland Avenue, St. Louis, MO 63108, (314)361-0475

MEDICATIONS

DRUG(S) OF CHOICE
• Aspirin or other non-narcotic analgesics
• Antibiotics, if other infection develops
• Parasympathomimetic (bethanechol) may help patient with urinary retention, 10-50 mg po bid-qid. Up to 100 mg qid may be required.
Contraindications: Refer to manufacturer's literature
Precautions: Bethanechol - adverse affects are rare, but may occur if dose increased. Includes colicky feeling, urinary urgency, skin flushing.
Significant possible interactions: Refer to manufacturer's literature

ALTERNATIVE DRUGS   N/A

FOLLOWUP

PATIENT MONITORING   Individualized depending on severity and long-term physical therapy requirements

PREVENTION/AVOIDANCE   Poliovirus vaccines. (NOTE: Use of these vaccines has effectively eliminated the disease in the industrialized world.)

POSSIBLE COMPLICATIONS
• Urinary tract infection
• Atelectasis
• Pneumonia
• Myocarditis
• Postpoliomyelitis progressive muscular atrophy (PPMA) - characterized by progressive weakness beginning 30 years or more after an attack of poliomyelitis
• Postpoliomyelitis motor neuron disease - occurs many years after acute poliomyelitis, less common than PPMA

EXPECTED COURSE AND PROGNOSIS
• Often irreversible paralysis; less than 5% mortality during acute disease
• Increased mortality over age 40
• Poor recovery for totally paralyzed muscle groups
• Good recovery for partially paralyzed muscle groups

MISCELLANEOUS

ASSOCIATED CONDITIONS   N/A

AGE-RELATED FACTORS
Pediatric: Most common in this age group. Polio is an extremely rare infection in U.S. since introduction of effective vaccines. (See vaccination instructions).
Geriatric: Extremely rare. Primary vaccination not recommended (except when traveling to endemic areas).
Others: N/A

PREGNANCY   A risk factor for developing polio

SYNONYMS
• Infantile paralysis
• Acute anterior poliomyelitis
• Acute lateral poliomyelitis

ICD-9-CM   045.1 acute poliomyelitis with other paralysis

SEE ALSO   Vaccination recommendations for inactivated Salk vaccine or Sabin live attenuated virus vaccine

OTHER NOTES   N/A

ABBREVIATIONS   N/A

REFERENCES
• Wyngaarden, J.B., Smith, L.H. (eds): Cecil Textbook of Medicine. 19th Ed. Philadelphia, W.B. Saunders Co., 1992
• Mandell, G.L. (ed.): Principles and Practice of Infectious Diseases. 3rd Ed. New York, Churchill Livingstone, 1990

Author   M. Dambro, M.D. & H. Griffith, M.D.

Polyarteritis nodosa

BASICS

DESCRIPTION Polyarteritis nodosa (PAN) presents pathologically as an ongoing segmental inflammatory response within the media of small and medium sized muscular arteries
• Organ involvement - kidney, GI tract, skin, muscles, joints, genitourinary tract, peripheral and central nervous system, heart, testes, epididymis and ovaries
• One of the vasculitic syndromes which vary in involvement from mild, self-limited skin lesions to severe systemic isolated and combined, multi-organ dysfunction and death
• Although heterogeneity and "overlap" manifestations abound, PAN is classified as a systemic necrotizing vasculitis
System(s) affected: Vascular, and may involve any tissue or organ in the body
Genetics: Unknown
Incidence/Prevalence in USA: No definite figures because of inclusive grouping of different types of vasculitic syndromes
Predominant age: Childhood to geriatric age groups. Mean is 45 years.
Predominant sex: Male > Female (2.5:1)

SIGNS AND SYMPTOMS
General (often nonspecific)
◊ Fever
◊ Weakness
◊ Weight loss
◊ Malaise
◊ Myalgia
◊ Livido reticularis
◊ Headache
◊ Abdominal pain and vague discomfort
Related to organ system involved (may dominate clinical picture and course)
◊ Renal - hypertension, hematuria (usually microscopic), proteinuria, progressive renal failure
◊ Musculoskeletal - myalgia, migratory arthralgia and arthritis
◊ Skin - purpura, urticaria, subcutaneous hemorrhages, polymorphic rashes, subcutaneous nodules (uncommon but characteristic), persistent livedo reticularis and Raynaud's phenomenon (rare)
◊ Gastrointestinal - recurrent and severe pain, hepatomegaly, nausea, vomiting and bleeding
◊ Lung - Hilar adenopathy, patchy infiltrates, reticular or nodular lesions, often fleeting
◊ CNS - seizures, CVA's, headache, papillitis, altered mental states
◊ Peripheral nervous system - mononeuritis multiplex
◊ Cardiac - pericarditis, CHF associated with hypertension and/or myocardial infarction
◊ Genitourinary - usually asymptomatic but may have testicular, epididymal, ovarian pain. Neutrogenic bladder reported.

CAUSES
Unclear. Suggestive evidence for immunological involvement.
◊ Tissue deposition of immune complexes
◊ Hepatitis B antigenemia in 30% of cases
◊ Hepatitis B antigen in circulating immune complexes
◊ Hepatitis B antigen, complement and IgM demonstrated in vascular walls

RISK FACTORS Included in Causes

DIAGNOSIS

DIFFERENTIAL DIAGNOSIS
• Systemic lupus erythematosis
• Cryoglobulinemia
• Subacute endocarditis
• Trichinosis
• Some rickettsial diseases
• The key differences from other necrotizing vasculitides are lack of granuloma formation, sparing of veins and pulmonary arteries

LABORATORY
Non specific:
◊ Abnormal urine sediment
◊ High neutrophil count
◊ Eosinophilia rare. Suggests granulomatous involvement when present
◊ Anemia of chronic disease
◊ Elevated sedimentation rate
◊ Hypergammaglobulinemia
◊ Hepatitis B surface antigen positive in 30% of cases (strong circumstantial evidence)
Specific
◊ Mainly based on pathological findings of biopsy material from involved organs
◊ Careful examinations of biopsies from "acute abdomens", especially in males between the second and fourth decade
Drugs that may alter lab results: Steroids
Disorders that may alter lab results: Allergic reactions and other immunologic disorders

PATHOLOGICAL FINDINGS
• Necrotizing inflammation, in various stages, of small and medium muscular arteries. Segmental in distribution, often seen at bifurcations and branchings. Involvement of venules not seen in classic PAN.
• Acute lesions show infiltration of polymorphonuclear cells through vessel wall and perivascular area
• Subsequent proliferation, degeneration, appearance of monocytes, necrosis with thrombosis and infarction of the involved tissue. Aneurysmal dilatations characteristic.
• Aortic dissection reported attributed to necrotizing vasculitis of the vasa vasorum

SPECIAL TESTS
Angiographic demonstration of aneursymal changes of small and medium sized arteries involving renal hepatic and mesenteric arteries represents strong evidence supporting the diagnosis

IMAGING Angiography: Mesenteric artery aneurysm, renal aneurysm, hepatic aneurysm, intestinal aneurysm

DIAGNOSTIC PROCEDURES N/A

TREATMENT

APPROPRIATE HEALTH CARE
Depends on extent and involvement of specific organs

GENERAL MEASURES The same as those needed for patients under treatment with steroids (high risk of infections), cytotoxic agents and plasmapheresis

ACTIVITY As tolerated

DIET Low salt if hypertension

PATIENT EDUCATION Arthritis Foundation, 1314 Spring Street N.W., Atlanta, GA 30309, (404)872-7100

MEDICATIONS

DRUG(S) OF CHOICE
• Favorable results reported with prednisone and cyclophosphamide. Reports differ as to the benefits of adding plasmaphoresis.
• Reports indicate plasmapheresis may increase favorable response
• Hepatitis B vaccine may be considered in at least the amelioration of any subsequent development of life-threatening complications of hepatitis B virus-associated polyarteritis nodosa
Contraindications: Refer to manufacturer's profile of each drug
Precautions: Refer to manufacturer's profile of each drug
Significant possible interactions: Refer to manufacturer's profile of each drug

ALTERNATIVE DRUGS   N/A

FOLLOWUP

PATIENT MONITORING
• Careful monitoring for infection
• Delayed appearance of neoplasms
• Angiographic changes may improve rapidly with combination steroid/cyclophosphamide therapy
• Acute phase reactants such as Interleukin-6 and C-reactive protein may be useful in diagnosis and monitoring activity level during treatment and followup

PREVENTION/AVOIDANCE   N/A

POSSIBLE COMPLICATIONS
• Glomerulonephritis
• Thrombosis
• Infarction
• Tissue/organ necrosis

EXPECTED COURSE AND PROGNOSIS
• Expected course of untreated polyarteritis nodosa is poor
• 5 year survival rate 13%
• Steroid treatment may increase percentage survival rate to 50-60% (prospective studies in progress)

MISCELLANEOUS

ASSOCIATED CONDITIONS
• Churg-Strauss syndrome
• Benign cutaneous periarteritis nodosa (bears watching and investigating because not necessarily benign)

AGE-RELATED FACTORS
Pediatric: N/A
Geriatric: N/A
Others: N/A

PREGNANCY   One case report suggests that if a patient attains remission before becoming pregnant, the chance of a successful delivery is reasonable

SYNONYMS
• Periarteritis
• Panarteritis
• Necrotizing arteritis

ICD-9-CM   446.0 polyarteritis nodosa

SEE ALSO   N/A

OTHER NOTES   N/A

ABBREVIATIONS   N/A

REFERENCES
• Braunwald, E. et.al., (eds.): Harrison's Principles of Internal Medicine, 12th Ed. New York, McGraw-Hill, 1991
• Wyngaarden, J.B. & Smith, L.H. (eds.): Cecil Textbook of Medicine., 18th Ed. Philadelphia, W.B. Saunders, 1992
• Iino, T., et al.: Polyarteritis nodosa. J Rheumatol. Oct 19(10):1632-36, 1992
• Nakayama, H.: Distinct response interleukin-6 and other laboratory parameters to treatment in a patient with polyarteritis nodosa. Angiology, 43(6):512-6, 1992

Author   J. Dix, M.D.

Polycystic kidney disease

 BASICS

DESCRIPTION Inherited disorders characterized by the development and growth of cysts in the kidneys
Incidence/Prevalence in USA: 100 per 100,000
System(s) affected: Renal/Urologic
Genetics: N/A
Predominant age: Usually diagnosed by age 45
Predominant race: Caucasian
Predominant sex: None

SIGNS AND SYMPTOMS
- Hypertension
- Hematuria; microscopic or macroscopic
- Palpable kidneys
- Hepatomegaly
- Abdominal pain
- Flank pain
- Headache
- Nocturia
- Dysuria
- Urinary frequency
- Polyuria

CAUSES Inherited autosomal dominant abnormality linked to chromosome 16. 90% penetrance by age 90 in gene carriers. Rare autosomal recessive form exists in neonates.

RISK FACTORS N/A

 DIAGNOSIS

DIFFERENTIAL DIAGNOSIS
- Renal cortical cysts
- Acquired cystic kidney disease

LABORATORY
- Hematocrit - elevated in 5% of cases
- Urinalysis - may have hematuria and mild proteinuria
- Serum creatinine - may be elevated
Drugs that may alter lab results: N/A
Disorders that may alter lab results: N/A

PATHOLOGICAL FINDINGS N/A

SPECIAL TESTS N/A

IMAGING
Ultrasonography or CT scan show either normal or enlarged kidneys with multiple cysts scattered throughout the cortices bilaterally. By age 25, 85% of patients with polycystic kidney disease can be detected.

DIAGNOSTIC PROCEDURES N/A

 TREATMENT

APPROPRIATE HEALTH CARE
Outpatient except for complicating emergencies (infected cyst)

GENERAL MEASURES No special measures

ACTIVITY Avoid contact activities that may damage enlarged organs.

DIET Low protein diet may retard progression of renal disease.

PATIENT EDUCATION
- Genetic counseling is critical
- Avoidance of nephrotoxic drugs

MEDICATIONS

DRUG(S) OF CHOICE No drug therapy available
Contraindications: N/A
Precautions: N/A
Significant possible interactions: N/A

ALTERNATIVE DRUGS N/A

FOLLOWUP

PATIENT MONITORING
• Serum creatinine and blood pressure monitoring twice a year; more frequently as disease progresses

PREVENTION/AVOIDANCE Genetic counseling

POSSIBLE COMPLICATIONS
• Progression to renal failure
• Renal calculi in up to 30%
• Cyst infection
• Cyst rupture

EXPECTED COURSE AND PROGNOSIS
• The disease is slowly progressive and has a variable outcome
• End stage renal disease occurs in 70% of patients by age 65

MISCELLANEOUS

ASSOCIATED CONDITIONS
• Cerebral aneurysms present in 10-40% of patients
• Colonic diverticuli in 80%
• Liver cysts in approximately 50%

AGE-RELATED FACTORS
Pediatric: N/A
Geriatric: N/A
Others: Hypertension is secondary to high renin. Responds to angiotensin converting enzyme inhibitors. May eventually require dialysis and/or renal transplantation.

PREGNANCY Higher frequency of new onset hypertension than in women without polycystic kidney disease. No adverse effect on the course of the polycystic kidney disease in asymptomatic patients. Patients with hypertension, proteinuria or renal insufficiency are at increased risk of complications.

SYNONYMS N/A

ICD-9-CM 753.13

SEE ALSO N/A

OTHER NOTES N/A

ABBREVIATIONS N/A

REFERENCES
• Welling, L.W., Granthem, J.J. Cystic and developmental diseases of the kidney. In Brenner, B.M., and Rector, F.C. (eds.): The Kidney. Philadelphia, W.B. Saunders, 1991
• Chapman, A.B., Johnson, A., Gabow, P.A., Schrier, R.W.: The renin-angiotensin-aldosterone system and autosomal dominant polycystic kidney disease. N Engl J Med 1990; 323:1091-1096

Author M. Siskind, M.D.

Polycystic ovarian disease

 BASICS

DESCRIPTION Polycystic ovarian disease (PCOD) is characterized by a state of chronic oligo-ovulation and/or anovulation culminating in oligomenorrhea and/or amenorrhea
Genetics: N/A
Incidence/Prevalence in USA: Unknown, but is a common cause of oligomenorrhea and/or amenorrhea
Predominant age: Women of reproductive age
Predominant sex: Female only

SIGNS AND SYMPTOMS
- Amenorrhea
- Oligomenorrhea
- Obesity
- Hirsutism
- Acne
- Dysfunctional uterine bleeding
- Infertility
- Acanthosis nigricans
- Hypertension
- Virilism
- Enlarged ovaries
- Enlarged clitoris
- Deep voice

CAUSES Disruption of hypothalamic-pituitary-ovarian axis (high normal luteinizing hormone and low normal follicle stimulating hormone leading to ovarian hyperandrogenism and follicular atresia and anovulation)

RISK FACTORS
- Endometrial hyperplasia
- Endometrial carcinoma
- Obesity
- Hypertension
- Diabetes mellitus
- Breast cancer
- Infertility

 DIAGNOSIS

DIFFERENTIAL DIAGNOSIS
- Cushing's syndrome
- Hairan syndrome (hyperandrogenism, insulin resistance, acanthosis nigricans)
- Testosterone-producing ovarian or adrenal tumor
- Prolactin-producing pituitary adenoma
- Hyperthecosis
- Adult-onset adrenal hyperplasia
- Partial congenital adrenal hyperplasia (21-hydroxylase deficiency)
- Other adrenal enzyme deficiencies
- Endometrial hyperplasia
- Endometrial carcinoma

LABORATORY
- Luteinizing hormone/follicle stimulating hormone (LH/FSH) $\geq$ 2.5-3.0/1
- Testosterone increased, but less than 200 ng/dl
- Dehydroepiandrosterone sulfate (DHEA-S) increased, but less than 800 mcg/dl
- Dehydroepiandrosterone (DHEA) increased
- 17-OH progesterone increased
- Estrone increased
- Androstenedione increased
- Sex hormone binding globulin decreased
- Prolactin
Drugs that may alter lab results: N/A
Disorders that may alter lab results: N/A

PATHOLOGICAL FINDINGS
- Ovary usually enlarged with a smooth white glistening capsule
- Ovarian cortex lined with follicles in all stages of development but most are atretic
- Theca cell proliferation with an increase in the stromal compartment

SPECIAL TESTS N/A

IMAGING Pelvis ultrasound revealing enlarged ovaries with multiple small follicular cysts

DIAGNOSTIC PROCEDURES
- History and physical examination
- Endometrial biopsy to rule out hyperplasia and or carcinoma

 TREATMENT

APPROPRIATE HEALTH CARE
- Outpatient
- Inpatient, if surgery for wedge resection recommended

GENERAL MEASURES No ideal treatment exists. Treatment must be individualized according to the needs and desires of the patient.

ACTIVITY Full activity

DIET Regular (weight loss recommended, if overweight)

PATIENT EDUCATION Counsel the patient regarding the risk of endometrial and breast carcinoma, insulin resistance and diabetes mellitus, obesity and infertility

MEDICATIONS

DRUG(S) OF CHOICE
<u>If pregnancy not desired:</u>
◊ Cyclic withdrawal bleeding with medroxyprogesterone acetate (Provera) 10 mg po x 12-14 days/month
or
◊ Low dose oral contraceptives
<u>If pregnancy desired:</u>
◊ Ovulation induction with clomiphene citrate (Clomid, Serophene)
or
◊ Human menopausal gonadotropins (Pergonal)
or
◊ Pure follicle stimulating hormone (Metrodin) with or without the addition of gonadotropin releasing hormone (GnRH) agonist (leuprolide acetate (Lupron) or nafarelin acetate (Synarel))
Contraindications: None, but if using oral contraceptive agents to prevent sequelae of anovulation, be aware of contraindications
Precautions:
• Risks of multiple fetuses with clomiphene citrate is 8%
• Risks of multiple fetuses with HMG, FSH is 25%
• Risk of severe ovarian hyperstimulation syndrome (OHS) is less than 1%
Significant possible interactions: Refer to manufacturer's profile of each drug

ALTERNATIVE DRUGS   N/A

FOLLOWUP

PATIENT MONITORING   Monitor patient frequently throughout the menstrual cycle depending upon which drug combination is utilized for ovulation induction

PREVENTION/AVOIDANCE   Prevent endometrial and breast carcinoma

POSSIBLE COMPLICATIONS
• Multiple pregnancies
• OHS
• Drug costs high
• Monitoring (ultrasounds, estradiols) costs high
• Oral contraceptives are not without risk

EXPECTED COURSE AND PROGNOSIS
• Prognosis for fertility is excellent depending upon other fertility factors
• Proper treatment and followup of chronic anovulation, can prevent endometrial hyperplasia and/or carcinoma

MISCELLANEOUS

ASSOCIATED CONDITIONS
• Obesity
• Hypertension
• Endometrial hyperplasia and/or carcinoma
• Breast carcinoma
• Diabetes mellitus
• Hairan syndrome
• Infertility
• Hyperthecosis

AGE-RELATED FACTORS
Pediatric: N/A
Geriatric: N/A
Others: N/A

PREGNANCY   N/A

SYNONYMS
• Stein-Leventhal syndrome
• Polycystic ovary syndrome

ICD-9-CM
• 256.4
• 628.0

SEE ALSO   N/A

OTHER NOTES   N/A

ABBREVIATIONS
• OHS = ovarian hyperstimulation syndrome
• HMG = human menopausal gonadotropins
• FSH = follicle stimulating hormone

REFERENCES   Danforth, D.M., Scott, J.R., et al. (eds.): Obstetric and Gynecology. 6th Ed. Philadelphia, J.B. Lippincott, 1990

Author   N. Spirtos, D.O. & M. Attaran, M.D.

Polycythemia vera

 BASICS

DESCRIPTION
A clonal cell hematologic malignant disorder with excessive erythroid, myeloid and megakaryocytic elements in the bone marrow. It is one of a group of myeloproliferative disorders.

System(s) affected:
Hemic/Lymphatic/Immunologic

Genetics: Unknown genetic pattern (some suggestion that a chromosomal abnormality may be involved)

Incidence/Prevalence in USA: 0.5 per 100,000

Predominant age: Middle to late years, mean is 60 years (range 15-90)

Predominant sex: Male > Female (slightly)

SIGNS AND SYMPTOMS
- Early stages may produce no symptoms
- Headaches
- Tinnitus
- Vertigo
- Blurred vision
- Epistaxis
- Increased blood viscosity
- Spontaneous bruising
- Upper GI bleeding
- Peptic ulcer disease
- Arterial and venous occlusive events
- Pruritis
- Sweating
- Weight loss
- Plethora (face, hands, feet)
- Splenomegaly
- Hepatomegaly
- Hyperhistaminemia
- Bone pain (ribs and sternum)
- Bone tenderness (ribs and sternum)

CAUSES
Unknown, origin of all three hematopoietic cell lines originate in a single clone

RISK FACTORS
- Jewish ancestry (may have increased frequency)
- Familial history (rare)

 DIAGNOSIS

DIFFERENTIAL DIAGNOSIS
- Secondary polycythemias
- Hemoglobinopathy
- Spurious polycythemia

LABORATORY
Tests used for diagnosis of polycythemia vera
◊ A1: Increased RBC mass - female ≥ 32 mL/kg, male ≥ 36 mL/kg
◊ A2: Normal arterial oxygen saturation (≥ 92%)
◊ A3: Splenomegaly
◊ B1: Thrombocytosis platelet count > 400,000μL
◊ B2: Leukocytosis > 12,000/μL
◊ B3: Leukocyte alkaline phosphatase increased
◊ B4: Increased serum B12 or increased unsaturated vitamin B12 binding capacity (UB12CB)
Diagnosis acceptable with following combinations:
◊ A1 + A2 + A3
◊ A1 + A2 + any 2 from B category (splenomegaly absent in about 25% of patients)
Other lab findings
◊ Hyperuricemia
◊ Hypercholesterolemia
◊ Elevated blood histamine level

Drugs that may alter lab results: Diuretics may cause a spurious polycythemia

Disorders that may alter lab results: Excessive use of alcohol or tobacco

PATHOLOGICAL FINDINGS
- Plethoric congestion in all organs and tissues
- Major vessels contain thick, viscous blood
- Sinuses of spleen packed with red blood cells

SPECIAL TESTS
Bone marrow aspiration (red cell hyperplasia, absent iron stores) and biopsy (fibrosis during spent phase of the disease)

IMAGING
CT - splenomegaly

DIAGNOSTIC PROCEDURES
Bone marrow aspiration - hyperplastic and panmyelosis

 TREATMENT

APPROPRIATE HEALTH CARE
Outpatient

GENERAL MEASURES
- Individualized management necessary. Dependent on many factors - age, disease duration, disease phenotype, complications, disease activity.
- Currently, phlebotomy is mainstay of therapy. Beyond that, differences exist among authorities about use and effectiveness of myelosuppressives.
Phlebotomy
◊ To reduce hematocrit to approximately 45%
◊ Performed as often as every 2 or 3 days until normal hematocrit reached. Phlebotomies of 250-500 m/L. Reduce to 250-350 m/L in elderly patients or patients with cardiovascular disease.
◊ Concomitant therapy possibilities, e.g., some form of myelosuppression, radioactive phosphorus (in elderly patients)
◊ Phlebotomy repeated as necessary for maintenance
◊ If patient cannot tolerate phlebotomy - chemotherapy (hydroxyurea is the least mutagenic agent) or radiation therapy
Other therapy
◊ Maintain hydration
◊ Pruritis therapy
◊ Manage thrombotic or hemorrhagic complications the same as with nonpolycythemic patient
◊ Uric acid reduction therapy

ACTIVITY
No restrictions

DIET
- No special diet (iron replacement not necessary)
- Phlebotomy regimen will produce pica, resulting in craving for crisp green vegetables (lettuce, celery) and ice

PATIENT EDUCATION
- Lifelong maintenance
- Complications to watch for

Polycythemia vera

MEDICATIONS

DRUG(S) OF CHOICE
Adjunctive
◊ Allopurinol 300 mg/day for uric acid reduction
◊ Cyproheptadine for pruritis, 4-16 mg as needed
◊ H2-receptor blockers or antacids for GI hyperacidity
Myelosuppression
◊ Radioactive phosphorous
◊ Chlorambucil or busulfan or hydroxyurea (alkylating agents)
◊ The use of low-dose aspirin is controversial in view of bleeding risk
◊ Note: Refer to hematologist/oncologist for dosages and instructions
Contraindications: Refer to manufacturer's literature
Precautions: Refer to manufacturer's literature
Significant possible interactions: Refer to manufacturer's literature

ALTERNATIVE DRUGS N/A

FOLLOWUP

PATIENT MONITORING
• Frequent during early treatment until satisfactory hematocrit is reached
• Monitor hematocrit often and phlebotomize when needed

PREVENTION/AVOIDANCE No known preventive measures

POSSIBLE COMPLICATIONS
• Uric acid stones
• Secondary gout
• Vascular thromboses (major cause of death)
• Transformation to leukemia
• Hemorrhage
• Peptic ulcer
• Increased risk for complications and mortality from surgery procedures. Assess risk-benefits and assure optimal control of disorder before any elective surgery.

EXPECTED COURSE AND PROGNOSIS
• Median survival without treatment - 6 to 18 months following diagnosis
• Survival up to 10 years with treatment
• Some patients live, symptom-free, for 20 or more years

MISCELLANEOUS

ASSOCIATED CONDITIONS
• Budd-Chiari Syndrome
• Mesenteric artery thrombosis

AGE-RELATED FACTORS
Pediatric: Rare in this age group
Geriatric: Phlebotomies and other therapies need to be adjusted for patients over 70
Others: N/A

PREGNANCY Treat with phlebotomy alone

SYNONYMS
• Primary polycythemia
• Vaquez disease
• Polycythemia, splenomegalic
• Vaquez-Osler disease

ICD-9-CM 238.4 polycythemia vera

SEE ALSO Myeloproliferative disorders

OTHER NOTES N/A

ABBREVIATIONS N/A

REFERENCES
• Williams, W.J., Beutler, E., Erslev, A.J., et al. (eds.): Hematology. 4th Ed. New York, McGraw-Hill, 1990
• Conley C.L.: Polycythemia vera, diagnosis and treatment. Hosp Practice 22:107, 1987

Author SG Smith

Polymyalgia rheumatica

BASICS

DESCRIPTION A clinical syndrome characterized by aching and stiffness of the shoulder and hip girdle muscles affecting older patients, associated with an elevated ESR, lasting over 1 month and responsive to low dose steroids
System(s) affected: Musculoskeletal, Hemic/Lymphatic/Immunologic
Genetics: Associated with HLA determinants
Incidence/Prevalence in USA:
Approximately 50/100,000 patients over age 50/year
Predominant age: 60 or older. Incidence increases with age (rare under 50 years old).
Predominant sex: Females > Male (2:1)

SIGNS AND SYMPTOMS
• Onset - abrupt or insidious
• Pain and stiffness proximal muscle girdles
• Usually symmetrical
• Symptoms more common in the morning
• Gel phenomena (stiffness after prolonged inactivity)
• Constitutional symptoms - fatigue, apathy, depression, weight loss, fevers
• Arthralgias/arthritis
• No weakness (pain may limit strength)
• Muscle tenderness rare, but may be seen
• No muscle atrophy
• Decreased range-of-motion of joints usually due to pain
• May see joint effusions
• May have signs and symptoms of giant cell arteritis (seen in approximately 15% of patients)

CAUSES
• Unknown
• May follow viral illness

RISK FACTORS
• Age greater than 50
• Presence of giant cell arteritis

DIAGNOSIS

DIFFERENTIAL DIAGNOSIS
• Rheumatoid arthritis
• Other connective tissue disease
• Fibromyalgia
• Depression
• Polymyositis
• Thyroid disease
• Viral myalgia
• Osteoarthritis
• Occult infection
• Occult malignancy

LABORATORY
• ESR (Westergren) elevation greater than 50
• Anemia - normochromic/normocytic
• Creatine phosphokinase - normal
• Rheumatoid factor (RF) - negative (5% patients over 60 will have positive RF without disease)
• Mild elevations in liver function tests
Drugs that may alter lab results:
Prednisone
Disorders that may alter lab results:
Disorders causing acute phase reactants can elevate ESR (e.g., infection, neoplasm, renal failure)

PATHOLOGICAL FINDINGS
• None in muscle biopsy
• There is no need to biopsy temporal artery unless symptoms/signs suggesting giant cell arteritis present. (Although the temporal artery biopsy may be positive, if there are no symptoms of giant cell arteritis, there is no reason to treat with high dose steroids. Increased morbidity has not been shown.
• Mild non-specific synovitis

SPECIAL TESTS N/A

IMAGING N/A

DIAGNOSTIC PROCEDURES None, unless giant cell arteritis suspected then temporal artery biopsy indicated

TREATMENT

APPROPRIATE HEALTH CARE
Outpatient unless needs temporal artery biopsy

GENERAL MEASURES Physical therapy for range-of-motion exercises if necessary

ACTIVITY No restrictions

DIET
• Appropriate salt restriction
• Adequate calcium intake

PATIENT EDUCATION
• Precautions regarding steroid use
• Instruct the patient about symptoms of giant cell arteritis and to report them immediately
• For patient education materials favorably reviewed on this topic, contact: American Academy of Family Physicians Foundation, P.O. Box 8418, Kansas City, MO 64114, (800)274-2237, ext. 4400
• Excellent materials also available from Arthritis Foundation, 1314 Spring Street, NW, Atlanta, GA 30309, (404)872-7100

MEDICATIONS

DRUG(S) OF CHOICE
Prednisone
◊ 10 mg/day initially (average initial affective dose 10-15 mg/d)
◊ Usually dramatic (diagnostic) response.
◊ May increase gradually to 20 mg if no response
◊ Begin slow taper at 4 weeks by only 1 mg every 1-4 weeks to a dose of 5-7.5 mg. Continue at this dose for approximately 18 months to 2 years, if no recurrence of symptoms.
◊ Then attempt to taper by 1 mg every 2-4 weeks until drug discontinued. Patient may, however, require steroids for 3 or more years.
◊ Increase prednisone for recurrence of symptoms (relapse common).
Contraindications: Avoid if possible in patients with chronic heart failure, diabetes mellitus, systemic fungal or bacterial infection. Must treat infections concurrently if steroids are absolutely necessary.
Precautions: Long term steroid use associated with several significant adverse effects including sodium and water retention, exacerbation of chronic heart failure, hypokalemia, increased susceptibility to infection, osteoporosis, cataracts, avascular necrosis. Gastrointestinal upset common, may lead to gastritis and/or peptic ulcer.
Significant possible interactions: Refer to manufacturer's literature

ALTERNATIVE DRUGS
NSAID's have been used, rarely successful

 FOLLOWUP

PATIENT MONITORING
• Follow monthly initially and during taper of medication, every 3 months otherwise
• Follow ESR as steroids tapered
• Followup with patient for symptoms of giant cell arteritis. Educate patient to report such symptoms immediately.

PREVENTION/AVOIDANCE N/A

POSSIBLE COMPLICATIONS
• Medication - complications related to steroid use
• Disease - exacerbation of disease with taper of steroids; development of giant cell arteritis

EXPECTED COURSE AND PROGNOSIS
• Average length disease is 3 years (range 1-4 years)
• Exacerbation if steroids tapered too fast
• Prognosis very good if treated (may gradually remit even if no treatment)
• Relapse common

 MISCELLANEOUS

ASSOCIATED CONDITIONS Giant cell arteritis

AGE-RELATED FACTORS
Pediatric: Does not occur in this age group
Geriatric: Incidence increases with age
Others: N/A

PREGNANCY N/A

SYNONYMS
• Senile rheumatic gout
• Anarthritic syndrome
• Forestier-Certonciny syndrome
• Polymyalgia rheumatica syndrome
• Rhizomelic pseudoarthrosis

ICD-9-CM 725 polymyalgia rheumatica

SEE ALSO Giant cell arteritis

OTHER NOTES Westergren ESR is the preferred laboratory technique. If other types of ESR studies are used (e.g., Wintrobe, or zeta sedimentation rate [ZSR]), the guidelines listed in this chapter cannot be used for abnormal levels.

ABBREVIATIONS PMR = polymyalgia rheumatica

REFERENCES
• Hunder, G.G.: Giant Cell Arteritis and Polymyalgia Rheumatica. In Textbook of Rheumatology. 3rd Ed. Edited by W.N. Kelly, E.D. Harris, S. Ruddy & C.B. Sledge. Philadelphia, W.B. Saunders Co., 1989
• Healey, L.A.: Polymyalgia Rheumatica and Giant Cell Arteritis. In Arthritis and Allied Conditions: A Textbook of Rheumatology. Edited by D.J. McCarty. Philadelphia, Lea and Febiger, 1989

Author B. Walsh, D.O. & E. Gall, M.D.

Polymyositis/Dermatomyositis

BASICS

DESCRIPTION Systemic connective tissue disease characterized by inflammatory and degenerative changes in muscles sometimes accompanied by characteristic skin rash.
• If skin manifestations are associated, it is designated as dermatomyositis
System(s) affected: Musculoskeletal, Pulmonary, Skin/Exocrine
Genetics: Unknown
Incidence in USA: Estimated at .5-.8 new cases/100,000
Prevalence in USA: 1-2 patients/100,000
Predominant age: 5-15 years, 40-60 years
Predominant sex: Female > Male (2:1)

SIGNS AND SYMPTOMS
• Difficulty when arising from sitting or lying positions
• Difficulty kneeling
• Difficulty climbing stairs
• Difficulty descending stairs
• Difficulty raising arms
• Joint pain/swelling
• Dysphagia
• Buttock pain
• Respiratory impairment
• Symmetrical proximal muscle weakness
• Decreased deep tendon reflexes
• Muscle swelling, stiffness, induration
• Rash over face (eyelids, nasolabial folds), upper chest, dorsal hands
• Periorbital edema

CAUSES
• Unknown
• Cell-mediated autoimmunity
• Viruses - possibly a participating factor

RISK FACTORS
Family history of autoimmune disease or vasculitis

DIAGNOSIS

DIFFERENTIAL DIAGNOSIS
• Vasculitis
• Progressive systemic sclerosis
• Systemic lupus erythematosus
• Rheumatoid arthritis
• Muscular dystrophy
• Eaton-Lambert syndrome
• Sarcoidosis
• Amyotrophic lateral sclerosis

LABORATORY
• Increased creatine phosphokinase (CPK)
• Increased aldolase
• Increased SGOT
• Increased LDH
• Myoglobinuria
• Increased ESR
• Positive rheumatoid factor (less than 50% of patients)
• Positive ANA (less than 50% of patients)
• Leukocytosis (less than 50% of patients)
• Anemia (less than 50% of patients)
• Hyperglobulinemia (less than 50% of patients)
• Increased creatinine (less than 50% of patients)
Drugs that may alter lab results: N/A
Disorders that may alter lab results: N/A

PATHOLOGICAL FINDINGS
• Micro - muscle fiber degeneration
• Micro - phagocytosis of muscle debris
• Micro - perifascicular muscle fiber atrophy
• Micro - inflammatory cell infiltrates in adult form
• Sarcoplasmic basophilia
• Muscle fiber increased in size

SPECIAL TESTS
• ECG - arrhythmias, conduction disturbances
• Electromyography (EMG) - muscle irritability, low amplitude potentials, polyphasic action potentials, fibrillations
• Muscle biopsy (deltoid or quadriceps femoris)

IMAGING Chest x-ray: pulmonary interstitial disease

DIAGNOSTIC PROCEDURES Diagnosis usually relies on 4 findings - weakness, CPK elevation, abnormal EMG, findings on muscle biopsy. Presence of skin rash of dermatomyositis also helpful.

TREATMENT

APPROPRIATE HEALTH CARE
Outpatient

GENERAL MEASURES
• Search for malignancy in all adults
• Follow serum muscle enzymes carefully

ACTIVITY
• Curtailed until after inflammation subsides
• Range-of-motion exercises to prevent contractures

DIET No special diet

PATIENT EDUCATION Muscular Dystrophy Association, 3561 E. Sunrise Dr., Tucson, AZ 85718. Telephone (800)221-1142.

MEDICATIONS

DRUG(S) OF CHOICE
• Prednisone 40-60 mg/day in divided doses. Reduce prednisone slowly when enzyme levels are normal. Probably need to continue 10-15 mg/day for maintenance.
• For patients resistant or intolerant to corticosteroids, azathioprine 1.0 mg/kg (arthritis dose) once or twice a day. Maintain at lowest possible dose.
• Methotrexate 10-25 mg weekly useful in some steroid-resistant cases

Contraindications: Refer to manufacturer's literature

Precautions:
• Prednisone: adverse effects associated with long-term steroid use include adrenal suppression, sodium, water retention, hypokalemia, osteoporosis, cataracts, increased susceptibility to infection
• Azathioprine: adverse effects include bone marrow suppression, increased LFT's, increased susceptibility to infection

Significant possible Interactions: Refer to manufacturer's literature

ALTERNATIVE DRUGS
Other immunosuppressant drugs such as cyclophosphamide, chlorambucil can be added to steroids. IV immunoglobulin being evaluated in resistant cases.

FOLLOWUP

PATIENT MONITORING
• Serial testing for muscle enzyme activity in serum
• Any adult should be studied for malignancy
• Monitor for steroid-induced metabolic complications (hypokalemia, hypertension, hyperglycemia, etc.)
• Monitor WBC, differential, platelets every week for the first month; then every 2 weeks for 2 months; then every month

PREVENTION/AVOIDANCE N/A

POSSIBLE COMPLICATIONS
• Pneumonia
• Infection
• Myocardial infarction
• Carcinoma (especially breast, lung)
• Severe dysphagia
• Respiratory impairment
• Aspiration pneumonitis
• Steroid myopathy
• Steroid induced diabetes, hypertension, hypokalemia, etc.

EXPECTED COURSE AND PROGNOSIS
• 30% residual weakness
• 20% persistent active disease
• 75% 5-year survival
• Survival worse for women and African-Americans
• Most patients improve with therapy
• 50% have full recovery
• Possibly relapsing

MISCELLANEOUS

ASSOCIATED CONDITIONS
• Malignancy
• Progressive systemic sclerosis
• Vasculitis
• Systemic lupus erythematosis
• Other connective tissue disorders

AGE-RELATED FACTORS
Pediatric:
• Childhood dermatomyositis occurs
• May be possible to discontinue prednisone gradually after a year or so
Geriatric:
• Rare after age 60
• Elderly patient with polymyositis more likely to have underlying neoplasm
Others: N/A

PREGNANCY N/A

SYNONYMS
• Neuromyositis
• Wagner-Unverricht syndrome

ICD-9-CM 710.4

SEE ALSO N/A

OTHER NOTES Classification of types of myositis: Childhood dermatomyositis, primary idiopathic dermatomyositis, dermatomyositis or polymyositis associated with malignancy, primary polymyositis, myositis associated with overlap syndrome

ABBREVIATIONS N/A

REFERENCES
• Kelley, W., et al.: Textbook of Rheumatology. 3rd Ed. Philadelphia, W.B. Saunders Co., 1989
• Kagen, L.J.: Polymyositis/dermatomyositis. In Arthritis and Allied Conditions. 11th Ed. Edited by D.J. McCarty, et al. Philadelphia, Lea & Febiger, 1989

Author C. M. Wise, M.D.

Porphyria

BASICS

DESCRIPTION Several heme synthesis pathway enzyme deficiencies with overproduction and accumulation of intermediate metabolic products and resultant neuropsychiatric-abdominal or dermatologic symptoms and syndromes. All more common in Caucasians than Blacks or Asians.
• Porphyria cutanea tarda (PCT) - dermatologic
• Acute intermittent porphyria (AIP) - pyrroloporphyria; neuropsychiatric-abdominal
• Protoporphyria (PP) - erythropoietic or hepatoerythropoietic; mild dermatologic
• Variegate porphyria (VP) - South African porphyria, prevalence in S. Africa is 1/400
• Hereditary coproporphyria (HCP) - neuropsychic, occasionally dermatologic
• Porphobilinogen synthetase deficiency (PBD) - delta-aminolevulinic aciduria; neuropsychiatric-abdominal
• Congenital erythropoietic porphyria (CEP) - Günther's disease; severe dermatologic
• Other rare genetic variants reported
System(s) affected: Gastrointestinal, Skin/Exocrine, Hemic/Lymphatic/Immunologic
Genetics:
• Autosomal dominant - PCT, AIP, PP, VP, HCP
• Autosomal recessive - PBD, CEP
• Latency common with variable expression, many asymptomatic or minimally symptomatic carriers
• PCT also sporadic and acquired
Incidence/Prevalence in USA:
• PCT - 1/10,000
• AIP, PP, VP - 1/10,000 to 1/100,000
• HCP - less than 1/100,000
• PBD, CEP - very rare
Predominant age:
• CEP - early childhood
• PP - older childhood
• AIP, VP, HCP, PBD - young adult
• PCT - middle age
Predominant sex:
• PP, CEP - male=female
• PCT - seen more commonly in male
• AIP, VP, HCP, PBD - seen more commonly in female

SIGNS AND SYMPTOMS
• All usually reversible, lasting days to weeks
• May be permanent
• Urine may turn dark red or brown on standing (word porphyria from Greek porphyra = purple)
Abdominal:
◊ Rather severe abdominal pain, occasionally in back and extremities
◊ Generalized more often than localized
◊ Often colicky
◊ Can mimic acute abdomen
◊ No fever should be present
◊ Chronic constipation common
◊ Severity of symptoms often out of proportion to physical findings
Neurologic:
◊ Essentially anything
◊ Includes sensory and motor systems
◊ Includes autonomic nervous system
◊ May include seizures
◊ May lead to quadriplegia and/or respiratory paralysis with death
Psychiatric:
◊ Essentially anything
◊ Psychosis most common
◊ Visual hallucinations common
◊ Disorientation frequent
◊ Chronic depression frequent
Dermatologic:
◊ Photosensitivity
◊ Scrapes, ulcerations, blisters with minimal trauma
◊ Hyperpigmentation, especially hands and face
◊ Scarring frequent
◊ CEP mutilating, with hemolysis, erythrodontia, splenomegaly
◊ PP occasional hepatic disease

CAUSES
• Genetic enzyme deficiencies
• PCT - uroporphyrinogen decarboxylase
• AIP - porphobilinogen deaminase
• PP - ferrochelatase
• VP - protoporphyrinogen oxidase
• HCP - coproporphyrinogen oxidase
• PBD - porphobilinogen synthetase
• CEP - uroporphyrinogen III synthetase (cosynthetase)
Acquired PCT causes:
◊ Decreased enzyme associated with alcohol, steroids, hormones
◊ Specific exposure to polyhalogenated hydrocarbons (e.g., hexachlorobenzene)
◊ Lead poisoning may alter pathways
◊ HIV
◊ Hepatitis C virus

RISK FACTORS
• Multiple precipitating factors, especially AIP, VP, HCP
• Drugs (e.g., barbiturates and sulfas in AIP)
• Estrogens, especially oral contraceptives
• Steroids
• Liver disease
• Menstrual cycles
• Infection
• Fasting

DIAGNOSIS

DIFFERENTIAL DIAGNOSIS Vast and protean

LABORATORY
• Urine for porphyrins during acute attack. Urine may be normal at other times.
• Individual enzyme activity in erythrocytes or other body cells/tissues
• Stool for porphyrins in PP, VP, HCP, CEP
• Bile for porphyrin in VP
• Erythrocyte uroporphyrin in CEP
• PP exception - urine unremarkable. Test erythrocyte protoporphyrin.
Drugs that may alter lab results: Unknown
Disorders that may alter lab results:
• Numerous conditions may cause slight increase in porphyrinuria, but patients asymptomatic
• Acute liver disease
• Hepatoma
• Hodgkin's lymphoma
• Multiple neurologic diseases

PATHOLOGICAL FINDINGS N/A

SPECIAL TESTS Genetic studies when applicable

IMAGING N/A

DIAGNOSTIC PROCEDURES N/A

TREATMENT

APPROPRIATE HEALTH CARE Outpatient, except for crises

GENERAL MEASURES
• Neuropsychiatric-abdominal - avoid drugs, alcohol, known toxins
• Dermatologic - shade, protective clothing; avoid skin trauma; PCT - phlebotomy weekly to monthly may help prevent
• CEP - consider bone marrow transplantation

ACTIVITY Normal, except dermatologic avoid sun

DIET Neuropsychiatric - large quantities of carbohydrates have been reported to help

PATIENT EDUCATION American Porphyria Foundation, P.O. Box 11163, Montgomery, AL 36111, (904)654-4754

MEDICATIONS

DRUG(S) OF CHOICE
Neuropsychiatric-abdominal
◊ Intravenous glucose 400 grams daily for one to two days
◊ Hematin (ferriprotoporphyrin IX, Panhematin) IV 1-4 mg/kg/d over 10-15 minutes x 3-14 days
◊ Epilepsy - consider clonazepam
◊ Depression - consider selective serotonin re-uptake inhibitors
Dermatologic:
◊ Oral carotenoids, e.g., beta-carotene (Solatene), 30 mg, 1-10 capsules per day
Contraindications: Known sensitivity to drug
Precautions: Hematin - phlebitis at IV site, reduced clotting ability
Significant possible interactions: None

ALTERNATIVE DRUGS
• PCT - chloroquine 125 mg twice weekly, or hydroxychloroquine 250 mg tid, in conjunction with phlebotomy
• Menstruating women - hematin premenstrual; cycle suppressors, e.g., luteinizing hormone releasing hormone (LHRH) analogues
• Autonomic manifestations - beta blockers
• Other symptoms - treat symptomatically

FOLLOWUP

PATIENT MONITORING Individualized

PREVENTION/AVOIDANCE
• Avoid precipitating drugs (alcohol, barbiturates, carbamazepine, chlorpropamide, danazol, ergots, estrogens and progestins, ethchlorvynol, glutethimide, griseofulvin, mephenytoin, meprobamate, methyprylon, phenytoin, pyrazolones, succinimides, sulfonamide antibiotics, valproic acid
• Eat an adequate diet with high carbohydrate intake

POSSIBLE COMPLICATIONS See list in
Signs and Symptoms

EXPECTED COURSE AND PROGNOSIS
• Patients who are asymptomatic or minimally symptomatic - unaffected longevity
• Patients who are more symptomatic - treatable and do well
• Neurologic complications (e.g., peripheral neuropathy, neurosis or hemiplegia) at times permanent
• In AIP, acute attacks have 25% mortality

MISCELLANEOUS

ASSOCIATED CONDITIONS
Acquired PCT:
• HIV
• Hepatitis C virus

AGE-RELATED FACTORS
Pediatric: N/A
Geriatric: N/A
Others: N/A

PREGNANCY Unpredictable disease
activity

SYNONYMS
• AIP
• IAP
• Pyrroloporphyria
• PP
• Erythropoietic porphyria
• Hepatoerythropoietic porphyria
• VP
• South African porphyria
• PBD
• Delta-aminolevulinic aciduria
• CEP
• Günther's disease

ICD-9-CM 277.1 disorders of porphyrin
metabolism

SEE ALSO N/A

OTHER NOTES Some drugs considered
safe - acetaminophen, aspirin, atropine, bromides, diazepam (in small doses), dicumarol, digoxin, diphenhydramine, ether, glucocorticoids, guanethidine, heparin, insulin, neostigmine, nitrous oxide, penicillin and derivatives, phenothiazines, narcotic analgesics, propranolol, streptomycin, succinylcholine, thiazides

ABBREVIATIONS N/A

REFERENCES
• Braunwald E., et al. (eds.): Harrison's Principles of Internal Medicine. 12th Ed. New York, McGraw-Hill, 1991
• Wyngaarden, J.B., Smith, L.H. (eds): Cecil Textbook of Medicine. 18th Ed. Philadelphia, W.B. Saunders Co., 1988

Author E. Dickstein, M.D.

Portal hypertension

BASICS

DESCRIPTION Increased portal vein pressure caused by extrahepatic vein obstruction, increased hepatic blood inflow, or increased resistance to hepatic blood outflow. Classification - presinusoidal, postsinusoidal. Usual course - progressive.
System(s) affected: Gastrointestinal, Cardiovascular
Genetics: No known genetic pattern
Incidence/Prevalence in USA: Unknown
Predominant age: Adult
Predominant sex: Male > Female

SIGNS AND SYMPTOMS
• Hematemesis
• Anorexia
• Abdominal pain
• Confusion
• Hemorrhoids
• Ascites
• Splenomegaly
• Black tarry stools
• Tachycardia
• Ascites
• Hepatomegaly
• Jaundice
• Confusion
• Asterixis
• Hyperreflexia
• Abdominal wall collaterals
• Abdominal bruit
• Stomach filled with blood

CAUSES
• Increased resistance to portal blood flow
• Alcoholic cirrhosis of the liver
• Portal vein thrombosis
• Schistosomiasis
• Congenital hepatic fibrosis
• Viral hepatitis with cirrhosis
• Budd-Chiari syndrome
• Chronic active hepatitis
• Right ventricular failure
• Splenic vein obstruction (e.g., thrombosis)
• Myeloproliferative disorders
• Lymphoproliferative disorders
• Cryptogenic

RISK FACTORS Any liver disease

DIAGNOSIS

DIFFERENTIAL DIAGNOSIS
• Any of the causes of:
  ◊ cirrhosis
  ◊ splenomegaly
  ◊ gastrointestinal bleeding
  ◊ ascites
• Sickle cell disease

LABORATORY
• Anemia
• Guaiac-positive
• Leukopenia
• Thrombocytopenia
• Decreased serum albumin
• Increased serum GGT
• Leukocytosis
• Increased alkaline phosphatase
• Increased SGOT
• Increased SGPT
Drugs that may alter lab results: N/A
Disorders that may alter lab results: N/A

PATHOLOGICAL FINDINGS
Arteriovenous or venous-venous anastomoses with collaterals

SPECIAL TESTS
• Galactose elimination capacity
• Antipyrine clearance

IMAGING
• Celiac angiography - varices; corkscrew configuration of intrahepatic vessels
• Barium meal - varices
• Ultrasound - increased portal vein diameter

DIAGNOSTIC PROCEDURES
• Endoscopy - esophageal varices and/or gastric varices
• Portal pressure measurement - increased wedged hepatic vein pressure

TREATMENT

APPROPRIATE HEALTH CARE
Inpatient

GENERAL MEASURES
• Administer NO sedatives, since encephalopathy can be expected
• Treat underlying cause (if due to alcohol, stop drinking)
• Surgery (portacaval or splenorenal shunt)
• Cleansing enemas
• Blood transfusion (as needed)
• Esophageal tamponade (balloon)
• Endoscopic sclerotherapy
• Transjugular intrahepatic porto-systemic shunt (TIPS) or banding

ACTIVITY Bedrest

DIET Restricted sodium and protein diet

PATIENT EDUCATION N/A

MEDICATIONS

DRUG(S) OF CHOICE
• For bleeding esophageal varices - vasopressin 0.2-0.4 units/min as a continuous drip; may increase to a maximum of 0.9 units/min
• Neomycin - orally, to reduce risk of encephalopathy
• Lactulose
Contraindications: Vasopressin - history of myocardial disease
Precautions: Vasopressin may cause hypertension, bradycardia, arrhythmias. Patient must be on a cardiac monitor while receiving this drug. Co-administration of nitroprusside may reduce cardiotoxicity.
Significant possible interactions: Refer to manufacturer's literature

ALTERNATIVE DRUGS
• Propranolol (results to date are contradictory)
• Somatostatin analogs

FOLLOWUP

PATIENT MONITORING Close followup of all functions until bleeding stops and underlying disorders are treated

PREVENTION/AVOIDANCE N/A

POSSIBLE COMPLICATIONS
• Transudative ascites
• Hypovolemic shock

EXPECTED COURSE AND PROGNOSIS
• 50% rebleed or develop recurrence of varices unless porto-systemic shunt is performed
• Dependent on cause

MISCELLANEOUS

ASSOCIATED CONDITIONS Cirrhosis of the liver

AGE-RELATED FACTORS
Pediatric: Unusual
Geriatric: Mortality and complication rate are high
Others: N/A

PREGNANCY N/A

SYNONYMS N/A

ICD-9-CM 572.3

SEE ALSO
• Cirrhosis of the liver
• Cirrhosis, alcoholic
• Hepatitis, viral

OTHER NOTES
Other treatment approaches (inadequately studied with non-control protocols)
  ◊ Transhepatic obliteration of varices
  ◊ Concomitant treatment with non-selective beta-adrenergic blockers

ABBREVIATIONS N/A

REFERENCES
• Sleisenger, M.H. and Fordtran, J.S. (eds.): Gastrointestinal Disease: Pathophysiology, Diagnosis, Management. 4th Ed. Philadelphia, W.B. Saunders Co., 1989
• Berkow, R., et al. (eds.): Merck Manual. 15th Ed. Rahway, NJ, Merck Sharp & Dohme, 1987

Author WH Schwesinger, M.D.

Post-traumatic stress disorder

 BASICS

DESCRIPTION A condition seen in people who experienced an event that would be extremely distressing to most human beings, e.g., serious threat to one's life, physical or psychological integrity; serious threat or harm to one's children, spouse, siblings, parents or other close relatives or friends; sudden destruction of one's home or community; seeing another person who has recently been (or is being) injured or killed as a result of a man-made violent act or natural disaster
• Symptoms of this condition did not exist prior to the trauma and symptoms persist for at least one month following the trauma
• There is a subtype of post-traumatic stress disorder (PTSD) with a delayed onset of the symptoms which starts at least six months after the trauma
System(s) affected: Nervous
Genetics: N/A
Incidence/Prevalence in USA: Up to 30% of victims of disasters develop PTSD
Predominant age: The elderly and the very young are more vulnerable
Predominant sex: Adult women are more inclined to ask for help. Young boys may be more vulnerable to trauma than girls.

SIGNS AND SYMPTOMS
The traumatic event is persistently re-experienced in at least one of the following ways:
◊ Recurrent and intrusive distressing recollections of the event
◊ Recurrent dreams relating to the trauma
◊ Sudden feeling or behavioral reenactment with a subjective sense of reliving the trauma (flashback)
Persistent avoidance of the stimuli associated with the trauma, or numbing of general responsiveness as indicated by at least three of the following:
◊ Efforts to void thoughts or feelings associated with the trauma
◊ Efforts to avoid activities or situations that arouse recollections of the trauma
◊ Inability to recall an important aspect of the trauma (psychogenic amnesia)
◊ Markedly diminished interest in significant activities (in young children, loss of recently acquired developmental skills such as toilet training or language skills)
◊ Feelings of detachment or estrangement from others
◊ Restricted range of affect, e.g., unable to have loving feelings
◊ Sense of a foreshortened future, e.g., does not expect to have a career, marriage, or children, or a long life

Persistent symptoms of increased arousal (not present before the trauma), as indicated by at least two of the following:
◊ Difficulty falling or staying asleep (insomnia)
◊ Irritability or outbursts of anger
◊ Difficulty in concentrating
◊ Hypervigilance
◊ Exaggerated startle response
◊ Physiologic reactivity upon exposure to events that symbolize or resemble an aspect of the traumatic event (e.g., a woman who was raped in an elevator breaks out in a sweat when entering an elevator)

CAUSES Events which are insults to one's personal integrity, self-esteem and security are psychologically traumatic and may lead to PTSD

RISK FACTORS Individuals with a history of childhood neglect or dysfunctional families, children of alcoholic parents, or childhood abuse, are predisposed and more susceptible to developing PTSD in response to trauma

 DIAGNOSIS

DIFFERENTIAL DIAGNOSIS
• Organic mental disorders
• Generalized anxiety disorder
• Phobic disorders
• Depressive disorder
• Panic disorder
• Conversion disorder
• Somatization disorder
• Personality disorders
• Substance and chemical dependency

LABORATORY N/A
Drugs that may alter lab results: N/A
Disorders that may alter lab results: N/A

PATHOLOGICAL FINDINGS Character pathology as shown on the Minnesota multiple personality inventory (MMPI)

SPECIAL TESTS
• Neuropsychological testing is helpful in cases of dementia and more subtle cognitive dysfunction
• EEG to rule out any brain damage (results may be altered by any drug affecting EEG patterns such as - sleeping pills, antidepressants, neuroleptics and other psychotropic medications)
• Psychological testing and a thorough mental status examination are valuable in a complete, thorough assessment of the patient
• Sleep lab studies of 8 hour EEG help in diagnosis of sleep disorders

• Through an examination and interview, assisted by Sodium amytal (given intravenously) or similar substances, one may uncover traumatic material in patients with amnesia. Similarly, an examination assisted by hypnosis may help in the diagnosis
• Tests may be affected by withdrawal or intoxication from drugs and alcohol; any organic brain syndromes such as multiple infarct dementia, other forms of dementia, and forms of epilepsy

IMAGING CT scan of the head, and MRI of the brain are valuable to rule out any brain damage

DIAGNOSTIC PROCEDURES
• Psychiatric examination
• Psychological testing

 TREATMENT

APPROPRIATE HEALTH CARE
• Most treatment is done on an outpatient basis
• In case of crisis such as a patient being suicidal or dysfunctional with activities of daily living, inpatient intensive treatment on a psychiatry unit is indicated

GENERAL MEASURES
• As indicated by the patient's physical condition, treatment includes individual psychotherapy, group therapy, hypnotherapy, narcoanalysis and narcosynthesis, and behavior therapy
• Crisis intervention shortly after the traumatic event is very valuable for the immediate distress and may prevent the development of a chronic or delayed form of Post-traumatic stress syndrome
• Relaxation exercises to help reduce anxiety and improve sleep have been found helpful.

ACTIVITY
• As indicated by patient's physical condition
• Restoration of regular sleep at night is essential in cases of insomnia

DIET No special diet

PATIENT EDUCATION
• Lenore Terr: Too Scared to Cry. Harper & Row, NY, 1990

Post-traumatic stress disorder

MEDICATIONS

DRUG(S) OF CHOICE
Tricyclic antidepressants:
◊ Doxepin 50-150 mg/day
◊ Nortriptyline 30-100 mg/day
◊ Imipramine 50-300 mg/day
◊ Desipramine 50-300 mg/day
◊ Amitriptyline 50-300 mg/day
◊ Trimipramine 50-300 mg/day
◊ Protriptyline 15-60 mg/ day
◊ Amoxapine 50-300 mg/day
◊ Maprotiline 50-225 mg/day (increased risk of seizures with higher doses)
Monoamine oxidase inhibitors
◊ Phenelzine 45-75 mg/day is useful especially in PTSD patients with panic attacks
Others
◊ Trazodone 100-400 mg/day, given mostly at bedtime is helpful in patients with insomnia
◊ Small doses of neuroleptics are helpful in selective patients
◊ Benzodiazepines should be used selectively and with caution
◊ Propranolol and clonidine have been used with limited results

Contraindications:
• Allergic reactions to specific drugs
• Use with caution in alcoholic patients with poor liver functions

Precautions:
• Do not mix tricyclic antidepressants with monoamine oxidase inhibitors
• Long-term use of benzodiazepines may lead to increased tolerance and dependency on the drug

Significant possible interactions:
Monoamine oxidase inhibitors may interact with other antidepressants, sympathomimetics such as pseudoephedrine and any foods with tyramine or its precursors

ALTERNATIVE DRUGS
• Clomipramine 75-250 mg/day in patients with obsessive compulsive symptoms has been helpful in some cases
• Selective serotonin reuptake inhibitors such as fluoxetine 20-80 mg/day, sertraline 50-200 mg/day, or paroxetine 20-50 mg/day have been found helpful in certain cases with depressive symptoms
• Buspirone 30-80 mg/day has been found helpful in cases with severe anxiety

FOLLOWUP

PATIENT MONITORING Psychotherapy for at least one hour per week is necessary in the first phase of treatment

PREVENTION/AVOIDANCE Crisis intervention immediately after the traumatic event involving intensive support and treatment may prevent the development of chronic PTSD later

POSSIBLE COMPLICATIONS
• Suicide
• Self-inflicted violence in reenactment of trauma

EXPECTED COURSE AND PROGNOSIS The lack of crisis intervention immediately following the trauma may lead to the persistence of symptoms. If they last beyond 4 to 6 weeks, acute PTSD develops. If symptoms persist over six months, patients may develop chronic PTSD which may lead to loss of job, marital conflicts, total disability and repeated and/or lengthy hospitalizations with severe morbidity.

MISCELLANEOUS

ASSOCIATED CONDITIONS Personality disorders such as borderline personality disorder, depression, panic disorder, anxiety disorder, and dissociative disorders

AGE-RELATED FACTORS
Pediatric: Young children are susceptible to abuse and neglect and can develop a chronic PTSD with failure to progress and grow in a healthy way
Geriatric: The elderly have fewer social support resources and their adjustment to trauma is less flexible. Also, they are more sensitive to medication and need dose adjustment.
Others: N/A

PREGNANCY Avoid psychotropics in the first trimester. Focus on non-pharmacologic treatment techniques such as psychotherapy, hypnotherapy, relaxation therapy, etc.

SYNONYMS
• Trauma syndrome
• Battle fatigue
• Shell shock
• Post-disaster syndrome
• Trauma survivor's syndrome
• Traumatic neurosis

ICD-9-CM 293.9

SEE ALSO N/A

OTHER NOTES N/A

ABBREVIATIONS N/A

REFERENCES
• Krystal, H.: Massive Psychic Trauma. New York, Int. Universities Press, 1984
• Terr, L.: Too Scared to Cry: Psychic Trauma in Childhood. New York, Harper & Row, 1990
• Van Der Kolk, B. (Ed.): Psychological Trauma. Washington, D.C., American Psychiatric Press, 1987
• Torem, M.S. & Curdue, K.: PTSD presenting as an eating disorder. Stress Med 4:139-142, 1988
• Torem, M.S.: Psychological sequelae in the rape victim. Stress Med 2:301-305, 1986
• Ulman, R.B. & Brothers, D.: The Shattered Self. Hillsdale, NJ, The Analytic Press, 1988
• Rowan, A.B. & Foy, D.W.: Post-Traumatic Stress Disorder in Child Sexual Abuse. J of Traumatic Stress, 6:3-31, 1993
• Briere, J.: Child Abuse Trauma: Theory and Treatment of the Lasting Effects. Newbury Park, CA, Sage, 1992

Author M. Torem, M.D.

Preeclampsia

 BASICS

DESCRIPTION Hypertension associated with proteinuria, edema, and acute excessive weight gain developing during pregnancy after 20 weeks gestation

System(s) affected: Reproductive, Cardiovascular, Nervous

Genetics: N/A

Incidence/Prevalence IN USA: 5-10% of all pregnancies

Predominant age:
• Young, primigravid women
• Women over 35 years of age

Predominant sex: Female only

SIGNS AND SYMPTOMS
• Elevated BP (> 140/90 or increased 30 systolic or increased 15 diastolic) recorded on 2 BP readings 6 hours apart
• Proteinuria (> 300 mg/24 hours or > 1 gram/L)
• Edema
• Rapid excessive weight gain (> 5 lbs/week)
• Epigastric pain
• Headache
• Hyperreflexia
• Visual disturbances
• Apprehension
• Retinal arteriola spasm
• Papilledema
• Retinal cotton-wool exudate
• Amnesia
• Oliguria
• Anuria

CAUSES
• Altered cardiovascular reactivity (current hypothesis)
• Increased capillary permeability
• Widespread vasospasm
• Microthrombi
• Hypertension

RISK FACTORS
• Familial incidence
• Lower socio-economic
• Multiple fetuses
• Teenage
• Collagen disorders
• Females > 35 years old
• Primigravida
• First subsequent pregnancy with a different father
• Diabetes mellitus of pregnancy
• Chronic hypertension
• Hydatid mole
• Fetal hydrops
• History of renal disease

 DIAGNOSIS

DIFFERENTIAL DIAGNOSIS
• Chronic hypertension
• Pregnancy worsened hypertension
• Pregnancy induced hypertension

LABORATORY
• Proteinuria (> 300 mg/24 hrs or > 1 gram/L)
• Uric acid increased (> 5.5 mg/dL [mild]); (> 9.5 mg/dL [severe])
• Thrombocytopenia
• CrCl < 90 mL/min
• Increased BUN (> 16)
• Increased creatinine (> 1.0)
• Abnormal increased liver function tests
• Increased fibrin degradation products
• Increased PT
• Decreased fibrinogen
• Granular casts in urine
• Red blood cell casts in urine
• Renal tubular cell casts in urine
• White blood cell casts in urine
• Increased urine specific gravity
• Increased T4
• Thrombocytopenia
• Decreased fibrinogen
• Disseminated intravascular coagulation
• Hyperbilirubinemia

Drugs that may alter lab results: N/A

Disorders that may alter lab results: Chronic renal disease

PATHOLOGICAL FINDINGS
• Fibrin deposits in kidneys
• Fibrin deposits in liver with necrosis and periportal hemorrhages
• Placental vascular abnormalities

SPECIAL TESTS N/A

IMAGING N/A

DIAGNOSTIC PROCEDURES 24 hour urine for protein

 TREATMENT

APPROPRIATE HEALTH CARE
• Outpatient care if mild
• Inpatient care if deterioration
• Delivery of fetus as soon as possible if severe
• Admit to hospital if blood pressure > 160/110, proteinuria > 5 gm/24 hr, oliguria, cerebral or visual disturbances (scotoma, blurred vision), severe headache, altered consciousness, pulmonary edema, thrombocytopenia, impaired liver function tests, epigastric pain

GENERAL MEASURES
• If outpatient, keep a daily weight record; use a home test to check for proteinuria
• If outpatient, twice a week blood pressure tests

ACTIVITY
• Bedrest on left side
• Ambulatory only to void

DIET
• Salt restriction is NOT good because the patient is in an intravascular contracted state
• Protein 80-100 gm/day

PATIENT EDUCATION Avoid excessive weight gain during pregnancy (> 25-30 lbs)

MEDICATIONS

DRUG(S) OF CHOICE For seizure prophylaxis - magnesium sulfate (MgSO4) loading dose 4 grams IV in 200 mL normal saline over 20-30 min. Maintenance dose - 1-2 grams/hr IV
Contraindications: Refer to manufacturer's profile of each drug
Precautions:
• Therapeutic magnesium levels are 4-7 mEq/L
• Toxicity (flushing, sweating, hyporeflexia, flaccid paralysis, CNS depression, oliguria, decreased cardiac function)
• Spinal/epidural anesthesia contraindicated
• Continue 24 hour postpartum
• Toxicity therapy with 10% calcium gluconate, 1 gram over 2-3 minutes plus oxygen
• Give oxytocin (Pitocin) postpartum to prevent bleeding (60 u/L at 50 cc/hr)
• Keep urine flow > 25 cc/hr
• Recheck reflexes often. They may be hypoactive, but should be present.
Significant possible interactions: Refer to manufacturer's profile of each drug

ALTERNATIVE DRUGS

Hypertension:
◊ Hydralazine (Apresoline) 5-10 mg IV q 20-30 minutes, or
◊ Diazoxide 30 mg minidose if refractory to hydralazine
◊ Avoid nitroprusside (decreased uterine blood flow plus possible lethal fetal cyanide levels)
Seizures:
◊ MgSO4 - not as effective for treatment of seizures as it is for prophylaxis
◊ Diazepam (Valium) 10 mg IV followed by 10 mg IM q 4 hrs if MgSO4 unavailable or ineffective

FOLLOWUP

PATIENT MONITORING
• Keep urine output > 25 cc/hr
• Continue MgSO4 for 24 hrs postpartum
• Give oxytocin (Pitocin) postpartum to prevent bleeding (60 u/L at 50 cc/hr)

PREVENTION/AVOIDANCE
• Weight control
• Recent data indicates that low dose ASA may sometimes prevent preeclampsia

POSSIBLE COMPLICATIONS
• Eclampsia (seizures)
• Hypertensive crisis
• Acute pyelonephritis
• Acute fatty liver
• Acute pulmonary edema

EXPECTED COURSE AND PROGNOSIS
• Prevention of seizures
• Delivery of viable fetus

MISCELLANEOUS

ASSOCIATED CONDITIONS Abruptio placenta

AGE-RELATED FACTORS
Pediatric: Increased incidence in teenagers
Geriatric: N/A
Others: Older pregnant females (> 35 years old) have increased incidence

PREGNANCY N/A

SYNONYMS
• Pregnancy-induced hypertension
• Toxemia of pregnancy

ICD-9-CM 624.4

SEE ALSO Eclampsia

OTHER NOTES N/A

ABBREVIATIONS MgSO4: magnesium sulfate

REFERENCES
• Family Practice Recertification (Jan 1988)
• Family Practice Recertification (Nov 1989)
• Cunningham, F.G., MacDonald, P.C.and Gant, N.F. (eds.): Williams Obstetrics. 18th Ed. Norwalk CT, Appleton and Lange, 1989

Author S. Abercrombie, M.D.

Premature labor

BASICS

DESCRIPTION Labor occurring prior to the completion of 36 weeks' gestation
Genetics: N/A
Incidence/Prevalence in USA: 8-12% of all births in the USA
Predominant age: Childbearing
Predominant sex: Female only

SIGNS AND SYMPTOMS
• Regular uterine contractions, with or without pain, continuing for 1 hour
• Dull, low backache, pressure, or pain
• Intermittent lower abdominal or thigh pain
• Intestinal cramping, with or without diarrhea or indigestion
• Change in vaginal discharge
• Palpable contractions on examination
• Dilatation of the cervix greater than 1 cm
• Effacement of the cervix more than 50%
• Signs of ruptured membranes (pH paper turns blue; fern positive)

CAUSES
• Infections (pyelonephritis)
• Subclinical chorioamnionitis (chlamydia or gonorrhea)
• Uterine abnormalities (incompetent cervix, leiomyomata; septa, diethylstilbestrol DES exposure)
• Over-distention (by multiple gestation or hydramnios)
• Premature rupture of membranes
• Unknown

RISK FACTORS
• Prior preterm delivery
• Multiple gestation
• Three or more first-trimester abortions
• Previous second-trimester abortion
• Cervical incompetence
• Abdominal surgery during pregnancy
• Uterine or cervical anomalies
• Placenta previa
• Premature placental separation (trauma or drug abuse - especially cocaine)
• Fetal abnormalities
• Hydramnios
• Serious maternal infection
• Second-trimester bleeding
• Prepregnancy weight less than 45 kg (100 lbs)
• Single parent
• No prenatal care

DIAGNOSIS

DIFFERENTIAL DIAGNOSIS
Dehydration, urinary tract infections, round ligament pain, viral gastroenteritis, lumbosacral muscular back pain, chlamydia vaginal infection, gonorrheal vaginal infection, yeast vaginitis, Braxton-Hicks contractions

LABORATORY
• Urinalysis and urine culture for evaluation of urinary tract infection
• Group B strep, gonorrhea, and chlamydial cultures for causes of chorioamnionitis
• Consider urine specific gravity and serum creatinine and BUN for dehydration
Drugs that may alter lab results: N/A
Disorders that may alter lab results: N/A

PATHOLOGICAL FINDINGS N/A

SPECIAL TESTS Consider amniocentesis
if 28-34 weeks' gestation for evaluation of lecithin/sphingomyelin (L/S) ratio and desaturated phosphatidylcholine (DSPC). If L/S ratio is greater than 2:1, and DSPC greater than 1000, hyaline membrane disease is unlikely.

IMAGING Consider uterine ultrasound to
quantitate gestational age, estimated fetal weight, multiple gestations, amount of amniotic fluid, and fetal growth

DIAGNOSTIC PROCEDURES
• Uterine monitoring for at least two hours
• Speculum vaginal examination for signs of infection and cultures
• pH and fern testing for ruptured membranes
• Digital cervical examination for effacement and dilatation

TREATMENT

APPROPRIATE HEALTH CARE
Outpatient or inpatient depending on circumstances

GENERAL MEASURES
• Treat underlying risk factors with appropriate measures (antibiotics for infections, hydration for dehydration)
• If delivery is inevitable, but not immediate, consider transport to a tertiary care center or hospital equipped with a neonatal intensive care unit
• If mother is at 27-34 weeks' gestation, consider administering glucocorticoids to reduce incidence of neonatal respiratory distress
• No sexual intercourse

ACTIVITY
• Bedrest. Discontinue work or other physical activities.
• Hospitalization may be necessary if on intravenous tocolysis or if bedrest is impossible at home

DIET Liquids only, if delivery becomes imminent

PATIENT EDUCATION Call any time for
contractions lasting over an hour, low back pain, change in vaginal discharge, "menstrual cramping", or intestinal cramping

MEDICATIONS

DRUG(S) OF CHOICE
• Hydrate with 500 mL D5NS for first half hour
<u>For tocolysis, protocols include:</u>
◊ Terbutaline 0.25-0.50 mg subcutaneously every 3 hours until contractions cease, or pulse is greater than 140. Change to oral terbutaline 2.5-5.0 mg every 3-6 hours if contractions have ceased.
◊ Ritodrine 150 mg per 500 mL of D5NS. Start at 100 micrograms/min, increase by 50 micrograms/min every 10 minutes. Stop for significant side effects or successful tocolysis. Decrease dose by 50 micrograms/min each hour to a minimum of 100 micrograms/min as long as tocolysis remains successful. Switch to po after 12-24 hours. Oral dose is 10 mg q 2 hours for the first 24 hours, then 10-20 mg q 4-6 hours. Total daily dose is 120 mg.
◊ Magnesium sulfate solution of 40 g per 1000 mL of D5NS. Bolus 4 g over 20 min, then begin infusion at 2 g/h, increasing by 0.5 g/h every 15-30 minutes; check serum magnesium levels (therapeutic is 6-8 mg/dL). Stop for significant side effects or when tocolysis occurs. Decrease dose by 0.5 g/h each hour to a minimum of 2 g/h and then switch to oral therapy after 12 hours.
<u>Glucocorticoids to reduce incidence of neonatal respiratory distress, protocols include:</u>
◊ Betamethasone 12 mg IM twice 24 hours apart
or
◊ Dexamethasone 5 mg IM bid x 4 doses
or
◊ Hydrocortisone 500 mg IM every 6 hours x 4 doses
◊ Doses are repeated every 7-10 days as long as preterm delivery is likely
Contraindications:
• Severe preeclampsia, hemorrhage, chorioamnionitis, advanced labor, intrauterine growth retardation, or fetal heart decelerations
• Relative contraindications to terbutaline or ritodrine include maternal cardiac rhythm disturbance or poorly controlled diabetes or thyrotoxicosis
• Relative contraindications to magnesium sulfate are myasthenia gravis, hypocalcemia, or renal failure
Precautions: Palpitations, nausea, intractable vomiting, pulse greater than 140
Significant possible interactions: Pulmonary edema from rehydration fluids and tocolytic agents

ALTERNATIVE DRUGS N/A

FOLLOWUP

PATIENT MONITORING
• Weekly office visits and cervical checks for those at high risk for preterm labor
• Ambulatory external tocodynamometry has not yet been proven efficacious for prevention of preterm labor

PREVENTION/AVOIDANCE
• Patient education
• Consider cerclage placement before 20 weeks, gestation for those at high risk because of an incompetent cervix

POSSIBLE COMPLICATIONS Labor resistant to tocolysis

EXPECTED COURSE AND PROGNOSIS If membranes are ruptured, delivery generally occurs within 3-7 days. If membranes are intact, treat until 37 weeks, gestational age.

MISCELLANEOUS

ASSOCIATED CONDITIONS See Risk factors

AGE-RELATED FACTORS N/A
Pediatric: N/A
Geriatric: N/A
Others: N/A

PREGNANCY By definition, a problem of pregnancy

SYNONYMS Preterm labor

ICD-9-CM N/A

SEE ALSO N/A

OTHER NOTES N/A

ABBREVIATIONS N/A

REFERENCES
• ACOG Technical Bulletin, No. 133, October 1989
• Hueston, W.J.: Prevention and treatment of preterm labor. In Am Fam Phys. 1989;40(5):139-146

Author C. Heath, M. D.

Premenstrual syndrome (PMS)

BASICS

DESCRIPTION Premenstrual syndrome is a constellation of symptoms that occurs prior to menstruation and is severe enough to interfere significantly with the patient's life
System(s) affected: Endocrine/Metabolic, Reproductive, Nervous
Genetics: Unknown, probably familial incidence
Incidence/Prevalence in USA: Almost all women have some symptoms prior to menses (this is not PMS). A low percentage have actual PMS.
Predominant age: Childbearing years
Predominant sex: Females only

SIGNS AND SYMPTOMS
Symptoms can involve any organ system but the following are more common:
- Depressed mood
- Mood Swings
- Irritability
- Difficulty concentrating
- Fatigue
- Edema
- Breast tenderness
- Headaches
- Sleep disturbances

CAUSES Unknown, presumed hormonal; perhaps interacting with neurotransmitters

RISK FACTORS
- Premenstrual exacerbations can occur with other diseases (i.e., depression)
- Caffeine and high fluid intake exacerbate PMS symptoms
- Stress may precipitate
- PMS increases with age

DIAGNOSIS

DIFFERENTIAL DIAGNOSIS The major differential are psychiatric syndromes, particularly depressive disorders and/or dysthymia. Other entities may be suggested by history or physical.

LABORATORY There are no laboratory tests which confirm or refute PMS. History and physical may disclose a need for specific laboratory tests.
Drugs that may alter lab results: N/A
Disorders that may alter lab results: N/A

PATHOLOGICAL FINDINGS N/A

SPECIAL TESTS N/A

IMAGING N/A

DIAGNOSTIC PROCEDURES Patients complete questionnaires over a minimum of two months to confirm premenstrual exacerbation of symptoms and lack of substantial symptoms in the follicular phase

TREATMENT

APPROPRIATE HEALTH CARE
Outpatient

GENERAL MEASURES
- Increase daily exercise
- Eat regular, balanced meals
- Stop smoking
- Get regular sleep
- Stress reduction techniques
- Individual or couples counseling
- Support groups

ACTIVITY
- No restrictions
- Exercise is recommended

DIET Low-salt; low-caffeine; low-fat; frequent, small meals; high complex carbohydrates

PATIENT EDUCATION Explain PMS and treatment

MEDICATIONS

DRUG(S) OF CHOICE
• No drugs are clearly indicated for PMS. Drugs that are used with varying degrees of success are listed
• Diuretics (usually spironolactone) at time of symptoms
• Symptomatic treatment of pain (ibuprofen or acetaminophen)
• Anti-depressants (fluoxetine, clomipramine or nortriptylene), particularly for patients with depressive symptoms
• Alprazolam 0.25 mg tid during symptoms
• Buspirone 5 -10 mg tid during luteal phase
• Magnesium 300-500 mg/day
• Elemental calcium 1000 mg/day
• Vitamin B-6 in modest doses (50 mg bid, may be toxic in higher doses)
• Vitamin E - up to 600 I.U./day
• Evening primrose oil (high content of fatty acids) 500 mg qd to 1000 mg tid for breast tenderness
• Bromocriptine 2.5 mg tid at time of symptoms and danazol 100 mg bid may also work for breast tenderness, but have more side effects
• Danazol for the total PMS symptom complex
• Oral contraceptives may help
• While progesterone (during luteal phase) has been used, recent research does not support much relief of symptoms
• In the future, a gonadotropin-releasing hormone agonist with or without concurrent estrogens/progestins may be used with more frequency
Contraindications: Refer to manufacturer's profile of each drug
Precautions: Refer to manufacturer's profile of each drug
Significant possible interactions: Refer to manufacturer's profile of each drug

ALTERNATIVE DRUGS   N/A

FOLLOWUP

PATIENT MONITORING   See patient to provide general support and further patient education

PREVENTION/AVOIDANCE   N/A

POSSIBLE COMPLICATIONS   N/A

EXPECTED COURSE AND PROGNOSIS   Many patients can have their symptoms adequately controlled

MISCELLANEOUS

ASSOCIATED CONDITIONS   N/A

AGE-RELATED FACTORS
Pediatric: N/A
Geriatric: N/A
Others: N/A

PREGNANCY   N/A

SYNONYMS   N/A

ICD-9-CM   625.4 premenstrual tension syndromes

SEE ALSO   N/A

OTHER NOTES   Treatment may need to be continued for a long time. PMS sometimes continues after hysterectomy. Effects of long-term hormonal treatment unknown.

ABBREVIATIONS   N/A

REFERENCES
• Johnson, S.R.: Clinician's Approach to Diagnosis and Management of Premenstrual Syndrome. Cl. Obst & Gyn. 35:637-657, 1992
• Chihal, H.J.: Premenstrual Syndrome: An Update for the clinician. Ob & Gyn Clinics of North America. 17:457-478,1990
• Severino, S.K., Moline, M.L.: Premenstrual syndrome. Ob & Gyn Clinics of North America.17:889-903,1990

Author   M. Bowman, M.D.

Pressure ulcer

BASICS

DESCRIPTION Skin breakdown is a common and serious complication affecting usually immobile elderly patients, especially within long-term care settings. Most common sites include elbows, hips, heels, outer ankles, and base of spine. Over 95% of sores develop on lower part of body. Median length of hospital stay to treat pressure sore is 46 days, with median cost $27,000. Risk of death in elderly patient increases fourfold when sores heal and sixfold when sores do not heal.

System(s) affected: Skin/Exocrine

Genetics: N/A

Incidence/Prevalence in USA:
• 3-30% of acute hospital and nursing home patients
• 2 million patients develop these pressure sores each year
• Incidence is 43/100,000 population every year
• Estimated prevalence in nursing home residents ranges from 2.6%-24%

Predominant age: 60-70% are elderly patients

Predominant sex: Female > Male (due to survival differential)

SIGNS AND SYMPTOMS
• Stage I - non-blanching erythema, warmth, tenderness
• Stage II - skin breakdown limited to dermis, excoriation, blistering, drainage, more sharply defined erythema, variable skin temperature, local swelling or edema
• Stage III - ulcer formation into subcutaneous tissues, crater formation, slough, eschar, and/or drainage
• Stage IV - ulcers extend beyond deep fascia into muscle or bone, decayed area may be larger than visibly apparent wound, osteomyelitis or sepsis may be present, granulation tissue and epithelialization may be present at wound margins

CAUSES
• Uneven application of pressure over a bony hard site; high pressure applied for two hours produces irreversible tissue ischemia and necrosis
• Shearing forces which develop when a seated person slides toward floor or toward foot of bed if supine
• Frictional forces which develop when pulling a patient across a bed sheet
• Moisture from incontinence or perspiration can increase the friction between two surfaces

RISK FACTORS
• Immobility (e.g., quadriplegia)
• Malnutrition and low body weight
• Hypoalbuminemia
• Fecal incontinence
• Urinary incontinence
• Bone fracture (especially femoral)
• Vitamin C deficiency

• Age-related skin changes, such as diminished pain perception, altered barrier properties, reduced immunity, and slowed wound healing
• Anemia
• Infections
• Peripheral vascular disease
• Dementia
• Malignancies
• Diabetes mellitus
• Cerebral vascular accidents
• Dry skin (low humidity, <40%, and cold)

DIAGNOSIS

DIFFERENTIAL DIAGNOSIS
• Stasis or ischemia ulcers
• Vasculitides
• Cancers
• Radiation injury
• Pyoderma gangrenosum and other dermatologic conditions

LABORATORY
• Culture of wound if there is evidence of infection (surrounding erythema, purulent drainage, foul odor)
• White blood cell count and differential if fever is present (greater than 37°)
• If leucocytosis present, urinalysis to identify causative agents
• If above tests positive, blood and urine cultures

Drugs that may alter lab results: N/A

Disorders that may alter lab results: N/A

PATHOLOGICAL FINDINGS Extensive necrosis of affected part

SPECIAL TESTS N/A

IMAGING If leukocytosis present, chest film to identify causative agents

DIAGNOSTIC PROCEDURES N/A

TREATMENT

APPROPRIATE HEALTH CARE
• An interdisciplinary approach usually indicated in nursing home, inpatient or home care settings if trained supervision available
• Complications will require inpatient setting to treat systemic infection, extensive debridement or skin grafting

GENERAL MEASURES
• Improve overall nutritional status (adequate protein intake)
• Débridement of necrotic pressure ulcers using occlusive dressings, hydrotherapy, proteolytic enzymes, and surgical or laser débridement

• Specialized beds and repositioning every two hours to relieve pressure at site of ulceration (air-fluidized or low-air-loss beds); static-pressure and foam mattresses are less expensive. Water mattresses, sheepskins, and egg-crate mattresses are other less expensive devices.
• Control of fecal and/or urine incontinence
• Specific measures by stage as follows:
Stage I
◊ Relieve pressure (flotation or airflow mattress/bed)
◊ Use skin cream or Granulex Spray on reddened areas
◊ Keep all skin areas clean and dry
◊ Assess skin every 8-12 hours
Stage II
◊ Use saline/peroxide soaked 4 x 4's to cleanse pressure sore
◊ Rinse with saline soaked 4 x 4's
◊ Pat dry with 4 x 4's
◊ Apply protective barrier film to unbroken skin surrounding pressure sore
◊ Apply occlusive hydrocolloid dressing
◊ Repeat every three days
Stage III
◊ Irrigate wound with peroxide/saline solution
◊ Scrub and debride with dry gauze
◊ Re-rinse wound
◊ Blot excess moisture with dry 4 x 4 gauze
◊ Apply protective barrier film
◊ Apply skin care product (occlusive hydrocolloid dressing, granules, or paste)
◊ If wound highly exudating, use absorption dressing and change daily
Stage IV
◊ Irrigate wound with peroxide/saline solution x 2
◊ Blot excess moisture with 4 x 4 dry gauze
◊ Apply protective barrier film to unbroken skin surrounding sore
◊ Moisten packing gauze (Kerlix) in saline and pack wound
◊ Apply outer dressing
◊ Surgical intervention for definitive treatment of deep and complicated pressure ulcers, such as myocutaneous flaps, split-thickness skin grafts and primary closure

ACTIVITY
• Any activity consistent with patient's ambulatory status and relief of pressure on wound
• Perform passive range-of-motion exercises for patient or encourage patient to do active exercises if possible

DIET
• Oral high-calorie and high-protein supplements
• Oral zinc sulfate, vitamin A and C, and iron

PATIENT EDUCATION
• Patient Care 1993; 27(7):65-66
• National Action Group for the Prevention and Treatment of Decubitus Ulcers, P.O. Box 1098, Union City, CT 06770
• ANCPR publication No. 92-0048, Preventing Pressure Ulcers: A Patient's Guide, May 1992.

MEDICATIONS

DRUG(S) OF CHOICE
• Clindamycin or gentamicin for complications such as cellulitis, osteomyelitis, or sepsis
• Supplements - vitamin C 500 mg twice a day, zinc sulfate
• Antibiotic prophylaxis for bacterial endocarditis if valvular lesions present
• Topical antimicrobials should be used only for superficial infections; cultures are necessary to determine whether antifungal (miconazole, clotrimazole, or haloprogin) or specific antibacterial agents (silver sulfadiazine, polymyxin B, neomycin, gentamicin, mupirocin 2%) are indicated
• Enzymatic debriding agents such as collagenase (Santyl), trypsin (Granulex), fibrinolysin and deoxyribonuclease (Elase), papain (Panafil) or sutilains (Travase) used with a moisture barrier to protect surrounding normal tissue
• Recommended dressings include polyurethane films (Op-site, Tegaderm), absorbent hydrocolloid dressings (Duoderm, Comfeel Ulcus)
Contraindications: Refer to manufacturer's literature
Precautions: Refer to manufacturer's literature
Significant possible interactions: Refer to manufacturer's literature

ALTERNATIVE DRUGS N/A

 FOLLOWUP

PATIENT MONITORING
• Frequent evaluation of all patients with history of pressure sores, especially if limited mobility. Include nutritional status and dietary intervention.
• Early identification of areas of skin redness to prevent subsequent breakdown
• Skin cleansing as soon as soiled and at routine intervals

PREVENTION/AVOIDANCE
• Early identification of at risk individuals and elimination of risk factors (risk asessment tools: Brader Scale for Predicting Pressure Sore Risk and The Norton Scale)
• Underpads (non-cloth) to absorb moisture
• Quality nursing care
• Early interdisciplinary supportive care - include staff, patient, family/caregiver
• Nutritional assessment of patient
• Frequent patient repositioning if immobile
• Functional assessment of patient and treatment of incontinence
• Frequent physical examination of skin areas affected by pressure, moisture, shearing or friction sources

POSSIBLE COMPLICATIONS
• Growth of resistant organisms if antibiotics used for local or systemic infection
• Gangrene

EXPECTED COURSE AND PROGNOSIS
• Though pressure ulcers are associated with an increased rate of mortality, with good medical care, most can be expected to heal
• In a recent study among long-term care hospital patients, 79% of pressure sores improved and 40% completely healed during a six-week followup period using ordinary therapies

 MISCELLANEOUS

ASSOCIATED CONDITIONS
• Malnutrition
• Fecal and/or urinary incontinence
• Immobility
• Impaired mental status
• Skin atrophy
• Low body weight

AGE-RELATED FACTORS
Pediatric: N/A
Geriatric: Over 60% occur in elderly
Others: N/A

PREGNANCY N/A

SYNONYMS
• Decubitus ulcer
• Bedsore
• Trophic ulcer
• Pressure sore

ICD-9-CM 707.0 decubitus ulcer

SEE ALSO N/A

OTHER NOTES N/A

ABBREVIATIONS N/A

REFERENCES
• Allman, R.M.: Pressure ulcers among the elderly. New Engl J Med. 1989; 320:850-853
• The Medical Letter. Treatment of Pressure Ulcers. Vol. 31 (Issue 812), Feb. 23, 1990
• Alvarez, O.M., Massac, E., Brown, B. & Grauer, K.: Management issues in the critical care of pressure ulcers. Family Practice Recertification 1990; 12(9):78-104
• Panel for the Prediction and Prevention of Pressure Ulcers in Adults. Pressure Ulcers in Adults: Predictin and Prevention. Clinical Practice Guidelines, No. 3. ANCPR Publication No. 92-0047, May, 1992.

Author E. Kligman, M.D.

Priapism

BASICS

DESCRIPTION Painful, abnormal penile erection not accompanied by sexual excitement or desire
System(s) affected: Reproductive
Genetics: N/A
Incidence/Prevalence in USA: Unknown
Predominant age: Young adult
Predominant sex: Male only

SIGNS AND SYMPTOMS
• Penile erection that is persistent, prolonged, painful, and tender
• Urination difficult during erection
• Loss of sexual function if treatment is not prompt and effective

CAUSES
• Pelvic vascular thrombosis
• Prolonged sexual activity
• Sickle cell anemia
• Leukemia
• Other blood dyscrasias
• Pelvic hematoma or neoplasia
• Cerebrospinal tumors
• Tertiary syphilis
• Bladder calculus
• Injury to penis
• Urinary tract infections, especially prostatitis, urethritis, cystitis
• Several drugs suspected as causing priapism, such as chlorpromazine, prazosin, trazodone, and certain corticosteroids, anticoagulants, antihypertensives

RISK FACTORS Listed with Causes

DIAGNOSIS

DIFFERENTIAL DIAGNOSIS N/A

LABORATORY Not helpful in diagnosis
Drugs that may alter lab results: N/A
Disorders that may alter lab results: N/A

PATHOLOGICAL FINDINGS
• Pelvic vascular thrombosis
• Partial thrombosis of corpora cavernosa
• Corpus spongiosum, glans penis: No involvement

SPECIAL TESTS N/A

IMAGING N/A

DIAGNOSTIC PROCEDURES Physical examination

TREATMENT

APPROPRIATE HEALTH CARE
Inpatient

GENERAL MEASURES
• Reassurance about outcome if warranted
• Continuous caudal or spinal anesthesia if etiology is neurogenic
• Introduction of 12 or 16 gauge needles into corpora cavernosa (best done by urologist if available)
• Create fistula between glans and corpus cavernosum (with biopsy needle by urologist)
• Semipermanent diversion by saphenous shunt from one or both corpora
• Cavernoso-spongiosum shunt to permit reestablishment of pelvic circulation
• Treat any underlying cause
• In sickle cell anemia: Intravenous hydration; partial exchange or repeated transfusions to reduce percent of sickle cells below 50%

ACTIVITY Bedrest until relieved

DIET N/A

PATIENT EDUCATION Information about long-term outlook, referral for counseling

MEDICATIONS

DRUG(S) OF CHOICE Narcotics for pain if needed
Contraindications: Refer to manufacturer's literature
Precautions: Refer to manufacturer's literature
Significant possible interactions: Refer to manufacturer's literature

ALTERNATIVE DRUGS N/A

FOLLOWUP

PATIENT MONITORING Close followup after surgery

PREVENTION/AVOIDANCE
- Avoid dehydration
- Avoid excessive sexual stimulation
- Avoid causative drugs (see Causes) when possible

POSSIBLE COMPLICATIONS Impotence

EXPECTED COURSE AND PROGNOSIS
- Even with excellent treatment, detumescence may require several weeks
- Impotence is likely

MISCELLANEOUS

ASSOCIATED CONDITIONS Sickle cell anemia

AGE-RELATED FACTORS
Pediatric: N/A
Geriatric: Treatment more difficult and less likely successful
Others: N/A

PREGNANCY N/A

SYNONYMS N/A

ICD-9-CM 607.3

SEE ALSO Sickle cell anemia

OTHER NOTES N/A

ABBREVIATIONS N/A

REFERENCES
- Smith, D.R.: General Urology. 12th Ed. Los Altos, CA, Lange Medical Publications, 1988
- Tanagho, E.A. & McAninch, J.W. (eds.): Smith's General Urology. 12th Ed. Norwalk, CT, Appleton & Lange, 1988

Author H. Griffith, M.D. & M. Dambro, M.D.

Primary pulmonary hypertension

 BASICS

DESCRIPTION Pulmonary arterial hypertension of unknown cause, where secondary causes have been ruled out. Three pathologic subtypes have been identified: (1) thrombotic, (2) plexogenic, (3) veno-occlusive.
System(s) affected: Pulmonary, Cardiovascular
Genetics: 7% familial; autosomal dominant with variable expression
Incidence/Prevalence in USA: Unknown
Predominant age: Mean age 34-36 years; second incidence peak in males 50-59 years
Predominant sex: Female > Male (3:1)

SIGNS AND SYMPTOMS
• Loud P2 (> 80%)
• Right ventricular lift (> 80%)
• Dyspnea (> 75%)
• Murmur of tricuspid insufficiency (50-80%)
• Increased jugular venous pressure (50-80%)
• Right ventricular S4 (50-80%)
• Chest pain (> 50%)
• Fatigue (> 50%)
• Palpitations (< 50%)
• Syncope (< 50%)
• Cough (< 50%)
• Raynaud's phenomenon (< 50%)
• Hepatomegaly (< 50%)
• Pulmonic ejection click (< 50%)
• Right ventricular S3 (< 50%)
• Murmur of pulmonic insufficiency (< 50%)
• Lower extremity edema (< 50%)

CAUSES
• Unknown; possible pulmonary arteriolar hyperactivity and vasoconstriction; occult thromboembolism; possible autoimmune (high frequency antinuclear antibodies)
• In Europe, reports of PPH associated with anorectic agent aminorex fumarate in late 1960's; tainted rapeseed oil

RISK FACTORS   Female sex

 DIAGNOSIS

DIFFERENTIAL DIAGNOSIS
◊ Pulmonary parenchymal disease (COPD, asthma, pulmonary fibrosis, granulomatous disease, malignancy)
◊ Pulmonary vascular disease (pulmonary thromboembolism, collagen vascular disease, pulmonary arteritis, schistosomiasis, sickle cell disease)
◊ Cardiac disease (cardiomyopathy, valvular heart disease, congenital heart disease)
◊ Other disorders of respiratory function (sleep apnea syndromes, neuromuscular diseases, pleural diseases, thoracic cage abnormalities)

LABORATORY
• ANA positive (1/3 of patients)
Drugs that may alter lab results:
Hydralazine, procainamide, isoniazid, etc.
Disorders that may alter lab results:
Many other diseases, e.g., lupus, scleroderma

PATHOLOGICAL FINDINGS
• Medial hypertrophy and arterial thrombosis are common in all subtypes
• Plexogenic pulmonary arteriopathy (30-70%): laminar "onion skin" intimal proliferation, focal medial disruption, aneurysmal dilatation
• Microthromboemboli (20-50%)
• Veno-occlusive disease (10-15%)

SPECIAL TESTS
• ECG - right ventricular hypertrophy and right axis deviation
• Pulmonary function testing - arterial hypoxemia, reduced diffusion capacity, hypocapnea
• VQ scan - must rule out proximal pulmonary artery emboli

IMAGING
• Chest x-ray - enlarged central pulmonary arteries. If interstitial markings, consider lung parenchymal disease or veno-occlusive disease.
• Echo-Doppler - right ventricular enlargement and overload; important to rule out underlying cardiac disease such as shunt or mitral stenosis

DIAGNOSTIC PROCEDURES
• Chest x-ray, pulmonary function tests, arterial blood gases, and VQ scan should be done
• Cardiac catheterization - right heart catheterization is necessary to measure pulmonary artery pressures and hemodynamics; rule out underlying cardiac disease
• Pulmonary angiography - should be done if segmental or larger defect on VQ scan. Caution in pulmonary hypertension; use low osmolar agents, subselective angiograms.
• Lung biopsy not recommended

 TREATMENT

APPROPRIATE HEALTH CARE
• Medical therapy is first line and primarily palliative; health care is guided by clinical status
• Hospitalization with invasive monitoring is needed to screen vasodilator responsiveness and initiate vasodilator therapy

GENERAL MEASURES
• Primary modalities are oxygen supplementation, vasodilators, anticoagulants, and treatment of heart failure
• Oxygen supplementation is indicated for rest, exercise, or nocturnal hypoxemia
• Surgical procedures - patients with documented large vessel thromboembolic disease should be considered for pulmonary thrombectomy
• Heart-lung or lung transplantation is an option for appropriate patients when medical therapy has failed

ACTIVITY   Restricted; Exercise worsens pulmonary vascular resistance

DIET   Low salt with heart failure

PATIENT EDUCATION   Need to discuss prognosis; options such as transplantation

MEDICATIONS

DRUG(S) OF CHOICE
Medical therapy may be guided by suspected subtype:
◊ Plexogenic (clear lung fields, normal perfusion scan) - vasodilators potentially useful. Vasodilators - calcium channel blockers, first line, may be more effective in high doses. Other agents: ACE-inhibitors, alpha-antagonists, hydralazine - none shown to improve survival.
◊ Thrombotic (clear lung fields, patchy perfusion scan) - anticoagulants potentially useful. Anticoagulants - warfarin, heparin, antiplatelet agents.
◊ Veno-occlusive (pulmonary venous congestion, patchy perfusion scan) - vasodilators probably useless
All types: Heart failure may be treated with diuretics. Dioxin use controversial - not shown to be beneficial or detrimental. Digoxin may adversely affect exercise capacity due to increase in pulmonary vascular resistance.
Contraindications: Avoid warfarin in patients with syncope or hemoptysis
Precautions: Vasodilator therapy and response should be evaluated with invasive monitoring. Short acting agents such as prostacyclin, adenosine, or acetylcholine are useful for screening.
Significant possible interactions: Refer to manufacturer's literature

ALTERNATIVE DRUGS
Continuous IV infusion of prostacyclin or its analogues (iloprost)

FOLLOWUP

PATIENT MONITORING
Frequent

PREVENTION/AVOIDANCE
None

POSSIBLE COMPLICATIONS
Thromboembolism, heart failure, sudden death

EXPECTED COURSE AND PROGNOSIS
Mean survival 2-3 years from time of diagnosis, 75% mortality at 5 years

MISCELLANEOUS

ASSOCIATED CONDITIONS
• Portal hypertension
• Systemic lupus erythematosus

AGE-RELATED FACTORS
Pediatric: N/A
Geriatric: N/A
Others: N/A

PREGNANCY
Must be avoided; high mother and fetal wastage

SYNONYMS
Primary pulmonary vascular disease

ICD-9-CM
416.0

SEE ALSO
• Cor pulmonale
• Pulmonary thromboembolism

OTHER NOTES
N/A

ABBREVIATIONS
VQ = ventilation/perfusion

REFERENCES
• Palevsky, H.E. & Fishman, A.P.: The Management of Primary Pulmonary Hypertension. JAMA 1991; 265:1014-1020
• Hawkins, J.W. & Dunn, M.I.: Primary Pulmonary Hypertension in Adults. Clinical Cardiology. 1990; 13:382-387
• Rich, S.: Primary Pulmonary Hypertension. In Harrison's Principles of Internal Medicine. 12th Ed. Edited by E. Braunwald, et al. McGraw-Hill, New York, 1991

Author A. Warner, M.D.

Proctitis

 BASICS

DESCRIPTION An acute or chronic inflammation of the rectal mucosa
System(s) affected: Gastrointestinal
Genetics: Higher incidence in Jews
Incidence in USA: 0.5-3/100,000 (ulcerative proctitis)
Prevalence in USA: 10-30/100,000 (ulcerative proctitis)
Predominant age: Adult
Predominant sex: Male > Female

SIGNS AND SYMPTOMS
• Rectal and/or perianal discomfort
• Rectal bleeding and/or mucus discharge
• Tenesmus
• Urgency
• Constipation
• Fever
• Weight loss

CAUSES
• Idiopathic
• Rectal gonorrhea
• Crohn's disease
• Syphilis (usually secondary)
• Nonspecific sexually transmitted infection
• Herpes simplex
• Chlamydia
• Papilloma virus
• Amebiasis
• Lymphogranuloma venereum
• Ischemia
• Radiation therapy
• Toxins (e.g., hydrogen peroxide enemas)
• Vasculitis

RISK FACTORS
• Rectal intercourse
• Radiation
• Rectal injury
• Rectal medications
• Jewish heritage

 DIAGNOSIS

DIFFERENTIAL DIAGNOSIS
• Traumatic proctitis
• Radiation proctitis
• Ulcerative colitis
• Crohn's disease
• Infections such as shigellosis or amebiasis

LABORATORY
• Serological tests for syphilis, ameba
• Smear, culture from rectal wall - many neutrophils
• Stool cultures
Drugs that may alter lab results: N/A
Disorders that may alter lab results: N/A

PATHOLOGICAL FINDINGS
• Inflammation of rectal mucosa
• Ulceration
• Disruption of crypts

SPECIAL TESTS N/A

IMAGING N/A

DIAGNOSTIC PROCEDURES
• Flexible sigmoidoscopy
• Biopsy for histology, culture, viral studies, chlamydia

 TREATMENT

APPROPRIATE HEALTH CARE
Outpatient, unless severe and refractory to usual measures

GENERAL MEASURES
• Treatment depends upon the cause
• Rectal gram stains have significant false-negative rate and if clinician has strong suspicion of gonorrheal proctitis, empiric treatment warranted while culture results pending
• Avoidance of causative factors
• Sitz baths may provide some relief

ACTIVITY No restrictions

DIET No special diet

PATIENT EDUCATION Counseling regarding HIV infection risk

MEDICATIONS

DRUG(S) OF CHOICE
• Ulcerative proctitis - topical steroids (enemas or foam), 5-ASA enemas or suppositories (Rowasa), oral 5-ASA (mesalamine, olsalazine [Dipentum], sulfasalazine); systemic steroids when refractory to above drugs
• Gonorrheal - IM ceftriaxone 250 mg in a single dose plus doxycycline 100 mg orally bid for 7 days
• Herpetic - oral acyclovir 200-400 mg 5 times a day for 10 days
• Chlamydial - oral tetracycline 500 mg tid or doxycycline 100 mg bid

Contraindications: Refer to manufacturer's literature
Precautions: Refer to manufacturer's literature
Significant possible interactions: Refer to manufacturer's literature

ALTERNATIVE DRUGS
For gonorrheal - in patients unable to take ceftriaxone - IM spectinomycin 2 g in a single dose or ciprofloxacin 500 mg orally in a single dose. Perform culture 4-7 days after treatment to verify efficacy of treatment.

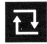
FOLLOWUP

PATIENT MONITORING
Follow until completely healed and monthly thereafter for 6 months

PREVENTION/AVOIDANCE
Safe sex, if sexually transmitted

POSSIBLE COMPLICATIONS
• Chronic ulcerative colitis
• Fistulae/abscess formation
• Treatment failure (may be as much as 35% in gonorrhea proctitis)
• Perforation

EXPECTED COURSE AND PROGNOSIS
Satisfactory cure or control with appropriate treatment

MISCELLANEOUS

ASSOCIATED CONDITIONS
• Syphilis
• Gonorrhea
• Other sexually transmitted disease
• Prostate cancer (radiation therapy)

AGE-RELATED FACTORS
Pediatric:
• Not common, but if found, is more apt to spread to full-blown disease in more proximal areas of the colon
• Consider sexual abuse, if gonorrheal infection
Geriatric: Slower to heal, consider ischemia
Others: N/A

PREGNANCY N/A

SYNONYMS N/A

ICD-9-CM 569.49

SEE ALSO
• Sexually transmitted diseases
• Ulcerative colitis
• Crohn's disease
• Syphilis
• Gonorrhea,
• Lymphogranuloma venereum
• Herpes simplex

OTHER NOTES N/A

ABBREVIATIONS N/A

REFERENCES
• Wexner, S.D.: Sexually transmitted diseases of the colon, rectum, and anus. The challenge of the nineties. Dis Colon Rectum 1990;33:1048-62
• Kirsner, J.B. & Shorter, G. (eds.): Diseases of the Colon, Rectum and Anal Canal. Baltimore, Williams & Wilkins, 1989

Author P. Jaffe, M.D.

Prostatic cancer

 BASICS

DESCRIPTION The prostate is composed of acinar glands and their ducts arranged in a radial fashion with the stroma containing blood vessels, lymphatics and nerves. 95% of prostate cancers are acinar adenocarcinomas.
<u>Degree of malignancy based on grading various stages:</u>
  ◊ A1A2 and B1B2 - confinement within the capsule
  ◊ C1 - extension beyond the capsule
  ◊ C2 - involving the seminal vesicles
  ◊ D1 - metastatic disease in regional lymph nodes
  ◊ D2 - metastatic disease in bone or other organs
System(s) affected: Reproductive
Genetics: Unknown
Incidence/Prevalence in USA: 69 per 100,000
Predominant Age: Sixth or seventh decade
Predominant sex: Male only

SIGNS AND SYMPTOMS
• May be asymptomatic early or late in the course of disease
• Induration of the prostate on digital rectal exam
• Hard prostate, localized or diffuse
• Bladder outlet symptoms
• Acute urinary retention
• Hematuria (rare)
• Urinary tract infection
• Bone pain
• Weight loss
• Anemia
• Shortness of breath
• Lymphedema
• Neurologic symptoms
• Lymphadenopathy

CAUSES   Unknown

RISK FACTORS
• Genetic predisposition
• Endogenous hormonal influences
• Exposure to chemical carcinogens
• Sexually transmitted diseases
• Male over 60 years of age
• Increased risk with vasectomy has been newly proposed but is unsupported

 DIAGNOSIS

DIFFERENTIAL DIAGNOSIS
• Benign nodule prostate growth
• Prostate stones
• Nodular whorls of adenoma
• Seminal vesicle enlargement

LABORATORY
• Prostate Specific Antigen (PSA), elevated
• Acid phosphatase, elevated with metastasis
• Alkaline phosphatase, elevated with metastasis
• Urine cytology, rarely helpful
Drugs that may alter lab results: None
Disorders that may alter lab results:
• Rectal manipulation will increase PSA
• Prior liver or bone disease

PATHOLOGICAL FINDINGS
• Size and shape of prostatic acini almost always altered
• Small closely packed interposed stroma
• Eosinophilic crystalloids present
• Architecture disrupted
• Cells invade perineural space

SPECIAL TESTS   Prostate Specific Antigen

IMAGING
• Bone scan, positive with metastasis
• Skeletal survey, positive with metastasis
• Lymph node aspiration, positive with metastasis
• Computerized tomography of pelvic lymph nodes, positive with metastasis
• Prostatic ultrasound
• Lymphoscintigraphy
• Magnetic resonance imaging

DIAGNOSTIC PROCEDURES
• Biopsy, fine needle aspiration or core
• Ultrasound
• Bone marrow aspiration
• Bone biopsy
• Lymph node aspiration
• Lymph node biopsy
• Lymphoscopic lymph node dissection

 TREATMENT

APPROPRIATE HEALTH CARE
Inpatient for surgery, outpatient for other treatment

GENERAL MEASURES
• Under age 70, aggressive surgery for cure
• Over 70 conservative or palliative treatment
• Surgical for stages A-B and selected C under 70
• Radiation, external beam or brachytherapy with implants
• Orchiectomy
• Total androgen ablation

ACTIVITY   Full activity

DIET   No special diet

PATIENT EDUCATION   Printed material available from:
• American Cancer Society
• National Kidney & Urologic Diseases Information Clearinghouse, Box NKUDIC, Bethesda, MD 20893, (301)468-6345

MEDICATIONS

DRUG(S) OF CHOICE
• None specific
• For androgen ablation:
  ◊ Flutamide (Eulexin) 250 mg tid
  ◊ Leuprolide (Lupron) 1 mg subcutaneously daily or 7.5 mg IM depot monthly

Contraindications: None

Precautions:
• Flare phenomenon with metastatic disease
• Fluid retention
• Nausea
• Vomiting
• Hot flashes
• Liver enzyme changes

Significant possible interactions: Refer to manufacturer's profile of each drug.

ALTERNATIVE DRUGS   None

FOLLOWUP

PATIENT MONITORING
• Routine clinical examination every 3 months for 1 year
• Routine clinical examination every 6 months for 1 year
• Annual examinations indefinitely
• PSA q 3 months for 1 year, q 6 months 1 year, then yearly
• Chest x-ray, bone scan, q 6 months for 1 year, then yearly

PREVENTION/AVOIDANCE   None

POSSIBLE COMPLICATIONS
• Cardiac failure
• Phlebitis
• Pathologic fracture

EXPECTED COURSE AND PROGNOSIS
• Early diagnosis and treatment of lesions should be curable
• Advanced disease favorable prognosis if endocrine sensitive
• Advanced unresponsive disease progresses in 18 months average

MISCELLANEOUS

ASSOCIATED CONDITIONS   N/A

AGE-RELATED FACTORS
Pediatric: N/A
Geriatric: N/A
Others: N/A

PREGNANCY   N/A

SYNONYMS
Cancer of the prostate

ICD-9-CM
185 Malignant neoplasm of prostate

SEE ALSO   N/A

OTHER NOTES   N/A

ABBREVIATIONS   PSA = Prostate specific antigen

REFERENCES   Walsh, P.C., Gittes, R.F. & Perlmutter, A.D.: Campbell's Urology. Philadelphia, W.B. Saunders Co., 1986

Author   J. Summers, M.D., Ph.D.

Prostatic hyperplasia, benign (BPH)

BASICS

DESCRIPTION Benign adenomatous growth of prostate which may result in bladder outlet obstruction
System(s) affected: Reproductive, Renal/Urologic
Genetics: Genetic factors may be involved
Incidence/Prevalence in USA:
• Universal pathologic phenomenon seen in older men
• No hard evidence suggesting racial predisposition
Predominant age:
• Rarely seen in men < 40
• Seen in 50% of men > 50; 80% of men > 70
Predominant sex: Male only

SIGNS AND SYMPTOMS
Prostate size correlates poorly with symptoms
Obstructive symptoms: Due to mechanical obstruction and/or detrusor muscle decompensation
◊ Decrease force or caliber of stream
◊ Hesitancy
◊ Post-void dribbling
◊ Sensation of incomplete bladder emptying
◊ Overflow incontinence
◊ Inability to voluntarily stop stream
◊ Urinary retention
Irritative symptoms: Due to incomplete bladder emptying and/or detrusor muscle instability
◊ Frequency
◊ Nocturia
◊ Urgency
◊ Urge incontinence
Other symptoms:
◊ Gross hematuria (terminal hematuria most common in men over 60 years of age)
◊ Observation of weak stream
◊ Distended bladder (> 150 cc in order to detect by percussion)
◊ Increased post-void residual (> 100 cc)
◊ Prostate enlarged (normal 20 gram prostate - size of horse chestnut)
◊ Alterations in perianal sensation, anal sphincter tone or bulbocavernosus reflex suggests a neurogenic component to voiding symptoms
◊ Clinical clues suggesting renal failure due to obstructive uropathy (edema, pallor, pruritis, ecchymoses, nutritional deficiencies, etc.)

CAUSES Exact etiology unknown, but evidence suggests BPH arises from a systemic hormonal alteration which may or may not act in combination with growth factors stimulating stromal or glandular hyperplasia

RISK FACTORS
• Intact testes (BPH rare in eunuchs)
• Aging (thus, rare in men < 40 years old)
• No dietary, environmental, or sexual practices implicated yet

DIAGNOSIS

DIFFERENTIAL DIAGNOSIS
Bladder outlet obstruction:
◊ Prostate cancer
◊ Urethral stricture
◊ Bladder neck contracture (acquired or congenital)
◊ Anterior or posterior urethral valves
◊ Mullerian duct cysts
◊ Inability of bladder neck or external sphincter to relax appropriately during voiding
Non-obstructive etiologies:
◊ Neurogenic bladder (detrusor denervation)
◊ Myogenic cause (detrusor muscle failure)
◊ Medications (parasympatholytics, sympathomimetics, etc.)
◊ Psychogenic
Irritative symptoms:
◊ Neurogenic bladder
◊ Inflammatory disorders (prostatitis, urethritis, radiation cystitis, interstitial cystitis, etc.)
◊ Neoplasm (bladder carcinoma, esp carcinoma in situ)

LABORATORY
• BPH is a pathologic diagnosis - lab data is only suggestive
• Urinalysis: pyuria, pH changes due to chronic residual urine
• Elevated serum creatinine (if obstructive uropathy present)
• Urine culture positive (sometimes due to chronic residual urine)
• Prostate specific antigen (PSA) may be elevated but usually <10
• Increased post-void residual (> 100 cc)
Drugs that may alter lab results: N/A
Disorders that may alter lab results:
Acute urinary retention or prostatitis may elevate the PSA

PATHOLOGICAL FINDINGS
Confirmation obtained by biopsy, resection or extirpation surgery. 5 types: Stromal (fibrous), fibromuscular, muscular ("leiomyoma"), fibroadenoma, fibromyoadenoma.

SPECIAL TESTS
• Transrectal prostate ultrasound. Gives volumetric estimate of gland
• Needle biopsy

IMAGING
• IVP: increased post-void residual, large prostatic impression on bladder, trabeculated bladder, bladder diverticula, upper tract dilation, bladder stones
• CT scan or MRI of pelvis: enlarged prostate

DIAGNOSTIC PROCEDURES
• Uroflow: amount voided per unit time. Peak flow < 10cc/sec suggests obstruction (accurate when voided volume is > 200cc).
• Pressure-flow curve (urine flow versus voiding pressures): decreased urine flow and increased pressure indicates obstruction
• Cystometrogram (CMG) for information about bladder compliance (volume vs pressure);

shows uninhibited contractions
• Cystoscopy shows occlusive prostatic lobes, bladder trabeculation

TREATMENT

APPROPRIATE HEALTH CARE
Inpatient or outpatient treatment required, either for surgery or medical treatment. Inpatient treatment required to manage fluid and electrolyte abnormalities of obstructive uropathy.

GENERAL MEASURES
• Avoid large boluses of oral or IV fluids
• Avoid prolonged periods of not voiding
• Avoid sympathomimetic or anticholinergic medications (e.g., cold preparations)
• If large post-void residual or retention, trial catheter either indwelling or intermittent until definitive treatment.
Surgery (indicators to determine necessity)
One of the following:
◊ Urinary retention due to prostatic obstruction
◊ Intractable symptoms due to prostatic obstruction (gauged by AVA symptom index)
◊ Obstructive uropathy
◊ Recurrent or persistent urinary tract infections due to prostatic obstruction
◊ Recurrent gross hematuria due to enlarged prostate
Surgical procedures
◊ Transurethral resection of prostate (TURP)
◊ Transurethral incision of prostate (TUIP), gland < 10 gms
◊ Open prostatectomy (glands > 40 grams)
◊ Transurethral (balloon) dilatation of prostate (TUDP)
◊ Transurethral microwave thermotherapy (TUMT)
◊ Transrectal prostatic hyperthermia
◊ Transurethral laser induced prostatectomy (TULIP)
◊ Visual laser assisted prostatectomy (VLAP)
◊ Prostatic urethral stenting

ACTIVITY No restriction

DIET
• Avoid caffeinated or alcoholic beverages
• Avoid excessively spiced foods

PATIENT EDUCATION
• The Prostate Book, published by Krames Communications, 312 90th St, Daly City, CA 94015-1898
• National Kidney & Urologic Diseases Information Clearinghouse, Box NKUDIC, Bethesda, MD 20893, (301)468-6345

MEDICATIONS

DRUG(S) OF CHOICE
Indicated when no strong indications of surgery exist, patient refuses or is a poor surgical risk.
- Alpha adrenergic antagonist: prazosin (Minipress), terazosin
- Hormonal (anti-androgens) agents: flutamide (a LHRH agonist), Leuprolide, finasteride (Proscar, a 5-alpha reductase inhibitor).

Contraindications: Use alpha adrenergic antagonists with caution in patients with cardiac or cerebrovascular disease

Precautions: Refer to manufacturer's profile of each drug

Significant possible interactions: Refer to manufacturer's profile of each drug

ALTERNATIVE DRUGS N/A

FOLLOWUP

PATIENT MONITORING
- Symptom index (AVA Symptom Index) monitored every 1-6 months
- Urodynamics every 3-12 months
- Digital rectal exam yearly
- PSA yearly

PREVENTION/AVOIDANCE Appears to be part of the aging process

POSSIBLE COMPLICATIONS
- Bladder stones
- Prostatitis
- Renal failure

EXPECTED COURSE AND PROGNOSIS
- Symptoms improve or stabilize in 70-80% of patients; 20-30% require treatment because of worsening symptoms
- 11-33% men with BPH have occult prostate cancer

MISCELLANEOUS

ASSOCIATED CONDITIONS N/A

AGE-RELATED FACTORS
Pediatric: N/A
Geriatric: Much more prevalent in elderly men
Others: N/A

PREGNANCY N/A

SYNONYMS
- Prostatic hyperplasia
- Prostatic hypertrophy

ICD-9-CM 600 hyperplasia of prostate

SEE ALSO N/A

OTHER NOTES N/A

ABBREVIATIONS
IVP = intravenous pyelogram

REFERENCES
- Grayhack, J.T.: Benign prostatic hypertrophy. In Adult and Pediatric Urology. Edited by J.Y. Gillenwater, J.T. Grayhack, S.S. Howard & J.W. Duckett. Chicago, Yearbook Medical Publishing, Inc., 1987
- Walsh, P.C.: Benign prostatic hypertrophy. In Campbell's Urology. Edited by P.C. Walsh, R.F. Gittes, A.D. Perlmutter, et al. Philadelphia, W.B. Saunders Co., 1986
- Mebust, W.K.: Surgical Management of Benign Prostatic Obstruction, Urology (Suppl.) 32(6):12, 1988.
- Blaivas, J.G.: Pathophysiology and Differential Diagnosis of Benign Prostatic Hypertrophy, Urology (Suppl.) 32(6):5, 1988.
- Kapoor, D.A., Reddy, P.K.: Surgical Alternatives to TURP in the management of BPH, AUA Update Series, Lession 3, Volume 12, 1993.

Author C. Jennings, M.D.

Prostatitis

BASICS

DESCRIPTION One of several inflammatory and/or painful conditions affecting the prostate gland
• Acute bacterial prostatitis: generally associated with urinary tract infection, has characteristically abrupt onset
• Chronic bacterial prostatitis: major cause of recurrent bacteriuria, less fulminant
• Nonbacterial prostatitis: findings similar to chronic bacterial, but no infection present
• Prostatodynia: symptoms and signs of prostatitis without evidence of inflammation
System(s) affected: Reproductive, Renal/Urologic
Genetics: No known genetic pattern
Incidence/Prevalence in USA: Common
Predominant age:
• Mostly ages 30-50, sexually active
• Chronic more common in ages over 50
Predominant sex: Male only

SIGNS AND SYMPTOMS
Acute bacterial
◊ Fever
◊ Chills
◊ Tense, boggy, very tender and warm prostate
◊ Low back pain
◊ Perineal pain
◊ Frequency
◊ Urgency
◊ Dysuria
◊ Nocturia
◊ Bladder outlet obstruction
Chronic bacterial
◊ Symptoms often absent
◊ Perineal pain
◊ Dysuria
◊ Irritative voiding
◊ Lower abdominal pain
◊ Low back pain
◊ Scrotal pain
◊ Penile pain
◊ Pain on ejaculation
◊ Hematospermia
Nonbacterial
◊ Similar to chronic prostatitis
Prostatodynia
◊ Abnormal flow
◊ Irritative voiding
◊ Pelvic pain

CAUSES
Acute and chronic bacterial
◊ Ascending infection through urethra
◊ Refluxing urine into prostate ducts
◊ Direct extension or lymphatic spread from rectum
◊ Hematogenous spread
◊ Calculi serving as nidus for infection
◊ Aerobic gram negative bacteria (Escherichia coli, pseudomonas, Klebsiella, Proteus)
◊ Gram positive bacteria (Streptococcus faecalis, Staphylococcus. aureus)
◊ Organisms suspected, but unproven (Staphylococcus epidermidis, Micrococci, Non-group D streptococcus, Diphtheroids)

Nonbacterial
◊ Currently unknown
◊ Ureaplasm and Chlamydia postulated, but not proven
Prostatodynia
◊ Unclear
◊ Stress, anxiety, depression possible

RISK FACTORS
• Male sex
• Age over 50
• Prostatic calculi
• Urinary tract infection

DIAGNOSIS

DIFFERENTIAL DIAGNOSIS
• Cystitis
• Urethritis
• Pyelonephritis
• Malignancy
• Obstructive calculus
• Foreign body
• Acute urinary retention

LABORATORY
• Fractional urine examination (initial 10 cc from urethra for voided bladder 1 (VB1) test, next 200 cc discarded, then midstream from bladder for VB2 test, then expressed prostate secretion (EPS), lastly urine after prostate massage for VB3 test. Some feel vigorous massage may lead to bacteremia.
• Urinalysis, culture, sensitivities on all samples
• Over 10-15 white cells per high powered field or positive culture in EPS or VB3 but not VB1 or VB2 diagnostic of bacterial prostatitis
• Bacteria count generally less in chronic than acute
• Nonbacterial will show white blood cells with a negative culture
• No abnormal findings with prostatodynia
Drugs that may alter lab results:
Antibiotics
Disorders that may alter lab results: N/A

PATHOLOGICAL FINDINGS
Inflammatory changes (except prostatodynia)

SPECIAL TESTS N/A

IMAGING CT or ultrasound, if malignancy or abscess suspected

DIAGNOSTIC PROCEDURES Needle biopsy or aspiration for culture

TREATMENT

APPROPRIATE HEALTH CARE
• Inpatient (proven or suspected abscess, urosepsis, immunocompromised)
• Outpatient, if nontoxic

GENERAL MEASURES
• Analgesics
• Antipyretics
• Stool softeners
• Hydration
• Sitz baths to relieve pain and spasm
• Avoid transrectal procedures
• Suprapubic catheter for severe urinary retention
• Surgical resection for intractable chronic disease, or to drain an abscess

ACTIVITY Bedrest in severe cases

DIET No special diet

PATIENT EDUCATION
Printed patient information available from:
• National Kidney & Urologic Diseases Information Clearinghouse, Box NKUDIC, Bethesda, MD 20893, (301)468-6345

MEDICATIONS

DRUG(S) OF CHOICE
• Acute bacterial:
Trimethoprim-sulfamethoxazole, double strength, two tablets, twice daily for 30 days. For parenteral therapy 8-10 mg/kg per day (trimethoprim).
• Chronic bacterial: A fluoroquinolone (norfloxacin 200 mg bid, ciprofloxacin 500 mg bid) at standard dose for periods as long as three months
• Nonbacterial: May benefit from erythromycin, doxycycline, trimethoprim-sulfa
• Prostatodynia: No drug therapy
• Analgesics
• Antipyretics
• Stool softeners
Contraindications: Drug allergies
Precautions:
• Renal disease
• Hepatic disease
• Elderly
• G-6-PD deficiency
Significant possible interactions:
Fluoroquinolones with magnesium/aluminum antacids, theophylline, and probenecid

ALTERNATIVE DRUGS Carbenicillin
with aminoglycoside, erythromycin, tetracycline, cephalexin

FOLLOWUP

PATIENT MONITORING
• Acute bacterial - urinalysis and culture 30 days after initiating treatment
• Chronic bacterial - Urinalysis and culture every 30 days (may take several months)

PREVENTION/AVOIDANCE
Suppression therapy may benefit patient with chronic bacterial prostatitis

POSSIBLE COMPLICATIONS
• Abscess
• Sepsis
• Urinary retention

EXPECTED COURSE AND
PROGNOSIS Often prolonged and difficult to cure. Studies with 55-97% cure rate depending on population and drug used.

MISCELLANEOUS

ASSOCIATED CONDITIONS
• Prostatic hypertrophy
• Cystitis
• Urethritis

AGE-RELATED FACTORS
Pediatric: None
Geriatric: Consider prostatic hypertrophy and urinary retention more seriously
Others: N/A

PREGNANCY N/A

SYNONYMS N/A

ICD-9-CM
• 601.0 acute
• 601.1 chronic

SEE ALSO N/A

OTHER NOTES None

ABBREVIATIONS
• VB = voided bladder
• EPS = expressed prostate secretion

REFERENCES
• Braunwald, E., et al. (eds.): Harrison's Principles of Internal Medicine. 12th Ed. New York, McGraw-Hill, 1991
• Edward, J.: Treatment of Bacterial Prostatitis. J of Fam Prac, 1991, Vol.44-6:2137-2141
• Crawford, D.E.: Benign and Malignant Prostatic Diseases. J of Fam Prac, 1991, Vol. 44-5 supplement: 65s-70s

Author T. Baker, M.D.

Pruritus ani

BASICS

DESCRIPTION Intense chronic itching in the anal and perianal skin. Usual course - acute. Chronic pruritis ani is a symptom, not a diagnosis or disease.
System(s) affected: Skin/Exocrine
Genetics: No known genetic pattern
Incidence/Prevalence in USA: Common
Predominant age: All ages
Predominant sex: Male > Female (4:1)

SIGNS AND SYMPTOMS
- Rectal and anal itching
- Anal erythema
- Anal fissures
- Maceration
- Lichenification
- Excoriations
- Candidiasis
- Tinea

CAUSES
Dermatologic disorders
  ◊ Allergies (soap, topical anesthetics, oral antibiotics)
  ◊ Fistulas
  ◊ Fissures
  ◊ Neoplasms
  ◊ Psoriasis
  ◊ Eczema
  ◊ Seborrheic dermatitis
  ◊ Contact dermatitis
  ◊ Eczema
  ◊ Psoriasis
Infections
  ◊ Pinworms and other worms
  ◊ Scabies
  ◊ Pediculosis
Other
  ◊ Poor hygiene (fecal material allowed to dry on the skin)
  ◊ Diabetes mellitus
  ◊ Chronic liver disease
  ◊ Diarrheic alkalotic irritation
  ◊ Trauma from scented toilet paper

RISK FACTORS
- Overweight
- Hairy, tendency to to perspire a great deal
- Anxiety-itch-anxiety cycle

DIAGNOSIS

DIFFERENTIAL DIAGNOSIS
- Allergies
- Psoriasis
- Atopic dermatitis
- Fungus infection
- Bacterial infection
- Parasites
- Hyperhidrosis
- Diabetes mellitus
- Liver disease
- Neoplasia
- Anxiety

LABORATORY
- Glycosuria
- Hyperglycemia
- Skin scraping, yeast
- Fungi
- Parasites
- Stool - ova plus parasites
Drugs that may alter lab results: N/A
Disorders that may alter lab results: N/A

PATHOLOGICAL FINDINGS Excoriation of epithelial layer of skin

SPECIAL TESTS Glucose tolerance test

IMAGING N/A

DIAGNOSTIC PROCEDURES
- Inspection
- Anuscopy biopsy (to exclude neoplasia)

TREATMENT

APPROPRIATE HEALTH CARE
Outpatient

GENERAL MEASURES
- Treat predisposing factors, such as parasites, diabetes, liver disease, cryptitis, scabies, pediculosis
- Resist over meticulous use of soap and rubbing
- Avoid tight clothing and under clothing
- Cleanse anal area after bowel movements with moistened absorbent cotton and plain water
- Dust anal area with non-medicated talcum powder
- If unable to completely empty rectum with defecation, use small plain water enema (infant bulb syringe) after each bowel movement. This may prevent post evacuation soilage and irritation.

ACTIVITY Avoid getting overheated

DIET If suspicious of food allergy, eliminate as a trial: Coffee, beer, cola, vitamin C tablets in excessive doses, spices, citrus fruits

PATIENT EDUCATION See information in General Measures

MEDICATIONS

DRUG(S) OF CHOICE
• Specific topical treatment for allergies, micro-organisms, bacteria
• For symptomatic treatment - hydrocortisone cream 0.5-1% applied sparingly, usually at night. If severe, may need to apply several times a day. Discontinue once itching stops.
Contraindications: Refer to manufacturer's literature
Precautions: Refer to manufacturer's literature
Significant possible interactions: Refer to manufacturer's literature

ALTERNATIVE DRUGS N/A

FOLLOWUP

PATIENT MONITORING As needed

PREVENTION/AVOIDANCE
• Avoid topical agents
• Avoid laxatives
• Avoid tight underclothing made from synthetic material
• Practice good hygiene
• Use talcum powder
• Possibly lactobacillus acidophilus (tablets or in milk); possibly malt soup extract
• Eat yogurt when taking broad-spectrum antibiotics

POSSIBLE COMPLICATIONS
• Secondary bacterial infection
• Chronicity
• Excoriation
• Lichenification

EXPECTED COURSE AND PROGNOSIS
• Depends upon etiology; usually good
• May be persistent and recurrent

MISCELLANEOUS

ASSOCIATED CONDITIONS
• Diabetes mellitus
• Psoriasis
• Hyperhidrosis
• Parasite infestations

AGE-RELATED FACTORS
Pediatric:
• Usually secondary to enterobiasis, anal fissures, other local inflammatory lesions, or coarse or moist undergarments. Nocturnal itching may be due to pinworms.
• Exposure to sunlight or dry heat may be helpful for infants with inflamed anal area
Geriatric: Common in this age group
Others: N/A

PREGNANCY N/A

SYNONYMS N/A

ICD-9-CM
698.0

SEE ALSO Anogenital pruritus

OTHER NOTES N/A

ABBREVIATIONS N/A

REFERENCES
• Sleisenger, M.H. & Fordtran, J.S. (eds.): Gastrointestinal Disease: Pathophysiology, Diagnosis, Management. 4th Ed. Philadelphia, W.B. Saunders Co., 1989
• Kirsner, J.B. & Shortet, G. (eds.): Diseases of the Colon, Rectum and Canal. Baltimore, Williams & Wilkins, 1988

Author S. Smith

Pruritus vulvae

BASICS

DESCRIPTION Pruritus vulvae is both a symptom and a pathologic process affecting the vulva. It is a symptom of underlying disease in the vast majority of the patients. As a primary diagnosis, it consists of irritation and vulvar itching without an underlying pathologic etiology.
System(s) affected: Skin/Exocrine
Genetics: Unknown
Incidence/Prevalence in USA: The exact incidence is unknown, although most women will complain of vulvar pruritus at some time during their life
Predominant age:
• Any age can be affected
• In young girls, it is usually caused by an infection
• Frequent in postmenopausal women
Predominant sex: Female only

SIGNS AND SYMPTOMS
• Constant itching of the vulva
• Constant burning of the vulva

CAUSES
• Infectious causes - vaginal yeast infections, Gardnerella, other vaginal infections, and yeast dermatitis of the vulva itself
• Urinary tract infections will produce vulvar burning on occasion
• Vulvar vestibulitis (inflammation of the vestibular glands) produces a constant burning with pruritus and dyspareunia
• Human papilloma virus (HPV) has been associated with burning and itching of the vulva
• Vulvar tissues are estrogen sensitive. Estrogen deprivation can produce burning and itching.
• A search for underlying malignancy should be paramount. Carcinoma in situ (Bowen's disease) and invasive malignancy will often be associated with pruritus.
• Changes in the epidermis, such as lichen sclerosis et atrophicus (LSA) (thinning of the vulvar tissues and homogenization at the basement membrane) or hyperkeratosis of the vulva produce pruritus
• Anal incontinence with fecal soilage produces pruritus
• Excessive heat produces symptoms from sweat and irritation
• Environmental and dietary irritants such as nylon, soaps, perfumes, and over-zealous cleansing can produce symptoms
• Dietary irritants include methylxanthines (coffee, cola), tomatoes, peanuts

RISK FACTORS Listed with Causes

DIAGNOSIS

DIFFERENTIAL DIAGNOSIS
• The diagnosis of primary idiopathic vulvar pruritus must be made by exclusion
• A search for infectious causes should be undertaken with treatment of yeast and other vaginitis
• Biopsy of any abnormal-appearing epithelium on the vulva to insure that malignant changes are not present
• Only when all other factors have been ruled out can the diagnosis primary idiopathic vulvar pruritus be established

LABORATORY
• Vaginal secretions can be evaluated by wet mount (NaCl for trichomonas or Gardnerella, and KOH for yeast). Cultures seldom required.
• Gram stain of the vagina is non-diagnostic as multiple organisms are present in the normal flora
Drugs that may alter lab results: N/A
Disorders that may alter lab results: N/A

PATHOLOGICAL FINDINGS These are related to the underlying etiology. In primary vulvar pruritus, no changes will be noted. If HPV is present, these changes will be seen in the cornified layer of the squamous epithelium.

SPECIAL TESTS Whenever necessary, biopsy of the vulva should be used to establish the primary diagnosis

IMAGING N/A

DIAGNOSTIC PROCEDURES Biopsy when needed

TREATMENT

APPROPRIATE HEALTH CARE
Outpatient

GENERAL MEASURES
• Treatment of any underlying cause must be undertaken
• Bowen's disease and premalignant changes are treated with excision or laser vaporization
• In cases of idiopathic primary vulvar pruritus, conservative measures include sitz baths, topical steroid creams, avoidance of chemical irritants and dietary changes
• When conservative measures fail, advanced cases can be treated with alcohol block or laser

ACTIVITY Unlimited

DIET A trial of dietary alteration should be attempted for idiopathic pruritus. Coffee and caffeine-containing beverages should be avoided. Other foods to avoid include tomatoes, peanuts.

PATIENT EDUCATION See Prevention/Avoidance

MEDICATIONS

DRUG(S) OF CHOICE
• Infectious sources should be treated with appropriate antimicrobials or antifungals
• Lichen sclerosis is treated with 2% testosterone in petrolatum
• Hyperkeratotic lesions are treated with topical steroid
• Idiopathic primary vulvar pruritus can be treated with topical steroids such as Kenalog or Topicort cream
Contraindications: N/A
Precautions: N/A
Significant possible interactions: N/A

ALTERNATIVE DRUGS N/A

FOLLOWUP

PATIENT MONITORING These women should be followed closely for the development of premalignant or malignant changes within the area of pruritus

PREVENTION/AVOIDANCE
• Irritants to the vulva such as perfumes, soaps (use non-allergenic) or perfume douches must be avoided
• Only cotton underwear should be worn
• No tight fitting clothes or nylon pantyhose

POSSIBLE COMPLICATIONS Chronic course

EXPECTED COURSE AND PROGNOSIS
• Vulvar pruritus can be kept under control with conservative measures and topical steroids
• When it advances to uncontrollable symptoms, alcohol block or laser may be necessary

MISCELLANEOUS

ASSOCIATED CONDITIONS N/A

AGE-RELATED FACTORS
Pediatric: N/A
Geriatric: More frequent
Others: N/A

PREGNANCY N/A

SYNONYMS
• Vulvar pruritus
• Vulvodynia
• Burning vulva syndrome

ICD-9-CM 698.1

SEE ALSO N/A

OTHER NOTES N/A

ABBREVIATIONS N/A

REFERENCES
• McKay, M.: Vulvodynia vs. Pruritus vulvae. Clin Obstet Gynecol 1985;28:123-133
• Smith, L., Henricks, D. & McCullah, R.: Prospective studies on the etiology and treatment of pruritus ani. Dis Colon Rectum 1982;25:258-363
• Hopkins, M.P.: Anatomy and pathology of the vulva and vagina. In Gynecology & Obstetrics, An Integrated Approach. Edited by R. Rebar & V. Baker. New York, Churchill Livingstone, 1993

Author M. Hopkins, M.D.

Pseudofolliculitis barbae

BASICS

DESCRIPTION Foreign body inflammatory reaction surrounding an ingrown hair (usually in beard area, especially submandibular region, but can occur on scalp, axilla, or pubic area if these sites are shaved or plucked). Characterized by red papule/pustule at point of entry. A mechanical problem.

System(s) affected: Skin/Exocrine

Genetics: Curly haired people, especially Blacks

Incidence in USA: N/A

Prevalence in USA: Widespread. Incidence of 45% in Black soldiers who shave. Adult male Blacks - 50,000/100,000; adult male Caucasians - 3000-5000/100,000.

Predominant age: Postpubertal, middle age (40-75)

Predominant sex: Male > Female

SIGNS AND SYMPTOMS
• Tender exudative, erythematous follicular papules or pustules in beard area (less commonly in scalp, axilla, pubic areas)
• Range from 2-4 mm in size
• Painful upon shaving
• Alopecia
• Lusterless brittle hair

CAUSES
• Reentry penetration of skin by external pointed tip of growing curved whisker, or sharped tipped whisker can grow into follicular wall if shaved too close
• Plucking of hair can cause abnormal hair growth in injured follicles

RISK FACTORS
• Possessing curly hair
• Shaving too close with multiple razor strokes
• Plucking hairs
• Black race

DIAGNOSIS

DIFFERENTIAL DIAGNOSIS
Bacterial/staphylococcal folliculitis

LABORATORY N/A
Drugs that may alter lab results: N/A
Disorders that may alter lab results: N/A

PATHOLOGICAL FINDINGS Clinical
pathology- follicular papules and pustules. Histopathology - because of its curvature, the advancing hair's sharp-tipped free end causes an epidermal invagination as it approaches the skin. This is accompanied by inflammation and often an intra-epidermal abscess. As hair enters dermis, more severe inflammation occurs with downgrowth of epidermis in an attempt to ensheath hair. An abscess forms within the pseudofollicle and a foreign body reaction forms at the tip of invading hair.

SPECIAL TESTS Culture of pustules -
usually sterile. May show coagulase-negative micrococcus (normal skin flora).

IMAGING N/A

DIAGNOSTIC PROCEDURES Clinical
diagnosis

TREATMENT

APPROPRIATE HEALTH CARE
Outpatient

GENERAL MEASURES
Acute treatment
◊ Dislodge embedded hair with sterile needle
◊ Discontinue shaving until red papules have resolved (minimum 3-4 weeks)
◊ Massage beard area with washcloths, coarse sponge or brush several times daily
◊ Systemic antibiotics if secondary infections present

ACTIVITY Unlimited

DIET No restrictions

PATIENT EDUCATION
• Dunn 88, Pseudofolliculitis Barbae, pages 170-172
• American Family Physician (see References)

MEDICATIONS

DRUG(S) OF CHOICE
Topical or systemic antibiotic for secondary infection
• Application of clindamycin solution (Cleocin-T) bid
• Low doses erythromycin or tetracycline (250 mg bid)
• Administer until papule/pustule resolution
Mild cases
◊ 5% benzoyl peroxide - apply after shaving
◊ 1% hydrocortisone cream - apply at bedtime
Moderate disease - chemical depilatories
◊ Disrupt cross-linking of disulfide bonds of hair causing blunt hair tip
◊ Apply no more frequently than every 3rd day - 2% barium sulfide (Magic Shave) or calcium thioglycolate (Surgex)
Moderate disease - adjunct treatment
◊ Tretinoin liquid/cream (Retin-A), applied daily or every other day
Contraindications:
• Clindamycin - history of regional enteritis or ulcerative colitis; history of antibiotic associated colitis
• Erythromycin, tetracycline, tretinoin hypersensitivity only
Precautions:
• Clindamycin - colitis, eye burning and irritation, skin dryness, pregnancy category B
• Erythromycin - cautious use in patients with impaired hepatic function, GI side effects especially abdominal cramping, pregnancy category B
• Tetracycline - permanent discoloration of teeth if given during last half of pregnancy
• Tretinoin - severe skin irritation, pregnancy category C
• Benzoyl peroxide - skin irritation and dryness, allergic contact dermatitis
• Hydrocortisone cream - local skin irritation, skin atrophy with prolonged use
Significant possible interactions:
• Erythromycin - increases theophylline and carbamazepine levels, decreases clearance of warfarin
• Tetracycline - depresses plasma prothrombin activity (therefore need to decrease warfarin dosages)

ALTERNATIVE DRUGS N/A

FOLLOWUP

PATIENT MONITORING As needed.
Educate patient on curative and preventive treatment.

PREVENTION/AVOIDANCE
Mild cases
◊ Use tiny plastic hook for removing ingrown hairs before shaving
◊ Shave either with a manual adjustable razor at coarsest settings (avoids close shaves), a twin blade razor (Trac-II, The Bump-Fighter), a foil guarded razor (PFB razor), or electric triple "O" head razor
◊ Shave beard in direction of hair growth
◊ Do not stretch skin when shaving
◊ Use correct shaving cream/gel (Ef-Kay Shaving Gel, Edge Shaving Gel, Easy Shave Medicated Shaving Cream)
◊ Consider 5% benzoyl peroxide after shaving and application of 1% hydrocortisone cream at bedtime
Moderate cases
◊ Chemical depilatories
◊ Consider 0.05% tretinoin (Retin-A) liquid or cream
Severe cases
◊ Avoidance of shaving completely
◊ Electrolysis to destroy remaining hair follicles

POSSIBLE COMPLICATIONS
• Scarring (occasionally keloidal)
• Foreign body granuloma formation
• Disfiguring postinflammatory hyperpigmentation
• Impetiginization of inflamed skin

EXPECTED COURSE AND PROGNOSIS
• Course is recurrent if preventative measures not followed
• Prognosis is poor in presence of progressive scarring and foreign body granuloma formation

MISCELLANEOUS

ASSOCIATED CONDITIONS Keloidal folliculitis

AGE-RELATED FACTORS
Pediatric: N/A
Geriatric: N/A
Others: N/A

PREGNANCY Do not use tretinoin (Retin-A), tetracycline, benzoyl peroxide

SYNONYMS
• Chronic sycosis barbae
• Pili incarnati
• Folliculitis barbae traumatica
• Razor bumps

ICD-9-CM 704.8

SEE ALSO Folliculitis

OTHER NOTES N/A

ABBREVIATIONS N/A

REFERENCES
• Lever, W.F. & Schaumburg-Lever, G.: Histopathology of the Skin. Philadelphia, J.B. Lippincott, 1990
• Dunn, J.F., Jr.: Pseudofolliculitis Barbae. Amer Fam Phys. Sept, 1988
• Habif, T.P.: Clinical Dermatology: A Color Guide to Diagnosis and Treatment. 2nd Ed. St. Louis, C.V. Mosby, 1990
• Sams, W., Jr., & Lynch, P.: Principles and Practice of Dermatology. New York, Churchill Livingstone, 1990

Author P. Slomiany, M.D.

Pseudogout (CPPD)

BASICS

DESCRIPTION An acute inflammatory arthritic disease usually involving large joints which primarily affects the elderly and is caused by calcium pyrophosphate dihydrate (CPPD) crystal deposition in joints. Associated with chondrocalcinosis.
• CPPD crystal deposition may cause a progressive degenerative arthritis in numerous joints
• CPPD crystal deposition may cause a more insidious, smoldering, symmetrical, polyarthritis which is similar to rheumatoid arthritis
System(s) affected: Musculoskeletal
Genetics:
• Uncommonly seen in familial pattern with autosomal dominant inheritance (less than 1% of cases)
• Most cases sporadic
Incidence in USA: Unknown, primarily a disease of the elderly
Prevalence in USA: Chondrocalcinosis is present 1 in 10 in ages 60-75, over age 80 in 1 in 3. Only a small percentage develop pseudogout.
Predominant age: 80% of patients are older than 60
Predominant sex: Female > Male (2:1)

SIGNS AND SYMPTOMS
• Acute pain and swelling of one or more joints. Knee is involved in one-half of all attacks, ankle, wrist and shoulder also common.
• Inflammation, joint effusion and limitation of motion
• 50% associated with fever
• Any other synovial joint may be involved including first metatarsophalangeal
• Progressive degenerative arthritis in numerous joints including: wrists, metacarpophalangeal, hips, shoulders, elbows, and ankles
• Low grade inflammatory arthritis with multiple symmetrical joint involvement (mimics rheumatoid arthritis) < 5% of cases

CAUSES
• Acute inflammatory reaction to CPPD crystals shed into synovial cavity
• Physical and chemical changes in aging cartilage that favor crystal growth

RISK FACTORS
• Aging
• Trauma
• Pseudogout will often occur as a complication in patients hospitalized for other medical and surgical illnesses
Metabolic diseases (10% or less of the cases)
◊ Hyperparathyroidism
◊ Hemochromatosis
◊ Gout
◊ Hypophosphatasia
◊ Hypothyroidism
◊ Ochronosis
◊ Wilson's disease
◊ Amyloidosis
◊ Hypomagnesemia

DIAGNOSIS

DIFFERENTIAL DIAGNOSIS
• Illness that may cause an acute inflammatory arthritis in a single or multiple joint(s): Gout, septic arthritis or trauma
• Other illnesses that may present with an acute inflammatory arthritis: Reiter's syndrome, Lyme disease, acute rheumatoid arthritis

LABORATORY
• Elevated sedimentation rate
• Leukocytosis with mild left shift
Drugs that may alter lab results: N/A
Disorders that may alter lab results: N/A

PATHOLOGICAL FINDINGS CPPD crystal deposition in articular cartilage, synovium, ligaments and tendons

SPECIAL TESTS
Synovial fluid analysis consistent with an inflammatory effusion:
◊ Cell count from 2000 to 100,000 WBC/mL
◊ Differential predominantly neutrophils (80-90%)
◊ Wet prep with polarized microscopy demonstrates small numbers of weakly positively birefringent crystals in the fluid and within neutrophils
Metabolic studies
◊ To exclude an underlying cause should always be obtained in patients under age 50 and considered in the elderly
◊ Serum calcium
◊ Serum phosphorous
◊ Serum alkaline phosphatase
◊ Serum parathormone
◊ Serum iron, total iron binding capacity, and serum ferritin
◊ Serum magnesium
◊ Serum thyroxine and thyroid stimulating hormone (TSH) level

IMAGING
X-rays of joints
◊ May demonstrate punctate and linear calcification in articular hyaline or fibrocartilage: Knees, hips, symphysis pubis, and wrists most often affected, may also be found in asymptomatic individuals
◊ In the chronic destructive indolent form of the disease: Subchondral cyst formation, fragmentation with formation of intra-articular radiodense bodies in joints not typically affected by degenerative joint disease.

DIAGNOSTIC PROCEDURES Aspiration of joint fluid with synovial fluid analysis required for proper confirmation of pseudogout; aspiration may relieve symptoms and speed resolution of inflammatory process

TREATMENT

APPROPRIATE HEALTH CARE
• If septic arthritis is considered possible, inpatient care may be required for empiric antibiotic therapy pending culture results
• If patient does not have adequate support system inpatient care may be required until patient is able to walk

GENERAL MEASURES
• Rest and elevate affected joint(s)
• Apply moist warm compresses to affected joints

ACTIVITY
• Non-weight bearing on affected joint while painful. Use crutches or walker.
• Perform isometric exercises to maintain muscle strength during the acute stage, i.e., quadriceps isometric contractions and leg lifts, if knee affected
• Begin range of motion of joint as inflammation and pain subside
• Resume weight bearing when pain subsides

DIET No special diet

PATIENT EDUCATION Specific instructions on exercise and activity

MEDICATIONS

DRUG(S) OF CHOICE
Nonsteroidal anti-inflammatory drugs (choose one of the following):
◊ Sulindac (Clinoril) 150-200 mg bid with food
◊ Ibuprofen (Motrin) 600-800 mg tid-qid with food. Maximum of 3.2 gm daily.
◊ Other NSAID's at anti-inflammatory doses are effective

Contraindications:
• History of hypersensitivity to NSAID's or aspirin
• Active peptic ulcer disease or history of recurrent upper gastrointestinal lesions
• Use with extreme caution when impaired renal function exists. Sulindac or piroxicam preferred for these patients. Monitor serum creatinine.

Precautions:
• May interfere with platelet aggregation and prolong bleeding time. This effect is much shorter lived than with aspirin.
• May cause fluid retention and worsen congestive heart failure
• Abnormal liver function tests may develop in approximately 15% of patients. Discontinue if findings worsen or systemic manifestations occur.
• Serious gastrointestinal bleeding can occur without warning. Follow patient carefully for internal bleeding. Administer misoprostol 200µg qid in patients with a history of peptic ulcer disease.

Significant possible interactions:
• May blunt the antihypertensive effects of angiotensin converting enzyme inhibitors
• May prolong the prothrombin time in patients taking oral anticoagulants
• Avoid concomitant usage of aspirin
• May blunt the diuretic effect of furosemide and hydrochlorothiazide
• May increase plasma lithium level in patients taking lithium carbonate
• May increase methotrexate levels.

ALTERNATIVE DRUGS
Intra-articular instillation of methylprednisolone acetate, 20-80 mg for large joints; 10-40 mg for medium joints. Available in 20, 40 and 80 mg/mL ampules.

FOLLOWUP

PATIENT MONITORING
Reevaluate patient for response to therapy 48-72 hours after treatment instituted. Reexamine 1 week later, then as needed.

PREVENTION/AVOIDANCE
None known

POSSIBLE COMPLICATIONS
• Erosive destructive arthritis in pattern of joints not usually affected by degenerative joint disease
• Recurrences may occur and a destructive arthritis may complicate CPPD

EXPECTED COURSE AND PROGNOSIS
Acute attack usually resolves in 10 days. Prognosis for resolution of acute attack is excellent.

MISCELLANEOUS

ASSOCIATED CONDITIONS
Consider in patients with pseudogout - hyperparathyroidism, hemochromatosis, gout, hypophosphatasia, hypothyroidism, ochronosis, Wilson's disease, amyloidosis, hypomagnesemia

AGE-RELATED FACTORS
Pediatric: Not seen in children
Geriatric: Most cases are in patients over 60
Others: N/A

PREGNANCY
N/A

SYNONYMS
• Calcium pyrophosphate deposition disease

ICD-9-CM
274.0

SEE ALSO
N/A

OTHER NOTES
N/A

ABBREVIATIONS
CPPD = calcium pyrophosphate deposition disease

REFERENCES
• McCarty, D.J.: Calcium Pyrophosphate Dihydrate Deposition Disease. In Primer on the Rheumatic Diseases. 9th Ed. Atlanta, Arthritis Foundation, 1988
• Braunwald E., et al. (eds.): Harrison's Principles of Internal Medicine. 12th Ed. New York, McGraw-Hill, 1991
• Reginato, A. & Schumacher, H.R.: Crystal-Associated Arthropathies. Clinics in Geriatric Medicine, Vol 4, No.2, May 1988

Author P. Cullen, M.D.

Pseudomembranous colitis

 BASICS

DESCRIPTION Inflammatory bowel disorder associated with antibiotic use. May be mild diarrhea, or move through several stages to a severe colitis. Usual course - acute, relapsing.
System(s) affected: Gastrointestinal
Genetics: No known genetic factors
Incidence/Prevalence in USA:
 • Epidemic or endemic in hospitals and nursing homes
 • 13.0/100 admissions - rate of asymptomatic carriage
 • 7.8/100 admissions - rate of C. difficile associated diarrhea
Predominant age: 40-75 years
Predominant sex: Male = Female

SIGNS AND SYMPTOMS
 • Diarrhea (watery and/or bloody)
 • Abdominal cramps
 • Lower abdominal tenderness
 • Fever

CAUSES
 • Antibiotic exposure particularly: clindamycin, lincomycin, ampicillin, cephalosporins. However, may also rarely occur with penicillins, erythromycin, sulfa-trimethoprim, chloramphenicol, tetracycline.
 • Cancer chemotherapy: fluorouracil, methotrexate, combination regimens.
 • Clostridium difficile and the toxins it liberates (A & B)

RISK FACTORS
 • Recent bowel surgery
 • Uremia
 • Intestinal ischemia
 • Shock
 • Tube feedings
 • Enemas
 • GI stimulants
 • Stool softener

 DIAGNOSIS

DIFFERENTIAL DIAGNOSIS
 • Other enteric pathogens
 • Nonspecific inflammatory bowel diseases

LABORATORY
 • Fecal leukocytosis
 • Leukocytosis
 • ELISA for Clostridium difficile toxin, positive
Drugs that may alter lab results: N/A
Disorders that may alter lab results: A high percentage of infants are normal carriers of Clostridium difficile

PATHOLOGICAL FINDINGS
 • Mild, nonspecific colitis without plaques
 • Gross - yellow-white plaques on colonic and small intestinal mucosa
 • Micro - pseudomembrane arising from point of superficial ulceration
 • Micro - fibrin
 • Micro - thick confluent pseudomembrane
 • Polymorphonuclear cells

SPECIAL TESTS
 • Sigmoidoscopy - may be normal in 10-33%
 • Colonoscopy may show involvement of the rectum and sigmoid colon and occasionally only right colon and/or distal ileum

IMAGING
 • Abdominal film - distorted haustral markings, colonic distention
 • CT - thickened or edematous colonic wall with pericolonic inflammation
Note: Avoid barium enemas

DIAGNOSTIC PROCEDURES
Endoscopic visualization

 TREATMENT

APPROPRIATE HEALTH CARE
 • Outpatient for mild cases
 • Inpatient for medical treatment

GENERAL MEASURES
 • Fluid replacement
 • Fluid plus electrolyte therapy
 • Discontinue antimicrobial agent
 • Successful in 25%

ACTIVITY Bedrest during acute phase

DIET Nothing by mouth during fulminant phase

PATIENT EDUCATION N/A

MEDICATIONS

DRUG(S) OF CHOICE
• Metronidazole 250 mg QID
• Oral vancomycin 125 mg QID (only for severe or resistant cases)
• Cholestyramine 4 grams orally qid (for mild symptoms); avoid with vancomycin
Note: Avoid antiperistaltic drugs such as diphenoxylate to reduce risk of toxic megacolon
Contraindications: Refer to manufacturer's literature
Precautions: Refer to manufacturer's literature
Significant possible interactions: Refer to manufacturer's literature

ALTERNATIVE DRUGS   N/A

FOLLOWUP

PATIENT MONITORING   Careful monitoring through fulminant phase

PREVENTION/AVOIDANCE
• Judicious use of antimicrobial agents
• Keep courses of antibiotics as brief as possible
Avoidance of recurrences
◊ Prolonged therapy
◊ Lactobacillus
◊ Repletion of other organisms which compete with C. Difficile
◊ In children, some success with IV gamma globulin

POSSIBLE COMPLICATIONS
• Dehydration
• Hypoalbuminemia
• Shock
• Perforation
• Toxic megacolon
• Death

EXPECTED COURSE AND PROGNOSIS
• If treated, virtually all patients recover
• Relapses do occur
• Untreated, 10-30% mortality
• In severely ill, colectomy sometimes required

MISCELLANEOUS

ASSOCIATED CONDITIONS
• Surgery
• Spinal fracture
• Intestinal obstruction
• Colon cancer

AGE-RELATED FACTORS
Pediatric:
• Unusual in children, but does occur
• Most infants are carriers; may become invasive in children with malignancy or Hirschsprung's disease
Geriatric: The elderly have a higher mortality rate from pseudomembranous colitis
Others: N/A

PREGNANCY   Serious complication if it occurs during pregnancy

SYNONYMS
• Antibiotic associated colitis
• Pseudomembranous enterocolitis

ICD-9-CM   564.1

SEE ALSO   N/A

OTHER NOTES   N/A

ABBREVIATIONS   N/A

REFERENCES
• Fekety, R. & Akshay, S.: Diagnosis and treatment of Clostridium difficile. JAMA, 269:71-75, Jan, 1993
• Leung, D., et al.: Treatment with intravenously administered gamma globulin of chronic relapsing colitis induced by Clostridium difficile toxin. Jour of Pediatr. 118:633-7, Apr, 1991
• Bartlett, J.G.: Antibiotic-associated diarrhea. Clinical Infect Dis. 15:573-81, Oct, 1992
• Fualman, S., et al.: Clostridial difficile invasion & toxin circulation in fatal pediatric pseudomembranous colitis. Amer J Clin Patholo. 94:410-6, Oct, 1990
• McFarland, L., Surawicz, C., & Stamm, W.: Risk factors for C. difficile carriage and C. difficile associated diarrhea in a cohort of hospitalized patients. Jour of Infect Dis. 162:678-84, 1990

Author   E. McCord, M.D.

Psittacosis

 BASICS

DESCRIPTION
Psittacosis is the clinical manifestation of a respiratory infection with the bacteria Chlamydia psittaci. The infection is virtually always contracted from an infected bird. Human to human transmission is rare.
• Pneumonia, bronchitis and fever of unknown origin (FUO) are most common diagnoses
• Can range from sub-clinical respiratory infection to severe systemic infection. Severity of illness may vary with strain of C. psittaci.

System(s) affected: Pulmonary

Genetics: No known genetic predisposition

Incidence in USA: .04-.08/100,000. 100-200 cases/year reported to Centers for Disease Control. True incidence probably greater.

Prevalence in USA:
• .003-.006/100,000
• Outbreaks may occur, usually associated with occupational exposure to infected turkeys or ducks

Predominant age: Adults

Predominant sex: Male = Female

SIGNS AND SYMPTOMS
• Onset usually acute but may be insidious
• Fever (often > 39° C)
• Chills
• Cough (may develop later, usually non-productive)
• Headache (may be severe)
• Malaise
• Anorexia
• Myalgias
• Confusion
• Vomiting and/or diarrhea
• Abdominal pain
• Pleuritic chest pain
• Hemoptysis
• Dyspnea without wheezing
• Arthralgias
• Sore throat
• Hoarseness
• Epistaxis
• Photophobia
• Tachycardia
• Retractions
• Flaring
• Cyanosis
• Crepitations more common than signs of consolidation
• Auscultation may be normal even with pneumonia
• Relative bradycardia
• Tender hepatomegaly and splenomegaly
• Horder's spots (faint, reddish brown, blanching rash)
• Petechiae

CAUSES
Infection with Chlamydia psittaci (Arthus type immunologic reaction to inhaled avian antigen)

RISK FACTORS
Exposure to infected bird(s), usually a pet pigeon or parakeet, or occupational exposure at a turkey or duck processing plant. Infected birds may appear healthy.

 DIAGNOSIS

DIFFERENTIAL DIAGNOSIS
• Consider other common bacterial respiratory pathogens including Streptococcus pneumoniae, Hemophilus influenzae, Klebsiella pneumoniae, Chlamydia pneumoniae, Mycoplasma pneumoniae, and Legionella species
• Early symptoms may suggest influenza, typhoid fever or mononucleosis

LABORATORY
• Leukocyte count often normal or low
• Erythrocyte sedimentation rate (ESR) usually elevated
• Sputum usually negative by gram stain and routine culture
• Proteinuria possible during febrile period
• Liver enzymes may be elevated
• Increased IgG, IgM, IgA
• Leukocytes with left shift
• Hypoxemia
• Hypocapnia
• Eosinophilia

Drugs that may alter lab results: Serologic response may be blunted by early treatment with tetracycline

Disorders that may alter lab results: N/A

PATHOLOGICAL FINDINGS
• Alveolar phagocyte and lymphocyte infiltrate
• Granuloma formation
• Bronchial wall thickening
• Type III and IV immune complex deposition
• Diffuse miliary nodules

SPECIAL TESTS
• Culture requires special facilities and is rarely done
• Sera for serology should be collected 2 to 3 weeks apart (3-4 weeks for micro-immunofluorescence, and a second convalescent sera at 6-8 weeks if the pattern is uninterpretable)
• Complement fixation (CF) test most common serologic test for psittacosis, but is also positive with C. pneumoniae (a much more common respiratory pathogen) and C. trachomatis infections
• A fourfold rise in CF titer is diagnostic of an acute infection with Chlamydia
• A single or stable CF titer of > 1:64 suggests a recent infection
• The species specific micro-immunofluorescence test for C. psittaci is preferred, but not as widely available as the CF test

IMAGING
• Chest radiograph often shows patchy alveolar infiltrates of interstitial pneumonitis and small nodular densities
• Lobar consolidation less common
• Hilar adenopathy
• Pleural effusion possible but usually scanty
• Radiographic abnormalities may persist for several months after successful treatment

DIAGNOSTIC PROCEDURES
None

 TREATMENT

APPROPRIATE HEALTH CARE
• Outpatient
• Patients with dyspnea, hypoxia, confusion or other signs or severe disease should be hospitalized

GENERAL MEASURES
• History of avian exposure (particularly to a sick bird) is key to making early diagnosis
• Treatment depends primarily on severity of respiratory symptoms. Severely ill patients may require oxygen, intravenous fluids and antibiotics.
• While human to human transmission is rare, sputum and respiratory secretion precautions should be observed

ACTIVITY
Based on disease severity. No disease-specific restrictions.

DIET
No special diet

PATIENT EDUCATION
American Lung Association, 1740 Broadway, New York, NY 10019, (212)315-8700

MEDICATIONS

DRUG(S) OF CHOICE
• Tetracycline 500 mg po qid for 14-21 days
• Doxycycline (Vibramycin) 100 mg po bid for 14-21 days or 100 mg IV q 12 hrs
Contraindications: History of allergic reaction to the medication
Precautions: Avoid dairy products and sun exposure. Reduce dosage in renal failure. Avoid using after the first trimester in pregnancy or in children less than 8 years old (causes permanent discoloration of teeth).
Significant possible interactions: Refer to manufacturer's profile of each drug

ALTERNATIVE DRUGS
• Erythromycin also has in vitro activity and can be used at doses of 500 mg po qid for 14 to 21 days
• Rifampin (Rifadin, Rimactane) has in vitro activity and has been used in doses of 600 to 1200 mg po per day with erythromycin to treat endocarditis due to C. psittaci
• Beta-lactam (penicillin based) antibiotics not effective
• Chloramphenicol may be effective, based on several case reports, but not generally recommended due to its association with severe and fatal blood dyscrasias. Better to use safer, effective drugs.

FOLLOWUP

PATIENT MONITORING
Determined by severity of illness in the acute period. No disease-specific monitoring.

PREVENTION/AVOIDANCE
• Report to local health department
• Identify source of the infection if possible
• Public health surveillance of poultry flocks and pet shops
• Prophylactic antibiotic treatment with doxycycline (100 mg po qd for 10 days) has been advocated for people with known exposure

POSSIBLE COMPLICATIONS
• Meningitis and encephalitis
• Endocarditis, pericarditis and myocarditis
• Renal failure
• Erythema nodosum
• Sinusitis
• Respiratory failure
• Reactive arthritis (rare)
• Disseminated intravascular coagulation (rare)
• Valvular heart disease (rare)
• Spontaneous abortion (rare)
• Thyroiditis (rare)
• Pancreatitis (rare)

EXPECTED COURSE AND PROGNOSIS
• Mortality rate less than 1% with appropriate treatment
• Patients usually respond within 24 to 48 hours following initiation of appropriate antibiotic therapy
• Full recovery may take weeks to months
• Relapse may occur necessitating second course of antibiotics
• Chest radiograph may not return to normal for up to 4 months

MISCELLANEOUS

ASSOCIATED CONDITIONS
None known

AGE-RELATED FACTORS
Pediatric: Uncommon in pediatric age group
Geriatric: Mortality rate may be higher in elderly or debilitated patients
Others: None

PREGNANCY
Spontaneous abortion has been reported with infection with some C. psittaci strains, primarily acquired from contact with sheep

SYNONYMS
• Ornithosis
• Bird breeder's disease
• Bird fancier's lung

ICD-9-CM
• 073.0 to 073.9
• 495.8 - other specified allergic alveolitis and pneumonitis

SEE ALSO
• Chlamydia pneumoniae
• Q fever

OTHER NOTES
• Incubation period ranges from 5 to 40 days; usually 7 to 15 days
• No persistent immunity to reinfection

ABBREVIATIONS
N/A

REFERENCES
• Macfarlane, J.T.and Macrae, A.D.: Psittacosis. Br Med Bull. 39:163-167, 1983
• Schachter, J., and Dawson, C.L.: Human Chlamydial Infections. Littleton, Massachusetts, PSG Publishing Company, 1978
• Meyer, K.F.: The ecology of psittacosis and ornithosis. Medicine. 21:175-206, 1942

Author D. Thom, M.D., Ph.D.

Psoriasis

 BASICS

 DIAGNOSIS

 TREATMENT

BASICS

DESCRIPTION Genetically determined common, chronic, epidermal proliferative disease. Clinically characterized by erythematous, dry scaling patches, recurring remissions and exacerbations. Flares may be related to systemic and environmental factors. Usual course - acute; chronic; unpredictable.
Clinical forms:
◊ Discoid or plaque psoriasis - most common, patches appear on scalp, trunk and limbs, nails may be pitted and/or thickened
◊ Guttate psoriasis - occurs most frequently in children, numerous small patches over wide area of skin, but greatest on the trunk
◊ Pustular psoriasis - small pustules over the body or confined to one area (i.e., palms and soles)
◊ Inverse flexural psoriasis - affects the flexural areas, lesions are moist and without scales (common in older people)
◊ Erythroderma (exfoliative psoriasis or red man syndrome) - patients skin turns red, may result from a flare of pre-existing dermatosis
◊ Ostraceous - grossly hyperkeratotic
Genetics:
• Genetic predisposition
• Higher incidence in Caucasians and atopic families
• Increased incidence of human leukocyte antigens (HLA antigens)
System(s) affected: Skin/Exocrine
Incidence/Prevalence in USA: 1000-2000 cases/100,000 people in the U.S.
Predominant age: Usually appears between ages 10 and 30, but can develop in infants and in the elderly
Predominant sex: Male = Female

SIGNS AND SYMPTOMS
• Arthritis
• Pruritus
• Silvery scales on red plaques
• Knee-elbow-scalp distribution
• Stippled nails and pitting
• Positive Auspitz's sign (underlying pinpoints of bleeding)
• Koebner's phenomenon (psoriatic response in previously unaffected area 1-2 weeks after skin injury)

CAUSES Possible genetic error in mitotic control

RISK FACTORS
• Local trauma
• Local irritation
• Infection (streptococcal pharyngitis can stimulate acute guttate psoriasis, HIV)
• Endocrine changes
• Stress (physical and emotional)
• Sudden withdrawal of systemic and/or potent topical steroids
• Alcohol use
• Obesity

DIAGNOSIS

DIFFERENTIAL DIAGNOSIS
• Scalp - seborrheic dermatitis
• Body folds - intertrigo or candidiasis
• Nails - onychomycosis
• Trunk - pityriasis rosea, pityriasis rubra pilaris, tinea corporis
• Squamous cell carcinoma
• Secondary and tertiary syphilis
• Cutaneous lupus erythematosus
• Eczema (nummular)
• Lichen planus
• Localized scratch dermatitis (lichen simplex chronicus)
• Mycosis fungoides
• Reiter's disease
• Subcorneal pustulosis

LABORATORY
• Negative rheumatoid factor
• Latex fixation test
• Leukocytosis and increased sedimentation rate often seen, especially in pustular psoriasis
• Fungal studies - may show a superimposed infection
• Uric acid increases in 10-20%
Drugs that may alter lab results: N/A
Disorders that may alter lab results: N/A

PATHOLOGICAL FINDINGS
• Parakeratosis (focal), especially with neutrophils
• Hyperkeratosis
• Hypogranulosis
• Epidermal hyperplasia
• Elongation and thickening of rete ridges
• Thin epidermis above dermal papillae
• Spongiform pustule of Kogoj
• Munro's microabscess
• Abnormal mitoses
• Dilated tortuous capillary loops
• "Squirting" papillae

SPECIAL TESTS Biopsy

IMAGING N/A

DIAGNOSTIC PROCEDURES Usually diagnosis accomplished by inspection, occasionally biopsy required.

TREATMENT

APPROPRIATE HEALTH CARE
• Outpatient usually
• May require inpatient for severe cases or for treatment. Emergency: Severe and unstable forms like acute pustular psoriasis (Von Zumbusch's) or acute erythroderma.

GENERAL MEASURES
• Solar radiation
• Mild disease - ultraviolet radiation (UVA, UVB)
• Medication to soften scale, followed by soft brush while bathing
• Oatmeal baths for itching
• Tar shampoos
• Avoid excessive sun exposure
• Desert climates provide a favorable effect for some patients
• Wet dressings may help relieve pruritis
• For extensive, recalcitrant psoriasis, a referral to a specialist in psoriatic therapy is suggested

ACTIVITY No restrictions

DIET No special diet

PATIENT EDUCATION
• Provide patient reassurance and anxiety relief to the extent possible
• Assurance to patient and family the condition is non-contagious
• For patient education materials favorably reviewed on this topic, contact: American Academy of Family Physicians Foundation, P.O. Box 8418, Kansas City, MO 64114, (800)274-2237, ext. 4400
• National Psoriasis Foundation, Suite 200, 6415 SW Canyon Court, Portland, OR 97221, (503)297-1545

MEDICATIONS

DRUG(S) OF CHOICE
Mild disease:
◊ Calamine or starch lotion - to start treatment
◊ Topical corticosteroid creams and ointments medium to high strength tid-qid (overnight occlusion with plastic wrap will hasten resolution). Switching from one product to another when efficacy diminishes prevents tachyphylaxis
◊ Tar compounds (Estar gel, PsoriGel) may be beneficial when alternated with topical steroids. Tar bath preparations for widespread involvement.
◊ Keratolytic agents - salicylic acid 6% gel may be alternated with topical steroids, especially with hyperkeratosis
◊ Corticosteroid solutions and tar shampoos - for treatment of scalp lesions
◊ Ultraviolet light including sunlight is effective. Lamps are available for home use.
◊ Anthralin ointment 1% may be useful for adjunctive treatment. Use prior to ultraviolet light (UVA, UVB). Mid-potency topical corticosteroid mometasone furoate is less atrophegenic. Three most potent steroids - halobetasol, betametharone dipronionate, or clobetasol are limited to 2 week use.
Severe disease:
◊ Goeckerman's regimen - patient receives tar and ultraviolet light in an outpatient treatment facility or as an inpatient
◊ Methotrexate - single weekly dose (25mg, ten 2.5mg tabs) or 2.5mg q12h for 3-4 days per week have proven effective, but precautions in its use are necessary. Also azathioprine and intralesional cyclosporine.
◊ Corticosteroids (po) only for severe or life-threatening diseaase
◊ PUVA (psoralen plus ultraviolet light) - very effective, but causes skin-aging and cataracts and increases risk of skin cancers
◊ Etretinate - for severe psoriasis (especially pustular) not responsive to standard treatments
◊ Isotretinoin - may work on some patients
◊ Triamcinolone (intralesional) - mix with procaine or normal saline for concentrate of 4 mg/mL. Administered with syringe or dermajet. Effective in treating solitary resistant plaques and psoriasis involving the nails.
◊ Vitamin D analogs (calcipotriol ointment not available in USA)
◊ Tacrolimus - only for recalcitrant psoriasis (possible nephrotoxicity)
Contraindications: Refer to manufacturer's literature
Precautions: Refer to manufacturer's literature
Significant possible interactions: Refer to manufacturer's literature

ALTERNATIVE DRUGS N/A

 ## FOLLOWUP

PATIENT MONITORING
• Continuous supportive care
• Medications used in treatment require close followup. Certain lab studies may be necessary. Long-term use of topicals is not recommended.

PREVENTION/AVOIDANCE
• Avoid irritating drugs
• Avoid stimulating drugs (lithium, beta-adrenergic blockers, antimalarials, tetracycline, NSAID's, and pustular flares with steroids, amiodarone, morphine, procaine, potassium iodide, salicylates, sulfapyridine, sulfonamides and penicillin)
• Avoid antimalarial medications (aminoquinolone compounds)

POSSIBLE COMPLICATIONS
• Pustular psoriasis
• Exfoliative erythrodermatitis
• Rebound of the psoriatic process after corticosteroids are discontinued

EXPECTED COURSE AND PROGNOSIS
• Usually benign
• Life-threatening forms do occur
• May be refractory to treatment

 ## MISCELLANEOUS

ASSOCIATED CONDITIONS
• Extensive erythrodermic psoriasis may accompany AIDS
• Arthritis
• Psoriatic arthritis
• Myopathy
• Enteropathy
• Spondylitic heart disease
• Acute anterior uveitis

AGE-RELATED FACTORS
Pediatric:
• Onset common before age 10, rarely before age 3
• Disease may be atypical in its course compared to adults
Geriatric:
• About 3% of psoriasis patients acquire the disease after age 65
• Detailed drug history important, since many drugs (e.g., beta-blockers) can exacerbate psoriasis
• If using cytotoxic medications for treatment of psoriasis, closely follow hepatic and renal functions, and creatinine clearance
• Elderly patients may have difficulty with application of topicals over all affected body parts
Others: N/A

PREGNANCY Unpredictable effect on disease

SYNONYMS N/A

ICD-9-CM 696.1 psoriasis

SEE ALSO N/A

OTHER NOTES N/A

ABBREVIATIONS N/A

REFERENCES
• Habif, T.: Clinical Dermatology. 2nd Ed. St. Louis, C.V. Mosby, 1990
• Abel, E.: Diagnosis of drug induced psoriasis. Seminars in Dermatology. Vol. 11, No. 4, Dec, 1992
• Jegsothy, B., et al.: Tacrolimus (FK 506): A new therapeutic agent for severe recalcitrant psoriasis. Arc Dermatol. Vol. 128, Jun, 1992
• Ho, V.C. & Zioty, D.: Immunosuppressive Agents in Dermatology. Dermatology Clinics. Vol. 11, No. 1, Jan, 1993
• Moschella, S., et al. (eds.): Dermatology. 3rd Ed. Philadelphia, W.B. Saunders Co., 1992

Author P. Jaster, M.D.

Psoriatic arthritis

 BASICS

DESCRIPTION Arthritis associated with psoriasis. Serologic tests for the rheumatoid factor are usually negative. Patients exhibit sausage-shaped digits and characteristic radiologic changes. Psoriatic arthropathy occurs in about 5% of individuals with psoriasis, especially those with psoriatic nail disease. There are several forms that have been described although the separation into these forms is not distinct. They are called by different descriptive terms by various authors.
Forms of psoriatic arthropathy:
◊ Psoriatic nail disease and distal interphalangeal involvement (classic psoriatic arthritis). Characteristics - nail pitting, transverse depressions, subungual hyperkeratosis, distal interphalangeal arthritis.
◊ Arthritis mutilans - a destructive, resorptive arthropathy. Produces the so-called opera-glass hand.
◊ Symmetric polyarthropathy resembling rheumatoid arthritis - may rarely be indistinguishable from RA and may represent coincidental rheumatoid arthritis in a patient who has psoriasis
◊ Asymmetric oligoarthropathy - little relationship between joint and skin activity; joints involved may be both large and small
◊ Psoriatic spondylitis - asymmetrical spondylitis and sacroiliitis
System(s) affected: Musculoskeletal, Skin/Exocrine
Genetics: HLA-B27 usually present in patients with spondylitis-type psoriatic arthropathy. Psoriasis itself is associated with HLA-B13, HLA-Bw17, HLA-Cw6, HLABw38, HLA-DR4 and HLA-DR7
Incidence in USA: Uncommon
Prevalence in USA: Uncommon, approximately 5% of individuals with psoriatic skin disease
Predominant age: Onset age 30-35
Predominant sex: Female > Male (slightly)

SIGNS AND SYMPTOMS
• Joint swelling, tenderness, warmth, restricted movement
• Distribution of arthritis - any joint, but most common in distal interphalangeal joints of the hands and sacroiliac
• Nail changes - pitting, transverse ridging, onycholysis, keratosis, yellowing and destruction of the entire nail
• Fever
• Malaise
• Other symptoms applying characteristically to the several types of psoriatic arthropathy. See description.

CAUSES
• Unknown
• Probably genetically related

RISK FACTORS
• Psoriasis
• Positive family history

 DIAGNOSIS

DIFFERENTIAL DIAGNOSIS
• Psoriasis
• Seropositive inflammatory polyarthritis
• Rheumatoid arthritis
• Osteoarthritis
• Gout
• Reiter's syndrome

LABORATORY
• Serum rheumatoid factor - negative
• Elevated erythrocyte sedimentation rate
• Elevated uric acid
• Anemia
Drugs that may alter lab results: N/A
Disorders that may alter lab results: N/A

PATHOLOGICAL FINDINGS Synovitis (resembling rheumatoid arthritis)

SPECIAL TESTS N/A

IMAGING
X-ray
◊ Gross destructive changes of isolated small joints
◊ Peripheral arthritis mutilans
◊ Fluffy periostitis
◊ Atypical spondylitis with syndesmophyte formation
◊ Absence of osteoporosis
◊ Erosions, ankylosis, sacroiliitis
◊ Acro osteolysis, "pencil-in-cup" appearance
◊ Extensive bone resorption to cause "opera-glass hand"
◊ Asymmetry sacroiliitis

DIAGNOSTIC PROCEDURES Special attention to nail pitting and distal interphalangeal joints

 TREATMENT

APPROPRIATE HEALTH CARE
Outpatient

GENERAL MEASURES
• Immobilizing splints
• Isometric exercises and swimming later
• Paraffin baths or other heat therapy
• Protect affected joints
• Regular, moderate exposure to sun

ACTIVITY Encourage exercise (particularly swimming) to maintain strength and flexibility

DIET No special diet

PATIENT EDUCATION
• Stress non-contagious
• Arthritis Foundation referral
• For patient education materials favorably reviewed on this topic, contact: American Academy of Family Physicians Foundation, P.O. Box 8418, Kansas City, MO 64114, (800)274-2237, ext. 4400 and/or Arthritis Foundation, 1314 Spring Street N.W., Atlanta, GA 30309, (404)872-7100

MEDICATIONS

DRUG(S) OF CHOICE
<u>Several options available depending on involvement of skin and joints:</u>
◊ Nonsteroidal anti-inflammatory drugs in usual doses. There is no evidence for superiority of any one NSAID in psoriatic arthritis
    ◊ Low-dose systemic steroids
    ◊ Topical steroids for skin
    ◊ PUVA therapy may be helpful for skin lesions
<u>Others sometimes useful:</u>
◊ Methotrexate (used only specific guidelines and by someone experienced with its use. Contraindicated in HIV positive patients).
    ◊ Gold salts
    ◊ Antimalarials (controversial)
    ◊ Immunosuppressives in resistant cases
    ◊ Sulfasalazine

Contraindications:
• Antimalarials can provoke exfoliative dermatitis
• NSAID's may flare psoriasis

Precautions: Phenylbutazone may cause bone marrow depression. NSAID's and ASA may cause gastritis. Refer to manufacturer's literature.

Significant possible interactions: NSAID's may impair methotrexate secretion and cause methotrexate toxicity. Refer to manufacturer's literature.

ALTERNATIVE DRUGS
Etretinate 0.5-1.0 mg/kg/day in 2 divided doses (severe side effects, avoid during pregnancy since it is highly teratogenic)

FOLLOWUP

PATIENT MONITORING
Frequent for medication adjustment and encouragement

PREVENTION/AVOIDANCE   N/A

POSSIBLE COMPLICATIONS
• Chronicity
• Severe deforming arthritis (arthritis mutilans)
• Spondylitic form of arthritis with sacroiliitis and spinal involvement

EXPECTED COURSE AND PROGNOSIS
• Course - acute, intermittent
• More favorable than rheumatoid arthritis (except for arthritis mutilans)
• Treatment of skin lesions often improves arthritic symptoms

MISCELLANEOUS

ASSOCIATED CONDITIONS   Psoriasis

AGE-RELATED FACTORS
Pediatric: Not seen in this age group
Geriatric: Arthritic symptoms worse
Others: N/A

PREGNANCY   N/A

SYNONYMS   Psoriasis, arthropathic

ICD-9-CM   696.0

SEE ALSO   N/A

OTHER NOTES   N/A

ABBREVIATIONS   N/A

REFERENCES
• Kelley, W.N., Harris, E.D. & Ruddy, S., et al.: Textbook of Rheumatology. 4th Ed. Philadelphia, W.B. Saunders, 1993
• McCarty, D.J. & Koopman, W.J. (eds.): Arthritis and Allied Disorders. 12th Ed. Philadelphia, Lea & Febiger, 1993

Author   J. Boyer, M.D.

Puerperal infection

BASICS

DESCRIPTION Bacterial infection of the genital tract following delivery. Includes perineal cellulitis, vaginal and cervical infections (all uncommon), necrotizing faciitis (rare), endomyometritis, pelvic cellulitis, septic pelvic thrombophlebitis, parametrial phlegmon.
System(s) affected: Reproductive
Genetics: N/A
Incidence in USA:
• Vaginal deliveries - 2% or 64,000 cases per year
• Cesarean sections - 13 %+ or 104,000 cases per year
Prevalence in USA: N/A
Predominant age: Teens at higher risk
Predominant sex: Female only

SIGNS AND SYMPTOMS
• Fever > 38°C (100.4°F)
• Localized pain and swelling
• Chills
• Abdominal pain
• Foul-smelling lochia
• Uterine tenderness on exam
• Peritonitis with severe pain, ileus
• Septic shock

CAUSES
• Puerperal infections often begin as wound infections following laceration of perineum, vagina, cervix, or the abdominal wound of C-section. Also, the entire endometrium is susceptible, especially at the site of placental attachment.
• Polymicrobial infections; primary pathogen often unclear
Commonly found bacteria include:
◊ Aerobes/ facultative aerobes - Group A, B, and D Streptococci, Enterococcus, gram-negative bacteria (E. coli, Klebsiella and Proteus sp), Staphylococcus aureus, Staph. epidermidis, Gardnerella vaginalis, Hemophilus influenza
◊ Anaerobes - Peptococcus sp., Peptostreptococcus sp., Bacteroides bivius, B. fragilis, B. disiens, Clostridium sp., Fusobacterium sp.
◊ Other - Mycoplasma hominis, Chlamydia trachomatis, Urea urealyticum

RISK FACTORS
• Bacterial contamination (cervical exams, fetal monitoring devices, or operative manipulation)
• Blood loss
• C-section - risk increased following prolapse of umbilical cord or fetal extremity
• Diabetes
• Drug addiction
• History of sexually transmitted diseases
• Immune deficiency
• Poverty

• Malnutrition
• Obesity
• Pre-existing chorioamnionitis
• Pre-term labor
• Premature rupture of membranes
• Prolonged labor
• Trauma
• Bacterial vaginosis
• Group B Streptococcus

DIAGNOSIS

DIFFERENTIAL DIAGNOSIS Fever from other sources - urinary tract infection, respiratory infection, mastitis or breast engorgement, thrombophlebitis, wound infection

LABORATORY
• CBC
• Genital tract cultures
• Amniotic fluid smear for WBC's and bacteria
• Blood cultures
Drugs that may alter lab results: Previous antibiotics may alter culture results
Disorders that may alter lab results: N/A

PATHOLOGICAL FINDINGS
• Microscopic sections show a superficial layer of infected necrotic material
• Peritonitis (caused by lymphatic spread)
• Phlegmon may form in the leaves of the broad ligament, usually after C-section. Rarely this forms an abscess.
• Thrombosis may involve any of the pelvic veins, including the inferior vena cava

SPECIAL TESTS N/A

IMAGING
• CT or MRI for thrombophlebitis
• Ultrasound (sensitive for abscess)

DIAGNOSTIC PROCEDURES
Culdocentesis with culture

TREATMENT

APPROPRIATE HEALTH CARE
Inpatient

GENERAL MEASURES
• IV antibiotics and close observation
• Infected wounds should be opened to establish drainage
• Necrotizing fasciitis requires wide débridement
• Peritonitis requires imaging to evaluate the cause
• Surgery may be needed to establish drainage or decompress the bowel
• Surgical drainage of a phlegmon is not advised unless suppurative
• Normalize fluid status

ACTIVITY As tolerated

DIET As tolerated, may be limited by ileus

PATIENT EDUCATION
• Avoidance of sexually transmitted diseases
• Prenatal discussion of premature rupture of membranes and preterm labor

MEDICATIONS

DRUG(S) OF CHOICE
Preferred:
◊ Ampicillin 1-2 gm IV q 6 hr, plus
◊ Metronidazole 7.5 mg/kg/q6h, plus
◊ Gentamicin 2 mg/kg/day in divided doses
Others have been shown to be effective:
◊ Beta-lactam antibiotic alone (ampicillin, cefoxitin, others)
◊ Clindamycin 1200-2700 mg/d in divided doses plus gentamicin
◊ Metronidazole plus gentamicin
◊ Chloramphenicol plus beta-lactam antibiotic for severe pelvic sepsis
Oral antibiotics
◊ Amoxicillin 500 mg TID has been used after patient afebrile for 24 hours. Not necessary in most cases.

Contraindications:
• Drug allergy
• Renal failure (aminoglycosides)
• Avoid chloramphenicol, sulfa, tetracyclines, fluoroquinolones before delivery or if breast-feeding

Precautions:
• Chloramphenicol rarely causes bone marrow suppression
• Clindamycin, others, occasionally cause pseudomembranous colitis
Significant possible interactions: Refer to manufacturer's literature

ALTERNATIVE DRUGS
• Piperacillin, mezlocillin, cefoperazone, ampicillin/sulbactam, cefotetan, cefotaxime, others
• Base therapy on cultures, sensitivities, and clinical response

FOLLOWUP

PATIENT MONITORING
Individualize according to severity

PREVENTION/AVOIDANCE
• Regular prenatal care
• Patient education regarding premature rupture of membranes and pre-term labor
• Minimize iatrogenic causes - cervical exams, fetal monitoring
• Prophylactic antibiotics for C-section if high risk

POSSIBLE COMPLICATIONS
• Infertility (uncommon)
• Need for surgery
• Shock
• Death

EXPECTED COURSE AND PROGNOSIS
• Depends on location and severity
• Most have dramatic response to therapy. If not, consider retained products of conception, abscess, hematoma, septic pelvic thrombophlebitis, or wound infection.

MISCELLANEOUS

ASSOCIATED CONDITIONS
See Risk Factors

AGE-RELATED FACTORS N/A
Pediatric: N/A
Geriatric: N/A
Others: Teen pregnancies at higher risk

PREGNANCY
A complication of pregnancy

SYNONYMS
• Endometritis
• Endoparametritis
• Endomyometritis
• Metritis with pelvic cellulitis

ICD-9-CM 615.9

SEE ALSO N/A

ABBREVIATIONS N/A

OTHER NOTES
Interpret WBC with care; may be as high as 20,000 as physiologic leucocytosis

REFERENCES
Cunningham, F.G., MacDonald, P.C. & Gant, N.F. (eds.): Williams Obstetrics. 18th Ed. Norwalk, CT, Appleton and Lange, 1989

Author R. Scott, M.D.

Pulmonary edema

BASICS

DESCRIPTION Pulmonary interstitial and/or alveolar fluid accumulation that results when the forces moving fluid out of the pulmonary capillary exceed the forces restraining that fluid
System(s) affected: Cardiovascular, Pulmonary
Genetics: Multifactorial
Incidence/Prevalence in USA:
Approximately 150,000 persons per year in U.S. affected with non-cardiogenic pulmonary edema
Predominant age: Middle age and elderly
Predominant sex: Male = Female

SIGNS AND SYMPTOMS
- Shortness of breath
- Dyspnea with exertion
- Anxiety
- Orthopnea, paroxysmal nocturnal dyspnea
- Cough
- Nocturnal angina
- Wheezing
- Weakness, fatigue
- Other symptoms depending on etiology
- Breathlessness, air hunger
- Noisy respirations
- Anxiety
- Cough, often accompanied by pink or blood-tinged and frothy sputum
- Tachycardia and tachypnea
- Dilated alae nasi
- Inspiratory retraction of the intercostal spaces and/or supraventricular fossae
- Cheyne-Stokes respirations
- Diaphoretic, cold, ashen, or cyanotic skin
- Moist, crepitant rales noted initially at bases and progressing to apices
- Rhonchi, wheezes, and gurgles
- Elevated jugular venous pulse
- Increased P2
- S3
- S4
- Pulsus alternans or presence of valvular heart disease
- Lower extremity edema
- Other signs depending on etiology

CAUSES
Cardiogenic
- ◊ Left heart failure
- ◊ Ischemic heart disease
- ◊ Acute myocardial infarction
- ◊ Aortic and mitral valvular disease
- ◊ Hypertensive heart disease
- ◊ Cardiomyopathy
- ◊ Volume overload
- ◊ Arrhythmias
- ◊ Endocarditis
- ◊ Myocarditis
- ◊ Congenital heart disease
- ◊ Acute rheumatic fever and rheumatic heart disease
- ◊ Septal defects
- ◊ Cardiac tamponade
- ◊ High cardiac output states (e.g., thyrotoxicosis, beriberi)

Noncardiogenic
- ◊ Shock
- ◊ Multiple trauma
- ◊ Infection/sepsis (especially pneumonia)
- ◊ Liquid aspiration (e.g., drowning, gastric contents)
- ◊ Inhaled toxic gases
- ◊ Pulmonary lymphatic obstruction
- ◊ Drug overdose (especially narcotics)
- ◊ High-altitude illness
- ◊ Pancreatitis
- ◊ Embolism (thrombus, fat, air, amniotic fluid)
- ◊ Neurogenic
- ◊ Hematologic and immunologic disorders
- ◊ Disorders associated with high negative pleural pressure
- ◊ Radiation pneumonitis
- ◊ Disseminated intravascular coagulation
- ◊ Eclampsia
- ◊ Decreased plasma oncotic pressure (e.g., hypoalbuminemia)
- ◊ Postcardioversion, postanesthesia, postcardiopulmonary bypass
- ◊ Oxygen toxicity
- ◊ ARDS

RISK FACTORS Dependent on etiology

DIAGNOSIS

DIFFERENTIAL DIAGNOSIS
- Most important distinction is cardiogenic versus noncardiogenic pulmonary edema
- Pneumonia
- Asthma
- COPD exacerbation
- Pulmonary embolism
- Hyperventilation syndrome

LABORATORY
- None specific for pulmonary edema; laboratory abnormalities (e.g., creatine kinase (CK), amylase, etc.) may point to underlying etiology
- Hypoxemia
- Hypocarbia
- Respiratory alkalosis
- Increased A-a gradient
- Leukocytosis
Drugs that may alter lab results:
Administered oxygen may complicate arterial blood gas interpretation
Disorders that may alter lab results:
Underlying pulmonary disease from an unrelated etiology may complicate arterial blood gas interpretation

PATHOLOGICAL FINDINGS
Cardiogenic
- ◊ Heavy, wet, subcrepitant lungs
- ◊ Intra-alveolar granular pink precipitate
- ◊ Alveolar microhemorrhages and hemosiderin-laden macrophages
- ◊ "Brown induration", chronic passive congestion
- ◊ Hypostatic bronchopneumonia

Noncardiogenic
- ◊ Heavy, firm, red, and boggy lungs
- ◊ Interstitial and intra-alveolar edema, inflammation, fibrin deposition, hemorrhage, and patchy atelectasis
- ◊ Hyaline membrane formation
- ◊ Interstitial and intra-alveolar fibrosis

SPECIAL TESTS
- Arterial blood gas
- Electrocardiogram
- Pulmonary function tests
- Mixed venous oxygen saturation

IMAGING
- Two-dimensional echocardiography with Doppler may be useful in some cases of cardiogenic pulmonary edema (e.g., valvular heart disease, systolic vs. diastolic dysfunction)
- Chest x-ray (may be difficult or impossible to differentiate cardiogenic from noncardiogenic pulmonary edema)
Cardiogenic chest x-ray
- ◊ Interstitial edema
- ◊ Cardiomegaly
- ◊ Pulmonary venous redistribution
- ◊ Kerley's B lines
- ◊ Alveolar edema, initially perihilar
- ◊ Pleural effusions
Noncardiogenic chest x-ray
- ◊ Alveolar edema
- ◊ Cardiomegaly absent
- ◊ Pulmonary venous redistribution absent
- ◊ Pleural effusions less common

DIAGNOSTIC PROCEDURES
- Swan-Ganz catheter placement may help differentiate cardiogenic from noncardiogenic pulmonary edema
- Cardiac catheterization may be beneficial in some subclasses of cardiogenic pulmonary edema

TREATMENT

APPROPRIATE HEALTH CARE
Generally inpatient or intensive care; outpatient for mildest forms

GENERAL MEASURES
- Treatment of the underlying condition
- Patient sitting, with legs dangling
- Oxygen via nasal cannula, ventimask, or endotracheal intubation
- Rotating tourniquets or phlebotomy in selected cases
- Mechanical ventilation, often requiring positive end-expiratory pressure support

ACTIVITY Bedrest in most cases

DIET Low sodium diet

PATIENT EDUCATION
- Diet
- Symptoms and signs of pulmonary edema
- Medical compliance

MEDICATIONS

DRUG(S) OF CHOICE
Acute cardiogenic pulmonary edema
◊ Morphine sulfate 2-5 mg IV
◊ Furosemide 20-80 mg IV
◊ Nitroglycerin paste 1-2 inches
◊ In selected cases: Nitroglycerin drip beginning at 5μg/min and increasing by 5-10 μg/min every few minutes, titrating to blood pressure, etc. Nitroprusside IV drip beginning at 10 μg/min and increasing by 5-10 μg/min every few minutes, titrating to blood pressure, etc. Dobutamine 2 μg/kg/min IV titrating to blood pressure, cardiac output, pulmonary capillary wedge pressure, etc.
Chronic management of cardiogenic pulmonary edema
◊ Furosemide 20-400 mg daily
◊ Angiotensin converting enzyme inhibitors (e.g., captopril 6.25-25 mg po tid, lisinopril 2.5-20 mg po qd, enalapril 2.5-15 mg po qd-bid)
◊ Digoxin 0.125-0.25 mg po qd
◊ Hydralazine 10-100 mg po qid
◊ Isosorbide dinitrate 10-60 mg po tid-qid
◊ Thiazide diuretics (e.g., HCTZ 25-50 mg po qd)
Noncardiogenic pulmonary edema
◊ Oxygen
◊ Selected cardiovascular drugs to optimize tissue oxygen delivery
Contraindications: Refer to manufacturer's profile of each drug
Precautions:
• Avoid liberal intravenous fluids, especially normal saline or lactated Ringer's
• Avoid negative inotropic agents such as calcium channel blockers or beta-blockers in the setting of cardiogenic pulmonary edema
• Avoid high forced inspiratory O2 (FiO2) > 50% for prolonged periods of time if possible
• Avoid prolonged administration of nitroprusside due to risk of cyanide toxicity. If nitroprusside administered for > 72 hrs, obtain a thiocyanate level.
Significant possible interactions: Additive hypotensive effects of nitrates, afterload reducers, diuretics, etc.

ALTERNATIVE DRUGS
• Chlorothiazide
• Metolazone
• Acetazolamide
• Bumetanide
• Potassium-sparing diuretics

FOLLOWUP

PATIENT MONITORING
Inpatient
◊ Serial arterial blood gases or pulse oximetry, often in the intensive care unit with one-on-one nursing
◊ Strict measurement of intake and output
◊ Attention to optimal fluid management
◊ Attention to optimal ventilator settings
◊ Serial chest x-rays
Outpatient
◊ Attention to clinical status
◊ Serial weights to assess fluid accumulation

PREVENTION/AVOIDANCE   Compliance with medications and diet

POSSIBLE COMPLICATIONS
• Death
• Reversible or irreversible organ ischemia
• Pulmonary fibrosis, particularly with noncardiogenic pulmonary edema

EXPECTED COURSE AND PROGNOSIS
• Dependent on underlying etiology
• Mortality approximately 50-60% for noncardiogenic pulmonary edema and up to 80% for cardiogenic shock

MISCELLANEOUS

ASSOCIATED CONDITIONS   (see Causes)

AGE-RELATED FACTORS
Pediatric: Usually secondary to lung immaturity, congenital heart disease, or associated with trauma
Geriatric: Higher mortality
Others: N/A

PREGNANCY   An obstetrician and cardiologist or pulmonologist should be involved in care

SYNONYMS   N/A

ICD-9-CM
• 428.1 acute pulmonary edema with heart disease
• 518.4 acute edema of lung, not otherwise specified

SEE ALSO
• Congestive heart failure
• Adult respiratory distress syndrome

OTHER NOTES   N/A

ABBREVIATIONS
ARDS = adult respiratory distress syndrome

REFERENCES
• Ingram, R.H. and Braunwald, E.: Pulmonary edema. In Heart disease - A Textbook of Cardiovascular Medicine. 3rd Ed. Edited by E. Braunwald. Philadelphia, W.B. Saunders, Co., 1988
• Ingram, R.H. and Braunwald, E.: Dyspnea and pulmonary edema. In Harrison's Principles of Internal Medicine. 12th Ed. Edited by E. Braunwald. New York, McGraw-Hill, Inc., 1991

Author G. Pennock, M.D.

Pulmonary embolism

BASICS

DESCRIPTION Pulmonary embolism occurs when venous thrombi in the deep venous system of the legs dislodge and enter the pulmonary arterial circulation
<u>Pulmonary embolism presents as three different syndromes</u>
◊ Acute cor pulmonale - due to massive pulmonary embolism, obstructing > 60-75% of the pulmonary circulation
◊ Pulmonary Infarction - occurs in patients with submassive pulmonary embolism with complete obstruction of a distal branch of the pulmonary circulation
◊ Acute unexplained dyspnea - occurs in patients who do not develop acute cor pulmonale or pulmonary infarction
System(s) affected: Pulmonary, Cardiovascular
Genetics: N/A
Incidence/Prevalence in USA:
• 600,000-700,000 cases/year
• 100,000-200,000 deaths/year
Predominant age: Very rare in children, incidence increases with advancing age
Predominant sex: Male = Female

SIGNS AND SYMPTOMS
<u>Acute cor pulmonale</u>
◊ Syncope
◊ Hypotension or cardiac arrest
◊ Dyspnea
◊ Anxiety
◊ Tachypnea
◊ Tachycardia
◊ Distended neck veins
◊ S3 gallop
◊ Clear lungs to auscultation
◊ ± signs of deep venous thrombosis
◊ ECG - SIQ3T3 pattern or incomplete right bundle branch block
◊ Chest x-ray - usually normal
◊ Arterial blood gases (room air) decreased P02, decreased PCo2
<u>Pulmonary infarction</u>
◊ Pleuritic chest pain
◊ Dyspnea
◊ ± hemoptysis
◊ Tachypnea
◊ Lungs - rales, wheezes and/or signs of pleural effusion
◊ ± signs of deep venous thrombosis
◊ ECG - normal
◊ Chest x-ray - elevated hemidiaphragm, infiltrate or small pleural effusion
◊ Arterial blood gases (room air) - normal or decreased P02, decreased PC02, alkalosis
<u>Acute unexplained dyspnea</u>
◊ Dyspnea
◊ ± anxiety
◊ ± tachycardia
◊ Tachypnea
◊ Clear lungs
◊ ± signs of deep venous thrombosis
◊ ECG - usually normal
◊ Chest x-ray - normal

CAUSES Hypercoagulability (difficult to document)

RISK FACTORS
• Prolonged bed rest
• Advanced age
• Congestive heart failure
• Carcinoma
• Stroke
• Pregnancy
• Oral contraceptives
• Postoperative
• Trauma to legs
• Obesity

DIAGNOSIS

DIFFERENTIAL DIAGNOSIS
• Pneumonia
• Myocardial infarction
• Congestive heart failure
• Viral pleuritis
• Pericarditis

LABORATORY N/A
Drugs that may alter lab results: N/A
Disorders that may alter lab results: N/A

PATHOLOGICAL FINDINGS Pulmonary infarction

SPECIAL TESTS N/A

IMAGING
• The diagnosis is confirmed by V/Q lung scan (multiple segmental or lobar perfusion defects with normal ventilation), or pulmonary angiogram (intraluminal filling defects and/or arterial cutoffs)
• Chest x-ray may reveal parachymal infiltrate, pleural effusion

DIAGNOSTIC PROCEDURES
• Lung scan
• Pulmonary angiogram
• Diagnosis suspected on basis of signs and symptoms consistent with one of the three syndromes in a patient with deep venous thrombosis (DVT) or with risk factors for DVT

TREATMENT

APPROPRIATE HEALTH CARE
Hospitalization, ICU if hemodynamically unstable

GENERAL MEASURES
• Designed to maintain adequate cardiovascular and pulmonary functions and to prevent recurrence of emboli
• Oxygen therapy as needed

ACTIVITY
• Bed rest, move legs frequently
• Range-of-motion exercises when patient stable

DIET No special diet, need to maintain adequate nutrition and fluids

PATIENT EDUCATION N/A

MEDICATIONS

DRUG(S) OF CHOICE
• Intravenous heparin by continuous infusion, at dose to prolong partial thromboplastin time to 1.5 -2.0 times control for five to ten days. Usual regimen requires beginning with 50-75 units/kg load followed by 20-30 u/kg/hr. Check PTT 6 hours after beginning infusion, then daily.
• Warfarin beginning day one or day two of hospitalization for at least three months. Warfarin dose adjusted to prolong prothrombin time to 2.0 to 3.0 INR.
• In event of hypotension requiring vasopressors in a patient with angiographically documented pulmonary embolism, pulmonary embolectomy or intravenous thrombolytic agents may be required
Contraindications: Refer to manufacturer's profile of each drug
Precautions:
• Refer to manufacturer's profile of each drug
• The major complication of heparin is the possibility of hemorrhage. If PTT is appropriately adjusted, the major hemorrhage rate should be low.
Significant possible interactions: Refer to manufacturer's profile of each drug

ALTERNATIVE DRUGS
Surgery to interrupt the inferior vena cava, if needed, in patients who have recurrent emboli, or can't take anticoagulants

FOLLOWUP

PATIENT MONITORING
After hospital discharge, prothrombin time should be prolonged to 2.0 to 3.0 (INR). Warfarin should be continued for at least three months. In patients with continuous predisposition to DVT, it should be continued indefinitely.

PREVENTION/AVOIDANCE
Recognition of hospitalized patients with multiple risk factors for deep venous thrombosis and implementation of prophylactic therapy including low dose heparin, warfarin or leg compression devices

POSSIBLE COMPLICATIONS
• Pulmonary infarction
• Cor pulmonale
• Recurrent deep venous thrombosis or pulmonary embolism, post phlebitic syndrome
• Treatment failure requiring surgical venous interruption

EXPECTED COURSE AND PROGNOSIS
With appropriate therapy hospital mortality is less than 10%. Long-term prognosis determined by coexisting disease.

MISCELLANEOUS

ASSOCIATED CONDITIONS
• Occult cancer (lung, GI tract, breast, uterus, prostate)
• Deep vein thrombosis

AGE-RELATED FACTORS
Pediatric: Quite rare
Geriatric: More common, more often fatal.
Others: N/A

PREGNANCY
Higher risk of occurrence during pregnancy and puerperium

SYNONYMS N/A

ICD-9-CM
415.1 pulmonary embolism and infarction

SEE ALSO Deep vein thrombosis

OTHER NOTES N/A

ABBREVIATIONS N/A

REFERENCES
• Braunwald E., et al. (eds.): Harrison's Principles of Internal Medicine. 12th Ed. New York, McGraw-Hill, 1991
• Rippe, J.M., et al.: (eds.): Intensive Care Medicine. 2nd Ed. New York, Little, Brown, 1991. Pages 308-316

Author J. Dalen, M.D.

Pulmonic valvular stenosis

 BASICS

DESCRIPTION A congenital deformity consisting of obstruction to right ventricular outflow at the pulmonic valve level
System(s) affected: Cardiovascular
Genetics: N/A
Incidence/Prevalence in USA: 10% of congenital heart disease
Predominant age: Newborn, but often asymptomatic for years
Predominant sex: Male = Female

SIGNS AND SYMPTOMS
• History of heart murmur since birth
• Acyanotic
• Dyspnea and fatigue are the most frequent symptoms
• Occasionally dizziness or syncope occurs, particularly exertional, due to the low fixed cardiac output
• Chest pain can occur
• Myocardial infarction of the hypertrophied right ventricle has been noted
• Prominent A wave of the jugular venous pulse
• Right ventricular impulse
• Midsystolic murmur (increased duration and later peaking with increased severity)
• Pulmonic ejection sound
• Soft, delay in P2
• Occasional tricuspid regurgitation

CAUSES
• Congenital
• Rubella embryopathy

RISK FACTORS Family history

 DIAGNOSIS

DIFFERENTIAL DIAGNOSIS
• Dysplastic pulmonic valve stenosis
• Discrete infundibular stenosis
• Subinfundibular obstruction
• Isolated pulmonary artery stenosis
• Supravalvar pulmonary stenosis
• Tetralogy of Fallot (Pink)

LABORATORY N/A
Drugs that may alter lab results: N/A
Disorders that may alter lab results: N/A

PATHOLOGICAL FINDINGS N/A

SPECIAL TESTS ECG - generally sinus rhythm, occasional supraventricular arrhythmias, tall peaked P waves, rightward axis, severity correlates with R/S ratio in leads VI and V6, right ventricular hypertrophy

IMAGING
• X-ray - post stenotic dilatation of the pulmonary trunk, prominence of right atrium and ventricle
• Echocardiogram - mobile dome, thickened pulmonic valve, post stenotic dilatation of the pulmonary trunk, small valve annulus; continuous wave Doppler provides an estimate of the transvalvular gradient
• Color-flow Doppler - delineates are of obstruction

DIAGNOSTIC PROCEDURES
Cardiac catheterization
  ◊ Not indicated in mild pulmonic stenosis
  ◊ Essential in severe pulmonic stenosis
  ◊ Used to assess morphology of the right ventricle, pulmonary outflow tract and the pulmonary arteries
  ◊ Also used to rule out associated lesions e.g., atrial septal defect (ASD)

 TREATMENT

APPROPRIATE HEALTH CARE Usually outpatient. Inpatient, if surgery indicated.

GENERAL MEASURES
• Though infective endocarditis is rare, SBE prophylaxis is advisable
• Diagnostic treatment for critical pulmonary stenosis in newborns
Intervention/surgery:
  ◊ None required for mild pulmonic stenosis
  ◊ Percutaneous balloon valvotomy (preferred) or surgical pulmonic valvotomy required for patient with severe obstruction
  ◊ Intervention of asymptomatic patients with moderate PS is controversial. At minimum, regular assessment is advisable.

ACTIVITY No specific prescription. The lesion, if significant, will limit activity.

DIET No specific regimen

PATIENT EDUCATION American Heart Association, 7320 Greenville Avenue, Dallas, TX 75231, (214)373-6300

MEDICATIONS

DRUG(S) OF CHOICE
• No specific regimen in the absence of congestive heart failure
• Endocarditis prophylaxis
Contraindications: Refer to manufacturer's literature
Precautions: Refer to manufacturer's literature
Significant possible interactions: Refer to manufacturer's literature

ALTERNATIVE DRUGS N/A

FOLLOWUP

PATIENT MONITORING
• Postoperative (or post-balloon valvotomy) Doppler ultrasound suggested at approximately 1 year after procedure
• Post valvotomy SBE prophylaxis still required
• Regular followup assessment for patients not undergoing surgical correction

PREVENTION/AVOIDANCE N/A

POSSIBLE COMPLICATIONS
• Up to 10% late mortality following valvotomy in critical pulmonary stenosis neonates
• Slower recovery in those with chronic severe right ventricular hypertrophy
• Post valvotomy pulmonic regurgitation reported in up to 50% (variable severity)
• Residual ASD or patent foramen ovale
• Persistent repolarization abnormalities on ECG associated with severe postoperative pulmonic regurgitation
• Late atrial arrhythmias

EXPECTED COURSE AND PROGNOSIS Outcome following either balloon or surgical valvotomy is excellent in general

MISCELLANEOUS

ASSOCIATED CONDITIONS Other cardiac abnormalities, e.g., ventricular and atrial septal defects

AGE-RELATED FACTORS
Pediatric: Congenital disorder
Geriatric: N/A
Others: N/A

PREGNANCY In asymptomatic young women with mild to moderate PS, pregnancy is generally well tolerated

SYNONYMS Pulmonic stenosis

ICD-9-CM 424.3; 746.02

SEE ALSO Tetralogy of Fallot

OTHER NOTES N/A

ABBREVIATIONS
• SBE = subacute bacterial endocarditis
• PS = pulmonic stenosis

REFERENCES
• Braunwald, E. (ed.): Heart Disease: A Textbook of Cardiovascular Medicine. 3rd Ed. Philadelphia, W.B. Saunders Co., 1988
• Liberthson, R.: Congenital Heart Disease: Diagnosis & Management in Children and Adults. Boston, Little Brown & Co., 1989
• Perloff, J.: Clinical Recognition of Congenital Heart Disease. 3rd Ed. Philadelphia, W.B. Saunders Co., 1987

Author S. Mamby, M.D.

Pyelonephritis

BASICS

DESCRIPTION
• Acute pyelonephritis is a syndrome that consists of localized flank or back pain combined with systemic symptoms such as fever, chills and prostration. It is caused by infection of the renal parenchyma and collecting system, accompanied by bacteriuria, and often by bacteremia, which can progress to "septic shock" and death.
• Chronic pyelonephritis is the pathological result of progressive inflammation on the renal interstitium and tubules, and the radiologic diagnosis of the renal scarring and destructive changes in the caliceal system that are presumed to be caused by bacterial infection, vesicoureteral reflux, or both.

System(s) affected: Renal/Urologic
Genetics: N/A
Incidence/Prevalence:
• Community acquired acute pyelonephritis - 15.7 per 100,000/per year
• Hospital acquired acute pyelonephritis - 7.3 per 10,000 hospital persons
Predominant age: All ages, especially > 50
Predominant sex: Female > Male

SIGNS AND SYMPTOMS
In adults
◊ Fever; above 38.5°C
◊ Chills
◊ Unilateral vs. bilateral pain in the lumbar flank area
◊ Malaise
◊ Myalgia
◊ Anorexia
◊ Nausea
◊ Vomiting
◊ Diarrhea
◊ Headache
◊ Dysuria
◊ Frequency
◊ Urgency
◊ Suprapubic discomfort
◊ Flank pain on palpation
◊ From no physical findings to septic shock
In infants and children
◊ Fever
◊ Inadequate weight gain or weight loss
◊ Gastrointestinal symptoms
◊ Meningitis
◊ Seizures
◊ Sepsis
◊ Jaundice to gray skin color
◊ Flank mass
◊ Hematuria
◊ Enuresis
◊ Vaginal discharge, vulval soreness or pruritus in girls

CAUSES
• E.Coli (75%)
• Other gram-negative rods, Proteus mirabilis, klebsiella and Enterobacter account for 10-15%
• Enterococcus
• Staphylococcus-epidermis, saprophyticus and aureus
• Leptospira
• Salmonella typhi
• Mycoplasma
• Anaerobes

RISK FACTORS
• Underlying urinary tract abnormalities
• Indwelling catheter
• Nephrolithiasis
• Diabetes mellitus
• Immunocompromised conditions
• Elderly, institutionalized women
• Acute pyelonephritis within the prior year

DIAGNOSIS

DIFFERENTIAL DIAGNOSIS
• Renal infarction
• Acute renal vein thrombosis
• Acute renal artery dissection
• Obstructive uropathy
• Acute glomerulonephritis
• Acute bacterial pneumonia
• Myocardial infarction
• Acute hepatitis
• Cholecystitis
• Acute pancreatitis
• Appendicitis
• A perforated viscus
• Splenic infarct
• Aortic dissection
• Acute pelvic inflammatory disease
• Zona

LABORATORY
• Urine culture > 100,000 colony-forming units (CFU/mL)
• Pyuria
• The leukocyte esterase test in the urine
• Leukocyte casts
• Hematuria and mild proteinuria
• Leukocytosis
• Blood culture(s)
Drugs that may alter lab results:
Antibiotics
Disorders that may alter lab results: N/A

PATHOLOGICAL FINDINGS
Acute:
◊ Abscess formation with neutrophils
◊ Glomeruli spared
◊ The area of the infection is wedge-shaped toward the medulla
Chronic:
◊ Fibrosis
◊ Reduction in renal tissue
◊ Scarring
◊ Calyceal clubbing, dilatation and distortion

SPECIAL TESTS
• Bladder washout
• Antibody coated bacteria or ACB test

IMAGING 67 Gallium or 131I-Hippuran scanning

DIAGNOSTIC PROCEDURES
• Cystoscopy with ureteral catheterization
• Ultrasound
• Intravenous pyelogram (IVP)

TREATMENT

APPROPRIATE HEALTH CARE
Inpatient, could be outpatient if toxic appearing with acute illness

GENERAL MEASURES
• Intravenous fluid when needed
• Treatment centers on antibiotic therapy according to culture and sensitivity studies

ACTIVITY As tolerated

DIET Encourage fluid

PATIENT EDUCATION Griffith, H. W.: Instructions for Patients; Philadephia, W.B. Saunders Co. 1988. p 211

MEDICATIONS

DRUG(S) OF CHOICE
• Gentamicin, tobramycin or netilmicin 1.5 mg/kg stat, then 1 mg/kg q8h if creatinine < 1.5 mg% and ampicillin 1 gm q4h IV or cefotaxime 1 gm q 6h, cefoperazone 1 gm q 12h, or piperacillin 2 gm q 6h. (The cephalosporins and piperacillin are probably not needed for community-acquired infections. Piperacillin for suspected Pseudomonas aeruginosa.)
• Response within 48 hours (95% of patients); discharge on appropriate oral medication (one of: trimethoprim (160 mg)/sulfamethoxazole [800 mg] bid, cephalexin 500 mg qid, amoxicillin 500 mg qid; nalidixic acid 1 g qid) after patient is afebrile for 48 hours, continue treatment 2 weeks for women, 6 weeks for men.
• No response within 48 hours (5% of patients) - reevaluate, review cultures, consider ultrasound or IVP if no alternative diagnosis, continue therapy
• In the case of outpatient treatment only - trimethoprim/sulfamethoxazole, cephalexin, or amoxicillin plus clavulanic acid
• With less symptomatic females - a single dose of trimethoprim/sulfamethoxazole (either two double-strength tablets or four regular-strength tablets) or amoxicillin 3 g

Contraindications:
• Allergies to penicillin-sulfa
• In impaired kidney function - nitrofurantoin, tetracyclines, sulfonamides

Precautions:
• Watch aminoglycoside levels carefully
• In impaired kidney function use aminoglycosides for 1-2 days only or use aztreonam

Significant possible interactions: N/A

ALTERNATIVE DRUGS As above

FOLLOWUP

PATIENT MONITORING At 2, 6, and 12 weeks with urine culture

PREVENTION/AVOIDANCE See Patient Education

POSSIBLE COMPLICATIONS
• Metastatic infection: skeletal system, endocardium, eye
• May complicate the pregnancy course and produce low weight babies
• Septic shock and death
• Chronic renal insufficiency
• Complications of antibiotics

EXPECTED COURSE AND PROGNOSIS 95% respond in 48 hours

MISCELLANEOUS

ASSOCIATED CONDITIONS N/A

AGE-RELATED FACTORS
Pediatric: Nonspecific systems, jaundice, enuresis, sepsis
Geriatric:
• May present as confusion
• Characteristics may change
Others: N/A

PREGNANCY The most common medical complications requiring hospitalization

SYNONYMS Acute upper urinary tract infection

ICD-9-CM
• Acute 590.10
• Chronic 590.0

SEE ALSO N/A

OTHER NOTES N/A

ABBREVIATIONS N/A

REFERENCES
• Schrier, R.W. & Gottschalk, C.W.: Diseases of the Kidney. 4th Ed. Boston, Little, Brown, 1988
• Kaye D.: The Medical Clinics of N. America, Philadelphia, W.B. Saunders Co., March, 1991

Author J. Asfoura, M.D.

Pyloric stenosis

 BASICS

DESCRIPTION A progressive stenosis of the pyloric canal occurring in infancy
System(s) affected: Gastrointestinal
Genetics: Unknown, sometimes familial
Incidence/Prevalence in USA: 1/300-1/1000 live births (male 1/150 live births; female 1/750 live births)
Predominant age: Infancy; onset usually at 3-4 weeks of age, rarely in the newborn period or as late as 5 months of age
Predominant sex: Male > Female (5:1)

SIGNS AND SYMPTOMS
• Intermittent, non-bilious, projectile vomiting of increasing frequency and severity
• Initially hunger, later weakness
• Epigastric distention
• Visible gastric peristalsis, sometimes retrograde
• Palpable tumor (olive) in right upper quadrant
• Jaundice, occasional
• Late signs: dehydration, weight loss

CAUSES
• Obscure, sometimes familial; 6% risk of recurrence if either parent had pyloric stenosis, much higher if the mother was affected

RISK FACTORS
• 2.5 times more common in Caucasians as in Blacks

 DIAGNOSIS

DIFFERENTIAL DIAGNOSIS
• Inexperienced or inappropriate feeding
• Gastroesophageal reflux
• Gastritis
• Congenital adrenal hyperplasia, salt-losing
• Pyloric diaphragm

LABORATORY
• Early - evidence hypochloremic alkalosis, with low serum chloride and high bicarbonate
• Later - may have acidosis with low bicarbonate and low potassium
• Elevated unconjugated bilirubin
Drugs that may alter lab results: N/A
Disorders that may alter lab results: N/A

PATHOLOGICAL FINDINGS Concentric hypertrophy of pyloric muscle

SPECIAL TESTS Abdominal ultrasound by experienced radiologist may outline the pyloric tumor

IMAGING
• Upright plain film of abdomen may reveal dilated stomach (filled with fluid and/or air) and relative lack of air in intestines
• Barium swallow (performed only when diagnosis is not clinically clear) reveals strong gastric contractions and elongated, narrow pyloric canal (string sign)
• Ultrasound (first choice if available)

DIAGNOSTIC PROCEDURES None

 TREATMENT

APPROPRIATE HEALTH CARE
• Inpatient
• Surgery: Fredet-Ramstedt pyloromyotomy

GENERAL MEASURES Surgery must be preceded by preoperative preparation, including: Empty stomach with nasogastric tube, fluid replacement, correction of electrolyte imbalance

ACTIVITY N/A

DIET
• No preoperative feeding
• No feeding for 8-16 hours postoperative
• Gradual increase in feedings thereafter
• Should reach full feedings 48-72 hours after surgery

PATIENT EDUCATION Instructions about preoperative and postoperative care

MEDICATIONS

DRUG(S) OF CHOICE N/A
Contraindications: N/A
Precautions: N/A
Significant possible interactions: N/A

ALTERNATIVE DRUGS N/A

FOLLOWUP

PATIENT MONITORING Routine pediatric health maintenance

PREVENTION/AVOIDANCE N/A

POSSIBLE COMPLICATIONS None; no long term morbidity

EXPECTED COURSE AND PROGNOSIS Complete recovery with catch-up growth and weight gain

MISCELLANEOUS

ASSOCIATED CONDITIONS Usually none; rarely hiatal hernia or esophageal atresia

AGE-RELATED FACTORS
Pediatric: N/A
Geriatric: N/A
Others: N/A

PREGNANCY N/A

SYNONYMS
• Infantile hypertrophic pyloric stenosis

ICD-9-CM
• 537.0 acquired hypertrophic pyloric stenosis
• 750.5 congenital hypertrophic pyloric stenosis

SEE ALSO N/A

OTHER NOTES N/A

ABBREVIATIONS N/A

REFERENCES
• Rudolph, A.M.: Pediatrics. 18th Ed. Norwalk, CT, Appleton and Lange, 1987
• Garcia, V.F. & Randolph, T.G.: Pyloric Stenosis: Diagnosis and Management. Pediatrics in Review 11:292-296, 1990

Author K. Wegner, M.D.

Rabies

BASICS

DESCRIPTION A rapidly progressive infection of the central nervous system caused by an RNA virus and affecting warm blooded mammals, including man
• The disease is essentially 100% fatal once symptoms develop
• Infection can be prevented by prompt, postexposure treatment of persons bitten by animals, known or suspected to be, carrying the disease.
Genetics: N/A
Incidence/Prevalence in USA: 0-3 cases per year in humans; about 8000 cases per year in animals; about 25,000 postexposure treatments. In US citizens, < 0.001/100,000/year.
Predominant age: Any
Predominant sex: Male = Female

SIGNS AND SYMPTOMS
• Usually proceed through four stages, although they may overlap
<u>Incubation</u>
◊ Initially no symptoms except bite trauma
◊ The incubation period is the time between bite and first symptoms of disease. This time is between one and three months in 2/3 of the cases. Sometimes can be as short as 5 days or longer than 5 years. It is shortest in patients with extensive bites about the head and trunk.
<u>Prodrome</u>
◊ Lasts 2 to 10 days
◊ Symptoms are often extremely variable and nonspecific, including fever, headache
◊ May be referable to any of a number of organ systems
◊ May suggest any of a number of common infections
◊ Diagnosis should considered if there is bite by an animal capable of transmitting the disease and pain or paraesthesia at the bite site; some patients do not recall exposure
<u>Acute neurologic period</u>
◊ Lasts 2 to 10 days
◊ Symptoms referable to central nervous system dominate clinical picture
◊ Generally takes one of two forms
◊ Furious rabies: Episodes of hyperactivity last about 5 minutes and include hydrophobia, aerophobia, hyperventilation, hypersalivation, interspersed with periods of normalcy
◊ Paralytic rabies: Paralysis dominates clinical picture, may be ascending (like Guillain-Barré syndrome) or affect one or more limbs differentially
<u>Coma</u>
◊ Last hours to days; with intensive care, may sometimes last months
◊ May slowly evolve following acute neurologic period
◊ May be sudden, with respiratory arrest
<u>Death</u>
◊ Usually occurs within three weeks of onset as result of a complications
◊ Only 3 survivors reported in the world's literature, none during past 15 years

CAUSES Rabies virus, a neurotropic virus present in saliva of infected animals

RISK FACTORS
For exposure to rabies:
• Professions or activities that may expose a person to wild animals, e.g., farm workers, forest rangers, some lab workers, veterinarians, spelunkers (cave explorers)
• International travel to countries where canine rabies is endemic (most common risk factor)

DIAGNOSIS

DIFFERENTIAL DIAGNOSIS Any rapidly progressive encephalitis; important to exclude treatable causes of encephalitis, especially herpes

LABORATORY WBC count in cerebrospinal fluid (CSF) exam may be normal or show moderate pleocytosis
Drugs that may alter lab results:
Immunosuppressive agents
Disorders that may alter lab results: None

PATHOLOGICAL FINDINGS
Encephalitis may be found in brain biopsy, but abnormal findings may be confined to parts (brainstem, midbrain, cerebellum) only examined postmortem

SPECIAL TESTS
• Only available in state and federal reference laboratories
• Rabies antibody titer should be obtained on serum and CSF
• Skin biopsy from nape of neck should be obtained for direct fluorescent antibody examination
• Saliva culture for rabies antibody

IMAGING Normal, or nonspecific findings consistent with encephalitis

DIAGNOSTIC PROCEDURES
• Spinal tap
• Skin biopsy
• Viral isolation from saliva or CNS

TREATMENT

APPROPRIATE HEALTH CARE
• Suspect rabies encephalitis - inpatient with isolation
• Exposure to rabies - inpatient if wounds serious; outpatient for prophylactic treatment

GENERAL MEASURES
• Since there is no treatment for clinical rabies, this section is directed at prevention of disease following exposure to potentially rabid animals
• Physicians should evaluate each possible exposure to rabies and consult with local or state public health officials about the need for rabies prophylaxis. In the United States, bats, skunks and raccoons are the animals most likely to be infected, but any carnivore can carry the disease. Outside the United States, dogs are a main reservoir in many developing countries.
• Before specific antirabies treatment is initiated, consider: Types of exposure (bite or nonbite), epidemiology of rabies in involved species, circumstances of biting incident and vaccination status of exposing animal

ACTIVITY As tolerated

DIET No restrictions

PATIENT EDUCATION
• Avoid wild and unknown domestic animals
• Seek treatment promptly if bitten
• Careful wound cleansing is first line of treatment

MEDICATIONS

DRUG(S) OF CHOICE
Postexposure prophylaxis regimen
• Essential components of rabies postexposure prophylaxis are local wound treatment and both passive and active vaccination

◊ Local wound treatment: Immediate and thorough washing of all bite wounds and scratches with soap and water

◊ Passive vaccination: Human rabies immune globulin (HRIG) is administered once, at the beginning of antirabies prophylaxis. Dose of HRIG is 20 IU/kg body weight (formula is applicable for all age groups, including children). If anatomically feasible, up to one-half the dose of HRIG should be thoroughly infiltrated in the area around the wound and the rest should be administered intramuscularly in the gluteal area. HRIG should never be administered in the same syringe or into the same anatomical site as vaccine.

◊ Active vaccination: Human Diploid Cell Rabies Vaccine (HDCV) or Rabies Vaccine Adsorbed (RVA) should be given intramuscularly in the deltoid. For children, the anterolateral aspect of the thigh is acceptable. Gluteal area should never be used for HDCV injections.
The first dose, 1mL, should be given as soon as possible after exposure; one additional dose should be given on days 3, 7, 14, and 28 after the first vaccination.
For the previously vaccinated, two intramuscular doses (1mL each) of vaccine should be administered, one immediately and one 3 days later. HRIG not necessary in these patients.
Preexposure vaccination
• Should be offered to persons in high risk groups, such as veterinarians, animal handlers, certain laboratory workers, and persons spending time (e.g., one month or more) in foreign countries where rabies is enzootic

◊ Primary preexposure: IM vaccination regimen consists of three 1.0 mL injections of HDCV or RVA given in deltoid area, one each on days 0, 7, and 28. HDCV may also be given in intradermal doses, administered with a special syringe developed for that purpose (Imovax Rabies I.D. Vaccine); the 0.1 mL dose is administered in the deltoid area, follow the same schedule as for IM doses.

◊ Preexposure boosters or serologic testing to determine antibody titer every 2 years thereafter for persons at continued risk of rabies exposures

Contraindications: None for postexposure treatment
Precautions: About 6% of persons develop mild serum sickness reaction following HDCV boosters. Mild local and systemic reactions are very common following vaccination. Mild reactions should not be a cause for interruption of immunization.
Significant possible interactions: Antibody response may be suppressed by diseases that suppress immune system

ALTERNATIVE DRUGS None

FOLLOWUP

PATIENT MONITORING After primary vaccination, serologic testing only necessary if patient has disease or takes medications that may suppress immune system

PREVENTION/AVOIDANCE See Treatment

POSSIBLE COMPLICATIONS None

EXPECTED COURSE AND PROGNOSIS No postexposure failures reported in the United States since the 1970's

MISCELLANEOUS

ASSOCIATED CONDITIONS N/A

AGE-RELATED FACTORS
Pediatric: N/A
Geriatric: N/A
Others: N/A

PREGNANCY N/A

SYNONYMS Hydrophobia

ICD-9-CM 071 (clinical rabies) or V01.5 (rabies exposure) or V04.5 (inoculation or prophylactic vaccination)

SEE ALSO Animal bites

OTHER NOTES N/A

ABBREVIATIONS
• HRIG = Human rabies immune globulin
• HDCV = Human Diploid Cell Rabies Vaccine
• RVA = Rabies Vaccine Adsorbed

REFERENCES
• Fishbein, D.B.: Rabies in humans. In Natural History of Rabies. 2nd Ed. Edited by G. Baer. Boca Raton, CRC Press, 1991: 519-549
• Bernard, K.W. & Fishbein, D.B.: Rabies virus. In Principles and Practice of Infectious Disease. Edited by G.L. Mandell, et al. New York, Churchill Livingstone, 1989
• Rabies Prevention - United States, 1991. Morbidity and Mortality Weekly Reports, 1991:40(RR-3):1-14

Author D. Fishbein, M.D.

Radiation sickness

BASICS

DESCRIPTION Any somatic or genetic disruption of function or form caused by electromagnetic waves or accelerated atomic particles
• Acute radiation sickness: Symptoms occurring within 24 hours of exposure
• Chronic radiation syndrome: Symptoms occurring greater than 24 hours after exposure, and generally over an extended time
Radiation measures
  ◊ 1 rad is the absorption of 100 ergs of energy by 1 gram of tissue
  ◊ 100 rads = 1 gray (Gy)
  ◊ The REM (Radiation Equivalent Man) unit was developed because different tissues have different sensitivities to radiation. 1 REM (Radiation Equivalent Man) is radiation dose in rads multiplied by a relative biologic effectiveness factor for the tissue involved. 100 REM = 1 sievert (Sv).
Radiation includes:
  ◊ Electromagnetic emissions. Energy (and hence penetration) is inversely proportional to wave length
  ◊ Particles. Alpha particles are the nuclei of helium atoms and beta particles are electrons. Both have low penetrance externally but are dangerous if ingested. Neutrons are damaging and penetrate well.
System(s) affected: Gastrointestinal, Endocrine/Metabolic, Skin/Exocrine, Reproductive, Hemic/Lymphatic/Immunologic, Pulmonary, Musculoskeletal
Genetics: Females tolerate better than males. The exception is pregnant females with risk of fetal injury at low dose.
Incidence/Prevalence in USA:
• Most acute radiation injury is related to accidents or radiation therapy
• 400,000 patients receive radiation therapy yearly for malignancies
• Accidents are sporadic and usually involve small numbers of individuals
Historically:
  ◊ 120,000 individuals developed acute radiation syndrome in Japan as a result of nuclear explosions
  ◊ 7,266 natives of the Marshall Islands were exposed to radiation due to errors in judging winds after a nuclear test in the South Pacific
  ◊ Chernobyl accident in Russia in 1986 where an estimated 50,000 individuals received at least 0.5 Sv of exposure.
Predominant age: N/A
Predominant sex: N/A

SIGNS AND SYMPTOMS
Acute radiation exposure is divided into several syndromes:
  ◊ Less than 200 rads = no disease. There may be some nausea more than 3 hours after the event. Nausea is not a reliable sign of exposure since most people involved in an accident of this type will complain of some nausea when questioned.
  ◊ 200-1000 rads = hematopoietic syndrome. Acute nausea and vomiting within 3 hours. Acute granulocyte elevation, then lymphopenia, then thrombocytopenia and neutropenia, then anemia. Peak lowering of platelets and granulocytes at 3 weeks (resolving in 12 weeks). Lymphopenia may last years. Survivors may get lung or kidney changes months after. Death rate 0-80% depending on dose received and treatment. Ld 50 for humans is 650 rads.
  ◊ 1000-5000 rads = gastrointestinal syndrome. Nausea and vomiting 30-60 minutes postexposure. Loss of the villus structure of small bowel. Severe GI bleeding, diarrhea and abdominal pain develop in 3 days and precede the hematopoietic syndrome. Death due to blood loss or gram negative sepsis. Survivors usually die late of bone marrow suppression. Death rate 80-100%.
  ◊ Over 5000 rads = neurovascular syndrome or "Spock syndrome". After a 15-30 minute asymptomatic period; tremors, ataxia, vomiting, hypotension, seizures and death. Death rate 100%.

CAUSES
• Nuclear weapons
• Industrial accidents
• Nuclear power accidents
• Radiation therapy

RISK FACTORS
• Young patients more susceptible than old
• Men more sensitive than women
• Debilitated more susceptible than healthy

DIAGNOSIS

DIFFERENTIAL DIAGNOSIS
Was the patient exposed to radiation?
• Acute viral illness or anxiety cause nausea and vomiting
• Blast or heat cause skin redness
• Chemical exposure causes blistering, pain

LABORATORY
Lymphocyte count at 48 hours post event
  ◊ Over 1500 = trivial or no exposure
  ◊ Over 1000 = survival without treatment
  ◊ 500-1000 = survival with treatment
  ◊ 100-400 = death without bone marrow transplant
  ◊ Under 100 = certain death
Drugs that may alter lab results:
Chemotherapeutic agents cause bone marrow suppression identical to radiation exposure
Disorders that may alter lab results: N/A

PATHOLOGICAL FINDINGS
• Hypocellular marrow with the hematopoietic syndrome
• The GI syndrome with loss of villus margin and sloughing of villus structure
• Late cases with fibrosis of lung, liver and kidney tissues
• Loss of hair indicates exposure of 350 rads and is complete at 700 rads

SPECIAL TESTS Total body dosimetry may suggest dose of compound ingested. Most radioisotopes are not excreted well.

IMAGING N/A

DIAGNOSTIC PROCEDURES N/A

TREATMENT

APPROPRIATE HEALTH CARE
Inpatient

GENERAL MEASURES
• Step 1 is decontamination to reduce external radiation and collateral exposure
• All wounds débrided to decontaminate
• All surgery within two days before loss of white cell and platelet function
• IV fluids, antinauseants and bedrest
• Platelet, RBC and WBC transfusion if needed
• Antibiotics for sepsis and neutropenia
• Bone marrow transplant for severe exposure
• Treatment of collateral injuries such as burns and lacerations only after decontamination

ACTIVITY Isolation techniques for immune system injury

DIET As tolerated. Hyperalimentation for severe GI syndromes.

PATIENT EDUCATION Recommend genetic counseling and screening to persons who have been exposed to significant amounts of radiation

MEDICATIONS

DRUG(S) OF CHOICE
Supportive therapy
◊ Antibiotics for enteric organisms for GI syndrome, e.g., sulfamethoxazole and trimethoprim, ciprofloxacin
◊ Broad spectrum antibiotics for infections common with bone marrow suppression, e.g., neutropenia
◊ If radioactive iodine - potassium iodide (SSKI) in doses proportional to the exposure
◊ If radioactive phosphorus - use parenteral magnesium sulfate
◊ Nonspecific ingestions - use laxatives to increase GI transit rate
Contraindications: Refer to manufacturer's literature
Precautions: Refer to manufacturer's literature
Significant possible interactions: Refer to manufacturer's literature

ALTERNATIVE DRUGS   N/A

FOLLOWUP

PATIENT MONITORING
• Daily CBC, platelet, granulocyte, lymphocyte counts
• Stools for blood
• Vital signs q4h looking for sepsis

PREVENTION/AVOIDANCE   Follow
safety procedures

POSSIBLE COMPLICATIONS
• Long-term fibrosis of kidneys, liver and lung. Occur within 6 months of acute exposure and with as little as 300 rads of exposure.
• Radiation exposure can induce malignancies
• Increased long-term risk of leukemia (acute lymphocytic or chronic myelogenous)
• Multiple myeloma and cancers of the breast, esophagus, stomach, colon, lung, ovary, bladder, thyroid
• Sterility

EXPECTED COURSE AND PROGNOSIS
• Patients surviving 12 weeks have excellent prognosis but should be monitored for long-term complications
• Hair lost usually returns within 2 months

MISCELLANEOUS

ASSOCIATED CONDITIONS   N/A

AGE-RELATED FACTORS
Pediatric: More sensitive to injury
Geriatric: Less sensitive to injury
Others: N/A

PREGNANCY   Injury to fetus likely

SYNONYMS   N/A

ICD-9-CM   990 radiation

SEE ALSO   N/A

OTHER NOTES   N/A

ABBREVIATIONS   N/A

REFERENCES
• Wyngaarden, J.B. & Smith, L.H. (eds.): Cecil Textbook of Medicine. 19th Ed. Philadelphia, W.B. Saunders Co., 1992
• Kissane, John M. (ed.): Anderson's pathology. 9th Ed. St. Louis, Mosby, 1990
• Cotran, Ramzi S. (and others) (eds.): Robbins Pathological Basis of Disease. 4th Ed. Philadelphia, Saunders 1989

Author   M. Essig, M.D.

Rape crisis syndrome

 BASICS

DESCRIPTION

<u>Definitions (legal definitions may vary slightly from state to state)</u>

◊ Sexual contact - intentional touching of a person's intimate parts (including thighs) or the clothing covering such areas, if it is construed as being for the purpose of sexual gratification

◊ Sexual conduct - vaginal intercourse between a male and female, or anal intercourse, fellatio, or cunnilingus between persons regardless of sex

◊ Rape - any sexual penetration, however slight, using force or coercion against the person's will

◊ Sexual imposition - similar to rape but without penetration or the use of force (i.e., non-consenting sexual contact)

◊ Gross sexual imposition - non-consenting sexual contact with the use of force

◊ Corruption of a minor - sexual conduct by an individual 18 years old or greater with an individual less than 15 years of age

System(s) affected: Nervous, Reproductive

Genetics: N/A

Incidence/Prevalence in USA:
• Over 100,000 cases of alleged rape reported in US every year
• Estimated that only 1 in 5 to 1 in 10 adult cases reported
• Estimated only 1 in 15 to 1 in 20 pediatric cases reported
• Estimated incidence of reported rape is 60/100,000 females

Predominant age:
• Majority of adult victims are female in teens and 20's, (reported as high as 97 years)
• Pediatric victims may be either gender with predominance of females. Reported as young as 2 months.
• Increasing numbers of adult male victims presenting for treatment

Predominant sex: Female > Male

SIGNS AND SYMPTOMS

<u>In adults</u>
◊ History of sexual penetration
◊ Sexual contact, or sexual conduct without consent and/or with the use of force

<u>In pediatrics</u>
◊ Actual observation of, or suspicion of, sexual penetration, sexual contact, or sexual conduct
◊ Signs include evidence of the use of force and/or evidence of sexual contact (e.g., presence of semen and/or sperm)

CAUSES Listed with Description

RISK FACTORS
• Numerous
• About 50% of rapes occur in the home, with 1/3 of these involving a male intruder

 DIAGNOSIS

DIFFERENTIAL DIAGNOSIS Consenting sex among adults

LABORATORY
• Record results of wet mount noting the presence or absence of sperm and, if present, whether or not it is motile or immotile
• If indicated, a serum or urine pregnancy test should be obtained and the results recorded

Drugs that may alter lab results: N/A
Disorders that may alter lab results: N/A

PATHOLOGICAL FINDINGS N/A

SPECIAL TESTS N/A

IMAGING N/A

DIAGNOSTIC PROCEDURES
<u>History:</u>
◊ Record in patient's own words in so far as possible. Include date, approximate time, and general location as best possible. Document physical abuse other than sexual. Describe all types of sexual contact whether actual/or attempted. History of alcohol and/or drugs before or after alleged incident.
◊ Document time of last activity which could possibly alter specimens (e.g., bath, shower, or douche). Thorough gynecologic history is mandatory including last menstrual period (LMP), last consenting sexual contact, contraceptive practice, and prior gynecologic surgery.
<u>Physical examination:</u>
◊ Use of drawings and/or photographs is encouraged. Use of UV light (Wood's lamp) to detect seminal stains on clothing or skin. Document all signs of trauma or unusual marks. Documentation of mental status/emotional state.
◊ Complete genital-rectal examination including evidence of trauma, secretions, or discharge. Use of a non-lubricated, water moistened speculum is mandatory since commonly used lubricants may destroy evidence.

 TREATMENT

APPROPRIATE HEALTH CARE
• Contact appropriate social services agency
• Majority of adult victims can be treated as outpatients unless associated trauma (physical or mental) requires admission
• Majority of pediatric sexual assault/abuse victims will require admission or outside placement until appropriate social agency can evaluate home environment

GENERAL MEASURES
• Providing health care to victims of sexual assault/abuse requires special sensitivity and privacy
• All such cases MUST be reported immediately to the appropriate law enforcement agency
• With the victim's permission, utilize personnel from local support agency(ies) (e.g., Rape Crisis Center). When available, use of in-house Social Services is extremely helpful to victim/family.
• Sedation and tetanus prophylaxis should be utilized when indicated
• Venereal disease prevention for gonorrhea/Chlamydia should be administered
• A discussion of possible pregnancy and pregnancy termination should be held with the victim. If hospital policy precludes such a discussion, then information about this option should be offered the victim via the followup mechanisms.
• Suspected HIV and hepatitis B exposure and testing should be discussed with the victim and be in keeping with hospital policies/protocols. The initial HIV test should be completed within seven days of the suspected exposure.

ACTIVITY No restrictions

DIET No restrictions

PATIENT EDUCATION
• Information and help available from local rape crisis support organizations
• National Institute of Mental Health, Public Inquiries Branch, Office of Scientific Information, Dept. of Health and Human Services, Parklawn Bldg., Room 15C-05, 5600 Fishers Lane, Rockville, MD 20857, (301)443-4513

MEDICATIONS

DRUG(S) OF CHOICE
• For gonorrhea - ceftriaxone 250 mg IM x 1. Alternative medications would include spectinomycin, ciprofloxacin, norfloxacin, ampicillin/probenecid, or amoxicillin/probenecid.
• For chlamydia - doxycycline 100 mg po bid, or tetracycline 250 mg qid for 10 days. If the patient is pregnant, erythromycin should be used, 500 mg every 6 hours
• Specific treatment for vulvovaginitis if present
• Note - gonorrhea and chlamydia medications may be given concomitantly
Contraindications: Refer to manufacturer's literature
Precautions: Refer to manufacturer's literature
Significant possible interactions: Refer to manufacturer's literature

ALTERNATIVE DRUGS N/A

FOLLOWUP

PATIENT MONITORING
• The patient should be seen in seven to ten days for followup care, including pregnancy testing, and counselling by a gynecologist or appropriate gynecologic clinic
• Close examination for vaginitis and treatment if necessary
• Followup test for syphilis and gonorrhea should occur in five to six weeks
• Followup testing for AIDS and hepatitis B should occur in six months
• Telephone numbers of counselling agency(ies) which can provide counselling/legal services to the patient should be provided

PREVENTION/AVOIDANCE
• Scope of rape prevention is too complex and too broad to be discussed in these pages. True prevention will require many changes.
• Women may benefit from assertiveness training and self-defense training

POSSIBLE COMPLICATIONS
• Sexually transmitted disease and subsequent treatment
• Pregnancy (with the possibility of abortion)
• Trauma (physical and mental)

EXPECTED COURSE AND PROGNOSIS
• Acute phase (usually 1-3 weeks following rape) - shaking, pain, wound healing, mood swings, appetite loss, crying. Also feelings of grief, shame, anger, fear, revenge or guilt.
• Late or chronic phase female victim may develop fear of intercourse, fear of men, nightmares , sleep disorders, daytime flashbacks, fear of being alone, loss of self-esteem, anxiety, depression, post-traumatic stress syndrome
• Recovery may be prolonged. Patients who are able to talk about their feelings seem to have a faster recovery.

MISCELLANEOUS

ASSOCIATED CONDITIONS N/A

AGE-RELATED FACTORS
Pediatric: Assurance to the child that he or she is a good person and was not the cause of the incident
Geriatric: N/A
Others: N/A

PREGNANCY Baseline pregnancy test conducted. Pregnancy prevention discussed with patient.

SYNONYMS
• Sexual assault
• Rape trauma

ICD-9-CM V71.5

SEE ALSO N/A

OTHER NOTES
• Rape is a legal term and the examining physician is encouraged to use terminology such as "alleged rape" or "alleged sexual conduct".
• In majority of states, wife may now accuse husband of rape if they are estranged and living apart
• Since "consent defense" is common, documentation of evidence supporting the use of force or the administration of drugs/alcohol is imperative
• The use of a protocol is encouraged to assure every victim a uniform, comprehensive evaluation regardless of the expertise of the examining physician. The protocol must ensure that all evidence is properly collected and labeled, chain-of-custody is maintained, and the evidence is sent to the most appropriate forensic laboratory.
• All medical records must be well documented and legible
• All medical personnel must be willing and able to testify on behalf of the patient

ABBREVIATIONS N/A

REFERENCES
• Harwood-Nuss, A. (ed.): The Clinical Practice of Emergency Medicine. Philadelphia, J.B. Lippincott, 1991
• Tintinalli, J.E. (ed): Emergency Medicine: A Comprehensive Study Guide. New York, McGraw-Hill, 1992
• Young, W.W., et al.: Sexual Assault: Review of a National Model Protocol for Forensic and Medical Evaluation. Obs & Gyn 80:5, 878-883, Nov, 1992

Author D. Schelble, M.D., FACEP

Raynaud's phenomenon

BASICS

DESCRIPTION Vasospastic disorder. Intermittent attacks of extreme pallor, then cyanosis of the fingers (rarely, of the toes) brought on by exposure to cold. With warming, vasodilatation and intense redness develops, followed by swelling, throbbing, paresthesia. Resolves with warming. May accompany emotional upset. Thumbs rarely involved. May progress to atrophy of digital fat pads, ischemic ulcers of fingertips. 50% idiopathic (disease), 50% secondary (phenomenon).
• Disease (primary) - progressive, symmetrical. Involves fingers. Almost always in women. Ages 15 to 45. Spasm more frequent, more severe with time. Rarely ulcerates. Diagnose only after 2-3 years with no underlying associated disease. May be associated with coronary vasospasm or primary pulmonary hypertension.
• Phenomenon (secondary) - may be unilateral, asymmetric; may affect only one or two fingers. Underlying condition usually identifiable with time. Usually worse morbidity and prognosis than primary disease.
System(s) affected: Skin/Exocrine, Musculoskeletal, Hemic/Lymphatic/Immunologic
Genetics: Probably hereditary, dominant
Incidence/Prevalence in USA: 1.9-4.6% of population (based on reporting of characteristic color changes, cold intolerance)
Predominant age: After 40
Predominant sex: Female > Male

SIGNS AND SYMPTOMS
• Pallor/whiteness of fingertips with cold exposure, followed by numbness, paresthesias, cyanosis, then redness and pain with warming
• Ulceration of finger pads, progressing to autoamputation in severe, prolonged cases
• May have no other findings, or may show signs of underlying vasospastic or autoimmune disease
• Attacks more frequent in cold weather

CAUSES
• Unknown
• Intrinsic vascular wall hyperactivity to cold
• Increased vasomotor tone due to sympathetic stimulation

RISK FACTORS
• Smoking
• Existing autoimmune or connective tissue disorder
• Exposure to cold
• Emotional stress with increased levels of epinephrine in blood

DIAGNOSIS

DIFFERENTIAL DIAGNOSIS
• Thromboangiitis obliterans (Buerger's disease) - men; involves legs and feet; less than 5% have hand involvement, 90% have Raynaud's; smoking related
• Rheumatoid arthritis
• Progressive systemic sclerosis (scleroderma) - 90% have Raynaud's; Raynaud's may precede other symptoms by years
• Systemic lupus
• Carpal tunnel syndrome
• Thoracic outlet syndrome
• CREST syndrome (calcinosis cutis, Raynaud's phenomenon, esophageal dysmotility, sclerodactyly and telangiectasia)
• Cryoglobulinemias
• Waldenström's macroglobulinemia
• Acrocyanosis
• Occupational injury (especially from vibrating tools)
• Drugs (beta-blockers, ergotamine, methysergide, bleomycin, vinblastine, cisplatin)

LABORATORY Tests for underlying secondary causes (CBC, ESR, RA, ANA, immunoelectrophoresis, etc.)
Drugs that may alter lab results: N/A
Disorders that may alter lab results: N/A

PATHOLOGICAL FINDINGS Histology of skin biopsy correlates poorly with clinical presentation. May show edema, necrotizing or non-necrotizing vasculitis, and/or perivasculitis, thrombosis with focal gangrene

SPECIAL TESTS Cold challenge test to elicit characteristic color changes in hands

IMAGING Osteolysis of distal metaphyseal portions of phalanges, tapering, calcification of soft tissue

DIAGNOSTIC PROCEDURES Diagnosis largely determined by history, provocative exposure to cold

TREATMENT

APPROPRIATE HEALTH CARE
Outpatient

GENERAL MEASURES
• Dress warmly, wear gloves, avoid cold
• No smoking
• Avoid beta-blockers, amphetamines, ergot alkaloids
• Biofeedback techniques to teach patients to increase hand temperature
• Sympathectomy - effect is transient; use only as last resort in extreme cases
• Finger guards over ulcerated fingertips

ACTIVITY Avoidance of situations in which exposure to cold is likely

DIET No special diet

PATIENT EDUCATION Emphasis on smoking cessation. Avoidance of aggravating factors (trauma, vibration, cold, etc.).

MEDICATIONS

DRUG(S) OF CHOICE Nifedipine 30-90 mg daily (sustained release form). (May only be needed during winter.)
Contraindications: Allergy to drug, pregnancy, congestive heart failure
Precautions: May cause headache, dizziness, lightheadedness, hypotension
Significant possible interactions:
• Increases serum level of digoxin - monitor digoxin levels closely after nifedipine added
• Cimetidine increases nifedipine level - may require dosage adjustment
• May increase prothrombin time in patients taking warfarin

ALTERNATIVE DRUGS
• Reserpine, prazosin, methyldopa, guanethidine, phenoxybenzamine, diltiazem have been used with varying success
• Response to ACE inhibitors has been inconsistent

FOLLOWUP

PATIENT MONITORING Management of fingertip ulcers, including rapid treatment of infection

PREVENTION/AVOIDANCE
• Avoid trauma to fingertips
• Avoid exposure to cold
• Avoid smoking

POSSIBLE COMPLICATIONS Gangrene, autoamputation of fingertips

EXPECTED COURSE AND PROGNOSIS
• Prolonged course with recurrent ischemia, ulceration
• In case of secondary phenomenon, may eventually develop hallmarks of underlying disease

MISCELLANEOUS

ASSOCIATED CONDITIONS
• Lupus
• Rheumatoid arthritis
• Scleroderma
• Polymyositis
• Sjögren's
• Occlusive arterial disease
• Cryoglobulinemia
• Cervical rib
• Carpal tunnel syndrome
• Use of pneumatic tool
• Crutch trauma
• Heavy metal intoxication

AGE-RELATED FACTORS
Pediatric: Associated with systemic lupus erythematosus and scleroderma in children
Geriatric: Appearance of Raynaud's after 40 almost always indicates an underlying disease
Others: N/A

PREGNANCY N/A

SYNONYMS N/A

ICD-9-CM 443.0

SEE ALSO N/A

OTHER NOTES N/A

ABBREVIATIONS N/A

REFERENCES
• Braunwald, E., et al. (eds.): Harrison's Principles of Internal Medicine. 12th Ed. New York, McGraw-Hill, 1991
• Maricq, H.R., et al.: Prevalence of Raynaud phenomenon in the general population. A preliminary study by questionnaire. J Chronic Dis 39:423, 1986

Author J. Perchalski, M.D.

Rectal prolapse

BASICS

DESCRIPTION Protrusion of the rectum through the anus
• Partial prolapse - involves only mucosa. This frequently follows anal operative procedures. (Radial rectal folds prolapsed through rectum).
• Complete prolapse - involves the entire rectal wall (procidentia). This type occurs most commonly as a spontaneous event in children and complication of other disorders in the elderly. (Concentric rectal folds prolapsed through anus).
Genetics: Unknown
Incidence/Prevalence in USA: 4.2:1000 overall; 10:1000 after age 65 years
Predominant age: 2 years in children, 60-70 years in adults
Predominant sex: Male > Female (5:1 in adults, and a slight predominance in children)

SIGNS AND SYMPTOMS
Children
    ◊ Sensation of anal mass
    ◊ Pain
    ◊ Rectal bleeding
    ◊ Protruding mass
Adults
    ◊ Anorectal pain or discomfort during defecation
    ◊ Feeling of incomplete evacuation
    ◊ Rectal and urinary incontinence
    ◊ Rectal bleeding or discharge

CAUSES
Children
    ◊ Idiopathic (most common)
    ◊ Abnormal innervation of levator ani muscle complex, puborectalis or anal sphincters or abnormal anatomic relationships of these muscle groups
Adults
    ◊ Diastasis of levator ani
    ◊ Loose endopelvic fascia
    ◊ Loss of normal horizontal position of rectum
    ◊ Weak anal sphincter

RISK FACTORS
• Myelomeningocele
• Exstrophy of the bladder
• Cystic fibrosis
• Chronic constipation or diarrhea
• Imperforate anus
• Multiple sclerosis
• Stroke/paralysis
• Dementia

DIAGNOSIS

DIFFERENTIAL DIAGNOSIS
• Intussusception
• Rectal polyps
• Hemorrhoids

LABORATORY   N/A
Drugs that may alter lab results: N/A
Disorders that may alter lab results: N/A

PATHOLOGICAL FINDINGS   N/A

SPECIAL TESTS   N/A

IMAGING   Barium enema is useful in selected cases of recurrent rectal prolapse

DIAGNOSTIC PROCEDURES
Sigmoidoscopy is useful in recurrent prolapse to rule out rectal lesions

TREATMENT

APPROPRIATE HEALTH CARE
Inpatient, unless easily reduced

GENERAL MEASURES
Acute
    ◊ Prompt manual reduction of prolapse
    ◊ Treatment of diarrhea or constipation
Recurrent
    ◊ Sub-mucosal injection of 5% phenol in glycerine in four quadrants under general anesthesia (outpatient)
    ◊ Linear electrocauterization (inpatient)
    ◊ Transabdominal Ripstein's procedure (suspension of rectum from sacrum by means of artificial material)
    ◊ Posterior sagittal rectal suspension and levator repair
    ◊ Ivalon sponge wrap procedure
    ◊ Anterior resection of rectum
    ◊ Transabdominal proctopexy (no artificial material used)
    ◊ Perineal rectosigmoidectomy
    ◊ Thiersch's wire (may be outpatient procedure and may be modified by using Marlex or Silastic strip instead of wire), has been used more commonly in children and elderly poor-risk adults
    ◊ Gracilis Sling procedure

ACTIVITY   Full activity, when able

DIET   High fiber

PATIENT EDUCATION
• Particular reassurance to parents of infants with prolapse regarding benign nature of problem and high rate of spontaneous resolution
• Diet instructions
• Teach measures to avoid constipation

MEDICATIONS

DRUG(S) OF CHOICE
• Mineral oil
• Stool softeners
Contraindications: N/A
Precautions: N/A
Significant possible interactions: N/A

ALTERNATIVE DRUGS N/A

FOLLOWUP

PATIENT MONITORING Monthly visits until possible need for surgery has been determined or until prolapse has resolved

PREVENTION/AVOIDANCE Avoid constipation and diarrhea

POSSIBLE COMPLICATIONS
• Mucosal ulcerations
• Necrosis of rectal wall

EXPECTED COURSE AND PROGNOSIS
• Spontaneous resolution expected in most children
• 5-10% recurrence rate for most procedures
• Good prognosis with treatment

MISCELLANEOUS

ASSOCIATED CONDITIONS
• Cystic fibrosis
• Myelomeningocele
• Exstrophy of the bladder
• Chronic constipation or diarrhea
• Imperforate anus
• Paraplegia
• Stroke
• Incontinence

AGE-RELATED FACTORS
Pediatric: Idiopathic most common type of rectal prolapse in children
Geriatric: Common problem in the elderly
Others: N/A

PREGNANCY N/A

SYNONYMS N/A

ICD-9-CM 569.1

SEE ALSO
• Intussusception
• Hemorrhoids

OTHER NOTES N/A

ABBREVIATIONS N/A

REFERENCES
• Holder, T.M. & Ashcraft, K.W., (eds.): Pediatric Surgery. 2nd Ed. Philadelphia, W.B. Saunders Co., 1993
• Schwartz, S.I., Shires, G.T., Spencer, F.C., et al. (eds.): Principles of Surgery. 4th Ed. New York, McGraw-Hill Book Co., 1984
• Welch, K.G., Randolph, J.G., Ravitch, M.M., et al. (eds.): Pediatric Surgery. 4th Ed. Chicago, Year Book Medical Publishers, 1986

Author T. Black, M.D. & J. Miller, M.D.

Reiter's syndrome

BASICS

DESCRIPTION A triad of features including arthritis, conjunctivitis, and urethritis or cervicitis. Epidemiologically similar to other reactive arthritis syndromes characterized by sterile inflammation of joints from infections originating at non-articular sites. A fourth feature may be buccal ulceration or balanitis. (It is possible for only two features to be present.)
• Two forms:
◊ Sexually transmitted, symptoms usually begin 7-14 days after exposure
◊ Post-dysentery
System(s) affected: Musculoskeletal, Skin/Exocrine, Renal/Urologic
Genetics: HLA-B27 tissue antigen present in 60-80% of patients
Incidence/Prevalence in USA: 0.24-1.5% incidence after epidemics of bacterial dysentery; complicates 1-2% cases of non-gonococcal urethritis
Predominant age: 20-40 years
Predominant sex: Male > Female

SIGNS AND SYMPTOMS
Musculoskeletal:
◊ Asymmetric arthritis (especially knees, ankles, MTP joints)
◊ Enthesopathy (inflammation at tendinous insertion into bone) such as plantar fasciitis, digital periostitis, Achilles tendinitis
◊ Spondyloarthropathy (spine and sacroiliac joint involvement)
Urogenital tract:
◊ Urethritis
◊ Prostatitis
◊ Occasionally cystitis
◊ Balanitis
◊ Cervicitis - usually asymptomatic
Eye:
◊ Conjunctivitis of one or both eyes
◊ Occasionally scleritis, keratitis, corneal ulceration
◊ rarely uveitis and iritis
Skin:
◊ Mucocutaneous lesions (small, painless, superficial ulcers on oral mucosa, tongue, glans penis)
◊ Keratoderma blennorrhagica (hyperkeratotic skin lesions of palms and soles and around nails)
Cardiovascular:
◊ Occasionally pericarditis, murmur, conduction defects, aortic incompetence
Nervous system:
◊ Rarely peripheral neuropathy, cranial neuropathy, meningoencephalitis, neuropsychiatric changes
Constitutional:
◊ Fever, malaise, anorexia, weight loss
◊ Can appear seriously ill (fever, rigors, tachycardia, exquisitely tender joints)

CAUSES
• Chlamydia trachomatis the usual causative organism of postvenereal variety
• Dysenteric form following enteric bacterial infection due to Shigella, Salmonella, Yersinia, and Campylobacter organisms. This form more likely in women, children and the elderly.

RISK FACTORS
• Sexual intercourse 7-14 days prior to illness
• Food poisoning or bacterial dysenteric outbreak

DIAGNOSIS

DIFFERENTIAL DIAGNOSIS
• For specific diagnosis, arthritis associated with urethritis for longer than one month
• Rheumatoid arthritis
• Ankylosing spondylitis
• Arthritis associated with inflammatory bowel disease
• Psoriatic arthritis
• Juvenile rheumatoid arthritis
• Bacterial arthritis including gonococcal

LABORATORY
Blood
◊ WBC 10,000-20,000
◊ Neutrophilic leukocytosis
◊ Elevated erythrocyte sedimentation rate
◊ Moderate normochromic anemia
◊ Hypergammaglobulinemia
Synovial fluid
◊ WBC 1000-8000 cells/mm3
◊ Bacterial culture negative
Collaborative tests
◊ Cultures or serology positive for Chlamydia trachomatis, or stools positive for Salmonella, Shigella, Yersinia or Campylobacter support the diagnosis
Drugs that may alter lab results: Antibiotics may affect isolation of the bacterial pathogens
Disorders that may alter lab results: N/A

PATHOLOGICAL FINDINGS
• A seronegative spondyloarthropathy (similar to ankylosing spondylitis, enteric arthritis and psoriatic arthritis)
• Villous formation in joints
• Joint hyperemia
• Joint inflammation
• Prostatitis
• Seminal vesiculitis
• Skin biopsy similar to psoriasis
• Non-specific conjunctivitis

SPECIAL TESTS Histocompatibility antigen HLA-B27 positive in 60-80% of cases

IMAGING
X-ray
◊ Periosteal proliferation, thickening
◊ Spurs
◊ Erosions at articular margins
◊ Residual joint destruction
◊ Syndesmophytes (spine)
◊ Sacroiliitis

DIAGNOSTIC PROCEDURES N/A

TREATMENT

APPROPRIATE HEALTH CARE
Inpatient possibly, during acute phase

GENERAL MEASURES
• Treatment is symptomatic
• No treatment necessary for conjunctivitis. Iritis may require treatment.
• Treatment unnecessary for mucocutaneous lesions
• Physical therapy during recovery phase
• Arthritis may be prominent and disabling during the acute phase

ACTIVITY Bedrest until joint inflammation subsides

DIET No special diet

PATIENT EDUCATION
• Teach home physical therapy techniques
• For patient education materials favorably reviewed on this topic, contact: American Academy of Family Physicians Foundation, P.O. Box 8418, Kansas City, MO 64114, (800)274-2237, ext. 4400
• Arthritis Foundation, 1314 Spring Street N.W., Atlanta, GA 30309, (404)872-7100

MEDICATIONS

DRUG(S) OF CHOICE
• Symptomatic management - NSAID's including indomethacin, Naprosyn; intraarticular or systemic corticosteroids for refractory arthritis and enthesitis
• For GI upset - antacids
• For iritis - intraocular steroids

Contraindications:
• Gastrointestinal bleeding
• Patients with peptic ulcer, gastritis, ulcerative colitis
• Renal insufficiency

Precautions: Refer to manufacturer's literature

Significant possible interactions: Refer to manufacturer's literature

ALTERNATIVE DRUGS
• Aspirin or other NSAID's
• Sulfasalazine is promising, but not yet approved
• Methotrexate or azathioprine in severe cases (still experimental and not approved or agreed to be effective. Contraindicated, if HIV related Reiter's).

FOLLOWUP

PATIENT MONITORING
Monitor clinical response to medications. Surveillance for complications of therapy, sulfasalazine, immunosuppressives.

PREVENTION/AVOIDANCE   N/A

POSSIBLE COMPLICATIONS
• Chronic or recurrent disease in 5-50%
• Ankylosing spondylitis develops in 30-50% of HLA-B27 positive patients
• Urethral strictures
• Cataracts and blindness
• Aortic root necrosis

EXPECTED COURSE AND PROGNOSIS
• Urethritis within 1-15 days after sexual exposure
• Onset of Reiter's syndrome within 10-30 days of infection
• Mean duration 19 weeks
• Poor prognosis associated with local disease involving heel, eye or heart

MISCELLANEOUS

ASSOCIATED CONDITIONS
• Prior shigellosis
• Salmonellosis
• Yersinia
• Mycoplasma
• Chlamydia urethritis
• HIV infection

AGE-RELATED FACTORS   N/A
Pediatric: Enteric etiology more likely than chlamydia
Geriatric: Enteric etiology more likely than sexually transmitted
Others: N/A

PREGNANCY
No special considerations other than usual precautions regarding drugs

SYNONYMS
• Idiopathic blennorrheal arthritis
• Arthritis urethritica
• Urethro-oculo-articular syndrome
• Fiessinger-Leroy-Reiter disease

ICD-9-CM   099.3 Reiter's disease

SEE ALSO
• Behçet's syndrome
• Ankylosing spondylitis
• Psoriatic arthritis

OTHER NOTES Effects of antibiotics on the development and long-term outcome of Reiter's syndrome not known

ABBREVIATIONS   N/A

REFERENCES
• Kean, W.F. & MacPherson, D.W.: Reiter's syndrome. In Prognosis in the Rheumatic Diseases. Edited by N. Bellamy. London, Kluwer Academic Publishers 1991
• Rein, M.F.: Urethritis. In Principles and Practice of Infectious Diseases. Edited by G.L. Mandell, R.G. Douglas & J.E. Bennett. 3rd Ed. New York, Churchill Livingstone, 1990

Author   E. R. Jeans, M.D. & D. W. MacPherson, M.D.

Renal calculi

 BASICS

DESCRIPTION Renal stones occur throughout the urinary tract and are common causes of pain, infection and obstruction. The pathogenesis is multifactorial. Stones are initially formed in the proximal urinary tract and pass distally. They usually become arrested at three points in the ureter - the ureteropelvic junction (UPJ), where the ureter crosses the iliac vessels, and the ureter-vesicular junction (UVJ). Renal stones consist of four basic types: 1) calcium stones - 80%, 2) uric acid stones - 5%, 3) cystine stones - 2%, 4) struvite stones.
System(s) affected: Renal/Urologic
Genetics: Genetic cause in production of cystine stones - inborn error in amino acid transport produces cystinuria
Incidence/Prevalence in USA:
 • Of all renal calculi, roughly 1:1000 annual frequency of hospitalization
 • Approximately 1% of autopsies
Predominant Age: 30-50 years, most common in third decade
Predominant sex:
 • Varies depending upon type of stone
 • Calcium stones - Male > Female (3:1)
 • Struvite stones - Female > Male

SIGNS AND SYMPTOMS
 • Back pain and "renal colic" - agonizing flank pain that waxes and wanes
 • Pain may radiate to groin, testicles, suprapubic area or labia
 • May be asymptomatic
 • Hematuria, dysuria, urinary frequency
 • Diaphoresis, tachycardia, tachypnea
 • Chills and fever if associated with acute infection due to obstruction
 • Hypertension due to pain
 • Gastrointestinal symptoms - nausea, vomiting, abdominal distention with associated reflex ileus
 • Costovertebral angle tenderness

CAUSES
 • Increased supersaturation of urine with stone-forming salts
 • Preformed crystals
 • Abnormal crystal growth inhibitors
 • Calcium stones - due to hypercalciuria, hyperparathyroidism, hyperoxaluria, hypocitruria
 • Uric acid stones - due to low urinary volume, overproduction of uric acid, acidic urinary pH
 • Cystine stones - inborn error in amino acid transport (cystinuria)
 • Struvite stones - due to alkalotic pH usually secondary to infection with urea splitting organisms (i.e., Proteus mirabilis)

RISK FACTORS
 • Intrinsic factors - renal tubular acidosis, cystinuria, genetic defects
 • Extrinsic factors - geographical, climatic and seasonal factors, low water intake, high animal protein diet, sedentary lifestyle

 DIAGNOSIS

DIFFERENTIAL DIAGNOSIS
 • Acute peritonitis
 • Gastroenteritis
 • Acute appendicitis
 • Colitis
 • Diverticulitis
 • Salpingitis
 • Cholecystitis
 • Peptic ulcer disease
 • Pancreatitis

LABORATORY
 • CBC with differential - look for signs of infection
 • BUN/creatinine - evaluate renal function
 • Urine culture and sensitivity if concerned about infection
 • Ca+, PO4, uric acid if recurrent problem
Urinalysis
  ◊ Microscopic or gross hematuria pyuria
  ◊ Bacteriuria
  ◊ Crystals
  ◊ PH-acidic = uric acid or cystine stones
  ◊ Alkaline = struvite stones
Drugs that may alter lab results: None
Disorders that may alter lab results: Other underlying infections or renal abnormalities

PATHOLOGICAL FINDINGS Calcium, uric acid, cystine and struvite stones

SPECIAL TESTS 24 hour urine collections for Ca+, uric acid, Mg+, oxalate, citrate and creatinine

IMAGING
 • Plain film x-ray of abdomen (may add oblique views) - 90% of stones are radiopaque. Ca+ phosphate stones most opaque followed by Ca+ oxalate, struvite and cystine stones. Uric acid stones radiolucent. Usually stones must be greater than 2 mm diameter to be seen on plain film.
 • Intravenous urography - to evaluate the extent of obstruction and detect radiolucent stones
 • Tomograms may reveal a stone obscured on plain film by gas or feces
 • Retrograde urography - rarely needed, only if diagnosis is suspect or patient allergic to intravenous contrast medium
 • Ultrasonography - if unable to obtain intravenous urography due to contrast allergy. Can assist in diagnosis of hydronephrosis.
 • CT - useful if filling defect to help differentiate ureteral calculi from other causes such as malignancy. Also helpful if non-opaque stone or tumor suspected.
 • MRI - not helpful

DIAGNOSTIC PROCEDURES Retrograde urography - rarely needed

 TREATMENT

APPROPRIATE HEALTH CARE
Generally outpatient (90%) unless associated with infection, excessive nausea or vomiting, or when stones are greater than 6 mm in diameter

GENERAL MEASURES
 • Pain relief
 • Aggressive fluid management
 • Strain urine for stone collection and analysis
 • Treatment includes percutaneous chemolysis, systemic chemolysis, endo-urologic stone extraction, extracorporeal shock wave lithotripsy, and rarely, open surgery

ACTIVITY As tolerated

DIET
 • Low animal fat diet
 • Increased fiber (especially bran)
 • Increased fluid intake to keep urine output greater than 3 liters a day
 • Other dietary restrictions depend upon specific type of stone formed

PATIENT EDUCATION
 • Follow dietary and fluid intake recommendations
 • Instruction on fitness

MEDICATIONS

DRUG(S) OF CHOICE
• Analgesia: Demerol 50-100 mg IM q 3-4 hrs or morphine 10-15 mg IM q 3-4 hrs
• For Ca+ stones due to hypercalciuria - hydrochlorothiazide 50 mg bid
• For Ca+ oxalate stones with hyperuricosuria - allopurinol 100 mg tid

Contraindications: Allergies to medications

Precautions: See manufacturer's profile of each drug

Significant possible interactions: See manufacturer's profile of each drug

ALTERNATIVE DRUGS
• Ketorolac tromethamine (Toradol) 30-60 mg IM, then 30 mg q 6 hrs prn (Note: very costly, and may cause GI bleeding in some patients)
• Percocet, Tylenol 3, other oral narcotics

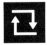

FOLLOWUP

PATIENT MONITORING
• Plain films of abdomen at 1-2 week intervals to monitor progress of stone in ureter
• Continue to strain urine until stone is passed
• Stone analysis required
• Usually resolved within 4 weeks
• Monitor K+ and blood pressure in patients taking hydrochlorothiazide

PREVENTION/AVOIDANCE
Follow dietary restrictions and fluid management

POSSIBLE COMPLICATIONS
• Complete obstruction
• Hydronephrosis
• Kidney failure
• Infection, death

EXPECTED COURSE AND PROGNOSIS
• Usually associated with complete return to previous baseline
• Recurrences common - up to 50% within 5 years

MISCELLANEOUS

ASSOCIATED CONDITIONS
• Hyperparathyroidism
• Gout
• Cystinuria
• Hyperuricemia
• Sarcoidosis
• Infections
• Immobilization from trauma or chronic illness

AGE-RELATED FACTORS
Pediatric: Rare in this age group
Geriatric: Complications more likely
Others: N/A

PREGNANCY
Approximately same prevalence

SYNONYMS
• Renal calculi
• Kidney stone
• Urologic stone

ICD-9-CM   592.0

SEE ALSO   Urolithiasis

OTHER NOTES   N/A

ABBREVIATIONS   N/A

REFERENCES
• Harvey, A.M.: The Principles and Practice of Medicine. 22nd Ed. Norwalk, CT, Appleton & Lange, 1988
• Rakel, R.E. (ed.): Conn's Current Therapy. Philadelphia, W.B. Saunders, Co., 1991
• Tanagho, E.A. & McAninch, J.W. (eds.): Smith's General Urology. 13th Ed. Norwalk, CT, Appleton & Lange, 1991

Author   L. Ralph, M.D.

Renal cell adenocarcinoma

 BASICS

DESCRIPTION
The most common solid renal neoplasm, renal cell adenocarcinoma, represents 2-3% of all adult malignancies; 9th most common male malignant tumor, 13th most common female malignant tumor
System(s) affected: Renal/Urologic
Genetics:
• Oncogenes localized to the short arm of chromosome 3 may have etiologic implications
• People with HLA antigen types Bw44 and DR8 are prone to develop renal cancer. These are rare familial renal carcinomas.
Incidence/Prevalence in USA:
• 15,000-18,000 new cases per year; 7,500 deaths per year
• Men: 9.4 per million
• Women: 4.6 per million
Predominant age: 5th and 6th decades
Predominant sex: Male > Female (2:1)

SIGNS AND SYMPTOMS
• Solid renal masses, most 6-7 cm (incidentally discovered in asymptomatic patient due to increased use of CT and MRI)
• Hematuria 50-60%
• Elevated erythrocyte sedimentation rate 50-60%
• Abdominal mass 24-45%
• Anemia 21-41%
• Flank pain 35-40%
• Hypertension 22-38%
• Weight loss 28-36%
• Pyrexia 7-17%
• Hepatic dysfunction 10-15%
• Classic triad (hematuria, abdominal mass, flank pain) 7-10%
• Hypercalcemia 3-6%
• Erythrocytosis 3-4%
• Varicocele 2-3%
• Patients with vena caval thrombus present with lower extremity edema, new varicocele, dilated superficial abdominal veins, albuminuria, pulmonary emboli, right atrial mass or non-function of the involved kidney

CAUSES Unknown

RISK FACTORS
• Smoking
• Obesity
• Urban environment
• Cadmium
• Asbestos
• Petroleum by-products
• Herpes simplex virus exposure
• Phenacetin or analgesic abuse for transitional cell of the renal pelvis

 DIAGNOSIS

DIFFERENTIAL DIAGNOSIS
• Hydronephrosis
• Polycystic kidneys
• Renal tuberculosis
• Renal calculi
• Renal infarction
• Benign renal cyst
• Transitional cell carcinoma

LABORATORY
• Anemia (21-41% of patients)
• Polycythemia
• Hematuria
• Alkaline phosphate may be elevated
• Increased erythrocyte sedimentation rate
• Urine - neoplastic cells
• Hypercalcemia
• Increased renin
• Transitional cell cancer (rare)
Drugs that may alter lab results: N/A
Disorders that may alter lab results: N/A

PATHOLOGICAL FINDINGS
• Renal cell tends to bulge out from the cortex producing a mass effect
• The average renal cell carcinoma measures 7-8 cm and is grossly yellow to yellow/orange due to its high lipid content in the clear cell variety. Average renal cell size has been decreasing due to incidental discovery.
• The granuloma cell type more likely gray to white
• Small tumors are homogenous
• Large tumors may have areas of necrosis and hemorrhage
• A pseudocapsule covers the tumors
• Tumor thrombi into the vena cava generally do not invade the vena caval wall
• Microscopically there is a mixture of clear granular and occasionally sarcomatoid cells

SPECIAL TESTS
• Arteriography (rarely needed) - for tumors larger than 10 cm, it may identify parasitic capsular vessels for early control
• Cystoscopy - to rule out bladder cancer
• ECG as needed

IMAGING
• Intravenous pyelography with infusion nephrotomography remains the primary screening test for renal malignancy
• Ultrasonography - if there appears to be a mass on IVP, confirms the presence of a lesion and determines whether it is solid or cystic. Cystic lesions may either be observed or subjected to percutaneous cyst puncture.
• CT scan and, occasionally, arteriography - if solid or complex masses upon ultrasonography require further evaluation. 3% of RCC are bilateral by CT scan.
• Rapid sequence CT can demonstrate tumor enhancement
• MRI has not been shown to be superior to CT for tumors smaller than 8 cm, for larger tumors it may have advantage in delineating the vena cava

• Bone scans are indicated if the alkaline phosphatase is elevated or the patient has bone pain
• Brain CT is indicated if the patient has neurologic symptoms

DIAGNOSTIC PROCEDURES
• Simple cyst need not be aspirated
• Calcified cysts may contain renal cell cancer and therefore require open renal biopsy of the wall of the cyst
• Hemorrhagic cyst - aspiration cytology may be helpful but needle biopsy of solid masses is to be discouraged, particularly if the patient has a normal contralateral kidney
• In solitary kidneys, open renal biopsy with wedge resection (not enucleation) can be performed
• Doppler flow ultrasound of the renal veins or CT (thin cuts) that shows the renal vein entering the vena cava can be used to rule out tumor thrombus
• Venogram - when tumor thrombus is identified. The venogram can demonstrate when the thrombus goes above the hepatic veins or diaphragm (i.e., rarely cardiopulmonary bypass needed to remove the thrombus above the diaphragm at the time of nephrectomy).

 TREATMENT

APPROPRIATE HEALTH CARE
Inpatient

GENERAL MEASURES
• Surgery is indicated. Drug therapy has been only erratically effective. Lesions are fairly radiation resistant.
• Maintain hydration during iodine injection diagnostic studies to prevent acute tubular necrosis
• Consider a mechanical bowel preparation to ease the nephrectomy
• Consider antibiotic bowel preparation for larger tumors (> 10 cm) where possible bowel injury or resection may be more likely
• Exploration wedge resection for solitary kidney or tumors less than 3 cm, otherwise radical nephrectomy in the face of a normal contralateral kidney is preferred
• Usual preoperative pulmonary toilet, pulmonary function tests if indicated
• Renal cell carcinoma (85% of renal parenchymal malignant tumors) - CT solid mass larger than 3 cm, radical nephrectomy if there is a normal contralateral kidney; smaller than 3 cm, wedge resection
• Angiomyolipoma (80% of tuberous sclerosis patients have these benign tumors) - classic CT findings, may be followed with CT
• Hemorrhage into a cyst - aspiration cytology
• Complex cyst (calcified cyst wall or irregular wall) - open cyst wall biopsy if cytology is inconclusive
• Transitional cell carcinoma of the renal pelvis or calyces - nephroureterectomy
• Oncocytoma - larger than 3 cm, radical nephrectomy

Renal cell adenocarcinoma

- Sarcoma - wide excision
- Adult Wilm's tumor - radical nephrectomy for unilateral disease
- Metastasis (lymphoma to lung to breast to stomach) - depends on prognosis of primary tumor; nephrectomy for uncontrolled bleeding
- Cortical adenoma smaller than 3 cm (7-22% at autopsy) - wedge resection

ACTIVITY
- No special preoperative activity
- Postoperatively - as tolerated

DIET
Total parenteral nutrition is seldom necessary

PATIENT EDUCATION
- Preoperative nursing education is indicated for pulmonary toilet
- Pre-anesthesia education is needed if the patient is to have a patient controlled analgesia pump or epidural catheter for postoperative pain relief
- Printed patient information available from: National Kidney & Urologic Diseases Information Clearinghouse, Box NKUDIC, Bethesda, MD 20893, (301)468-6345

MEDICATIONS

DRUG(S) OF CHOICE None
Contraindications: N/A
Precautions: N/A
Significant possible interactions: N/A

ALTERNATIVE DRUGS
- For advanced renal cell carcinoma - interleukin (IL)-2 plus LAK, or IL-2 alone
- Hormones - progesterone agents yield a 5-10% response rate
- Chemotherapy - vinblastine alone or with CCNU yields a 10-15% response rate

FOLLOWUP

PATIENT MONITORING
- One CT scan of the abdomen and renal fossa can be done 3-6 months later, particularly if the capsule or lymph nodes are positive, to monitor recurrences and repeat resection if needed for flank pain or mass
- Chest x-rays are performed quarterly to rule out pulmonary metastasis
- Skeletal x-rays and bone scan can be useful in detecting skeletal metastasis but should only be obtained if patient complains of bone pain or an alkaline phosphatase elevation
- Postoperative followup may be possible with plasma transcobalamin II or serum haptoglobin level to detect or monitor recurrences

PREVENTION/AVOIDANCE
- Do not smoke
- Eat a sensible diet
- Avoid stress, asbestos, cadmium, and petroleum distillates

POSSIBLE COMPLICATIONS
- Paraplegia can result with little warning from spinal vertebral metastasis
- CNS metastasis are not uncommon
- Approximately 30% of patients with RCC have metastatic disease when the diagnosis is established. The most common sites of metastasis are the lung (50-60%), bone (30-40%), regional nodes (15-30%), brain (10%) and adjacent organs (10%).

EXPECTED COURSE AND PROGNOSIS

```
---STAGING--------------------
                  Robson's  5 year
                  staging   survival
Small tumor       I         60-70%
Large tumor       I         60-70%
Perinephric fat   II        50-65%
Renal vein        IIIa      50-60%
IVC involvement†  IIIa      5-35%
Adjacent structure IVa      0-5%
Single node       IIIb      35%
Multiple node     III       5-35%
Fixed nodes       IIIb      5%
Distant metastases IVb      0-5%
------------------------------
                  TNM       5 year
                  staging   survival
Small tumor       T1        60-70%
Large tumor       T2        60-70%
Perinephric fat   T3        50-65%
Renal vein        T3b       50-60%
IVC involvement†  T3c       5-35%
Adjacent structure T4a      0-5%
Single node       N1        35%
Multiple node     N2        5-35%
Fixed nodes       N3        5%
Distant metastases M1       0-5%
------------------------------
†Infradiaphragmatic vena caval
```

MISCELLANEOUS

ASSOCIATED CONDITIONS
- Von Hippel-Lindau disease (30-45% of these patients develop renal cell)
- Adult polycystic kidney disease
- Horseshoe kidney
- Acquired renal cystic disease from chronic renal failure

AGE-RELATED FACTORS
Pediatric: Extremely rare in children
Geriatric: Most commonly presents in the 5th and 6th decade
Others: N/A

PREGNANCY
N/A

SYNONYMS
- Kidney cancer
- Hypernephroma
- Grawitz's tumor
- Hypernephroid cancer

ICD-9-CM 189.0 malignant neoplasm of the kidney

SEE ALSO N/A

OTHER NOTES N/A

ABBREVIATIONS RCC = renal cell carcinoma

REFERENCES
- Williams, R.D.: Renal, perirenal and ureteral neoplasms, In Adult and Pediatric Urology. Edited by J.Y. Gillenwater. Chicago, Year Book Medical Publishers, 1987
- Resnick, M.Y.: Current Therapy in Genitourinary Surgery. 2nd Ed. St. Louis, Mosby-Year Book Publishers, 1992
- Novick, A.C.: Partial nephrectomy for renal carcinoma. Urol Clin N Am, 14:419, 1987
- Spencer, W., Novick, A.C., et al.: Conservative surgery for transitional cell carcinoma of the renal pelvis. J Urol, 139:507, 1988
- Montie, J., Jackson, C., Cosgrove, D., Streem, S. & Novick, A.C.: Resection of large inferior vena cava thrombi from renal cell carcinoma with the use of circulatory arrest. J Urol, 139:25, 1988
- Novick, A.C., Streem, S.B., et al.: Conservative surgery for renal cell carcinoma; A single center experience with 100 patients. J Urol, 141:835, 1989

Author M. Thomas, M.D.

Renal failure, acute (ARF)

BASICS

DESCRIPTION A syndrome of rapidly deteriorating kidney function with the accumulation of nitrogenous wastes
Systems affected: Initial renal/urological; later all
Genetics: No known genetic pattern
Incidence/Prevalence in USA: 5% of patients admitted to the hospital develop ARF; 10-15% of ICU patients develop ARF; 2-7% post open heart patients develop ARF; 50% of hospital ARF is iatrogenic.
Predominant age: All ages (average age increasing)
Predominant sex: Male = Female

SIGNS AND SYMPTOMS
- Anorexia
- Asterixis
- Back pain
- Coma
- Delirium
- Diarrhea
- Dyspnea
- Ecchymosis
- Edema
- Encephalopathy
- Epistaxis
- Fasciculation
- Fatigue
- GI hemorrhage
- Headache
- Hiccups
- Hyperpnea
- Hypertension
- Left ventricular failure
- Lethargy
- Muscle cramps
- Myoclonus
- Nausea
- Oliguria
- Pericarditis
- Petechiae
- Purpura (vasculitis)
- Rales
- Rash (acute interstitial nephritis)
- Retinopathy
- Seizure
- Somnolence
- Tachycardia
- Tachypnea
- Uriniferous odor
- Vomiting
- Weakness
- Xerostomia

CAUSES
Pre-renal
  ◊ Hypovolemia
  ◊ Ineffective circulating volume: Congestive heart failure, cirrhosis, nephrotic syndrome and early sepsis
Renal
  ◊ Tubular, interstitial: Acute interstitial nephritis (AIN) (drugs, infection); nephrotoxins; acute tubular necrosis
  ◊ Glomerular: Rapidly progressive (crescentic) glomerulonephritis (RPGN) (Immunofluorescence biopsy staining: linear, immune complex or pauci-immune); pregnancy (2%); systemic lupus erythematosus
Vascular
  ◊ Ischemic nephropathy (renal artery stenosis)
  ◊ Dissecting aortic aneurysm
  ◊ Ruptured abdominal aortic aneurysm
Post-renal
  ◊ Obstruction (See hydronephrosis)

RISK FACTORS
- Surgery (especially with increased age, elevated creatinine, simultaneous cardiac valve and bypass surgery)
- Volume depletion (especially in diabetes)
- Aminoglycoside therapy, congestive heart failure, contrast exposure, septic shock
- Nephrotoxic drugs (e.g., ACE inhibitors in renal artery stenosis)

DIAGNOSIS

DIFFERENTIAL DIAGNOSIS See causes

LABORATORY
Urinalysis
  ◊ Proteinuria
  ◊ Hematuria
  ◊ Brown granular urinary casts
  ◊ Urinary renal tubular epithelial cells
Urine sediment
  ◊ Coarse granular casts
  ◊ Renal tubular epithelial cells
  ◊ Eosinophils (AIN?)
  ◊ Red cell or hemoglobin casts (RPGN)
  ◊ Crystals (lithiasis, obstruction)
Urine electrolytes/osmolality
  ◊ Increased urine sodium (> 20 meq/L), increased fractional excretion of sodium (> 3%) (e.g. renal).
Calculation: Fractional excretion of sodium = [(Urine Na+/Serum Na+) / (Urine creatinine/Serum creatinine)] X 100
  ◊ Urine isotonic to plasma
  ◊ Low urine sodium (< 10 meq/L), low fractional excretion of sodium (≤ 1%), concentrate urine osmolality (≥ 500 mOsm/liter) (e.g., pre-renal)
Other
  ◊ Azotemia
  ◊ Decreased creatinine clearance
  ◊ Hyperosmolarity
  ◊ Hyperphosphatemia
  ◊ Hyperkalemia
  ◊ Decreased serum bicarbonate
  ◊ Increased plasma volume

  ◊ Decreased hemoglobin
  ◊ Decreased hematocrit
  ◊ Hypocapnia
  ◊ Increased serum magnesium
  ◊ Acidemia (increased anion gap)
  ◊ Increased serum amylase/lipase
  ◊ Hyponatremia
  ◊ Hypocalcemia
  ◊ Increased serum uric acid
  ◊ Increased bleeding time
Drugs that may alter lab results: Too many to list
Disorders that may alter lab results: Too many to list

PATHOLOGICAL FINDINGS Kidney biopsy: Not particularly helpful in acute tubular necrosis (ATN). Diagnostic in AIN and RPGN.

SPECIAL TESTS
- Angiogram (renal vascular disease)
- Cystoscopy - retrograde
- Bleeding time

IMAGING
- Obstruction - renal scan, CT scan
- Kidney ultrasound
  ◊ Renal cause: "Medical" renal disease (renal echogenicity = liver), normal size kidneys, kidney size disparity: ischemia
  ◊ Post renal cause - hydronephrosis

DIAGNOSTIC PROCEDURES Renal biopsy (ARF, unknown cause), diagnostic for AIN, RPGN

TREATMENT

APPROPRIATE HEALTH CARE
Inpatient and intensive care

GENERAL MEASURES
- Correction of underlying hemodynamic abnormalities
- Hemodialysis as soon as diagnosis of uremia is established
- Decrease catabolism
- Convert oliguria to nonoliguria
- Daily weight
- Correct reversible causes (volume and mannitol)
- Modify dosages of renal excreted drugs
- If drug induced, discontinue offending agent
- Meticulous aseptic technique
- Continuous arteriovenous hemofiltration
- Intravenous human immunoglobulin G
- Correct easy bleeding with DDAVP, estrogen and cryoprecipitate
- Question prednisone in AIN

ACTIVITY As tolerated

DIET
• Restrict protein
• Restrict fluids to volume of urine output plus 500 mL/day
• Eliminate potassium if serum level increased
• Oral and IV amino acids
• Increase carbohydrates to decrease catabolism

PATIENT EDUCATION
National Kidney & Urologic Diseases Information Clearinghouse, Box NKUDIC, Bethesda, MD 20893, (301)468-6345 and The National Kidney Foundation, Inc., 30 East 33rd Street, NY, NY 10016. "What Everyone Should Know About Kidneys and Kidney Disease" (Order #01-01BP - English), (Order #01-02BP -Spanish).

MEDICATIONS

DRUG(S) OF CHOICE Prior to fixed renal failure: IV volume expansion with normal saline followed by mannitol, Lasix, and calcium channel blockers
Contraindications: N/A
Precautions:
• Pharmokinetics of all drugs used in renal failure should be reviewed for appropriate adjustment
For example, antiarrhythmic drugs:
◊ Quinidine - decrease dose, closely monitor drug level
◊ Procainamide - avoid in renal failure
◊ Disopyramide - reduction in maintenance dose
◊ Mexiletine - no dose adjustment-liver metabolized, etc.
Significant possible interactions: Refer to manufacturer's literature

ALTERNATIVE DRUGS N/A

FOLLOWUP

PATIENT MONITORING As needed

PREVENTION/AVOIDANCE
• See risk factors
• Allopurinol prior to chemotherapy for hematologic malignancy
• Hydration most important, especially prior to contrast and chemotherapy.

POSSIBLE COMPLICATIONS
• Sepsis - infection (leading cause of mortality)
• Convulsions
• Edema
• Pulmonary edema
• Congestive heart failure
• Hyperkalemia
• Paralysis
• Arrhythmias
• Death (50%)
• Pericarditis/tamponade
• Uremia
• Bleeding

EXPECTED COURSE AND
PROGNOSIS Recover usually in days to 6 weeks. High mortality rate (5-80%) depending on cause/multi-organ involvement, and age.

MISCELLANEOUS

ASSOCIATED CONDITIONS
• Hyperphosphatemia
• Hydronephrosis
• Muscle injury
• Congestive heart failure
• Cirrhosis
• Malignant hypertension
• Vasculitis
• Bacterial infections
• Drug reactions
• Hypercalcemia
• Hyperuricemia
• Sepsis
• Severe trauma
• Burns
• Transfusion reactions
• Internal bleeding

AGE-RELATED FACTORS
Pediatric: Congenital
Geriatric: Greater occurrence in this age group especially after surgery
Others: N/A

PREGNANCY N/A

SYNONYMS N/A

ICD-9-CM 584.9 acute renal failure unspecified

SEE ALSO
• Myeloma
• Hepatorenal syndrome
• Reye's syndrome
• Malignant hypertension
• Rocky Mountain spotted fever
• Hydronephrosis
• Chronic renal failure

OTHER NOTES N/A

ABBREVIATIONS
• ATN - acute tubular necrosis
• AIN - acute interstitial nephritis
• RPGN - rapidly progressive glomerulonephritis
• ACE = angiotensin converting enzyme

REFERENCES
• Schrier, R.W. (ed.): Renal and Electrolyte Disorders. 4th Ed. Boston, Little Brown & Co., 1992, p.495.
• Rutecki, G.W. & Whittier, F.C.: The Rules of Three in Oliguria. Consultant, 1993;33-43

Author G. Rutecki, M.D.

Renal failure, chronic

BASICS

DESCRIPTION The results of any renal injury that decreases renal excretory and regulatory function chronically. Characteristic findings: nitrogen retention, acidosis, and anemia.

System(s) affected: Renal/Urologic

Genetics:
• Hereditary renal diseases can lead to chronic renal failure in children and some adults (Alport's syndrome)
• Autosomal dominant polycystic kidney disease is a relatively common cause of chronic renal failure in adults affecting approximately 10% of dialysis population. Inherited in an autosomal dominant pattern with mutation on short arm chromosome 16.

Incidence/Prevalence in USA: Common (estimated that 160,000 persons per year are treated for end stage renal disease). Prevalence in the USA: 2.8/100,000 people in USA (estimate) with a chronic elevation of creatinine greater than 2.0 mg/dl.

Predominant age: All ages - much more common in adults. In children, chronic renal failure affects between 2 and 6 per 1 million population.

Predominant sex: Male = Female

SIGNS AND SYMPTOMS
• Anemia (normochromic, normocytic)
• Anorexia
• Confusion (late sign)
• Emotional lability
• Encephalopathy
• Fatigue on slight exertion
• Hypertension
• Insomnia
• Intractable hiccups
• Lassitude
• Mental depression
• Metallic taste in mouth
• Muscle cramps
• Muscle twitching
• Nausea
• Neuropathy
• Nocturia
• Pallor
• Polyuria
• Pruritus
• Seizures (late sign)
• Serositis
• Skin dry
• Stomatitis
• Slight breathlessness
• Vomiting

CAUSES
• Renal parenchymal: Glomerular: membranous nephropathy, membrano-proliferative glomerulonephritis, systemic lupus erythematosus, focal glomerulosclerosis, diabetes mellitus, proliferative glomerulonephritis, amyloidosis, Alport's syndrome, connective tissue disease.
• Interstitial-tubular: Heavy metals, drugs, nephrotoxins, multiple myeloma, hypertension, gout(?), thrombotic microangiopathies, oxalate deposition, infection, renal artery stenosis, connective tissue disease, autosomal dominant polycystic kidney disease, congenital.
• Post-renal: See hydronephrosis causes
• Pre-renal: Cirrhosis, cardiac, volume, nephrotic, drugs (e.g., NSAID's)

RISK FACTORS
• Contrast (diabetes, myeloma)
• Circulatory failure
• Urinary tract obstruction
• Analgesic abuse
• Untreated hypertension
• Diabetes mellitus

DIAGNOSIS

DIFFERENTIAL DIAGNOSIS See causes

LABORATORY
Blood:
◊ Smear - normochromic, normocytic anemia
◊ Decreased immune responsiveness
◊ Thrombocytopenia
◊ Decreased hematocrit
◊ Increased capillary fragility
◊ Increased bleeding time
Chemistry:
◊ Azotemia
◊ Elevated ammonia
◊ Type IV hyperlipidemia
◊ Decreased active Vitamin D
◊ Increased parathyroid hormone
◊ Elevated glucose, insulin resistance
◊ Elevated phosphate
◊ Elevated potassium
◊ Elevated sulfate
◊ Elevated uric acid
◊ Reduced calcium
◊ Serum CO_2 content - 15-20 mEq/L
Urine
◊ Proteinuria
◊ Casts

Drugs that may alter lab results:
• Cimetidine
• Trimethoprim
• Cefazolin: increase creatinine

Disorders that may alter lab results:
Ketosis may artifactually raise creatinine

PATHOLOGICAL FINDINGS
• Kidney biopsy
• Glomerulonephritis
• Interstitial nephritis

SPECIAL TESTS
• 24 hour urine studies (protein, clearance)
• Glofil clearance
• Complement studies
• Antinuclear antibody
• Serum protein electrophoresis
• Urine immune electrophoresis
• Hepatitis B surface antigen

IMAGING
• Ultrasound - shows decreased kidney size, may show obstructed ureter and bladder outlet
• CT scan

DIAGNOSTIC PROCEDURES Kidney biopsy

TREATMENT

APPROPRIATE HEALTH CARE
Inpatient or outpatient depending on severity

GENERAL MEASURES
• Treat any aggravating cause aggressively (salt and water depletion, nephrotoxins, congestive heart failure, infection, hypercalcemia, urinary obstruction)
• Drugs may exacerbate chronic renal failure
• Pay careful attention to dosing, and avoid use of nephrotoxic agents. When possible treat anemia with erythropoietin
• Dialysis: hemo, peritoneal, transplant
• Vitamin D (active) and calcium supplements

ACTIVITY Restricted only by patient's condition

DIET
• Adequate caloric intake
• Restricted protein intake
• Restricted intake of phosphate
• Water intake limited to maintain serum sodium concentration of 135 to 145 mEq/L
• Sodium restriction if volume expanded
• Potassium restriction if hyperkalemic
• Vitamin supplementation (avoid extra-dietary intake of magnesium)
• Strict dietary restrictions in the elderly may not be necessary, since they often have a low protein and salt intake

PATIENT EDUCATION
• For patient education materials favorably reviewed on this topic, contact: National Kidney and Urologic Diseases Information Clearinghouse, Box NKUDIC, Bethesda MD 20893. (301)468-6345
• The National Kidney Foundation, Inc. 30 East 33rd Street, New York, New York 10016. "Bone Disease in Chronic Renal Failure" (Order #02-27CP), "Diabetes and Kidney Disease" (Order #02-09CP). "Drug Abuse Can Hurt Your Kidneys" (Order #02-22N) or "Nutrition and Changing Kidney Function" (Order #0401).

MEDICATIONS

DRUG(S) OF CHOICE
• Multivitamin
• Lipid lowering agents appropriate for disorder (cholesterol lowering specifically for nephrotic syndrome)
• Erythropoietin for anemia
• Salt restriction and diuretics for edema
• Calcium acetate and oral vitamin D for renal failure osteodystrophy
• Hypertension: drugs to lower blood pressure
• Muscle cramps: Vitamin E or quinine
• Pruritus: Skin moisturizes, diphenhydramine, activated charcoal
• Bleeding: DDAVP, cryoprecipitate, dialysis in uremia
Contraindications: Refer to manufacturer's literature
Precautions:
• Monitor serum electrolytes carefully
• Monitor loop diuretic use to avoid volume depletion
• Decrease the dose of all medications with a renal route of excretion
Significant possible interactions: Refer to manufacturer's literature

ALTERNATIVE DRUGS
• Multivitamin preparation excluding fat-soluble vitamins and magnesium containing products
• Angiotensin converting enzyme inhibitors may prevent or slow progression to end stage renal failure (non renal vascular)

FOLLOWUP

PATIENT MONITORING
• Blood, urine, chemistries and clinical status
• Blood pressure, volume monitored frequently

PREVENTION/AVOIDANCE
• Avoid nephrotoxic drugs when possible (especially iodinated contrast, NSAID's)
• Treat all disorders known to lead to chronic renal failure
• Many drugs require dosage reduction to prevent toxicity
• Avoid volume depletion

POSSIBLE COMPLICATIONS
• Anemia
• Changes in calcium and phosphorous metabolism
• Lipid disorders
• Pericarditis
• Serositis
• Pseudogout
• Hypothyroidism
• Infections
• Hyperkalemia
• Acidosis
• Hyponatremia
• Gout
• Accelerated hypertension
• Metabolic calcification
• Spontaneous abortion
• Infertility
• Impotence
• Bleeding
• GI mucosal ulcerations
• GI A-V malformations
• Seizures
• Fractures

EXPECTED COURSE AND PROGNOSIS
Serious, chronic, mortality 50% despite careful attention to fluid and electrolyte balance or other treatment

MISCELLANEOUS

ASSOCIATED CONDITIONS
See conditions listed under Risk factors

AGE-RELATED FACTORS
Pediatric:
• Main causes in children include congenital renal and urinary tract malformations (signs appear before age 5), glomerular and hereditary renal diseases (signs appear between ages 5-15)
• Medical management much more difficult in children
• When it develops in infancy, growth impairment more profound than when disease develops in an otherwise healthy teenager
Geriatric:
• Highest incidence, highest morbidity, highest mortality. Renal disease is secondary to many age-dependent illnesses.
• Rule out such potentially reversible causes as urinary tract obstruction (particularly in men), renal arterial occlusion, hypercalcemia, use of nephrotoxic agents
• Older patients may tolerate dialysis quite well
Others: N/A

PREGNANCY N/A

SYNONYMS
• Uremia
• CRF

ICD-9-CM 585

SEE ALSO
• Acute renal failure
• Hydronephrosis
• Nephrotic syndrome
• Polycystic kidney disease

OTHER NOTES N/A

ABBREVIATIONS N/A

REFERENCES
• Chronic Renal Failure: Manifestations and Pathogenesis. In Renal and Electrolyte Disorders. 4th Ed. Edited by R.W. Schrier. Boston, Little Brown Co., 1992

Author G. Rutecki, M.D.

Renal tubular acidosis (RTA)

 BASICS

DESCRIPTION A group of disorders characterized by abnormal renal tubular acidification mechanisms, with glomerular function preserved, resulting in metabolic acidosis. These disorders are divided into three types:
• RTA-1: classic, distal, hypokalemic - due to inability to maintain H+ ion gradient
• RTA-2: proximal - due to decreased bicarbonate reabsorption. This is a limited acidosis because of the distal tubule resorptive capacity.
• RTA-3: no longer considered a distinct entity
• RTA-4: generalized, distal, hyperkalemic - due to primary or secondary aldosterone deficiency, or aldosterone resistance
Incidence/Prevalence in USA: N/A
System(s) affected: Renal/Urologic, Endocrine/Metabolic
Genetics: RTA-1 in children is autosomally dominant
Predominant age:
• RTA-1 and 2 mostly children
• RTA-4 mostly adults
Predominant sex: Male = Female

SIGNS AND SYMPTOMS
• Failure to thrive in RTA 1 and 2
• Emesis
• Polyuria
• Dehydration
• Weakness due to potassium loss
• Respiratory distress, hyperventilation in attempt to compensate for acidosis
• Gait disturbance and bone pain from disturbed calcium metabolism in RTA 2

CAUSES
• RTA 1
  ◊ Drug induced - amphotericin B, toluene, lithium, NSAID's
  ◊ Hypergammaglobulinemic syndromes
  ◊ Cirrhosis of liver
  ◊ Pyelonephritis
• RTA 2
  ◊ Drug induced - deteriorated tetracycline, acetazolamide, sulfonamides, diachrome heavy metals
  ◊ Amyloidosis
  ◊ Multiple myeloma
• RTA 4
  ◊ Lupus nephropathy
  ◊ Diabetic nephropathy
  ◊ Nephrosclerosis due to hypertension
  ◊ Tubulo-interstitial nephropathies
  ◊ Addison's disease
  ◊ Acute adrenal insufficiency

RISK FACTORS
• Hyperparathyroidism
• Chronic renal failure (CRF)

 DIAGNOSIS

DIFFERENTIAL DIAGNOSIS
• Metabolic acidosis of other causes - RTA has hyperchloremic non-anion gap acidosis
• Diarrhea with bicarbonate loss in stools
• CRF acidosis
• Respiratory acidosis

LABORATORY
• ABG - metabolic acidosis picture
• Serum electrolytes - potassium is increased in RTA 4, and normal or decreased in RTA 1 and 2. Chloride is increased. Bicarbonate is decreased.
• Serum BUN and creatinine - to rule out renal failure
• Urine pH - not acidified with metabolic acidosis present in RTA 1
• Urine Ca++ elevated
• Urine culture - to rule out UTI with urea splitting organisms
• Renin and aldosterone levels - decreased in most types RTA 4 caused by aldosterone deficiency, aldosterone resistant type RTA 4 have high levels
• Anion gap - normal
Drugs that may alter lab results:
• Diuretics
• NaHCO3 (sodium bicarbonate)
Disorders that may alter lab results: N/A

PATHOLOGICAL FINDINGS Tubular transport dysfunction

SPECIAL TESTS
• Maximize metabolic acidosis and monitor for urine acidification. Give po NH4Cl (ammonium chloride), and monitor urine pH. Beware for problems associated with exacerbating metabolic acidosis.
• Bicarbonate titration curves

IMAGING
• Intravenous pyelogram (IVP) - nephrocalcinosis, nephrolithiasis, intrinsic renal disease
• Renal sonograms - to evaluate for renal size, cysts or stones
• Bone films - osteomalacia with pseudo-fractures

DIAGNOSTIC PROCEDURES N/A

 TREATMENT

APPROPRIATE HEALTH CARE
Outpatient

GENERAL MEASURES
• Treatment with appropriate medications to correct acidosis
• May need respiratory support till acidosis corrected

ACTIVITY As tolerated

DIET NaCl (sodium chloride) restriction

PATIENT EDUCATION For patient education materials on this topic, contact: National Kidney & Urologic Diseases Information Clearinghouse, Box NKUDIC, Bethesda, MD 20893, (301)468-6345

MEDICATIONS

DRUG(S) OF CHOICE
RTA 1
◊ Sodium bicarbonate - 1-4 mEq/kg/day starting and titrate up as needed. Bicarbonate wasting forms will need more. Dosing is 2 or 3 times daily.
◊ Potassium bicarbonate - if hypokalemia is a problem. Amount of HCO3 (the bicarbonate radical) given in this form depends on severity of hypokalemia.
RTA 2
◊ Sodium bicarbonate - 5-20 mEq/kg/day titrated as necessary, with frequency of dosing 4-6 times a day
RTA 4
◊ Sodium bicarbonate - 1-4 mEq/kg/day titrated as necessary with 2 or 3 times daily dosing
◊ Furosemide - to lower potassium levels, except if salt wasting is also occurring
◊ Kayexalate - initially to bring down very high potassium levels
◊ Fludrocortisone - 0.1-0.3 mg/day, if the patient is mineralocorticoid deficient, or in some cases of end organ resistance
Contraindications: Refer to manufacturer's literature
Precautions: Refer to manufacturer's literature
Significant possible interactions: N/A

ALTERNATIVE DRUGS
Hydrochlorothiazide (HCTZ) as an adjunct in RTA 2 after maximal NaHCO3. Shohl's solution (sodium citrate) can be used if large doses of bicarbonate are needed. Citrate is metabolized to bicarbonate in the liver, avoiding distention and flatulence caused by the gastric CO2 production.

FOLLOWUP

PATIENT MONITORING Electrolytes, serum pH, urine pH, renal function studies

PREVENTION/AVOIDANCE Careful use or avoidance of causative agents listed above

POSSIBLE COMPLICATIONS
• Nephrocalcinosis
• RTA-1 - pyelonephritis

EXPECTED COURSE AND PROGNOSIS
• Permanent disorder, but prognosis is good with therapy if irreversible renal damage has not yet occurred
• Good, if not associated with any other autoimmune disease. Otherwise, prognosis dependent on the associated disease.

MISCELLANEOUS

ASSOCIATED CONDITIONS
• RTA-1 in children - hypercalciuria leading to rickets, nephrocalcinosis, and nephrolithiasis
• RTA-1 in adults - autoimmune diseases such as Sjögren's disease
• RTA-2 - Fanconi's syndrome

AGE-RELATED FACTORS
Pediatric: N/A
Geriatric: N/A
Others: N/A

PREGNANCY N/A

SYNONYMS N/A

ICD-9-CM
• 588.8 other specified disorder resulting from impaired renal function
• 270.0 disorder of amino acid transport (Fanconi's syndrome)

SEE ALSO N/A

OTHER NOTES N/A

ABBREVIATIONS
• NaHCO3 = sodium bicarbonate
• RTA = renal tubular acidosis
• CRF = chronic renal failure

REFERENCES
• Braunwald, E., et al. (eds.): Harrison's Principles of Internal Medicine. 12th Ed. New York, McGraw-Hill, 1991
• Oski, F.A.: Principles and Practice of Pediatrics. 3rd Ed. Philadelphia, J.B. Lippincott, 1990

Author R. Ram, M.D.

Respiratory distress syndrome, adult

BASICS

DESCRIPTION A patient with previously normal lungs who suffers a catastrophic pulmonary or nonpulmonary event followed by a cascade of events that occur at the alveolar-arteriolar capillary membrane. Reduction in functional residual capacity and lung compliance are hallmarks.
• Hypoxemia, decreased pulmonary compliance, and an increasing shunt forms as the proteinaceous material collects in the interstitium and alveoli. Hypoxemic respiratory failure secondary to noncardiogenic pulmonary edema almost always requires mechanical ventilation
System(s) affected: Pulmonary
Genetics: N/A
Incidence/Prevalence in USA: 150,000/year
Predominant age: All ages
Predominant sex: Male = Female

SIGNS AND SYMPTOMS Most patients demonstrate similar clinical and pathologic features regardless of the cause of the acute lung injury.
There are 4 phases:
◊ Phase 1: Acute injury - normal physical exam, normal chest x-ray, tachypnea, tachycardia, and respiratory alkalosis
◊ Phase 2: Latent phase - 6-48 hours after injury: Hyperventilation, hypocapnia, increase in work of breathing, widening alveolar-arterial oxygen gradient
◊ Phase 3: Acute respiratory failure, tachypnea and dyspnea, decreased lung compliance, diffuse infiltrates on chest roentgenogram, high-pitched diffusely scattered crackles
◊ Phase 4: Severe abnormalities, severe hypoxemia unresponsive to therapy, increased intrapulmonary shunting, metabolic and respiratory acidosis
Signs and symptoms common to all 4 phases:
◊ Tachypnea and tachycardia during the first 12 to 24 hours
◊ Moist and cyanotic skin
◊ Breathing difficulty with intercostal and accessory respiratory muscles
◊ Dramatic increase in work of breathing
◊ High-pitched end-expiratory crackles are heard throughout all lung fields
◊ Increased agitation
◊ Lethargy, then obtundation
◊ Hypoxemia may be present long before clinical signs

CAUSES

Recent studies have revealed a number of mediators are involved in the initiation and perpetuation of ARDS
◊ Cytokines (tumor necrosis factor, interleukin 1, interleukin 6)
◊ Complement activation
◊ Coagulation activation
◊ Platelet - activating factor
◊ Oxygen radicals
◊ Lipoxygenase pathways (Leukotrienes C4, D4 and E4)
◊ Neutrophil proteases
◊ Nitric oxide - may be deleterious or advantageous
◊ Endotoxin
◊ Cyclooxygenase pathway products (thromboxane A2, prostacyclin)
All of the following causes can initiate a systemic inflammatory response with activation of the previous mediators
◊ Aspiration
◊ Pulmonary and systemic infections (bacterial, fungal, viral and protozoan)
◊ Sepsis (gram negative, gram positive, fungi, tuberculous, pneumocystis pneumonia)
◊ Pulmonary contusion
◊ Near-drowning
◊ Multiple fractures, especially long bones (fat embolism)
◊ Multiple transfusions
◊ Pancreatitis, severe
◊ Head injury
◊ Inhalation of toxic gases (oxygen, smoke, NH3, chlorine, plastics, phosgene, cadmium)
◊ Burns
◊ Shock (hemorrhage, cardiogenic, septic, anaphylactic)
◊ Eclampsia
◊ Carcinomatosis
◊ Leukoagglutinin reaction
◊ Air or amniotic fluid emboli

RISK FACTORS
• Systemic sepsis
• Pulmonary contusion
• Aspiration
• Inhalation of toxic substances
• Diffuse pneumonia
• Multiple emergency blood transfusions

DIAGNOSIS

DIFFERENTIAL DIAGNOSIS Cardiogenic pulmonary edema

LABORATORY
• PaO2 < 50 mm Hg with FiO2 > 0.6
• Overall compliance < 50 ml/cm H2O (usually 20-30 ml/cm H20)
• Increased shunt fraction Q's/Q't and dead space ventilation VD/VT
Drugs that may alter lab results: N/A
Disorders that may alter lab results:
• Multiple pulmonary embolism
• Cardiogenic pulmonary edema
• Severe chronic obstructive pulmonary disease
• Severe pneumonia

PATHOLOGICAL FINDINGS
• Lungs show exudative phase, early proliferative phase or late proliferative phase
• Interstitial and alveolar edema
• Inflammatory cells and erythrocytes spill into interstitium and the alveolus
• Type I cells are destroyed, leaving a denuded basement membrane
• Protein-rich fluid fills the alveoli
• Type II alveolar cells appear unaltered initially
• Type II cells begin to proliferate within 72 hours of initial insult
• The type II cells cover the denuded basement membrane
• Aggregates of plasma proteins, cellular debris, fibrin and surfactant remnants form hyaline membranes
• Over next 3-10 days, alveolar septum thickens by proliferating fibroblasts, leukocytes and plasma cells
• Capillary injury begins to occur
• Hyaline membranes begin to reorganize
• Fibrosis becomes apparent in respiratory ducts and bronchioles

SPECIAL TESTS
• Pulmonary artery catheter
• Measure pulmonary edema fluid content

IMAGING Chest roentgenogram

DIAGNOSTIC PROCEDURES
Pulmonary artery catheterization to demonstrate:
◊ Normal pulmonary arterial occlusion pressure (PAOP)
◊ Note: The main point of this study is to determine if the PAOP is inconsistent with cardiogenic pulmonary edema. A low PAOP with low serum albumin may lead to cardiogenic etiology. The patient with chronic congestive heart failure may have high wedge, but still develop adult respiratory distress syndrome.

TREATMENT

APPROPRIATE HEALTH CARE
Intensive care unit

GENERAL MEASURES
• Treat underlying etiology as appropriate
• Corticosteroids have theoretical, but not proven, benefit. This is still controversial. Do not use if occult infection exists.
• Support ventilation mechanically as necessary
• Support oxygenation with positive end-expiratory pressure (PEEP) with an amount that allows adequate hemoglobin saturation (90-95%) with an FiO2 of ≤ 60%. PaO2 is less important than oxygen delivery.
Maintain oxygen delivery:
   ◊ Increase O2 content with packed red blood cell transfusion as necessary
   ◊ Optimize cardiac output with fluid or inotropes. Measure CO with each PEEP change. If CO decreases, give fluids to regain adequate CO and allow additional PEEP adjustments if necessary.
• Avoid over-ventilation
• Avoid large tidal volumes (> 10 cc/kg) if peak airway pressures are high
• A pulmonary artery catheter may be helpful in assessing left ventricular function, CO, oxygen delivery and consumption. It is necessary if high levels of PEEP are used.
• Be aware of possible respiratory superinfection
• Deep vein thrombosis prophylaxis is essential
• Consider paralyzing agents (to improve compliance and decrease barotrauma) if patient is fighting ventilator. (Initiate anxiolytics when instituting treatment with paralytics.)
• Ulcer prophylaxis
Extraordinary management
   ◊ 1. Extracorporeal membrane oxygenation (ECMO) is conceivable in children
   ◊ 2. High-frequency ventilation - it achieves adequate gas exchange; however, there is no improvement on outcome
   ◊ 3. Pressure controlled inverse ratio ventilation (PCIRV)
   ◊ 4 Extracorporeal CO2 removal with low frequency ventilation. (Used in Europe and Salt Lake City on NIH trial.)

ACTIVITY
Bedrest

DIET
Nutritional support - avoid excess carbohydrates (could increase respiratory quotient)

PATIENT EDUCATION
N/A

MEDICATIONS

DRUG(S) OF CHOICE
• Inotropic agents - dobutamine to maintain adequate cardiac output
• Vasodilators - nitroprusside, ACE inhibitors, hydralazine. (Only if BP is adequate.)
• Corticosteroids (controversial)
• Anxiolytics
• Heparin 5000 units q12h for deep-vein thrombosis prophylaxis
• Ulcer prophylaxis with H2 blockers or sucralfate
Contraindications: See manufacturer's profile of each drug
Precautions: See manufacturer's profile of each drug
Significant possible interactions: See manufacturer's profile of each drug

ALTERNATIVE DRUGS
Specific mediator inhibitors: Are being evaluated in animal models and humans
   ◊ Xanthine oxidase inhibitors (early in burn patients)
   ◊ Monoclonal derived antibodies to released monokines, i.e. Tumor necrosis factor
   ◊ NSAID's, i.e., ibuprofen
   ◊ High-dose corticosteroids are still being studied and reviewed
   ◊ Pentoxifylline - has shown to be of some benefit
   ◊ Maximizing gut barrier function by using early enteral feeds
   ◊ Surfactant replacement is being reviewed
   ◊ Ventilator management by using permissive hypercapnea with low tidal volumes to prevent extensive barotrauma from mechanical ventilation

FOLLOWUP

PATIENT MONITORING
• Vital capacity and static lung compliance are important measures of mechanics
• Daily labs until no longer critical
• Chest x-rays to assess - endotracheal tube placement; the possible development of barotrauma; the presence of infiltrates; PA cath migration
• Swan-Ganz catheter - to help assess O2 delivery and consumption; monitor cardiac output

PREVENTION/AVOIDANCE
N/A

POSSIBLE COMPLICATIONS
• Multiple organ dysfunction syndrome (MODS)
• Death
• Permanent lung disease
• Oxygen toxicity
• Barotrauma
• Superinfection

EXPECTED COURSE AND PROGNOSIS
• 50% mortality rate; the syndrome is heterogeneous and mortality runs from 15-90%, depending on multiple factors; mainly, underlying cause, age of patient, number of failed organs.
• There is a decrease in diffusing capacity due to fibrosis and restrictive lung disease. Many people will have abnormal pulmonary function tests up to 6 months after illness. Most who survive will reveal abnormalities only with sensitive function testing, such as pulmonary exercise tests.

MISCELLANEOUS

ASSOCIATED CONDITIONS
See Causes

AGE-RELATED FACTORS
N/A
Pediatric: N/A
Geriatric: Increasing mortality with increasing age
Others: N/A

PREGNANCY
N/A

SYNONYMS
• Shock Lung
• Wet Lung
• Noncardiac pulmonary edema

ICD-9-CM
786.09

SEE ALSO
N/A

OTHER NOTES
N/A

ABBREVIATIONS
PEEP = positive end expiratory pressure

REFERENCES
• Civetta, J.M.: Critical Care. Philadelphia, J.B. Lippincott, 1988
• Matthay,M.A.: JAMA 6/19/91; Volume 265, No. 23:3109-3110
• Murray, J.F., Matthay,M.A., et al.: Amer. Review Resp. Disease. 1988;138:720-723.1
• Wyngaarden, J.B., Smith, L.H. (eds): Cecil Textbook of Medicine. 19th Ed. Philadelphia, W.B. Saunders Co., 1992
• Demling, R.: Adult Respiratory Distress Syndrome; Current Concepts. New Horizons, 1993. Vol. 1, No. 3; 388-401

Author M. Ferrebee, M.D. & D. Heiselman, D.O.

Respiratory distress syndrome, neonatal

BASICS

DESCRIPTION Serious disorder of prematurity, with clinical manifestation of respiratory distress. Pulmonary surfactants that are deficient at birth cause diffuse lung atelectasis. Must differentiate from pneumonia, sepsis.
System(s) affected: Pulmonary
Genetics: No known genetic pattern
Incidence/Prevalence in USA: Common
Predominant age: Neonatal
Predominant sex: Male = Female

SIGNS AND SYMPTOMS
• Onset within few hours after birth
• Delayed, weak cry
• Expiratory grunt
• Frothing at lips
• Positive chin reflex
• Intercostal, sternal retractions
• Nasal flaring
• Rapid respiratory rate
• Chest contracted
• Respiratory excursions decreased
• Rales
• Cyanosis
• Peripheral edema
• Oliguria

CAUSES
• Prematurity
• Deficient pulmonary surfactants in the neonatal period
• Possible pulmonary ischemia

RISK FACTORS
• Premature infants born prior to 37 weeks gestation
• Infants born of diabetic mothers

DIAGNOSIS

DIFFERENTIAL DIAGNOSIS
• Early group B streptococcal pneumonia
• Transient tachypnea of newborn
• Meconium aspiration pneumonia
• Sepsis with Beta streptococcus pneumonia

LABORATORY
• Amniotic fluid:
  ◊ Lecithin/sphingomyelin ratio (L:S ratio < 2)
  ◊ Absence of phosphotidyl glycerol
  ◊ Surfactant production
• Features of respiratory, metabolic acidosis
• Arterial blood gases - hypoxemia and hypercarbia
Drugs that may alter lab results: Artificial or human surfactant; betamethasone
Disorders that may alter lab results: N/A

PATHOLOGICAL FINDINGS
• Voluminous, noncrepitant, purplish red lungs
• Dilatation right heart and vena cava
• Possible patent ductus
• Extensive resorptive atelectasis

SPECIAL TESTS
• Monitor arterial blood gases

IMAGING
• X-ray - reticulogranular appearance of lung fields demonstrating:
  ◊ diffuse atelectasis
  ◊ air bronchograms

DIAGNOSTIC PROCEDURES N/A

TREATMENT

APPROPRIATE HEALTH CARE
Inpatient - intensive care

GENERAL MEASURES
• Positive pressure ventilation
• Warm, humidified, oxygen enriched gases by hood
• Monitor respiratory and circulatory status carefully
• Umbilical artery catheter placed for monitoring blood pressure and sampling arterial blood gases
• Transcutaneous monitors to measure O2 and CO2 tension
• Pulse oximetry
• Radiant infant warmer
• Tube feedings or hyperalimentation
• High-frequency ventilation. Choices include conventilation at faster-than-normal rates; high-frequency jet ventilation; high-frequency oscillation
• Relationship between using surfactant and high-frequency ventilation still being studied
• Extracorporeal membrane oxygenation (EMCO) measure of last resort. Its use is still uncommon and there are risks associated

ACTIVITY None; may require sedation or paralysis while on ventilator

DIET Special from neonatologist

PATIENT EDUCATION For patient education materials favorably reviewed on this topic, contact: American Lung Association, 1740 Broadway, New York, NY 10019, (212)315-8700

MEDICATIONS

DRUG(S) OF CHOICE Synthetic surfactant (Exosurf) given directly into the tracheobronchial tree via endotracheal tube. Prophylaxis 5 mL/kg ASAP after birth, then 2nd and 3rd doses at 12 and 24 hours.
Contraindications: Refer to manufacturer's literature
Precautions: Refer to manufacturer's literature
Significant possible interactions: Refer to manufacturer's literature

ALTERNATIVE DRUGS
• Calf-lung surfactant (Survanta) recently approved in the U.S.

FOLLOWUP

PATIENT MONITORING Continuous monitoring in an intensive care nursery

PREVENTION/AVOIDANCE Systemic betamethasone given to mother when fetal lung profile is immature; at least 24 hours before delivery

POSSIBLE COMPLICATIONS
• Intraventricular hemorrhage
• Intracranial pathology
• Tension pneumothorax
• Retinopathy of prematurity
• Apnea

EXPECTED COURSE AND PROGNOSIS
• Course: acute, possibly fatal within 48 hours in 20%-30%, increasing with lower birth weights, especially < 1,000 grams.
• Prognosis:
 ◊ Successful outcome expected in tertiary care centers in children older than 28 weeks gestation
 ◊ Chronic lung disease, bronchopulmonary dysplasia (BPD), frequent in severe cases, especially after prolonged artificial ventilation.

MISCELLANEOUS

ASSOCIATED CONDITIONS N/A

AGE-RELATED FACTORS
Pediatric: A disorder of the neonatal period
Geriatric: N/A
Others: N/A

PREGNANCY N/A

SYNONYMS
• Hyaline membrane disease
• Respiratory distress syndrome, perinatal

ICD-9-CM 770.8

SEE ALSO N/A

OTHER NOTES N/A

ABBREVIATIONS N/A

REFERENCES
• Pons, P.T.: Respiratory Emergencies. Emergency Care Quarterly 5(1) 1989
• Freezer, N.J., et al.: Pulmonary mechanics of neonates on EMCO. Pediatr Pulmonal 1991; 11(2):108-12
• Bhutan, V.K., et al.: Pulmonary mechanics and energetics in preterm infants who had respiratory distress syndrome treated with synthetic surfactant. J Pediatr. 1992 Feb;120:518-24

Author K. Wegner, MD

Retinal detachment

BASICS

DESCRIPTION A retinal detachment is the separation of the sensory retina from the underlying retinal pigment epithelium, with an accumulation of fluid between them
• Rhegmatogenous detachment: Occurs when the fluid gains access to the subretinal space from the vitreous through a break in the retina (Greek rhegma, rent). This is the most common form and is usually the type referred to as "retinal detachment".
• Exudative detachment: Occurs when there is a breakdown of the blood/retinal barrier with consequent accumulation of fluid /exudate beneath the retina
• Traction detachment: Occurs when traction on the retina, usually from abnormal fibrous or fibro-vascular tissue, elevates the retina from the underlying pigment epithelium
System(s) affected: Nervous
Genetics: No specific genetic pattern unless related to underlying inheritable condition. Patients with a family history of retinal detachment are at increased risk.
Incidence/Prevalence in USA:
• Incidence - 10 per 100,000 persons per year without preceding eye surgery or trauma will have a rhegmatogenous retinal detachment
• 1-3% of patients undergoing cataract surgery will have a rhegmatogenous retinal detachment
Predominant age:
• Posterior vitreous detachment (separation of the vitreous gel from the retina) which is critical in the development of retinal tears (see below), is rare before age 30 and seen in 63% of patients over age 70
• Younger patients usually have underlying vitreoretinal disorders or degenerations
Predominant sex: Male = Female

SIGNS AND SYMPTOMS
• Flashes (photopsia)
• Floaters (entopsia)
• Visual field loss (typically, a "curtain" across portion of the visual field)
• Central vision and reasonable acuity may be preserved if there is no macular detachment
• Poor visual acuity when macula is detached (typically, counting fingers)
• If the detachment is large, an afferent pupillary defect may be detected (Marcus-Gunn pupil)
• Dilated fundus examination with binocular indirect ophthalmoscopy shows elevation of the neurosensory retina associated with one or more retinal tears in rhegmatogenous detachment or bullous elevation of the retina without tears in exudative detachment

CAUSES
Rhegmatogenous detachment:
◊ Acute posterior vitreous detachment (PVD), a normal aging phenomenon caused by liquefaction of the vitreous, may exert traction on the retina where the vitreous is firmly attached and cause a retinal tear
◊ Symptoms of acute PVD include sudden onset of floaters (typically a "cobweb") and flashes
◊ 15% of patients with acute PVD will have a retinal tear, but most will not develop retinal detachment
Exudative detachment:
◊ Tumors
◊ Inflammatory diseases (Harada's, posterior scleritis)
◊ Miscellaneous (uveal effusion, malignant hypertension)
Traction detachment:
◊ Proliferative retinopathies (diabetes)
◊ Intraocular foreign bodies

RISK FACTORS
• Myopia
• Aphakia (no crystalline lens)
• Trauma
• Retinal detachment in fellow eye
• Predisposing retinal degeneration (lattice)

DIAGNOSIS

DIFFERENTIAL DIAGNOSIS
Retinoschisis (splitting of the retina)

LABORATORY N/A
Drugs that may alter lab results: N/A
Disorders that may alter lab results: N/A

PATHOLOGICAL FINDINGS Elevation of neurosensory retina from underlying retinal pigment epithelium

SPECIAL TESTS N/A

IMAGING N/A

DIAGNOSTIC PROCEDURES Binocular indirect ophthalmoscopy

TREATMENT

APPROPRIATE HEALTH CARE Referral to retina specialist for examination and definitive repair

GENERAL MEASURES
• Eye shield (Fox's metal shield) if trauma was inciting event and ruptured globe cannot be excluded
• Repair of rhegmatogenous detachment is surgical with a scleral buckling procedure (external plombage) being the most common technique employed
• Exudative detachments are usually managed by work-up and treatment of the underlying disorder

ACTIVITY In rhegmatogenous detachment, some ophthalmologists advocate bilateral patching and bedrest if the macula is not detached and surgery is delayed. This may lessen the likelihood of macular detachment, since this alters the prognosis (see below).

DIET Nothing by mouth if surgical intervention imminent

PATIENT EDUCATION Printed material available from the American Academy of Ophthalmology (415)561-8500

Retinal detachment

MEDICATIONS

DRUG(S) OF CHOICE N/A
Contraindications: N/A
Precautions: N/A
Significant possible interactions: N/A

ALTERNATIVE DRUGS N/A

FOLLOWUP

PATIENT MONITORING This depends on type of detachment, response to treatment and occurrence of complications, and should therefore be individualized

PREVENTION/AVOIDANCE
• Patients at risk should have regular ophthalmoscopic examination by a trained ophthalmologist
• Patients with an acute posterior vitreous detachment (see above) should be given the warning symptoms of retinal detachment: Increased flashes; sudden shower of floaters; enlarging curtain across visual field. If any of these develop, patients should be re-examined promptly.

POSSIBLE COMPLICATIONS Partial or total loss of vision, usually due to macular detachment or proliferative vitreoretinopathy

EXPECTED COURSE AND PROGNOSIS
Rhegmatogenous detachment:
◊ Left untreated visual loss progresses and ultimately complete blindness results
◊ Overall 50% of patients will have vision of 20/50 or better
◊ If the macula is detached for less than 1 week duration, 75% will obtain a postoperative vision of 20/70 or better as apposed to 50% with macular detachment of 1-8 weeks duration
◊ The prognosis for cases of retinal detachment without macular detachment is far better than those with macular involvement
◊ With current techniques 90-95% of retinal detachments can be repaired (anatomical restoration)
Exudative and traction detachment:
◊ Prognosis depends on severity of underlying disorder

MISCELLANEOUS

ASSOCIATED CONDITIONS Numerous heritable vitreoretinal disorders

AGE-RELATED FACTORS
Pediatric: Usually associated with underlying vitreoretinal disorders and retinopathy of prematurity
Geriatric: N/A
Others: N/A

PREGNANCY Pre-eclampsia/eclampsia may be associated with exudative retinal detachment. No intervention is indicated and provided hypertension is controlled, prognosis is usually good.

SYNONYMS Retinal separation

ICD-9-CM 361.00

SEE ALSO N/A

OTHER NOTES N/A

ABBREVIATIONS N/A

REFERENCES Benson, W.E.: Retinal Detachment: Diagnosis and Management. Philadelphia, Harper and Row Publishers, 1980

Author D. Metrikin, M.D.

Retinitis pigmentosa

 BASICS

DESCRIPTION Retinitis pigmentosa (RP) is the name given to a group of retinal diseases which may be exclusively ocular or associated with systemic disease. Characteristics include 1) progressive visual field loss 2) night blindness and 3) abnormal or non-recordable electroretinogram (ERG).
System(s) affected: Nervous
Genetics:
• Autosomal dominant - 22%
• Autosomal recessive - 16%
• X-linked recessive - 9%
• Approximately half of the cases have no family history
Incidence/Prevalence in USA: 29 cases per 100,000
Predominant age: Onset varies. First two decades for X-linked and autosomal recessive. 40's and 50's for autosomal dominant.
Predominant sex: Male > Female

SIGNS AND SYMPTOMS
• Night blindness from early childhood years
• Progressive peripheral visual field loss through the twenties
• Severe visual disability with tubular fields in the forties
• No functional vision at age sixty to seventy
• Searching nystagmus in children
• Localized, peripheral, perivascular retinal pigment deposits ("bone spicules")
• Sclerosis of retinal vessels and vascular attenuation
• "Waxy pallor" of the optic nerve

CAUSES
• Inherited disorders
• Role of environmental factors difficult to ascertain

RISK FACTORS
• Family member with RP
• Syndrome or disease associated with RP

 DIAGNOSIS

DIFFERENTIAL DIAGNOSIS
• Infectious retinopathies; viral (rubella) or bacterial (syphilis)
• Following resolution of exudative detachment
• "Atypical" retinitis pigmentosa; sectoral, unilateral or pericentral
• Toxic retinopathies secondary to chloroquine or phenothiazines
• Miscellaneous - ophthalmic artery occlusion, trauma

LABORATORY Fluorescent treponemal antibody absorption (FTA-ABS)
Drugs that may alter lab results: N/A
Disorders that may alter lab results: N/A

PATHOLOGICAL FINDINGS
• Bone spicule-like pigmentation seen on ophthalmoscopy is due to the retinal pigment epithelium filled with melanin granules
• Depigmentation and atrophy of the retinal pigment epithelium
• Atrophy of the photoreceptor layer of the retina

SPECIAL TESTS
• Electrophysiological and psychophysical testing
• Automated visual field testing
• Fluorescein angiography and fundus photography
• Audiograms in patients with slurred speech or stutter

IMAGING N/A

DIAGNOSTIC PROCEDURES See Special tests

 TREATMENT

APPROPRIATE HEALTH CARE
Outpatient

GENERAL MEASURES
• Supportive
• Genetic counselling in cooperation with trained geneticist
• Counselling on dealing with narrow visual fields
• Low vision clinics and visual aids
• When legally blind (visual field ≤ 20 degrees) may qualify for governmental or corporation support
• Educating the patient
• Maintaining optimal vision
• Emphasize chronicity and slow progression

ACTIVITY Full activity

DIET No special diet

PATIENT EDUCATION Information, services, and fund raising for research from - Retinitis Pigmentosa Foundation Fighting Blindness, 1401 Mt. Royal Avenue, 4th Floor, Baltimore, MD 21217, (800)638-2300

MEDICATIONS

DRUG(S) OF CHOICE
• A recent study suggests that daily administration of 15,000 IU of Vitamin A is associated with retardation of the rate of ERG changes in RP and that Vitamin E may have adverse effects
• Vitamin A replacement in RP associated with Vitamin A deficiency
• Animal studies suggest the use of radical oxygen quenchers such as vitamin E and carotene. Vitamin C has slowed retinal dystrophy in mice.
Contraindications: None
Precautions: Avoid toxic doses of vitamins
Significant possible interactions: None

ALTERNATIVE DRUGS   None

FOLLOWUP

PATIENT MONITORING
• Individualize depending on severity of disease and rate of progression
• Screen for other ocular disorders (cataract/glaucoma)

PREVENTION/AVOIDANCE   Genetic counseling

POSSIBLE COMPLICATIONS
• Slightly less than half develop cataract at late stages
• Macular changes (surface wrinkling, edema, atrophy)
• Do not appear to be at increased risk for retinal detachment
• Blindness

EXPECTED COURSE AND PROGNOSIS
• Symptomatic in childhood; incapacitating in adulthood
• Poorer prognosis if childhood onset
• Mostly chronic and slowly progressive
• Difficult to predict how individual patients will progress so avoid estimating when the patient will be classified as "blind"

MISCELLANEOUS

ASSOCIATED CONDITIONS
• Numerous syndromes (e.g., Fanconi's, Friedreich's ataxia) with associated systemic pathology, most of which can be recognized early in life
• Congenital deafness is rarely associated with RP (Usher's syndrome) but is frequently a concern of patients with RP

AGE-RELATED FACTORS
Pediatric:
• Congenital blindness may be secondary to many different causes including cortical blindness, optic atrophy, inflammatory diseases and neuronal storage diseases
• Age of onset, fundus findings, ERG and visual evolved response (VER) results and associated systemic pathology will help in arriving at a diagnosis
Geriatric: N/A
Others: N/A

PREGNANCY   N/A

SYNONYMS   Rod-cone or cone-rod degenerations

ICD-9-CM   362.74

SEE ALSO   N/A

OTHER NOTES   N/A

ABBREVIATIONS
• RP = retinal pigmentosa
• ERG = electroretinogram

REFERENCES   Heckinlively, J.R.: Retinitis Pigmentosa. Philadelphia, J.B.Lippincott Company, 1988

Author   D. Metrikin, M.D.

Retinopathy, diabetic

 BASICS

DESCRIPTION Noninflammatory retinal disorder characterized by intraretinal capillary closure and microaneurysms. Retinal ischemia leads to release of a vasoproliferative factor stimulating neovascularization on the retina, optic nerve head, or iris.
• Most patients with diabetes mellitus will develop diabetic retinopathy. It is the leading cause of new cases of legal blindness among Americans between the ages of 20-64.
Diabetic retinopathy can be divided into three stages:
  ◊ Background diabetic retinopathy
  ◊ Preproliferative diabetic retinopathy
  ◊ Proliferative diabetic retinopathy
Genetics: N/A
Incidence/Prevalence in USA:
• Approximately 6.6% of the population between ages 20-74 has diabetes
• Approximately 25% of the diabetic population have some form of diabetic retinopathy
• Diabetic retinopathy accounts for approximately 10% of new cases of blindness each year
Predominant age:
• Peak incidence of Type I, juvenile onset diabetes mellitus, is between the ages of 12-15
• Peak incidence of Type II, adult onset, between the ages of 50-70
Predominant sex:
• Male = Female - juvenile onset diabetes mellitus
• Female > Male - non-insulin-dependent diabetes mellitus

SIGNS AND SYMPTOMS
Background diabetic retinopathy
  ◊ Microaneurysms
  ◊ Intraretinal hemorrhage
  ◊ Macular edema
  ◊ Lipid deposits
Preproliferative diabetic retinopathy
  ◊ Nerve fiber layer infarctions (cotton wool spots)
  ◊ Venous beading
  ◊ Venous dilation
  ◊ Intraretinal microvascular abnormalities (IRMA)
  ◊ Extensive retinal hemorrhage
Proliferative diabetic retinopathy
  ◊ New blood vessel proliferation (neovascularization) on the retinal surface, optic nerve, and iris

CAUSES Related to the development of diabetic microaneurysms and microvascular abnormalities.

RISK FACTORS
• Duration of diabetes mellitus (usually over 10 years)
• Poor glycemic control
• Pregnancy
• Renal disease
• Systemic hypertension

 DIAGNOSIS

DIFFERENTIAL DIAGNOSIS Other causes of retinopathy, i.e., radiation retinopathy, retinal venous obstruction, and hypertensive retinopathy.

LABORATORY N/A
Drugs that may alter lab results: N/A
Disorders that may alter lab results: N/A

PATHOLOGICAL FINDINGS
• Increased capillary permeability
• Microaneurysms
• Hemorrhages in retina
• Exudates in retina
• Capillary nonperfusion

SPECIAL TESTS Fluorescein angiography: Demonstrates retinal nonperfusion, retinal leakage, and proliferative diabetic retinopathy

IMAGING N/A

DIAGNOSTIC PROCEDURES
Eye examination: Measurement of visual acuity and documentation of the status of the iris, lens, vitreous and fundus

 TREATMENT

APPROPRIATE HEALTH CARE
Inpatient or outpatient surgery for vitrectomy; inpatient or outpatient for laser treatment

GENERAL MEASURES
• Laser treatment: Recommended for patients with proliferative diabetic retinopathy and for patients with clinically significant macular edema
• The Diabetic Retinopathy Study demonstrated panretinal photocoagulation overall reduced the rate of severe visual loss from 15.9% in untreated eyes to 6.4% in treated eyes. In certain subgroups of eyes with proliferative diabetic retinopathy, the incidence of severe visual loss in untreated eyes was as high as 36.9% with a follow-up of 2 years.
• The Early Treatment Diabetic Retinopathy Study (ETDRS) demonstrated that eyes with clinically significant diabetic macular edema benefitted from focal laser treatment. Clinical significant diabetic macular edema is defined as the following:
  ◊ 1 Thickening of the retina within 500 microns of the center of the macula
  ◊ 2 Hard exudates within 500 microns of the center of the macula associated with thickening of the adjacent retina
  ◊ 3 A zone of retinal thickening 1 disc area or larger within 1 disc diameter of the center of the macula
• The Early Treatment Diabetic Retinopathy Study demonstrated that systemic aspirin did not prevent the development of proliferative diabetic retinopathy, or reduce the risk of visual loss associated with diabetic retinopathy
• Cryoretinopexy can be used instead of laser treatment in certain cases to decrease the neovascular stimulus and treat proliferative diabetic retinopathy
• Vitrectomy: Recommended for patients with severe proliferative diabetic retinopathy, traction retinal detachment involving the macula, and nonclearing vitreous hemorrhage. In eyes undergoing vitrectomy for severe proliferative diabetic retinopathy, the percentage of eyes with a visual acuity of 10/20 or better was greater in the group that underwent early vitrectomy versus conventional management.
• The relationship between glycemic control and the microvascular complications of diabetic retinopathy is unclear

ACTIVITY As tolerated

DIET Follow prescribed diabetic diet

PATIENT EDUCATION Patient information available from the American Diabetes Association - (800)232-3472 or local office

MEDICATIONS

DRUG(S) OF CHOICE None are helpful for retinopathy
Contraindications: N/A
Precautions: N/A
Significant possible Interactions: N/A

ALTERNATIVE DRUGS N/A

FOLLOWUP

PATIENT MONITORING
Scheduled eye examinations by an ophthalmologist:
◊ The diabetic patient with a normal exam should be followed yearly
◊ Patients with background diabetic retinopathy should be followed at least every six months
◊ Patients with preproliferative diabetic retinopathy should be followed at least every three to four months
◊ Patients with proliferative diabetic retinopathy should be followed at least every two to three months

PREVENTION/AVOIDANCE
• Careful monitoring and control of blood glucose
• Routine visits to an ophthalmologist

POSSIBLE COMPLICATIONS Blindness

EXPECTED COURSE AND PROGNOSIS If treated early, outlook good. If treatment delayed, blindness may result.

MISCELLANEOUS

ASSOCIATED CONDITIONS
• Glaucoma
• Cataracts
• Retinal detachment
• Vitreous hemorrhage

AGE-RELATED FACTORS
Pediatric: N/A
Geriatric: Prevalence will increase as population ages and diabetic patients live longer
Others: N/A

PREGNANCY
• Pregnancy can exacerbate diabetic retinopathy
• Any woman with diabetes who becomes pregnant should be examined in the first trimester. She should be examined at least every three months until parturition.

SYNONYMS N/A

ICD-9-CM 362.0

SEE ALSO Diabetes mellitus

OTHER NOTES N/A

ABBREVIATIONS
• BDR = background diabetic retinopathy
• PPDR = preproliferative diabetic retinopathy
• PDR = proliferative diabetic retinopathy

REFERENCES
• Diabetic Retinopathy Study Research Group: Indications for photocoagulation treatment of diabetic retinopathy. DRS Report No. 14. Int Ophthal Clin, 1987, 27:239-253
• Early Treatment Diabetic Retinopathy Study Research Group: Photocoagulation for Diabetic Macular Edema. ETDRS Report No. 1. Arch Ophthalmol, 1985; 103:1796-1806
• Early vitrectomy for severe proliferative diabetic retinopathy in eyes with useful vision: results of a randomized trial diabetic retinopathy vitrectomy study. Report No. 3. The Diabetic Retinopathy Vitrectomy Study Research Group. Ophthalmol 1988;95:1307-1320

Author R. Allinson, M.D.

Retrolental fibroplasia

BASICS

DESCRIPTION Retrolental fibroplasia (RLF) is a proliferative disorder of the retinal blood vessels in premature infants. The normal retinal vascularization occurs nasally at approximately 36 weeks of gestation and temporally at approximately 40 weeks of gestation. Also referred to as retinopathy of prematurity (ROP).
System(s) affected: Nervous, Cardiovascular
Genetics: Black infants appear less susceptible
Incidence/Prevalence in USA:
• 65.8% of infants weighing less than 1251 grams at birth, and 81.6% of those weighing less than 1000 grams
• Of babies born with a birth weight of 1001-1500 grams, 2.2% will develop cicatricial changes as a complication of retrolental fibroplasia and 0.5% of them will be blind
• Approximately one third of all infants weighing less than 1500 grams at birth may show evidence of retrolental fibroplasia
Predominant age: Premature infants
Predominant sex: Male = Female

SIGNS AND SYMPTOMS
• The development of a demarcation line between the vascularized and nonvascularized retina is the earliest ophthalmoscopic sign
• The demarcation line may develop neovascularization
• The retinal neovascularization can lead to retinal detachment and vitreous hemorrhage
• Gray, nonvascular, peripheral retina
• Retinal vessel tortuosity

CAUSES N/A

RISK FACTORS
• Low birth weight
• Prematurity
• Supplemental oxygen. Once the retina becomes fully vascularized, oxygen will not affect the retina.

DIAGNOSIS

DIFFERENTIAL DIAGNOSIS
• Retinoblastoma
• Congenital cataracts
• Norrie's disease
• Incontinentia pigmenti
• Familial exudative vitreoretinopathy

LABORATORY N/A
Drugs that may alter lab results: N/A
Disorders that may alter lab results: N/A

PATHOLOGICAL FINDINGS
• Retinal capillary destruction
• Retinal neovascularization
• Retinal hemorrhages
• Retinal detachment

SPECIAL TESTS N/A

IMAGING N/A

DIAGNOSTIC PROCEDURES
• An ophthalmologist skilled in the detection of this disorder should examine all infants who weigh less than 1,251 grams
• The initial eye exam should be performed at 4 to 6 weeks of age
• Follow-up exams are performed until the retina is noted to be fully vascularized

TREATMENT

APPROPRIATE HEALTH CARE
Treatment usually is performed in the neonatal intensive care unit or as an outpatient as the child grows older

GENERAL MEASURES
• The multicenter trial of cryotherapy demonstrated a favorable outcome for eyes treated at threshold (Stage 3+ retinopathy of prematurity) versus control eyes
• Threshold disease was defined as at least 5 contiguous or 8 cumulative clock hours of Stage 3 associated with retinal vascular tortuosity in the posterior segment of the eye
• Transscleral cryotherapy to the avascular retina when applied to high risk eyes can reduce the incidence of sight threatening complications. The multicenter trial of cryotherapy has shown that treatment of high risk eyes reduces the incidence of unfavorable outcomes by 46%
• Photocoagulation applied to the avascular retina in high risk eyes can reduce the incidence of sight-threatening complications
• Vitrectomy and/or scleral buckling can be used to treat retinal detachment associated with retrolental fibroplasia
• The role of vitamin E administration for the prophylaxis is controversial. It may reduce the severity, but not the incidence of retrolental fibroplasia
• Extremely low birth weight infants receiving prophylactic treatment with calf lung surfactant extract demonstrated a lower incidence of any stage when compared with control infants

ACTIVITY N/A

DIET N/A

PATIENT EDUCATION Expectant mothers should avoid behavioral and environmental risk factors associated with low birth weight. These include smoking, alcohol and other substance abuse, and poor nutrition.

MEDICATIONS

DRUG(S) OF CHOICE None
Contraindications: N/A
Precautions: N/A
Significant possible interactions: N/A

ALTERNATIVE DRUGS N/A

FOLLOWUP

PATIENT MONITORING Close followup of patients with retrolental fibroplasia is required

PREVENTION/AVOIDANCE See Patient Education

POSSIBLE COMPLICATIONS
- Retinal detachment
- Retinal fold involving the macula
- Vitreous hemorrhage
- Angle closure glaucoma
- Amblyopia
- Strabismus
- Myopia

EXPECTED COURSE AND PROGNOSIS Spontaneous regression occurs over a period of weeks or months in most cases. Spontaneous regression occurs in approximately 85% of eyes.

MISCELLANEOUS

ASSOCIATED CONDITIONS Neonatal respiratory distress syndrome

AGE-RELATED FACTORS
Pediatric: N/A
Geriatric: N/A
Others: N/A

PREGNANCY N/A

SYNONYMS
- ROP
- Retinopathy of prematurity

ICD-9-CM 362.21 retrolental fibroplasia

SEE ALSO N/A

OTHER NOTES N/A

ABBREVIATIONS
- RLF = retrolental fibroplasia
- ROP = retinopathy of prematurity

REFERENCES
- Cryotherapy for retinopathy of prematurity cooperative group. Multicenter trial of cryotherapy for retinopathy of prematurity: one year outcome - structure and function. Arch Ophthalmology, 1990; 108:1408-1416
- Ben-Sira, I., Nissenkorn, I. & Kremer, I: Retinopathy of Prematurity. Surv Ophthalmol. 1988; 33:1-16

Author R. Allinson, M.D.

Reye's syndrome

 BASICS

DESCRIPTION A rare but potentially fatal disease characterized by encephalopathy with cerebral edema and fatty infiltration of the liver. Occurs acutely in previously healthy children. Often associated with an antecedent viral infection such as varicella or influenza. Evidence of a link between the disease and aspirin use during the prodromal illness. Reye's syndrome is not contagious nor does natural immunity develop.

System(s) affected: Nervous

Genetics: No known genetic pattern

Incidence/Prevalence in USA:
0.3-3.5/100,000 children under 18 annually. There has been a dramatic decrease in the incidence during the past 10 years.

Predominant age: Infants, children, adolescents. Peak incidence at 6 years of age. Most cases between 5-10 years of age.

Predominant Sex: Male = Female

SIGNS AND SYMPTOMS

- Protracted vomiting
- Lethargy, drowsiness
- Delirium, stupor, coma
- Irritability, combativeness
- Altered muscle tone
- Hyperpnea, irregular respirations

Symptoms reflected in clinical staging system
 ◊ I: Vomiting, sleepy, lethargic, Type 1 EEG
 ◊ II: Confusion, delirium, hyperventilation, combative Type 2 EEG
 ◊ III: Obtunded, light coma, decorticate rigidity, loss of oculocephalic reflexes, fixed pupils, Type 3 or 4 EEG
 ◊ IV: Coma, decerebrate posturing spontaneously or in response to painful stimuli, sluggish pupillary response to light
 ◊ V: Coma, flaccid paralysis, loss of deep tendon reflexes, convulsions, respiratory arrest, isoelectric EEG

CAUSES

Remains unknown - several etiologies suggested:
 ◊ Varicella, influenza A and B, echo virus, Coxsackie A virus have been cultured from some patients
 ◊ Toxic causes - insecticides, herbicides, aflatoxins
 ◊ Drugs - salicylates
 ◊ Metabolic causes - defects in the urea cycle or in lipid metabolism

RISK FACTORS

- Pediatric age group
- Viral illness with associated use of preparations containing aspirin, salicylates, and/or salicylamides

 DIAGNOSIS

DIFFERENTIAL DIAGNOSIS

- Acute toxic encephalopathy
- Hepatic coma
- Fulminant hepatitis
- Drug poisoning
- Sudden obstruction to cerebral spinal fluid flow by tumor
- Encephalitis without pleocytosis

LABORATORY

- Moderate to severe elevation of AST (SGOT), ALT (SGPT)
- Normal or slightly elevated bilirubin or alkaline phosphatase
- Elevated ammonia
- Prolonged prothrombin time
- Hypoglycemia
- Increased CSF pressure without pleocytosis (< 8 leukocytes per cubic millimeter)
- Mixed respiratory alkalosis and metabolic acidosis
- Elevated BUN
- Hyperaminoacidemia (glutamine, alanine, lysine)
- Hypocitrullinemia

Drugs that may alter lab results: N/A
Disorders that may alter lab results: N/A

PATHOLOGICAL FINDINGS

- Cerebral swelling
- Slightly enlarged, firm, yellow liver with fat droplets throughout
- Pallor
- Slight widening of the renal cortex
- Uniformly severe mitochondrial injury

SPECIAL TESTS EEG

IMAGING N/A

DIAGNOSTIC PROCEDURES Liver biopsy

 TREATMENT

APPROPRIATE HEALTH CARE Medical emergency requiring immediate hospitalization

GENERAL MEASURES

- Supportive depending on severity of illness
- Nasogastric tube, foley catheter, arterial and central venous pressure lines
- Hyperventilation, mannitol, barbiturates and/or decompression craniotomy to reduce intracranial pressure
- Mechanical ventilation
- Dialysis to reduce high ammonia levels
- IV glucose and close monitoring with dextrostixs (to prevent severe hypoglycemia)

ACTIVITY Complete bedrest

DIET Nothing by mouth

PATIENT EDUCATION Printed material from the National Reye's Syndrome Foundation, (800)233-7393

MEDICATIONS

DRUG(S) OF CHOICE
• Neomycin 100 mg/kg/day
• Vitamin K, 5 mg/day IM
• For increased intracranial pressure -
mannitol 0.5-1.0 gm/kg IV and dexamethasone
0.5 mg/kg/day
Contraindications: Mannitol - do not use if
patient has no renal output. May result in
vascular overload, pulmonary edema.
Precautions: Refer to manufacturer's literature
Significant possible interactions: Refer to
manufacturer's literature

ALTERNATIVE DRUGS   N/A

FOLLOWUP

PATIENT MONITORING   Will depend on
specific residual effects; may require care of
doctors; nurses; psychologists; physical,
occupational and/or speech therapists

PREVENTION/AVOIDANCE
• Avoidance of salicylates in children with
viral illness
• Recognition of early symptoms of the
disease

POSSIBLE COMPLICATIONS
• Aspiration pneumonia
• Respiratory failure
• Cardiac dysrhythmia/arrest
• Inappropriate vasopressin excretion
• Diabetes insipidus
• Cerebral edema

EXPECTED COURSE AND
PROGNOSIS
• Majority will have mild illness without
progression. Prognosis related to degree of
cerebral edema and ammonia level on
admission.
• Possible neurologic sequelae include
problems with attention, concentration, speech,
language, fine and gross motor skills

MISCELLANEOUS

ASSOCIATED CONDITIONS   N/A

AGE-RELATED FACTORS
Pediatric: In infants, Reye's syndrome does
not always follow typical pattern. Vomiting may
not occur. There may be diarrhea or respiratory
distress.
Geriatric: N/A
Others: N/A

PREGNANCY   N/A

SYNONYMS   White liver disease

ICD-9-CM   331.81

SEE ALSO   N/A

OTHER NOTES   N/A

ABBREVIATIONS   N/A

REFERENCES
• Behrman, R.E. & Kliegman, R.M. (eds.):
Nelson Textbook of Pediatrics. Philadelphia,
W.B. Saunders Co., 1992
• Maheady, D.C.: Reye's syndrome: review and
update. J Pediatr Health Care 1989 Sep-Oct;
3(5):246-50

Author   L. Olafson, M.D.

Rh incompatibility

BASICS

DESCRIPTION
Antibody-mediated destruction of red blood cells that bear Rh surface antigens by individuals who lack the antigens and have become isoimmunized ("sensitized") to them. Can occur with transfusion of incompatible blood. More commonly seen in the Rh-positive fetus or infant of an Rh-negative mother.

System(s) affected:
Hemic/Lymphatic/Immunologic

Genetics:
Complex autosomal inheritance of Rh antigens. Three closely-linked loci on chromosome 1 are known as C, D, and E; each may have alleles: Cc, Dd, Ee. Individuals who express the D antigen (also called Rho or Rho[D]) or its Du variant are considered Rh positive. Individuals lacking the D antigen are Rh negative. Antibodies may be produced to C, c, D, E, or e in individuals lacking the specific antigen; only D is strongly immunogenic. Isoimmunization to Rh antigens is not inherited.

Incidence/Prevalence in USA:
• 15% of Caucasian population and smaller fractions of other races are Rh negative
• Risk of isoimmunization during or after an Rh-positive pregnancy is about 15%
• Only 1-2% of isoimmunizations occur antepartum
• With Rho(D) immune globulin prophylaxis, risk of sensitization is reduced to less than 1% of susceptible pregnancies

Predominant age: Childbearing
Predominant sex: Female only

SIGNS AND SYMPTOMS
• Hemolytic transfusion reaction in recipient of Rh-incompatible blood
• Jaundice of newborn
• Kernicterus
• Congenital or fetal anemia
• Fetal hydrops
• Fetal death in utero

CAUSES
• Transfusion of Rh-positive blood to Rh-negative recipient
• Maternal exposure to fetal Rh antigens, either antepartum or intrapartum

RISK FACTORS
• Any Rh-positive pregnancy in Rh-negative woman
• Induced abortion
• Spontaneous abortion
• Ectopic pregnancy
• Amniocentesis, chorionic villus sampling
• Fetomaternal hemorrhage (fetal death in utero)
• Fetal manipulation, external version
• Cesarean delivery
• Maternal trauma
• Placental abruption
• Placenta previa
• Manual placental removal

DIAGNOSIS

DIFFERENTIAL DIAGNOSIS
• ABO incompatibility
• Other blood group (non-Rh) isoimmunization
• Nonimmune fetal hydrops
• Hereditary spherocytosis
• Red cell enzyme defects

LABORATORY
Positive indirect Coombs' test (antibody screen) during pregnancy

Drugs that may alter lab results:
Prior administration of Rho(D) immune globulin may lead to weakly (false) positive indirect Coombs' test in mother and direct Coombs' test in infant

Disorders that may alter lab results: N/A

PATHOLOGICAL FINDINGS N/A

SPECIAL TESTS
• Paternal blood typing
• Kleihauer-Betke test to quantify an acute feto-maternal bleed

IMAGING N/A

DIAGNOSTIC PROCEDURES N/A

TREATMENT

APPROPRIATE HEALTH CARE
Outpatient, ambulatory management in most cases. Because of the specialized, somewhat hazardous treatment measures involved, pregnancies usually managed at tertiary care level.

GENERAL MEASURES
• See Patient Monitoring also
• Depending on severity of involvement, treatment of newborn or fetus may include:
  ◊ Phototherapy
  ◊ Transfusion after delivery
  ◊ Exchange transfusion
  ◊ Diuretics and digoxin for hydrops
  ◊ Early delivery
  ◊ Intrauterine transfusion

ACTIVITY N/A

DIET N/A

PATIENT EDUCATION
Griffith: Instructions for Patients; Philadelphia, 1988 W.B. Saunders Co.

MEDICATIONS

DRUG(S) OF CHOICE
For prophylaxis:
Rho(D) immune globulin (RhIG, RhoGAM, Gamulin Rh) given to unsensitized, Rh-negative women following:
• Spontaneous abortion
• Induced abortion
• Ectopic pregnancy
• Antepartum hemorrhage
• Amniocentesis
• Chorionic villus sampling
• Routinely at 28 weeks
• Within 72 hours after delivery of Rh-positive infant
Dose:
• 50 mcg dose for events up to 12 weeks gestation
• 300 mcg dose for events after 12 weeks
• Higher doses may be required in the event of a large fetal - maternal hemorrhage (> 30 mL whole blood)
Contraindications: Patient with known severe reaction to human globulin. Refer to manufacturer's profile.
Precautions: Refer to manufacturer's profile
Significant possible interactions: N/A

ALTERNATIVE DRUGS N/A

FOLLOWUP

PATIENT MONITORING
• Antibody titer measured every few weeks during pregnancy. A titer of 1:16 or greater indicates need for further testing.
• Amniocentesis for amniotic fluid bilirubin levels
• Umbilical blood sampling (cordocentesis) for fetal blood type, hematocrit, reticulocyte count, presence of erythroblasts
• Fetal heart rate testing/ultrasonography to assess fetal status
• Amniocentesis for fetal lung maturity

PREVENTION/AVOIDANCE
• Blood typing (ABO and Rh) on all pregnant women
• Antibody screening early in pregnancy
• Rh immune globulin prevents only sensitization to the D antigen
• Follow prophylaxis routine listed in Medications for unsensitized, Rh-negative women

POSSIBLE COMPLICATIONS
• Pregnancy loss from umbilical blood sampling
• Pregnancy loss from intrauterine transfusion
• Fetal distress requiring emergent delivery

EXPECTED COURSE AND PROGNOSIS
• With appropriate monitoring and treatment, infants born of severely affected pregnancies have a survival rate of greater than 80%
• Hydropic fetuses have poor salvage rate
• Disease is likely to be more severe in affected subsequent pregnancies

MISCELLANEOUS

ASSOCIATED CONDITIONS
• Hemolytic disease of newborn
• Hydrops fetalis
• Neonatal jaundice
• Kernicterus

AGE-RELATED FACTORS
Pediatric: N/A
Geriatric: N/A
Others: N/A

PREGNANCY N/A

SYNONYMS
• Rh isoimmunization
• Rh alloimmunization
• Rh sensitization

ICD-9-CM
• 656.10-656.13 Rh isoimmunization in pregnancy
• 656.20-656.23 Other isoimmunization in pregnancy
• 773.0 Rh hemolytic disease in fetus or newborn
• 773.1 ABO hemolytic disease in fetus or newborn
• 773.2 Other hemolytic disease in fetus or newborn
• 773.3 Isoimmune hydrops fetalis
• 773.4 Isoimmune kernicterus
• 773.5 Isoimmune late anemia

SEE ALSO
• Jaundice
• Hemolytic anemia
• Erythroblastosis

OTHER NOTES N/A

ABBREVIATIONS N/A

REFERENCES
• Perkins, J.T.: Hemolytic Disease of the Newborn. In Principles and Practice of Medical Therapy in Pregnancy. 2nd Ed. Edited by N. Gleicher. Norwalk, CT, Appleton & Lange, 1992
• Socol, M.L.: Management of Blood Group Isoimmunization. In Principles and Practice of Medical Therapy in Pregnancy. 2nd Ed. Edited by N. Gleicher. Norwalk, CT, Appleton & Lange, 1992
• Management of Isoimmunization in Pregnancy. ACOG Technical Bulletin, 148, Oct 1990
• Prevention of Rho(D) Isoimmunization. ACOG Technical Bulletin, 79, Aug 1984
• Giblett, E.R.: Blood Groups and Blood Transfusion. In Harrison's Principles of Internal Medicine. 12th Ed. Edited by E. Braunwald, et al. New York, McGraw-Hill Inc., 1991

Author D. Nelson, M.D.

Rheumatic fever

BASICS

DESCRIPTION Rheumatic fever is an inflammatory disease, possibly autoimmune in nature. Rheumatic fever involves many tissues, including the heart, joints, skin, and central nervous system. Preceding infection of the upper tract with group A Streptococcus is a prerequisite to the development of acute rheumatic fever.
• Rheumatic fever can cause permanent cardiac valvular disease as well as acute cardiac decomposition.
• Recurrences are common if not prevented with "prophylactic" antibiotic treatment. In recent years there have been multiple reports of recurrences in adults as well as children.
System(s) affected: Cardiovascular, Hemic/Lymphatic/Immunologic, Nervous, Musculoskeletal, Skin/Exocrine
Genetics: A specific genetic marker that correlates with susceptibility to rheumatic fever has not been found, but the disease is known to occur in families
Incidence/Prevalence in USA:
• The incidence of rheumatic fever in the United States has been showing an overall decline for decades. In the 1970's it was a rare disease with an incidence of 0.5-1.88 cases per 100,000. However, since the mid-1980's there has been a resurgence of cases with multiple "outbreaks" having been reported in the U. S.
• The incidence calculated based on recent outbreaks has been as high as 18.1 per 100,000 in children aged 5-17 years
Predominant age: Most common in children aged 5-15. Recurrences can be seen in adulthood.
Predominant sex: Male = Female

SIGNS AND SYMPTOMS
• Joint symptoms ranging from arthralgias to frank arthritis (75%)
• Joints involved are medium to large, e.g., ankles, knees, wrists
• Joint involvement is classically migratory
• Joint symptoms usually disappear in 3-4 weeks without permanent deformities
• Carditis (65%), mild or severe with murmurs
• Cardiac involvement may include pericarditis, myocarditis, and/or valvular insufficiency. Appears within 2 weeks and lasts 6 weeks to 6 months.
• Valvular damage may be permanent
• P-R prolongation on ECG
• Erythema marginatum (classic rash) < 5%
• Subcutaneous nodules (painless, hard swellings overlying bony prominences) 5-10%
• Chorea is often a late finding but may be a presenting complaint. It occurs in 10-15% of patients, and its duration is not altered by treatment.
• Fever 101-104°F
• Abdominal pain is common. It may be severe.
• Epistaxis (historically important, but rarely seen in acute rheumatic fever)
• Facial tics
• Facial grimace

CAUSES
• Autoimmune mechanisms
• A preceding upper respiratory infection with group A Streptococcus is a prerequisite

RISK FACTORS
• Crowded living, school or working conditions
• Tendency to upper respiratory infections

DIAGNOSIS

DIFFERENTIAL DIAGNOSIS Lupus, juvenile rheumatoid arthritis, infectious arthritis, viral myocarditis, innocent murmurs, Tourette's syndrome, Kawasaki syndrome

LABORATORY
• Increased acute phase reactants, including sedimentation rate (ESR) and C-reactive protein (CRP)
• Bacteriological or serological evidence of group A streptococcal infection, antistreptolysin O (ASO), Streptozyme, or anti-deoxyribonuclease B (DNase)
• Anemia
Drugs that may alter lab results: Prior treatment with aspirin or steroids
Disorders that may alter lab results: N/A

PATHOLOGICAL FINDINGS
• Subcutaneous nodules have a characteristic histological appearance
• Pericardial effusion
• Fibrinous pericardium

SPECIAL TESTS   N/A

IMAGING
• Chest x-ray
• Echocardiogram (reveals pericardial effusion)

DIAGNOSTIC PROCEDURES
• Throat cultures for beta-hemolytic streptococci
• Diagnosis is dependent on fulfilling the modified Jones criteria of two major manifestations or one major and two minor manifestations. In either case, there must be evidence of preceding group A streptococcal infection. The five major criteria are carditis, arthritis, chorea, erythema marginatum, subcutaneous nodules. The minor criteria include fever, arthralgia (cannot use if arthritis was used as a major criteria), previous rheumatic fever, acute phase labs, prolonged P-R interval on EKG.

TREATMENT

APPROPRIATE HEALTH CARE
• Outpatient
• Initial hospitalization may be helpful to diagnose and establish stability of the patient

GENERAL MEASURES
• Patients with arthritis - therapy for relief of pain
• Patients with carditis - suppress inflammation
• Patients with arrhythmias - treat with appropriate agents

ACTIVITY
• Initial bedrest with activity increasing gradually as tolerated
• Advance activity cautiously if there is evidence of carditis

DIET   Regular; low sodium initially if the patient has carditis

PATIENT EDUCATION   Information available from the American Heart Association

MEDICATIONS

DRUG(S) OF CHOICE
• If patient has carditis with cardiomegaly, start prednisone, 2 mg/kg/day (maximum 60 mg) for two weeks then taper over two weeks. Start aspirin at beginning of steroid taper. Continue aspirin for 6 weeks.
• If no cardiomegaly, start aspirin 60 mg/kg/day (to maintain salicylate level of 20-25µg/mL) for 4-6 weeks
• Treat initially with penicillin as if active streptococcal infection is present, then begin prophylaxis. See Followup.
• Chorea may require treatment with haloperidol
Contraindications: Specific drug allergies
Precautions:
• Usual steroid side effects
• Extrapyramidal effects can occur with haloperidol
Significant possible interactions: Refer to manufacturer's profile of each drug

ALTERNATIVE DRUGS
Sulfadiazine may be used for prophylaxis in penicillin allergic patients. Patients who take sulfadiazine should take at least 2 liters of fluid daily to guard against sulfadiazine crystalluria.

FOLLOWUP

PATIENT MONITORING
Each week initially, then every 6 months

PREVENTION/AVOIDANCE
• Patients will need to be on prophylactic penicillin throughout childhood and possibly indefinitely during adulthood. Monthly injections of 1.2 million units of benzathine penicillin intramuscularly is the preferred treatment.
• Adults should be treated for a minimum of five years after an attack. Some treat adults indefinitely if there has been valvular disease. Oral penicillin V-K, 125 mg twice daily is an alternative to monthly injections. In the event of penicillin allergy, Sulfadiazine, 500 mg daily for children weighing less than 30 kg or 1 gr daily for all. Others may be used.
• If patients have valvular damage from acute rheumatic fever, they will require bacterial endocarditis prophylaxis for dental and other high risk procedures

POSSIBLE COMPLICATIONS
• Subsequent attacks of acute rheumatic fever secondary to streptococcal reinfection
• Carditis
• Mitral stenosis
• Congestive heart failure

EXPECTED COURSE AND PROGNOSIS
Sequelae limited to the heart and dependent of severity of carditis during an acute attack

MISCELLANEOUS

ASSOCIATED CONDITIONS N/A

AGE-RELATED FACTORS
Pediatric: More common in children
Geriatric: N/A
Others: N/A

PREGNANCY
Residual valvular disease may be exacerbated by pregnancy. Refer pregnant patient to cardiologist for assistance in management.

SYNONYMS N/A

ICD-9-CM 390

SEE ALSO N/A

OTHER NOTES N/A

ABBREVIATIONS N/A

REFERENCES
• Vaughn, V.C. & McKay, R.J. (eds.): Nelson's Textbook of Pediatrics. Philadelphia, W.B. Saunders Co., 1992
• Ferrieri, P.: AJDC 141 (7): 125-7. 1987 July
• Quinn, R.W.: Review Infect Dis 11: 128-153, 1989

Author H. Smith, M.D.

Rheumatoid arthritis (RA)

BASICS

DESCRIPTION A chronic systemic inflammatory disease of unknown etiology that has a predilection for joint involvement. Articular inflammation may be remitting, but if continued usually results in joint damage and disability. Certain extra-articular manifestations are characteristic, including rheumatoid nodules, arteritis, neuropathy, scleritis, pericarditis, and splenomegaly.
System(s) affected: Musculoskeletal, Hemic/Lymphatic/Immunologic, Pulmonary, Cardiovascular, Nervous
Genetics: Seropositive RA aggregates in families. Genetic factors versus their interaction with environmental facilitators is unclear. HLA-DR4 is found in 70% of Caucasian seropositive patients compared to 25% of controls. Increased relative risk of 4-5 times for the DR4 positive person, although a minority are affected. African Americans tend not to exhibit this predilection.
Incidence/Prevalence in USA:
• 0.3-1.5%; women affected 2-3 times more often, but men and women have equal prevalence of erosive disease
• Prevalence in Native Americans is 3.5-5.3%
Predominant age: Third to sixth decades
Predominant sex:
• Female > Male (overall incidence and prevalence of articular manifestations)
• Male > Female (exhibit more systemic disease)

SIGNS AND SYMPTOMS
• Morning stiffness, joint swelling, pain on passive motion, joint heat, typical joint deformity, fatigue, depression, malaise, anorexia, rheumatoid nodules, lymphadenopathy, splenomegaly, ocular disease, entrapment neuropathies

CAUSES Arthritogenic stimuli activate both humoral and cellular immune systems in the susceptible host. Antibodies (IgG, IgM, IgA anti-immunoglobulins) made by B cells and plasma cells in the joint space are complexed and fix complement, resulting in an inflammatory process. Infiltrating lymphocytes; primarily CD4 helper T-cells. Infectious etiology unproven.

RISK FACTORS
• HLA-DR4
• Family history
• Native American ethnicity
• Female gender, age 20-50 years

DIAGNOSIS

DIFFERENTIAL DIAGNOSIS
Sjögren's syndrome, sarcoidosis, polymyositis, erosive osteoarthritis, seronegative polyarthritis, vasculitis, gout, pseudogout, inflammatory bowel disease, hypersensitivity reactions, Reiter's syndrome, Behçet's syndrome, psoriatic arthritis, systemic lupus erythematosus, Lyme disease, scleroderma, chronic infection, occult malignancy

LABORATORY
• Hematocrit - mild anemia common
• Sedimentation rate (ESR) - usually elevated; helpful adjunct to follow disease activity
• Rheumatoid factor (RF) - titer > 1:80 detectable in 70-80% of patients with RA
• ANA - present in 20-30%.
• Complement (CH50), C3, C4 - normal or increased; most useful to detect persons with early RA from those with early lupus, in whom C levels are decreased
• Other: electrolytes, creatinine, liver function
Synovial fluid
• Yellowish-white, turbid, poor viscosity
• "Mucin clot" poor due to degradation of hyaluric acid by lysosomal enzymes
• Synovial WBC increased (3500-50,000)
• Synovial CH50 is lower than serum
• Synovial protein - approximately 4.2
• Serum-synovial glucose difference ≥ 30

SPECIAL TESTS None; biopsy of nodules is not indicated in diagnosis
Drugs that may alter lab results: Prior treatment with immunosuppressives may "normalize" results
Disorders that may alter lab results: N/A

PATHOLOGICAL FINDINGS
• Synovial infiltration by lymphocytes, plasma cells, and macrophages
• Hypertrophy and hyperplasia of synovial lining cells
• Local production of "self-associating" IgG

SPECIAL TESTS N/A

IMAGING
• X-rays rarely necessary in diagnosis, but useful in following the progression of disease
• Arthrography - to define joint abnormalities or injury to a supporting structure
• Bone scan - if aseptic necrosis is suspected
• CT/MRI - useful in specific situations such as cervical spine symptoms

DIAGNOSTIC PROCEDURES
American college of Rheumatology criteria:
Note: 4 of the 7 must be present. Numbers 1-4 must be present for at least 6 weeks.
• 1. Morning stiffness > 1 hour's duration
• 2. Arthritis of at least three joint groups with soft tissue swelling or fluid
• 3. Arthritis involving at least one of the following joint groups: proximal interphalangeal, metacarpophalangeal, or wrists
• 4. Symmetrical joint swelling

• 5. Subcutaneous nodules
• 6. Positive rheumatoid factor test
• 7. Radiographic changes consistent with RA

TREATMENT

APPROPRIATE HEALTH CARE
Outpatient except for complicating emergencies or orthopedic procedures

GENERAL MEASURES
• Emphasis on exercise and mobility; general health care
• Special emphasis should be placed on 1) reduction of joint stress, 2) physical and occupational therapy

ACTIVITY
• Encourage full activity, but avoid heavy work and vigorous exercise during active phases due to risk of intensifying joint inflammation
• Hydrotherapy or water exercise is effective and soothing

DIET No special diet

PATIENT EDUCATION Printed materials available from American Rheumatism Association (800)282-7023

MEDICATIONS

DRUG(S) OF CHOICE
There is controversy regarding the "pyramid of therapy" (beginning with anti-inflammatories and moving to disease modifying regimens) and the use of treatment combinations.
Early disease or acute/chronic inflammation
◊ Aspirin or other NSAID
Severe disease or as a "bridging agent" to remission-inducing agents
◊ Corticosteroids (5-15 mg prednisone or equivalent, each day). For short-term use only.
Persistent disease activity (chronic synovitis) - remission-inducing agents
◊ Antimalarials: hydroxychloroquine (Plaquenil) 400 mg q hs for 2-3 months, then 200 mg/hs; 6 month trial usual
◊ Gold: auranofin 6-10 mg/d po; reevaluate after 4-6 months or 1 gram total. Injectable gold given weekly until 1 gram total dose given, then reevaluate
◊ Sulfasalazine: 500 mg/d, increasing to 2 g/d over one month; maximum dosage is 2-3 g/day; 4-6 month trial
◊ D-penicillamine: 250 mg/d initially, increasing slowly to a maximum of 750-1000 mg/day; 6-9 month trial of at least 8-12 weeks at maximum dosage
◊ Methotrexate: 5-15 mg/wk po; 3-6 month trial

Contraindications: Various, depending on medication used

Precautions: Careful monitoring of disease activity and signs of drug toxicity

Significant possible interactions:

Drug interactions with NSAIDs:

◊ Antacids: Reduce the rate and extent of absorption of NSAID's; variable effect

◊ Anticoagulants: Phenylbutazone and oxyphenbutazone enhance warfarin activity. All NSAID's increase the risk of bleeding in an anticoagulated patient.

◊ Oral hypoglycemic agents (OHA): Aspirin, phenylbutazone, and oxyphenbutazone may potentiate the activity of OHA's; others currently available do not

◊ Antihypertensive/diuretics: NSAID's may attenuate the effect of diuretics, beta-blockers, hydralazine, prazosin, and ACE inhibitors

◊ Lithium: Elevation of plasma lithium levels may occur, especially with indomethacin and diclofenac

◊ Methotrexate: Salicylate inhibits the renal clearance of methotrexate, and toxic levels may occur

◊ Phenytoin: Phenylbutazone inhibits metabolism of phenytoin. Salicylates displace phenytoin from albumin and increase the concentration of free drug.

◊ Probenecid: Inhibits renal clearance of several NSAID's

◊ Combination of NSAID's: Avoid

ALTERNATIVE DRUGS N/A

FOLLOWUP

PATIENT MONITORING

- Duration of morning stiffness
- Time of onset of fatigue
- NSAID need/day
- Grip strength
- Number of joints that are tender or painful on passive range-of-motion
- Degree of swelling of affected joints
- Sedimentation rate - often best laboratory test of disease activity
- Other laboratory testing as indicated, depending on medication used and degree of disease progression
- Hydroxychloroquine: Major toxicity is retinopathy - ophthalmological exam every 6 months
- Auranofin: Major toxicity is rash, diarrhea, thrombocytopenia, granulocytopenia, proteinuria (rare) - CBC, platelet count, urinalysis monthly
- IM gold: Major toxicity is rash, thrombocytopenia, granulocytopenia, proteinuria - CBC, platelets, urinalysis before each injection
- D-penicillamine: Major toxicity is rash, GI intolerance, proteinuria, thrombocytopenia, granulocytopenia - CBC, platelets, urinalysis every 2 weeks x 6 months, then every month

- Methotrexate: Major toxicity is liver dysfunction, possible bone marrow toxicity - CBC, platelets, liver function every 1-3 months depending on dose and experience with drug
- Corticosteroids: Cushing's syndrome, osteoporosis
- NSAID's: GI problems, ? role of methotrexate with concomitant administration

PREVENTION/AVOIDANCE

- Possible association of oral contraceptive use with decreased risk of RA
- Specific types presented and specific types of individuals protected still being defined

POSSIBLE COMPLICATIONS

- Erosive arthritis and joint destruction
- Skin vasculitis
- Pericarditis
- Intracardiac rheumatoid nodules causing valvular, conduction abnormalities
- Pleural, subpleural disease; interstitial fibrosis
- Mononeuritis multiplex, median nerve entrapment
- Sjögren's syndrome, scleral rheumatoid nodules
- Felty's syndrome (splenomegaly, anemia, thrombocytopenia, neutropenia) - almost entirely restricted to seropositive patients with active arthritis
- Treatment induced complications (e.g., gastric complications with NSAID's, Cushing's syndrome with long term steroid use, liver abnormalities with methotrexate, ocular manifestations with Plaquenil)

EXPECTED COURSE AND PROGNOSIS

Progressive decline in function has been the usual course; this may be altered significantly with proper medical, surgical, and physiotherapeutic interventions. Management plan must take into account all aspects of a patient's life. Use of ARA Database helpful (see Reference).

MISCELLANEOUS

ASSOCIATED CONDITIONS Sjögren's, Felty's

AGE-RELATED FACTORS

Pediatric: See juvenile RA

Geriatric:

- Onset in geriatric population less common (20% of persons over age 60 with the disease)
- Despite improved treatment, expect increased contribution/interaction of other age-related comorbidities. Pericarditis, septic arthritis, Sjögren's syndrome more common in elderly.
- Elderly have less tolerance to medications; increased incidence of hydroxychloroquine-associated-maculopathy, D-penicillamine rash, and sulfasalazine induced nausea and vomiting. Toxicity from parenteral gold not age-related.

Others: N/A

PREGNANCY

- Labor and delivery pose no serious problems, unless severe mechanical joint disease (e.g., hips)
- Over 75% of RA patients who become pregnant experience improvement; 50% during the first trimester, with maximum improvement occurring in the third trimester, in spite of discontinuing medications such as gold and methotrexate. Occasionally first episodes occur during pregnancy (questionable significance). Cause of improvement unclear. Relapse invariably occurs after delivery (within six months).
- No increased number of fetal abnormalities have been reported due to RA per se. Presence of Sjögren's syndrome and anti-Ro antibody associated with congenital complete heart block (not all affected, however; most cases reported are with mothers with lupus).

SYNONYMS N/A

ICD-9-CM 714.0

SEE ALSO N/A

OTHER NOTES

Functional ability - general classification

◊ Class I: No restriction of ability to perform normal activities

◊ Class II: Moderate restriction but adequate to perform normal activities

◊ Class III: Marked restriction, inability to perform most duties of the patient's usual occupation or self-care

◊ Class IV: Incapacitation or confinement to a bed or wheelchair

Functional ability - proposed by Pincus, et al.:

◊ To dress self

◊ To get in and out of bed

◊ To eat and drink with utensils

◊ To walk outside on flat ground

◊ To wash and dry entire body

◊ To bend down & pick up clothing from floor

◊ To turn regular faucets on and off

◊ To get in and out of car

ABBREVIATIONS N/A

REFERENCES

- McCarty, D.J.: Clinical assessment of arthritis. In Arthritis and Allied Conditions. 9th Ed. Edited by D.J. McCarty. Philadelphia, Lea and Febiger, 1979
- Schumacher, H.R. (ed.): Primer on Rheumatic Diseases. 9th Ed. Atlanta, Arthritis Foundation, 1988
- American Rheumatism Association: A Uniform Database for Rheumatic Diseases, 1985 (obtainable from ARAMIS, Suite 3301, Welch Road, Palo Alto, CA 94304)
- Pincus, T., Callahan, L.F., Brooks, R.H., et al.: Self-report questionnaire scores in rheumatoid arthritis compared with traditional physical, radiographic, and laboratory measures. Ann Intern Med 110:259, 1989
- Koepsell et al., Br J Rheumatol 1989; 28 [suppl 1]:41

Author K. Elward, M.D.

Rhinitis, allergic

BASICS

DESCRIPTION Immediate and delayed reactions to airborne allergens, beginning with the generation and presence of specific antigen-responsive IgE antibody receptors on mast cells of the nasal mucosa
• An antigen-antibody chemical union initiates a cascade of events in the mast cell culminating in its degranulation and production of inflammatory mediators including histamine, leukotrienes, prostaglandins, proteases and platelet activating factor
• An immediate symptomatic response occurs followed by a more prolonged, persistent late phase reaction. This involves the infiltration into the reactive region of eosinophils, neutrophils, basophils and mononuclear cells
• May be seasonal or perennial depending on climate and individual response
• Seasonal responses usually to grasses, trees and weeds
• Perennial responses exampled by house dust mites, mold antigens and animal body products
System(s) affected: Pulmonary, Skin/Exocrine, Hemic/Lymphatic/Immunologic
Genetics: Complex, but strong genetic determination present
Incidence/Prevalence in USA: 8-12% of the population affected
Predominant Age:
• Onset usually before the age of 30 with tendency to diminish with time
• Mean age onset approximately 10 years
Predominant sex: Male = Female

SIGNS AND SYMPTOMS
• Nasal stuffiness and congestion
• Pale, boggy mucous membranes
• Nasal polyps
• Sneezing, often paroxysmal
• Watery eyes
• Dark circles under eyes, "allergic shiners"
• Long eye lashes often associated
• Sensation of plugged ears
• Symptom associated sleeping difficulties
• Fatigue
• Mouth breathing
• Scratchy throat
• Voice change
• Irritating cough
• Post nasal drip
• Loss or alteration of smell
• Itchy nose, eyes, ears and palate
• Transverse nasal crease from rubbing nose upwards
• Dull facies

CAUSES
Animal and plant proteins: Pollens, molds, mite dust, animal danders, dried saliva and urine
Insect debris: Cockroach, locusts, fish food (thirps)

RISK FACTORS
• Family history
• Repeated exposure to offending antigen
• Exposure to multiple offending allergens
• Presence of other allergies, e.g., atopic dermatitis, asthma, urticaria
• Non-compliance to appropriate therapeutic measures

DIAGNOSIS

DIFFERENTIAL DIAGNOSIS
• Nonallergic rhinitis with eosinophilia syndrome (NARES)
• Vasomotor rhinitis
• Chronic sinusitis
• IgA deficiency with recurrent sinusitis
• Nasal polyps and tumor
• Reactive rhinitis of recumbency
• Cribiform plate defect with cerebrospinal fluid leakage (rule out by testing watery discharge for sugar)
• Foreign body
• Medications
  ◊ Rebound effect associated with continued use of topical decongestant drops and sprays
  ◊ Aldosterone converting enzyme inhibiters
  ◊ Chronic aspirin use
• Septal/anatomical obstruction
• Chronic rhinitis digitorum

LABORATORY
• CBC with differential. May have slight increase in eosinophils but often normal with uncomplicated rhinitis.
• Nasal probe smear with cytologic exam for eosinophils
• Increase IgE level. May do RAST determinations for specific suspected allergens.
Drugs that may alter lab results:
• Corticosteroids will ablate eosinophilia
Disorders that may alter lab results:
• Secondary infections may alter differential and decrease nasal eosinophils
• Parasitic infestations with more marked eosinophilia

PATHOLOGICAL FINDINGS
Nasal washing/scraping
• Eosinophils predominate
• Basophils
• May see mast cells
Nasal mucosa
• Submucosal edema but intact without evidence of destruction
• Eosinophilic infiltration
• Granulocytes to lesser extent
• Increased amount of tissue water with poor staining of ground substance
• Congested mucous glands and goblet cells

SPECIAL TESTS
Skin tests using suspected antigens
Either technique manifests a positive reaction by inducing an expanding wheal and flare reaction. Special training recommended and available treatment for anaphylaxis mandatory
  ◊ Scratch or prick: a superficial injury to the epidermis with application of diluted test antigen
  ◊ Intradermal: Introduction of diluted material between layers of skin raising a 4 mm wheal using a 25 gauge needle
Radioallergosorbent test (RAST)
  ◊ More expensive and used especially in cases where skin testing not practical, e.g., in atopic dermatitis and dermatographia
Audiometry
  ◊ For deficits and base line evaluation
  ◊ Rhinoscopy (optional)- excellent visual advantages.

IMAGING Sinus film when indicated. Check for complete opacity, fluid level and mucosal thickening.

DIAGNOSTIC PROCEDURES See special lab tests. Appropriate diagnostic prick test kits available.

TREATMENT

APPROPRIATE HEALTH CARE
Outpatient

GENERAL MEASURES
• Patient education, assurance and understanding important
• Limit exposure to offending allergen
• Try to establish specific cause(s) - history and appropriate skin testing
• Intensity of treatment determined by severity of disease
• Septoplasty when deviation significant enough to interfere with benefits of medication.
Immunotherapy:
• Usually reserved for seasonal allergies uncontrollable with drugs and not responding to environmental adjustment.
• Specific allergen extract is injected subcutaneously in increasing doses to patient tolerance as determined by local reaction
• Patient response should be evaluated each season or year

ACTIVITY No specific restrictions. Emphasize avoiding activity in areas of allergen exposure.

DIET No special diet unless concomitant food reactions suspected and evaluated

PATIENT EDUCATION Printed material available from many sources including: Asthma & Allergy Foundation of America. 1717 Massachusetts Ave., Suite 305, Washington, DC 20036, (800)7-ASTHMA

MEDICATIONS

DRUG(S) OF CHOICE
Most patients present because of inability to control symptoms and improve life style with avoidance of allergens or with over the counter medications.
Antihistamines:
Classification charts available. Five major classes: Ethanolamines (Benadryl, Tavist), alkylamines (chlorpheniramine, brompheniramine), ethylenediamines (PBZ), piperazines (Atarax), phenothiazines (Phenergan, Tacaryl).
• Those with sedating side effects cheaper and often non-prescription. May start using at bedtime. Drowsiness often lessens with continued, regular dosage.
• Non-sedating type, e.g., terfenadine (Seldane) and astemizole (Hismanal) widely used. Emphasize that prescribed dosage NOT be exceeded. Be aware of drug interactions.
Decongestants
• Oral, e.g., pseudoephedrine
• Topical drops or sprays, e.g., phenylephrine
• Topical ophthalmic vasoconstrictors for annoying conjunctival itching
Nasal sprays
• Physiologic saline solution
• Cromolyn (Nasalcrom)
• Beclomethasone (Beconase AQ or Vancenase AQ), flunisolide (Nasalide, AeroBid), triamcinolone (Nasacort).
Systemic steroids
Only in urgent, selected cases and only for short-term use.
Contraindications:
• Antihistamines may precipitate urinary retention in males with prostatism and/or hypertrophy
• Decongestants if congestion is a "rebound" phenomenon
• Discourage decongestants if hypertension a problem
• Non-sedating antihistamines (Seldane and Hismanal) should not be used in patients with liver disease or in situations in which potassium channeling is a problem
Precautions: The elderly often require less aggressive treatment and will more frequently present with non-allergic rhinitis
Significant possible interactions:
• Refer carefully to manufacturer's literature
• Always mention antihistamine associated somnolence
• Terfenadine or astemizole
◊ Ketoconazole, erythromycin, quinidine: may precipitate ventricular arrhythmias

ALTERNATIVE DRUGS
• Combinations with decongestants

FOLLOWUP

PATIENT MONITORING
• Emphasize that you wish to do the most for, but the least to the patient
• Initiate patient education, supplementing with available videotapes and/or literature

PREVENTION/AVOIDANCE
• Avoidance - most patients with inhalant allergy have problems controlling their symptoms totally with allergen avoidance
• Air conditioning and limited outside exposure during season helpful
• Instructions as to the best housekeeping tactics and control for mite dust in patients sensitive to this allergen helpful
• Exposure to all animal contacts minimized. Discourage house pets.
• Avoid environmental irritants, e.g., smoke and fumes
• Air cleaners
• Use of allergy control covers especially on mattresses and pillows

POSSIBLE COMPLICATIONS
• Secondary infection
• Otitis media
• Sinusitis
• Epistaxis
• Nasopharyngeal lymphoid hyperplasia
• Decreased pulmonary function
• Continue to suspect effects of medications
• Facial changes (see Signs and Symptoms)

EXPECTED COURSE AND PROGNOSIS
• Maximal, beneficially acceptable control of symptoms should be the goal
• Treatment tailored to each individual case.
• Immune system changes over time often associated with lessening of symptoms of allergic rhinitis. Therefore early, adequate control important.

MISCELLANEOUS

ASSOCIATED CONDITIONS
• Other IgE mediated conditions, e.g., asthma and atopic dermatitis

AGE-RELATED FACTORS
Pediatric:
• Consider allergy as principle cause of persistent rhinitis
• Family understanding and involvement important
• Environmental control a cooperative effort and may include carpet and drape removal, removal of house plants, pet control, etc.
Geriatric:
• Increased medication side effects
• Number and specific allergens causing symptoms may change
• Symptoms may decrease by 4th-5th decade (not a hard rule)
Others: N/A

PREGNANCY Physiological changes of pregnancy may aggravate all types of rhinitis including allergic, vasomotor, nonallergic rhinitis with eosinophilia and chronic irritable airways

SYNONYMS
• Hay fever
• Pollinosis, seasonal and perennial
• IgE mediated rhinitis

ICD-9-CM 477 allergic rhinitis

SEE ALSO N/A

OTHER NOTES N/A

ABBREVIATIONS N/A

REFERENCES
• Middleton, E., JR., Reed, C.E. & Ellis, E.F.: Allergy Principles and Practice. 4th Ed. St. Louis, C.V. Mosby Co, 1993
• JAMA. Primer on Allergic and Immunologic Diseases. 1992
• Wyngaarden, J.B. & Smith, L.H. (eds): Cecil Textbook of Medicine. 18th Ed. Philadelphia, W.B. Saunders Co., 1992

Author J. Dix, M.D.

Rocky Mountain spotted fever

 BASICS

DESCRIPTION Rocky Mountain spotted fever (RMSF) is an acute, potentially fatal febrile illness caused by Rickettsia rickettsii and transmitted by tick bite. The primary pathology is a vasculitis due to direct endothelial cell invasion by rickettsiae. The cardinal clinical features are headache, fever, and a centripetal rash which is often petechial.

Genetics: N/A

Incidence/Prevalence in USA: About 600 new cases are reported each year in the USA. There is considerable geographic variability; most cases are reported from south Atlantic (229 cases in 1989) and south central states (105 cases in 1989). Peak incidence is in late spring and summer.

Predominant age: Highest incidences occur among children and young adults, primarily due to environmental exposure patterns. All ages are susceptible.

Predominant sex: Males > Female (due to greater male outdoor activity)

SIGNS AND SYMPTOMS
- Fever (100%)
- Rash (macular, maculopapular, petechial) (90-100%)
- Headache (65%)
- Rash (petechial) (50%)
- Headache, fever, rash (50-60%)
- Other neuropsychiatric symptoms (40-50%)
- Nausea, vomiting (30-50%)
- Headache, fever, petechial rash (33%)
- Abdominal pain (30%)
- Myalgias (30%)
- Hepatosplenomegaly (30%)
- Lymphadenopathy (25%)
- Arthralgias (10%)
- Cough (15%)
- Central nervous system dysfunction (stupor, confusion, coma, focal abnormalities) (10-30%)

CAUSES RMSF is caused by Rickettsia rickettsii which is transmitted by the bite of ticks (Dermacentor andersoni, Dermacentor variabilis). Rarely by direct inoculation of tick blood into open wounds or conjunctivae.

RISK FACTORS
- Outdoor activity during warm months
- Contact with dogs

 DIAGNOSIS

DIFFERENTIAL DIAGNOSIS
- Viral exanthems (measles, rubella, etc.)
- Meningoencephalitis (viral meningitis or encephalitis, bacterial meningitis)
- Typhus, rickettsialpox
- Ehrlichiosis
- Lyme disease
- Meningococcemia
- Leptospirosis

LABORATORY
Nonspecific laboratory changes
- ◊ Thrombocytopenia
- ◊ WBC normal, increased, or decreased
- ◊ Anemia (mild)
- ◊ Hyponatremia (usually mild)
- ◊ CSF protein and WBC modestly elevated (lymphocytic predominance), glucose usually normal
- ◊ Prolonged PT, PTT; decreased fibrinogen; elevated fibrin degradation products (FDP) (uncommon)

Specific laboratory diagnosis
- ◊ Serum Proteus Ox-19 antibody; fourfold increase (acute and convalescent) or solitary titer > 1:320 (relatively specific)
- ◊ Serum complement fixation (CF) antibody: fourfold increase or solitary titer > 1:16
- ◊ Serum indirect fluorescent antibody (IFA): fourfold increase or solitary titer > 1:64
- ◊ Direct fluorescent antibody (DFA) test on skin biopsy (not widely available)

Drugs that may alter lab results: N/A

Disorders that may alter lab results: Early treatment may blunt antibody response

PATHOLOGICAL FINDINGS
- The principal pathological abnormality is a systemic vasculitis
- Rickettsiae may be demonstrated within endothelial cells by DFA or electron microscopy
- Petechiae due to the vasculitis may be seen on various organ surfaces (e.g., liver, brain, epicardium)
- Secondary thromboses and tissue necrosis may be seen

SPECIAL TESTS N/A

IMAGING Other than nonspecific pneumonic infiltrates which may be seen on routine chest x-ray, imaging procedures are rarely helpful

DIAGNOSTIC PROCEDURES
- Tissue (primarily skin) biopsy can be helpful if rapid DFA or electron microscopy are available
- Diagnosis is usually presumptive, based upon a compatible syndrome in a patient with exposure history in an endemic area; confirmation is obtained by subsequent serology

 TREATMENT

APPROPRIATE HEALTH CARE
- Patients with the full clinical presentation or who are moderately ill should usually be hospitalized
- Patients with mild disease are treated presumptively as outpatients. Close followup is important in identifying complications.

GENERAL MEASURES
- Oxygen therapy and assisted ventilation for pulmonary complications, if necessary
- Good mouth care
- Blood transfusions for anemia
- Turning bed-confined patient frequently
- Watch patient closely for signs of renal failure

ACTIVITY Bed rest until symptoms subside

DIET Critically ill patients may require IV nutrition. In others, small frequent meals may be necessary to maintain nutritional levels.

PATIENT EDUCATION See information in Prevention/avoidance

MEDICATIONS

DRUG(S) OF CHOICE
For adults (choose one of the following)
• Doxycycline (Vibramycin) 200 mg po initially, followed by 100 mg po bid for 7-10 days; same dosage IV; 100 mg q 24 h in renal failure
• Tetracycline 500 mg po q6h for 7-10 days; should not be used in renal failure
• Chloramphenicol 500-750 mg po q6h for 7-10 days; 20 mg per kg IV q6h (4 gm per day maximum); same dose in renal failure
For children (choose one of the following)
• Doxycycline (Vibramycin) 2.0-2.5 mg/kg po q12h for 7-10 days; 4.4 mg/kg IV initially, followed by 2.2 mg per kg IV every 12 h
• Tetracycline 10 mg per kg po q6h for 7-10 days
• Chloramphenicol 20 mg per kg po q6h; same dosage IV

Contraindications:
• Children less than 9 years old - doxycycline and tetracyclines are generally not used because of the risk of tooth staining
• Pregnant women - doxycycline and tetracyclines are contraindicated because they may cause severe hepatic disease in the mother and retarded bone growth in the fetus

Precautions:
• Patients taking doxycycline or tetracyclines should minimize sun exposure to avoid photosensitization
• Infants or children with liver disease taking chloramphenicol should have serum drug levels monitored

Significant possible interactions:
Absorption of tetracyclines may be inhibited if they are ingested with milk products, iron preparations, or antacids containing aluminum or magnesium

ALTERNATIVE DRUGS
There are no currently available or adequately studied alternative drugs

FOLLOWUP

PATIENT MONITORING
• If patients are not hospitalized, they should be seen every 2-3 days until symptoms have fully resolved
• CBC, creatinine, electrolytes should be monitored

PREVENTION/AVOIDANCE
People who go into tick-infested areas can take measures to prevent infection
◊ Occlusive clothing should be worn and insect repellants applied
◊ After possible exposure, all body areas should be carefully inspected for ticks, especially legs, groin, external genitalia, belt lines. Likelihood of infection increases with the duration of tick attachment.
◊ Ticks should be removed from humans or animals with caution; gloves should be worn or instruments used to minimize direct contact. Place a drop of oil, alcohol, gasoline or kerosine on the tick first. Hands should be washed thoroughly afterwards.

POSSIBLE COMPLICATIONS
• Encephalopathy, usually transient (30-40%)
• Seizures, focal neurologic signs (10%)
• Renal insufficiency (10%)
• Hepatitis (10%)
• Congestive heart failure (5%)
• Respiratory failure (5%)

EXPECTED COURSE AND PROGNOSIS
• The usual prognosis is excellent with resolution of symptoms over several days and no sequelae
• Mortality is rare with prompt institution of appropriate therapy
• If complications develop (see above), the course may be more severe and long-term sequelae may be present

MISCELLANEOUS

ASSOCIATED CONDITIONS N/A

AGE-RELATED FACTORS
Pediatric: N/A
Geriatric: Mortality risk higher
Others: N/A

PREGNANCY N/A

SYNONYMS Tick typhus

ICD-9-CM
082.0

SEE ALSO N/A

OTHER NOTES
Treatment should be initiated on the basis of clinical diagnosis or skin biopsy. Treatment should not be delayed for serologic confirmation.

ABBREVIATIONS N/A

REFERENCES
• Kirk, J.L., Fine, D.P., Sexton, D.J. & Muchmore, H.G.: Rocky Mountain spotted fever. A clinical review based on 48 confirmed cases, 1943-1986. Medicine 69:35-45,1990
• Melnick, C.G., Bernard, K.W. & D'Angelo, L.J.: Rocky Mountain spotted fever: Clinical, laboratory, and epidemiological features of 262 cases. J Infect Dis 150:480-488,1984
• Linnemann, C.C., Jr. & Janson, P.J.: The clinical presentations of Rocky Mountain spotted fever. Clin Pediatr 17:673-679, 1978

Author D. Fine, M.D. & R. Greenfield, M.D.

Roseola

BASICS

DESCRIPTION An acute disease of infants or very young children with an incubation period of about 5-15 days. Characteristically, it causes first a high fever, followed by the appearance of an eruption (whose appearance is similar to that of measles) simultaneously with, or following defervescence. Both cause and transmission mode are unknown, but presumably it is a communicable virus.

System(s) affected: Endocrine/Metabolic, Skin/Exocrine

Genetics: No known genetic pattern

Incidence in USA: Unknown

Prevalence in USA:
• Estimated that 30% of all children
• More likely to occur in spring and fall

Predominant age: Infants and very young children (6 months to 3 years)

Predominant sex: Male = Female

SIGNS AND SYMPTOMS
• Abrupt fever without apparent cause (103-105°F) for 3-5 days
• Sudden drop of fever. As fever disappears, skin rash begins.
• Anorexia
• Irritability
• Listlessness
• Does not appear seriously ill
• Maculopapular, nonpruritic rash, first appearing on the trunk, that blanches on pressure
• Rash appears as very slightly elevated, rose-pink papules that appear profusely on trunk, arms and neck; mild on face and legs
• Rash fades within a few hours to 2 days
• Febrile convulsions during height of fever (uncommon)
• Lymphadenopathy in cervical and posterior auricular regions
• Spleen enlarged (uncommon)

CAUSES
A communicable virus, human herpes virus type 6 (HHV-6), leads list of possible viruses (neurodematopic)

RISK FACTORS
• Day care center
• Exposure to infected infant

DIAGNOSIS

DIFFERENTIAL DIAGNOSIS
• Sepsis
• Pyelonephritis
• Otitis media
• Meningitis
• Bacterial pneumonia
• Drug eruption

LABORATORY
• Urinalysis
• CBC - leukopenia with relative lymphocytosis

Drugs that may alter lab results: N/A
Disorders that may alter lab results: N/A

PATHOLOGICAL FINDINGS None

SPECIAL TESTS N/A

IMAGING Chest x-ray negative

DIAGNOSTIC PROCEDURES Careful physical examination. Roseola should be suspected if it is known to be in the community and the child presents with a high temperature.

TREATMENT

APPROPRIATE HEALTH CARE
Outpatient

GENERAL MEASURES
• Symptomatic
• Tap water baths to cool excess temperature elevation
• Lightweight clothing
• Maintain normal room temperature

ACTIVITY Rest until rash appears and fever breaks

DIET Encourage fluids

PATIENT EDUCATION
• Infection is self-limiting
• If seizures occur, they will not cause brain damage and will cease after fever subsides

MEDICATIONS

DRUG(S) OF CHOICE
• Antipyretics for excessively high fever. Avoid aspirin. Instead use acetaminophen, 10-15 mg/kg/q 4 h to a maximum of 2.6 g/24 hr. (Aspirin may enhance the risk of Reye's syndrome.)
• Phenobarbital if needed for seizure
Contraindications: N/A
Precautions: N/A
Significant possible interactions: N/A

ALTERNATIVE DRUGS N/A

FOLLOWUP

PATIENT MONITORING None after typical rash appears

PREVENTION/AVOIDANCE None

POSSIBLE COMPLICATIONS
• Febrile seizures
• Encephalitis (rare)

EXPECTED COURSE AND PROGNOSIS
• Course - acute, benign, complete recovery without sequelae
• One attack confers permanent immunity

MISCELLANEOUS

ASSOCIATED CONDITIONS N/A

AGE-RELATED FACTORS
Pediatric: A disease of infants and very young children
Geriatric: N/A
Others: N/A

PREGNANCY N/A

SYNONYMS
• Exanthem subitum
• Pseudorubella
• Sixth disease

ICD-9-CM
• 056.9 roseola
• 056.8 roseola complicated

SEE ALSO N/A

OTHER NOTES N/A

ABBREVIATIONS N/A

REFERENCES
• Mandell, G.L. (ed.): Principles and Practice of Infectious Diseases. 3rd Ed. New York, Churchill Livingstone, 1990
• Barlett, J.: 1991-92 Pocketbook of Pediatric Infectious Disease Therapy. Baltimore, Williams & Wilkins, 1991
• Krugman, S.,Katz, S.L., Gershon, A.A. & Wilfert, C.M. (eds.): Infectious Diseases of Children. 9th Ed. St. Louis, C.V. Mosby, 1992

Author J. Kirchner, D.O.

Roundworms, intestinal

BASICS

DESCRIPTION Intestinal roundworms (nematodes) have adult stages infecting the intestinal tract of man. Larval stages may exist elsewhere in the body. Except for Trichinella spiralis, which is encysted in muscle; egg and/or larval stages can be isolated from the intestinal canal.

<u>Nematodes parasitizing the intestinal tract of man:</u>
  ◊ Enterobius vermicularis (pinworm)
  ◊ Trichuris trichiura (whipworm)
  ◊ Ascaris lumbricoides (large roundworm of man)
  ◊ Necator americanus (hookworm)
  ◊ Ancylostoma duodenale (hookworm)
  ◊ Strongyloides stercoralis
  ◊ Trichostrongylus
  ◊ Trichinella spiralis (trichinosis)

System(s) affected: Gastrointestinal, Cardiovascular, Pulmonary, Nervous, Renal/Urologic, Musculoskeletal
Genetics: N/A
Incidence/Prevalence in USA:
• Up to 40% of children may have pinworms
• Trichinella 4-20%
• Others mostly in Southern regions
• Incidence of intestinal obstruction with ascaris is 2/1000
• Incidence of ascaris reportedly decreasing in the US, presumably due to improved sanitation

Predominant age: All ages; pinworm infestations more common in children
Predominant sex: Male = Female

SIGNS AND SYMPTOMS

<u>Lung Invasion:</u>
  ◊ Fever
  ◊ Cough
  ◊ Blood-tinged sputum
  ◊ Wheezing
  ◊ Rales
  ◊ Dyspnea
  ◊ Substernal pain
  ◊ Pulmonary consolidations
  ◊ Eosinophilia
  ◊ Urticaria
  ◊ Asthma
  ◊ Angioneurotic edema
  ◊ Brain, kidney, eye, spinal cord, etc. (rare)
<u>Intestinal invasion:</u>
  ◊ May be asymptomatic (small number)
  ◊ Abdominal pain (usually vague)
  ◊ Abdominal cramps/colic
  ◊ Diarrhea
  ◊ Rarely vomiting
  ◊ Occasionally constipation

<u>Muscle and other tissue invasion:</u> (Trichinosis)
  ◊ Myalgias
  ◊ Fever
  ◊ Edema and spasm
  ◊ Periorbital and facial edema
  ◊ Photophobia
  ◊ Sweating
  ◊ Conjunctivitis
  ◊ Weakness or prostration
  ◊ Pain on swallowing
  ◊ Subconjunctival, retinal and nail hemorrhages
  ◊ Rashes and formication
  ◊ Encephalitis, myocarditis, nephritis
  ◊ Pneumonia, meningitis, neuropathy

CAUSES
• Ingestion of mature eggs in fecally contaminated food or drink
• Larval penetration of skin (hookworm)

RISK FACTORS
• Low standard of hygiene
• Poor sanitation
• Human feces fertilizer

DIAGNOSIS

DIFFERENTIAL DIAGNOSIS
• Pulmonary ascariasis with eosinophilia - consider asthma, Löffler's syndrome, eosinophilic pneumonia, systemic lupus erythematosus, Hodgkin's disease, and other parasitic causes (tropical pulmonary eosinophilia, toxocariasis, strongyloidiasis, hookworm, paragonimiasis)
• Worm-induced GI diseases - consider other causes of pancreatitis, appendicitis, diverticulitis, duodenitis, esophagitis, cholecystitis

LABORATORY
• Based on characteristics of eggs or larvae in stool or adult worm, if passed
• Cellophane-tape impression for pinworms
• Eosinophilia
• Larvae in sputum or adult worms seen on radiologic studies (uncommon)
Drugs that may alter lab results: N/A
Disorders that may alter lab results: N/A

PATHOLOGICAL FINDINGS
Characteristic eggs/worms

SPECIAL TESTS Serologic tests not useful

IMAGING N/A

DIAGNOSTIC PROCEDURES
• Stool exams
• Cellophane-tape impression

TREATMENT

APPROPRIATE HEALTH CARE
Outpatient

GENERAL MEASURES None other than medications to eradicate the worms

ACTIVITY No restrictions

DIET No special diet

PATIENT EDUCATION Avoid fecally contaminated food, water, and soil

MEDICATIONS

DRUG(S) OF CHOICE
• Enterobius vermicularis (pinworm) -
mebendazole 100 mg single dose, or pyrantel
pamoate 11 mg/kg once (maximum of 1 g),
repeat after 2 weeks (all dosages for adult and
pediatrics)
• Trichuris trichiura (whipworm) - mebendazole
100 mg bid x 3 days or albendazole 400 mg
once (all dosages for adult and pediatrics).
Note - albendazole available in the US only
from manufacturer.
• Ascaris lumbricoides (large roundworm of
man), mebendazole 100 mg bid x 3 days or
pyrantel pamoate 11 mg/kg once (maximum of
1 g) (all dosages for adult and pediatrics)
• Necator americanus (hookworm),
Ancylostoma duodenale (hookworm) -
mebendazole 100 mg bid x 3 days or pyrantel
pamoate 11 mg/kg (maximum of 1 g) x 3 days
(all dosages for adult and pediatrics)
• Trichostrongylus - pyrantel pamoate 11
mg/kg once (maximum of 1 g) or mebendazole
100 mg bid x 3 day (all dosages for adult and
pediatrics)
• Trichinella spiralis - mebendazole 200-400
mg tid x 3 days, then 400-500 mg tid x 10 days
(adult dosage) plus steroids if severe
• Strongyloides stercoralis - thiabendazole 50
mg/kg/d in 2 doses (maximum of 3 g a day) for
2 days (adult and pediatric)
• Note: FDA may consider certain uses of
above drugs investigational, consult Medical
Letter or appropriate drug reference
Contraindications: Refer to manufacturer's
profile of each drug
Precautions: Refer to manufacturer's profile of
each drug
Significant possible interactions: Refer to
manufacturer's profile of each drug

ALTERNATIVE DRUGS N/A

FOLLOWUP

PATIENT MONITORING Followup stool
studies at 2 weeks and retreat if necessary

PREVENTION/AVOIDANCE Good
hygiene and sanitation

POSSIBLE COMPLICATIONS
• Vomiting worms
• Cholangitis - migration to common bile duct
• Pancreatitis - migration to pancreatic duct
• Appendicitis - migration to appendix
• Diverticulitis - migration to diverticuli
• Liver abscess
• Intestinal obstruction
• Volvulus
• Intussusception
• Bowel penetration

EXPECTED COURSE AND
PROGNOSIS Good for light to moderate
infections. Ascariasis should always be
treated due to the risk of migrating adult worms.

MISCELLANEOUS

ASSOCIATED CONDITIONS N/A

AGE-RELATED FACTORS Affects all
ages
Pediatric: Children commonly infected
Geriatric: N/A
Others: N/A

PREGNANCY Mebendazole should not be
used

SYNONYMS Nematodes

ICD-9-CM 127.0

SEE ALSO
• Tissue roundworms
• Intestinal parasites

OTHER NOTES N/A

ABBREVIATIONS N/A

REFERENCES
• Markell, E.K., Voge, M. & John, D.T.: Medical
Parasitology. 6th Ed. Philadelphia, W.B.
Saunders Co., 1986
• Schroeder, S.A., Krupp, M.A., Tierney, L.M. &
McPhee, S.J. (eds.): Current Medical Diagnosis
and Treatment. Norwalk, CT, Appleton &
Lange, 1989
• Strickland, G.T.: Hunter's Tropical Medicine.
6th Ed. Philadelphia, W.B. Saunders Co., 1984
• Drugs for Parasitic Infections. The Medical
Letter. Vol 34 (issue 865) March 6, 1992
• Tietze, P.E. & Tietze, P.H.: Roundworms,
Ascaris Lumbricoides. Primary Care; Clinics in
Office Practice. 16(1):25-41 (VI:9118002), Mar,
1991

Author R. Weston, M.D.

Roundworms, tissue

BASICS

DESCRIPTION Tissue roundworms (nematodes) affect man when the adults or larval stages infect certain tissues. Infective larval stages are transmitted to man by arthropod vectors or from the soil. Once in human tissue, worms mature over 6-12 months and survive as long as 15 years. Symptoms depend on tissue infected.
Filarial infections
◊ Wuchereria bancrofti (bancroftian filariasis)
◊ Brugia malayi (Malayan filariasis)
◊ Brugia timori (Timorian filariasis)
◊ Loa loa (eye worm)
◊ Onchocerca volvulus (river blindness, onchocerciasis)
◊ Mansonella perstans
◊ Mansonella ozzardi (Ozzard's filariasis)
◊ Mansonella streptocerca
Other Tissue nematode infections
◊ Dracunculus medinensis (guinea worm, dracunculosis)
◊ Ancylostoma braziliense (cutaneous larva migrans, creeping eruption)
◊ Toxocara canis or cati (visceral larva migrans, toxocariasis)
Distribution
◊ Over 300 million people are exposed to lymphatic filariasis in India and SE Asia; 30 million to onchocerciasis
◊ W. bancrofti: Tropics worldwide
◊ B. malayi: Southeast Asia
◊ B. timori: Indonesia
◊ L. loa: Africa
◊ O. volvulus: Africa, Central and South America
◊ M. perstans: Africa, South America
◊ M. ozzardi: Africa
◊ M. streptocerca: Central and South America
◊ D. medinensis: Africa, Asia
◊ A. braziliense: Tropics and Subtropics worldwide
◊ T. canis/cati: Over 50 countries worldwide, especially warmer tropical and subtropical regions
System(s) affected: Skin/Exocrine, Nervous, Gastrointestinal, Musculoskeletal, Hemic/Lymphatic/Immunologic, Cardiovascular, Renal/Urologic
Genetics: N/A
Incidence/Prevalence in USA:
• Visceral larva migrans - 4-30% seroprevalence has been reported, highest in southeastern United States
• Others - unknown
Predominant age: All ages, but children more commonly infected
Predominant sex: Male = Female

SIGNS AND SYMPTOMS
Lymphatic filariasis (W. bancrofti, B. malayi, B. timori)
◊ Inflammatory signs - pain, tenderness, swelling, erythema
◊ Filarial adenolymphangitis
◊ Filarial orchitis
◊ Funiculitis and epididymitis
◊ "Filarial" and "Elephantoid" fever
◊ Filarial abscess
◊ Obstructive signs - lymph varices, lymph scrotum, hydrocele
◊ Lymphedema and elephantiasis
◊ Chyluria
◊ Filarial hypereosinophilia (tropical pulmonary eosinophilia)
Loiasis (L. loa)
◊ Calabar swellings - recurrent subcutaneous inflammation/swelling
◊ Eye worm - adult or larvae migrate under conjunctiva
◊ Eosinophilia (may exceed 70%)
◊ Fever, irritability, urticaria and pruritis
Onchocerciasis (O. volvulus)
◊ Dermatitis
◊ Nodules
◊ Lymphadenitis
◊ Occular changes - intraocular microfilariae, punctate keratitis, sclerosing keratitis, anterior uveitis chorioretinitis, optic neuritis, optic atrophy, glaucoma, blindness (river blindness)
Other filarial syndromes (M. ozzardi, M. perstans, M. streptococci)
◊ Headaches, coldness, pruritis, and articular swelling/arthritis
◊ Eosinophilia and vague allergic signs
◊ Chronic dermatitis and macules can be confused with leprosy
◊ Lymphadenopathy
Dracunculiasis (D. medinensis, guinea worm disease)
◊ Allergic manifestations - erythema, urticaria, pruritis, nausea, vomiting, giddiness, syncope, and occasional fever)
◊ Local lesions - papule, sterile blister, ulceration, abscesses
◊ Worm protrusion
Toxocariasis (T. canis/cati, visceral or ocular larva migrans)
◊ Eosinophilia
◊ Visceral larva migrans
◊ Ocular larva migrans
Cutaneous larva migrans (A. braziliense, creeping eruption)
◊ Itching and red papules
◊ Serpiginous track
◊ Edema and acute inflammation
◊ Scars
◊ Secondary infection

CAUSES Larvae introduced into human host by arthropod vector or infected soil

RISK FACTORS
• Geographic exposure to arthropod vectors
• Fishermen or women washing clothes have increased risk of 'river blindness'
• Contact with infected soil in cutaneous larva migrans (hence plumber's itch, sandworm, duckhunter's itch)

DIAGNOSIS

DIFFERENTIAL DIAGNOSIS
• Other causes of tissue inflammation (i.e., lymphangitis, epididymitis, dermatitis, conjunctivitis, blisters, pleuritis, peritonitis, pericarditis, encephalitis, nephropathy, cardiomyopathy, etc.)
Nonfilarial causes of lymphangitis:
◊ Acute bacterial lymphangitis
◊ Phlebitis
◊ Unusual - plague, anthrax, TB, lymphogranuloma inguinale
Nonfilarial causes of lymphedema, chyluria, and elephantiasis:
◊ Infiltrative or granulomatous process: Tumor, fungus, TB, leprosy
◊ Chronic venostasis or phlebitis
◊ Cardiac insufficiency
◊ Nutritional deficiencies
◊ Hereditary (Milroy's disease)
◊ Lateritious soil obstructing lymphatics

LABORATORY Examination of larvae or adult worms taken from the tissue; characteristic microfilariae on blood smear; eosinophilia
Drugs that may alter lab results: N/A
Disorders that may alter lab results: N/A

PATHOLOGICAL FINDINGS
Characteristic eggs/worms/larvae in tissue

SPECIAL TESTS Skin snip, nodulectomy, slit-lamp exam, and Mazzotti, test may be helpful in onchocerciasis

IMAGING Occasional worms seen on x-ray

DIAGNOSTIC PROCEDURES
Microfilariae on blood smear or other body fluids; clinical observations; serologies (e.g., ELISA)

TREATMENT

APPROPRIATE HEALTH CARE
Outpatient

GENERAL MEASURES
• Identify cause and treat accordingly
• Best treatment - direct removal of worm from tissue with caution not to break the worm
• Treat secondary infections

ACTIVITY
No restrictions. If edema a problem, may want to elevate legs while sitting.

DIET
No special diet

PATIENT EDUCATION
• Avoid bites by arthropod vectors, insect repellants and other protective measures, e.g., proper clothing
• Avoid rivers and streams and soils known to be infected

MEDICATIONS

DRUG(S) OF CHOICE
• Visceral larva migrans (Toxocara) - diethylcarbamazine (DEC) 6 mg/kg/d in 3 doses x 7-10 days for adult and pediatric, or thiabendazole 50 mg/kg/d in 2 doses x 5 days (max 3 grams/day) for adult and pediatric
• Cutaneous larva migrans (Ancylostoma) - thiabendazole topical and/or oral 50 mg/kg/d in 2 doses x 2-5 days (max 3 grams/day) for adult and pediatric
• Filariasis (Wuchereria, Bancrofti, Loa) - diethylcarbamazine, adult - day 1) 50 mg po after meals, day 2) 50 mg tid, day 3) 100 mg tid, days 4-21) 6 mg/kg/d in 3 doses; pediatric - day 1) 1 mg/kg po after meals, day 2) 1 mg/kg tid, day 3) 1-2 mg/kg tid, days 4-21) 6 mg/kg/d in 3 doses
• Onchocerciasis - ivermectin (available from the CDC Drug Services 404-639-3670) 150 µg/kg po once, repeated every 6-12 months for adult and pediatric
• Mansonella ozzardi - ivermectin (see above) 25-200 µg/kg in single dose (reported to be effective)
• Mansonella perstans - mebendazole 100 mg bid x 30 days (approved drug, but considered investigational for this condition)
• Guinea worm (Dracunculus) - metronidazole 250 mg tid x 10 days for adult; 25 mg/kg/d (max 750 mg/d) in 3 doses x 10 days for pediatric
• Note: FDA may consider certain uses of above drugs investigational and some may not be available in USA. Contact Parasitic Disease Drug Service, Parasitic Diseases Branch, Center for Disease Control, Atlanta 30333, (404)488-4240.
Contraindications: Refer to manufacturer's information

Precautions: Children, pregnancy, lactation
Significant possible interactions: Refer to manufacturer's profile of each drug

ALTERNATIVE DRUGS
Albendazole (available in USA only from the manufacturer)

FOLLOWUP

PATIENT MONITORING
N/A

PREVENTION/AVOIDANCE
• Avoid sources of infection (arthropod bites, rivers/streams, or contaminated soils)
• Diethylcarbamazine (DEC) once weekly has been used successfully in Peace Corps' workers for prophylaxis against L. loa
• Prophylaxis with ivermectin is under investigation
• Public health activities such as vector control

POSSIBLE COMPLICATIONS
• Depends upon type of worm
• Eye worms - blindness
• Visceral worms - hepatitis, splenomegaly, pleuritis, peritonitis, eosinophilic granuloma or other organ damage as larvae migrate for up to 6 months
• Filariasis - lymphatic destruction leading to severe edema (elephantiasis)

EXPECTED COURSE AND
PROGNOSIS   Good for light to moderate infections; depends on organ infected and extent of infection

MISCELLANEOUS

ASSOCIATED CONDITIONS N/A

AGE-RELATED FACTORS
Pediatric: Children commonly infected
Geriatric: N/A
Others: N/A

PREGNANCY N/A

SYNONYMS
• Creeping eruption
• Cutaneous larva migrans
• Dracunculosis
• Elephantiasis
• Filariasis
• Guinea worm
• Larva migrans
• Loiasis
• Nematodes
• River blindness
• Toxocariasis
• Visceral larva migrans

ICD-9-CM   127.0

SEE ALSO   Roundworms, intestinal

OTHER NOTES   N/A

ABBREVIATIONS   N/A

REFERENCES
• Markell, E.K., Voge, M. & John, D.T.: Medical Parasitology. 6th Ed. Philadelphia, W.B. Saunders Co., 1986
• Schroeder, S.A., Krupp, M.A., Tierney, L.M. & McPhee, S.J. (eds.): Current Medical Diagnosis and Treatment. Norwalk, CT, Appleton & Lange, 1989
• Strickland, G.T.: Hunter's Tropical Medicine. 7th Ed. Philadelphia, W.B. Saunders Co., 1991
• Warren, K.S. & Mahmoud, A.A.F.: Tropical and Geographic Medicine. New York, McGraw-Hill, 1990
• Drugs for Parasitic Infections. Medical Letter. New Rochelle, NY, Medical Letter, Inc. 34:865, 1992

Author   R. Weston, M.D.

Salivary gland calculi

BASICS

DESCRIPTION The presence of stones within the ducts of any of the major salivary glands
System(s) affected: Gastrointestinal, Skin/Exocrine
Genetics: No known genetic pattern
Incidence/Prevalence in USA: Not uncommon
Predominant age: Middle to geriatric age groups. Uncommon in children.
Predominant sex: Male > Female (2:1)

SIGNS AND SYMPTOMS
• Mass palpable within the mouth or in the neck or face
• May be associated with sialadenitis
• Most stones are unilateral and tend to be recurrent

CAUSES
• Related to inflammation, trauma or factors that alter secretion
• Stones felt to be due to calcifications that occur around impacted food particles and organic debris. Increased with conditions that result in stasis of saliva. Examples include chronic parotitis, Sjögren's syndrome, cystic fibrosis, poor oral hygiene.

RISK FACTORS Existing chronic, debilitating illness

DIAGNOSIS

DIFFERENTIAL DIAGNOSIS
• Lymphadenitis
• Sialadenitis
• Oral or cervical carcinoma
• Foreign body
• Dental abscess
• Salivary carcinoma. Patients present with mass in the neck with or without intermittent swelling of the affected salivary gland.

LABORATORY Nonspecific except for factors altered by inflammation. If associated with sialadenitis there may be elevation of serum amylase.
Drugs that may alter lab results: N/A
Disorders that may alter lab results: N/A

PATHOLOGICAL FINDINGS
Submandibular glands are affected 90% of cases; parotid about 10%; other glands rarely

SPECIAL TESTS N/A

IMAGING
• Plain film of the head and neck
• Sialogram
• CT of head and neck
• 80% of stones are radiopaque and contain inorganic calcium and phosphate

DIAGNOSTIC PROCEDURES N/A

TREATMENT

APPROPRIATE HEALTH CARE
Inpatient or outpatient surgery

GENERAL MEASURES
• Stone(s) within 2 cm of the end of the duct - the stone is removed intraorally by massage or by sectioning the duct
• Stone(s) in the submandibular gland more than 2 cm from the orifice - treated by removal of the gland and the associated duct
• Parotid stones are almost always removed intraorally
• Massage of the gland may cause expulsion of the stone if in the distal duct
• Look for primary diseases causing stasis such as Sjögren's syndrome
• Treat associated infections or conditions

ACTIVITY No restriction

DIET Avoid sour substances that may cause salivation

PATIENT EDUCATION Relate the general management and diet as listed above

MEDICATIONS

DRUG(S) OF CHOICE If infection, use an antistaphlococcus antibiotic
Contraindications: Hypersensitivity to drug chosen
Precautions: Refer to manufacturer's literature
Significant possible interactions: Refer to manufacturer's literature

ALTERNATIVE DRUGS N/A

FOLLOWUP

PATIENT MONITORING Patients should be followed clinically approximately every 6 months for recurrence of the stone. Stones tend to be recurrent in the same gland in which the original stone was found.

PREVENTION/AVOIDANCE Treat primary disease; good oral hygiene

POSSIBLE COMPLICATIONS
Postsurgery salivary fistula is possible. Sialadenitis may be caused by stones or they may cause stones and need separate treatment.

EXPECTED COURSE AND PROGNOSIS
• Most patients have permanent recovery after the stone is removed
• Recurrence is possible

MISCELLANEOUS

ASSOCIATED CONDITIONS
• Sjögren's syndrome
• Cystic fibrosis
• Sialadenitis
• Oral trauma

AGE-RELATED FACTORS
Pediatric: N/A
Geriatric: N/A
Others: N/A

PREGNANCY N/A

SYNONYMS N/A

ICD-9-CM 527.5

SEE ALSO Sialadenitis

OTHER NOTES Multiple calculi in 20% of cases. In past, stones were felt to be secondary to diseases of calcium metabolism but this has been disproven.

ABBREVIATIONS N/A

REFERENCES
• Cotran, R.S., et al: Robbins Pathologic Basis of Disease. 4th Ed. Philadelphia, W.B. Saunders, Co., 1989
• Paparella, M.M. & Shunrick, D.A.: Otolaryngology. Philadelphia, W.B. Saunders Co., 1980

Author M. Essig, M.D.

Salivary gland tumors

BASICS

DESCRIPTION Neoplasms benign or malignant of the major (parotid, submaxillary, sublingual) salivary glands or the minor (intra-oral, pharyngeal, nasal) salivary glands. Most tumors are discrete masses although some may manifest as diffuse enlargement of the gland or submucosal intraoral swelling. Malignant tumors are characterized by local recurrence and perineural spread (adenoid cystic), or local recurrence and lymph node metastases (mucoepidermoid, adenocarcinoma, squamous cell carcinoma).
Types
◊ Pleomorphic adenoma (most common tumor) - 45% overall
◊ Monomorphic adenoma - 12% overall
◊ Mucoepidermoid carcinoma - 12% overall
◊ Adenoid cystic - 6% overall
◊ Less frequent lesions are - adenocarcinoma, squamous cell carcinoma, acinic cell carcinoma, oxyphilic adenomas, Warthin's tumor
Distribution of neoplasms
◊ Parotid (80% benign, 20% malignant) - 70% are pleomorphic adenoma; 10% are monomorphic adenoma; 12% are mucoepidermoid carcinoma; 5% are adenoid cystic
◊ Submandibular (60% benign, 40% malignant) - 40% are pleomorphic adenoma; 10% are mucoepidermoid carcinoma; 20% are adenoid cystic carcinoma
◊ Minor salivary glands (40% benign, 60% malignant) - 40% are pleomorphic adenoma; 25% are mucoepidermoid carcinoma; 25% are adenoid cystic carcinoma
System(s) affected: Nervous, Digestive
Genetics: Increased incidence of adenocarcinoma of parotid in Eskimos, otherwise no known genetic pattern
Incidence/Prevalence in USA: 3% of new tumors; 6% of head and neck neoplasms
Predominant age: Malignant - age 55; benign - age 45
Predominant sex:
• Pleomorphic adenoma: Female > Male
• Other adenomas: Male = Female

SIGNS AND SYMPTOMS
• Discrete mass in anatomic area - 96% (malignant)
• Elevation of earlobe
• Pain 12-25% (malignant); 2.5% (benign)
• Trigeminal paresthesias
• Facial nerve palsy or dysfunction 8-26% (malignant)
• Fixation to masseter and pterygoids 17% (malignant)
• Skin ulceration 9% (malignant)
• Cervical lymph node metastases 20% (malignant)
• Pharyngeal mass (representing deep lobe tumors of the parotid gland)

CAUSES
• Unknown
• Possible ionizing radiation

RISK FACTORS None known

DIAGNOSIS

DIFFERENTIAL DIAGNOSIS
• Inflammatory masses
• Parotid and submandibular lymph nodes
• Mikulicz's syndrome
• Salivary gland stones
• Torus palatinus (minor)
• Necrotizing sialometaplasia (minor)
• Cervical lymph nodes
• Sjögren's syndrome

LABORATORY
• Autoimmune studies
• Fractionated amylase (inflammation)
Drugs that may alter lab results: None known
Disorders that may alter lab results: None known

PATHOLOGICAL FINDINGS Of 100 parotid masses, 70 will be non-neoplastic, 21 will be benign neoplasms, and 9 will be malignant neoplasms

SPECIAL TESTS
• Technetium-99 (Warthin's tumor)
• Ultrasound (inflammatory or malignant)
• Sialography (for calculi or chronic parotitis)

IMAGING
• CT/MRI. Both provide anatomic detail and diagnostic information.
• Chest x-ray - Sjögren's, metastases

DIAGNOSTIC PROCEDURES
• Fine needle aspiration (some authors would not utilize this procedure in fear of disseminating a malignant tumor)
• Superficial lobectomy

TREATMENT

APPROPRIATE HEALTH CARE
Inpatient

GENERAL MEASURES
• Inpatient procedures with usual nursing care
• Drain parotid bed
• Usually 2-4 day hospitalization
• Benign tumors - superficial or total conservative (nerve-sparing) parotidectomy depending on site of tumor
• Malignant tumors - total parotidectomy, or sialadenectomy with adjuvant radiotherapy to parotid base of skull with/without neck depending on histology. Preservation of facial nerve unless involved by tumor.
• Cervical lymphadenectomy if palpable nodes or elective neck dissection in squamous cell carcinoma, high grade mucoepidermoid carcinoma or high grade adenocarcinoma
• Elevate head of bed postoperative
• Suction drainage x 1-2 days
• Suture line care with antibiotic ointment

ACTIVITY Moderate restriction for 1 day

DIET Non-stimulating liquid

PATIENT EDUCATION
• Basic cancer followup
• Recurrent masses
• Trigeminal nerve symptoms
• Frey's syndrome (gustatory sweating)
• Facial nerve symptoms (paresis)

MEDICATIONS

DRUG(S) OF CHOICE N/A
Contraindications: N/A
Precautions: N/A
Significant possible interactions: N/A

ALTERNATIVE DRUGS N/A

FOLLOWUP

PATIENT MONITORING
• For malignancy - once every 4 months the first year, once every six months subsequent 3 years, once per year subsequently
• For benign tumors - once per year for five years

PREVENTION/AVOIDANCE No known etiologic agents

POSSIBLE COMPLICATIONS
• Frey's syndrome (gustatory sweating) occurs symptomatically in about 20% of patients undergoing parotidectomy
• Facial neurapraxia from surgery should resolve within six months, even with use of adjuvant radiotherapy
• Cosmetic deformity of moderate facial flattening on side of parotidectomy
• Injury to hypoglossal or lingual nerve during submandibular resection
• Pleomorphic adenoma may recur, if inadequately excised, since it has pseudopods throughout the lobe

EXPECTED COURSE AND PROGNOSIS
• Parotid pleomorphic adenoma untreated will demonstrate malignant degeneration in 2-10% over 20 years. Treated adequately, parotid pleomorphic adenoma has 1.5% recurrence rate. Malignancy prognosis depends on stage.
• Adenoid cystic - parotid 5 year survival 73%, 15 year 21%; submandibular 5 year 50%, 15 year 0%; palate 5 year 80%, 15 year 38%
• Adenocarcinoma - 5 year survival 78%, 20 year 41%
• Mucoepidermoid - low grade 5 year survival 81%, 15 year 48%, high grade 5 year survival 46%, 15 year 25%

MISCELLANEOUS

ASSOCIATED CONDITIONS None known

AGE-RELATED FACTORS
Pediatric: Hemangioma is the most common benign tumor in pediatric population followed by pleomorphic adenoma. Mucoepidermoid most common malignant.
Geriatric: N/A
Others: N/A

PREGNANCY Not affected

SYNONYMS N/A

ICD-9-CM 142-142.9 malignant neoplasm of major salivary glands

SEE ALSO N/A

OTHER NOTES N/A

ABBREVIATIONS N/A

REFERENCES
• Coleman, J.J.: Salivary gland disorders. In Fundamentals of Plastic Surgery. Edited by M.J. Jurkiewicz, T.J. Krizek, S. J. Mathews & S. Ariyan. St. Louis, C.V. Mosby Co., 1990
• Rankow, R.M. & Polayes, I.M.: Diseases of the Salivary Glands, Philadelphia, W.B. Saunders, 1976
• Batsakis, J.G.: Tumors of the head and neck. Clinical and Pathological Considerations. 2nd Ed. Baltimore, Williams and Wilkins, 1979

Author J. Coleman, M.D.

Salmonella infection

BASICS

DESCRIPTION Disease caused by any serotype of the genus Salmonella. Clinical syndromes include enterocolitis (75%), bacteremia (10%), enteric fever (10%) (see Typhoid fever), localized infection outside gastrointestinal tract (5%) and an asymptomatic carrier state (< 1%). Organisms invade gut mucosa, producing inflammatory, cytotoxic response. Organisms can then disseminate into systemic circulation via lymphatics. Infective dose and host defenses dictate extent of disease.
Genetics: A condition similar to Reiter's syndrome may follow Salmonella Enterocolitis in patients with the HLA-B27 histocompatibility antigen
Incidence in USA:
800 cases/100,000 population/year. Peak frequency July-November. Salmonella isolations represent only 1-10% of actual yearly incidence.
Prevalence in USA:
• Infants: 130/100,000
• Adults: 6/100,000
Predominant age: High prevalence in persons > 70 or < 20. Highest in infants < 1 year.
Predominant sex: Male = Female

SIGNS AND SYMPTOMS
Acute uncomplicated illness
◊ Nausea, vomiting, diarrhea
◊ Abdominal cramps
◊ Headache, myalgias
◊ Fever to 102°F (39°C)
Protracted disease
◊ Persistent fever
◊ Arthritis, reactive or septic
◊ Osteomyelitis
◊ Sacroiliitis
◊ Wound infection, soft tissue abscesses
◊ Meningitis
◊ Arteritis
◊ Endocarditis, pericarditis
◊ Pneumonia, lung abscess, empyema
◊ Hypovolemia
◊ Splenic (abscess)
◊ Hepatic (abscess)
◊ Urogenital tract infection

CAUSES
• Ingestion of contaminated food - (poultry, meat, eggs, dairy products) or water
• Person-to-person and/or fecal-oral spread
• Contact with animal reservoirs - poultry, cows, pigs, birds, sheep, seals, donkeys, lizards, snakes, pets (turtles, cats, dogs, mice, guinea pigs, hamsters)
• Iatrogenic contamination - blood transfusion, endoscopy
• Contact with asymptomatic chronic carrier
• Achlorhydria - gastroduodenal surgery, idiopathic
• Ulcerative colitis
• Systemic lupus erythematosis
• Schistosomiasis
• Cholelithiasis
• Nephrolithiasis
• Drugs - antibiotics, purgatives, opiates

RISK FACTORS
• Hemolytic anemias - sickle-cell, malaria, bartonellosis
• Malignancy - lymphoma, leukemia, disseminated carcinoma
• Immunosuppression - AIDS, steroids, other immunosuppressants, chemotherapy, radiation

DIAGNOSIS

DIFFERENTIAL DIAGNOSIS
• Viral gastroenteritis
• Other bacterial enteritises (e.g., shigellosis, cholera)
• Other bacterial sources or systemic and localized sepsis (e.g., meningococci, staphylococci)
• Pseudomembranous colitis
• Inflammatory or granulomatous bowel disease
• Appendicitis
• Cholecystitis
• Perforated viscus

LABORATORY
Enterocolitis
◊ Fecal leukocytes positive
◊ Stool culture positive for Salmonella species
◊ WBC normal or decreased
◊ Blood cultures negative
Bacteremia
◊ Blood cultures positive
◊ Stool cultures negative
Local infections
◊ Polymorphonuclear leukocytosis
◊ Tissue site culture positive
Asymptomatic carrier state
◊ Stool culture positive for more than 1 year
◊ Urine culture may be positive with certain serotypes
Drugs that may alter lab results:
Antibiotics used early may lead to false-negative cultures and blunted immunologic response
Disorders that may alter lab results: N/A

PATHOLOGICAL FINDINGS
• Mucosal ulceration, hemorrhage and necrosis
• Reticuloendothelial hyperplasia and hypertrophy
• Focal organ and soft tissues abscesses

SPECIAL TESTS Serologic tests identify particular clinical syndromes and serve as epidemiologic markers

IMAGING Angiography in patients over 50 with bacteremia. To rule out presence of infected aneurysm, particularly of aorto-iliac vessels.

DIAGNOSTIC PROCEDURES N/A

TREATMENT

APPROPRIATE HEALTH CARE
• Outpatient for uncomplicated enterocolitis and carrier state
• Inpatient for bacteremia and extra-intestinal infection

GENERAL MEASURES
• Correct fluid and electrolyte deficits
• Control symptoms (pain, nausea, vomiting)
• Surgical drainage and vascular bypass procedures for infected tissue sites

ACTIVITY As tolerated

DIET Oral rehydration solution during diarrhea phase; advance to normal diet as tolerated

PATIENT EDUCATION Food Safety and Inspection Service, Office of Public Awareness, Dept. of Agriculture, Rm. 1165-S, Washington, DC 20205, (202)447-9351

MEDICATIONS

DRUG(S) OF CHOICE
<u>Enterocolitis uncomplicated:</u>
◊ None recommended
<u>Enterocolitis complicated:</u> (by age extremes, immunosuppression, underlying cardiovascular abnormalities, prosthetic orthopedic devices, hemolytic anemia)
◊ Ampicillin po for 10-14 days - pediatric dose 50-100mg/kg/day in 4 divided doses; adult dose 500mg qid, or
◊ Trimethoprim-sulfamethoxazole (Bactrim, Septra suspension) po for 14 days - pediatric dose 10mg/kg/day trimethoprim, 50mg/kg/day sulfamethoxazole in 2 divided doses (maximum 320 mg/day trimethoprim; 1600 mg/day sulfamethoxazole); adult dose 1 double strength tablet q12h
<u>Bacteremia:</u>
◊ Ampicillin IV for 10-14 days - pediatric dose 200-300 mg/kg/day in 4 divided doses; adult dose 1-2 gm q4h; or
◊ Cefotaxime (Claforan) IV for 14 days - pediatric dose 200 mg/kg/day q8h; adult dose 1-2 gm q8hr, maximum 12 gm/day
<u>Localized infection:</u>
◊ Same as for bacteremia with additional option of chloramphenicol 25-75 mg/kg/day (maximum 4 gm/day) IV in 4 divided doses for 14 days
◊ In sustained bacteremia or prolonged local infection, antibiotics can be given po for 4-6 weeks (substitute trimethoprim-sulfamethoxazole for cefotaxime, using 2-4 double strength (DS) tablets given 3 times a day)
<u>Chronic carrier state:</u>
◊ Ampicillin 2-4 gm/day plus probenecid 1-2 gm/day, both divided into 4 oral doses, for 6 weeks; or
◊ 40-160 mg/day trimethoprim and 200-800 mg/day sulfamethoxazole divided into 2 doses for 6 weeks
Contraindications: None
Precautions:
• Use bowel motility inhibitors (Lomotil, Imodium) with caution, if at all
• Monitor blood levels of chloramphenicol in neonates and infants
Significant possible interactions:
Ampicillin failure rate is 75% in chronic carriers with gallbladder disease

ALTERNATIVE DRUGS
Fluoroquinolones (Cipro, Floxin) gaining favor in management of gastroenteritis, osteomyelitis and carrier state. Use is restricted to adults only.

FOLLOWUP

PATIENT MONITORING
Repeat stool culture at 5 months (40% of children negative, 90% of adults negative) and at 1 year (> 99% of all patients negative)

PREVENTION/AVOIDANCE
• Proper hygiene in production, transport and storage of food
• Control of animal reservoir
• Hand washing emphasized
• No vaccine available to oppose salmonellosis

POSSIBLE COMPLICATIONS
• Toxic megacolon
• Hypovolemic shock
• Metastatic abscess formation
• Acute or chronic hydrocephalus

EXPECTED COURSE AND PROGNOSIS
• Prognosis for enterocolitis is excellent. Exceptions - in the very young (7.0% fatal), the very old (8.7% fatal) and the debilitated and/or institutionalized (2.3% fatal)
• Prognosis for meningitis or endocarditis is poor, unless effective treatment given early

MISCELLANEOUS

ASSOCIATED CONDITIONS N/A

AGE-RELATED FACTORS
Pediatric: Children, especially neonates, more likely to become chronic carriers
Geriatric: Patients over 60 also have high carrier rate presumably due to biliary sequestration of organisms
Others: Contaminated marijuana is important source of infection, particularly in young adults

PREGNANCY Consult obstetrician regarding antibiotics

SYNONYMS N/A

ICD-9-CM 003

SEE ALSO
• Typhoid fever
• Gasteroenteritis, viral

OTHER NOTES
If one member of a household becomes infected with salmonellosis, the chance of at least one other member becoming infected is 60%

ABBREVIATIONS N/A

REFERENCES
• Rubin, RH: Infections due to gram-negative bacilli. Scientific American Medicine, 1992
• Sleisenger, M.H. & Fordtran, J.S. (eds.): Gastrointestinal Disease: Pathophysiology, Diagnosis, Management. 5th Ed. Philadelphia, W.B. Saunders Co., 1993
• Mandell, G.L. (ed.): Principles and Practice of Infectious Diseases. 3rd Ed. New York, Churchill Livingstone, 1990

Author R. Viken, M.D.

Sarcoidosis

 BASICS

DESCRIPTION Non-infectious multisystem disease of unknown cause, commonly affecting young and middle-age adults. Frequently presents with bilateral hilar adenopathy, pulmonary infiltrates, ocular and skin lesions. Other organs may be involved, including liver, spleen, lymph nodes, heart, and central nervous system.
System(s) affected:
Hemic/Lymphatic/Immunologic, Pulmonary, Cardiovascular, Gastrointestinal
Genetics: Although world-wide in distribution, increased prevalence found in Scandinavians, Japanese, Irish females, and African American women
Incidence/Prevalence in USA: 30-80 per 100,000
Predominant age: 20-60 years
Predominant sex: Female > Male

SIGNS AND SYMPTOMS
- Patients may be asymptomatic
- Cough
- Shortness of breath)
- Skin (new lesions)
- Pain or irritation of eyes
- General fatigue, malaise
- Fever
- Night sweats

CAUSES Unknown

RISK FACTORS None known

 DIAGNOSIS

DIFFERENTIAL DIAGNOSIS
- Infectious granulomatous disease such as tuberculosis and fungal infections
- Foreign body reactions
- Lymphoma
- Other malignancies associated with lymphadenopathy
- Berylliosis

LABORATORY
- Lymphopenia, anemia, or leukopenia can be seen in over half of the patients
- Abnormal liver function, especially increased alkaline phosphatase is frequently encountered
- Hypercalciuria occurs in up to 10% of patients, with hypercalcemia less frequent
Drugs that may alter lab results:
Prednisone will lower serum-angiotensin converting enzyme and normalize Gallium scan
Disorders that may alter lab results: None known

PATHOLOGICAL FINDINGS
Noncaseating epithelioid granulomas without evidence of fungal or mycobacterial infection

SPECIAL TESTS
- Serum angiotensin converting enzyme (ACE) is elevated in over 60% of patients
- Gallium scan uptake in chest, lymph nodes, and parotids may be seen in active disease
- Characteristically in active disease, bronchoalveolar lavage (BAL) fluid has an increased percentage of lymphocytes, specifically CD4 positive (T-helper/inducer lymphocytes)
- Ophthalmologic exam

IMAGING
- Routine chest roentgenograms are staged using Scadding's classification: Stage 0=normal; Stage 1=hilar adenopathy alone; Stage 2=hilar adenopathy plus parenchymal infiltrates; Stage 3= parenchymal infiltrates alone; Stage 4=pulmonary fibrosis
- Gallium scan will be positive in areas of acute disease
- Computerized tomography may enhance appreciation of lymph nodes and high resolution CT scan shows peribronchial disease

DIAGNOSTIC PROCEDURES
- Bronchoscopy with transbronchial biopsy and bronchoalveolar lavage is often performed to diagnose lung disease
- Mediastinoscopy, skin or lymph node biopsy (if needed to establish diagnosis)
- When available, Kveim-Silzbach skin test can be performed. This test is fairly sensitive (approximately 80%) and highly specific (> 95%). Unfortunately, the antigen is not generally available.

 TREATMENT

APPROPRIATE HEALTH CARE
Outpatient

GENERAL MEASURES
- The disease may require no specific therapy in the asymptomatic individual or may treat for specific indications, such as cardiac, central nervous system, ocular, or hypercalcemia
- Treatment of pulmonary and skin manifestations usually done on the basis of impairment

ACTIVITY Generally no limitations

DIET
- Avoid high calcium diets
- In patients on corticosteroids, avoid high salt foods

PATIENT EDUCATION Generally stress the benign nature of the disease and the fact that it is not contagious to others and is not malignant

Sarcoidosis

MEDICATIONS

DRUG(S) OF CHOICE
• Systemic corticosteroids in the symptomatic individual, usually prednisone initially 40 mg every day or every other day. Treatment with tapering doses of prednisone for at least one year.
• In patients with skin or ocular disease, topical steroids may be effective
Contraindications: Patients with known problems with corticosteroids
Precautions: Careful monitoring in patients with diabetes mellitus and/or hypertension
Significant possible interactions: Refer to manufacturer's profile of each drug

ALTERNATIVE DRUGS
Methotrexate (10 mg per week), hydroxychloroquine (Plaquenil) (100-200 mg per day), and chlorambucil (0.1-0.2 mg/kg). May increase risk of carcinogenicity.

FOLLOWUP

PATIENT MONITORING
• Patients on prednisone for symptoms should be seen every month or two while on therapy
• Patients not requiring therapy should be seen regularly (every three months) for at least the first two years after diagnosis
• Chest roentgenograms and pulmonary function tests are useful for monitoring for pulmonary changes
• Serum angiotensin converting enzyme level is used by some to follow disease activity. In patients with an initially elevated ACE level, it should fall towards normal while on therapy or when the disease resolves.

PREVENTION/AVOIDANCE   None known

POSSIBLE COMPLICATIONS
• Patients may develop significant respiratory involvement including cor pulmonale
• Other organs, especially the heart (congestive heart failure, arrhythmias), eyes (rarely blindness) and central nervous system can be involved with serous consequences. Fortunately, cardiac, ocular, and CNS involvement usually manifests itself early on in patients with these manifestations of the disease.

EXPECTED COURSE AND PROGNOSIS
• 80% of patients will have spontaneous resolution within two years
• 10% will have significant fibrosis but no further worsening of disease after two years
• 10% (higher in some populations, including African Americans) will have chronic disease

MISCELLANEOUS

ASSOCIATED CONDITIONS   None known

AGE-RELATED FACTORS
Pediatric: Rare
Geriatric: Less than 5% of patients with active disease are 60 years or older
Others: Sarcoidosis is a disease of youth to middle age

PREGNANCY   No increased incidence

SYNONYMS
• Löfgren's syndrome (erythema nodosum, hilar adenopathy plus uveitis)
• Besnier-Boeck disease
• Boeck's sarcoid
• Schaumann's disease

ICD-9-CM   135

SEE ALSO   None

OTHER NOTES   N/A

ABBREVIATIONS   N/A

REFERENCES
• Thomas, P.D. & Hunninghake, G.W.: Current concepts of the pathogenesis of sarcoidosis. Am Rev Respir Dis. 1987; 135:747-760
• Sharma, O.P.: Sarcoidosis. Dis Month. 1990; 36:469-535.3
• Lower, E.E. & Baughman, R.P.: The use of low dose methotrexate for refractory sarcoidosis. Am J Med Sci. 1990; 299:153-157

Author   R. Baughman, M.D. & E. Lower, M.D.

Scabies

BASICS

DESCRIPTION A contagious disease caused by infestation of the skin by the mite Sarcoptes scabiei, var. hominis
System(s) affected: Skin/Exocrine
Genetics: N/A
Incidence in USA: Common, although number of cases per year is declining as the epidemic, which began in 1971, passed its peak (1986). Worldwide incidence is 300 million cases per year.
Prevalence in USA: N/A
Predominant age: Children and young adults
Predominant sex: Male = Female

SIGNS AND SYMPTOMS
• Generalized itching
• Nocturnal pruritus
• Burrows in finger webs, wrists, hands, feet, penis, scrotum, buttocks, waistline
• Vesicles and papules (discrete)
• Secondary erosions
• Pustules (if secondarily infected)
• Scaling
• Erythema
• Nodules in covered areas (buttocks, groin, axillae)
• Atypical infestations in immunosuppressed patients

CAUSES Skin infestation by the mite Sarcoptes scabiei, var. hominis

RISK FACTORS Personal skin-to-skin contact, e.g., sexual promiscuity, crowding, poverty, nosocomial infection

DIAGNOSIS

DIFFERENTIAL DIAGNOSIS
• Atopic dermatitis
• Dermatitis herpetiformis
• Eczema
• Insect bites
• Pityriasis rosea
• Prurigo
• Seborrheic dermatitis
• Syphilis

LABORATORY N/A
Drugs that may alter lab results: N/A
Disorders that may alter lab results: N/A

PATHOLOGICAL FINDINGS Skin biopsy of a nodule (although rarely performed) will reveal portions of the mite in the corneal layer

SPECIAL TESTS N/A

IMAGING N/A

DIAGNOSTIC PROCEDURES
• Examination of skin with magnifying lens - look for typical burrows in finger webs, on flexor aspects of the wrists, and penis. Look for a dark point at the end of the burrow (the mite). The mite can be extracted with a 25 gauge needle and examined microscopically.
• Mineral oil mounts - place a drop of mineral oil over a suspected lesion. Non-excoriated papules or vesicles may also be sampled. Scrape the lesion with a #15 surgical blade. Examine under a microscope for mites, eggs, egg casings or feces. Scraping from under fingernails may often be positive.
• Potassium hydroxide wet mount - transfer skin scrapings directly to a glass slide, add a drop of KOH (potassium hydroxide), and apply a cover slip. Examine the slide for diagnostic material. If none is evident, heat slide gently to separate squamous cells and reexamine.
• Burrow ink test - if burrows are not obvious, apply blue black ink to an area of rash. Wash off the ink with alcohol. A burrow should remain stained and become more evident. Then apply mineral oil, scrape and observe microscopically as previously noted.

TREATMENT

APPROPRIATE HEALTH CARE
Outpatient

GENERAL MEASURES
• Treat all intimate contacts and close household and family members
• Wash all clothing, bed linen, and towels in a normal wash cycle

ACTIVITY Full activity

DIET No special diet

PATIENT EDUCATION
• Patient instruction sheet "Scabies" in Epstein: Common Skin Disorders (see References)
• Pamphlet titled "Questions and Answers About Scabies", available through Reed & Carnick, Piscataway, NJ 08854

MEDICATIONS

DRUG(S) OF CHOICE
• Permethrin (Elimite cream) - considered by many to be the drug of choice for scabies. Cream is applied into the skin from the head to the soles of the feet and left on for 8 to 14 hours, then thoroughly washed off. Thirty grams is usually adequate for an adult.
• Lindane (Kwell, Scabene) - available in lotion, cream and shampoo. The cream or lotion should be applied to all skin surfaces from the neck down and washed off 8 to 12 hours later. Some dermatologists routinely retreat in 7 days.
• Crotamiton (Eurax) - cream is applied into the skin from the head to the soles of the feet and left on for 8 to 14 hours, then thoroughly washed off. It is felt to be less toxic than lindane, but perhaps slightly less effective, therefore, application 2 nights in a row is advised.
• 5% sulfur ointment applied to the entire body from the neck down. It is malodorous and messy, but is thought to be safer than lindane.

Contraindications: Lindane should be avoided in children who are premature, malnourished or emaciated and those with severe underlying skin disease or a history of seizure disorders.

Precautions:
• Patients should be cautioned not to overuse the medication when applying it to the skin
• Patients should use a second application only when specifically advised to do so by their physician.

Significant possible interactions: N/A

ALTERNATIVE DRUGS   N/A

FOLLOWUP

PATIENT MONITORING   Recheck patient at weekly intervals only if rash or itching persists

PREVENTION/AVOIDANCE   N/A

POSSIBLE COMPLICATIONS
• Eczema
• Pyoderma
• Postscorbutic pruritus
• Nodular scabies

EXPECTED COURSE AND PROGNOSIS
• Lesions begin to regress in 1 to 2 days along with the worst itching
• Some itching and dermatitis commonly persists for 10 to 14 days and can be treated with antihistamines and/or topical or oral corticosteroids

MISCELLANEOUS

ASSOCIATED CONDITIONS   N/A

AGE-RELATED FACTORS
Pediatric: Infants often have more widespread involvement. They are occasionally infested on the face and scalp (rare for adults). Vesicular lesions on the palms and soles are also more commonly seen.
Geriatric: The elderly often itch more severely, despite fewer cutaneous lesions. Elderly at risk for extensive infestations, perhaps related to a decline in cell-mediated immunity.
Others: N/A

PREGNANCY   Lindane should be used cautiously and no more than twice during pregnancy due to its potential to cause neurotoxicity and convulsions

SYNONYMS   N/A

ICD-9-CM   133.0 scabies

SEE ALSO   N/A

OTHER NOTES   N/A

ABBREVIATIONS   N/A

REFERENCES
• Epstein, E.: Common Skin Disorders. 3rd Ed., Montvale, NJ, Med. Econ. Books, 1988
• Habif, T.: Clinical Dermatology. 2nd Ed. St. Louis, C.V. Mosby, 1990
• Reeves, J. and Maibach, H.: Clinical Dermatology Illustrated. 2nd Ed. Philadelphia, F.A. Davis, 1991

Author   G. Silko, M.D.

Scarlet fever

BASICS

DESCRIPTION "Streptococcal sore throat with a rash". A childhood disease characterized by high fever, vomiting, and rash caused by Group A beta-hemolytic streptococci (GAS) pyogenes that elaborate erythrogenic toxin. Incubation period 1-7 days, duration of illness 4-10 days.
System(s) affected: Gastrointestinal, Skin/Exocrine
Genetics: N/A
Incidence/Prevalence in USA: Up to 10% of GAS pharyngitis
Predominant age: 6-12 years
Predominant sex: Male = Female

SIGNS AND SYMPTOMS
Prodrome 1-2 days
◊ Sore throat
◊ Headache
◊ Vomiting
◊ Abdominal pain (may mimic acute abdomen)
◊ Fever (up to 40° C or 103.6° F)
Oral exam
◊ "Beefy red" tonsils and pharynx with or without exudate
◊ Petechiae on palate
◊ White coating on tongue "White strawberry tongue" appears on days 1-2. This sheds by day 4-5 leaving a "Red strawberry tongue" - shiny, red with prominent papillae.
Exanthem (appears within 12-24 hours)
◊ Orange-red punctate skin eruption with sandpaper-like texture - "sunburn with goose pimples"
◊ Rash begins on chest and axillae and spreads to abdomen and extremities; prominent in skin folds (axillae, groin, buttocks)
◊ Flushed face with circumoral pallor
◊ Transverse red streaks in skin folds of abdomen, antecubital space, and axillae: "Pastia's lines"
◊ Desquamation begins on face after 7-10 days and proceeds over trunk to hands and feet; may persist for 6 weeks

CAUSES
• Hypersensitivity to erythrogenic toxins produced by GAS
• Site of GAS infection: Usually tonsils, may be surgical wound infection
• Erythrogenic toxin produced by Staphylococcus aureus can produce staphylococcal "scarlet fever" - may actually be a mild form of toxic shock syndrome or scalded skin syndrome

RISK FACTORS
Age - most commonly affects school age children - by age 10, 80% have antibodies to erythrogenic toxin

DIAGNOSIS

DIFFERENTIAL DIAGNOSIS
• Measles
• Rubella
• Infectious mononucleosis
• Roseola
• Severe sunburn
• Secondary syphilis
• Corynebacterium hemolyticus pharyngitis
• Toxic shock syndrome
• Staphylococcal scalded skin syndrome
• Kawasaki disease
• Drug hypersensitivity

LABORATORY
• Throat culture definitive diagnosis
• Rapid strep antigen tests - diagnostic if positive
• Serologic tests (includes anti-streptolysin O titer and streptozyme tests) - confirm recent GAS infection; not helpful for diagnosis of acute disease
Drugs that may alter lab results:
• Prior antibiotic therapy may result in negative throat culture
• Penicillin within 5 days of symptoms can delay/abolish anti-streptolysin O response
Disorders that may alter lab results: N/A

PATHOLOGICAL FINDINGS   N/A

SPECIAL TESTS   N/A

IMAGING   N/A

DIAGNOSTIC PROCEDURES   N/A

TREATMENT

APPROPRIATE HEALTH CARE
Outpatient except for severe suppurative complications

GENERAL MEASURES
• Warm soaks to relieve pain in swollen glands
• Rest
• Drink plenty of fluids

ACTIVITY   Fully active

DIET   No special diet

PATIENT EDUCATION   Must take antibiotics for full 10 days

MEDICATIONS

DRUG(S) OF CHOICE
• Penicillin V - 125 mg po 3-4 times/day for under 60 lb/27 kg; 250 mg po 3-4 times/day for over 60 lb/27 kg; (maximum 3.0 gm/day). If compliance questionable, use benzathine penicillin - single IM dose 900,000-1,200,000 units for under 60 lb/27 kg; 1,200,000 million units for over 60 lb/27 kg. (Note: some authorities claim satisfactory results, with better compliance, using a regimen of bid penicillin dosage with same total daily dose.)
• Acetaminophen for fever and comfort
Contraindications: Penicillin allergy
Precautions: Refer to manufacturer's profile of each drug
Significant possible interactions: Refer to manufacturer's profile of each drug

ALTERNATIVE DRUGS
• Erythromycin 40 mg/kg po divided q6h, do not exceed 1 gm/day
• Oral cephalosporins (e.g., Cephalexin 40 mg/kg po divided qid, up to 1 gm/day)
• Clindamycin 20 mg/kg/day po divided tid for 10 days. Effective therapy for penicillin treatment failures.
• Tetracyclines and sulfonamides should not be used
• Sulfamethoxazole-trimethoprim is not effective against group A beta-hemolytic streptococci

FOLLOWUP

PATIENT MONITORING   Repeat throat cultures if symptoms persist after therapy

PREVENTION/AVOIDANCE
• GAS spread by contact with respiratory secretions. Avoid if possible.
• Children should not return to school or day care until after 24 hours of antibiotic therapy
• Prophylactic penicillin not recommended after exposure to scarlet fever

POSSIBLE COMPLICATIONS
Suppurative
   ◊ Sinusitis
   ◊ Otitis media/mastoiditis
   ◊ Cervical adenitis
   ◊ Peritonsillar abscess/retropharyngeal abscess
   ◊ Pneumonia
   ◊ Septicemia/meningitis/osteomyelitis
Non-suppurative
   ◊ Rheumatic fever (penicillin prevents RF when started as long as 10 days after onset of acute GAS infection)
   ◊ Glomerulonephritis (prevention even after adequate treatment of GAS is less certain)
   ◊ "Streptococcal toxic shock syndrome": Fever, hypotension, disseminated intravascular coagulation (DIC); cardiac, liver, kidney dysfunction.

EXPECTED COURSE AND PROGNOSIS
• With penicillin, defervescence in 24 hours
• Can have recurrent attacks

MISCELLANEOUS

ASSOCIATED CONDITIONS
• Pharyngitis
• Impetigo
• Puerperal sepsis

AGE-RELATED FACTORS
Pediatric: Rare in infancy
Geriatric: N/A
Others: N/A

PREGNANCY   N/A

SYNONYMS   Scarlatina

ICD-9-CM   034.1

SEE ALSO   N/A

OTHER NOTES   Asymptomatic carriers can spread disease

ABBREVIATIONS   N/A

REFERENCES
• Committee on Infectious Diseases of Amer Acad Ped. (Red Book). 436-7,1991
• Krugman, T. & Ward, R.: Infectious Diseases of Children . 7th Ed. 1981. St. Louis, C.V. Mosby Co, 1981

Author   M. Kelliher, M.D. & C. Marchant, M.D.

Schizophrenia

 BASICS

DESCRIPTION Major psychiatric psychotic (out of touch with reality) disorder with prodromal, active and residual symptoms involving delusions, hallucinations, disturbed affect (emotion) and impaired thought processes, lasting at least six months
System(s) affected: Nervous
Genetics: Genetic predisposition necessary for development
Incidence/Prevalence in USA: Lifetime (1%). Highest prevalence in lower socioeconomic classes.
Predominant age: Onset before age 45
Predominant sex: Male = Female

SIGNS AND SYMPTOMS
• Withdrawal from reality
• Delusions (fixed false unreal beliefs - paranoid (people persecuting or after you)
• Reference (people or things have unusual significance)
• Others can hear your thoughts, put thoughts into you or control you; grandiose or religious delusions
• Hallucinations - usually auditory
• Affect - flat or inappropriate emotion
• Thought processes - loose associations (thoughts don't follow)
• Much speech but convey little information
• Extremes of gross overactivity to stupor with mutism

CAUSES Unknown - not initiated or maintained by an organic factor. Probably a complex interaction between inherited and environmental factors.

RISK FACTORS Biologic relative with schizophrenia

 DIAGNOSIS

DIFFERENTIAL DIAGNOSIS
• Organic mental disorder - characterized by JOMAC (a mnemonic that stands for impaired Judgment, Orientation, Memory, Affect and Concentration). Disorientation, in particular indicates organicity. Organic mental disorders may be due to trauma, infection, tumor, metabolic, endocrine, intoxication (psychoactive substance use), epilepsy, neurological disorders, etc.
• Organic delusional syndrome - secondary to substance use/abuse (e.g., amphetamines, LSD, or phencyclidine) may have identical symptoms
• Mood disorders - especially bipolar disorder (manic depressive disorder); schizoaffective disorder

LABORATORY
• No test available to indicate schizophrenia
• Laboratory tests needed to rule out organicity - may include CBC, blood chemistries, thyroid screen, urinalysis, vitamins (B12, folate, thiamin), blood and urine for drugs and alcohol
• Others for: heavy metals - ceruloplasmin, urine porphobilinogen
Drugs that may alter lab results: N/A
Disorders that may alter lab results: N/A

PATHOLOGICAL FINDINGS N/A

SPECIAL TESTS
• Psychological - Bender Gestalt, intelligence testing (WISC-R) thematic apperception test (TAT), and Rorschach
• EEG - to rule out seizure disorder, brain damage, etc.
• Glucose tolerance

IMAGING CT and MRI to rule out organicity

DIAGNOSTIC PROCEDURES Lumbar puncture

 TREATMENT

APPROPRIATE HEALTH CARE
• Usually hospitalize initially for organic workup and for treatment of psychotic symptoms
• Outpatient if not dangerous to self or others, able to cooperate with treatment, and supportive family

GENERAL MEASURES Ensure safety of patient and others - may act on delusional thinking

ACTIVITY Establish safe hospital environment

DIET No special diet

PATIENT EDUCATION Education and support groups for patient and family available from National Alliance for the Mentally Ill (NAMI)

MEDICATIONS

DRUG(S) OF CHOICE
• Benzodiazepines and/or neuroleptics
• While evaluating for organicity, may treat agitation with benzodiazepines - lorazepam (Ativan) 1, 2 or 4 mg po or IM every 2-6 hrs up to 10 mg/day
• If violent or severely disruptive - rapid neuroleptization - haloperidol 5 mg IM every 4-8 hrs up to 30 mg/day or chlorpromazine 10-25 mg IM test dose (check for hypotension in one hour) then 25 mg IM every 4 hr up to 150 mg day for low dose
• After stable - change to oral medicines and titrate dosage
• After 6 months in remission, may withdraw from neuroleptics. If relapse, reinstitute medications.
Contraindications: Refer to manufacturer's profile of each drug
Precautions:
• For acute side effects of neuroleptic - dystonic reaction (especially of head and neck) - diphenhydramine (Benadryl) 25-50 mg IM
• For pseudoparkinsonism reaction - trihexyphenidyl (Artane) 2 mg bid (may be increased to 15 mg/day if needed) or benztropine (Cogentin) 0.5 bid (range: 1-4 mg/day)
• Neuroleptic malignant syndrome-hyperthermia, severe extrapyramidal effect and autonomic dysfunction (hypertension, tachycardia, diaphoresis and incontinence)
Significant possible interactions: Refer to manufacturer's profile of each drug

ALTERNATIVE DRUGS
• Thioridazine (Mellaril) - only by mouth. Do not exceed 800 mg/day.
• Trifluoperazine (Stelazine) 4-30 mg/day for maintenance
• Thiothixene (Navane) 4-30 mg/day for maintenance
• Clozapine (Clozaril) 25 mg qd or bid. Increase slowly to dose of 300-400mg given tid. Serious toxicity of agranulocytosis mandates weekly CBC; reserve for therapy resistant patients.

FOLLOWUP

PATIENT MONITORING
Continue neuroleptic as well as psychiatric therapies (individual, group, family), vocational rehabilitation, day hospital

PREVENTION/AVOIDANCE   N/A

POSSIBLE COMPLICATIONS
• Side effects of neuroleptics especially risk of tardive dyskinesia with chronic use
• Self-inflicted trauma
• Combative behavior toward others

EXPECTED COURSE AND PROGNOSIS
• Chronic course - remission and exacerbations
• Guarded prognosis, although 30% recover completely
• The negative symptoms (consisting of decreased ambition, energy and emotional responsiveness) are often most difficult to treat

MISCELLANEOUS

ASSOCIATED CONDITIONS   N/A

AGE-RELATED FACTORS
Onset in 30's - more paranoid type
Pediatric: Unusual before puberty
Geriatric: Those who survive enter into a chronic phase
Others: N/A

PREGNANCY
Complications of being on neuroleptic medication

SYNONYMS   N/A

ICD-9-CM
295 schizophrenic disorders

SEE ALSO   N/A

OTHER NOTES
Schizophrenic patients occupy about half the beds in mental hospitals and 1/4 of all hospital beds

ABBREVIATIONS   N/A

REFERENCES
Schatzberg, A.F. and Cole, J.O.: Manual of Clinical Psychopharmacology, 2nd Ed. APA Press, Inc. Washington, D.C., 1991

Author   S. Jaffe, M.D.

Scleritis

DESCRIPTION   Scleritis is an inflammation of the scleral outer coat of the eye
System(s) affected: Nervous
Genetics: None
Incidence/Prevalence in USA: Scleritis is uncommon
Predominant age: None
Predominant sex: Male = Female

SIGNS AND SYMPTOMS
• Redness and inflammation of the sclera
• Pain ranging from mild discomfort to extreme localized tenderness

CAUSES   The most common causes of scleritis is in association with collagen vascular diseases such as rheumatoid arthritis

RISK FACTORS   Individuals with autoimmune disorders, and chronic rheumatoid arthritis are most at risk

DIFFERENTIAL DIAGNOSIS
• Conjunctivitis
• Episcleritis
• "Pink eye"
• Iritis
• Trauma

LABORATORY
• Rheumatoid factor
• ANA, and HLA serotyping may help aid in the diagnosis
• Elevated sedimentation rate
Drugs that may alter lab results: None
Disorders that may alter lab results: None

PATHOLOGICAL FINDINGS
• Nodules can form on the sclera which demonstrate fibrinoid necrosis of the sclera
• There may or may not be adjacent inflammation
• The scleritis may be diffuse, nodular, or necrotizing
• If the posterior region of the globe is involved, adjacent swelling of orbital tissues may occur

SPECIAL TESTS   N/A

IMAGING   CT scan of the orbit may help differentiate the extensiveness and location of scleritis

DIAGNOSTIC PROCEDURES   History and physical examination

APPROPRIATE HEALTH CARE
Outpatient

GENERAL MEASURES
• Treatment of the inflammation usually with systemic steroids is required
• All of the immunosuppressants and antimetabolites used for autoimmune and collagen vascular disorders may be of help in active scleritis

ACTIVITY   No restrictions

DIET   No special diet

PATIENT EDUCATION   N/A

MEDICATIONS

DRUG(S) OF CHOICE Prednisone is the mainstay of treatment including both topical, periocular, and systemic administration
Contraindications: None
Precautions: Scleritis can progress to ocular perforation which may be hastened with periocular steroid injection
Significant possible interactions: Refer to manufacturer's literature

ALTERNATIVE DRUGS Nonsteroidal anti-inflammatory medications

FOLLOWUP

PATIENT MONITORING The patient should be followed very closely in the active stage of inflammation to assess the effectiveness of therapy

PREVENTION/AVOIDANCE None

POSSIBLE COMPLICATIONS
• Increased intraocular pressure
• Cataract and glaucoma can result as a result of treatment
• Ocular perforation can occur in severe stages

EXPECTED COURSE AND PROGNOSIS
• Scleritis is indolent, chronic, and often times progressive
• Recurrent bouts of inflammation occur

MISCELLANEOUS

ASSOCIATED CONDITIONS
• Sjögren's syndrome
• Pseudo tumor

AGE-RELATED FACTORS
Pediatric: N/A
Geriatric: N/A
Others: N/A

PREGNANCY N/A

SYNONYMS N/A

ICD-9-CM 379.0

SEE ALSO N/A

OTHER NOTES N/A

ABBREVIATIONS N/A

REFERENCES Merrill, G.M.: Diseases of The Cornea. Boston, Little, Brown, 1990

Author R. Kershner, M.D., F.A.C.S.

Scleroderma

BASICS

DESCRIPTION Scleroderma (progressive systemic sclerosis [PSS]) is a chronic disease of unknown etiology, characterized by diffuse fibrosis, degenerative changes, and vascular abnormalities in the skin, articular structures and other organs (kidneys, lung, heart, gastrointestinal and skeletal muscles). The majority of manifestations have vascular features (e.g., Raynaud's phenomenon), but frank vasculitis is rarely seen. It can range from a mild disease, affecting the skin, to a systemic disease that can cause death in a few months.
Genetics: Familial clustering has been seen
System(s) affected: Skin, Kidneys, Heart, Gastrointestinal, Skeletal muscle, Vascular
Incidence in USA: Unknown
Prevalence in USA: 1/100,000
Predominant age:
 • Young adult (16-40 years); middle age (40-75 years)
 • Symptoms usually appear in the 3rd to 5th decade
Predominant sex: Female > Male (4:1)

SIGNS AND SYMPTOMS
 • CREST syndrome (calcinosis, Raynaud's phenomenon, esophageal dysmobility, sclerodactyly, telangiectasia)
 • Diarrhea
 • Digital ulcerations
 • Dry crackles at lung bases
 • Dysphagia
 • Dyspnea
 • Facial pain
 • Finger tightness, swelling, thickening
 • Flexion contractures
 • Friction rub on tendon movement
 • Hand swelling
 • Hyperpigmentation
 • Hypertension
 • Joint stiffness
 • Narrowed oral aperture
 • Nausea and vomiting
 • Peripheral neuropathy
 • Polyarthralgia
 • Proximal muscle weakness
 • Pruritus
 • Raynaud's phenomenon
 • Scaling of skin
 • Sclerodactyly
 • Subcutaneous calcinosis
 • Substernal fullness
 • Telangiectasia
 • Weakness
 • Weight loss
 • Xerostomia

CAUSES
 • Unknown
 • Possible alterations in immune response
 • Possibly some association with quartz mining, quarrying, vinyl chloride, hydrocarbons
 • Treatment with bleomycin has caused a scleroderma-like syndrome

RISK FACTORS Unknown

DIAGNOSIS

DIFFERENTIAL DIAGNOSIS
 • Sclerodermatomyositis
 • Mixed connective tissue disease
 • Toxic oil syndrome (Madrid, 1981, affecting 20,000 people)
 • Eosinophilia-myalgia syndrome

LABORATORY
 • Increased ESR
 • Normocytic anemia
 • Normochromic anemia
 • Positive ANA
 • Positive nucleolar immunofluorescence
 • Albuminuria
 • Microscopic hematuria
 • Eosinophilia
 • Hemolysis
 • Hypergammaglobulinemia
 • Decreased maximum breathing capacity
 • Increased residual volume
 • Diffusion defect
 • Positive rheumatoid factor test (33%)
Drugs that may alter lab results: N/A
Disorders that may alter lab results: N/A

PATHOLOGICAL FINDINGS
 • Skin - edema
 • Lymphocytic infiltrate around sweat glands
 • Loss of capillaries
 • Endothelial proliferation
 • Hair follicle atrophy
 • Subcutaneous tissue replaced by thick collagen bundles
 • Synovium - pannus formation, fibrin deposits in tendons
 • Inflammatory process
 • Kidney - small kidneys, intimal proliferation in interlobular arteries
 • Heart - endocardial thickening, myocardial interstitial fibrosis
 • Enlarged heart
 • Cardiac hypertrophy
 • Lung - interstitial pneumonitis, cyst formation
 • Interstitial fibrosis
 • Bronchiectasis
 • Esophagus - esophageal atrophy, fibrosis

SPECIAL TESTS
 • ECG - low voltage; possibly nonspecific abnormalities
 • Lung function tests - decreased diffusion and vital capacity
 • Skin biopsy - marked thickening of the dermis, occlusive vessel changes
 • Nail fold capillary loop abnormalities

IMAGING
 • Hand x-ray - absorption of tufts from terminal phalanges, soft tissue atrophy, subcutaneous calcinosis
 • Upper GI - esophageal dilatation, atonic esophagus
 • Barium enema - colonic diverticula, megacolon
 • Chest x-ray - diffuse reticular pattern, bilateral basilar pulmonary fibrosis
 • Gallium-67 lung scan - can be positive in early interstitial disease

DIAGNOSTIC PROCEDURES N/A

TREATMENT

APPROPRIATE HEALTH CARE
Outpatient. Inpatient possibly for some surgical procedures.

GENERAL MEASURES
 • Treatment is symptomatic and supportive
 • Esophageal dilatation
 • Avoid cold, dress appropriately for the weather
 • Avoid smoking (crucial)
 • For chronic digital ulcerations - débridement after soaking in half-strength hydrogen peroxide solution, digital plaster to immobilize
 • Physical therapy to maintain function and promote strength
 • Avoid finger sticks (e.g., blood tests)
 • Be wary of air conditioning
 • Heat therapy to relieve joint stiffness
 • Some success with gastroplasty for correction of gastroesophageal reflux
 • Elevation of the head of the bed during sleep may help relieve gastrointestinal symptoms
 • Skin - use softening lotions, ointments, bath oils to help prevent dryness and cracking
 • Dialysis may be necessary as disease progresses

ACTIVITY Stay as active as possible, but avoid fatigue

DIET
 • Soft, bland diet with frequent small meals
 • Drink plenty of fluids with meals

PATIENT EDUCATION
 • Printed patient information available from: Scleroderma Federation, 1725 York Avenue, No. 29F, New York, NY 10128, (212)427-7040
 • Advise patient to report any abnormal bruising or non-healing abrasions
 • Assist patient in smoking cessation, if needed

Scleroderma

MEDICATIONS

DRUG(S) OF CHOICE
• There are no drug therapies of proven value, except for ACE inhibitors for hypertensive renal crisis
• Corticosteroids - for disabling myositis or mixed connective tissue disease
• Antibiotics - for secondary infections in bowel
• Antacids or cimetidine - for gastric reflux
• Dipyridamole (Persantine) or aspirin - antiplatelet therapy
• Hydrophilic skin ointments - skin therapy
• Topical clindamycin or erythromycin or Silvadene cream - prevent recurrent infection (following systemic antibiotic therapy for infection)
• Consider immunosuppressives - used alone or with plasmapheresis for treatment of life-threatening or potentially crippling scleroderma
• Vasoactive agents and antihypertensives - for Raynaud's phenomenon
• D-penicillamine - reduce skin thickening and delay the rate of new visceral involvement
• Angiotensin-converting enzyme (captopril) - for kidney disease
Contraindications: Refer to manufacturer's literature
Precautions: Refer to manufacturer's literature
Significant possible interactions: Refer to manufacturer's literature

ALTERNATIVE DRUGS
Many other drugs are currently under investigation, but no evidence of real benefits as yet

FOLLOWUP

PATIENT MONITORING
Frequent to monitor medications and offer encouragement

PREVENTION/AVOIDANCE
None

POSSIBLE COMPLICATIONS
• Renal failure
• Death
• Respiratory failure
• Flexion contractures
• Disability
• Esophageal dysmotility
• Reflux esophagitis

EXPECTED COURSE AND PROGNOSIS
• Variable
• Possible improvement, but incurable
• Prognosis is poor if cardiac, pulmonary or renal manifestations present early

MISCELLANEOUS

ASSOCIATED CONDITIONS
• Rheumatoid arthritis
• Systemic lupus erythematosus
• Polymyositis

AGE-RELATED FACTORS
Pediatric: Rare in this age group
Geriatric: Not rare until after age 75
Others: N/A

PREGNANCY
N/A

SYNONYMS
• Progressive systemic sclerosis
• Morphea
• PSS

ICD-9-CM
710.1 systemic sclerosis

SEE ALSO
N/A

OTHER NOTES
N/A

ABBREVIATIONS
N/A

REFERENCES
• Kelley, W.N., Harris, E.D. & Ruddy, S., et al.: Textbook of Rheumatology. 4th Ed. Philadelphia, W.B. Saunders, 1993
• McCarty, D.J. & Koopman, W.J. (eds.): Arthritis and Allied Disorders. 12th Ed. Philadelphia, Lea & Febiger, 1993

Author J. Boyer, M.D.

Seizure disorders

BASICS

DESCRIPTION A sudden alteration of behavior, characterized by a sensory perception or motor activity without or with change in awareness or consciousness, due to aberrant cortical electrical activity
Classification of seizures
◊ I. Partial seizures (seizures begin locally) - A) without impairment of consciousness, B) with complex symptoms (with impairment of consciousness)
◊ II. Generalized seizures (bilaterally symmetrical and without local onset)
◊ III. Unclassified epileptic seizures
System(s) affected: Nervous
Genetics: Three times the prevalence of seizures in close relatives of seizure patients
Incidence/Prevalence in USA:
• 1.5 million for epilepsy
• The age adjusted prevalence is 0.625% or 6.25/1000
• Isolated seizures may occur in 10% of the general population
• 10-20% of all patients have intractable epilepsy
Predominant age: All ages
Predominant sex: Male = Female

SIGNS AND SYMPTOMS
General
◊ Fever - indicative of infectious etiology
◊ Focal neurologic finding - may indicate tumor or localized injury to the brain
◊ Papilledema - suggestive of increased intracranial pressure
◊ Hemorrhagic eye grounds - suggests underlying hypertension
◊ Meningismus - may be present with meningitis
◊ Headache - sometimes associated with infectious or hemorrhagic causes of seizures
Generalized seizures
◊ Absence - loss of consciousness or posture
◊ Myoclonic - repetitive muscle contractions
◊ Tonic-clonic - sustained contraction followed by rhythmic contractions of all four extremities
Partial seizures
◊ Simple - Focal seizures without alteration of awareness/consciousness
◊ Complex - Focal seizures with alteration of awareness/consciousness
Febrile seizures (see separate chapter on febrile seizures)
◊ Occurs between three months and five years of age
◊ Fever without evidence of any other defined cause for seizures
◊ If febrile seizures occur in the first year, the recurrence rate is 51%
◊ If febrile seizures occur in the 2nd year, the recurrence rate is 25%.
◊ 88% of all recurrences of febrile seizures occur in the first 2 years
◊ The earlier the age of onset, the more likely repetitive febrile seizures will occur

◊ Recurrent febrile seizures probably do not increase the risk of epilepsy
Status epilepticus (see separate chapter)
◊ Repetitive generalized seizures without return to consciousness between seizures
◊ Considered a neurological emergency

CAUSES
• Brain tumor
• Cerebral hypoxia (breath holding, carbon monoxide poisoning, anesthesia)
• Cerebrovascular accident (infarct or hemorrhage)
• Convulsive or toxic agents (lead, alcohol, picrotoxin, strychnine)
• Eclampsia
• Exogenous factors (sound, light, cutaneous stimulation)
• Fever (see chapter on febrile seizures)
• Head injury
• Heat stroke
• Infection
• Metabolic disturbances
• Withdrawal from, or hereditary intolerance of, alcohol

RISK FACTORS
• Susceptibility to seizures determined by a complex interplay between genetic factors and acquired brain disorders
• Children delivered breech have a prevalence rate of 3.8% compared with 2.2% in children delivered vertex

DIAGNOSIS

DIFFERENTIAL DIAGNOSIS
Infancy (0-2)
◊ Perinatal hypoxia
◊ Birth injury
◊ Metabolic - hypoglycemia, hypocalcemia, hypomagnesemia, vitamin B6 deficiency, phenylketonuria
◊ Acute infection
Childhood (2-10)
◊ Febrile seizure
◊ Idiopathic
◊ Acute infection
◊ Trauma
Adolescent (10-18)
◊ Idiopathic
◊ Trauma
◊ Drug and alcohol withdrawal
◊ Arteriovenous malformations
Early adulthood (18-25)
◊ Idiopathic
◊ Drug and alcohol withdrawal
◊ Trauma
Middle age (25-60)
◊ Drug and alcohol withdrawal
◊ Trauma
◊ Tumor
◊ Vascular disease
Late adulthood (over 60)
◊ Vascular disease
◊ Tumor
◊ Degenerative disease
◊ Metabolic - hypoglycemia, uremia, hepatic failure, electrolyte abnormality

LABORATORY
• Serum tests - glucose, sodium, potassium, calcium, phosphorus, magnesium, BUN, ammonia
• Anticonvulsant levels - inadequate level of anticonvulsant medication is the most common cause of recurrent seizures in children, and many adults
• Drug and toxic screens - include alcohol
• Complete blood count - helpful in evaluating infection
Drugs that may alter lab results:
• Anticonvulsant therapy may dramatically affect the EEG results
• Levels of anticonvulsants may be altered by a variety of common medications such as erythromycin, sulfonamides, warfarin, and cimetidine, as well as alcohol
Disorders that may alter lab results:
Pregnancy decreases serum concentration. Frequent monitoring and dosage adjustments are necessary.

PATHOLOGICAL FINDINGS None

SPECIAL TESTS
• Electroencephalogram (EEG). A negative EEG does not rule out a seizure disorder. Sensitivity, specificity and predictive value of the test depends on the underlying cause and anatomic location of the seizure focus.
• 24-hour ambulatory EEG - allows for continuous monitoring of cortical activity during regular activities
• Video-monitoring - useful in conjunction with simultaneous EEG monitoring in separating true events from pseudoseizures

IMAGING
• MRI of brain - superior in evaluation of the temporal lobes
• CT scan of brain - indicated routinely in work-up of tonic-clonic seizures

DIAGNOSTIC PROCEDURES None

TREATMENT

APPROPRIATE HEALTH CARE
Outpatient therapy except for status epilepticus

GENERAL MEASURES Protect the patient's airway

ACTIVITY As tolerated

DIET Regular

PATIENT EDUCATION
• Stress the importance of compliance with anticonvulsant therapy
• Printed patient information available from: Epilepsy Foundation of America, 4351 Garden City Drive, Landover, MD 20785, (800)EFA-1000

MEDICATIONS

DRUG(S) OF CHOICE
• To avoid a particular side effect, one drug may be preferred within one of the seizure groups listed below
<u>Generalized seizures - absence</u>
◊ Phenytoin (Dilantin) - therapeutic range: 10-20 mcg/mL
◊ Phenobarbital - therapeutic range: 10-30 mcg/mL
◊ Carbamazepine (Tegretol) - therapeutic range:4-12 mcg/mL
<u>Generalized seizures - absence</u>
◊ Ethosuximide (Zarontin) - therapeutic range: 40-100 mcg/mL
◊ Valproate (Depakene) - therapeutic range: 50-100 mcg/mL
◊ Clonazepam (Klonopin) - therapeutic range: 20-80 nanograms/mL
<u>Partial seizures</u>
◊ Phenytoin (Dilantin)
◊ Carbamazepine (Tegretol)
◊ Phenobarbital
Contraindications: Refer to manufacturer's profile of each drug
Precautions: Doses should be individualized according to the patient's age and weight. Refer to manufacturer's profile of each drug.
Significant possible interactions: Refer to manufacturer's profile of each drug

ALTERNATIVE DRUGS
• felbamate
• Several additional drugs awaiting FDA approval

FOLLOWUP

PATIENT MONITORING
• Regular monitoring of anticonvulsant levels
• CBC once a month
• Monitor medication side effects and adverse reactions

PREVENTION/AVOIDANCE   Maintain adequate epileptic drug therapy

POSSIBLE COMPLICATIONS   Drug toxicity

EXPECTED COURSE AND PROGNOSIS
• Depends on the pathophysiology of seizure within particular patient
• Seizure activity may become quiescent. If a patient has been seizure-free for two years, withdrawal of therapy may be considered. Relapse rate after three years of being off medications is 33%.

MISCELLANEOUS

ASSOCIATED CONDITIONS
• Infections
• Tumors
• Drug abuse
• Metabolic disorders

AGE-RELATED FACTORS
Pediatric: Breastfeeding is not contraindicated in mothers receiving epileptic medication, although drug concentration in the infant may require monitoring if problems such as sedation occur
Geriatric: N/A
Others: N/A

PREGNANCY   There is a two-fold increased risk of congenital malformation in mothers taking anticonvulsant medication

SYNONYMS
• Convulsions
• Epilepsy
• Fits
• Spells

ICD-9-CM   780.3

SEE ALSO   N/A

OTHER NOTES   N/A

ABBREVIATIONS   N/A

REFERENCES
• Beignat, J.L.: Getting a handle on an adult's first seizure. Emergency Med. 20:20-28, 1989
• Schewer, M.L. & Pedley, T.A.: The evaluation and treatment of seizures. New Engl J Med. 323(21):1468-1474, 1990
• Applegate, M.S. & Lo, W.: Febrile seizures: current concepts concerning prognosis and clinical management. Journal of Fam Prac. 299(4):422-428, 1989
• Freeman, J. & Vinny, E.: Decision making and the child with afebrile seizure. Pediatrics in Review.13(8):305-310, 1992

Author   W. Toffler, M.D & S. Fields, M.D.

Seizures, febrile

BASICS

DESCRIPTION Seizure occurring with fever in infancy or childhood without evidence of other underlying cause. Seizures secondary to other CNS events like meningitis, tumor, or afebrile convulsive history excluded from this topic.
• Simple febrile seizure - single episode in 24 hours, lasting less than 15 minutes and generalized tonic/clonic activity. Accounts for 85% of febrile seizures.
• Complex febrile seizure - multiple episodes in 24 hours with focalizing findings and lasting more than 15 minutes. Accounts for 15% of febrile seizures.
System(s) affected: Nervous
Genetics: Uncertain but may be autosomal dominant with variable expression and incomplete penetrance
Incidence in USA: Unknown
Prevalence in USA: Approximately 2500/100,000. 2-5% of all children, comprising 30% of all childhood seizures.
Predominant age: 95% occur by 5 years; peak at 2 years
Predominant sex: Male > Female (slightly)

SIGNS AND SYMPTOMS
• Fever usually 39° C (102.2° F) or over
Tonic/clonic convulsive activity
  ◊ Generalized with simple seizure or focal with complex event
  ◊ Usually occurs within hours of fever onset
  ◊ The seizure is the initial sign of illness in 25% of patients
  ◊ Duration is less than 15 minutes with simple seizures; longer with complex episodes
  ◊ Average frequency is once in 24 hours with simple; more with complex

CAUSES
• Fever may lower seizure threshold in susceptible children
• Temperature usually greater than 39° C (102.2° F), but rate of change may be more important than temperature
• Viral illnesses: URI's, roseola infantum, influenza A, gastroenteritis
• Bacterial infections: Shigella, salmonella, otitis media
• Mumps, measles, rubella immunization (MMR) within prior 7-10 days or diphtheria, pertussis, tetanus immunization (DPT) within prior 48 hours

RISK FACTORS Febrile seizure in sibling raises risk 2-3 times

DIAGNOSIS

DIFFERENTIAL DIAGNOSIS
• Febrile delirium
• Febrile shivering with pallor and peri-oral cyanosis
• Breath holding spell during fever event
• Afebrile seizure occurring during fever event
• Acute meningitis presenting with seizure
• Head injury and fever
• Drug induced seizures
• Sudden discontinuance of anticonvulsants

LABORATORY
• First episode: CBC, calcium, glucose, magnesium, electrolytes, urinalysis, blood culture, BUN, creatinine
• A toxologic screen may be indicated in unclear cases
• First episode or under 1 year old, a lumbar puncture for meningitis
Drugs that may alter lab results: N/A
Disorders that may alter lab results: Infections

PATHOLOGICAL FINDINGS N/A

SPECIAL TESTS EEG may be indicated: If recurrent frequent febrile seizures, those with focal findings, complex type, underlying neurological disorder, family history of afebrile seizures, delayed awakening after event, or if this is first event after age 3. Perform EEG 2-4 weeks after event. EEG not indicated for simple febrile seizure when there is a ready explanation for fever and recovery is quick.

IMAGING CT scan of brain for complex types, focal findings, underlying neurological disorder, or prolonged recovery phase

DIAGNOSTIC PROCEDURES Lumbar puncture

TREATMENT

APPROPRIATE HEALTH CARE
Emergency room or extended observation based on clinical situation, seizure type and whether first or subsequent event

GENERAL MEASURES
• Supportive care
• If seizure ended and simple type with recovery progressing, determine fever source so underlying cause can be treated
• Tepid sponge bath to lower temperature
• If seizure less than 10 minutes, supportive measures with laying on side, protecting from injury, maintaining airway, low flow oxygen

ACTIVITY Bedrest during observation interval

DIET Nothing by mouth until status clarified

PATIENT EDUCATION
• Parents need much support
• Febrile seizures do not cause developmental delay
• Febrile seizures do not cause retardation
• Febrile seizures do not cause behavioral abnormalities
• Febrile seizures do not cause death
• Recurrence risk 33%, with 95% occurring within next 1 year

MEDICATIONS

DRUG(S) OF CHOICE
• Rectal or oral acetaminophen for fever 10-15 mg/kg/dose
• Anticonvulsants rarely indicated. See topic Status epilepticus for treatment of prolonged seizures.
• Oxygen
Contraindications: Allergy to drug
Precautions: Respiratory compromise needing support or intubation
Significant possible interactions: N/A

ALTERNATIVE DRUGS
• Phenobarbital 10-15 mg/kg IV, slower onset of action and may cause respiratory depression and hypotension
• Phenytoin 10-15 mg/kg IV, slower onset of action and may cause cardiac arrhythmias and hypotension
• Valproic acid 40-60 mg/kg in equal parts water - 5 cm rectally is longer acting but may cause hepatotoxicity in under 2 year age group, slower onset of action
• Paraldehyde - 0.2 ml/kg up to 2 ml at one site IM, but slower onset of action, or paraldehyde in rectal dosage form - 0.3 cc (300 mg)/kg/dose in 1:1 dilution with cottonseed oil or olive oil (maximum dose 5 mL)

FOLLOWUP

PATIENT MONITORING
Based on the site, severity, and origin of the fever.

PREVENTION/AVOIDANCE
• Acetaminophen 10 mg/kg orally or rectally, temperature greater than 100.5° F rectal
• May use intermittent prophylactic rectal diazepam for fever greater than 38.5° C (101.3° F); 5 mg if under 3 years or 7.5 mg 3 to 6 years or 0.5 mg/kg (up to 15 mg), repeated every 12 hours for 4 doses total
• Continuous prophylaxis is controversial; may consider for high risk child with strong family history, multiple recurrences, complex events, or underlying neurological abnormalities until 1 year after last seizure. Phenobarbital 3-5 mg/kg/day may be used but often causes behavioral problems; valproic acid 30-40 mg/kg/day may be tried but may cause severe hepatotoxicity

POSSIBLE COMPLICATIONS
• Febrile seizures do not cause death, retardation, behavioral problems nor developmental delays
• Children with febrile seizures are at greater than average risk to develop epilepsy later in life

EXPECTED COURSE AND PROGNOSIS
• 33% develop recurrent febrile seizures, 50% if first episode before 12 months, 45% if two involved siblings
• 95% of recurrences occur within 1 year
• Epilepsy occurs in 0.5% of general population but 3-4% of population with prior febrile seizure
• Risks for epilepsy include: Complex initial event with risk climbing with each complex feature independently, age at first episode under 6 months, three or more recurrences, pre-seizure neurological abnormalities, and family history of epilepsy

MISCELLANEOUS

ASSOCIATED CONDITIONS
• Examine child for port wine stain over trigeminal nerve with Sturge-Weber syndrome, adenoma sebaceum and hypopigmented skin of tuberous sclerosis, and café-au-lait spots and subcutaneous nodules of neurofibromatosis
• 13-18% of meningitis cases present with seizures

AGE-RELATED FACTORS
Pediatric: Range 3 months to 5 years with 95% by age 5 and peak incidence at age 2 years
Geriatric: N/A
Others: N/A

PREGNANCY N/A

SYNONYMS
• Febrile convulsions
• Febrile fits

ICD-9-CM 780.3

SEE ALSO Status epilepticus

OTHER NOTES
• Intermittent phenobarbital prophylaxis not recommended
• Phenytoin and carbamazepine are ineffective for prophylaxis
• No evidence that preventing recurrent febrile seizures prevents epilepsy
• Critical to distinguish between simple and complex events
• Post-ictal sleepiness is mild; if marked may indicate underlying pathology

ABBREVIATIONS N/A

REFERENCES
• Leung, A.K.C.: Febrile Convulsions: How dangerous are they? Postgraduate Medicine, April 1991, Vol 89; 5:217-224
• Applegate, M.S. & Lo, W.: Febrile Seizures: Current Concepts Concerning Prognosis and Clinical Management. Journal of Family Practice, 1989, Vol. 29, 4:422-428
• Sexton, M.E.: Childhood Seizures. AAFP Home Study Audio Series, Sept. 1991

Author M. Sexton, M.D.

Septicemia

BASICS

DESCRIPTION The presence of microorganisms in the blood; most commonly refers to the clinical consequences of bacteremia. However, it encompasses a broad array of clinical manifestations.
• Bacteremia: bacteria in the blood; may have no accompanying symptoms
• Sepsis: the systemic response to the presence of microorganisms in the blood or tissues
• Early septic shock (warm shock): sepsis and hypotension which is responsive to fluid replacement
• Late, or refractory, septic shock (cold shock): sepsis and hypotension which is unresponsive to fluid replacement
System(s) affected: Cardiovascular, Endocrine/Metabolic, Hematologic, Renal, Neurologic, Pulmonary, Gastrointestinal
Genetics: N/A
Incidence in USA: 176/100,000 persons/year
Prevalence in USA: Unknown
Predominant age: All ages
Predominant sex: Male = Female

SIGNS AND SYMPTOMS
• Fever
• Chills, rigors
• Myalgias
• Changes in mental status - restlessness, agitation, confusion, delirium, lethargy, stupor, coma
• Tachycardia
• Tachypnea
• Hypotension
• Skin lesions - erythema, petechiae, ecthyma gangrenosum, embolic lesions
Signs and symptoms related to site of primary infection:
  ◊ Respiratory tract - cough, sputum production, dyspnea, chest pain
  ◊ Urinary tract - dysuria, flank pain, frequency, urgency
  ◊ Intra-abdominal source - nausea, vomiting, diarrhea, constipation, abdominal pain
  ◊ Central nervous system - stiff neck, headache, photophobia, focal neurologic signs
Signs and symptoms related to end organ failure:
  ◊ Pulmonary - cyanosis
  ◊ Renal - oliguria, anuria
  ◊ Hepatic - jaundice
  ◊ Cardiac - congestive heart failure

CAUSES
Specific etiologic agents include:
  ◊ Gram positive organisms - most commonly Staphylococcus sp, Streptococcus sp, Enterococcus sp
  ◊ Gram negative organisms - most commonly Escherichia coli, Klebsiella sp, Proteus sp, Pseudomonas sp
  ◊ Fungi - most commonly Candida sp
  ◊ Other agents - anaerobes. Also, see Differential diagnosis.

Common sources of septicemia include:
  ◊ Lungs
  ◊ Urinary tract
  ◊ Intra-abdominal focus - biliary tree, abscess, peritonitis
  ◊ Intravascular catheters
  ◊ Skin - cellulitis, decubitus ulcer, gangrene
  ◊ Heart valves

RISK FACTORS
• Age extremes (very old and very young)
• Impaired host (see associated conditions)
• Indwelling catheters - intravascular, urinary, biliary, etc.
• Complicated labor and delivery - premature and/or prolonged rupture of membranes, etc.
• Certain surgical procedures

DIAGNOSIS

DIFFERENTIAL DIAGNOSIS
• Viral diseases (influenza, dengue and other hemorrhagic viruses, Coxsackie B virus)
• Rickettsial diseases (Rocky Mountain spotted fever, endemic typhus)
• Spirochetal diseases (leptospirosis, relapsing fever [Borrelia sp], Jarisch-Herxheimer reaction in syphilis)
• Protozoal diseases (Toxoplasma gondii, Trypanosoma cruzi, Pneumocystis carinii, Plasmodium falciparum)
• Collagen vascular diseases, vasculitides, myocardial infarction, pulmonary embolus, thrombotic thrombocytopenic purpura/hemolytic-uremic syndrome, thyrotoxicosis, adrenal insufficiency (Addison's disease), dissecting aortic aneurysm

LABORATORY
• Positive blood cultures
• Positive cultures from other sites (sputum, urine, cerebrospinal fluid [CSF], etc.)
• Gram stain of clinical specimens (sputum, urine, CSF, etc.)
Common:
  ◊ Leukocytosis
  ◊ Proteinuria
  ◊ Hypoxemia
  ◊ Eosinopenia
  ◊ Hypoferremia
  ◊ Hyperglycemia
  ◊ Hypocalcemia
  ◊ Mild hyperbilirubinemia
Less common:
  ◊ Lactic acidosis
  ◊ Leukopenia
  ◊ Azotemia
  ◊ Thrombocytopenia
  ◊ Prolonged prothrombin time
  ◊ Anemia
  ◊ Hypoglycemia
Drugs that may alter lab results: Prior antibiotic use
Disorders that may alter lab results: N/A

PATHOLOGICAL FINDINGS
• Inflammation at primary site of infection
• Disseminated intravascular coagulation
• Noncardiogenic pulmonary edema

SPECIAL TESTS
• Antigen detection systems - counterimmune electrophoresis (CIE) and latex agglutination tests (pneumococcus, H. influenzae type B, group B streptococcus, meningococcus)
• Gram stain of buffy coat smears occasionally useful

IMAGING
• X-rays (e.g., chest)
• Ultrasound, CT scan, or MRI may be useful in delineating sites of infection

DIAGNOSTIC PROCEDURES
• Aspiration of potentially infected body fluids (pleural, peritoneal, CSF) when appropriate
• Biopsy, drainage of potentially infected tissues (abscess, biliary tree, etc.) when appropriate

TREATMENT

APPROPRIATE HEALTH CARE
• Hospitalization
• Intensive care treatment of patients with shock, respiratory failure

GENERAL MEASURES
• Removal or drainage of septic foci
• Correction of metabolic abnormalities (hypoxemia, hyperglycemia, hypoglycemia, severe acidemia [pH < 7.10])
• Mechanical ventilation for respiratory failure
• Transfusion of RBC, platelets, and/or fresh frozen plasma for bleeding
• Volume replacement followed by pressors for hypotension

ACTIVITY Bedrest

DIET NPO initially; intravenous hyperalimentation appropriate in some severely malnourished patients and in patients who will be unable to receive enteral alimentation within the week

PATIENT EDUCATION N/A

MEDICATIONS

DRUG(S) OF CHOICE
• Antibiotic coverage should be broad initially and directed against organisms associated with identified septic foci. After culture results are available, treatment should be more organism-specific. Knowledge of the antibiotic susceptibility patterns of local pathogens extremely important.
• Neonatal (< 7 days old) sepsis - ampicillin (200 mg/kg/d in 4 divided doses) and gentamicin (Garamycin) 5-7.5 mg/kg/d in 2-3 divided doses
• Non-immunocompromised child - cefotaxime (Claforan) 200 mg/kg/d in 4 divided doses
• Non-immunocompromised adult - ampicillin/sulbactam (Unasyn) 1.5-3 gm q6h
• Neutropenic host - vancomycin (Vancocin) 1 gm q 12h, ceftazidime (Fortaz) 1-2 gm q8-12h, and gentamicin (Garamycin) or tobramycin 3-5 mg/kg/d in 2-3 divided doses

Contraindications: History of anaphylaxis or other allergic reaction to the antibiotic

Precautions: Dose adjustments required in renal failure

Significant possible interactions:
• Aminoglycosides - increased nephrotoxicity with enflurane, cisplatin and possibly vancomycin; increased ototoxicity with loop diuretics; increased paralysis with neuromuscular blocking agents
• Ampicillin - increased frequency of rash with allopurinol

ALTERNATIVE DRUGS
Many other drug combinations are possible to get adequate coverage

FOLLOWUP

PATIENT MONITORING
• Depends upon source of infection, underlying disease(s)
• Peak and trough drug levels for aminoglycosides, vancomycin
• BUN, creatinine, electrolytes and complete blood counts at least twice weekly; more frequently if unstable

PREVENTION/AVOIDANCE
• Vaccination - pneumococcal (geriatric patients, patients with certain chronic diseases), Hemophilus influenzae type B (infants, young children)
• Gamma globulin (for hypo- or agammaglobulinemic patients)
• Hand washing by hospital personnel, appropriate catheter care, etc., for hospitalized patients

POSSIBLE COMPLICATIONS
• Death
• Adult respiratory distress syndrome (ARDS)
• Multi-organ failure (cardiac, pulmonary, renal, hepatic)
• Disseminated intravascular coagulation (DIC)
• Gastrointestinal hemorrhage

EXPECTED COURSE AND PROGNOSIS
Even with optimal care, mortality will be 10-50% overall; this is increased in patients with neutropenia, diabetes, alcoholism, renal failure, respiratory failure, hypogammaglobulinemia, certain etiologic agents (e.g., Pseudomonas aeruginosa), a delay in appropriate antimicrobial therapy, and those patients at the age extremes

MISCELLANEOUS

ASSOCIATED CONDITIONS
• Neutropenia
• Diabetes mellitus
• Alcoholism
• Leukemia, lymphoma, and solid tumors
• Cirrhosis
• Burns
• Multiple trauma
• Intravenous drug abuse
• Malnutrition
• Complement deficiencies
• Hypo- or agammaglobulinemia
• Splenectomy
• HIV infection

AGE-RELATED FACTORS
Pediatric: Screen newborns for infection for prolonged rupture of membranes (> 24 h), maternal fever, prematurity
Geriatric:
• Often more difficult to diagnose clinically in the elderly
• Change in mental status/behavior may be only early manifestation
Others: N/A

PREGNANCY Beta lactam antibiotics, aminoglycosides, erythromycin are considered safe

SYNONYMS
• Sepsis
• Septic shock
• Sepsis neonatorum

ICD-9-CM 038

SEE ALSO
• Bacterial pneumonia
• Pyelonephritis
• Bacterial meningitis
• Endocarditis
• Toxic shock syndrome
• Rocky Mountain spotted fever
• Candidiasis
• Listeriosis
• Tularemia

OTHER NOTES High dose steroids of no benefit

ABBREVIATIONS N/A

REFERENCES
• Bone, R.C.: The pathogenesis of sepsis. Ann Intern Med. 115:457-469, 1991
• Harris, R.L., et al.: Manifestations of sepsis. Arch Intern Med. 147:1895-1906, 1987
• Center for Disease Control: Increase in National Hospital Discharge Rates for Septicemia-United States. 1979-1987. MMWR 39:31-34, 1990

Author R. Atmar, M.D.

Serum sickness

BASICS

DESCRIPTION Allergic reaction to foreign serum or drugs, usually appearing 5-14 days after administration of the allergen. Characterized by fever, arthralgias, skin rash and lymphadenopathy.
System(s) affected: Musculoskeletal, Gastrointestinal, Skin/Exocrine, Hemic/Lymphatic/Immunologic, Cardiovascular
Genetics: N/A
Incidence/Prevalence in USA: Common
Predominant age: All ages
Predominant sex: Male = Female

SIGNS AND SYMPTOMS
• History of antibiotic therapy (especially penicillin and related drugs)
• History of injection of horse serum or other species serum
• Fever
• Arthralgias (particularly TM joint)
• Malaise
• Pruritus
• Nausea
• Vomiting
• Abdominal pain
• Splenomegaly
• Myalgias
• Extremity weakness
• Sneezing
• Coughing
• Dyspnea
• Melena
• Cutaneous eruptions
• Facial swelling
• Lymphadenopathy
• Urticaria
• Joint effusion
• Myocarditis (rare)

CAUSES
• IgG antibodies that form soluble complexes with the antigen to cause an immune complex (type III) reaction
• Drugs (penicillin, cephalorsporins, sulfanamides, thiouracils, iodinated dyes, streptomycin)
• Tetanus toxoid
• Rabies antiserum
• Release of vasoactive substance
• Rabbit antiserum
• Crotalidae antivenin

RISK FACTORS
Previous exposure to injection of foreign protein (reaction usually occurs sooner than the expected 5-14 days)

DIAGNOSIS

DIFFERENTIAL DIAGNOSIS
• Periarteritis nodosa
• Anaphylaxis
• Drug hypersensitivity

LABORATORY
• Proteinuria
• Decreased C3
• Decreased C4
• Increased ESR
• Mixed IgG-IgM cryoprecipitates
Drugs that may alter lab results: N/A
Disorders that may alter lab results: N/A

PATHOLOGICAL FINDINGS Nodular lesions in segments of arteries resembling periarteritis nodosa

SPECIAL TESTS Test all persons prior to receiving a foreign serum (see Prevention/avoidance)

IMAGING N/A

DIAGNOSTIC PROCEDURES N/A

TREATMENT

APPROPRIATE HEALTH CARE
Inpatient, if severe; outpatient for mild cases

GENERAL MEASURES Treat symptomatically. Usually self-limited.

ACTIVITY Bed rest during acute illness

DIET No special diet

PATIENT EDUCATION N/A

MEDICATIONS

DRUG(S) OF CHOICE
• Antihistamine of choice for urticaria and generalized pruritis
• Aspirin 0.6-1.5 grams orally q 4h
Contraindications: Refer to manufacturer's literature
Precautions: Refer to manufacturer's literature
Significant possible interactions: Refer to manufacturer's literature

ALTERNATIVE DRUGS
Prednisone - 40 mg/day orally if simpler medicines do not bring symptomatic relief. Prednisone also used if peripheral neuritis or myocarditis (rare) develops.

FOLLOWUP

PATIENT MONITORING
During acute illness, monitor closely for signs of myocarditis or peripheral neuritis

PREVENTION/AVOIDANCE
• Special caution in patients who need foreign serum if they have history of asthma, hay fever, urticaria or other allergic symptoms
• Testing in patients with no previous exposure or allergic history: Before administering a foreign protein - prick test with 1:10 dilution. If this is negative, 0.02 mL of 1:10 dilution given intracutaneously.
• Testing in patients with previous exposure or allergic history: Test first with 1:1000 dilution
• If skin test is positive and serum treatment is essential, then desensitization is necessary

POSSIBLE COMPLICATIONS
• Vasculitis
• Neuropathy
• Glomerulonephritis (rare)
• Anaphylaxis
• Shock
• Death

EXPECTED COURSE AND PROGNOSIS
• Favorable; self-limiting with 2-3 weeks for recovery

MISCELLANEOUS

ASSOCIATED CONDITIONS
Drug hypersensitivity

AGE-RELATED FACTORS
Pediatric: N/A
Geriatric: N/A
Others: N/A

PREGNANCY N/A

SYNONYMS
• Inoculation reaction
• Protein sickness

ICD-9-CM 999.5

SEE ALSO N/A

OTHER NOTES
Horse antiserum still used in treatment of botulism, diptheria, venomous snake bites, spider bites. Antilymphocyte or antilymphocyte serum is used to suppress immune reactions to transplanted organs.

ABBREVIATIONS N/A

REFERENCES
• Rodnam, G.P. & Schumacker, H.R. (eds.): Serum sickness and drug reactions. In Primer on Rheumatic Diseases. 8th Ed. Atlanta, Arthritis Foundation, 1983
• Virella, G.: Hypersentivity reactions. Immunology Series, 1993;58:329

Author B. Murray, M.D.

Sexual dysfunction in women

BASICS

DESCRIPTION Difficulty getting or staying sexually aroused, reaching orgasm too quickly, difficulty or inability to reach orgasm, inability to relax, lack of interest in sex, distaste or revulsion with sex, too little foreplay, too little tenderness after intercourse.
• Most women who have orgasms do not do so invariably during intercourse, and some mistakenly think this is dysfunction
Four major types:
◊ Disorder of desire - both hypo- and hyper-(initiation and response), global desire disorder, couple desire discrepancy, situational desire disorder - these must be evaluated in the context of the relationship overall
◊ Disorder of arousal
◊ Dyspareunia, vaginismus
◊ Orgasmic disorders - primary and secondary, during masturbation or coitus, situational or partner specific
System(s) affected: Reproductive, Nervous
Genetics: N/A
Incidence in USA: Unknown
Prevalence in USA:
• 1 in 5 women is sexually dissatisfied, and two thirds of women report some degree of sexual dysfunction. Only one third of anorgasmic women in general think it is a problem.
• Overall prevalence for dysfunction is 15-30% of all women. Desire disorders are complaint of 30-55% of individual patients presenting to clinics, and 31% of couples; arousal disorders present in about 14-48% in community studies. Orgasmic disorders probably the most common; about 10% primary, and up to 65-80% secondary in community studies.
• There are many barriers to seeking help, so data for prevalence incomplete; barriers include stigma of exposing sexual inadequacy, fear of unknown therapy, e.g., of having to perform before a therapist.
Predominant age: Can occur in post-pubertal age group; women's ability to experience orgasm increases gradually from puberty; in later teens nearly half have not had orgasm; by mid-thirties, about 10% have not
Predominant sex: Female (heterosexual, homosexual, and bisexual women)

SIGNS AND SYMPTOMS
• Complaint to health care provider (if the clinician inquires, over twice as many are revealed than if clinician waits for patient to mention)
• Infertility
• Marital conflict
• Family dysfunction

CAUSES
• Interrelational difficulties and conflict regarding intimacy
• Anxiety
• Survivor of sexual abuse, including incest
• Alcohol
• Drug use, including prescription medications (e.g., MAO inhibitors, tricyclic antidepressants, beta-blockers, especially SSRI antidepressants [Prozac, Paxil, Zoloft, etc.])
• Proximity of other people in household (mother-in-law)
• Anorgasmia can be due to diabetes
• Spinal cord damage
• Hormonal imbalance?
• Thyroid disease
• Sexual frequency myths
• Control issues in the relationships
• Dyspareunia, including vaginal dryness causing interference with lubrication, secondary to infection or endocrine
• There is little endocrine data on women with sexual dysfunction

RISK FACTORS Couple discrepancies in - expectations, cultural backgrounds, attitudes toward sexuality in family of origin, previous sexual trauma, low self-esteem

DIAGNOSIS

DIFFERENTIAL DIAGNOSIS
• Medications including psychotropics (monoamine oxide inhibitors, tricyclic and other antidepressants)
• Marital dysfunction including domestic violence
• Decreased sensation secondary to back or nerve disease
• Multiple sclerosis
• Abdominal surgery (can interfere with pelvic innervation)
• Depression
• Vaginitis
• Decreased vaginal lubrication secondary to hormonal imbalance
• Pregnancy
• Anatomic or congenital abnormalities
• Pseudodyspareunia (use of complaint of pain to distance from partner)

LABORATORY As needed to identify infections and other medical causes
Drugs that may alter lab results: N/A
Disorders that may alter lab results: N/A

PATHOLOGICAL FINDINGS Varied if any

SPECIAL TESTS May need life experiences or some other psychological inventory to evaluate couple. (Alcohol, marijuana or other illicit drug use may make these evaluations unreliable.)

IMAGING N/A

DIAGNOSTIC PROCEDURES N/A

TREATMENT

APPROPRIATE HEALTH CARE
Outpatient

GENERAL MEASURES
• For childhood trauma - scripting, psychotherapy, cognitive restructuring
• For anorgasmia - directed masturbation and "homework" with partners
• For prescription drug causes - reduced dosages, or change to different medication
• Other - family therapy, sensate conditioning; referral to specialized sex therapy

ACTIVITY Varies with couple

DIET Weight reduction if needed for either partner

PATIENT EDUCATION Information about normal sexual function and human reproductive anatomy and function and changes expected with aging

MEDICATIONS

DRUG(S) OF CHOICE These are usually multifactorial psychosocial conditions. Using medications doesn't address the cause of the problem and can make it worse.
Contraindications: N/A
Precautions: N/A
Significant possible interactions: N/A

ALTERNATIVE DRUGS N/A

FOLLOWUP

PATIENT MONITORING Varies with patient

PREVENTION/AVOIDANCE Sex education starting in elementary years, early intervention in dysfunctional family or incest

POSSIBLE COMPLICATIONS Marital or family stress, breakup and divorce

EXPECTED COURSE AND PROGNOSIS Desire is the most difficult to treat (less than 50% successful by patient report), and success is sometimes less optimal than patient's initial wish. Best predictors are desire to change and overall healthy relationship.

MISCELLANEOUS

ASSOCIATED CONDITIONS Marital stress

AGE-RELATED FACTORS
Pediatric: N/A
Geriatric:
• Societal expectations about geriatric sexuality, (especially the myth older women aren't sexually active) can cause distress if patient has sexual desires or sexual experience
• Normal physiologic changes in aging are misinterpreted as dysfunction
Others: Sex role stereotypes

PREGNANCY Often affects but the effect varies depending on the patient and couple's beliefs about pregnancy and the problem

SYNONYMS
• Hypoactive sexual desire disorder
• Sexual aversion disorder
• Female sexual arousal disorder
• Inhibited female orgasm
• Dyspareunia and vaginismus

ICD-9-CM
• 302.70 sexual function psychogenic
• 301.72 frigidity

SEE ALSO Vaginismus

OTHER NOTES
• Women must feel safe in order to let go and lose some control to experience orgasm
• Performance anxiety makes males ejaculate prematurely, while it inhibits orgasm in women
• Simple lack of knowledge about anatomy and physiology of sex can lead to problems

ABBREVIATIONS N/A

REFERENCES
• Leiblum, S.R. & Rosen, R.C.: Principles and Practice of Sex Therapy: Update for the 1990's. New York, The Guilford Press, 1989
• Wincze, J.P. & Carey, M.P.: Sexual Dysfunction: A Guide for Assessment and Treatment. New York, The Guilford Press, 1991
• Bancroft, J.: Human Sexuality and Its Problems. 2nd Ed. New York, Churchill Livingstone, 1989

Author S. Duiker, M.D. & J. Graves-Moy, M.D.

Shock, circulatory

BASICS

DESCRIPTION Inadequate perfusion (oxygen supply) of tissues which results in organ dysfunction, cellular and organ damage and, if not corrected quickly, death of the patient. Classification of shock:
- Hypovolemic shock - cardiac output is severely reduced due to loss of intravascular volume which results in reduced return of venous blood to the heart. Most often caused by blood loss.
- Cardiogenic shock - cardiac output is severely reduced due to a loss of myocardial muscle function, valvular dysfunction or arrhythmia. Most often caused by large myocardial infarctions.
- Obstructive shock - cardiac output is severely reduced by vascular obstruction to venous return to the heart (vena cava syndrome), compression of the heart, (pericardial tamponade) or outflow from the heart (aortic dissection, pulmonary embolism)
- Distributive shock - maldistribution of blood flow
- Venous pooling (most often due to spinal shock or drug overdose) behaves much like hypovolemic shock, cardiac output severely reduced because blood is pooled in peripheral veins rather than being returned to the heart
- High output or vasodilating shock (most often due to sepsis or septic like states such as toxic shock) is unique in that cardiac output is normal or elevated, but not distributed appropriately, resulting in over perfusion of some tissues and underperfusion (to the point of critical ischemia) of other tissues.

System(s) affected: Cardiovascular
Genetics: Unknown
Incidence/Prevalence in USA: N/A
Predominant age: All ages. Determined by underlying diseases causing shock. More frequent and less well tolerated in the elderly.
Predominant sex: Male = Female

SIGNS AND SYMPTOMS
Underlying disease:
◊ Upper gastrointestinal (UGI) bleeding (ulcer pain, hematemesis, melena)
◊ Sepsis (fever, chills, dysuria and/or costovertebral angle [CVA] tenderness with urinary tract infection)
◊ Myocardial infarction (chest pain, diaphoresis, nausea, vomiting, S4 or S3 gallop, new heart murmur, rales due to pulmonary edema)
Underperfusion of organ systems:
◊ Brain: confusion, anxiety, agitation, coma only if severe
◊ Kidney: oliguria
◊ Skin: peripheral cyanosis, sluggish capillary refill, mottling, coolness, may be overperfused (flushed) in high output (septic) shock
◊ GI: absence of bowel sounds
◊ Circulation: thready pulses, tachycardia, hypotension (mean arterial pressure < 60 torr or systolic pressure < 90 torr or blood pressure > 40 torr less than usual blood pressure in chronic hypertension), secondary cardiac

ischemia (ST depression) or heart failure may occur due to underperfusion of the heart during shock. Jugular-venous distention (JVD), pulsus paradoxus in pericardial tamponade.

CAUSES
Hypovolemic shock
◊ Blood loss due to trauma or gastrointestinal bleeding
◊ Third space loss of plasma volume (pancreatitis, bowel obstruction, infarction, anaphylaxis)
◊ Diarrhea (e.g., in cholera like states)
◊ Burns
Cardiogenic shock
◊ Acute myocardial infarction (> 40% of LV mass)
◊ Arrhythmia (heart block, ventricular tachycardia, atrial fibrillation with rapid ventricular response, etc.)
◊ Acute valvular dysfunction (mitral valve due to papillary muscle rupture following inferior MI's or chordal rupture) aortic or mitral valve due to bacterial endocarditis
◊ Ventricular septal rupture following anterior/septal MI's
Obstructive shock
◊ Pericardial tamponade
◊ Inferior/superior vena caval obstruction usually due to neoplasms
◊ Aortic dissection
◊ Massive pulmonary embolism
Distributive shock
◊ Venous pooling is due to a loss of venous tone caused by loss of sympathetic nervous system activity due to acute spinal injury, general or spinal anesthesia or overdose of sedative drugs
◊ High output shock is due to sepsis, toxic shock or anaphylaxis (once plasma volume normalized)

RISK FACTORS Included with Causes

DIAGNOSIS

DIFFERENTIAL DIAGNOSIS N/A

LABORATORY
Specific to shock
◊ Elevated lactate (> 2 m moles/liter) indicates anaerobic metabolism due to underperfusion of tissues
◊ Reduced mixed venous P02 (< 28 torr) obtained from the pulmonary artery indicates vigorous extraction of oxygen from tissues due to underperfusion
Underlying diseases responsible to shock
◊ ECG, CPK (serial)
◊ Chest x-ray
◊ Arterial blood gases
◊ Gram stain and culture of infected sites
◊ Blood cultures
◊ CBC (serial determination of HB/HCT in bleeding patients)
Drugs that may alter lab results: N/A
Disorders that may alter lab results: N/A

PATHOLOGICAL FINDINGS N/A

SPECIAL TESTS
- Certain tests are essential to making correct and prompt diagnosis in order to dictate specific therapy of disease states producing shock. For example:
- Endoscopy/Radioisotope bleeding scans enable localization of ongoing bleeding which may direct surgical intervention. The endoscopist may intervene directly via the endoscope. (e.g., injection of sclerosants into varices or ulcers).
- Echocardiograms may detect and/or quantify pericardial effusions in shock due to pericardial tamponade. Pericardiocentesis can then be performed under echocardiographic guidance. Also useful for detection of valvular failure.
- Lung scans and/or pulmonary arteriography for the detection of massive pulmonary embolism
- Pulmonary artery (Swan-Ganz) catheterization allows for serial measurement of cardiac output, central venous, pulmonary arterial and pulmonary arterial occlusion pressures (left atrial pressure) and vascular resistance. Mixed venous blood gases can be drawn from the catheter. Indicated when the etiology of shock is uncertain, in cardiogenic and septic shock, or when initial therapy of shock fails to provide for rapid correction of perfusion failure.

IMAGING See Special tests

DIAGNOSTIC PROCEDURES See Special tests

TREATMENT

APPROPRIATE HEALTH CARE
- Emergency room or intensive or coronary care unit
- Continuous electrocardiographic monitoring with frequent assessment of blood pressure, respiratory status, and urine output

GENERAL MEASURES
- Therapy must proceed quickly before extensive damage to vital organs occur. Therapy is directed simultaneously to correct both the deficit in tissue perfusion and the underlying disease causing shock (see Associated conditions).
- Maintain SaO2 > 95% with supplemental oxygen. Intubate and mechanically ventilate patient if patient cannot be oxygenated with 100% oxygen or has markedly increased breathing effort (excessive oxygen cost of breathing).

• Maintain pH above 7.3 (but less than 7.5) to preserve vascular responsiveness to endogenous or exogenous catecholamines.
• Correct plasma volume deficits rapidly by volume expanders consisting of isotonic saline (.9Ns or Ringer's lactate) with or without colloid (albumin 5% or hydroxyethyl starch 6%)
• Packed red blood cell transfusion to correct or prevent anemia. HB maintained at or above 10 grams/dl.
• Administer coagulation factors (fresh frozen plasma, cryoprecipitate) and platelets if coagulopathy (prolonged PT, PTT or platelet count < 50,000) is present in a patient who is bleeding
• Tachyrrhythmias (other than sinus tachycardia) should be promptly corrected by electrocardioversion. Transvenous pacemakers should be placed to correct bradyrhythmias.
• Vasopressors (see Medications) to correct hypotension or low cardiac output due to myocardial failure or hypotension due to low vascular resistance
• End points of resuscitation: adequate blood pressure (> 60 torr mean or > 90 torr systolic or within 40 mm of patient's normal blood pressure). Patient is awake/alert, urine output adequate, heart rate < 100, warm skin with brisk capillary refill, bowel sounds present. Lactate < 2 m moles/L, mixed venous PO2 > 30 torr.

ACTIVITY None

DIET N/A

PATIENT EDUCATION N/A

MEDICATIONS

DRUG(S) OF CHOICE
• Dopamine (low dose 1-4 µg/kg/min) augments contractility and cardiac output (beta-1) and increases heart rate. This provides increased blood flow to kidneys and gut. Also acts directly on dopaminergic receptors in the renal vasculature to enhance renal blood flow.
• Dopamine (> 4 µg/kg/min): augments contractility, and cardiac output (beta-1) and increased heart rate. Increases blood pressure by a combination of increased cardiac output and vasoconstriction (alpha).
• Norepinephrine (2-12 µg/min): augments blood pressure by increased vascular resistance (alpha). Reduced blood flow to splanchnic bed can be reversed by low dose dopamine.
• Phenylephrine (20-200 µg/min): see norepinphrine
• Dobutamine (5-10 µg/kg/min) augments contractility and cardiac output (beta-1). Has both vasoconstrictive (alpha) and vasodilator (beta-2) properties. These effects have a minimal effect on systemic vasculature.
Contraindications: Refer to manufacturer's profile of each drug

Precautions:
• Myocardial oxygen consumption is increased by increased heart rate, afterload, and contractility
• Pressors can increase myocardial ischemia if present
• May precipitate or worsen tachyarrhythmias
• Should be used in lowest possible dose for as limited period of time as possible
Significant possible interactions: Refer to manufacturer's profile of each drug

ALTERNATIVE DRUGS N/A

FOLLOWUP

PATIENT MONITORING Careful monitoring of all life functions in intensive care

PREVENTION/AVOIDANCE Shock is best avoided by prompt recognition and treatment of underlying diseases which cause shock (e.g., early antibiotic therapy for infections)

POSSIBLE COMPLICATIONS
• Multiple organs may be damaged by underperfusion during shock
• Acute tubular necrosis
• Ischemic hepatitis
• Ischemic bowel
• Disseminated intravascular coagulopathy
• Adult respiratory distress syndrome (ARDS)
• Encephalopathy and/or cerebrovascular accident

EXPECTED COURSE AND PROGNOSIS
• Mortality is determined by a complex interaction of primary disease causing shock, age, coexisting chronic disease and shock severity as marked by the number of acute organ system failures that follow shock
• Best outcome (> 90% survival) in young patient with transient shock due to trauma or gastrointestinal blood loss without chronic irreversible illnesses
• Poor outcome (> 90% mortality) in elderly patient with septic shock, underlying chronic liver disease, who develops acute renal failure, ARDS, and coagulopathy

MISCELLANEOUS

ASSOCIATED CONDITIONS
• Gastrointestinal blood loss: may require endoscopic or surgical intervention if bleeding doesn't spontaneously cease, e.g., electrocoagulation or injecting sclerosant for bleeding peptic ulcers, sclerotherapy in esophageal varices
• Sepsis: empiric antibiotic therapy, based on the patient's underlying illnesses, age, site of infection, and hospital sensitivity patterns.

After hemodynamic stabilization, surgical drainage of abscesses, if present. Antibodies directed against gram negative cell wall antigens (endotoxin) may reduce mortality in patients with gram negative bacteremia.
• Cardiogenic shock: therapy should help reduce cardiac ischemia (oxygen, nitrates) and accomplish rapid reperfusion of injured, but potentially viable, myocardium (thrombolysis with fibrinolytic agents, balloon angioplasty of stenotic vessels or surgical bypass grafting) A balloon pump may temporize by providing improved coronary blood flow during and following diagnostic testing and revascularization therapy. If shock is due to acute failure of the mitral or aortic valve, surgical valve replacement may be lifesaving.
• Pulmonary embolism: reduction in the obstruction to pulmonary outflow is accomplished by infusion of thrombolytics (streptokinase, urokinase, tissue plasminogen activator [TPA]). If fibrinolytic therapy is contraindicated (e.g., recent surgery, intracerebral lesion) then pulmonary embolectomy may be life saving although mortality may be 50% or higher.
• Pericardial tamponade: shock due to tamponade is best treated by prompt removal of pericardial fluid either by catheter or surgical drainage

AGE-RELATED FACTORS
Pediatric: N/A
Geriatric: N/A
Others: N/A

PREGNANCY N/A

SYNONYMS N/A

ICD-9-CM
• 785.50, 785.51 (Cardiogenic)
• 785.59 (Septic, hypovolemic)

SEE ALSO N/A

OTHER NOTES N/A

ABBREVIATIONS N/A

REFERENCES
• Parillo, J.E.: Shock. In Harrison's Principles of Internal Medicine. 12th Ed. Edited by E. Braunwald, et al. New York, McGraw-Hill, Inc, 1991
• Schuster, D.P. & Lefrah, S.S.: Shock. In Critical Care. Edited by J.F. Civetta, et al. Philadelphia, J.B. Lippincott Corp, 1988, pp 891-908

Author S. Traeger, M.D

Sialadenitis

 BASICS

DESCRIPTION Inflammation of the salivary glands from nonspecific bacterial infection or inflammation most often arises in the excretory duct. The parotid is the most commonly affected gland with invasion of bacteria from the oral cavity. Inflammation may also follow trauma, spread of infection from adjoining tissues, and via hematogenous routes during bacteremia. Inflammation may lead to stone formation (sialolithiasis) or an obstructed duct may lead to inflammation of the gland. Stones are more commonly associated with the submaxillary glands. Recurrent infections or other chronic inflammatory processes can lead to decreased gland function with resulting xerostomia.
System(s) affected: Skin/Exocrine, Gastrointestinal
Genetics: Unknown
Incidence/Prevalence in USA: N/A
Predominant age: N/A
Predominant sex: N/A

SIGNS AND SYMPTOMS
• Enlarged, painful salivary gland
• Purulent discharge from duct orifice
• Red, painful duct orifice
• Fever
• Xerostomia
• Decreased salivary secretion (aptyalism)

CAUSES
• Bacteria from the oral cavity are the most common infectious cause of sialadenitis.
• The causative agents of the following diseases may also infect a salivary gland to cause sialadenitis:
  ◊ Mumps
  ◊ Actinomycosis
  ◊ Tuberculosis
  ◊ Syphilis
  ◊ CMV
  ◊ Cat-scratch disease

RISK FACTORS
• Dehydration
• Fever

 DIAGNOSIS

DIFFERENTIAL DIAGNOSIS
Decreased salivary secretion is associated with:
• Drugs:
  ◊ Tricyclic antidepressants (amitriptyline, etc.)
  ◊ Phenothiazines (chlorpromazine, fluphenazine, thioridazine, prochlorperazine, etc.)
• Myxedema
• Plummer-Vinson disease
• Pernicious anemia
• Febrile diseases
• Neuropsychiatric disorders
• Mikulicz's disease (benign lymphoepithelial lesion)
Enlarged glands may be the result of a variety of neoplasms including:
• Pleomorphic adenoma
• Mucoepidermoid carcinoma
• Other tumor types can also occur very rarely (lipoma, neurofibroma, fibrosarcoma, melanoma, lymphocytoma, Hodgkin's, etc.)
Also, obesity results in what appears to be enlarged parotids, but the bilateral nature and non-progressive course should help differentiate this from malignant neoplasms.

LABORATORY
Drugs that may alter lab results: N/A
Disorders that may alter lab results: N/A

PATHOLOGICAL FINDINGS
With chronic infection of the gland:
• Enlarged gland
• Ductal dilatation with retention of saliva
• Acinar atrophy or dilated and filled with mucus
• Purulent/seropurulent exudate within the duct
• Glandular replacement by fibrotic tissue
• Infiltration with leukocytes

SPECIAL TESTS N/A

IMAGING Radiographs may reveal a stone in sialolithiasis

DIAGNOSTIC PROCEDURES
Digital manipulation of the duct may express pus from the ductal orifice

 TREATMENT

APPROPRIATE HEALTH CARE
Outpatient

GENERAL MEASURES Heating pad and/or cool compresses may be comforting

ACTIVITY Unrestricted

DIET Avoid pain-producing sialagogues (lemon, etc.) during an acute episode

PATIENT EDUCATION N/A

MEDICATIONS

DRUG(S) OF CHOICE
• Antibiotics: Pencillin (Pen VK) 250-500mg QID or erythromycin 250mg QID
• Analgesic: codeine, NSAID, etc
Contraindications: N/A
Precautions: N/A
Significant possible interactions: N/A

ALTERNATIVE DRUGS N/A

FOLLOWUP

PATIENT MONITORING N/A

PREVENTION/AVOIDANCE N/A

POSSIBLE COMPLICATIONS
Occasional loss of salivary function

EXPECTED COURSE AND PROGNOSIS Complete recovery and good prognosis

MISCELLANEOUS

ASSOCIATED CONDITIONS
• Rheumatoid arthritis (Sjögren's syndrome)
• Sarcoidosis (Herrfordt's syndrome)

AGE-RELATED FACTORS
Pediatric: Rare in children
Geriatric: N/A
Others: N/A

PREGNANCY N/A

SYNONYMS N/A

ICD-9-CM 527.2 sialadenitis

SEE ALSO N/A

OTHER NOTES N/A

ABBREVIATIONS
CMV = cytomegalovirus

REFERENCES Cotran, R.S. et al.(eds.): Robbins Pathological Basis of Disease, 4th Ed. Philadelphia, W.B. Saunders Co., 1989

Author MR Dambro, M.D

Silicosis

BASICS

DESCRIPTION Pneumoconiosis (fibrogenic) caused by inhaling silica dust (quartz dust). Characteristics include discrete nodular pulmonary fibrosis (conglomerate fibrosis later) and impaired respiration.
System(s) affected: Pulmonary
Genetics: No known genetic pattern
Incidence/Prevalence in USA: Unknown
Predominant age: 40-75
Predominant sex: Male > Female

SIGNS AND SYMPTOMS
- Exertional dyspnea
- Chest tightness
- Cough
- Expectoration
- Increased anteroposterior chest diameter
- Hyperresonance
- Rales
- Decreased breath sounds

CAUSES Chronic inhalation of high concentrations of silica, usually requires 20-30 years of exposure, but possibly less than 10 years for tunnelers, sandblasters and abrasive soap makers

RISK FACTORS
Working in any of these industries:
◊ Metal mining (copper, silver, gold, lead, hard coal)
◊ Foundries
◊ Pottery making
◊ Sandstone cutting
◊ Granite cutting
◊ Smoking

DIAGNOSIS

DIFFERENTIAL DIAGNOSIS
- Miliary tuberculosis
- Welder's siderosis
- Hemosiderosis
- Coal worker's pneumoconiosis

LABORATORY
- Hypoxemia
- Hypercarbia
Drugs that may alter lab results: N/A
Disorders that may alter lab results: N/A

PATHOLOGICAL FINDINGS
Lung
◊ Pleural adhesions
◊ Pleural thickening
◊ Gray-black subpleural nodules
◊ Blackened lung
◊ Leathery lung
◊ Concentric layers of dense connective tissue
◊ Cellular infiltrate
◊ Ischemic degeneration of central nodule
◊ Metachromatic silica particles

SPECIAL TESTS
Pulmonary function test - decreased pulmonary compliance, decreased lung volumes, decreased diffusing capacity

IMAGING
Chest x-ray
◊ Egg shell calcification in hilar and mediastinal lymph nodes
◊ Large shadows in upper pulmonary fields
◊ Discrete nodular shadows (< 2 mm)
◊ Coalescent nodules
◊ Cavitation

DIAGNOSTIC PROCEDURES
- Bronchoscopy
- Careful history and physical examination

TREATMENT

APPROPRIATE HEALTH CARE
Outpatient

GENERAL MEASURES
- No known effective treatment
- Postural drainage
- Mist inhalation
- Chest physical therapy
- Breathing exercises
- Lung transplantation

ACTIVITY Maintain regular exercise program

DIET
- No special diet
- Increase fluid intake

PATIENT EDUCATION Printed patient information available from: American Lung Association, 1740 Broadway, New York, NY 10019, (212)315-8700

MEDICATIONS

DRUG(S) OF CHOICE
• None specific for silicosis
• Broad spectrum antibiotics (e.g., erythromycin) for recurrent bronchial infection or purulent sputum
• Bronchodilators (e.g., albuterol or metaproterenol inhaler) - 1-2 puffs every 6 hours for bronchospasm

Contraindications: Avoid sedatives and hypnotics

Precautions: Refer to manufacturer's literature

Significant possible interactions: Refer to manufacturer's literature

ALTERNATIVE DRUGS   N/A

FOLLOWUP

PATIENT MONITORING
• Monitor for heart failure and hypoxemia
• Treat intercurrent infections aggressively

PREVENTION/AVOIDANCE
• Avoid dust exposure; substitute other materials for silica
• If tuberculin test is positive, at least one year of isoniazid

POSSIBLE COMPLICATIONS
• Progressive massive fibrosis
• Respiratory infection
• Pneumothorax
• Emphysema

EXPECTED COURSE AND PROGNOSIS   Poor, chronic respiratory impairment

MISCELLANEOUS

ASSOCIATED CONDITIONS
Tuberculosis

AGE-RELATED FACTORS
Pediatric: Unusual
Geriatric: Symptoms and complications more severe
Others: N/A

PREGNANCY   N/A

SYNONYMS   N/A

ICD-9-CM   502 silicosis

SEE ALSO   N/A

OTHER NOTES   Silica - formula for calculating the threshold limit value (TLV) for respirable dust: TLV (threshold limit value) = (10 mg per cu meter/% SiO2) + 2

ABBREVIATIONS   N/A

REFERENCES
• Silicosis and Silicate Disease Committee. Diseases associated with exposure to silica and non-fibrous silicate materials. Arch Pathol Lab Med 112:673, 1988
• Murray, J.F. & Nadel, J.A. (eds.): Textbook of Respiratory Medicine. Philadelphia, W.B. Saunders Co., 1988

Author   H. Griffith, M.D. & M. Dambro, M.D.

Sinusitis

 BASICS

DESCRIPTION
Inflammation of the paranasal sinuses. Classified as acute or chronic depending on duration of infection. Occurs when an undrained collection of pus accumulates in the sinus.

System(s) affected: Pulmonary
Genetics: No known genetic pattern
Incidence/Prevalence in USA: Common
Predominant age: All ages
Predominant sex: Male = Female

SIGNS AND SYMPTOMS
- Nasal congestion (acute sinusitis)
- Gradual buildup of pressure feeling in sinus area with tenderness
- Nasal discharge - blood tinged, becoming purulent
- Malaise
- Sore throat (sometimes)
- Headache
- Fever
- Pain over cheeks and upper teeth (maxillary sinusitis) worse with bending
- Pain over eyebrows (frontal sinusitis)
- Pain over eyes (ethmoid sinusitis)
- Pain behind eyes (ethmoid)
- Cough (occasional)
- Post nasal discharge
- Periorbital edema
- Symptoms aggravated by air travel

CAUSES
- Bacterial infection (H. influenza, pneumococci, streptococci, catarrhalis)
- Viral infections
- Fungal infections (Aspergillus, bipolaris, mucormycosis)
- Preceding upper respiratory infection
- Predisposing factors - chronic nasal edema, viscous mucous, polyps, nasal allergy, sudden temperature changes

RISK FACTORS
- Allergic diathesis
- Immunosuppression
- Continuous positive airway pressure
- Air travel during upper respiratory infection
- Tooth abscess
- Swimming in contaminated water

 DIAGNOSIS

DIFFERENTIAL DIAGNOSIS
- Viral rhinitis
- Allergic rhinitis
- Vasomotor rhinitis
- Tumors
- Cysts
- Foreign bodies
- Wegener's granulomatosis

LABORATORY
- Elevated WBC
- Culture for identification of infecting organism

Drugs that may alter lab results: N/A
Disorders that may alter lab results: N/A

PATHOLOGICAL FINDINGS
- Inflammation
- Edema
- Thickened mucosa
- Nasal polyps
- Ulcerations

SPECIAL TESTS
- Endoscopy - identify areas of persistent infection
- Maxillary sinuscopy - for biopsy and cyst removal
- Sphenoid sinuscopy - rarely needed

IMAGING
- Sinus x-rays - cloudiness, air-fluid levels, thick mucosa in affected sinuses
- CT scan - for ostiomeatal complex pathology; aids in diagnosing local underlying causes of chronic sinusitis
- MRI - not current choice for evaluation

DIAGNOSTIC PROCEDURES
Transillumination reveals opacity in affected sinus cavities

 TREATMENT

APPROPRIATE HEALTH CARE
Outpatient except for surgery (rarely indicated). Consider hospitalization for frontal or sphenoid sinusitis.

GENERAL MEASURES
- Early treatment is medical
- Steam inhalations can aid comfort and draining
- Avoid smoke and other environmental pollutants if possible
- Avoid smoking cigarettes
- If medical treatment fails, can perform irrigation to wash out the inspissated material
- Surgery for sinusitis that persists despite medical treatment. Numerous techniques available for cleaning the different sinuses (nasal window procedure, Caldwell-Luc procedure, ethmoidectomy, external ethmoidectomy, fronto-ethmoidectomy, osteoplastic flap)

ACTIVITY
No restrictions. May need additional rest during acute phase.

DIET
No special diet. Drink plenty of fluids.

PATIENT EDUCATION
For patient education materials favorably reviewed on this topic, contact: Asthma & Allergy Foundation of America, 1717 Massachusetts Avenue, Suite 305, Washington, DC 20036, (800)7-Asthma

MEDICATIONS

DRUG(S) OF CHOICE
• Antibiotics - amoxicillin 500 mg tid for 14-21 days or trimethoprim-sulfa. If no response, switch to antibiotics with activity against B-lactamase producing bacteria.
• Analgesics
• Vasoconstrictors
• Antihistamines

Contraindications: Refer to manufacturer's literature

Precautions: Refer to manufacturer's literature

Significant possible interactions: Refer to manufacturer's literature

ALTERNATIVE DRUGS
Consider 3-5 days of topical decongestants at start of treatment. Chronic nasal steroid use indicated if sinusitis is secondary to allergic rhinitis.

FOLLOWUP

PATIENT MONITORING
Follow until clinically clear of disease

PREVENTION/AVOIDANCE
Treat nasal congestion prior to sinusitis

POSSIBLE COMPLICATIONS
• Meningitis
• Abscess (extradural, subdural, brain, retrobulbar)
• Osteomyelitis
• Orbital infection
• Septic cavernous thrombosis

EXPECTED COURSE AND PROGNOSIS
• Acute - favorable prognosis with timely treatment and avoidance of complications
• Chronic - may improve if causative allergen is removed or drainage is feasible

MISCELLANEOUS

ASSOCIATED CONDITIONS
• Rhinitis
• Barosinusitis
• Pansinusitis

AGE-RELATED FACTORS
Pediatric:
• Incidence of both acute and chronic sinusitis increases in the latter part of childhood
• May be more prevalent in children who have had tonsils and adenoids removed
• Chronic sinusitis indicates a need to search for underlying cause, e.g., nasal deformities or infected and hypertrophied adenoids
Geriatric:
• Incidence increases up to age 75 and then decreases
• More difficult to heal when it occurs in this age group
Others: N/A

PREGNANCY N/A

SYNONYMS N/A

ICD-9-CM
• 461.9 acute
• 473.9 chronic

SEE ALSO N/A

OTHER NOTES N/A

ABBREVIATIONS N/A

REFERENCES
• Adams, G.L., et al.: Fundamentals of Otolaryngology. 6th Ed. Philadelphia, W.B. Saunders Co., 1989
• Alberti, P.W. & Ruben, R.J. (eds.): Otologic Medicine and Surgery. New York, Churchill Livingstone, 1988

Author C. Zucker, M.D.

Sleep apnea, obstructive

BASICS

DESCRIPTION Repetitive episodes of upper airway occlusion during sleep, often with oxygen desaturation. Nearly always associated with snoring. Apneas often terminate with a snort or gasp. Repetitive apneas produce sleep disruption, leading to excessive daytime sleepiness (EDS). Usual course is chronic.
Genetics: Hereditary factors unknown. Familial patterns sometimes seen.
Incidence/Prevalence in USA: 1-2% of general adult population
Predominant age: Middle-age
Predominant sex: Males > Females

SIGNS AND SYMPTOMS
• Cardinal symptom is excessive daytime sleepiness (EDS)
• Loud snoring
• Complaints of disrupted sleep
• Repetitive awakenings with transient sensation of shortness of breath or for unclear reasons
• Tired and unrefreshed upon A.M. awakening
• Witnessed apneas at night
• Complaints of poor concentration, memory problems, irritability
• Morning headaches
• Short-tempered
• Decreased libido is also common
• Depression

CAUSES Upper airway narrowing due to enlarged tonsils, adenoids, uvula, low soft palate, large or posteriorly located tongue or craniofacial abnormalities superimposed upon a coexistent abnormality of neurological control of upper airway muscle tone or ventilatory control during sleep

RISK FACTORS
• Obesity
• Nasal obstruction (due to polyps, rhinitis or deviated septum)
• Hypothyroidism
• Acromegaly
• Persons with hypertension, cardiovascular or arteriovascular disease or alveolar hypoventilation have a much higher risk of OSA

DIAGNOSIS

DIFFERENTIAL DIAGNOSIS
• Other causes of EDS such as narcolepsy, idiopathic daytime hypersomnolence, depressive episodes with EDS
• Respiratory disorders with nocturnal awakenings such as asthma, COPD, CHF
• Central sleep apnea may mimic OSA
• Sudden nocturnal awakenings due to panic attacks
• Sleep-related choking or laryngospasm
• Gastroesophageal reflux may also present with similar symptoms

LABORATORY
• Polycythemia (occasional) reflects the degree of nocturnal hypoxemia due to OSA
• Thyroid function should be evaluated to rule out concomitant hypothyroidism
• Daytime hypercapnia occasionally seen
Drugs that may alter lab results: N/A
Disorders that may alter lab results: N/A

PATHOLOGICAL FINDINGS
• Anatomically small upper airway common
• CNS abnormalities rare

SPECIAL TESTS
• Echocardiography may demonstrate right and/or left ventricular enlargement or pulmonary hypertension
• Polysomnogram (nighttime sleep study) including O2 saturation
• Multiple sleep latency testing (MSLT) provides an objective measurement of daytime sleepiness

IMAGING
• Cephalometric measurements from lateral head and neck x-rays
• MRI, CT scans or fiberoptic evaluation of upper airway occasionally helpful

DIAGNOSTIC PROCEDURES
Nighttime sleep study (polysomnogram)
◊ Shows repetitive episodes of cessation or marked reduction in airflow despite continued respiratory efforts
◊ These apneic episodes must last at least 10 seconds and occur at least 10-15 times per hour to be considered clinically significant
◊ Polysomnogram demonstrates severity of hypoxemia, sleep disruption and cardiac arrhythmias associated with OSA

TREATMENT

APPROPRIATE HEALTH CARE
Outpatient for treatment or sleep study; inpatient for surgery

GENERAL MEASURES
• An OSA present only when supine - keep patient off the back (e.g., tennis ball sewn on nightshirt)
• Mild to moderate OSA - surgery (tonsillectomy or uvulopalatopharyngoplasty [UPPP]), dental appliances or nasal continuous positive airway pressure (CPAP)
• Moderate to severe OSA - CPAP is the standard therapy
• Severe OSA that is not controllable with nasal CPAP or UPPP - tracheostomy or craniofacial surgery (mandibular advancement)
• Avoid driving if EDS significant
• No alcohol within 6 hours of bedtime
• Avoid sedatives and sleeping pills

ACTIVITY No restrictions

DIET Obese patients must lose weight. All patients must avoid weight gain and alcohol.

PATIENT EDUCATION
• Stress the fact that obesity can be the cause of OSA and weight loss may "cure" the condition
• Necessity to avoid alcohol and sedatives
• Stress the dangers of driving while suffering EDS

Sleep apnea, obstructive

 MEDICATIONS

DRUG(S) OF CHOICE Protriptyline (10-30 mg/d) can be useful adjunct in the management of OSA (especially OSA in REM sleep) and to improve EDS
Contraindications: None
Precautions: May cause or exacerbate narrow angle glaucoma or urinary retention. Use with caution in patients with supraventricular tachycardia.
Significant possible interactions: See manufacturer's profile of each drug

ALTERNATIVE DRUGS
Medroxyprogesterone is helpful in Pickwickian patients with both daytime alveolar hypoventilation and OSA

 FOLLOWUP

PATIENT MONITORING Physician followup improves compliance with CPAP therapy. Observe for return of snoring, EDS, or sleep disruption which may indicate inadequate control of apneas.

PREVENTION/AVOIDANCE See Patient education

POSSIBLE COMPLICATIONS
• Untreated OSA can be associated with development of pulmonary hypertension, ventricular arrhythmias, cor pulmonale, CHF
• Significant morbidity and mortality due to accidents caused by EDS and inattentiveness
• Acute blood pressure elevations

EXPECTED COURSE AND PROGNOSIS
• With appropriate control of apneas, EDS dramatically improves within a week
• All therapeutic measures other than surgery and aggressive weight loss in obese patients are methods of apnea control, rather than cure. Lifelong compliance with weight loss or nasal CPAP are necessary for therapy of OSA.
• Untreated, OSA appears to progress in severity
• Death due to OSA usually secondary to arrhythmias, cardiac ischemia or hypertensive complications

 MISCELLANEOUS

ASSOCIATED CONDITIONS
• Hypertension
• Arteriosclerotic vascular disease
• Coronary arterial disease
• Diabetes
• Obesity
• Nasal obstructive problems
• Acromegaly
• Hypothyroidism

AGE-RELATED FACTORS
Pediatric: OSA uncommon in pediatric age group. If present, often due to tonsillar enlargement, response to tonsillectomy often good.
Geriatric: OSA appears to increase in frequency after middle age and after the menopause in women. Often coexists with other health problems in the elderly.
Others: N/A

PREGNANCY Rare

SYNONYMS
• Pickwickian syndrome
• Sleep apnea syndrome
• Nocturnal upper airway occlusion

ICD-9-CM 306.1 psycogenic apnea

OTHER NOTES OSA rare in premenopausal women unless there is coexistent morbid obesity or neurologic/craniofacial abnormalities

SEE ALSO N/A

OTHER NOTES N/A

ABBREVIATIONS
• CPAP = continuous positive airway pressure
• UPPP = uvulopalatopharyngoplasty
• EDS = excessive daytime sleepiness
• OSA = obstructive sleep apnea

REFERENCES
• Kryger, M.H.: Principles and Practice of Sleep Medicine. Philadelphia, W.B. Saunders Co., 1989
• Thorpy, M.J.: Handbook of Sleep Disorders. New York, Marcel Dekker Inc., 1990

Author M. Klink, M.D.

Snake envenomations: Crotalidae

BASICS

DESCRIPTION Symptom complex occurring following human envenomation by a snake of the family Crotalidae (pit vipers)
• These include those of the genus Crotalus (rattlesnakes), Agkistrodon (moccasins) and Sistrurus (pygmy rattlesnakes). Occurs most commonly in southeastern and southwestern US.
• These snakes characteristically have triangular-shaped heads, eyes with elliptical pupils, and small heat-sensing facial pits located between the nostril and the eye
Genetics: N/A
Incidence in USA: 3.2/100,000. 8,000 bites/year (20-25% of bites do not result in envenomation)
Prevalence in USA: N/A
Predominant age: 19-30 years
Predominant sex: Male > Female

SIGNS AND SYMPTOMS
• These vary by species; prevalence as stated refers to family as whole
• Fang marks (may be two or only one) (> 90%)
• Pain out of proportion to puncture wound (> 50%)
• Edema of site, progressing proximally up extremity (> 50%)
• Weakness, dizziness (> 50%)
• Numbness/tingling in extremity, in mouth, tongue (> 50%)
• Ecchymosis of skin, vesiculations around bite (> 50%)
• Tachycardia (> 50%)
• Nausea/vomiting (< 50%)
• Hypo/Hypertension (< 50%)
• Muscle fasciculations (< 50%)
• Mental status changes including coma (< 25%)
• Elevated creatine kinase (CPK)

CAUSES Pit viper venom is a complex mixture which contains cytotoxins, hemotoxins, neurotoxins, and cardiotoxins

RISK FACTORS
• Risk taking behaviors
• Acute ethanol intoxication or intoxication with other drugs which impair judgment

DIAGNOSIS

DIFFERENTIAL DIAGNOSIS Bite of non-venomous snake, bite of venomous species other than from Crotalidae family

LABORATORY
• CBC (Hgb/Hct decreased in < 50%)
• PT/PTT (prolonged in > 50%)
• Fibrinogen (decreased in < 50%), fibrin degradation products (increased in < 50%)
• Urinalysis - glycosuria (< 50%), proteinuria (< 25%), hematuria (< 25%)
• Decrease in blood platelets (< 50%)
• Type and crossmatch "to hold" in severe envenomations
• Electrolytes, blood urea nitrogen, creatinine
• Creatine kinase in severe envenomations
• Serum ethanol level if suspicious
Drugs that may alter lab results:
Anticoagulants
Disorders that may alter lab results: N/A

PATHOLOGICAL FINDINGS N/A

SPECIAL TESTS N/A

IMAGING N/A

DIAGNOSTIC PROCEDURES If suspicious of developing compartment syndrome, measure compartment pressures (rarely needed)

TREATMENT

APPROPRIATE HEALTH CARE
Patients with true envenomations and resulting signs/symptoms need Emergency Department evaluation with admission if necessary

GENERAL MEASURES
• Support vital signs
• Reassurance
• Remove rings and constrictive items proximal to site of envenomation
• Place affected injured part at level of heart
• Evaluate all pre-hospital care. If tourniquet has been placed in pre-hospital setting, sudden removal could "bolus" patient with venom.
• Obtain toxicology consultation by contacting American Association of Poison Center (AAPCC) Regional Poison Information Center for your area
Level 1:
◊ If local signs of edema are confined to area of bite without any other symptom of envenomation, place intravenous line of crystalloid at maintenance rates (if no history of renal or heart disease requiring fluid restriction) and draw laboratory studies
◊ Place reference marks for measuring circumference of extremity at 10 cm and 20 cm proximal to site of envenomation
◊ Measure every 15 minutes and trace leading edge of swelling
◊ Give tetanus toxoid
◊ Pain relief with opiate or acetaminophen (avoid aspirin)
◊ Repeat laboratory studies in six hours. If all remain normal and swelling does not progress, observe 8-12 hours then follow as outpatient.
◊ If swelling progresses or systemic signs and symptoms appear will need admission and further therapy (progresses to Level 2)
Level 2:
◊ If edema, vesiculations, erythema progress beyond the immediate bite area and there are associated systemic signs/symptoms or laboratory abnormalities (as above), all therapy as in Level 1 above plus intravenous antivenom
◊ Intensive care monitoring may be necessary in most institutions
◊ Repeat laboratory evaluations every 6 hours initially until stable, then less frequently
◊ Continue to monitor vital signs and circumference of affected part

ACTIVITY Bedrest with extremity elevated to level of atria

DIET Nothing by mouth initially

PATIENT EDUCATION Snake bite prevention and first aid.

MEDICATIONS

DRUG(S) OF CHOICE
Polyvalent Crotalidae antivenin
◊ First administer skin test according to product brochure. If negative, prepare five vials of antivenin in 250 mL normal saline IV fluid.
◊ Begin infusion at 3-5 mL/hr and, if no systemic reaction occurs, increase until a rate of 180-240 mL/hr is achieved (one vial every 15-20 minutes)
◊ Give by continuous infusion, not IV push
◊ If signs/symptoms continue to progress rapidly following the first 5 vials, repeat dose of 5 vials. Severe envenomations may require up to 30 vials.

Contraindications:
• History of allergy to horse serum product
• If skin test positive, and antivenin is necessary to save life or limb, contact Poison Information Center. Pretreatment with antihistamines, steroids, etc., in ICU setting may make antivenin administration possible.

Precautions:
• Have equipment and medications readily at hand to treat anaphylaxis
• Avoid aspirin or other anticoagulants
Significant possible interactions: N/A

ALTERNATIVE DRUGS
• Blood products only necessary for coagulopathies with clinical bleeding, not for treatment of laboratory abnormalities
• Steroid use is controversial.

FOLLOWUP

PATIENT MONITORING
• First return visit within 48 hours, then as clinically indicated
• Physical therapy referral should be made early for optimal outpatient intervention

PREVENTION/AVOIDANCE
• Use of preventive measures if handling snakes
In snake-infested areas
• Wear protective shoes and clothing when walking
• Do not insert hands or feet into cracks or crevices or hollow logs
• Carry a flashlight if walking at night

POSSIBLE COMPLICATIONS
• Serum sickness from antivenom therapy (perhaps in > 50%)
• Local wound infection

EXPECTED COURSE AND
PROGNOSIS If properly treated, mortality is very rare. Morbidity rare.

MISCELLANEOUS

ASSOCIATED CONDITIONS Underlying health of patient

AGE-RELATED FACTORS
Pediatric: Course may be more severe
Geriatric: Course may be more severe
Others: N/A

PREGNANCY N/A

SYNONYMS
• Snakebite
• Venomous snakebite
• Pit viper snake bite

ICD-9-CM 989.5 venomous snake bite

SEE ALSO Snake envenomations: Elapidae

OTHER NOTES N/A

ABBREVIATIONS N/A

REFERENCES
• Ellenhorn, M.J. & Barceloux, D.G.: Medical Toxicology: Diagnosis and Treatment of Human Poisoning. New York, Elsevier, 1988; 1113-1126
• Russell, F.E.: Snake Venom Poisoning. Philadelphia, J.B. Lippincott, 1980
• Kurecki, B.A. & Brownlee, H.J.: Venomous snakebites in the United States. J Fam Prac, 1987; 25(4):386-392

Author G. Gaar, M.D.

Snake envenomations: Elapidae

 BASICS

 DIAGNOSIS

 TREATMENT

BASICS

DESCRIPTION Symptom complex occurring following human envenomation by a snake of the family Elapidae
• In the United States these include the genera Micrurus and Micruroides, commonly called "Coral Snakes." The Sonoran or Arizona coral snake is found mainly in Arizona (Micruroides euryxanthus), the Texas coral snake (Micrurus fulvius tenere) in Texas, Arkansas, and Louisiana, and the eastern coral snake (Micrurus fulvius fulvius) throughout the Southeastern United States.
• The snakes have a characteristic rounded head with round pupils. Coloration is important in that in the U.S. broad rings of red and black are separated by narrow rings of yellow. ("Red on yellow, kill a fellow; red on black, venom lack.")
• Unlike Crotalidae envenomations, local signs and symptoms are mild in envenomation of Elapidae, even those which prove to be severe envenomations. Neurologic symptoms may be delayed; they have been reported to develop up to 12 or more hours after the envenomation.
Genetics: N/A
Incidence/Prevalence in USA: Unknown
Predominant age: 19-30 years
Predominant sex: Male > Female

SIGNS AND SYMPTOMS
• Fang marks; may be shallow or appear as scratch (> 75%)
• Local swelling (<50%)
• Numbness/change in sensation (< 50%)
• Nausea/vomiting (< 50%)
• Weakness (< 25%)
• Dizziness (< 15%)
• Diplopia (< 15%)
• Muscle fasciculations (< 15%)

CAUSES Venom is primarily a neurotoxin. Little or no cytotoxin to cause local tissue reaction.

RISK FACTORS Coral snakes are nocturnal and timid. Therefore they rarely bite humans. They must be deliberately provoked to bite.

DIAGNOSIS

DIFFERENTIAL DIAGNOSIS
• Bite of other venomous snake (Crotalidae) without envenomation ("dry bite")
• Bite of a non-venomous snake

LABORATORY
• Creatine kinase (CPK) often elevated
• Blood ethanol level often elevated
• Laboratory not diagnostic
Drugs that may alter lab results: N/A
Disorders that may alter lab results: N/A

PATHOLOGICAL FINDINGS N/A

SPECIAL TESTS None

IMAGING N/A

DIAGNOSTIC PROCEDURES N/A

TREATMENT

APPROPRIATE HEALTH CARE All patients with suspected coral snake envenomation need Emergency Department evaluation

GENERAL MEASURES
• All patients who have 1) confirmed bite by a snake identified as a coral snake, 2) history of the snake's having chewed on the person, and, 3) visible fang marks which pierce the epidermis, should be admitted to hospital for intensive care monitoring
• In this group of patients, perform a skin test for horse serum sensitivity. If negative, antivenom to Micrurus fulvius should be given early, even if there are no neurologic signs or symptoms present.
• If skin test is positive, and neurological symptoms are rapidly progressing, admission to ICU is indicated
• Pretreatment with IV diphenhydramine, steroids, and other antihistamines may allow for infusion of antivenom, although it is not clear from the literature if antivenom should be administered in light of a positive skin test. In this instance, obtain toxicology consultation from the American Association of Poison Control Centers (AAPCC) certified Poison Information Center for your area.
• Support vital signs, intubation may be necessary if respiratory compromise ensues
• Good supportive care with cardiac, respiratory, neurological monitoring
• Reassurance
• Immobilize extremity and keep at level of atria
• Contact AAPCC Regional Center for your area

ACTIVITY Bedrest initially. May need physical therapy in severe cases of envenomation.

DIET Nothing by mouth initially

PATIENT EDUCATION N/A

MEDICATIONS

DRUG(S) OF CHOICE
• There is no antivenom available for Micruroides euryxanthus
• Tetanus booster if necessary
• Antivenom to the North American coral snake (Micrurus fulvius)

◊ Is available commercially. It is a horse serum product and is effective only for the envenomation of the Texas and eastern coral snakes (Micrurus fulvius tenere and Micrurus fulvius fulvius).

◊ If patients meet the criteria above (see General Measures), skin test should be performed according to directions taken from package insert. If negative, 4-6 vials of the antivenom should be reconstituted and diluted into 250 mL of normal saline. Begin infusion at 3-5 mL/hr and, if no systemic reaction occurs, increase until a rate of 1 diluted vial is being given every thirty minutes.

◊ Envenomations with more severe sequelae or prolonged sequelae may require larger doses of antivenom. Unfortunately it is impossible to specify dosage more specifically.

Contraindications: History of allergy to horse serum
Precautions: Have equipment and medications readily at hand to treat anaphylaxis
Significant possible interactions: N/A

ALTERNATIVE DRUGS
Steroid use is controversial.

FOLLOWUP

PATIENT MONITORING
First return visit within 48 hours, then as clinically indicated

PREVENTION/AVOIDANCE
• Use of preventive measures if handling snakes
In snake-infested areas:
◊ Wear protective shoes and clothing when walking
◊ Do not insert hands or feet into cracks or crevices or hollow logs
◊ Carry a flashlight if walking at night

POSSIBLE COMPLICATIONS
• Serum sickness from antivenom therapy (perhaps in 10% or more)
• Local wound infection
• Aspiration pneumonia

EXPECTED COURSE AND PROGNOSIS
• Neurologic deterioration may progress despite antivenom administration. Complete paralysis can occur.
• Early, elective intubation during progression of paralysis may help to prevent aspiration pneumonia
• Discharge should not occur until the patient has made neurologic recovery to the point that there is no concern of respiratory failure
• Muscle strength may not return to normal for 4-6 weeks
• Long-term morbidity rare
• Mortality does occur even with antivenom therapy

MISCELLANEOUS

ASSOCIATED CONDITIONS
N/A

AGE-RELATED FACTORS
Pediatric: Not well described
Geriatric: Morbidity and danger of mortality is greater
Others: N/A

PREGNANCY
N/A

SYNONYMS
• Neurotoxic snake bite
• Snakebite

ICD-9-CM
989.5 venomous snake bite

SEE ALSO
Snake envenomation: Crotalidae

OTHER NOTES
N/A

ABBREVIATIONS
N/A

REFERENCES
• Kitchens, C.S. & Van Mierop, L.H.S.: Envenomation by the eastern coral snake (Micrurus fulvius fulvius). JAMA, 1987; 258(12):1615-1618
• Russell, F.E.: Snake Venom Poisoning. Philadelphia, J.B. Lippincott, 1980
• Ellenhorn, M.J. & Barceloux, D.G.: Medical Toxicology: Diagnosis and Treatment of Human Poisoning. New York, Elsevier, 1988; 1127-1128

Author G. Gaar, M.D.

Sporotrichosis

 BASICS

DESCRIPTION
Subacute or chronic fungal infection occurring in 4 forms: cutaneous or lymphocutaneous, pulmonary, osteo-articular, or disseminated and rarely musculoskeletal (joint and tendon by puncture wounds). Most likely to occur in farmers, horticulturists, gardeners. Cutaneous lesions occur 20-90 days after cutaneous inoculation.

System(s) affected: Skin, Hemic/Lymphatic/Immunologic, Bone/Joint

Genetics: No known genetic pattern

Incidence/Prevalence in USA: N/A

Predominant age: Adults

Predominant sex: Male > Female (mostly due to occupational exposure)

SIGNS AND SYMPTOMS
Cutaneous or lymphocutaneous:
◊ Characteristic skin lesions, beginning as an inoculation chancre, or erythematous plaque with satellite, small papule, painless, movable, subcutaneous nodules in a linear distribution. Progress to larger nodules which may ulcerate and drain. Affects primarily upper extremities.
◊ Additional lesions spread proximally along lymphatics
Pulmonary
◊ Cough, occasionally productive
◊ Cavitary lung disease
◊ Hilar adenopathy
◊ Signs and symptoms indistinguishable from other chronic pneumonias
Osteo-articular
◊ Subacute or chronic inflammatory arthritis, often monoarticular, may persist for many years
◊ Signs and symptoms of osteomyelitis
◊ Generally afebrile
Disseminated
◊ Multifocal skin lesions
◊ Polyarticular arthritis
◊ Weight loss
◊ Chronic lymphocytic meningitis

CAUSES
Infection with Sporothrix schenckii, a fungus found in soil, sphagnum peat moss, and decaying vegetation. Infection acquired by direct inoculation (usual) or inhalation (rare).

RISK FACTORS
• Gardening - contact with mulch, sphagnum moss, hay, timber, thorny bushes
• Occupations handling gardening materials, such as nursery workers, landscapers, florists, carpenters
• Animal handlers (transmission from animals to humans has been documented, especially cats)
• Immunocompromised (drugs or HIV infection)
• Alcoholism (pulmonary and disseminated)

 DIAGNOSIS

DIFFERENTIAL DIAGNOSIS
Cutaneous or Lymphocutaneous
◊ Sporotrichoid nocardiosis
◊ Leishmaniasis
◊ Atypical mycobacterial infection (M. marinum, M chelonae, M. kansasii)
◊ Tularemia
Pulmonary
◊ Tuberculosis
◊ Sarcoidosis
◊ Chronic fungal pneumonia
◊ Neoplasm
Osteo-articular
◊ Rheumatoid arthritis
◊ Bacterial arthritis/osteomyelitis

LABORATORY
• Culture of S. schenckii in sputum, pus, or bone drainage
• Organism found with difficulty with PAS and Gomori stains of skin or other biopsied lesions
• Serum antibody tests may be useful for extracutaneous disease

Drugs that may alter lab results:
Antifungal drugs

Disorders that may alter lab results: N/A

PATHOLOGICAL FINDINGS
Granulomas with central necrosis

SPECIAL TESTS
Immunohistochemical staining of biopsy specimens

IMAGING
Chest and skeletal x-rays

DIAGNOSTIC PROCEDURES
• Careful history and physical
• Culture of draining lesions
• Culture of inflammatory joint effusions or sputum
• Biopsy if diagnosis not confirmed

 TREATMENT

APPROPRIATE HEALTH CARE
• Many patients can be managed on outpatient basis
• Hospitalization for adjunctive surgical procedures or initiation of amphotericin B therapy

GENERAL MEASURES
• Local heat application useful for cutaneous and lymphocutaneous disease
• Keep cutaneous lesions clean
• Repeated drainage of infected joints may be indicated
• Synovectomy of infected joints may be indicated
• Surgical debridement of osteomyelitis usually indicated

ACTIVITY
No restrictions

DIET
No special diet

PATIENT EDUCATION
Patients should be advised of the nature of the infection, the toxicities associated with therapy, and the need for sustained therapy

MEDICATIONS

DRUG(S) OF CHOICE
• Cutaneous or lymphocutaneous: Potassium iodide saturated solution (SSKI), initially 10 drops orally tid increased by 1 drop each dose to maximum tolerated dose or 120 drops/day. Dilute in a beverage to disguise taste. Continue for 1-2 months after all lesions have healed
• Extracutaneous disease: IV amphotericin B, 1.5-2.5 g total dose
Contraindications: SSKI contraindicated in tuberculosis
Precautions:
• Amphotericin B can cause fever, chills, nausea and vomiting. Dosage varies for sex and age groups. Refer to manufacturer's literature for precautions, adverse effects and interactions.
• SSKI requires extra care if patient also has tuberculosis, kidney disease or hyperthyroidism
Significant possible interactions:
Hyperpotassemia if SSKI taken concurrently with amiloride, spironolactone or triamterene

ALTERNATIVE DRUGS
• Ketoconazole 400 mg orally daily may be effective alternative therapy in immunocompetent hosts
• Fluconazole 800 mg per day orally or intravenously is a potential alternative agent currently under investigation
• Itraconazole 200 to 400 mg orally daily is promising but inadequately studied for a definitive recommendation

 FOLLOWUP

PATIENT MONITORING
Check for compliance with long-term drugs (SSKI should be continued for 1-2 months after lesions heal)

PREVENTION/AVOIDANCE
• Avoid endemic areas
• Wear gloves when working in soil

POSSIBLE COMPLICATIONS
• Secondary bacterial infection
• Bone and joint deformities from osteo-articular disease

EXPECTED COURSE AND PROGNOSIS
• Prognosis is excellent for complete recovery from cutaneous or lymphocutaneous infections
• Other disease forms demonstrate a chronic indolent course and are variably responsive to therapy

 MISCELLANEOUS

ASSOCIATED CONDITIONS
See Risk Factors

AGE-RELATED FACTORS
Pediatric: Rare
Geriatric: N/A
Others: N/A

PREGNANCY N/A

SYNONYMS
• Schenck's disease
• Beurmann's disease
• Rose gardener's disease

ICD-9-CM 117.1

SEE ALSO N/A

OTHER NOTES
Rare ocular disease due to direct inoculation

ABBREVIATIONS N/A

REFERENCES
• Winn, R.E.: Sporotrichosis. Infect Dis Clinic North Am 2:899, 1988
• Mandell, G.L. (ed.): Principles and Practice of Infectious Diseases. 3rd Ed. New York, Churchill Livingstone, 1990

Author E. Scott, M.D. & R. Greenfield, M.D.

Sprains and strains

 BASICS

DESCRIPTION

• A sprain is a complete or partial ligamentous injury, either within the body of the ligament or at the site of attachment to bone. It may be classified as Grade I, II, or III. Grades I and II are incomplete tears and differ in severity; Grade III is complete dissolution of the ligamentous connection. Physical exam is key to the diagnosis.
• A strain is partial or complete disruption of the muscle or tendon
• Strains usually are associated with overuse injuries whereas sprains usually occur secondary to trauma (falls, twisting injuries, or motor vehicle accidents)

Genetics: N/A

Incidence/Prevalence in USA:
• Total incidence including spine, upper and lower extremities probably occurs in close to 80% of all atheletes at one point in their career
• Prevalence - approximately 30,000

Predominant age:
• Sprains- any age where patient is physically active
• Strains - usually 15-40

Predominant sex: Male > Female

SIGNS AND SYMPTOMS
• Swelling
• Pain
• Erythema and/or ecchymosis
• Tenderness
• Gait disturbances if severe
• Decreased range of motion of joint and joint instability

CAUSES
• Falls
• Motor vehicle accident
• Trauma
• Excessive exercise or inadequate warm-up and stretching prior to activity
• Poor conditioning

RISK FACTORS
• Improper shoe gear
• Improper or excessive training

 DIAGNOSIS

DIFFERENTIAL DIAGNOSIS
• Sprains must be differentiated from strains, although this is difficult and often the diagnosis is strain/sprain
• Tendonitis
• Bursitis
• Bony injuries
• Rarely, muscle hematomas account for some of the signs and symptoms of strains

LABORATORY N/A
Drugs that may alter lab results: N/A
Disorders that may alter lab results: N/A

PATHOLOGICAL FINDINGS N/A

SPECIAL TESTS
• Exam under anesthesia
• Arthroscopy in some cases
• For ankle, anterior drawer test, which tests the integrity of the anterior talofibular ligament

IMAGING
• X-rays to rule out bony injury and stress views may be helpful
• CT scan of the affected area
• MRI

DIAGNOSTIC PROCEDURES
Sprains
  ◊ Grade I - pain/tenderness of joint without lax ligaments
  ◊ Grade II - pain/tenderness; ecchymosis with lax ligaments but intact joint
  ◊ Grade III - pain/tenderness; swelling and ecchymosis and no end point felt when joint is stressed
Strains
  ◊ Pain and tenderness localized to sight of injury with weakness of involved musculotendinous unit

 TREATMENT

APPROPRIATE HEALTH CARE
Outpatient

GENERAL MEASURES
• Includes initial history and physical exam and treatment of worst possible suspected injury
• RICE therapy - Rest, Ice, Compression, Elevation
• Wrapping with elastic (Ace) bandage, Jone's dressing for more severe injuries
• Casting for Grade III sprains which may require surgery
• "Air Cast" type devices are extremely effective in providing stability and pain relief
• Patient may need crutches and crutch gait training

ACTIVITY
• Bedrest for acute injuries
• Physical therapy for more severe injuries
• Elevate joint while sleeping

DIET No special diet

PATIENT EDUCATION
• Instructions on how to wrap with elastic bandage
• Prevention of injury

MEDICATIONS

DRUG(S) OF CHOICE Nonsteroidal anti-inflammatories (NSAID's)
Contraindications: Refer to manufacturer's profile of each drug
Precautions: Refer to manufacturer's profile of each drug
Significant possible interactions: Refer to manufacturer's profile of each drug

ALTERNATIVE DRUGS Painkillers acutely for severe pain (non-narcotics and/or narcotics as warranted)

FOLLOWUP

PATIENT MONITORING After initial treatment, consider rehabilitation. Direct emphasis towards limiting swelling and providing a pain-free full range of motion.

PREVENTION/AVOIDANCE
• Maintaining a reasonable level of physical fitness
• Avoidance of excessive physical stresses and wearing of proper exercise gear (particularly shoes). Using proper equipment for the activity.
• Knowledge of the risks associated with the intended activity
• Appropriate conditioning, warm-up and cool-down exercises

POSSIBLE COMPLICATIONS
• Chronic joint instability
• Arthritis

EXPECTED COURSE AND PROGNOSIS
With appropriate treatment and rest, 6-8 weeks or longer for recovery, depending on severity of injury

MISCELLANEOUS

ASSOCIATED CONDITIONS
Hemarthrosis, stress, avulsion, or other fractures, syndesmotic injuries, contusions, wounds, dislocations

AGE-RELATED FACTORS
Pediatric: Sprains and strains accounted for 24% of injuries in an analysis of 1,124 sports injuries of children in a study done in West Germany, 1980-82
Geriatric: More likely to see associated bony injuries due to decreased joint flexibility and prevalence of osteoporosis and osteopenia
Others: N/A

PREGNANCY N/A

SYNONYMS N/A

ICD-9-CM 848.9

SEE ALSO N/A

OTHER NOTES N/A

ABBREVIATIONS N/A

REFERENCES
• Kvist, M., Kujala, V.M., Heinonen, O.J., Vuori, I.V., Aho, A.J., Pajulo, O., Hintsa, A. & Parvinen, T.: Sports related injuries in children. IJSM 1989;10(2):81-86
• Strong, W.B., Stanitski, E.L., Smith, R.E. & Wilmore, J.H.: Diagnosis and treatment of ankle sprains. AJDC 1990;144:809-814
• Ruda, S.: Sports Nursing. In Nursing Clinics of North America. Philadelphia, W.B. Saunders Co., Mar, 1991

Author T. Robinson, D.O. & R. Birrer, M.D.

Status epilepticus

BASICS

DESCRIPTION Epileptic seizures that are so frequently repeated or so prolonged as to create a fixed and lasting epileptic condition. Tonic-clonic (grand mal) status epilepticus (SEp) is the most common and most serious form. SEp is a life-threatening emergency
System(s) affected: Nervous
Genetics: Unknown
Incidence/Prevalence in USA: 25-60 new cases/100,000/yr
• 1/3 as unprovoked first seizure
• 1/3 in patients with known epilepsy
• 1/3 secondary to an acute CNS insult
Predominant age: 85% of new cases of SEp occur in patients under age five. Risk is also increased in those over age 60
Predominant sex: Male = Female

SIGNS AND SYMPTOMS
• Depend on the duration and type of seizure
• Recurrent tonic-clonic convulsions: May be preceded by aura. Tonic phase (stiffening) for 30 to 45 seconds. Clonic phase (rhythmic jerking) for 2-5 minutes. No intervening consciousness before seizure recurs. (For additional seizure types see Other Notes).
• Associated autonomic phenomena: Excess catecholamines, glandular hypersecretion, piloerection, cyclic pupillary dilation, and prolonged apnea (may lead to cyanosis)
• Metabolic changes: Lactic acidosis, carbon dioxide narcosis, hyperkalemia, hyperglycemia - followed by hypoglycemia
• Cardiopulmonary changes: Hypertension, arrhythmias, high output failure, pulmonary edema, aspiration pneumonia
• Renal complications: Acute tubular necrosis resulting from myoglobinuria after rhabdomyolysis
• Cerebrovascular changes: Loss of autoregulation, focal ischemia, cerebral edema
• Postictal findings: Fever, tachycardia, mydriasis, conjugate deviation of eyes, decreased corneal reflex, positive Babinski's sign, fecal and urinary incontinence and tongue lacerations

CAUSES
• Search for the primary pathology is essential
• Febrile convulsions (especially in children)
• Acute CNS injury - trauma, infection, mass lesion or metabolic disorder (includes anticonvulsant withdrawal)
• Idiopathic
• Intoxication - multiple agents
• Chronic CNS injury - previous trauma, stroke, infection, encephalopathy (hypoxic or other chronic or degenerative type)

RISK FACTORS
Known seizure disorder plus any precipitating insult. Prior history of SEp (recurrence rate is 17% in children; 50% in those with neurologic abnormality).

DIAGNOSIS

DIFFERENTIAL DIAGNOSIS
• Pseudostatus may occur in a patient with pseudoseizures; avoid potentially dangerous therapy
• Tonic/clonic status is usually apparent. Other forms of status may require detailed neurologic examination and EEG analysis. (See Other Notes).
• Primary diagnostic problem is differentiation of the underlying pathology

LABORATORY
Glucose, electrolytes, calcium and osmolarity; arterial blood gases; toxicology screen; serum levels of anticonvulsants; liver and renal function.
Drugs that may alter lab results: N/A
Disorders that may alter lab results: N/A

PATHOLOGICAL FINDINGS Variable

SPECIAL TESTS
EEG will differentiate pseudoseizures and prolonged seizures not classically recognized as status.

IMAGING
CT scan, MRI may detect mass lesions or injuries

DIAGNOSTIC PROCEDURES
Lumbar puncture may detect subarachnoid bleeding or infection. CAUTION - intra cranial pressure may be increased.

TREATMENT

APPROPRIATE HEALTH CARE
Tonic-clonic status epilepticus is an emergency and should be stopped within 60 minutes. Patients with status seizures require hospitalization to rule out underlying pathology and to assure seizure control. An anesthesiologist, intensivist, neurologist, and/or neurosurgeon may be required.

GENERAL MEASURES
• Assure adequate airway and oxygenation
• Monitor circulation and respiration: ECG, blood pressure, pulse oximetry, end-tidal CO2
• Observe and confirm fit is SEp
• Establish intravenous access (or for child: intraosseous) and obtain initial lab studies
• Evaluate by history and physical exam
• Initiate anticonvulsant therapy to end seizure; then add maintenance therapy
• Diagnose and treat any underlying pathology

ACTIVITY Protect the patient from injury

DIET NPO, maintenance IV of lactated Ringer's or normal saline

PATIENT EDUCATION N/A

MEDICATIONS

DRUG(S) OF CHOICE
• Depend on the type of seizure
• Tonic-clonic SEp is the most serious and may be approached as follows (For other types, see Other Notes)
Stabilization:
Clear the airway and give nasal oxygen. Monitor: ECG, blood pressure, oximetry. Prepare for endotracheal intubation. Give:
• Thiamin: 100mg IV or IM
• 50% Glucose: 50ml IV [for child: use D25W give 2-4ml/kg (0.5-1 g/kg) IV slowly]
• Naloxone (Narcan): 2 mg IV (for child: 0.1 mg/kg IV, up to 2 mg)
To stop seizure (IV available):
Give BOTH:
• Diazepam (Valium): up to 0.25mg/kg IV at 5mg/min; may repeat q5-10 min up to 30mg total. (For child: Max = 10mg for age > 5 years, Max = 5mg for age < 5 years)
AND
• Phenytoin (Dilantin): 18mg/kg IV at a rate of < 50mg/min with ECG monitoring (slow to 25mg/min in patients > 60 years old or with cardiac history). Repeat 100-150mg q30min, up to 1.5gm. (for child: 15-20mg/kg IV at a rate of 0.5-1.5mg/kg/min. May repeat 1.5 mg/kg IV q30min up to 20mg/kg).

To stop seizure (IV not available):
Give BOTH:
• Midazolam (Versed): 0.20 mg/kg IM, (onset is rapid)
• Intraosseous infusion may be used in small children for benzodiazepines, phenytoin, and phenobarbital - doses are the same as IV
If seizures persist:
• Perform nasal or oral endotracheal intubation; monitor EEG and end-tidal CO2; then give:
• Phenobarbital (Luminal): 10-20 mg/kg IV at a rate of < 50 mg/min (decrease to 25 mg/min for old age or cardiac history). If no response in 20 min, repeat dose of 120-240 mg IV, to a maximum of 1-2 g/24 hr. (For child: 20 mg/kg IV at a rate of 25-50 mg/min. If no response in 20 min, repeat dose of 6 mg/kg IV, up to total of 40 mg/kg/24 hr.)
OR
• Give Diazepam: IV drip at 4-8 mg/hr
If seizures still persist:
• Administer general anesthesia with a short acting barbiturate adjusted to obtain a burst suppression pattern EEG
• Requires continuous respiratory and cardiovascular monitoring and support
• Alternatives include:
◊ pentobarbital: induction dose 5 mg/kg IV or until EEG seizure activity is suppressed. Maintenance dose: 1-3 mg/kg/hr, adjusted according to the EEG response
◊ thiopental: induction dose: 3-6 mg/kg IV, then add 50mg IV q 2-5 min to produce EEG burst suppression. Maintenance dose: IV drip of 0.2% solution adjusted to keep EEG at burst suppression.

Contraindications:
• Review current package inserts
• Benzodiazepines (diazepam, lorazepam, midazolam) - in acute narrow-angle glaucoma
• Barbiturates - in acute intermittent porphyria

Precautions:
• Endotracheal intubation may be necessary
• Reduce dosage of depressants in patients with shock, coma or alcoholic intoxication
• Diazepam: apnea may occur with rapid IV injection, especially in patients receiving barbiturates. Venous thrombosis and phlebitis can occur at injection site. Reduce dose in the elderly and hepatic insufficiency. Reduced dose not required in renal failure.
• Phenobarbital: caution in pulmonary insufficiency, hepatic disease and pregnancy. Withdrawal seizures may occur following abrupt termination of high doses. Increase the dosing interval in renal failure. Reduce dose in severe liver disease.
• Phenytoin - monitor ECG for arrhythmias, prolonged QT interval, and hypotension. If these occur, decrease the rate of administration. Use with caution in pregnancy (increased risk of malformations), liver disease, hyperglycemia, and elderly patients. Abrupt withdrawal may precipitate status. Use in normal or half normal saline to prevent precipitation that occurs in dextrose solutions. Overdose may cause paradoxical inefficacy

Significant possible interactions:
• Each of the drugs listed may potentiate the effects of other CNS depressants.
• Phenobarbital - may reduce the efficacy of quinidine and warfarin; induces metabolism of phenytoin
• Phenytoin - increased serum levels and toxicity may occur with concomitant warfarin, disulfiram, phenylbutazone, and isoniazid

ALTERNATIVE DRUGS
Alternate benzodiazepines:
◊ Lorazepam (Ativan) (longer acting) 4 mg IV over 2 min (0.1 mg/kg) (pediatric: 0.05 to 0.1 mg/kg IV at rate of 1 mL/min)
◊ Midazolam (Versed) (more rapidly acting); sedation - 0.125 mg/kg IV(< 2 mg/min); anesthesia induction dose - 0.2-0.5 mg/kg IV
Second line drugs:
◊ Lidocaine (Xylocaine): 1 to 3 mg/kg IV bolus; maintenance 3 to 10 mg/kg/hr
◊ Valproic acid: 500 mg via nasogastric tube or 500 mg with 300 mL water via rectal tube (clamp for 15 minutes)
◊ Paraldehyde: 0.3 mL (300 mg)/kg (usual dose is 4-8mL) per rectum diluted in an 2 volumes of cotton seed or olive oil to prevent mucosal irritation (mix in glass only since paraldehyde will decompose plastic). Rectal adsorption is slow; peak levels may not occur for 2-4hrs. May also be given by gastric tube. (Though sometimes recommended IV or IM, no parenteral preparation is commercially available in the US)
Investigational drugs:
◊ Isoflurane by inhalation
◊ Phenytoin prodrug (ACC-9653) IV and IM
◊ Propofol by continuous IV infusion
◊ Etomidate by continuous IV infusion
◊ Chlormethiazol by IV infusion
◊ Resection of the epileptogenic zone

 ## FOLLOWUP

PATIENT MONITORING Therapeutic blood levels of anticonvulsants

PREVENTION/AVOIDANCE Once seizures are controlled, establish a maintenance regimen of anticonvulsants

POSSIBLE COMPLICATIONS
• Morbidity and mortality are related to the acute CNS insult, stress, injury from repeated seizures
• Causes of death - cardiopulmonary arrest, renal failure, hyperthermia, aspiration pneumonia, the underlying pathology or the treatment instituted
• Anticonvulsants cause both respiratory and cardiovascular depression

EXPECTED COURSE AND PROGNOSIS Mortality is 6-18% (lower in children), usually related to the underlying cause. Prolonged seizures (> 30-60 min) may cause neurologic injury or even death.

 ## MISCELLANEOUS

ASSOCIATED CONDITIONS
Etiology or underlying pathology associated with SEp varies significantly by age group. In adults, usually related to a known condition: e.g., established epilepsy, alcohol withdrawal or acquired CNS lesion (especially frontal).

AGE-RELATED FACTORS
Pediatric:
• Lower mortality rate
More likely present in SEp as their first seizure due to:
◊ Febrile seizure
◊ New onset epilepsy (idiopathic)
◊ CNS infection
◊ Metabolic derangement
Geriatric: More likely to have SEp secondary to a change in drug therapy (noncompliance, drug interaction or toxicity); tend to have localized (often frontal lobe) CNS lesions.
Others: Neonatal status is most often related to meningitis or metabolic disorders (deficiencies of calcium, magnesium, or pyridoxine) and deserves careful workup for the underlying cause

PREGNANCY
• Phenytoin - use with caution (increased risk of malformations in first trimester)
• Phenobarbital - use with caution

SYNONYMS   N/A

ICD-9-CM
• 345.3 grand mal status and status epilepticus NOS
• 345.7 epilepsia partialis continua, psychomotor status and temporal lobe status

SEE ALSO
• Seizure disorders
• Seizures, febrile

OTHER NOTES
Additional forms of status include:
◊ Focal motor status - starts distally with clonic jerking in ascending pattern; eyes and head deviate to side opposite the focus; may progress to generalized status; underlying CNS pathology is common. Treat like tonic-clonic SEp. May respond to carbamazepine.
◊ Epilepsia partialis continua - rapid focal jerking; no loss of consciousness; worsened by voluntary movements; may persist for hours to days; poor response to therapy; often associated with underlying pathology. Pentobarbital and diazepam recommended.
◊ Myoclonic status - sudden spasmodic contraction of limbs; usually secondary to widespread neurologic or metabolic dysfunction; consciousness usually maintained. Treat with diazepam.
◊ Complex partial status (psychomotor status): short seizures with automatisms (e.g., lip smacking, random eye movements, chewing, staring); followed by post ictal confusion. With status, first line treatment is diazepam and phenytoin.
◊ Absence status - varies from mild lethargy to severe confusion, 10 second duration, with no aura, eyes flutter and turn upward, with irregular myoclonic jerks, automatisms, no post ictal confusion; may progress to generalized status. If so, treat as tonic-clonic status.
◊ Neonatal status epilepticus - subtle multifocal, clonic, tonic, and myoclonic features; risk of intracerebral hemorrhage; meningitis and metabolic disorders (deficiencies of calcium, magnesium, pyridoxine) more common. Begin with phenobarbital and diazepam.

ABBREVIATIONS SEp = status epilepticus

REFERENCES
• Honigman, B.: Status Epilepticus (Disease & Trauma Monograph for Acute Care). In EMERGINDEX(R) Information System. Edited by B. Honigman & B.H.Rumack. Denver, Micromedex, Inc., (Edition expired March, 1993)
• Tunik, M.G. & Young, G.M.: Status Epilepticus in Children. Pediatric Clinics of North America, 1992, 39(5):1007-1030
• Engel, J.: Status Epilepticus. In Seizures and Epilepsy. Contemporary Neurology Series; Vol. 31. Philadelphia, F.A. Davis Co., 1989, 256-280
• Uthman, B. & Wilder, B.: Emergency management of seizures: an overview. Epilepsia, 1989; 30(suppl 2):S33-S37

Author J. Gibson, Jr., M.D.

Stevens-Johnson syndrome

BASICS

DESCRIPTION A severe variant of erythema multiforme. Acute, severe, generally self-limited hypersensitivity reaction involving the skin and mucous membranes. It may involve multiple organ systems as complications of the disease.
System(s) affected: Skin/Exocrine
Genetics: Possible association with HLA-B15
Incidence in USA: 0.1/100,000/year
Prevalence in USA: Unknown
Predominant Age: More common in children and young adults
Predominant sex: Males > Females (2:1)

SIGNS AND SYMPTOMS
• Variable and nonspecific prodrome, often with features of upper respiratory tract infection
• Sudden onset, rapidly progressive, pleomorphic rash, with vesicles and bullae
• Nikolsky's sign absent
• Mucous membrane with characteristic vesicles/ulcers
• Stomatitis
• Rash may have features of erythema multiforme
• Burning sensation to skin/mucous membranes, sometimes tenderness of skin also
• Pruritus usually absent
• Fever to 39-40°C (102-104°F)
• Headache
• Malaise
• Arthralgias
• Rhinitis
• Epistaxis
• Crusting of nares
• Conjunctivitis
• Corneal ulcerations
• Erosive vulvovaginitis, or balanitis
• Cough
• Thick mucopurulent sputum
• Tachypnea/respiratory distress
• Hematuria
• Albuminuria
• Arrhythmias
• Pericarditis
• Congestive heart failure
• Mental status changes
• Seizures
• Coma
• Sepsis
• Electrolyte disturbances

CAUSES
Idiopathic in up to 50% of cases. The remaining 50% may represent a hypersensitivity response to one of the following:
• Viral infections - particularly herpes simplex; also Epstein-Barr, Coxsackie, echovirus, varicella, mumps and poliovirus
• Bacterial infections - especially mycoplasma pneumoniae; also brucellosis, diphtheria, Yersinia, tuberculosis, tularemia, and gonorrhea
• Protozoan infections
• Collagen vascular disease

• Medications - especially sulfonamides, penicillins, anticonvulsants, salicylates
• Vaccines - diphtheria/typhoid, bacillus Calmette-Guerin (BCG), oral polio vaccine (OPV)
• Malignancy
• Pregnancy
• Premenstrual hormonal changes
• Consumption of beer
• Reiter's syndrome
• Sarcoidosis

RISK FACTORS
• Previous history of erythema multiforme/Stevens-Johnson syndrome
• Male sex

DIAGNOSIS

DIFFERENTIAL DIAGNOSIS
• Bullous impetigo
• Graft vs. host disease
• Pemphigus vulgaris
• Pemphigoid
• Septicemia
• Serum sickness
• Hand-foot-mouth disease
• Collagen vascular diseases
• Meningococcemia
• Behçet's syndrome
• Staphylococcal scalded skin syndrome

LABORATORY Culture for suspected sources of infection
Drugs that may alter lab results: N/A
Disorders that may alter lab results: N/A

PATHOLOGICAL FINDINGS Epidermal necrolysis is characteristic. Spongiosis, intracellular edema, vacuolar changes at the dermal-epidermal junction, edema and extravasated erythrocytes in the dermis may also be seen on biopsy specimen.

SPECIAL TESTS None

IMAGING N/A

DIAGNOSTIC PROCEDURES Skin biopsy

TREATMENT

APPROPRIATE HEALTH CARE
Inpatient care, often in the intensive care setting

GENERAL MEASURES
• Withdrawal of any implicated medications or treatment of any identified underlying infection/disease
• Meticulous wound care - use Burow's solution or Domeboro solution dressings
• With extensive skin involvement - reverse isolation and treatment of skin (similar to burn care)
• Supportive care for maintenance of fluid, electrolyte and protein balance
• Empiric antibiotic use not recommended
• Oral lesions: To provide symptomatic relief, oral hygiene; to facilitate oral intake, treat with mouthwashes of warm saline, or a solution of diphenhydramine, Xylocaine, and Kaopectate
• Ophthalmologic consultation for eye care

ACTIVITY Bedrest, until clinically stabilized

DIET As tolerated. Increased fluid intake should be encouraged in those with more extensive skin involvement. Intravenous nutritional support may be required.

PATIENT EDUCATION
• Patients should be reassured that the disease is self-limited
• Recurrences are possible, and avoidance of any identified etiologic agent should be encouraged

MEDICATIONS

DRUG(S) OF CHOICE
• Systemic corticosteroids may provide benefit, particularly in rapidly evolving or more severe cases. Initial dosage equivalent to prednisone 1-2 mg/kg/day with subsequent tapering.
• Provide treatment to any underlying infection or disease
• Empiric antibiotic use not recommended
Contraindications: Any infectious process in which use of steroids would be contraindicated
Precautions: Refer to manufacturer's profile of each drug
Significant possible interactions: Refer to manufacturer's profile of each drug

ALTERNATIVE DRUGS
Acyclovir may be given to suppress recurrent herpetic disease if herpes is identified as the underlying cause

 ## FOLLOWUP

PATIENT MONITORING
The disease is generally self-limited. During the course of the disease, patients should be monitored for signs of secondary infections, dehydration, electrolyte imbalances, and malnutrition.

PREVENTION/AVOIDANCE
• Known or suspected etiologic agents should be avoided
• Acyclovir (used to treat viral infections) may help prevent herpes-related erythema multiforme
• Tamoxifen has been shown to prevent premenstrual related disease

POSSIBLE COMPLICATIONS
• Secondary infections
• Sepsis
• Pneumonia (10-20%)
• Dehydration/electrolyte disturbances
• Acute tubular necrosis
• Ophthalmic complications of corneal ulcerations or iritis
• Arrhythmias
• Death in up to 15% of untreated cases

EXPECTED COURSE AND PROGNOSIS
• Disease may have a rapid onset or evolve over 1-2 weeks with subsequent resolution over 4-6 weeks
• Scarring may result from the skin involvement
• Blindness or corneal opacities may occur in 7-20% of patients
• The mortality rate for untreated cases is 5-15%
• Risk of recurrence may be as high as 37%

 ## MISCELLANEOUS

ASSOCIATED CONDITIONS
• Any of the infections or diseases listed under Causes may be associated with Stevens-Johnson Syndrome
• Toxic epidermal necrolysis
• Erythema multiforme (directly related, but a milder form of the disease)
• Mycoplasma pneumonia

AGE-RELATED FACTORS
Pediatric: More severe forms of the disease tend to occur in younger males. Rare under age 3 years.
Geriatric: Rare over age 50 years
Others: N/A

PREGNANCY
Reported as a possible etiologic condition

SYNONYMS
• Ectodermosis erosiva pluriorificialis
• Febrile mucocutaneous syndrome
• Herpes iris
• Erythema polymorphe

ICD-9-CM 695.1 Stevens-Johnson syndrome

SEE ALSO
• Erythema multiforme
• Bullous impetigo
• Pemphigus vulgaris
• Pemphigoid bullous
• Serum sickness

OTHER NOTES
Because it is an immunologic reaction, drug related disease will not occur until 7-14 days after first exposure to the offending agent. Subsequent exposure may cause reaction to occur more quickly.

ABBREVIATIONS
N/A

REFERENCES
• Fitzpatrick, T.B., et al. (eds.): Dermatology. In General Medicine. 3rd Ed. New York, McGraw-Hill, 1987
• Moschella, S.L. & Hurley, H.J.: Dermatology. 2nd Ed. Philadelphia, W.B. Saunders Co., 1985
• Domonkos, A.N., Arnold, H.L., & Odom, R.B.: Andrews' Diseases of the Skin. 8th Ed. Philadelphia, W.B. Saunders Co., 1990

Author M. LeDuc, M.D. & M. King, M.D.

Stokes-Adams attacks

 BASICS

DESCRIPTION Syncope due to transient complete heart block and resulting severe bradycardia or asystole with hypotension
System(s) affected: Cardiovascular, Nervous
Genetics: No known genetic pattern
Incidence/Prevalence in USA: Undocumented
Predominant age: Most commonly, greater than 40 years of age
Predominant sex: Male = Female

SIGNS AND SYMPTOMS
• Acute bradycardia
• Hypotension
• Paleness
• Altered sensorium or loss of consciousness, unrelated to position or exertion
• Acute onset of syncopal or near syncopal symptoms (with or without palpitations)

CAUSES
Medications:
  ◊ Calcium channel blockers
  ◊ Beta blockers
  ◊ Digoxin
  ◊ Ouabain
  ◊ Propafenone
  ◊ Clonidine
Other causes:
  ◊ Myocardial ischemia involving the AV node
  ◊ Infiltrative or fibrosing diseases involving the heart and its conduction system
  ◊ Degeneration of the AV node secondary to aging
  ◊ Neuromuscular diseases (e.g., myotonic muscular dystrophy or Kearns-Sayre syndrome)

RISK FACTORS
• Use of the above mentioned medications
• Coronary artery disease
• History of previous AV nodal dysfunction
• Acute myocardial infarction (especially acute right coronary artery occlusion)
• Amyloidosis
• Chagas' disease
• Connective tissue diseases involving the heart (e.g., systemic lupus erythematosus, rheumatoid arthritis)

 DIAGNOSIS

DIFFERENTIAL DIAGNOSIS
• Seizures
• Transient ischemia attacks
• Orthostatic hypotension
• Vasovagal attacks
• Neurocardiogenic syncope
Cardiac arrhythmias
  ◊ Ventricular tachycardia
  ◊ Supraventricular tachycardia
  ◊ Re-entrant tachycardia
  ◊ Wolff-Parkinson-White syndrome
  ◊ Sinus arrest
  ◊ Sinus exit block
  ◊ "Sick-sinus syndrome"
  ◊ Transition from normal sinus rhythm to atrial fibrillation or from atrial fibrillation to normal sinus rhythm

LABORATORY Serum digoxin level, cardiac enzymes
Drugs that may alter lab results: None
Disorders that may alter lab results: Transient or long-standing renal failure may falsely elevate cardiac enzymes (creatinine kinase)

PATHOLOGICAL FINDINGS
• Elevated serum digoxin levels
• Elevated serum cardiac enzymes
• EKG, event monitor or Holter monitor demonstrating (transient) complete heart block with slow or no ventricular escape

SPECIAL TESTS ECG, event monitor, Holter monitor

IMAGING Transthoracic cardiac 2d-echo Doppler if infiltrative disease is suspected

DIAGNOSTIC PROCEDURES
• Cardiac coronary catheterization to rule out coronary ischemia
• Electrophysiologic testing to assess status of AV nodal conduction
• Myocardial biopsy if infiltrative disease is suspected

 TREATMENT

APPROPRIATE HEALTH CARE
• Inpatient assessment in a monitored setting
• Continuing treatment - ambulatory

GENERAL MEASURES
• Cardiac monitoring during workup
• Trans-thoracic pacer availability during workup
• Atropine by the bedside during workup
• Possible temporary pacemaker placement during workup
• Permanent pacemaker placement if etiology of transient complete heart block not reversible

ACTIVITY As tolerated after assessment

DIET Regular

PATIENT EDUCATION Once the diagnosis has been made and pacemaker has been implanted (if indicated) patient should be instructed in pacemaker guidelines

MEDICATIONS

DRUG(S) OF CHOICE
• Atropine, one (1) milligram IV push to be given during the complete heart block with hypotension; may be repeated once for a total dosage of two (2) milligrams
• Epinephrine, one (1) milligram 1:10,000 IV push to be given during the complete heart block if associated with asystole; may be repeated every 5 minutes
• Isoproterenol drip, one (1) milligram in 250 cc D5W or normal saline to be started at 5 micrograms per minute if patient maintains bradycardia and hypotensive after atropine given; may titrate drip as necessary
Contraindications: Use of epinephrine in bradycardia patient with a normal blood pressure may precipitate hypertensive crisis
Precautions: Possible tachycardiac response to the above mentioned medications
Significant possible Interactions: None

ALTERNATIVE DRUGS N/A

 ## FOLLOWUP

PATIENT MONITORING
• Routine pacemaker checks, if permanent pacemaker implanted
• Followup Holter and/or event, monitor within two weeks after causal medications have been discontinued
• Discontinuation of driving, heavy machinery operation and being at unprotected heights pending normal followup

PREVENTION/AVOIDANCE Avoidance of taking any drug similar to those causing the complete heart block

POSSIBLE COMPLICATIONS
• Protracted bradycardia with hypotension leading to end-organ damage or death
• Loss of consciousness while operating machinery or at unprotected heights

EXPECTED COURSE AND PROGNOSIS Once diagnosis is made and appropriate treatment is implemented (e.g., pacemaker insertion), prognosis is excellent and further difficulty not expected

 ## MISCELLANEOUS

ASSOCIATED CONDITIONS
• Myocardial ischemia
• Acute myocardial infarction
• Systemic manifestations of connective tissue disease
• Unreliable self-administration of medications
• Neuromuscular disease

AGE-RELATED FACTORS
Pediatric: N/A
Geriatric: More common problem in this age group
Others: N/A

PREGNANCY Rare during pregnancy

SYNONYMS Drop attacks

ICD-9-CM 426.9

SEE ALSO N/A

OTHER NOTES N/A

ABBREVIATIONS N/A

REFERENCES
• Brandenburg, R.O., Fuster, V., Giuliani, E.R. & McGoon, D.C.: Cardiology: Fundamentals and Practice. Chicago, Year Book Medical Publishers, 1987
• Braunwald, E. (ed): Heart Disease: A Textbook of Cardiovascular Medicine. 3rd Ed. Philadelphia, W.B. Saunders Co., 1988

Author D. Framm, M.D.

Stomatitis

BASICS

DESCRIPTION Generalized inflammation of the oral mucosa of many possible etiologies
System(s) affected: Skin/Exocrine
Genetics: N/A
Incidence/Prevalence in USA:
• Herpetic stomatitis, hand-foot-and-mouth disease, and recurrent aphthous stomatitis are very common
• Herpangina is fairly common as are nicotinic and denture related stomatitis. The remaining causes are uncommon or rare.
Predominant age:
• Herpetic-primary infections - children
• Hand-foot-and-mouth disease - children
• Vincent's stomatitis - teenagers and young adults
• Behçet's disease - young adults
• Herpangina - children
• Others - N/A
Predominant sex: Male = Female

SIGNS AND SYMPTOMS
General:
◊ Depends on etiology
◊ Varies from minimal to severe pain
◊ Many have multiple intraoral ulcers from 1 mm to several centimeters in diameter
◊ Some with constitutional symptoms - fever, malaise, headache
Allergic stomatitis:
◊ Intense shiny erythema
◊ Slight swelling
◊ Itching
◊ Dryness
◊ Burning
Vincent's infection:
◊ Necrotic ulceration of interdental papillae and mucous membrane
Thrush (candidiasis):
White patches, slightly raised (resembling milk curds)
◊ Distribution - tongue, buccal mucosa, palate, gums, tonsils, larynx, pharynx, GI tract, skin; commonly seen in infants, immunocompromised patients; patients on long-term antibiotics, corticosteroids, and neoplastic treatment
Pseudomembraneous stomatitis:
◊ Membrane-like exudate
Mucous lesions accompanying systemic disease:
Mucous patches (syphilis)
◊ Strawberry (measles)
◊ Koplik's spots (measles)
◊ Ulcers (erythema multiforme)
◊ Smooth, fire-red, painful (pellagra)

CAUSES
• Allergy - foods, drugs, contact (some erythema multiforme)
• Vitamin deficiency - riboflavin (angular stomatitis)
• Viral - herpes simplex I and II (herpetic stomatitis), Coxsackie A (herpangina and hand-foot-and-mouth disease)
• Smoking (nicotinic stomatitis)
• Hormonal (possibly recurrent ulcerative stomatitis)
• Uncertain (recurrent aphthous stomatitis, Vincent's stomatitis, recurrent scarifying stomatitis, Behçet's disease, angular stomatitis, gangrenous stomatitis, erythema multiforme)
• Bacterial (scarlatina)
• Uremic (uremic/nephritic)
• Dentures

RISK FACTORS Listed with Causes

DIAGNOSIS

DIFFERENTIAL DIAGNOSIS
• Herpetic stomatitis
• Hand-foot-and-mouth disease
• Recurrent aphthous stomatitis
• Vincent's stomatitis
• Nicotinic stomatitis
• Denture related stomatitis
• Erythema multiforme/Stevens-Johnson syndrome
• Recurrent ulcerative stomatitis
• Recurrent scarifying stomatitis
• Behçet's disease
• Angular stomatitis
• Noma (gangrenous stomatitis)
• Scarlatina (scarlet fever)
• Herpangina
• Uremic

LABORATORY
• Hematologic profile
• Tzanck test of historic interest only
• Serologic test for syphilis
Drugs that may alter lab results: N/A
Disorders that may alter lab results: N/A

PATHOLOGICAL FINDINGS Biopsy suspicious lesions or lesions that fail to heal or chronically recur to rule out cancer or vasculitis

SPECIAL TESTS N/A

IMAGING N/A

DIAGNOSTIC PROCEDURES Biopsy if persistent/recurrent/suspicious

TREATMENT

APPROPRIATE HEALTH CARE
Outpatient, unless severe

GENERAL MEASURES
• In most cases treatment is symptomatic only
• Severe cases may require parenteral fluids, particularly in children
• Topical anesthesia
• Analgesics
• Oral rinses such as 1/2 strength hydrogen peroxide
• Mycostatin, if superinfected with candida
• Stop smoking

ACTIVITY As tolerated by patient

DIET May need to avoid spicy, sharp, hard, and dry foods

PATIENT EDUCATION Griffith: Instructions for Patients; Philadelphia, W.B. Saunders Co.

MEDICATIONS

DRUG(S) OF CHOICE
• Steroids and cytotoxic drugs for Behçet's disease
• 2% viscous lidocaine (Xylocaine) for local discomfort
• Liquid diphenhydramine (Benadryl) po, or swish and spit
• Antibiotics for gangrenous stomatitis
• Antifungal ointment (Mycostatin) for candida complicating angular stomatitis
• For candidiasis - nystatin oral suspension 400,000 units (4 mL) qid for 10 days. Use as oral rinse, then swallow.
Contraindications: Allergy to specific medication
Precautions: Toxic dose of topical Xylocaine uncertain, but likely only 25-33% of infiltration dose - may have significant absorption from open ulcers or mucous membrane
Significant possible interactions: Refer to manufacturer's literature

ALTERNATIVE DRUGS N/A

FOLLOWUP

PATIENT MONITORING Lesions need to be followed until resolved. If they fail to resolve, continuously recur, or appear suspicious, biopsy may be needed to establish a diagnosis.

PREVENTION/AVOIDANCE Avoid causative factors

POSSIBLE COMPLICATIONS
• Recurrent scarifying stomatitis may result in intraoral scarring with restriction of oral mobility
• Behçet's disease may result in visual loss, pneumonia, colitis, vasculitis, large artery aneurysms, thrombophlebitis, or encephalitis
• Gangrenous stomatitis may lead to death
• Scarlet fever may result in cardiac disease
• Herpetic stomatitis may be complicated by ocular or CNS involvement

EXPECTED COURSE AND PROGNOSIS
• Herpetic - self-limited with resolution in 7-14 days
• Hand-foot-and-mouth disease - same as herpetic
• Recurrent aphthous - 7-14 day course per episode
• Vincent's - may progress to fascial space infection with airway compromise or sepsis
• Nicotinic - will resolve with cessation of smoking
• Denture - will resolve with careful oral hygiene and daytime denture wear only
• Erythema multiforme - resolution in 2-3 weeks
• Stevens-Johnson - resolution in about 6 weeks with adequate supportive care
• Recurrent ulcerative - as the name implies, these recur over time, but the overall prognosis is good
• Recurrent scarifying - occasional patients suffer continuous ulcers, others recur with eventual scarring. The prognosis is otherwise good.
• Behçet's disease - may recur for several years. Prognosis for vision is poor. Overall prognosis is related to other aspects of the disease.
• Angular - after correction of mechanical problems, allergic disorders, and nutritional deficiencies the prognosis is good
• Gangrenous - this is the most serious stomatitis, requiring aggressive treatment with IV antibiotics and débridement to avoid death
• Scarlatina - the prognosis is related to other manifestations of the disease
• Herpangina - 7-14 day course with total resolution
• Uremic - depends on the underlying renal disease

MISCELLANEOUS

ASSOCIATED CONDITIONS N/A

AGE-RELATED FACTORS
Pediatric: Certain etiologies more likely in the pediatric population: Herpetic-primary, hand-foot-and-mouth disease, herpangina
Geriatric: Certain etiologies more likely in the geriatric population, e.g., dentures
Others: N/A

PREGNANCY May bring on recurrent ulcerative stomatitis

SYNONYMS N/A

ICD-9-CM 528.0
• Herpetic - 054.2
• Hand-foot-and-mouth disease - 282.61
• Aphthous - 528.2
• Vincent's - 101
• Denture - 528.9
• Erythema multiforme/Stevens-Johnson syndrome - 695.1
• Ulcerative - 101
• Behçet's syndrome - 136.1
• Angular - 528.5
• Gangrenous - 528.1
• Scarlet Fever - 034.1
• Herpangina - 074.0
• Viral (epidemic) - 078.4
• Candidal - 112.0
• Secondary to vitamin or dietary deficiency - 266.0

SEE ALSO N/A

OTHER NOTES N/A

ABBREVIATIONS N/A

REFERENCES
• Moran W.J.: Diseases of the mouth. In Conn's Current Therapy. Edited by R.E. Rakel. Philadelphia, W.B. Saunders Co., 1990
• Teele D.W.: Inflammatory diseases of the mouth and pharynx. In Otolaryngology. Edited by M.M. Paparella & D.A. Shumrick. Philadelphia, W.B. Saunders Co., 1980 pp 974-1017

Author A. Namon, M.D. & W. Moran, M.D.

Stroke rehabilitation

 BASICS

DESCRIPTION Stroke rehabilitation involves restoration of function after medical and neurologic stability have been achieved
• Cerebrovascular diseases and/or disorders that affect central nervous system function by compromising delivery of blood or by hemorrhage resulting in ischemia, necrosis, gliosis
• Anterior lesions in the cerebrovascular system affect the arteries that supply the cerebral hemispheres and cause thrombotic strokes
• Posterior lesions affect arteries that supply the brain stem and yield crossed motor and/or sensory signs and symptoms
• Both anterior and posterior lesions can cause sudden death, but the lower in the central nervous system the lesion, or the more incomplete the lesion, or the more hemorrhagic the lesion, the higher the chance for neurologic return
System(s) affected: Nervous, Cardiovascular
Genetics: Similar to the probability of developing hypertension or coronary artery disease
Incidence/Prevalence in USA: 459/100,000
Predominant age: Over 45
Predominant sex: Male > Female

SIGNS AND SYMPTOMS
• Variable - depends upon the arterial system affected
• Hemiparesis
• Hemianesthesia
• Unilateral central facial palsy
• Homonomous hemianopsia
• Aphasia, apraxia (if the dominant cerebral hemisphere is involved)

CAUSES
• Coronary artery disease
• Hypertension
• Cerebral atherosclerosis
• Cardiac thrombus embolus
• Foreign body embolus
• Frequently, the combination of gout, diabetes, hypertension has been untreated for some 5-10 years before the onset of the stroke disorder

RISK FACTORS
• Many are lifestyle oriented and preventable. Factors include coffee ingestion, cigarette smoking, obesity, inactivity, hyperactivity to the point of exhaustion, emotional lability, sexual hyperactivity, starvation, antidepressant or diet reduction medication, alcohol or recreational drug habituation, unusual stress states.
• Ethnicity may be a risk factor but relationships to factors above first must be clarified

 DIAGNOSIS

DIFFERENTIAL DIAGNOSIS
• Infection, tumor, bleeding disorders, endocrinologic, metabolic, gastrointestinal, toxic, etc.
• Different types of stroke disorders can occur in one patient

LABORATORY
• CBC
• Spinal fluid for routine studies (only if indicated)
• Urinalysis
• RPR
• ANA for collagen vascular disorders
• Consider quantitative immunoelectrophoresis with the combination of stroke disorders, anemia, hypertension
• Carotid flow studies
Drugs that may alter lab results: N/A
Disorders that may alter lab results: N/A

PATHOLOGICAL FINDINGS Thrombotic, hemorrhagic, mixed, combinations can be present

SPECIAL TESTS
• Somatosensory, auditory, and visual evoked potential technology can monitor neurologic recovery.
• EEG sometimes useful in evaluating seizure disorders

IMAGING
• Scanning - CT, MRI and PET scanning give good data about anatomy, blood flow, and metabolic activity
• Serial exams can delineate the course of this disease

DIAGNOSTIC PROCEDURES
• Spinal taps, myelography, pneumoencephalography, angiography all have special indications and contraindications at this time. none are routinely used.
• Electrodiagnosis for neuritis, radiculitis in specialized centers if available

 TREATMENT

APPROPRIATE HEALTH CARE
Referral to a full service rehabilitation center - a rehabilitation medicine team can make the difference between independence and dependency. Refer when medically and neurologically stable.

GENERAL MEASURES
• Full service rehabilitation center characteristics: Comparison with national standards for admission, process, discharge, and followup care; closed units; regular team meetings to discuss long and short term objectives; quality assurance system in place; accreditation by Commission on Accreditation of Rehabilitation Facilities.
• Use heat with caution in patients with stroke or atherosclerotic vascular disease because of reduced sensation
• Use hydrotherapy and/or isometric exercise cautiously in patients with limited cardiopulmonary reserve
• In patients able to respond to the protocols after surgery, restorative, tendon transplant, or nerve transplants may be of value
• Cardiac precautions and a CPR team may be required during exercise programs since obese, hypertensive, or patients with coronary artery disease are at increased risk. Real-time monitoring might be required.

ACTIVITY
• Physical therapy, occupational therapy, speech pathology, psychology, nursing therapy should be delivered to the patient for at least three hours/day throughout the inpatient stay.
• The patient must be able to tolerate this vigorous activity level. If the patient becomes medically or neurologically unstable during the inpatient stay, a 48 hour leeway is usually built into the system. After that period, therapy must resume or the patient must be returned to an acute hospital bed. Most stroke rehabilitation units are usually able to deliver this type of functional return within one month of inpatient stay, although length of stay is individually determined.
• While most rehabilitative efforts take place within a very short time after ictus, successful rehabilitative efforts have taken place as long as five years later

DIET Depends upon other medical conditions

PATIENT EDUCATION
• Stroke is usually an unnecessary illness. Major risk factors are nearly all preventable. The difficulty that arises is that the patient's life style must be changed. Patients mount a great deal of active and passive resistance.
• The progressive physical and mental deterioration noted with hypertension and/or coronary artery disease is not inevitable
• Family pressure and support is helpful to interest the patient in his/her health in a consistent and sustained manner
• Disuse will add subsequent complications and sequellae

MEDICATIONS

DRUG(S) OF CHOICE As needed for underlying disorders (e.g., hypertension, heart disease) or for complications (e.g., seizures, deep vein thrombosis, pneumonitis)
Contraindications: Refer to manufacturer's profile of each drug
Precautions:
• Four or more medications will often have interactions; polypharmacy is frequent
• Antihypertensive medication can generate orthostatic hypotension
• Antidepressant medication can lower the seizure threshold
• Muscle relaxants, tranquilizers, major neuroleptic medication can confuse, delay return of memory and cognition, sedate, occasionally agitate, and obliterate spontaneous thought
• Unnecessary medications should be withdrawn
• Elderly patients regularly require lower dosages
Significant possible interactions: Refer to manufacturer's profile of each drug

ALTERNATIVE DRUGS N/A

FOLLOWUP

PATIENT MONITORING
• Within the month following discharge, the patient and family should be seen in an outpatient group "alumni" day coordinated with an interdisciplinary outpatient clinic appointment
• If outpatient therapy is rendered, the team therapist(s) should meet with the physician regularly to rate progress and discuss long and short term objectives

PREVENTION/AVOIDANCE   See Risk factors and Patient education

POSSIBLE COMPLICATIONS
• Reflex sympathetic dystrophy syndromes - such as hand/shoulder syndrome - are nonspecific complications and last for 12 weeks before subsiding to adhesive capsulitis
• Tendonitis-bursitis-capsulitis may coexist with prolonged paralysis. Prolonged range-of-motion and neuromuscular re-education exercises help retard functional deterioration of the limb. Electrical stimulation and biofeedback for control and relaxation have also been used, but the treatment of choice is restoration of function.
• Diabetes, alcohol intake will add peripheral neuritis
• Many patients develop osteoporosis - especially on side of paresis. The normal side can develop osteoarthritis.

EXPECTED COURSE AND PROGNOSIS   Generally good, although pneumonia, respiratory failure, heart failure, and myocardial infarction occur more frequently after stroke

MISCELLANEOUS

ASSOCIATED CONDITIONS
• Hypertension
• Coronary artery disease
• Diabetes mellitus
• Gout
• Atherosclerosis

AGE-RELATED FACTORS
Pediatric: Aneurysms, hypertension, tumors, trauma
Geriatric: Heart disease, vascular disease, hypertension
Others: See Risk factors

PREGNANCY   Hypertension in pregnancy can lead to stroke

SYNONYMS   N/A

ICD-9-CM   438/(3429)/(7843)

SEE ALSO   N/A

OTHER NOTES   N/A

ABBREVIATIONS   N/A

REFERENCES
• Brandstater, M.E. & Basmajian, J.V. (eds.): Stroke Rehabilitation. Baltimore, Williams & Wilkins, 1987
• Kaplan, P.E. & Cerullo, L.J. (eds.): Stroke Rehabilitation. Boston, Butterworth, 1986

Author   P. Kaplan, M.D.

Subarachnoid hemorrhage

 BASICS

DESCRIPTION Subarachnoid hemorrhage is the extravasation of blood into the subarachnoid space particularly of the basal cisterns and into the cerebral spinal fluid pathways.
<u>Traumatic:</u> More common and it is related to head trauma
<u>Spontaneous:</u> Rare. 60-75% of spontaneous subarachnoid hemorrhages are due to intracranial saccular aneurysms.
Incidence/Prevalence in USA:
Spontaneous: Incidence is 10.9/100,000 per year
System(s) affected: Nervous
Genetics: N/A
Predominant age: The majority of subarachnoid hemorrhages due to aneurysms occur in the fourth to seventh decades whereas subarachnoid hemorrhage due to arterio-venous (A-V) malformation appears more commonly in the second, third, and fourth decades.
Predominant Sex: Subarachnoid hemorrhage due to aneurysm occurs slightly more commonly in females (55%).

SIGNS AND SYMPTOMS
• Abrupt onset of headache associated with stiff neck and photophobia
• May or may not lose consciousness
• May develop focal neurological deficits such as hemiparesis or a dilated pupil
• Subhyaloid hemorrhages are more common in anterior communicating artery aneurysms

CAUSES
Causes of subarachnoid hemorrhages are trauma, intracranial saccular aneurysm, intracranial A-V malformation, hypertension, rarely tumors and blood dyscrasias.

RISK FACTORS
• Intracranial aneurysms associated with coarctation of the aorta
• A-V malformations
• Polycystic disease of the kidneys
• Fibromuscular dysplasia of the renal arteries
• Hypertension is not necessarily associated with saccular aneurysms, but is associated with rupture of an existing aneurysm

 DIAGNOSIS

DIFFERENTIAL DIAGNOSIS
Differential diagnosis of subarachnoid hemorrhage includes intracerebral hematomas, meningitis, and benign cephalalgia

LABORATORY N/A
Drugs that may alter lab results: N/A

PATHOLOGICAL FINDINGS N/A

SPECIAL TESTS N/A

IMAGING
The diagnosis is established in better than 95% of the cases with a CT scan. This demonstrates blood in the basal cisterns and may help in localizing the source of hemorrhage. It also can rule out mass effect so that if this study is negative a spinal puncture can be safely performed. A small percentage of subarachnoid hemorrhages will be missed on the CT scan. Following the establishment of the diagnosis of subarachnoid hemorrhage it is imperative to find out the source of bleeding, therefore, cerebral angiography is used to identify the source of hemorrhage such as a saccular aneurysm or A-V malformation. It must be remembered that occasional hemorrhage may occur from an A-V malformation of the spinal cord or a vascular tumor in the spinal arachnoid space. Therefore, if no source of subarachnoid hemorrhage is found intracranially, consideration might be made for studies involving the subarachnoid space which would include MRI spinal scanning or myelography.

DIAGNOSTIC PROCEDURES See above

 TREATMENT

APPROPRIATE HEALTH CARE Initial therapy is carried out in the Intensive Care Unit

GENERAL MEASURES
• The treatment is directed to prevent complications of subarachnoid hemorrhage which include rebleeding, hydrocephalus, and cerebral vasospasm
• If the source of hemorrhage such as an aneurysm can be readily obliterated, this reduces the risk of rebleeding and allows more vigorous treatment with fluid and hypertensive therapy of cerebral vasospasm
• Hydrocephalus should be treated with cerebral spinal fluid drainage and may require permanent shunting procedures
• A-V malformations may be obliterated with embolization and surgery
• Vasospasm is treated with generous volume expansion and hypertension to promote cerebral perfusion after the aneurysm has been obliterated. This is not wise if an aneurysm is untreated.
• Once the patient has stabilized and recovered from the initial hemorrhage, then a vigorous rehabilitation program is indicated

ACTIVITY Strict bedrest until source of hemorrhage is eliminated

DIET N/A

PATIENT EDUCATION N/A

MEDICATIONS

DRUG(S) OF CHOICE
Nimodipine
◊ Has been used at 60-90 mg q 4 h for the prevention of cerebral vasospasm
◊ Therapy should begin as soon as possible
◊ The capsule contents may be given via NG tube if patient can't swallow
Contraindications: Hypotension is contraindication in patients with vasospasm
Precautions:
• Quiet room
• Reduce stress
• Control blood pressure until source of hemorrhage eliminated
• Stool softeners to prevent straining
Significant possible interactions: Refer to manufacturer's profile

ALTERNATE DRUGS   Nicardipine

FOLLOWUP

PATIENT MONITORING   As needed

PREVENTION/AVOIDANCE   Incidental aneurysms have a risk of hemorrhage of 2-3% per year so prophylactic surgery may be indicated

POSSIBLE COMPLICATIONS
• Death
• Paralysis

EXPECTED COURSE AND PROGNOSIS
• Unfortunately, approximately 25-30% of the patients will die from a spontaneous subarachnoid hemorrhage due to an aneurysm. The highest morbidity is secondary to cerebral vasospasm.
• If the aneurysm can be successfully clipped and the vasospasm treated effectively, satisfactory outcome occurs in approximately 50-65% of patients.
• It should be remembered that approximately 25-30% of aneurysms will be multiple. It is advisable to treat multiple aneurysms during the same operative procedure, but if this is not possible, surgery is directed at the aneurysm most likely to have hemorrhaged.
• Further surgical procedures may be necessary to obliterate additional aneurysms
• A-V malformations do not have as high morbidity and mortality associated with the hemorrhage. On the other hand, both untreated aneurysms and A-V malformations are likely to bleed at about 2-3% per year. Therefore in the younger age groups, incidentally found A-V malformations and aneurysms may require aggressive treatment.

MISCELLANEOUS

ASSOCIATED CONDITIONS   N/A

AGE RELATED FACTORS
Pediatric: N/A
Geriatric: In the elderly patient, incidental aneurysms and A-V malformations may best be followed since the chance of hemorrhage is only 2-3% per year.
Others: In younger and middle-aged people, surgery is recommended.

PREGNANCY
In the pregnant female, increased blood pressure and blood volume may predispose to hemorrhages. Under life-threatening situations, surgical procedures can be performed on a pregnant patient. However, with A-V malformations, a less lethal lesion compared to aneurysms it may be worthwhile to allow the pregnancy go to term.

SYNONYMS   N/A

ICD-9-CM
430 subarachnoid hemorrhage
852 subarachnoid, subdural, and extradural hemorrhage, following injury

OTHER NOTES   N/A

ABBREVIATIONS   A-V: arterio-venous

REFERENCES
• Weir, B. ed. Aneurysm Affecting the Nervous System. Baltimore, Williams and Wilkins, 1987.
• Sahs, Perret, & Nishioka (eds.): Intracranial and Subarachnoid Hemorrhage A Cooperative Study. Philadelphia, Lippincott Co, 1969
• Youmans, J.R. (ed.): A Comprehensive Reference Guide to the Diagnosis and Management of Neurosurgical Problems, 3rd Ed. Philadelphia, W.B. Saunders Co., 1990

Author   L. Carter, M.D.

Subclavian steal syndrome

BASICS

DESCRIPTION Origin of the subclavian artery becomes compromised causing a reversal of flow in the branches of the first portion of the subclavian artery as a means of supplying blood to the upper extremity, especially during exercise. This may result in symptoms of vertebral-basilar insufficiency.
System(s) affected: Cardiovascular, Musculoskeletal, Nervous

Genetics N/A
Incidence in USA: Unknown, not common
Prevalence in USA: Unknown, 70% of the time, the left subclavian artery is involved
Predominant age: > 55 years
Predominant sex: Male > Female (2:1)

SIGNS AND SYMPTOMS
• Most common - vertigo or presyncope following upper extremity exercise. The reversal of flow down the ipsilateral vertebral artery results in a relative vertebral-basilar insufficiency
• Less common: - weakness and clumsiness of an extremity, loss of vision, homonymous hemianopsia, ataxia and drop attacks
• Arm claudication following minimal exercise.
• Reduced blood pressure of > 20 mmHg in involved arm
• Symptoms should be reproducible by exercising the arm

CAUSES
• Arteriosclerosis obliterans of the proximal subclavian artery in 95% of cases
• Less common causes of obstruction: dissecting aneurysm of aortic arch, embolus and Takayasu's arteritis

RISK FACTORS
• Smoking
• Hypertension
• Diabetes

DIAGNOSIS

DIFFERENTIAL DIAGNOSIS
• Intracranial vascular disease
• Carotid artery disease
• Vertebral artery disease
• Brain tumor
• Subdural hematoma

LABORATORY
• Noninvasive measurement of blood pressure in upper extremities
• Arteriogram of arch vessels with delayed films of vertebral arteries
Drugs that may alter lab results: N/A
Disorders that may alter lab results: N/A

PATHOLOGICAL FINDINGS
• Absent or diminished pulses in ipsilateral arm
• Reduced blood flow (> 20 mmHg) in same arm

SPECIAL TESTS Pulse volume recording of upper extremities

IMAGING
• Duplex scanning of extracranial vessels
• Arteriography

DIAGNOSTIC PROCEDURES
Arteriography

TREATMENT

APPROPRIATE HEALTH CARE
Surgical correction of problem by carotid-subclavian bypass

GENERAL MEASURES None

ACTIVITY Reduced exercise of arms

DIET None

PATIENT EDUCATION
• Prevent injury to arm
• Reduce exercise to arm

MEDICATIONS

Drug of choice None
Complications: N/A
Precautions: N/A
Significant possible interactions: N/A

ALTERNATE DRUGS N/A

 FOLLOWUP

PATIENT MONITORING Annual physical to include blood pressure in both arms

PREVENTION/AVOIDANCE N/A

POSSIBLE COMPLICATIONS
Completed stroke

EXPECTED COURSE AND PROGNOSIS Good

 MISCELLANEOUS

ASSOCIATED CONDITIONS
• Carotid artery disease
• Heart disease
• Arteriosclerosis

AGE-RELATED FACTORS
Pediatric: N/A
Geriatric: Older patient more likely to have arteriosclerosis
Others: N/A

PREGNANCY N/A

SYNONYMS N/A

ICD-9-CM 435.2

SEE ALSO N/A

OTHER NOTES N/A

ABBREVIATIONS N/A

REFERENCES
• Rutherford, R.B.: Vascular Surgery. Philadelphia, W.B. Saunders Co., 1984
• Sabiston, Jr., D.C.: Essentials of Surgery. Philadelphia, W.B. Saunders Co., 1987

Author W. V. Sharp, M.D.

Subdural hematoma

BASICS

DESCRIPTION The accumulation of blood in the subdural space
Acute subdural hematoma: The most severe form, usually the result of trauma involving acceleration or deceleration head injury and commonly associated with parenchymal brain injury. Hematoma age is three days or less.
Chronic subdural hematoma: Often the result of trivial head injury in older patients, one-fourth to one-half have no history of head trauma. Hematoma is classically older than three weeks and is associated with an encapsulating membrane.
Subacute subdural hematoma: Appearing 4-21 days from maturation of acute subdural hematoma
System(s) affected: Nervous, Cardiovascular
Genetics: N/A
Incidence in USA:
• Acute subdural hematoma: 1-2/100,000
• Chronic subdural hematoma: 1-2/100,000
Prevalence in USA: Acute subdural hematoma in newborn infants and children are relatively infrequent, occurring approximately 25% as often as in adults. Chronic subdural hematomas occur in children of all ages. However, chronic subdural hematomas present a peak incidence at approximately six months of age and rarely after one year of age.
Predominant age:
• Acute subdural hematoma - less than 60 years
• Chronic subdural hematoma - greater than 50 years
Predominant sex: Male > Female

SIGNS AND SYMPTOMS
Acute subdural hematoma:
◊ Altered level of consciousness 99%
◊ Pupillary irregularity (usually it is unilateral to hematoma) 47-53%
◊ Hemiparesis (usually contralateral to hematoma) 34-47%
◊ Decerebrate posturing or flaccid motor exam 47%
◊ Papilloedema 16%
◊ Cranial nerve VI palsy 5%
Chronic subdural hematoma:
◊ Impaired consciousness 53%
◊ Hemiparesis 45%
◊ Papilledema 24%
◊ Cranial nerve III abnormality 11%
◊ Hemianopsia 7%

CAUSES
Acute subdural hematoma
◊ High velocity acceleration or deceleration head injury resulting in tearing of the bridging veins between cerebral cortex and the dural venous sinuses
◊ Due to bleeding from injured cortical vessels

Chronic subdural hematoma
◊ Often from a trivial head injury in adults and birth trauma or abuse in children. A balance between recurrent bleeding from the hematoma membrane and resorption determines the ultimate size of the hematoma. The osmotic theory of fluid accumulation within the hematoma cavity has been discredited.

RISK FACTORS
Acute subdural hematoma
◊ 0.5-1% of severe head trauma
◊ High velocity acceleration or deceleration head injury (motor vehicle accidents, falls, blunt head trauma)
Chronic subdural hematoma
◊ Chronic alcoholism
◊ Epilepsy
◊ Coagulopathy/anticoagulation therapy
◊ Cerebral spinal fluid shunt for hydrocephalus
◊ Rarely metastatic carcinoma to subdural space

DIAGNOSIS

DIFFERENTIAL DIAGNOSIS
• Acute subdural hematoma and other forms of intracranial hematoma (epidural hematoma, cerebral contusion/hematoma)
• Chronic subdural hematoma
• Dementia
• Stroke
• Transient ischemic attack
• Brain tumor
• Subdural empyema
• Meningitis

LABORATORY
• Acute subdural hematoma - consumptive coagulopathy due to underlying parenchymal injury diagnosed with elevated PT and PTT, elevated fibrin degradation products, decreased fibrinogen, decreased platelet level, and extended bleeding time
• Chronic subdural hematoma - predisposing factors such as coagulopathy or anticoagulation therapy producing appropriate abnormalities in bleeding time or coagulation parameters. Subtherapeutic anticonvulsant levels in patients with epilepsy. Serum ethanol level in alcoholics.
Drugs that may alter lab results:
Anticoagulants (e.g., Coumadin)
Disorders that may alter lab results: DIC and other coagulopathies (e.g., hemophilia)

PATHOLOGICAL FINDINGS
• Acute subdural hematoma - this is a fresh hemorrhage
• Chronic subdural hematoma - there is a liquefied hematoma, an outer membrane beneath the dura after one week, and an inner membrane between the hematoma and arachnoid after three weeks. Cytology examination may reveal metastatic carcinoma cells on rare occasions to be associated with the hemorrhage.

SPECIAL TESTS EEG for seizures and intensive care consisting of continuous cardiac monitoring often in conjunction with continuous monitoring of intra-arterial pressure and intracranial pressure (ventriculostomy or intraparenchymal or subdural pressure monitoring probe)

IMAGING
• Acute subdural hematoma - the imaging study of choice is the CT head scan (with intravascular contrast if hemoglobin is less than or equal to 9 gm/dL)
• Chronic subdural hematoma - a CT head scan is also preferred. An MRI head scan is often necessary for hematomas isodense with brain due to the mixture of chronic hematoma with recurrent hemorrhage.

DIAGNOSTIC PROCEDURES   N/A

TREATMENT

APPROPRIATE HEALTH CARE
• Acute subdural hematoma - medically, the management consists of controlling elevated intracranial pressure with osmotic and loop diuretics and hyperventilation to induce hypocapnia (PaCO2 of 22-28). Emergent craniotomy is indicated for evacuation of hematomas causing significant mass effect.
• Chronic subdural hematoma - burr hole drainage of hematoma

GENERAL MEASURES
Subacute subdural hematoma
◊ If patient is neurologically stable, surgery may be delayed until hematoma matures and becomes chronic at which time a burr hole drainage can be performed
◊ Subacute hematomas causing significant mass effect and neurological deficit may require craniotomy for evacuation
◊ Maintenance of adequate airway and ventilation and support of cardiovascular system to promote normal cerebral perfusion
◊ Treatment of multi-system trauma and precautions for cervical and other spine injury

ACTIVITY
• Acute subdural hematoma - the patient will need the head of the bed elevated to reduce intracranial pressure and flexion of lower body avoided until thoracic, lumbar, or sacral spine injuries are ruled out. The patient should be maintained in a rigid cervical collar until the cervical spine is cleared radiographically.
• Chronic subdural hematoma - the head of the bed is flat and appropriate precautions are taken if a spinal injury is present

DIET

• Most patients with acute subdural hematoma require enteral or total parenteral nutrition initially
• Depending on level of consciousness, patients with chronic subdural hematoma can usually have the diet advanced to regular food as tolerated

PATIENT EDUCATION
The National Institute of Neurological and Communicative Disorders and Stroke (NINDS), The National Institutes of Health, Bethesda, Maryland 20892

MEDICATIONS

DRUG(S) OF CHOICE
Acute subdural hematoma:
◊ Prior to surgical therapy, management of cerebral edema and elevated intracranial pressure may require mannitol 20% solution 0.5-1.0 gm/kg followed by 0.25-0.75 gm/kg every 4-6 hours. If a loop diuretic is used in conjunction with mannitol, furosemide (Lasix) 0.5 mg/kg IV is administered. Check serum osmolality every 8 hours and serum electrolytes at least daily. A 5% or 25% albumin preparation (Plasmanate) may be used either as a continuous or an intermittent infusion to augment osmotherapy as needed.
◊ Seizure prophylaxis includes phenytoin (Dilantin) 1000 mg load (50 mg/min IV) with ECG monitoring followed by 100 mg IV every 8 hours or as needed to maintain therapeutic blood levels (10-20 μg/mL). Dilantin therapy should be converted to the oral route as soon as possible to avoid cardiovascular complications of IV Dilantin administration.
◊ In the chronic subdural hematoma medical management alone is frequently unsuccessful and entails risks of neurological deterioration. When small and asymptomatic, however, it may be appropriate to treat such patients conservatively with observation as some chronic subdural hematomas have been known to resolve spontaneously.
Contraindications: Refer to manufacturer's literature
Precautions: Refer to manufacturer's literature
Significant possible interactions: Refer to manufacturer's literature

ALTERNATIVE DRUGS N/A

FOLLOWUP

PATIENT MONITORING
• Anticonvulsant levels should be checked approximately every 3-6 months after initiation
• Consider discontinuing anticonvulsant if patient has no seizures for at least one year
• EEG may be complimentary in the decision making process for discontinuation of anticonvulsants

PREVENTION/AVOIDANCE
Acute subdural hematoma
◊ Trauma prevention programs
Chronic subdural hematoma
◊ Alcoholism prevention
◊ Medical and surgical management of epilepsy
◊ Conservative use of anticoagulation therapy
◊ Medium or high pressure ventriculoperitoneal shunt valves in at risk patients with hydrocephalus

POSSIBLE COMPLICATIONS
• Acute subdural hematoma - immediate postoperative complications include elevated intracranial pressure and brain edema, new or recurrent hematoma, infection, and seizures (in approximately one-third of cases)
• Chronic subdural hematoma - recurrent hematoma in up to 50% of cases (can be alleviated by the use of subdural drainage catheters), infection (subdural empyema, wound), and seizures in up to 10% of cases

EXPECTED COURSE AND PROGNOSIS
• Acute subdural hematoma - mortality is greater then 50%. Significant neurological disability and impairment of function is seen in most surviving patients. Seizure prophylaxis is usually required for at least one year.
• Chronic subdural hematoma - mortality is less than 10%. Most patients resume preoperative functional status. Outcome highly dependent on pre-surgical neurological status.

MISCELLANEOUS

ASSOCIATED CONDITIONS
Acute subdural hematoma
◊ Multi-system trauma
◊ Cervical spinal cord injury
◊ Injury to the thoracic, lumbar, or sacral spine
◊ Disseminated intravascular coagulation
◊ Epilepsy
Chronic subdural hematoma
◊ Alcoholism
◊ Epilepsy
◊ Coagulopathy
◊ Cerebral spinal fluid shunt
◊ Birth trauma
◊ Child abuse
◊ Rarely metastatic carcinoma

AGE-RELATED FACTORS
Pediatric: N/A
Geriatric:
• Cerebral atrophy common
• Can be confused clinically with senile dementia
Others:
• Acute subdural hematoma - lower mortality in patients less than 40 years of age compared to those older then 40 years of age
• Chronic subdural hematoma - majority of patients are older than 50 years of age

PREGNANCY N/A

SYNONYMS Subdural hemorrhage

ICD-9-CM 852.30 subdural hemorrhage following injury with open cranial wound

OTHER NOTES N/A

ABBREVIATIONS N/A

REFERENCES
• Cooper, P.: Traumatic intracranial hematomas. In Neurosurgery. Edited by R. Wilkins & S. Rengachary. New York, McGraw-Hill, 1985, pp 1657-1666
• Fogelholm, R. & Waltimo, O.: Epidemiology of chronic subdural hematoma. Acta Neurochir 32:247-250, 1975.
• Seeling, J., Becker, D., Miller, J., et al.: Traumatic acute subdural hematoma. New Engl J Med 304: 1511-1518, 1981
• McLaurin, R. & Tobin, R.: Diagnosis and Treatment of Head Injury in Infants and Children. In Neurological Surgery. Edited by J. Youmans. Philadelphia, W.B. Saunders, 1992

Author M. Weinand, M.D.

Subphrenic abscess

 BASICS

DESCRIPTION Any localized collection of pus below the diaphragm and in contact with the diaphragm
System(s) affected: Gastrointestinal, Pulmonary
Genetics: N/A
Incidence/Prevalence in USA: N/A
Predominant age: N/A
Predominant sex: N/A

SIGNS AND SYMPTOMS
- High spiking fever with chills and sweating
- Abdominal tenderness
- Ileus
- Anterior abdominal wall erythema
- Abdominal pain
- Tachycardia
- Chest pain
- Nausea
- Dyspnea
- Localized tenderness on palpation
- Pleural effusion
- Elevation of diaphragm
- Shoulder pain
- Hiccups
- Tenderness when compressing lower ribs
- Rales at lung base

CAUSES
- Complications of abdominal surgery cause 50%
- Penetrating trauma
- Gastrointestinal perforations - appendicitis, diverticulitis

RISK FACTORS
- Operative procedure with significant contamination
- Patients with chronic disease - cirrhosis, renal failure, malnutrition
- Patients on corticosteroids, chemotherapy, radiotherapy
- Myelosuppression

 DIAGNOSIS

DIFFERENTIAL DIAGNOSIS
- Other intra-abdominal abscesses
- Empyema

LABORATORY
- White blood count
- Blood cultures
- Automated chemical profile
Drugs that may alter lab results: N/A
Disorders that may alter lab results: N/A

PATHOLOGICAL FINDINGS
- Pus under diaphragm
- Organisms: Escherichia, Streptococcus, Proteus, Klebsiella, Bacteroides fragilis, cocci, Clostridium

SPECIAL TESTS N/A

IMAGING
- CT scan
- Ultrasound
- Plain films of chest and abdomen display elevation and immobility of right diaphragm, fluid in right costophrenic sulcus; air-fluid level in subphrenic space
- Gallium scan

DIAGNOSTIC PROCEDURES CT or ultrasound directed aspiration

 TREATMENT

APPROPRIATE HEALTH CARE
Inpatient

GENERAL MEASURES
- Adequate drainage of abscess - percutaneous and/or surgical
- Percutaneous drainage not advised if 1) abscess is multiloculated, 2) drainage route would traverse bowel, uncontaminated peritoneal or pleural space, 3) source of continued contamination still present, 4) fungal infection, 5) pus too viscous
- Surgical drainage mandated if patient fails to respond to percutaneous drainage in 24 to 48 hours
- Antibiotics
- Supportive care - nutrition, monitoring, oxygenation, hydration
- Swan-Ganz catheter if unstable
- Mechanical ventilation if necessary
- Vasopressors if indicated

ACTIVITY As tolerated

DIET NPO until intestinal function returns

PATIENT EDUCATION N/A

MEDICATIONS

DRUG(S) OF CHOICE
• Broad spectrum antibiotics based on culture and sensitivity
• Aminoglycosides (tobramycin or gentamicin) 1.5-2.0 mg/kg loading dose
• Amikacin 5-7.5 mg/kg loading dose (very expensive)
• Plus clindamycin 600 mg IV q6h,
or
• Metronidazole (Flagyl) loading dose 15 mg/kg and maintenance dose 7.5 mg/kg q6h
Contraindications: Known allergy to antibiotics
Precautions:
• Aminoglycosides are ototoxic and nephrotoxic - follow BUN, creatinine and serum blood levels (peak and trough)
• Prolong dosing interval to achieve appropriate trough level; especially in renal failure
• Adjust dose for desired peak level
• Dosage adjustments in renal failure not needed for metronidazole since it is metabolized by the liver
Significant possible interactions: N/A

ALTERNATIVE DRUGS
• Cefoxitin 2 gm IV q4-6h
• Cefoperazone 1-2 gm IV q12h
• Cefotaxime 1 gm IV q 6-8 h
• Mezlocillin 3 gm IV q 4 h

FOLLOWUP

PATIENT MONITORING
• Frequent evaluation after discharge up to six weeks
• White blood counts regularly
• Chest x-rays until normal

PREVENTION/AVOIDANCE N/A

POSSIBLE COMPLICATIONS
• Mortality - 10 to 90% if not adequately drained
• Multi-system organ failure
• Recurrent abscess
• Hemorrhage
• Bowel obstruction
• Wound dehiscence
• Continuing sepsis
• Pneumonia
• Pleural effusion
• Suppurative pylephlebitis

EXPECTED COURSE AND PROGNOSIS
• Death if abscess is not adequately drained or patient vigorously supported

MISCELLANEOUS

ASSOCIATED CONDITIONS
• Multi-system organ failure
• Systemic sepsis
• Fistula

AGE-RELATED FACTORS
Pediatric: N/A
Geriatric: Worse prognosis
Others: N/A

PREGNANCY N/A

SYNONYMS Subdiaphragmatic abscess

SEE ALSO N/A

ICD-9-CM 998.5

OTHER NOTES N/A

ABBREVIATIONS N/A

Reference Hau, T., et al.: Diagnosis and Treatment of Abdominal Abscesses, Current Problems in Surgery, Vol. XXI No. 7, Chicago, Year Book Medical Publishers, 1984

Author G. Williams, M.D.

Sudden infant death syndrome (SIDS)

BASICS

DESCRIPTION The sudden death of an infant under one year of age which remains unexplained after a thorough case investigation, including performance of a complete autopsy, examination of the death scene, and review of the clinical history. SIDS was first formally defined in 1969 and the definition was revised in 1989.
 • Apparent Life Threatening Events (ALTEs) is a related entity.
System(s) affected: Endocrine/Metabolic, Pulmonary, Nervous, Cardiovascular
Genetics: No genetic association has been identified
Incidence/Prevalence in USA:
 • All races: 130/100,000 live births; 5,400 cases per year
 • White: 110/100,000 live births; 3,600 cases per year
 • Black: 230/100,000 live births; 1,600 cases per year
Predominant age: Rare in first month of life, peak occurs in infants between 2 and 4 months, 90% of deaths occur by 6 months
Predominant sex: Males > Females (52-60% of SIDS cases are males)

SIGNS AND SYMPTOMS These babies generally appear healthy, or may have had a minor upper respiratory or gastrointestinal infection in the last 2 weeks of life

CAUSES
There are many theories about the cause of SIDS. There may be subtle developmental abnormalities resulting from pre- and/or perinatal brain injury.
Possible causes:
 ◊ Abnormalities in respiratory control
 ◊ Upper airway obstruction
 ◊ Bronchospasm
 ◊ Central and peripheral nervous system abnormalities
 ◊ Cardiac arrhythmias
 ◊ SIDS may occur when a combination of factors coincide; such triggers may include infectious agents, climatic changes, or environmental factors

RISK FACTORS
 • Most SIDS deaths occur in children who are "low-risk." However, there are several risk factors associated with SIDS:
 ◊ Race: Native Americans and African Americans have highest incidence
 ◊ Season - late fall and winter months
 ◊ Time of day - between midnight and 6 AM
 ◊ Activity - during sleep
 ◊ Low birth weight; intrauterine growth retardation (IUGR)
 ◊ Poverty

 • Maternal factors: Teenage mothers; maternal use of cigarettes or drugs (cocaine, opiates) during pregnancy; higher parity; maternal anemia during pregnancy
 • Respiratory or gastrointestinal infection in recent past
 • Previous SIDS death in sibling (the risk of recurrence in a subsequent child is estimated to be 1%)
 • Sleep practices - prone sleep position, heavier clothing and bedding
 • Lack of breast-feeding
 • Passive cigarette smoke exposure after birth

DIAGNOSIS

DIFFERENTIAL DIAGNOSIS
 • Suffocation
 • Abnormalities of fatty acid metabolism (e.g., deficiency of medium-chain acyl-CoA dehydrogenase, or of carnitine)
 • Homicide
 • Dehydration/electrolyte disturbance
 • Infant botulism

LABORATORY
 • Pneumocardiograms have been abandoned in the workup
 • For ALTEs: ABGs, X-rays, EKG, EEG, esophageal pH.
 • Postmortem laboratory tests are done to rule out other cause of death (e.g., electrolytes to rule out dehydration and electrolyte imbalance). In SIDS, there are no consistently abnormal laboratory tests.
Drugs that may alter lab results: N/A
Disorders that may alter lab results: N/A

PATHOLOGICAL FINDINGS
Characteristic findings on postmortem examination:
 ◊ Frothy discharge, sometimes blood-tinged, from nostrils and mouth in majority
 ◊ Petechiae on surface of lungs, heart and thymus gland in 50-85%
 ◊ Pulmonary congestion and edema often present
 ◊ Morphologic markers of hypoxia: Increased gliosis in brain stem, retention of periadrenal brown fat, and hematopoiesis in the liver - present to varying degrees, not confirmed by all studies

SPECIAL TESTS N/A

IMAGING X-rays are taken to rule out possible child abuse

DIAGNOSTIC PROCEDURES N/A

OTHER Because the diagnosis of SIDS is often one of "exclusion", it is crucial to do a thorough death scene investigation and case review, in addition to the autopsy and lab tests

TREATMENT

APPROPRIATE HEALTH CARE
Because a SIDS death is sudden and the cause is unknown, SIDS cannot be "treated." However, there are some measures that may be effective in preventing SIDS: Maternal avoidance of cigarette and illicit drug use during pregnancy; breast-feeding; avoidance of the prone sleep position, excessive bed clothing, avoidance of passive cigarette smoke exposure.
Recent studies from Europe suggest some risk reduction with sleeping on back or side. (Because of concern over aspiration, the side position may be best.)

GENERAL MEASURES N/A

ACTIVITY N/A

DIET N/A

PATIENT EDUCATION
 • Family counseling (see Expected Course and Prognosis)
 • American Sudden Infant Death Syndrome Institute: 800-232-SIDS in Atlanta, Georgia
 • SIDS Alliance/National SIDS Foundation, Columbia, MD, (800)221-SIDS

MEDICATIONS

DRUG(S) OF CHOICE N/A
Contraindications: N/A
Precautions: N/A
Significant possible interactions: N/A

ALTERNATIVE DRUGS N/A

FOLLOWUP

PATIENT MONITORING Some authorities recommend cardiopulmonary monitoring in siblings of prior SIDS victims

PREVENTION/AVOIDANCE N/A

POSSIBLE COMPLICATIONS N/A

EXPECTED COURSE AND PROGNOSIS
• SIDS deaths have a powerful impact on families and their functioning. Physicians play an important role in providing immediate information about SIDS and sensitive counseling to limit parents' misinformation and feelings of guilt.
• Counseling needs of families vary from short-term to long-term; support groups are helpful to many couples. Physicians need to be familiar with resources available in their communities to help families mourning a SIDS death. Parents need to be counseled about subsequent pregnancies.
• Follow-up counseling, including review of the autopsy report with the family after some time has passed, will be important to help with understanding this condition and to clear the tremendous guilt these families experience.

MISCELLANEOUS

ASSOCIATED CONDITIONS N/A

AGE-RELATED FACTORS N/A
Pediatric: Occurs in infants only
Geriatric: N/A
Others: N/A

PREGNANCY N/A

SYNONYMS
• Crib death
• Cot death

ICD-9-CM 798.0

SEE ALSO N/A

OTHER NOTES N/A

ABBREVIATIONS N/A

REFERENCES
• Corr, C.A., Fuller, H., Barnickol, C.A. & Corr, D.M. (eds.): Sudden Infant Death Syndrome. Who Can Help and How. New York, Springer Publishing Co., 1991
• Hoffman, H.J., Damus, K., Hillman, L. & Krongrad, E.: Risk factors for SIDS. Results of the National Institute of Child Health and Human Development SIDS Cooperative Epidemiological Study. Annals NY Acad Sciences 1988, 533:13-30
• Peterson, D.R.: Evolution of the epidemiology of sudden infant death syndrome. Epidemiol Reviews 1980;2:97-112
• Willinger, M., James, L.S. & Catz, C.: Defining the Sudden Infant Death Syndrome (SIDS): Deliberations of an expert panel convened by the National Institute of Child Health and Human Development. Pediatr Pathol 1991;11:677-684
• AAP News Release, 4/15/92.

Author F. Hauck, M.D., M.S.

Suicide

BASICS

DESCRIPTION Completed suicide refers to self-inflicted death. Attempted suicide refers to potentially lethal acts which do not result in death and non-lethal, attention-seeking gestures (e.g., superficial cuts on wrists).
System(s) affected:
Genetics: No known genetic pattern
Incidence in USA:
• 10-12 in 100,00. Ninth leading cause of death in US adults. Second leading cause of death among children and adolescents.
• Approximately 28,000 completed suicides yearly in US accounting for 2% of all deaths
• Attempted suicide is ten times more frequent than completed suicides
Subpopulation incidence
  ◊ Ages 5-14 - 8/100,000
  ◊ Ages 15-24 - 13.1/100,000
Prevalence in USA: N/A
Predominant age: Highest in elderly (> 65 years) and adolescent age period (15-24 years)
Predominant sex:
• Men > Female - complete suicide (3:1)
• Female > Male - attempted suicide (3:1)

SIGNS AND SYMPTOMS
• Hopelessness about future
Suicidal thoughts with organized plan and intent
  ◊ Suicide note
  ◊ Giving away personal possessions
  ◊ Quitting a job
Major depression (screen for symptoms)
  ◊ Change in sleep
  ◊ Loss of interest
  ◊ Loss of energy
  ◊ Loss of concentration
  ◊ Loss of appetite
  ◊ Diminished psychomotor activity
  ◊ Guilt
  ◊ Suicidal ideations
Psychosis
  ◊ Ask about command auditory hallucinations to kill oneself

CAUSES
• Combination of psychiatric illness and social circumstances. Most patients have active psychiatric illness.
• Major depression and bipolar disorder account for 50% of completed suicides
• Alcoholism and drug abuse disorders account for 25% of completed suicides
• Schizophrenia and other psychotic disorders account for 10% of completed suicides

RISK FACTORS
Psychiatric
  ◊ Mood disorders (major depression, bipolar), alcoholism, drug abuse, psychotic disorders, personality disorders
    ◊ Family history of suicide
    ◊ History of previous suicide attempt

  ◊ Medical diagnosis of terminal illness (cancer, AIDS), chronic intractable pain, chronic and disabling illness (renal dialysis patient)
  ◊ Hopelessness about future
Epidemiologic
  ◊ Sex - males three times females
  ◊ Age - adolescent and geriatric population (males peaking at 75 years, females peaking at 55 years)
  ◊ Race - American Indian, Caucasian
  ◊ Marital status - single > divorced, widowed > married
Psychologic
  ◊ History of recent loss (loved one, job, etc.)
  ◊ Loss of social supports
  ◊ Important dates (holidays, birthdays, anniversaries, etc.)
Review mnemonic for risk factors = SAD PERSONS
  ◊ S=sex
  ◊ A-age
  ◊ D=depression
  ◊ P=previous attempt
  ◊ E=ethanol abuse
  ◊ R=rational thinking loss
  ◊ S=social support loss
  ◊ O=organized plan
  ◊ N=no spouse
  ◊ S=sickness
  ◊ If five risk factors present, consider very high suicidal risk

DIAGNOSIS

DIFFERENTIAL DIAGNOSIS
Psychiatric
  ◊ Mood disorders (major depression, bipolar)
  ◊ Alcohol intoxication and other drug abuse
  ◊ Psychotic disorders (e.g., schizophrenia)
  ◊ Personality disorder (e.g., borderline)
  ◊ Organic mental disorders (e.g., dementia, delirium)
  ◊ Adjustment disorders
  ◊ Panic disorders
  ◊ Post-traumatic stress disorder
Medical
  ◊ Hypothyroidism
  ◊ Cushing's disease/syndrome
  ◊ Addison's disease
  ◊ Hypopituitarism
Other (medications associated with depression)
  ◊ Anti-hypertensives (methyldopa, reserpine, clonidine)
  ◊ Corticosteroids
  ◊ Opiates
  ◊ Anti-tuberculous agents (isoniazid, ethionamide, cycloserine)
  ◊ Anabolic steroid withdrawal
  ◊ Barbiturates
  ◊ Benzodiazepines
  ◊ Cocaine withdrawal
  ◊ Amphetamine withdrawal

LABORATORY There are no laboratory tests to determine who will commit suicide. Patients who have completed violent suicides were found to have low CSF levels of 5-Hydroxyindoleacetic acid (5-HIAA), a serotonin metabolite. Other findings have included: increased CSF methoxyhydroxyphenylglycol (MHPG), nonsuppression of dexamethasone suppression test (DST), low platelet MAO (mono amine oxidase), low platelet serotonin, high platelet serotonin-2 receptor responsivity.
Drugs that may alter lab results: N/A
Disorders that may alter lab results: N/A

PATHOLOGICAL FINDINGS N/A

SPECIAL TESTS N/A

IMAGING N/A

DIAGNOSTIC PROCEDURES N/A

TREATMENT

APPROPRIATE HEALTH CARE
• Admit to psychiatric ward (voluntarily/involuntarily) if patient is severely depressed, intoxicated, psychotic or status post serious suicide attempt
• Admit to general hospital for acute medical care with psychiatric consultation
• Consider outpatient treatment with scheduled followup appointment if patient has social support system and no evidence of severe depression, psychosis or intoxication
• If unsure or patient is high risk (i.e., five positive risk factors - SAD PERSONS), admit to hospital for further observation and evaluation

GENERAL MEASURES
• All patients with suicide threats, gestures or attempts should be screened for suicide risk factors and have a full mental status exam and psychiatric consultation
• Ensure patient safety by least restrictive method (i.e., remove potentially dangerous objects, provide one-to-one constant observation, medication, 2-4 point restraints)
• Diagnose and treat underlying psychiatric and medical disorder
• Electroconvulsive therapy provides rapid, safe, and effective treatment option for severely depressed, acutely suicidal patients

ACTIVITY Suicide precautions; q 15 minute checks; one-to-one observation; 2-4 point restraints

DIET N/A

PATIENT EDUCATION American Academy of Family Physicians Foundation, P.O. Box 8418 Kansas City, MO 64114 (800)274-2237, ext. 4400

MEDICATIONS

DRUG(S) OF CHOICE
• Treat underlying psychiatric and medical illness
• Antidepressants, psychostimulants, and lithium for mood disorders
• A minimum of two weeks required to obtain response from antidepressants
• Neuroleptic medications (e.g., haloperidol, chlorpromazine) for psychotic symptoms
• Benzodiazepines (e.g., lorazepam) for anxiety symptoms
Agitated, combative and intoxicated patients in the emergency room
◊ May require sedation with neuroleptics (e.g., haloperidol 2-5 mg IM/IV) and/or benzodiazepines (e.g., lorazepam 2 mg IM/IV)
◊ Clinical response typically seen within 20-30 minutes
◊ If no response, increase previous dose (e.g., 4-10 mg haloperidol)
Contraindications: Avoid tricyclic antidepressants in patient with evidence of 2°, 3° AV block or left bundle branch block ECG
Precautions: Use smaller doses in elderly patients
Significant possible interactions:
Hypertensive crisis if MAO inhibitor antidepressants given in combination with medications containing sympathomimetic amines; tyramine-rich food; Demerol; tricyclic antidepressants

ALTERNATIVE DRUGS N/A

FOLLOWUP

PATIENT MONITORING
• Weekly outpatient followup appointments
• Prescribe only a weekly supply of antidepressants or other psychotropic medications at each appointment

PREVENTION/AVOIDANCE
• Provide crisis hot-line phone number and nearest crisis emergency room location
• Mobilize social support system and inform family and friends of options if patient becomes more suicidal
• Instruct patient to avoid any alcohol consumption

POSSIBLE COMPLICATIONS Brief
period of increased suicide risk as depression resolves and patient's energy and initiative returns

EXPECTED COURSE AND PROGNOSIS
• 15% of suicidal, depressed patients will ultimately complete suicide
• 82% of suicide victims have seen a doctor within the previous six months
• Approximately one-half of suicide victims have seen a doctor within one month of their death
• The key to a favorable course and prognosis is early recognition of risk factors, early diagnosis and treatment of a psychiatric disorder, and appropriate intervention and followup

MISCELLANEOUS

ASSOCIATED CONDITIONS Depression

AGE-RELATED FACTORS
Pediatric: Increasing suicide rate in adolescents. Suicide is second leading cause of death in adolescents.
Geriatric: Increasing rate with increasing age (women peak at 55 years, men peak at 75 years)
Others: N/A

PREGNANCY N/A

SYNONYMS N/A

ICD-9-CM N/A

SEE ALSO N/A

OTHER NOTES
• Overdose is the most common method for suicide attempts
• Shooting is the most common method for completed suicides
• Men prone to more violent suicides (i.e., shooting, jumping, hanging)
• Jumping most common method of suicide among patients in a general medical/surgical hospital

ABBREVIATIONS N/A

REFERENCES
• Hackett, T.P. & Cassem, N.H.: MGH Handbook of General Hospital Psychiatry. 2nd Ed. New York, PSG Publishing Company, Inc., 1987
• Talbott, J.A., Hales, R.E. & Yudofsky, S.C.: Textbook of Psychiatry. Washington, DC, American Psychiatric Press, Inc., 1988
• Patterson, W.M., Dohn, H.H., et al: Evaluation of suicidal patients, THE SAD PERSONS Scale, Psychosomatics, 1983

Author B. Currier, M.D. & E. Olsen, M.D.

Superior vena cava syndrome

BASICS

DESCRIPTION Partial or complete obstruction of the superior vena cava, 90% extrinsic, 70% from neoplasm (most frequently bronchogenic carcinoma), also thrombosis, fibrosis, invasion and aneurysm causing suffusion, varying degrees of airway obstruction and/or cyanosis of the face, neck, arms and occasionally chest and upper abdomen. Usual course - acute onset; chronic onset: often progressive.
System(s) affected: Cardiovascular, respiratory
Genetics: N/A
Incidence/Prevalence in USA: N/A
Predominant age: Young adult (16-40 years); middle age (40-60 years)
Predominant sex: Male > Female

SIGNS AND SYMPTOMS
• Dyspnea
• Facial swelling
• Truncal swelling
• Arm swelling
• Easy fatigability
• Orthopnea
• Chest pain
• Cough
• Headache
• Visual disturbances
• Altered consciousness
• Dysphagia
• Hoarseness
• Thoracic vein distention
• Neck vein distention
• Facial edema
• Chest vein distention
• Wheezing
• Tachypnea
• Facial plethora
• Cyanosis
• Arm edema
• Paralyzed vocal cord
• Conjunctival edema
• Proptosis
• Stridor
• Horner's syndrome
• Dilated retinal vessels
• Enlarged tongue
• Non-pitting edema of the neck (Stoke's collar)
• Fullness or stuffiness in ears/eyes
• Symptoms worse with lying down or leaning forward

CAUSES
• Obstruction of venous drainage of upper part of chest and neck. Sudden occlusion can cause rapid development of cerebral edema, intracranial thrombosis and death.
• Lung cancer, bronchogenic carcinoma/small cell
• Lymphoma
• Thymoma
• Fungus infections
• Breast cancer
• Other malignancies
• Iatrogenic
• Thyroid goiter
• Syphilitic aneurysm
• Tuberculous mediastinitis
• Primary superior vena caval thrombosis
• Pericardial constriction
• Idiopathic sclerosing mediastinitis

RISK FACTORS HIV infection

DIAGNOSIS

DIFFERENTIAL DIAGNOSIS
• Aortic aneurysm
• Tuberculosis, Histoplasmosis
• Fungal infections

LABORATORY Sputum cytology-malignant cells
Drugs that may alter lab results: N/A
Disorders that may alter lab results: N/A

PATHOLOGICAL FINDINGS Sputum cytology, occasionally thoracentesis, bone marrow, lymph node biopsy, bronchoscopy or thoracotomy confirm - malignant cells.

SPECIAL TESTS Increased central venous pressure (CVP), usually 20-50 mm Hg.

IMAGING
• Tc 99m scan - block to flow of contrast material into right heart, large collateral veins
• Chest x-ray, MRI, CT scan, and/or tomography - mediastinal mass, superior mediastinal mass, pulmonary lesion, superior vena cava obstruction, hilar adenopathy, pleural effusion.
• Venography - superior vena cava obstruction

DIAGNOSTIC PROCEDURES
• Bronchoscopy
• Thoracentesis, thoracotomy, lymph node biopsy, as indicated

TREATMENT

APPROPRIATE HEALTH CARE
• Inpatient, intensive care
• Surgical - superior vena cava reconstruction for benign processes may be considered

GENERAL MEASURES Radiotherapy

ACTIVITY Bedrest (head of bed elevated)

DIET As tolerated, possibly salt restriction

PATIENT EDUCATION As appropriate

MEDICATIONS

DRUG(S) OF CHOICE
• Chemotherapy for cancer
• Steroids for some malignancies, esp. if cerebral or laryngeal edema
• Antifungal or antitubercular medications according to underlying cause
• Consider diuretics
• Anticoagulation role unclear
• Fibrinolytics (e.g., urokinase) for thrombosis
Contraindications: Refer to manufacturer's literature
Precautions: Refer to manufacturer's literature
Significant possible interactions: Refer to manufacturer's literature

ALTERNATIVE DRUGS   N/A

FOLLOWUP

PATIENT MONITORING   Linked to cause. If infection, monitor for evaluation of antimicrobial treatment. If malignant, monitor response to radiotherapy or chemotherapy.

PREVENTION/AVOIDANCE   No preventive measures known

POSSIBLE COMPLICATIONS
Complications of underlying disease

EXPECTED COURSE AND PROGNOSIS   High probability of response; prognosis linked to cause; 20% 1-year survival for lung cancer; 50% 2-year survival for lymphoma. 85% neoplastic causes better in 3 weeks with radiation therapy, but symptoms usually recur.

MISCELLANEOUS

ASSOCIATED CONDITIONS
• Breast cancer
• Lung cancer
• HIV infection
• Hyperthyroidism
• Tuberculosis, histoplasmosis
• Lymphoma

AGE-RELATED FACTORS
Pediatric: N/A
Geriatric: Occurs in geriatric patients
Others: N/A

PREGNANCY   Must treat underlying condition despite pregnancy

SYNONYMS
• Superior mediastinal syndrome
• Superior vena cava obstruction

ICD-9-CM   459.2

SEE ALSO   N/A

OTHER NOTES   N/A

ABBREVIATIONS   N/A

REFERENCES
• Sculier, J.P. & Feld, R.: Superior Vena Cava Obstruction Syndrome: Recommendations for Management. In Cancer Treat Rev, 1985; 12:209
• DeVita, V.T., Jr., Hellman, S. & Rosenberg, S.A. (eds.): Cancer: Principles and Practices of Oncology. 3rd Ed. Philadelphia, J.B. Lippincott, 1989
• Wyngaarden, J.B., et al. (eds.): Cecil Textbook of Medicine.19th Ed. Philadelphia, W.B. Saunders Co.,1992
• Schwartz, S.I. (ed): Principles of Surgery. 4th Ed. New York, McGraw-Hill, 1984

Author   P. Jaster, M.D.

Syncope

BASICS

DESCRIPTION Approximately 5-20% of adults will have one or more episodes of syncope by age 75. The disorder accounts for about 1% of hospital admissions and about 3% of emergency room visits. Its annual incidence in the institutionalized elderly is about 6%.

System(s) affected: Nervous, Cardiovascular
Genetics: N/A
Incidence in USA: 6% in persons over age 75
Prevalence in USA: UNknown
Predominant age: Elderly
Predominant sex: N/A

SIGNS AND SYMPTOMS
Transient loss of consciousness characterized by unresponsiveness, loss of postural tone, and spontaneous recovery

CAUSES
• Cardiac - obstruction to outflow:
  ◊ Aortic stenosis
  ◊ Hypertrophic cardiomyopathy
  ◊ Pulmonary embolus
• Cardiac - arrhythmias:
  ◊ Ventricular tachycardia
  ◊ Sick sinus syndrome
  ◊ 2nd and 3rd degree AV block
• Non-cardiac:
  ◊ Vasovagal, situational (micturition, defecation, cough)
  ◊ Orthostatic hypotension
  ◊ Drug induced
  ◊ Seizures
  ◊ Transient ischemic attack
  ◊ Carotid sinus
  ◊ Psychogenic

RISK FACTORS
• Patients with heart disease
• Patients taking following drugs:
  ◊ Antihypertensives
  ◊ Vasodilators (including calcium channel blockers, ACE inhibitors, and nitrates)
  ◊ Phenothiazines
  ◊ Antidepressants
  ◊ Antiarrhythmics
  ◊ Diuretics

DIAGNOSIS

DIFFERENTIAL DIAGNOSIS
• Drop attacks
• Coma
• A careful history, physical examination and an ECG are more important than other investigations in determining a diagnosis. Make sure that the patient or witness (if present) is not talking about vertigo, coma, or drop attacks. Prodromal manifestations of sudden weakness, nausea, and sweating, especially in circumstances provoking strong emotion, are diagnostic of vasovagal syncope. Syncope of sudden onset with no prodrome or brief premonitory symptoms suggest a cardiac cause. Vasovagal syncope does not occur when the patient is horizontal; cardiac syncope can occur in any position. Syncope with exertion suggestions a cardiac cause. Physical exam should be directed to blood pressure and pulse, both lying and standing. Check for a cardiac murmur or a focal neurologic abnormality.
After a careful evaluation, including diagnostic procedures and special tests, the cause of syncope will be found in only 50-60% of patients.

LABORATORY Rarely helpful. Less than 2% have hyponatremia, hypocalcemia, hypoglycemia or renal failure causing seizures.
Drugs that may alter lab results: N/A
Disorders that may alter lab results: N/A

PATHOLOGICAL FINDINGS N/A

SPECIAL TESTS
• If history and physical suggestive of ischemic, valvular or congenital heart disease - echocardiogram, cardiac catheterization
• If CNS disease suspected - EEG, head CT, head MRI

IMAGING Lung scan if history and physical examination suggestive of pulmonary embolism

DIAGNOSTIC PROCEDURES
• ECG monitoring, either in the hospital or ambulatory (Holter), is useful in 2-17% of patients. Arrhythmias are frequently documented, but rarely associated with syncope. Monitoring should be done in patients with heart disease, and in patients with recurrent syncope. Patient activated intermittent loop recorders, which the patient activates after regaining consciousness, can record 4-5 minutes of retrograde ECG rhythm. These have been helpful in patients with recurrent syncope
• Electrophysiologic studies (EPS) have been positive in 18-75% of patients. Induction of ventricular tachycardia and dysfunction of the His-Purkinje system are the two most common abnormalities. Although there is the problem of knowing whether the arrhythmia noted or induced during the study is the cause of syncope, EPS should be done in patients with heart disease and recurrent syncope.
• The following findings are probable causes of syncope:
  ◊ Sustained ventricular tachycardia
  ◊ Sinus node recovery time 3 seconds or more
  ◊ Pacing-induced infranodal block
  ◊ H-V interval greater than 100 msec
• Carotid hypersensitivity should be considered in patients with syncope on head turning, especially with head turning while wearing tight collar, and in patients with neck tumors and neck tissue scars. The technique is not standardized. One side should be massaged at a time for 20 seconds with constant monitoring of pulse and blood pressure. Atropine should be readily available.
• Tilt testing, with and without isoproterenol infusion, is a new provocative test for vasovagal syncope which is not standardized, but has been reported positive (symptomatic hypotension and bradycardia) in 26-87% of patients. However, the test has been reported positive in 0-45% of control subjects. The role of this test in the workup of patients with syncope of unknown origin is not known. Patients with a positive tilt test often respond to beta-blocker treatment.
• Psychiatric evaluation should be considered in patients with multiple episodes of syncope (greater 5/year) who do not have heart disease. Anxiety, depression, alcohol and drug abuse can be associated with syncope.

TREATMENT

APPROPRIATE HEALTH CARE
• Patients with heart disease should be admitted to the hospital for evaluation
• Elderly patients without previously recognized heart disease should be admitted if the physician thinks that a cardiac cause of syncope is likely
• Patients without heart disease, especially young patients (less 60 years old), can be safely worked up as outpatients

GENERAL MEASURES
No specific measures

ACTIVITY
Fully active unless severe cardiac disease

DIET
No specific diet unless heart disease

PATIENT EDUCATION
Reassure the patient that most cardiac causes of syncope can be treated, and that patients with non-cardiac causes do well, even if the cause of syncope is never discovered

 MEDICATIONS

DRUG(S) OF CHOICE
Antiarrhythmic drugs should be used to treat arrhythmias documented during monitoring which occur simultaneously with syncope or symptoms of presyncope. Asymptomatic arrhythmias found on monitoring usually do not require treatment.
The decision to treat patients on the basis of arrhythmias or conduction abnormalities provoked or detected during EPS is even more problematic. Does the arrhythmia or conduction abnormality have anything to do with the patient's symptoms? Most would treat a patient with provoked sustained ventricular tachycardiac with an antiarrhythmic drug that suppressed the arrhythmia during the study. Many recommend pacemaker implantation in patients with H-V intervals greater than 100 msec, pacing induced infranodal block, or sinus node recovery time of 3 sec or more. The rationale basis for such treatment is that recurrent syncope is less frequent in those patients with positive EPS who are treated than it is in those who have negative EPS.
Contraindications: N/A
Precautions: N/A
Significant possible interactions: N/A

ALTERNATIVE DRUGS
N/A

 FOLLOWUP

PATIENT MONITORING
• Frequent followup visits for patients with cardiac causes of syncope, especially patients on antiarrhythmic drugs
• Patients with an unknown cause of syncope rarely (5%) have a diagnosis made during followup

PREVENTION/AVOIDANCE
Avoid Risk factors

POSSIBLE COMPLICATIONS
• Trauma from falling
• Death - see prognosis

EXPECTED COURSE AND PROGNOSIS
Cumulative mortality at 2 years:
◊ Low (2-5%) - young patients (< 60) with a non-cardiac cause or unknown cause of syncope.
◊ Intermediate (20%) - older patients (> 60) with a non-cardiac or unknown cause of syncope.
◊ High (32-38%) - patients with cardiac cause of syncope.

 MISCELLANEOUS

ASSOCIATED CONDITIONS
See Causes

AGE-RELATED FACTORS
Pediatric: Rare in this age group
Geriatric: More common in this age group, prognosis worse in older patients
Others: N/A

PREGNANCY
N/A

SYNONYMS
N/A

ICD-9-CM
780.2 syncope and collapse

SEE ALSO
• Aortic valvular stenosis
• Carotid sinus syndrome
• Stokes-Adams attacks
• Idiopathic hypertrophic subaortic stenosis
• Ventricular tachycardia
• Complete heart block
• Pulmonary embolism

ABBREVIATIONS
N/A

REFERENCES
Kapoor, W.N.: Diagnosis and management of the patient with syncope. JAMA.268:2553-2560, 1992

Author J. Smith, M.D.

Synovitis, pigmented villonodular

 BASICS

DESCRIPTION
A proliferative disorder of unknown etiology affecting synovial lined joints, tendon sheaths or bursa. Occurs in diffuse or focal forms which have a quite different prognosis.

System(s) affected: Musculoskeletal
Genetics: N/A
Incidence/Prevalence in USA: Two occurrences per 1 million population
Predominant age:
• Diffuse form appears more commonly in the 3rd and 4th decades
• Focal is more common in the 5th and 6th decades
Predominant sex:
• Diffuse form: Male = Female
• Focal form: Female > Male

SIGNS AND SYMPTOMS
Diffuse form:
◊ Unilateral and monoarticular with 80% occurring in the knee and affecting the hip, ankle and shoulder in decreasing order
◊ Mild and progressive pain in involved joint
◊ History of trauma (30% of cases)
◊ Recurrent swelling and tenderness to palpation of involved joint
◊ Increased skin temperatures over involved joint
Focal form:
◊ More common in tendon than joints
◊ Involves the tendons of the hand and feet, usually, rarely the wrist and ankle or a major joint
◊ Presents as slow growing, painless mass
◊ Most common cause of tumor in hand, second to ganglion
Chronic, inflammatory:
Unusual monoarticular presentation

CAUSES
Unknown, possibly repeated local hemorrhages

RISK FACTORS
N/A

 DIAGNOSIS

DIFFERENTIAL DIAGNOSIS
Diffuse form (if soft tissue swelling is the main finding):
◊ Synovioma - frequently calcifies
◊ Synovial hemangioma - usually occurs in childhood and often associated with cutaneous hemangioma
◊ Lipoma - boggy fullness to palpation and absence of serosanguinous fluid on aspiration
◊ Unusual mono-articular presentation for other forms of chronic, inflammatory arthritis
Diffuse form (if multiple subchondral cysts on x-ray are the main finding):
◊ Degenerative joint disease - cysts occur on weight bearing surfaces only, while cysts of PVNS may occur anywhere in joints. Osteophytes common in degenerative arthritis, absent in PVNS.
◊ Tuberculous arthritis is characterized by severe juxta-articular osteoporosis
◊ Amyloid arthropathy is usually symmetrical and more common in the upper extremities. The joint space is preserved.
◊ Synovial chondromatosis - presence of punctate calcifications along the margin. (Occurs 60-70% of time.)
Focal form:
◊ Ganglion - contains jelly-like fluid on aspiration
◊ Dupuytren's nodules - not attached to tendon sheath and therefore does not move with tendon

LABORATORY
Aspiration of a serosanguineous fluid from a joint in the absence of trauma is highly suggestive of diffuse pigmented villonodular synovitis (fluid can be clear, however). Aspirated joint fluid may contain high cholesterol.
Drugs that may alter lab results: N/A
Disorders that may alter lab results: N/A

PATHOLOGICAL FINDINGS
The synovium shows proliferation into villi or nodules with subsynovial cellular infiltrate that includes fibroblasts, lymphocytes and lipid-laden macrophages (foam cells)

SPECIAL TESTS
N/A

IMAGING
• The CT scan may be helpful, but MRI has the best potential for being diagnostic due to the presence of hemosiderin and fat within the abnormal tissue present in the joint
• X-ray shows soft tissue swelling of involved joints. Subchondral cysts and pressure erosions are limited mostly to the hip. The absence of osteophytes and juxta-articular osteoporosis is significant.

DIAGNOSTIC PROCEDURES
• Arthroscopy usually reveals characteristic synovial changes and allows definitive biopsy
• An arthrogram is not usually diagnostic
• Radioisotopes and ultrasound studies are also usually not definitive

 TREATMENT

APPROPRIATE HEALTH CARE
Inpatient or outpatient surgery

GENERAL MEASURES
• Diffuse form - total synovectomy is the usual recommended treatment, but has a recurrence rate of 25-40%. X-ray therapy alone or combined with synovectomy has been tried, again with high recurrence rate. Recently, intra-articular injections of radioisotopes, in particular yttrium-90, has been tried and shows some early promise, but evaluation of this is incomplete.
• Focal form - local excision results in cure

ACTIVITY
No restrictions

DIET
No special diet

PATIENT EDUCATION
N/A

MEDICATIONS

DRUG(S) OF CHOICE None
Contraindications: N/A
Precautions: N/A
Significant possible interactions: N/A

ALTERNATIVE DRUGS N/A

FOLLOWUP

PATIENT MONITORING Patients should be followed twice annually after treatment of the diffuse form by history and physical examination. X-rays yearly, especially if the hip is involved.

PREVENTION/AVOIDANCE N/A

POSSIBLE COMPLICATIONS
Osteoarthritis, especially in the hip joint

EXPECTED COURSE AND PROGNOSIS
• Good in focal type
• Guarded in the diffuse form with recurrences of disease common as well as joint dysfunction

MISCELLANEOUS

ASSOCIATED CONDITIONS N/A

AGE-RELATED FACTORS
Pediatric: N/A
Geriatric: N/A
Others: N/A

PREGNANCY N/A

SYNONYMS
• Xanthoma
• Benign synovioma
• Giant cell tumor of tendon sheath
• Fibro xanthoma
• PVNS

ICD-9-CM 719.20

SEE ALSO Rheumatoid arthritis

OTHER NOTES N/A

ABBREVIATIONS N/A

REFERENCES
• Flandry, J.B. & Hughston, J.S.: Pigmented Villonodular Synovitis. Current Concepts and Review. 1987

Author F. Johnston, M.D.

Syphilis

BASICS

DESCRIPTION An infection, characterized by sequential stages (acute, subacute or chronic), with the spirochete, Treponema pallidum
• Infectious (primary or early syphilis) consists of a primary stage and a secondary stage. It may include neurosyphilis (central nervous system involvement). If the patient is untreated, the infectious stage may be followed by a latent stage.
• Latent stage syphilis (secondary) is an asymptomatic phase. If it occurs up to one year after the infectious stage, it is described as early latent. If it occurs 2 or more years after the infectious stage, it is termed late latent.
• Tertiary (or late syphilis) stage is late generalized syphilis
• Congenital is syphilis acquired in utero
System(s) affected: Reproductive, Skin/Exocrine, Nervous, Cardiovascular
Genetics: Unknown, however Caucasians more likely to develop CNS complications, African-Americans to develop cardiac problems
Incidence/Prevalence in USA:
• 1989 - nationally 18.4/100,000 new cases
• In urban African-American populations, as high as 124/100,000
• Cases reported are rapidly rising
Predominant age: Sexually active years
Predominant sex: Male > Female

SIGNS AND SYMPTOMS
Infectious syphilis - primary
◊ Chancre begins as a papule which erodes to a 0.3 to 2 cm non-tender ulcer with a hard edge and clean, yellow base (unless secondarily infected) 9 to 90 days after exposure (median 3 weeks)
◊ Usually found on genitalia, frequently solitary, may be multiple, may have regional lymphadenopathy
◊ Heals with scarring in 3 to 6 weeks with 75% of patients having no further symptoms
Infectious syphilis - secondary
◊ 25% of patients enter this stage 2-6 weeks after exposure, may overlap with chancre
◊ Resolves spontaneously in 2-6 weeks in most patients
◊ May wax and wane between secondary and latent stages
◊ Rash is bilaterally symmetric, polymorphic, palpable lesions with "fresh cut ham" color, non-pruritic, usually not bullous or vesicular, frequently on palms and soles
◊ Patchy alopecia of scalp, eyebrows and beard common
◊ Mucous patches - thin gray smears - and condyloma lata - moist, flat, pink, peripheral warty lesions - may be present on glans, vulva, perianal, vulva areas
◊ Generalized lymphadenopathy and flu-like symptoms occur early with rash
◊ Rarely may be accompanied by nephritis, meningitis, uveitis, hepatitis
◊ Mild hepatosplenomegaly often noticeable

Latent syphilis
◊ Characterized by positive serology but no signs or symptoms
◊ Patient is not infectious after one year, but may relapse to infectious secondary stage in untreated patients (25% in first year, small percent second year, none after that)
Tertiary syphilis
◊ Marked by cardiovascular (aortic valve disease or aneurysms)
◊ Neurological (meningitis, encephalitis, tabes dorsalis)
◊ Dementia (paresis)
◊ Deep cutaneous (gummas which are destructive granulomatous pockets)
◊ Orthopedic (Charcot's joints, osteomyelitis) complications (rare with antibiotics)
◊ Serologies often negative
Congenital syphilis
◊ Failure to thrive
◊ Rhinitis
◊ Lymphadenopathy
◊ Jaundice
◊ Anemia
◊ Hepatosplenomegaly
◊ Nephrosis
◊ Meningitis
◊ Rash (the hallmark) similar to secondary syphilis in adults, but may be bullous or vesicular

CAUSES
• Exposure through sexual contact
• Exposure to infected body fluids
• Transplacentally
• Treponema pallidum

RISK FACTORS
• Multiple sexual partners
• IV drug use
• Male homosexuality

DIAGNOSIS

DIFFERENTIAL DIAGNOSIS
• Primary syphilis - chancroid, lymphogranuloma venereum, granuloma inguinale, herpes, Behçet's syndrome, trauma
• Secondary syphilis - pityriasis rosea, guttate psoriasis, drug eruption
• Positive serology and/or negative clinical signs and symptoms - previously treated syphilis, biological false positive, other spirochetal disease (yaws, pinta)

LABORATORY
• Requires either demonstration of organisms on microscopy or positive serology on blood or cerebrospinal fluid (CSF)
• Organism cannot be cultured, but diagnosis is never made on clinical signs and symptoms alone

Nonspecific treponemal tests: Venereal Disease Research Laboratory (VDRL) or rapid plasma reagin (RPR) are characterized as follows:
◊ Relatively inexpensive, primary screening test
◊ Positive within 7 days of exposure
◊ Titer decreases with time or treatment
◊ Used to monitor therapy: fourfold rise in titer indicates new infection while failure to decrease fourfold within one year is treatment failure
◊ False-positive common but positives are highly suggestive even without clinical signs and symptoms (confirm with fluorescent treponemal antibody absorption [FTA-ABS])
◊ Titer >= 1:64 even without confirming test is probably diagnostic of acute syphilis or other treponematoses
◊ Labs need to titer tests to final end point (not report as ">1:512" for example) to make best use of results in monitoring therapy response
◊ Beware of prozone phenomenon - negative results due to very high titers of antibody. Test diluted serum sample, as well, to declare a given specimen as negative.
Specific treponemal tests: Fluorescent treponemal antibody absorption (FTA-ABS), microhemagglutination treponema pallidum (MHA-TP)
◊ More expensive, used to confirm diagnosis
◊ Usually positive for life after treatment
◊ Due to unusual nonspecific test results in HIV infected patients, these tests may be needed to absolutely rule out syphilis
Lumbar puncture for CSF serologies should be done:
◊ In cases of latent syphilis where duration is unknown or non-penicillin therapy is planned
◊ Whenever neurological symptoms are present
◊ VDRL, not RPR is used on CSF, may be negative in neurosyphilis
◊ Negative FTA-ABS or MHA-TP on CSF excludes neurosyphilis
Drugs that may alter lab results: Many drugs reported to cause false-positive, but this is relatively uncommon with a good history
Disorders that may alter lab results:
• Rheumatoid disorders
• Acute febrile illness
• HIV infection
• Pregnancy

PATHOLOGICAL FINDINGS Aneurysm, osteomyelitis, gummas in late cases

SPECIAL TESTS
• Dark field microscopy
• Immunofluorescence
• Skin biopsy

IMAGING Only in late cases as indicated

DIAGNOSTIC PROCEDURES
Specialized test available from Center for Disease Control (CDC) to confirm false-positive if necessary

TREATMENT

APPROPRIATE HEALTH CARE
Outpatient, except for initiating IV penicillin or desensitization

GENERAL MEASURES
• Baseline serologies prior to treatment to monitor its success
• Symptomatic treatment of the chancres and rash of secondary syphilis (for patient's comfort only) prior to definitive antibiotic therapy

ACTIVITY
• Full activity, but no sexual contacts until declared cured

DIET No special diet

PATIENT EDUCATION
• Need to trace and treat all sexual contacts of the patient
• Keep followup appointments to monitor success of therapy
• Advise patient to avoid intercourse until treatment is complete
• Local health department can provide literature and contact tracing

MEDICATIONS

DRUG(S) OF CHOICE
• Primary, secondary and latent less than one year - benzathine penicillin G, 2.4 million units IM for 1 dose
• Latent > 1 year - benzathine penicillin G, 2.4 million units IM weekly for 3 doses
• Neurosyphilis - aqueous procaine penicillin G (APPG) 2-4 million units IM daily for 10-14 days with probenecid 500 mg q6h, or 2-4 million units penicillin GK IV every 4 hours for at least 10 days. Follow each therapy with benzathine penicillin G 2.4 million units IM weekly for 3 doses.
• Epidemiologic treatment for contacts without symptoms, treat as primary after baseline serologies are obtained
• Congenital - with abnormal CSF, 50,000 units/kg of aqueous procaine penicillin G (APPG) IM for at least 10 days. With negative CSF serologies, 50,000 units/kg benzathine penicillin G in one IM injection.
Contraindications: Allergy to penicillin
Precautions:
• HIV infected and pregnant patients may show poor response to recommended IM doses. Use IV therapy for all treatment failures in these patients.
• Do NOT give benzathine or procaine penicillins IV

Significant possible interactions: None, however, Jarisch-Herxheimer reaction, marked by fever, chills, headache, myalgias, new rash is common on starting treatment due to the lysis of treponemes and should not be confused with a reaction to antibiotics. It is managed with antihistamines and antipyretics.

ALTERNATIVE DRUGS
• Erythromycin, tetracyclines, ceftriaxone (Rocephin) may be used. However, in penicillin allergic patients, desensitization is easily accomplished and is recommended for HIV infected and pregnant patients so that penicillin can be used.
• Standard treatment with ceftriaxone and tetracycline used for gonorrhea is usually therapeutic for incubating syphilis

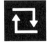
FOLLOWUP

PATIENT MONITORING Repeat serologies for 3 months, then yearly to confirm treatment. Do serological studies more frequently in HIV infected patients.

PREVENTION/AVOIDANCE
• Discuss safe sex
• Use of condoms

POSSIBLE COMPLICATIONS
• Cardiovascular disease
• Central nervous system disease
• Membranous glomerulonephritis
• Paroxysmal cold hemoglobinemia
• Organ damage that cannot be reversed
• Many other disorders

EXPECTED COURSE AND PROGNOSIS Excellent in all cases except late syphilis complications and a few HIV infected patients

MISCELLANEOUS

ASSOCIATED CONDITIONS
• Other sexually transmitted diseases
• HIV infection and hepatitis B (strongly urge patients treated for syphilis to obtain screenings for both)

AGE-RELATED FACTORS
Pediatric: In non-congenital cases, must consider possible child abuse
Geriatric: N/A
Others: N/A

PREGNANCY Early detection is imperative, all expectant mothers should have serologies as part of routine prenatal care

SYNONYMS
• Lues
• The Great Imitator

ICD-9-CM 090.0-097

SEE ALSO N/A

OTHER NOTES Many experts urge more aggressive treatment than standard regimens in all patients and strongly advocate the use of penicillin rather than any alternative antibiotic

ABBREVIATIONS
• CSF = cerebrospinal fluid
• FTA-ABS = fluorescent treponemal antibody absorption
• MHA-TP = microhemagglutination treponema pallidum
• VDRL = Venereal Disease Research Laboratory
• RPR = rapid plasma reagin

REFERENCE
Centers for Disease Control: Sexually transmitted diseases: Treatment for, Guidelines 1985. MMWR 34:94S, 1985

Author K. Hepler, M.D.

Systemic lupus erythematosus (SLE)

 BASICS

DESCRIPTION
A multi-system, autoimmune inflammatory condition characterized by a fluctuating, chronic course. Varies from mild to severe and may be lethal (CNS and renal forms).

System(s) affected: Hemic/Lymphatic/Immunologic, Nervous, Renal/Urologic, Endocrine/Metabolic, Skin/Exocrine, Gastrointestinal, Musculoskeletal

Genetics: Markers: HLA-B8; HLA-DR2; HLA-DR3

Incidence in USA: Unknown

Prevalence in USA: 20/100,000

Predominant age: All ages, but 30-50 are most common

Predominant sex: Female > Male (10:1)

SIGNS AND SYMPTOMS
- Arthritis
- Fever
- Anorexia
- Malaise
- Weight loss
- Skin lesions
- Oral ulcers
- Eye pain and/or redness
- Chest pain and/or shortness of breath
- Pallor
- Nausea, vomiting, diarrhea
- Muscles - tenderness, aching and stiffness
- Headaches and visual problems
- Psychosis/delirium

CAUSES
- Most cases are idiopathic
- Drugs - drug induced lupus is clinically different from idiopathic SLE

RISK FACTORS
- Race - Blacks, Hispanics, Asians, and Native Americans have higher prevalence than Whites.
- Genetic markers - HLA-B8, HLA-DR2, HLA-DR3.
- Hereditary complement deficiency especially C2 and C4

 DIAGNOSIS

DIFFERENTIAL DIAGNOSIS
- SLE mimics numerous systemic conditions, especially those involving inflammation
- Many other disorders mimic SLE - rheumatoid arthritis, mixed connective tissue disease (MCTD), scleroderma, metastatic malignancy, fever of unknown origin, psychogenic rheumatism and many cutaneous rashes. No one test or biopsy is pathognomonic.

LABORATORY
- Positive antinuclear antibody (ANA)
- Anti-double standard DNA (dsDNA), anti-Sm, false-positive VDRL, or positive LE preparation. These tests have either high sensitivity (ANA, false-positive VDRL) or specificity (anti-dsDNA, anti-Sm and LE preparation) and are included as American Rheumatology Association (ARA) criteria for the diagnosis of SLE along with the clinical features.
- Sedimentation rate is nonspecific, but valuable in assessing activity of SLE
- Anemia
- Leukopenia
- Lymphopenia
- Abnormal urinary sediment
- Proteinuria
- Increased prothrombin time
- Positive anticardiolipin
- Hypoalbuminuria
- Thrombocytopenia
- Increased serum creatinine
- Positive Coombs test

Drugs that may alter lab results: N/A

Disorders that may alter lab results: N/A

PATHOLOGICAL FINDINGS
Connective tissue disorders affecting skin, blood vessels, serous and synovial membranes
- Collagenous swelling
- Fibrinoid change
- Cellular necrosis
- Periarterial sclerosis
- Granulomatous reaction
- Infiltration of polymorphonuclear leukocytes, plasma cells, lymphocytes in walls of small vessels, arterioles of skin, spleen, glomeruli, endocardium pericardium, brain
- Hematoxylin bodies resembling those in LE cells
- Vegetation on heart valves

SPECIAL TESTS
- Complement levels, immune complex assays (cryoglobulins, Raji cell test, C1q precipitins)
- Coagulation studies (lupus anticoagulant)
- Biopsy of skin, kidney and peripheral nerves may reveal typical histopathology

IMAGING
- Cerebral angiography in CNS lupus
- Chest x-ray for pulmonary infiltration, pleural effusion
- MRI to detect CNS lupus
- Echocardiogram for pericardial effusion

DIAGNOSTIC PROCEDURES
American Rheumatology Association (ARA) criteria are a combination of any 4 manifestations of the 11 listed
- ◊ 1 Malar (butterfly) rash
- ◊ 2 Discoid rash
- ◊ 3 Photosensitivity
- ◊ 4 Oral/nasopharyngeal ulcers
- ◊ 5 Nonerosive arthritis
- ◊ 6 Pleuritis or pericarditis
- ◊ 7 Renal disorder - proteinuria or cylindruria
- ◊ 8 Neurologic disorder - psychosis or seizures
- ◊ 9 Hematologic disorder - hemolytic anemia, leukopenia (less than 4,000), lymphopenia (less than 1,500), thrombocytopenia (less than 100,000)
- ◊ 10 Immunologic disorder
- ◊ 11 Positive antinuclear antibody (ANA) in absence of drugs known to cause positive ANA
- ◊ Note: While the above criteria are required for proper epidemiologic classification of SLE, in practical situations, the combination of a multi-system inflammatory illness, positive antinuclear antibody (ANA) and absence of a better diagnosis often represents the most practical way to make a clinical diagnosis

 TREATMENT

APPROPRIATE HEALTH CARE
Outpatient with regular monitoring

GENERAL MEASURES
- Avoidance of or protection from ultraviolet light by using sunscreens, hats, etc.
- Early intervention when infections occur
- Energy conservation
- Stress avoidance/management

ACTIVITY
- As active as possible
- Those with arthritis may be limited by their pain, but active exercises are to be encouraged

DIET No special diet unless for complications such as renal failure

PATIENT EDUCATION Printed materials available on lupus from the Arthritis Foundation, 1314 Spring Street N.W., Atlanta, GA 30309, (404)872-7100 and from the Lupus Foundation of America, 1717 Massachusetts Avenue, NW, Suite 203, Washington, D.C. 20036, (800)558-0121

MEDICATIONS

DRUG(S) OF CHOICE
• No one drug of choice available. Treatment is symptomatic with certain exceptions. Use of local steroids for cutaneous manifestations, nonsteroidal anti-inflammatory drugs for minor arthritis symptoms, low dose steroids for minor discomfort and high dose steroids for major inflammatory disease.
• Use of immunosuppressants is indicated for renal disease and severe disease in other organs
• Minor arthritis - NSAID's
• More significant arthritis or dermal lupus - hydroxychloroquine 310 mg (400 mg of the sulfate salt) qd
• Major symptoms in any organ system or combination of organ systems - prednisone 30-60 mg qd
• Glomerulonephritis - cyclophosphamide 0.5 gm/m2 IV monthly together with prednisone 60 mg po qd tapering to 10 mg every other day after 4 months
Contraindications: Refer to manufacturer's profile of each drug
Precautions: Ensure good hydration when administering cyclophosphamide due to possibility of hemorrhagic cystitis
Significant possible interactions: Refer to manufacturer's profile of each drug

ALTERNATIVE DRUGS   Included in Drug(s) of choice

FOLLOWUP

PATIENT MONITORING
• Follow acute flares frequently, (weekly to monthly) for adjustment of medication based on clinical impression. Laboratory parameters are of limited value. CBC useful in hematologic lupus. Serum creatinine or renal clearance tests of value in renal lupus. Sedimentation rate often helps determine adequate suppression of symptoms or development of a remission.
• The confirming tests for lupus (ANA titers, anti-DNA titers, complement levels, etc.) are usually not helpful in Followup assessment
• Use of continuing medication depends upon symptoms. Exception is in the case of renal lupus for which it has been shown that a defined course of monthly IV cyclophosphamide has been of value.

PREVENTION/AVOIDANCE
• Avoiding sun exposure is only necessary for approximately one sixth of SLE patients (those who self report such sensitivity)
• Routine vaccinations are safe and appropriate for SLE patients
• Drugs known to induce SLE in normal individuals are not necessarily contraindicated in patients who have idiopathic SLE

POSSIBLE COMPLICATIONS   Fever, vasculitis, panniculitis, myositis, avascular necrosis of bone, endocarditis, pulmonary fibrosis, renal failure, organic brain syndromes, peripheral neuropathy, stroke syndromes, pancreatitis and elevated liver enzymes, infertility, ascites, venous thrombosis, seizures

EXPECTED COURSE AND PROGNOSIS
• Most patients with lupus follow a course of remissions and exacerbations. Many experience spontaneous permanent remission.
• Treatment of renal lupus (the most serious form) with immunosuppressors, renal dialysis, and renal transplantation, has increased the five year life expectancy to over 90%. For those patients surviving the first two years of disease, life expectancy is essentially normal.
• In patients with drug-induced lupus, symptoms should gradually decrease upon discontinuation of the suspected agent.

MISCELLANEOUS

ASSOCIATED CONDITIONS   Other autoimmune diseases - rheumatoid arthritis, hypothyroidism, diabetes

AGE-RELATED FACTORS
Pediatric: Stroke syndromes frequently seen in children
Geriatric:
• Higher percentage of males involved among the elderly
• Since "false-positive ANA" reaches 15% in the elderly, caution in interpretation is required in this age group
Others: N/A

PREGNANCY
• Onset of lupus and lupus flares are more common during pregnancy
• Fetal loss is increased for mothers with lupus
• Newborns of mothers who have lupus are more likely to have cardiac arrhythmias
• Specialists' collaboration during pregnancy is indicated

SYNONYMS
• SLE
• Disseminated lupus erythematosus

ICD-9-CM   710.0

SEE ALSO
• Autoimmune hemolytic anemia
• Glomerulonephritis

OTHER NOTES   N/A

ABBREVIATIONS   N/A

REFERENCE   Kelley, W.N., Harris, E.D., Ruddy S. & Sledge, C.B.: Textbook of Rheumatology. 4th Ed. Philadelphia, W.B. Saunders Co., 1993

Author   J. Boyer, M.D.

Tapeworm infestation

BASICS

DESCRIPTION Tapeworms (t.) are segmented intestinal cestodes (worms). Its head is called the scolex; its chain-like body is the strobila. Each segment of the strobila is a proglottid. The body chain of proglottides may vary in length from 3 mm to 25 meters.
• The majority of the tapeworm's life cycle requires an intermediate host before man becomes involved. Man usually acquires an infection by eating the cyst form in tissue (pork, beef, fresh water fish) or by eating an infected arthropod (rat fleas, beetles, cockroaches, dog fleas or lice) that may he found in dry or bulk cereals, or stored products. Small children or adults playing with a friendly dog or cat may get an infected intermediate host on their hands, from table food or snacks eaten from a playroom floor or den. With the extra intestinal tapeworm, Echinococcosis granulosis, humans become infected by contact with contaminated dog feces.
System(s) affected: Gastrointestinal, Nervous
Genetics: N/A
Incidence in USA: Unknown
Prevalence in USA:
• Not known with precision. Overall, tapeworms occur infrequently in the U.S.
• Most of the cestodes that infect man are endemic to the northern temperate regions of the West. Endemic foci in the U.S. appear to be related to immigrant population and ethnic groups with selected cultural habits.
Predominant age: All ages affected
Predominant sex: Male = Female

SIGNS AND SYMPTOMS
Taenia saginata
◊ Mild abdominal cramps
◊ Anal irritation from passage of proglottid
◊ Intestinal phase - minor abdominal complaints
Taenia solium
◊ Intestinal phase - minor abdominal complaints
◊ Larval migration - human cysticercosis; alteration of CNS function; headache, decreased vision, seizures, intracranial hypertension, mental disturbance, visual deterioration
Diphyllobothrium latum
◊ Intestinal phase competes with and prevents Vitamin B12 from being absorbed by humans; megaloblastic anemia with glossitis, loss of tongue papillae and neurologic symptoms occur
Hymenolepis nana (with heavy worm burdens)
◊ Abdominal cramps
◊ Diarrhea
◊ Vomiting
◊ Weight loss
Echinococcosis (hydatid disease)
◊ Symptoms related to the growth of the cyst. Most common location is the right lobe of the liver. Splenic, renal, cerebral, ocular and osseous hydatid cysts have been reported.
◊ Allergic symptoms are rare
◊ Eosinophilia mild to moderate

Dipylidium caninum
◊ Mild abdominal distress
◊ Restlessness
◊ Eosinophilia

CAUSES
• Important tapeworms that may infect man include: Taenia saginata (beef t.), Taenia solium (pork t.), Diphyllobothrium latum (fish t.), Hymenolepis nana (dwarf t.), Hymenolepis diminuta (rodent t.), and Dipylidium caninum (dog t.)
• Extra intestinal tapeworm cause Echinococcosis. There are three species that may affect man: E. granulosis (hydatid disease of the liver, spleen, etc.), E. multilocularis (alveolar hydatid disease) and E. vogeli (polycystic hydatid disease).

RISK FACTORS Travel to Far East, Russia, Africa and eating undercooked foods (T. saginata); travel to Mexico, Latin America, Africa, India, Spain, Portugal, China and eating undercooked pork (T. solium); travel to Alaska, Canada, Japan, Middle East and eating inadequately cooked freshwater fish (D. latum); indiscriminate play with dogs (D. caninum); contact with dogs particularly those involved in herding sheep (E. granulosis)

DIAGNOSIS

DIFFERENTIAL DIAGNOSIS
• The majority of tapeworm intestinal infections are asymptomatic. A patient may become aware only by passing a proglottid in the stool.
• Differential diagnosis of general intestinal symptoms are legion
• Differential diagnosis of cysts depends upon location. A wide variety of malignant and non-malignant cysts exist.
• Pernicious anemia (D. latum)

LABORATORY
• Microscopic examination of proglottid in stool
• Recognition of eggs in stool
Drugs that may alter lab results: N/A
Disorders that may alter lab results: N/A

PATHOLOGICAL FINDINGS
• T. saginata: N/A
• T. solium: Cysticercus can develop in almost any body tissue. Cysts 5-10 mm in soft tissue. Calcified cysts in CNS, striated muscle (cysticercus).
• D. latum: Macrocytic megaloblastic anemia
• H. nana: N/A
• H. diminuta: N/A
• D. caninum: N/A
• E. granulosa: Hydatid cyst found most commonly in right lobe of liver

SPECIAL TESTS
• T. saginata - perianal cellophane tests for ova, stool ova and parasites (O&P)
• T. solium -stool exam for proglottides

• D. latum - stool O&P
• H. nana - stool O&P
• H. diminuta - stool O&P
• D. caninum - proglottides in stool
• E. granulosa - scolex in cyst aspiration

IMAGING
• T. saginata: Occasionally seen on GI and small bowel x-rays with contrast media
• T. solium: Plain x-rays may show calcified cysts in subcutaneous or cerebral tissues. CT may detect both non-calcified and calcified cysts. MRI may also be useful.
• D. latum: N/A
• H. nana: N/A
• H. diminuta: N/A
• D. caninum: N/A
• E. granulosa: Liver scan, CT and ultrasonography helpful to indicate cysts

DIAGNOSTIC PROCEDURES
• T. saginata: N/A
• T. solium: Excisional biopsy of subcutaneous tissues. Several immunodiagnostic tests available (ELISA and EITB).
• D. latum: Characteristic opercular eggs in stool
• H. nana: Double membrane eggs in stool
• H. diminuta: N/A
• D. caninum: N/A
• E. granulosa: Several serologic tests are available. False negative and false positive tests occur.

TREATMENT

APPROPRIATE HEALTH CARE
Outpatient

GENERAL MEASURES
• Awareness of transmission and general supportive care during treatment
• Hygienic disposal of feces during and after treatment
• For neurocysticercosis, consider steroids (for cerebral edema) and anticonvulsants

ACTIVITY As tolerated

DIET As tolerated

PATIENT EDUCATION
• Taenia species, thoroughly cooked beef and pork (especially when traveling out of country)
• Avoid raw and undercooked fish
• Be careful of dogs as pets, especially if they are used in herding sheep with endemic hydatid disease
• Careful washing of hands after using toilet
• Avoid eating food directly off floor (H. nana)
• Ensure that pets are free of fleas and lice, and if infected, avoid contact with young children (D. caninum)
• Avoid feeding waste products of butchered animals to dogs (hydatid disease)

MEDICATIONS

DRUG(S) OF CHOICE
• Intestinal stage of D. latum (fish), T. saginata (beef), D. caninum (dog) and T. solium (pork) tapeworms: Niclosamide (Niclocide) chewable tablets. Adults 4 tablets (2 grams) chewed thoroughly. Children 25 to 75 lbs 2 tablets (1 gram). Children more than 75 lbs 3 tablets (1.5 grams). Give both adults and children a single dose.
• H. nana (dwarf tapeworm): Praziquantel (Biltricide) 25 mg/kg in one dose
• Larval tissue stage E. granulosis (hydatid cysts): Test with albendazole (Zentel). Adults 400 mg bid x 28 days. Children: > 2 years use adult dose; age 1-2 years 200 mg/day
• Cysticercus cellulosae (larval from T. solium), (cysticercosis): Praziquantel (Biltricide) 50 mg/kg/day in 3 doses x 14 days for both children and adults
Contraindications: Previous sensitivity, none specifically reported
Precautions:
• Niclosamide: Occasional nausea and abdominal pain
• Praziquantel: Malaise, headache and dizziness occur frequently; occasionally sedation, abdominal discomfort, fever, sweating, nausea, eosinophilia and fatigue. Rarely pruritus and rash occur.
• Albendazole (Zentel): Occasionally diarrhea and pain, and rarely leukopenia. Increased serum transaminase levels occur.
Significant possible interactions: No data reported

ALTERNATIVE DRUGS
• For intestinal stage of D. latum, T. saginata, T. solium and D. caninum - praziquantel 10-20 mg/kg in a single dose (an investigational drug in the U.S. for this condition). For H. nana, a single dose of 4 tablets (2 gm), then 2 tablets daily for 6 days may be used for adults.
• For cysticercosis in adults and children, albendazole 15 mg/kg/day in 3 doses x 30 days
• Dichlorophen may be used for treatment of taeniasis

FOLLOWUP

PATIENT MONITORING Examine stool for O&P within two weeks after treatment for intestinal stages of tapeworm

PREVENTION/AVOIDANCE
• Patient instruction in those ethnic cultural traditions that favor dietary exposure
• When traveling in Far East, Africa and Russia, avoid undercooked beef
• The pork tapeworm is prevalent in Mexico, Latin American, Asia, India, and China
• Humans infected by eating undercooked beef and by accidentally ingesting eggs in human wastes from poor sanitary practices. Inadequately cooked fish (including salmon) from fresh or brackish water in Europe, Asia, Canada, Alaska and Africa.
• Avoid sampling of gefilte fish during its preparation
• Dog tapeworm can be avoided by instructing children in sanitary habits when playing with pets
• Control deposition of human excrement and continued control by meat inspection. In sheep-raising areas, dogs should be dewormed regularly. Carcasses of sheep should not be fed to dogs to prevent access to hydatid cysts.
• Fresh water fish frozen at 14°F for 48 hours will kill parasite of D. latum
• Families living abroad in endemic areas, wishing to hire cooks and support personnel, should have them appropriately examined.

POSSIBLE COMPLICATIONS
• Larval form of T. solium - diffuse system-wide cysticercosis may occur. CNS involvement, neurocysticercosis with epilepsy, meningoencephalitis and muscle involvement may be seen.
• E. granulosis - single or multiple cysts may occur. Cysts may rupture intra-abdominally. Hepatic, splenic, ocular, ventricular, cerebral cysts have been reported.
• D. latum - vitamin B-12 deficiency anemia occurs predominantly among the people from Finland. Neurological symptoms including numbness, paresthesias, unsteady gait and weakness.

EXPECTED COURSE AND PROGNOSIS
• The majority of adult intestinal tapeworms are adequately treated with current medications. Cure rates of 95% have been reported.
• A second treatment course may be required
• In alveolar hydatid disease, if the pulmonary cyst is not resected intact, death rates of over 90% within 10 years have been reported

MISCELLANEOUS

ASSOCIATED CONDITIONS N/A

AGE-RELATED FACTORS
Pediatric: Poor personal hygiene habits and willingness to play indiscriminately with dogs can lead to infection
Geriatric: N/A
Others: N/A

PREGNANCY N/A

SYNONYMS
• Taeniasis
• Cysticercosis
• Diphyllobothriasis
• Echinococcosis hydatid disease
• Cysticercus cellulosae
• Hymenolepiasis
• Coenurosis
• Unilocular hydatid disease

ICD-9-CM
123 Other cestode infection (specific organisms coded separately)

SEE ALSO N/A

OTHER NOTES N/A

ABBREVIATIONS N/A

REFERENCES
• Brown, H.W. & Neva, F.A.: Basic Clinical Parasitology. 3rd Ed. New York, Appleton-Century-Crofts, 1964
• Berkow, R.B., et al. (eds.): Merck Manual. 15th Ed. Rahway, NJ, Merck & Co., 1987. pp. 229, 231
• Schroeder, S.A., Krupp, M.A., Tierney, L.M. & McPhee, S.J. (eds.): Current Medical Diagnosis and Treatment. Norwalk, CT, Appleton & Lange, 1989
• Medical Letter on Drugs and Therapeutics, Vol. 32, pp. 23-29, 1990
• Last, J.M. & Wallace, R.B.: Public Health and Preventive Medicine. Norwalk, CT, Appleton & Lange, 1992

Author A. Vuturo, M.D., M.P.H.

Teething

BASICS

DESCRIPTION Teething is the eruption of the deciduous teeth which most children experience without difficulty. It is a natural, gradual and predictable process but the timetable varies from baby to baby.

Deciduous teeth

◊ Most deciduous teeth begin to erupt at 5-7 months of age and teething is completed by 2-3 years

◊ The mandibular central incisors erupt first, then the two or four maxillary incisors followed by the lower lateral incisors

◊ After a few months, the four molars appear (lower ones at 12 months, the upper ones at 14 months)

◊ After the cuspid teeth appear at 16-18 months of age the second molars erupt at 20-24 months

◊ About 25% normal babies may have delayed eruption of teeth until 4 or 6 teeth simultaneously appear after their first birthday

◊ Premature babies erupt teeth according to their gestational age rather than chronological age. If teething seems particularly delayed, refer patient to a pedodontist.

Teeth in neonates

◊ One in 2000 neonates are born with a tooth (appears to be familial)

◊ These neonatal teeth may be loose but most are the normal deciduous lower central incisors and can persist

◊ Mild ulceration in the sublingual area has been reported in 18% of these babies

◊ Because of the potential for aspiration there is some controversy about elective removal of the loose teeth (most pediatric dentists would remove these teeth if they are loose)

System(s) affected: Gastrointestinal
Genetics: N/A
Incidence/Prevalence in USA: N/A
Predominant age: Birth to 2 years
Predominant sex: N/A

SIGNS AND SYMPTOMS

• A large percent of babies have no signs or symptoms of teething

• Excessive drooling and chewing on fingers begins at 3-4 months of age. This is also the time that normal hand-mouth stimulation increases salivation.

• A small red or white spot may appear over the swollen gum just prior to tooth eruption

• Local inflammation, swelling and occasional hemorrhage can be found on the involved gums

• Discomfort may be noted more with the eruption of the first tooth, the molars and/or with the simultaneous eruption of multiple teeth

• Restlessness, irritability, disturbed sleep, changes in feeding patterns, nasal discharge, mild cough, chin rash, fever, diarrhea, pulling of ear and rubbing of the cheeks have been reported by parents. It is impossible to document that these are caused by teething, so parents and health providers should consider other possible etiologies so as not to miss or delay diagnosing an illness.

CAUSES N/A

RISK FACTORS N/A

DIAGNOSIS

DIFFERENTIAL DIAGNOSIS N/A

LABORATORY N/A
Drugs that may alter lab results: N/A
Disorders that may alter lab results: N/A

PATHOLOGICAL FINDINGS N/A

SPECIAL TESTS N/A

IMAGING N/A

DIAGNOSTIC PROCEDURES N/A

TREATMENT

APPROPRIATE HEALTH CARE
Outpatient

GENERAL MEASURES N/A

• Treatment for teething include reassurance for the parents and symptomatic relief, if needed

• Provide the infant with a safe, one piece teething ring, clean cloth or pacifier for gumming

• Rub the involved swollen gums if the baby appears to be comforted

• Cool fluids may be offered but avoid frozen foods or objects. These could cause thermal damage to the tissues.

• Toast, cookies, bagels and crackers are offered by some parents for teething, but parents must observe carefully to prevent choking

• Avoid over-the-counter preparations for teething such as Xylocaine 2%, Baby Ora-Gel, Num-zit Gel, Num-zit Liquid, Ambesol. Misuse, overuse and sensitivity have been reported.

• Avoid the use of alcohol

• For the infant with low grade fever, irritability and/or inflamed gums (where other comforting measures have not been of help) - acetaminophen, in proper doses (10-15 mg/kg/dose every 4 hours prn), can be used intermittently

• Gum hematomas that erupt appear as a blue cyst. Most do not require medical intervention. Be sure there are no other signs of a bleeding disorder.

• Breast feeding babies may attempt to chew on the nipple at the end of sucking while teething but can be taught not to bite. Breast feeding can continue after teeth are present.

• Advise parents to avoid: Sugared pacifiers, painted furniture which may contain lead, tying teething ring with cord around the infant's neck, and imported fluid-filled teething rings

ACTIVITY No restrictions

DIET No special diet

PATIENT EDUCATION
• Parents should be cautioned not to misinterpret teething as the cause of any systemic manifestation. The health provider should be consulted for any systemic complaints.

• The ABC's of Teething, Am Academy of Pediatric Dentistry, Public Relations Manual

MEDICATIONS

DRUG(S) OF CHOICE N/A
Contraindications: N/A
Precautions: N/A
Significant possible interactions: N/A

ALTERNATIVE DRUGS N/A

FOLLOWUP

PATIENT MONITORING N/A

PREVENTION/AVOIDANCE N/A

POSSIBLE COMPLICATIONS N/A

EXPECTED COURSE AND PROGNOSIS Normal progression through the teething process without illness

MISCELLANEOUS

ASSOCIATED CONDITIONS N/A

AGE-RELATED FACTORS
Pediatric: N/A
Geriatric: N/A
Others: N/A

PREGNANCY N/A

SYNONYMS N/A

ICD-9-CM N/A

SEE ALSO N/A

OTHER NOTES N/A

ABBREVIATIONS N/A

REFERENCES
• King, N.M. & Lee, A.: Prematurely erupted teeth in the newborn infant. J Ped, 1989, 114:807
• Gardiner, J.: Erupted teeth in the newborn. Proc Roy Soc Med, 1961, 4:504
• Falkner, F.: Deciduous tooth eruption. Archives Disease of Childhood, 1957, 32:386-391
• Seward, M.: General disturbances attributed to the eruption of human primary dentition. J of Dent for Children, 1972, 39(3):178-183
• Golden, N., Takieddine, F. & Hirsch, V.: Teething age - prematurely born infants. Am J of Dis of Child, 1981, 135:903-904
• McDonald, R.E.: Eruption of the teeth, local, systematic and congenital factors that influence the process. In Dentistry for the Child and Adolescent. 5th Ed. St. Louis, C.V. Mosby Co., 1987, 189-196

Author N. Fawcett, M.D. & D. Varon, D.D.S., M.S.

Temporomandibular joint (TMJ) syndrome

 BASICS

DESCRIPTION Syndrome characterized by pain and tenderness in the jaw muscles, sound and/or pain over the temporomandibular joint (TMJ), with limitation of mandibular movement
System(s) affected: Musculoskeletal
Genetics: N/A
Incidence in USA: Unknown
Prevalence in USA: Symptoms or signs of TMJ dysfunction are present in up to one half of the population but only 5-25% seek treatment
Predominant age: Symptoms more common age 30-50
Predominant sex: Female > Male (3:1)

SIGNS AND SYMPTOMS
• Facial and/or TMJ pain
• Locking or catching of the jaw
• TMJ noises - clicking, grinding, popping
• Headache
• Earache
• Neck pain

CAUSES
• TMJ synovitis
• TMJ disc derangement
• Hyper- or hypomobile TMJ
• Occluso-muscular dysfunction
• Masticatory muscle spasm
• Trauma
• Poorly fitting dentures

RISK FACTORS
• Chronic oral habits such as clenching or grinding of the teeth
• Osteoarthritis, rheumatoid arthritis
• Dental malocclusion
• Fibrositis
• Psychosocial stress

 DIAGNOSIS

DIFFERENTIAL DIAGNOSIS
• Condylar fracture/dislocation
• Trigeminal neuralgia
• Dental or periodontal conditions
• TMJ neoplasm

LABORATORY N/A
Drugs that may alter lab results: N/A
Disorders that may alter lab results: N/A

PATHOLOGICAL FINDINGS
• Condylar head displacement
• Anterior disc displacement
• Posterior capsulitis
• Loosening of disc and capsular attachments
• Chondroid metaplasia of disc leading to disc perforation and degeneration

SPECIAL TESTS Jaw range of motion
(opening, closing, lateral, protrusive) and masticatory muscle strength

IMAGING
• Single-contrast videoarthrography demonstrates joint dynamics and disc movement
• Panoramic dental radiographs
• MRI - noninvasive study for disc position. Information gained helps in deciding conservative versus surgical management.

DIAGNOSTIC PROCEDURES
Arthroscopy

 TREATMENT

APPROPRIATE HEALTH CARE
Outpatient treatment

GENERAL MEASURES
• Jaw rest
• Local heat therapy
• Anti-inflammatory medications
• Muscle relaxants
• Analgesics
• Correction of malocclusion with orthodontic appliance
• Stress reduction
• Behavior modification to eliminate tension-relieving oral habits

ACTIVITY Jaw rest

DIET Soft diet to reduce chewing

PATIENT EDUCATION
• Be aware of any teeth-clenching or grinding habits, and relax the jaw by disengaging the teeth
• Avoid wide uncontrolled opening such as yawning
• Management of stress. Behavioral modification counseling may be helpful.

MEDICATIONS

DRUG(S) OF CHOICE Nonsteroidal anti-inflammatory drugs (NSAID's) - no single drug more efficacious than another

Contraindications:
• History of anaphylaxis to aspirin
• Peptic ulcer disease
• Renal insufficiency

Precautions:
• Peptic ulcers, gastritis or GI bleeding may occur with chronic use
• May cause acute interstitial nephritis
• Drug accumulation with renal insufficiency
• Liver function abnormalities in up to 15% of patients

Significant possible interactions:
• Albumin-bound drugs - displacement of either drug
• Warfarin - increased prothrombin time
• Lithium - increased lithium plasma level
• Furosemide - decreased natriuretic effect
• Propranolol - decreased anti-hypertensive effect

ALTERNATIVE DRUGS N/A

FOLLOWUP

PATIENT MONITORING
• Ongoing assessment of clinical response to conservative therapies (NSAID's, behavior modification, occlusal splints) is necessary
• A surgical procedure to correct disc displacement or replace a damaged disc may be indicated only if the patient has not responded to conservative treatment

PREVENTION/AVOIDANCE Elimination of tension-relieving oral habits and reducing overall muscle tension

POSSIBLE COMPLICATIONS
• Secondary degenerative joint disease
• Chronic TMJ dislocation
• Loss of joint range of motion
• Depression and chronic pain syndromes

EXPECTED COURSE AND PROGNOSIS
• With conservative therapy, symptoms resolve in 3/4 of the cases within three months
• Patients benefit the most from a comprehensive treatment approach including correction of occlusal discrepancies, restoration of normal muscle function, pain control, stress management and behavior modification

MISCELLANEOUS

ASSOCIATED CONDITIONS
Cranio-mandibular disorders

AGE-RELATED FACTORS
Pediatric: N/A
Geriatric: N/A
Others: N/A

PREGNANCY No association

SYNONYMS Myofascial pain-dysfunction (MPD) syndrome

ICD-9-CM 524.6

SEE ALSO N/A

OTHER NOTES N/A

ABBREVIATIONS N/A
REFERENCES:
• Guralnick, W., Kaban L.B. & Merrill, R.G.: Temporomandibular joint afflictions. New Engl J Med. 299(3):123-29, 1978
• Bronstein, S.L.: Update on temporomandibular joint problems: Diagnosis and treatment. Res & Staff Phys. 34(1):71-87, 1988
• Sickels, J.E. & Dolwick, M.F.: Temporomandibular-joint pain. Hosp Phys. 26-32, Jul 1983

Author P. Eiff, M.D. & S. Fields, M.D.

Tendinitis

BASICS

DESCRIPTION Inflammation of tendon occurring usually at its point of insertion into bone or at the point of muscular origin. The inflammation can extend to adjacent bursal tissue.
System(s) affected: Musculoskeletal
Genetics: N/A
Incidence/Prevalence in USA: Common
Predominant age: None
Predominant sex: Male > Female (slightly)

SIGNS AND SYMPTOMS
• Pain overlying the point of inflammation. This is usually worsened by active motion, but can be present at rest.
• Tenderness over the affected tendon
• Mild erythema and increased heat of overlying skin, especially if the tendon is superficial as in the case of the tendo Achilles

CAUSES Usually related to repetitive activity or trauma, but can be without obvious cause

RISK FACTORS Professional athletes and manual laborers are especially prone to tendinitis due to repetitive use

DIAGNOSIS

DIFFERENTIAL DIAGNOSIS
• Avulsion of the tendon - may occur with loss of function of the affected muscle. X-rays may show a portion of bone avulsed with the tendon, though this is not constant.
• Bursitis - can be impossible to differentiate, especially since the two conditions may coexist
• Infectious tenosynovitis - this occurs largely in the hand. The tenderness and swelling are located along the synovial lines proximally, instead of the insertion. Pain is more marked as is swelling and erythema. The sedimentation rate and white count will usually be elevated.
• Arthritis - the joint may be swollen. Tenderness and pain are in the joint proper in contrast to tendinitis which will be localized to the side of the joint where tendon insertion occurs.

LABORATORY Normal
Drugs that may alter lab results: N/A
Disorders that may alter lab results: N/A

PATHOLOGICAL FINDINGS Tendinitis is usually associated with some degenerative changes in the tendon under microscopic examinations with presence of fibrinoid, mucoid or hyaline degeneration of the connective tissue

SPECIAL TESTS Sonogram - this can be an accurate examination when done with real-time machines. Dynamics of the tendon during contraction may be obtained. Exert care that the ultrasound beam does not cross the tendon obliquely.

IMAGING The CT scan and MRI have replaced even arthrography of the shoulder in most instances. In case where diagnosis is in doubt, especially as regards tendon integrity, an MRI can be obtained and this will usually identify tears, partial tears, inflammation, or tumors. MRI cannot show irregularities of the tendon sheath itself however, and will not diagnose stenosing tenosynovitis or minimal tenosynovitis, unless fluid is present.

DIAGNOSTIC PROCEDURES N/A

TREATMENT

APPROPRIATE HEALTH CARE
Outpatient

GENERAL MEASURES Treatment goals are to relieve pain, reduce inflammation, rest the joint

ACTIVITY
• In acute phases the involved muscle and tendon should be put at rest. Use slings and splints for the upper extremity. Use braces, canes and/or crutches for the lower limbs.
• Physical therapy, once patient is free of pain

DIET No special diet

PATIENT EDUCATION
• Explanation of the problem
• Instructions for use of supportive devices (e.g., crutches, slings)

MEDICATIONS

DRUG(S) OF CHOICE
Anti-inflammatory drugs:
◊ NSAID's - all have about the same efficacy and the one which is most familiar to the prescriber can be used e.g., piroxicam (Feldene) 10 mg daily or indomethacin (Indocin) 25 or 50 mg tid after meals. Ibuprofen is a low-cost NSAID available over-the-counter.
◊ Corticosteroids - injectable, 40 mg of Depo-Medrol accompanied by 4-6 cc of 1% or 2% Xylocaine often results in dramatic relief. Never inject tendon, only into tendon sheath or surrounding bursa. (Careful preparation of the skin using Betadine or similar surgical prep is mandatory to prevent infection).
Contraindications: A tendon should never be injected with a local anesthetic and/or cortisone to allow participation in an athletic event. This can result in complete rupture of the tendon.
Precautions: See manufacturer's profile of each drug
Significant possible interactions: See manufacturer's profile of each drug

ALTERNATIVE DRUGS N/A

FOLLOWUP

PATIENT MONITORING Symptoms will usually subside within a few days after treatment

PREVENTION/AVOIDANCE After adequate rest and treatment, prevention of recurrences is important. Splints such as circular bands for forearm extension tendinitis or patella tendinitis may be useful.

POSSIBLE COMPLICATIONS
• Tendon rupture or avulsion fractures may occur
• Repeated exacerbations of pain. This is probably the most common indication for MRI to confirm the diagnosis and determine the extent of attenuation of the tendon.

EXPECTED COURSE AND PROGNOSIS The great majority subside without complications

MISCELLANEOUS

ASSOCIATED CONDITIONS Bursitis, arthritis - osteophytes may be a factor in traumatizing tendons if located adjacent to a tendon

AGE-RELATED FACTORS
Pediatric: A prevalent form of tendinitis is patellar tendinitis associated with inflammation of the tibial apophysis. Known as Osgood-Schlatter disease, it is seen in adolescents especially during a growth spurt. Splinting with a patella band and restricted activity usually alleviate symptoms. However, some are recalcitrant and may require steroid injections and even surgery with splitting of the patella tendon.
Geriatric: N/A
Others: N/A

PREGNANCY N/A

SYNONYMS N/A

ICD-9-CM 762.90

SEE ALSO Osgood-Schlatter disease

OTHER NOTES N/A

ABBREVIATIONS N/A

REFERENCES
• Forrage & Rifkin: Ultrasonic examinations of tendons. Radiologic Clinics of North America, January, 1988; Vol. 26, No.1, p. 87
• Baker, et al: Current Role of Tenorrhaphy and Bursoghraphy. In American Journal of Roentgenography, January 1990; Vol 154: 7, pp. 120-33
• Lawrence, B.D., et al.: Recent Advances in Magnetic Resonance Imaging of the Knee. In Radiologic Clinics of North America, March 1990; Vol. 28, No.1

Author F. Johnston, M.D.

Testicular malignancies

BASICS

DESCRIPTION Primary testicular neoplasms may arise from any testicular or adnexal cell component. They are divided into germinal (90-95%) and non-germinal tumors. The germinal tumors, discussed here, are further divided into seminomatous and non-seminomatous types (embryonal, teratoma, choriocarcinomas, yolk sac).
Clinical staging
◊ A - tumor limited to testis and cord
◊ B - tumor of testis and retroperitoneal nodes
◊ B1 - Nodes less than 2cm
◊ B2 - positive retroperitoneal nodes 2-6 cm in diameter (seen on imaging studies)
◊ B3 - positive retroperitoneal nodes > 6 cm in diameter
◊ C - metastases above diaphragm or involving abdominal solid organs
System(s) affected: Reproductive
Genetics: No solid evidence of familial connection
Incidence/Prevalence in USA:
• 1-2% of all neoplasms in male
• 2.3-6.3 cases/year per 100,000 men (less common in African-Americans - 0.9 cases/year per 100,000)
• In adults, germ cell types comprise 90-95% of testicular cancers; in children, they represent only 60-75%
Predominant age: Peak incidence - age 20-40; smaller peaks between age 0-10 years and > 60
Predominant sex: Male only

SIGNS AND SYMPTOMS
In adults
◊ Scrotal nodule or swelling most common
◊ Sensation of fullness or heaviness of scrotum, may be interpreted as "pain"
◊ Previously "small" testicle enlarging to size of "normal" contralateral one
◊ Firm, non-tender mass within confines of tunica albuginea usually palpably distinct from cord structures
◊ Acute or chronic epididymitis/epididymo-orchitis resulting in delay of diagnosis (10%)
◊ Manifestations due to metastasis e.g., neck mass (supraclavicular node), respiratory symptoms (lung metastasis), low back pain (nerve root or psoas irritation), uni- or bilateral lower extremity swelling (iliac or caval thrombosis or obstruction) palpable abdominal mass.
◊ Hydrocele (10-20%)
◊ Gynecomastia (may or may not be due to elevated hormones) (5%)
◊ Rapid tumor growth resulting in hemorrhage and necrosis
In children
◊ Non-tender, non-painful scrotal mass
◊ Non-transilluminable, large, non-tender testicle
◊ Hydrocele (15-20%)
◊ With hormonally active tumors, the scrotal exam may be unrevealing

CAUSES No real clear cause and effect relations identified

RISK FACTORS
• Caucasian race; especially Scandinavian background
• Higher social status
• Unmarried
• Rural resident
• History of cryptorchism (even if previously repaired) - only undisputed risk factor
• Weak associations - maternal ingestion of hormones during 1st trimester, intersex disorders in genotypic male with dysgenetic gonad, trauma (no hard evidence of significant risk factor)

DIAGNOSIS

DIFFERENTIAL DIAGNOSIS
• Hernia
• Hydrocele
• Hematoma
• Spermatocele
• Syphilitic gumma
• Varicocele
• In children - epidermoid/dermoid cyst, para-testicular rhabdomyosarcoma, macroorchidism, torsion

LABORATORY
• Alpha fetoprotein (AFP) - levels elevated by pure embryonal carcinoma, teratocarcinoma, yolk sac tumor or combinations of these three, but not by pure choriocarcinoma or seminoma
• Beta human chorionic gonadotropin (beta-HCG) - elevated by all choriocarcinoma, 40-60% embryonal carcinoma; 5-10% pure seminomas have detectable levels of beta-HCG (usually < 500 ng/mL)
• Placental alkaline phosphatase (PLAP) - may be marker of choice for seminoma. 70-90% patients with recurrent or disseminated seminomas have elevated PLAP.
• Lactate dehydrogenase (LDH) - too ubiquitous to be specific. May be direct relationship between elevated LDH levels and tumor burden. Elevated LDH may be sole biochemical abnormality in 10% of patients with persistent or recurrent non-seminomatous tumors.

Drugs that may alter lab results: N/A
Disorders that may alter lab results:
• AFP alterations may be caused by - benign liver disease; telangiectasia and tyrosinemia; malignancies of the liver, pancreas, stomach and lung; heavy marijuana smoking
• PLAP may be elevated by heavy tobacco smoking
• Beta-HCG can also be produced by liver, lung, pancreatic and stomach malignancies; and by kidney, breast and bladder tumors

PATHOLOGICAL FINDINGS Basically, two different groups based on germinal vs. non-germinal and seminomatiour vs. non-seminomatous types.

SPECIAL TESTS Scrotal ultrasound - see mass clearly originating within testis with echotexture pattern (hypoechoic) distinct from surrounding normal testicular tissue

IMAGING
• Chest x-ray - good PA and lateral
• CT scan - very accurate; able to define pelvic retroperitoneal and mediastinal lymphadenopathy as well as to detect abdominal visceral and lung metastases
• Pedal lymphangiography (LAG) - is sensitive in picking up lymph node involvement intra-abdominally but not as accurate as CT scan in picking up upper para aortic nodes or visceral involvement
• MRI - still largely experimental

DIAGNOSTIC PROCEDURES
• Transinguinal scrotal exploration with biopsy and/or radical orchiectomy (testicle and spermatic cord excised) makes definite diagnosis
• Transcrotal open or percutaneous biopsy or transcrotal orchiectomy contraindicated secondary to anatomical trespassing into different lymph drainage system

TREATMENT

APPROPRIATE HEALTH CARE
Inpatient for surgery

GENERAL MEASURES
• Both seminomatous and non-seminomatous tumors are chemosensitive and have good chemotherapeutic response. Seminomas are extremely radiosensitive; more so than non-seminomas
• All patients receive radical orchiectomy for diagnosis and excellent local control
Treatment for seminomas stages
◊ A - irradiation, 2500 R to ipsilateral inguinal, iliac chains and bilateral periaortic/pericaval nodes to level of diaphragm
◊ B2 - same as A, with irradiation using 600-1000 R to positive nodes
◊ B3 - chemotherapy - if post-chemotherapy lymph nodes persists more than 3 cm in diameter, then a retroperitoneal lymph node dissection is added (43% of cases have viable tumor present)
◊ C - primary chemotherapy
Treatment for non-seminomatous germ cell tumor stages
◊ A - nerve sparing staging and therapeutic retroperitoneal lymph node dissection (RPLND) alone
◊ B1 (microscopic metastasis in 1-6 nodes, <2cm) - observation
◊ B2 (microscopic metastases in more than 6 nodes or grossly positive nodes, 2-6cm) - observation or two courses of chemotherapy
◊ B3 (nodes > 6 cm or tumor extension outside nodes) - initially 4 courses of chemotherapy. If complete response based on CT scan, serum markers, and no teratoma seen in original specimen, then observe. If partial response, do retroperitoneal lymph node dissection and tumor excision plus 2 more courses of chemotherapy. If tumor cannot all be excised, salvage chemotherapy.

ACTIVITY As tolerated

DIET No special diet

PATIENT EDUCATION
• Discuss patient's concerns about sterility, impotence, testicular prostheses, hormone supplements
• Patient education material available from American Cancer Society

 MEDICATIONS

DRUG(S) OF CHOICE
• Commonly used chemotherapeutic agents include cisplatin + etoposide ± bleomycin
• Salvage chemotherapy includes cyclophosphamide (Cytoxan) or ifosfamide based protocols
Contraindications: N/A
Precautions:
• Cisplatin - nephrotoxicity, neurotoxicity
• Etoposide - thrombocytopenia
• Cytoxan/ifosfamide - hemorrhagic cystitis (patients must be well-hydrated to minimize hemorrhage cystitis). Patients receiving ifosfamide should also receive mesna to reduce risk.
• Bleomycin - pulmonary fibrosis
Significant possible interactions: Refer to manufacturer's literature

ALTERNATIVE DRUGS
• Carboplatin

 FOLLOWUP

PATIENT MONITORING
• First year - markers and chest x-ray every month, physical exam (emphasizing nodes) every 2 months
• After 1 year - markers and chest x-ray every 2 months and physical exam every 4 months
• After 2 years - markers and chest x-ray and physical exam every 6-12 months
• If patient had teratoma at diagnosis, need to followup for at least 5 years and get CT scan every year for 3 years

PREVENTION/AVOIDANCE N/A

POSSIBLE COMPLICATIONS
• RPLND treatment - loss of seminal emission (prevented by using nerve-sparing RPLND), atelectasis, hypoalbuminemia
• Radiation treatment - radiation nephritis, enteritis
• Non-seminomatous tumors are more likely to have metastatic disease than seminomas (50-70% vs. 25%, respectively)

EXPECTED COURSE AND
PROGNOSIS Usually complete cure in patients with limited disease, 70-80% cure in patients with advanced disease

 MISCELLANEOUS

ASSOCIATED CONDITIONS N/A

AGE-RELATED FACTORS
Pediatric: Rare in childhood (only 2% of all solid tumors in childhood)
Geriatric: N/A
Others: N/A

PREGNANCY N/A

SYNONYMS N/A

ICD-9-CM 186.9

SEE ALSO N/A

OTHER NOTES N/A

ABBREVIATIONS
• AFP = alpha fetoprotein
• Beta-HCG = beta human chorionic qonadotropin
• LDH = lactate dehydrogenase
• PLAP = placental alkaline phosphatase
• RPLND = retroperitoneal lymph node dissection

REFERENCES
• Rowland RG, Donohue JP: Scrotum and Testis, in Adult and Pediatric Urology, edited by JY Gillenwater, JT Grayhack, SS Howards and JW Duckett, St. Louis Mosby Yearbook, Inc. 1991.
• Morse MJ, Whitmore WF: Campbell's Urology, edited by PC Walsh, RF Gittes, AD Perlmutter, et al. WB Saunders Co., 1986.
• Klein EA: Tumor Markers in Testis Cancer, The Urologic Clinics of North America, 20(1):67, 1993.
• Motzer RJ, Bosl GJ: Role of Adjuvant Chemotherapy in patients with Stage II, non-seminomatiour germ cell tumors, The Urologic clinics of North America. 20(1):111, 1993.

Author C. Jennings, M.D.

Testicular torsion

BASICS

DESCRIPTION Twisting of testis and spermatic cord resulting in acute ischemia.
• Intravaginal torsion: occurs within tunica vaginalis
• Extravaginal torsion: involves twisting of testis, cord and processus vaginalis (especially in newborns) and in undescended testes
Genetics: Unknown
Prevalence in USA: 1:160 males
Predominant age: Occurs from newborn period to 7th decade; 2/3 of cases occur in 2nd decade, with peak at age 14 years; 2nd peak in neonates
Predominant sex: Males only

SIGNS AND SYMPTOMS
• Scrotum is enlarged, red, and edematous
• First symptom is pain (sudden or gradual onset, increasing in severity)
• Nausea and vomiting are common
• Fever may occur
• Testicle exquisitely tender
• Testis may be high in scrotum with a transverse lie
• Absence of cremasteric reflex

CAUSES
• Torsion is usually spontaneous and idiopathic
• History of trauma in 20% of patients
• 1/3 have had prior episodic testicular pain
• Contraction of cremasteric muscle or dartos may play a role and is stimulated by trauma, exercise, cold, sexual stimulation
• Possible alterations in testosterone levels during nocturnal sex response cycle; possible elevated testosterone levels in neonates
• Testis must have inadequate, incomplete or absent fixation within scrotum

RISK FACTORS
• May be more common in winter
• Paraplegia

DIAGNOSIS

DIFFERENTIAL DIAGNOSIS
• Epididymo-orchitis
• Incarcerated/strangulated inguinal hernia
• Acute hydrocele
• Traumatic hematoma
• Idiopathic scrotal edema
• Torsion appendix testis
• Acute varicocele
• Testicular tumor
• Henoch-Schonlein purpura
• Scrotal abscess
• Leukemic infiltrate

LABORATORY Urinalysis may be helpful (usually not)
Drugs that may alter lab results: N/A
Disorders that may alter lab results: N/A

PATHOLOGICAL FINDINGS
• Venous thrombosis
• Tissue edema and necrosis
• Arterial thrombosis

SPECIAL TESTS N/A

IMAGING CT scan or ultrasound may confirm testicular swelling, but are rarely indicated

DIAGNOSTIC PROCEDURES
• Doppler ultrasonic flow detection demonstrates absent or reduced pulse with torsion, increased flow with inflammatory process (only reliable in 1st 12 hrs.)
• Radionuclide testicular scintigraphy with technectium 99m. pertechnetate demonstrates absent/decreased vascularity in torsion, increased vascularity with inflammatory processes (including torsion of appendix testes)

TREATMENT

APPROPRIATE HEALTH CARE
• Manual reduction - may be successful, facilitated by Lidocaine 1% (Plain) injection at level of external ring. Must always be followed by orchidopexy.
• Surgical exploration via scrotal approach with detorsion, evaluation of testicular viability, orchidopexy of viable testicle, orchiectomy of non-viable testicle.

GENERAL MEASURES
• Bilateral testicular fixation is recommended
• At least 3-4 point fixation with non-absorbable sutures
• Excision of window of tunica albuginea with suture to dartos fascia
• Any testis that is not clearly viable (and obvious) should be removed.

ACTIVITY As tolerated

DIET Regular

PATIENT EDUCATION Possibility of testicular atrophy in salvaged testis with depressed sperm counts

MEDICATIONS

DRUG (S) OF CHOICE N/A
Contraindications: N/A
Precautions: N/A
Significant possible interactions: N/A

ALTERNATIVE DRUGS N/A

 FOLLOWUP

PATIENT MONITORING
• Postoperative visit at 1-2 weeks
• Yearly visits until puberty to evaluate for atrophy

PREVENTION/AVOIDANCE N/A

POSSIBLE COMPLICATIONS
• Possible testicular atrophy
• Abnormal spermatogenesis
• Infertility

EXPECTED COURSE AND PROGNOSIS
• Testicular salvage directly related to duration of torsion (85-97% if less than 6 hours, less than 10% if greater than 24 hrs)
• 80-94% may have depressed spermatogenesis related to duration of ischemic injury (possibly related to autoimmune - mediated injury)
• As many as 2/3 of salvaged testicles may atrophy in first 2-3 years post torsion

 MISCELLANEOUS

ASSOCIATED CONDITIONS N/A

AGE-RELATED FACTORS N/A
Pediatric: Most common at age 14
Geriatric: Rare in this age group
Others: N/A

PREGNANCY N/A

SYNONYMS N/A

ICD-9-CM
608.2

SEE ALSO N/A

OTHER NOTES N/A

ABBREVIATIONS N/A

REFERENCES
• Ashcraft, K.W.: Pediatric Urology. Philadelphia, W.B. Saunders Co, 1990.
• Ashcraft, K.W. & Holder, T.M.: Pediatric Surgery. 2nd Ed. Philadelphia, W.B. Saunders Co., 1993.
• Kelalis, P.P., King, L.R., & Belman, A.B.: Clinical Pediatric Urology. 3rd Ed. Philadelphia, W.B. Saunders Co, 1992.

Author T. Black, M.D.

Tetanus

 BASICS

DESCRIPTION
Severe illness characterized by intermittent tonic spasms of voluntary muscles. Toxin enters the central nervous system along the peripheral nerves or is blood borne. Tetanospasmin binds at synapses and blocks inhibitors. Usual course is acute.

System(s) affected: Nervous
Genetics: N/A
Incidence/Prevalence in USA: Rare
Predominant age: Over 70% of cases in persons > 50 years of age
Predominant sex: Male = Female

SIGNS AND SYMPTOMS
- Arrhythmias
- Asphyxia
- Convulsions
- Cyanosis
- Drooling
- Dysphagia
- Fluctuating hypertension
- Hydrophobia
- Hyperhidrosis
- Hyperpyrexia
- Hyperreflexia
- Hypotension
- Irritability
- Low-grade fever
- Muscular rigidity
- Muscular spasticity
- Nuchal rigidity
- Opisthotonos
- Pain at wound site
- Painful tonic convulsions
- Risus sardonicus (fixed smile)
- Stiffness of the jaw
- Sudden bradycardia
- Sudden cardiac arrest
- Tachycardia
- Tingling at wound site
- Trismus
- Wound history (may be absent)

CAUSES
- Infection with Clostridium tetani
- Neurotoxin produced by Clostridium tetani
- Tetanospasmin (an exotoxin)

RISK FACTORS
- Burns
- Drug addiction (parenteral)
- Ear infection (with tympanic membrane perforation)
- Early postpartum with an infected uterus
- Exposure of open wounds to soil and animal feces
- Frostbite
- Newborn (umbilicus stump entry)
- Skin ulcers
- Surgical wounds
- Age > 50 years
- Traumatic wound

 DIAGNOSIS

DIFFERENTIAL DIAGNOSIS
- Dental abscess
- Subarachnoid hemorrhage
- Seizure disorder
- Meningoencephalitis
- Peritonsillar abscess
- Dystonic reaction to phenothiazines
- Hypocalcemic tetany
- Strychnine poisoning
- Alcohol withdrawal

LABORATORY
- Polymorphonuclear leukocytosis
- Culture of Clostridium tetani from wound (may not be positive even if tetanus is the problem)

Drugs that may alter lab results: N/A
Disorders that may alter lab results: N/A

PATHOLOGICAL FINDINGS   N/A

SPECIAL TESTS
- ECG - supraventricular tachycardia
- Multifocal ventricular ectopia
- Bradycardia
- EEG sleeping pattern
- Culture of wound infrequently recover C. tetani

IMAGING   N/A

DIAGNOSTIC PROCEDURES   N/A

 TREATMENT

APPROPRIATE HEALTH CARE
Intensive care

GENERAL MEASURES
- Wound excision
- Quiet observation
- Intubation
- IV hydration
- Catheterize the bladder
- Prevent jarring of bed or drafts
- Tracheostomy if needed

ACTIVITY   Absolute bedrest with sedation

DIET   Nothing by mouth until well

PATIENT EDUCATION   Griffith: Instructions for Patients, p 300. Philadelphia, W.B. Saunders Co.,1988

MEDICATIONS

DRUG(S) OF CHOICE
- Anticonvulsants
- Diazepam (to counter muscle rigidity)
- Pancuronium bromide (administered by anesthesiologist) plus ventilation
- Tetanus toxoid (in a previously immunized patient)
- Tetanus immune human globulin 3000 units to 6000 units IM. May infiltrate the area around the wound with a portion of the dose.
- Penicillin G-2 million units IV q 6 h. In a penicillin allergic patient, use doxycycline 100 mg q12h, or clindamycin 150-300 mg I.V. q6h.

Contraindications: Refer to manufacturer's literature

Precautions: Refer to manufacturer's literature. Do not use tetanus immune globulin intravenously.

Significant possible interactions: Refer to manufacturer's literature

ALTERNATIVE DRUGS
Equine tetanus antitoxin 50,000 units IM - only if tetanus immune globulin (human) is not available

FOLLOWUP

PATIENT MONITORING
Careful observation in intensive care

PREVENTION/AVOIDANCE
Active immunization with tetanus toxoid; wound débridement; passive immunization with tetanus immune globulin; benzathine penicillin; penicillin G; erythromycin

POSSIBLE COMPLICATIONS
- Respiratory arrest
- Cardiac failure
- Pulmonary emboli
- Bacterial infection
- Dehydration
- Vertebral fractures
- Airway obstruction
- Anoxia
- Urinary retention
- Constipation
- Pneumonia
- Rhabdomyolysis

EXPECTED COURSE AND PROGNOSIS
- 25-50% mortality

Poor prognostic factors:
  ◊ Form of tetanus
  ◊ Incubation period
  ◊ Onset period
  ◊ Patient's age
  ◊ Severity of symptoms
  ◊ Heart wound
- Recovery is complete if patient survives

MISCELLANEOUS

ASSOCIATED CONDITIONS
N/A

AGE-RELATED FACTORS
Pediatric:
- Mortality high in young
- Infection may enter through umbilical cord

Geriatric: Mortality high in elderly

Others: N/A

PREGNANCY
- Must treat vigorously despite pregnancy
- Infection may enter uterus postpartum

SYNONYMS
Lockjaw

ICD-9-CM
037

SEE ALSO
Meningitis

OTHER NOTES
N/A

ABBREVIATIONS
N/A

REFERENCES
- Centers for Disease Control, Tetanus: United States 1981-1984. MMWR, 1985;34:602
- Mandell, G.L. (ed.): Principles and Practice of Infectious Diseases. 3rd Ed. New York, Churchill Livingstone, 1990

Author A. Abyad, M.D.

Tetralogy of Fallot

BASICS

DESCRIPTION Large ventricular septal defect (VSD) associated with right ventricular outflow obstruction (infundibular and/or valvular pulmonic stenosis), right ventricular (RV) hypertrophy and an overriding aorta
• Pathophysiology dependent primarily on severity of right ventricular outflow tract obstruction
• Right and left ventricular pressures are generally equal (VSD is proximal to level of RV obstruction, therefore, RV pressures are elevated)
• Right to left shunting is typical
Genetics: Familial occurrence, components indicating dominant hereditary
Incidence in USA:
• 5-10% of all congenital heart disease. Most common cardiac cyanotic anomaly after age 1.
• 40 per 100,000 live births
Prevalence in USA: N/A
Predominant age: Newborn
Predominant sex: Male > Female (slightly)

SIGNS AND SYMPTOMS
• With mild RV outflow tract obstruction a left to right shunt predominates, and the patient is acyanotic = ("Pink" tetralogy of Fallot)
• Cyanosis with severe RV outflow tract obstruction (generally recognized early)
• Exertional dyspnea, poor exercise tolerance
• Lower birth weight, retarded growth
• Clubbing and polycythemia commonly in children
• Squatting position, typical following exertion (allows increased systemic vascular resistance, lessening right to left shunting)
• No typical facies
• Scoliosis is common
• Normal arterial and jugular venous pulses
• Systolic thrill along the left sternal border
• Early systolic ejection sound (aortic)
• Single S2 (decreased P2)
• Systolic ejection murmur due to flow across narrowed RV outflow tract
• May auscultate the continuous diminished murmur of bronchial collateral vessels
• Right aortic arch in 30%
• Atrial septal defect (ASD) in 15%
• Anomalous coronary arteries in 2-10%
• Retinal engorgement
• Hemoptysis
• Aortic ejection click

CAUSES Unknown

RISK FACTORS
• Documented increased incidence with increased maternal age
• Occasional familial occurrence

DIAGNOSIS

DIFFERENTIAL DIAGNOSIS
• Fallot's tetralogy with absent pulmonic valve
• Fallot's tetralogy with absent pulmonary artery
• Pseudotruncus arteriosus

LABORATORY N/A
Drugs that may alter lab results: N/A
Disorders that may alter lab results: N/A

PATHOLOGICAL FINDINGS
• Anterior deviation of the infundibular septum, resulting in malalignment with the muscular septum, creating a ventricular septal defect
• Malposition of the infundibular septum, which encroaches on the right ventricular outflow tract, resulting in an increased aortic root size
• Aortic root rotated into overriding position

SPECIAL TESTS
ECG
◊ Right axis deviation, right ventricular hypertrophy, subsequent right ventricular conduction abnormality
◊ Sinus rhythm in general, however, some may develop atrial fibrillation or flutter

IMAGING
Chest x-ray
◊ In children, typically a small boot-shaped heart (coeur en sabot) with diminished pulmonary blood flow
◊ Prominent right ventricle
◊ Possibly a right sided aortic arch and knob
◊ Normal (or perhaps decreased) pulmonary vascularity in approximately 50% adults
2D echocardiogram/Doppler echocardiogram
◊ 2D images demonstrate the VSD, overriding aorta, extent and location of the infundibular obstruction, assessment of pulmonic valve, right ventricular hypertrophy, and coronary anatomy, additional ventricular septal defects, and peripheral branch pulmonic arteries
◊ Doppler echocardiogram allows quantification of the outflow gradient
◊ Colorflow Doppler provides assessment of the VSD
◊ Coronary anatomy

DIAGNOSTIC PROCEDURES
Cardiac catheterization
◊ Assesses pulmonary annulus size and pulmonary arteries
◊ Assesses severity of right ventricular outflow obstruction
◊ Locates position of VSD and its size
◊ Rules out possible coronary artery anomalies

TREATMENT

APPROPRIATE HEALTH CARE
Inpatient for diagnosis and surgery

GENERAL MEASURES
• Good dental hygiene
• Endocarditis prophylaxis
Palliative surgical therapy
◊ It is important to emphasize that complete repair is the preferable modality of treatment
◊ Blalock-Taussig shunt or modified shunt (subclavian to pulmonary artery)
◊ Pott's procedure (descending aorta to pulmonary artery)
◊ Waterston's shunt (ascending aorta to pulmonary artery)
Total correction surgical therapy
◊ Includes patch closure of VSD and relief of right ventricular outflow obstruction

ACTIVITY As tolerated

DIET Salt restriction

PATIENT EDUCATION American Heart Association, 7320 Greenville Avenue, Dallas, TX 75231, (214)373-6300

MEDICATIONS

DRUG(S) OF CHOICE No specific drug therapy in the absence of heart failure
Contraindications: N/A
Precautions: N/A
Significant possible interactions: N/A

ALTERNATIVE DRUGS N/A

FOLLOWUP

PATIENT MONITORING
• Postoperative (or post-balloon valvotomy) Doppler ultrasound suggested at approximately 1 year from procedure
• Post-valvotomy SBE prophylaxis still required
• Regular followup assessment for patients not undergoing surgical correction

POSSIBLE COMPLICATIONS
• Erythrocytosis may develop secondary to chronic hypoxemia (risk for thrombosis, thrombotic CVA and paradoxical emboli)
• Increased risk for brain abscess, acute gouty arthritis
• Infective endocarditis
• Cerebrovascular thrombosis
• Delayed puberty
Postoperatively
◊ Residual right ventricular outflow obstruction
◊ Residual VSD
◊ Pulmonic regurgitation
◊ Ventricular arrhythmias
◊ Right bundle branch block quite common
◊ Left anterior hemiblock
◊ Infective bacterial endocarditis
◊ Ventricular arrhythmias

PREVENTION/AVOIDANCE N/A

EXPECTED COURSE AND PROGNOSIS Fatal if not surgically corrected

MISCELLANEOUS

ASSOCIATED CONDITIONS
• Stenotic pulmonary artery
• Patent ductus arteriosus
• Atrial septal defect
• Iron deficiency anemia

AGE-RELATED FACTORS
Pediatric: Congenital disorder
Geriatric: N/A
Others: N/A

PREGNANCY Well tolerated after total surgical correction

SYNONYMS N/A

ICD-9-CM 745.2

SEE ALSO N/A

OTHER NOTES N/A

ABBREVIATIONS
• VSD = ventricular septal defect
• RV = right ventricle

REFERENCES
• Braunwald, E. (ed.): Heart Disease: A Textbook of Cardiovascular Medicine. 3rd Ed. Philadelphia, W.B. Saunders Co., 1988
• Liberthson, R.: Congenital Heart Disease: Diagnosis & Management in Children and Adults. Boston, Little Brown, 1989
• Perloff. J.: Clinical Recognition of Congenital Heart Disease. 3rd Ed. Philadelphia, W.B. Saunders Co., 1987

Author S. Mamby, M.D.

Thalassemia

 BASICS

DESCRIPTION A group of inherited disorders that affect the synthesis of hemoglobin. In beta-thalassemia, there is deficient synthesis of beta globin, while in alpha-thalassemia, there is deficient synthesis of alpha globin. This leads to deficient hemoglobin accumulation, resulting in hypochromic and microcytic red cells. Abnormality of the red cells is the most characteristic feature of the thalassemias.
• Thalassemia is prevalent in the Mediterranean region, Middle East and Southeast Asia, and among ethnic groups originating from these areas

Types
◊ Beta-thalassemia major (Cooley's anemia) - severe anemia growth retardation, hepatosplenomegaly, bone marrow expansion and bone deformities. Transfusion therapy necessary to sustain life.
◊ Thalassemia intermedia - milder form. Transfusion therapy may not be needed.
◊ Thalassemia trait (alpha or beta) - mild anemia with microcytosis and hypochromia. No transfusion therapy needed.

Genetics:
• Inherited in an autosomal recessive pattern
• Inheritance of one defective gene = milder type of thalassemia, two defective genes = severe type of thalassemia

Incidence/Prevalence in USA:
• Approximately 1000 patients with severe thalassemia
• The incidence of thalassemia trait within the ethnic groups involved ranges from 3-5%

Predominant age: Symptoms start to appear 3-6 months after birth

Predominant sex: Male = Female

SIGNS AND SYMPTOMS
• Pallor
• Poor growth
• Inadequate food intake
• Fatigue
• Shortness of breath
• Splenomegaly
• Jaundice
• Leg ulcers
• Cholelithiasis
• Pathologic fractures

CAUSES Genetic

RISK FACTORS Family history

 DIAGNOSIS

DIFFERENTIAL DIAGNOSIS
• Iron deficiency
• Other hemoglobinopathies
• Other hemolytic anemias

LABORATORY
Hemoglobin
◊ Elevated Hb A2 levels in beta-thalassemia trait
◊ Elevated Hb A2, elevated Hb F, reduced or absent Hb A1 in beta-thalassemia major or intermedia
Peripheral blood
◊ Pronounced microcytosis
◊ Anisocytosis
◊ Hypochromia
◊ Punctate basophilic stippling
◊ High percentage of target cells
◊ Reticulocyte count elevated
Hematocrit
◊ 28-40% in alpha-thalassemia trait and beta-thalassemia trait
◊ May fall to less than 10% in beta-thalassemia major
Drugs that may alter lab results: N/A
Disorders that may alter lab results: N/A

PATHOLOGICAL FINDINGS
• Bone marrow hyperactivity
• Iron deposits in heart muscle
• Hepatic siderosis

SPECIAL TESTS Bone marrow aspiration

IMAGING Chest x-ray - thickened diploë of skull, osteoporosis

DIAGNOSTIC PROCEDURES Family history

 TREATMENT

APPROPRIATE HEALTH CARE
Outpatient for mild cases. Inpatient for transfusion therapy.

GENERAL MEASURES
• Mild cases require no therapy
• Thalassemia intermedia - normally no therapy necessary unless hemoglobin levels fall to a dangerous level, then may need transfusion therapy
Patients with severe thalassemia
◊ Maintain the mean hemoglobin level of at least 9.3 grams per dL with a regular transfusion schedule (transfusions of about 15 mL per kg at 3-5 week intervals)
◊ Folate supplementation
◊ Treat infections promptly
Splenectomy
◊ May be needed if hypersplenism causes a marked increase in the transfusion requirement
◊ Recommendation is to defer surgery until patient is 4-6 years of age (due to increased infection risk)
◊ Administer polyvalent pneumococcal vaccine one month prior to splenectomy
◊ Prophylaxis with a daily regimen of penicillin
Iron overload
◊ Patients receiving transfusion therapy increase total body iron 4 times over the normal amount
◊ Therapy is iron chelation
Bone marrow transplantation
◊ Cures the disease, but associated with significant mortality and morbidity

ACTIVITY
• Avoid strenuous activities (e.g., football, soccer)
• Acceptable activity levels will need to be determined on an individual basis depending on severity of disorder

DIET
• Avoid iron-rich foods (meats such as liver, and and some cereals)
• Drinking tea may possibly help reduce iron

PATIENT EDUCATION
• Genetic counseling
• Teach parents signs of hepatitis, iron overload
• Printed patient information available from: Cooley's Anemia Foundation, 105 E. 22nd St., Suite 911, New York, NY 10010, (212)598-0911

MEDICATIONS

DRUG(S) OF CHOICE
• Antibiotics for infection
• Folic acid supplements
• Iron chelation with deferoxamine (Desferal). Continuous subcutaneous or intravenous infusion with a small infusion pump 40 mg per kg per day (about a 10 hour period). Usually started before 5-8 years of age.
Contraindications: Refer to manufacturer's literature
Precautions: Refer to manufacturer's literature
Significant possible interactions: Refer to manufacturer's literature

ALTERNATIVE DRUGS N/A

FOLLOWUP

PATIENT MONITORING Life-long monitoring necessary because both the therapy and disease progression have numerous possible complications

PREVENTION/AVOIDANCE
Prenatal information
◊ Genetic counseling
◊ Prenatal diagnosis - study of beta globin genes performed on fetal cell DNA obtained by amniocentesis after 14 weeks
Complication prevention
◊ Evaluation for thalassemia by 1 year of age for offspring of adult thalassemia patients
◊ Avoidance of infections
◊ Prompt treatment of infections (after splenectomy, patients should maintain a supply of ampicillin to take if symptoms of infection appear)
◊ Periodic dental checkups
◊ Avoidance of activities that could result in bone fractures

POSSIBLE COMPLICATIONS
• Chronic hemolysis
• Susceptibility to infections after splenectomy
• Infections from blood transfusion
• Intercurrent infections
• Worsening of anemia during infections
• Jaundice
• Leg ulcers
• Cholelithiasis
• Pathologic fractures
• Impaired growth rate
• Delayed or absent puberty
• Hepatic siderosis
• Hemolytic anemia
• Splenomegaly
• Cardiac disease from iron overload
• Aplastic and megaloblastic crises

EXPECTED COURSE AND PROGNOSIS
• Outlook varies depending on type
• Thalassemia major patients live an average of 17 years, some into their mid-twenties.
• Thalassemia minor patients live a normal life span

MISCELLANEOUS

ASSOCIATED CONDITIONS See Possible complications

AGE-RELATED FACTORS
Pediatric: A disorder of childhood
Geriatric: N/A
Others: N/A

PREGNANCY Genetic counseling - advised for parents or other relatives of a child with thalassemia and for any individual with beta-thalassemia minor

SYNONYMS
• Mediterranean anemia
• Hereditary leptocytosis
• Thalassemia major and minor
• Cooley's anemia

ICD-9-CM 282.4

SEE ALSO N/A

OTHER NOTES N/A

ABBREVIATIONS N/A

REFERENCES
• Nathan, D.G. & Oski, F. (eds.): Hematology of Infancy and Childhood. Philadelphia, W.B. Saunders Co., 1991
• Fosburg, M.T. & Nathan, D.G.: Treatment of Cooley's anemia. Blood. 76:435, 1990

Author H. Griffith, M.D. & M. Dambro, M.D.

Thoracic outlet syndrome

 BASICS

DESCRIPTION A constellation of symptoms that affect the head, neck, shoulders and upper extremities caused by compression of the neurovascular structures (viz. cords of brachial plexus and subclavian artery and vein) at the thoracic outlet
• May be due to congenital bony muscular or tendonous anomalies; post traumatic, following clavicular or cervical spine injures; or idiopathic, without discernible cause
System(s) affected: Nervous, Musculoskeletal, Cardiovascular
Genetics: N/A
Incidence/Prevalence in USA: Unknown
Predominant age:
• Neurologic type (95%) - 20-60 years
• Venous type (4%) - 20-35 years
• Arterial type (1%) (atherosclerosis) - young adult or older than 50
Predominant sex:
• Neurologic type - Female > Male (3:1)
• Venous type - Male > Female
• Arterial type - Male = Female

SIGNS AND SYMPTOMS
General symptoms
◊ Positive costoclavicular maneuver
◊ Positive hyperabduction maneuver
◊ Positive Adson's maneuver
◊ Positive elevated arm stress test
◊ Tenderness to percussion or palpation of supraclavicular area
◊ Worsening of symptoms with elevation of arm, overhead extension of arms, or with arms extended forward (e.g., driving a car, typing, carrying objects). Prompt disappearance of symptoms with arm returning to neutral position.
◊ Supraventricular bruit
Neurologic type. upper plexus (c4-c7)
◊ Pain and paresthesias in head, neck, mandible, face, temporal area, upper back/chest, outer arm & hand in a radial nerve distribution
◊ Occipital headache
Neurologic type. lower plexus (c8-t1)
◊ Pain and paresthesias in axilla, inner arm and hand in an ulnar nerve distribution
◊ Hypothenar and interosseous muscle atrophy
Venous type
◊ Arm claudication
◊ Cyanosis
◊ Swelling
◊ Distended arm veins
Arterial type
◊ Digital vasospasm
◊ Thrombosis/embolism
◊ Aneurysm
◊ Gangrene

CAUSES
• Upper thoracic neurovascular bundle compression
• Cervical rib
• Taut anomalous scalene muscles
• Elongated c7 transverse process
• Poor posture
• Pancoast's tumor
• Atherosclerotic plaques within vessels
• Subclavian muscle
• Costocoracoid tendon
• Callous bone formation from fractured clavicle or first rib
• Aberrant tissue

RISK FACTORS
• Exuberant callus after fracture of clavicle or first rib
• Exostosis of clavicle or first rib
• Postural abnormalities (e.g., drooping of shoulders, scoliosis)
• Body building, with increased muscular bulk in thoracic outlet area
• Rapid weight loss combined with vigorous physical exertion and/or exercise

 DIAGNOSIS

DIFFERENTIAL DIAGNOSIS
• Cervical disk syndrome
• Carpal tunnel syndrome
• Orthopedic shoulder problems (shoulder strain, rotator cuff injury, tendinitis)
• Cervical spondylitis
• Ulnar nerve compression at the elbow
• Multiple sclerosis
• Spinal cord tumor or disease
• Angina pectoris
• Migraine

LABORATORY N/A
Drugs that may alter lab results: N/A
Disorders that may alter lab results: N/A

PATHOLOGICAL FINDINGS
• Bony abnormalities (cervical rib, anomalous first thoracic rib)
• Abnormal muscles
• Congenital fibromuscular bands

SPECIAL TESTS
• Plethysmography with previously mentioned maneuvers
• Doppler and duplex ultrasound if venous obstruct suspected
• Nerve conduction studies (< 70 m/sec is abnormal)

IMAGING
• X-ray (chest x-ray, oblique C-spine)
• Arteriogram - if arterial obstruction, aneurysm or emboli are suspected
• Phlebogram - if signs of venous obstruction
• CT scan - if cord compressive lesions (disc and/or tumor) are suspected

DIAGNOSTIC PROCEDURES TOS is a clinical diagnosis

 TREATMENT

APPROPRIATE HEALTH CARE
• Outpatient for conservative treatment
• Inpatient if surgery required

GENERAL MEASURES
Conservative
◊ If no vascular involvement is present and/or if no loss of function or lifestyle is present due to severity of symptoms, conservative therapy may be undertaken for 2-3 months
◊ Improvement can be expected in 60% of patients
◊ Exercise program to promote shoulder muscle function
◊ Physical therapy for postural faults
◊ Cervical collar, traction
◊ Weight loss if axillary folds are causing compression
Surgery
◊ Operative - if vascular involvement is present and/or if there is loss of function or lifestyle secondary to severity of symptoms and if conservative therapy fails after 2-3 months
◊ Removal of first rib or cervical ribs (transaxillary, supraclavicular, posterior approaches)
◊ Removal of adhesive bands
◊ Anterior scalenectomy (not scalenotomy)

ACTIVITY
• Light activity with arm and hand encouraged
• No straining or heavy activity for 3 months

DIET N/A

PATIENT EDUCATION Physical therapy following surgery

MEDICATIONS

DRUG(S) OF CHOICE
• Analgesics
• Muscle relaxants
• Antispasmodics
Contraindications: Refer to manufacturer's profile of each drug
Precautions: Refer to manufacturer's profile of each drug
Significant possible interactions: Refer to manufacturer's profile of each drug
ALTERNATIVE DRUGS: N/A

FOLLOWUP

PATIENT MONITORING
Office follow-up visits e.g., q3 weeks x 2

PREVENTION/AVOIDANCE N/A

POSSIBLE COMPLICATIONS
• Postoperative shoulder, arm, hand pain and paresthesias in 10%, usually responds to physiotherapy
• 1.5 to 2% of patients will have symptomatic recurrences 1 month to 7 years postoperatively (usually within 3 months)
• 0.5-1% of patients have brachial plexus injury, probably due to intraoperative traction
• Re-operation indicated for symptomatic recurrence with long posterior remnant of first rib (posterior approach) or with disrupted fibrous adhesions (transaxillary approach)

EXPECTED COURSE AND PROGNOSIS
• 60% improve with appropriate physiotherapy program
• 90% have excellent or good early results with surgery
• 70-80% have no recurrence at 5 years and 10 years

MISCELLANEOUS

ASSOCIATED CONDITIONS N/A

AGE-RELATED FACTORS N/A
Pediatric: N/A
Geriatric: N/A
Others: N/A

PREGNANCY
Generalized tissue fluid accumulations and postural changes could aggravate symptoms

SYNONYMS
• Scalenus anticus syndrome
• Cervical rib syndrome
• Costoclavicular syndrome
• TOS

SEE ALSO N/A

ICD-9-CM 353.0

OTHER NOTES
2-3 months trial of physiotherapy always indicated except in presence of obvious bony abnormality

ABBREVIATIONS N/A

REFERENCES
• Ursche, H.C. & Rassuk, M.A.: Thoracic Outlet Syndromes. In Surgery of the Chest. 5th Ed. Edited by D.C. Sabiston & F.C. Spencer. Philadelphia, W.B. Saunders Co.,1990
• Roos, D.B.: Thoracic Outlet Nerve Compression. In Vascular Surgery. 3rd Ed. Edited by R.B. Ruthford. Philadelphia, W.B. Saunders Co.,1989
• Dale, W.Q.: Thoracic outlet compression syndrome. Arch Surg. 117:1437, 1982
• Stallworth, J.M.: Thoracic Outlet Compression Syndromes. In Vascular Surgery. 3rd Ed. Edited by H. Haimoviei. Norwalk, Appleton & Lange,1989

Author K. Magliato, M.D., M. Oddi, M.D., D. Moorman, M.D., F.A.C.S.

Thromboangiitis obliterans (Buerger's disease)

 BASICS

DESCRIPTION Occlusion of small and medium sized arteries and veins caused by inflammatory changes of these vessels. It occurs almost exclusively in men who smoke.
System(s) affected: Cardiovascular
Genetics: Greater prevalence of HLA-A9 and HLA-B5. Familial cases reported rarely.
Incidence in USA: 13/100,000
Prevalence in USA: Unknown
Predominant age: 20 to 40 years
Predominant sex: Male > Female (3:1). Increasing numbers of women are being diagnosed, presumably due to increased smoking.

SIGNS AND SYMPTOMS
Symptoms tend to wax and wane in early disease and are often asymmetric. Symptoms may be gradual or have a sudden onset related to impaired vasculature.
• Ulceration of digits; pain may be disabling
• Coldness in feet and/or fingers
• Cold sensitivity
• Paresthesias (numbness, tingling, burning, hypoesthesia) of feet and/or fingers
• Intermittent claudication in arch of foot or leg (rarely hand, forearm)
• Persistent extremity pain (may be worse at rest)
• Paroxysmal "electric shock" pain of ischemic neuropathy
• Raynaud's phenomenon
• Postural color changes (pallor on elevation; rubor on dependency)
• "Buerger's colour" - cyanosis of hands and feet
• Migratory superficial phlebitis
• Tender skin nodules on extremities
• Impaired distal pulses; proximal pulses normal
• Foot edema
• Gangrene

CAUSES (postulated)
• Smoking
• Genetic factors
• Autoimmune disorder with cell mediated sensitivity to types I and III human collagens (both are constituents of blood vessels)

RISK FACTORS
• Smoking tobacco
• Incidence higher in Israel, Eastern Europe, Japan, India, Far East

 DIAGNOSIS

DIFFERENTIAL DIAGNOSIS
• Peripheral neuropathy
• Peripheral atherosclerotic disease
• Arterial embolus and thrombosis
• Idiopathic peripheral thrombosis
• Other causes of vasculitis
• Scleroderma
• Occupational trauma
• Cervical rib
• Livedo reticularis
• Raynaud's disease
• Acrocyanosis
• Ergotism
• Frostbite
• Neurotrophic ulcers
• Reflex sympathetic dystrophy
• Metatarsalgia
• Gout
• Periarteritis nodosa

LABORATORY Routine laboratory studies show no changes characteristic of this disorder. Auto-antibodies to collagen and circulating immune complexes may be present, but are considered a research tool only.
Drugs that may alter lab results: N/A
Disorders that may alter lab results: N/A

PATHOLOGICAL FINDINGS
• Segmental nonsuppurative panarteritis or panphlebitis with thrombosis
• Histologic findings may vary between acute, subacute, and chronic stages of the disease
• Histologic sine qua non - granulomas with collections of neutrophils in the organizing thrombus. Inflammation reaction permeates the entire thickness of the vessel wall.
• Chronic lesions show recanalized thrombus and perivascular fibrosis.

SPECIAL TESTS Doppler ultrasound (not specific)

IMAGING
Arteriogram or digital-subtraction angiography (DSA)
◊ Multiple areas of segmental occlusion of small to medium arteries of arms and legs
◊ "Skip" areas may be demonstrated
◊ Numerous collateral vessels around occluded segments may give a characteristic "cork screw" appearance
◊ Larger arteries are spared

DIAGNOSTIC PROCEDURES
• History and physical examination
• Studies of nerve conduction velocity (to exclude neuropathy)

 TREATMENT

APPROPRIATE HEALTH CARE
• Outpatient
• Inpatient if surgery needed for gangrene
• Inpatient for dorsal or lumbar sympathectomy if indicated

GENERAL MEASURES
• Stop smoking (mandatory)
• Protect against trauma (poor fitting shoes)
• Protect against infections (fungal)
• Protect against vasoconstriction from cold or drugs
• Eliminate exposure to thermal damage
• Eliminate exposure to chemical damage (iodine, carbolic acid, salicylic acid)
• Amputation (rare) for non-healing ulcers, gangrene or intractable pain. Should preserve as much limb as possible.
• Thrombolytic therapy of occlusive thrombus and angioplasty are experimental
• Omental autotransplantation has been successful in treating ulcers
• In severe disease, a lumbar sympathectomy to increase blood supply to the skin
• Direct revascularization of distal arteries is not practical unless coexistent atherosclerotic disease

ACTIVITY Restricted by symptoms. Use a bed cradle (non-heated) to prevent pressure from bed linens.

DIET No restrictions

PATIENT EDUCATION
• Must stop smoking
• Remove possibilities of exposure to others in the environment who smoke
• Use heel pads or foam rubber boots
• See General Measures

Thromboangiitis obliterans (Buerger's disease)

MEDICATIONS

DRUG(S) OF CHOICE
• Medications are not a substitute for discontinuance of smoking
• Antibiotics for infected digital ulcers and osteomyelitis
• Iloprost (a prostacyclin analogue) promotes ulcer healing
• No form of medical treatment has been shown to be effective (including steroids, calcium channel blockers, reserpine, pentoxifylline, vasodilators, antiplatelet drugs, anticoagulants)
Contraindications: Refer to manufacturer's literature
Precautions: Refer to manufacturer's literature
Significant possible interactions: Refer to manufacturer's literature

ALTERNATIVE DRUGS
Calcium channel blocking agents such as nifedipine may allow vasodilatation, but have not been proven effective.

FOLLOWUP

PATIENT MONITORING
Frequent history and physical examinations

PREVENTION/AVOIDANCE
Never smoke

POSSIBLE COMPLICATIONS
• Ulcerations
• Gangrene
• Need for amputation
• Rare involvement of cerebral, coronary, renal or mesenteric arteries

EXPECTED COURSE AND PROGNOSIS
• Occasional remissions
• Unremitting progression if patient continues to smoke
• Death rare; normal survival curve

MISCELLANEOUS

ASSOCIATED CONDITIONS N/A

AGE-RELATED FACTORS
Pediatric: Not a problem in this age group
Geriatric: Not common in this age group, but diagnosis in the elderly is increasing
Others: N/A

PREGNANCY N/A

SYNONYMS
• Buerger's disease
• TAO

ICD-9-CM 443.1

SEE ALSO N/A

OTHER NOTES
May be difficult to differentiate from some types of atherosclerosis, systemic emboli or idiopathic peripheral thromboses

ABBREVIATIONS N/A

REFERENCES
• Hurst, J.W., et al.: The Heart. 7th Ed. New York, McGraw-Hill, 1990
• Case records of the Mass. General Hospital. Weekly clinicopathological exercises. case 16-1989. A 36 year-old man with peripheral vascular disease. New Eng J Med. April 20;320(16):1068-76, 1989
• Olin, J.W., et al.: The changing clinical spectrum of thromboangiitis obliterans (Buerger's disease). Circulation. Supplement IV. 82(5), 1990
• Juergens, J.L.: Thromboangiitis Obliterans (Buerger's disease, TAO). In Peripheral Vascular Disease. Edited by J.L. Juergens. Philadelphia, W.B. Saunders Co., 1980

Author R. Kellerman, M.D.

Thrombophlebitis, superficial

BASICS

DESCRIPTION Superficial thrombophlebitis is an inflammatory condition of the veins with secondary thrombosis.
Septic (suppurative) thrombophlebitis types:
  ◊ Iatrogenic
  ◊ Infectious, mainly syphilis and psittacosis
Aseptic thrombophlebitis types:
  ◊ Primary hypercoagulable states - disorders with measurable defects in the proteins of the coagulation and/or fibrinolytic systems
  ◊ Secondary hypercoagulable states - clinical conditions with a risk of thrombosis
System(s) affected: Cardiovascular
Genetics:
• Septic - no known genetic pattern
• Antithrombin III deficiencies - autosomal dominant
• Proteins C and S deficiency - autosomal dominant with variable penetrance
• Disorders of fibrinolytic system - congenital defects inheritance variable
• Dysfibrinogenemia - autosomal dominant
• Factor XII deficiency - autosomal recessive
Incidence in USA:
Septic
  ◊ Up to 10% of all nosocomial infections
  ◊ Incidence of catheter-related thrombophlebitis is 88/100,000
  ◊ Develops in 4-8% if cut down is performed
Aseptic primary hypercoagulable state
  ◊ Antithrombin III and heparin cofactor II deficiency incidence is 50/100,000
Aseptic secondary hypercoagulable state
  ◊ Trousseau incidence in malignancy 5-15%
  ◊ Trousseau in pancreatic carcinoma 50%
  ◊ In pregnancy 49-fold increased incidence of phlebitis
  ◊ Superficial migratory thrombophlebitis in 27% of patients with thromboangiitis obliterans
Prevalence in USA: Unknown
Predominant age:
Septic
  ◊ More common in childhood
Aseptic primary hypercoagulable state
  ◊ Antithrombin III and heparin cofactor II deficiency - neonatal period, but first episode usually at age 20-30 years
  ◊ Proteins C and S - before age 30
Aseptic secondary hypercoagulable state
  ◊ Mondor's disease: women, ages 21-55 years
  ◊ Thromboangiitis obliterans onset: 20-50 years
Predominant sex:
Suppurative:
  ◊ Male = Female
Aseptic
  ◊ Mondor's - Female > Male (2:1)
  ◊ Thromboangiitis obliterans - Female > Male (1-19% of clinical cases)

SIGNS AND SYMPTOMS
• Swelling, tenderness, redness along the course of the veins
• May look like cellulitis or erythema nodosa
• Fever in 70% of patients
• Warmth, erythema, tenderness, or lymphangitis in 32%
• Sign of systemic sepsis in 84% in suppurative
• Red, tender cord
• Pain

CAUSES
Septic
  ◊ Staphylococcus aureus in 65-78%
  ◊ Enterobacteriaceae, especially Klebsiella
  ◊ Multiple organisms in 14%
  ◊ Anaerobic isolate rare
  ◊ Candida spp.
  ◊ Cytomegalovirus in AIDS patients
Aseptic primary hypercoagulable state
  ◊ Antithrombin III and heparin II deficiency
  ◊ Protein C and protein S deficiency
  ◊ Disorder of tissue plasminogen activator
  ◊ Abnormal plasminogen and co-plasminogen
  ◊ Dysfibrinogenemia
  ◊ Factor XII deficiency
  ◊ Lupus anticoagulant and anticardiolipin antibody syndrome
Aseptic secondary hypercoagulable states
  ◊ Malignancy (Trousseau syndrome: Recurrent migratory thrombophlebitis)
  ◊ Pregnancy
  ◊ Oral contraceptive
  ◊ Infusion of prothrombin complex concentrates
  ◊ Behçet's disease
  ◊ Buerger's disease
  ◊ Mondor's disease

RISK FACTORS
Nonspecific
  ◊ Immobilization
  ◊ Obesity
  ◊ Advanced age
  ◊ Postoperative states
Septic
  ◊ Intravenous catheter
  ◊ Duration of intravenous catheterization (68% of cannulae have been left in place for 2 days)
  ◊ Cutdowns
  ◊ Cancer, debilitating diseases
  ◊ Steroid
  ◊ Incidence is 40 times higher with plastic cannula (8%) than with steel or scalp cannulas (0.2%)
  ◊ Thrombosis
  ◊ Dermal infection
  ◊ Burned patients
  ◊ Lower extremities intravenous catheter
  ◊ Intravenous antibiotics
  ◊ AIDS
  ◊ Varicose veins
Antithrombin II and heparin cofactor II deficiency
  ◊ Pregnancy
  ◊ Oral contraceptives
  ◊ Surgery
  ◊ Trauma
  ◊ Infection

In pregnancy
  ◊ Increased age
  ◊ Hypertension
  ◊ Eclampsia
  ◊ Increased parity
Thromboangiitis obliterans
  ◊ Persistent smoking
Mondor's disease
  ◊ Breast abscess
  ◊ Antecedent breast surgery
  ◊ Breast augmentation
  ◊ Reduction mammoplasty

DIAGNOSIS

DIFFERENTIAL DIAGNOSIS
• Cellulitis
• Erythema nodosa
• Cutaneous polyarteritis nodosa
• Sarcoid
• Kaposi's sarcoma
• Hyperalgesic pseudothrombophlebitis

LABORATORY
Septic
  ◊ Bacteremia in 80-90%
  ◊ Culture of IV fluid bag
  ◊ Leukocytosis
Aseptic
  ◊ Acute phase reactant
  ◊ Factor levels
  ◊ Thrombin activity
  ◊ Platelet function test
Drugs that may alter lab results: In septic, broad spectrum antibiotics
Disorders that may alter lab results: N/A

PATHOLOGICAL FINDINGS
• The affected vein is enlarged, tortuous, and thickened
• Associated perivascular suppuration and/or hemorrhage
• Vein lumen may contain pus and thrombus
• Endothelial damage, fibrinoid necrosis and thickening of the vein wall

SPECIAL TESTS   Leukocyte imaging

IMAGING
Septic and aseptic
  ◊ Ultrasound of veins reveal an increase in the diameter of the lumen
  ◊ Chest x-ray - multiple peripheral densities or a pleural effusion consistent with pulmonary embolism, abscess, or empyema
  ◊ Bone and gallium scan - for associated subperiosteal abscess in septic thrombophlebitis
  ◊ Evaluation of complications (deep vein thrombosis and others)

DIAGNOSTIC PROCEDURES   Skin biopsy

TREATMENT

APPROPRIATE HEALTH CARE
• Septic - inpatient
• Aseptic - outpatient

GENERAL MEASURES
• Heat application
• Extremity elevation
Septic
◊ Excision of the involved vein segment and all involved tributaries
◊ Excision from ankle to groin may be required in some burn patients
◊ If systemic symptoms persist after vein excision, re-exploration is necessary with removal of all involved veins
◊ Drainage of contiguous abscesses
◊ Remove all cannulae
Aseptic
◊ Mondor's disease, consider surgical transection of the phlebitic cord
◊ Management of underlying conditions

ACTIVITY Bedrest

DIET No restrictions

PATIENT EDUCATION
• Avoid trauma
• Be alert to change in skin color
• Be alert to tenderness over extremities

MEDICATIONS

DRUG(S) OF CHOICE
Septic
◊ Initially: semisynthetic penicillin (e.g., nafcillin 2 g IV q6h) plus an aminoglycoside (e.g., gentamicin, 1.0-1.7 mg/kg IV)
◊ Duration of therapy is empiric
◊ If due to Candida albicans, consider a short course of amphotericin B (approximately 200 mg cumulative dose)
◊ If osteomyelitis documented, antibiotic therapy for at least 6 weeks
Aseptic general
◊ Nonsteroidal anti-inflammatories
◊ Oral anticoagulant warfarin
◊ Systemic anticoagulant heparin
Antithrombin III and heparin cofactor II deficiency
◊ IV heparin
◊ Antithrombin III concentrate
◊ Prophylaxis: warfarin, oxymetholone
Proteins C and S
◊ Long-term warfarin, lower dose, no loading
Tissue plasminogen activate
◊ Phenformin and ethylestrenol
◊ Stanozolol and phenformin
◊ Stanozolol alone
◊ Ethylestrenol alone
Dysfibrinogemia
◊ Acute attack - anticoagulation
◊ Prophylaxis - stanozolol

Abnormal plasminogen and plasminogenemia
◊ Acute attack - anticoagulation
◊ Prophylaxis - warfarin
Factor XII deficiency
◊ Standard therapy
Lupus anticardiolipin
◊ Prophylaxis - warfarin
Trousseau's syndrome
◊ Heparin
For pregnancy
◊ Heparin
Behcet's disease
◊ Phenformin
◊ Ethylestrenol
◊ Stanozolol
Thromboangiitis obliterans
◊ Stop smoking
◊ Pentoxifylline
Contraindications: Refer to manufacturer's literature
Precautions: Refer to manufacturer's literature
Significant possible interactions:
Refer to manufacturer's literature

ALTERNATIVE DRUGS
• Factor XII deficiency - streptokinase or TPA
• Behcet's - oral anticoagulants plus cyclosporine
• Thromboangiitis obliterans - corticosteroid, antiplatelets and vasodilating drugs

FOLLOWUP

PATIENT MONITORING
Septic
◊ Routine WBC and differential and culture
◊ Repeat culture from the phlebitic vein
Aseptic
◊ Clinical followup to rule out secondary complications
◊ Repeat of blood studies for fibrinolytic system, platelets and factors

PREVENTION/AVOIDANCE
• Use of scalp vein cannulae
• Avoidance of lower extremity cannulations
• Insertion under aseptic conditions
• Secure anchoring of the cannulae
• Replacement of cannulae, connecting tubing, and IV fluid every 48-72 hrs
• Neomycin-polymyxin B-bacitracin ointment in cutdown

POSSIBLE COMPLICATIONS
Septic
◊ Systemic sepsis, bacteremia (84%)
◊ Septic pulmonary emboli (44%)
◊ Metastatic abscess formation
◊ Pneumonia (44%)
◊ Subperiosteal abscess of adjacent long bones in children
Aseptic
◊ Deep vein thrombosis
◊ Thromboembolic phenomena

EXPECTED COURSE AND PROGNOSIS
Septic
◊ High mortality (50%), if untreated
Aseptic
◊ Usually benign course with recovery in 7-10 days
◊ Antithrombin III and heparin cofactor deficiency; recurrence rate is 60%
◊ Proteins C and S, recurrence rate 70%
◊ Prognosis depends on development of DVT and early detections of complications
◊ Aseptic thrombophlebitis can be isolated, recurrent or migratory

MISCELLANEOUS

ASSOCIATED CONDITIONS Varicose
veins, manifestation of systemic disease, hypercoagulable states, surgery, trauma, burns, obesity, pregnancy

AGE-RELATED FACTORS
Pediatric: Subperiosteal abscesses of adjacent long bone may complicate
Geriatric: Septic thrombophlebitis is more common, prognosis poorer
Others: N/A

PREGNANCY
• Associated with increased risk of aseptic superficial thrombophlebitis
• Warfarin and NSAID's are contraindicated

SYNONYMS
• Phlebitis
• Phlebothrombosis

ICD-9-CM
• Phlebitis and thrombophlebitis - 451
• Phlebitis and thrombophlebitis of superficial vessels of lower extremities - 451.0
• Phlebitis and thrombophlebitis of deep vessels of lower extremities - 451.1

SEE ALSO Deep vein thrombosis

OTHER NOTES N/A

ABBREVIATIONS DVT = deep vein thrombosis

REFERENCES
• Samlaskie, C.P. & James, W.D.: Superficial thrombophlebitis II. Secondary hypercoagulable states. J Am Acad Dermatol 1990 Jul; 23(1)1-18
• Samlaskie, C.P. & James, W.D.: Superficial thrombophlebitis I. Primary hypercoagulable states. J Am Acad Dermatol 1990, Jun; 22:975-89
• Mandell, G.L. (ed.): Principles and Practice of Infectious Diseases. 3rd Ed. New York, Churchill Livingstone, 1990

Author A. Abyad, M.D., M.P.H.

Thrombosis, deep vein (DVT)

 BASICS

DESCRIPTION
Development of single or multiple blood clots within the deep veins of the extremities or pelvis, usually accompanied by inflammation of the vessel wall. The major clinical consequence is embolization, usually to the lung, that is frequently life-threatening.

System(s) affected: Cardiovascular

Genetics: N/A

Incidence/Prevalence in USA: Common (approximately 2 million cases per year)

Predominant age: Usually over 40

Predominant sex: Female > Male (1.2:1)

SIGNS AND SYMPTOMS
- Many cases are completely asymptomatic, diagnosed retrospectively after embolization
- Limb pain (common)
- Limb swelling (common)
- Leg pain on dorsiflexion of the foot (Homan's sign; common)
- Palpable tender cord in affected limb (uncommon)
- Warmth of skin over area of thrombosis (uncommon)
- Redness of skin over area or thrombosis (uncommon)
- Fever (uncommon, except in septic thrombophlebitis)
- Non-tender swelling of collateral superficial veins (uncommon)
- Massive edema with cyanosis and ischemia (Phlegmasia cerulea dolens, rare)

CAUSES
- Venous stasis
- Injury to vessel wall
- Abnormalities of coagulation

RISK FACTORS
Clinical risk factors:
- ◊ Trauma, especially long bone fractures or crush injuries
- ◊ Surgery, particularly hip surgery
- ◊ Prolonged immobility
- ◊ Pregnancy, especially the puerperium
- ◊ Indwelling central venous catheters
- ◊ Oral contraceptive use (risk is confined to current usage and is proportional to estrogen content)
- ◊ Extreme high altitude (> 14,000 feet)

Pathological risk factors:
- ◊ Carcinoma
- ◊ Deficiencies of protein C, protein S, antithrombin III, all endogenous anticoagulants
- ◊ Presence of anti-phospholipid antibodies (also known as lupus anticoagulant or anti-cardiolipin antibodies)
- ◊ Nephrotic syndrome
- ◊ Polycythemia vera
- ◊ Homocystinuria (rare)
- ◊ Campylobacter jejuni bacteremia (very rare)

 DIAGNOSIS

DIFFERENTIAL DIAGNOSIS
- Cellulitis
- Ruptured synovial cyst (Baker's cyst)
- Lymphedema
- Extrinsic compression of vein by tumor or enlarged lymph nodes
- Pulled, strained, or torn muscle

LABORATORY
- No specific laboratory test is available for DVT
- Protein C, protein S, antithrombin III and anti-phospholipid antibodies can be measured in some laboratories. But as these are rare causes of DVT they are not routinely indicated and should be ordered only when the clinical circumstances suggest such a disorder.

Drugs that may alter lab results:
- Heparin, estrogens may lower antithrombin III levels
- Coumadin affects protein C and protein S function so may interfere with functional assays of these proteins

Disorders that may alter lab results:
- Thrombosis itself lowers antithrombin III levels so any workup for antithrombin III deficiency must be performed after patient has completed therapy
- Syphilis and systemic lupus erythematosus are associated with increased anti-phospholipid antibodies

PATHOLOGICAL FINDINGS
- Clot consisting predominantly of red blood cells, with some platelets and fibrin attached to vessel wall at one end with proximal end floating free in the lumen. Varying degrees of inflammation of the vessel wall are present.
- Biochemical abnormalities such as proteins S, C or antithrombin III deficiency, anti-phospholipid antibody or homocystinuria are found in only a small minority of cases

SPECIAL TESTS   N/A

IMAGING
- Imaging studies are necessary to diagnose or rule out suspected DVT
- Contrast venography is the gold standard test (i.e., most sensitive and specific). Disadvantages include discomfort, technical difficulty and small risk of morbidity.
- B-mode ultrasound combined with Doppler flow detection (duplex ultrasound); noninvasive, highly sensitive and specific for popliteal and femoral thrombi. Disadvantages include poor ability to detect calf vein thrombi; it is a highly operator-dependent technique; and its inability to reliably distinguish extrinsic compression of the vein from intrinsic clot.
- Impedance plethysmography (IPG); probably as accurate as duplex ultrasound, less operator dependency, but poor at detecting calf vein thrombi
- 125 I-fibrinogen scan; detects only active clot formation; very good at detecting ongoing calf thrombi. Major disadvantage is that it takes 4 hours for results. This test has generally been supplanted by duplex ultrasound and IPG.

DIAGNOSTIC PROCEDURES   N/A

 TREATMENT

APPROPRIATE HEALTH CARE
Patients with DVT confined to the calf (i.e., distal to the popliteal system) can be managed conservatively as outpatients. All others must be admitted.

GENERAL MEASURES
- For hospitalized patient - intravenous anticoagulation, bedrest, and close observation for embolic events
- Non-drug therapy - if anticoagulants and thrombolytics are contraindicated, filtering devices ("umbrellas") can he inserted into the vena cava to "trap" emboli before reaching the lungs

ACTIVITY
Bedrest for 1-5 days, then gradual resumption of normal activity, with avoidance of prolonged immobility

DIET   No special diet

PATIENT EDUCATION
- Advise women taking oral contraceptives of the risks, and the common symptoms of thromboembolic disease
- Discourage prolonged immobility

MEDICATIONS

DRUG(S) OF CHOICE
• Immediate therapy: Heparin 5,000-10,000 units intravenous bolus followed by continuous IV infusion at 1,000 units per hour. Adjust dosage based on activated partial thromboplastin time (APTT) to achieve APTT of approximately 2 x control value.
• Maintenance therapy: Warfarin (Coumadin) beginning 1-5 days after starting heparin, in a single daily dose starting at 5-10 mg daily and adjusting based on prothrombin time (PT) with a target value of PT of 1.3-1.5 x control value. Patient should remain on heparin until target PT level is achieved.

Contraindications:
• Absolute contraindications: Severe active bleeding, recent neurosurgical procedure (within 30 days), pregnancy (Coumadin only), previous adverse reaction to the drug (other than bleeding, which is a known side effect)
• Relative contraindications: Recent severe hemorrhage, recent surgical procedure other than neurosurgery, history of significant peptic ulcer disease, recent non-embolic stroke

Precautions:
• Observe patient carefully for signs of embolization, further thrombosis or bleeding
• While on anticoagulant therapy avoid intramuscular injections. Periodically check stool and urine for occult blood, monitor complete blood counts.
• Heparin - other possible but rare adverse reactions include thrombocytopenia and/or paradoxical thrombosis with thrombocytopenia
• Coumadin - necrotic lesions of the skin (Warfarin necrosis) occasionally result from treatment

Significant possible interactions:
• Agents that may prolong or intensify the response to oral anticoagulants: Alcohol, allopurinol, amiodarone, anabolic steroids, androgens, many antimicrobials, cimetidine chloral hydrate, disulfiram, all nonsteroidal anti-inflammatory drugs (NSAID's), sulfinpyrazone, tamoxifen, thyroid hormone, vitamin E, ranitidine, salicylates
• Agents that may diminish the response to anticoagulants: Aminoglutethimide, antacids, barbiturates, carbamazepine, cholestyramine, diuretics, griseofulvin, rifampin, oral contraceptives

ALTERNATIVE DRUGS
• Thrombolytic agents (urokinase, streptokinase, tissue plasminogen activator) are effective in dissolving clots and are currently investigational for treatment of DVT. In current clinical practice they should he reserved for massive thromboembolic disease. The same contraindications apply as to anticoagulants.
• If Coumadin is contraindicated, heparin can be given in the ambulatory setting by intermittent subcutaneous self-injection (see Pregnancy)

FOLLOWUP

PATIENT MONITORING
• APTT must be monitored several times a day while on IV heparin until dose stabilizes. Platelets should also be monitored and heparin discontinued if platelets fall below 75,000
• While on Coumadin, PT must be monitored daily until target achieved, then weekly for several weeks, then (if stable) monthly as long as patient is on the drug
• For first episode of DVT patients should be treated for 3-6 months. Subsequent episodes should be treated for at least a year.
• Significant bleeding such as hematuria or gastrointestinal hemorrhage should be thoroughly investigated since anticoagulant therapy frequently unmasks a pre-existing lesion such as cancer, peptic ulcer disease, or arteriovenous malformation

PREVENTION/AVOIDANCE
• General preventive measures such as avoiding prolonged immobility and using low-estrogen birth control pills when possible
• Surgical patients need active prophylaxis. Low dose subcutaneous heparin with dosage adjusted to slightly prolong the APTT, low dose Coumadin, and intermittent mechanical compression of the legs have all been effective in reducing the risks of DVT following various types of surgery.

POSSIBLE COMPLICATIONS
• Pulmonary embolism (fatal in 10-20% of cases)
• Systemic embolism ("paradoxical embolization") in cases where there is arteriovenous shunting (rare)
• Chronic venous insufficiency
• Post-phlebitic syndrome, i.e., pain and swelling in affected limb without new clot formation
• Treatment induced hemorrhage
• Soft tissue ischemia associated with massive clot and very high venous pressures - phlegmasia cerulea dolens (very rare but should be considered a surgical emergency)

EXPECTED COURSE AND PROGNOSIS
• About 20% of untreated proximal (i.e., above the calf) DVT's progress to pulmonary emboli and 10-20% of those are fatal. With aggressive anticoagulant therapy the mortality is decreased five to tenfold.
• DVT confined to the calf virtually never causes clinically significant emboli so does not require anticoagulation. However calf DVT's do sometimes propagate into the proximal system so known or suspected calf DVT's should be followed with IPG or duplex ultrasound every 3-5 days for 10 days and treated aggressively if they propagate into the popliteal or femoral system.

MISCELLANEOUS

ASSOCIATED CONDITIONS
• Budd-Chiari syndrome (hepatic vein thrombosis)
• Renal vein thrombosis
• Homocystinuria
• Anti-phospholipid antibody syndrome

AGE-RELATED FACTORS
Pediatric: In this age group patients with DVT, in absence of preceding trauma, should be worked up for congenital coagulopathy
Geriatric: More common because predisposing conditions are more common
Others: N/A

PREGNANCY
• Coumadin is a known teratogen so is contraindicated in pregnancy. Treat pregnant women with DVT with full dose heparin initially followed by subcutaneous heparin starting at 15,000 units twice daily with target APTT of 1.5-2 x control value.
• Septic thrombophlebitis, usually associated with childbirth, requires antibiotic therapy as well as anticoagulation

SYNONYMS Deep venous thrombophlebitis

SEE ALSO N/A

ICD-9-CM 451.19

OTHER NOTES N/A

ABBREVIATIONS
• DVT = deep vein thrombophlebitis
• IPG = impedance plethysmography

REFERENCES
• Rubenstein, E.: Thromboembolism. In Scientific American Medicine. Edited by E. Rubenstein & D.D. Federman. New York, Scientific American, 1990
• Kontos, H.A.: Vascular Diseases of the Limbs. In Cecil Textbook of Medicine. Edited by J.B. Wyngaarden & L.H. Smith. Philadelphia, W.B. Saunders Co., 1992

Author R. Sliman, M.D.

Thyroglossal duct cyst

 BASICS

DESCRIPTION Cystic remnant of thyroid descent in the neck
Genetics: N/A
Incidence/Prevalence in USA: N/A
Predominant age: 50% less than 10 years, 65% less than 20 years of age
Predominant sex: Male = Female

SIGNS AND SYMPTOMS
• Midline neck mass
• Non-tender, unless infected
• Rises in the neck with tongue protrusion
• 80% juxtaposed to the hyoid bone

CAUSES Failure of obliteration of the thyroglossal duct following descent of the thyroid in the 6th week of fetal life

RISK FACTORS None

 DIAGNOSIS

DIFFERENTIAL DIAGNOSIS
• Ectopic midline thyroid
• Dermoid cyst
• Thyroid adenoma of isthmus or pyramidal lobe
• Lymphadenitis

LABORATORY None
Drugs that may alter lab results: N/A
Disorders that may alter lab results: N/A

PATHOLOGICAL FINDINGS Cyst lined with stratified squamous or pseudostratified ciliated columnar epithelium. Thyroid tissue seen in 10-45% of cysts.

SPECIAL TESTS N/A

IMAGING
• Ultrasound
• Thyroid scan if midline ectopic thyroid or thyroid nodule is suspected

DIAGNOSTIC PROCEDURES N/A

 TREATMENT

APPROPRIATE HEALTH CARE
Outpatient surgery

GENERAL MEASURES
• Once diagnosed, the excision can be done with Sistrunk procedure. This requires removal of the center portion of the hyoid bone to minimize recurrence.
• If the cyst is infected, it should be initially treated (antibiotics and local heat) or drained. After resolution of the inflammation, excision should be performed.

ACTIVITY Unrestricted

DIET Unrestricted

PATIENT EDUCATION
• Reassurance to family about absence of malignancy
• Patient may require thyroid medication for life, if ectopic, midline thyroid mistakenly removed

MEDICATIONS

DRUG(S) OF CHOICE None. All thyroglossal duct cysts should be surgically removed.
Contraindications: N/A
Precautions: N/A
Significant possible interactions: N/A

ALTERNATIVE DRUGS N/A

 FOLLOWUP

PATIENT MONITORING 1-2 weeks after drainage or resection

PREVENTION/AVOIDANCE N/A

POSSIBLE COMPLICATIONS Infection and malignant degeneration if not excised

EXPECTED COURSE AND PROGNOSIS Resolution with resection (less than 5% recurrence using the Sistrunk procedure)

 MISCELLANEOUS

ASSOCIATED CONDITIONS None

AGE-RELATED FACTORS
Pediatric: N/A
Geriatric: N/A
Others: N/A

PREGNANCY N/A

SYNONYMS N/A

ICD-9-CM 759.2

SEE ALSO N/A

OTHER NOTES N/A

ABBREVIATIONS N/A

REFERENCES Welch, K.J., Randolph, J.G., Ravitch, M.M., et al. (eds.): Pediatric Surgery, 4th Ed. New York, Year Book Medical Publishers, 1986

Author J. Miller, M.D. & T. Black, M.D.

Thyroid malignant neoplasia

 BASICS

DESCRIPTION Autologous growth of
thyroid nodules with potential for metastases
• Papillary carcinoma - most common variety, 60-70% of thyroid tumors. May be associated with radiation exposure. Tumor contains psammoma bodies. Metastasizes by lymphatic route.
• Follicular carcinoma - 10-20% of thyroid tumors. The incidence has been decreasing since the addition of dietary iodine. It occurs usually in females over 40 years of age. Metastasizes by the hematogenous route.
• Hürthle cell carcinoma - usually in patients over 60 years of age. Radioresistant. Composed of distinct large eosinophilic cells with abundant cytoplasmic mitochondria.
• Medullary carcinoma - arises from parafollicular cells, C-cells. 2-5% of all thyroid tumors. Associated with multiple endocrine neoplasia (MEN) syndromes which can be familial or sporadic. Calcitonin is a chemical marker.
• Anaplastic carcinoma - 3% of thyroid tumors, usually in patients over 60 years of age
• Other - lymphoma, sarcoma, or metastatic (renal, breast or lung)
System(s) affected: Endocrine/Metabolic
Genetics:
• Medullary - autosomal dominant with MEN syndrome
• Others - none known
Incidence in USA: 0.0051/100,000 (10,500 new cases per year)
Prevalence in USA: Unknown
Predominant age: Usually over 40 years of age
Predominant sex: Female > Male (2.6:1)

SIGNS AND SYMPTOMS
• Painless hard, fixed neck mass (in advanced cases; otherwise soft to hard masses)
• Hoarseness
• Dysphagia
• Cervical lymphadenopathy
• Dyspnea

CAUSES Unknown

RISK FACTORS
• Neck irradiation (6-2000 rads) - papillary carcinoma
• Iodine deficiency - follicular carcinoma
• MEN syndrome - medullary carcinoma
• Previous history of less than a total thyroidectomy for malignancy - anaplastic carcinoma

 DIAGNOSIS

DIFFERENTIAL DIAGNOSIS
• Multinodular goiter
• Thyroid adenoma
• Thyroglossal duct cyst
• Thyroiditis
• Thyroid cyst
• Ectopic thyroid

LABORATORY Thyroid function tests
usually normal
Drugs that may alter lab results: N/A
Disorders that may alter lab results: N/A

PATHOLOGICAL FINDINGS
• Papillary - psammoma bodies, anaplastic epithelial papillae
• Follicular - anaplastic epithelial cords with follicles
• Hürthle cell - large eosinophilic cells with granular cytoplasm
• Medullary - large amounts of amyloid stroma
• Anaplastic - small cell and giant cell undifferentiated tumors

SPECIAL TESTS
• Medullary carcinoma - calcitonin level (normal is less than 300 pg/mL)
• Thyroglobulin level - post operative tumor marker
• DNA content of tumors from biopsy specimen. Diploid content has a better prognosis.

IMAGING
• Thyroid scan - cold nodules are more suspicious of malignancy
• Ultrasound - solid mass is more suspicious of malignancy
• CT and MRI can be useful to evaluate large substernal masses

DIAGNOSTIC PROCEDURES
• Fine needle aspiration
• Surgical biopsy
• Laryngoscopy, if vocal cord paralysis is suspected

 TREATMENT

APPROPRIATE HEALTH CARE
Inpatient

GENERAL MEASURES
• Papillary carcinoma - lobectomy with isthmectomy or total thyroidectomy, and removal of suspicious lymph nodes
• Follicular carcinoma and Hurthle cell - total thyroidectomy and removal of suspicious lymph nodes
• Medullary carcinoma - total thyroidectomy with central node dissection. Unilateral or bilateral modified radical neck dissection if lateral nodes are histologically positive.
• Anaplastic carcinoma - aggressive en bloc thyroidectomy. Often times tracheostomy required.

ACTIVITY As tolerated

DIET Avoid iodine deficiency

PATIENT EDUCATION
National Cancer Institute
Building 31, Room 101-18
9000 Rockville Pike
Bethesda, MD 20892
(301)496-5583

MEDICATIONS

DRUG(S) OF CHOICE Post operatively will require thyroid replacement to suppress serum TSH level: Levothyroxine (T4) (Synthroid) 100-200 mcg/day or liothyronine (T3) (Cytomel) 50-100 mcg/day
Contraindications: N/A
Precautions: N/A
Significant possible interactions:
- Amphetamines
- Anticoagulants
- Tricyclic antidepressants
- Antidiabetic medications
- Aspirin
- Barbiturates
- Beta adrenergic blockers
- Cholestyramine
- Colestipol
- Oral contraceptives
- Digitalis preparation
- Ephedrine
- Estrogens
- Methylphenidate
- Phenytoin

ALTERNATIVE DRUGS N/A

FOLLOWUP

PATIENT MONITORING
- Thyroid scan at 6 weeks and administration of I131 for any visible uptake
- At 6 months and then yearly the patient should have a thyroid scan and chest x-ray
- Papillary and follicular - a thyroglobulin level should be done yearly
- Medullary - calcitonin level should be done yearly
- The thyroid scan and thyroglobulin level should be done with the patient in the hypothyroid state induced by 6 week withdrawal of levothyroxine or 2-3 week withdrawal of liothyronine

PREVENTION/AVOIDANCE
- Physical exam in high risk group
- Calcium infusion or pentagastrin stimulation test in high risk MEN patients

POSSIBLE COMPLICATIONS
Recurrence of tumor

EXPECTED COURSE AND PROGNOSIS
- Papillary carcinoma - overall mortality 3-8%
- Follicular carcinoma - overall 80% 5 year survival rate, 77% 10 year survival rate. Histologically microinvasive tumors parallel papillary tumor results while grossly invasive tumors do far worse.
- Hürthle cell carcinoma - 93% 5 year survival rate, and 83% survival rate overall. Grossly invasive tumors - survival is less than 25%.
- Medullary carcinoma - negative nodes 90% 5 year survival rate and 85% 10 year survival rate; with positive nodes 65% 5 year survival rate and 40% 10 year survival rate
- Anaplastic carcinoma - survival unexpected

MISCELLANEOUS

ASSOCIATED CONDITIONS Medullary carcinoma - pheochromocytoma, hyperparathyroidism, ganglioneuroma of the GI tract, neuromata of mucosal membranes

AGE-RELATED FACTORS
Pediatric: Over 60% of thyroid nodules are malignant
Geriatric: Risk of malignancy increases over age 60
Others: N/A

PREGNANCY N/A

SYNONYMS
- Follicular carcinoma of the thyroid
- Papillary carcinoma of the thyroid
- Hürthle cell carcinoma of the thyroid
- Anaplastic cell carcinoma of the thyroid

ICD-9-CM
- Primary 193
- Metastatic 198.89

SEE ALSO N/A

OTHER NOTES N/A

ABBREVIATIONS MEN = multiple endocrine neoplasia

REFERENCES
- Bell, R.M.: Thyroid carcinoma. Surg Clin North Am. 66:13, 1986
- Lennquist, S.: The Thyroid Nodule, Surg Clin North Am. 66:213-232, 1987

Author J. Miller, M.D. & T. Black, M.D.

Thyroiditis

BASICS

DESCRIPTION A variety of inflammatory thyroid disorders that can cause thyroid enlargement and thyroid atrophy. May lead to hypothyroidism or hyperthyroidism. Complete resolution can occur.
- Lymphocytic thyroiditis - the most common form, an autoimmune disease, often presenting as an asymptomatic diffuse goiter. Often first detected after thyroid atrophy and hypothyroidism have occurred and occasionally as hyperthyroidism (Hashimoto's thyroiditis).
- Granulomatous thyroiditis - probably related to viral infection and usually presenting with thyroid pain (which may be severe), involving one or both thyroid lobes, accompanied by hyperthyroidism, going through a phase of mild hypothyroidism and then to permanent resolution to normal
- "Silent" thyroiditis - one form is characterized by spontaneously resolving hypothyroidism and/or hyperthyroidism often associated with pregnancy. Another form has the characteristics of .granulomatous thyroiditis without the pain.
- Rare forms of thyroiditis - suppurative, due to bacterial infection and radiation due to ingested radionuclides or external irradiation
System(s) affected: Endocrine/Metabolic
Genetics: N/A
Incidence/Prevalence in USA:
- Not known definitively
- Lymphocytic thyroiditis increases with age, probably up to 10% over age 65
- Granulomatous thyroiditis much less common, has an epidemic pattern
Predominant age: All ages, postpuberty
Predominant sex: Female > Male

SIGNS AND SYMPTOMS
Lymphocytic thyroiditis
  ◊ Insidious onset of goiter, often detected incidentally
  ◊ Slow onset of hypothyroidism
  ◊ Association with other autoimmune diseases
Granulomatous thyroiditis
  ◊ Pain, tenderness and enlargement of one or both thyroid lobes
  ◊ Malaise, fever
  ◊ Mild to moderate symptoms of hyperthyroidism
  ◊ History of recent respiratory infection

CAUSES
Lymphocytic thyroiditis
  ◊ Autoimmune response of thyroid tissue
  ◊ Genetic susceptibility
Granulomatous thyroiditis
  ◊ Chronic inflammatory response of thyroid tissue
  ◊ Preceding infection with any of a variety of viruses

RISK FACTORS
Lymphocytic thyroiditis
  ◊ Positive family history of thyroid disease
  ◊ Preceding autoimmune diseases including type I diabetes, primary adrenal insufficiency, rheumatoid arthritis, pregnancy/delivery
Granulomatous thyroiditis
  ◊ Recent viral respiratory infection
  ◊ Other known cases in the community

DIAGNOSIS

DIFFERENTIAL DIAGNOSIS
Lymphocytic thyroiditis
  ◊ Simple goiter
  ◊ Iodine-deficient goiter (especially in endemic areas)
  ◊ Early Graves' disease
  ◊ Lithium induced goiter
Granulomatous thyroiditis
  ◊ Infections of oropharynx and trachea
  ◊ Hemorrhage into a thyroid cyst
  ◊ Subacute systemic illness
  ◊ Suppurative thyroiditis

LABORATORY
Lymphocytic thyroiditis
  ◊ Elevated anti-thyroid antibodies (especially high titers of anti-microsomal anti-TP) antibodies)
  ◊ Free thyroxine index (FTI, normal 4.5-12) less than 5 with TSH greater than 5 mcg/dl (normal 0.5-5 mcg/dl)
  ◊ Thyroid radioactive iodine uptake (RAIU) variable with scintiscan showing patchy distribution of radioiodine
  ◊ Positive cytopathology of fine needle aspirate or positive formal biopsy
Granulomatous thyroiditis
  ◊ Elevated erythrocyte sedimentation rate
  ◊ Normal or moderately elevated WBC without a granulocyte shift to band forms
  ◊ FTI greater than 12, TSH undetectable, RAIU less than 5% in 24 hours (often nil) early in course. FTI less than 4.5 with RAIU above normal (greater than 35% in 24 hours in USA) late in course
Drugs that may alter lab results:
- Thyroid
- Corticosteroids
- Iodine containing drugs and contrast media
- Lithium
Disorders that may alter lab results:
- Iodine-deficiency
- Non-thyroidal illness

PATHOLOGICAL FINDINGS
Lymphocytic thyroiditis
  ◊ Lymphocytic infiltration
  ◊ Oxyphilic changes in follicular cells
  ◊ Fibrosis
  ◊ Atrophy
Granulomatous thyroiditis
  ◊ Giant cells
  ◊ Mononuclear cell infiltrate

SPECIAL TESTS
- Radioimmunoassays
- Anti-thyroid antibody titers
- Complete blood count with differential count
- Erythrocyte sedimentation rate

IMAGING
- Thyroid radioiodine uptake and scan in granulomatous thyroiditis
- Ultrasonography if hemorrhage into thyroid cyst suspected

DIAGNOSTIC PROCEDURES Needle biopsy in confusing cases

TREATMENT

APPROPRIATE HEALTH CARE
Outpatient

GENERAL MEASURES No special measures

ACTIVITY Fully active

DIET No special diet

PATIENT EDUCATION N/A

MEDICATIONS

DRUG(S) OF CHOICE
• Lymphocytic thyroiditis: Levothyroxine if hypothyroid or goitrous. Begin with 25 or 50 mcg/day and titrate to TSH suppression to lower limit of assay normal range. Propylthiouracil and propranolol if thyrotoxic and symptomatic.
• Granulomatous thyroiditis: Analgesics/codeine for pain. Propranolol 40 mg q6h for symptomatic hyperthyroidism. Levothyroxine 100 mcg per 100 lbs body wt/day if hypothyroid phase is symptomatic. Prednisone once daily in lowest effective dose for severe symptoms.
• Maintenance: Optimal dose can be established by measuring TSH at 6-8 week intervals until dosage level causes TSH to be at the lower level of normal for the assay used

Contraindications:
• Propylthiouracil - allergy or hypersensitivity to analgesics/narcotics
• Propranolol - insulin therapy, asthma
• Prednisone - adverse reactions
• Levothyroxine - none

Precautions: Reduce doses of corticosteroids, propranolol and narcotics as soon as feasible

Significant possible interactions: None unique to this condition. Refer to manufacturer's profile of each drug.

ALTERNATIVE DRUGS
Methimazole for propylthiouracil

FOLLOWUP

PATIENT MONITORING
• Repeat thyroid function tests every 3-12 months in lymphocytic thyroiditis
• Repeat thyroid function tests every 3-6 weeks in granulomatous thyroiditis until permanently euthyroid

PREVENTION/AVOIDANCE N/A

POSSIBLE COMPLICATIONS
Treatment induced hypothyroidism or hyperthyroidism

EXPECTED COURSE AND PROGNOSIS
• Lymphocytic thyroiditis - persistent goiter, eventual thyroid failure
• Granulomatous thyroiditis - eventual return to normal over weeks or months

MISCELLANEOUS

ASSOCIATED CONDITIONS
Other autoimmune diseases with lymphocytic thyroiditis including type I diabetes, primary adrenal insufficiency, premature ovarian failure

AGE-RELATED FACTORS
Pediatric: N/A
Geriatric: Remission of granulomatous thyroiditis may be slower in the elderly
Others: N/A

PREGNANCY
• Avoid radio-isotope scanning
• Avoid hypothyroidism
• Minimize use of antithyroid drugs

SYNONYMS
• Lymphocytic thyroiditis
• Granulomatous thyroiditis
• Silent thyroiditis
• Hashimoto's disease

ICD-9-CM 245

SEE ALSO N/A

OTHER NOTES N/A

ABBREVIATIONS
• RAIU = radioactive iodine uptake
• FTI = free thyroxine index
• TSH = thyroid stimulating hormone

REFERENCES
• Degroot, L.J. (ed.): Endocrinology. 2nd Ed. Philadelphia, W.B. Saunders Co., 1989
• Bardin, C.W. (ed.): Current Therapy In Endocrinology and Metabolism, 4th Ed. Philadelphia, B.C. Decker, 1991

Author R. Levy, M.D.

Tinea capitis

 BASICS

DESCRIPTION
A fungal infection of the scalp often called "ringworm". The infection results from contact with infected persons or animals. It is contagious and may become epidemic. Affected areas of the scalp can show characteristic black dots resulting from broken hairs.

System affected: Skin

Genetics: N/A

Incidence/Prevalence in USA: Although still common the incidence and prevalence have been rapidly dropping over the past 30 years

Predominant age: Children particularly ages 3 to 9. Adult infection is rare.

Predominant sex: Male = Female

SIGNS AND SYMPTOMS
• Infection commonly begins with round patches of scale or alopecia
• These patches can become multiple and show the characteristic black dot pattern of broken hairs. Less frequently, infection will take on the patterns of chronic scaling with little inflammation or marked inflammation and alopecia. Extreme inflammation results in kerion, a nodular exudative pustule.

CAUSES
• 90% Trichophyton tonsurans
• 10% Microsporum species (canis, audouini, gypseum)

RISK FACTORS
• Day-care centers or schools
• Living in confined quarters
• Poor hygiene
• Immunosuppression

 DIAGNOSIS

DIFFERENTIAL DIAGNOSIS
• Psoriasis and seborrhea dermatitis are most often confused with tinea capitis
• Pyoderma
• Alopecia areata and trichotillomania

LABORATORY
• Microscopy of a KOH preparation of hairs from affected area can show arthrospores that appear within hair shafts
• Fungal culture of hairs from affected areas allows the infection to be confirmed and the causative organism to be identified

Drugs that may alter lab results: N/A

Disorders that may alter lab results: N/A

PATHOLOGICAL FINDINGS
• Chronic inflammation
• Superficial infection producing lesions with follicular pustules, abscess
• Hyphae in follicles, keratin of skin

SPECIAL TESTS
Viewed under a Wood's lamp, the 10% of infections caused by Microsporum species will fluoresce a light green. 90% of tinea capitis infections, those caused by Trichophyton, will NOT fluoresce.

IMAGING N/A

DIAGNOSTIC PROCEDURES N/A

 Treatment

APPROPRIATE HEALTH CARE
Outpatient

GENERAL MEASURES
• Careful hand washing
• Launder towels, clothing, head wear of infected individual
• Check other family members

ACTIVITY No restrictions

DIET
No special diet except persons treated with Griseofulvin should not be on a restricted fat diet

PATIENT EDUCATION See General Measures

MEDICATIONS

DRUG(S) OF CHOICE
Griseofulvin- preferred treatment
◊ Microsized preparation
◊ Available in 125 mg, 250 mg and 500 mg tablets and 125 mg/5 mL suspension
◊ Dose at 10 mg/kg/day taken bid or as single daily dose
Ketoconazole - alternative treatment for cases that do not respond to Griseofulvin
◊ Available in 200 mg tablets
◊ Dose 3.3 - 6.6 mg/kg/day up to 200 mg per day
• Treat with oral medication for 6 to 8 weeks
• Selenium sulfide (2.5%) shampoo used concurrently will reduce spore shedding
Contraindications:
• Known hypersensitivity to the medications.
• Griseofulvin contraindicated in patients with porphyria due to hepatotoxicity
Precautions:
Griseofulvin
◊ Headache in up to 10% of patients initially but generally resolves after first week of treatment
◊ Abdominal bloating, dyspepsia, and diarrhea also common
◊ Hypersensitivity and liver toxicity rare. The manufacturer recommends monitoring liver functions while on Griseofulvin but due to rarity of hepatotoxicity many physicians choose to forgo any testing.
Ketoconazole
◊ Hepatotoxicity is common with 10% of exposed patients experiencing elevations in liver enzymes. 1 in 10,000 develops severe hepatotoxicity and rarely death. Monitor liver functions if course of therapy exceeds 14 days.
Significant possible interactions:
• Griseofulvin accentuates the effect of alcohol and increases the metabolism of warfarin and oral contraceptives.
• Ketoconazole requires an acid gastric pH so antacids and H2 blockers will decrease absorption
• Concomitant use of terfenadine (Seldane) or astemizole (Hismanal) with ketoconazole can cause ventricular tachycardia

ALTERNATIVE DRUGS   N/A

FOLLOWUP

PATIENT MONITORING   Recheck after two weeks of therapy to document improvement and after the 6 week course of therapy. Patients might need liver function monitoring - see medication precautions.

PREVENTION/AVOIDANCE
• Good personal hygiene
• Don't share head wear
• Identification and treatment of infected individuals and household pets

POSSIBLE COMPLICATIONS
Permanent scarring and hair loss from kerion

EXPECTED COURSE AND PROGNOSIS   Without treatment lesions will usually spontaneously heal in 6 months. Lesions with marked inflammation will spontaneously resolve much more rapidly but are more likely to leave scarring.

MISCELLANEOUS

ASSOCIATED CONDITIONS   N/A

AGE-RELATED FACTORS
Pediatric: Highest incidence in this age group
Geriatric: N/A
Others: N/A

PREGNANCY   Oral antifungals are contraindicated in pregnancy

SYNONYMS
• Ringworm, scalp

ICD-9-CM   110.0 dermatophytosis of scalp and beard

SEE ALSO   N/A

OTHER NOTES   N/A

ABBREVIATIONS   N/A

REFERENCES
• Rook, A. & Dawber, R. (eds): Diseases of the Hair and Scalp. St Louis, Mosby-Year Book, 1991
• Habif, T.P.: Clinical Dermatology. 2nd Ed. St. Louis, Mosby Company, 1990
• Bergus, G.R. & Johnson, J.S.: Superficial fungal infections. Am Family Physician, in press, 1993

AUTHOR   G. Bergus, M.D.

Tinea corporis

 BASICS

DESCRIPTION Scaling plaque characterized by a sharply defined annular pattern with peripheral activity and central clearing. Papules and occasionally pustules/vesicles present at border, and less commonly in center. Affects face, trunk, and extremities.
• Zoophilic infections (found in children and adults) are acquired from animals
• Anthropophilic infections (found only in adults) acquired from personal contact or fomites
System(s) affected: Skin/Exocrine
Genetics: There is evidence for genetic susceptibility in some people
Incidence in USA: Fairly common
Prevalence in USA: Fairly common
Predominant age: All ages
Predominant sex: Male = Female

SIGNS AND SYMPTOMS
• Characteristic rash and mild pruritus
• Scaling plaques that are circular, bright red, sharply marginated, occur singly or in groups of 3-4
• Each plaque is less than 5 cm in diameter
• Plaques are solid, but annular forms occur
• Patient may experience intense itching

CAUSES Fungal infection due to dermatophyte, e.g., Trichophyton rubrum

RISK FACTORS
• Warm climates
• Direct contact with an active lesion on a human, an animal, or rarely from soil
• Working with animals
• Immunosuppression including prolonged use of topical steroids

 DIAGNOSIS

DIFFERENTIAL DIAGNOSIS
• Pityriasis rosea
• Eczema
• Contact dermatitis
• Syphilis
• Psoriasis
• Subacute lupus erythematosus
• Elastosis perforans serpiginosa
• Erythema annulare
• Gyrate erythemas, especially centrifugium

LABORATORY Potassium hydroxide preparation of skin scrapings. Fungal culture may be obtained, but is not generally necessary.
Drugs that may alter lab results: N/A
Disorders that may alter lab results: N/A

PATHOLOGICAL FINDINGS Branching hyphae with septa on potassium hydroxide preparation

SPECIAL TESTS Tinea corpora does not fluoresce with Wood's light

IMAGING N/A

DIAGNOSTIC PROCEDURES
Skin scraping:
◊ Use No.15 blade and place several small scrapings of the active border on glass slide with coverslip
◊ Apply 10-20% potassium hydroxide and heat gently without boiling
◊ Let stand for 5 minutes and examine for septate, branching hyphae. Use lowered condenser and dim light to enhance contrast. Hyphae may be accentuated with a commercial fungal stain or a drop of blue ink.

 TREATMENT

APPROPRIATE HEALTH CARE
Outpatient

GENERAL MEASURES Proper hygiene

ACTIVITY Full activity

DIET Unrestricted diet

PATIENT EDUCATION Avoid contact with suspected lesions. Be careful with animal contacts.

MEDICATIONS

DRUG(S) OF CHOICE
• Topical antifungal creams - miconazole (Monistat-Derm) or clotrimazole (Lotrimin, Mycelex) applied bid for 2 weeks. Also ketoconazole (Nizoral) applied qd for 2 weeks. To prevent relapse should use for one week after resolution. Also econazole (Spectazole and allylamines (Naftin, Lamisil)
• For resistant, extensive and/or invasive infections, oral agents are recommended for 4 weeks. Oral ultramicrosize griseofulvin (e.g., Gris-PEG) 7 mg/kg/day in children over 2 years; 375 mg/day in adults. Oral itraconazole (in lieu of ketaconazole - less toxic and less drug side effects)..

Contraindications: Known hypersensitivity to agent

Precautions: Ketoconazole contains a sulfite and should be avoided in sulfite sensitive people. There is a 1:10,000 reported incidence of hepatotoxicity with oral ketoconazole. Baseline liver function tests should be obtained prior to initiating oral ketoconazole and patients should be followed closely.

Significant possible interactions: Griseofulvin induces hepatic enzymes that metabolize warfarin and other drugs. H2 blockers and antacids reduce ketoconazole absorption. Ketoconazole is an enzyme inhibitor and may cause drug toxicity (case report of apparent terfenadine toxicity causing ventricular arrhythmia). Ketoconazole also significantly increases cyclosporine levels.

ALTERNATIVE DRUGS N/A

FOLLOWUP

PATIENT MONITORING Necessary for invasive disease or prolonged treatment with oral ketoconazole

PREVENTION/AVOIDANCE Avoid contact with suspicious lesions

POSSIBLE COMPLICATIONS
• Bacterial super-infection
• Generalized, invasive dermatophyte infection

EXPECTED COURSE AND PROGNOSIS Resolution without sequelae in 1-2 weeks of therapy

MISCELLANEOUS

ASSOCIATED CONDITIONS Other tineas - pedis, cruris, capitis, barbae, and manus

AGE-RELATED FACTORS
Pediatric: N/A
Geriatric: N/A
Others: N/A

PREGNANCY N/A

SYNONYMS Ringworm

ICD-9-CM 110.5

SEE ALSO
• Tinea capitis
• Tinea cruris
• Tinea pedis

OTHER NOTES N/A

ABBREVIATIONS N/A

REFERENCES
• Habif, T.: Clinical Dermatology. 2nd Ed. St. Louis, C.V. Mosby, 1990
• Fitzpatrick, T.B. et al.: Color Atlas and Synopsis of Clinical Dermatology. New York, McGraw-Hill, 1983

Author W. Williams, M.D.

Tinea cruris

BASICS

DESCRIPTION A superficial fungal infection of the groin area caused by a group of fungi known as dermatophytes, also called ringworm fungi. These dermatophyte infections may result from three genera of fungi: Microsporum, Trichophyton, and Epidermophyton.
• Tinea cruris is characterized by development of well marginated erythematous half-moon shaped plaques in the crural folds which spread to the upper thighs. The advancing border is well-defined often with fine scaling and sometimes includes vesicular eruptions. The skin within the border often heals to a red-brown with occasional red papules. The lesions are usually bilateral and do not include the scrotum or penis, but may migrate to the buttock and gluteal cleft area.
System(s) affected: Skin/Exocrine
Genetics: N/A
Incidence/Prevalence in USA: Common
Predominant age: Any age (rare prior to puberty)
Predominant sex: Males > Females

SIGNS AND SYMPTOMS
• Lesions may be asymptomatic but more frequently are quite pruritic
• Acute inflammation may result from wearing occlusive clothing
• Chronic scratching may result in an eczematous appearance
• Previous application of topical steroids may alter the appearance causing a more extensive eruption with irregular borders and erythematous papules. This modified form is called tinea incognito.

CAUSES
• Trichophyton rubrum
• Trichophyton interdigitale
• Trichophyton verrucosum
• Trichophyton tonsurans
• Trichophyton mentagrophytes
• Epidermophyton floccosum
• Microsporum canis

RISK FACTORS
• Summer months and/or increased sweating
• Wearing wet clothing
• Wearing multiple layers of clothing
• Depression of cell mediated immune response (atopic individuals, AIDS, etc.)
• Obesity

DIAGNOSIS

DIFFERENTIAL DIAGNOSIS
• Intertrigo - inflammatory process of moist opposed skin folds, often including infection with bacteria, yeast, and fungi. Painful longitudinal fissures occur in the creases of skin folds.
• Erythrasma - diffuse brown scaly noninflammatory plaque with irregular border often involving the groin. Caused by bacterial infection with Corynebacterium minutissimum. Fluoresces coral-red with Wood's lamp.
• Seborrheic dermatitis of the groin
• Psoriasis of the groin
• Candidiasis of the groin

LABORATORY
• Fungal culture using Sabouraud's dextrose agar or dermatophyte test medium (DTM)
• Potassium hydroxide preparation of skin scrapings from the dermatophyte leading border shows translucent branching, rod-shaped hyphae
Drugs that may alter lab results:
• Partial treatment with antifungal preparations
• Topical steroid treatment may confuse diagnosis by causing tinea incognito
Disorders that may alter lab results:
Pruritis with extensive itching

PATHOLOGICAL FINDINGS Skin biopsy showing fungal hyphae in the epidermis

SPECIAL TESTS Wood's lamp exam reveals no fluorescence

IMAGING N/A

DIAGNOSTIC PROCEDURES Potassium hydroxide, KOH preparation of skin scrapings form leading border

TREATMENT

APPROPRIATE HEALTH CARE
Outpatient

GENERAL MEASURES
• Avoid predisposing conditions, keep area as dry as possible
• Topical steroid preparations should not be used

ACTIVITY Full activity

DIET No restrictions

PATIENT EDUCATION Explanation of the causative agents, predisposing factors, and prevention measures

MEDICATIONS

DRUG(S) OF CHOICE
• Topical antifungals including - naftifine, oxyconazole, clotrimazole (Lotrimin, Mycelex), ciclopirox (Loprox), econazole (Spectazole), haloprogin (Halotex), tolnaftate (Tinactin), miconazole (Monistat-Derm, Micatin) and undecylenic acid (Desenex). These should be applied twice daily for 10-14 days.
• If agents listed above are unsuccessful, a 10 day course of topical ketoconazole (Nizoral) applied once a day may be tried
• Absorbent powders may help to avoid excess moisture
Contraindications: Refer to manufacturer's literature
Precautions: Must continue therapy for at least 10 days even if symptoms resolve earlier
Significant possible interactions: N/A

ALTERNATIVE DRUGS
Oral antifungal agents are effective, but not indicated in uncomplicated tinea cruris. If there is no response to topical therapy, or there is significant irritation, then griseofulvin (ultramicrosize) 500 mg daily with food for 3-4 weeks, or ketoconazole 200 mg qd for 2-3 months may be used.

FOLLOWUP

PATIENT MONITORING
• Liver function testing prior to therapy and at regular intervals during the course of therapy for those patients requiring oral ketoconazole
• Monitor CBC, renal, and hepatic function of patients on griseofulvin.

PREVENTION/AVOIDANCE
Avoidance of risk factors

POSSIBLE COMPLICATIONS
Secondary bacterial infection

EXPECTED COURSE AND PROGNOSIS
Excellent prognosis for cure with therapy

MISCELLANEOUS

ASSOCIATED CONDITIONS
None

AGE-RELATED FACTORS
Pediatric: Rare in pediatric population prior to puberty
Geriatric: More common due to increase in risk factors
Others: N/A

PREGNANCY
Rare

SYNONYMS
• Jock itch
• Ring worm

ICD-9-CM
110.3

SEE ALSO
N/A

OTHER NOTES
N/A

ABBREVIATIONS
N/A

REFERENCES
• Fitzpatrick, Thomas B., et al.: Color Atlas and Synopsis of Clinical Dermatology. New York, McGraw-Hill, Inc., 1992
• Habif, T.P.: Clinical Dermatology. St. Louis, C.V. Mosby Co., 1985
• Lynch, P.J.: Dermatology for the House Officer. 2nd Ed. Baltimore, Williams & Wilkins, 1987

Author M. Boespflug, M.D.

Tinea pedis

BASICS

DESCRIPTION Tinea pedis is a superficial infection of the feet caused by dermatophytes
System(s) affected: Skin/Exocrine
Genetics: No known genetic pattern
Incidence/Prevalence in USA: Extremely common
Predominant age: All ages, but most common in teens and young adults
Predominant sex: Male = Female

SIGNS AND SYMPTOMS
• Itching
• Scaling
• Maceration
• Vesicles/bullae
• Primarily in interdigital spaces
• May also involve sole and arch

CAUSES
• Trichophyton mentagrophytes
• Trichophyton rubrum
• Epidermophyton floccosum

RISK FACTORS
• Hot, humid weather
• Occlusive footwear
• Immunosuppressed patients
• Prolonged application of topical steroids

DIAGNOSIS

DIFFERENTIAL DIAGNOSIS
• Interdigital psoriasis
• Intertrigo
• Hyperkeratosis
• Contact dermatitis
• Eczema
• Dyshidrosis

LABORATORY
• Direct microscopic examination (KOH)
• Culture
Drugs that may alter lab results: N/A
Disorders that may alter lab results: N/A

PATHOLOGICAL FINDINGS
• Septate and branched mycelia on KOH
• Culture - dermatophyte

SPECIAL TESTS N/A

IMAGING N/A

DIAGNOSTIC PROCEDURES Culture

TREATMENT

APPROPRIATE HEALTH CARE
Outpatient

GENERAL MEASURES
• Treatment is generally with topical medications
• After soaking or bathing, patient should carefully remove or debride dead or thickened tissues

ACTIVITY Avoid sweating feet

DIET No restrictions

PATIENT EDUCATION See Prevention/Avoidance

MEDICATIONS

DRUG(S) OF CHOICE
• Acute vesicular stage - Burow's wet dressings, followed by clotrimazole 1%
• Subacute (maceration, scaling) - clotrimazole cream or lotion bid for 4 weeks. Use antifungal powders between the toes and in the shoes.
• Chronic - same as treatment of subacute. Griseofulvin 500 mg orally bid for 3-6 months.

Contraindications:
• Clotrimazole - do not use in any individual who has shown hypersensitivity to any of drugs' components
• Griseofulvin - patients with porphyria, hepatocellular failure, and in patients with a history of hypersensitivity to griseofulvin

Precautions:
• Clotrimazole - if irritation or sensitivity develop, treatment should be discontinued
• Griseofulvin - periodic monitoring of organ system functioning, including renal, hepatic, and hematopoietic. Possible photosensitivity reactions. Lupus erythematosus, lupus-like syndromes, or exacerbation of existing lupus erythematosus have been reported.

Significant possible interactions:
• Clotrimazole - none
• Griseofulvin - decreases the activity of warfarin-type anticoagulants. Barbiturates usually depress griseofulvin activity. The effect of alcohol may be potentiated, producing such effects as tachycardia and flush.

ALTERNATIVE DRUGS
• Topicals - imidazole, ketoconazole, sulconazole, miconazole, econazole, oxiconazole
• Allylamine topicals - naftifine, terbinafine
• Ketoconazole 200 mg daily by mouth, for griseofulvin-resistant dermatophytosis. (Hepatotoxicity has been reported from its use. There is also a risk of cardiovascular events for patients taking terfenadine (Seldane) or astemizole (Hismanal) concomitantly with ketoconazole). Itraconazole is an alternative.

FOLLOWUP

PATIENT MONITORING As needed

PREVENTION/AVOIDANCE
• Good personal hygiene
• Wearing rubber or wooden sandals in community showers or bathing places
• Careful drying between the toes after showering or bathing
• Changing socks frequently
• Applying drying or dusting powder

POSSIBLE COMPLICATIONS
• Secondary bacterial infections
• Eczematoid changes

EXPECTED COURSE AND PROGNOSIS Control, but not completely cured. Symptoms continue indefinitely with periods of relative quiescence.

MISCELLANEOUS

ASSOCIATED CONDITIONS
Hyperhidrosis

AGE-RELATED FACTORS
Pediatric: Rare in younger children (common in teens)
Geriatric: Elderly are more susceptible to outbreaks because of changes in the distal tissues resulting from peripheral vascular disease and the aging process
Others: N/A

PREGNANCY N/A

SYNONYMS Athlete's foot

ICD-9-CM 110.4

SEE ALSO
• Dyshidrosis
• Dermatitis, contact

OTHER NOTES N/A

ABBREVIATIONS N/A

REFERENCES Fitzpatrick, T.B. et al.: Color Atlas and Synopsis of Clinical Dermatology. New York, McGraw-Hill, 1989

Author R. Daigneault, M.D.

Tinea versicolor

 BASICS

DESCRIPTION Multiple patches on skin, generally asymptomatic. Ranges in color, usually white to brown. In Blacks, lesions may be hyperpigmented.. Probably the most common superficial mycosis.
System(s) affected: Skin/Exocrine
Genetics: No known genetic pattern
Incidence/Prevalence in USA: Common
Predominant age: Teenagers and young adults
Predominant sex: Male = Female

SIGNS AND SYMPTOMS
• Versicolor = various colors. Sun exposed areas - lesions usually white; on covered areas - they are often brown or red-brown.
• Distribution - (sebum-rich areas) chest, shoulders, back
• Appearance - sharply marginated 3 or 4 mm in diameter with centrifugal growth and coalescence
• Scale - fine, visible only with scraping
• Itching (rare)
• More prominent in summer
• Periodic recurrence

CAUSES
• Pityrosporon orbiculare (formerly Malassezia furfur)
• Variations in skin lipid formation

RISK FACTORS
• High heat
• High humidity
• Excessive sweating

 DIAGNOSIS

DIFFERENTIAL DIAGNOSIS Other skin diseases with white patches and plaques such as pityriasis alba, vitiligo, seborrheic dermatitis, nummular eczema

LABORATORY Routine lab not usually necessary
Drugs that may alter lab results: N/A
Disorders that may alter lab results: N/A

PATHOLOGICAL FINDINGS
• Short stubby fungal hyphae
• Y-shaped hyphae
• Small round spores in clusters on hyphae

SPECIAL TESTS KOH preparation to visualize budding yeast forms and club-shaped hyphae

IMAGING N/A

DIAGNOSTIC PROCEDURES Wood's lamp - golden fluorescence or pigment changes

 TREATMENT

APPROPRIATE HEALTH CARE
Outpatient

GENERAL MEASURES
• Apply prescribed medications to affected parts with cotton balls
• Repeat treatment each spring prior to tanning

ACTIVITY No restrictions

DIET No special diet

PATIENT EDUCATION For patient education materials favorably reviewed on this topic, contact: American Academy of Dermatology, 930 N. Meacham Rd., P.O. Box 4014, Schaumberg, IL 60168-4014, (708)330-0230

MEDICATIONS

DRUG(S) OF CHOICE
• Selenium sulfide shampoo (Excel and Selsun), allowed to dry for 40 minutes prior to showering daily for 1 week or allowed to remain on body for 12-24 hours before showering once a week for 4 weeks
or
• Clotrimazole topical (Lotrimin) bid for several weeks,
or
• Miconazole (Micatin, Monistat) bid for several weeks,
or
• Ketoconazole cream (Nizoral) bid for several weeks
Contraindications: Ketoconazole contraindicated in pregnancy
Precautions: N/A
Significant possible interactions: N/A

ALTERNATIVE DRUGS Oral ketoconazole (rarely needed and has significant adverse reactions) 400 mg/day x 2 days is as effective as longer courses

FOLLOWUP

PATIENT MONITORING Recheck each spring

PREVENTION/AVOIDANCE N/A

POSSIBLE COMPLICATIONS None expected

EXPECTED COURSE AND PROGNOSIS Recurs almost routinely

MISCELLANEOUS

ASSOCIATED CONDITIONS N/A

AGE-RELATED FACTORS
Pediatric: Usually occurs after puberty
Geriatric: Not common in this age group
Others: N/A

PREGNANCY N/A

SYNONYMS Pityriasis versicolor

ICD-9-CM 111.0

SEE ALSO N/A

OTHER NOTES
• Warn patients that whiteness will remain for several months after treatment
• Treat again each spring prior to tanning season

ABBREVIATIONS N/A

REFERENCES
• Lynch, P.J.: Dermatology for the House Officer. 2nd Ed. Baltimore, Williams & Wilkins, 1987
• Rausch, L.J., Jacobs, P.H.: Tinea versicolor: treatment and prophylaxis. Cutis 34:470, 1984

Author K. Reilly, M.D.

Torticollis

BASICS

DESCRIPTION Rotation and tilting of head caused by primary pathology of the neck muscles or secondary to head and neck disorders. The condition may be congenital or acquired.
System(s) affected: Musculoskeletal, Nervous
Genetics: No known genetic pattern
Incidence/Prevalence in USA: Uncommon
Predominant age:
• Congenital - newborn
• Acquired - under age 10, and adults 30-60
Predominant sex: Male = Female

SIGNS AND SYMPTOMS
• Rotation and tilting of the head to the affected side, chin rotates to the opposite side
• Intermittent painful spasms of sternomastoid, trapezius and other neck muscles
• With congenital form, the first sign may be a firm, nontender, palpable enlargement of the sternocleidomastoid muscle that is visible at birth
• An early sign in acquired form is stiffness of neck muscles

CAUSES
Congenital
 ◊ Injury to sternocleidomastoid muscle on one side at birth
 ◊ Possible malposition of head in utero
 ◊ Prenatal injury
 ◊ Fibroma
Acquired
 ◊ Muscular damage from inflammatory disease (myositis, lymphadenitis, tuberculosis)
 ◊ Cervical spine injuries that produce scar tissue contracture
 ◊ Ocular muscle palsy
 ◊ Organic CNS disorder causing rhythmic muscle spasms
 ◊ Psychogenic inability to control neck muscles
 ◊ Tumor
 ◊ Cervical spondylosis
 ◊ Trauma
 ◊ Medications

RISK FACTORS
• Traumatic delivery, including breech
• Psychiatric illness, neurosis, stress, hypochondriasis
• Medications - phenothiazines and butyrophenones
Acquired
 ◊ Inflammation
 ◊ Neurologic disorder
 ◊ Optical disorder
 ◊ Trauma

DIAGNOSIS

DIFFERENTIAL DIAGNOSIS
• Central nervous system infections
• Tumors of soft tissue or bone
• Basal ganglia disease
• Abscess of cervical glands
• Myositis of cervical muscles
• Cervical disk lesions

LABORATORY N/A
Drugs that may alter lab results: N/A
Disorders that may alter lab results: N/A

PATHOLOGICAL FINDINGS N/A

SPECIAL TESTS N/A

IMAGING X-ray (appearence may be subtle), CT or MRI of cervical spine to aid in differential diagnosis, especially for acquired cases

DIAGNOSTIC PROCEDURES Physical examination, history

TREATMENT

APPROPRIATE HEALTH CARE
Outpatient

GENERAL MEASURES
• Physical therapy
• Massage
• Local heat
• Analgesics
• Sensory biofeedback
• Congenital - operative division of involved muscle if physical therapy (i.e., passive stretching) is unsuccessful by one year of age
• Psychiatric treatment if there is an emotional disorder
Acquired
 ◊ If less than 1 week in duration - soft collar and rest
 ◊ If less than 1 month duration - traction

ACTIVITY No restrictions

DIET No special diet

PATIENT EDUCATION For congenital, training of parents to perform massage and range-of-motion exercises

Torticollis

MEDICATIONS

DRUG(S) OF CHOICE None indicated, other than analgesics for pain. If the torticollis has been drug induced, treatment can include diphenhydramine or diazepam.
Contraindications: N/A
Precautions: N/A
Significant possible interactions: N/A

ALTERNATIVE DRUGS N/A

FOLLOWUP

PATIENT MONITORING For support during physical therapy, biofeedback, or counseling

PREVENTION/AVOIDANCE No preventive measures known

POSSIBLE COMPLICATIONS
• Movement disorders
• Postural disorders
• May recur or persist throughout life
• Facial asymmetry in congenital

EXPECTED COURSE AND PROGNOSIS Good prognosis for correctable pathology

MISCELLANEOUS

ASSOCIATED CONDITIONS Difficult delivery

AGE-RELATED FACTORS
Pediatric: Congenital variety, associated with injury at time of birth that without treatment, becomes a fibrous cord
Geriatric: N/A
Others: N/A

PREGNANCY Associated with breech birth

SYNONYMS
• Spasmodic torticollis
• Wryneck

ICD-9-CM
• 333.83 spasmodic
• 754.1 congenital
• 300.11 hysterical

SEE ALSO N/A

OTHER NOTES Torticollis means "rotation", anterocollis means "tilting"

ABBREVIATIONS N/A

REFERENCE
• Tachdjian, M.: Pediatric Orthopedics. 2nd Ed. Philadelphia, W.B. Saunders Co., 1990
• Wenger, D.R. & Rang, M.: Art and Practice of Childrens Orthopedics. New York, Raven Press, 1992

Author F. Valencia, M.D.

Toxic shock syndrome

BASICS

DESCRIPTION An acute multisystem illness associated with Staphylococcus aureus infections and characterized by the sudden onset of high fever, peculiar skin rash with desquamation, and shock
• Menstrual toxic shock - associated with menstruation and tampon use
• Nonmenstrual toxic shock - more common than the menstrual form; associated with postoperative wounds, barrier contraception, etc. Can occur in children, men, and women.
Incidence/Prevalence in USA: 0.22 to 1.23 cases per 100,000
System(s) affected: Cardiovascular, Endocrine/Metabolic, Skin/Exocrine
Genetics: No specific mode of inheritance is recognized
Predominant age: All ages, but especially 30-60 years
Predominant sex: Female > Male (3:2)

SIGNS AND SYMPTOMS
Almost always present (> 80%)
◊ Temperature > 38.9°C
◊ Erythroderma
◊ Diffuse macular rash
◊ Skin desquamation a few days after rash appears
◊ Shock, orthostatic hypotension or syncope
◊ Nausea or vomiting
Commonly present (20-80%)
◊ Headache
◊ Confusion or agitation
◊ Adult respiratory distress syndrome
◊ Meningismus
◊ Pharyngeal erythema
◊ Vaginitis or vaginal discharge
◊ Conjunctivitis
◊ Periorbital edema
◊ Strawberry tongue
◊ Non-pitting edema
◊ Myalgia
◊ Oliguria
◊ Arthralgia
◊ Diarrhea
Rarely present (< 20%)
◊ Arthritis
◊ Lymphadenopathy
◊ Hepatosplenomegaly
◊ Cardiomyopathy
◊ Pericarditis
◊ Photophobia
◊ Seizure

CAUSES Staphylococcus aureus exotoxins, especially toxic shock syndrome toxin-1 (TSST-1), and staphylococcal enterotoxins A, B and C

RISK FACTORS
High
◊ Absence of antibody to TSS toxin-1
◊ Infection with Staphylococcus aureus which produces TSST-1
◊ Continuous use of super absorbency tampons during menstruation
◊ Nasal surgery with packing
Moderate
◊ Use of regular absorbency tampons during menstruation
◊ Use of contraceptive sponge
Low
◊ Alternating use of tampons and pads during menstruation
◊ Intrauterine contraceptive device
◊ Surgical wound infections
◊ Early postpartum state

DIAGNOSIS

DIFFERENTIAL DIAGNOSIS
• Streptococcal scarlet fever
• Toxic strep syndrome
• Drug reactions
• Rocky Mountain spotted fever
• Leptospirosis
• Kawasaki disease
• Staphylococcal scalded skin syndrome
• Meningococcal or possibly gram negative sepsis

LABORATORY
Microbiologic:
◊ Positive culture for Staphylococcus aureus from vagina or surgical wound (> 90%)
◊ Nasal or perineal carriage of Staphylococcus aureus
◊ Positive blood culture for Staphylococcus aureus (uncommon)
Hematologic: (50-90%)
◊ Granulocytosis with increased band forms
◊ Lymphopenia
◊ Normocytic, normochromic anemia
◊ Thrombocytopenia
◊ Coagulopathy
Biochemical: (50-90%)
◊ Hypoalbuminemia
◊ Abnormal electrolytes
◊ Hypocalcemia
◊ Hypomagnesemia
◊ Hypophosphatemia
◊ Increased SGOT
◊ Increased SGPT
◊ Increased CPK
◊ Increased BUN
◊ Increased serum creatinine
◊ Increased calcitonin
◊ Increased serum bilirubin
◊ Abnormal urine sediment
Drugs that may alter lab results: N/A
Disorders that may alter lab results: N/A

SPECIAL TESTS
• Absent serum antibodies to TSST-1
• Detection of TSST-1 in Staphylococcus aureus isolate

PATHOLOGICAL FINDINGS
• Subepidermic cleavage plane in the skin
• Minimal inflammatory reaction in tissues
• Lymphocyte depletion in lymph nodes
• Cervico-vaginal ulcerations

IMAGING No unusual or characteristic findings

DIAGNOSTIC PROCEDURES No specific diagnostic test is currently available

TREATMENT

APPROPRIATE HEALTH CARE
Inpatient, admission to intensive care for monitoring

GENERAL MEASURES
• Removal of tampon or other vaginal foreign bodies
• Surgical drainage of loculated infections
• Fluid resuscitation
• Management of renal or cardiac insufficiency
• Mechanical ventilation if necessary

ACTIVITY Bed rest throughout acute illness

DIET As tolerated

PATIENT EDUCATION Advise patient regarding possible sequelae or recurrence

MEDICATIONS

DRUG(S) OF CHOICE
Treatment of shock or hypotension
◊ Fluid replacement
◊ Dopamine
◊ Steroids or naloxone have not been proven to be of value
Eradication of Staphylococcus aureus
◊ Oxacillin or nafcillin 100 mg/kg/day every 6 hours
Contraindications: Penicillin allergy
Precautions:
• Rash, diarrhea, seizures
• Reduce oxacillin dosage in patients with severe renal failure. Not necessary to reduce nafcillin dose for renal dysfunction.
Significant possible interactions: See manufacturer's profile of each drug

ALTERNATIVE DRUGS
• Clindamycin 25 mg/kg/day every 8 hours for patients allergic to penicillin
• Vancomycin 30 mg per kg per day every 6 hours
• Toxin neutralization. Benefit in humans is unproven, but animal and in vitro studies support this approach.
◊ Intravenous immunoglobulin (IVIG) 0.4g/kg over 6 hours

 FOLLOWUP

PATIENT MONITORING
• Admit to intensive care if in shock
• Daily vital signs until patient is afebrile and normotensive

PREVENTION/AVOIDANCE
• Avoidance of continuous tampon use during menstruation
• Avoidance of super absorbency tampons
• Encourage frequent tampon changes during the day
• Use sanitary napkins at night
• Early medical attention to infected wounds

POSSIBLE COMPLICATIONS
Common (> 20%)
◊ Acute renal failure
◊ Adult respiratory distress syndrome
◊ Menorrhagia
◊ Alopecia
◊ Nail loss
Rare (< 20%)
◊ Disseminated intravascular coagulation
◊ Ataxia, toxic encephalopathy
◊ Memory impairment
◊ Cardiomyopathy
◊ Protracted malaise

EXPECTED COURSE AND PROGNOSIS
• Mortality 3-9%
• Recurrence 10-15%

MISCELLANEOUS

ASSOCIATED CONDITIONS
Staphylococcal infections

AGE-RELATED FACTORS
Pediatric: May occur as a complication of chickenpox
Geriatric: Cellulitis or surgical wound infections
Others: None

PREGNANCY
Postpartum infections, especially postcesarean section wound infection, or episiotomy infections

SYNONYMS
Staphylococcal scarlet fever

ICD-9-CM
• 785.5 shock without mention of trauma
• 785.59 septic shock

SEE ALSO
• Scarlet fever
• Rocky Mountain spotted fever
• Measles
• Acute pancreatitis

OTHER NOTES
Streptococcal toxic shock syndrome or toxic strep syndrome may be clinically indistinguishable from staphylococcal toxic shock

ABBREVIATIONS
N/A

REFERENCES
• Whiting, J.L. & Chow, A.W.: Toxic shock syndrome. In Conn's Current Therapy. Edited by R.E. Rakel. Philadelphia, W.B. Saunders Co., 1990, pp 972-975
• See, R.H. & Chow, A.W.: Microbiology of TSS: overview. In Rev Infect Dis, 1989;11(suppl 1):S55-S60
• Reingold, A.L.: Toxic shock syndrome: An update. In Am J Obstet Gynecol, 1991;165(suppl):1236-1239
• Barry W., et al.: Intravenous immunoglobulin therapy for Toxic Shock Syndrome. JAMA, 1992;267:3315-3316.

Author A. W. Chow, M.D.

Toxoplasmosis

BASICS

DESCRIPTION Infection with the protozoan Toxoplasma gondii. Four types:
Congenital toxoplasmosis: Acute infection of mother during gestation that is passed to fetus. Often asymptomatic, effects on fetus are more severe in first trimester infection.
Ocular toxoplasmosis: Important cause of chorioretinitis, usually resulting from congenital infection but remaining asymptomatic until second or third decade of life
Acute toxoplasmosis in immunocompetent host: Acute self-limiting asymptomatic or mildly symptomatic infection in normal host
Acute toxoplasmosis in immunocompromised host: Primary or reactivation infection that can be a life-threatening disseminated infection involving many organ systems such as heart, lung, liver, but especially the central nervous system
System(s) affected: Nervous, Cardiovascular, Pulmonary, Gastrointestinal, Skin/Exocrine
Genetics: No known genetic pattern
Incidence/Prevalence in USA:
• Up to 70% of healthy adults are seropositive
• Seroconversion rate for women of childbearing age is 0.8% per year
• Affects more than 3500 newborns in U.S. each year
Predominant age: All ages
Predominant sex: Male = Female

SIGNS AND SYMPTOMS
Congenital toxoplasmosis
◊ Most severe when maternal infection occurs early in pregnancy
◊ No signs or symptoms of infection (67%)
◊ Chorioretinitis (15%)
◊ Intracranial calcifications (10%)
◊ Cerebrospinal fluid pleocytosis and elevated protein (20%)
◊ Anemia, thrombocytopenia, jaundice at birth
◊ Microcephaly
◊ Affected survivors may have mental retardation, seizures, visual defects, spasticity, other severe neurologic sequelae
Ocular toxoplasmosis
◊ Chorioretinitis - focal necrotizing retinitis
◊ Yellowish white elevated cotton patch with indistinct margins
◊ May be small clusters of lesions
◊ Congenital disease is usually bilateral
◊ Acquired disease is usually unilateral
◊ Symptoms include blurred vision, scotoma, pain, photophobia

Acute toxoplasmosis in immunocompetent host
◊ 80-90% are asymptomatic
◊ Cervical lymphadenopathy with discrete, usually non-tender nodes, less than 3 cm in diameter
◊ Fever, malaise, night sweats, myalgias
◊ Sore throat
◊ Maculopapular rash
◊ Retroperitoneal and mesenteric lymphadenopathy with abdominal pain may occur
◊ Chorioretinitis
Acute toxoplasmosis in immunocompromised host
◊ May be newly acquired or reactivation disease
◊ Central nervous system disease (50%)
◊ Encephalitis, meningoencephalitis or mass lesions
◊ Hemiparesis, seizures, mental status changes
◊ Visual changes
◊ May have signs and symptoms as seen in immunocompetent host
◊ Myocarditis, pneumonitis

CAUSES
• Etiologic agent for each of the clinical syndromes is Toxoplasma gondii
• Congenital disease is passed transplacentally from newly infected mother to fetus during pregnancy
• Other syndromes may result from newly acquired infection reactivation of latent infection
• Ingestion of meats or foods containing cysts or oocysts present in cat feces
• Infection can be transmitted by blood transfusion

RISK FACTORS
• Immunocompromised hosts especially those with defects in cellular immunity such as AIDS
• Risk of transplacental transmission is greatest during third trimester

DIAGNOSIS

DIFFERENTIAL DIAGNOSIS
• Congenital toxoplasmosis: Other members of TORCH syndrome (rubella, cytomegalovirus, herpes simple), syphilis, Listeria, other infectious encephalopathies, erythroblastosis fetalis, sepsis
• Ocular toxoplasmosis: Tuberculosis, syphilis, leprosy, ocular histoplasmosis
• Acute toxoplasmosis (normal and immunocompromised): Must consider lymphoma, infectious mononucleosis, cytomegalovirus, cat scratch disease, sarcoidosis, tuberculosis, tularemia, metastatic carcinoma, leukemia
• Toxoplasma encephalitis: Tuberculosis, fungal diseases, vasculitis, progressive multifocal leukoencephalopathy (PML), brain abscess, tumor, herpes encephalitis

LABORATORY
• Demonstration of Toxoplasma organism in blood, body fluids or tissue is evidence of infection
• Isolation of Toxoplasma from placenta is diagnostic of congenital infection
• Lymphocyte transformation to Toxoplasma antigens is indicator of previous Toxoplasma infection in adults
• Increased T suppressor lymphocyte count in adults with acquired disease
• Detection of Toxoplasma antigen in blood or body fluids by ELISA technique indicates acute infection
• Several serologic tests used in diagnosis, some measuring IgM and others IgG antibody
• Sabin-Feldman dye test is a sensitive and specific neutralization test, measures IgG antibody, is the standard reference test for toxoplasmosis, but requires live Toxoplasma organisms, so is not available in most labs. High titers suggest acute disease.
• Indirect fluorescent antibody test (IFA) measures same antibodies as dye test. Titers parallel dye test titers.
• IgM fluorescent antibody test detects IgM antibodies with first week of infection but titers fall within a few months
• Indirect hemagglutination test measures a different antibody than dye test. Titers tend to be higher and remain elevated longer.
• Double-sandwich IgM ELISA is more sensitive and specific than other IgM tests
Drugs that may alter lab results: None
Disorders that may alter lab results:
• Antinuclear antibodies and rheumatoid factor may cause false positive serologic test
• Pregnancy may cause false negative hemagglutination test

PATHOLOGICAL FINDINGS
Lymph node histology shows triad of:
◊ Reactive follicular hyperplasia
◊ Irregular clusters of epithelioid histiocytes encroaching on and blurring the margins of the germinal centers
◊ Focal distention of sinuses with monocytoid cells

SPECIAL TESTS
• Skin test showing delayed skin hypersensitivity to Toxoplasma antigens may be useful as a screening test
• Antibody levels in aqueous humor or cerebrospinal fluid may reflect local antibody production and infection at these sites
• Amniocentesis at 20-24 weeks in suspected congenital disease

IMAGING
• CT scan of head in cerebral toxoplasmosis
• Ultrasound of fetus at 20-24 weeks

DIAGNOSTIC PROCEDURES
• Lymph node biopsy showing characteristic pathologic triad
• Brain biopsy in CNS disease and demonstration of organisms by peroxidase-antiperoxidase technique

TREATMENT

APPROPRIATE HEALTH CARE
• Outpatient for acquired disease in immunocompetent host and ocular toxoplasmosis
• Inpatient initially for CNS toxoplasmosis and acute disease in immunocompromised host

GENERAL MEASURES
• Usually no treatment in asymptomatic hosts except in child under 5
• Symptomatic patients should be treated until immunity is assured

ACTIVITY
Level of activity dependent on severity of disease and organ systems involved

DIET
No special diet

PATIENT EDUCATION
• Infected mother must be completely informed of potential consequences to fetus
• Explain prevention methods, e.g., protecting children's play area from cat litter
• Additional materials available from:
• National Institute of Allergy and Infectious Disease, Dept. of Health and Human Services, Bldg. 31, Rm 7A-32, 9000 Rockville Pike, Bethesda, MD 20892, (301)496-5717

MEDICATIONS

DRUG(S) OF CHOICE
• Acute toxoplasmosis in immunodeficient host:
Sulfadiazine (Microsulfon) 100 mg/kg/day up to 8 grams/day plus pyrimethamine (Daraprim) 200 mg the first day, then 25-50 mg/day for several months
• Ocular toxoplasmosis: Above regimen for 1-2 months
• Acute toxoplasmosis in pregnant women: Above regimen may be used after the 16th week of pregnancy
• Congenital toxoplasmosis: Sulfadiazine 100 mg/kg/day plus pyrimethamine I mg/kg every 2 days plus folinic acid 5 mg every 2 days
Contraindications:
• Pyrimethamine should not be used in first trimester of pregnancy
• Known hypersensitivity to pyrimethamine or sulfadiazine (Note: many HIV positive patients have a sulfa sensitivity)

Precautions:
• Bone marrow toxicity an important problem while treating toxoplasmosis
• Use with caution in patients with possible folate deficiency
• Use with caution in patients with renal or hepatic dysfunction
• Sulfonamides may increase anticoagulant effect of coumadin
• Sulfonamides may increase phenytoin (Dilantin) levels
• Sulfonamides may increase hypoglycemic effect of oral hypoglycemic agents
• Adequate hydration is essential since sulfadiazine is poorly soluble and may crystallize in the urine
Significant possible interactions:
Sulfonamides may interact with phenytoin, coumadin and oral hypoglycemic agents

ALTERNATIVE DRUGS
• In pregnancy - Spiramycin 3g/day for 3 weeks, then 2 weeks off, then repeat 5 week cycles throughout pregnancy
• Clindamycin 900-1200mg tid IV has been used for ocular and CNS toxoplasmosis alone and in combination with pyrimethamine. May be as effective as the sulfa/pyrimethamine combination, but with fewer adverse effects.
• Corticosteroids (prednisone 1-2 mg/kg/day) may be added for macular chorioretinitis or CNS infection

FOLLOWUP

PATIENT MONITORING
• Followup visits every 2 weeks until stable, then monthly during therapy
• CBC weekly for first month, then every 2 weeks
• Renal and liver function tests monthly

PREVENTION/AVOIDANCE
Prevention is important in seronegative pregnant women and immunodeficient patients. Avoid eating raw meat, unpasteurized milk, uncooked eggs and avoid contact with cat feces.

POSSIBLE COMPLICATIONS
• Seizure disorder or focal neurologic deficits in CNS toxoplasmosis
• Partial or complete blindness with ocular toxoplasmosis
• Multiple complications may occur with congenital toxoplasmosis including mental retardation, seizures, deafness and blindness

EXPECTED COURSE AND PROGNOSIS
• Immunodeficient patients often relapse if treatment is stopped
• Treatment may prevent the development of untoward sequelae in both symptomatic and asymptomatic infants with congenital toxoplasmosis

MISCELLANEOUS

ASSOCIATED CONDITIONS
Cellular immune compromised patients, especially those with AIDS, have a higher incidence of toxoplasmosis

AGE-RELATED FACTORS
Pediatric: With acute congenital toxoplasmosis, children often die in the first month of life. Subacute congenital disease may not be observed until some time after birth, when symptoms start to appear.
Geriatric: Acquired infection. Often reactivation disease more likely.
Others: None

PREGNANCY
• Have serum examined for Toxoplasma antibodies. Those with negative titers should take extra precautions to avoid contact with cats, not to eat raw meat and wash all fruits and vegetables carefully.
• For toxoplasmosis infection during pregnancy, refer patient to specialist

SYNONYMS N/A

ICD-9-CM
• 130.9 Toxoplasmosis, unspecified
• 771.2 Other congenital infections

SEE ALSO N/A

OTHER NOTES N/A

ABBREVIATIONS N/A

REFERENCE
Mandell, G.L. (ed.): Principles and Practice of Infectious Diseases. 3rd Ed. New York, Churchill Livingstone, 1990

Author W. Gardner, M.D.

Tracheitis

 BASICS

DESCRIPTION
• Bacterial tracheitis, also called pseudomembranous croup, is an uncommon disease of childhood, with rapid onset and severe, progressive course. Characteristics include stridor in both younger and older children. Children appear more ill than they do with croup. Usual course - insidious onset; acute deterioration; rapidly progressive.
• Acute viral tracheitis, an entirely different disease, is a common inflammatory condition. As compared with bacterial tracheitis, this disease most often takes a benign course. It is often linked with bronchitis (tracheobronchitis) or laryngitis (laryngotracheobronchitis).

System(s) affected: Pulmonary
Genetics: No known genetic pattern
Incidence in USA:
• Bacterial tracheitis - uncommon
• Acute viral tracheitis - common
Prevalence in USA: 2-5% of children hospitalized with acute infectious upper airway obstruction
Predominant age: 1 month-6 years, can occur at any age
Predominant sex: Male = Female

SIGNS AND SYMPTOMS
• Fever
• Barking cough
• Hoarse voice
• Upper respiratory infection symptoms
• Toxic appearance
• Inspiratory stridor
• Upper airway obstruction
• Copious, thick tracheal secretions
• Subglottic edema

CAUSES
Bacterial tracheitis
   ◊ Staphylococcus aureus
   ◊ Haemophilus influenzae
   ◊ Streptococcus species (usually Beta-hemolytic group A)
   ◊ Gram negative enterovirus
Viral laryngotracheitis
   ◊ Parainfluenza
   ◊ Influenza
   ◊ Enterovirus

RISK FACTORS
Existing or recent viral infection

 DIAGNOSIS

DIFFERENTIAL DIAGNOSIS
• Croup or laryngotracheobronchitis
• Epiglottitis
• Spasmotic croup
• Diphtheria

LABORATORY
• Leukocytosis
• Left shift of the WBC
• Positive secretion culture
Drugs that may alter lab results: N/A
Disorders that may alter lab results: N/A

PATHOLOGICAL FINDINGS
• Micro - gram-positive cocci
• Micro - pleomorphic gram-negative bacilli

SPECIAL TESTS N/A

IMAGING
Lateral and anteroposterior neck x-rays:
   ◊ Subglottic narrowing
   ◊ Shaggy laryngeal wall
   ◊ Hypopharyngeal distention
   ◊ Adherent membrane

DIAGNOSTIC PROCEDURES
Laryngoscopy (direct or indirect) - shaggy exudative membrane on larynx; inflammation in the subglottic area

 TREATMENT

APPROPRIATE HEALTH CARE
• Outpatient for mild cases of viral disease only
• Inpatient for bacterial tracheitis

GENERAL MEASURES
Acute viral tracheitis:
   ◊ Usually short-lived
   ◊ Normally no treatment necessary
Bacterial tracheitis:
   ◊ Intubation
   ◊ Tracheal suctioning
   ◊ Rare tracheostomy
   ◊ Air humidification
   ◊ Blood gases (for monitoring)
   ◊ Oxygen
   ◊ Intravenous hydration
   ◊ Parenteral broad-spectrum antibiotics

ACTIVITY Complete rest

DIET
• Acute viral tracheitis - increase fluids (fruit sherbets or ices)
• Bacterial tracheitis - IV hydration

PATIENT EDUCATION N/A

MEDICATIONS

DRUG(S) OF CHOICE
For acute or bacterial tracheitis:
◊ Cough may be relieved by codeine or dextromethorphan
◊ If proven bacterial infection present or in patients with co-existing cardiopulmonary disease, antibiotics (amoxycillin 250 mg q 8 hours or erythromycin 250 mg q 6 hours)
Bacterial tracheitis
◊ IV antibiotics including Staphlyococcal coverage
◊ Oxygen
Contraindications: Refer to manufacturer's literature
Precautions: Refer to manufacturer's literature
Significant possible interactions: Refer to manufacturer's literature

ALTERNATIVE DRUGS
• Corticosteroids (controversial)

FOLLOWUP

PATIENT MONITORING
• Arterial blood gases
• Monitor for cyanosis and accelerated respiratory rate

PREVENTION/AVOIDANCE   None

EXPECTED COURSE AND PROGNOSIS
• Acute viral tracheitis - recovery complete after about 7 days
• Bacterial tracheitis - complete recovery, but complications may occur

POSSIBLE COMPLICATIONS
• Sudden respiratory arrest
• Subglottic stenosis
• Airway granulomas
• Airway webs
• Pneumonia
• Toxic shock syndrome

MISCELLANEOUS

ASSOCIATED CONDITIONS
• Parainfluenza laryngotracheobronchitis
• Epiglottitis

AGE-RELATED FACTORS
Pediatric: Common age group is 1 month to 6 years
Geriatric: N/A
Others: N/A

PREGNANCY   N/A

SYNONYMS
• Bacterial tracheitis
• Pseudomembranous croup

ICD-9-CM   464.1 acute tracheitis

SEE ALSO
• Laryngotracheobronchitis
• Epiglottitis
• Diphtheria

OTHER NOTES   N/A

ABBREVIATIONS   N/A

REFERENCES
• Grad, R.. & Taussig, L.M.: Kendig's Disorders of the Respiratory Tract in Children. 5th Ed. Philadelphia, W.B. Saunders Co., 1990
• Berkow, R., et al. (eds.): Merck Manual, 14th Ed. Rahway, NJ, Merck Sharp & Dohme, 1986
• Seaton, A., Seaton, D. & Leitch, A.G.: Crofton & Douglas's Respiratory Diseases. 4th Ed. London/Boston, Blackwell Scientific Publications, 1989

Author   E. Bailey, M.D.

Transfusion reaction, hemolytic

BASICS

DESCRIPTION A cytotoxic, hemolytic reaction that occurs with IV administration of blood or blood components. Reactions may be immune or nonimmune, and can vary from a mild to fatal consequence. (Infection risks outweigh immune risks.)
System(s) affected:
Hemic/Lymphatic/Immunologic, Cardiovascular
Genetics: No known genetic pattern
Incidence/Prevalence in USA: Uncommon
Predominant age: All ages
Predominant sex: Male = Female

SIGNS AND SYMPTOMS
• Chills
• Restlessness
• Anxiety
• Nausea
• Vomiting
• Tingling sensation
• Tachycardia
• Pain in back
• Pain in thighs
• Precordial oppression
• Precordial pain
• Urticaria
• Facial flush
• Rapid, feeble pulse
• Cyanosis
• Shock (cold, clammy skin)
• Fever
• Delirium
• Pulmonary edema
• Note: symptoms are masked in anesthetized patient
• Delayed findings - anemia within 2 weeks

CAUSES
• Immune reactions - incompatibility within ABO system
• A nonhemolytic febrile reaction due to immune sensitivity to leukocytes, platelets, plasma constituents
<u>Hemolytic reactions:</u>
◊ Transfusion of mismatched blood
◊ Destruction of donor erythrocytes by recipient incompatible isoantibodies
◊ Isosensitization by repeated transfusions
◊ Isosensitization by prior pregnancies
◊ Universal blood donor type considered dangerous unless thoroughly checked for agglutination titer

RISK FACTORS
• Multiple blood transfusions
• Rh negative mother
• Multiple pregnancies

DIAGNOSIS

DIFFERENTIAL DIAGNOSIS Other causes of hemolysis: autoimmune disease, uremia, defective hemoglobin, red blood cell defects

LABORATORY
<u>Intravascular hemolysis:</u>
◊ Plasma obtained 2-4 hours after lysis is red or pink, indicating free hemoglobin
◊ Increased BUN
◊ Elevated bilirubin in serum
<u>Extravascular hemolysis:</u>
◊ Plasma pink, dark red or brown
◊ Increased conjugated bilirubin
◊ Hemoglobinuria
◊ In blood - decreased WBC, platelets, fibrinogen
Drugs that may alter lab results: N/A
Disorders that may alter lab results: N/A

PATHOLOGICAL FINDINGS N/A

SPECIAL TESTS N/A

IMAGING N/A

DIAGNOSTIC PROCEDURES N/A

TREATMENT

APPROPRIATE HEALTH CARE
Inpatient

GENERAL MEASURES
• Stop transfusion immediately upon first sign of reaction
• Substitute infusion with normal saline at 150-300 ml per hour
• Check paperwork for any clerical error (usual cause of an ABO-incompatible transfusion)
• Monitor vital signs
• Increase hydration and diuresis
• Maintain urine flow at 100 ml/hr for 6-8 hours or until hemoglobinuria clears
• Preventive measures for congestive heart failure and renal failure
• Recognize and treat disseminated intravascular coagulation if it occurs

ACTIVITY Bedrest

DIET As tolerated

PATIENT EDUCATION N/A

MEDICATIONS

DRUG(S) OF CHOICE
• 1000 mL 0.9% NaCl/h for 2-3 hours
• Oxygen as needed
• 5% albumin for hypotension shock (maintain systolic pressure above 100 mm Hg)
• Epinephrine for wheezing and/or dyspnea
• Diphenhydramine to combat cellular histamine release from mast cells
• Diuretic - furosemide 40 mg IV or ethacrynic acid 50 mg IV
• Appropriate IV antibiotics for bacterial contamination
• Corticosteroids to reduce inflammation
Contraindications: Refer to manufacturer's literature
Precautions: Refer to manufacturer's literature
Significant possible interactions: Refer to manufacturer's literature

ALTERNATIVE DRUGS   N/A

FOLLOWUP

PATIENT MONITORING   Until hemolytic signs are gone

PREVENTION/AVOIDANCE
• History of patient's responses to previous transfusions
• Risk/benefit of any transfusion needs to favor benefit
• Autologous transfusion
• Careful typing and crossmatch, double-check all data available
• Identity of unit of blood is carefully checked before administered
• Close observation of the patient during the transfusion
• Consider leukocyte depleted blood in people with history of recurrent febrile reactions

POSSIBLE COMPLICATIONS
• Uremia, oliguria, anuria
• Right heart failure

EXPECTED COURSE AND PROGNOSIS
• Usual course - acute
• Usually no harm if transfusion is stopped at onset of manifestations
• Severe - mortality 50%

MISCELLANEOUS

ASSOCIATED CONDITIONS
Disseminated intravascular coagulation

AGE-RELATED FACTORS
Pediatric: Reaction greater and outlook poorer in the very young
Geriatric: Outlook more grave in the elderly
Others: N/A

PREGNANCY   N/A

SYNONYMS   N/A

ICD-9-CM   999.8

SEE ALSO   N/A

OTHER NOTES   N/A

ABBREVIATIONS   N/A

REFERENCES
• Mollison, P.L., Engelfriet, C.P. & Contreas, M.: Blood Transfusion in Clinical Medicine. 8th Ed. Oxford, Blackwell Scientific Publications, 1987
• Huestis, D.W., Bove, J.R. & Case, S.: Practical Blood Transfusion. 4th Ed. Boston, Little, Brown and Co., 1988

Author   H. Griffith, M.D. & M. Dambro, M.D.

Transient ischemic attack

 BASICS

DESCRIPTION The sudden onset of a focal and transient (< 24 hours) neurological deficit due to brain ischemia
System(s) affected: Nervous
Genetics: Inheritance is polygenic with a tendency to clustering of risk factors within families
Incidence/Prevalence in USA: Incidence 160/100,000; prevalence 135 per 100,000
Predominant age: Risk increases over age 45 and is highest in the seventh and eighth decades
Predominant sex: Male > Female (3:1)

SIGNS AND SYMPTOMS
• Carotid circulation (hemispheric) - hemiplegia, hemianesthesia, neglect, aphasia, visual field defects; less often headaches, seizures, amnesia, confusion
• Vertebrobasilar (brainstem or cerebellar) - diplopia, vertigo, ataxia, facial paresis, Horner's syndrome, dysphagia, dysarthria
• Cerebellar or brainstem lesion in patients with headache, nausea, vomiting and ataxia

CAUSES
• Carotid atherosclerotic disease with artery to artery thromboembolism
• Small, deep, vessel disease associated with hypertension
• Cardiac - cardioembolism secondary to valvular (mitral valve) pathology; mural hypo- or akinesias with thrombosis (acute anterior myocardial infarctions or congestive cardiomyopathies); cardiac arrhythmia (atrial fibrillation)
• Hypercoagulable states - antiphospholipid antibodies, deficiency of protein S, protein C. Presence of antithrombin 3, oral contraceptives.
• Other causes - spontaneous and post-traumatic (i.e., chiropractic manipulation) arterial dissection, fibromuscular dysplasia

RISK FACTORS
• Age
• Hypertension
• Cardiac disease
• Smoking
• Diabetes
• Antiphospholipid antibodies
• Family History

 DIAGNOSIS

DIFFERENTIAL DIAGNOSIS
• Migraine (hemiplegic)
• Focal seizure (Todd's paralysis)
• Hypoglycemia
• Todd's paralysis

LABORATORY N/A
Drugs that may alter lab results: N/A
Disorders that may alter lab results: N/A

PATHOLOGICAL FINDINGS N/A

SPECIAL TESTS
• Duplex carotid ultrasonography
• Cerebral angiography
• ECG
• Transthoracic echocardiogram (TTE); if normal and a cardiac source is suspected, follow with transesophageal echocardiogram
• Holter monitoring
• EEG for suspected seizure
• Prothrombin time (PT) and partial thromboplastin time (PTT) (Coumadin prolongs PT)
• Antiphospholipid antibodies

IMAGING
• Acute phase - CT of head to rule out hemorrhage
• Angiography - carotid arterial stenosis
• Digital substraction - stenosis

DIAGNOSTIC PROCEDURES N/A

 TREATMENT

APPROPRIATE HEALTH CARE
• Acute phase: Outpatient for investigations; inpatient for surgery

GENERAL MEASURES
• Strict control of medical risk factors, e.g., diabetes, hypertension, hyperlipidemia, cardiac disease
• Counseling towards cessation of smoking
• Surgical therapy: In medically fit patients with non-disabling stroke, carotid endarterectomy is indicated for stenosis of >70% on side ipsilateral to stroke; medical therapy for < 30% stenosis. Best therapy for stenosis of 30-70% is unknown, therefore it is best to refer the patient to a center involved in North American Symptomatic Carotid Endarterectomy Trial (NASCET).

ACTIVITY No restrictions

DIET As appropriate to underlying medical problems (diabetic diet, low fat diet, low salt diet etc.)

PATIENT EDUCATION National Stroke Association, 300 East Hampden Ave., Suite 240, Engle Wood, CO 80110-2622

MEDICATIONS

DRUG(S) OF CHOICE
• Enteric coated aspirin (EC ASA) 325 mg daily,
or
• Ticlopidine 250 mg po bid

Contraindications:
• EC ASA - active peptic ulcer disease, hypersensitivity to aspirin, patients who had bronchospastic reaction to ASA or other nonsteroidal anti-inflammatory drugs
• Ticlopidine - known hypersensitivity to the drug, presence of hematopoietic disorders, presence of a hemostatic disorder, conditions associated with active bleeding, severe liver dysfunction

Precautions:
• EC ASA - may aggravate pre-existing peptic ulcer disease , may worsen symptoms in some patients with asthma
• Ticlopidine - 2.4% of patients develop neutropenia (0.8% severe neutropenia) which is reversible with cessation of drug. Monitor blood counts every 2 weeks for the first 3 months.

Significant possible interactions:
• EC ASA - may potentiate effects of anticoagulants and sulfonylurea, hypoglycemic agents
• Ticlopidine - digoxin plasma levels decreased 15%, theophylline half-life increased from 8.6 to 12.2 hours

ALTERNATIVE DRUGS
• Dipyridamole (Persantine) of no proven benefit
• Sulfinpyrazone (Anturane) of no proven benefit

FOLLOWUP

PATIENT MONITORING
Followup every 3 months for first year then yearly

PREVENTION/AVOIDANCE
• Stop smoking
• Control blood pressure, diabetes, hyperlipidemia
• EC ASA 650 mg bid or ticlopidine 250 mg po bid for patients with prior transient ischemic attack

POSSIBLE COMPLICATIONS
• Stroke
• Seizure
• Trauma if patient experiences sudden fall due to weakness

EXPECTED COURSE AND PROGNOSIS
5-20% risk of stroke on ipsilateral side within one year and cumulative thereafter. Frequency increases with addition of multiple risk factors and severity of carotid stenosis.

MISCELLANEOUS

ASSOCIATED CONDITIONS
• Atrial fibrillation
• Major cause of death in first five years after a TIA is cardiac disease

AGE-RELATED FACTORS
Pediatric:
• Cardiac (especially developmental abnormalities)
• Metabolic - homocystinuria, Fabry's disease
Geriatric: Atrial fibrillation is a frequent cause of TIA among the elderly
Others: Adults < 45 years old most likely to have a cardiac source of embolism

PREGNANCY
A hypercoagulable state is associated with pregnancy and parturition

SYNONYMS
Mini-stroke

ICD-9-CM
435.9

SEE ALSO
Stroke

OTHER NOTES
N/A

ABBREVIATIONS
EC ASA = enteric coated aspirin

REFERENCES
• Hachinski, V.C. & Norris, J.W.: The Acute Stroke. Philadelphia, F.A. Davis, 1985
• Barnett, J.H.M., Mohr J.P., Stein, B.M. & Yatsu, F.M. (eds.): Stroke. New York, Churchill Livingstone, 1986
• Norris, J.W. & Hachinski, V.C.: Prevention of Stroke. Philadelphia, F.A. Davis, 1991

Author C. Graffagnino, M.D. & V. Hachinski, M.D., D.Sc.

Trichinosis

BASICS

DESCRIPTION A parasitic disease caused by the tissue dwelling roundworm Trichinella spiralis. Humans are infected by eating the encysted larvae stage in improperly cooked pork, bear, walrus, horse and other wild animal meats. Clinical symptoms occur during the parasite's life cycle. Larvae are eaten and the intestinal phase of the adult form develops. This phase occurs from five days to two weeks following ingestion. The larval migration and muscle invasion phase occurs from one to six weeks after ingestion of improperly cooked meat. The final stage is the period of larval encystment within the human muscle and occurs from the third to the ninth week post ingestion.
System(s) affected: Musculoskeletal
Genetics: N/A
Incidence/Prevalence in USA: Between 20-50 cases were reported annually to the CDC from 1983-1989. In 1990, 129 cases were reported, of which 79 cases were from Iowa and 16 cases were from Virginia.
Predominant age: Cases have been reported from all age groups. It occurs most frequently in ages 20-49.
Predominant sex: Male = Female

SIGNS AND SYMPTOMS
• Symptoms depend upon organ involved and the total worm burden. Skeletal muscles most likely involved are masseter, tongue, diaphragm, deltoid, biceps, gluteus and gastrocnemius muscles. Phases I and II, and II and III may occur concurrently.
Phase I, intestinal
  ◊ Vomiting
  ◊ Cramps
  ◊ Diarrhea
  ◊ Abdominal pain
  ◊ Chills
  ◊ Fever
Phase II, larval migration
  ◊ Eosinophilia
  ◊ Periorbital edema
  ◊ Myalgia
  ◊ Muscle soreness
  ◊ Joint pain
  ◊ Conjunctivitis
  ◊ Subconjunctival hemorrhage
  ◊ Retinal hemorrhage
  ◊ Photophobia
  ◊ Thirst
  ◊ Pneumonitis
Phase III, muscle encystment
  ◊ Dyspnea
  ◊ Hoarseness
  ◊ Malaise
  ◊ Prostration

CAUSES Eating pork, walrus, bear, horse, or wild game that is partially cooked

RISK FACTORS
• Access to wild game, homemade pork products, noncommercial sources of meat
• Ethnic groups from Southeast Asia raising their own pork or favoring partially cooked pork products
• Groups living on small farms failing to use modern hog management techniques

DIAGNOSIS

DIFFERENTIAL DIAGNOSIS
• Acute rheumatic fever
• Arthritis, angioedema
• Collagen vascular diseases
• Encephalitis
• Eosinophilic leukemia
• Dermatomyositis
• Gastroenteritis
• Influenza
• Glomerulonephritis
• Myositis
• Meningitis
• Myocarditis
• Pneumonitis
• Polyarteritis nodosa
• Typhoid fever
• Tuberculosis
• Undulant fever

LABORATORY
• Marked hypergammaglobulinemia
• Eosinophilia
• Increased creatine phosphokinase (CPK)
• Increased lactate dehydrogenase (LDH)
• Normal sedimentation rate
Drugs that may alter lab results: Rare increases in SGOT with thiabendazole
Disorders that may alter lab results: N/A

PATHOLOGICAL FINDINGS Living larvae in muscle, adult worm in stool (rare)

SPECIAL TESTS
• Complement fixation
• Indirect immunofluorescence
• Bentonite flocculation
• ELISA (enzyme linked immunosorbent assay)

IMAGING
• Chest x-ray may detect patchy infiltrate
• CT may be helpful in calcified muscle cysts

DIAGNOSTIC PROCEDURES Muscle biopsy of gastrocnemius or deltoid

TREATMENT

APPROPRIATE HEALTH CARE
Outpatient. May call the CDC in Atlanta, Georgia for appropriate diagnostic tests (404-639-3311).

GENERAL MEASURES No special measures. Bed rest may relieve muscular pain.

ACTIVITY As tolerated

DIET As tolerated

PATIENT EDUCATION
• Depends upon complications, if any
• Education about usual methods to interrupt further transmission, i.e., cook pork and game thoroughly, proper hog raising practices, proper preparation, storage and disposal of game

MEDICATIONS

DRUG(S) OF CHOICE
• For early intestinal phase and treatment of adult worms, thiabendazole 25 mg/kg orally for 5-10 days, maximal dose 1.5 gm. Clinical response variable. For tissue larvae, mebendazole may be used in a dose of 200-400 mg tid x 3 days followed by 400-500 tid for 10 days. All stages, intestinal, larval, migration and muscle encystment are reported to respond.
• Call CDC for current dosage and recommendation, (404)639-3311
• Treat allergic reactions with corticosteroids, 20-60 mg/day for five days, then taper over a one month period
• Treat muscle plain with salicylates

Contraindications: Corticosteroids have been reported to be contraindicated in the intestinal phase

Precautions: Minimal experience exists with use of medications in small children and in pregnancy

Significant possible interactions:
Thiabendazole may compete for binding sites in liver with theophylline. Theophylline may be elevated to toxic levels.

ALTERNATIVE DRUGS
Albendazole 400 mg bid x 15 days (not yet available in the US)

FOLLOWUP

PATIENT MONITORING
Monitor for signs and symptoms of complications

PREVENTION/AVOIDANCE
Avoid undercooked pork and game meat. Prolonged freezing is also effective, although less reliable.

POSSIBLE COMPLICATIONS
• Meningitis
• Encephalitis
• Myocarditis
• Nephritis
• Sinusitis
• Glomerulonephritis

EXPECTED COURSE AND PROGNOSIS
Most infections asymptomatic or short-lived. Prognosis good in most cases. Occasional death reported (usually the result of cardiac failure or pneumonia).

MISCELLANEOUS

ASSOCIATED CONDITIONS N/A

AGE-RELATED FACTORS
Pediatric: N/A
Geriatric: Not enough data
Others: N/A

PREGNANCY
No information available

SYNONYMS
• Trichinellosis
• Trichinelliasis

ICD-9-CM 124

SEE ALSO N/A

OTHER NOTES N/A

ABBREVIATIONS N/A

REFERENCES
• Bailey, T. & Schantz, P.: Trends in the Incidence and Transmission Patterns of Trichinosis in Humans in the United States: Comparisons of the Period 1975-1981 and 1982-86. Reviews of Infectious Diseases, Vol. 12, No. 1, Jan-Feb, pp. 5-10, 1990
• Brown, H.W. & Neva, F.A.: Basic Clinical Parasitology. 3rd Ed. New York, Appleton-Century-Crofts, 1964

Author A. Vuturo, M.D., M.P.H.

Trichomoniasis

 BASICS

DESCRIPTION
Trichomonas is a protozoan parasite found in men and women at genitourinary sites
System(s) affected: Reproductive, Renal/Urologic
Genetics: N/A
Incidencee in USA: 300/100,000 women/year for first time diagnosis of trichomoniasis; 600/100,000 women/year for any diagnosis for trichomoniasis
Prevalence in USA: In sexually active adult women: 2,000/100,000 in a family planning clinic; 35,000/100,000 in a STD clinic
Predominant age:
• Young and middle aged adults
• Rare until onset of sexual activity
• Not uncommon in postmenopausal women
Predominant sex: Both affected, but women more commonly symptomatic

SIGNS AND SYMPTOMS
Female
◊ 40% can be asymptomatic at time of diagnosis
◊ Symptoms typically begin or worsen at time of menstrual period
◊ Vaginal discharge (75%, usually copious and pooling, can be frothy)
◊ Vulvovaginal irritation (50%)
◊ Dysuria (50%)
◊ Vaginal odor (10%)
◊ A "strawberry cervix" from punctate hemorrhages (5% of cases)
◊ Vaginal hyperemia
◊ Dyspareunia
◊ Suprapubic discomfort
◊ Cervical erosion
Male
◊ Many are asymptomatic
◊ Urethral discharge (50%)
◊ Dysuria
◊ Epididymitis (rare)

CAUSES
• Trichomonas vaginalis is a pear shaped protozoan which is a facultative anaerobe. It is usually sexually transmitted although a non-venereal route is possible as the organism survives for several hours in a moist environment.
• Transmission is seen in up to 15% of female children of infected women
• Incubation period is 5 to 28 days

RISK FACTORS
Multiple sexual partners

 DIAGNOSIS

DIFFERENTIAL DIAGNOSIS
• Female - vaginal candidiasis, bacterial vaginosis. Cervical inflammation can lead to the mistaken diagnosis of cervicitis.
• Male - chlamydia urethritis

LABORATORY
Female
◊ Wet prep is 60-70% sensitive and highly specific. Sensitivity is reduced with loss of motility due to cooling, low inoculum size and rapid scanning of the slide. Specificity is about 100%.
Male
◊ A wet prep and culture of urethral discharge after prostatic exam is 50-80% sensitive
Drugs that may alter lab results: N/A
Disorders that may alter lab results: N/A

PATHOLOGICAL FINDINGS   N/A

SPECIAL TESTS
• Culture has a sensitivity of greater than 95% but takes 4-7 days
• ELISA and direct fluorescent antibody tests are available and are 80-90% sensitive
• Pap smear has a 60% sensitivity and 99% specificity

IMAGING   N/A

DIAGNOSTIC PROCEDURES   N/A

 TREATMENT

APPROPRIATE HEALTH CARE
Outpatient

GENERAL MEASURES
Education about the venereal aspect of the infection

ACTIVITY
Sexual activity should not be resumed until patient and partner are both treated

DIET
Should abstain from alcohol if metronidazole used for therapy

PATIENT EDUCATION
• Vaginitis, Questions and Answers Planned Parenthood Federation of America, Inc (212)541-7800
• Roses Have Thorns, RAJ Publications, P.O. Box 150720, Lakewood, CO 80215
• American College of Obstetricians & Gynecologists (ACOG), 409 12th St., SW, Washington, DC 20024-2188, (800)762-ACOG

MEDICATIONS

DRUG(S) OF CHOICE Metronidazole - adult dose 2 grams at one time, or 250 mg tid for 7 days, or 500 mg bid for 5 days. The routines are effective in women but the one time dose has a higher failure rate in men. All sexual partners need treatment.
Contraindications: First trimester pregnancy or allergy to the antibiotic
Precautions: Avoid metronidazole or reduce the dosage in patients with liver failure
Significant possible interactions: Ethanol, warfarin, disulfiram, phenobarbital

ALTERNATIVE DRUGS
 • Clotrimazole 100 mg vaginal tablets q/hs for 14 days. Cure rate is 20-25% but symptoms will be reduced in most women.
 • Alternatively saline or vinegar dosing can be tried

FOLLOWUP

PATIENT MONITORING Monitor target symptoms. No followup is needed if symptoms resolve with treatment.

PREVENTION/AVOIDANCE Practice safe sex by using condoms

POSSIBLE COMPLICATIONS Recurrent infections

EXPECTED COURSE AND PROGNOSIS Prognosis is good but recurrent infection raises possibility of non-compliance with therapy, re-infection, or infection with a resistant organism. If resistance is suspected, try metronidazole 500 mg tid for 14 days along with acetic acid vaginal douches twice weekly.

MISCELLANEOUS

ASSOCIATED CONDITIONS Other sexually transmitted diseases

AGE-RELATED FACTORS
Pediatric: Very uncommon in prepuberty (confirmed diagnosis should raise concern of sexual abuse)
Geriatric: Older people remain at risk for Trichomonas
Others: N/A

PREGNANCY Do not use metronidazole in the first trimester

SYNONYMS
 • Trick
 • Trichomonal urethritis

ICD-9-CM
 • 131.9
 • Vulva or vagina 131.01
 • Urogenitalis 131.00

SEE ALSO N/A

OTHER NOTES N/A

ABBREVIATIONS N/A

REFERENCE
 • McCue, J.D.: Evaluation and Management of Vaginitis, An Update for Primary Care Practitioners. Arch Intern Med.149:565-8, 1989
 • Lossick, J.G. & Kent, H.L.: Trichomoniasis: rends in diagnosis and management. Am J Obstet & Gynol. 165;1217-22, 1991
 • Krieger JN: Clinical Manifestations of Trichomoniasis in Men. Ann Int Med, 118:844-849, 1993.

Author G. Bergus, M.D.

Trigeminal neuralgia

 BASICS

DESCRIPTION A disorder of the sensory nucleus of the 5th cranial nerve (trigeminal nerve), producing bouts of severe lancinating pain in the distribution of one or more divisions. Often precipitated by stimulation of well-defined trigger paths, usually perioral, perinasal, occasionally intraoral, ipsilaterally.
Systems(s) affected: Nervous
Genetics: N/A
Incidence in USA: 16/100,000
Prevalence in USA: N/A
Predominant age: Over age 50, peak age 60
Predominant sex: Male > Female (1.6:1)

SIGNS AND SYMPTOMS
• Unilateral (< 4% bilateral), symptoms rarely present at night
• Excruciating lip pain
• Excruciating gum pain
• Excruciating cheek pain
• Paroxysmal facial pain
• Wincing
• Pain elicited by tickle
• Flushing
• Lacrimation
• Salivation
• Pain elicited by touch
• Pain "bursts" several seconds with refractory period after
• Right > left side preference
• 2nd and/or 3rd division trigeminal nerve most commonly affected

CAUSES Most commonly compression of the trigeminal nerve by arteries or veins of the posterior fossa.

RISK FACTORS Unknown

 DIAGNOSIS

DIFFERENTIAL DIAGNOSIS
• Other forms of neuralgia usually have sensory loss. The presence of sensory loss nearly excludes the diagnosis of trigeminal neuralgia.
• Neoplasia in the cerebellopontine angle
• Vascular malformation of the brain stem
• Demyelinating lesion
• Vascular insult
• Migraine
• Chronic meningitis
• Acute polyneuropathy

LABORATORY N/A
Drugs that may alter lab results: N/A
Disorders that may alter lab results: N/A

PATHOLOGICAL FINDINGS
• Semilunar ganglion - inflammatory changes
• Degenerative changes

SPECIAL TESTS N/A

IMAGING N/A

DIAGNOSTIC PROCEDURES MRI or CT scan - neoplasm in cerebellopontine angle must be ruled out

 TREATMENT

APPROPRIATE HEALTH CARE
Outpatient

GENERAL MEASURES
• Drug treatment is first approach. Invasive procedures for patients who cannot tolerate, or fail to respond to, drug treatment.
• Microvascular decompression of the 5th cranial nerve at its entrance to (or exit from) the brainstem (73% relief)
• Peripheral block or section of 5th nerve proximal to the Gasserian ganglion
• Alcohol, glycerol or radio-frequency gangliolysis
• Avoidance of stimulation (air, heat, cold) of trigger zones (lips, cheeks, gums)

ACTIVITY Full activity

DIET No special diet

PATIENT EDUCATION Instruct regarding medication dosage and side effects

MEDICATIONS

DRUG(S) OF CHOICE Carbamazepine 100-1200 mg/day (maximum)
Contraindications: MAO inhibitors taken concurrently
Precautions: Use with caution in presence of liver disease
Significant possible interactions:
Macrolide antibiotics with Carbamazepine. Oral anticoagulants, anticonvulsants, tricyclics, oral contraceptives, steroids, digitalis, INH, MAO inhibitors, methyprylon nabilone, nizatidine, other H2 blockers, phenytoin, propoxyphene, benzodiazepines, calcium, channel blockers.

ALTERNATIVE DRUGS
• Phenytoin 400 mg/day and synergistic with carbamazepine
• Baclofen 10-80 mg/day

FOLLOWUP

PATIENT MONITORING
• Carbamazepine and/or phenytoin serum levels
• Liver and hematopoietic functions if carbamazepine is prescribed

PREVENTION/AVOIDANCE Reduce drugs after 4-6 weeks to determine if condition is in remission, resume at previous dose if pain recurs. Withdraw drugs slowly after several months again to check for remission or if lower dose of drugs can be tolerated.

POSSIBLE COMPLICATIONS Mental and physical sluggishness, dizziness with carbamazepine

EXPECTED COURSE AND PROGNOSIS Exacerbations in fall and spring; otherwise good

MISCELLANEOUS

ASSOCIATED CONDITIONS
• Sjogren's syndrome
• Rheumatoid arthritis
• Chronic meningitis
• Facial migraine
• Acute polyneuropathy
• Multiple sclerosis
• Hemifacial spasm
• Pretrigeminal neuralgia

AGE-RELATED FACTORS
Pediatric: Unusual in childhood
Geriatric: N/A
Others: N/A

PREGNANCY N/A

SYNONYMS
• Tic douloureux
• Fothergill's neuralgia
• Trifocal neuralgia

ICD-9-CM 350.1

SEE ALSO N/A

OTHER NOTES N/A

ABBREVIATIONS N/A

REFERENCES
• Bell, W.E. Orofacial Pain. 4th Ed. Chicago, Year Book Medical Publishers, 1989
• Adams, R.D. & Victor, M.: Principles of Neurology. New York, McGraw-Hill, 1986
• Sweet, W.H.: The Treatment of Trigeminal Neuralgia (Tic Douloureux), New Engl J Med, July 17, 1986 Pg. 174-177
• Moller, A.R.: The Cranial Nerve Vascular Compression Syndrome: A Review of Treatment, Acta Neurochirurgica (1991) 113: 18-23
• Merrill, R., Graff-Radford, S.B.: Trigeminal Neuralgia: How to Rule Out the Wrong Treatment, JADA (1992) 123: 63-68
• Smith, L.H., Jr. & Bennett, C.: Trigeminal neuralgia. In Cecil Textbook of Medicine. 19th Ed. Edited by J.B. Wyngaarden. Philadelphia, W.B. Saunders Co., 1992

Author P. Jaster, M.D.

Tropical sprue

BASICS

DESCRIPTION Malabsorption syndrome of unknown etiology that occurs primarily in the tropics and subtropics. Characteristics include protein malnutrition and folic acid anemia. Usual course - relapsing without treatment. Symptoms may appear years after leaving an endemic area.
• Endemic areas - tropical regions only, Far East, India, Caribbean. Distribution is sporadic.
• The presence of normal jejunal biopsy nearly excludes this diagnosis
System(s) affected: Gastrointestinal, Hemic/Lymphatic/Immunologic
Genetics: N/A
Incidence/Prevalence in USA: Unknown
Predominant age: None
Predominant sex: Male = Female

SIGNS AND SYMPTOMS
• Fatigue
• Asthenia
• Weight loss
• Diarrhea
• Abdominal cramps
• Borborygmus
• Night blindness
• Stomatitis
• Glossitis
• Cheilosis
• Anorexia
• Steatorrhea
• Hyperkeratosis
• Edema
• Abdominal distension
• Hyperpigmentation
• Koilonychia

CAUSES
• Unknown
• Possible dietary deficiency
• Possible infectious agent
• Vitamin deficiency (folate)
• Food toxins (rancid fats)

RISK FACTORS Parasitic infestation

DIAGNOSIS

DIFFERENTIAL DIAGNOSIS
• Other causes of megaloblastic anemia
• Other malabsorption syndromes
• Celiac disease
• Inflammatory bowel disease
• Giardiasis
• Strongylosis

LABORATORY
• Megaloblastic anemia in 60% of cases
• Steatorrhea
• Decreased D-xylose
• Decreased serum iron
• Decreased calcium
• Decreased folic acid
• Decreased serum vitamin B12
Drugs that may alter lab results: N/A
Disorders that may alter lab results: N/A

PATHOLOGICAL FINDINGS Jejunal biopsy - mild villous atrophy, increased villous crypts, mononuclear cell infiltration

SPECIAL TESTS Serum vitamin B12

IMAGING
• Mild jejunal dilatation
• Jejunal fold coarsening

DIAGNOSTIC PROCEDURES
• Jejunal biopsy - not specific
• Malabsorption of at least two nutrients is considered essential for diagnosis
• D- Xylose, fat and radiolabelled vitamin B12 are used to test for absorptive capacity
• Stool microscopy

TREATMENT

APPROPRIATE HEALTH CARE
Outpatient

GENERAL MEASURES
• Replace deficiencies, such as vitamin B12 and folic acid
• Control of diarrhea
• Fluid and blood replacement

ACTIVITY No restrictions

DIET No special diet (gluten-free diets do not improve this disease)

PATIENT EDUCATION Written patient information available from:
National Digestive Diseases Information Clearinghouse
Box NDDIC
Bethesda, MD 20892
(301)468-6344

MEDICATIONS

DRUG(S) OF CHOICE
 • Vitamin B12 1000 mg IM for several days, then monthly thereafter for 6 months
 • Tetracycline 250 mg qid for 1-2 months, then half doses for up to 6 months. Occasionally, longer course is required.
Contraindications: Allergy to tetracycline or oxytetracycline
Precautions:
 • Use with caution in patients with lupus, myasthenia gravis, kidney or liver disease
 • Don't take with milk, antacids or iron preparations
 • Don't use during pregnancy
 • Don't use in children under age 8
Significant possible interactions:
 • Antacids, anticoagulants, bismuth subsalicylate
 • Oral contraceptives
 • Lithium

ALTERNATIVE DRUGS
 • Oxytetracycline
 • Nonabsorbable sulfonamides

FOLLOWUP

PATIENT MONITORING As needed for symptoms

PREVENTION/AVOIDANCE N/A

POSSIBLE COMPLICATIONS
 • Malabsorption
 • Relapse if medication regimen is stopped too soon

EXPECTED COURSE AND PROGNOSIS Good with appropriate treatment

MISCELLANEOUS

ASSOCIATED CONDITIONS N/A

AGE-RELATED FACTORS
Pediatric: Don't treat with tetracycline
Geriatric: N/A
Others: N/A

PREGNANCY Don't treat with tetracycline during pregnancy

SYNONYMS N/A

ICD-9-CM 579.1

SEE ALSO
 • Whipple disease
 • Diarrhea, chronic
 • Celiac disease

OTHER NOTES N/A

ABBREVIATIONS N/A

REFERENCE
 • Sleisenger, M.H. & Fordtran, J.S. (eds.): Gastrointestinal Disease: Pathophysiology, Diagnosis, Management. 4th Ed. Philadelphia, W.B. Saunders Co., 1989
 • Mandell, G.L. (ed.): Principles and Practice of Infectious Diseases. 3rd Ed. New York, John Wiley & Sons, 1990

Author A. Abyad, M.D.

Tuberculosis

 BASICS

DESCRIPTION
Tuberculosis is an increasingly common infection in the 1990's. After inhalation of organisms, pulmonary inoculation can lead to involvement of multiple other areas of the body including middle ear, bones, joints, meninges, kidney, and skin. Inhaled organisms not successfully killed by cell-mediated immunity can spread through lymphatic, blood or contiguous tissues. Adenopathy of hilar, mediastinal and cervical regions is common. Incubation is 2-10 weeks.
• Organisms can survive many years and recrudescent, post-primary disease can become manifest with pregnancy, stress, other diseases, or old age. Recrudescence most commonly occurs in the lung apices (85%).
• Highest risk for active disease is within the first two years after exposure

System(s) affected: Pulmonary, Hemic/Lymphatic/Immunologic, Renal/Urologic, Gastrointestinal, Nervous, Endocrine/Metabolic

Genetics: N/A

Incidence/Prevalence in USA: Varies greatly, may be 32-100 per 100,000

Predominant age:
• Primary disease - infant and adolescence
• Post primary or recrudescent disease - adults and elderly
• At any age - immunosuppressed

Predominant Sex: Male > Female

SIGNS AND SYMPTOMS
• Cough
• Hemoptysis
• Fever and night sweats
• Weight loss
• Decreased activity
• Adenopathy
• Pleuritic pain
• Hepatosplenomegaly
• Renal, bone or CNS disease are late findings

CAUSES
Mycobacterium tuberculosis, Mycobacterium bovis, and Mycobacterium africanum

RISK FACTORS
• Urban, homeless, minority
• Institutionalized (e.g., correctional facility)
• Immunosuppressed (especially HIV)
• Hodgkin's
• Lymphoma
• Diabetes
• Chronic renal failure
• Malnutrition
• Chronic high dose steroids
• Close contact with an infected individual

 DIAGNOSIS

DIFFERENTIAL DIAGNOSIS
• Other pneumonias
• Lymphomas
• Fungal infections, especially other atypical Mycobacteria or Nocardia

LABORATORY
• OT (old tuberculin) skin test - multiple puncture tests for screening, 10 to 20% false positive rate
• Purified protein derivative (PPD) the Mantoux skin test method - 5 units intermediate strength, 0.1 cc volar forearm. Intradermal wheal should be read at 48 to 72 hours. Greater than 10 mm is positive (> 5 mm in HIV positive patient)
• Nonspecific laboratory includes anemia, monocytosis, thrombocytosis, hypergammaglobulinemia, syndrome of inappropriate antidiuretic hormone (SIADH) and sterile pyuria

Drugs that may alter lab results:
• Past vaccination with bacillus Calmette-Guerin (BCG) causes a false-positive skin test
• Inactive vaccine or improper placement may cause a false-negative skin test
• Steroids may cause a false-negative skin test

Disorders that may alter lab results:
Recent viral infections, new infection, 6 to 8 weeks, severe malnutrition may cause a false-negative skin test

PATHOLOGICAL FINDINGS
• Granulomatous process with foci of caseating necrosis surrounded by epithelioid histiocytes and giant cells, in turn surrounded by lymphocytes
• Acid-fast bacillus (AFB) stains show red rods in necrotic area of phagocytes

SPECIAL TESTS
• Lumbar puncture, if meningitis suspected
• Bone marrow biopsy and liver biopsy for culture
• Fluorescent staining and DNA probes for rapid diagnosis

IMAGING
Chest x-ray may show infiltrate with or without effusion with primary disease. Cavitary lesions and upper lobe disease with hilar adenopathy common. Diffuse miliary pattern possible with appearance of "millet seeds." Right upper lobe atelectasis with hilar adenopathy common in primary infection of children.

DIAGNOSTIC PROCEDURES
Ziehl-Neelsen or auramine-rhodamine stain of sputum, gastric aspirate (esp. in children), bronchoalveolar lavage fluids, peritoneal fluids, pleural fluids, bone marrow aspirates, cerebrospinal fluid (CSF). Culture is positive within 3-6 weeks. Tuberculous organisms are slow growing, obligate, intracellular aerobes.

 TREATMENT

APPROPRIATE HEALTH CARE
• Prophylaxis for all ages with positive PPD skin test without disease, use isoniazid for minimum six months
• For active disease, use minimum of two drugs for 9 months, or 3-4 drugs for 2 months, then 2 drugs to complete 6 months
• Pediatrics with active pulmonary disease - three drugs for two months using isoniazid, rifampin and pyrazinamide, then four months with isoniazid and rifampin
• HIV positive patients should be treated with a minimum of 3 drugs
• Severe disease any age, use four drugs for the first two to three months

GENERAL MEASURES
Careful reevaluation required. Only change to twice weekly dosing if health professional personally documents drug administration.

ACTIVITY
• As tolerated
• Coughing children may be contagious
• Coughing patients with AFB positive sputum usually not contagious after a few days of treatment

DIET
Regular. If meat/milk deficient, as child, adolescent or pregnant woman, give isoniazid plus pyridoxine.

PATIENT EDUCATION
Teach pathogenesis, emphasize importance of medical drug therapy, warn of effects and/or interactions, find contacts

MEDICATIONS

DRUG(S) OF CHOICE
Isoniazid: scored tabs 100 mg, 300 mg or syrup 10 mg/mL
◊ Daily dose - adult 300 mg; pediatric 10-20 mg/kg (maximum 300 mg)
◊ Twice weekly - adult 15 mg/kg; pediatric 20-40 mg/kg (maximum 900 mg)
◊ Note: Peripheral neuritis and hypersensitivity reactions may be decreased or prevented with adequate daily doses of pyridoxine
Rifampin capsules (150/300 or syrup 10 mg/mL)
◊ Daily dose - adult 600 mg; pediatric dose 10-20 mg/kg (maximum 600 mg)
◊ Twice weekly - adult 600 mg; pediatric 10-20 mg/kg (maximum 600 mg)
Pyrazinamide (scored 500)
◊ Daily dose - adult 20-35 mg/kg (maximum 1-3 gm); pediatric 20-30 mg/kg (maximum 2 gm)
Streptomycin (IM only, vials 1,4 gm)
◊ Daily dose - 20-40 mg/kg (maximum 1 gm); pediatric 20-40 mg/kg (maximum 1 gm)
◊ Twice weekly - 25 mg/kg; pediatric 25-30 mg/kg
Contraindications: Streptomycin - never use longer than 12 weeks secondary to ototoxicity
Precautions:
• Follow liver function if the patient has history of liver dysfunction or develops new signs of liver disorder
• GI distress possible with rifampin
• Pyrazinamide should be used only if the patient can be closely monitored for abnormal liver function tests
Significant possible interactions:
• Rifampin - colors urine, tears and secretions orange. Can permanently stain contact lenses, may inactivate birth control pills.
• Isoniazid - peripheral neuritis and hypersensitivity possible. Be sure to prescribe adequate pyridoxine.

ALTERNATIVE DRUGS
• Ethambutol - tablets 100/400 bacteriostatic - daily dose 15-25 mg/kg, with maximum of 2.5 gm a week or twice weekly dose 50 mg/kg, with maximum of 2.5 gm. Because of side effect of optic neuritis, never use ethambutol unless patient old enough to cooperate for visual acuity and color testing. GI distress is also possible with ethambutol.
• Steroids - use only if concurrent anti-TB therapy is ongoing. Consider for meningitis, effusions, severe miliary disease or endobronchial disease.

FOLLOWUP

PATIENT MONITORING
• See every 2-3 months for duration of treatment
• Follow chest x-ray at 2-3 month intervals and again if symptoms change
• If symptoms of liver disease, check liver enzymes, modify drugs if needed

PREVENTION/AVOIDANCE
• PPD screening at 15 months and annually, and persons with high contact
• Careful tracking to identify and treat contagious persons is mandatory. Notify public health department.

POSSIBLE COMPLICATIONS
• Cavitary lesions can be secondarily infected
• Spread to susceptible persons of all ages
• Drug resistance

EXPECTED COURSE AND PROGNOSIS
Generally few complications and full resolution if drugs taken regularly as prescribed for full course

MISCELLANEOUS

ASSOCIATED CONDITIONS
HIV infection

AGE-RELATED FACTORS
Pediatric:
• See every 2-4 weeks
• Children on medications can attend day care and school
• TB more common in infants, pubertal adolescent
• Congenital infection rare with maternal pulmonary disease, more common with miliary disease of maternal bacillemia, endometritis or amniotic aspiration. Consider BCG.
Protocol for newborn contact with infected mother or infected household member
◊ Mother/household member with positive PPD, but no disease: Give newborn PPD check at 1 and 3 months. Treat mother and/or household member with isoniazid.
◊ Mother/household member with positive PPD who has disease and has been treated for more than 2 weeks: For newborn, a chest x-ray and a PPD at 1 month, then a PPD at 3 and 6 months. Treat mother and/or household member and newborn with isoniazid.
◊ Mother/household member with positive PPD who has disease but no treatment to date: Separate newborn until mother and/or household member has been treated for more than 2 weeks. Treat newborn with isoniazid. Evaluate infant as above.

Geriatric:
• Symptoms may be more subtle and may be attributed to associated conditions or to aging
• Should have a PPD prior to entering a chronic-care facility
• Side effects of isoniazid are more pronounced
Others: N/A

PREGNANCY
• Treat pregnant woman with isoniazid, pyridoxine and rifampin. Ethambutol only for active disease after first trimester. Use isoniazid, rifampin for 9 months or ethambutol, rifampin for 18 months.
• Use isoniazid, pyridoxine for skin test converters without disease

SYNONYMS
• TB
• Consumption

ICD-9-CM
• 011.9 tuberculosis
• Multiple modifiers, check carefully for specific type

SEE ALSO
N/A

OTHER NOTES
Bacillus Calmette-Guerin (BCG) vaccine, live attenuate Mycobacterium bovis, only considered in USA for uninfected children at unavoidable risk for whom isoniazid has failed or is not feasible. Severe ulcerations, regional lymphadenitis, lupus vulgaris occurs in 1-10%. Fatal infection in severely immunosuppressed patients can occur. If used in developing country, it is effective for about 10 years, causes a false-positive PPD.

ABBREVIATIONS
PPD = purified protein derivative

REFERENCES
• Centers for Disease Control; Screening for tuberculosis and tuberculosis infection in high risk populations. MMWR 1990;39:1-12
• American Thoracic Society: Treatment of tuberculosis and tuberculosis infections in adults and children. Am rev Respir Dis 1986;134:355
• Red Book, 1993

Author K. Hardy, M.D.

Tuberous sclerosis complex

 BASICS

DESCRIPTION
A genetic, neurocutaneous developmental disorder with variable presentations, a broad clinical spectrum and multi-organ involvement. Included as one of the phakomatoses along with neurofibromatosis, Sturge-Weber disease, von Hippel-Lindau syndrome and ataxia telangiectasia.

Systems affected: May be few and subtle but can encompass multiple types of cutaneous lesions and tumor formation in the central nervous system and one or more areas including the skin, brain, retina, heart, lung, viscera, liver, kidney, bone, teeth, and nails

Genetics:
• Transmitted as an autosomal dominant gene
• Cytosine,adenine repeats on chromosome 16 implicate strongly a gene locus

Incidence/prevalence in USA:
• Reported to affect 1 in 9400 subjects in the population
• A detailed study in Olmstead County, Minnesota reported the point prevalence on December 31, 1989 to be 6.9 per 100,000 persons, and the incidence at birth 6.0 per 100,000 live births

Predominant age: Clinical expression varies so that recognition and diagnosis may be delayed to well after birth

Predominant sex:
• If a parent has the gene, there is a 50-50 chance that each child will have the gene
• Equal sex ratio among probands, but male probands with autism more than female

SIGNS AND SYMPTOMS
• Most cases of tuberous sclerosis complex have more than one feature of the disorder
• Angiofibromata (labeled as adenoma sebaceum) ranging from 0.1-1.0 cm characteristic and often present as facial lesions in a "butterfly" distribution
• Hypopigmented areas mainly on trunk and extremities often the first sign
• Infantile spasms
• Seizure disorders
• Renal cysts
• Pulmonary lymphangiomatosis
• Multiple periventricular calcifications
• Retinal astrocytomas/hamartomas
• Cardiac rhabdomyomas associated with a variety of nonspecific clinical signs
• Mental retardation
• Autism
• Ungual fibromas, multiple
• Dental pits
• Liver hamartomas

CAUSES
An inherited autosomal dominant genetic disorder

RISK FACTORS
Family history

 DIAGNOSIS

DIFFERENTIAL DIAGNOSIS
• Clinical diagnostic criteria are being periodically reviewed and updated
• Polycystic kidney disease
• Other causes for seizure disorders, mental retardation, autistic behavior, traumatic ungual fibromata
• Other neurocutaneous syndromes (see above)

LABORATORY
• Present day diagnostic criteria mainly confined to clinical evaluations
• Abnormal electroencephalogram
• Search for reliable molecular marker and gene appears fruitful

Drugs that may alter lab results: N/A
Disorders that may alter lab results: N/A

PATHOLOGICAL FINDINGS
• Nodular lesions made up largely of irregular groups of glial fibrils, ganglion cells and atypical cells seeming to result from faults in developing tissue combinations as in hamartomas
• Lesions may be sparse at birth
• Calcification of subependymal lesions may not occur until several months after birth
• Facial angiofibromas, ungual fibromas, renal angiomyolipomas are quite specific lesions which may develop months after birth
• Not practical to have age specific criteria. Periodic reassessment in at risk-families necessary.

SPECIAL TESTS
Must rely on clinical diagnostic criteria pending development of reliable molecular marker

IMAGING
• Magnetic resonance imaging (MRI) has become a major diagnostic technique
• With gadolinium enhancement, MRI provides more detailed imaging of characteristic subependymal nodules and cortical white matter tubers

DIAGNOSTIC PROCEDURES
• Biopsy and pathological evaluation often of highest importance. May not be necessary if lesions clinically obvious.
• Hypopigmented spots more clearly seen under ultraviolet light (Wood's lamp)

 TREATMENT

APPROPRIATE HEALTH CARE
• Outpatient except for more severely involved cases and uncontrollable seizures

GENERAL MEASURES
• Team approach with neurological, orthopedic, dermatological, surgical and radiological involvement
• Surgical excision of tumors where and when appropriate
• Physical, occupational and speech therapy
• Social worker, home care, support and genetic counseling important

ACTIVITY
Determined by degree and complexity of involvement

DIET
Balanced nutrition. A ketogenic diet has been used for seizure control.

PATIENT EDUCATION
• Swim alert for seizure prone children
• Seizure frequency changes with fever
• Updated information available from: National Tuberous Sclerosis Association, Inc., 8000 Corporate Drive, Suite 120, Landover, MD. 20785

MEDICATIONS

DRUG(S) OF CHOICE
• Anticonvulsants to control seizures
• Surgeons choice of antibiotic prophylaxis if indicated
Contraindications: N/A
Precautions: See patient education
Significant possible interactions:
• Knowledge of anticonvulsant used is necessary to avoid drug interactions especially with antibiotics
• Refer to manufacturer's profile of each drug

ALTERNATIVE DRUGS N/A

FOLLOWUP

PATIENT MONITORING
• Periodic reassessment of at-risk individuals very important in establishing clinical diagnosis
• Clinical features of patients periodically reviewed and updated

PREVENTION/AVOIDANCE Genetic counseling

POSSIBLE COMPLICATION See above

EXPECTED COURSE AND PROGNOSIS Variable. Decreased survival curves compared with general population.

MISCELLANEOUS

ASSOCIATED CONDITIONS N/A

AGE-RELATED FACTORS
Pediatric: N/A
Geriatric: N/A
Others: Stigmata may be present at or shortly after birth or may become apparent in late childhood or adulthood

PREGNANCY Genetic counseling

SYNONYMS Bourneville's disease

ICD-9-CM
SEE ALSO: N/A

OTHER NOTES N/A

ABBREVIATIONS
• TS = tuberous sclerosis
• TSC = tuberous sclerosis complex

REFERENCES
• Shepherd, C.W., et al.: Tuberous sclerosis complex in Olmsted County, Minnesota, 1950-1989 Department of Health Sciences Research, Mayo Clinic, Rochester, MN 55905. Arch Neurol 1991 Apr;48(4):400-1
• Wilson, J.D., et al.(eds.): Harrison's Principles of Internal Medicine. 12th Ed. New York, McGraw-Hill, 1991
• Perspective Newsletter, National Tuberous Sclerosis Association, Inc.Spring/Summer, Fall, Winter publications

Author J. Dix, M.D. & D. Lowder, R.N.

Tularemia

BASICS

DESCRIPTION Acute infection with Francisella tularensis. Incubation averages 3 to 4 days. May be ulceroglandular, glandular, typhoidal, oculoglandular, or oropharyngeal.
System(s) affected: Skin/Exocrine, Pulmonary, Cardiovascular, Hemic/Lymphatic/Immunologic
Genetics: N/A
Incidence/Prevalence in USA: (Incidence) 0.1 per 100,000
Predominant age: All ages
Predominant sex: Male > Female

SIGNS AND SYMPTOMS
• Nearly all cases have fever, chills, fatigue, malaise
Ulceroglandular (3/4 of cases)
 ◊ Non-healing ulcer
 ◊ Regional adenopathy
 ◊ Failure of cephalosporin treatment
Glandular
 ◊ Localized adenopathy
 ◊ No ulcer
Typhoidal
 ◊ Systemic febrile illness
 ◊ Fulminating sepsis
 ◊ Pleuropulmonary disease
 ◊ No ulcer
Oropharyngeal
 ◊ Exudative pharyngitis
 ◊ Membranous pharyngitis
 ◊ Cervical adenopathy
Oculoglandular
 ◊ Purulent conjunctivitis
 ◊ Preauricular adenopathy
 ◊ Cervical adenopathy

CAUSES
Inoculation of F. tularensis via:
 ◊ Tick bite
 ◊ Deer fly bite
 ◊ Cat bite
 ◊ Aerosol inhalation
 ◊ Contact with infected carcass (can penetrate unbroken skin)
 ◊ Ingestion

RISK FACTORS
• Location in endemic area (> 50% cases in AR, MO, OK, TN, TX)
• Outdoor work
• Rural residence
• Game handling (butchers, hunters, farmers, fur-handlers)
• Laboratory work

DIAGNOSIS

DIFFERENTIAL DIAGNOSIS
Ulceroglandular/glandular
 ◊ Staphylococcal infections
 ◊ Streptococcal infections
 ◊ Pasteurella infections
 ◊ Lymphogranuloma venereum
 ◊ Cat-scratch disease
 ◊ Sporotrichosis
 ◊ Plague
 ◊ Toxoplasmosis
 ◊ Viral pneumonia
Typhoidal
 ◊ Typhoid fever
 ◊ Infectious mononucleosis
 ◊ Non-typhoid salmonellosis
 ◊ Brucellosis
 ◊ Q fever
 ◊ Psittacosis
 ◊ Legionellosis
 ◊ Rocky Mountain spotted fever
 ◊ Ehrlichiosis
 ◊ Borreliosis (including Lyme disease)
 ◊ Tick-borne typhus
 ◊ Viral pneumonia
Oropharyngeal
 ◊ Streptococcal pharyngitis
 ◊ Viral pharyngitis
 ◊ Diphtheric pharyngitis
 ◊ Infectious mononucleosis
 ◊ Viral pneumonia

LABORATORY
• Fourfold rise in antibody titer (peak in 4-8 weeks)
• Convalescent titer of 160 or greater
• Delayed growth on specific media or blood culture
• Elevated ESR
• Normal WBC, but increased percentage of polymorphonuclear neutrophils (PMN)
Drugs that may alter lab results: N/A
Disorders that may alter lab results: Brucella antibodies may cross-react

PATHOLOGICAL FINDINGS
• Necrotic areas in liver, spleen, other organs
• Caseating granulomata
• Microscopic foci with PMN's, macrophages, giant cells

SPECIAL TESTS
• Referral to specialized lab
• Pleomorphic Gram-negative coccobacilli on smear
• Metabolic profile of isolate
• Specific immunofluorescent stain of smear
• Foshay's skin test
• Culture ulcer

IMAGING
Chest x-ray may show ill-defined infiltrates, lobar consolidation, or pleural effusion

DIAGNOSTIC PROCEDURES
• Lymph node aspiration
• Thoracentesis
• Thorough history of patient's contact with wild rodents or exposure to arthropod vectors

TREATMENT

APPROPRIATE HEALTH CARE
Inpatient during work-up and early treatment. Outpatient as soon as possible, depending on severity.

GENERAL MEASURES
• Isolation not needed for patient, but handle secretions carefully
• Hydration, fever control, antibiotics
• Wet saline dressings for skin lesions
• Incision and drainage of abscesses

ACTIVITY
As tolerated

DIET
As tolerated, high caloric, easily digestible

PATIENT EDUCATION
• Person-to-person transmission not documented
• See Prevention/avoidance
• Vaccine for high-risk persons

MEDICATIONS

DRUG(S) OF CHOICE Streptomycin 15-20 mg/kg IM per day, divided bid for 7-14 days (drug may not be available commercially)
Contraindications: Known hypersensitivity, pregnancy
Precautions:
• Long-term therapy may produce eighth nerve damage
• Reduce dose in renal dysfunction
• Long-term therapy may produce renal dysfunction
• Use with care post-anesthesia (respiratory paralysis), and in patients with myasthenia gravis
Significant possible interactions: Other aminoglycosides, cephaloridine, polymyxin B, amphotericin B, colistin, muscle relaxants, paralyzing anesthetic agents

ALTERNATIVE DRUGS
• Gentamicin
• Tetracycline
• Doxycycline
• Chloramphenicol

FOLLOWUP

PATIENT MONITORING
• Monitor eighth nerve function in long-term therapy
• Monitor renal function in long-term therapy

PREVENTION/AVOIDANCE
• Tick repellents
• Remove tick by grasping near mouthparts and lifting
• Avoid squeezing body of embedded tick
• Wear gloves while dressing game
• Avoid contact if game appeared ill
• Lab workers - vaccine possibly protective. Wear protective hoods.
• Cooking wild game and birds thoroughly

POSSIBLE COMPLICATIONS
• Lung abscess
• Adult respiratory distress syndrome
• Hepatic dysfunction
• Rhabdomyolysis
• Renal failure
• Osteomyelitis, meningitis, endocarditis, pericarditis, peritonitis
• Mediastinitis

EXPECTED COURSE AND PROGNOSIS
• Cure is usually complete if treated early and vigorously
• Immunity is lifelong
• Mortality is 1-3%, higher in typhoidal-type disease

MISCELLANEOUS

ASSOCIATED CONDITIONS
• Other arthropod-borne diseases
• Conjunctivitis tularemic
• Bacteremia
• Atypical pneumonia

AGE-RELATED FACTORS
Pediatric: N/A
Geriatric: Complications more likely, mortality rate higher
Others: More likely to occur in outdoor-type, young adult males

PREGNANCY Streptomycin may cause fetal 8th nerve damage

SYNONYMS
• Rabbit fever
• Deer-fly fever
• Pasteurella tularensis
• Bacterium tularense
• Tick fever
• Ohara's disease
• Francis' disease

ICD-9-CM 021.0-021.9

SEE ALSO N/A

OTHER NOTES N/A

ABBREVIATIONS N/A

REFERENCES
• Mandell, G.L. (ed.): Principles and Practice of Infectious Diseases. 3rd Ed. New York, Churchill Livingstone, 1990
• Feigin, R.D. & Cherry J.D.: Textbook of Pediatric Infectious Disease. 2nd Ed. Philadelphia, W.B. Saunders Co., 1987

Author G. Elders, M.D.

Turner's syndrome

 BASICS

DESCRIPTION Edema of hands and feet and excess skin of the neck are presenting features during infancy. As children, girls are short and may have left sided heart or aortic abnormalities. Primary amenorrhea or delayed onset of puberty with short stature are important clues during adolescence.
System(s) affected: Nervous, Reproductive, Endocrine/Metabolic, Cardiovascular, Musculoskeletal, Renal/Urologic
Genetics: usually sporadic
Incidence in USA: 40 per 100,000 female births
Prevalence in USA: Unknown
Predominant age: All ages
Predominant sex: Female only

SIGNS AND SYMPTOMS
• Frequencies are for classic 45,X and vary somewhat with other chromosomal abnormalities associated with Turner's syndrome
• Short stature (98%)
• Gonadal dysgenesis (95%)
• Lymphedema (70%)
• Broad chest (75%)
• Hypoplastic, wide-spaced nipples (78%)
• Prominent, anomalous ears (70%)
• High palate (82%)
• Short neck (80%)
• Webbing of neck (65%)
• Low hairline (80%)
• Cubitus valgus (75%)
• Short fourth metacarpal (65%)
• Nail hypoplasia (75%)
• Excess nevi (70%)
• Renal anomalies (60%)
• Heart malformations (30%)
• Hearing impairment (70%)

CAUSES Monosomy for all or part of the X chromosome can result in symptoms consistent with Turner's syndrome

RISK FACTORS Familial chromosome translocations involving the X chromosome can increase the risk that an individual will conceive a child with Turner's syndrome

 DIAGNOSIS

DIFFERENTIAL DIAGNOSIS
<u>Short stature</u>
◊ Noonans syndrome
◊ Hypothyroidism
◊ Familial short stature
◊ Léri-Weil syndrome
◊ Brachydactyly E
◊ Growth hormone deficiency
◊ Glucocorticoid excess
◊ Klippel-Feil anomaly
◊ Short stature due to chronic disease
<u>Amenorrhea or delayed puberty</u>
◊ Pure gonadal dysgenesis
◊ Stein-Leventhal syndrome
◊ Primary/secondary amenorrhea
<u>Lymphedema</u>
◊ Hereditary congenital lymphedema
◊ Milroy's disease
◊ Lymphedema with recurrent cholestasis
◊ Lymphedema with intestinal lymphangiectasia
<u>Other</u>
◊ Multiple pterygium syndrome
◊ Pseudohypoparathyroid

LABORATORY
• Chromosome analysis (a buccal smear is not an adequate test to rule out the diagnosis)
• At puberty FSH and LH levels may approach castration levels. FSH may be transiently high in infancy
Drugs that may alter lab results: N/A
Disorders that may alter lab results: N/A

PATHOLOGICAL FINDINGS
• Ovarian dysgenesis (> 90%)
• Renal - horseshoe kidney, double collecting system (60%)
• Cardiac - bicuspid aortic valve, coarctation of aorta, valvular aortic stenosis (70% with heart defects also have coarctation)
• Bone dysplasia (> 50%)
• Gonadoblastomas in X/XY mosaics

SPECIAL TESTS
• Upper/lower extremity blood pressures
• ECG

IMAGING
• Renal ultrasound
• Cardiac ultrasound

DIAGNOSTIC PROCEDURES N/A

 TREATMENT

APPROPRIATE HEALTH CARE
Outpatient

GENERAL MEASURES
Once diagnosis is confirmed by karyotype, the following measures are appropriate:
• Cardiology evaluation to include upper and lower extremity blood pressures, and echocardiography. If an abnormality exists, prophylactic antibiotics may be indicated (e.g., dental procedures).
• Renal ultrasound or intravenous pyelography
• Thyroid function test and antithyroid antibodies
• Routine hearing examination
• Removal of gonads in X/XY individuals
• Therapy for gonadal failure is necessary for girls who do not enter puberty spontaneously to start at an age appropriate time. Replacement therapy usually begins with one to two years of low dose estrogen replacement followed by larger dose estrogens cycled with progesterone. Birth control pills can be used as maintenance therapy once menses and secondary sexual characteristics have been established. Therapy should continue into the late forties. Routine gynecologic evaluation is indicated. Infertility is the general rule, but alternatives such as in vitro fertilization and embryo transfer may be an option.
• Growth retardation has been managed with sex hormone replacement, anabolic agents, and most recently human recombinant growth hormone (hrGH). Current data shows that some Turner's syndrome patients increase final height attainment with hrGH treatment. Ideally, if hrGH therapy is provided, it is best started before significant growth deceleration occurs (between 3-10 years of age) and in a daily subcutaneous dose of approximately 0.05 mg/kg.
• Physical appearance may be enhanced by plastic surgery for inner canthal folds, protruding auricles and webbed neck.
• Intelligence is usually normal. Problems may exist in non-verbal areas such as imagining objects in relationship to one another. If concerns about school performance arise, they should be appropriately evaluated and treated.
• Regular check-ups are recommended to detect problems early. Physicians and health care givers should be aware of the social problems and emotional problems associated with issues such as short stature and infertility.

ACTIVITY Normal other than limitations that may be placed on individuals with similar cardiac or renal abnormalities.

DIET Normal, but there is a tendency toward obesity

PATIENT EDUCATION
• Both families and patients need a thorough explanation of the condition and its management especially in regards to sexual development and growth. Jones/Smith suggest advising patient between age 8 and adolescence that she will probably not bear children.

Excellent patient educational materials include:

◊ Plumridge, D.: Good things come in small packages: the whys and hows of Turner's Syndrome. Crippled Children's Division, University of Oregon Health Sciences Center, Portland, OR 97203.

◊ Rieser, P.A., Underwood, L.E.: Turner's syndrome: a guide for families. Turner's Syndrome Society, York University, ASB 006, 4700 Keele St., Downsview, Ontario, Canada, M3J 1P3, (416)667-3773 or Turner's Syndrome Society, 3539 Tonkawood Rd., Minnetonka, MN 55345, (612)938-3118

MEDICATIONS

DRUG(S) OF CHOICE N/A
Contraindications: N/A
Precautions: N/A
Significant possible interactions: N/A

ALTERNATIVE DRUGS N/A

FOLLOWUP

PATIENT MONITORING
• Regular measurement of growth parameters
• Regular blood pressure checks
• Annual urine analysis if renal abnormality is present
• Monitor for signs of hypothyroidism
• Regular hearing testing
• Regular eye exams
• Monitor for blood in stool

PREVENTION/AVOIDANCE Prenatal
detection is available for couples who carry chromosomal translocations which would put them at high risk or for couples who have had an affected child. There is no in utero treatment, but pregnancy termination is an option if a fetus with Turner's syndrome is identified

POSSIBLE COMPLICATIONS
Complications are related to associated abnormalities

EXPECTED COURSE AND
PROGNOSIS Most girls with Turner's syndrome can be expected to lead reasonably normal lives with appropriate medical management

MISCELLANEOUS

ASSOCIATED CONDITIONS
• Hashimoto's thyroiditis
• Hypothyroidism
• Alopecia
• Vitiligo
• Gastrointestinal disorders
• Carbohydrate intolerance

AGE-RELATED FACTORS
Pediatric: N/A
Geriatric: N/A
Others: N/A

PREGNANCY N/A

SYNONYMS
• Ullrich-Turner syndrome
• Bonnevie-Ullrich
• XO syndrome
• Monosomy X
• Short stature-sexual infantilism
• Gonadal dysgenesis

ICD-9-CM 758.6

SEE ALSO
• Amenorrhea
• Coarctation of the aorta
• Hypothyroidism, adult
• Thyroiditis

OTHER NOTES N/A

ABBREVIATIONS N/A

REFERENCES
• Buyse, M.L. (ed.): Birth Defects Encyclopedia. Cambridge, Massachusetts, Blackwell Scientific Publications, 1990
• Hall, J.G. & Gilchrist, D.M.: Turner's Syndrome and Its Variants. Pediatr Clinics NA, 37(6):1421-1440, 1990
• Jones, K.L.: Smith's Recognizable Patterns of Human Malformation. Philadelphia, W.B. Saunders Co., 1988

Author J. Waterson, M.D., Ph.D.

Typhoid fever

 BASICS

DESCRIPTION
Typhoid fever is an acute systemic illness unique to humans caused by Salmonella typhi. It is a classic example of enteric fever caused by the Salmonella family of bacteria.
• It is endemic in Third World countries where sanitation is suboptimal. Majority of cases in North America are acquired after travel to endemic areas.
• Mode of transmission is fecal-oral through ingestion of contaminated food (commonly poultry), water and milk. Incubation period varies from 7 to 21 days.
System(s) affected: Gastrointestinal, Pulmonary, Skin/Exocrine
Genetics: N/A
Incidence in USA: 300-500 cases per year
Prevalence in USA: N/A
Predominant age: All ages
Predominant sex: Male = Female

SIGNS AND SYMPTOMS
• Fever
• Headache
• Malaise
• Abdominal discomfort/bloating/constipation
• Diarrhea (less common)
• Dry cough
• Confusion/lethargy
• Rose spot (transient erythematous maculopapular rash in anterior thorax or upper abdomen)
• Splenomegaly
• Hepatomegaly
• Cervical adenopathy
• Relative bradycardia
• Conjunctivitis

CAUSES
Salmonella typhi

RISK FACTORS
Must be considered in any patient presenting with fever after tropical travel or exposed to chronic carrier

 DIAGNOSIS

DIFFERENTIAL DIAGNOSIS
• Malaria
• "Enteric fever-like" syndrome caused by Yersinia enterocolitica, Yersinia pseudotuberculosis, and Campylobacter fetus
• Enteric fever caused by non-typhi Salmonella
• Infectious hepatitis
• Atypical pneumonia
• Infectious mononucleosis
• Subacute bacterial endocarditis
• Tuberculosis
• Brucellosis
• Q fever

LABORATORY
• Definitive diagnosis by isolation of S. typhi from blood. Isolation of S. typhi in sputum, urine or stool is presumptive diagnosis in typical clinical presentation.
• Serology is nonspecific and usually not useful
• If multiple blood cultures are negative or in patients with prior antibiotic therapy, diagnostic yield is better with bone marrow culture
• Anemia, leukopenia (neutropenia), thrombocytopenia or evidence of DIC (disseminated intravascular coagulopathy) are supportive evidence. Elevated liver enzymes are commonly seen.
Drugs that may alter lab results
• Prior antibiotic therapy
• Vaccination
Disorders that may alter lab results: N/A

PATHOLOGICAL FINDINGS
Classically, mononuclear proliferation involving lymphoid tissue of intestinal tract especially Peyer's patch in terminal ileum

SPECIAL TESTS
N/A

IMAGING
Serial plain abdominal films for evidence of intestinal perforation

DIAGNOSTIC PROCEDURES
• Bone marrow aspirate for culture is rarely indicated
• String test (Enterotest) may increase diagnostic yield

 TREATMENT

APPROPRIATE HEALTH CARE
• Inpatient if acutely ill
• Outpatient for less ill patient or for carrier

GENERAL MEASURES
• Fluid and electrolyte support
• Strict isolation of patient's linen, stool and urine
• Monitor clinically with aid of serial plain abdominal films for evidence of perforation, usually in the third to fourth week of illness
• Indication for treatment must be determined on an individual basis. Factors to be considered are age, public health (food handler, chronic care facilities, medical personnel), intolerance to antibiotics, and evidence of biliary tract disease.
• Cholecystectomy may be warranted in carriers with cholelithiasis, relapse after therapy, or intolerance to antimicrobial therapy
• For hemorrhage - need blood transfusion and shock management

ACTIVITY
Bedrest initially, then as tolerated

DIET
If abdominal symptoms severe, nothing by mouth. With improvement, normal low-residue diet, possibly enriched in calories.

PATIENT EDUCATION
• Discussion of chronic carrier state and its complications
• For family members, travelers or workers at risk, provide hygiene education, possibly vaccination

MEDICATIONS

DRUG(S) OF CHOICE
• Chloramphenicol: Children - 50 mg/kg/d po qid x 2 weeks; adult dose - 50 mg/kg per day, divided each 6 hours x 2 weeks,
or
• Ampicillin: Children - 100 mg/kg/d qid po x 2 weeks; adults - 500 mg each 6 hours x 2 weeks,
or
• Ciprofloxacin 500 mg po bid x 2 weeks (avoid in children),
or
• Ceftriaxone 1-2 gm IV qd x 2 weeks,
or
• Cefoperazone 2-4 g IV q 6-12 hours x 2 weeks
<u>Chronic carrier state</u>
   ◊ Is treated with ampicillin 4-5 gram/day plus probenecid 2 grams/day qid x 6 weeks (for patients with normal functioning gallbladder without evidence of cholelithiasis)
   ◊ Ciprofloxacin 500 mg po bid x 4-6 weeks is also efficacious
Note: Chloramphenicol resistance - reported in Mexico, South America, Central America, Southeast Asia, India, Pakistan, Middle and Africa
Contraindications: Refer to manufacturer's profile of each drug
Precautions: Rarely, Jarisch-Herxheimer reaction post antimicrobial therapy
Significant possible interactions: Refer to manufacturer's profile of each drug

ALTERNATIVE DRUGS
Trimethoprim-sulfamethoxazole

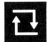

FOLLOWUP

PATIENT MONITORING

PREVENTION/AVOIDANCE
• For travel to an endemic area, consider vaccination for typhoid, parenterally (phenol-killed or Vi vaccines) or live oral vaccine (Ty21a)
• Avoid tap water, salad/raw vegetables, unpeeled fruits, dairy products in tropical travel
• Avoid poultry or poultry products left unrefrigerated for prolonged period of time

POSSIBLE COMPLICATIONS
• Intestinal hemorrhage and perforation in distal ileum
• Patient may become chronic carrier state (up to 3%) defined as persistent stool excretor for greater than 1 year
• Predilection for seeding in the biliary tract exists and may become a focus for relapse of typhoid fever. Most common in female and the elderly (> 50 years old).
• Osteomyelitis especially in sickle cell anemia, systemic lupus erthyematosus, hematologic neoplasms and immunosuppressed hosts
• Endovascular infection in the elderly and in patients with history of by-pass operation or aneurysm
• Rarely, endocarditis or meningitis

EXPECTED COURSE AND
PROGNOSIS   Overall prognosis good with therapy. 2% mortality rate, 15% relapse rate

MISCELLANEOUS

ASSOCIATED CONDITIONS   N/A

AGE-RELATED FACTORS
Pediatric: Disease more critical in infants, but may be milder in children
Geriatric: Disease more serious in elderly
Others: N/A

PREGNANCY   Ciprofloxacin not
recommended for pregnant women

SYNONYMS
• Typhoid
• Typhus abdominalis
• Enteric fever

ICD-9-CM   002.0

SEE ALSO   N/A

OTHER NOTES   N/A

ABBREVIATIONS   N/A

REFERENCES   Mandell, G.L. (ed.):
Principles and Practice of Infectious Diseases. 3rd Ed. New York, Churchill Livingstone, 1990

Author   D.W. MacPherson, M.D., & T.C. Yang, M.D.

Typhus fevers

BASICS

DESCRIPTION Acute infectious diseases caused by three species of rickettsiae
• Epidemic typhus - human to human transmission by body louse. Primarily in unclean circumstances such as refugee camps, war, famine and disaster. Recrudescent disease, occurring years after initial infection can be source of human outbreak. Flying squirrels also reservoir.
• Endemic (murine) typhus - infection of rodents. To humans by rat flea.
• Scrub typhus - infection of chiggers and of rodents. To humans by the chigger. Primarily in Asia and the Western Pacific.
System(s) affected: Endocrine/Metabolic, Pulmonary, Skin/Exocrine, Hemic/Lymphatic/Immunologic
Genetics: N/A
Incidence/Prevalence in USA:
• Epidemic typhus - rare
• Endemic typhus - fewer than 100 cases annually, primarily in gulf states, especially South Texas, under-reporting suspected
• Scrub typhus - none except for travelers returning from endemic areas
Predominant age: N/A
Predominant sex: N/A

SIGNS AND SYMPTOMS
General
  ◊ Acute onset
  ◊ Fever
  ◊ Chills
  ◊ Headache
  ◊ Myalgia
  ◊ Malaise
  ◊ Diffuse organ involvement, e.g., intestine, liver, heart, kidneys, brain
Epidemic typhus
  ◊ Incubation period about 1 week
  ◊ Macular or maculopapular rash beginning on trunk about fifth day of illness
  ◊ Nonproductive cough
  ◊ Pulmonary infiltrates
Endemic typhus
  ◊ Incubation period 1-2 weeks
  ◊ Macular or maculopapular rash beginning on trunk third to fifth day of illness
Scrub typhus
  ◊ Incubation period 1-3 weeks
  ◊ Eschar at bite site
  ◊ Regional lymphadenopathy
  ◊ Generalized lymphadenopathy
  ◊ Splenomegaly
  ◊ Macular or maculopapular rash beginning on trunk about the fifth day of illness
  ◊ Relative bradycardia early in disease
  ◊ Ocular pain
  ◊ Conjunctival injection

CAUSES
• Epidemic typhus by Rickettsia prowazekii
• Endemic typhus by R. typhi
• Scrub typhus by R. tsutsugamushi

RISK FACTORS
• Exposure to vectors, e.g., travel to certain countries
• Elderly may have more severe disease
• Laboratory worker

DIAGNOSIS

DIFFERENTIAL DIAGNOSIS
• Any acute febrile disease
• Rocky Mountain spotted fever
• Meningococcemia
• Bacterial meningitis
• Measles
• Rubella
• Toxoplasmosis
• Leptospirosis
• Typhoid fever
• Dengue
• Relapsing fever
• Secondary syphilis
• Infectious mononucleosis

LABORATORY
• WBC usually normal
• Abnormalities reflecting the particular organs affected
• Weil-Felix serological reaction may be positive; test limited to mid-illness or after, and by low sensitivity and non-specificity. Epidemic and endemic typhus, fourfold titer rise or titer > 1/320 to OX-19. Scrub typhus, fourfold rise in titer to OX-K.
• Hyponatremia in severe cases
• Hypoalbuminemia in severe cases
Drugs that may alter lab results:
Antibiotics
Disorders that may alter lab results: N/A

PATHOLOGICAL FINDINGS Diffuse vasculitis

SPECIAL TESTS Specific serological test showing a rising antibody titer. Isolation of rickettsia should be undertaken only in special laboratories to minimize risk of laboratory-acquired infection.

IMAGING N/A

DIAGNOSTIC PROCEDURES N/A

TREATMENT

APPROPRIATE HEALTH CARE
Outpatient unless severely ill

GENERAL MEASURES
• Protect agitated patient from injury
• Skin and mouth care
• Supportive care for the severely ill, directed to the complications

ACTIVITY Bedrest during acute stages, otherwise as tolerated

DIET As tolerated

PATIENT EDUCATION
• Prevention information to travelers
• Vaccination information

Typhus fevers

 MEDICATIONS

DRUG(S) OF CHOICE
• Treatment should begin when diagnosis is reasonably likely and continue until improved and afebrile for a minimum of 48 hours
Children over 8 years and adults:
◊ Tetracycline (Achromycin), or a congener, orally 25 mg per kg initially, and then 25 mg per kg daily in equally divided doses every 6 hours
◊ If severely ill, may use doxycycline IV, adults 100 mg every 12 hours, children >8 years 5 mg per kg in 24 hours (maximum of 200 mg/24 hrs)
Children under 8 years, pregnant women or if typhoid fever is possible cause of illness:
◊ Chloramphenicol (Chloromycetin) orally 50 mg per kg initially, and then 50 mg per kg daily in equally divided doses every 6 hours
◊ If severely ill, chloramphenicol (Chloromycetin) sodium succinate intravenously 20 mg per kg initially infused in 30-45 minutes, and then 50 mg per kg daily infused in equally divided doses every 6 hours until orally tolerable.
Contraindications: N/A
Precautions: Refer to manufacturer's profile of each drug
Significant possible interactions: Refer to manufacturer's profile of each drug

ALTERNATIVE DRUGS
• Doxycycline (Vibramycin) single oral dose of 100 or 200 mg in refugee camps, disasters or limited medical services
• Isolated reports indicate that erythromycin and ciprofloxacin are effective

 FOLLOWUP

PATIENT MONITORING Severely ill patients should be observed regularly in hospital. Outpatients checked periodically as improvement is evident.

PREVENTION/AVOIDANCE
• Avoid vectors for each disease, e.g., scrub typhus; wear protective clothing and use insect repellents, endemic typhus; practice ectoparasite and rodent control, and epidemic typhus; delousing
• Epidemic typhus vaccine considered for persons at high risk of exposure

POSSIBLE COMPLICATIONS
Consequences of specific organ system involvement in the second week, e.g., azotemia, meningoencephalitis, seizures, delirium, coma, myocardial failure, hyponatremia, hypoalbuminemia, hypovolemia, and shock

EXPECTED COURSE AND PROGNOSIS
• Recovery expected if treatment is instituted before complications
• Relapses may follow treatment, especially if initiated within 48 hours of onset (this is not an indication to delay treatment). Relapses treated same as primary disease.
• Without treatment the mortality is 40-60% in epidemic, 1-2% in endemic, and up to 30% in scrub typhus. Mortality higher among the elderly.

 MISCELLANEOUS

ASSOCIATED CONDITIONS N/A

AGE-RELATED FACTORS
Pediatric: N/A
Geriatric: N/A
Others: N/A

PREGNANCY N/A

SYNONYMS
• Louse-borne typhus
• Brill-Zinsser disease
• Murine typhus

ICD-9-CM
• Epidemic typhus 080.0
• Endemic typhus 081.0

SEE ALSO N/A

OTHER NOTES
• Severe headache often intractable and not eased by the usual drugs
• Report case to Health Department

ABBREVIATIONS N/A

REFERENCES
• Mandel, G.L., Douglas, R.G. & Bennett, J.E., (eds.): Principles and Practice of Infectious Diseases. 3rd Ed. New York, Churchill Livingstone, 1990
• Dumlev, J.S., Taylor, J.P. & Walker, D.H.: Clinical and laboratory features of murine typhus in south Texas, 1980 through 1987. JAMA 266: 1365-1370, 1991

Author W. Sawyer, M.D.

Ulcerative colitis

 BASICS

DESCRIPTION One of a group of inflammatory bowel diseases of unknown etiology characterized by intermittent bouts of inflammation of all or portions of the colon. Manifested by recurrences of rectal bleeding and various constitutional symptoms.
System(s) affected: Gastrointestinal
Genetics: Family aggregates common, positive family history in 8-11%. More likely vertical than horizontal. More common in Jews.
Incidence/Prevalence in USA: 70-150 per 100,000. Incidence 6-8 new cases per 100,000 population.
Predominant age: Between ages of 15 and 35 years. There is a second and smaller peak in the 7th decade.
Predominant sex: Male = Female

SIGNS AND SYMPTOMS
• Bloody diarrhea
• Abdominal pain
• Fever
• Weight loss
• Arthralgias and arthritis (15-20%)
• Spondylitis (3-6%)
• Ocular complications (4-10%) includes episcleritis, uveitis, cataracts, keratopathy, marginal corneal ulceration, and central serous retinopathy
• Erythema nodosum
• Pyoderma gangrenosum
• Aphthous ulcers of mouth (5-10%)
• Asymptomatic fatty liver common - occasional hepatomegaly
• Pericholangitis (uncommon)
• Primary sclerosing cholangitis (1-4%)
• Cirrhosis of liver (1-5%)
• Bile duct carcinoma
• Thromboembolic disease (1-6%)
• Pericarditis (rare)
• Amyloidosis (rare)

CAUSES Unknown (genetic, infectious, immunologic, and psychological factors have all been suggested)

RISK FACTORS
• None known
• Higher incidence in Jews and those with positive family history
• Negative association with smoking

 DIAGNOSIS

DIFFERENTIAL DIAGNOSIS
• Other sources of rectal bleeding including hemorrhoids, neoplasms, colonic diverticuli, A-V malformation, Crohn's disease
• Infectious causes of diarrhea including bacteria (Enterotoxigenic E.Coli, E.Coli 0157:H7, Salmonella, Shigella, Aeromonas, Plesiomonas), parasitic (entamoeba histolytica)
• "Gay bowel" syndrome causes (herpes simplex, Chlamydia trachomatous, Cryptosporidium, Isospora belli, cytomegalovirus, and other infectious causes as listed above)
• Antibiotic associated diarrhea
• Radiation proctitis
• Ischemic proctitis

LABORATORY
• Nonspecific. Usually reflects the degree of severity of the bleeding and inflammation.
• Anemia may reflect chronic disease as well as iron deficiency from blood loss
• Leukocytosis during exacerbation
• Elevated sedimentation rate
• Electrolyte abnormalities, especially hypokalemia
• Hypoalbuminemia
• Elevated liver function tests (if there is associated hepatobiliary disease)
Drugs that may alter lab results: N/A
Disorders that may alter lab results: N/A

PATHOLOGICAL FINDINGS
Inflammation of the colonic mucosa with ulcerations. These appear hyperemic and hemorrhagic. Rectum involved 95% of time. The inflammation extends proximally in a continuous fashion, but for a variable distance. May affect terminal ileum - referred to as "backwash ileitis."

SPECIAL TESTS None

IMAGING Air contrast barium enema

DIAGNOSTIC PROCEDURES
• Sigmoidoscopy, may include biopsy
• Colonoscopy, may include biopsy for evaluation for premalignant features; also used to differentiate from Crohn's disease, and to investigate abnormalities that appear on radiography, such as stricture or mass lesions. Colonscopy useful to define the extent of involvement and specific segments involved as this has bearing on therapy and prognosis.

 TREATMENT

APPROPRIATE HEALTH CARE
Outpatient, except for severe exacerbations which may require hospitalization

GENERAL MEASURES
• Goal is to control inflammation, prevent complications, replace nutritional losses and blood volume
• Complications or refractory disease may require surgical intervention

ACTIVITY Full activity as tolerated

DIET No specific diet; milk products not withheld unless an associated lactase deficiency exists

PATIENT EDUCATION
• Close doctor/patient relationship encouraged
• Self-help organizations such as:
National Foundation for Ileitis and Colitis 444 Park Avenue S., 11th Floor, New York, NY 10016-7374, (800)343-3637

MEDICATIONS

DRUG(S) OF CHOICE
• Sulfasalazine is treatment of choice both for mild flare-ups and for the chronic treatment used to decrease the frequency of relapses (dosage range 1-4 grams daily)
• Disease limited to the rectum (proctitis) or to the left side of the colon and rectum (proctosigmoiditis) may be treated topically (steroid enemas or the new 5-Aminosalicylic acid (5-ASA) enemas or suppositories - dosages and dosage schedules are not yet well standardized)
• Oral or parenteral corticosteroids are used for more severe flare-ups (e.g., prednisone 40-60 mg qd, gradually tapered off over two months)
• Approximately 10% of patients have chronic disease activity and require continuous low - moderate steroid doses
• Newer agents include oral 5-ASA derivatives. Topical use of sodium cromoglycate and sucralfate being studied.
• Immunomodulators such as azathioprine, 6-mercaptopurine, methotrexate, levamisole, and cyclosporine A are controversial in a disease potentially curable by colectomy. However, have been shown to be effective in patients who either refuse surgery or are poor surgical candidates.
• Antimicrobial agents (anti-mycobacteriums and metronidazole) sometimes useful in Crohn's disease but not in ulcerative colitis
• Antidiarrheal agents, diphenoxylate and loperamide may be used to help control diarrhea, but require careful monitoring since they may precipitate toxic megacolon
Contraindications:
• Allergy to any of above agents
• Refer to manufacturer's profile of each drug
Precautions: Use of antidiarrheal agents in severe disease could precipitate toxic megacolon
Significant possible interactions: Refer to manufacturer's profile of each drug

ALTERNATIVE DRUGS   Included in Drug(s) of Choice

FOLLOWUP

PATIENT MONITORING   Regularly scheduled appointments are important to evaluate for disease activity, appearance of complications, and the psychological and social well being of the patient

PREVENTION/AVOIDANCE
Colonoscopic evaluation for cancer surveillance with biopsy evaluation of the mucosa for evidence of dysplasia must be performed every 1-2 years after the disease has been present for 7-8 years. This is particularly important in pancolitis. Low grade dysplasia warrants more frequent evaluation (e.g., every 3-6 months) and high grade dysplasia (or low grade dysplasia within a mass) warrant consideration of colectomy.
• Annual liver tests
• Cholangiography for cholestasis

POSSIBLE COMPLICATIONS
• Perforation
• Toxic megacolon
• Liver disease
• Stricture formation (less than Crohn's disease)
• Colon cancer (may occur in as many as 30% of those with pancolitis for 25 years). Incidence of cancer is cumulative and begins after 7-8 years of disease; risk may be considerably less in left sided disease.

EXPECTED COURSE AND PROGNOSIS
• Course extremely variable; mortality for initial attack approximately 5%. Approximately 75-85% of patients experience relapse, and up to 20% in some studies eventually require colectomy.
• Colon cancer risk is the single most important risk factor affecting long-term prognosis
• Left-sided colitis and ulcerative proctitis have very favorable prognosis with probable normal life span

MISCELLANEOUS

ASSOCIATED CONDITIONS   Ankylosing spondylitis

AGE-RELATED FACTORS
Pediatric:
• Approximately 20% of patients are 21 years or younger
• Cancer surveillance is important since occurrence of cancer relates to the duration and extent of disease, whether frequently symptomatic or not
Geriatric: Increased mortality with initial attack in patients over 60
Others: N/A

PREGNANCY
• Outcome of pregnancy similar to general population. One study showed 30% of those with inactive disease at onset of pregnancy relapsed and 14% did so in first trimester.
• Treatment with sulfasalazine does not seem to affect outcome of pregnancy
• Recommend patient delay pregnancy until time when disease is inactive

SYNONYMS   Idiopathic proctocolitis

ICD-9-CM   556

SEE ALSO
• Crohn's disease of the colon
• Diarrhea, acute
• Diarrhea, chronic
• Intestinal parasites

OTHER NOTES   N/A

ABBREVIATIONS   N/A

REFERENCES
• Braunwald, E., et al. (eds.): Harrison's Principles of Internal Medicine. 12th Ed. New York, McGraw-Hill, 1991
• Farmer, R.G.: Inflammatory Bowel Disease. Medical Clinics Issue, Volume 74/number 1. Philadelphia, W.B. Saunders Co., January 1990

Author   M. Worshtil, M.D.

Urethritis

BASICS

DESCRIPTION Syndrome of urethral inflammation marked by painful urination and discharge. Usually a sexually transmitted disease (STD); other causes not uncommon. Two types: Gonorrhea (GC) found usually in males, rarely in women, and nongonococcal urethritis (NGU).
- In males - gonorrhea marked by a yellow purulent discharge, abrupt onset of symptoms 3 to 5 days after exposure to Neisseria gonorrhea. Nongonococcal urethritis marked by clear to white scanty discharge developing gradually at least a week after exposure, waxing and waning in intensity from a variety of other organisms, most commonly Chlamydia trachomatis
- In females, classic urethral syndrome present when patient complains of dysuria, urinalysis is clear, urine cultures are negative and patient fails to respond to regimens for simple cystitis. However, females with GC or other infections which cause simple urethritis in males will often have symptoms besides dysuria, including vaginal discharge and suprapubic pain.
- Untreated cases will gradually resolve, but complications, especially urethral stricture in males or pelvic inflammatory disease (PID) in women, may then ensue

System(s) affected: Renal/Urologic
Genetics: N/A
Incidence/Prevalence in USA: Very common - annually 2 million cases of gonorrhea, probably many more cases of Chlamydia. Highest incidence in urban, non-white populations.
Predominant age: Sexually active, postpubertal
Predominant sex: Classic symptoms more commonly reported by males; incidence in females probably equal

SIGNS AND SYMPTOMS
- Both sexes may be asymptomatic carriers of the causative organisms
- Dysuria - pain throughout urination
- Urethral discharge - may be profuse and purulent in acute GC, or scanty, evident only with milking of the urethra in NGU
- Suprapubic discomfort
- Urethral itching or tenderness
- Tenderness, edema and inflammation of the urethral meatus, especially in women
- Dyspareunia
- Vaginitis, cystitis, cervicitis in women
- Proctitis, pharyngitis, conjunctivitis may also be present (sexual history is important)
- Lymphadenopathy or fever are not part of the syndrome and suggest another diagnosis
- Bloody discharge - rarely seen and suggests another diagnosis

CAUSES Sexual contact with carrier of causative organisms. Most common are N. gonorrhea, C. trachomatis, Ureaplasma urealyticum, Trichomonas vaginalis, viruses (including herpes, cytomegalovirus [CMV], human papilloma virus), many other bacteria, rarely fungi

RISK FACTORS
- Multiple sexual partners
- History of other STD's

DIAGNOSIS

DIFFERENTIAL DIAGNOSIS
- Postgonococcal urethritis (PGU) - following adequate treatment of acute GC, patient continues to have symptoms, due to a second organism resistant to original medication (see Treatment)
- Other urinary tract infections - cystitis, epididymitis, prostatitis, etc.
- Trauma - frequent milking of the urethra in males, caused by concern about possible infection may lead to dysuria and a clear discharge. Young girls may occasionally develop symptoms from external irritation.
- Atrophy, especially in postmenopausal women
- Intraurethral foreign bodies or growths, e.g., venereal warts, congenital polyps
- Allergic or sensitivity reactions - vaginal douches and lubricants, foods, other medications (rare)
- Substance abuse - frequent heavy users of amphetamines or other stimulants may develop a scant, clear discharge without white cells and mild dysuria
- Stevens-Johnson syndrome
- Reiter's syndrome - probably an immunological reaction to Chlamydial infection

LABORATORY
- Gram stain of discharge: Polymorphic neutrophils with intracellular gram-negative diplococci strongly indicates GC; sheets of polymorphonuclear leukocytes without organisms suggests NGU, few to no polymorphonuclear leukocytes suggests other etiologies
- Discharge cultures or slide reagins for GC: False-negatives can occur, so treatment should be directed by physical exam and Gram stain results and should not wait for culture results. Conjunctiva, pharynx, rectum cultured as indicated by history and symptoms. Labs should test positives for drug resistances.
- Cultures or reagin detection for Chlamydia: Negatives may be false results or indicate another infecting organism

- Urinalysis: If indicated, sample discharge before patient voids, usually normal in cases of simple urethritis
- Urine culture: Performed only if Gram stain of discharge is unremarkable or unobtainable
- Wet prep of discharge: may reveal Trichomonas, unusual to demonstrate trichomoniasis in infected males
- Syphilis, HIV serology as indicated to rule out concomitant STD's
Drugs that may alter lab results: Previous recent treatment with antibiotics may lead to false negative results
Disorders that may alter lab results: N/A

PATHOLOGICAL FINDINGS Urethral strictures (untreated GC), intraurethral lesions (venereal warts, congenital anomalies)

SPECIAL TESTS Viral cultures if typical lesions are present

IMAGING Urethrogram for persistent symptoms, rarely indicated

DIAGNOSTIC PROCEDURES
Urethrocystoscopy for persistent cases with suspected foreign body, intraurethral warts

TREATMENT

APPROPRIATE HEALTH CARE All cases can be treated as outpatients except females with severe symptoms of PID

GENERAL MEASURES Identification and treatment of sexual partners

ACTIVITY Full activity, except no sexual intercourse until treatment is completed

DIET No special diet

PATIENT EDUCATION
- Many handouts available from local health departments on avoidance, causes and treatments
- Most important to emphasize need for compliance with therapy and treatment of sexual partners. Also, patients should be urged to undergoing screening for other STD's.

MEDICATIONS

DRUG(S) OF CHOICE
• Note: There is an ever-increasing incidence of multiple drug resistances
• Gonorrhea - ceftriaxone (Rocephin) 250 mg IM x 1 dose. All cases of GC need to be treated additionally with a regimen specific for Chlamydia due to the high incidence of mixed infections.
• Chlamydia - doxycycline 100 mg po bid for at least 7 days. Patients who continue with symptoms after treatment (and their sexual partners) should be retreated with erythromycin.
• NGU (especially U. urealyticum) - doxycycline 100 mg po bid for at least 7 days
• Trichomonas - 2 grams metronidazole (Flagyl) po for 1 dose or 250 mg tid for 7 days
Contraindications: Sensitivity to any of the indicated medications. Pregnant patients should not receive tetracyclines
Precautions: Patients taking tetracyclines need to be told of the possibility of increased sensitivity to sunlight
Significant possible interactions:
Tetracyclines should not be taken with milk products or antacids. Oral contraceptives may be rendered ineffective by oral antibiotics. Patients and partners should use a back-up method of birth control for remainder of the cycle.

ALTERNATIVE DRUGS
• Gonorrhea - spectinomycin 2 grams IM once. Ciprofloxacin (Cipro) 500 mg po once. Amoxicillin 3 grams with 1 gram probenecid (Benemid) po once.
• Chlamydia - erythromycin 500 mg po qid x 7 days. Azithromycin (Zithromax), a new azalide may also be effective.

FOLLOWUP

PATIENT MONITORING
• Patients with positive cultures should have cultures repeated several days after completing treatment as a test of cure
• Ensure that sexual partners were treated

PREVENTION/AVOIDANCE   Safer sex
protection techniques, urinating immediately after intercourse, treatment of all sexual partners

POSSIBLE COMPLICATIONS
• Stricture formation in untreated patients, PID in women
• When urethritis is accompanied by suprapubic discomfort, consider prostatitis in males, PID in females

EXPECTED COURSE AND
PROGNOSIS   If diagnosis is firmly established, appropriate medications prescribed and patient is compliant with treatment, there will be relief of symptoms within 24 hours and the problem will resolve without sequelae

MISCELLANEOUS

ASSOCIATED CONDITIONS   Other STD's
- patients should be strongly urged to undergo testing for syphilis and HIV

AGE-RELATED FACTORS
Pediatric: Proven cases of GC or Chlamydia, trichomoniasis should raise the question of sexual abuse
Geriatric: N/A
Others: None

PREGNANCY   Tetracyclines are
contraindicated. Use erythromycin instead but not the estolate form because of an increased risk of cholestatic jaundice.

SYNONYMS   N/A

ICD-9-CM
• 098.0 gonorrhea
• 099.4 nongonococcal urethritis
• 131.02 trichomonas infections
• 99.3 Reiter's syndrome

SEE ALSO   Gonorrhea, chlamydia, PID,
vaginitis, urinary tract infections, prostatitis, epididymitis

OTHER NOTES   For patients who present
without symptoms stating that a sexual partner was treated for this problem: Obtain specimens for lab tests, but treat this patient before the results are available (due to the high prevalence of the illness and the possibility of false-negative test results). Use any of the regimens discussed in Medications section.

ABBREVIATIONS
• STD = sexually transmitted disease
• GC = gonococcus infection
• NGU = nongonococcal urethritis
• PGU = postgonococcal urethritis

REFERENCES
• Centers for Disease control: Sexually transmitted diseases: Treatment guidelines. MMWR 1985:34:75S
• Drugs for Sexually transmitted Diseases. Medical Letter, Vol. 23, Issue 860, Dec, 1991

Author   K. Hepler, M.D.

Urinary incontinence

 BASICS

DESCRIPTION
Urinary incontinence is the involuntary loss of urine from the bladder. It can occur while asleep or awake. The amount of urine lost can vary greatly. The condition comes to medical attention when it is perceived to be a social and/or health problem by the patient or family.

System(s) affected: Renal/Urologic
Genetics: Unknown
Incidence/Prevalence in USA:
• 5-15% in community-dwelling elderly (over age 65)
• Up to 50% in nursing home populations
Predominant age: Geriatric populations. Increases with age.
Predominant sex: Female > Male

SIGNS AND SYMPTOMS
• Involuntary loss of urine
• Urinary urgency
• Burning with urination
• Perineal irritation

CAUSES
• Pelvic floor muscle weakness
• Urethral sphincter weakness
• Bladder irritation (cystitis, tumors, stones, diverticula)
• Detrusor motor/sensory instability (stroke, dementia, parkinsonism)
• Anatomic obstruction (prostate, stricture, cystocele)
• Neurogenic bladder (diabetes, spinal cord injury, multiple sclerosis)
• Loss of central nervous system control (severe dementia)

RISK FACTORS
• Increasing age
• Female sex/estrogen deficiency
• Prostatic hypertrophy (males)
• Multiparity (females)
• Dementia
• Diabetes
• Spinal cord injury
• Multiple sclerosis
• General debilitated condition

 DIAGNOSIS

DIFFERENTIAL DIAGNOSIS
• Urinary tract infection
• Vaginal discharge (women)
• Urethral discharge (men)
• Medication effect (diuretics)

LABORATORY
• Urinalysis - generally normal. May show glycosuria (diabetes), proteinuria (glomerular disease), white blood cells (infection), red blood cells (tumor), or bacteria (infection).
• Urine culture - will be positive in urinary tract infection
• IVP - may show renal pathology
Drugs that may alter lab results:
• Diuretics (low urine specific gravity)
• Antibiotics (negative urine culture)
Disorders that may alter lab results: Not applicable. Disorders producing abnormal lab results generally contribute to the problem of incontinence.

PATHOLOGICAL FINDINGS
• Relate to the primary cause of incontinence
• Urinary sphincter incompetence
• Prostatic hypertrophy
• Neurogenic bladder
• Bladder tumors
• Urinary tract infection

SPECIAL TESTS
• Voiding cystourethrogram - may show bladder and/or urethral pathology
• Cystometrograms - may show abnormal sphincter pressure or bladder physiology
• Post - voiding residual measurement

IMAGING
• Renal ultrasound - may show renal pathology
• Pelvic ultrasound - may show pelvic pathology
• Transrectal ultrasound - may show prostate pathology

DIAGNOSTIC PROCEDURES
• The diagnosis is generally made on history
• Physical examination of men should include palpation of abdomen (for distended bladder), digital rectal exam (for prostatic hypertrophy), and neurological exam
• Physical exam of women should include palpation of abdomen (for distended bladder), vaginal speculum and bimanual pelvic exam (for genitourinary pathology), and neurologic exam
• It is sometimes helpful to ask the patient to reproduce the activities (e.g., coughing, sneezing, laughing) which result in loss of urine

 TREATMENT

APPROPRIATE HEALTH CARE
Outpatient

GENERAL MEASURES
• All primary conditions relating to urinary incontinence should be identified and treated specifically (e.g., urinary tract infection, bladder tumors, prostatic hypertrophy)
• Good perineal hygiene
• Pelvic floor (Kegel) exercises
• Biofeedback/behavioral training
• Intermittent catheterization (selected patients)
• Incontinence pads
• Indwelling catheterization (selected patients)

ACTIVITY
Full activities should be encouraged

DIET
• No special diet
• In situations where access to bathroom facilities is limited, may want to avoid high volume fluid intake and reduce intake of caffeine or alcohol-containing beverages

PATIENT EDUCATION
• Should be directed at the general problem, as well as any underlying diseases
• Should include instructions regarding good general nutrition and exercise practices
• Rational toileting schedule, based on the patient's pattern of incontinence
• Easy access to toilet facilities
• Pelvic floor (Kegel) exercises
• Examples of specific instructions can be found in Clinics in Geriatric Medicine, November, 1986, pages 841-855

MEDICATIONS

DRUG(S) OF CHOICE
Detrusor instability
◊ Oxybutynin (Ditropan) 2.5-5 mg qid
◊ Propantheline (Pro-Banthine) 15-30 mg tid
◊ Dicyclomine (Bentyl) 10-20 mg qid
◊ Flavoxate (Urispas) 100-200 mg tid
◊ Imipramine (Tofranil) 25-50 mg tid
Sphincter incompetence
◊ Pseudoephedrine (Sudafed) 30-60 mg tid
◊ Phenylpropanolamine (Ornade) 75 mg bid
◊ Imipramine (Tofranil) 25-50 mg tid
Overflow/atonic bladder
◊ Bethanechol (Urecholine) 10-30 mg tid
Overflow/prostatic enlargement
◊ Prazosin (Minipress) 1-2 mg tid
◊ Finasteride (Proscar) 5 mg q day

Contraindications:
• Should be reviewed for each specific medication prior to initiating
• Anticholinergic agents are contraindicated in patients with glaucoma or prostatic hypertrophy

Precautions:
• Use smallest dose possible in elderly patients
• Common side effects include: Dry mouth, blurred vision, constipation, postural hypotension, mental confusion

Significant possible interactions: Will vary for each of the drugs listed

ALTERNATIVE DRUGS
• Oral or topical estrogens for stress incontinence associated with atrophic vaginitis
• Prostaglandin inhibitors (investigational)
• Calcium antagonists (investigational)
• DDAVP nasal spray (nocturnal enuresis)

FOLLOWUP

PATIENT MONITORING
• Biweekly at first (while exercises are being learned and medication dosage is being adjusted)
• Quarterly, once incontinence is under control and medication doses are stable
• Ask about side effects of medication
• Check for orthostatic hypotension
• Consider measuring intraocular pressure in high risk patients
• Periodic urinalysis to detect early urinary tract infection

PREVENTION/AVOIDANCE
• Instruct women in routine use of Kegel exercises after birth of children
• Regular pelvic examination of female patients to detect pelvic pathology
• Regular rectal examination in male patients to pick up early prostatic pathology. Treatment for hypertrophy.

POSSIBLE COMPLICATIONS
• Urinary tract infection
• Hydronephrosis (with atonic bladder or outlet obstruction)
• Renal failure (with obstructive hydronephrosis)
• Adverse drug reactions

EXPECTED COURSE AND
PROGNOSIS Prognosis is generally good. Most patients can achieve an increase in bladder control with appropriate medical management.

MISCELLANEOUS

ASSOCIATED CONDITIONS N/A

AGE-RELATED FACTORS
Pediatric: N/A
Geriatric: This problem is most commonly seen in the aging population
Others: N/A

PREGNANCY N/A

SYNONYMS
• Transient incontinence
• Urge incontinence
• Overflow incontinence
• Stress incontinence

ICD-9-CM 788.3 incontinence of urine

SEE ALSO N/A

OTHER NOTES N/A

ABBREVIATIONS N/A

REFERENCES
• Hazard, W.R., et al. (eds.): Principles of Geriatric Medicine and Gerontology. 2nd Ed. New York, McGraw-Hill Co, 1990
• Ouslander, J.G. (ed.): Clinics in Geriatric Medicine; 2:4. Philadelphia, W.B. Saunders Co., November, 1986
• Brocklehurs, J.C. (ed.): Gerontology; 36/52/90. Basel, Switzerland, S. Karger Publisher, September, 1990

Author A. Costa, M.D

Urinary tract infection in men

BASICS

DESCRIPTION Cystitis is an infection of the lower urinary tract, usually resulting from a single gram-negative enteric bacteria. (See separate chapters for information on prostatitis, pyelonephritis, and non-gonococcal urethritis.)
System(s) affected: Renal/Urologic
Genetics: No specific genetic pattern
Incidence/Prevalence in USA: Not common
Predominant age: Increases with age. Uncommon in men under 50.
(Predominant sex:) Male only (for this discussion)

SIGNS AND SYMPTOMS
• Urinary frequency
• Urinary urgency
• Dysuria
• Hesitancy
• Slow urinary stream
• Dribbling of urine
• Nocturia
• Suprapubic discomfort
• Low back pain
• Hematuria
• Systemic symptoms (chills, fever) present with concomitant pyelonephritis or prostatitis

CAUSES
• Escherichia coli (80% of infections)
• Klebsiella
• Enterobacter
• Proteus
• Pseudomonas
• Serratia
• Streptococcus faecalis and Staphylococcus

RISK FACTORS
• Benign prostatic hypertrophy
• Cognitive impairment
• Fecal incontinence
• Urinary incontinence
• Anal intercourse
• Recent urologic surgery, catheterization
• Infection of the prostate or kidney
• Urinary tract instrumentation
• Immunocompromised host
• Outlet obstruction

DIAGNOSIS

DIFFERENTIAL DIAGNOSIS
• Anatomic or functional pathology
• Urethritis
• Infections in other sites of the genitourinary tract (e.g., epididymis)

LABORATORY
• Pyuria
• Bacteriuria
• Urine dipstick leukocyte esterase (75-90%, sensitivity, 95% specificity), and nitrate (35-85% sensitivity, 70% specificity)
• Urine culture - 10/higher power colonies of pathogens (or counts > 100,000 bacteria/mL of urine) confirms diagnosis (Escherichia coli, Klebsiella, Pseudomonas, other agents). Lower counts can also be indicative of infection, especially in presence of pyuria.
<u>Segmented bacteriologic localization cultures</u>
  ◊ VB1 - collect 5-10 mL of urine of patient's initial voiding
  ◊ VB2 - then a sample of sterile midstream urine is obtained
  ◊ EPS - prostatic massage performed, and expressed prostatic secretion is collected from the meatus
  ◊ VB3 - patient completes voiding and 4th sample is collected
  ◊ Cultures and sensitivity collected from each specimen
Drugs that may alter lab results:
Antibiotics prior to culture
Disorders that may alter lab results: N/A

PATHOLOGICAL FINDINGS Depends on site of infection

SPECIAL TESTS Urologic investigations necessary to rule out other disorders

IMAGING Intravenous pyelography, cystoscopy, ultrasound

DIAGNOSTIC PROCEDURES Careful history and physical

TREATMENT

APPROPRIATE HEALTH CARE
Outpatient, except for acute illness with toxicity or kidney failure

GENERAL MEASURES
• Hydration and analgesia if required
• Discontinue sexual activity until cured
<u>Patient with indwelling catheters</u>
  ◊ If asymptomatic bacterial colonization - no need to treat (sterilization of urine not possible and resistant organisms can take up residence)
  ◊ If symptomatic of acute infection - institute treatment

ACTIVITY Activity as tolerated.

DIET No special diet

PATIENT EDUCATION For patient education materials favorably reviewed on this topic, contact: National Kidney Foundation, 30 E. 33rd Street, Suite 1100, New York, NY 10016, (212)889-2210

MEDICATIONS

DRUG(S) OF CHOICE
• Acute UTI , first infection, no risk factors for treatment: 7-10 days of oral antibiotics either empirically or based on cultures and sensitivity results. For empiric therapy, SMX/TMP BID will usually treat the most likely pathogens.
• Complicated or recurrent UTI: 14-21 days of antibiotics based on antimicrobial sensitivities with repeat urine check after treatment
Contraindications: Refer to manufacturer's information
Precautions: Refer to manufacturer's information
Significant possible interactions: Refer to manufacturer's information

ALTERNATIVE DRUGS
According to culture and sensitivity results and patient's history

FOLLOWUP

PATIENT MONITORING
Close followup until clinically well and repeat urinalysis after treatment

PREVENTION/AVOIDANCE
• Prompt treatment of predisposing factors
• Catheter use only when necessary. If needed, use aseptic technique and closed system, with removal as soon as possible.

POSSIBLE COMPLICATIONS
• Pyelonephritis
• Ascending infection
• Recurrent infection

EXPECTED COURSE AND PROGNOSIS
Clearing of infections with appropriate antibiotic treatment

MISCELLANEOUS

ASSOCIATED CONDITIONS
• Acute bacterial pyelonephritis
• Chronic bacterial pyelonephritis
• Urethritis
• Prostatitis
• Prostatic hypertrophy
• Prostate cancer

AGE-RELATED FACTORS
Pediatric: Usually associated with obstruction to normal flow of urine, such as vesicoureteral reflux
Geriatric: Bacteriuria is common in the elderly, appears related to functional status and is usually transient. If asymptomatic bacteriurea is noted, no treatment is needed.
Others: N/A

PREGNANCY N/A

SYNONYMS
• UTI
• Cystitis

ICD-9-CM
• 595 cystitis
• 595.1 acute cystitis
• 595.2 chronic cystitis

SEE ALSO Associated conditions

OTHER NOTES N/A

ABBREVIATIONS N/A

REFERENCES
• Lipsky, B.A.: Urinary tract infections in men. Epidemiology, pathophysiology, diagnosis, and treatment. Ann Intern Med 1989;110:138-150
• Smith, D.R.: General Urology. 12th Ed. Los Altos, CA, Lange Medical Publications, 1988
• Finn, S.D.: Urinary tract infections - diagnosis and treatment in women and men. Consultant. 10:43-58, 1992

Author S. Fields, M.D.

Urinary tract infection in women

BASICS

DESCRIPTION Inflammation of the bladder mucosa caused by bacterial infection
System(s) affected: Renal/Urologic
Genetics: N/A
Incidence/Prevalence in USA: 3-8% of women have bacteriuria at any given time. 43% of females aged 14-61 have had at least one UTI.
Predominant age: Young adults and older
Predominant sex: Female

SIGNS AND SYMPTOMS
• Note: Any or all may be present
• Burning during urination
• Pain during urination
• Urgency (sensation of need to urinate frequently)
• Sensation of incomplete bladder emptying
• Blood in urine
• Lower abdominal pain or cramping

CAUSES
Acute infection, almost always with gram negative bacteria

RISK FACTORS
• Previous urinary tract infection
• Diabetes mellitus
• Pregnancy
• More frequent or vigorous sexual activity than usual
• Underlying abnormalities of the urinary tract such as tumors, calculi, strictures, incomplete bladder emptying, etc.

DIAGNOSIS

DIFFERENTIAL DIAGNOSIS
• Vaginitis
• Sexually transmitted diseases causing urethritis
• Hematuria from causes other than infection (e.g., neoplasia, calculi)
• Psychological dysfunction

LABORATORY
• Urinalysis demonstrating pyuria (more than 5-8 neutrophils per high power field on microscopic exam). Leukocyte esterase dipsticks also useful for detecting pyuria but false positives occur from vaginal leukocytes.
• Urinalysis demonstrating bacteriuria (any amount). Nitrate dipsticks also useful but fail to detect bacteriuria in 10-30 percent of patients.
• Urine culture demonstrating growth of single type of bacteria. Suspect contaminated specimen when culture shows multiple types of bacteria.
Drugs that may alter lab results: N/A
Disorders that may alter lab results: N/A

PATHOLOGICAL FINDINGS   N/A

SPECIAL TESTS   N/A

IMAGING
• Radiographic, ultrasound, and/or endoscopic imaging of upper and lower urinary tract indicated for all infants and may be indicated for older patients with recurrent infections

DIAGNOSTIC PROCEDURES
• Suprapubic bladder aspiration or urethral catheterization to obtain urine specimen from infants
• Urethral catheterization to obtain urine specimen from children and adults if voided urine suspected of being contaminated
• Classic symptoms in non-pregnant young adult female with first episode of UTI require no laboratory testing for diagnosis. Obtain urinalysis and culture in other age groups, if repeat episode, if pregnant, or if symptoms not classic.

TREATMENT

APPROPRIATE HEALTH CARE
Outpatient, except for complicating upper tract infections

GENERAL MEASURES
• Maintain good hydration
• One-fourth of women with simple UTI experience a second UTI within six months. Patients with multiple recurrent UTI and no underlying urinary tract abnormality may receive long-term prophylactic antibiotic treatment. Trimethoprim-sulfamethoxazole and nitrofurantoin commonly used.
• Patients with chronic indwelling urinary catheters always have infections that should not be treated unless symptomatic with fever, sepsis, etc.

ACTIVITY   Avoid sexual intercourse when symptoms present

DIET   No special diet

PATIENT EDUCATION
• Take antibiotic as directed
• Return if symptoms not resolved within 48 hours
• Return if fever, chills, or flank pain develop

MEDICATIONS

DRUG(S) OF CHOICE
• First UTI in adolescents and adults who are not pregnant, not diabetic, not febrile, not immunosuppressed, and have no known abnormality of urinary tract: Single dose treatment with double-strength trimethoprim-sulfamethoxazole, two tablets taken at once, or 10 days of oral amoxicillin, cephalosporin, sulfisoxazole, nitrofurantoin, ciprofloxacin (note: only for patients with recurrent or chronic urinary tract infections)
• Pregnant patients: 10 to 14 day treatment with pregnancy-safe antibiotic chosen based on culture/sensitivity results. May begin with cephalosporin, amoxicillin, or other antibiotic while awaiting culture/sensitivity results.
• All other patients: 10-14 day treatment with antibiotic chosen based on culture/sensitivity results. May begin with trimethoprim-sulfamethoxazole, cephalosporin, ciprofloxacin, amoxicillin, nitrofurantoin, or other antibiotic while awaiting culture/sensitivity results.
Contraindications: Refer to manufacturer's literature
Precautions: Refer to manufacturer's literature
Significant possible interactions: Refer to manufacturer's literature

ALTERNATIVE DRUGS
Change to other antibiotic if indicated by culture/sensitivity results

FOLLOWUP

PATIENT MONITORING
• First UTI - in young or middle-age, non pregnant adult female requires no followup if patient cured after single dose therapy. If not resolved within two to three days after single dose therapy, obtain culture/sensitivity and change antibiotic accordingly.
• All other patients should have post-treatment urine culture to document eradication of infection

PREVENTION/AVOIDANCE
• Maintain good hydration
• Women with frequent or intercourse-related UTI should empty bladder immediately following intercourse

POSSIBLE COMPLICATIONS
• Pyelonephritis
• Renal abscess
• Gram-negative sepsis

EXPECTED COURSE AND PROGNOSIS
Symptoms resolve within 2-3 days after starting treatment in almost all patients

MISCELLANEOUS

ASSOCIATED CONDITIONS
Described above under Risk factors

AGE-RELATED FACTORS
Pediatric: Infants and young children at higher risk of pyelonephritis
Geriatric:
• Elderly may have bacteriuria without symptoms; generally does not require treatment if urinary tract otherwise normal
• Elderly more apt to have underlying urinary tract abnormality
• UTI often associated with incontinence in the elderly
Others: N/A

PREGNANCY
UTI during pregnancy always requires culture/sensitivity and always requires 10-14 day treatment. Following treatment of acute infection, pregnant women often receive prophylactic antibiotics for the remainder of pregnancy.

SYNONYMS
Cystitis

ICD-9-CM
• 595 cystitis
• 595.1 acute cystitis
• 595.2 chronic cystitis

SEE ALSO   N/A

OTHER NOTES   N/A

ABBREVIATIONS   N/A

REFERENCES
• Kunin, C.M.: Detection, Prevention and Management of Urinary Tract Infections. Philadelphia, Lea & Febiger, 1987
• Maskell, R.: Urinary Tract Infection in Clinical and Laboratory Practice. London, Edward Arnold Publishers, 1988
• Fowler, J.E.: Urinary Tract Infection and Inflammation. Chicago, Yearbook Medical Publishers, 1989

Author B. Weiss, M.D.

Urolithiasis

BASICS

DESCRIPTION The state describing the presence of calculi within the urinary system. Commonly known as kidney stones.
System(s) affected: Renal/Urologic
Genetics: Familial tendency
Incidence in USA: Unknown
Prevalence in USA: 70-210 in 100,000 population. 2%-5% of population in lifetime.
Predominant age: Peak 20-30. Range 20-60.
Predominant sex: Male > Female (4:1)

SIGNS AND SYMPTOMS
- Usually sudden onset
- Severe agonizing pain, costovertebral angle to groin depending on stone location
- Patient in constant motion, no comfort
- Nausea with or without vomiting
- Diaphoresis
- Tachycardia
- Intestinal ileus
- Abdominal guarding and rebound (rare)
- Tenderness to deep abdominal palpation, usually at CVA
- Lower tract stone with frequency, urgency, dysuria
- Fever, with infection
- Hematuria
- Pyuria, with infection
- May be asymptomatic if stone stays within kidney

CAUSES
<u>Calcium oxalate/calcium phosphate 65%-85%</u>
- ◊ Supersaturation from any cause
- ◊ Dehydration
- ◊ Increased absorption
- ◊ Increased calcium excretion - familial
- ◊ Renal tubular acidosis
- ◊ Hyperparathyroidism
- ◊ Chronic bowel disease with absorptive disorders
- ◊ Poor GI citrate absorption
- ◊ Excessive oral vitamin D or C
- ◊ Alkaline urinary pH
- ◊ Chronic use of calcium antacids
- ◊ Diet high in calcium or oxalate
- ◊ Malignancy
<u>Struvite (staghorn calculus) 15%-20%</u>
- ◊ Infection
- ◊ Alkaline urine
<u>Uric acid 5%</u>
- ◊ Hereditary
- ◊ Gout
- ◊ Chronic bowel disease
- ◊ High purine diet
- ◊ Acidic urine, very low pH
- ◊ Malignancy with chemotherapy
<u>Cystine 1%-3%</u>
- ◊ Hereditary homocystinuria

RISK FACTORS
- Family history
- Climate, hot
- Work in hot environment
- Poor fluid consumption
- Diet high in oxalate, purine, calcium
- Excessive vitamins
- Malignancy
- Sarcoidosis
- Gout
- Thiazide diuretics
- Bowel or kidney disease

DIAGNOSIS

DIFFERENTIAL DIAGNOSIS
- Pyelonephritis
- Clot or sloughed papillae (secondary to diabetes, infection, analgesic abuse)
- Drug-seeking addiction
- Acute abdomen
- Gynecological problems
- Diverticulitis

LABORATORY
- Urinalysis: Hematuria nearly 100%; if pH < 5.5 means uric acid, if pH > 7.5 means struvite
- Chemistries: Calcium, phosphorus, lytes, uric acid, creatinine
- Parathyroid hormone: If serum calcium high
- Urine cystine: If stone not visible on plain x-ray
- Urine culture: If pyuria or fever
Drugs that may alter lab results: N/A
Disorders that may alter lab results: See Causes and Risk Factors

PATHOLOGICAL FINDINGS Stone analysis: 60-80% calcium base, 15-20% struvite, 5% uric acid, 1-3% cystine

SPECIAL TESTS Stone analysis

IMAGING
- Plain kidney, ureter and bladder (KUB) x-ray: 80%-90% visible with some calcium
- Intravenous pyelogram (IVP): Primary study for urolithiasis
- Ultrasound: Technique varies, if good has equal sensitivity and specificity to IVP

DIAGNOSTIC PROCEDURES Retrograde pyelogram, if necessary

TREATMENT

APPROPRIATE HEALTH CARE
- 80% outpatient only, most will pass in 48 hours. 20% hospitalization and urology referral.
- Refer to urologist for: Intractable pain, obstruction, size > 6 mm, infection, dehydration, failure to progress, stone growth, single kidney, persistent gross hematuria, pregnancy, severe renal disease
<u>Surgical procedures:</u>
- ◊ Extracorporeal shock wave lithotripsy: Stone in renal pelvis or upper 2/3 ureter, size < 2 cm, noninfected, no coagulopathy
- ◊ Urethroscopy: Lower 1/3 ureter, normal anatomy present
- ◊ Percutaneous nephrolithotomy: Renal collecting system or upper 2/3 ureter, size > 2 cm, ureter stricture, cystine or uric acid stones, struvite, infection, obesity
- ◊ Open surgery: Less than 5% of patients, complex anatomy, obstruction, large infected struvite stone

GENERAL MEASURES
- Reassurance
- Strain urine
- Hydration
- Pain control

ACTIVITY Bedrest, if necessary during acute phase. No restrictions after stone passes.

DIET
- Normal diet, 8 oz. water every 1 hour while awake, and if possible every 2 hours during sleep hours
- If uric acid stones, less protein in diet and take sodium bicarbonate to alkalinize urine

PATIENT EDUCATION
- Instructions on urine straining, dietary advice
- See Patient Care, August 15, 1990, p.42

MEDICATIONS

DRUG(S) OF CHOICE
Acute therapy:
◊ Pain control (in office) - IM meperidine (Demerol)or morphine or buprenorphine (Buprenex), etc.
◊ 3 day supply pain control - oxycodone (Percocet), pentazocine (Talwin), hydrocodone and acetominophen (Vicodin), etc.
◊ Uric acid stone - potassium citrate (Urocit-K), 60-80 mEq/d to keep urine pH 6.5-7.0. Check urine pH qid.
◊ Cystine stone - penicillamine (Cuprimine, Depen) 1-4 g/d, K-citrate (Urocit-K) 60 mEq/d
◊ Infected stones - antibiotics for complicated pyelonephritis
Maintenance therapy:
◊ Hypercalciuria - sodium cellulose phosphate 10-15 g/d (2.5-5.0 grams with each meal), HCTZ 50 mg bid, K-citrate 15-20 mEq bid
◊ Uric acid - allopurinol (Zyloprim) 300 mg/d, K-citrate 20-30 mEq bid
◊ Cystine - K-citrate 30 mEq bid, penicillamine 1-4 g/d
Contraindications: Penicillamine with pregnancy, renal failure, aplastic anemia, hypersensitivity reaction
Precautions: Penicillamine requires regular CBC with differential counts, urinalysis, liver function tests
Significant possible interactions: Refer to manufacturer's profile of each drug

ALTERNATIVE DRUGS
Individualize to any underlying metabolic etiology found

FOLLOWUP

PATIENT MONITORING
Acute urolithiasis:
◊ Strain urine until stone or 72 hours after symptoms cease
◊ Repeat urinalysis 2-3 days
◊ Repeat KUB x-ray and or IVP/Ultrasound if no stone passed
◊ Stone analysis
◊ KUB x-ray at 3-6 months and at 1 year, if no new stone, then no further followup needed
Recurrent urolithiasis:
◊ 24 hour urine: volume, pH, calcium, phosphorus, sodium, uric acid, oxalate, citrate, creatinine clearance
◊ Measure parathyroid hormone (PTH)
◊ Calcium restricted diet test for urine calcium level

PREVENTION/AVOIDANCE
Hydration with urine > 2 liters a day (including nocturia once nightly). Dietary calcium < 1 g/d.

POSSIBLE COMPLICATIONS
• Hydronephrosis or kidney damage
• Infection and sepsis

EXPECTED COURSE AND PROGNOSIS
80% will pass in 48-72 hours with outpatient therapy, 60% no recurrence at 10 years

MISCELLANEOUS

ASSOCIATED CONDITIONS
See Causes section

AGE-RELATED FACTORS
Pediatric: Homocystinuria or other hereditary disorder
Geriatric: N/A
Others: N/A

PREGNANCY
Urology referral

SYNONYMS
• Nephrolithiasis
• Kidney stone
• Renal colic

ICD-9-CM
592.9

SEE ALSO
Renal calculi

OTHER NOTES
N/A

ABBREVIATIONS
• KUB = kidney, ureter and bladder
• IVP = intravenous pyelogram

REFERENCES
• NIH Consensus Development Conference on Prevention and Treatment of Kidney Stones. J of Urology. March, 1989, 141;3(2):705-804
• O'Brien, W.M., Rotolo, J.E. & Pahirz, J.J.: New Approaches in the Treatment of Renal Calculi. AFP, Nov, 1987, 36(5):181-194
• Stewart, C.: Nephrolithiasis. Emer Med Cl Nor Am. August, 1988, 6(3):617-630

Author W. Billica, M.D.

Urticaria

BASICS

DESCRIPTION Itchy rash. Single or multiple superficial raised pale macules with red halo. Subside rapidly; no scars or change in pigmentation. May be recurrent.
Acute urticaria
◊ Subsides over several hours
◊ Response to many stimuli
◊ IgE-mediated histamine release from mast cells
◊ Sometimes idiosyncratic response to drug exposure
Chronic urticaria (persists > 6 weeks (30% of cases). Not mediated by IgE. Multiple types:
◊ Cold urticaria: from cooling, rewarming. Can be fatal (cold immersion with massive histamine release). Also a familial form with fever, chills, arthralgia, myalgia, headache, lymphocytosis.
◊ Cholinergic urticaria - heat urticaria. Wheals on upper trunk from overheating, hot shower.
◊ Exercise-induced urticaria - from extreme exercise; presents as cholinergic urticaria, angioedema, wheezing, hypotension. Often associated with eating food to which patient is allergic.
◊ Dermatographism - linear wheal and flare resulting from scratching the skin
◊ Solar urticaria - result of exposure to sunlight. Several types, by wavelength of light which induces reaction. Majority react to ultraviolet. Onset in minutes; subsides in 1-2 hours.
◊ Delayed pressure urticaria - occurs 4-6 hours after pressure to skin (elastic, shoes, etc.)
◊ Aquagenic urticaria - rare. Small wheals after contact with water at any temperature.
Idiopathic urticaria
◊ Acute or chronic
System(s) affected: Skin/Exocrine
Genetics: No consistent genetic pattern known
Incidence/Prevalence in USA: 1 in 1000. Affects 15-20% of population at some time during life.
Predominant age: All ages. Acute form mainly in children, young adults.
Predominant sex: Male = Female (chronic forms more often in older women)

SIGNS AND SYMPTOMS
• Seen alone or with angioedema
• May occur with generalized anaphylactic reaction, potentially fatal
• Single or multiple raised, blanched, central wheals surrounded by red flare
• Intensely pruritic
• May occur anywhere on body
• Variably sized, 1-2 mm to 15-20 cm or larger; sometimes confluent
• Rapid onset, resolves spontaneously in less than 48 hours

CAUSES
• Allergic or non-allergic; massive histamine release from mast cells in superficial dermis
• Drug reaction (any drug) either from allergy or idiosyncrasy
• Aspirin, NSAID's seem to trigger by inhibiting cyclo-oxygenase, without IgE
• Food or food additive allergy
• Inhalant, contact, or ingestant allergy
• Transfusion reaction
• Insect bite, sting
• Infection - bacterial, viral (infectious mononucleosis, hepatitis), fungal, helminthic
• Collagen vascular disease (cutaneous vasculitis, serum sickness, lupus)
• Physical trauma (heat, cold, sunlight, etc.)
• Emotional stress (reported; little supporting evidence)

RISK FACTORS Listed with Causes

DIAGNOSIS

DIFFERENTIAL DIAGNOSIS
• Insect bites
• Morbilliform drug eruptions
• Erythema multiforme
• Vasculitis and polyarteritis
• Systemic lupus erythematosus
• Urticaria pigmentosa (mastocytosis). Pink lesions urticate when scratched (Darier's sign).
• Bullous pemphigoid (urticarial stage)

LABORATORY
• Cause found in 10-25% of chronic cases
• Food and drug reactions - elimination diets, challenges with suspected agents
• Inhalant allergens - skin tests, radioallergosorbent (RAST)
• Idiopathic for > 6 weeks - CBC, skin biopsy, ESR, urinalysis, ANA
Drugs that may alter lab results:
Antihistamines, H2-blockers, tricyclic antidepressants
Disorders that may alter lab results: N/A

PATHOLOGICAL FINDINGS Edema, vasculitis and/or perivasculitis involving only superficial dermis

SPECIAL TESTS
• Cold urticaria: ice cube test (place ice cube on skin 5 minutes, observe 10-15 minutes)
• Cholinergic or exercise-induced: exercise challenge; methacholine skin test (local reaction to 0.01 mg in 0.05 ml saline intradermally. 50% false negatives).
• Dermatographism: scratch skin with piece of tongue blade, observe
• Solar: expose to defined wavelengths of light. Must rule out erythropoietic protoporphyria.
• Delayed pressure: apply 5-10 pound sandbag for 3 hours, observe
• Aquagenic: apply tap water at different temperatures
• Vibratory: apply vibration 4-5 minutes with a lab mixing device, observe
• Infection: pharyngeal culture, antistreptolysin (ASO) titer, rapid plasma reagin (RPR), parasitology, liver function tests, mononucleosis test
• Autoimmune: antinuclear antibody (ANA), rheumatoid arthritis (RA), complement, cryoglobulins, serum protein electrophoresis

IMAGING N/A

DIAGNOSTIC PROCEDURES Skin biopsy (correlates poorly with clinical picture)

TREATMENT

APPROPRIATE HEALTH CARE Don't work up acute cases (results usually inconclusive)

GENERAL MEASURES Cool moist compresses help to control itching

ACTIVITY As desired. Avoid overheating.

DIET As desired. Avoid foods implicated as possible etiologic agents.

PATIENT EDUCATION Avoidance if etiology is apparent. Antihistamines if accidentally re-exposed.

MEDICATIONS

DRUG(S) OF CHOICE
• Older children and adults - hydroxyzine HCl 25-50 mg q6h or diphenhydramine 25-50 mg q6h for 2-3 days
• Children over 6 - hydroxyzine HCl 0.6 mg/kg q6h or diphenhydramine 12.5-25 mg q6h (available over-the-counter in liquid or capsules)
• Children under six - diphenhydramine 12.5 mg (elixir) q 6-8 hours (5 mg/kg/day)
Contraindications: Early pregnancy, history of hypersensitivity to drug
Precautions: Drowsiness (usually transient), dry mouth, urinary retention, paradoxical hyperactivity in some children
Significant possible interactions: Can potentiate other CNS depressants

ALTERNATIVE DRUGS
• Doxepin (Sinequan), tricyclic antidepressant with strong H1 and H2 blocking properties
• H2-blockers (cimetidine, ranitidine, etc.) may be helpful in chronic urticaria
• Terfenadine, astemizole (more expensive). Astemizole has slower onset, less helpful acutely.
• Corticosteroids for unresponsive cases (not for use acutely). 6-day taper. (Prednisone dose pack.)
• Cyproheptadine (Periactin) - especially for cold urticaria, children 0.25 mg/kg/day divide bid or tid; adults 0.5 mg/kg/day (maximum), divide bid or tid

FOLLOWUP

PATIENT MONITORING
No followup for initial episode. Evaluate if symptoms persist or recur.

PREVENTION/AVOIDANCE
If etiology identified, avoidance is best solution

POSSIBLE COMPLICATIONS
Severe systemic allergic reaction (bronchospasm, anaphylaxis)

EXPECTED COURSE AND PROGNOSIS
70% better in < 72 hours. 30% chronic. 20% have attacks for > 20 years. Becomes chronic in 75% of patients with both urticaria and angioedema.

MISCELLANEOUS

ASSOCIATED CONDITIONS
Angioedema, anaphylaxis

AGE-RELATED FACTORS
Pediatric: Acute isolated incidents are more frequent, chronic urticaria is rare
Geriatric: Less likely to occur in this age group
Others: N/A

PREGNANCY
Chronic urticaria

SYNONYMS
Hives

ICD-9-CM
708.8 other specified urticaria

SEE ALSO
• Anaphylaxis
• Angioedema

OTHER NOTES
Same pathophysiology for urticaria and angioedema - localized anaphylaxis causes vasodilatation, vascular permeability of skin (urticaria) or subcutaneous tissue (angioedema)

ABBREVIATIONS
N/A

REFERENCES
• Lockey, R.F. & Bukantz, S.C.: Principles of Immunology and Allergy. Philadelphia, W.B. Saunders Co., 1987
• Cooper, K.D.: Urticaria and angioedema: Diagnosis and evaluation. J Am Acad Dermatol 25(1):166, 1991

Author J. Perchalski, M.D.

Uterine malignancy

 BASICS

DESCRIPTION
Endometrial cancer:
◊ Malignancy of the endometrial lining of the uterus. Tumor grade - low, moderate, high. Cell types - adenocarcinoma, adenosquamous (benign or malignant squamous elements), clear cell, papillary serous.
Sarcomas:
◊ Mixed müllerian sarcoma - heterologous elements not native to the müllerian systems, such as cartilage or bone; homologous elements native to the mullerian system
◊ Endometrial stromal sarcoma develops from the stromal component of the endometrium
◊ Leiomyosarcoma develops in the myometrium or in a myoma (fibroid)
System(s) affected: Reproductive
Genetics: Unknown
Incidence/Prevalence in USA: Most common gynecologic malignancy, 35,000 new cases per year
Predominant age:
• Endometrial cancer - postmenopausal (mid fifties to mid sixties). Also can occur in young women in their twenties and thirties with polycystic ovarian disease or chronic anovulation.
• Sarcomas - forties to sixties
Predominant sex: Female only

SIGNS AND SYMPTOMS
Endometrial cancer:
◊ Postmenopausal bleeding is the most frequent sign. Any spotting should lead to evaluation.
◊ Pap smear is rarely positive
◊ Occasionally a patient will pass tissue that will render a diagnosis
Sarcoma:
◊ Mixed müllerian sarcoma - bleeding and prolapsing tissue
◊ Leiomyosarcoma - increasing size of presumed uterine myomas
◊ D & C rarely diagnostic

CAUSES
Endometrial cancer - unopposed estrogen due to:
◊ Polycystic ovarian disease
◊ Obesity
◊ Chronic anovulation
◊ Estrogen replacement therapy. (Estrogen replacement without concomitant progesterone increases the risk 70 times. When progesterone is added the risk does not decrease to zero but decreases to that of the population in general).
Sarcomas:
◊ Etiology unknown

RISK FACTORS
• Early menarche
• Late menopause
• Nulliparity
• Hypertension and diabetes are probably associated with underlying obesity

 DIAGNOSIS

DIFFERENTIAL DIAGNOSIS
• Atypical complex hyperplasia (a premalignant lesion of the endometrium)
• Bleeding from cervical cancer
• Ovarian cancer invading the uterus
• Adenocarcinoma of the cervix
• Endometriosis

LABORATORY
• Liver function tests
• CA-125 can be elevated when intra-abdominal disease is present
Drugs that may alter lab results: N/A
Disorders that may alter lab results: A biopsy of a pregnant uterus can produce tissue which has a hyperplastic or premalignant appearance

PATHOLOGICAL FINDINGS
Stage I
◊ A. Confined to endometrium
◊ B. Less than 50% myometrial invasion
◊ C. More than 50% myometrial invasion
Stage II
◊ A. Endocervical involvement (microscopic)
◊ B. Cervical stromal invasion (macroscopic)
Stage III
◊ A. Uterine serosal/adnexal involvement/positive peritoneal cytology
◊ B. Vaginal metastases
◊ C. Involved pelvic/para aortic lymph nodes
Stage IV
◊ A. Extension to involve the mucosa of the bladder or rectum
◊ B. Distant metastatic disease or inguinal node involvement
Stages are also subgrouped according to histologic grade:
◊ GI - Well differentiated
◊ G2 - Moderately differentiated
◊ G3 - Poorly differentiated

SPECIAL TESTS
Any that may be indicated preoperatively

IMAGING
• Chest x-ray - the most common site of metastases is the lungs. Rarely does this malignancy go to the bone or the liver except in advanced disease.
• CT scan, bone scan, liver spleen scan - not part of the routine evaluation, but may be needed occasionally
• Mammogram (endometrial cancer is associated with breast cancer)
• Barium enema (endometrial cancer is associated with colon cancer)
• MRI has been reported to accurately show the depth of myometrial penetration, but this is not always cost-effective
• Vaginal ultrasound can show increased endometrial echoes prior to D & C which will lead to the diagnosis

DIAGNOSTIC PROCEDURES
• Office endometrial biopsy (90% accurate). If this is negative, a D & C is necessary. Endometrial stromal sarcoma and leiomyosarcoma are rarely diagnosed preoperatively.
• D & C (99% accurate)

 TREATMENT

APPROPRIATE HEALTH CARE
Inpatient surgery

GENERAL MEASURES
• Surgical procedure is abdominal exploration with extrafascial total abdominal hysterectomy, bilateral salpingo-oophorectomy, cytology, pelvic and para-aortic node sampling
• Surgery is followed by radiation therapy in high-risk patients who have Stage 1B disease or greater, or for patients with poorly differentiated tumors regardless of stage. There is no adjuvant therapy that has been shown to be effective after surgery and radiation.
• Radiation is used to prevent the recurrence of tumor at the vaginal cuff
• When distant metastatic disease occurs, progesterone produces a 30% response rate. Active chemotherapeutic agents are cisplatin and Adriamycin.

ACTIVITY Patients are usually ambulatory and able to resume full activity by six weeks after surgery

DIET Unrestricted unless they are undergoing radiation

PATIENT EDUCATION
• The American Cancer Society in the local community
• American College of Obstetricians & Gynecologists (ACOG), 409 12th St., SW, Washington, DC 20024-2188, (800)762-ACOG

MEDICATIONS

DRUG(S) OF CHOICE
• There are no drugs as adjuvant therapy
• Premalignant lesions in young women or in patients unsuitable for hysterectomy can be treated with Megace, 160 mg qd x 3 months. This is followed by repeat D & C to ascertain whether the hyperplasia has resolved.
• Metastatic disease is treated with high dose progesterone, or Adriamycin or cisplatin

Contraindications:
• Progestational agents can cause significant fluid retention in 5-10% of patients
• Patients with congestive heart failure must be observed closely

Precautions: Usual precautions with chemotherapeutic agents. Refer to manufacturer's profile of each drug.

Significant possible interactions: Refer to manufacturer's profile of each drug

ALTERNATIVE DRUGS N/A

FOLLOWUP

PATIENT MONITORING
• Pap smear every 3 months for two years, then every 6 months for 3 years
• Chest x-ray once a year

PREVENTION/AVOIDANCE
• In young women taking birth control pills, endometrial cancer can be reduced by cyclic progesterone to prevent unopposed estrogen
• Estrogen replacement therapy should always include progestational agents unless the woman has undergone hysterectomy

POSSIBLE COMPLICATIONS Those
attendant upon major abdominal surgery

EXPECTED COURSE AND
PROGNOSIS Five year survival is based on stage and tumor grade

```
Grade        5 yr survival (%)
-----------------------------
  IAG1          98
  IBG2          85
  ICG3          60
  IIA/B         60
  III           40
  IV            15
-----------------------------
```

MISCELLANEOUS

ASSOCIATED CONDITIONS
• Obese patients with endometrial cancer should be screened annually because of increased risk of breast and colon cancer
• Patients who have breast or colon cancer are at increased risk for endometrial cancer. Granulosa cell tumors of the ovary produce estrogen and these patients will have an increased risk of endometrial cancer.

AGE-RELATED FACTORS
Pediatric: N/A

Geriatric: Older (especially obese) patients may be at high risk for surgery. Alternative radiation therapy can be considered.

Others: If preserving fertility is desired - young anovulatory women, polycystic ovarian patients with atypical complex hyperplasia, or patients with well differentiated endometrial cancer can be treated with progestational agents x 3 months followed by D & C

PREGNANCY This malignancy is not
associated with pregnancy

SYNONYMS
• Uterine cancer
• Endometrial cancer
• Corpus cancer

ICD-9-CM
• 182.0 Malignant neoplasm of body of uterus, corpus uteri, except isthmus
• 182.8 Malignant neoplasm of body of uterus, other specified sites of body of uterus
• 182.1 Malignant neoplasm of body of uterus, isthmus
• 180.0 Malignant neoplasm of body of cervix uteri, endocervix

SEE ALSO N/A

OTHER NOTES N/A

ABBREVIATIONS N/A

REFERENCES Hopkins, M.P.: Benign and
Malignant Diseases of the Uterus. In Obstetrics and Gynecology. Edited by J.R. Willson. St. Louis, Mosby Year Book,

Author M. Hopkins, M.D. & E.L. Jenison, M.D.

Uterine myomas

BASICS

DESCRIPTION Uterine leiomyomas or fibroleiomyomas are well circumscribed, pseudo-encapsulated benign tumors composed mainly of smooth muscle but with varying amounts of fibrous connective tissue

<u>Three major types:</u>
◊ Submucous: 5% of total, susceptible to abnormal uterine bleeding, infection and occasionally protrude from cervix
◊ Subserous: Common, may become pedunculated and rarely parasitic
◊ Intramural: Common, may cause marked uterine enlargement

System(s) affected: Reproductive
Genetics: N/A
Incidence/Prevalence in USA: 4-11% of all women, 20% of all women over 35 years of age and 40% of women over 50 years of age
Predominant age: Fourth and fifth decades
Predominant sex: Female only

SIGNS AND SYMPTOMS
• Majority are asymptomatic and are only suspected from pelvic examination
• Most common symptom is abnormal uterine bleeding. Hypermenorrhea most common. Secondary anemia with associated symptomatology may result.
• Pressure on bladder may result in suprapubic discomfort, urinary frequency, urinary retention or hydronephrosis
• Pressure on rectosigmoid may result in constipation, low back pain
• Edema and varicosities of the lower extremities may result from large tumors
• Pain may result from twisted, pedunculated myomas or degenerating, hemorrhagic or infected myomas
• Sterility may result from submucous myomas with distortion of uterine cavity
• Rapid growth particularly in perimenopausal or postmenopausal may indicate sarcoma

CAUSES
• May arise from totipotential primitive cells normally giving rise to muscle and connective tissue cells
• May arise from small immature smooth cell nests
• Positive correlation with estrogen stimulation, i.e., not seen before menarche, grow rapidly during pregnancy, with use of oral estrogen, and seen with estrogen producing tumors. The myomas regress following pregnancy and after menopause.

RISK FACTORS
• Later reproductive and perimenopausal age groups
• 3-9 times higher among African-Americans

DIAGNOSIS

DIFFERENTIAL DIAGNOSIS
• Intrauterine pregnancy
• Ovarian tumor
• Cecal or sigmoid tumor
• Appendiceal abscess
• Diverticulitis
• Pelvic kidney
• Urachal cyst

LABORATORY
• Pregnancy test
• CBC, differential count
• SED rate
• CA-125 - may be slightly elevated in some cases of uterine myomas, but generally is more useful in differentiating myomas from various gynecologic adenocarcinomas
Drugs that may alter lab results: N/A
Disorders that may alter lab results: Pregnancy may also slightly elevate CA-125 antigen level

PATHOLOGICAL FINDINGS
• Myomas are usually multiple and vary in size and location. Have been reported up to 100 pounds.
• Gross pathology reveals firm tumors with characteristic whorl-like trabeculated appearance. A thin psuedocapsular layer is present.
• Microscopic appearance reveals bundles of smooth muscle mixed with varying amounts of connective tissue elements running in different directions
• Cellular variant has a preponderance of muscle cells. Mitoses are rare.
<u>May undergo various types of degeneration:</u>
◊ I Hyaline degeneration. Very common, eventually results in liquification and cyst formation.
◊ II Calcification. Late result of circulatory impairment to myomas.
◊ III Infection and suppuration. Submucous myomas most prone to infection and may lead to sepsis.
◊ IV Necrosis. Pedunculated subserous fibroids most prone to necrosis secondary to torsion.
◊ V Sarcomatous change. Incidence ranges from 1.0 to 0.1% of myomas.

SPECIAL TESTS N/A

IMAGING
• Ultrasonography shows characteristic hypoechoic appearance
• CT scan, MRI may help to differentiate complex cases
• Intravenous pyelogram (IVP)
• Barium enema

DIAGNOSTIC PROCEDURES
• Presumptive diagnosis by abdominal and pelvic examination: Firm, smooth nodules or masses arising from uterus. Masses are mobile without pain.
• Fractional D & C aids in ruling out cervical carcinomas
• Hysteroscopy may help diagnose submucous myomas
• Laparoscopy may be useful in complex cases in ruling out other pelvic pathology

TREATMENT

APPROPRIATE HEALTH CARE
Outpatient usually; inpatient for some surgical procedures

GENERAL MEASURES
• Treatment must be individualized
• Patients with minimal symptoms may be managed with iron preparations and analgesics
• Conservative management: Asymptomatic myomas of less than 12 weeks' size gestation should be closely observed with pelvic examinations and ultrasonography at 3-6 month intervals. Observation continued as long as size stable.
• Asymptomatic myomas greater than 12 week gestation may be observed if the patient is perimenopausal and size remains stable. Usually regress after menopause.
• Luteinizing hormone releasing hormone (LHRH) agonists induce an abrupt artificial menopause with cessation of bleeding and shrinkage of myomas. Not recommended for more than six months. May be useful in perimenopausal patients or as an adjunct in preparation for surgery.
<u>Surgical management is indicated in the following situations:</u>
◊ Excessive uterine size (> 12-14 weeks gestation) or excessive rate of growth (except during pregnancy)
◊ Submucous location if associated with hypermenorrhea
◊ Pedunculated myomas may undergo torsion, pain, necrosis and hemorrhage
◊ Symptomatic from pressure symptoms on bladder or rectum
◊ If differentiation from ovarian mass is not possible
◊ If there is associated pelvic disease, i.e., endometriosis, pelvic inflammatory disease, etc.
◊ If infertility or habitual abortion is likely due to the anatomic location of the myoma

Surgical procedures:
◊ Hysteroscopic loop cautery or yttrium-argon-garnet (YAG) laser myoma resection can be performed in selected cases (outpatient procedure)
◊ Myomectomies may be performed in younger women desiring to maintain fertility
◊ Hysterectomy, either vaginal or abdominal, is procedure of choice for women no longer desiring fertility (inpatient procedure)
◊ Preliminary Pap smear and endometrial sampling or D & C must be performed to rule out malignant or premalignant conditions in all cases

ACTIVITY
• Following hysteroscopic myoma resection, bedrest 24 hours, no sexual intercourse for one month
• Following myomectomy and hysterectomy, 3-5 days hospital, followed by limited activity and no sexual intercourse for one month

DIET No restrictions

PATIENT EDUCATION ACOG (American College of Obstetricians and Gynecologists) pamphlet entitled "Uterine Fibroids", ACOG p-074

MEDICATIONS

DRUG(S) OF CHOICE
Luteinizing hormone releasing hormone (LHRH) agonists (Synarel Nasal Spray, Zoladex Depot, Lupron Depot)
◊ Induce abrupt, artificial menopause and render patients asymptomatic
◊ Induce atrophy of myomas by 60% within 2-3 months
◊ May be valuable as a preoperative adjunct to myomectomy or hysterectomy by allowing recovery of anemia, donation of autologous blood and possibly converting abdominal to vaginal hysterectomy, thereby decreasing postoperative pain, hospitalization, and morbidity. Generally used two to three months prior to surgery.
◊ Not recommended for use longer than six months
◊ Following discontinuation, myomas return within 60 days to pretherapy size
Patients with minimal symptoms
◊ May be managed conservatively with iron preparations and analgesics
◊ Progestins such as norethindrone, 10 mg daily, or medroxyprogesterone acetate (Depo-Provera) 200 mg IM, once monthly, may reduce the amount of blood flow. They do not reduce myoma size.

Contraindications:
• Progestins - history of thromboembolic phenomenon
• LHRH agonists - history of osteoporosis
Precautions: LHRH agonists induce acute menopausal symptoms: hot flashes, night sweats, insomnia, emotional lability, and osteoporosis
Significant possible interactions: Refer to manufacturer's profile of each drug

ALTERNATIVE DRUGS N/A

FOLLOWUP

PATIENT MONITORING
• Newly diagnosed uterine myoma, if symptomatic or excessive size, 2-3 months with pelvic exam and ultrasonography
• Consider CA-125 antigen
• Monitor hemoglobin and hematocrit, if uterine bleeding excessive
• If uterine size and symptoms stable, monitor every 6 months

PREVENTION/AVOIDANCE
• 10% myoma recurrence rate following myomectomy
• Excessive growth during estrogen stimulation, i.e., birth control pills, postmenopausal estrogen replacement therapy and pregnancy

POSSIBLE COMPLICATIONS
• Complications during pregnancy include - abortion; premature labor second trimester rapid myoma growth leading to degeneration and pain third-trimester fetal dystocia during labor and delivery
• Previous myomectomy patients in labor may develop uterine rupture. C-section is recommended if myomectomy entered endometrial cavity.
• May mask other gynecologic malignances, i.e., uterine sarcoma, ovarian cancer

EXPECTED COURSE AND PROGNOSIS
• Following myomectomy, 40% pregnancy rate in patients previously infertile
• At least 10% myomas recur following myomectomy

MISCELLANEOUS

ASSOCIATED CONDITIONS Endometrial carcinoma, associated with high unopposed estrogen stimulation

AGE-RELATED FACTORS
Pediatric: N/A
Geriatric: In postmenopausal patients with newly diagnosed uterine myoma or enlarging uterine myomas, highly suspect uterine sarcoma or other gynecologic malignancy
Others:
• Not seen in premenarchal females
• Incidence increases with each decade during reproductive years and is highest in perimenopausal age group

PREGNANCY See associations above

SYNONYMS
• Fibroids
• Fibromyoma
• Myofibroma
• Fibroleiomyoma

ICD-9-CM 218.0

SEE ALSO N/A

OTHER NOTES N/A

ABBREVIATIONS N/A

REFERENCES
• Cunningham, F.G., MacDonald, P.C. & Gant, N.F. (eds.): Williams Obstetrics. 18th Ed. Norwalk CT, Appleton and Lange, 1989
• Novak, E. & Woodruff, J.D.: Novak's Gynecologic and Obstetric Pathology: With Clinical and Endocrine Relations. 8th Ed. Philadelphia, W.B. Saunders Co., 1979
• Ryan, K.J., Berkowitz, R. & Barbieri, R.L.: Kistners' Gynecology: Principles & Practice. 5th Ed. Chicago, Year Book Publishers, 1990
• Jones, H.W., III, Wentz, A.C. & Burnett, L.S.: Novak's Textbook of Gynecology. 11th Ed. Baltimore, Williams and Wilkins, 1988

Author E. Jenison, M.D. & M. Hopkins, M.D.

Uterine prolapse

 BASICS

DESCRIPTION
Uterine prolapse occurs when the integrity of supporting structures is lost. This allows the uterus to descend into the vagina. In advanced cases, complete protrusion with inversion of the vagina occurs.
• Prior to menopause, the degree and severity of prolapse is usually related to the number of children and the difficulty of childbirth. After menopause, atrophy and loss of tissue integrity leads to prolapse.
System(s) affected: Reproductive, Renal/Urologic
Genetics:
• Common among Caucasian races
• Much less common among Orientals and African Americans and particularly uncommon in the South African Bantu and West Africans
Incidence/Prevalence in USA:
Approximately 1 in 10 women will experience some degree of prolapse
Predominant age: Aging female
Predominant sex: Female only

SIGNS AND SYMPTOMS
• Pelvic pressure and low back pain
• As prolapse progresses, the woman will eventually feel a bulging as a result of protrusion
• Dyspareunia
• Difficulty with urination or defecation

CAUSES
• Advancing age and vaginal childbirth are the most important factors
• The incidence of prolapse increases with the frequency and difficulty of vaginal deliveries. Less than 2% of prolapse occurs in nulliparous women.
• Other causes of prolapse include connective tissue disorders with lax tissue, i.e., Marfan's syndrome and neurogenic disorders, i.e., multiple sclerosis, and the rare disorder of cloacal agenesis
• Patients who have undergone radical vulvectomy with loss of the external supporting structures have a higher rate of prolapse

RISK FACTORS
• Childbirth, particularly multiple parity
• Advancing age
• Caucasian
• Gynecoid type pelvis
• Various connective tissue and neurogenic disorders
• Conditions resulting in increased intra-abdominal pressure, such as obesity, abdominal or pelvic tumors, pulmonary disease with chronic coughing, chronic constipation
• Occupations requiring heavy lifting

 DIAGNOSIS

DIFFERENTIAL DIAGNOSIS
Diagnosis is by physical and pelvic examination. With coughing and straining, the cervix will prolapse toward introitus or beyond. The patient may need to be examined in the standing as well as lying position for diagnosis and better demonstration of the disorder. Herniations of the bladder (cystocele or urethrocele), rectum (rectocele) and small bowel (enterocele) are associated conditions that may be simultaneously diagnosed.

LABORATORY
• Evaluation of renal function to rule out ureteral obstruction
• Urinalysis to rule out urinary tract infection
Drugs that may alter lab results: N/A
Disorders that may alter lab results: N/A

PATHOLOGICAL FINDINGS
• Hyperkeratosis of the cervical and vaginal tissues occur with prolapse beyond the introitus due to chronic irritation and drying. As the irritation becomes more pronounced, bleeding and ulceration occur.
<u>Degrees of prolapse:</u>
◊ First degree prolapse - to the ischial spines
◊ Second degree prolapse - to the introitus
◊ Third degree prolapse - just beyond the introitus
◊ Fourth degree prolapse - complete uterine and vaginal inversion involving bladder and bowel

SPECIAL TESTS N/A

IMAGING
• Intravenous pyelogram should be obtained to rule out ureteral obstruction in complete uterine prolapse
• Pelvic ultrasound or CT scan to rule out pelvic pathology, if suspected

DIAGNOSTIC PROCEDURES
If ulceration or bleeding is present, Pap smears and appropriate cervical and endometrial biopsies should be done to rule out concomitant malignancies

 TREATMENT

APPROPRIATE HEALTH CARE
• Outpatient
• Inpatient when surgery is necessary

GENERAL MEASURES
• Treatment depends on multiple variables including the severity of prolapse, age, sexual activity, associated pelvic pathology and desire for future fertility
• Treatment of first and second degree prolapse is expectant unless patient is symptomatic
• Mildly symptomatic patients and poor surgical candidates - can be treated nonoperatively with perineal (Kegel) exercises, estrogen replacement and vaginal pessaries. Estrogen replacement restores healthy vaginal mucosa and promotes healing.
• Elderly, non-sexually active women - can be treated with a colpocleisis or vaginal obliteration procedure
• Surgically able patients without additional pelvic pathology - vaginal hysterectomy with or without enterocele, cystocele, rectocele repair and vaginal vault suspension. Provides excellent results.

ACTIVITY
Heavy lifting or significant increases in intra-abdominal pressure will lead to worsening of prolapse or recurrence after surgical correction. Lifting should therefore be restricted.

DIET
Unlimited. Avoid constipation.

PATIENT EDUCATION
• Kegel exercises when applicable
• American College of Obstetricians & Gynecologists (ACOG), 409 12th St., SW, Washington, DC 20024-2188, (800)762-ACOG

MEDICATIONS

DRUG(S) OF CHOICE Estrogen replacement therapy can increase the blood supply to the vaginal tissues and in mild cases increase supporting tissue strength to a point where surgery or pessary use may be avoided

Contraindications: Those associated with the use of estrogen. Refer to manufacturer's literature.

Precautions: If estrogen therapy is utilized and the uterus is present, progesterone should be utilized to offset the potential adverse effects of estrogen on the uterus

Significant possible interactions: Refer to manufacturer's literature

ALTERNATIVE DRUGS None

FOLLOWUP

PATIENT MONITORING
• Expectant management is appropriate with periodic followup examinations
• If a pessary is placed, it should be removed, cleaned and replaced each month

PREVENTION/AVOIDANCE
• The instruction of Kegel exercises will increase the strength of the pelvic diaphragm muscles and may provide some pelvic support
• Weight loss and proper management of conditions that would increase abdominal pressure help to prevent prolapse

POSSIBLE COMPLICATIONS
• Ureteral obstruction and renal failure
• Incarceration of bowel herniations
• Pessary use - may not always be effective, and may cause discomfort

EXPECTED COURSE AND PROGNOSIS
• It is expected that as patients age, the incidence and severity of prolapse will increase
• Surgical correction usually successful

MISCELLANEOUS

ASSOCIATED CONDITIONS Cystocele, rectocele, enterocele and vaginal vault prolapse are often associated with uterine prolapse

AGE-RELATED FACTORS
Pediatric: Prolapse in newborn has been reported, but is rare and usually associated with congenital disorders and neuropathies
Geriatric: This is largely a disease of aging and will be much higher as the population ages
Others: N/A

PREGNANCY This disorder in large part results from vaginal childbirth and the distention and distortion of supporting tissues with childbirth

SYNONYMS
• Uterine prolapse
• Genital prolapse
• Genital relaxation
• Uterine descensus
• Total or partial procidentia
• Dropped uterus

SEE ALSO N/A

OTHER NOTES N/A

ICD-9-CM 618. (fourth digits 1-9)

ABBREVIATIONS N/A

REFERENCES
• Nichols, D.H. & Randall, C.L.: Vaginal Surgery. 3rd Ed. Baltimore, Williams & Wilkins, 1989
• Ryan, K.J., Berkowitz, R. & Barbieri, R.L.: Kistner's Gynecology: Principles and Practice. 5th Ed. Chicago, Year Book Medical Publishers, Inc., 1986
• Friedman, E.A. (ed.): Gynecologic Decision Making. St. Louis, C.V. Mosby Company, 1983

Author E. Jenison, M.D. & M. Hopkins, M.D.

Uveitis

BASICS

DESCRIPTION Uveitis is a nonspecific term used to describe any intraocular inflammatory disorder. Symptoms vary depending on depth of involvement and associated conditions.
• Anterior uveitis - refers to ocular inflammation limited to the iris (iritis) alone or iris and ciliary body (iridocyclitis)
• Intermediate uveitis - refers to inflammation of the structures just posterior to the lens (pars planitis or peripheral uveitis)
• Posterior uveitis - refers to inflammation of the choroid (choroiditis), retina (retinitis), or vitreous near the optic nerve and macula
System(s) affected: Nervous, Ophthalmologic
Genetics: No specific pattern for uveitis in general; iritis: 50- 70% of patients are HLA-B27 positive
Incidence in USA: Anterior uveitis most common (8.2 cases/100,000 annual incidence)
Prevalence in USA: Iritis is 4 times more prevalent than posterior uveitis
Predominant age: All ages
Predominant sex: Male = Female (except for HLA-B27 anterior uveitis male > female (2.5:1)

SIGNS AND SYMPTOMS
Anterior uveitis (approximately 80% of patients with uveitis)
◊ Decreased visual acuity
◊ Generally acute in onset
◊ Deep eye pain
◊ Photophobia (consensual)
◊ Conjunctival vessel dilation
◊ Perilimbal (circumcorneal) dilation of episcleral and scleral vessels (ciliary flush)
◊ Small pupillary size of affected eye
◊ Frequently unilateral (95% of HLA-B27 associated cases)
◊ Bilateral involvement and systemic symptoms (fever, fatigue, abdominal pain) may be associated with interstitial nephritis
◊ Systemic disease is most likely to be associated with anterior uveitis (53% of patients found to have systemic disease in one study)
Intermediate and posterior uveitis
◊ Decreased visual acuity
◊ Generally insidious in onset
◊ More commonly bilateral
◊ Posterior inflammation will generally cause minimal pain or redness unless associated with an iritis

CAUSES
• Infectious - may result from viral, bacterial, parasitic, or fungal etiologies
• Suspected immune-mediated - possible autoimmune or immune-complex mediated mechanism postulated in association with systemic (especially rheumatologic) disorders
• Isolated eye disease
• Idiopathic (approximately 25%)
• Masquerade syndromes - diseases such as malignancies that may be mistaken for inflammation of the eye

RISK FACTORS No specific risk factors. Higher incidence seen with specific associated conditions.

DIAGNOSIS

DIFFERENTIAL DIAGNOSIS
• Conjunctivitis
• Episcleritis
• Scleritis
• Keratitis
• Acute angle-closure glaucoma

LABORATORY
• No specific test for the diagnosis of uveitis. Tests for etiologic factors or associated conditions should be based on history and physical examination.
• CBC, BUN, creatinine (interstitial nephritis)
• HLA-B27 typing (ankylosing spondylitis, Reiter's syndrome)
• ANA, ESR (SLE, Sjögren's syndrome)
• VDRL, FTA (syphilis)
• PPD (tuberculosis)
• Lyme serology (Lyme disease)
Drugs that may alter lab results: N/A
Disorders that may alter lab results: Immune deficiency

PATHOLOGICAL FINDINGS Keratic precipitates, inflammatory cells in anterior chamber or vitreous, synechiae (fibrous tissue scarring between iris and lens), macular edema, perivasculitis of retinal vessels

SPECIAL TESTS Slit lamp examination and indirect ophthalmoscopy are necessary for precise diagnosis

IMAGING
• Chest x-ray - (sarcoidosis, histoplasmosis, tuberculosis, lymphoma)
• Sacroiliac x-ray (ankylosing spondylitis)

DIAGNOSTIC PROCEDURES Slit lamp examination

TREATMENT

APPROPRIATE HEALTH CARE
Outpatient with urgent ophthalmologic consultation

GENERAL MEASURES
• Medical therapy best initiated following full ophthalmologic evaluation
• Treatment of underlying cause, if identified
• Cycloplegia
• Anti-inflammatory therapy

ACTIVITY Full activity

DIET No special diet

PATIENT EDUCATION
• Instructions on proper method for instilling eye drops
• Wear dark glasses, if photophobia a problem
• Medication side effects to watch for and report

MEDICATION

DRUG(S) OF CHOICE
• Homatropine hydrobromide 2% ophthalmic solution (Isopto) - 2 gtts to the affected eye bid, or as often as every 3 hours if necessary, plus
• Prednisolone acetate 1% ophthalmic suspension - 2 gtts to the affected eye every 1 hour initially, tapering to qid with improvement
Contraindications:
• Hypersensitivity to the medication or component of the preparation
• Cycloplegia is contraindicated in patients known to have, or predisposed to, glaucoma
• Topical corticosteroid therapy is contraindicated in uveitis secondary to infectious etiologies
Precautions:
• Homatropine hydrobromide may produce adverse systemic antimuscarinic effects. Use extreme caution in infants and young children because of increased susceptibility to systemic effects.
• Topical corticosteroids may increase intraocular pressure. Prolonged use may cause cataract formation and exacerbate existing herpetic keratitis which may masquerade as iritis.
Significant possible interactions: Refer to manufacturer's profile of each drug

ALTERNATIVE DRUGS
• Cycloplegia - scopolamine hydrobromide 0.25% (Isopto Hyoscine) up to 3 times daily, or cyclopentolate hydrochloride 1% (Cyclogyl)
• Anti-inflammatory - prednisolone sodium phosphate 1% (Ocu-Pred Forte), dexamethasone sodium phosphate 0.1% (Ocu-Dex), and dexamethasone suspension
• Systemic nonsteroidal anti-inflammatory agents may provide some benefit

FOLLOWUP

PATIENT MONITORING
• Ophthalmologic followup as recommended by consultant
• Schedule for complete history and physical to evaluate for associated systemic disease

PREVENTION/AVOIDANCE   N/A

POSSIBLE COMPLICATIONS
Loss of vision as a result of the following:
◊ Keratic precipitate deposition on the corneal or lens surfaces
◊ Increased intraocular pressure, acute angle-closure glaucoma
◊ Formation of synechiae
◊ Cataract formation
◊ Vasculitis with vascular occlusion, retinal infarction
◊ Macular edema
◊ Optic nerve damage

EXPECTED COURSE AND PROGNOSIS
• Dependent upon the presence of causal diseases, or associated conditions
• Uveitis resulting from infections (systemic or local) tend to resolve with eradication of the underlying infection
• Uveitis associated with seronegative arthropathies tend to be acute (lasting less than 3 months) and frequently recurrent

MISCELLANEOUS

ASSOCIATED CONDITIONS
• Viral infections: HIV, herpes simplex, herpes zoster, cytomegalovirus
• Bacterial infections: Tuberculosis, leprosy, Propionibacterium, syphilis, leptospirosis, brucellosis, Lyme disease, Whipple's disease
• Parasitic infections: Toxoplasmosis, acanthamebiasis, toxocariasis, cysticercosis, onchocerciasis
• Fungal infections: Histoplasmosis, coccidioidomycosis, candidiasis, aspergillosis, sporotrichosis, blastomycosis, cryptococcosis
• Suspected immune-mediated: Ankylosing spondylitis, Behçet's disease, Crohn's disease, drug or hypersensitivity reaction, interstitial nephritis, juvenile rheumatoid arthritis, Kawasaki disease, multiple sclerosis, psoriatic arthritis, Reiter's syndrome, relapsing polychondritis, sarcoidosis, Sjögren's syndrome, systemic lupus erythematosus, ulcerative colitis, vasculitis, vitiligo, Vogt-Koyanagi (Harada's) syndrome

• Isolated eye disease: Acute multifocal placoid pigmentary epitheliopathy, acute retinal necrosis, bird-shot choroidopathy, Fuch's heterochromatic cyclitis, glaucomatocyclitic crisis, lens-induced uveitis, multifocal choroiditis, pars planitis, serpiginous choroiditis, sympathetic ophthalmia, trauma
• Masquerade syndromes: Leukemia, lymphoma, retinitis pigmentosa, retinoblastoma

AGE-RELATED FACTORS
Pediatric: Infection should be the primary consideration. Allergies and psychological factors (depression, stress) may serve as a trigger factor.
Geriatric: The inflammatory response to systemic disease may be suppressed
Others: N/A

PREGNANCY   May be of importance in the selection of medications

SYNONYMS
• Iritis, iridocyclitis
• Choroiditis, retinochoroiditis, chorioretinitis
• Anterior uveitis, posterior uveitis
• Pars planitis, panuveitis

ICD-9-CM
364.3 uveitis nos

SEE ALSO
• Iritis
• Retinitis

OTHER NOTES
• Synonyms are anatomic descriptions of the focus of the uveal inflammation
• Severe or unresponsive uveitis may require therapy including periocular injection of corticosteroids, systemic corticosteroids, cytotoxic agents (azathioprine, cyclophosphamide, chlorambucil and methotrexate), or immunosuppressive agents (cyclosporine)

ABBREVIATIONS
gtt = drop

REFERENCES
• Rosenbaum, J.T.: Uveitis: an internist's view. Arch Intern Med., V149, N5; P1173-6; May, 1989
• Rosenbaum, J.T.: An algorithm for the systemic evaluation of patients with uveitis: guidelines for the consultant. Semin Arthritis Rheum., V19; N4; 248-57; Feb, 1990
• Herman, D.C.: Endogenous uveitis: current concepts of treatment. Mayo Clin Proc; V65; N5; 671-83; May, 1990

Author   D. Peterson, M.D. & W. Toffler, M.D.

Vaginal adenosis

BASICS

DESCRIPTION Adenosis is a term used to describe non-epithelialized columnar glandular epithelium in the vagina. At approximately the 15th week of embryological development, the müllerian system, which forms the upper two-thirds of the vagina, fuses with the invaginating cloaca, which forms the lower vagina. Squamous metaplasia from the cloacal region then produces a squamous epithelium through the vagina. Adenosis occurs when this squamous epithelium fails to completely epithelialize the vagina.

System(s) affected: Reproductive

Genetics: Unknown

Incidence/Prevalence in USA: Adenosis is relatively common, affecting 10-20% of young females studied. As maturation progresses with puberty, epithelialization occurs.

Predominant age:
• Teenage years. From puberty to approximately age twenty, epithelialization occurs.
• By age thirty, it is extremely rare to have adenosis present

Predominant sex: Female only

SIGNS AND SYMPTOMS A clear, watery vaginal discharge which is the glandular epithelium producing a small amount of mucus

CAUSES
• In the vast majority of young females, the etiology is incomplete squamous metaplasia. This occurs as a natural phenomenon and resolves with age.
• In diethylstilbestrol (DES) exposed females, the incidence of adenosis is higher and the etiology presumably is from the effect of the DES on the developing embryological system

RISK FACTORS Diethylstilbestrol (DES) exposed females

DIAGNOSIS

DIFFERENTIAL DIAGNOSIS A thorough evaluation for adenocarcinoma of the vagina arising in adenosis should be done. A biopsy may be necessary to ensure that the process represents only benign adenosis. Colposcopy of the upper vagina aids in choosing the areas for biopsy. On visual inspection, adenosis appears as a fine, raised, reddened, granular type tissue.

LABORATORY
When extensive adenosis is present
◊ Four-quadrant Pap smear of the vagina should be obtained
◊ Initial colposcopy performed
◊ Once squamous metaplasia is complete, four quadrant pap smear need not be performed
Drugs that may alter lab results: N/A
Disorders that may alter lab results: N/A

PATHOLOGICAL FINDINGS Biopsy will show benign glandular epithelium, which has not yet undergone squamous metaplasia. Biopsies in the areas of ongoing squamous metaplasia will be typical for this process.

SPECIAL TESTS N/A

IMAGING N/A

DIAGNOSTIC PROCEDURES
• Four quadrant Pap smear should be liberally utilized to isolate quadrants of the vagina which may contain abnormalities. This can be followed by colposcopy and biopsy.
• Colposcopy should be used to outline areas of adenosis and insure that no malignancy is present

TREATMENT

APPROPRIATE HEALTH CARE
Outpatient

GENERAL MEASURES
• Unless malignancy is present, conservative treatment is indicated
• In the vast majority of young females with this condition, it will resolve with expectant management
• Aggressive therapy such as laser or surgical excision is only necessary if premalignant or malignant changes arise

ACTIVITY
• No limitations
• It is not necessary to avoid intercourse or placing objects in the vagina

DIET No special diet

PATIENT EDUCATION The patient should be educated that in the vast majority of situations this is benign and expectant management is all that is necessary
• American College of Obstetricians & Gynecologists (ACOG), 409 12th St., SW, Washington, DC 20024-2188, (800)762-ACOG

MEDICATIONS

DRUG(S) OF CHOICE N/A
Contraindications: N/A
Precautions: N/A
Significant possible interactions: N/A

ALTERNATIVE DRUGS N/A

FOLLOWUP

PATIENT MONITORING
• Initial evaluation consists of four-quadrant vaginal pap smear, cervical pap smear and colposcopy of the upper vagina and cervix
• If the initial colposcopy is normal, a yearly four-quadrant pap smear of the vagina and pap smear of the cervix is all that is necessary

PREVENTION/AVOIDANCE N/A

POSSIBLE COMPLICATIONS N/A

EXPECTED COURSE AND PROGNOSIS
• It is expected that the vast majority of patients will have squamous metaplasia with complete resolution of the adenosis
• The rare patient, 1:1,000 to 1:10,000, may develop adenocarcinoma in the adenosis and will require definitive therapy as for vaginal cancer

MISCELLANEOUS

ASSOCIATED CONDITIONS
DES exposure
◊ Adenosis from DES exposure should lead to an evaluation of other DES related abnormalities
◊ The greatest risk to the patient is from müllerian tract anomalies of the reproductive tract. These include cervical abnormalities with cervical hood, ridges, shortened cervix and incompetent cervix.
◊ Patients with a known DES exposure should have the reproductive tract evaluated prior to conception
◊ The vast majority of patients with adenosis have not been DES exposed and do not require evaluation of the reproductive system
◊ DES was last used to prevent spontaneous abortion in approximately 1970. This is a problem of decreasing importance.

AGE-RELATED FACTORS
Pediatric: N/A
Geriatric:
• Adenosis is a disorder of the young female. By the time of menopause the vagina and cervix should be completely epithelialized.
• The presence of glandular epithelium in the postmenopausal patient is an indication for excision and close evaluation for the possibility of a well-differentiated adenocarcinoma
Others: N/A

PREGNANCY Pregnancy produces a wide eversion of the transformation zone of the cervix. This will occasionally become so widely everted that it will extend onto the vaginal fornices leading to the impression of adenosis. This will resolve after the pregnancy is completed.

SYNONYMS N/A

ICD-9-CM 752.49

SEE ALSO N/A

OTHER NOTES N/A

ABBREVIATIONS N/A

REFERENCES
• Sandberg, E.C.: The incidence and distribution of occult vaginal adenosis. Am J Obstet Gynecol 1968;101:322-34
• Hopkins, M.P.: Vaginal Neoplasms. In Textbook of Gynecology. Edited by L.J. Copeland. Philadelphia, W.B. Saunders Co., 1993

Author M. Hopkins, M.D. & E. Jenison, M.D.

Vaginal bleeding during pregnancy

 BASICS

DESCRIPTION Vaginal bleeding during pregnancy has many etiologies and ranges in severity from mild (with normal pregnancy outcome) to life-threatening for both infant and mother. The bleeding can vary from scant to excessive, from brown to bright red, and can be painless or painful. The different causes can be divided into vaginal, cervical and uterine factors. The differential diagnosis is guided by the gestational age of the pregnancy.

System(s) affected: Reproductive, Cardiovascular
Genetics: No known genetic pattern
Incidence in USA: Common
Prevalence in USA: Common
Predominant age: Childbearing
Predominant sex: Female only

SIGNS AND SYMPTOMS
• Bleeding can vary from scant to excessive
• Color of blood varies from brown to bright red
• May be painless or painful

CAUSES
• Vaginal infection or trauma
• Cervicitis
• Cervical polyp
• Cervical neoplasia
• Hyperemia of cervix
• Postcoital bleeding
• Ectopic pregnancy
• Molar pregnancy
• Implantation bleeding
• Spontaneous abortion
• Placenta previa
• Placental abruptio
• Bloody show
• Unknown - 50% of first trimester bleeding, no cause ever found

RISK FACTORS Varies, based on individual causes

 DIAGNOSIS

DIFFERENTIAL DIAGNOSIS
• Vaginal or cervical causes can occur throughout the pregnancy
• First trimester bleeding - ectopic pregnancy, molar pregnancy, or spontaneous abortion
• Second or third trimester bleeding - placenta previa, placental abruptio, or bloody show

LABORATORY
• CBC
• Quantitative beta human chorionic gonadotropin (HCG) - in early pregnancy bleeding; follow serially every couple of days. Levels fall in spontaneous abortion, are extremely high in molar pregnancy, and rise gradually in ectopic or intrauterine pregnancy.
• Blood type and screen - Rh negative patients need Rho(D) immune globulin (RhoGAM). If bleeding profuse, a transfusion may be required.
• Coagulation studies (fibrinogen, fibrin split products, platelets) - useful in late pregnancy bleeding and missed abortion
Drugs that may alter lab results: N/A
Disorders that may alter lab results: N/A

PATHOLOGICAL FINDINGS Depends on cause

SPECIAL TESTS N/A

IMAGING
• Ultrasound - gestational sac seen at 5-6 weeks, fetal heart tones at 8-9 weeks. Diagnostic of molar pregnancy with 98% accuracy, locates placenta, may show degree of placenta separation in abruptio.
• Serial ultrasound may be required in early pregnancy to make diagnosis

DIAGNOSTIC PROCEDURES
• In first trimester bleeding - pelvic exam, culdocentesis, laparoscopy, laparotomy
• In second or third trimester bleeding - locate placenta by ultrasound prior to pelvic exam. If placenta previa, do not perform bimanual or speculum exam unless set up for immediate cesarean delivery.

 TREATMENT

APPROPRIATE HEALTH CARE
• In first trimester bleeding most patients can be managed as outpatient
• In late pregnancy bleeding, most patients need inpatient monitoring

GENERAL MEASURES
• Once ectopic or molar pregnancy is diagnosed immediate surgical treatment is appropriate
• In late pregnancy bleeding, the amount of bleeding and presence of maternal or fetal compromise indicates whether emergent cesarean section is performed or whether conservative measures are appropriate until greater fetal maturity can be obtained

ACTIVITY Bedrest, no coitus, no douching

DIET No restrictions

PATIENT EDUCATION
• Patient should be instructed to report any increase in the amount and frequency of bleeding and should seek immediate care if experiencing abdominal pain or sudden increased bleeding. She should bring for examination any tissue passed vaginally.
• Grief counselling is appropriate if pregnancy loss is inevitable
• American College of Obstetricians & Gynecologists (ACOG), 409 12th St., SW, Washington, DC 20024-2188, (800)762-ACOG

MEDICATIONS

DRUG(S) OF CHOICE None
Contraindications: N/A
Precautions: N/A
Significant possible interactions: N/A

ALTERNATIVE DRUGS N/A

FOLLOWUP

PATIENT MONITORING Daily to weekly depending on diagnosis and severity of bleeding

PREVENTION/AVOIDANCE N/A

POSSIBLE COMPLICATIONS
• Anemia
• Shock
• Fetal or maternal death
• Infection
• Choriocarcinoma or invasive mole in the case of hydatidiform mole
• Premature delivery of infant with associated complications
• Coagulopathy

EXPECTED COURSE AND PROGNOSIS Depends on the cause of vaginal bleeding, the severity of bleeding and the rapidity of diagnosis. Maternal mortality is 1 in 826 of ectopic pregnancies.

MISCELLANEOUS

ASSOCIATED CONDITIONS Depends on cause of vaginal bleeding

AGE-RELATED FACTORS
Pediatric: N/A
Geriatric: N/A
Others: N/A

PREGNANCY A complication of pregnancy

SYNONYMS N/A

ICD-9-CM
• Molar pregnancy 630
• Ectopic pregnancy 633.9
• Spontaneous abortion 634.9
• Placenta previa 641.1
• Placental abruptio 641.2

SEE ALSO
• Abortion, spontaneous
• Abruptio placenta
• Cervical cancer
• Cervical dysplasia
• Cervical polyps
• Cervicitis
• Cervicitis ectropion and true erosion
• Ectopic pregnancy
• Premature labor
• Vagina, malignancy
• Vulvovaginitis, monilial

OTHER NOTES N/A

ABBREVIATIONS N/A

REFERENCES
• Cunningham, F.G., MacDonald, P.C. & Gant, N.F. (eds.): William's Obstetrics. 18th Ed. Norwalk, CT, Appleton & Lange, 1989
• Danforth, D.M., Scott, J.R., et al. (eds.): Obstetrics and Gynecology. 6th Ed. Philadelphia, J.B. Lippincott, 1990

Author K. Vore, M.D.

Vaginal malignancy

BASICS

DESCRIPTION
• Vaginal intraepithelial neoplasia (carcinoma in situ): A premalignant phase with full thickness neoplastic changes in the superficial epithelium. However there is no invasion through the basement membrane.
• Invasive malignancies: Vaginal malignancies are squamous cell in 90% of the patients and the remaining 10% are adenocarcinomas, sarcomas and melanomas. The clear cell carcinoma is a subtype of adenocarcinoma.
• To be classified as a vaginal malignancy, only the vagina can be involved. If the cervix or the vulva is involved, then the tumor is classified as a primary cancer arising from the cervix or the vulva.
System(s) affected: Reproductive
Genetics: No known genetic pattern
Incidence/Prevalence in USA: This is the rarest of all gynecological malignancies
Predominant age:
• Carcinoma in situ - mid-forties to sixties
• Invasive squamous cell malignancy - mid-sixties to seventies
• Adenocarcinoma - any age range, fifties is mean age
• Mixed müllerian sarcomas and leiomyosarcomas in the adult population - mean age sixty
• Sarcoma botryoides and embryonal sarcomas - occur in the pediatric population
Predominant sex: Female only

SIGNS AND SYMPTOMS
• Abnormal bleeding is the most common symptom. This results from a fungating tumor present in the vagina.
• Dyspareunia
• Postcoital bleeding can result from direct trauma to the tumor
• Pain along with symptoms and signs of hydroureter are late findings when tumor has spread into the paravaginal tissues and extends to the pelvic side wall
• In the pediatric population, sarcomas can present either as a mass protruding from the vagina or as abnormal genital bleeding

CAUSES
• Women with a history of cervical malignancy have a higher probability of developing squamous cell malignancy in the vagina after hysterectomy
• The human papilloma virus (HPV) has been associated with vulvovaginal, cervical, adenocarcinoma and squamous cell carcinoma
• Smokers have a higher incidence
• Clear cell adenocarcinoma of the vagina in young women has been associated with diethylstilbestrol (DES) exposure. The incidence, however, is exceedingly rare estimated at 1:1,000 to 1:10,000 DES exposed females.
• Metastatic lesions can involve the vagina from the other gynecologic organs

• Renal cell carcinoma and breast cancer can metastasize to the vagina (rarely)

RISK FACTORS
• History of squamous cell cancer of the cervix or vulva
• Smoking
• Multiple sex partners

DIAGNOSIS

DIFFERENTIAL DIAGNOSIS
• Vaginal intraepithelial neoplasia (VAIN) involves premalignant changes that do not infiltrate beyond the basement membrane
• Adequate biopsies ensure that invasive lesions are not overlooked. Invasive lesions penetrate the basement membrane and cannot be treated conservatively. Other malignancies such as endometrial, cervix, bladder or colon cancer can invade directly into the vagina or metastasize to the vagina.
• In the childbearing age, female trophoblastic disease should be considered. The vagina is a common site of metastases. Biopsy will usually provide a clue to the primary site.

LABORATORY
Cytology will usually be positive when an obvious lesion is present
Drugs that may alter lab results: N/A
Disorders that may alter lab results: N/A

PATHOLOGICAL FINDINGS
• Stage 0 - carcinoma in situ
• Stage I - infiltrative tumor not involving the paravaginal tissues
• Stage II - paravaginal extension but not to the side wall
• Stage III - paravaginal extension to the side wall
• Stage IVA - tumor involving the bladder or the rectum
• Stage IVB - distant metastatic disease

SPECIAL TESTS   N/A

IMAGING
• Chest x-ray - lung metastases are a late finding.
• IVP - to evaluate for ureteral obstruction
• CAT scan to evaluate the retroperitoneum and especially the lymph nodes in the pelvic and periaortic area
• Lymphangiography is also useful for evaluation of the lymph node status
• Cystoscopy and cystograms to rule out bladder invasion
• Barium enema to rule out rectal invasion

DIAGNOSTIC PROCEDURES
• Colposcopy with directed biopsies for small lesions
• Wide excision under anesthesia of superficial disease may be necessary to insure that invasive cancer is not present
• Cystoscopy to rule out bladder invasion
• Sigmoidoscopy to rule out rectal invasion

TREATMENT

APPROPRIATE HEALTH CARE
Outpatient or inpatient depending on treatment

GENERAL MEASURES
• Carcinoma in situ can be treated by a variety of methods: Laser vaporization under microscopic guidance; Efudex intravaginal cream; partial vaginectomy
• Whenever there is a doubt as to the presence or absence of invasive disease, vaginectomy must be performed
• Invasive lesions are usually treated by radiation therapy, however, stage I lesions can be treated with radical hysterectomy, radical vaginectomy with pelvic lymph node dissection
• If the lesion involves the lower vagina, inguinal node dissection must also be done as cancer involving the lower vagina can metastasize to the groin region
• There is no effective chemotherapy for squamous cell malignancy of the vagina
• Sarcomas are treated by radiation therapy followed by pelvic exenteration if persistent disease is present
• Childhood sarcomas are treated with chemotherapy followed by local resection. Childhood sarcomas are responsive to multiagent combination chemotherapies.
• In all tumor types, metastatic disease from the vagina to other sites is only minimally responsive to chemotherapy

ACTIVITY
• The patients are usually ambulatory and able to resume full activity by six weeks after surgery
• Most patients are fully active while receiving radiation therapy

DIET
Unrestricted unless they are undergoing radiation

PATIENT EDUCATION
• This is a rare malignancy and these patients should be treated by a physician familiar and experienced with this malignancy
• Printed patient information available from: American College of Obstetricians & Gynecologists, 409 12th St., SW, Washington, DC 20024-2188, (800)762-ACOG

MEDICATIONS

DRUG(S) OF CHOICE
• With one exception, there are no chemotherapeutic agents to which this tumor is responsive. The exception is the childhood sarcomas, which have been treated with combinations of vincristine/Actinomycin/Cytoxan/cisplatin/VP-16.
• Adjuvant chemotherapy has no proven benefit in squamous cell or adenocarcinoma of the vagina
• Carcinoma in situ can be eradicated in 90% of patients with Efudex cream 5% applied bid x 2 hours x 7 days, then qd x 7 days, repeated in six weeks

Contraindications:
• Prior to treatment the diagnosis must be established with certainty
• If there is any doubt that a process beyond in situ disease exists, vaginectomy must be performed. Because these patients are often elderly, aggressive therapy is limited by the patient's performance status and ability to tolerate radical surgery, chemotherapy or radiation.

Precautions: Refer to manufacturer's literature
Significant possible interactions: Refer to manufacturer's literature

ALTERNATIVE DRUGS N/A

FOLLOWUP

PATIENT MONITORING
• Pelvic examination and Pap smear every 3 months for 2 years and then every 6 months for subsequent 3 years
• Chest x-ray once a year

PREVENTION/AVOIDANCE
• A Pap smear should be performed for all women on a yearly basis, even after hysterectomy
• Premalignant changes discovered on Pap smear screening should be followed up with colposcopy, biopsy and treatment. This needs to be undertaken by a physician well trained in the diagnosis and treatment of vaginal disease.
• Patients with a history of in situ or invasive disease of the cervix and/or the vulva should be followed at close intervals for development of disease in the vagina

POSSIBLE COMPLICATIONS Those
associated with major abdominal surgery or radiation therapy

EXPECTED COURSE AND PROGNOSIS
<u>Survival is based on stage</u>
Stage and 5 year survival
◊ I - 60%
◊ II - 40%
◊ III - 20%
◊ IVA - 5%
◊ IVB - 0%

MISCELLANEOUS

ASSOCIATED CONDITIONS Due to the field effect, patients with vaginal cancer are more likely to develop malignancy in the cervix or vulva and should be followed closely

AGE-RELATED FACTORS
Pediatric: Childhood sarcomas can be treated in a conservative fashion with multi-modality therapy. This avoids the loss of the young child's bladder and/or rectum.
Geriatric: Older patients, many with a long smoking history are at a higher risk for surgery
Others:
• Younger patients, who have not completed their family, can occasionally be treated with limited resection and localized radiation to the area
• Premenopausal women, who desire to retain ovarian function, are better candidates for radical surgery for early stage disease

PREGNANCY This malignancy is not associated with pregnancy

SYNONYMS
• Bowen's disease
• Vaginal intraepithelial neoplasia (VAIN)

ICD-9-CM 184.0

SEE ALSO N/A

OTHER NOTES N/A

ABBREVIATIONS N/A

REFERENCES
• Hopkins, M.P.: Vaginal Neoplasms. In Textbook of Gynecology. Edited by L.J. Copeland. Philadelphia, W.B. Saunders Co., 1993
• Peters, W.A., Kumar, N.B. & Morley, G.W.: Carcinoma of the vagina: Factors influencing treatment outcome. Cancer 1985;55(4):892-97

Author M. Hopkins, M.D. & E. Jenison, M.D.

Vaginismus

BASICS

DESCRIPTION Involuntary painful contraction of perineal muscles prior to or during insertion of any object into vagina. The experience or even the anticipation of pain on vaginal entry causes these muscles to contract, occluding the vaginal opening and causing further pain when penetration is attempted.
System(s) affected: Reproductive
Genetics: N/A
Incidence/Prevalence in USA: Unknown
Predominant age: Postpubertal
Predominant sex: Female only

SIGNS AND SYMPTOMS
• Pain with vaginal sexual intercourse
• Reluctance or avoidance of pelvic examination
• Infertility
• Small and non-distensible vaginal opening
• Rigid hymen
• Anatomic or congenital abnormalities

CAUSES
• History of genital or psychic trauma, especially incest
• Previous traumatic gynecologic examination
• Vaginal infections
• Skin disorders involving vulva
• Bartholin's cysts or abscess
• Scarring following episiotomy or vaginal repair operations
• PID and endometriosis
• Vaginitis
• Decreased vaginal lubrication secondary to hormonal imbalance

RISK FACTORS
• Previous sexual trauma
• Incest
• Rape

DIAGNOSIS

DIFFERENTIAL DIAGNOSIS N/A

LABORATORY As needed to identify infections and other medical causes
Drugs that may alter lab results: N/A
Disorders that may alter lab results: N/A

PATHOLOGICAL FINDINGS Varied if any

SPECIAL TESTS Psychiatric consultation or psychologic tests. May be invalidated by any axis I from American Psychiatric Association's Diagnostic and Statistical Manual of Mental Disorders (DSM-III-R).

IMAGING N/A

DIAGNOSTIC PROCEDURES
• Careful pelvic examination
• General and sexual history

TREATMENT

APPROPRIATE HEALTH CARE
Outpatient

GENERAL MEASURES
• Trusting and non-judgmental attitude on part of physician and all office staff
• Treatment of medical problems such as infections, cystocele, episiotomy scarring
• Referral to psychiatrist or counselor, if appropriate
• If patient has insufficient lubrication for intercourse, suggest use of lubricating creams or jellies

ACTIVITY Simple techniques of gentle, progressive, patient-controlled vaginal dilation

DIET No special diet

PATIENT EDUCATION
• Education about reproductive biology, normal adult sexual function, link between past trauma and current symptoms
• Instruction in techniques for vaginal dilatation
• American College of Obstetricians & Gynecologists (ACOG), 409 12th St., SW, Washington, DC 20024-2188, (800)762-ACOG

MEDICATIONS

DRUG(S) OF CHOICE None
Contraindications: Anxiolytics, especially benzodiazepines
Precautions: Anxiolytics can disinhibit and lead to traumatic memories of incest, possible suicide
Significant Possible Interactions: N/A

ALTERNATIVE DRUGS N/A

FOLLOWUP

PATIENT MONITORING When possible, initiate preventive health care such as Pap smear

PREVENTION/AVOIDANCE Societal action against incest, rape

POSSIBLE COMPLICATIONS
Precipitation of memory of incest prior to patient's readiness to deal with it

EXPECTED COURSE AND PROGNOSIS Some progress generally made if physician and therapist allow patient to proceed at her own pace

MISCELLANEOUS

ASSOCIATED CONDITIONS
• Marital stress, family dysfunction
• Dyspareunia

AGE-RELATED FACTORS Vaginismus is generally primary, e.g., happens with first attempt at intercourse (if previous incest, first attempt after puberty is time of onset)
Pediatric: N/A
Geriatric: N/A
Others: N/A

PREGNANCY Pregnancy can occur in patients with vaginismus via perineal ejaculation

SYNONYMS N/A

ICD-9-CM 306.51

SEE ALSO Sexual dysfunction in women

OTHER NOTES N/A

ABBREVIATIONS N/A

REFERENCES
• Leiblum, S.R. & Rosen, R.C.: Principles and Practice of Sex Therapy: Update for the 1990's. New York, The Guilford Press, 1989
• Wincze, J.P. & Carey, M.P.: Sexual Dysfunction: A Guide for Assessment and Treatment. New York, The Guilford Press, 1991
• Bancroft, J.: Human Sexuality and Its Problems. 2nd Ed. New York, Churchill Livingstone, 1989

Author J. Graves-Moy, M.D. & S. Duiker, M.D.

Varicose veins

BASICS

DESCRIPTION Elongated, dilated, tortuous superficial veins with congenitally absent valves, or valves that have become incompetent. Affects legs where reverse flow occurs when dependent.
System(s) affected: Cardiovascular, Skin/Exocrine
Genetics: Familial, dominant, x-linked
Incidence/Prevalence in USA: About 20% of adults
Predominant age: Middle age
Predominant sex: Female > Male (5:1)

SIGNS AND SYMPTOMS
- Sometimes asymptomatic
- Leg muscular cramp
- Dilatation, tortuosity of superficial veins chiefly in the lower extremities
- Edema of affected limb
- Leg aching
- Fatigue
- Symptoms worse during menses
- Pain if varicose ulcer develops

CAUSES
- Faulty valves in one or more perforator veins in the lower leg causing secondary incompetence at the saphenofemoral junction
- Deep thrombophlebitis
- Increased venous pressure from any cause
- In many individuals, no cause or precipitating factor found

RISK FACTORS
- Pregnancy
- Occupations requiring prolonged standing, restrictive clothing (e.g., very tight girdles)

DIAGNOSIS

DIFFERENTIAL DIAGNOSIS
- Nerve root compression
- Arthritis
- Peripheral neuritis

LABORATORY None helpful
Drugs that may alter lab results: N/A
Disorders that may alter lab results: N/A

PATHOLOGICAL FINDINGS
- Elongation and tortuosity of veins
- Medial fibrosis of veins
- Disappearance or atrophy of valves

SPECIAL TESTS Trendelenburg's test

IMAGING N/A

DIAGNOSTIC PROCEDURES Clinical inspection

TREATMENT

APPROPRIATE HEALTH CARE
Outpatient

GENERAL MEASURES
Conservative methods
◊ Frequent rest periods with legs elevated
◊ Lightweight, elastic compression hosiery. Best put on before getting out of bed.
◊ Avoid girdles and other restrictive clothing
◊ If stasis ulcers present, use warm, wet dressings
Surgical and other methods
◊ If there is pain, recurrent phlebitis, skin changes, or for cosmetic improvement for severe cases
◊ Ligation and stripping of the saphenous vein
◊ Injection of sclerosing solution
◊ Stab evulsion phlebectomy - newer procedure with shorter recovery time
◊ For extensive fibrosis - excision of the entire area, followed by skin graft may be necessary
Spider veins (idiopathic telangiectases)
◊ Fine intracutaneous angiectasis
◊ May be extensive/unsightly
◊ Eliminate with intracapillary injections of 1% solution of sodium tetradecyl sulfate (or hypertonic saline 23.4%) using a fine-bore needle
◊ Subsequent treatments may be required until optimal results attained

ACTIVITY
- Avoid long periods of standing
- Appropriate exercise routine as part of conservative treatment
- Walking regimen after sclerotherapy is important to help promote healing
- Apply elastic stockings before lowering legs from the bed
- Never sit with legs hanging down

DIET
- No special diet
- Weight loss diet recommended, if obesity a problem

PATIENT EDUCATION
- Inform patients that the surgery or sclerotherapy may not prevent development of varicosities and that the procedure may need to be repeated in later years
- For patient education materials favorably reviewed on this topic, contact: National Heart, Lung & Blood Institute, Communications & Public Information Branch, National Institutes of Health, Building 31, Room 41-21, 9000 Rockville Pike, Bethesda, MD 20892, (301)496-4236

MEDICATIONS

DRUG(S) OF CHOICE Injection sclerotherapy with compression to totally obliterate the vein by fibrosis. Sclerosant is sodium tetradecyl sulfate 1-3% solution. Bandages remain 3 weeks or longer.
Contraindications: Refer to manufacturer's literature
Precautions: No oral contraceptives for at least 6 weeks prior to sclerotherapy because of their thrombogenic effect
Significant possible interactions: Refer to manufacturer's literature

ALTERNATIVE DRUGS N/A

FOLLOWUP

PATIENT MONITORING Until surgery or conservative therapy brings maximal benefit

PREVENTION/AVOIDANCE N/A

POSSIBLE COMPLICATIONS
- Petechial hemorrhages
- Chronic edema
- Superimposed infection
- Varicose ulcers
- Pigmentation
- Eczema
- Recurrence after surgical treatment
- Scarring or nerve damage from stripping technique

EXPECTED COURSE AND PROGNOSIS
- Usual course - chronic
- Prognosis - favorable with appropriate treatment

MISCELLANEOUS

ASSOCIATED CONDITIONS
- Stasis dermatitis
- Stasis ulcer

AGE-RELATED FACTORS
Pediatric: Unlikely in this age group
Geriatric:
- More common, usually valvular degeneration, but may be secondary to chronic venous deficiency
- Recommended therapy - elastic support hose and frequent rests with legs elevated rather than ligation and stripping
Others: N/A

PREGNANCY Frequent problem. Use of elastic stockings recommended for individuals who have a history of varicosities or when activities involve a great deal of standing.

SYNONYMS N/A

ICD-9-CM 454.1

SEE ALSO Dermatitis stasis

OTHER NOTES N/A

ABBREVIATIONS N/A

REFERENCES Berkow, R., et al. (eds.): Merck Manual. 15th Ed. Rahway, NJ, Merck Sharp & Dohme, 1987

Author J. Florence, M.D.

Ventricular septal defect (VSD)

 BASICS

DESCRIPTION Congenital or acquired defect of the interventricular septum that allows communication of blood between the left and right ventricles. Other than bicuspid aortic valve, this is the most common congenital heart malformation reported in infants and children. It also occurs as a complication of acute myocardial infarctions (MI).
Genetics: Multifactorial etiology; autosomal dominant and recessive transmission have been reported
Incidence/Prevalence in USA:
• Congenital - 100-500 of 100,000 live births
• Acute myocardial infarctions - estimated to complicate 1-3%
Predominant age: Infants and children
Predominant sex: Male = Female (male > female if secondary to myocardial infarction)

SIGNS AND SYMPTOMS
• Respiratory distress, tachypnea
• Forceful apical impulse
• Thrill along the left lower or midsternal borders
• High-frequency holosystolic murmur
• S3
• Increased intensity of P2
• Elevated jugular venous pressure

CAUSES
• Congenital
• In adults, secondary to myocardial infarction

RISK FACTORS
Congenital
  ◊ 4.2% risk of sibling being affected
  ◊ 4.0% of offspring being affected
Post-acute myocardial infarctions
  ◊ First MI
  ◊ Limited coronary artery disease
  ◊ Hypertension
  ◊ Most frequent within first week after myocardial infarction (MI)

 DIAGNOSIS

DIFFERENTIAL DIAGNOSIS
• Any disease with left-to-right shunt, such as large patent ductus arteriosus or atrial septal defect
• Children - tetralogy of Fallot
• Adults - acute mitral regurgitation

LABORATORY None specific
Drugs that may alter lab results: None
Disorders that may alter lab results: None

PATHOLOGICAL FINDINGS
Congenital VSD's (4 major anatomical types):
  ◊ Membranous (75%)
  ◊ Muscular (10%)
  ◊ Atrioventricular canal type (10%)
  ◊ Supracristal (5%; higher percent in Oriental population)
Postmyocardial infarction VSD's
  ◊ Involve predominantly the muscular septum

SPECIAL TESTS None

IMAGING
• Chest x-ray may demonstrate increased pulmonary vascularity and/or cardiomegaly
• Two-dimensional echocardiogram for visualization
• Color-flow Doppler, for detection of ventricular septal defect jet

DIAGNOSTIC PROCEDURES
• Electrocardiogram may demonstrate left ventricular hypertrophy initially, with right ventricular hypertrophy occurring later in the course
• Cardiac catheterization (left and right heart) can establish the diagnosis
• Demonstration of an oxygen saturation step-up (> 8 mm Hg) from the right atrium to the distal pulmonary artery with Swan-Ganz catheter

 TREATMENT

APPROPRIATE HEALTH CARE
• Outpatient, until surgical repair is indicated
• Inpatient in setting of acute MI
• Inpatient for treatment of severe congestive heart failure

GENERAL MEASURES
• In most cases, surgical closure of the VSD is the treatment of choice
• In adults, intra-aortic balloon pump placement may be a temporizing measure prior to surgery
• Congenital VSD - surgery is usually performed electively before the child enters school, or before, if hemodynamically indicated
• Post-MI VSD's - the timing of surgery is disputed and dependent on the clinical setting

ACTIVITY As tolerated

DIET Low sodium

PATIENT EDUCATION
• Endocarditis prophylaxis
• Parents need support and instructions for prevention of complications until the child is ready for surgery
• Possible side effects of medications

MEDICATIONS

DRUG(S) OF CHOICE
Pediatric
◊ Nitroglycerin 0.5-5 mcg/kg/min IV (max 60 mcg/kg/min)
◊ Hydralazine 0.5 mg/kg/day po q6-8h (max 200 mg/day)
◊ Captopril 0.1-0.4 mg/kg/dose po given q6-24h. (max 6 mg/kg/24h)
◊ Nitroprusside 0.5-8 mcg/kg/min IV
◊ Prazosin first dose 5 mcg/kg po (max 25 mcg/kg/dose q6h)
Adult
◊ Nitroglycerin drip beginning at 5 mcg/kg/min and increasing by 5 mcg/kg/min every few minutes, then by up to 20 mcg/kg/min and titrate effect blood pressure, cardiac output, etc.
◊ Nitroprusside beginning at 10 mcg/min and increasing by 5-10 mcg/min every few minutes, titrating to blood pressure, cardiac output, etc.
◊ Angiotensin converting enzyme (ACE) inhibitors (e.g., captopril 6.25-25 mg po tid or lisinopril 2.5-20 mg po qd or enalapril 2.5-15 mg po qd or bid)
◊ Hydralazine 10-100 mg po qid
Contraindications: Drugs that increase peripheral vascular resistance may increase right-to-left shunting
Precautions: Hypotension
Significant possible interactions: Refer to manufacturer's profile of each drug

ALTERNATIVE DRUGS   Diuretics and digoxin may also be beneficial in certain circumstances

FOLLOWUP

PATIENT MONITORING   Close followup (at least every 6 months) of a congenital VSD is necessary until primary intracardiac repair is performed to ensure that significant pulmonary hypertension does not develop

PREVENTION/AVOIDANCE   For adults, avoiding risk factors for myocardial infarction

POSSIBLE COMPLICATIONS
• Congestive heart failure
• Infective endocarditis
• Sudden death
• Hemoptysis
• Chest pain
• Cerebral abscess
• Paradoxical emboli
• Cardiogenic shock
• Heart block may rarely accompany surgical closure

EXPECTED COURSE AND PROGNOSIS
Congenital
◊ Course is variable depending on the size of the VSD
◊ 4% of patients with VSD develop infective endocarditis by the third or fourth decade of life
◊ Progressive pulmonary vascular disease and pulmonary hypertension are the most feared complications of VSD caused by left-to-right shunting, and may eventually lead to reversal of the shunt (Eisenmenger's complex)
◊ Death usually occurs in the fourth decade of life if untreated
Post-myocardial infarction
◊ Variable course
◊ Dependent on right ventricular function
◊ Cardiogenic shock in 55% in one series

MISCELLANEOUS

ASSOCIATED CONDITIONS
Congenital
◊ Tetralogy of Fallot
◊ Aortic valvular deformities, especially aortic insufficiency
◊ Down's syndrome (Trisomy 21)
◊ Transposition of the great arteries
◊ Tricuspid atresia
◊ Truncus arteriosus
◊ Patent ductus arteriosus
◊ Atrial septal defect
◊ Pulmonic stenosis
◊ Subaortic stenosis
Adult
◊ Coronary artery disease

AGE-RELATED FACTORS
Pediatric: 30% of VSD's in children close spontaneously by age 3
Geriatric: Almost entirely associated with myocardial infarction
Others: N/A

PREGNANCY
• May exacerbate symptoms and signs with a congenital VSD
• Tolerated during pregnancy if the septal defect is small

SYNONYMS   VSD

ICD-9-CM   745.4

SEE ALSO
• Tetralogy of Fallot
• Myocardial infarction

OTHER NOTES   N/A

ABBREVIATIONS   N/A

REFERENCES
• Friedman, W.F.: Congenital heart disease in infancy and childhood. In Heart disease - A Textbook of Cardiovascular Medicine. 3rd Ed. Edited by E. Braunwald. Philadelphia, W.B. Saunders Co., 1988, pp. 920-923, 985-988
• Radford, M.J., et al.: Ventricular septal rupture: a review of clinical and physiologic features and an analysis of survival. Circulation 64(3), 1981

Author   G. Pennock, M.D.

Vitamin deficiency

BASICS

DESCRIPTION Vitamin deficiency syndromes develop slowly and are difficult to diagnose. Multiple deficiencies of vitamins occur more frequently than a deficiency in a single vitamin.
- Vitamin classifications: Fat-soluble (A, D, E, and K) and water-soluble (B group and C)
- Vitamin A (retinol)
- Vitamin B1 (thiamine)
- Vitamin B2 (riboflavin)
- Vitamin B3 (niacin, nicotinic acid, niacinamide)
- Vitamin B6 (pyridoxine)
- Vitamin B12 (cobalamin)
- Vitamin C (ascorbic acid)
- Vitamin D (vitamin D2 = ergocalciferol; vitamin D3 = cholecalciferol)
- Vitamin K (K1 = phytomenadione; K2 = menaquinone; K3 = menadione)

Genetics:
- Hereditary vitamin D-dependent rickets - autosomal recessive syndrome
- Thiamine-dependent beriberi - rare hereditary metabolic disorder

Incidence/Prevalence in USA: Unknown
Predominant age: Elderly
Predominant sex: Male = Female

SIGNS AND SYMPTOMS
Vitamin A (retinol)
- ◊ Night blindness
- ◊ Hyperkeratosis
- ◊ Xerophthalmia
- ◊ Growth retardation, loss of appetite, and anemia commonly found in children
- ◊ Bitot's spots (superficial foamy patches on exposed bulbar conjunctiva)

Vitamin B1 (thiamine)
- ◊ Beriberi (peripheral neuropathy, muscular weakness, anorexia, congestive heart failure and generalized edema)
- ◊ Infantile beriberi (heart failure, aphonia, and absent deep tendon reflex; occurs in infants breast-fed by thiamine-deficient mothers
- ◊ Wernicke-Korsakoff syndrome (brain hemorrhage, mental confusion and aphonia are early symptoms followed by weakness of sixth nerve, total ophthalmoplegia, coma, and death)

Vitamin B2 (riboflavin)
- ◊ Angular stomatitis
- ◊ Corneal vascularization
- ◊ Amblyopia
- ◊ Cheilosis
- ◊ Sebaceous dermatitis
- ◊ During pregnancy, deficiency leads to fetal skeletal abnormalities such as shortened bones and deformed growth

Vitamin B3 (niacin, nicotinic acid, niacinamide)
- ◊ Pellagra (dermatosis, glossitis, GI dysfunction, CNS dysfunction, organic psychosis)

Vitamin B6 (pyridoxine)
- ◊ Convulsions in infants
- ◊ Anemias
- ◊ Neuropathy
- ◊ Seborrhea-like skin lesions

Vitamin B12 (cobalamin)
- ◊ Peripheral neuropathy
- ◊ Megaloblastic anemia
- ◊ Pernicious anemia
- ◊ Some psychiatric syndromes

Vitamin C (ascorbic acid)
- ◊ Scurvy (loose teeth, gingivitis, hemorrhages)

Vitamin D (vitamin D2 = ergocalciferol; vitamin D3 = cholecaliferol)
- ◊ Rickets
- ◊ Osteomalacia

Vitamin E (alpha-tocopherol)
- ◊ RBC hemolysis
- ◊ Creatinuria
- ◊ Ceroid deposition in muscle

Vitamin K (K1 = phytomenadione; K2 = menaquinone; K3 = menadione)
- ◊ Hemorrhage from deficient prothrombin

CAUSES
- Inadequate dietary intake
- Impaired absorption or storage

RISK FACTORS
- Alcoholism
- Parenteral nutrition
- Malabsorption
- Bile deficiency
- Dialysis
- Chronic protein-calorie undernutrition
- Deficiencies of other vitamins
- Interactions with medications
- Infants
- Elderly
- Lower socioeconomic status
- Laxative abuse
- Genetic disorder - abetalipoproteinemia (vitamin E)
- Prolonged lactation (vitamin C)
- Intestinal parasites
- Drug abuse
- Food faddism or bizarre nutritional practices
- Gastrointestinal surgery

DIAGNOSIS

DIFFERENTIAL DIAGNOSIS
- Vitamin A deficiency - retinitis pigmentosa
- Vitamin B1 deficiency - polyneuropathy
- Vitamin B2 deficiency - other causes of seborrheic dermatitis and ocular lesions
- Vitamin D - infantile scurvy; congenital syphilis; chondrodystrophy; readily distinguishable disorders (creatinism, hydrocephalus, poliomyelitis, etc.); convulsions due to other causes
- Vitamin K - liver damage, anticoagulant or salicylate therapy, other disorders that produce hemorrhagic symptoms (scurvy, allergic purpura, leukemia, thrombocytopenia)
- Niacin - other causes of stomatitis, glossitis, diarrhea, dementia

LABORATORY
- Vitamin A - serum levels below normal
- Vitamin B1 - elevated blood pyruvate, decreased urinary thiamine excretion
- Vitamin B2 - serum level < than 2 mcg/100 mL, urinary excretion of < 30 mcg of riboflavin/gm of creatinine
- Vitamin B3 - none
- Vitamin B6 - may be decreased serum levels or RBC transaminases (no generally accepted test to determine a deficiency)
- Vitamin B12 - serum levels < 150 pg/mL (Schilling test)
- Vitamin C - serum levels < 0.4 mg/mL; WBC ascorbic levels < 25 mg/100 mL
- Vitamin D - plasma calcium level < 7.5 mg/100 mL; low plasma vitamin D sterolsinorganic phosphate serum levels < 3 mg/100 mL; serum citrate levels, 2.5 mg/100 mL; alkaline phosphate < 4 Bodansky units/100 mL
- Vitamin E - serum levels < 0.8 mg/100 mL (adults)
- Vitamin K - prothrombin time 25% longer than normal range (diagnostic for vitamin deficiency after ruling out other disorders), PIUKA II test

Drugs that may alter lab results: Refer to laboratory test reference
Disorders that may alter lab results: Refer to laboratory test reference

PATHOLOGICAL FINDINGS N/A

SPECIAL TESTS N/A

IMAGING N/A

DIAGNOSTIC PROCEDURES History and physical

TREATMENT

APPROPRIATE HEALTH CARE
Outpatient usually. Inpatient in severe cases.

GENERAL MEASURES
- Treatment of any underlying causes
- Oral or parenteral vitamin therapeutic replacement
- Maintenance vitamin supplement as required
- For vitamin D deficiency - adequate exposure to sunlight

ACTIVITY As tolerated

DIET
- For dietary deficiencies - provide nutritional counseling with emphasis on appropriate foods and the proper methods for their preparation
- Abstain from alcohol

PATIENT EDUCATION
- Refer patients to appropriate social service agencies if socioeconomic factors contribute to deficient diet
- Emphasis on compliance with vitamin supplementation regimens
- Help with alcohol or smoking cessation

MEDICATIONS

DRUG(S) OF CHOICE
• Vitamin A - cod liver or halibut liver oil. Acute deficiencies require aqueous vitamin A solution IM.
• Vitamin B1 - oral thiamine 5-30 mg tid depending on deficiency. Maintenance - supplemental B complex vitamin.
• Vitamin B2 - oral riboflavin 10-30 mg/day in divided doses until patient response is evident, then decrease to 2-4 mg/day until recovered. May be given IM 5-20 mg/day.
• Vitamin B3 - confirmed deficiencies require niacinamide 300-500 mg/day in divided doses by mouth or IV. Supplemental B complex vitamins and dietary increase in foods high in niacin.
• Vitamin B6 - oral or parenteral replacement for confirmed deficiency. Prophylactic doses for epileptic children. Women on oral contraceptives may need supplement (2.5-10 mg po).
• Vitamin B12 - for severe deficiency, parenteral cobalamin 30 mcg IM or subcutaneous for 5-10 days. Supplements as needed for maintenance.
• Vitamin C - daily doses of 100-200 mg in synthetic form or in orange juice for mild scurvy, doses up to 500 mg/day in severe disease
• Vitamin D - oral doses of vitamin D or cod liver oil. For rickets refractory to vitamin D, include 25-hydroxycholecalciferol (active form of vitamin D).
• Vitamin E - oral or parenteral replacement with a water soluble vitamin E supplement, 60-70 units/day for adult, 1 unit/kg/day for children
• Vitamin K - 10 mg (adult dose) phytonadione (vitamin K) for hypoprothrombinemia given subcutaneously or IM. For nonemergency, give oral dose 5-20 mg.
Contraindications: Refer to manufacturer's literature
Precautions: Refer to manufacturer's literature
Significant possible interactions: Refer to manufacturer's literature

ALTERNATIVE DRUGS N/A

FOLLOWUP

PATIENT MONITORING As needed depending on severity of problem

PREVENTION/AVOIDANCE
• Proper nutrition
• Supplemental vitamins if needed
• Reduce risk factors that lead to deficiency where possible
• Vitamin D deficiency - adequate exposure to sunlight (30 minutes several times a week)
• Postoperative vitamin K for patients who receive nothing by mouth
• Neonates - should receive vitamin K1 IM, subcutaneously or orally to prevent hemolytic disease of the newborn

POSSIBLE COMPLICATIONS
• Vitamin A deficiency - mortality high in advanced cases; eye lesions are a threat to vision
• Vitamin B1 (thiamine) deficiency - cardiac beriberi and Wernicke-Korsakoff syndrome may be fatal if left untreated
• Vitamin B6 chronic deficiency - may increase risk of kidney stone formation
• Vitamin D deficiency - skeletal deformities, greenstick fractures, bone pain
• Excessive synthetic vitamin K may lead to hemolytic anemia and kernicterus in infants

EXPECTED COURSE AND
PROGNOSIS With proper diagnosis and adequate therapy, expect full recovery without complications

MISCELLANEOUS

ASSOCIATED CONDITIONS N/A

AGE-RELATED FACTORS
Pediatric:
• Vitamin D deficiency rickets is now rare in the U.S., but may occur in breast-fed infants who do not receive a vitamin D supplement, or in infants fed a formula with a nonfortified milk base
• Vitamin E deficiency in infants usually results from formulas high in polyunsaturated fatty acids that are fortified with iron but not vitamin E
• Vitamin K deficiency - common among newborns
Geriatric: More likely to have multiple risk factors that can lead to vitamin deficiencies
Others: N/A

PREGNANCY Women should take a supplemental multivitamin tablet that contains at least 60 mg of elemental iron and 1.0 mg of folic acid

SYNONYMS N/A

ICD-9-CM
• Multiple deficiency 269.2
• Vitamin A deficiency 264.9
• Vitamin B complex 266.9
• Vitamin B1 265.1
• Vitamin B2 266.0
• Vitamin B6 266.1
• Vitamin B12 266.2
• Vitamin C 267
• Vitamin D 268.9
• Vitamin E 269.1
• Vitamin K 269.0
• Vitamin K newborn 776.0

SEE ALSO N/A

OTHER NOTES N/A

ABBREVIATIONS N/A

REFERENCES
• Machlin, L.J. (ed.): Handbook of Vitamins. 2nd Ed. New York, Marcel Dekker, 1990
• Shils, M.E. & Young, V.R.: (eds.): Modern Nutrition in Health and Disease. 7th Ed. Philadelphia, Lea & Febiger, 1988

Author J. Florence, M.D.

Vitiligo

BASICS

DESCRIPTION An acquired, slowly progressive depigmenting condition in small or large areas of the skin due to the disappearance of previously active melanocytes.
• Type A is non-dermatomal and widespread. It represents 75% of cases.
• Type B is dermatomal or segmental. It represents the remaining 25% of cases.
System(s) affected: Skin/Exocrine
Genetics: Autosomal dominant with variable expression and incomplete penetrance. Positive family history in 30% of cases.
Incidence in USA: Unknown
Prevalence in USA: 1000-2000/100,000
Predominant age: All ages: 50% begin before age 20
Predominant sex: Male = Female

SIGNS AND SYMPTOMS
• Loss of pigment
• Locally increased sunburning
• Pruritus (10%)
• Premature greying (35%)
• Koebner's Phenomenon (aggravation by trauma)

CAUSES Etiology is unclear, but is thought to be an autoimmune reaction to preexisting melanocytes

RISK FACTORS
• Positive family history
• Autoimmune disorders

DIAGNOSIS

DIFFERENTIAL DIAGNOSIS Any condition that causes acquired hypomelanosis, including tinea versicolor, leprosy, lupus erythematosis, pityriasis alba, atopic dermatitis, albinism, alopecia areata, chemical exposure (phenols, arsenic, chloroquine, hydroquinone) steroid exposure, retinoic acid use, tuberous sclerosis, neurofibromatosis, melanocytic nevi (halo nevi), tumor regression of malignant melanoma, Addison's disease, hypopituitarism, hyperthyroidism

LABORATORY Routine blood and urine studies are usually normal in the absence of associated disease
Drugs that may alter lab results: N/A
Disorders that may alter lab results: N/A

PATHOLOGICAL FINDINGS Complete absence of melanocytes in skin biopsy. At the margins one may see a few lymphocytes and large melanocytes with abnormal melanosomes.

SPECIAL TESTS N/A

IMAGING N/A

DIAGNOSTIC PROCEDURES
• Examination under Wood's light accentuates the hypopigmented areas, especially in light-skinned individuals
• Skin scraping and a potassium hydroxide (KOH) preparation can be examined microscopically to rule out tinea versicolor

TREATMENT

APPROPRIATE HEALTH CARE
Outpatient except in rare cases of surgical skin-grafting or transplantation

GENERAL MEASURES
• Sun exposure can accentuate the difference between normal and abnormal skin, so for cosmetic reasons patients may wish to avoid this
• Skin dyes and cosmetics may be used as cover-ups

ACTIVITY Full Activity

DIET No special diet

PATIENT EDUCATION Reassure patient that in absence of associated autoimmune illness the problem is purely cosmetic. Successful cosmetic cover-up is usually quite simple.

Vitiligo

MEDICATIONS

DRUG(S) OF CHOICE
• Localized vitiligo: High potency topical steroids, e.g. clobetisol propionate (Temovate) cream applied qd for 2 months (qod on the face). Treatment may be resumed following a 1 to 4 month respite. Alternatively topical psoralens applied in a 1% solution followed in 90 minutes by ultraviolet exposure (UVA).
• Widespread vitiligo: Oral trimethylpsoralen or -8 methoxysoralen methoxsalen (Oxsoralen-Ultra) and UVA over a 12 to 24 month period. Alternatively depigmenting the remaining normal skin with hydroquinone cream (Benoquin) may be elected.

Contraindications:
• Absolute contraindications to use of psoralen compounds: Idiosyncratic reaction to psoralens, photosensitive disease (e.g., systemic lupus erthyematosus, albinism, porphyria), invasive squamous cell carcinoma, melanoma, aphakia
• Relative contraindications to use of psoralen compounds: Cardiac disease, hepatic dysfunction, multiple basal cell carcinomas, prior radiation therapy, prior arsenic therapy

Precautions:
• Watch for skin atrophy and telangiectasias when using topical steroids, especially on the face
• Watch for photosensitizers with UVA treatment
• Severe burns possible with topical psoralens
• Psoralen plus UVA (PUVA) cannot be used for children less than 12 years of age
• Patients undergoing PUVA therapy should have a screening ophthalmologic examination to rule out subclinical retinal pigmentary disease that is frequently associated with vitiligo

Significant possible interactions: Other
photosensitizers, e.g., tetracyclines and retinoic acid

ALTERNATIVE DRUGS N/A

FOLLOWUP

PATIENT MONITORING   If patient
receives PUVA therapy, a complete blood count, liver and renal function tests, and an ANA should be repeated at 6 month intervals

PREVENTION/AVOIDANCE   While
undergoing all therapies, excessive sun exposure should be avoided

POSSIBLE COMPLICATIONS
• Phototoxic reactions ranging from mild to severe with PUVA
• Skin atrophy and telangiectasias with topical steroids
• Contact dermatitis can occur with use of depigmenting agents and cosmetic covers

EXPECTED COURSE AND PROGNOSIS
• Only 5% spontaneously repigment
• Best results are with PUVA therapy where 70% have repigmentation of head and neck area, less in other body areas. Lower percentages respond to topical therapy
• There is no response in at least 20% of cases
• Once repigmentation occurs it usually persists.

MISCELLANEOUS

ASSOCIATED CONDITIONS
• Addison's disease
• Alopecia Areata
• Chronic Mucocutaneous candidiasis
• Diabetes mellitus
• Hypoparathyroidism
• Melanoma
• Pernicious anemia
• Polyglandular autoimmune syndrome
• Thyroid disorders (hyper and hypothyroidism)
- 30% of patients with vitiligo
• Uveitis

AGE-RELATED FACTORS
Pediatric: Childhood vitiligo is a distinct subset of vitiligo. Higher incidence of Type B (segmental) vitiligo. Also higher incidence of autoimmune and endocrine disease. Response is poor to topical PUVA therapy, but can be tried, or topical steroids may be prescribed.
Geriatric: NA
Others: N/A

PREGNANCY   Treatment with topical or oral
psoralens is pregnancy class C

SYNONYMS
• Hypomelanosis
• Depigmentation

ICD-9-CM   709.0

SEE ALSO   N/A

OTHER NOTES   If PUVA therapy
considered, dermatologic consultation should be considered

ABBREVIATIONS   N/A

REFERENCES
• Habif, T.: Clinical Dermatology. 2nd Ed. St. Louis, C.V. Mosby, 1990
• Reeves, J. & Maibach, H.: Clinical Dermatology Illustrated. 2nd Ed. Philadelphia, F.A. Davis, 1991

Author G. Silko, M.D.

Vulvar cancer

BASICS

DESCRIPTION
• Carcinoma in situ (Bowen's disease). Premalignant changes involving the squamous epithelium of the vulva.
• Squamous cell carcinoma - invasive squamous cell carcinoma is the most common malignancy involving the vulva in 85% of the patients. The malignancy can be well, moderately or poorly differentiated.
• Other invasive cell types include melanoma, Paget's disease, adenocarcinoma, adenocystic carcinoma, small cell carcinoma and sarcomas. Sarcomas are usually leiomyosarcoma and probably arise at the insertion of the round ligament in the labium majus.
System(s) affected: Reproductive
Genetics: No known genetic pattern
Incidence/Prevalence in USA: Invasive vulvar malignancy is a rare gynecologic malignancy accounting for approximately 2,000 new cases per year in the USA
Predominant age:
• In situ disease - mean age, forties
• Invasive malignancy - mean age, sixties with a range of twenties to nineties
Predominant sex: Female only

SIGNS AND SYMPTOMS
• In situ disease - a small raised area associated with pruritus
• Invasive malignancy - an ulcerated, non-healing area; as lesions become large, bleeding occurs with associated pain and foul smelling discharge
• In far advanced diseases - the patients can develop rectal bleeding or urethral obstruction
• Large involved inguinal lymph nodes are also associated with advanced disease

CAUSES
• Patients with cervical cancer are more likely to develop vulvar cancer at a later date. This is due to the so-called field effect with a carcinogen involving the lower genital tract.
• Human papilloma virus (HPV) has been associated with squamous cell abnormalities of the cervix, vagina and the vulva but has not been proven to be the causative agent
• Smoking is associated with squamous cell disease of the vulva possibly from direct irritation of the vulva by the transfer of tars and nicotine on the patient's hands

RISK FACTORS
• Old age. Invasive disease is rarely seen before age forty and the majority of the patients are elderly.
• In situ disease can occur at any age but is rarely seen before the age of twenty-five

DIAGNOSIS

DIFFERENTIAL DIAGNOSIS
• The definitive diagnosis for vulvar lesions is made by biopsy. Infectious processes can present as ulcerative lesions and include syphilis, lymphogranuloma venereum and granuloma inguinale
• Crohn's disease can present as an ulcerative area on the vulva
• Rarely, lesions can metastasize to the vulva

LABORATORY
• Squamous cell antigen can be elevated with invasive disease
• Hypercalcemia can occur when metastatic disease is present
Drugs that may alter lab results: N/A
Disorders that may alter lab results: N/A

PATHOLOGICAL FINDINGS
A surgical staging system is used for vulva cancer - TNM Classification = tumor, mode, and metastases:
◊ T1 - tumor less than or equal to 2.0 cm
◊ T2 - tumor greater than 2.0 cm
◊ T3 - lower urethra or vagina involved
◊ T4 - upper urethra, bladder, or rectum involved
◊ N0 - nodes negative
◊ N1 - unilateral positive lymph nodes
◊ N2 - bilateral positive lymph nodes
◊ M0 - no metastatic disease
◊ M1 - distant metastatic disease, positive pelvic lymphs node
International Federation of Obstetrics and Gynecology Classification using TNM:
◊ Stage I - T1, N0, M0
◊ Stage II - T2, N0, M0
◊ Stage III - T1-3, N1, M0; T3, N0-I, M0
◊ Stage IVA - T1-3, N2, M0
◊ Stage IVB - any T, any N, any M

SPECIAL TESTS N/A

IMAGING
• Chest x-ray to evaluate for metastatic disease to lungs
• CAT scan to evaluate pelvic lymph node status and periaortic lymph node status

DIAGNOSTIC PROCEDURES
• Office vulvar biopsy; vulvar punch biopsy should be done to establish the diagnosis
• Wide excision can be performed for carcinoma in situ and any lesion where there is doubt should be further excised for definitive diagnosis to insure that invasive disease is not coexistent with the carcinoma in situ
• Cystoscopy and sigmoidoscopy should be performed if there is a question of invasion into the urethra, bladder or rectum

TREATMENT

APPROPRIATE HEALTH CARE
Inpatient for treatment

GENERAL MEASURES
• In situ disease can be treated with wide excision or laser vaporization of the affected area. Laser vaporization is preferable in the younger patient while wide excision is preferable in the elderly patient where the risk of invasive disease is also higher.
• Invasive disease is treated primarily by radical vulvectomy and bilateral groin node dissection
• Radiation therapy is used as adjuvant therapy for patients with positive inguinal lymph nodes
• In selected patients, pelvic lymphadenectomy can be performed. If the pelvic lymph nodes are negative, radiation therapy can be avoided.
• In advanced malignancy involving the urethra and rectum, concomitant cisplatin/5-FU chemotherapy with radiation produces significant decrease in size of the primary tumor, usually obviating the need for pelvic exenteration
• Pelvic exenteration provides effective therapy for advanced or recurrent malignancies involving the bladder or rectum after radiation
• Radical vulvectomy and bilateral groin node dissection can be performed through three separate incisions
• Unilateral lesions can be treated with radical hemivulvectomy and unilateral groin node dissection. These modified techniques provide fewer complications and better cosmetic results.

ACTIVITY The patients are usually ambulatory and able to resume full activities by six weeks after surgery unless wound breakdown occurs

DIET Unrestricted, unless undergoing radiation

PATIENT EDUCATION Two complications are common with radical vulvectomy and bilateral groin node dissection, which is the usual treatment of this disease. In the immediate postoperative period, approximately 50% of patients will experience breakdown of the wound. This requires aggressive wound care by visiting nurses approximately twice a day. The wounds usually will granulate and heal over a period of six to ten weeks. Approximately 15-20% of the patients experience some form of mild to moderate lymphedema after the groin node dissection. The patients should be instructed in use of leg elevation and support hose. Less than 1% of the patients will experience severe debilitating lymphedema.
• American College of Obstetricians & Gynecologists (ACOG), 409 12th St., SW, Washington, DC 20024-2188, (800)762-ACOG

MEDICATIONS

DRUG(S) OF CHOICE
• There are no curative drugs
• As an adjuvant therapy, Efudex cream for in situ disease can produce occasional results, but the regimen is not well tolerated because of the excoriation and irritation of the vulva. Adjuvant chemotherapy has not proven to be effective in this disease.
• Metastatic disease, especially in the subcutaneous tissues of the leg or abdomen will produce hypercalcemia, which is treated in the usual medical fashion for hypercalcemia
Contraindications: Elderly patients - if chemotherapeutic agents are used, pay close attention to the patient's performance status and ability to tolerate aggressive chemotherapy
Precautions: The usual precautions for chemotherapy agents. Refer to manufacturer's literature.
Significant possible interactions: Refer to manufacturer's literature

ALTERNATIVE DRUGS   N/A

FOLLOWUP

PATIENT MONITORING
• Clinical examination of the groin nodes and vulvar area every 3 months for 2 years, then every 6 months for 3 years
• Chest x-ray should be obtained once a year

PREVENTION/AVOIDANCE
• Any woman complaining of symptoms related to the vulva should have a close examination and biopsies made of appropriate areas
• The vulva can be washed with 3% acetic acid to highlight areas. Areas of white raised epithelium should be biopsied.
• Patients with new onset of pruritus should be biopsied in the area of pruritus
• Liberal biopsy must be used to diagnose in situ disease prior to invasion and to diagnose early invasive disease
• The patient should not be treated for presumed benign conditions of the vulva without full examination and biopsy
• When symptoms persist, reexamination and rebiopsy should be undertaken
• The treatment of benign condyloma of the vulva has not been shown to decrease the eventual incidence of in situ or invasive disease of the vulva

POSSIBLE COMPLICATIONS   The major
complications from radical vulvectomy and groin node dissection are wound breakdown, lymphedema and urinary stress incontinence

EXPECTED COURSE AND PROGNOSIS
The five year survival is based on stage:
   ◊ Stage I 90%
   ◊ Stage II 85%
   ◊ Stage III 70%
   ◊ Stage IVA 25%
   ◊ Stage IVB 5%

MISCELLANEOUS

ASSOCIATED CONDITIONS
• The patients with invasive vulvar cancer are often times elderly and have associated medical conditions
• High rate of other gynecologic malignancies. Patients should be evaluated for these.

AGE-RELATED FACTORS
Pediatric: N/A
Geriatric:
• Older patients with associated medical problems are at high risk for radical surgery. The surgery, however, is external, usually well-tolerated and is the treatment of choice.
• In the very elderly, palliative vulvectomy provides relief of symptoms for ulcerating symptomatic advanced disease
Others:
More limited surgery
   ◊ Has been undertaken for invasive lesions especially in young patients to preserve the clitoris and sexual function
   ◊ Radical vulvectomy with groin node dissection through separate incisions provides better cosmetic results than the en bloc technique
   ◊ Radical hemivulvectomy can also be utilized for smaller lesions

PREGNANCY   This malignancy is not
associated with pregnancy

SYNONYMS
• Bowen's disease
• Cancer of the vulva
• Vulvar cancer

ICD-9-CM   184.4

SEE ALSO   N/A

OTHER NOTES   N/A

ABBREVIATIONS   N/A

REFERENCES
• Hopkins, M.P.: Disease of the vulva. In Obstetrics & Gynecology. Edited by J.R. Willson. St. Louis, C.V. Mosby Co., 1991
• Hopkins, M.P., Reid, G.C., Vettrano, I. & Morley G.W.: Squamous cell carcinoma of the vulva: Prognostic factors influencing survival. Gynecol Oncol 1991;43:113-7

Author   M. Hopkins, M.D. & E. Jenison, M.D.

Vulvovaginitis, bacterial

BASICS

DESCRIPTION Infectious disease affecting the vagina, only rarely affecting the vulva
Genetics: N/A
Incidence/Prevalence in USA: As low as 4% in unselected populations; up to 33% in STD clinics; up to 44% in patients with vaginitis
Predominant age: N/A
Predominant sex: Female

SIGNS AND SYMPTOMS
• Unpleasant vaginal odor, musty or fishy, exacerbated immediately after intercourse
• Thin gray-white vaginal discharge, mildly adherent to vaginal walls
• 10-30% with vaginal/vulvar irritation
• 10% with frothy discharge.

CAUSES
• Polymicrobial; Gardnerella vaginalis, Mobiluncus species, Mycoplasma hominis, Peptostreptococcus, other various anaerobes, including Prevotella, Bacteroides, and Fusobacterium
• There is a shift from a healthy lactobacilli based endogenous flora to an anaerobically based endogenous flora

RISK FACTORS
• Controversial regarding multiple sexual partners
• IUD

DIAGNOSIS

DIFFERENTIAL DIAGNOSIS
• N. gonorrhea
• Chlamydia
• Trichomonas
• E. coli
• Staphylococci
• Fungal
• Trophic

LABORATORY
• PH paper (pH > 4.5)
• Wet prep - clue cells in > 10-20% of epithelial cells, fewer WBC's than epithelial cells
• 10% KOH - "whiff test" transient amine or fishy odor
• Gram stain indicating absence of lactobacilli
• May be seen on cytology
• Culture difficult for mycoplasma, not useful
Drugs that may alter lab results: Recent douching
Disorders that may alter lab results: N/A

PATHOLOGICAL FINDINGS
Biopsies demonstrate no histologic evidence of inflammation

SPECIAL TESTS N/A

IMAGING N/A

DIAGNOSTIC PROCEDURES N/A

TREATMENT

APPROPRIATE HEALTH CARE
Outpatient

GENERAL MEASURES Consider repletion of lactobacilli

ACTIVITY No restrictions

DIET No restrictions

PATIENT EDUCATION N/A

MEDICATIONS

DRUG(S) OF CHOICE
• Metronidazole (95% cure) 500 mg bid for 7 days
• Clindamycin 450 mg q 6 hr for 7 days, or topical 2% vaginal cream for 7 days, or metronidazole vaginal cream for bacterial vaginosis
Contraindications: Refer to manufacturer's literature
Precautions: Refer to manufacturer's literature
Significant possible interactions:
Metronidazole and alcohol

ALTERNATIVE DRUGS
• Augmentin 500 mg q 8 hr for 7 days
• Cephradine 500 mg q 6 hr for 7 days
• Less effective - Ampicillin (66% cure rate) 500 mg q 6 hr
• Consider treating partner, especially in recurrent cases

FOLLOWUP

PATIENT MONITORING None indicated

PREVENTION/AVOIDANCE
• Good hygiene
• Use of condoms for sexual intercourse

POSSIBLE COMPLICATIONS
Uncommon but include adnexal tenderness, PID, intrauterine infections, chorioamnionitis, post abortion PID, post partum endometritis, pelvic abscesses, vaginitis emphysematous; rare extravaginal disease; implicated in some pre-term labor, premature rupture of membranes, chorioamnionitis, rare newborn infections, including scalp electrode sites, abscesses, and 1 reported case of meningitis;

EXPECTED COURSE AND PROGNOSIS Relapses fairly common, can be decreased by increased colonization of lactobacilli

MISCELLANEOUS

ASSOCIATED CONDITIONS N/A

AGE-RELATED FACTORS
Pediatric: N/A
Geriatric: N/A
Others: N/A

PREGNANCY N/A

SYNONYMS
• Gardnerella Vaginosis
• Bacterial vaginosis/ vaginitis,
• Nonspecific vaginitis
• Haemophillis vaginalis
• Corynebacterium vaginalis

ICD-9-CM 616.0

SEE ALSO N/A

ABBREVIATIONS N/A

REFERENCES
• Herbst, A., Mishell, D., Jr., Stenchever, A. & Droegueller, W.: Comprehensive Gynecology. 2nd Ed. C.V. Mosby Yearbook, 1992
• Catlin, B.: Gardnerella vaginalis: Characteristics, clinical considerations, and controversies. Clinical Microbiology Reviews, 5(3) July 1992
• Reed, B. & Eyler, A.: Vaginal infections: Diagnosis and management", Amer Fam Phys. 47(8), June, 1993
• Holst, E.: Reservoir of Four organisms associated with bacterial vaginosis suggests lack of sexual transmission. J of Clin Microbiolgy. 28(9), Sept, 1990
• Ray,A., et al.: Non-specific vaginitis vis-a-vis Gardnerella vaginalis. J of Communicable Dis. 22(4), Dec, 1990
• Livengood, C., Thomason, J. & Hill, G.: Bacterial vaginosis: Diagnostic and pathogenetic findings during topical clindamycin therapy. Amer J of Obs and Gynecol. 163(2), Aug 1990

AUTHOR E. McCord, M.D.

Vulvovaginitis, estrogen deficient

 BASICS

DESCRIPTION Decreased blood flow with a thinning and atrophy of the female genital tissue. Changes from estrogen deficiency occur throughout the body. The genital tissues are hormone responsive. Estrogen deficient vulvovaginitis is frequently associated with urinary incontinence.

System(s) affected: Reproductive

Genetics: No known genetic pattern

Incidence/Prevalence in USA: This disorder will affect all women, to some degree, unless estrogen replacement therapy is provided

Predominant age: This is predominantly a problem of the postmenopausal female. The average age of menopause in the United States is 52.5 years.

Predominant sex: Female only

SIGNS AND SYMPTOMS
- Vaginal dryness
- Decreased vaginal secretions
- Dyspareunia
- Vulva undergoes a thinning of the epidermis along with decreased integrity of the supporting structures. The thinning and atrophy often produces pruritus.

CAUSES
Estrogen deficiency
 ◊ Menopause (surgical or natural)
 ◊ Ovariectomy
 ◊ Radiation of the pelvis

RISK FACTORS
- Estrogen deficient states accompanying metabolic disorders
- Vaginal infections with bacteria and fungi

 DIAGNOSIS

DIFFERENTIAL DIAGNOSIS
- Malignancy
- Vulvar dystrophies

LABORATORY
- Cytology for maturation index will show a low maturation index, signifying a decreased turnover of the cells from the decreased estrogen effect
- In the perimenopausal or menopausal female, follicle stimulating hormone (FSH) will be elevated and estradiol will be decreased

Drugs that may alter lab results:
- Estrogen therapy will alter the maturation index
- Digoxin has estrogen-like properties
- Tamoxifen (Nolvadex) can produce menopausal type symptoms but also can act on genital tissues as a weak estrogen agonist. Symptoms can vary.
- Drugs used to treat endometriosis or uterine bleeding such as progestins, Danazol or gonadotropin releasing hormone (GnRH) agonists can produce a pseudomenopause which is reversible

Disorders that may alter lab results: N/A

PATHOLOGICAL FINDINGS Thinning of the cornified squamous layer of both the vulva and the vagina

SPECIAL TESTS N/A

IMAGING N/A

DIAGNOSTIC PROCEDURES
- Examination of the vagina and the vulva with maturation index
- FSH level to confirm menopause
- Estradiol level to evaluate circulating estrogen level

 TREATMENT

APPROPRIATE HEALTH CARE
Outpatient

GENERAL MEASURES
- Estrogen replacement therapy (ERT) will alleviate and reverse the symptoms and the thinning of the squamous epithelial layer. Replacement therapy leads to an increased blood supply to the genital tissues.
- Symptomatic relief, if needed, e.g., cool baths or compresses

ACTIVITY No restriction

DIET No special diet

PATIENT EDUCATION
- American College of Obstetricians & Gynecologists (ACOG), 409 12th St., SW, Washington, DC 20024-2188, (800)762-ACOG

MEDICATIONS

DRUG(S) OF CHOICE
A wide variety of preparations are available:
◊ Premarin 0.625 mg daily
◊ Estrace 1 mg daily
◊ Estraderm patch 0.05 mg, changed twice weekly
◊ If the uterus is not removed, progesterone should be added. This can be added as Provera 2.5 mg daily or 10 mg for 10 days of each month.
◊ Conjugated estrogen vaginal cream (2-4 g/day intravaginally)

Contraindications:
• Estrogen therapy is contraindicated in patients with a history of breast cancer or estrogen positive tumor receptors
• A history of uterine malignancy is a relative contraindication

Precautions: Refer to manufacturer's literature
Significant possible interactions: Refer to manufacturer's literature

ALTERNATIVE DRUGS N/A

FOLLOWUP

PATIENT MONITORING The patient should be instructed that symptoms should resolve within 30-60 days. If they do not, reevaluation and reexamination for other causes should be undertaken.

PREVENTION/AVOIDANCE N/A

POSSIBLE COMPLICATIONS Those associated with estrogen replacement - postmenopausal bleeding, nausea, headache, libido changes, thrombophlebitis

EXPECTED COURSE AND PROGNOSIS Excellent. The vast majority of symptoms will be relieved with estrogen replacement therapy.

MISCELLANEOUS

ASSOCIATED CONDITIONS None

AGE-RELATED FACTORS
Pediatric: N/A
Geriatric: N/A
Others: N/A

PREGNANCY The lactating postpartum woman with high levels of prolactin are in a hypo-estrogenic state. These women should be instructed to use lubrication for symptoms of dyspareunia. The symptoms will resolve when breast-feeding is stopped.

SYNONYMS N/A

ICD-9-CM 616.10

SEE ALSO N/A

OTHER NOTES The obese patient, especially those weighing more than 100 pounds more than ideal body weight, have higher levels of circulating estrogen and thus may have fewer symptoms. (Androstenedione is converted to estrone in peripheral adipose tissue and when there is an abundance of adipose, higher estrone levels are present.)

ABBREVIATIONS N/A

REFERENCES
• Cunningham, F.G., MacDonald, P.C. & Gant, N.F. (eds.): Williams Obstetrics. 18th Ed. Norwalk CT, Appleton & Lange, 1989
• Novak, E.R., et al. (eds.): Novak's Textbook of Gynecology. 11th Ed. Baltimore, Williams & Wilkins, 1988

Author M. Hopkins, M.D. & E. Jenison, M.D.

Vulvovaginitis, monilial

 BASICS

DESCRIPTION Abnormal vaginal discharge with associated vulvar irritation
System(s) affected: Reproductive
Genetics: N/A
Incidence/Prevalence in USA:
• 40% of vulvovaginitis is caused by Candida
• 16% of non-pregnant premenopausal women are asymptomatic carriers
Predominant Age: Menarche to menopause
Predominant sex: Female only

SIGNS AND SYMPTOMS
• Intense vulvar itching
• Thick curd-like vaginal discharge
• Dyspareunia at times
• Erythema of vulva
• Erythema, pain and pruritus of crural and perineal area
• Thick white patches appear attached to vaginal mucosa
• Inflamed, angry vulvar skin

CAUSES Overgrowth of Candida albicans in vagina

RISK FACTORS
• Pregnancy
• Diabetes mellitus
• Antibiotic therapy
• Corticosteroid therapy
• Immunosuppressed states
• Occlusive synthetic underpants and undergarments
• Hypoparathyroidism
• Oral contraceptive medications

 DIAGNOSIS

DIFFERENTIAL DIAGNOSIS
• Trichomonas vaginitis
• Gonorrheal vaginitis - in prepubertal girls
• Bottenal vaginosis

LABORATORY
• Finding of yeast and pseudohyphae on smear with 10% KOH solution
• Culture findings on Nickerson's media
Drugs that may alter lab results: N/A
Disorders that may alter lab results: N/A

PATHOLOGICAL FINDINGS N/A

SPECIAL TESTS N/A

IMAGING N/A

DIAGNOSTIC PROCEDURES
• Smear of discharge with 10% KOH solution
• Pap smear

 TREATMENT

APPROPRIATE HEALTH CARE
Outpatient

GENERAL MEASURES
• Remove foreign body if one present
• Consider providone iodine douche 15 to 30 mL/L (2 tbsp/qt) of water for symptomatic relief until specific therapy is effective
• If urination causes burning, have the patient urinate through a tubular device such as a toilet-paper roll or plastic cup with the end cut out. Or pour warm water over vaginal area while urinating.
• Insist on strict diabetic control if patient is diabetic

ACTIVITY
• Avoid overexertion, heat, and excessive sweating
• Delay sexual relations until symptoms clear

DIET No restrictions

PATIENT EDUCATION
• Keep the genital area clean. Use plain unscented soap.
• Take showers rather than tub baths
• Wear cotton underpants with a cotton crotch. Avoid clothing made from non-ventilating materials, including most synthetic underclothing.
• Don't sit around in in wet clothing - especially a wet bathing suit
• Avoid frequent douches
• Limit intake of sweets and alcohol
• Avoid broad-spectrum antibiotics when possible
• After urinating or bowel movements, cleanse by wiping or washing from front to back (vagina toward anus)
• Lose weight, if obese
• American College of Obstetricians & Gynecologists (ACOG), 409 12th St., SW, Washington, DC 20024-2188, (800)762-ACOG

Vulvovaginitis, monilial

MEDICATIONS

DRUG(S) OF CHOICE
• Miconazole nitrate (Monistat) - one suppository q night x 3, or miconazole vaginal cream q night x 7, or
• Butoconazole nitrate (Femstat) - vaginal cream q night x 3, or
• Terconazole (Terazol) - one suppository or vaginal cream q night x 3, or
• Clotrimazole (Gyne-Lotrimin) - two 100 mg tablets intravaginally x 3 days or cream each night x 7 days
Contraindications: N/A
Precautions: Refer to manufacturer's profile of each drug
Significant possible interactions: Refer to manufacturer's profile of each drug

ALTERNATIVE DRUGS
• Retreat with different agent, if recurrence
• Course of oral nystatin, 100,000 units tid X 2 weeks

FOLLOWUP

PATIENT MONITORING Repeat pelvic exam and culture at end of treatment

PREVENTION/AVOIDANCE
• Follow instructions under patient education
• Exam and treat sex partner for Candida balanitis and oral Candida if vaginitis recurs
• Check for risk factors

POSSIBLE COMPLICATIONS
Secondary bacterial infections of the vagina or pelvic organs

EXPECTED COURSE AND PROGNOSIS
• Complete cure with vigorous treatment
• Recurrences are common

MISCELLANEOUS

ASSOCIATED CONDITIONS STD

AGE-RELATED FACTORS
Pediatric: Less common before puberty
Geriatric: N/A
Others: N/A

PREGNANCY Common

SYNONYMS Vaginitis, monilial

ICD-9-CM 112.1

SEE ALSO N/A

OTHER NOTES N/A

ABBREVIATIONS N/A

REFERENCES Jones, H.W. & Wentz-Colston, A. (eds.): Novak's Textbook of Gynecology. 11th Ed. Baltimore, Williams & Williams Co., 1988

Author H. Chevlen, M.D.

Vulvovaginitis, prepubescent

 BASICS

DESCRIPTION Irritation and/or inflammation of the vulva and/or vagina frequently associated with vaginal discharge
System(s) affected: Reproductive, Skin/Exocrine
Genetics: Not well studied
Incidence/Prevalence in USA: Common
Predominant age: Toddlers to menarche
Predominant sex: Female only

SIGNS AND SYMPTOMS
- Irritation and erythema of vulva
- Vaginal discharge
- Offensive odor
- Itching
- Excoriation
- Bleeding

CAUSES
- Most often secondary or concurrent with infection elsewhere in body, e.g., otitis media, pharyngitis

Specific organisms:
  ◊ Group A beta-hemolytic streptococci - Streptococcus pyogenes, Streptococcus pneumoniae
    ◊ Neisseria meningitidis
    ◊ Candida sp.
    ◊ Shigella
    ◊ Staphylococcus aureus
    ◊ Hemophilus influenzae
    ◊ Neisseria gonorrhea
    ◊ Trichomonas vaginalis
    ◊ Chlamydia trachomatis
    ◊ Gardnerella vaginalis
    ◊ Herpes viruses
    ◊ Human papilloma virus
    ◊ Pinworms
    ◊ Scabies
Systemic illnesses:
    ◊ Measles
    ◊ Chickenpox
    ◊ Stevens-Johnson syndrome
Localized vulvar disease:
    ◊ Seborrheic dermatitis
    ◊ Psoriasis
    ◊ Atopic dermatitis
    ◊ Contact dermatitis
    ◊ Lichen sclerosis
Other:
    ◊ Sexual abuse
    ◊ Other trauma
    ◊ Foreign body
    ◊ Tumors or polyps
    ◊ Poor hygiene
    ◊ Masturbation

RISK FACTORS
- Co-existing pharyngitis or other systemic conditions
- Faulty hygiene
- Trauma or abuse
- Diabetes mellitus

 DIAGNOSIS

DIFFERENTIAL DIAGNOSIS
- Contact dermatitis
- Eczema

LABORATORY
- Gram stain
- Potassium hydroxide and saline smears
- Culture for bacteria, fungi or viruses
Drugs that may alter lab results: N/A
Disorders that may alter lab results: N/A

PATHOLOGICAL FINDINGS   N/A

SPECIAL TESTS Exploration of vagina for foreign body may be necessary in long-standing vaginal discharge

IMAGING   N/A

DIAGNOSTIC PROCEDURES
Visualization of the vagina may be necessary using a nasal speculum or infant laryngoscope. If blood or foul-smelling discharge is present, visualization is mandatory.

 TREATMENT

APPROPRIATE HEALTH CARE
Outpatient (except where systemic illness requires hospital care)

GENERAL MEASURES
Hygiene:
  ◊ Wipe front-to-back after elimination
  ◊ Avoid bubble baths and other irritating products
  ◊ Clean daily with mild soap and water, drying thoroughly with soft towel
  ◊ Apply bland ointments for protection of the skin, if necessary

ACTIVITY Normal

DIET N/A

PATIENT EDUCATION As noted above under General measures

MEDICATIONS

DRUG(S) OF CHOICE
• Group A beta-streptococcus, Streptococcus pneumoniae - penicillin V (Pen Vee K) 125-250 mg qid x 10 days
• C. trachomatis - erythromycin 50 mg/kg/d po x 10 days
• N. gonorrhoea - ceftriaxone IM x 1, 125 mg if < 45 kg; 250 mg if > 45 kg
• Candida sp - topical nystatin (Mycostatin), miconazole, clotrimazole or terconazole
• Shigella - trimethoprim/sulfamethoxazole 8/40 mg/kg/day po x 7 days
• Staphylococcus aureus - cephalexin 25-50 mg/kg/day, divided qid x 7-10 days or dicloxacillin 12 5-25 mg/kg/day x 7-10 days
• H. influenzae - amoxicillin 20-40 mg/kg/day x 7 days; amoxicillin/clavulanic acid 20 mg/kg/day
• Trichomonas vaginalis - metronidazole 125 mg (15 mg/kg/day) tid x 7-10 days
• Estrogen deficiency with labial adhesion/agglutination - conjugated estrogen cream to fused area nightly for two weeks
Contraindications: Allergy to proposed treatment
Precautions: Avoid potential allergens/topical sensitizers if possible
Significant possible interactions: See manufacturer's profile of each drug

ALTERNATIVE DRUGS   Topical corticosteroids for pruritis

FOLLOWUP

PATIENT MONITORING   Only if symptoms do not respond to treatment

PREVENTION/AVOIDANCE
• Perineal hygiene
• Avoidance of irritants and tight or occlusive, non-breathable clothing

POSSIBLE COMPLICATIONS   Labial agglutination or adhesions

EXPECTED COURSE AND PROGNOSIS   Usually clears with appropriate treatment with no permanent sequelae (if not due to underlying disease such as psoriasis, etc.)

MISCELLANEOUS

ASSOCIATED CONDITIONS   N/A

AGE-RELATED FACTORS
Pediatric:
• Usual adult vulvitis/vaginitis organisms are rare in the prepubertal child
• Lack of estrogen causing thin vaginal mucosa which is more susceptible to trauma and infection
Geriatric: N/A
Others: N/A

PREGNANCY   N/A

SYNONYMS   Vaginitis, vulvitis

ICD-9-CM   616.1

SEE ALSO   N/A

OTHER NOTES   N/A

ABBREVIATIONS   N/A

REFERENCES
• Emans, S.J.: Vulvovaginitis in the child and adolescent. Pediatr Rev 1986;8:13
• Dewhurst, C.J.: Practical Pediatric and Adolescent Gynecology. New York, Marcel Dekker Inc., 1980

Author   J. Daugherty, M.D.

Warts

BASICS

DESCRIPTION Warts are painless, benign skin tumors characterized by an area of well circumscribed epithelial thickening. The DNA papillomavirus is causative and is passed by direct contact with an infected person or from recently shed virus kept intact in a moist, warm environment. Five types of warts are caused by specific genotypes of HPV:
• Common wart (verruca vulgaris)
• Plantar wart (verruca plantaris)
• Flat wart (verruca plana)
• Venereal wart (condyloma acuminatum)
• Epidermodysplasia verruciformis
System(s) affected: Skin/Exocrine
Genetics: N/A
Incidence/Prevalence in USA: 7-10% of the population
Predominant age: Young adults and children
Predominant sex: Female > Male

SIGNS AND SYMPTOMS
• Verruca vulgaris: Rough surfaced, raised, skin-colored papules 5-10 mm in diameter. They may coalesce into a mosaic 1-3 cm in diameter.
• Vurruca plantaris: Rough surfaced (although smoother than the common wart), flat, skin-colored papules not infrequently attaining 2-3 cm in diameter
• Verruca plana: Slightly elevated, flat-topped, skin-colored papules 1-3 mm in diameter sometimes in a linear arrangement
• Condyloma acuminatum: thin, flexible, tall, papules sometimes demonstrating a confluent growth resembling cauliflower. They do not have the visible or palpable keratin of the previous warts.
• Epidermodysplasia verruciformis: Flat, reddish lesions on the hands and shoulders presenting in childhood with lifelong persistence

CAUSES Human papillomavirus (HPV)

RISK FACTORS
• Locker room use
• Skin trauma

DIAGNOSIS

DIFFERENTIAL DIAGNOSIS
• Corns (on paring, a single "eye" of keratin is observed, whereas the wart shows hemorrhagic spots or "roots")
• Scar tissue
• Molluscum contagiosum (central umbilication and, after curettage, the characteristic pearl)
• Condyloma lata (flat warts of syphilis)
• Seborrheic keratoses

LABORATORY HPV cannot be cultured
Drugs that may alter lab results: N/A
Disorders that may alter lab results: N/A

PATHOLOGICAL FINDINGS
• Papilloma virus found in the nuclei and nucleoli of the stratum granulosum and keratin layers of the epidermis.
• Plantar warts have rete pegs (a downward proliferation of epidermal ridges).

SPECIAL TESTS
Definitive diagnosis can be achieved with the following, but are not clinically relevant for most presentations:
• Electron microscopy
• Immunohistochemical study
• Nucleic acid hybridization

IMAGING N/A

DIAGNOSTIC PROCEDURES Paring or débridement and simple visualization will be diagnostic in most cases.

TREATMENT

APPROPRIATE HEALTH CARE
Outpatient

GENERAL MEASURES Spontaneous remissions are common, probably related to a host immune response. Conservative, non-scarring treatments are preferred. Each treatment is associated with a 60-70% cure rate. Cure is achieved when skin lines are restored to a normal pattern.

ACTIVITY Plantar warts occasionally cause significant discomfort requiring a decrease in activity

DIET N/A

PATIENT EDUCATION Infectious nature should be discussed; keep warts covered while under treatment to avoid auto-innoculation and transmission to others.

MEDICATIONS

DRUG(S) OF CHOICE
Destructive treatments
◊ Cryotherapy - often preferred because scar formation is minimized. Freezing of periungual warts may injure the nail matrix leading to a deformed nail.
◊ Surgery including excision with electrocautery, laser ablation, curettage (the virus may be found in smoke so that masks should be worn)
Chemotherapy
◊ All treatments begin by paring the wart as closely as possible, then soaking the area in warm water to moisten the wart
◊ Duofilm - daily treatment for about 3 months
◊ Trans-Ver-Sal (salicylic acid in a transdermal delivery system) - daily treatment for about 6 weeks
◊ Keralyt (salicylic acid in propylene glycol); rub into warts each night
◊ Topical retinoids (Retin-A) - for flat warts, less scarring than cryotherapy or surgical approaches; may be best for warts on the face. Apply bid for 4-6 weeks
◊ Benzoyl peroxide - apply bid for 4-6 weeks
◊ Others - dichloroacetic acid, trichloroacetic acid, podophyllin, 5-fluoruracil, silver nitrate, idoxuridine (Herplex Liquifilm)
◊ Occlusion - the easiest and least expensive; cover the wart with a waterproof tape and leave on for a week. Remove and leave open for 12 hours then re-tape if wart is still present. The environment under the tape does not foster viral growth. May be the best for periungual warts.
◊ Bleomycin - intradermal injection, is expensive and causes severe pain, but has a 75% cure rate
Immunotherapy
◊ Dinitrochlorobenzene (DNCB) - should be considered a last resort because of side effects and possible mutagenicity
◊ Interferon - intralesional for venereal warts
Contraindications: See specific treatments
Precautions: Avoid normal skin when using the topical chemicals
Significant possible interactions: N/A

ALTERNATIVE DRUGS N/A

FOLLOWUP

PATIENT MONITORING
One third of the warts of epidermodysplasia may become malignant

PREVENTION/AVOIDANCE Cover warts under treatment. Avoid the wound fluid after cryotherapy.

POSSIBLE COMPLICATIONS
• Auto-innoculation
• Scar formation
• Chronic pain after plantar wart removal and scar formation
• Nail deformity after injury to nail matrix

EXPECTED COURSE AND PROGNOSIS Good; complete resolution with or without treatment

MISCELLANEOUS

ASSOCIATED CONDITIONS
• Acquired immunodeficiency syndrome
• Renal transplantation
• Other conditions with immunosuppression
• Lewandowsky-Lutz disease (associated with epidermodysplasia)

AGE-RELATED FACTORS
Pediatric: Generally more prevalent in children
Geriatric: Less common in non-immunocompromised adults
Others: N/A

PREGNANCY Podophyllin is contraindicated

SYNONYMS N/A

ICD-9-CM 078.1 viral warts

SEE ALSO
• Venereal warts
• Plantar warts

OTHER NOTES N/A

ABBREVIATIONS
HPV = Human papillomavirus

REFERENCES
• Bolton, R.A.: Warts. Am Fam Phys, June 1991, p. 2049-2056
• Lynch, P.J.: Dermatology for the House Officer. 2nd Ed. Baltimore, Williams & Wilkins, 1987

Author MR Dambro, M.D.

Warts, plantar

 BASICS

DESCRIPTION Discrete or grouped firm keratotic masses on the sole of the foot initiated by a viral infection of keratinocytes
System(s) affected: Skin/Exocrine
Genetics: Unknown
Incidence in USA: Widespread
Prevalence in USA: 2000/100,000
Predominant age: Any age, although more common in children and young adults
Predominant sex: Female > Male (slightly)

SIGNS AND SYMPTOMS
• Foot pain
• Discrete or grouped masses on sole of foot
• Callus formation
• Foot, leg, or back pain (distortion of posture)

CAUSES Human papilloma viruses, types 1, 2 and 4

RISK FACTORS
• AIDS
• Atopic dermatitis
• Lymphomas
• Patient taking immunosuppressive drugs

 DIAGNOSIS

DIFFERENTIAL DIAGNOSIS
• Corns (clavi)
• Calluses
• Black heel (ruptured capillaries)

LABORATORY N/A
Drugs that may alter lab results: N/A
Disorders that may alter lab results: N/A

PATHOLOGICAL FINDINGS N/A

SPECIAL TESTS N/A

IMAGING N/A

DIAGNOSTIC PROCEDURES
• Inspection usually confirms the diagnosis
• If cannot distinguish between callus and wart, can examine with a magnifying lens. The wart should demonstrate a highly organized mosaic pattern.

 TREATMENT

APPROPRIATE HEALTH CARE
• Outpatient cryotherapy at weekly intervals
• Repeated parings at weekly intervals with or without use of a keratolytic is also an option. Most successful appears to be curettage and chemical cautery (with phenol or trichloroacetic acid) or light electrocautery. (Note: extreme care must be exercised with this procedure because excessive cautery or curettage can cause a painful scar.)

GENERAL MEASURES
• If warts are asymptomatic, no treatment is necessary. However patient may be at risk for spread of warts.
• Warm soaks followed by patient's paring of the top layer of skin on repeated occasions may speed disappearance
• Patient may use pumice stone, emery board or a blade
• Over-the-counter keratolytics containing salicylic acid may help. The advised procedure is paring of skin followed by warm soaks, and finally application of a few drops of keratolytic.
• Other measures include use of a heel bar or appropriate padding to relieve pressure points where warts tend to aggregate

ACTIVITY Ambulatory unless warts or treatment is painful

DIET No special diet

PATIENT EDUCATION
• In Epstein: Common Skin Disorders, patient instructions, pages 105-107 (see References)
• In Reeves and Mailbach: Clinical Dermatology Illustrated, patient guide - "All About Warts", page 22
• American Academy of Dermatology (708)330-0230

MEDICATIONS

DRUG(S) OF CHOICE
• No effective antiviral wart medications currently exist. Keratolytics (over-the-counter or prescription) and a variety of chemotherapeutic acids may be used
• Salicylic acid - see General measures for instructions
• 40% salicylic acid plasters - available as Mediplast. It is supplied in 3 by 4 inch sheets which are cut to the size of the wart and the sticky surface applied to the wart. They are removed every 1 to 2 days, the white keratin peeled and a fresh plaster applied.
• Chemotherapy, bi- and trichloroacetic acid kits are available. Callus is pared and the surrounding skin is protected by a ring of petrolatum. The wart(s) are coated with acid which is then worked into the wart with a sharp toothpick. Procedure should be repeated at weekly intervals.
• Cryotherapy - application of liquid nitrogen is often effective. It usually requires at least 4 applications at weekly or biweekly intervals.
• Transdermal salicylates (Trans-Plantar)
• Vesicants containing cantharidin (Cantharone, Verrusol)
Contraindications: Infection, vascular insufficiency
Precautions:
• If the dermis is damaged with any of the above procedures, a scar may result which can be permanently painful
• Care should be taken to avoid excessive contact with normal skin when using keratolytics or chemotherapy
Significant possible interactions: N/A

ALTERNATIVE DRUGS   N/A

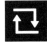
FOLLOWUP

PATIENT MONITORING   With any treatment modality, followup weekly

PREVENTION/AVOIDANCE   Use rubber footwear in communal shower areas

POSSIBLE COMPLICATIONS   Scarring with overly aggressive treatment

EXPECTED COURSE AND PROGNOSIS   The course of plantar warts is like that of other varieties of warts, i.e., highly variable. Most resolve spontaneously in weeks to months.

MISCELLANEOUS

ASSOCIATED CONDITIONS   N/A

AGE-RELATED FACTORS
Pediatric: Duration of warts is generally shorter in children than in adults
Geriatric: N/A
Others: N/A

PREGNANCY   N/A

SYNONYMS   Verruca plantaris

ICD-9-CM   078.1

SEE ALSO
• Warts
• Venereal warts

OTHER NOTES   N/A

ABBREVIATIONS   N/A

REFERENCES
• Epstein, E.: Common Skin Disorders. 3rd Ed. Oradell, N.J. Medical Economics Books, 1988
• Habif, T.: Clinical Dermatology. 2nd Ed. St. Louis, C.V. Mosby, 1990
• Reeves, J. & Maibach, H.: Clinical Dermatology Illustrated. 2nd Ed. Philadelphia, F.A. Davis, 1991

Author   G. Silko, M.D.

Wegener's granulomatosis

BASICS

DESCRIPTION A multisystem disease characterized by granulomatous vasculitis involving multiple organs. The characteristic "triad" of involvement includes the upper airway (otitis, sinusitis, nasal mucosa), lung, and kidney. Other organ systems involved include skin, joints, nervous system (peripheral or central).
• As the condition progresses untreated, upper airway erosions, necrotic pulmonary nodules, and renal failure are common, and, without treatment, mortality rate is high
System(s) affected: Cardiovascular, Pulmonary, Renal/Urologic, Gastrointestinal, Nervous, Skin/Exocrine
Genetics:
• Increased presence in HLA-B8
• Increased presence in HLA-DR2
Incidence in USA: Estimated at approximately 0.4/100,000
Prevalence in USA: Uncommon
Predominant age: Mean age of onset in mid-40's, but has been described in all age groups
Predominant sex: Male > Female (3:2)

SIGNS AND SYMPTOMS
• Pulmonary infiltrates (71%)
• Sinusitis (67%)
• Arthralgia/arthritis (44%)
• Fever (34%)
• Cough (34%)
• Otitis (25%)
• Rhinitis (22%)
• Hemoptysis (18%)
• Ocular inflammation (16%)
• Weight loss (16%)
• Skin rash (13%)
• Epistaxis (11%)
• Renal failure (11%)
• Chest pain, anorexia, proptosis, dyspnea, oral ulcers, hearing loss, headache (all < 10%)

CAUSES No known etiology. Autoimmune phenomena and immune complex deposition in arterial walls are implicated as pathogenetic factors. Triggering infectious agents, yet unidentified, may be involved.

RISK FACTORS None identified

DIAGNOSIS

DIFFERENTIAL DIAGNOSIS
• Infectious otitis and sinusitis (bacterial or fungal)
• Midline granuloma or other upper airway malignancy
• Relapsing polychondritis
• Fungal or tuberculous pulmonary infections, (Goodpasture's syndrome)
• Other vasculitic syndromes (including polyarteritis nodosa, lymphomatoid granulomatosis, Churg-Strauss vasculitis, and overlap vasculitis syndromes)
• Any disease associated with necrotizing and crescentic glomerulonephritis, sarcoidosis

LABORATORY
• Anemia, leukocytosis, and thrombocytosis common during active phases of disease
• Erythrocyte sedimentation rate (ESR) usually markedly elevated (75%)
• Rheumatoid factor present in low to moderate titer in up to 50%
• Hematuria and/or cellular casts with moderate range proteinuria
• Renal insufficiency, mild to moderate at first, but frequently progresses to end-stage renal disease
Drugs that may alter lab results: Corticosteroids and cytotoxic drugs, used to treat the disease, may cause normalization of most abnormal laboratory findings
Disorders that may alter lab results: See disorders listed under Differential Diagnosis

PATHOLOGICAL FINDINGS
• Upper airways: Granulomatous inflammation frequently seen, although not specific unless showing actual vasculitis
• Lung: Granulomatous arteritis involving vessels of all sizes, classically medium-sized arteries
• Kidney: Necrotizing and crescentic glomerulonephritis without immunofluorescent staining (pauci-immune) is common, granulomatous vasculitis rarely seen
• Skin: Vasculitic lesions, from leukocytoclastic vasculitis of small vessels; granulomatous arteritis seen occasionally

SPECIAL TESTS
Antibodies to neutrophilic cytoplasmic antigens with a cytoplasmic pattern of staining (c-ANCA) are detected in a majority (60-90%) of patients. Such pattern of staining is highly specific (90+%) for this diagnosis. A similar finding, with perinuclear staining (p-ANCA), is nonspecific, but frequently seen in patients with other vasculitic syndromes or isolated necrotizing glomerulonephritis.

IMAGING
• Upper airways: Chronic otitis and sinusitis, often with evidence of erosion into bony structures - seen on plain x-rays
• CT scans of sinuses useful in demonstrating mucosal and bony involvement
• Lungs: X-rays show nodular pulmonary densities, often with central necrosis and cavitation. Local infiltrates, or more diffuse interstitial involvement also described, as are radiographic findings of pulmonary hemorrhage.

DIAGNOSTIC PROCEDURES
• Renal biopsy may give findings consistent with diagnosis, although not always definitive
• Sinus or upper airway mucosal biopsy often helpful, although findings are often nonspecific
• Open lung biopsy most likely to confirm granulomatous arteritis
• Diagnosis best made by demonstration of granulomatous arteritis of involved organ, although compatible renal lesion in setting of chronic destructive sinusitis and/or pulmonary nodules can be used to make a presumptive diagnosis
• A positive serologic test for c-ANCA in proper clinical setting felt to be diagnostic by many

TREATMENT

APPROPRIATE HEALTH CARE
• Patients are usually ill enough with fever, sinus or pulmonary involvement, or renal disease to require hospitalization for diagnostic tests (to rule out infectious causes) and appropriate biopsies
• An occasional patient can be managed as an outpatient

GENERAL MEASURES Careful attention to upper airway drainage, and supportive measures for pulmonary, renal, or neurologic involvement

ACTIVITY No specific restrictions. Fatigue, fever, and weight loss usually limit activity.

DIET Vigorous nutritional support may be needed early in illness

PATIENT EDUCATION Nutritional and drug counseling when patient is able to return home

Wegener's granulomatosis

MEDICATIONS

DRUG(S) OF CHOICE
• Prednisone - given initially in high doses (60-100 mg/day). After initial 2-4 weeks may be tapered to alternate-day regimen. Then gradually discontinued over 2-6 months in most patients, depending on clinical course.
• Cyclophosphamide - in critically ill patient, may be given initially at a dose of 4 mg/kg/day IV for 2-3 days, then continued at 2 mg/kg/day orally. In stable patient, may be started at 2 mg/kg/day orally. Dosage may need to be adjusted, based on patient response and toxicity (usually bone marrow suppression). Usually continued for 1-2 years after patient felt to be in remission, and tapered slowly, with careful monitoring for re-activation of disease.
Contraindications: No absolute contraindications, although diabetes, hypertension, metabolic bone disease are relative contraindications to prednisone
Precautions:
• Careful monitoring if taking corticosteroids
• Consider reducing dose of cyclophosphamide in patient with baseline leukopenia, renal insufficiency
Significant possible interactions:
• Prednisone may interfere with hypoglycemics, anti-hypertensives
• Cyclophosphamide may increase risk of other drugs with potential for bone marrow toxicity

ALTERNATIVE DRUGS
• Azathioprine has been used in patients with history of severe bone marrow toxicity or hemorrhagic cystitis from cyclophosphamide
• Trimethoprim/sulfamethoxazole (TMP/SMX) has been used alone with success in some patients with limited (usually upper airway) disease, and has some potential as adjunctive therapy with prednisone and cyclophosphamide
• Methotrexate has also been used.

FOLLOWUP

PATIENT MONITORING
• Early, careful monitoring of upper airway, pulmonary, and renal manifestations for response to therapy
• Monitor blood pressure, glucose, potassium for steroid effects
• Frequent (every 2-4 weeks) CBC with differential to monitor for bone marrow toxicity from cyclophosphamide. Leukopenia most common. Dose needs to be reduced if peripheral WBC < 3000/ mm3.
• Monitor urinalysis for potential of hemorrhagic cystitis from cyclophosphamide. Consider cystoscopy for persistent or recurrent hematuria, especially later in course of treatment.

PREVENTION/AVOIDANCE
• Calorie and salt reduction in patients on prednisone
• High fluid intake to prevent hemorrhagic cystitis from cyclophosphamide
• Give cyclophosphamide dose in morning to decrease amount of drug present overnight in bladder.

POSSIBLE COMPLICATIONS
Disease related
◊ Destructive nasal lesions with "saddle nose" deformity
◊ Deafness from refractory otitis
◊ Necrotic pulmonary nodules with hemoptysis
◊ Interstitial lung disease
◊ Renal failure
◊ Foot drop from peripheral nerve disease
◊ Skin ulcers, digital and limb gangrene from peripheral vascular involvement
Drug related
◊ Prednisone - weight gain, hyperglycemia, hypertension, hypokalemia, skin thinning and bruising, infection, osteoporosis
◊ Cyclophosphamide - bone marrow suppression (especially leukopenia, neutropenia), alopecia, hemorrhagic cystitis, mucosal membrane irritation, sterility and premature gonadal failure, secondary malignancies (especially leukemias) with long term therapy

EXPECTED COURSE AND PROGNOSIS
• Without treatment, almost uniformly fatal with 10% 2 year survival and mean survival of 5 months
• With aggressive treatment, survival improved to 75-90% at 5 years
• Treatment-related toxicity is significant, especially from long-term cyclophosphamide. After 1-2 years of disease-free interval, cyclophosphamide is usually tapered, although some patients demonstrate disease re-activation during this phase.

MISCELLANEOUS

ASSOCIATED CONDITIONS None

AGE-RELATED FACTORS
Pediatric: N/A
Geriatric: N/A
Others: N/A

PREGNANCY
• Rarely reported. Pregnancy should be considered only when patient is disease-free and off therapy.
• Cyclophosphamide often causes sterility and is potentially teratogenic

SYNONYMS N/A

ICD-9-CM 446.4

SEE ALSO
• Polyarteritis nodosa
• Goodpasture's syndrome

OTHER NOTES N/A

ABBREVIATIONS
• c-ANCA = antibodies to neutrophilic cytoplasmic antigens with cytoplasmic staining pattern
• p-ANCA = antibodies to neutrophilic cytoplasmic antigens with perinuclear staining pattern

REFERENCES
• Cupps, T.R. & Fauci, A.S.: The vasculitides. Philadelphia, W.B. Saunders Co., 1981
• Fauci, A.S., et al.: Wegener's granulomatosis: Prospective clinical and therapeutic experience with 85 patients for 21 years. Ann Intern Med. 98 76-85, 1983
• Nolle, B., et al.: Anticytoplasmic autoantibodies: Their immunodiagnostic value in Wegener's granulomatosis. Ann Intern Med. 111:28, 1989

Author C. M. Wise, M.D.

Wilms' Tumor

 BASICS

DESCRIPTION An embryonal renal neoplasm containing blastema, stromal or epithelial cell types usually affecting children before the 5th year.

Genetics: Several congenital anomalies are known to be associated with Wilms' tumor. A two stage mutational model has been proposed: occurrence in either hereditary form or sporadic form. Patients with aniridia have a deletion of the short arm of chromosome 11 (11p13).

System(s) affected: Renal/urological

Incidence in USA: N/A

Prevalence in USA: 0.69/100,000 people in the U.S. 8 cases/100,000 children under 15 year of age

Predominant age: Median age of 36.5 months

Predominant sex: Female > Male (1.1 : 1)

SIGNS AND SYMPTOMS
- Usually asymptomatic
- Palpable upper abdominal mass
- Abdominal Pain
- Fever
- Anemia
- Rarely, signs of acute abdomen with free intraperitioneal rupture
- Cardiac murmur
- Hepatosplenomegaly
- Ascites
- Prominent abdominal wall veins
- Varicocele
- Gonadal metastases

CAUSES
- Hereditary or sporadic forms of genetic mutation
- Familial form: autosomal dominant trait with incomplete penetrance (1%)
- Potential of paternal occupational exposure (machinists, welders, motor vehicle mechanics, autobody repairmen)

RISK FACTORS
- Aniridia (600 times greater than normal risk)
- Hemihypertrophy (100 times greater than normal risk)
- Cryptorchidism
- Hypospadias
- Duplicated renal collecting systems
- Wiedemann - Beckwith syndrome
- Drash's syndrome
- Klippel - Trenaunay syndrome
- Familial occurrence
- Paternal occupation (see causes)

 DIAGNOSIS

DIFFERENTIAL DIAGNOSIS
- Neuroblastoma
- Hepatic tumors
- Sarcoma
- Rhabdoid tumors

LABORATORY
- Urinalysis (occasional hematuria)
- CBC (anemia)
- LDH
- Plasma renin (rarely helpful)
- Urine catecholamines

Drugs that may alter lab results: N/A
Disorders that may alter lab results: N/A

PATHOLOGICAL FINDINGS
Favorable Findings (mortality of 7%)
- Bulky lesion, well-encapsulated
- Focal areas of hemorrhage and necrosis
- Absence of anaplasia and sarcomatous cell types
- Presence of blastema, stomal and epithelial elements

Unfavorable histology (mortality rate of 57%)
- Anaplasia - markedly enlarged and multipolar mitotic figures 3-fold enlargement of nuclei in compasrison with adjacent similar nuclei, hyperchromasia of enlarge nuclei. Anaplasia may be diffuse or focal.
- Sarcomatous changes - are now considered to be separate from Wilms, not subtypes. (Mortality of 64%)

Nephroblastomatosis
- Considered premalignant

SPECIAL TESTS N/A

IMAGING
- Chest x-ray
- KUB (presence of linear calcifications)
- Abdominal ultrasound - gives best information about extension into IVC
- CT with IV and oral contrast of chest and abdomen
- IVP rarely helpful

DIAGNOSTIC PROCEDURES
Occasionally bone marrow aspiration necessary to distinguish from neuroblastoma

 TREATMENT

APPROPRIATE HEALTH CARE
- In-patient work-up and treatment until stable postoperative and induction chemotherapy completed

GENERAL MEASURES
- Examination (visual and manual) of contralateral kidney
- Radical nephroureterectomy and biopsies as needed to provide precise staging information
- Sampling of any enlarged lymph nodes
- Identification of any retained tumor with titanium clips
- Tumor should be given to pathologist fresh, not on formalin
- Vertical midline incision if tumor extension to right atrium present (possible use of cardiopulmonary bypass)
- With bilateral Wilms' tumors, biopsy, then chemotherapy and 2nd look operation 6 weeks to 6 month later for partial bilateral nephrectomy if possible
- Chemotherapy
- Radiation therapy in Stage II, unfavorable histology, Stage III and Stage IV

ACTIVITY As tolerated

DIET No special diet

PATIENT EDUCATION
- Patient and family teaching regarding long-term outlook
- Possibility of second malignancy
- Side effects of chemotherapy, radiation therapy

MEDICATIONS

DRUG(S) OF CHOICE
• Actinomycin - D
• Vincristine
• Doxorubicin
• Cytoxan

Contraindications: Refer to manufacturer's literature

Precautions: Refer to manufacturer's literature

Significant possible interactions: Refer to manufacturer's literature

ALTERNATIVE DRUGS
• Adriamycin
• Cyclophosphamide

FOLLOWUP

PATIENT MONITORING
• Multidrug chemotherapy every 3-4 weeks for 16 weeks - 15 months depending on stage
• Every 4 months for 1 year, every 6 months for 2nd - 3rd year, yearly after that
• CBC, CT chest and abdomen with each visit

PREVENTION/AVOIDANCE N/A

POSSIBLE COMPLICATIONS
• 1-2% will develop second malignant neoplasms (leukemia, lymphoma, hepatocellular carcinoma, soft tissue sarcoma)
• High risk of low birth weight infants, perinatal mortality in offspring of female survivors of Wilms' tumor
• Chest is usual site of recurrence

EXPECTED COURSE AND PROGNOSIS
• With favorable histology, 91% survival
• With diffuse anaplasia, 20% survival
• With focal anaplasia, 64% survival
• Staging
 ◊ I - tumor limited to kidney, completely excised
 ◊ II - Tumor extends beyond kidney, completely excised
 ◊ III - Residual non-hematogenous tumor confined to abdomen (lymph nodes positive, spillage of tumor, peritoneal implants, extension beyond resection region)
 ◊ IV - Hematogenous metastases
 ◊ V - Bilateral renal involvement

MISCELLANEOUS

ASSOCIATED CONDITIONS See risk factors

AGE-RELATED FACTORS occurs only in children
Pediatric: N/A
Geriatric: N/A
Others: N/A

PREGNANCY N/A

SYNONYMS
• Nephroblastoma

ICD-9-CM
189.0 malignant neoplasm of kidney

SEE ALSO N/A

OTHER NOTES
• Mesoblastic nephroma - distinguished only by histology. Age usually under 6 months. Essentially benign although metastases have been reported tends to be locally invasive. Operative spillage may lead to recurrence. No chemotherapy or radiotherapy needed with complete excision.
• Nephroblastomatosis - considered premalignant; may present as nodularity as one or both kidneys; treated with biopsy and local excision (renal tissue sparing)

ABBREVIATIONS N/A

REFERENCES
• Ashcraft, K.W. & Holder, T.M.: Pediatric Surgery. 2nd Ed. Philadelphia, W.B. Saunders Co., 1993.
• Shochat, S.J.: Wilms' Tumor: Diagnosis and Treatment in the 1990's. Seminars in Pediatric Surgery, 2(1): 59-68, 1993.
• Welch, K.J., Randolph, J.G., Ravitch, M.M., O'Neill, S.A. & Rowe, M.I.: Pediatric Surgery. 4th Ed. Chicago, Year Book Medical Publishers, 1986.

Author T. Black, M.D.

Wiskott-Aldrich syndrome

BASICS

DESCRIPTION An x-linked recessive disorder of male infants. Characteristics include eczema, thrombocytopenia, and recurrent infection. B and T cell functions are defective. This syndrome may cause early death.

System(s) affected:
Hemic/Lymphatic/Immunologic, Skin/Exocrine

Genetics: X-linked recessive

Incidence/Prevalence in USA: Rare

Predominant age: Newborns (symptoms develop as infants get older)

Predominant sex: Males (exclusively)

SIGNS AND SYMPTOMS
Neonatal:
◊ Bloody diarrhea
◊ Petechiae
◊ Purpura
Childhood:
◊ Eczema (at about 1 year)
◊ Secondary skin infections
◊ Pneumonia
◊ Otitis media
◊ Herpes infections (skin and eyes)
◊ Hepatosplenomegaly
◊ Leukemia or lymphoma likely to develop

CAUSES
• X-linked recessive trait
• Inherited defect in both B and T cell functions that compromise the child's immune system
• Platelet storage pool defect

RISK FACTORS Family history of congenital defects

DIAGNOSIS

DIFFERENTIAL DIAGNOSIS
• Eczema
• Other causes of thrombocytopenia
• Bronchitis
• Lymphoma
• Acute lymphoblastic anemia

LABORATORY
• Thrombocytopenia (platelets below 100,000/cubic millimeter)
• Low IgM in serum
• Low isohemagglutinins
• IgE and IgA normal or elevated
• Normal IgG

Drugs that may alter lab results:
Antibiotics

Disorders that may alter lab results:
Infections

PATHOLOGICAL FINDINGS
• Multiple thromboses of small arterioles of kidneys, lungs, pancreas
• Hyperplasia of the spleen, lymph nodes
• Inflammatory changes in skin

SPECIAL TESTS N/A

IMAGING N/A

DIAGNOSTIC PROCEDURES Bone marrow aspiration. Although not diagnostic, it helps by excluding marrow aplasia and/or leukemia.

TREATMENT

APPROPRIATE HEALTH CARE
Inpatient

GENERAL MEASURES
• Crossmatched platelet transfusions
• Splenectomy, if there is special indication of severe thrombocytopenia
• Aggressive antibiotic therapy for any infection
• Bone marrow transplant (with HLA-matched sibling)

ACTIVITY
• Plan levels of activity to help in normal development, e.g., bike-riding (with acceptable protective gear) or swimming
• No contact sports
• Avoid crowds

DIET No special diet

PATIENT EDUCATION
• Genetic counseling
• Patient teaching for coping with the disorder and expected outcome

MEDICATIONS

DRUG(S) OF CHOICE
 • Immune globulin infusions
 • Topical corticosteroids
 • Continuous antibiotics as indicated by cultures and/or postsplenectomy
Contraindications: Refer to manufacturer's literature
Precautions: Refer to manufacturer's literature
Significant possible interactions: Refer to manufacturer's literature

ALTERNATIVE DRUGS   N/A

FOLLOWUP

PATIENT MONITORING   As needed for therapy, infection treatment, progression of the disorder

PREVENTION/AVOIDANCE   Genetic counseling

POSSIBLE COMPLICATIONS
 • Severe infections - especially following splenectomy
 • Hemorrhage
 • Fatal malignancy

EXPECTED COURSE AND PROGNOSIS
 • Usual course - acute, chronic
 • Usually fatal before age 10 (average life span is about 4 years)

MISCELLANEOUS

ASSOCIATED CONDITIONS   N/A

AGE-RELATED FACTORS
Pediatric: A disease of male newborns
Geriatric: No patient survives this long
Others: N/A

PREGNANCY   N/A

SYNONYMS
 • Immunodeficiency with eczema and thrombocytopenia
 • Aldrich's syndrome

ICD-9-CM
279.12 Wiskott-Aldrich syndrome

SEE ALSO   N/A

OTHER NOTES   N/A

ABBREVIATIONS   N/A

REFERENCES
 • Wyngaarden, J.B., Smith, L.H. (eds): Cecil Textbook of Medicine. 19th Ed. Philadelphia, W.B. Saunders Co., 1992
 • Joklik, W.K., Willett, H.P. & Amos, D.B. (eds.); Zinsser Textbook of Microbiology and Immunology. 19th Ed. New York, Appleton-Century-Crofts, 1988

Author   H. Griffith, M.D. & M. Dambro, M.D.

Zinc deficiency

BASICS

DESCRIPTION Constellation of growth retardation, hypogonadism, cell mediated immune dysfunction, and skin changes related to decreased zinc
Genetics: Usually acquired, but rarely acrodermatitis enteropathica (autosomal recessive) and associated with sickle cell anemia (autosomal recessive)
Incidence/Prevalence in USA: Unknown
Predominant age: All ages, most often adolescent
Predominant sex: Male = Female

SIGNS AND SYMPTOMS
Mild deficiency
  ◊ Hypogeusia
  ◊ Decreased dark adaptation
  ◊ Decreased lean body mass
Moderate deficiency
  ◊ All of the above
  ◊ Diarrhea
  ◊ Growth retardation
  ◊ Hypogonadism (especially male)
  ◊ Mental lethargy
  ◊ Anergy
  ◊ Rough skin
  ◊ Delayed wound healing
  ◊ Glucose intolerance
  ◊ Impaired cell mediated immunity
Severe deficiency
  ◊ All of the above
  ◊ Bullous pustular dermatitis
  ◊ Weight loss
  ◊ Dwarfism
  ◊ Emotional instability
  ◊ Tremors
  ◊ Ataxia
  ◊ Alopecia
  ◊ Death

CAUSES
Increased requirements
  ◊ Pregnancy
  ◊ Lactation
  ◊ Rapid growth phase of childhood
  ◊ Burns
  ◊ Major trauma
Increased losses
  ◊ Diabetes
  ◊ Cirrhosis
  ◊ Renal disease
  ◊ Malabsorption states, e.g., inflammatory bowel diseases
  ◊ Sickle cell anemia
Decreased absorption
  ◊ Acrodermatitis enteropathica, an autosomal recessive deficiency in the enzyme required for intestinal absorption
  ◊ Geophagia
  ◊ Chelating agents
  ◊ Parasitism
  ◊ Diet high in phytates

Insufficient dietary intake
  ◊ Vegetarianism
  ◊ Parenteral hyperalimentation without supplementation
  ◊ Breast feeding
  ◊ Suboptimal zinc conditions in diet (rare)
  ◊ Alcoholism

RISK FACTORS
• High milk consumption
• Low socioeconomic status

DIAGNOSIS

DIFFERENTIAL DIAGNOSIS
• Congenital dwarfism
• Failure to thrive in infants
• Primary hypogonadism
• Mental retardation

LABORATORY
• Plasma zinc levels decreased (in moderate to severe zinc deficiency)
• Erythrocyte or leukocyte zinc levels more adequately assess tissue stores, but these are more costly and not widely available
• Hair or fingernail zinc levels not useful
Drugs that may alter lab results: N/A
Disorders that may alter lab results: N/A

PATHOLOGICAL FINDINGS N/A

SPECIAL TESTS N/A

IMAGING N/A

DIAGNOSTIC PROCEDURES N/A

TREATMENT

APPROPRIATE HEALTH CARE
Outpatient

GENERAL MEASURES N/A

ACTIVITY Full activity

DIET
• Balanced omnivorous diet
• Avoid excessive intake of foods with high phytate content, (e.g., cereals)

PATIENT EDUCATION Dietary consultation

MEDICATIONS

DRUG(S) OF CHOICE
• Zinc gluconate or zinc sulfate 25-50 mg po qd for 6-9 months
• 4-6 mg of elemental zinc qd added to hyperalimentation in adult patient, may increase to 12 mg qd if suspect ongoing heavy zinc losses, e.g., burns or major trauma
• In pediatric patients, 0.02-0.04 mg zinc/kg/day in hyperalimentation
• Prenatal vitamins with minerals during pregnancy and lactation to prevent deficiency
Contraindications: None
Precautions: Avoid large (> 20 mg elemental zinc) parenteral doses
Significant possible interactions: N/A

ALTERNATIVE DRUGS N/A

FOLLOWUP

PATIENT MONITORING Clinical status such as improved outlook, weight gain, resolution of symptoms

PREVENTION/AVOIDANCE
• Adequate diet
• Supplementation when indicated (see Medications)

POSSIBLE COMPLICATIONS N/A

EXPECTED COURSE AND PROGNOSIS Immediate improvement in clinical status. Full resolution of signs and symptoms.

MISCELLANEOUS

ASSOCIATED CONDITIONS
• Sickle cell anemia
• Pregnancy and lactation
• Alcoholism
• Malabsorption
• Parenteral hyperalimentation
• In the older patient, diabetes, cirrhosis, those taking diuretics

AGE-RELATED FACTORS
Pediatric: Zinc deficiency may cause failure to thrive, impair growth and development of secondary sexual characteristics
Geriatric:
• Zinc deficiency may cause poor night vision leading to falls; poor wound healing or chronic skin ulcer; loss of taste which may cause worsening nutrition
• Elderly persons living in institutions may have low zinc intake
Others: N/A

PREGNANCY Requirements increase; deficiency may cause spontaneous abortion, inadequate weight gain

SYNONYMS N/A

ICD-9-CM 269.3

SEE ALSO N/A

OTHER NOTES N/A

ABBREVIATIONS N/A

REFERENCES
• Tasman-Jones, C.: Disturbances of trace mineral metabolism. In Cecil Textbook of Medicine. Edited by J.B Wyngaarden, et al. Philadelphia, W.B. Saunders Co., 1992
• Ronaghy, H.: World Review Nutr. Diet, 54:1987

Author C. Harris, M.D.

Zollinger-Ellison syndrome

 BASICS

DESCRIPTION
• A triad of
◊ Marked elevated gastric acid secretion
◊ Peptic ulcer disease
◊ A non-beta islet cell tumor of the pancreas
(and sometimes other sites)
• Gastrin producing tumor, single or multiple, large or small, benign or malignant: 80% sporadic, 20% associated with multiple endocrine neoplasia (MEN I)
System(s) affected: Gastrointestinal, Endocrine/Metabolic
Genetics: Associated with MEN I
Incidence/Prevalence in USA: 0.1% of patients with duodenal ulcer
Predominant age: Middle age (40-75)
Predominant sex: Male > Female (3:2)

SIGNS AND SYMPTOMS
• Abdominal pain
• Epigastric pain
• Reflux esophagitis
• Vomiting unresponsive to standard therapy
• 25% have diarrhea which persists with fasting
• Complications of severe peptic ulcer disease (hemorrhage, perforation, obstruction)
• Signs related to MEN I (hyperparathyroidism, hypercalcemia)
• Weight loss
• Enlarged liver when metastasized
• Endoscopic (esophagitis, duodenal ulceration with multiple ulcers)
• Steatorrhea

CAUSES
Gastrinoma - found in the gastric triangle in 90%

RISK FACTORS
• MEN I
• Family history of ulcer disease
• Over age 60

 DIAGNOSIS

DIFFERENTIAL DIAGNOSIS
Elevated serum gastrin with hypochlorhydria/achlorhydria
◊ Atrophic gastritis
◊ Drug induced
◊ Gastric cancer
◊ Gastric ulcer
◊ Pernicious anemia
◊ Postvagotomy
◊ Vitiligo
Elevated serum gastrin with normal or increased gastric acid
◊ Antral G-cell hyperfunction
◊ Chronic renal failure
◊ Gastric outlet obstruction
◊ Pheochromocytoma (rare)
◊ Retained gastric antrum
◊ Rheumatoid arthritis
◊ Small bowel resection

LABORATORY
• Elevated serum gastrin - fasting
• Elevated basal gastric acid output >15 mEq/hr
• Elevated maximal acid output >150 mEq/hr
• Gastric pH <2.0
• Increased pancreatic polypeptides
Drugs that may alter lab results: N/A
Disorders that may alter lab results: N/A

PATHOLOGICAL FINDINGS
• Gastrinoma found in gastric triangle (60-70% in head of pancreas)
• 50% of tumors stain for VIP, ACTH, insulin, neurotensin
• In addition, 50% will have multiple metastases to liver, bone, lymph nodes, or with blood vessel invasion
• Duodenal ulcer
• Jejunal ulcer
• Gastric ulcer

SPECIAL TESTS
• Secretion stimulation test - gastrin level increases > 200 pg/mL
• Calcium infusion test

IMAGING
• Used to localize tumor
• Abdominal CT scan
• Abdominal ultrasound
• Abdominal angiography
• Selective venous sampling of gastrin from portal venous tributaries

DIAGNOSTIC PROCEDURES
Endoscopy to look for tumors

 TREATMENT

APPROPRIATE HEALTH CARE
Advise daily care based on symptoms

GENERAL MEASURES
• Medical treatment alone in some cases
• Medical treatment plus laparotomy to search for resectable tumors
• Definitive therapy - removal of gastrinoma when found
• Total gastrectomy (is no longer used in most patients)
• Vagotomy in some patients to reduce acid secretion and add to inhibitory effect of medication
• In MEN I, parathyroidectomy

ACTIVITY
As tolerated

DIET
Restrict only foods which aggravate symptoms

PATIENT EDUCATION
Inform as to nature of disease and prognosis

MEDICATIONS

DRUG(S) OF CHOICE
H2-receptor antagonists
◊ Note: Dosages may exceed maximum recommended daily dose. Start at the recommended doses as listed below, and titrate up to maximum as listed.
◊ Cimetidine start 300 mg q6h, up to maximum of 1.25-5.0 gm/day
◊ Ranitidine 150 mg q 12 hrs, up to maximum of 6 gm/day
◊ Famotidine 20 mg at bedtime, up to maximum of 800 mg/day
Proton pump inhibitors:
◊ Omeprazole 60-120 mg/d
Anticholinergics:
◊ Note: These are rarely recommended because doses needed for effectiveness are associated with many adverse effects
◊ Propantheline
or
◊ Isopropamide

Contraindications:
• H2-receptor antagonists - anti-androgen effects; drug interactions due to hepatic oxides system
• Proton pump inhibitor/omeprazole - none
• Anticholinergics - prostate enlargement, glaucoma, gastric outlet obstruction, chronic renal failure in elderly

Precautions: Refer to manufacturer's literature. Gynecomastia reported with high doses of cimetidine (> 2.4 gm/day).

Significant possible interactions: Refer to manufacturer's literature

ALTERNATIVE DRUGS N/A

FOLLOWUP

PATIENT MONITORING
• Close followup necessary following any surgical procedure
• Careful dose titration required with medical therapy
• Gastric analysis to measure acid secretion rates for dose adjustment of H2-receptor antagonists

PREVENTION/AVOIDANCE None

POSSIBLE COMPLICATIONS
• The complications of ulcer disease, e.g., bleeding or perforation
• Approximately two thirds of Zollinger-Ellison tumors are malignant with metastases
• Multiple hormone production and related syndromes such as Cushing's and others

EXPECTED COURSE AND PROGNOSIS
• Survival rate - 5 year = 62-75%, 10 year = 47-53%
• Prognosis improves with complete resection
• If tumor inoperable due to metastases, 5 year = 43%, 10 year = 25%

MISCELLANEOUS

ASSOCIATED CONDITIONS
• Hyperparathyroidism
• Prolactinoma
• Insulinoma
• Carcinoid tumors

AGE-RELATED FACTORS
Pediatric: N/A
Geriatric:
• One third of patients with Z-E are over age 50
• Consider this diagnosis for any patient with persistent or recurring peptic ulcer disease
Others: N/A

PREGNANCY N/A

SYNONYMS
• Z-E syndrome
• Pancreatic ulcerogenic tumor syndrome
• Multiple endocrine neoplasia, partial
• Ulcerogenic islet cell tumor

ICD-9-CM 251.5, other codes based on related diagnosis

SEE ALSO N/A

OTHER NOTES N/A

ABBREVIATIONS N/A

REFERENCES McGuigan, J.E.: The Zollinger-Ellison Syndrome. In Gastrointestinal Disease. 4th Ed. Edited by M.H. Sleisenger & J.S. Fordtran. Philadelphia, W.B. Saunders Co., 1989

Author L. Deranek, M.D.

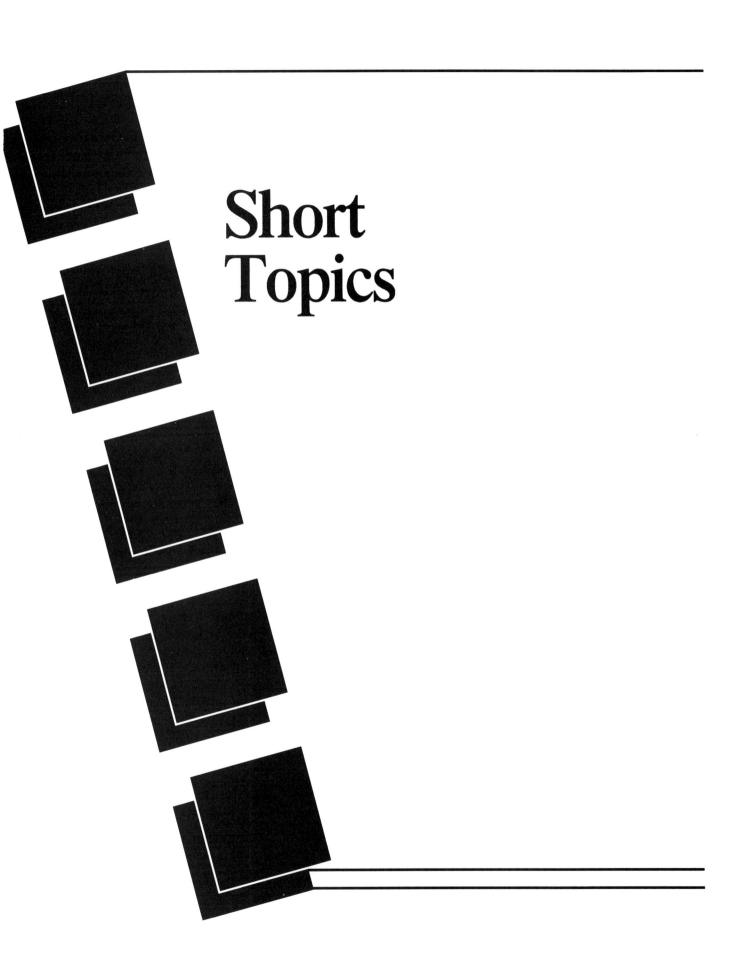

Short
Topics

Acanthosis nigricans

DESCRIPTION A circumscribed melanosis consisting of a brown pigmented velvety verrucosity or fine papillomatosis appearing in the axillae and other body folds. Occurs in association with endocrine disorders, underlying malignancy, administration of certain drugs, or as in inherited disorder. Usual course - chronic.

CAUSES
- congenital
- associated with malignant disease
- obesity
- idiopathic

TREATMENT
- treat underlying cause
- malignancy workup

ICD-9-CM
701.2 acquired acanthosis nigricans

 ## Acquired adrenogenital syndrome

DESCRIPTION A condition of adults that is acquired or congenital in which excessive output of adrenal androgenic hormones causes virilization. The effects depend on age. Usual course - chronic; progressive.

CAUSES
- androgen producing tumors
- adrenal adenoma
- adrenal adenocarcinoma

TREATMENT
- surgery

ICD-9-CM
255.2 adrenogenital disorders

 ## Acrodermatitis enteropathica

DESCRIPTION Previously fatal disorder resulting from malabsorption of zinc. Characteristics: psoriasiform dermatitis, hair loss, paronychia, diarrhea, and growth retardation. Symptoms begin in infants just after weaning.

SYNONYMS
- Danbolt-Closs syndrome
- Brandt syndrome

CAUSES
- zinc deficiency
- defective zinc absorption

TREATMENT
- oral elemental zinc

ICD-9-CM
686.8 acrodermatitis enteropathica

 ## Acromegaly

DESCRIPTION A disorder due to excessive secretion of pituitary growth hormone, characterized by progressive enlargement of the head and face, hands and feet, and thorax. Usual course - progressive.

SYNONYMS
- Acromegalia
- Eosinophilic adenoma syndrome

CAUSES
- growth hormone excess from pituitary adenoma

TREATMENT
- transsphenoidal resection
- heavy particle irradiation
- radiotherapy
- bromocriptine

ICD-9-CM
253.0 acromegaly and gigantism

 ## Actinomycosis of the kidney

DESCRIPTION Infectious bacterial disease that appears in 4 clinical forms - abdominal, cervicofacial, thoracic, and generalized. The generalized form can involve the kidneys as well as other organs. Characteristics - back pain, lethargy, weight loss, fever, hematuria. Usual course - acute.

CAUSES
- retrograde infection by actinomyces israelii

TREATMENT
- antibiotics
- drainage

ICD-9-CM
039.2 abdominal actinomycotic infection

 ## Actinomycosis of the thorax

DESCRIPTION Infectious bacterial disease affecting the thorax and lungs. It also occurs in three other forms that include abdominal, cervicofacial and generalized. Usual course - progressive.

CAUSES
- actinomyces infection
- oral commensal
- aspiration of infected material
- impaired consciousness
- alcoholism

TREATMENT
- prolonged antibiotic therapy
- surgical drainage of suppurative lesions

ICD-9-CM
039.1 actinomycosis, thoracic

 ## Adenocarcinoma of the bladder

DESCRIPTION Malignant growth in the bladder with characteristic hematuria, dysuria, urinary frequency, weight loss and suprapubic mass. Usual course - progressive.

CAUSES
- cystitis glandularis
- exstrophy of the bladder

TREATMENT
- segmental bladder resection
- total cystectomy

ICD-9-CM
188.9 malignant neoplasm of bladder, part unspecified

 ## Adenocarcinoma of the colon

DESCRIPTION The colon and rectum account for more new cases of cancer each year than any other site, exclusive of the lung. The incidence increases with age and peaks at 60-75. Characteristics - melena, diarrhea, rectal mass, iron deficiency anemia. Usual course - progressive.

CAUSES
- familial polyposis
- chronic ulcerative colitis
- possibly low fiber, high fat diet
- granulomatous colitis

TREATMENT
- surgery
- radiotherapy
- palliative chemotherapy

ICD-9-CM
153.9 malignant neoplasm of colon, unspecified

 ## Adenocarcinoma of the endometrium

DESCRIPTION Third rank in frequency of malignancies affecting women after breast and colon. Usually postmenopausal. Peak incidence between 50 and 60 years. Characteristics - positive Pap smear, menometrorrhagia, postmenopausal bleeding, perimenopausal bleeding. Usual course - progressive.

SYNONYMS
- Fundal carcinoma
- Corpus carcinoma
- Endometrial cancer

CAUSES
- irregular menses
- late menopause
- obesity
- diabetes mellitus
- hypertension
- infertility
- prolonged unopposed exogenous estrogen
- polycystic ovary disease

TREATMENT
- hysterectomy
- radiotherapy
- hormonal therapy with progesterone

ICD-9-CM
182.0 malignant neoplasm of corpus uteri, except isthmus

Adenocarcinoma of the gallbladder

DESCRIPTION The most frequent cause of extrabiliary obstruction. Characteristics - nausea, vomiting, abdominal pain, anorexia, jaundice, hepatomegaly, enlarged gallbladder.

CAUSES
• cholelithiasis
• calcified gallbladder

TREATMENT
• surgical resection
• palliative radiotherapy
• palliative chemotherapy

ICD-9-CM
156.0 malignant neoplasm of gallbladder

 ## Adenocarcinoma of the rectum

DESCRIPTION A slow-growth rate malignancy that depends on routine examination to discover before symptom-producing size. Most common symptom is blood passage at the time of bowel movement. All rectal bleeding should raise suspicion of cancer until proven otherwise. Usual course - progressive; surgical cure.

CAUSES
• ulcerative colitis
• previous rectal cancer
• familial polyposis

TREATMENT
• surgery
• radiotherapy

ICD-9-CM
154.1 malignant neoplasm of the rectum

 ## Adrenoleukodystrophy

DESCRIPTION A sphingolipidosis which combines the features of leukodystrophy and Addison's disease. A rare, sex-linked recessives metabolic disorder that occurs in boys. Characteristics include - adrenal atrophy and widespread cerebral demyelinization. Usual course - progressive.

SYNONYMS
• sudanophilic leukodystrophy with adrenal atrophy
• Addison-Schilder disease
• Siemerling-Creutzfeldt disease
• diffuse cerebral sclerosis with adrenocortical atrophy
• Addison disease with cerebral sclerosis
• Sex-linked metachromatic leukodystrophy

CAUSES
• unknown biochemical enzyme defect

TREATMENT
• hormone replacement therapy
• dietary therapy

ICD-9-CM
330.0 leukodystrophy

 ## Afibrinogenemia, congenital

DESCRIPTION Hereditary recessive disorder characterized by failure of synthesis of adequate amounts of fibrinogen causing blood to be incoagutable. Symptoms include easy posttraumatic bleeding.

CAUSES
• No fibrinogen
• No factor I

TREATMENT
• transfusion
• cryoprecipitate
• plasma
• whole blood

 ## Agammaglobulinemia, acquired

DESCRIPTION Heterogenous disorder characterized by onset of recurrent bacterial infections in 2nd and 3rd decade, resulting from drastic decrease in Ig and antibody levels. It affects males and females equally and does not interfere with normal lifespan. Usual course - chronic.

SYNONYMS
• late-onset agammaglobulinemia
• common variable immunodeficiency

CAUSES Unknown, but most patients have defective synthesis or release of immunoglobulins.

TREATMENT
• maintenance gamma globulin
• fresh frozen plasma acutely

ICD-9-CM
279.06 common variable immunodeficiency

 ## Agranulocytosis

DESCRIPTION Reduction of blood neutrophile (granulocyte) count, leading to increased susceptibility to bacterial and fungal infection. Acute, severe neutropenia due to impaired production is often life-threatening. Characteristics - fever, fatigue, sore throat, buccal ulcers, dyspnea, tachycardia. Usual course - acute.

SYNONYMS
• malignant neutropenia
• primary granulocytopenia
• agranulocytic angina

CAUSES
• ionizing radiation, benzene, antimetabolites, nitrogen mustards, aminopyrine, phenothiazines, sulfonamides, chloramphenicol
• typhoid, paratyphoid, influenza, measles, rickettsia, cachexia, septicemia

TREATMENT
• eliminate etiological agent
• antibiotics
• supportive measures

ICD-9-CM
288.0 agranulocytosis

 ## Agranulocytosis, infantile genetic

DESCRIPTION Rare, hereditary and congenital disease, including familial neutropenia, cyclic neutropenia, pancreatic insufficiency with neutropenia, and several other disorders combining impaired neutrophil production and severe immune deficiency. Characteristics include fever, recurrent skin and respiratory infections, cough. Usual course - progressive; chronic; spontaneous remission.

SYNONYMS
• Kostmann's syndrome

CAUSES
• defective bone marrow microenvironment
• progenitor defect

TREATMENT
• antibiotics
• bone marrow transplantation

ICD-9-CM
288.0 agranulocytosis

 ## Ainhum

DESCRIPTION A condition occuring chiefly in Black people in tropical countries. Characteristics - linear constriction of a toe, especially the little toe, which by its contraction gradually amputates the toe. Usual course - progressive; leading to amputation. Endemic areas - tropics; Africa.

SYNONYMS
• dactylolysis spontanea
• dactylysis spontanea
• fibrous bands

CAUSES
• unknown

TREATMENT
• surgery
• Z-plasty
• relaxing incision
• amputation
• control infection

ICD-9-CM
136.0 ainhum

 ## Albright's syndrome with precocious puberty

DESCRIPTION Fibrous dysplasia (cystic bone lesion) involving several bones plus cutaneous pigmentation and endocrine abnormalities. Usual course - chronic; progressive.

SYNONYMS
• polyostotic fibrous dysplasia
• McCune-Albright syndrome
• osteitis fibrosa cystica

TREATMENT

ICD-9-CM
756.54 polyostotic fibrous dysplasia of bone

Alcaptonuria

DESCRIPTION Inborn aminoacidopathy due to defective homogentisate 1,2-dioxygenase. The accumulation of homogentistic acid leads to homogentistic aciduria causing the urine to turn dark brown on standing or alkinization. Other characteristics include ochronosis and arthritis Usual course - asymptomatic until adulthood; progressive.

SYNONYMS
• homogentisicaciduria

CAUSES
• No homogentisic acid oxidase activity
• INCR homogentisic acid

TREATMENT
• supportive rehabilitation

ICD-9-CM
270.2 other disturbances of aromatic amino acid metabolism

 Alveolar proteinosis of the lung

DESCRIPTION Rare disease of unknown etiology characterized by filling of alveolar spaces with granular, periodic acid-Schiff (PAS)- positive material consisting of phospholipids and proteins. Age predilection is 20 to 60 years. It predominantly occurs in previously healthy males or females. Usual course - progressive.

SYNONYMS
• pulmonary alveolar proteinosis

TREATMENT
• total lung lavage under general anesthesia
• No steroids

ICD-9-CM
516.0 pulmonary alveolar proteinosis

 Amaurosis fugax

DESCRIPTION Acute, transient episode of blindness or partial blindness, lasting ten minutes or less.

CAUSES
• retinal arteriolar emboli

TREATMENT
• medical: control hypertension
• antithrombotic medications
• aspirin
• dipyridamole
• surgical: carotid endarterectomy

ICD-9-CM
362.34 transient arterial occlusion

 Amaurosis, congenital

DESCRIPTION A cone-rod abiotrophy causing blindness or amblyopia at birth; frequently found in Holland and Sweden. Usual course - stable; gradual deterioration.

SYNONYMS
• congenital retinal blindness
• amaurosis congenita of Leber
• heredoretinopathia congenita

CAUSES
• unknown

TREATMENT
• NONE

ICD-9-CM
362.76 dystrophies primarily involving the retinal pigment epitheluim

 Amebiasis of the bladder

DESCRIPTION Amebiasis usually affects the gastrointestinal tract, but may involve the kidney, bladder, and male or female genitalia, usually by blood-borne spread. Usual course: acute; chronic; relapsing. Endemic areas: worldwide

CAUSES
• entamoeba histolytica

TREATMENT
• anti-parasitics

ICD-9-CM
006.8 amebic infection of other sites

 Amebic abscess of the liver

DESCRIPTION A complication of amebiasis. It may develop during the acute attack of dysentery or one to three months later. (Occasionally will not be associated with dysentery). Abscesses occur most frequently in male adults. Amebic abscesses develop insidiously, but symptoms may begin abruptly and include pain over the liver, intermittent fever, sweats, chills, nausea, vomiting, weakness and weight loss. The abscess may perforate into the subphrenic space, right pleural cavity or other nearby organs.
Usual course - acute; progressive. Endemic areas: Southern rural USA; Indian reservations; migrant farm camps; Asia.

SYNONYMS
• hepatic amebiasis

CAUSES
• entameba histolytica
• fecal-oral transmission
• amebic colitis

TREATMENT
• metronidazole
• chloroquine plus emetine
• metronidazole plus iodoquinal

ICD-9-CM
006.3 amebic liver abscess

 Amebic colitis

DESCRIPTION An infection of the colon caused by Entamoeba histolytica with characteristic diarrhea or dysentery. It is spread either from person to person or by eating contaminated food. Usual course: acute; relapsing. Endemic areas - Southern rural USA; Indian reservations; migrant farm camps; Asia.

SYNONYMS
• dientamoebal diarrhea
• intestinal amebiasis

CAUSES
• entamoeba histolytica
• fecal-oral transmission

TREATMENT
• metronidazole plus iodoquinal
• metronidazole plus emetine

ICD-9-CM
006.0 acute amebic dysentery without mention of abscess

 Amebic meningoencephalitis

DESCRIPTION A rare and often fatal, acute, febrile, purulent meningoencephalitis caused by usually free-living soil and water amebas of the genera Naegleria, Acanthamoeba, or Hartmannella. Generally seen in young persons who swim in contaminated fresh water. Also seen in a less fulminant form in older persons and in immunocompromised persons. Usual course -acute.

CAUSES
• naegleria
• acanthamoeba
• hartmanella
• swimming in infected water

TREATMENT
• amphotericin
• miconazole
• rifampin

ICD-9-CM
006.5 amebic brain abscess

 Aminoaciduria

DESCRIPTION Impairment of renal tubular transport of amino acids.

SYNONYMS
• cystinuria
• dibasic aminoaciduria
• Hartnup disease
• iminoglycinuria
• dicarboxylate aminoaciduria

TREATMENT
• diet management
• high fluid intake
• lithotomy
• penicillamine
• nicotinamide

ICD-9-CM
270.9 unspecified disorder of amino-acid metabolism

Amyloid heart disease

DESCRIPTION A disease characterized by an accumulation in the heart of the fibrillar protein amyloid in amounts sufficient to impair normal heart function. May produce dizziness, syncope, dyspnea, and weight loss. Usual course - chronic; progressive.

SYNONYMS
• cardiac amyloidosis

CAUSES
• unknown

TREATMENT
• alkylating agents
• bilateral nephrectomy
• dimethyl sulfoxide

ICD-9-CM
277.3 amyloidosis

Amyloid neuropathy

DESCRIPTION Accumulation in the kidney of the fibrillar protein amyloid in amounts sufficient to impair normal function. The nephrotic syndrome due to amyloid is characterized by anasarca, hypoproteinemia, and massive proteinuria. Usual course - chronic.

CAUSES
• amyloid deposition in nerve roots

TREATMENT
• colchicine

ICD-9-CM
277.3 amyloidosis

Anemia due to chronic disease

DESCRIPTION The second most common anemia in the world. The major characteristic is that the marrow erythroid mass fails to expand appropriately in response to microcytic anemia from whatever cause. The defect, then, is one of decreased red blood cell production. The symptoms are primarily those of the underlying disease, such as rheumatoid arthritis, infections, or cancer. Usual course - chronic.

CAUSES
• chronic inflammation: iron metabolism abnormality
• defective RBC production
• inability to compensate for decreased red blood cell life span

TREATMENT
• treat underlying condition

ICD-9-CM
285 other and unspecified anemias

Anemia due to folate deficiency

DESCRIPTION Decreased red blood cells and hemoglobin content due to impaired production. This is one form of megaloblastic anemia charcterized by decreased red blood cells and decreased serum folate.

SYNONYMS
• nutritional macrocytic anemia
• tropical macrocytic anemia

CAUSES
• malnutrition
• inadequate folate intake
• malabsorption of folate
• increased demand for folate
• drugs

TREATMENT
• folic acid supplements
• avoid precipitating drug

ICD-9-CM
281.2 folate-deficiency anemia

Anemia, acquired sideroblastic

DESCRIPTION A microcytic (or normocytic), hypochromic anemia due to inadequate or abnormal utilization of intracellular iron for hemoglobin synthesis, despite adequate or increased amounts of iron within the mitochondria of the developing red blood cell precursors. Peripheral blood shows polychromatic, stippled, targeted red blood cells. Usual course - slowly progressive.

CAUSES
• idiopathic
• antituberculous drugs
• alcohol
• chloramphenicol

TREATMENT
• avoid precipitating drug
• avoid alcohol
• treat consequences

ICD-9-CM
285.0 sideroblastic anemia

Anemia, myelophthisic

DESCRIPTION Anemia characterized by appearance of immature myeloid and nucleated erythrocytes in the peripheral blood, resulting from infiltration of the bone marrow by foreign or abnormal tissue. Usual course - progressive.

SYNONYMS
• myelopathic anemia
• leukoerythroblastosis
• secondary myelofibrosis

CAUSES
• hematologic consequences of marrow infiltration
• lymphoma
• leukemias
• myelomas
• metastatic carcinoma
• tuberculosis
• lipid storage diseases
• fungus infection
• granulomatous disorders

TREATMENT
• treat underlying condition
• supportive measures
• splenectomy if hypersplenism

ICD-9-CM
285.8 other specified anemias

Aneurysym, abdominal aortic

DESCRIPTION Localized dilatation of the abdominal aorta that commonly passes unnoticed until it becomes large enough to be felt (4-6 cm) as a pulsating mass. Pain from leaking or bleeding is usually felt in the left side. Rupture can lead to death. Usual course - acute; progressive.

CAUSES
• aortic dissection, trauma, tuberculosis, mycotic aneurysm, atherosclerosis, hypertension, congenital Marfan's syndrome, relapsing polychondritis, Takayasu's aortitis, syphilis, infective carditis, cystic medial necrosis

TREATMENT
• trimethaphan
• propranolol
• beta-adrenergic blockers
• surgery
• aortic graft
• aneurysmectomy
• nitroprusside

ICD-9-CM
441.4 abdominal aneurysm without mention of rupture

Angina variant

DESCRIPTION A clinical syndrome characterized by development of chest pain at rest with concomitant transient ST segment elevation in the electrocardiogram. Exercise capacity is well preserved. Usual course - intermittent

SYNONYMS
• Prinzmetal's angina pectoris
• anterior chest wall syndrome

CAUSES
• coronary artery spasm

TREATMENT
• calcium antagonists
• nifedipine
• verapamil

ICD-9-CM
413.1 Prinzmetal angina

Anhidrosis

DESCRIPTION Abnormal deficiency of sweat. Other characteristics - malaise, easy fatiguability, headache, nausea, warmth, dry skin, tachcardia.

CAUSES
• senile skin
• radiodermatitis
• acrodermatitis chronica atrophica
• scleroderma
• lichen sclerosis et atrophica
• spinal cord lesions
• fabry's disease
• quinacrine toxicity
• miliaria
• sympathectomy
• peripheral neuropathy
• sympathetic ganglion antagonists
• hereditary anhidrotic ectodermal dysplasia
• acetylcholine antagonists
• hysteria
• brainstem tumors
• pontine tumors
• medulla tumors
• franceschetti-judassohn syndrome
• fabry's disease

TREATMENT
• Symptomatic

ICD-9-CM
705.0 anhidrosis

Anorectal fissure

DESCRIPTION An acute tear or chronic ulcer in the stratified squamous epithelium of the anal canal. Symptoms include rectal pain and bleeding with defecation.

SYNONYMS
- Anal fissure
- Fissure in ano
- Anal ulcer

CAUSES Unknown. Probably traumatic laceration from a hard or large stool with secondary infection.

Anthracosis

DESCRIPTION Usually asymptomatic form of pneumoconiosis caused by deposition of coal dust in the lungs. Usual course - progressive; chronic. Endemic areas - urban areas.

CAUSES
- inhalation of atmospheric particles
- inhalation of soot

TREATMENT
- NONE

ICD-9-CM
500 coal worker's pneumoconiosis

Anthrax of the intestine

DESCRIPTION Highly infectious disease of animals, (especially ruminants) that is rarely transmitted to man by contact with the animals or their products. Anthrax infection also occurs in a cutaneous form. Characteristics - fever, malaise, hematemesis, anorexia, abdominal pain, blody diarrhea. Usual course - acute.

CAUSES
- bacillus anthracis
- ingestion of bacillus
- contaminated meat

TREATMENT
- penicillin
- tetracycline

ICD-9-CM
022.2 gastrointestinal anthrax

Anthrax of the lung

DESCRIPTION Highly infectious disease of animals (especially ruminants) that is rarely transmitted to man by contact with the animals or their products. Caracteristics - fever, malaise, cough, myalgia, dyspnea, headache. This infection can be severe enough to be fatal. Usual course - acute; 3-4 day incubation. (Rare in U.S.)

SYNONYMS
- woolsorter disease
- anthrax pneumonia

CAUSES
- bacillus anthracis
- inhalation

TREATMENT
- penicillin
- streptomycin
- hydration

ICD-9-CM
022.1 pulmonary anthrax

Anthrax of the skin

DESCRIPTION Highly infectious disease of animals, especially ruminants. Transmitted to man by contact with the animals or their products. Cutaneous form begins as a red-brown papule that enlarges with peripheral erythema, vesiculation, and induration, followed by ulceration and local lymphadenopathy. Usual course - acute. Endemic areas - Haiti; South Africa; Asia.

SYNONYMS
- cutaneous anthrax
- charbon
- malignant pustule
- siberian ulcer
- malignant edema
- splenic fever
- milzbrand
- ragpicker's disease

CAUSES
- bacillus anthracis
- skin contact

TREATMENT
- penicillin
- tetracycline
- erythromycin
- hydrocortisone

ICD-9-CM
022.0 cutaneous anthrax

Aortic regurgitation

DESCRIPTION Retrograde flow from the aorta into the left ventricle through incompetent aortic cusps. Usual course - acute; chronic.

SYNONYMS
- aortic valve insufficiency

CAUSES
- bacterial endocarditis, aortic dissection, ankylosing spondylitis, aortic stenosis, rheumatic fever, giant cell arteritis, syphilis, marfan's syndrome, osteogenesis imperfection, reiter's syndrome, rheumatoid arthritis, cystic medial necrosis, sinus of valsalva aneurysm, hypertension, arteriosclerosis, myxomatous degeneration of valve, dissection of aorta, bicuspid aortic valve

TREATMENT
- aortic valve replacement

ICD-9-CM
424.1 Aortic valve disorders

Apert's syndrome

DESCRIPTION Autosomal dominant mutation characterized by acrocephalosyndactyly and mental retardation. Usual course - chronic; progressive.

SYNONYMS
- acrocephalosyndactyly

CAUSES
- unknown
- probable early bridging of mesenchymal blastema
- probable early bridging of bone hypoplasia

TREATMENT
- supportive
- orthopedic surgery
- maxillofacial surgery
- neurosurgery

ICD-9-CM
755.55 acrocephalosyndactyly

Argininosuccinicaciduria

DESCRIPTION Presence in urine of argininosuccinic acid, characteristic of a condition resulting from an inborn error of metabolism (autosomal recessive) and accompanied by mental retardation, failure to thrive, ataxia, seizures. Usual course - progressive.

SYNONYMS
- arginosuccinicaciduria
- arginosuccinicacidemia
- argininosuccinase deficiency

CAUSES
- argininosuccinase deficiency

TREATMENT
- DECR urea precursors
- DECR ureapoiesis
- DECR nitrogen waste production

ICD-9-CM
270.6 Disorders of urea cycle metabolism

Arsenic poisoning

DESCRIPTION Toxic condition caused by exposure to arsenic. Characteristics - throat constriction, dysphagia, burning gastrointestinal pain, vomiting, diarrhea, dehydration, pulmonary edema, renal failure, liver failure. Usual course - acute; chronic.

CAUSES
- pentavalent arsenic salt
- trivalent arsenic salt
- arsine gas

TREATMENT
- dimercaprol
- induce vomiting
- gastric lavage
- milk
- penicillamine
- hemodialysis

ICD-9-CM
985.1 Toxic effect of arsenic and its compounds

Arterial embolus and thrombosis

DESCRIPTION Acute ischemia produced by obstruction of blood flow due to embolization or clot formation. Characteristics - sudden onset of severe pain, coldness, numbness, pallor, absent pulses distal to obstruction. Arteriography and digital subtraction angiography to provide details of precise location and extent of clot.

SYNONYMS N/A

CAUSES
• Embolization from the heart
• Occlusion by a proximal atherosclerotic plaque
• Acute thrombosis
• Pre-existing atherosclerotic disease

ICD-9-CM
958.0 Air embolism
444.9 Arterial embolism and thrombosis of unspecified artery

 ## Arteriosclerosis obliterans

DESCRIPTION Arteriosclerosis in which proliferation of the intima leads to occlusion of the lumen of the arteries. Usual course - progressive

CAUSES
• atherosclerosis

TREATMENT
• exercise
• pentoxifylline
• weight loss
• avoid tobacco smoking
• angioplasty
• surgery
• lumbar sympathectomy

ICD-9-CM
440.9 generalized and unspecified arteriosclerosis

 ## Ascites, chylous

DESCRIPTION The presence of chyle in the peritoneal cavity as a result of anomalies, injuries, or obstruction of the thoracic duct. Characteristics - abdominal pain, fullness, discomfort, distention, shortness of breath, nausea, weight gain.

SYNONYMS
• chylous peritonitis

CAUSES
• abdominal neoplasm
• lymphoma
• abdominal lymphatic obstruction
• trauma
• intestinal obstruction
• chylous cyst rupture
• hodgkin's disease

TREATMENT
• paracentesis

ICD-9-CM
789.5 ascites

 ## Astrocytoma

DESCRIPTION A tumor composed of astrocytes characterized by hemiparesis, cranial nerve palsy, personality changes, headache, seizures, and mentation change. Usual course - progressive.

SYNONYMS
• Astrocytic glioma
• Astroglioma

CAUSES
• tuberous sclerosis

TREATMENT
• grade I: surgery
• combined surgery plus radiotherapy
• grade II: combined surgery plus radiotherapy
• grade III: combined surgery plus radiotherapy

 ## Ataxia-telangiectasia

DESCRIPTION Autosomal recessive progressive multisystem disorder characterized by cerebellar ataxia, skin and conjunctival teleangiectasia, recurrent infections of sinuses and lungs, and variable immunologic disease. Usual course - progressive.

SYNONYMS
• Louis-Bar syndrome
• cerebello-oculocutaneous telangiectasia

CAUSES
• immunoglobulin metabolic disorder
• defective mesodermal differentiation

TREATMENT
• treat complications

ICD-9-CM
334 spinocerebellar disease
334.8 other spinocerebellar ataxia

 ## Atrial fibrillation

Description Atrial rate greater than 400 beats per minute, ventricular rate varies. "Irregular irregularity" with QRS complexes uniform in shape at irregular intervals. P-R interval cannot be discerned. No P waves or erratic P waves. Irregular QRS rate.

Causes Enlarged atrium secondary to congestive heart failure, chronic obstructive pulmonary disease, pulmonary embolus, mitral stenosis, hyperthyroidism, sepsis, digitalis toxicity, postcoronary by-pass surgery, or valve replacement surgery.

ICD-9-CM
427.31 Atrial fibrillation

 ## Atrial flutter

DESCRIPTION Atrial rate 240-400 beats per minute. QRS complexes uniform in shape, irregular in rate. P waves may have saw-toothed configuration.

CAUSES Postoperative revascularization, digitalis toxicity, pulmonary embolism, valvular heart disease, congestive heart failure

ICD-9-CM
427.32 Atrial flutter

 ## Atrial myxoma

DESCRIPTION A benign tumor composed of primitive connective tissue cells forming a gelatinous growth, usually pedunculated. Symptoms include dyspnea of effort, weight loss, fatigue, low-grade fever, polyneuritis, nausea, syncopal attacks. Usual course: progressive.

CAUSES
• unknown

TREATMENT
• surgical excision of mass

ICD-9-CM
212.7 benign neoplasm of heart

 ## Attention deficit disorder

DESCRIPTION Inappropriate inattention and impulsivity with or without hyperactivity. Affects 5-10% of school-aged children. 10 times more frequent in boys than girls.
• Characteristics - symptoms include restlessness, inattention, hyperactivity, motor incoordination, nonlocalized neurological findings, EEG abnormalities, emotional lability, anxiety, aggressiveness, low tolerance to frustration. Children do not grow out of this difficulty.

SYNONYMS
• ADD
• Hyperactivity
• Hyperkinesis
• Minimal brain dysfunction

CAUSES Unknown

Treatment
• Controversial

Atypical mycobacterial infection

DESCRIPTION Disease caused by mycobacteria other than the tubercle and lepra bacillus. The illnesses are similar both pathlogically and clinically to tuberculosis. Usual course - acute; progressive.
Endemic areas: central USA; texas; england; wales; southeastern USA

CAUSES
• mycobacterium ulcerans
• mycobacterium kansasii
• mycobacterium avium intracellulare
• mycobacterium xenopi
• mycobacterium szulgai

TREATMENT
• rifampin
• ethambutol
• isoniazid
• surgery
• minocycline
• trimethoprim sulfa
• ethionamide
• pyrazinamide
• cycloserine

ICD-9-CM
031.9 Unspecified diseases due to mycobacteria

 Autism

DESCRIPTION A syndrome of early childhood. Thge condition of being dominated by self-centered trendsof thought or behavior which are not subject to correction by external information. Characteristics:
◊ Abnormal social relationships
◊ Language disorder with impaired understanding
◊ Rituals and compulsive phenomena
◊ Uneven intellectual development
◊ Male to female ratio 4:1
◊ Pronominal reversal
◊ Labile mood
◊ Aggressive, self-destructive behavior

SYNONYMS
• Infantile autism
• Kanner's syndrome

CAUSES Mostly unclear. Relationship to schizophrenia is controversial. Predisposing factors include maternal rubella, phenylketonuria, encephalitis, meningitis.

 Babesiosis

DESCRIPTION A group of tick-borne diseases of cattle, sheep, goats, horses, swine, dogs and cats; caused by protozoans of the genus Babesia, which parasitize the red blood cells, producing hemolysis.
Usual course - acute
Endemic areas: cape cod; nantucket island; martha's vineyard; fire island; shelter island; long island

SYNONYMS
• piroplasmosis

CAUSES
• babesia microti
• tick bite
• blood transfusion
• ixodes dammini

TREATMENT
• quinine
• clindamycin
• pentamidine isethionate
• exchange transfusion

ICD-9-CM
NA

 Balantidiasis

DESCRIPTION Infection by protozoan parasites of the genus Balantidium. B. coli may cause diarrhea and dysentery in man, with ulceration of the colon mucosa. Usual course - acute. Endemic areas - tropical areas.

CAUSES
• balantidium coli

TREATMENT
• tetracycline
• iodoquinol

ICD-9-CM
007.0 balantidiasis

 Balkan nephritis syndrome

DESCRIPTION A chronic progressive nephritis seen in a large percentage of the population living in the endemic areas of Yugoslavia, Romania, Bulgaria.

CAUSES
• Unknown
• Possible environmental toxin

TREATMENT
• treat renal failure
• avoid endemic areas

ICD-9-CM
582.89 nephritis, interstitial, chronic

 Barbiturate dependence

DESCRIPTION A dependence on barbiturates that is characterized by inability to stop the barbiturate use, social and occupational impairment, sluggishness, and difficulty in thinking. Usual course - chronic; progressive; relapsing.

CAUSES
• chronic use of barbiturates

TREATMENT
• hospitalization
• mild doses of phenobarbital
• fluids
• psychotherapy

ICD-9-CM
304.10 barbiturate and similarly acting sedative or hypnotic dependence

 Bartonellosis

DESCRIPTION Infection with Bartonella bacilliformis, transmitted by sandflies found in Andean valleys in Peru, Ecuador, and Colombia. Usual course - acute; chronic; incubation 2-6 weeks.

SYNONYMS
• carrion disease
• oroya fever
• verruga peruana

CAUSES
• bartonella bacilliformis
• phlebotomus fly

TREATMENT
• antibiotics
• surgical excision of larger verrugas

ICD-9-CM
088.0 bartonellosis

 Bartter's syndrome

DESCRIPTION Hypertrophy and hyperplasia of the juxtaglomerular cells producing hypokalemic alkalosis and hyperaldosteronism. Characteristics - absence of hypertension in the presence of markedly increased plasma renin concentrations and insensitivity to the pressor effects of angiotensin. It usually affects children, is perhaps hereditary, and may be associated with other congenital anomalies, such as short stature and mental retardation. Usual course - chronic.

CAUSES
• unknown
• primary renal potassium wasting
• defective renal tubular potassium transport
• defective renal tubular chloride transport

TREATMENT
• liberal dietary potassium
• liberal dietary sodium chloride
• potassium supplementation
• spironolactone
• indomethacin
• ibuprofen
• aspirin
• captopril
• propranolol

ICD-9-CM
255.1 bartter's syndrome

 Beckwith-Wiedemann syndrome

DESCRIPTION A syndrome of multiple defects characterized primarily by umbilical hernia, macroglossia, and gigantism and secondarily by visceromegaly, hypoglycemia, ear abnormalities, etc. Also called Exomphalos-Macroglossia-Gigantism (EMG) syndrome. Usual course - acute.

SYNONYMS
• Beckwith syndrome
• Wiedemann II syndrome
• Exomphalos-macroglossia-gigantism syndrome

CAUSES
• unknown

TREATMENT
• steroids
• feeding manipulations
• non-ketogenic diet high in calories
• surgery

ICD-9-CM
759 other and unspecified congenital anomalies
759.8 other specified anomalies

Beribethen heart disease

DESCRIPTION A form of beriberi caused by a deficiency of thiamine characterized by cardiac failure and edema, but without extensive nervous system involvement.

SYNONYMS
• vitamin B1 deficiency heart disease
• wet beriberi

CAUSES
• chronic alcoholism
• thiamine deficiency
• malnutrition

TREATMENT
• thiamine
• diuretics
• digitalis

ICD-9-CM
265.0 beriberi

 Beriberi nervous system syndrome

DESCRIPTION Usual course - chronic; progressive; generally associated with beriberi heart disease; often progresses to cerebral beriberi

CAUSES
• thiamine deficiency
• malnutrition
• chronic alcoholism
• fever
• high carbohydrate intake
• thyrotoxicosis
• dialysis
• diuresis

TREATMENT
• intramuscular thiamine
• water-soluble vitamin repletion

ICD-9-CM
265.0 beriberi

 Bezoar

DESCRIPTION Concretions of swallowed hair, fruit or vegetable fibers, or similar substances found in the alimentary canal. Usual course - acute.

CAUSES
• partial gastrectomy
• autonomic neuropathy
• accumulation of vegetable fibers
• accumulation of hairs

TREATMENT
• phytobezoars: cellulose digestion
• papain digestion
• lavage
• surgery
• trichobezoars: lavage
• surgery

ICD-9-CM
938 bezoar

 Bezold abscess

DESCRIPTION Sore throat and nuchal rigidity caused by insufficiently treated otitis media. Named after Frederich Bezold, an otologist from Munich. Usual course - chronic.

SYNONYMS
• subperiosteal abscess of the temporal bone
• bezold mastoiditis

CAUSES
• insufficiently treated otitis media

TREATMENT
• antibiotics
• surgical drainage

ICD-9-CM
383.01 subperiosteal abscess of mastoid

 Bladder tumors

DESCRIPTION
• The second most common site for tumors of the urinary tract. Most bladder tumors occur in men aged 50 and over. Common types include transitional cell carcinoma (the most common) type), epidermoid tumors, adenocarcinoma, and sarcoma with systemic disease
• Characteristics - symptoms include hematuria, urinary frequency, urgency, dysuria, reduced force and size of the urinary stream, suprapubic pain, and sometimes a palpable suprapubic mass. Should rule out renal calculi, cystitis, nephritis. Measures to confirm diagnosis include cystoscopy, biopsy, CT scan, ultrasound.

SYNONYMS N/A

CAUSES Unknown. Risk factors include alcoholism, tobacco smoking, radiation exposure.

 Bloom's syndrome

DESCRIPTION Autosomal recessive syndrome developing during infancy. Characteristics include erythema and telangiectasia (in a butterfly distribution the face), photosensitivity, and dwarfism. Usual course - chronic; onset in infancy; decreased infection rate with age.

SYNONYMS
• congenital telangiectatic erythema

CAUSES
• chromosomal breakage
• chromosomal instability
• sister chromatid exchanges
• chromosomal aberrations

TREATMENT

ICD-9-CM
NA

 Blue diaper syndrome

DESCRIPTION Defect in tryptophan absorption in which the urine contains abnormal indoles, giving it a blue color. This is similar to Hartnup's disease. Usual course - chronic.

SYNONYMS
• familial hypercalcemia; with nephrocalcinosis and indicanuria
• tryptophan malabsorption

CAUSES
• defective tryptophan absorption

TREATMENT
• low tryptophan diet
• definitive treatment unknown

ICD-9-CM
275.4 disorders of calcium metabolism

 Boutonneuse fever

DESCRIPTION A febrile disease of the Mediterranean area, the Crimea, Africa and India, due to infection with Rickettsia conorii.
Usual course - acute; 5-7 day incubation period
Endemic areas: mediterranean littoral; africa; indian subcontinent

SYNONYMS
• african tick typhus
• african tick-borne fever

CAUSES
• rickettsia conorii
• tick bite
• rodent reservoir
• dog reservoir

TREATMENT
• chloramphenicol
• tetracycline

ICD-9-CM
082.1 boutonneuse fever
087.1 tick-borne relapsing fever

 Bowen's disease

DESCRIPTION An epidermal hyperplasia (often occurring in multiple primary sites), which may progress to squamous cell carcinoma

SYNONYMS
• precancerous dermatosis
• intradermal epidermoid carcinoma
• carcinoma in-situ
• intraepidermal squamous cell carcinoma

CAUSES
• sun damage
• arsenic

TREATMENT
• surgical excision

ICD-9-CM
NA

Brill's disease

DESCRIPTION Recrudescence of epidemic typhus occurring years after the initial infection in which the etiologic agent Rickettsia prowazekii persists in body tissues in an inactive state (up to 70 Years). Usual course - relapsing. Endemic areas - worldwide.

SYNONYMS
• Brill-Zinsser disease
• recrudescent typhus
• recrudescent typhus fever

CAUSES
• persistent rickettsia prowazekii in human reservoirs
• prior epidemic typhus fever
• No lousiness

TREATMENT
• tetracycline
• chloramphenicol
• pediculocides

ICD-9-CM
081.1 brill's disease

 Broncholithiasis

DESCRIPTION Condition in which calculi (broncholiths) are present within the lumen of the tracheobronchial tree.

SYNONYMS
• calculi of bronchus
• bronchopulmonary lithiasis

CAUSES
• usually a late complication of a granulomatous disease

TREATMENT
• antibiotics
• endoscopic removal
• surgery

ICD-9-CM
518.8 broncholithiasis

 Brown-Sequard syndrome

DESCRIPTION Syndrome due to damage of one half of the spinal cord, resulting in ipsilateral paralysis and loss of discriminatory and joint sensation, and contralateral loss of pain and temperature sensation.

SYNONYMS
• hemiparaplegic syndrome
• spastic spinal monoplegia syndrome

CAUSES
• spinal trauma
• unilateral spinal cord lesion
• spinal cord tumors
• spinal cord radiation
• spinal cord compression

TREATMENT
• surgery
• decompression

ICD-9-CM
344.8 brown-sequard syndrome

 Budd-Chiari's syndrome

DESCRIPTION Symptomatic occlusion or obstruction of the hepatic veins, causing hepatomegaly, abdominal pain and tenderness, intractable ascites, mild jaundice, portal hypertension and liver failure. The onset may be acute. In cases of complete occlusion, death may occur within days of onset. More often, there is a chronic course with survival for months or years.

SYNONYMS
• hepatic vein thrombosis

CAUSES
• trauma
• oral contraceptives
• polycythemia rubra vera
• paroxysmal nocturnal hemoglobinuria
• hypercoagulable state
• pyrrolizidine alkaloids

TREATMENT
• portacaval shunt

ICD-9-CM
453.0 budd-chiari syndrome

 Carcinoid syndrome

DESCRIPTION A symptom complex associated with carcinoid tumors (argentaffinoma). Characteristics - attacks of severe cyanotic flushing of the skin that lasts from minutes to days; watery stools; bronchoconstrictive attacks; sudden drop in blood pressure; edema; ascites. Symptoms are caused by the tumor secreting serotonin prostaglandins, and other biologically active substances.

SYNONYMS
• Thorson-Bioerck syndrome
• argentaffinoma syndrome
• flush syndrome
• Cassidy-Scholte syndrome

TREATMENT
• medical management of symptoms
• appropriate treatment of tumor

ICD-9-CM
259.2 carcinoid syndrome

 Carcinoid tumor

DESCRIPTION Yellow, circumscribed tumor occurring in the small intestine, appendix, stomach or colon. Usual course - progressive.

SYNONYMS
• argentaffinoma
• carcinoid
• argentaffin carcinoid tumor

TREATMENT
• surgical excision
• antihormonal therapy as needed

ICD-9-CM
238.9 neoplasm of uncertain behavior, nos

 Carcinoma of the male breast

DESCRIPTION A malignant disease of the male breast that is progressive if not cured. There is some familial distribution. Usual course - progressive if not cured.

CAUSES
• hyperestrogenism, bilharziasis, klinefelter's syndrome, adult mumps, steelwork, possibly gynecomastia

TREATMENT
• radical mastectomy
• metastatic disease: orchiectomy
• radiotherapy
• adrenalectomy
• metastatic disease: hypophysectomy

ICD-9-CM
175 malignant neoplasm of male breast

 Cardiogenic shock, acute

DESCRIPTION Shock resulting from primary failure of the heart in its pumping action, as in myocardial infarction, severe cardiomyopathy, or mechanical obstruction of the heart. Usual course - acute.

CAUSES
• myocardial infarction
• myocarditis
• myocardial depression
• acute valvular insufficiency
• myocardial rupture
• septal perforation
• arrhythmias
• severe bradycardia
• severe tachycardia
• fibrillation
• pericardial effusion
• cardiac tamponade
• tension pneumothorax
• positive pressure breathing
• pulmonary embolism
• atrial myxoma
• ball valve myxoma

TREATMENT
• intravenous fluid
• vasopressors
• vasodilator
• inotropic agents
• intra-aortic balloon counterpulsation

ICD-9-CM
785.51 cardiogenic shock

 Cardiomyopathy

DESCRIPTION Cardiomyopathy is usually manifested by dyspnea and palpitations with cardiomegaly and congestive heart failure.

SYNONYMS
• idiopathic myocardiopathy

CAUSES
• Alcohol, amyloidosis, hemosiderosis, glycogen storage disease, idiopathic hypertrophic subaortic stenosis, sarcoidosis, endomyocardial fibrosis, Loeffler's eosinophilia, radiation, peripartum, adriamycin, beriberi, kwashiorkor, potassium deficiency, cobalt, Pompe's disease, Hurler's syndrome, Hunter's syndrome, Fabry's disease, Duchenne's muscular dystrophy, Friedreich's ataxia, Coxsackie virus, poliomyelitis, diphtheria, toxoplasmosis, trichinosis, trypanosomiasis, giant cell myocarditis, acute rheumatic fever

TREATMENT
• digitalis
• diuretics

ICD-9-CM
425.5 cardiomyopathy, nos

Cardiomyopathy, alcoholic

DESCRIPTION Cardiomyopathy resulting from: 1) a toxic effect of alcohol on the myocardium; 2) thiamine deficiency due to malnutrition in alcoholics; or 3) a toxic effect of cobalt additives in beer in heavy beer drinkers. This disease is usually manifested by dyspnea and palpitations with cardiomegaly and congestive heart failure. Usual course - chronic; progressive

SYNONYMS
• alcoholic myocardiopathy

CAUSES
• ethanol

TREATMENT
• avoid alcohol
• symptomatic
• supportive

ICD-9-CM
425.5 alcoholic cardiomyopathy

 Cardiospasm

DESCRIPTION Failure to relax the smooth muscle fibers of the esophagus. Usual course - chronic; progressive.

SYNONYMS
• achalasia
• megaesophagus
• esophageal dyssynergia

CAUSES
• unknown
• impairment of postganglionic innervation of esophagus

TREATMENT
• soft foods
• sedatives
• nitrates
• anticholinergics
• calcium channel blockers
• balloon dilatation
• myotomy

ICD-9-CM
530.0 achalasia and cardiospasm

 Caroli's disease

DESCRIPTION Congenital dilatation of the intrahepatic bile ducts. Characteristics - abdominal pain, fever, intermittent jaundice, hepatomegaly. Usual course - chronic; progressive; relapsing.

CAUSES
• congenital dilatation of intrahepatic bile ducts
• intrahepatic stones
• biliary obstruction

TREATMENT
• antibiotics
• No surgery

ICD-9-CM
751.69 other congenital anomalies of gallbladder, bile ducts, and liver

 Cat-scratch disease

DESCRIPTION Usually a benign, self-limited infectious disease of the regional lymph nodes, chiefly characterized subacute painful regional lymphadenitis and mild fever of short duration. It is most often associated with close contact to a cat, the primary symptom being a papule or pustule at the site of a scratch.

SYNONYMS
• cat-scratch fever
• benign inoculation lymphoreticulosis
• nonbacterial regional lymphadenitis

CAUSES
• pleomorphic gram-negative bacilli

TREATMENT
• analgesia
• node aspiration
• excision

ICD-9-CM
078.3 cat-scratch disease

 Cauda equina syndrome

DESCRIPTION Dull aching pain of the perineum, bladder, and sacrum, generally radiating in a sciatic fashion, with associated paresthesias and paralysis, due to compression of the spinal nerve roots. Usual course - chronic.

SYNONYMS
• cauda equina pseudo-claudication

CAUSES
• lumbar spondylosis with cauda equina compression
• congenital narrowing of lumbar canal

TREATMENT
• decompressive laminectomy
• rest

ICD-9-CM
344.60 cauda equina syndrome without mention of neurogenic bladder
344.61 cauda equina syndrome with neurogenic bladder

 Cavernous sinus thrombosis

DESCRIPTION Infection of the venous channels that drain the orbit and face. Characteristics - symptoms include exophthalmos, papilledema, headache, convulsions, septic temperature curve. Prognosis is grave.

SYNONYMS N/A

CAUSES Direct extension of infection from the orbit and face. Risk factors include diabetes mellitus and immunosuppression.

 Celiac disease of childhood

DESCRIPTION Disease characterized by intestinal malabsorption and precipitated by gluten-containing foods. The intestinal mucosa shows loss of villous structure. The infantile form of celiac disease may begin as early as three months of age. There is a possible genetic predisposition.

SYNONYMS
• celiac sprue
• gluten-induced enteropathy
• nontropical sprue

CAUSES
• gluten intolerance

TREATMENT
• gluten-free diet

ICD-9-CM
579.0 celiac disease

 Cervical extension injury

DESCRIPTION Sometimes called "whiplash" - an ambiguous term with confusing medicolegal implications. Whiplash indicates only the mechanism, not the nature or extent of possible injury. Extension injuries may include dislocations, fractures, fracture-dislocations.
• Characteristics - symptoms include pain (frequently vague), soreness, tenderness, dizziness. X-rays are usually negative, but may show organic changes.

SYNONYMS Whiplash

CAUSES Hyperextension, hyperflexion of neck, usually occurring in rear-end automobile collision. Mechanism - a sudden change in speed of hit car throwing head backward, then forward.

 Chagas' disease

DESCRIPTION An acute, subacute or chronic form of trypanosomiasis occurring widely in Central and South America, transmitted by bites of reduviid bugs. Usual course - acute; chronic; progressive.
Endemic areas: western hemisphere; mexico to central america; south america; identified mammalian reservoirs in USA

SYNONYMS
• brazilian trypanosomiasis

CAUSES
• inoculation of trypanosoma cruzi
• congenital breast milk
• transfusion-related infection

TREATMENT
• nifurtimox in acute phase
• No definitive treatment
• metronidazole
• pacemaker
• esophageal dilatation
• gastrointestinal surgery

ICD-9-CM
086.2 chagas' disease without mention of organ involvement

Charcot joint

DESCRIPTION Neuropathic arthropathy associated with certain chronic disorders. Usual course - chronic; progressive.

SYNONYMS
• neuropathic arthropathy
• tabetic osteoarthropathy
• neuropathic joint disease

CAUSES
• peripheral neuropathy
• diabetes
• tertiary syphilis
• tabes dorsalis
• syringomyelia
• myelomeningocele

TREATMENT
• immobilization
• reduction of weight-bearing
• surgical arthrodesis

ICD-9-CM
094.0 tabes dorsalis
713.5 arthropathy associated with neurological disorders

 Charcot-Marie-Tooth

disease

DESCRIPTION Progressive neuropathic (peroneal) muscular atrophy, usually autosomal dominant. Characteristics - cramps, paresthesias, leg and hand weakness, difficulty in walking. Usual course - chronic; progressive.

SYNONYMS
• peroneal muscular atrophy
• charcot-marie-tooth atrophy
• charcot-marie-tooth disease
• charcot-marie disease

CAUSES
• hereditary

TREATMENT
• leg braces

ICD-9-CM
356.1 charcot-marie-tooth disease

 Cheese-worker's lung

DESCRIPTION A pathologic condition caused by inhalation of mold that grows on cheese. Usual course - acute; subacute; chronic.

SYNONYMS
• cheese-washer's lung

CAUSES
• antigens of aspergillus clavatus
• antigens of penicillium casei
• breathing cheese mold

TREATMENT
• avoid causative agents
• tapered steroids suppress alveolitis
• chronic disease: long-term steroids

ICD-9-CM
495.8 cheese washers' lung

 Chiari-Frommel syndrome

DESCRIPTION Persistent lactation and amenorrhea following pregnancy.
Usual course - chronic

SYNONYMS
• Frommel's Disease
• Persistent postpartum amenorrhea-galactorrhea syndrome
• Pregnancy-related A-G syndrome

CAUSES
• microadenoma of the pituitary

TREATMENT

ICD-9-CM
676.6 galactorrhea associated with childbirth

 Chikungunya

DESCRIPTION A self-limited dengue-like illness caused by an alphavirus transmitted by mosquitoes of the genus Aedes, principally occurring in Southeast Asia and Africa. Usual course - acute.

CAUSES
• group A arbovirus
• alphavirus
• arthropod-borne
• mosquito vector
• aedes aegypti

TREATMENT
• supportive
• bed rest
• non-salicylate antipyretics
• analgesics
• anti-inflammatory agents
• physiotherapy
• anticonvulsants
• rehydration

ICD-9-CM
066.3 chikungunya fever

 Chloasma

DESCRIPTION Sharply demarcated, blotchy, brown, macules found in a symmetric distribution over the cheeks and forehead and sometimes on the neck or upper lip. Frequently occurs during pregnancy, at menopause, and in patients taking oral contraceptives. Same type may be seen in patients with chronic liver disease. Usual course - variable; chronic; relapsing.

SYNONYMS
• melasma
• mask of pregnancy

CAUSES
• oral contraceptives plus ultraviolet light
• pregnancy plus ultraviolet light
• endocrine dysfunction
• cosmetics
• Mesantoin
• diphenylhydantoin

TREATMENT
• avoid sun exposure
• avoid oral contraceptives
• delivery
• discontinue implicated drug
• discontinue implicated cosmetic
• topical bleaching agents

ICD-9-CM
709.0 chloasma

 Chondroma

DESCRIPTION Benign tumor of cartilage cells. Usual course - progressive; curable

SYNONYMS
• true chondroma
• enchondroma
• chondromyxoma

CAUSES
• cartilaginous exostoses

TREATMENT
• block excision of tumor
• combined surgery plus radiotherapy
• palliative radiotherapy for advanced disease

ICD-9-CM
213.9 neoplasm, cartilage, benign

 Chordoma

DESCRIPTION Rare malignant bone tumor that develops from the remnants of the primitive notochord. May be located in the sacrum or near the base of the skull. Usual course - slowly progressive; recurrent; cure possible.

TREATMENT
• surgical resection
• radiotherapy if positive margins

ICD-9-CM
170.2 neoplasm, malignant of spine

Choriocarcinoma of the

testes

DESCRIPTION Malignant tumor of the testes composed of syncytiotrophoblastic cells. This is a solid testicular tumor. Characteristics - testicular mass, testicular pain. Usual course - progressive.

CAUSES
• cryptorchidism

TREATMENT
• cis-platin for nonmetastatic disease
• cis-platin
• vinblastine
• bleomycin
• radical orchiectomy
• possibly radical retroperitoneal lymphadenectomy

ICD-9-CM
186.9 choriocarcinoma, nos, male

Chromomycosis

DESCRIPTION Systemic infectious fungus disease caused by Hormodendrum pedrosoi, H. compactum, or Phialophora verrucosa. Characteristics - slowly develop into large papillomatous vegetations that frequently ulcerate. Usual course - chronic. Endemic areas - worldwide; most common in tropical and subtropical areas; Brazil; Costa Rica.

SYNONYMS
• dermatomycosis
• verrucous dermatitis
• phaeohyphomycosis
• cystic chromomycosis
• cerebral chromomycosis

CAUSES
• traumatic inoculation of saprophytic soil fungi
• phialophora fungi
• fonsecaea fungi
• cladosporium fungi

TREATMENT
• successful in inverse relation to duration of infection
• successful in inverse relation to extent of infection
• antifungals
• amphotericin B
• flucytosine
• ketaconazole
• anthelmintic
• thiabendazole

ICD-9-CM
117.2 chromoblastomycosis

 Chromophobe adenoma of the pituitary

DESCRIPTION Tumor of anterior lobe of the pituitary gland whose cells do not stain with either acid or base dyes. The tumor may be non- functioning or may be associated with hyperpituitarism including acromegaly or Cushing's syndrome. Usual course - progressive.

CAUSES
• increased incidence after bilateral adrenalectomy

TREATMENT
• radiotherapy for small tumors
• surgery with postoperative radiotherapy for large tumors

ICD-9-CM
227.3 benign neoplasms of pituitary gland and craniopharyngeal duct

 Cirrhosis, alcoholic

DESCRIPTION Cirrhosis in the patient with alcoholism. Probably attributable to chronic nutritional deficiency or to exposure to alcohol as a hepatotoxic. Usual course - progressive.

SYNONYMS
• portal liver cirrhosis
• Laennec's cirrhosis

CAUSES
• alcoholism
• jejunoileal bypass

TREATMENT
• supportive
• treat complications
• treat consequences
• diet
• multivitamins
• complete abstinence from alcohol

ICD-9-CM
571.2 alcoholic cirrhosis of liver

 Cirrhosis, cardiac

DESCRIPTION Fibrosis of the liver following central hemorrhagic necrosis associated with congestive heart failure. Usual course - chronic.

SYNONYMS
• posthepatic cirrhosis

CAUSES
• right ventricular failure
• tricuspid stenosis
• rheumatic heart disease
• cardiomyopathy
• constrictive pericarditis

TREATMENT
• fluid restriction
• diuretics
• sodium restriction
• digitalis
• rest

ICD-9-CM
571.5 posthepatic cirrhosis

 Cirrhosis, macronodal

DESCRIPTION Disorganization of liver structure by widespread fibrosis characterized by connective tissue bands of varying thickness and by nodules that vary in size and contain portal spaces and terminal hepatic veins. Characteristics - anorexia, fatigue, jaundice, right upper quadrant pain, ascites. Usual course - chronic; progressive.

SYNONYMS
• postnecrotic liver cirrhosis
• toxic cirrhosis
• posthepatic cirrhosis
• necrotic liver cirrhosis

CAUSES
• unknown
• possible sequela of viral hepatitis
• phosphorus intoxication
• poisons
• infection
• metabolic disorders

TREATMENT
• treat complications
• avoid drugs
• protein restriction

ICD-9-CM
571.5 postnecrotic cirrhosis

 Cirrhosis, primary biliary

DESCRIPTION Fibrosis of the liver due to obstruction or infection of the major extra- or intrahepatic bile ducts. Characteristics include jaundice, abdominal pain, steatorrhea, and enlargement of the liver and spleen.

SYNONYMS
• Hypertrophic cirrhosis of Hanot
• Hanot syndrome
• Cholangiolitic biliary cirrhosis

CAUSES
• autoimmune

TREATMENT
• corticosteroids
• azathioprine
• penicillamine
• colchicine

ICD-9-CM
571.6 biliary cirrhosis

 Colorado tick fever

DESCRIPTION A febrile illness characterized by chills, aches, vomiting, leucopenia, and sometimes encephalitis; caused by a retrovirus transmitted by the tick Dermacentor andersoni. Usual course - 3 to 7 day incubation period after tick bite; acute onset; brief symptom-free interval; second febrile illness. Endemic areas - Rocky Mountain area; western Canada.

SYNONYMS
• American mountain tick fever
• mountain tick fever

CAUSES
• arbovirus transmitted by bite of hard-shelled wood tick (dermacentor andersoni)

TREATMENT
• supportive therapy

ICD-9-CM
066.1 colorado tick fever

 Complete heart block

DESCRIPTION Characteristics - QRS interval normal (nodal pacemaker); wide and bizarre (ventricular pacemaker). No relationship between P waves and QRS complexes. No constant P-R interval.

SYNONYMS N/A

CAUSES Myocardial infarction or ischemic heart disease, postsurgical valve replacement, hypoxia with syncope as with Stokes-Adams syndrome, digitalis toxicity

Treatment Pacemaker

 Congestive heart failure, right

DESCRIPTION Right ventricular congestive heart failure. Characteristics - venous hypertension and edema. Fatigue and low cardiac output are late manifestations. Commonly associated with left ventricular failure, which causes pulmonary arterial hypertension induced by pulmonary vascular changes and by elevated pulmonary venous pressure.

CAUSES
• pulmonic stenosis
• primary pulmonary hypertension
• pulmonary embolism
• left ventricular failure
• tricuspid stenosis
• tricuspid atresia
• pericardial constriction
• anomalous pulmonary venous connection
• chronic obstructive pulmonary disease
• restrictive lung disease
• upper airway obstruction
• diminished ventilatory drive
• severe liver disease
• sarcoidosis
• collagen vascular diseases
• aminorex ingestion

TREATMENT
• digitalis
• treat underlying condition

ICD-9-CM
428.0 congestive heart failure

Cor triloculare biatriatum

DESCRIPTION Three chambered heart

SYNONYMS
• single ventricle
• univentricular heart
• double inlet ventricle

TREATMENT
• palliative surgery
• corrective surgery
• medical treatment of cardiac failure

ICD-9-CM
745.3 cor triloculare biatriatum

 Cornelia de Lange's syndrome

DESCRIPTION A congenital syndrome in which severe mental retardation is associated with many abnormalities such as short stature, brachycephaly, low-set ears, webbed neck, bushy eyebrows and flat hands. Possible autosomal dominant; autosomal recessive; chromosomal mutation.

SYNONYMS
• typus degenerativus amstelodamensis
• Amsterdam dwarf syndrome of deLange
• Brachman de Lange syndrome

TREATMENT

ICD-9-CM
NA

 Cowden's syndrome

DESCRIPTION Autosomal dominant hereditary disease. Characteristics - ectodermal neoplasia, microstomia, trichilemmomas of the face, acral verrucous papules. Usual course - chronic; progressive.

SYNONYMS
• cowden's disease
• multiple hamartoma syndrome

CAUSES
• ectodermal neoplasia
• mesodermal neoplasia
• malignant transformation

TREATMENT
• surgical
• chemotherapy when applicable

ICD-9-CM
NA

 Craniopharyngioma

DESCRIPTION A tumor arising from cell rests derived from the hypophyseal stalk, frequently associated with increased intracerebral pressure, and showing calcium deposits in the capsule or the tumor proper. Usual course - progressive.

SYNONYMS
• rathke pouch tumor
• suprasellar cyst
• pituitary epidermoid tumor
• ameloblastoma
• pituitary adamantinoma

TREATMENT
• surgery
• radiotherapy
• hormone replacement therapy

ICD-9-CM
237.0 craniopharyngioma

 Creutzfeldt-Jakob disease

DESCRIPTION Rare, usually fatal, transmissible spongiform encephalopathy, occurring in middle life in which there is partial degeneration of the pyramidal and extrapyramidal systems accompanied by progressive dementia, tremor, muscle wasting, athetosis and spastic dysarthria. Usual course - progressive; 15-20 months incubation; 6 months average duration.

SYNONYMS
• spastic pseudosclerosis
• corticostriatal-spinal degeneration
• transmissible virus dementia

CAUSES
• risk factors: neurosurgery
• surgery
• trauma
• risk factors: intraocular pressure testing
• risk factors: ingestion of animal brains

TREATMENT
• effective treatment unknown
• experimentally amantadine
• experimentally vidarabine

ICD-9-CM
046.1 jakob-creutzfeldt disease

 Crigler-Najjar disease

DESCRIPTION An autosomal recessive form of nonhemolytic jaundice due to the absence of the hepatic enzyme glucuronosyltranferase. Characteristics include presence in the blood of unconjugated bilirubin and by kernicterus and severe disturbances of the central nervous system. Usual course - acute; progressive.

SYNONYMS
• congenital hyperbilirubinemia
• glucuronyl transferase deficiency type I
• familial unconjugated hyperbilirubinemia

CAUSES
• No uridine diphosphoglucuronic transferase

TREATMENT
• exchange transfusion
• phototherapy
• cholestyramine

ICD-9-CM
277.4 disorders of bilirubin excretion

 Dehydration

DESCRIPTION Extracellular fluid volume depletion. Routes of loss are from the gastrointestinal tract, urinary tract, and skin.
• Characteristics - signs and symptoms include diminished skin turgor, diminished intraocular tension, dry shrunken tongue, low central venous pressure (measured from neck veins), postural hypotension, tachycardia, disorientation, shock, increased hematocrit.

SYNONYMS N/A

CAUSES Excessive loss of fluid from the gastrointestinal tract, urinary tract and skin. Conditions favoring excess loss include vomiting, diarrhea, gastric suction, excessive sweating, dialysis, chronic renal failure, salt-wasting renal disease, interstitial nephritis, myeloma, acute real failure, diuretic therapy, diabetes mellitus with ketoacidosis or extreme glycosuria, Bartter's syndrome, adrenal disease (glucocorticoid deficiency), hypoaldosteronism.

 Delirium tremens

DESCRIPTION Severe alcohol withdrawal syndrome characterized by agitation, violence, anxiety, insomnia, muscle cramps, tremor, delusion, hallucinations, ataxia, fever, with clearing beginning in 12-24 hours up to 2-10 days. Usual course - acute; relapsing.

SYNONYMS
• alcohol withdrawal delirium

CAUSES
• cessation in alcohol consumption after heavy alcohol ingestion

TREATMENT
• benzodiazepines
• barbiturates
• beta-adrenergic blockers

ICD-9-CM
291.0 alcohol withdrawal delirium

Dengue fever

DESCRIPTION Acute, self-limited disease. Characteristics include fever, prostration, headache, myalgia, rash, lymphadenopathy, leukopenia, Caused by four antigenically related but distinct types of the dengue virus. Endemic areas are tropics and subtropics.

SYNONYMS
• breakbone fever

CAUSES
• aedes aegypti mosquito vector
• group B arbovirus
• flavivirus

TREATMENT
• symptomatic
• supportive if hemorrhagic

ICD-9-CM
061 dengue

Diabetes insipidus, nephrogenic

DESCRIPTION A rare congenital and familial form of diabetes insipidus, resulting from failure of the renal tubules to resorb water. There is excessive production of antidiuretic hormone, but the tubules fail to respond to it. Genetics - usually X-linked; possibly dominant male to male.

SYNONYMS
• diabetes insipidus, vasopressin resistant

CAUSES
• lithium
• interstitial nephritis
• renal amyloidosis
• renal sarcoidosis

TREATMENT
• thiazide

ICD-9-CM
588.1 nephrogenic diabetes insipidus

Diabetic coma

DESCRIPTION The coma of severe diabetes mellitus Acute - hypoglycemic coma. Subacute - nonketotic hyperglycemic coma. Progressive - ketoacidotic coma. Usual course - acute (hypoglycemic coma); subacute (nonketotic hyperglycemic coma); progressive (ketoacidotic coma).

SYNONYMS
• diabetes related coma

CAUSES
• hypoglycemia
• ketoacidosis
• nonketotic hyperglycemia
• lactic acidosis

TREATMENT
• hypoglycemic coma: glucose
• fluid plus electrolyte therapy
• hyperglycemic coma: insulin
• fluid replacement
• fluid plus electrolyte therapy
• lactic acidotic coma: fluid replacement
• vasopressor agents
• oxygen
• lactic acidotic coma: antibiotics
• bicarbonate
• hemodialysis
• dichloroacetate

ICD-9-CM
250.3 diabetic coma

Diffuse esophageal spasm

DESCRIPTION Retching, chest pain, dysphagia, and regurgitation associated to esophageal motor dysfunction. Usual course - progressive; intermittent.

CAUSES
• esophageal motor dysfunction

TREATMENT
• anticholinergics
• nitrates
• esophageal dilatation

ICD-9-CM
530.5 diffuse spasm of the esophagus

Diphtheria of the skin

DESCRIPTION Occurs when any disruption of the skin becomes colonized by C. Diphtheriae. Poor personal and community hygiene are particular risk factors. Lesions are punched out ulcers and appear on extremities. Usual course - acute. Endemic areas - tropics; Pacific Northwest; Southwest USA.

SYNONYMS
• cutaneous diphtheria

CAUSES
• corynebacterium diphtheriae
• skin trauma
• poor hygiene

TREATMENT
• intramuscular diphtheria antitoxin
• penicillin
• erythromycin
• quarantine

ICD-9-CM
032.85 Cutaneous diphtheria

Dubin-Johnson syndrome

DESCRIPTION Rare autosomal recessive disorder characterized by various organic anions as well as bilirubin. The hyperbilirubinemia is conjugated and bile appears in the urine. Usual course - intermittent.

SYNONYMS
• chronic idiopathic jaundice
• Dubin-Sprinz disease

CAUSES
• impaired intrahepatic bilirubin secretion
• conjugated hyperbilirubinemia

TREATMENT
• NONE
• DECR bilirubin with phenobarbital

ICD-9-CM
277.4 Dubin-Johnson syndrome

Dyslexia

DESCRIPTION Disparity between intellectual potential and achievement in reading and spelling. Characteristics - normal, intelligent child 2 years behind expected reading level for his grade. Affects children in all socioeconomic levels. Affects more boys than girls.

SYNONYMS
• Congenital word blindness
• Primary reading disability

CAUSES Unknown

Echinococcosis of the liver

DESCRIPTION Infection involving the liver caused by a genus of small tapeworms of the family Taeniidae. Its larvae may form hydatid cysts in the liver. Usual course - slowly progressive; 5-20 year latency. Endemic areas: ranching areas; Middle East; Australia; South Africa; Central Europe.

SYNONYMS
• hydatid cyst of the liver

CAUSES
• larval echinococcus granulosus
• canine fecal contamination
• fecal-oral transmission

TREATMENT
• surgery

ICD-9-CM
122.0 echinococcus granulosus infection of liver

Echinococcosis of the lung

DESCRIPTION Infection of the lung with hydatid cysts of the larvae of small tapeworms of the family Taeniidae. Usual course - progressive; 5-20 year latency. Endemic areas - Middle East; Australia; South Africa; South America; Central Europe.

CAUSES
• larval echinococcus granulosus
• canine fecal contamination
• childhood ingestion of contaminated material

TREATMENT
• surgical cystectomy

ICD-9-CM
122.1 echinococcus granulosus infection of lung

Ecthyma

DESCRIPTION An ulcerative pyoderma usually caused by group A beta-hemolytic streptococcal infection at the site of minor trauma, predominantly of the shins and feet. Healing is with variable scar formation. Usual course - acute; progression of vesiculopustule to crusts to ulceration.

CAUSES
• bacterial infection (streptococcal, staphylococcal)
• poor hygiene
• minor injuries

TREATMENT
• antibiotics
• good hygiene
• proper nutrition

ICD-9-CM
686.8 ecthyma

Ectrodactyly, ectodermal dysplasia, clefting syndrome

DESCRIPTION A congenital ectodermal dysplasia. Characteristics - lobster claw deformity, cleft lip, cleft palate, decreased hair growth, photophobic ectrodactyly, syndactyly. Usual course - chronic; progressive.

SYNONYMS
• EEC syndrome

CAUSES
• unknown

TREATMENT
• oral surgery
• ophthalmologic surgery
• orthopedic surgery

ICD-9-CM
757.31 congenital ectodermal dysplasia

Ehlers-danlos syndrome

DESCRIPTION A group of inherited disorders of the connective tissue occurring in many types based on clinical, genetic and biochemical evidence, varying in severity from mild to lethal. Transmitted as autosomal recessive, autosomal dominant, or X-linked recessive traits. The major manifestations include hyperextensibility of skin and joints, easy brusability, friability of tissues with bleeding and poor wound healing, calcified subcutaneous spheroids and pseudotumors, and cardiovascular, gastrointestinal, orthopedic, and ocular defects. Usual course: chronic; progressive.

SYNONYMS
• Ehlers-Danlos syndrome gravis

CAUSES
• probable defective cross-linkage of collagen

TREATMENT
• symptomatic
• preventive
• prolonged wound fixation
• conservative surgical repair

ICD-9-CM
756.83 Ehlers-Danlos syndrome

Elephantiasis of the scrotum

DESCRIPTION A chronic tropical disease with inflammation and obstruction of the lymphatics of the scrotum causing hypertrophy and swelling. Usual course - chronic; progressive. Endemic areas - tropical South America; subtropical South America; Africa; Asia; North america.

CAUSES
• adult worms
• wuchereria bancrofti
• brugia malayi
• prolonged lymphatic obstruction

TREATMENT
• diethylcarbamazine citrate
• surgery for hydrocele
• elastic stockings

ICD-9-CM
457.1 elephantiasis, scrotal

Elephantiasis, filarial

DESCRIPTION A chronic disease of the tropics due to infection of the lymphatic channels characterized by inflammation and obstruction of the lymphatics and hypertrophy of the skin and subcutaneous tissues. Usual course - acute; chronic; progressive. Endemic areas - South America; Africa; Asia; tropics; subtropics.

SYNONYMS
• filariasis
• wuchereriasis
• lymphatic filariasis

CAUSES
• microfilariae
• wuchereria bancrofti
• brugia malayi
• mosquito vector

TREATMENT
• diethylcarbamazine citrate
• plastic surgery
• fulguration
• elastic stockings

ICD-9-CM
125.9 elephantiasis, filarial, nos

Empyema

DESCRIPTION Presence of pus in a hollow organ or body cavity, particularly the pleural cavity. Usual course - acute.

CAUSES
• purulent inflammatory exudate of pleural cavity
• pulmonary infection
• thoracic surgery
• esophageal perforation
• hematogenous spread from other sites
• idiopathic
• subphrenic abscess

TREATMENT
• drainage
• antimicrobial therapy

ICD-9-CM
510.9 empyema without mention of fistula

Encephalitis, Saint Louis

DESCRIPTION A viral disease first observed in Illinois in 1932, closely similar to western equine encephalomyelitis. It occurs in late summer and early fall. Transmitted usually by mosquitoes of the genus Culex. It ranges from an abortive type of infection to severe disease. Endemic areas - Eastern USA; Midwestern USA.

CAUSES
• group B arbovirus
• transmitted by culex mosquito

TREATMENT
• supportive

ICD-9-CM
062.3 st. louis encephalitis

Encephalitis, viral

DESCRIPTION Acute inflammation of the brain due to direct viral invasion or to hypersensitivity initiated by a virus or other foreign protein. Encephalomyelitis is the same disorder that affects the spinal cord structures as well as the brain. Some viruses may be borne by mosquitoes and infect man only during warm weather.
• Characteristics - signs and symptoms include CSF pleocytosis, normal glucose, no bacteria, fever, headache, vomiting, malaise, stiff neck and back, cranial nerve abnormalities, seizures, personality change

CAUSES
• Epidemic - arbo, polio, echo, and Coxsackie viruses
• Sporadic - herpes simplex, herpes zoster viruses
• Secondary - those following measles, chickenpox, rubella, smallpox vaccination, vaccinia

Endomyocardial fibrosis, eosinophilic

DESCRIPTION Idiopathic myocardiopathy occurring endemically in various regions of Africa, characterized by cardiomegaly, marked thickening of the endocardium with dense, white fibrous tissue that frequently extends to involve the inner third or half of the myocardium.

SYNONYMS
• loeffler endomyocardial fibrosis
• loeffler fibroplastic parietal endocarditis

CAUSES
• unknown
• possibly eosinophil disorder

TREATMENT
• inotropic support
• fluid restriction plus diuretics
• anticoagulants
• immunosuppression
• endomyocardiectomy
• valve replacement
• glenn shunt

ICD-9-CM
425.0 endomyocardial fibrosis

Eosinophilic adenoma of the pituitary

DESCRIPTION A tumor of the eosinophilic cells of the anterior lobe of the pituitary gland whose presence is associated with acromegaly and gigantism. Usual course - slowly progressive.

TREATMENT
• transsphenoidal surgery
• frontal craniotomy
• radiotherapy
• bromocriptine
• combined therapy

ICD-9-CM
194.3 malignant neoplasms of pituitary gland

Eosinophilic fasciitis

DESCRIPTION Inflammation of the fascia of the extremities caused by unusual strenuous exercise. Usual course - acute; progressive; relapsing.

CAUSES
• unusual strenuous physical exercise
• inflammatory reaction due to chemotactic collagen breakdown products

TREATMENT
• corticosteroids
• nonsteroidal anti-inflammatory drugs

ICD-9-CM
729.4 fasciitis, unspecified

Eosinophilic gastroenteritis

DESCRIPTION A disorder characterized by infiltration of the mucosa of the small intestine by eosinophils, with edema but without vasculitis. Symptoms include diarrhea, abdominal pain, nausea, fever, malabsorption. The stomach is also frequently involved. This disorder is commonly associated with intolerance to specific foods. Usual course: -chronic; recurrent.

CAUSES
• food allergy
• idiopathic

TREATMENT
• exclusionary diets
• prednisone

ICD-9-CM
558.9 other noninfectious gastroenteritis and colitis

Epilepsy, grand mal

DESCRIPTION Paroxysmal transient disturbances of brain function. Symptoms are due to paroxysmal electrical disturbances of the brain. Grand mal episodes are frequently preceded by an aura, in which the sudden loss of consciousness is immediately followed by generalized convulsions. Usual course - chronic; recurrent; intermittent.

SYNONYMS
• primary generalized tonic-clonic seizures
• generalized convulsive epilepsy

CAUSES
• idiopathic, birth injury, metabolic disturbances, head trauma sequelae, CNS infection sequelae, congenital cerebral malformation, drug withdrawal, alcohol withdrawal, brain tumor, cerebrovascular disease, secondary generalization of partial seizures

TREATMENT
• anticonvulsant medication
• phenytoin
• diphenylhydantoin
• carbamazepine
• neurosurgery for treatable structural lesions
• intravenous benzodiazepines for status epilepticus

ICD-9-CM
345.1 grand mal, idiopathic

Epilepsy, Jacksonian

DESCRIPTION Epilepsy characterized by unilateral clonic movements that start in one group of muscles and spread systematically to adjacent groups, reflecting the march of epileptic activity through the motor cortex.. Usual course - chronic; recurrent; intermittent.

SYNONYMS
• simple partial seizures

CAUSES
• head trauma sequelae
• CNS infection sequelae
• birth injury
• congenital cerebral malformation
• cerebrovascular disease
• brain tumor
• idiopathic

TREATMENT
• anticonvulsant medication
• phenytoin
• diphenylhydantoin
• carbamazepine
• phenobarbital
• neurosurgery for treatable structural lesions

ICD-9-CM
345.5 jacksonian epilepsy

Epilepsy, petit mal

DESCRIPTION Epilepsy in which there is a sudden loss of consciousness with only minor myoclonic jerks, seen especially in children. These episodes are accompanied by 3-c.p.s. spike and wave discharges on the electroencephalogram. Usual course - chronic; recurrent; intermittent; may resolve spontaneously with increasing age. Familial predisposition.

SYNONYMS
• primary generalized absence epilepsy
• absence epilepsy
• pyknolepsy

CAUSES
• idiopathic

TREATMENT
• anticonvulsant medications
• ethosuximide
• valproic acid

ICD-9-CM
345.0 petit mal, idiopathic

Epithelial mesothelioma

DESCRIPTION A malignant tumor derived from mesothelial tissue of the pleura, with some regions containing spindle-shaped, sarcoma-like cells and other regions showing adenomatous patterns. Usual course - progressive.

CAUSES
• asbestos
• tobacco smoking

TREATMENT
• surgical resection for solitary lesion
• palliative radiotherapy for advanced disease
• palliative chemotherapy for advanced disease
• pleurocentesis for pleural effusion

ICD-9-CM
163.9 malignant neoplasm of the pleura

Erythema marginatum

DESCRIPTION Superficial, often asymptomatic, form of gyrate erythema associated with some cases of rheumatic fever. Characterized by presence on the trunk and extensor surfaces of the extremities of a transient eruption of flat to slightly indurated, non-scaling multiple lesions. Usual course - acute.

CAUSES
• rheumatic fever

TREATMENT Treat underlying disease

ICD-9-CM
695.0 erythema marginatum

Ewing's sarcoma

DESCRIPTION Malignant tumor of bone arising in medullary tissue, occurring more often in cylindrical bones. Prominent symptoms include pain, fever and leukocytosis. Usual course - acute; relapsing probable.

CAUSES
• enchondroma
• aneurysmal bone cyst

TREATMENT
• cyclophosphamide
• possibly surgery
• megavoltage radiotherapy
• vincristine
• actinomycin D
• adriamycin

ICD-9-CM
170.9 malignant neoplasms of the bone

Fabry's disease

DESCRIPTION An x-linked lysosomal storage disease of glycosphingolipid catabolism. Usual course - progressive.

SYNONYMS
• glycosphingolipidosis
• angiokeratoma corporis diffusum
• ceramide trihexoside lipoidosis

CAUSES
• alpha-galactosidase a deficiency
• ceramide trihexosidase deficiency

TREATMENT
• analgesic
• phenytoin
• carbamazepine
• corticosteroid

ICD-9-CM
272.7 Fabry's disease

Factor IX deficiency

DESCRIPTION Deficiency of Factor IX, the plasma thromboplastin component of substances in the blood essential to the clotting process and hence to the maintenance of normal hemostasis. Usual course - intermittent.

SYNONYMS
- hemophilia B
- christmas disease

CAUSES
- factor IX deficiency
- inherited error of metabolism

TREATMENT
- fresh frozen plasma for mild hemorrhage
- factor IX plasma concentrate for severe hemorrhage

ICD-9-CM
286.1 congenital factor IX disorder

 Factor X deficiency

DESCRIPTION Deficiency of Factor X, a storage-stable factor essential to the clotting process that participates both in the intrinsic and extrinsic pathways of blood coagulation. Usually inherited as an autosomal recessive trait, though it can be acquired. It is characterized by defective activity in both the intrinsic and extrinsic pathways, impaired thromboplastin time, and impaired prothrombin consumption. Usual course - chronic; intermittent.

SYNONYMS
- Stuart-Prower factor deficiency

CAUSES
- inherited metabolic abnormality

TREATMENT
- fresh frozen plasma for hemorrhagic episodes

ICD-9-CM
286.3 congenital deficiency, factor X

 Familial Mediterranean fever

DESCRIPTION Hereditary disease transmitted in an autosomal recessive manner, usually occurring in Armenians and Sephardic Jews. Characteristics include short, recurrent attacks of fever with pain in the abdomen, chest, or joints and erythema resembling that seeen in erysipelas. It is sometimes complicated by amyloidosis. Usual course - intermittent.

SYNONYMS
- paroxysmal polyserositis
- familial recurrent polyserositis
- periodic fever
- periodic disease

CAUSES
- stress

TREATMENT
- colchicine

ICD-9-CM
277.3 familial mediterranean fever

 Familial neonatal hyperbilirubinemia

DESCRIPTION Transient familial form of hyperbilirubinemia with onset of jaundice within four days after birth. This form can lead to kernicterus.

SYNONYMS
- transient familial neonatal hyperbilirubinemia

TREATMENT
- exchange transfusion

ICD-9-CM
774.6 unspecified fetal and neonatal jaundice

 Fanconi's syndrome

DESCRIPTION A general term for a disorder marked by dysfunction of the proximal tubules of the kidney, with generalized hyperaminoaciduria, renal glycosuria, hyperphosphaturia, and water and bicarbonate loss. It occurs in genetic and acquired forms.

CAUSES
- multiple myeloma
- amyloidosis
- sjogren's syndrome
- nephrotic syndrome
- renal transplantation
- vitamin D deficiency
- lead
- mercury
- cadmium
- uranium
- strontium
- tetracycline
- maleic acid
- cystinosis
- wilson's disease
- galactosemia
- hereditary fructose intolerance
- tyrosinemia
- lowe's syndrome

TREATMENT

ICD-9-CM
270.0 fanconi syndrome

 Fascioliasis

DESCRIPTION Infection with a trematode worm found in the small intestines of residents in many parts of Asia. Intermediate hosts are snails. Characteristics include nausea, diarrhea, and malabsorption. Usual course - acute; chronic; progressive; 3 month incubation.

CAUSES
- fasciola hepatica

TREATMENT
- praziquantel

ICD-9-CM
121.3 fascioliasis

 Fasciolopsiasis

DESCRIPTION The state of being infected with flukes of the trematode worm genus Fasciolopsis. Characteristics - asymptomatic. Usual course - chronic; progressive. Endemic areas - Southern China; Southeast Asia; Indian subcontinent.

CAUSES
- fasciolopsis buski

TREATMENT
- praziquantel

ICD-9-CM
121.4 fasciolopsiasis

 Fatigue

Description A state of discomfort and decreased efficiency resulting from prolonged or excessive exertion or loss of power (from any cause) to respond appropriately to stimulation.
- Characteristics - closely related to approximately equal terms: Lassitude, tiredness, lethargy, malaise, and ennui

Synonyms N/A

Causes Drugs, overexertion, Addison's disease, alcohol, anemia, chronic fatigue syndrome (Epstein-Barr virus infection has unclear, possible association), diabetes mellitus, emotional problems (depression, somatization disorder), emphysema, endocarditis, environmental toxins, hepatitis, inadequate nutrition, inadequate rest, infectious mononucleosis, intestinal parasites, malignancies, myasthenia gravis, obesity, poor physical conditioning, rheumatoid arthritis, sedative-hypnotics, systemic lupus erythematosis, thyroid disease, tuberculosis, and others.

 Fatty liver due to pregnancy, acute

DESCRIPTION A serious complication of pregnancy that can lead to encephalopathy, bleeding and shock. Usual course - acute.

CAUSES
- unknown

TREATMENT
- delivery

ICD-9-CM
646.7 pregnancy complicated by fatty metamorphosis of liver

Favism

DESCRIPTION Hemolytic anemia due to the ingestion of fava beans or after inhalation of pollen from the Vicia fava plant by person with glucose-6-phosphate dehydrogenase deficient erythrocytes. Usual course - acute; chronic; intermittent; relapsing. Endemic areas - malarial endemic areas; worldwide.

CAUSES
• acute hemolysis
• fava bean ingestion
• vicia faba ingestion
• mediterranean type glucose-6-phosphate dehydrogenase deficiency

TREATMENT
• supportive
• transfusion
• folic acid
• maintain adequate urine output
• alkalinize urine

ICD-9-CM
282.2 favism

 Felty's syndrome

DESCRIPTION Chronic rheumatoid arthritis with leukopenia, splenomegaly, pigmented skin spots on the extremities, anemia, and thrombocytopenia. Usual course - chronic.

SYNONYMS
• rheumatoid arthritis-hypersplenism syndrome

CAUSES
• rheumatoid arthritis

TREATMENT
• splenectomy

ICD-9-CM
714.1 Felty's syndrome

 Filariasis

DESCRIPTION Infection with the filarial worm, Wuchereria bancrofti. The adult worms migrate to the lymphatic system producing recurrent lymphangitis with obstruction and fibrosis. Edema progresses to elephantiasis. Transmitted by mosquitoes, which harbor the larval forms. Usual course - chronic; relapsing; 8-12 month incubation. Endemic areas - Africa; Pacific islands; Southeast Asia; West Indies; Central America; eastern coastal plains of South America.

SYNONYMS
• bancroftian filariasis
• Malayan filariasis
• lymphatic filariasis
• Filarioidea infection

CAUSES
• adult filarial worms
• wuchereria bancrofti
• brugia malayi
• brugia timori
• lymphatic obstruction

TREATMENT
• diethylcarbamazine
• treat hypersensitivity to dying parasite
• aspirin
• antihistamine
• steroids

ICD-9-CM
125.9 filariasis, nos

 First degree AV block

DESCRIPTION P-R interval prolonged to greater than .20 seconds. Normal QRS complex.

SYNONYMS N/A

CAUSES Anterior or inferior myocardial infarction, hypothyroidism, digitalis toxicity, potassium imbalance

 Floppy infant syndrome

DESCRIPTION Congenital myopathy marked by hypotonia and muscle weakness

CAUSES
• CNS diseases, atonic diplegia, congenital cerebellar ataxia, kernicterus, chromosomal defects, oculocerebrorenal syndrome, cerebral lipidoses, Prader-Willi syndrome, spinal cord diseases, spinal cord trauma, Werdnig-Hoffmann disease, peripheral nerve diseases, polyneuritis, familial dysautonomia, congenital sensory neuropathy, neuromuscular junction diseases, myasthenia gravis, infantile botulism, muscle diseases, congenital muscular dystrophy, myotonic dystrophy, glycogen storage disease of muscle and heart, central core disease, nemaline myopathy, mitochondrial myopathies

TREATMENT

ICD-9-CM
781.9 other symptoms involving nervous and musculoskeletal systems

 Forbes-Albright syndrome

DESCRIPTION Galactorrhea-amenorrhea syndrome usually associated with a pituitary tumor. There is no relationship to pregnancy. Usual course - chronic; indolent.

SYNONYMS
• amenorrhea-galactorrhea syndrome
• nonpuerperal galactorrhea

CAUSES
• pituitary prolactinoma

TREATMENT
• bromocriptine
• surgery

ICD-9-CM
253.1 forbes-albright syndrome

 Formaldehyde poisoning

DESCRIPTION Unusual poisoning with formaldehyde due to occupational exposure. Toxic symptoms include gastrointestinal upsets, vascular collapse and coma. 60 mL of 40% formalin can cause fatality. Usual course - acute; chronic; progressive. Endemic areas - occupational exposure.

CAUSES
• cytotoxicity
• conversion to formic acid

TREATMENT
• activated charcoal
• supportive
• bicarbonate infusion
• avoid emetics
• avoid lavage

ICD-9-CM
989.8 formaldehyde poisoning

 Friedreich's ataxia

DESCRIPTION Antosomal recessive disease beginning in childhood or youth. Characteristics include sclerosis of the dorsal and lateral columns of the spinal cord. symptoms include ataxia, speech impairment, lateral curvature of the spinal column, peculiar swaying and irregular movements, and paralysis of the muscles of the lower extremities. Usual course - chronic; progressive.

SYNONYMS
• spinocerebellar ataxia
• familial ataxy
• Friedreich's ataxy
• familial ataxia
• hereditary ataxia of Friedreich
• hereditary spinal ataxia

CAUSES
• usually hereditary

TREATMENT
• NONE

ICD-9-CM
334.0 Friedreich's ataxia
334.2

 Gardner's syndrome

DESCRIPTION An autosomal dominant disorder characterized by familial polyposis of the large bowel, with supernumerary teeth, fibrous dysplasia of the skull, osteomas, fibromas and epithelial cysts. The polyps of the large bowel have malignant potential. Usual course - progressive.

CAUSES
• genetic

TREATMENT
• total colectomy

ICD-9-CM
NA

Gastroenteritis, viral

DESCRIPTION Acute inflammation of the lining of the stomach and intestines accompanied by fever and caused by any one of a number of viruses. Usual course - acute.

SYNONYMS
• acute infectious nonbacterial gastroenteritis
• epidemic diarrhea
• winter vomiting disease

CAUSES
• rotavirus
• adenovirus
• astrovirus
• norwalk-like agents
• coxsackievirus
• echovirus

TREATMENT
• fluid replacement
• bismuth subsalicylate

ICD-9-CM
008.8 viral gastroenteritis

 Gaucher's disease

DESCRIPTION Hereditary disorder of glucocerebroside metabolism, usually occurring in infancy, and characterized by mental retardation, bulbar palsy, opisthotonus and enlargement of the spleen and liver. Usual course - acute; progressive.

SYNONYMS
• cerebroside lipoidosis

CAUSES
• beta-glucosidase deficiency
• glucocerebroside accumulation

TREATMENT
• splenectomy for hemorrhage
• orthopedic immobilization
• bone marrow transplantation
• analgesics

ICD-9-CM
272.7 gaucher's disease

 Gestational trophoblastic neoplasm

DESCRIPTION A tumor usually arising in the uterus developing from hydatidiform mole,(50%), following abortion (24%), or during normal pregnancy (22%). Usual course - slow onset; curable. Endemic areas - Asia.

SYNONYMS
• choriocarcinoma
• chorioadenoma destruens
• hydatidiform mole

CAUSES
• increasing age

TREATMENT
• hydatidiform mole: removal of mole
• hysterectomy
• stage I: chemotherapy with optional hysterectomy
• stage II: chemotherapy with recommended hysterectomy
• stage III: combination chemotherapy with optional hysterectomy
• stage IV: combination chemotherapy with local radiotherapy plus optional surgery

ICD-9-CM
239.5 unspecified neoplasm of the placenta

 Giant hypertrophic gastritis

DESCRIPTION Excessive proliferation of the gastric mucosa, producing diffuse thickening of the stomach wall. Frequently associated with inflammatory changes. Usual course - chronic. The presence of diffuse carcinoma; diffuse lymphoma; Zollinger-Ellison syndrome nearly excludes this diagnosis.

SYNONYMS
• Menetrier's disease
• protein-losing gastroenteropathy

CAUSES
• idiopathic

TREATMENT
• observation
• H2-receptor blockers
• anticholinergic medications
• vagotomy
• antifibrinolytic medications
• partial gastrectomy

ICD-9-CM
535.2 hypertrophic gastritis

 Glioblastoma multiforme

DESCRIPTION Astrocytoma of grade III or IV. Characteristics include rapid growth, confinement to the cerebral hemispheres and cell types of a mixture of spongioblasts, astroblasts, and astrocytes. Headache, vomiting, and personality changes comprise prominent symptoms. Most likely in males ages 40-75 years. Usual course - progressive over months.

SYNONYMS
• grade 3 and 4 astrocytoma
• spongioblastoma multiforme

TREATMENT
• surgical excision plus radiotherapy plus chemotherapy

ICD-9-CM
191.9 malignant neoplasm of the brain, unspecified

 Glomerulonephritis, membranous

DESCRIPTION A disease of the glomerulus manifested clinically by proteinuria, and sometimes by other features of the nephrotic syndrome. Histologically characterized by deposits in the glomerular capillary wall between the epithelial cell and the basement membrane and a thickening of the membrane. Also characteristic are outward projections of the membrane between the epithelial deposits in the form of "spikes". There is some agreement that the deposits are antigen-antibody complexes. Usual course - progressive.

SYNONYMS
• membranous glomerulopathy
• membranous nephropathy
• extramembranous glomerulopathy
• idiopathic membranous glomerulonephritis
• idiopathic membranous nephropathy
• membranous glomerulonephropathy
• MGN

CAUSES
• idiopathic
• circulating antigen-antibody complexes

TREATMENT
• steroids
• cytotoxic drugs

ICD-9-CM
583.1 nephritis and nephropathy, not specified as acute or chronic, with lesion of membranous glomerulonephritis

 Glomerulonephritis, rapidly progressive

DESCRIPTION Acute glomerulonephritis marked by a rapid progression to end-stage renal failure and, histologically, by profuse epithelial proliferation. The principal signs are anuria, proteinuria, hematuria, and anemia. Usual course - progressive.

SYNONYMS
• extracapillary glomerulonephritis

CAUSES
• idiopathic

TREATMENT
• corticosteroids
• azathioprine
• cyclophosphamide
• anticoagulants
• plasmapheresis
• renal transplantation

ICD-9-CM
583.4 nephritis and nephropathy, not specified as acute or chronic, with lesion of rapidly progressive glomerulonephritis

 Glomerulopathy, membranous

DESCRIPTION A noninflammatory disease of the renal glomerulus. Characteristics - edema, hypertension, subendothelial immune deposits, thickened glomerular basement membrane.

SYNONYMS
• membranous nephropathy

CAUSES
• idiopathic
• drugs
• penicillamine
• gold
• captopril
• hepatitis B
• parasitic infestation
• SLE
• malignancy
• NSAID

TREATMENT
• corticosteroids
• anti-metabolites
• antiplatelet drugs
• anticoagulants

ICD-9-CM
583.1 nephritis and nephropathy, not specified as acute or chronic, with lesion of membranous glomerulonephritis

 Glossopharyngeal neuralgia

DESCRIPTION Rare disease of the 9th cranial nerve (glossopharyngeal). Characteristics - paroxysms of sharp, darting pain affecting the posterior pharynx, base of tongue, jaw.

SYNONYMS N/A

CAUSES Rare tumor (nasopharyngeal or other intracranial tumor), trauma, usually no known cause

Glucagonoma

DESCRIPTION Glucagon-secreting tumor of the pancreatic alpha cells characterized by a distinctive rash, weight loss, stomatitis, glossitis, diabetes, hypoaminoacidemia, and normochromic normocytic anemia. Usual course - progressive.

SYNONYMS
• alpha cell tumor
• alpha-cell adenoma

TREATMENT
• surgical enucleation to partial pancreatectomy
• fluorouracil plus streptozotocin for unresectable tumor

ICD-9-CM
235.5 neoplasm of the pancreas

 Goodpasture's syndrome, pulmonary component

DESCRIPTION Glomerulonephritis associated with pulmonary hemorrhage and circulating antibodies against basement membrane antigens. This condition exists most frequently in young men. It has a course of rapidly progressive renal failure with hemoptysis, pulmonary infiltrates, and dyspnea. Usual course - chronic.

TREATMENT
• corticosteroids
• cytotoxic agents
• plasmapheresis

ICD-9-CM
446.2 goodpasture's syndrome

 Goodpasture's syndrome, renal component

DESCRIPTION Glomerulonephritis occurring most often in young men accompanied by rapidly progressive renal failure. Other characteristics include hemotysis, dyspnea, and pulmonary infiltrates. Usual course - progressive.

CAUSES
• anti-glomerular basement membrane antibody

TREATMENT
• corticosteroids
• plasmapheresis
• cyclophosphamides
• renal transplantation

ICD-9-CM
446.2 goodpasture's syndrome

 Granuloma inguinale

DESCRIPTION Genital ulcers (not to be confused with lymphogranuloma inguinale) caused by Donovania granulomatis; also called donovanosis. Diagnosis is by demonstration of typical intracellular Donovan bodies in crushed-tissue smears. Usual course - acute; progressive; relapsing; indolent. Endemic areas - tropics; subtropics.

SYNONYMS
• donovanosis
• donovania
• granuloma venereum

CAUSES
• sexual transmission
• calymmatobacterium granulomatous
• fomites
• autoinoculation

TREATMENT
• antibiotics

ICD-9-CM
099.2 granuloma inguinale

 Granulomatous disease of childhood, chronic

DESCRIPTION A group of immunodeficiency of X-linked or autosomal recessive inheritance, caused by failure of the respiratory or metabolic burst resulting in deficient microbacidal activity. Characteristics - patients sustain frequent, severe, and prolonged bacterial and fungal infections. Usual course - chronic.

SYNONYMS
• congenital dysphagocytosis
• familial chronic granulomatosis
• septic progressive granulomatosis

CAUSES
• bacterial infection
• fungal infection
• defective phagocytic cell microbicidal activity
• abnormal oxidative metabolism during phagocytosis

TREATMENT
• antibiotics

ICD-9-CM
NA

 Graves' disease

DESCRIPTION Disorder of the thyroid of unknown but probably autoimmune etiology, occurring most often in women. Characteristics include thyrotoxicosis with diffuse goiter, exophthalmos, or pretibial myxedema or any combination of the three. See hyperthyroidism.

SYNONYMS
• exophthalmic goiter
• diffuse toxic goiter
• thyrotoxicosis
• Basedow's disease
• Parry's disease

CAUSES
• idiopathic
• autoimmune

TREATMENT
• subtotal thyroidectomy
• radioactive iodine
• propylthiouracil
• methimazole
• propranolol

ICD-9-CM
242.0 graves' disease

 Halitosis

DESCRIPTION Unpleasant odor to the breath. Characteristics - gastrointestinal disorders do not generally cause halitosis, so breath odor does not reflect the state of digestive system or bowel function

SYNONYMS N/A

CAUSES
• Inhaled substances
• Ingested substances
• Gingival disease
• Dental disease
• Food fermentation in mouth
• Systemic disease (tonsillitis, pneumonia, bronchiectasis, lung abscess)
• Hepatic encephalopathy
• Diabetic acidosis
• Infectious diseases
• Neoplastic disease of the respiratory tract
• Hypochondriasis

 Hallervorden-Spatz disease

DESCRIPTION Autosomal recessive hereditary disorder usually beginning in first or second decade. Characteristics include marked reduction in the number of myelin sheaths of the globus pallidus and substantia nigra, progressive rigidity in legs, dyarthria, choreoathetoid movements, and progressive mental degeneration. Usual course - chronic; progressive.

SYNONYMS
• pigmentary pallidal degeneration syndrome
• progressive pallidal degeneration syndrome
• late infantile neuroaxonal dystrophy

TREATMENT
• L-dopa
• tryptophan
• megavitamins

ICD-9-CM
333.0 hallervorden-spatz disease or syndrome

 Hand-foot-and-mouth disease

DESCRIPTION Usually mild and self-limited exanthematous eruption most often caused by Coxsackievirus. It occurs primary in preschool children. Characteristics include vesicles on the buccal mucosa, tongue, soft palate, gingivae, and hand and feet, including the palms and soles. Usual course - subacute; chronic; recurrent.

SYNONYMS: N/A

CAUSES
• coxsackie virus

TREATMENT

ICD-9-CM
074.3 hand, foot, and mouth disease

Hand-Schueller-Christian syndrome

DESCRIPTION Disseminated, chronic form of Langerhans-cell histiocytosis. May exhibit the classic triad of exophthalmos, diabetes insipidus and bone destruction. Usual course - chronic; remission.

SYNONYMS
• craniohypophyseal xanthoma
• idiopathic chronic xanthomatosis
• multifocal eosinophilic granuloma
• multifocal eosinophilic granuloma
• histiocytosis x
• Schueller-Christian Disease

CAUSES
• eosinophilic infiltration

TREATMENT
• chemotherapy
• access to free water

ICD-9-CM
277.8 hand-schueller-christian disease

 Hartnup disease

DESCRIPTION Familial syndrome characterized clinically by a pellagrous rash, cerebellar ataxia, and mental retardation and biochemically by the loss of renal tubular and intestinal transport of neutral amino acids. Usual course - intermittent

CAUSES
• abnormal intestinal amino acid transport
• abnormal renal tubular amino acid transport

TREATMENT
• nicotinamide
• high protein diet

ICD-9-CM
270.0 Hartnup disease

 Heat cramp

DESCRIPTION A form of heat exhaustion characterized by muscle spasm attended by pain, dilated pupils, and weak pulse. It occurs in people who lose much salt and water by working intensely in excessive heat. Usual course - acute; intermittent. Endemic areas: tropics; subtropics.

CAUSES
• electrolyte depletion

TREATMENT
• rest
• adequate salt replacement
• isotonic saline solution

ICD-9-CM
992.2 heat cramps

 Hemangioma of the liver

DESCRIPTION Benign tumor made of newly formed blood vessels resulting from malformation of angioblastic tissue of fetal life. Usual course - stable; usually asymptomatic.

SYNONYMS
• cavernous hemangioma of the liver
• cavernoma of the liver

TREATMENT
• none for small asymptomatic lesions
• surgical excision
• radiotherapy has been used for massive hemangiomas

ICD-9-CM
228.04 hemangioma of intraabdominal structures

 Hemiplegia, acute infantile

DESCRIPTION Hemiparesis, weakness, seizures present at or before birth, due to cerebral thrombosis. Numerous causes for cerebral thrombosis. Usual course - acute.

CAUSES
• cerebral artery embolism
• cerebral artery thrombosis
• vasculitis
• tonsillar infection
• cervical adenitis
• trauma
• arteriosclerosis
• fibromuscular hyperplasia
• sickle cell disease
• lupus
• polyarteritis nodosa
• cyanotic heart disease

TREATMENT
• treat underlying condition
• control seizures
• treat INCR intracranial pressure if present

ICD-9-CM
343.4 infantile hemiplegia

 Hemoglobin C disease

DESCRIPTION A disease characterized by compensated hemolysis with a normal hemoglobin level or a mild to moderate anemia. There may be intermittent abdominal discomfort, splenomegaly, and slight jaundice. Hereditary, autosomal recessive. Usual course - chronic.

CAUSES
• point mutation in hemoglobin beta gene

TREATMENT

ICD-9-CM
282.7 hemoglobin C disease

 Hemolytic anemias

DESCRIPTION A general term covering a large group of anemias in which there is a shortened life span of the red blood cells (normal = 120 days). Most hemolysis occurs extravascularly in the spleen, liver, and bone marrow.
• Characteristics - signs and symptoms include chills, fever, pain in the back and abdomen, prostration, shock, jaundice, splenomegaly, hemoglobinuria, hemosiderinuria, reticulocytosis
• Designations are as follows:
◊ Anemia, hemolytic, acquired autoimmune
◊ Anemia, hemolytic, acquired infectious
◊ Anemia, hemolytic acquired, physical, chemical agents
◊ Anemia, hemolytic elliptocytic
◊ Anemia, hemolytic, G-6-PD deficiency
◊ Anemia, hemolytic, hereditary nonspherocytic
◊ Anemia, hemolytic, microangiopathic
◊ Anemia, hemolytic, sickle cell
◊ Anemia, hemolytic, thalassemia major
◊ Anemia, hemolytic, thalassemia minor

SYNONYMS N/A

CAUSES
• G-6-PD deficiency
• Intrinsic abnormalities of red blood cell contents (hemoglobin or enzymes) or membrane
• Serum antibodies, trauma in circulation, infectious agents
• Temporary failure of red blood cell production
• Autoantibodies against red cell antigens, idiopathic or secondary to autoimmune diseases
• Drug-induced (penicillin type or methyldopa type)

 Hemosiderosis, pulmonary

DESCRIPTION Rare disease of unknown etiology. Must be distinguished from Goodpasture's syndrome and from lung hemorrhage in systemic lupus erythematosus.
• Characteristics - episodes of hemoptysis, hemorrhage into the lung, pulmonary infiltration, secondary iron deficiency anemia. Most common in children. Pathology shows diffuse infiltration with hemosiderin-containing macrophages. Death may occur from massive hemorrhage, although patients may live for several years with pulmonary fibrosis and insufficiency.

SYNONYMS N/A

CAUSES Unknown

 Hemothorax

DESCRIPTION A collection of blood in the pleural cavity. Characteristic signs and symptoms include chest pain, dyspnea, weakness, tachycardia, and asymmetrical chest movement. Usual course - acute.

CAUSES
• frank bleeding into pleural space
• penetrating chest trauma
• blunt chest trauma
• hematologic disorders

TREATMENT
• drainage by catheter
• thoracotomy if continuous serious bleeding

ICD-9-CM
511.8 hemothorax
860.2

Hepatic artery aneurysm

DESCRIPTION Aneurysmal dilatation of a portion of the hepatic artery. Characteristics - right upper quadrant pain, bruit in right upper quadrant, jaundice. Usual course - progressive.

CAUSES
• weakening of vessel wall by stone eliciting aneurysmal dilatation

TREATMENT
• surgery

ICD-9-CM
442.84 hepatic artery aneurysm

 Hepatic fibrosis, congenital

DESCRIPTION Developmental disorder of the liver characterized by irregular broad bands of fibrous tissue containing multiple cysts formed by disordered terminal bile ducts, chiefly in the portal areas, which leads to portal hypertension. Symptoms include splenomegaly, hepatomegaly, and gastrointestinal bleeding.

TREATMENT
• splenectomy
• splenorenal shunt

ICD-9-CM
571.5 cirrhosis of liver without mention of alcohol

 Hepatitis, alcoholic

DESCRIPTION An acute or chronic degenerative and inflammatory lesion of the liver in the alcoholic patient which is potentially progressive or reversible; it does not necessarily include steatosis, fibrosis, or cirrhosis of alcoholics, although it is frequently associated with these conditions. Usual course - acute; chronic.

SYNONYMS
• alcoholic steatonecrosis
• sclerosing hyaline necrosis

CAUSES
• alcoholism

TREATMENT
• well-balanced diet
• intravenous alimentation
• avoid alcohol

ICD-9-CM
571.1 acute alcoholic hepatitis

 Hepatorenal syndrome

DESCRIPTION Functional renal failure associated with cirrhosis and ascites or with obstructive jaundice. There are no pathological renal changes. Characteristics include low urinary sodium concentration and oliguria. The presence of prerenal azotemia; acute tubular necrosis nearly excludes this diagnosis.

SYNONYMS
• urohepatic syndrome
• Heyd's syndrome
• bile nephrosis

CAUSES
• severe liver disease
• hepatitis
• liver cirrhosis
• hepatic encephalopathy

TREATMENT
• fluid restriction

ICD-9-CM
572.4 hepatorenal syndrome

 Hereditary angioneurotic edema

DESCRIPTION Inherited C1 inhibitor deficiency. An autosomal dominant disorder characterized by recurrent episodes of edema of the skin, upper respiratory tract, and gastrointestinal tract. Frequently mediated by minor trauma, sudden changes in environmental temperature, and sudden emotional stress. Usual course - acute; intermittent; relapsing.

SYNONYMS
• hereditary angioedema

CAUSES
• No complement C1 esterase inhibitor

TREATMENT
• antifibrinolytic agent
• epsilon-aminocaproic acid

ICD-9-CM
277.6 hereditary angioneurotic edema

 Hereditary anhidrotic ectodermal dysplasia

DESCRIPTION A congital ectodermal defect that is x-linked recessive; autosomal recessive. Only males fully express the condition; female carriers may have mild symptoms in x-linked recessive form; both sexes are equally affected in the autosomal recessive form. Symptoms include heat intolerance, anhidrosis, hypotrichosis, facial anomalies, short stature, dry skin, no mammary glands, and mental retardation. Usual course - chronic.

SYNONYMS
• Christ-Siemens-Touraine syndrome
• Siemens syndrome

CAUSES
• defective ectodermal structures
• inherited disease

TREATMENT
• dental reconstruction

ICD-9-CM
757.31 congenital ectodermal dysplasia

 Hereditary hemorrhagic telangiectasia

DESCRIPTION Autosomal dominant vascular anomaly. Characteristics - multiple small telangiectases of the skin, mucous membranes, gastrointestinal tract and other organs; recurrent episodes of bleeding; gross or occult melena. Usual course - very slowly progressive.

SYNONYMS
• Osler-Weber-Rendu disease

TREATMENT
• symptomatic

ICD-9-CM
448.0 hereditary hemorrhagic telangiectasia

 Herpes simplex keratitis

DESCRIPTION Infection of the cornea with herpes simplex virus leading to chronic inflammation, vascularization, scarring, and loss of vision. Initial infection usually as a conjunctivitis with vesicular blepharitis. Recurrence may be dendritic keratitis or disciform keratitis.
• Characteristics - signs and symptoms include foreign body sensation, photophobia, lacrimation and conjunctival injection followed by corneal anesthesia or decreased response to pain

SYNONYMS N/A

CAUSES Herpes simplex virus

 Herpes zoster ophthalmic

DESCRIPTION Virus infection of the Gasserian ganglion and its nerve branches. Characteristics - pain, vesicular eruption with much lid swelling. Ocular involvement is usually heralded by a vesicle on the tip of the nose.

SYNONYMS N/A

CAUSES Reactivation of latent virus from dorsal root ganglia, Refsum's syndrome (hereditary mental deficiency and spastic paralysis), involvement of ophthalmic branch of trigeminal nerve, lymphoma

ICD-9-CM 053.2 herpes zoster with ophthalmic complications

Histiocytosis, pulmonary

DESCRIPTION A disorder of the mononuclear phagocyte system caused by tobacco smoking. Characteristics - cough, dyspnea, chest pain, weight loss. No known treatment except to stop smoking. Usual course - chronic; progressive in some cases.

SYNONYMS
- histiocytosis X
- pulmonary eosinophilic granuloma

CAUSES
- disorder of the mononuclear phagocyte system
- tobacco smoking

TREATMENT
- unknown

ICD-9-CM
277.8 histiocytosis X

 Hutchinson-Gilford syndrome

DESCRIPTION Premature old age. Characteristics - small stature; absence of facial and genital hair; wrinkled skin; gray hair; and appearance, manner, and attitude of old age. Usual course - progressive; fatal. Possibly autosomal recessive.

SYNONYMS
- childhood progeria
- premature senility syndrome

CAUSES
- unknown

TREATMENT
- NONE

ICD-9-CM
259.8 hutchinson-gilford syndrome

 Hyperbilirubinemia, physiologic neonatal

DESCRIPTION A mild, transient physiological hyperbilirubinemia of unconjugated type occurring in the normal neonate.

SYNONYMS
- icterus neonatorum
- hyperbilirubinemia in the newborn

CAUSES
- fetal hemolysis
- inadequate bilirubin conjugation
- prematurity

TREATMENT
- phototherapy

ICD-9-CM
774.6 transient neonatal jaundice

 Hyperhidrosis

DESCRIPTION Excessive perspiration due to over-activity of the sweat glands. Distribution - general or confined to palms, soles, axillas, inframammary region, groin. Symptoms include skin maceration, fissuring, scaling. A bad odor may be produced by decomposition of sweat and cellular debris resulting from yeast and bacteria infection.

SYNONYMS
- Xeroderma
- Dry skin

CAUSES Various skin diseases, such as pyogenic or fungal infections, contact dermatitis, fever, hyperthyroidism, central nervous system disorders, psychogenic

 Hyperprolactinemia

DESCRIPTION Elevated level of prolactin (one of the hormones of the anterior pituitary gland that normally stimulates and sustains lactation in postpartum mammals) - Characteristics - hyperprolactinemia leads to galactorrhea, hypogonadotropism, and hypogonadism. Any one of these requires investigation to rule out drug ingestion, primary hypothyroidism, and prolactinomas.

SYNONYMS N/A

CAUSES Bronchogenic carcinoma, chronic renal failure, drugs (phenothiazines, tricyclic antidepressants, haloperidol, metoclopramide, reserpine, methyldopa, oral contraceptives, thyroid releasing hormone), Hand-Schuller-Christian disease (histiocytosis X), herpes zoster, hypernephroma, hypoglycemia, hypothalamic tumors, idiopathic galactorrhea, neoplasms of the chest wall, post-encephalitis, postpartum, primary hypothyroidism, prolactin secreting pituitary tumors, pituitary stalk lesions, sarcoidosis, sexual intercourse, sleep, stress, surgical scars, trauma, pregnancy.

 Hyperthermia, malignant

DESCRIPTION Autosomal inherited condition occurring in patients undergoing general anesthesia. Characteristics - sudden, rapid temperature rise, tachycardia, tachypnea, sweating, cyanosis, muscle rigidity. Usual course - acute.

SYNONYMS
- fulminating hyperpyrexia
- malignant hyperpyrexia

CAUSES
- general anesthesia
- sukamethonium
- succinylcholine
- halothane
- duchenne muscular dystrophy

TREATMENT
- cooling
- cessation of anesthesia
- correct acidosis
- dantrolene
- mannitol

ICD-9-CM
995.89 hyperpyrexia, malignant, due to anesthetic

 Hyphema

DESCRIPTION Hemorrhage within the anterior chamber of the eye. Usual course - acute; recurrent.

CAUSES
- traumatized iris roof
- traumatized stromal vessels
- spontaneous bleeding

TREATMENT
- strict bed rest
- keep upright
- binocular patching
- mydriatics
- miotics
- antifibrinolytic agents
- surgery
- sedation
- ocular hypotensives

ICD-9-CM
364.41 hyphema of iris and ciliary body

 Hypocalcemia

DESCRIPTION Calcium level of 8.5 mg/dL or less (with a normal albumin) - Characteristics - symptoms include neuromuscular irritability, weakness, weight loss, diarrhea, abdominal cramping, bone pain, paresthesias, headache, seizures, dry skin. Signs include Chvostek's sign and Trousseau's sign.

SYNONYMS N/A

CAUSES Surgically induced hyperparathyroidism, Addison's disease, candidiasis, carcinoma of the thyroid, chronic liver disease, hyperphosphatemia, idiopathic, malabsorption, malnutrition, nephrosis, pancreatitis, pernicious anemia, pseudohypoparathyroidism, renal disease, rickets and osteomalacia

 Hypohidrotic ectodermal dysplasia syndrome

DESCRIPTION Inherited, ectodermal hypoplasia disorder characterized by decreased or no sweating, hairlessness, thin skin, anodontia, mental deficiency, hyperthermia. Usual course - chronic.

CAUSES
- ectodermal hypoplasia

TREATMENT
- cool climate
- water cooling
- dentures
- wig

ICD-9-CM
757.31 congenital ectodermal dysplasia

Hypophosphatasia

DESCRIPTION Genetic metabolic disorder resulting from serum and bone alkaline phosphatase deficiency leading to ethanolamine phosphaturia and ethanolamine phosphatemia. Clinical characteristics include severe skeletal defects resembling rickets, failure of the calvarium to calcify, dyspnea, cyanosis, and gastrointestinal symptoms, renal calcinosis, failure to thrive. Usual course - chronic; progressive.

SYNONYMS
- juvenile Paget's disease
- hyperostosis corticalis juvenilis deformans
- Rathbun's syndrome

CAUSES
- unknown

TREATMENT
- symptomatic
- sodium fluoride
- calcitonin
- corticosteroids

ICD-9-CM
275.3 hypophosphatasia

Hypoprothrombinemia

DESCRIPTION Deficiency of prothrombin (coagulation Factor II) in the blood. Characteristics - epistaxis, gingival bleeding, hematuria, melena, excessive bleeding with injury. Usual course - chronic.

SYNONYMS
- prothrombin deficiency
- factor II deficiency

CAUSES
- genetic deficiency
- vitamin K deficiency

TREATMENT
- fresh frozen plasma
- vitamin K

ICD-9-CM
286.3 hypoprothrombinemia

Hypovolemic shock

DESCRIPTION Shock resulting from insufficient blood volume for the maintenance of adequate cardiac output, blood pressure and tissue perfusion. Usually refers to shock caused by excessive fluid loss or acute hemorrhage.

CAUSES
- external hemorrhage
- vomiting
- diarrhea
- intestinal obstruction
- diabetes
- burns
- excessive sweating
- fractures
- ascites
- hemothorax
- hemoperitoneum

TREATMENT
- restoration of blood volume
- metabolic correction

ICD-9-CM
785.59 hypovolemic shock

Ichthyosis

DESCRIPTION A symptom in several rare hereditary syndromes - ichthyosis vulgaris; X-linked ichthyosis; lamellar ichthyosis (nonbullous congenital ichthyosiform erythroderma), epidermolytic hyperkeratosis (bullous congenital ichthyosiform erythroderma). Also occurs in several systemic disorders. Xeroderma, the mildest form is neither congenital nor associated with systemic disease. Characteristics - skin is dry, scaling, thick over widespread parts of the body.

SYNONYMS
- Xeroderma
- Dry skin

CAUSES Inherited, Refsum's syndrome (hereditary mental deficiency and spastic paralysis), Sjogren-Larrson syndrome, leprosy, hypothyroidism, AIDS

Treatment Skin lubricants

Icterohemorrhagic leptospirosis

DESCRIPTION A severe form of leptospirosis. Characterized by jaundice usually accompanied by azotemia, hemorrhages, anemia, continued fever, and disturbances of consciousness. Usual course - acute; biphasic.
Endemic areas: worldwide

SYNONYMS
- Weil's syndrome
- leptospiral jaundice
- spirochetal jaundice
- spirochaetosis icterohemorrhagica

CAUSES
- spirochetes of genus leptospira
- systemic infectious disease
- zoonosis
- contact with infected animal tissues
- contact with infected animal urine

TREATMENT
- supportive therapy
- antibiotics

ICD-9-CM
100.0 leptospirosis icterohemorrhagica

Idiopathic edema

DESCRIPTION Swellings of unknown cause affecting women, occurring intermittently over a period of years. Usually worse during premenstrual phase. Associated with increased aldosterone secretion. Usual course - intermittent; relapsing.

SYNONYMS
- cyclic edema
- periodic edema
- stress edema
- distress edema
- periodic swelling

CAUSES
- unknown
- abnormal albumin metabolism
- hormonal imbalance

TREATMENT
- DECR salt intake
- elastic stockings
- captopril
- bromocriptine
- diuretics

ICD-9-CM
782.3 edema

IgG heavy chain disease

DESCRIPTION A rare malignant neoplasm of lymphoplasmacytic cells consisting of monoclonal immunoglobulin heavy chains. Usual course - progressive; fatal.

SYNONYMS
- gamma chain disease
- franklin disease

CAUSES
- secretion of free gamma immunoglobulin chains

TREATMENT
- unresponsive to chemotherapy

ICD-9-CM
273.2 heavy chain disease

IgM heavy chain disease

DESCRIPTION Rarest heavy chain disease. Found in patients with chronic lymphocytic leukemia. Characteristics - hepatomegaly, splenomegaly. Usual course - slowly progressive.

SYNONYMS
- mu chain disease

CAUSES
- secretion of free mu chains

TREATMENT

ICD-9-CM
273.2 heavy chain disease

Insulinoma

DESCRIPTION Tumor of beta cells of islets of Langerhans, usually benign. An important cause of hypoglycemia. Usual course - progressive.

SYNONYMS
- insuloma
- nesidioblastoma
- beta cell tumor
- beta cell adenoma

TREATMENT
- surgical enucleation
- partial pancreatectomy
- fluorouracil plus streptozotocin for unresectable tumor
- pharmacologic palliation with diazoxide

ICD-9-CM
157.4 malignant neoplasm of the islets of langerhans

Interstitial keratitis

DESCRIPTION Chronic, non-ulcerative infiltration of the deep layers of the cornea, rare in the USA. Characteristics - signs and symptoms include photophobia, pain, lacrimation, gradual loss of vision.

SYNONYMS N/A

CAUSES Congenital or acquired syphilis; tuberculosis

 Intrahepatic cholestasis due to pregnancy

DESCRIPTION A benign disorder of pregnancy causing jaundice, pruritus, and hepatomegaly that clears upon delivery. Usual course - intermittent.

SYNONYMS
• cholestatic jaundice of pregnancy

CAUSES
• sensitivity to hormones normally produced in pregnancy

TREATMENT
• unnecessary
• cholestyramine for pruritus

ICD-9-CM
646.7 icterus gravis of pregnancy

 Iron intoxication, acute

DESCRIPTION Acute iron overload. Characteristics - vomiting, upper abdominal pain, pallor, cyanosis, diarrhea, drowsiness, shock. Usual course - acute.

SYNONYMS
• iron poisoning

CAUSES
• excessive iron ingestion

TREATMENT
• induce vomiting
• gastric lavage with sodium bicarbonate
• treat shock
• chelation with deferoxamine
• hemodialysis
• peritoneal dialysis
• exchange transfusion

ICD-9-CM
964.0 poisoning by iron and its compounds

 Jaundice

DESCRIPTION A descriptive term implying deposition of bile pigment in the skin and mucous membranes with resulting yellow appearance of the patient. Yellow skin and sclerae appear whenever bilirubin reaches 3 mg/mL. Characteristics - jaundice is usually brought about by hemolysis, virus infection, alcoholism, drugs, stones in the bile ducts, cancer of the pancreas or liver.

SYNONYMS N/A

 Jaundice, breast milk

DESCRIPTION Self-limited hyperbilirubinemia in a healthy vigorous neonate. Cause unknown. Usual course - progressive; self-limiting.

CAUSES
• unknown
• possibly maternal estrogen isomer interference with infant bilirubin conjugation

TREATMENT
• NONE
• interrupt nursing as diagnostic trial

ICD-9-CM
774.3 neonatal jaundice due to delayed conjugation from other causes

 Juvenile amaurotic familial idiocy

DESCRIPTION Neuronal ceroid lipofuscinosis. Characteristics - loss of vision, onset 5-10 years, death during late adolescence, atypical retinitis pigmentosa, cerebellar ataxia, dementia. Genetics - autosomal recessive. Usual course - progressive.

SYNONYMS
• Spielmayer-Sjogren chronic neuronal ceroid lipofuscinosis
• Spielmayer-Vogt disease
• Batten disease

CAUSES
• neuronal accumulation of ceroid
• neuronal accumulation of lipofuscin

TREATMENT
• rehabilitation as needed

ICD-9-CM
330.1 spielmayer-vogt disease

 Kala-azar

DESCRIPTION Classic form of visceral leishmaniasis. A chronic (fatal if untreated) infectious disease affecting the liver, spleen, bone marrow, lymph nodes and skin. Characteristics - hepatosplenomegaly, fever, chills, vomiting, emaciation, hypergammaglobulinemia. Transmission is by phlebotomus sandflies.

SYNONYMS
• visceral leishmaniasis
• black fever

CAUSES
• leishmania donovani
• phlebotomus sandflies

TREATMENT
• pentavalent antimonial
• amphotericin B
• pentamidine
• allopurinol
• transfusion
• sodium antimony gluconate
• meglumine antimoniate

ICD-9-CM
085.0 kala-azar

 Kartagener's syndrome

DESCRIPTION An inherited disorder involving a combination of situs inversus, bronchiectasis, and sinusitis. Genetics - familial; autosomal recessive; 1/70 persons of those involved are heterozygous. Usual course - chronic; variable onset.

SYNONYMS
• Kartagener triad

TREATMENT
• chest physiotherapy
• antibiotics
• bronchodilators

ICD-9-CM
759.3 Kartagener's syndrome

 Kearns-Sayre syndrome

DESCRIPTION Inherited disorder (autosomal dominant with onset before age 15). Characteristics - progressive ophthalmoplegia, pigmentary degeneration of the retina, ataxia, myopathy, cardiac conduction defect. Usual course - progressive; ophthalmic onset at ages 5-20; retinal onset at ages 8-40; cardiac onset at ages 10-40.

SYNONYMS
• oculocraniosomatic neuromuscular disease
• ragged red fiber disease
• ophthalmoplegia-plus
• hereditary external ophthalmoplegia

CAUSES
• unknown

TREATMENT
• folic acid
• coenzyme Q10
• pacemaker

ICD-9-CM
NA

Keratitis, superficial punctate

DESCRIPTION Loss of epithelium from the corneal surface of one or both eyes. Often associated with trachoma, staphylococcus blepharitis, conjunctivitis, or a respiratory tract infection.
• Characteristics - symptoms include photophobia, pain, lacrimation, diminished vision, conjunctival injection

SYNONYMS N/A

CAUSES ultraviolet light exposure, bacterial infection, viral infection

Kernicterus

DESCRIPTION A condition characterized by high levels of nonconjugated bilirubin in the blood with biliary pigmentation of certain nuclei in the brain and spinal cord and frequently resulting in cerebral palsy, mental retardation, and hearing deficit. It is commonly a sequel to icterus gravis neonatorum. Usual course - acute; progressive; chronic.

SYNONYMS
• bilirubin encephalopathy
• nuclear jaundice

CAUSES
• isoimmunization
• erythrocyte biochemical defects
• erythrocyte structural abnormalities
• infection
• sequestered blood

TREATMENT
• physical therapy

ICD-9-CM
773.4 kernicterus due to isoimmunization
774.7 kernicterus not due to isoimmunization

Klinefelter's syndrome

DESCRIPTION Congenital disorder. Characteristics - small testes, azoospermia, infertility, increased urinary excretion of gonadotropin, tall long legs, gynecomastia. Associated with an abnormality of the sex chromosomes. Usual course - chronic; manifestations begin at puberty.

SYNONYMS
• seminiferous tubule dysgenesis
• XXY syndrome

CAUSES
• congenital
• supernumerary X chromosome
• mosaicism
• advanced maternal age predisposes

TREATMENT
• mastectomy for disfiguring gynecomastia
• supplemental androgens for delayed secondary sexual characteristics
• supplemental androgens for impotence

ICD-9-CM
758.7 klinefelter's syndrome

Korsakoff's psychosis

DESCRIPTION Anterograde and retrograde amnesia with confabulation associated with alcoholic or nonalcoholic polyneuritis. Usual course - subacute; possibly acute; possibly chronic.

SYNONYMS
• korsakoff's amnesia
• alcohol amnestic syndrome

CAUSES
• alcoholism
• thiamine deficiency
• malnutrition

TREATMENT
• parenteral thiamine replacement
• vitamin supplementation

ICD-9-CM
291.1 korsakoff's psychosis

Krabbe leukodystrophy, infantile form

DESCRIPTION Lysosomal storage disease. Characteristics - begins in infancy, fretfulness, rigidity, followed by tonic seizures, convulsions, quadriplegia, deafness, progressive mental deterioration. Usual course - progressive.

SYNONYMS
• globoid cell leukodystrophy; Krabbe's disease
• Krabbe's brain leukodystrophy
• globoid cell brain sclerosis

CAUSES
• galactocerebrosidase deficiency

TREATMENT
• NONE

ICD-9-CM
330.0 leukodystrophy

Kuru

DESCRIPTION Progressive nervous system disorder of melanesian tribes of central New Guinea thought to be associated with cannibalism. Usual course - progressive.

CAUSES
• unknown
• slow virus of central nervous system

TREATMENT
• NONE

ICD-9-CM
046.0 kuru

Kwashiorkor

DESCRIPTION Syndrome produced by severe protein deficiency. Characteristics - retarded growth, skin and hair pigment changes, edema, liver pathology, mental apathy, pancreatic atrophy, gastrointestinal disorders, anemia, low serum albumin, dermatoses. Usual course - chronic; prolonged. Endemic areas - third world countries.

SYNONYMS
• protein-calorie malnutrition

CAUSES
• prolonged dietary malnutrition followed by acute stress

TREATMENT
• nutrient replacement
• proper nutrition

ICD-9-CM
260 kwashiorkor

Kyasanur forest disease

DESCRIPTION Severe hemorrhagic fever. Tick-borne arbovirus infection occurring in the Kyasanur Forest in India. Characteristics - fever, hemorrhagic manifestations and rash. Usual course - recurrent.

CAUSES
• ixodes
• haemaphysalis spinigera
• tick-borne flavivirus
• rodent hosts
• monkey hosts

TREATMENT
• symptomatic
• fluid replacement
• transfusion

ICD-9-CM
065.2 kyasanur forest disease

Lassa fever

DESCRIPTION Acute, possible fatal infectious disease occurring in West Africa. Characteristics - high fever, pharyngitis, vomiting, abdominal pain, dyspnea followed by hemorrhages and shock. Usual course - acute; gradual defervescence.

CAUSES
• lassa virus form of arenavirus found in excreta of wild rodents

TREATMENT
• supportive care
• fluid plus electrolyte therapy

ICD-9-CM
078.89 lassa fever

Lathyrism

DESCRIPTION A morbid condition resulting from eating leguminous plants (includes many kinds of peas). characteristics - spastic paraplegia, pain, hyperesthesia, paresthesia. Usual course - progressive. Endemic areas - Africa; Asia.

SYNONYMS
• neurolathyrism

CAUSES
• beta-aminopropionitrile ingestion
• sweet peas of species Lathyrus sativus

TREATMENT
• NONE

ICD-9-CM
988.2 lathyrism

Laurence-Moon-Biedl syndrome

DESCRIPTION A hereditary syndrome of childhood, transmitted as an autosomal recessive trait, with obesity, retinitis pigmentosa, mental retardation, polydactyly, and hypogonadism as the main features. Usual course - progressive.

SYNONYMS
• Laurence-Moon syndrome
• Bardet-Biedl syndrome

TREATMENT

ICD-9-CM
759.8 laurence-moon-biedl syndrome

Laxative abuse

DESCRIPTION The presence of fever; recurrent diarrhea; stool mucus; bloody stool; sigmoidoscopy: friable mucosa; fluoroscopy: abnormal distensibility; barium enema demonstrates rigid segments colon, fistula formation, longitudinal ulcerations. Usual course - chronic.

SYNONYMS
• cathartic colon

CAUSES
• irritant laxative abuse

TREATMENT
• discontinue laxative use
• treat constipation

ICD-9-CM
305.9 laxative habit

Left ventricular failure, acute

DESCRIPTION Left heart failure. Characteristics - dyspnea, cough, sense of suffocation, frothy sputum, cyanosis, rales, wheezing, tachycardia, Cheyne-Stokes respiration. Usual course - acute.

SYNONYMS
• ventricular failure
• left heart failure

CAUSES
• hypertension
• coronary artery disease
• incompetent mitral valve
• incompetent aortic valve
• myocardial infarction

TREATMENT
• diuretics
• vasodilators
• digitalis

ICD-9-CM
428.1 left heart failure

Leprosy, dimorphous

DESCRIPTION Slowly progressive chronic infectious disease. Characteristics - granulomatous or neurotrophic lesions in the skin, mucus membranes, nerves, bones, and viscera. Endemic areas - tropical regions; Mexico; India; Hawaii; USA Gulf Coast.

SYNONYMS
• borderline leprosy

CAUSES
• mycobacterium leprae
• human-to-human transmission via prolonged close contact
• variable cell-medicated immunity to mycobacterium leprae

TREATMENT
• combination antibiotic therapy for several years
• dapsone plus rifampin plus clofazimine
• other antibiotic combinations for resistant strains
• isolation unnecessary, walking casts, physical therapy, plastic surgery

ICD-9-CM
030.3 dimorphous leprosy

Leprosy, lepromatous

DESCRIPTION The most malignant and infectious polar type of leprosy. Characteristics - a chronic, progressive disorder with widespread dissemination of leprosy bacilli, cutaneous lesions, (papules, plaques, nodules) causing tissue destruction and deformities. Nerve involvement is seen in advanced disease. Endemic areas - tropical regions; Mexico; Hawaii; USA Gulf Coast.

SYNONYMS
• cutaneous leprosy
• nodular leprosy

CAUSES
• mycobacterium leprae
• human-to-human transmission via prolonged close contact
• impaired cell-mediated immunity to mycobacterium leprae

TREATMENT
• combination antibiotic therapy for many years
• dapsone plus rifampin plus clofazimine
• other antibiotic combinations for resistant strains
• isolation unnecessary, physical therapy, plastic surgery for facial disfigurement

ICD-9-CM
030.0 lepromatous leprosy

Leptospirosis

DESCRIPTION Infection by leptospira organisms transmitted to man from dogs, swine, and rodents or by contact with contaminated water. Characteristics - lymphocytic meningitis, hepatitis, nephritis. Weil's syndrome is severe leptospirosis with jaundice, bleeding and renal failure. Usual course - acute; abrupt; biphasic; relapsing. Endemic areas - Southern USA; tropics.

SYNONYMS
• autumnal fever
• Fort Bragg fever
• mud fever
• pea-picker's disease
• European swamp fever
• seven day fever
• wycon fever
• Bushy Creek fever
• cane field fever
• swineherd disease

CAUSES
• leptospira interrogans
• spirochete
• contact with infected animal tissues
• contact with infected animal excrement

TREATMENT
• antibiotics, supportive care, fluid replacement, electrolyte therapy, possibly steroids if hepatic coma

ICD-9-CM
100.9 leptospirosis, unspecified

Lesch-Nyhan syndrome

DESCRIPTION An X-linked disease caused by a deficiency of an enzyme of purine metabolism, hypoxanthine-guanine phosphoribosyl transferase, and characterized by physical and mental retardation, hyperuricemia, self-mutilation, and choreoathetosis.

SYNONYMS
• hypoxanthine-guanine phosphoribosyltransferase deficiency syndrome
• HG-PRT deficiency syndrome

CAUSES
• hypoxanthine-guanine phosphoribosyltransferase deficiency

TREATMENT
• sedation

ICD-9-CM
277.2 lesch-nyhan syndrome

Letterer-Siwe disease

DESCRIPTION Acute, disseminated, rapidly progressive form of Langerhans-cell histiocytosis. Genetics - Some familial predisposition. Characteristics include - hemorrhage tendency, eczematoid skin eruption, hepatosplenomegaly, progressive anemia, lymphadenopathy. Usual course - acute; fulminant; progressive; chronic.

SYNONYMS
• acute diffuse histiocytosis
• acute infantile reticuloendotheliosis
• acute reticulosis of infancy
• generalized histiocytosis
• non-lipid reticuloendotheliosis

CAUSES
• nonneoplastic proliferation of langerhans cells

TREATMENT
• irradiation, chemotherapy, steroids, vasopressin replacement, antibiotics

ICD-9-CM
202.50 letterer-siwe disease, unspecified site

Leukemia, acute monocytic

DESCRIPTION Leukemia in which the predominating leukocytes are identified as monocytes. Characteristics - fever, fatigue, bleeding, lymphadenopathy, hepatosplenomegaly, anemia. Usual course - acute; possibly relapsing.

SYNONYMS
- acute monocytoid leukemia
- monoblastic leukemia
- acute monoblastic leukemia

CAUSES
- chloramphenico, phenylbutazone, ionizing radiation, benzene, down's syndrome, alkylating agents

TREATMENT
- cytosine arabinoside
- daunorubicin
- 6-thioguanine

ICD-9-CM
206.0 monocytic leukemia, acute

Leukemia, acute myeloblastic

DESCRIPTION An acute nonlymphoblastic leukemia occurs at all ages and is the more common leukemia among adults. Usually associated with irradiation as a causative agent and occurring as a second malignancy following cancer chemotherapy. Characteristics - bleeding, pallor, fever, headaches, vomiting, weakness, lethargy, pallor, joint pain. Usual course - acute; progressive; relapsing.

SYNONYMS
- acute granulocytic leukemia
- acute myelocytic leukemia

CAUSES
- idiopathic
- retroviral infection
- ionizing radiation
- genetic defect
- chemical poisoning

TREATMENT
- chemotherapy
- immunotherapy
- bone marrow transplantation

ICD-9-CM
205.0 myeloid leukemia, acute

Leukemia, acute myelogenous

DESCRIPTION Leukemia arising from myeloid tissue in which the granular, polymorphonuclear leukocytes and their precursors predominate. Characteristics - fever, anorexia, bleeding, hepatosplenomegaly, anemia, lymphadenopathy. Usual course - acute; possibly relapsing.

CAUSES
- bloom's syndrome
- philadelphia chromosome
- chloramphenicol
- ionizing radiation
- benzene
- down's syndrome
- fanconi's syndrome
- phenylbutazone
- alkylating agents

TREATMENT
- cytosine arabinoside, daunorubicin, 6-thioguanine, prednisone, vincristine, intrathecal methotrexate, cranial radiotherapy

ICD-9-CM
205.0 myeloid leukemia, acute

Leukemia, chronic myelogenous

DESCRIPTION Clonal myoloproliferation caused by malignant transformation of a pluripotent cell. Characteristics - extraordinary overproduction of granulocytes. Usual course - slowly progressive.

SYNONYMS
- chronic granulocytic leukemia

CAUSES
- unknown
- possibly ionizing radiation

TREATMENT
- busulfan, allopurinol, leukophoresis, localized radiotherapy, vincristine, prednisone, cytosine arabinoside, doxorubicin

ICD-9-CM
205.1 myeloid leukemia, chronic.

Leukemia, hairy cell

DESCRIPTION A neoplastic disease of the lymphoreticular cells which is considered to be a rare type of chronic leukemia. It is characterized by an insidious onset, splenomegaly, anemia, granulocytopenia, thrombocytopenia, little or no lymphadenopathy, and the presence of "hairy" or "flagellated" cells in the blood and bone marrow. Usual course - chronic; progressive.

SYNONYMS
- leukemic reticuloendotheliosis

TREATMENT
- splenectomy
- interferon

ICD-9-CM
202.4 hairy-cell leukemia

Lichen sclerosis of the vulva

DESCRIPTION Thickened skin and accentuated markings affecting the vulva. Characteristics - external genital itching and pain. Usual course - chronic; progressive; may have spontaneous regression.

SYNONYMS
- lichen sclerosis et atrophicus
- lichen albus
- csillag's disease
- white spot disease
- circumscribed scleroderma

TREATMENT
- vitamin A ointment
- intralesional corticosteroids
- topical corticosteroids
- oral estrogen

ICD-9-CM
701.0 circumscribed scleroderma

Lipoid nephrosis

DESCRIPTION Nephrosis characterized by edema, albuminuria, changes in lipids and proteins in the blood, accumulation of globules of cholesterol esters in the tubular epithelium of the kidney.

SYNONYMS
- minimal change disease
- foot process disease
- nil disease
- minimal change nephropathy
- minimal change glomerulopathy

CAUSES
- loss of negative charge in glomerular capillary wall

TREATMENT
- steroids
- antibiotics
- cyclophosphamide
- chlorambucil

ICD-9-CM
581.3 lipoid nephrosis

Loiasis

DESCRIPTION A parasitic infection caused by the nematode Loa loa. The vector in the transmission of this infection is the horsefly (Tabanus) or the deerfly or mango fly (Chrysops). The larvae may be seen just beneath the skin or passing through the conjunctiva. Eye lesions are not uncommon. The disease is generally mild and painless. Usual course - chronic; progressive; 10-15 year incubation period. Endemic areas - West Africa; Central Africa.

SYNONYMS
- calabar swellings

CAUSES
- loa loa filaria

TREATMENT
- diethylcarbamazine

ICD-9-CM
125.2 loiasis

Ludwig's angina

DESCRIPTION Severe form of cellulitis affecting the submandibular, submental, and sublingual spaces. Characteristics - tongue elevation, difficult eating and swallowing, edema of the glottis, fever, tachypnea, and moderate leukocytosis. Usual course - acute.

CAUSES
- oral trauma
- aerobic infection of submandibular space
- anaerobic infection of submandibular space

TREATMENT
- broad-spectrum intravenous antibiotics
- maintain airway
- tracheostomy if necessary

ICD-9-CM
528.3 Ludwig's angina

Lupus nephritis

DESCRIPTION Glomerulonephritis associated with systemic lupus erythematosus. Characteristics - hematuria, a fulminant or chronic progressive course. Hypertension does not occur until late in the course of the disease. Usual course - relapsing; progressive.

SYNONYMS
• focal glomerulonephritis
• lupus glomerulonephritis

CAUSES
• SLE

TREATMENT
• steroids
• renal transplantation

ICD-9-CM
710.0 lupus nephritis

Lymphangitis

DESCRIPTION Inflammation of a lymphatic vessel or vessels. Characteristics - painful subcutaneous streaks along the course of the vessels. Usual course - acute; relapsing.

CAUSES
• beta-hemolytic streptococci
• staphylococcus

TREATMENT
• antibiotics
• drainage
• heat
• moisture

ICD-9-CM
457.2 lymphangitis

Lymphoma, non-Hodgkin's

DESCRIPTION Heterogenous group of malignant lymphomas with absence of giant Reed-Sternberg cells characteristic of Hodgkin's disease. Characteristics - widespread disease, painless enlargement of one or more peripheral lymph nodes. Usual course - progressive.

CAUSES
• malignant tumors of lymphoid tissues with the exception of hodgkin's disease

TREATMENT
• radiotherapy
• chemotherapy

ICD-9-CM
202.8 non-hodgkin's lymphoma, nos

Lymphoma, pulmonary

DESCRIPTION Malignant disease of the lung. Characteristics - cough, weight loss, chest pain. Usual course - progressive.

CAUSES
• tumor of the immune system
• hodgkin's lymphoma
• lymphocytic lymphoma

TREATMENT
• radiotherapy
• chemotherapy

ICD-9-CM
202.8 malignant lymphoma, nos

Macular degeneration

DESCRIPTION Atrophy or degeneration of the macular disk, a leading cause of visual diminution in the elderly. Despite being legally blind, good peripheral and color vision survive.

SYNONYMS Senile macular degeneration

CAUSES Unknown. More common in whites than in African-Americans

Magnesium deficiency syndrome

DESCRIPTION Abnormally low magnesium content of the blood plasma. Characteristics - neuromuscular hyperirritability. Usual course - progressive; acute; relapsing.

SYNONYMS
• hypomagnesemia

CAUSES
• dietary deficiency
• DECR absorption
• INCR excretion
• alcoholism
• uremia
• diuretics
• parathyroid disease
• eclampsia

TREATMENT
• magnesium

ICD-9-CM
275.2 magnesium deficiency

Mallory-Weiss syndrome

DESCRIPTION Mucosal tears usually linear and confined to the esophagogastric junction but may be located in the fundus of the stomach or in the distal esophagus. Upper gastrointestinal bleeding from these lacerations is often precipitated by retching or vomiting. Usual course - acute.

SYNONYMS
• gastroesophageal laceration-hemorrhage syndrome

CAUSES
• retching after alcoholic bout
• hiatus hernia
• atrophic gastritis
• esophagitis
• straining at stool

TREATMENT
• vasopressin
• gastrotomy with sutures

ICD-9-CM
530.7 mallory-weiss syndrome

Maple bark stripper's disease

DESCRIPTION Granulomatous, interstitial pneumonitis caused by a mold found under the bark of maple logs. Usual course - acute; relapsing.

SYNONYMS
• maple bark stripper's pneumonitis
• maple bark stripper's granulomatosis

CAUSES
• hypersensitivity reaction to spores of cryptostroma corticale

TREATMENT
• eliminate etiological agent

ICD-9-CM
495.6 maple bark-strippers' lung

Maple syrup urine disease

DESCRIPTION Familial cerebral degenerative disease caused by a defect in branched chain amino acid metabolism and characterized by severe mental and motor retardation and urine with a maple-syrup-like odor. Usual course - progressive.

SYNONYMS
• branched chain ketoaciduria

CAUSES
• deficiency of branched chain alpha-ketoacid decarboxylase

TREATMENT

ICD-9-CM
270.3 maple syrup urine disease

Marburg virus disease

DESCRIPTION Severe, acute often fatal viral hemorrhagic fever. Characteristics - prostration, fever, pancreatitis, hepatitis. The Marburg virus first infected laboratory workers handling infected African green monkeys. Usual course - acute. Endemic areas: Germany; Yugoslavia; Africa.

SYNONYMS
• green monkey virus disease

CAUSES
• Marburg virus

TREATMENT
• isolation
• treat dehydration
• nasogastric suction
• heparin

ICD-9-CM
078.89 marburg virus disease

 Marchiafava-Bignami syndrome

DESCRIPTION Progressive degeneration of the corpus callosum. Characteristics - progressive intellectual degeneration, confusion, hallucinations, tremor, rigidity, and convulsions. Usual course - chronic; progressive.

SYNONYMS
• marchiafava disease
• callosal demyelinating encephalopathy

CAUSES
• chronic alcoholism
• addiction to crude red wine

TREATMENT
• avoid alcohol

ICD-9-CM
341.8 marchiafava-bignami disease or syndrome

 Meckel's diverticulum

DESCRIPTION Sacculation or appendage of the ileum derived from an unobliterated yolk stalk. Symptoms of infection may resemble those of appendicitis. Usual course - acute; intermittent; chronic.

CAUSES
• vestigial remnant of omphalomesenteric duct

TREATMENT
• surgery

ICD-9-CM
751.0 Meckel's diverticulum

 Meigs' syndrome

DESCRIPTION Ascites and hydrothorax associated with ovarian fibroma or other pelvic tumors. Usual course - acute; relapsing.

SYNONYMS
• ovarian ascites-pleural effusion syndrome
• Demons-Meigs syndrome
• Meigs-Coss syndrome

CAUSES
• benign fibroma
• ovarian tumor
• movement of the ascitic fluid across the diaphragm

TREATMENT
• tumor excision

ICD-9-CM
789.5 ascites

 Melanoma, lentigo maligna

DESCRIPTION A cutaneous lesion that is the slowest growing malignant melanoma and has the least tendency to metastasize. Other characteristics: occurs most often on the face, begins as a circumscribed macular patch of mottled pigmentation showing shades of dark brown, tan, or black. Usual course: insidious onset; progressive.

SYNONYMS
• melanoma of the skin

CAUSES
• hutchinson's freckle
• lentigo maligna

TREATMENT
• local excision
• radiotherapy

ICD-9-CM
172.9 malignant melanoma of skin, site unspecified

 Melanoma, ocular

DESCRIPTION A malignant progressive lesion of the eye. Usual course: chronic; progressive.

SYNONYMS
• intraocular melanoma

CAUSES
• nickel subsulfide
• platinum
• methylcholanthrene
• ethionine
• N-2-fluorenylacetamide
• radium

TREATMENT
• local excision
• enucleation
• proton beam radiotherapy
• brachytherapy
• photocoagulation

ICD-9-CM
190.9 malignant neoplasm of the eye

 Meningioma

DESCRIPTION Hard, slow growing, vascular tumor arising along the meningeal vessels and superior longitudinal sinus. It invades the dura and skull and leads to thinning and erosion of the skull. Usual course - progressive; surgical cure.

SYNONYMS
• arachnoidal fibroblastoma
• leptomeningioma
• dural endothelioma
• meningeal fibroblastoma

TREATMENT
• surgical excision
• radiotherapy for incomplete removal
• radiotherapy for recurrence

ICD-9-CM
225.2; 225.4 benign neoplasm of meninges

 Meningococcemia

DESCRIPTION Invasion of the blood stream by meningococci. Usual course - acute.

CAUSES
• neisseria meningitidis

TREATMENT
• antimicrobials
• supportive therapy
• chemoprophylaxis

ICD-9-CM
036.2 meningococcemia

 Mesenteric adenitis, acute

DESCRIPTION Inflammation of lymph glands located in the mesentery. It causes a clinical picture at times that is difficult to differentiate from acute appendicitis.

SYNONYMS
• acute mesenteric lymphadenitis

CAUSES
• yersinia enterocolitica
• yersinia pseudotuberculosis
• streptococcus viridans
• giardia lamblia
• staphylococcus aureus

TREATMENT
• antibiotics

ICD-9-CM
289.2 acute mesenteric lymphadenitis

Metachromatic leukodystrophy, late infantile form

DESCRIPTION A form of leukoencephalopathy transmitted autosomal recessive. Characteristics - accumulation of sphingolipid in neural and non-neural tissues with a diffuse loss of myelin in the central nervous system. The infantile form begins in the second year of life with blindness, motor disturbances, mental deterioration. Usual course - progressive.

SYNONYMS
- metachromatic brain leukodystrophy
- metachromatic leukoencephalopathy
- sulfatidosis
- greenfield disease
- arylsulfatase A deficiency

CAUSES
- arylsulfatase A deficiency

TREATMENT
- NONE

ICD-9-CM
330.0 leukodystrophy

Metastatic neoplasm of the liver

DESCRIPTION Progressive form of hepatic cancer that has metastasized from malignancies arising primarily from other locations. Usual course - progressive.

CAUSES
- colon metastases
- rectal metastases
- gastric metastases
- pancreatic metastases
- breast metastases

TREATMENT
- palliative chemotherapy
- palliative radiotherapy
- surgical resection in rare cases

ICD-9-CM
197.7 secondary malignant neoplasm to the liver

Milker's nodules

DESCRIPTION A disease caused by paravaccinia virus, transmitted to humans during milking. Characteristics - purple nodules on fingers or adjacent areas. Lesions break down and crust and heal without scarring. It can be retransmitted to uninfected cows. Usual course - acute; relapsing. Endemic areas - dairy farms.

SYNONYMS
- pseudocowpox
- paravaccinia

CAUSES
- paravaccinia virus of poxviridae family
- transmitted through direct contact
- cutaneous disease of cow teats
- oral lesions in suckling calves

TREATMENT
- NONE

ICD-9-CM
051.9 paravaccinia, nos

Millard-Gubler syndrome

DESCRIPTION Paralysis caused by infarction of the pons involving the 6th and 7th cranial nerves and fibers of the corticospinal tract. Characteristics - crossed paralysis affecting the limbs on one side of the body and the face on the opposite side. Additionally, paralysis of outward movement of the eye. Usual course - acute; chronic; progressive.

SYNONYMS
- alternating inferior hemiplegia
- gubler paralysis
- abducens-facial syndrome

CAUSES
- basal pontine infarction
- basal pontine tumor

TREATMENT
- supportive plus rehabilitative
- treat underlying cause of infarction

ICD-9-CM
344.8 millard-gubler syndrome

Mitral regurgitation due to papillary muscle dysfunction

DESCRIPTION Retrograde blood flow from the left ventricle in the left atrium through an incompetent mitral valve. Characteristics - fatigue, orthopnea, systolic murmur, left ventricular hypertrophy, S3 gallop. Usual course: chronic; progressive; acute (after myocardial infarction).

CAUSES
- coronary artery disease
- infiltrative diseases
- cardiac tumors

TREATMENT
- dental endocarditis prophylaxis
- surgical endocarditis prophylaxis
- nitrates
- calcium channel blockers
- diuretics
- digitalis
- inotropic agents
- afterload reducing agents
- mitral valve replacement

ICD-9-CM
394.9 other and unspecified mitral valve diseases

Mitral regurgitation due to rheumatic fever

DESCRIPTION Retrograde blood flow from the left ventricle into the left atrium through an incompetent mitral valve. Characteristics - history of rheumatic fever, fatigue, dyspnea, holosystolic murmur, left ventricular hypertrophy. Usual course - chronic; progressive disability.

CAUSES
- autoimmune cross reaction between streptococcal antigens and heart tissue

TREATMENT
- medical endocarditis prophylaxis
- dental endocarditis prophylaxis
- surgical endocarditis prophylaxis
- afterload reducing agents
- nitrates
- calcium channel blockers
- digitalis
- diuretics
- mitral valve replacement

ICD-9-CM
394.1 rheumatic mitral insufficiency

Munchausen's syndrome

DESCRIPTION A chronic disorder characterized by habitual presentation for medical care. Often requires hospitalization. The patient gives a plausible and dramatic history, all of which is factitious.

SYNONYMS
- chronic factitious disorder with physical symptoms
- hospital-addiction syndrome

CAUSES
- factitious
- No external incentives

TREATMENT
- psychotherapy
- behavior modification techniques

ICD-9-CM
301.51 munchausen syndrome

Mushroom poisoning, Amanita phalloides

DESCRIPTION Characteristics include: nausea, vomiting, abdominal pain, diarrhea, followed by a period of improvement up to 48 hours. Then culminating in severe renal, hepatic, and central nervous system damage. Usual course - progressive. Endemic areas - Western USA; Europe.

CAUSES
- cyclic octapeptide amatoxin
- hepatic cytotoxicity by interference with RNA polymerase
- renal cytotoxicity by interference with RNA polymerase

TREATMENT
- intragastric activated charcoal
- intensive supportive care
- charcoal hemoperfusion
- thiotic (alpha-lipoic acid)

ICD-9-CM
988.1 toxic effect of mushrooms eaten as food

Mushroom-worker's disease

DESCRIPTION Allergic respiratory disease, resembling farmer's lung, developing in persons working with moldy compost prepared for growing mushrooms. Characteristics - fever, dyspnea, dry cough, chills, malaise, myalgia, tachypnea. Usual course - acute; chronic; intermittent; progressive; relapsing.

SYNONYMS
- pulmonary granulomatosis of mushroom pickers

CAUSES
- immunological reaction to inhaled antigens
- micropolyspora faeni
- thermoactinomyces vulgaris

TREATMENT
- corticosteroids
- eliminate etiological agent

ICD-9-CM
495.5 mushroom workers' lung

Mussel poisoning

DESCRIPTION Food poisoning due to ingestion of toxin from dinoflagellate Gonyaulax. Characteristics - dysesthesias of tongue, lips, fingertips, dysphagia, abdominal cramps, ascending weakness, seizures. Usual course - acute; progressive. Endemic areas - Mid-Pacific coast from May to October; Northeastern seaboard; Western European coast.

SYNONYMS
• mytilotoxism
• paralytic shellfish poisoning

CAUSES
• alkaloid saxitoxin of dinoflagellate gonyaulax catanella
• alkaloid saxitoxin of dinoflagellate gonyaulax tamarensis
• neuromuscular blockade by preventing depolarization
• aerosolized ingestion has been reported

TREATMENT
• emergent gastrointestinal decontamination
• supportive
• mechanical ventilation

ICD-9-CM
988.0 toxic effect of fish and shellfish eaten as food

Myiasis

DESCRIPTION The invasion of living tissues of man and other mammals by dipterous larvae (fly maggots). Usual course - acute. Endemic areas - tropical America; Africa; South America; Mexico; California.

SYNONYMS
• maggot infestation

CAUSES
• ingestion of fly eggs
• eggs deposited in open wounds

TREATMENT
• surgery
• local anesthesia
• mineral oil
• ether bath

ICD-9-CM
134.0 myiasis

Myxedema heart disease

DESCRIPTION Heart disease associated with primary hypothyroidism. Usual course - acute; progressive.

CAUSES
• DECR thyroid hormone
• congenital developmental defect
• idiopathic
• postablative
• postradiation
• iodine deficiency

TREATMENT
• thyroid hormone replacement

ICD-9-CM
244.9 myxedema

Necrobiosis lipoidica diabeticorum

DESCRIPTION Degenerative disease of dermal connective tissue. Characteristics - erythematous papules or nodules in the pretibial area that extend to form waxy, yellowish red plaques covered with telangiectatic vessels. The plaques have a red-violet border and depressed atrophic center. Usual course - chronic.

SYNONYMS
• oppenheim-urbach disease

CAUSES
• unknown

TREATMENT
• triamcinolone acetonide

ICD-9-CM
250.8 necrobiosis lipoidica diabeticorum
709.3

Nephropathy, analgesic

DESCRIPTION Kidney damage due to massive intake of analgesics, particularly phenacetin. Usual course - chronic.

CAUSES
• phenacetin
• aspirin
• acetaminophen

TREATMENT
• cessation of analgesic use

ICD-9-CM
965 poisoning by analgesics, antipyretics, and antirheumatics

Nephropathy, chronic lead

DESCRIPTION Kidney damage due to lead poisoning. Particularly present in Queensland, Australia. Usual course - chronic.

SYNONYMS
• lead related hyperuricemia
• hyperuricemic nephropathy
• saturnine gout

CAUSES
• lead poisoning
• lead paint ingestion
• lead vapor inhalation
• moonshine alcohol

TREATMENT
• EDTA

ICD-9-CM
984 toxic effect of lead and its compounds (including fumes)

Nephrosclerosis

DESCRIPTION Hardening of the kidney due to overgrowth and contraction of interstitial connective tissue. Characteristics - edema, headache, hypertension, retinal hemorrhages. Usual course - chronic; progressive.

CAUSES
• unknown
• essential hypertension
• diabetes

TREATMENT
• antihypertensive medication

ICD-9-CM
403.9 nephrosclerosis

Neuritis/neuralgia

DESCRIPTION Degeneration of peripheral nerves
• Characteristics - insidious onset, muscle weakness with sensory loss, muscle atrophy, decreased tendon reflexes, paresthesias, hyperesthesias in hands and feet. Electromyography shows delayed action potential.

SYNONYMS
• Multiple neuritis
• Peripheral neuropathy
• Polyneuritis

CAUSES
◊ Chronic intoxication (alcohol, arsenic, lead, other drugs)
◊ Infections
◊ Metabolic and inflammatory (diabetes) gout, rheumatoid arthritis, systemic lupus erythematosus
◊ Nutritive (vitamin deficiencies, cachexia)

Treatment
◊ Supportive
◊ Physical therapy
◊ Analgesics
◊ Treat underlying specific disorders if possible
◊ Drugs - amitriptyline, carbamazepine, phenytoin (uneven and unpredictable response, but helpful for some)

Neutropenia, autoimmune

DESCRIPTION Decreased number of neutrophilic leukocytes in the blood due to an autoimmune mechanism. Usual course - acute; chronic; intermittent; progressive; relapsing.

CAUSES
• antineutrophil antibodies

TREATMENT
• antibiotics
• prednisone
• splenectomy
• supportive

ICD-9-CM
NA

Neutropenia, chronic idiopathic

DESCRIPTION An autosomal dominant, familial disorder with a chronic decrease in number of neutrophilic granulocytes. Characteristics - repeated non-life-threatening infections of skin, oral cavity, and sometimes upper respiratory tract. Usual course - chronic; relapsing.

SYNONYMS
• chronic benign neutropenia

CAUSES
• abnormal homeostasis of mitosis of granulocyte precursors

TREATMENT
• symptomatic

ICD-9-CM
NA

 Neutropenia, cyclic

DESCRIPTION Autosomal dominant disorder of children and young adults characterized by cyclical neutropenia, producing fever, malaise, mouth ulcers and cervical lymphadenopathy. Usual course - relapsing; 21-day cycles.

SYNONYMS
• cyclic agranulocytosis
• periodic neutropenia
• cyclic leukopenia
• periodic myelocytic dysplasia

CAUSES
• defective regulation of hematopoietic cell proliferation

TREATMENT
• glucocorticoids
• androgens
• splenectomy
• antibiotics

ICD-9-CM
288.0 agranulocytosis

 Nevus of ota

DESCRIPTION A macular lesion on the side of the face (usually lifelong and unilateral), involving the conjunctiva and lids, as well as the adjacent facial skin, sclera, ocular muscles, and periosteum. Histological features vary from those of a mongolian spot to those of a blue nevus. Usual course - chronic.

SYNONYMS
• oculodermal melanocytosis
• nevus fusco-caeruleus ophthalmo-maxillaris

CAUSES
• unknown

TREATMENT
• cosmetic cover up

ICD-9-CM
NA

 Niemann-Pick disease

DESCRIPTION Sphingolipidosis due to sphingomyelinase deficiency with sphingomyelin accumulation in the reticuloendothelial system. There are 5 types (A, B, C, D, and E) with differing ages of onset and differing amounts of CNS involvement and sphingomyelinase activity. Genetics - autosomal recessive. Usual course - acute; chronic; progressive.

SYNONYMS
• sphingomyelin lipidosis
• sphingomyelinase deficiency

CAUSES
• sphingomyelinase deficiency

TREATMENT
• supportive
• splenectomy
• bone marrow transplantation

ICD-9-CM
272.7 niemann-pick disease

 Nitrobenzene poisoning

DESCRIPTION Poisoning due to excessive exposure to nitrobenzene, a benzene derivative used in the manufacture of aniline. Complete recovery from pathologic changes can be expected if survival greater than 24 hours.

SYNONYMS
• nitrobenzol toxicity
• oil of mirbane toxicity

CAUSES
• direct mucous membrane irritation
• methemoglobin formation

TREATMENT
• cutaneous plus gastric decontamination
• oxygen
• 1% methylene blue
• exchange transfusion
• hemodialysis

ICD-9-CM
983.0 poisoning, nitrobenzene

 Osteochondritis dissecans

DESCRIPTION A type of osteochondritis in which articular cartilage and associated bone becomes partially or totally detached to form joint loose bodies. Affects mainly the knee, ankle, and elbow joints. Usual course - progressive. There is some genetic predisposition.

CAUSES
• trauma
• vascular occlusion with insufficient collateral circulation

TREATMENT
• surgery

ICD-9-CM
732.7 osteochondritis dissecans

 Osteopetrosis

DESCRIPTION Excessive formation of dense trabecular bone leading to pathological fractures, osteitis, splenomegaly with infarct, anemia and extramedullary hemopoiesis. Genetics: malignant form: autosomal recessive; benign form: autosomal dominant. Usual course - progressive; chronic.

SYNONYMS
• marble bone disease
• Albers-Schonberg disease
• osteosclerosis fragilis generalisata

CAUSES
• replacement of marrow space with bone
• No carbonic anhydrase II in erythrocytes
• defective osteoclast function

TREATMENT
• bone marrow transplantation
• calcitriol

ICD-9-CM
756.52 osteopetrosis

 Ovarian mucinous cystadenocarcinoma

DESCRIPTION Carcinoma and cystadenoma of the ovary. Characteristics — multilocular tumor produced by the epithelial cells of the ovary having mucin-filled cavities. Symptoms include abdominal pain and distention, menstrual disturbances, weight loss, dyspareunia, ascites. Clinical findings are the same as those with ovarian serous cystadenocarcinoma.

SYNONYMS
• pseudomucinous ovarian cystadenocarcinoma

TREATMENT
• hysterectomy
• stage I: bilateral salpingo-oophorectomy plus omentectomy if high grade
• stage II: add radiotherapy or chemotherapy
• stage III: surgical debulking

ICD-9-CM
183.0 malignant neoplasm of ovary

 Paralysis of the recurrent laryngeal nerve

DESCRIPTION Paralysis may be unilateral or bilateral with many possible underlying causes. Characteristics — dysphagia, stridor, dyspnea, and aphonia. Usual course: acute; insidious.

CAUSES
• innominate artery aneurysm
• right subclavian artery aneurysm
• neck surgery
• thyroid goiter
• trauma
• aortic aneurysm
• left atrial enlargement
• laryngeal tuberculosis

TREATMENT
• treat underlying condition

ICD-9-CM
478.31 partial unilateral paralysis of vocal cords

Parapsoriasis

DESCRIPTION A group of slowly evolving erythrodermas. common characteristics: chronicity, resistance to treatment. The group includes chronic and acute lichenoid pityriasis and large and small plaque parapsoriasis. Usual course - chronic; relapsing; benign forms; premalignant forms.

SYNONYMS
• maculopapular erythroderma

TREATMENT

ICD-9-CM
696.2 parapsoriasis

Paratyphoid

DESCRIPTION An infection due to any of the salmonella serotypes except S. typhi and salmonellosis. Characteristics — prolonged febrile illness less severe than typhoid fever, frequently follows an attack of salmonella food poisoning.

SYNONYMS
• paratyphoid fever
• enteric fever

CAUSES
• salmonella paratyphi A
• salmonella paratyphi B
• salmonella paratyphi C
• salmonella sendai
• enteric pathogens

TREATMENT
• fluid replacement
• antibiotics in elderly at greatest risk
• antibiotics in infants at greatest risk

ICD-9-CM
002.9 paratyphoid fever, nos

Paroxysmal atrial tachycardia

DESCRIPTION Heart rate greater than 140 beats per minute. May increase up to 250. P waves regular but aberrant. Onset may be sudden. Symptoms include light-headedness and palpitations.

SYNONYMS
• Premature atrial tachycardia
• Paroxysmal supraventricular tachycardia

CAUSES Abnormal AV conduction system. Physical or psychological stress, hypokalemia, hypoxia, caffeine, marijuana, digitalis toxicity, sympathomimetics

Paroxysmal cold hemoglobinuria

DESCRIPTION A rare disease in which blood hemolyzes minutes to hours after exposure to cold (atmospheric, drinking cold water, handwashing in cold water). Usually occurs following a non-specific viral type illness. Usual course - acute; progressive; relapsing.

SYNONYMS
• Donath-Landsteiner hemolytic anemia
• Dressler syndrome
• Harley syndrome

CAUSES
• immune-mediated hemolysis upon rewarming after cold exposure

TREATMENT
• supportive
• transfusion
• oxygen
• maintain adequate urine output
• alkalinize urine
• steroids

ICD-9-CM
283.2 paroxysmal cold hemoglobinuria

Paroxysmal hemoglobinuria following exercise

DESCRIPTION A benign disorder characterized by red urine, hemoglobinuria, myoglobinuria and abdominal pain. Usual course - acute.

SYNONYMS
• march hemoglobinuria

CAUSES
• strenuous exercise
• running on hard ground
• poorly cushioned shoes

TREATMENT
• unnecessary

ICD-9-CM
283.2 march hemoglobinuria

Paroxysmal nocturnal hemoglobinuria

DESCRIPTION Chronic acquired blood cell dysplasia with proliferation of a clone of stem cells producing erythrocytes, platelets, and granulocytes that are abnormally susceptible to lysis by complement. Characteristics — episodic intravascular hemolysis, particularly following infections, and by various thromboses, particularly of the hepatic veins. Usual course - chronic. Genetics - genetic mutation

SYNONYMS
• Marchiafava-Micheli syndrome

CAUSES
• intrinsic erythrocyte defect
• unusual complement sensitivity

TREATMENT
• transfusion
• androgens
• corticosteroids
• anticoagulants

ICD-9-CM
283.2 paroxysmal nocturnal hemoglobinuria

Pellagra

DESCRIPTION Clinical deficiency syndrome. Characteristics — dermatitis, diarrhea, dementia, inflammation of mucus membranes. Skin lesions appear in area exposed to light and/or trauma. Mental symptoms include depression, irritability, anxiety, confusion, disorientation, delusions and hallucinations. Usual course - progressive. Endemic areas - Southern USA.

SYNONYMS
• niacin deficiency disease

CAUSES
• nicotinic acid deficiency
• tryptophan deficiency
• folic acid deficiency
• carcinoma
• isoniazid

TREATMENT
• nicotinic acid

ICD-9-CM
265.2 pellagra

Pemphigus, benign chronic familial

DESCRIPTION Benign, persistently recurrent bullous dermatitis (autosomal dominant; 66% positive family history). Characteristics — crops of lesions (may remain localized or become generalized), that rupture, undergo erosion and become thickly crusted. sites: sides of the neck, axillae, groin, and flexural and opposing surfaces of the body. Usual course - intermittent; spontaneous exacerbations with remissions.

SYNONYMS
• Hailey-Hailey disease

CAUSES
• defective intercellular cohesion
• defective tonofilament attachment to desmosomes
• precipitated by infection
• precipitated by trauma

TREATMENT
• antibiotics
• dapsone
• systemic steroids for severe cases
• topical steroids of limited value
• complete excision with split thickness skin graft

ICD-9-CM
694.4 pemphigus

Pemphigus, Brazilian

DESCRIPTION Progressive and sometimes fatal variant of pemphigus foliaceus endemic in south central Brazil. Most frequently in children and adolescents. Characteristics — flaccid blisters that rupture easily, forming erosions with peripheral rolls of epidermis, associated with a burning sensation. Usual course - progressive; variable. Endemic areas - South Central Brazil.

SYNONYMS
• fogo selvagem

CAUSES
• unknown
• possibly infectious agent

TREATMENT
• topical corticosteroids for localized disease
• systemic corticosteroids for generalized disease

ICD-9-CM
694.4 pemphigus

Peptic ulcer with hemorrhage

DESCRIPTION One of the complications of peptic ulcer. Characteristics — coffee-ground emesis, melena, syncope, nausea, abrupt abdominal pain. Usual course: -acute.

CAUSES
• erosion of ulcer into blood vessel
• aspirin
• alcohol
• tobacco
• corticosteroid

TREATMENT
• antacids
• histamine H2 blockers
• surgery
• anticholinergics
• sucralfate
• avoid tobacco smoking
• intravenous fluid
• transfusion if needed

ICD-9-CM
533.40 chronic or unspecified peptic ulcer of unspecified site with hemorrhage, without mention of obstruction
533.9

 ## Peptic ulcer with penetration

DESCRIPTION Peptic ulcer that extends beyond the serosa. May lead to encroachment on the pancreas. May cause choledochoduodenal fistula or a giant duodenal ulcer. Characteristics — intractable ulcer pain and other peptic ulceration symptoms. Usual course - acute; chronic.

CAUSES
• aspirin
• alcohol
• tobacco
• corticosteroids
• ulcer erosion into a solid abdominal organ
• ulcer confinement by a solid abdominal organ

TREATMENT
• antacids
• histamine H2 blockers
• surgery
• nasogastric suction
• may require IV hyperalimentation

ICD-9-CM
533.50 chronic or unspecified peptic ulcer of unspecified site with perforation, without mention of obstruction

 ## Pericholangitis

DESCRIPTION Inflammation of the tissues that surround the bile ducts. Characteristics — fever, mild icterus, hepatomegaly, mild pruritus. Usual course - progressive.

TREATMENT
• NONE

ICD-9-CM
576.9 biliary tract disorder, nos

 ## Perleche

DESCRIPTION Single or multiple fissures and cracks at corners of the mouth. In advanced stages may extend to lips and cheeks. Usual course - chronic; relapsing; acute.

SYNONYMS
• angulus infectiosus

CAUSES
• poorly fitting dentures
• monilia infection
• dietary deficiency

TREATMENT
• antimonilial drugs
• vitamins
• refit dentures

ICD-9-CM
686.8 perleche

 ## Peutz-Jeghers syndrome

DESCRIPTION Multiple pigmented (melanin) macules of the skin and mouth mucosa and multiple polyposis of the small intestine. Usual course - chronic.

SYNONYMS
• intestinal polyposis II
• intestinal polyposis-cutaneous pigmentation syndrome
• periorificial lentiginosis syndrome

CAUSES
• hereditary

TREATMENT

ICD-9-CM
759.6 peutz-jeghers syndrome

 ## Phlyctenular keratoconjunctivitis

DESCRIPTION Conjunctivitis and keratitis with discrete nodules of inflammation (phlyctenules).
• Characteristics - signs and symptoms include blepharospasm, severe lacrimation, photophobia, and pain

SYNONYMS N/A

CAUSES Atopic reaction of a hypersensitive conjunctiva to an unknown allergen, perhaps the protein of staphylococcal, tuberculous or other bacteria

 ## Phosphine poisoning

DESCRIPTION Poisoning by hydrogen phosphide, PH3, a malodorous gas. Usual course - acute; progressive

CAUSES
• acid on phosphorus-contaminated metals
• water on phosphorus-contaminated metals
• acetylene to release phosphine gas
• phosphides to release phosphine gas

TREATMENT
• gastric decontamination
• irrigate eyes
• supportive
• excise sequestered jaw bone

ICD-9-CM
987.8 poisoning, phosphine

 ## Phosphorus poisoning

DESCRIPTION Condition resulting from inhalation or ingestion of phosphorous. Characteristics — garlic breath odor, mandibular necrosis, toothache, anemia, anorexia, weakness, luminescent vomitus. Usual course - acute; progressive.

SYNONYMS
• yellow phosphorous poisoning

CAUSES
• cytotoxicity

TREATMENT
• gastric decontamination
• irrigate eyes
• supportive
• bone excision

ICD-9-CM
983.9 poisoning, phosphorus

 ## Pick's disease

DESCRIPTION Rare progressive degenerative disease of the brain. Clinically similar to Alzheimer's with impaired reasoning, poor insight, memory loss, apathy, amnesia, aphasia, incontinence, and extrapyramidal signs. Pathologically, cortical atrophy is confined to frontal and temporal lobes. Usual course - chronic; progressive.

SYNONYMS
• lobar atrophy
• circumscribed brain atrophy
• presenile dementia

CAUSES
• degenerative disease

TREATMENT

ICD-9-CM
331.1 pick's disease

Pickwickian syndrome

DESCRIPTION Extreme obesity with polycythemia, somnolence, hypoventilation, arterial unsaturation and hypercapnia, and pulmonary hypertension. Usual course - chronic; intermittent.

SYNONYMS
• hypoventilation associated with extreme obesity

CAUSES
• marked obesity

TREATMENT
• caloric restriction
• progesterone
• tracheostomy

ICD-9-CM
278.8 pickwickian syndrome

 Pilonidal cyst

DESCRIPTION Hair-containing sacrococcygeal dermoid cyst or sinus that opens at a post anal dimple. Usual course - acute; chronic.

SYNONYMS
• pilonidal sinus
• jeep driver's disease
• coccygeal sinus
• pilliferous cyst

CAUSES
• ingrown broken hair
• stocky body build
• trauma

TREATMENT
• drainage
• excision

ICD-9-CM
685.1 pilonidal cyst without mention of abscess

 Pituitary basophilic adenoma

DESCRIPTION Small tumor of the anterior lobe whose cells stain with basic dyes and give rise to excessive secretion of ACTH resulting in Cushing's syndrome. Characteristics include truncal obesity, hypertension, visual disturbances, menstrual irregularity, impotence, muscle atrophy, osteoporosis, psychic disturbances. Usual course - chronic; progressive.

CAUSES
• unknown

TREATMENT
• transsphenoidal resection
• pituitary irradiation
• bromocriptine

ICD-9-CM
227.3 benign neoplasm of the pituitary

 Pituitary chromophobe adenoma

DESCRIPTION Anterior lobe of the pituitary gland tumor. Characteristics — hypopituitarism, headache, lassitude, visual disturbances, galactorrhea, hypogonadism. Usual course - chronic; progressive.

CAUSES
• unknown

TREATMENT
• transsphenoidal resection
• irradiation
• bromocriptine

ICD-9-CM
227.3 benign neoplasm of the pituitary

 Pituitary dwarfism

DESCRIPTION Dwarfism caused by hypofunction of the anterior pituitary gland with decreased secretion of growth hormone.

SYNONYMS
• ateliotic dwarfism
• panhypopituitary dwarfism
• hypopituitary dwarfism

CAUSES
• idiopathic
• pituitary tumor
• intrathecal methotrexate
• trauma
• CNS irradiation
• hemochromatosis
• sarcoidosis
• hypothalamic failure
• hypothalamic tumor
• CNS infection
• histiocytosis
• septo-optic dysplasia
• holoprosencephaly
• biologically inactive growth hormone
• growth hormone receptor insensitivity
• deficiency insulin-like growth factor I
• psychosocial dwarfism

TREATMENT
• exogenous growth hormone
• counseling

ICD-9-CM
253.3 pituitary dwarfism

 Pituitary eosinophilic adenoma

DESCRIPTION A tumor of the anterior lobe of the pituitary associated with acromegaly and gigantism Usual course - chronic; progressive.

SYNONYMS
• pituitary acidophilic adenoma

CAUSES
• unknown

TREATMENT
• transsphenoidal resection
• pituitary irradiation
• bromocriptine

ICD-9-CM
227.3 benign neoplasm of the pituitary

 Pituitary gigantism

DESCRIPTION Giantism due to excessive pituitary secretion occurring before puberty and before epiphyses close. May be caused by eosinophilia or chromophobe adenoma. Usual course - insidious.

CAUSES
• somatotropic cell adenoma of the pituitary
• somatotropic cell adenoma of mixed cell
• somatotropic cell adenoma of stem cell
• bronchial adenoma
• pancreatic islet cell tumor
• carcinoid tumor
• ectopic growth hormone production

TREATMENT
• surgery
• irradiation
• bromocriptine

ICD-9-CM
253.0 pituitary gigantism

 Pituitary hypothyroidism

DESCRIPTION Hypothyroidism caused by deficiency of thyrotropin secretion. Usual course - chronic.

CAUSES
• pituitary irradiation
• pituitary ablative surgery
• failure of anterior pituitary due to infarction

TREATMENT
• thyroid hormone replacement

ICD-9-CM
244.9 pituitary hypothyroidism

Placental insufficiency syndrome

DESCRIPTION Malnutrition and hypoxia of the fetus due to degenerative changes in the placenta.

TREATMENT
• good perinatal care

ICD-9-CM
762.2; 656.5 placental insufficiency

Pleural malignant mesothelioma

DESCRIPTION Malignant tumor derived from mesothelial tissue. Characteristics — chest pain, dyspnea, weight loss, asthenia, cough, hemoptysis. Usual course - progressive; insidious onset.

CAUSES
• primary tumor of the pleura
• asbestos
• first exposure 20 to 60 years prior to diagnosis

TREATMENT
• surgery
• radiotherapy
• chemotherapy

ICD-9-CM
163.9 malignant neoplasm of the pleura

Pneumonia, aspiration

DESCRIPTION Infection of the lung due to the aspiration of food, liquid, or gastric contents into the upper respiratory tract. Usual course - acute; intermittent.

SYNONYMS
• aspiration bronchopneumonia
• inhalation bronchopneumonia
• aspiration pneumonitis
• acid aspiration syndrome

CAUSES
• oropharyngeal aspiration
• altered consciousness
• general anesthesia
• esophageal carcinoma
• achalasia
• botulism
• tetanus

TREATMENT
• pulmonary suctioning
• penicillin
• clindamycin
• oxygen
• intubation
• mechanical ventilation

ICD-9-CM
482 other bacterial pneumonia
507.0

Pneumonia, Staphylococcal

DESCRIPTION Pneumonia caused by Staphylococcus aureus; a frequent complication of viral influenza. Usual course - acute.

CAUSES
• staphylococcus aureus

TREATMENT
• antibiotics
• drainage

ICD-9-CM
482.4 pneumonia due to staphylococcus

Pneumonitis, allergic

DESCRIPTION Inflammation of the lung due to hypersensitivity to inhaled organic particles. Usual course - acute.

SYNONYMS
• extrinsic interstitial alveolitis
• allergic interstitial pneumonitis

CAUSES
• hypersensitivity to inhaled organic particles
• moldy hay
• corn
• oats
• barley beet pulp
• sugar cane residue
• wood dust
• bird dust
• excreta
• enzyme detergents
• heated air

TREATMENT
• discontinue antigen exposure
• corticosteroids

ICD-9-CM
495.9 unspecified allergic alveolitis and pneumonitis

Portal vein thrombosis

DESCRIPTION Clotting of the portal vein of the liver usually from unknown cause. Characteristics — hematemesis, melena splenomegaly, pancytopenia, encephalopathy, portal hypertension. It occurs in pregnancy (especially eclampsia) chronic heart failure, constrictive pericarditis, malignancies. Diagnosis established by angiography. Usual course - chronic; progressive.

CAUSES
• usually idiopathic
• neonatal septicemia
• omphalitis
• hepatocellular cancer
• umbilical vein catheterization for exchange transfusion

TREATMENT
• treat underlying condition
• possible shunt surgery

ICD-9-CM
452 portal vein thrombosis

Postconcussion syndrome

DESCRIPTION Signs and symptoms that develop after concussion of the brain. Characteristics — amnesia, headache, dizziness, tinnitus, irritability, insomnia, difficulty in concentrating, sweating, heart palpitations. Usual course - acute; intermittent.

SYNONYMS
• posttraumatic brain syndrome

CAUSES
• mild head injury
• severe head injury

TREATMENT
• benzodiazepines

ICD-9-CM
310.2 postconcussion syndrome

Prader-Willi syndrome

DESCRIPTION A congenital disorder of unknown etiology characterized by mental retardation, muscular hypotonia, obesity, short stature, hypogonadism and frequently developing insulin-resistant diabetes. Genetics - occasional small deletion of chromosome 15; sporadic; possible autosomal recessive. Usual course - progressive.

CAUSES
• hypothalamic dysfunction

TREATMENT
• dietary restrictions
• testosterone
• gastric bypass
• jaw wiring
• progesterone

ICD-9-CM
759.8 prader-willi syndrome

Premature atrial contraction (PAC)

DESCRIPTION Premature, abnormal P waves. QRS complexes follow except in very early or blocked PAC. P wave may be buried in the preceding T wave or may be identified in the preceding T wave.

CAUSES Congestive heart failure, coronary artery disease with ischemia, acute respiratory failure, chronic obstructive pulmonary disease, digitalis toxicity, aminophylline, adrenergic drugs, anxiety, caffeine

Premature ventricular contraction (PVC)

DESCRIPTION Irregular pulse. Ventricular beat occurs prematurely, followed by a compensatory pause after the premature ventricular contraction. QRS complex is wide and distorted. Most ominous when clustered, multifocal, with R wave on T pattern.

CAUSES Multiple causes can include psychological stress, physiologic stress, drug toxicity (digitalis, aminophylline, tricyclic antidepressants, beta adrenergics (isoproterenol or dopamine)), caffeine, tobacco, electrolyte imbalances (especially hypokalemia)

Primary hyperlipoproteinemia, Type I

DESCRIPTION A form of hyperlipoproteinemia that may be caused by genetic factors. Genetic form - rare, autosomal recessiveor associated with secondary causes. The risk for atherosclerosis for this form is not increased, although plasma cholesterol level is normal or slightly increased and plasma triglyceride level is greatly increased. Characteristics - the non-genetic form may be clinically associated with eruptive xanthomas, hepatosplenomegaly, pancreatitis, lipemia retinalis

SYNONYMS
- Hyperchylomicronemia
- Exogenous hypertriglyceridemia
- Familial chylomicronemia
- Fat-induced hyperlipidemia

CAUSES Genetic (rare, autosomal recessive), plus secondary causes that may include systemic lupus erythematosus, dysgammaglobulinemia, insulinopenic diabetes mellitus

Primary hyperlipoproteinemia, Type II

DESCRIPTION A form of hyperlipoproteinemia that may be caused by genetic factors or associated with secondary causes. The risk for atherosclerosis for this form is strong, especially for coronary artery disease. Plasma cholesterol level is greatly increased and plasma triglyceride level is either normal or slightly increased.
- Characteristics - the non-genetic form may be clinically associated with xanthelasma, tendon and tuberous xanthomas, and juvenile corneal arcus

SYNONYMS
- Familial hypercholesterolemia
- Familial hypercholesterolemic xanthomatosis
- Familial hyperbetalipoproteinemia

CAUSES Genetic (common, autosomal dominant), plus secondary causes that may include excess dietary cholesterol, hypothyroidism, multiple myeloma, porphyria, obstructive liver disease, nephrosis and hypothyroidism

Primary hyperlipoproteinemia, Type III

DESCRIPTION A form of hyperlipoproteinemia that may be caused by genetic factors or associated with secondary causes. The risk for atherosclerosis for this form is strong, especially in peripheral arteries and coronary arteries. Plasma cholesterol level is greatly increased and plasma triglyceride level is greatly increased.
- Characteristics - the non-genetic form may be clinically associated with plantar xanthomas, tuberoeruptive and tendon xanthomas, as well as accelerated atheroscleroses of coronary and peripheral vessels

SYNONYMS
- Broad beta disease
- Familial dysbetalipoproteinemia
- Floating betalipoproteinemia

CAUSES Genetic (uncommon, mode of inheritance not determined), plus secondary causes that may include hypothyroidism, dysgammaglobulinemia

Primary hyperlipoproteinemia, Type IV

DESCRIPTION A form of hyperlipoproteinemia that may be caused by genetic factors or associated with secondary causes. There is possible risk for atherosclerosis, perhaps for coronary artery disease. The plasma cholesterol level is normal or slightly increased and plasma triglyceride level is greatly increased.
- Characteristics - the non-genetic form may be clinically associated with glucose intolerance, hyperuricemia, and possible accelerated atherosclerosis

SYNONYMS
- Carbohydrate-induced triglyceridemia
- Familial hyperbetalipoproteinemia
- Endogenous hypertriglyceridemia

CAUSES Genetic (rare, autosomal recessive), plus secondary causes that may include excess alcohol consumption, oral contraceptives, glycogen storage disease, diabetes mellitus, pregnancy, nephrotic syndrome, stress

Primary hyperlipoproteinemia, Type V

DESCRIPTION A form of hyperlipoproteinemia that may be caused by genetic factors or associated with secondary causes. The risk for atherosclerosis for this form is not clearly increased. Plasma cholesterol level is normal or slightly increased and plasma triglyceride level is greatly increased.
- Characteristics - the non-genetic form may be clinically associated with pancreatitis, eruptive xanthomas, sensory neuropathy, lipemia retinalis, hyperuricemia, glucose intolerance, hepatosplenomegaly

SYNONYMS
- Mixed hyperlipemia
- Combined exogenous and endogenous hypertriglyceridemia
- Mixed hypertriglyceridemia

CAUSES Genetic (rare, autosomal recessive), plus secondary causes that may include alcoholism, nephrosis, insulin-dependent diabetes mellitus, dysgammaglobulinemia

Primary lateral sclerosis

DESCRIPTION Degeneration of the lateral columns of the spinal cord. Characteristics — spastic paraplegia, rigidity of limbs, increased tendon reflexes, absence of nutritive and sensory disturbance. Usual course - chronic; slowly progressive.

CAUSES
- unknown
- existence as separate clinical entity questioned

TREATMENT
- NONE

ICD-9-CM
335.24 primary lateral sclerosis

Progressive external ophthalmoplegia

DESCRIPTION Slowly progressive bilateral myopathy affecting the extraocular muscles. Characteristics — weakness of levators of the upper lids, ptosis, followed by total ocular paresis. Usual course - chronic; progressive.

SYNONYMS
- chronic dystrophic ophthalmoplegia

CAUSES
- unknown

TREATMENT
- NONE

ICD-9-CM
378.72 progressive external ophthalmoplegia

Progressive hemiatrophy face

DESCRIPTION Atrophy of one half of the face which is usually progressive, but may eventually become stationary.

SYNONYMS
- Romberg's disease
- Parry-Romberg syndrome
- progressive hemifacial atrophy

CAUSES
- unknown
- possible lipodystrophy

TREATMENT
- plastic reconstructive surgery
- skin transplantation
- subcutaneous fat transplantation

ICD-9-CM
349.89 hemiatrophy, face, progressive.

Progressive multifocal leukoencephalopathy

DESCRIPTION Serious, usually fatal viral disease. Characteristics — demyelination in white matter of the brain, but may be seen in the brain stem and cerebellum. It occurs secondary to lymphosarcoma and lymphatic myeloid leukemia. Usual course - progressive.

CAUSES
- latent papovavirus

TREATMENT
- cytosine arabinoside

ICD-9-CM
046.3 progressive multifocal leukoencephalopathy

Prolactinoma

DESCRIPTION A pituitary adenoma which secretes prolactin, leading to increased serum levels of prolactin. Prolactinomas in women are presented with galactorrhea associated with amenorrhea. Though much less common for men, prolactinomas in men rarely produce galactorrhea and are later presented as larger, space-occupying tumors. Usual course - progressive.

SYNONYMS
- prolactin secreting pituitary adenoma
- PRL secreting pituitary adenoma

CAUSES
- prolactin-secreting pituitary microadenoma

TREATMENT
- transsphenoidal resection
- bromocriptine
- irradiation

ICD-9-CM
253.1 forbes-albright syndrome

Pseudocyst pancreas

DESCRIPTION Unilocular cyst of the pancreas. Characteristics — tender mass in left upper quadrant, abdominal pain, weight loss, nausea, anorexia, jaundice. Usual course - acute; progressive.

SYNONYMS
- pancreatic pseudocyst

CAUSES
- acute pancreatitis
- trauma
- pancreatic enzymes released into lesser omentum

TREATMENT
- serial ultrasound
- needle aspiration
- internal drainage surgery
- external drainage

ICD-9-CM
577.2 cyst and pseudocyst of pancreas

Pulmonary artery thrombosis

DESCRIPTION Blood clot in the pulmonary artery. Characteristics — dyspnea, weakness, chest pain, tachycardia, tachypnea.

CAUSES
- reduction in blood flow of pulmonary artery
- organization of previous embolism
- malignancy
- infection
- trauma
- intrinsic disease

TREATMENT
- anticoagulants

ICD-9-CM
415.1 pulmonary artery thrombosis

Pulmonary hypertension, secondary

DESCRIPTION Increased pressure in the pulmonary circulation above 30 millimeters of mercury systolic, and 12 millimeters of mercury diastolic, secondary to any of the listed causes.

CAUSES
- CHF, left ventricular failure, mitral stenosis, mitral regurgitation, myxoma, pulmonary embolism, interstitial fibrosis, sarcoidosis, asbestosis, radiation, alveolar hypoventilation, chronic obstructive pulmonary disease, chronic bronchitis, emphysema, ventricular septal defect, atrial septal defect, silicosis, anthrosilicosis, tuberculosis, SLE, scleroderma, dermatomyositis, connective tissue disorder, cystic fibrosis

TREATMENT
- corticosteroids, oxygen, cardiac catheterization, nitroprusside, hydralazine, diazoxid, isoproterenol, phentolamine, prazosin, verapamil, nifedipine, captopril

ICD-9-CM
416.8 secondary pulmonary hypertension

Pulmonary infarction

DESCRIPTION Hemorrhagic consolidation of lung parenchyma resulting from thromboembolic pulmonary arterial occlusion. Usual course - acute.

SYNONYMS N/A

CAUSES
- stasis, vein injury, hypercoagulable state, phlebitis, phlebothrombosis, thrombus, deep vein thrombosis, burn, surgery, oral contraceptives, trauma, hip fracture, immobilization, congestive heart failure, cardiomyopathy, subacute bacterial endocarditis, atrial myxoma, polycythemia rubra vera, sickle cell anemia, pancreatic carcinoma

TREATMENT
- anticoagulation
- heparin
- coumadin
- warfarin
- thrombolytic agent
- urokinase
- streptokinase
- embolectomy
- vena cava clip

ICD-9-CM
415.1 pulmonary embolism and infarction

Pulmonary interstitial fibrosis, idiopathic

DESCRIPTION Interstitial pneumonia, "nonspecific," or "usual." The term used when etiology leading to pulmonary fibrosis cannot be defined (about 50% of cases). Usual course - chronic; progressive.

SYNONYMS
- alveolocapillary block
- fibrosing alveolitis

CAUSES
- unknown
- loss of functional alveolarcapillary units
- inflammation

TREATMENT
- corticosteroids

ICD-9-CM
516.3 diffuse interstitial pulmonary fibrosis

Pyogenic abscess liver

DESCRIPTION Bacterial abscess of the liver. Characteristics - fever, abdominal pain, anorexia, jaundice, hepatomegaly, elevated hemidiaphragm. Usual course - acute; relapsing.

CAUSES
- portal vein bacteremia
- systemic bacteremia
- ascending cholangitis
- direct extension
- trauma

TREATMENT
- aspiration
- antibiotics
- surgical drainage

ICD-9-CM
572.0 abscess of liver

Pyrogenic shock

DESCRIPTION Shock associated with overwhelming infection, most commonly with gram-negative bacteria. Characteristics — fever, tachycardia, chills myalgia, confusion, tachypnea, hypotension, nausea. Usual course - acute.

SYNONYMS
- septic shock
- endotoxic shock

CAUSES
- inadequate tissue perfusion following bacteremia
- escherichia coli
- klebsiella
- pseudomonas
- serratia
- neisseria meningitidis
- staphylococci
- pneumococci
- streptococci
- bacteroides

TREATMENT
- respiratory support
- fluid replacement
- antibiotics
- vasoactive drugs

ICD-9-CM
785.59 septic shock

Q fever

DESCRIPTION Acute, generally self-limited rickettsial infection. Characteristics — fever, chills, headache, myalgia, malaise, rash (rarely), pneumonitis, hepatitis, and endocarditis. No vector involved. Infection by inhalation of dust or aerosols derived from infected domestic animals. Usual course - abrupt; relapsing; chronic; usually mild. Endemic areas - Western USA; Australia; Africa; England; Mediterranean countries.

SYNONYMS
- Australian Q fever
- Balkan grippe
- nine mile fever
- hibemo-vernal bronchopneumonia
- Derrick-Burnet disease
- Query fever

CAUSES
- coxiella burnetii (rickettsia)
- aspiration of infected material
- contaminated raw milk ingestion
- infected animal conceptional product exposure

TREATMENT
- antibiotics

ICD-9-CM
083.0 Q fever

Rat-bite fever, spirillary

DESCRIPTION Infection caused by a rat or mouse bite. Characteristics — wound heals promptly; inflammation recurs at bite site after 10 or more days, accompanied by relapsing fever and regional lymphadenitis; WBC elevated; myalgia, skin rash, chills, malaise, headache. Usual course - relapsing. Endemic areas - Asia; Europe; USA.

SYNONYMS
• sodoku

CAUSES
• spirillum minor-a spirochete
• rodent bite
• rodent scratch
• rodent-ingesting animal bite

TREATMENT
• antibiotics
• rapid bite cleaning

ICD-9-CM
026.9 rat-bite fever

Rat-bite fever, streptobacillary

DESCRIPTION Bacterial infection caused by a rat or mouse bite, although occasionally associated with ingestion of contaminated milk or with the bite of a different rodent. Characteristics (10 or more days following the bite) — abrupt illness with chills, fever, vomiting, headache, arthralgia, backache, elevated WBC, morbilliform petechial skin rash. Usual course - relapsing. Endemic areas - Asia; Europe; USA.

CAUSES
• streptobacillus moniliformis
• rodent bite
• rodent scratch
• contaminated raw milk ingestion

TREATMENT
• antibiotics
• rapid bite cleansing

ICD-9-CM
026.9 rat-bite fever

Renal artery stenosis

DESCRIPTION Occlusive disease of the renal arteries. This problem occurs in about 5% of patients with hypertension and is one form of hypertension that is surgically correctable. The disease is most often unilateral. Usual course - progressive.

CAUSES
• atherosclerosis
• fibromuscular dysplasia

TREATMENT
• surgery
• angioplasty
• antihypertensives

ICD-9-CM
440.1 renal artery stenosis

Renal infarction

DESCRIPTION Localized area of kidney necrosis caused by either renal arterial or venous occlusion. Characteristics - steady, aching, flank pain, fever, nausea, vomiting, hypertension, leukocytosis, proteinuria, microscopic hematuria. Renal imaging confirms the diagnosis. Usual course - acute.

CAUSES
• renal artery thrombosis
• renal emboli
• arteriosclerosis
• renal artery aneurysm
• fibrous dysplasia
• aortic dissection
• periarteritis nodosa
• vasculitis
• sickle cell disease
• scleroderma
• polycythemia
• trauma
• surgery
• cardiomegaly
• subacute bacterial endocarditis
• atrial myxoma
• rheumatic heart disease

TREATMENT
• surgery
• balloon angioplasty

ICD-9-CM
593.81 renal infarction

Renal vein thrombosis

DESCRIPTION Clotting within the renal vein. Characteristics — lumbar pain; dysuria; enlarged, tender kidney. Usual course - acute; chronic.

CAUSES
• abdominal operation
• CHF
• dehydration
• renal disease
• reduction in renal blood flow
• pregnancy
• constrictive pericarditis
• morbid obesity

TREATMENT
• anticoagulants
• corticosteroids

ICD-9-CM
453.3 embolism and thrombosis of renal vein

Respiratory syncytial virus infection

DESCRIPTION Serious, lower respiratory viral illness of infants and young children. It includes bronchiolitis and pneumonia. May be a factor in sudden death of a baby with respiratory disease. Characteristics — rapid, shallow breathing; cough; nasal congestion; tachycardia; cyanosis. Usual course - acute.

CAUSES
• respiratory syncytial virus

TREATMENT
• oxygen
• bronchodilators
• ribavirin

ICD-9-CM
480.1 pneumonia due to respiratory syncytial virus

Reticulum cell sarcoma

DESCRIPTION Malignant histiocytic lymphoma made of a substance like embryonic connective tissue. Characteristics — fatigue, anorexia, weight loss, excessive sweating, fever, painless adenopathy, hepatosplenomegaly. Usual course - chronic; progressive; relapsing.

SYNONYMS
• reticulum cell lymphosarcoma
• diffuse histiocytic lymphoma
• reticulosarcoma

CAUSES
• unknown

TREATMENT
• chemotherapy
• radiotherapy
• surgery

ICD-9-CM
200.00 reticulosarcoma, nos

Retinal vein occlusion

DESCRIPTION One of the causes of sudden unilateral vision loss. Characteristics — extensive retinal hemorrhages; dilated, tortuous retinal veins. Usual course - acute.

SYNONYMS
• central retinal vein occlusion
• CRVO

TREATMENT
• panretinal photocoagulation

ICD-9-CM
362.35 central retinal vein occlusion

Retinoblastoma

DESCRIPTION Malignant congenital hereditary blastoma (autosomal dominant with high penetrance). Characteristics — appears in one or both eyes in children under 5 years of age, diagnosed initially by a bright white or yellow pupillary reflex. Usual course - progressive.

SYNONYMS
• glioma retina

TREATMENT
• radiotherapy to preserve vision
• photocoagulation to preserve vision
• cryotherapy to preserve vision
• brachytherapy to preserve vision
• enucleation
• palliative radiotherapy for extraocular disease

ICD-9-CM
190.5 malignant neoplasm of the retina

Rhabdomyosarcoma

DESCRIPTION Highly malignant tumor of striated muscle. There are 3 forms - pleomorphic affecting predominantly the extremities of adults; alveolar form, occurring primarily in adolescents and young adults affecting muscles of extremities, trunk, and orbital region; embryonal form, occurring mainly in infants and children, affecting the head and neck, lower genitourinary tract, pelvis and extremities. Usual course - progressive.

SYNONYMS
• rhabdosarcoma

CAUSES
• fetal alcohol syndrome

TREATMENT
• surgical excision
• add radiotherapy in most cases
• group 2: add chemotherapy with vincristine plus dactinomycin
• group 3: add chemotherapy with vincristine plus dactinomycin
• combination chemotherapy for advanced disease

ICD-9-CM
171.9 malignant neoplasm of connective and soft tissue

Rheumatoid pneumoconiosis

DESCRIPTION Pneumoconiosis associated with rheumatoid arthritis. Characteristics — multiple spherical modular lesions with clearly demarcated borders found throughout both lungs. Usual course: chronic; progressive.

SYNONYMS
• caplan syndrome
• rheumatoid lung with silicosis
• silicoarthritis

CAUSES
• unknown
• immune mechanism

TREATMENT
• manage complications

ICD-9-CM
714.81 caplan's syndrome

Rhinosporidiosis

DESCRIPTION Chronic, localized granulomatous infection of mucocutaneous tissues, especially the nose. Characteristics — nasal polyps, tumors, papillomas, or wart-like lesions. Other (rare) areas of infection include the conjunctiva, penis, anus, vagina, ears, pharynx, larynx. Usual course - progressive. Endemic areas - India; Sri-Lanka.

SYNONYMS
• rhinosporosis

CAUSES
• rhinosporidium seeberi

TREATMENT
• surgery

ICD-9-CM
117.0 rhinosporidiosis

Riboflavin deficiency

DESCRIPTION Deficiency of vitamin B2. Deficiency characteristics — cheilosis, photophobia, sore throat, glossitis, fissure tongue, seborrheic dermatitis. Usual course - acute; progressive.

SYNONYMS
• vitamin B2 deficiency
• ariboflavinosis

CAUSES
• inadequate dietary intake
• intestinal malabsorption

TREATMENT
• riboflavin administration

ICD-9-CM
266.0 ariboflavinosis

Rickettsialpox

DESCRIPTION Mild, self-limited disease transmitted by a mite that is an ectoparasite of the house mouse. Characteristics — eschar-like primary skin lesion, generalize papulovesicular rash, headache, and backache. Usual course - acute; incubation period 10 days to 3 weeks after bite. Endemic areas - USA; Europe; Africa.

CAUSES
• rickettsia akari
• bite from mite (vector) infected by rodent

TREATMENT
• tetracycline
• chloramphenicol

ICD-9-CM
083.2 rickettsialpox

Rubella syndrome, congenital

DESCRIPTION Transplacental infection of the fetus with rubella usually in the first trimester of pregnancy as a consequence of maternal infection, resulting in various developmental abnormalities in the newborn, including cardiac and ocular lesions, microcephaly, deafness, mental retardation. Usual course - transient; chronic; progressive.

SYNONYMS
• Gregg's syndrome

CAUSES
• maternal rubella primary infection
• rarely reinfection between 0-20 weeks gestation
• RNA virus

TREATMENT
• strict isolation of infected babies
• care by rubella immune workers
• health department reporting

ICD-9-CM
771.0 congenital rubella

Ruptured chordae tendineae

DESCRIPTION Rupture of a tendinous chord that connects each cusp of atrioventricular valves to approximate papillary muscles in the heart ventricles. Characteristics include a dramatic wholosystolic apical murmur, precordial thrill, chest pain, dyspnea. Rupture of the chordae of the mitral valve is not uncommon. Usual course - acute; progressive.

SYNONYMS N/A

CAUSES
• endocarditis
• trauma
• thoracic compression
• myxomatous perforation

TREATMENT
• diuretics
• surgical repair

ICD-9-CM
429.5 rupture of chordae tendineae

Ruptured mitral papillary muscle

DESCRIPTION Rupture of conical muscular projections from walls of the cardiac ventricles, attached to cusps of the mitral arterioventricular valves by the chordae tendinae. Characteristics — pansystolic murmur, apical thrill, signs and symptoms of congestive heart failure. Usual course - acute; progressive.

SYNONYMS
• papillary muscle rupture

CAUSES
• myocardial infarction
• myocardial necrosis
• trauma

TREATMENT
• diuretics
• surgery

ICD-9-CM
429.6 rupture of papillary muscle

Schatzki's ring

DESCRIPTION Ring-like narrowing of the distal esophagus at the squamo-columnar junction. It is probably congenital and measures 2-4 mm in the submucosa. Characteristics — dysphagia. X-ray with barium swallow confirms the diagnosis by displaying the annular constriction of the lower esophagus. Usual course - chronic; progressive.

SYNONYMS
• esophagogastric ring syndrome
• lower esophageal ring syndrome

CAUSES
• unknown

TREATMENT
• rubber dilatation of ring

ICD-9-CM
530.3 ; 750.3 schatzki's ring

Schistosomiasis haematobium

DESCRIPTION Parasitic disease caused by blood flukes of the genus Schistosoma haematobium. S. Haematobium causes symptoms in the genitourinary system or lower colon and rectum. Endemic in Africa, India, Middle East, Indian Ocean islands. Usual course - acute; chronic; intermittent; progressive.

SYNONYMS
- endemic hematuria
- urogenital schistosomiasis

CAUSES
- trematode schistosoma haematobium
- fresh water snail reservoir

TREATMENT
- praziquantel
- metrifonate
- niridazole

ICD-9-CM
120.0 schistosomiasis due to schistosoma haematobium

Schistosomiasis japonica

DESCRIPTION Parasitic disease caused by blood flukes of Schistosoma japonica causing disturbances in the small intestine, colon, and rectum. Characteristics — may be asymptomatic, melena, diarrhea, hepatosplenomegaly. Endemic area - Africa, India, Middle East, Indian Ocean islands. Usual course - acute; chronic; intermittent; progressive.

SYNONYMS
- eastern schistosomiasis
- katayama disease
- yangtze river disease

CAUSES
- trematode schistosoma japonica
- fresh water snail reservoir

TREATMENT
- praziquantel
- niridazole
- stibocaptate

ICD-9-CM
120.2 schistosomiasis due to schistosoma japonicum

Schistosomiasis mansoni

DESCRIPTION Parasitic disease caused by blood flukes of Schistosoma mansoni causing disturbances in the small intestine, colon, and rectum. Characteristics — diarrhea, weight loss, anorexia, melena, jaundice, hepatosplenomegaly. Endemic areas - Africa, South America, Caribbean, Middle East. May occur in Americans who lived in Puerto Rico. Usual course - acute; chronic; intermittent; progressive.

SYNONYMS
- intestinal bilharziasis
- schistosomal dysentery
- katayama fever
- Manson's schistosomiasis
- Schistosoma mansonii infection
- intestinal schistosomiasis

CAUSES
- trematode schistosoma mansoni
- fresh water snail reservoir

TREATMENT
- praziquantel
- oxamniquine

ICD-9-CM
120.1 schistosomiasis due to schistosoma mansoni

Schistosomiasis of the liver, chronic

DESCRIPTION Parasitic disease caused by blood flukes of the genus Schistosoma that penetrate the skin and develop in the liver, causing fever, eosinophilia, urticaria, hepatosplenomegaly, lymphadenopathy, ascites, esophageal varices. Endemic areas - Africa, Asia, South America, Caribbean Islands.

SYNONYMS
- bilharziasis

CAUSES
- schistosoma mansoni
- schistosoma japonicum
- fresh water snails

TREATMENT
- oxamniquine
- praziquantel
- niridazole
- splenorenal anastomosis surgery

ICD-9-CM
120.9 schistosomiasis, unspecified

Schistosomiasis, cutaneous

DESCRIPTION Parasitic disease caused by blood flukes of the genus Schistosoma. Fresh and salt water mollusks are intermediate hosts. Characteristics — intense pruritus, stinging, macules, papules, and vesicles. Endemic areas - Hawaii, Florida, Great Lakes area. Usual course - acute; intermittent; relapsing.

SYNONYMS
- swimmer's itch
- clam digger's itch

CAUSES
- nonspecific schistosome cercaria
- snail reservoir
- skin penetration
- abnormal host foreign body reaction

TREATMENT
- antipruritics
- antibiotics for secondary bacterial infections

ICD-9-CM
120.3 cutaneous schistosomiasis

Scleredema

DESCRIPTION Diffuse, symmetrical, wooden-like, non-pitting induration of the skin of face, head, shoulders, arms, thorax. Usually preceded by an infectious process. It occurs in association with diabetes mellitus. Resolves in 6 months to 2 years. Usual course - acute; chronic.

SYNONYMS
- scleredema adultorum of buschke

CAUSES
- unknown
- following streptococcal infection

TREATMENT
- self-limited
- unnecessary

ICD-9-CM
710.1 scleredema adultorum

Sclerosis of the brain

DESCRIPTION Familial form of leukoencephalopathy occurring in early life and running a slowly progressive course into adolescence or adulthood. Characteristics — nystagmus, ataxia, tremor, choreoathetotic movements, dyarthria, and mental deterioration.

SYNONYMS
- Pelizaeus-Merzbacher disease
- diffuse familial cerebral sclerosis
- aplasia axialis extracorticalis congenita

TREATMENT
- supportive

ICD-9-CM
330.0 leukodystrophy

Scurvy, infantile

DESCRIPTION Nutritional disease of children caused by ascorbic acid deficiency. Characteristics — weakness, anemia, spongy gums, mucocutaneous hemorrhages, brawny induration of calves and legs.

SYNONYMS
- vitamin C deficiency
- barlow disease
- subperiosteal hematoma syndrome

TREATMENT
- ascorbic acid
- fruit juice

ICD-9-CM
267 infantile scurvy

Second degree AV block

DESCRIPTION Two subtypes:
- Type I or Wenckebach: P-R interval becomes progressively longer with each cycle until a non-conducted atrial beat occurs. After the dropped beat the P-R interval is shorter.
- Type II: Constant P-R intervals preceding a non-conducted atrial beat.
Ventricular rate is irregular. Atrial rhythm is regular.

SYNONYMS
- Mobitz type 1
- Wenckebach's period

CAUSES Inferior wall myocardial infarction, digitalis toxicity, vagal stimulation

Seminoma of the testes

DESCRIPTION Radiosensitive malignant neoplasm of the testes. Occurs in 3 types - classical, anaplastic, and spermatocystic. Characteristics — testicular mass, palpable retroperitoneal nodes.

SYNONYMS
• germinoma of the testes
• dysgerminoma of the testes

CAUSES
• cryptorchid testes

TREATMENT
• stage I: radical inguinal orchiectomy followed by radiotherapy
• chemotherapy for bulky tumors
• stage II: radical inguinal orchiectomy followed by radiotherapy
• chemotherapy for bulky tumors
• stage III: orchiectomy plus multidrug chemotherapy

ICD-9-CM
186.9 malignant neoplasm of the testis

Sheehan's syndrome

DESCRIPTION Postpartum pituitary necrosis resulting form hypovolemia and shock in the immediate peri-partem period. Characteristics — endocrine deficiency syndromes due to loss of anterior lobe pituitary function. Usual course - progressive; acute.

SYNONYMS
• postpartum panhypopituitary syndrome
• postpartum hypopituitarism

CAUSES
• intrapartum hemorrhage
• postpartum hemorrhage
• postpartum infection
• peripheral vascular collapse
• vascular spasm
• DIC

TREATMENT
• hormone replacement therapy
• new pregnancy

ICD-9-CM
253.2 sheehan's syndrome

Shigellosis

DESCRIPTION Acute infection of the bowel. Source of infection: excreta of infected individuals that may be indirectly spread by contaminated food. Incubation period - 1 to 4 days. Characteristics — sudden onset of fever, irritability, drowsiness, anorexia, nausea, vomiting, diarrhea, abdominal pain and distention. Stools show blood, pus and mucus.

CAUSES
• shigella ingestion

TREATMENT
• fluid replacement
• ampicillin
• tetracycline
• sulfamethoxazole-trimethoprim
• chloramphenicol

ICD-9-CM
004.9 shigellosis, unspecified

Short-bowel syndrome

DESCRIPTION A malabsorption syndrome resulting from massive resection of small bowel. Characteristics — diarrhea, steatorrhea, malnutrition. Usual course - chronic; progressive.

SYNONYMS
• massive bowel resection syndrome

CAUSES
• excessive resection of small bowel

TREATMENT
• parenteral nutrition
• low fat diet
• trace metal replacement
• mineral replacement
• vitamin replacement
• parenteral bile-salt sequestering agent
• H-2 receptor antagonist

ICD-9-CM
579.2 short bowel syndrome

Shoulder-hand syndrome

DESCRIPTION Clinical disorder of the upper extremity. Characteristics — pain and stiffness in the shoulder with puffy swelling and pain in the ipsilateral hand, sometimes occurring after myocardial infarction. Usual course - chronic; acute exacerbations.

SYNONYMS
• Steinbrocker syndrome
• reflex sympathetic dystrophy syndrome
• coronary-scapular syndrome
• postinfarction sclerodactylia

CAUSES
• reflex sympathetic stimulation
• cerebral vascular accident
• myocardial infarction
• upper extremity trauma

TREATMENT
• physical therapy
• analgesics
• oral steroids
• stellate ganglion block
• steroid injections

ICD-9-CM
337.9 shoulder-hand syndrome

Siderosis of the lung

DESCRIPTION Pneumoconiosis due to inhalation of iron particles. X-rays are abnormal, but there is no functional impairment and there are no symptoms. Usual course - chronic; acute; progressive.

SYNONYMS
• silver polisher lung
• welder lung

CAUSES
• inhalation of iron oxide dust

TREATMENT
• unnecessary

ICD-9-CM
503 siderosis of the lung

Silo filler disease

DESCRIPTION Pulmonary edema caused by nitrogen dioxide intoxication, which may take place among welders or silo fillers. Symptoms may not appear for 12 hours after exposure. Usual course - progressive; acute.

SYNONYMS
• nitrogen dioxide toxicity
• silage gas poisoning
• silo filler pneumoconiosis

CAUSES
• inhalation of nitrogen dioxide

TREATMENT
• bronchodilators
• mechanical ventilation
• supplemental oxygen

ICD-9-CM
506.9 silo fillers' disease

Silver poisoning

DESCRIPTION Permanent ashen-gray discoloration of the skin, conjunctiva, and internal organs resulting from long over-exposure to silver. Usual course - acute; chronic.

SYNONYMS
• argyria
• argyriasis

CAUSES
• absorption through skin
• inhalation of dust fumes
• accidental ingestion
• abuse of silver nose drops
• mining
• silver plating
• handling of metallic silver

TREATMENT
• emesis
• hydration
• gastric lavage
• activated charcoal

ICD-9-CM
985.8 argyria

Sinoatrial arrest or block

DESCRIPTION Unexpectedly long P-P interval interrupting normal sinus rhythm. Often terminated by a junctional escape beat or return to normal sinus rhythm. QRS complexes uniform, but irregular.

SYNONYMS
• Sinus arrest

CAUSES Digitalis toxicity, quinidine toxicity, sick sinus syndrome

Sinus bradycardia

DESCRIPTION Rate of less than 60 beats per minute. A QRS complex follows each P wave.

CAUSES Sick sinus syndrome, hypothyroidism, mechanical ventilation, inferior myocardial infarction, increased intracranial pressure, increased vagal tone (straining at stool), vomiting, intubation, treatment with beta-blockers and sympatholytic drugs

 Sinus tachycardia

Description Cardiac rate greater than 100 beats per minute. May rarely increase to exceed 160 beats per minute. Every QRS complex follows a P wave.

Causes Cardiac response to fever, anxiety, vigorous exercise, pain, dehydration, shock, left ventricular heart failure, cardiac tamponade, anemia, hyperthyroidism, hypovolemia, pulmonary embolus, myocardial infarction

 Small cell carcinoma of the lung

DESCRIPTION Malignancy of the lung with characteristic pathologic findings of small cells. Has poor outlook, although combination chemotherapy has produced some cures. Usual course - progressive in almost all cases.

SYNONYMS
• oat cell carcinoma of the lung

CAUSES
• tobacco smoking
• radioisotopes
• asbestos
• polycyclic aromatic hydrocarbons
• tuberculosis
• halogen ethers
• nickel
• chromium
• inorganic arsenic
• iron ore
• printing inks
• pollutants

TREATMENT
• combination chemotherapy
• cyclophosphamide
• doxorubicin
• vincristine
• etoposide
• may add prophylactic cranial irradiation
• may add chest radiotherapy

ICD-9-CM
162.9 malignant neoplasm of the lung

 Smallpox

DESCRIPTION An acute infectious disease caused by pox virus. This disease is now extinct worldwide due to successful inoculation. Alastrim, a mild form of the disease is known as variola minor.

SYNONYMS
• variola
• variola major

CAUSES
• double-stranded DNA virus transmitted by inhalation
• rare family transmission

TREATMENT
• isolation, report to health department, meticulous fluid management, skin hygiene, antihistamines, antibiotics for secondary bacterial infections

ICD-9-CM
050.9 smallpox, nos

 Sparganosis

DESCRIPTION Infection of animals, including fish and man, with a developmental stage of Diphyllobothrium. This stage has recently been referred to as a plerocercoid but the name sparganum has persisted. Therefore, infection of fish or other animals with the plerocercoid larvae is sparganosis. Fish-eating mammals, including man, are the final hosts. Usual course - chronic.

SYNONYMS
• larval diphyllobothriasis
• sparganosis (larval diphyllobothriasis)

CAUSES
• spirometra species
• larval diphyllobothrium ingestion from undercooked flesh
• animal flesh poultices

TREATMENT
• surgical excision only

ICD-9-CM
123.5 sparganosis

 Spinal cord compression

DESCRIPTION Impingement on the spinal cord, usually by an extramedullary neoplasm. Characteristics — local back pain, hyperreflexia, Babinski's sign, weakness of lower extremities, sensory loss, loss of sphincter control. Back pain and weakness may last hours to days, but total loss of function control to the site of compression may take only minutes. Usual course - acute onset; chronic onset; often progressive primary disease.

CAUSES
• carcinoma of the lung
• breast carcinoma
• carcinoma of the prostate
• lymphoma
• neural malignancy
• herniated disk
• extradural abscess
• spinal tuberculosis
• rheumatoid arthritis
• cervical spondylosis

TREATMENT
• high dose corticosteroids
• radiotherapy
• surgery
• chemotherapy for primary tumor

ICD-9-CM
336.9 spinal cord compression, nos

 Splenic agenesis syndrome

DESCRIPTION Congenital absence of the spleen, partial situs inversus viscerum accompanied by cardiac defects (right type atria, endocardial cushion defect). This is a familial disorder that is autosomal recessive with sporadic penetrance. Usual course - acute; chronic; progressive.

SYNONYMS
• Ivemark syndrome
• asplenia

CAUSES
• failure of normal asymmetry in morphogenesis

TREATMENT
• antibiotics
• cardiac surgery
• gastrointestinal surgery

ICD-9-CM
759.0 agenesis of the spleen

 Squamous cell carcinoma, anterior tongue

DESCRIPTION Malignancy of the oral tongue that does not include the base of the tongue. Characteristics — located on lateral aspects of the undersurface of the tongue.

TREATMENT
• stage I: surgery plus radiotherapy
• stage II: surgery plus radiotherapy
• stage III: radiotherapy
• surgery plus radiotherapy
• stage IV: radiotherapy
• surgery plus radiotherapy

ICD-9-CM
141.4 malignant neoplasm of anterior two-thirds of tongue

 Squamous cell carcinoma, anus

DESCRIPTION These malignancies comprise 3-5% of rectal and anal cancers. Characteristics — fungating anal mass, tight sphincter, perineal pain and pressure. Usual course - insidious onset; surgical cure; progressive if untreated.

CAUSES
• condylomata
• rectal fistulae
• rectal fissures
• rectal abscesses
• leukoplakia of the anus
• irradiation

TREATMENT
• surgery
• radiotherapy

ICD-9-CM
154.3 malignant neoplasm of anus

Squamous cell carcinoma, bladder

DESCRIPTION Bladder malignancy frequently associated with parasitic infection or chronic mucosal irritation. Characteristics — highly infiltrative, poor prognosis, gross hematuria, dysuria. Usual course - progressive.

SYNONYMS
• epidermoid bladder carcinoma

CAUSES
• beta-naphthylamine
• 4-aminodiphenyl
• tobacco smoking
• chronic schistosoma haematobium infection
• aniline dye

TREATMENT
• endoscopic resection
• segmental bladder resection
• total cystectomy
• methotrexate
• cis-platin
• doxorubicin
• intravesical thiotepa
• preoperative radiotherapy
• supervoltage radiotherapy
• intracavitary radium
• interstitial implantations

ICD-9-CM
188.9 malignant neoplasm of the bladder

 Squamous cell carcinoma, esophagus

DESCRIPTION Characteristics — dysphagia, weight loss, cough, hematemesis, malaise, cervical lymphadenopathy. Usual course - progressive.

CAUSES
• betel nut chewing
• bidi smoking
• tylosis palmaris et plantaris
• lye stricture
• women with plummer-vinson syndrome
• tobacco smoking
• alcohol

TREATMENT
• surgical resection
• bypass
• radiotherapy
• chemotherapy possible

ICD-9-CM
150.9 malignant neoplasm of the esophagus

 Squamous cell carcinoma, floor of the mouth

DESCRIPTION These account for 20,000 new cases of oral cancer each year. Appears most often as a red (erythroblastic) lesion at first appearing as an inflammatory lesion. Characteristics — lump in floor of the mouth; chronic, non-healing ulcer; foul breath odor; very few are indurated or raised. Usual course - progressive if not cured.

CAUSES
• tobacco
• alcohol
• poor oral hygiene
• epstein-barr virus
• chronic oral trauma
• plummer-vinson virus
• betel nut chewing

TREATMENT
• surgery plus radiotherapy depending on stage
• surgery plus radiotherapy depending on location

ICD-9-CM
144.9 malignant neoplasm of the floor of the mouth

 Squamous cell carcinoma, lung

DESCRIPTION A type of bronchogenic carcinoma. Characteristics — cough, hemoptysis, chest pain, dyspnea, weight loss, fever. Usual course - usually progressive.

SYNONYMS
• epidermoid carcinoma of the lung

CAUSES
• tobacco smoking
• radioisotopes
• asbestos
• halogen ethers
• polycyclic aromatic hydrocarbons
• tuberculosis
• nickel
• chromium
• inorganic arsenic
• iron ore
• printing inks
• other pollutants

TREATMENT
• stage I: surgery
• radiotherapy
• stage II: surgery
• radiotherapy
• stage III: surgery
• radiotherapy

ICD-9-CM
162.9 malignant neoplasm of the lung

 Squamous cell carcinoma, nasopharynx

DESCRIPTION Malignancy associated with tobacco consumption and the Epstein-Barr virus. Characteristics — nasal obstruction, epistaxis, tinnitus, facial pain, painless upper neck mass, occipital and temporal headache. Usual course - relapsing; early cure.

CAUSES
• nitrosamines
• ebstein barr virus
• salted fish

TREATMENT
• high dose external beam radiotherapy
• surgical resection in selected patients

ICD-9-CM
147.9 malignant neoplasm of the nasopharynx

 Staphylococcal food poisoning

DESCRIPTION Bacterial food poisoning caused by ingestion of food contaminated by staphylococcal enterotoxin. Characteristics — 2 to 8 hours incubation period with abrupt onset of severe nausea and vomiting, abdominal cramps, diarrhea, headache, fever. Usual course - acute.

SYNONYMS
• staphylococcal gastroenteritis

CAUSES
• coagulase positive staphylococcus aureus

TREATMENT
• fluids

ICD-9-CM
005.0 staphylococcal food poisoning

 Strabismus

DESCRIPTION Deviation of one eye from parallelism with the other

SYNONYMS
• Squint
• Cross eyes
• Heterotropia

CAUSES Paralytic (nonconcomitant) strabismus - paralysis of one or more ocular muscles. Nonparalytic (concomitant) - unequal muscle tone.

 Strongyloidiasis

DESCRIPTION Infection with Strongyloides stercoralis occurring widely in tropical and subtropical countries. Larvae develop in the soil and penetrate the human skin on contact. They travel to the lungs via the bloodstream and thence to the trachea and esophagus and intestines. Usual course - intermittent.

CAUSES
• parasitic infection caused by strongyloides stercorous
• penetration of the skin by larvae
• contaminated food ingestion
• autoinfection

TREATMENT
• thiabendazole

ICD-9-CM
127.2 strongyloidiasis

 Subacute combined degeneration

DESCRIPTION The neurologic manifestations of pernicious anemia. Characteristics — peripheral paresthesias, weakness, leg stiffness, unsteadiness, lethargy, fatigue. Usual course - progressive.

SYNONYMS
• subacute combined degeneration of spinal cord
• combined system disease
• posterolateral sclerosis
• ataxic paraplegia
• neuroanemic syndrome
• funicular spinal disease
• Dana syndrome
• Putnam-Dana syndrome
• Lichtheim syndrome

CAUSES
• vitamin B12 deficiency
• pernicious anemia
• No intrinsic factor in gastric secretion

TREATMENT
• intramuscular cobalamin

ICD-9-CM
336.2 subacute combined degeneration of spinal cord in diseases classified elsewhere

Sulfur dioxide poisoning

DESCRIPTION Irritant gas poisoning as an industrial accident. Characteristics — cough, hemoptysis, wheezing, retching, dyspnea, X-ray findings of diffuse mottled infiltrates indicating pulmonary edema. Usual course - acute; chronic; progressive; relapsing.

CAUSES
• cytotoxicity due to reactions between organic compounds and nitrogen oxides
• oxidation to form sulfuric acid
• occupational exposure
• industrial cleaners

TREATMENT
• supportive
• oxygen
• bronchodilators
• eye dilution plus irrigation
• acid dilution
• analgesia
• corticosteroids
• dilute skin contact
• treat shock
• antibiotics

ICD-9-CM
987.3 poisoning, sulfur dioxide

 Sunburn

DESCRIPTION
• Characteristics - mild erythema with subsequent scaling, pain, swelling, skin tenderness, blisters, fever, chills, weakness, shock, secondary infections, miliaria-like eruptions, exfoliation

SYNONYMS N/A

CAUSES Exposure to sunlight (or other ultraviolet light source) following administration of phototoxicity-producing drugs. Overexposure to ultraviolet rays of UVB (2800 to 3200A). Danger increases proportionately to high altitude.

Treatment Prophylaxis with sunscreens rated 15 or better. Avoid additional exposure until well. Use tap-water compresses. Avoid topical anesthetic lotions and ointments. Use oral corticosteroids for extensive, severe sunburn (prednisone 10 mg qid for 4-6 days).

 Superior sagittal sinus thrombosis

DESCRIPTION Blood clotting in the superior sagittal sinus, a single venous sinus of the dura mater beginning in front of the crista galli and extending backward in the convex border of the falx cerebri. Characteristics — fever, prostration, headache, obtundation, engorged scalp veins, seizure, aphasia, hemiplegia. Usual course - acute.

SYNONYMS
• superior longitudinal sinus thrombosis

CAUSES
• infection
• extension from osteomyelitis
• dehydration
• trauma
• tumors

TREATMENT
• antimicrobials
• drainage
• surgery

ICD-9-CM
437.6 nonpyogenic thrombosis of intracranial venous sinus

 Syringomyelia

DESCRIPTION Often associated with syringobulbia. Fluid-filled cavity (syrinx) within the substance of the spinal cord or brainstem.
• Characteristics - lack of sensation for noxious stimuli in fingers (painless cut or burn). Capelike sensory defect over shoulders and back. Spasticity and weakness of the lower extremities. Muscular atrophy and fasciculations. Vertigo, nystagmus

SYNONYMS N/A

CAUSES Congenital (50%), intramedullary tumors

 Tabes dorsalis

DESCRIPTION Parenchymatous neurosyphilis in which there is slowly progressive degeneration of the posterior columns and roots and ganglia of the spinal cord. Occurs 15 to 20 years after initial syphilitic infection. Characteristics — lancinating lightning pains, urinary incontinence, ataxia, impaired position and vibratory sense, optic atrophy, hypotonia, hyporeflexia and trophic joint degeneration (Charcot's joints).

SYNONYMS
• tabetic neurosyphilis
• locomotor ataxia
• Duchenne's disease
• spinal cord syphilis

CAUSES
• treponema pallidum

TREATMENT
• penicillin
• tetracycline
• erythromycin
• anticonvulsants
• carbamazepine
• phenytoin
• surgery

ICD-9-CM
094.0 tabes dorsalis
094.89 other specified neurosyphilis

 Takayasu syndrome

DESCRIPTION Pulseless disease. Progressive obliteration of the brachiocephalic trunk and the left subclavian and left common carotid arteries above their origin in the aortic arch. Characteristics — loss of pulse in both arms and carotids; symptoms associated with ischemia of the brain (synope, transient hemiplegia), eyes (transient blindness), face and arms. Usual course - progressive. Endemic areas - Orient.

SYNONYMS
• pulseless disease
• young female arteritis
• reverse coarctation
• Martorell syndrome
• brachiocephalic ischemia
• aortic arch syndrome
• Takayasu arteritis
• Takayasu's disease

CAUSES
• unknown
• autoimmune
• hypersensitivity

TREATMENT
• corticosteroids
• surgery

ICD-9-CM
446.7 takayasu's disease

 Thallium poisoning

DESCRIPTION Poisoning due to ingestion of thallium compounds. Characteristics — vomiting, alopecia, neurologic and psychicsymptoms, (ataxia, restlessness, delirium, hallucinations, semicoma, blindness), liver and kidney damage. Thallium is commonly found in ant, rat, and roach poisons. Symptoms usually begin approximately 3 weeks after poisoning. Usual course - acute; progressive.

CAUSES
• thallium ingestion

TREATMENT
• gastric decontamination
• potassium ferric hexacyanoferrate
• skin decontamination
• forced diuresis
• hemoperfusion
• hemodialysis
• urine output maintenance
• supportive

ICD-9-CM
985.8 poisoning, thallium

 Thrombocythemia (adult), idiopathic

DESCRIPTION Hemorrhagic thrombocythemia (one of the myeloproliferative syndromes). Characteristics — repeated spontaneous hemorrhages, either external or into the tissues and an extraordinary increase in the number of circulating platelets. Usual course - chronic; progressive.

SYNONYMS
• primary thrombocythemia
• essential thrombocythemia
• primary hemorrhagic thrombocythemia
• essential thrombocytosis
• primary thrombohemorrhagic thrombocytosis

CAUSES
• clonal megakaryocytic disorder

TREATMENT
• chemotherapy
• radiotherapy
• iron replacement
• plateletpheresis
• platelet anti-aggregating agents

ICD-9-CM
238.7 idiopathic thrombocythemia

 Thymoma, malignant

DESCRIPTION Tumor derived from the epithelial or lymphoid elements of the thymus. Characteristics — cough, dyspnea, dysphagia, chest pain, weakness. Usual course - possibly acute; otherwise progressive.

TREATMENT
• surgical thymectomy
• radiotherapy for invasive thymoma
• corticosteroids if radiotherapy fails
• chemotherapy for advanced disease

ICD-9-CM
164.0 malignant neoplasm of the thymus

Thyrotoxic heart disease

DESCRIPTION Heart disease associated with hyperthyroidism. Characteristics — atrial fibrillation, cardiac enlargement, congestive heart failure. Usual course - progressive; relapsing.

SYNONYMS
• hyperthyroid heart disease

CAUSES
• hyperthyroidism

TREATMENT
• treat underlying hyperthyroidism
• radioactive iodine
• surgery
• beta-adrenergic blockers

ICD-9-CM
242.9; 425.7 thyrotoxic heart failure<

 Thyrotoxic storm

DESCRIPTION Severe thyrotoxicosis accompanied by organ system decompensation. Characteristics — fever, severe tachycardia, dehydration, mental status abnormalities representing dysfunction of the cardiovascular and central nervous systems. Usual course - acute.

SYNONYMS
• thyrotoxicosis
• thyrotoxic crisis
• basedow crisis

CAUSES
• exacerbation of hyperthyroidism
• thyroid surgery
• infection
• trauma

TREATMENT
• fluids
• propylthiouracil
• iodine
• hydrocortisone
• external cooling
• beta-adrenergic blockers
• oxygen
• treat precipitating factors

ICD-9-CM
242.91 thyrotoxicosis without mention of goiter or other cause, with mention of thyrotoxic crisis or storm

 Tinea barbae

DESCRIPTION Fungal infection involving the bearded area of the face and neck. Characteristics — kerion-like swellings and nodular swellings with marked crusting. Usual course - acute; chronic.

SYNONYMS
• tinea sycosis
• barber's itch
• beard ringworm

CAUSES
• fungal infection of coarse facial hair
• zoophilic dermatophytes

TREATMENT
• systemic antifungal agents
• systemic steroid added in severe inflammatory infections

ICD-9-CM
110.0 tinea barbae

 Toluene poisoning

DESCRIPTION A form of poisoning from toluene, a colorless liquid obtainable from coal tar. Toluene is an organic solvent used in rubber, plastic cements, paint removers, etc. Poisoning may result from inhalation or ingestion. Usual course - acute; chronic; progressive.

SYNONYMS
• toluol poisoning
• methylbenzene poisoning
• methylbenzol poisoning
• phenylmethane poisoning

CAUSES
• cytotoxicity

TREATMENT
• supportive
• oxygen
• bicarbonate
• CPR
• gastric decontamination
• skin decontamination
• eye irrigation
• epinephrine contraindicated

ICD-9-CM
982.0 poisoning, toluene

 Tonsillitis

DESCRIPTION Inflammation of the palatine tonsils • Characteristics - symptoms vary with type of disturbance. Bacterial infections cause pain in the throat (frequently referred to the ears) chills, headache, malaise, dysphagia, nausea, vomiting, and arthralgia. Signs of bacterial tonsillitis include abrupt onset with swelling and hyperemia of the tonsils with purulent exudate, edema of the uvula, cervical adenopathy. Adenovirus infections are milder and may be accompanied with conjunctivitis. Complications include diffuse pharyngitis, peritonsillar abscess, sinusitis, otitis media, mastoiditis. Streptococcal tonsillitis can lead to rheumatic fever and glomerulonephritis if not adequately treated. Culture may determine infecting organism.

CAUSES Infection by hemolytic streptococcus or by any adenovirus. Also associated with diphtheria, pneumococcus infection, infectious mononucleosis, and Vincent's angina.

 Toxaphene poisoning

DESCRIPTION Poisoning among agricultural workers using DDT. Characteristics — vomiting, paresthesias, malaise, course tremors, convulsions, pulmonary edema, ventricular fibrillation, respiratory failure. Usual course - acute; chronic; progressive.

SYNONYMS
• chlorinated camphene poisoning

CAUSES
• direct cytotoxicity
• diffuse neuronal excitation

TREATMENT
• gastric decontamination
• skin decontamination
• oxygen
• anticonvulsants
• avoid sympathomimetics
• supportive

ICD-9-CM
989.2 poisoning, toxaphene

 Trachoma

DESCRIPTION Chronic infectious disease of the conjunctiva and cornea. Characteristics — photophobia, pain, lacrimation. The organism is a bacterium, Chlamydia trachomatis. Usual course - acute; progressive. Endemic areas - Africa; Middle East; Asia; Central America.

SYNONYMS
• granular conjunctivitis
• egyptian ophthalmia

CAUSES
• chlamydia trachomatis
• transmission through birth canal

TREATMENT
• tetracyclines
• erythromycin
• sulfonamides

ICD-9-CM
076 trachoma
076.0 trachoma, initial stage
076.9 trachoma, unspecified

 Transposition of the great vessels

DESCRIPTION A congenital heart defect where the great arteries are reversed - the aorta arises from the right ventricle and the pulmonary artery from the left ventricle. This produces two noncommunicating circulatory systems (pulmonary and systemic). It often coexists with other congenital anomalies and affects boys 2 to 3 times more than females. Usual course - acute.

SYNONYMS
• complete dextrotransposition of the great arteries

CAUSES
• abnormal embryogenesis

TREATMENT
• balloon septostomy
• surgical redirection

ICD-9-CM
745.10 complete transposition of the great vessels

 Trichloroethylene poisoning

DESCRIPTION Trichloroethylene is a widely used industrial solvent and formerly used as an inhalation anesthetic. Poisoning characteristics: dizziness, headache, delirium, vomiting, abdominal pain, jaundice, flush. Usual course - acute; chronic; progressive.

CAUSES
• decomposition to dichloroethylene
• decomposition to phosgene
• decomposition to carbon monoxide
• hepatotoxicity
• renal toxicity

TREATMENT
• supportive
• gastric decontamination
• remove contaminated clothing
• epinephrine contraindicated
• volume expanders
• diuretics for urine output maintenance

ICD-9-CM
982.3 poisoning, trichloroethylene

Trichostrongyliasis

DESCRIPTION Infection by nematodes of the genus Trichostrongylus whose eggs are frequently mistaken for hookworms. Endemic areas - Middle East; Far East; Iran. Usually asymptomatic but may cause cramps and diarrhea. Usual course - acute.

SYNONYMS
• trichostrongyloidiasis

CAUSES
• trichostrongylus larvae ingestion

TREATMENT
• thiabendazole
• pyrantel pamoate

ICD-9-CM
127.6 trichostrongyliasis

 Tricuspid atresia

DESCRIPTION Absence of the orifice between the right atrium and ventricle. Circulation made possible by presence of an atrial septal defect, allowing blood to pass from the right to left atrium and then to the left ventricle and aorta. Intra-atrial communication due to anomalous embryonal development.
• Signs and symptoms include marked underdevelopment, severe cyanosis, clubbing of fingers, prominent jugular A wave, apical heave, pulmonic second sound absent, systolic murmur, enlarged liver, presystolic pulsation. EKG shows left axis deviation, left ventricular hypertrophy, tall P waves. Transposition of great vessels, patent foramen ovale and ventricular septal defect all may accompany tricuspid atresia.

CAUSES Unknown

 Tricuspid regurgitation

DESCRIPTION Retrograde blood flow from the right ventricle to the right atrium due to inadequate apposition of the tricuspid valves. Characteristics — low output symptoms plus pulsations in the neck due to high jugular regurgitant waves from the transmitted right ventricular pressure. Usual course - acute; chronic.

SYNONYMS
• tricuspid valve insufficiency

CAUSES
• marked dilatation of right ventricle
• right ventricular failure
• rheumatic heart disease
• cor pulmonale
• congenital heart disease

TREATMENT
• treat underlying condition
• surgery
• tricuspid annuloplasty
• tricuspid valve replacement

ICD-9-CM
424.2 tricuspid valve insufficiency (nonrheumatic)

 Tricuspid stenosis

DESCRIPTION Narrowing of the tricuspid orifice obstructing blood flow from the right atrium to the right ventricle. Characteristics — fatigue, enlarged liver, fluttering discomfort in the neck caused by giant A waves in the jugular pulse. Usual course - chronic; progressive.

SYNONYMS
• tricuspid valve stenosis

CAUSES
• rheumatic fever
• bacterial vegetations
• atrial thrombi
• tumors
• carcinoid heart disease
• fibroelastosis

TREATMENT
• sodium restriction
• digitalization
• diuretics
• surgery
• valvulotomy

ICD-9-CM
397.0 disease of tricuspid valve
424.2 tricuspid valve disorders, specified as nonrheumatic
746.1 tricuspid atresia and stenosis, congenital

 Tropical eosinophilia

DESCRIPTION Subacute or chronic form of filariasis. Characteristics — episodic nocturnal wheezing and coughing, strikingly elevated eosinophilia and lung infiltrations. Usual course - chronic; progressive.

CAUSES
• adult wuchereria bancrofti worms
• adult brugia malayi worms

TREATMENT
• diethylcarbamazine

ICD-9-CM
518.3 tropical eosinophilia

 Truncus arteriosus

DESCRIPTION Congenital anomaly in which there is a single arterial trunk arising from the heart, receiving blood from both ventricles and supplying blood to the coronary, pulmonary, and systemic circulations. Frequently co-exists with malformations of other organ systems.
• Characteristics - signs and symptoms begin during the first week of life and include poor development, minimal or absent cyanosis, marked hypertrophy of the heart, loud and clear second sound, harsh systolic murmur at the base and along the left sternal border, continuous bruit over the upper sternum, thrill with maximum intensity over base of the heart, dyspnea, wide pulse pressure.

SYNONYMS Persistent truncus arteriosus

CAUSES Unknown

 Trypanosomiasis, East African

DESCRIPTION Acute, severe, sometimes fatal form of African trypanosomiasis, transmitted by bites of tsetse flies. Usual course - acute; progressive; lethal within 1 year. Endemic areas - tropical East Africa.

SYNONYMS
• sleeping sickness
• Rhodesian sleeping sickness

CAUSES
• trypanosoma brucei rhodesiense
• tsetse fly bites
• bushbuck antelope reservoir of infection

TREATMENT
• suramin prior to CNS involvement
• pentamidine prior to CNS involvement
• melarsoprol plus suramin pretreatment for CNS disease

ICD-9-CM
086.4 rhodesian trypanosomiasis

 Trypanosomiasis, West African

DESCRIPTION Chronic, less severe form of African trypanosomiasis. Disease persists for several months or years with central nervous system involvement late in its course. Usual course - chronic; intermittent; relapsing; progressive; delayed onset; successive bouts; intervening latent periods; may persist many years. Endemic areas - tropical West Africa; Central Africa.

SYNONYMS
• sleeping sickness
• Gambian sleeping sickness

CAUSES
• trypanosoma brucei gambiense
• tsetse fly bites
• transplacental transmission
• human reservoir

TREATMENT
• suramin prior to CNS involvement
• pentamidine prior to CNS involvement
• melarsoprol plus suramin pretreatment for CNS disease

ICD-9-CM
086.3 gambian trypanosomiasis

 Tuberculoid leprosy

DESCRIPTION Relatively benign, least infectious, and usually self-limited polar type of leprosy. Characteristics — early severe damage to nerves and sharply demarcated skin lesions. Usual course - chronic; intermittent. Endemic areas - tropical regions; India; Hawaii; USA Gulf Coast.

SYNONYMS
• tuberculoid hansen's disease

CAUSES
• mycobacterium leprae
• human-to-human transmission via close contact
• intense cell-mediated immunity to mycobacterium leprae

TREATMENT
• combination antibiotic therapy for 1 year with dapsone plus rifampin
• dapsone for additional year
• other antibiotic combinations for resistant strains
• isolation unnecessary
• walking casts
• physical therapy
• plastic surgery

ICD-9-CM
030.1 tuberculoid leprosy

Tuberculosis of the kidney

DESCRIPTION Begins as a small focus in the renal cortex (where it has been seeded by hematogenous spread) and progresses to the medulla. Patients may be asymptomatic until late stages when inflammation or other genitourinary disorders develop. Usual course: progressive.

CAUSES
• mycobacterium tuberculosis
• hematogenous seeding
• debilitation

TREATMENT
• isoniazid plus second antituberculous drug for 2 years

ICD-9-CM
016.00 tuberculosis of kidney, unspecified examination

Tuberculosis, miliary

DESCRIPTION Early postprimary tuberculous septicemia due to hematogenous spread. Characteristics — high fever and general toxicity, sign of meningitis kidney infection, positive liver and bone marrow culture. Usual course: acute; chronic; intermittent.

SYNONYMS
• disseminated tuberculosis

CAUSES
• hematogenous dissemination of primary tuberculosis
• dissemination of reactivated old tuberculosis infection

TREATMENT
• antituberculous chemotherapy

ICD-9-CM
018 miliary tuberculosis
018.0 acute miliary tuberculosis
018.9 miliary tuberculosis, unspecified

Tuberculous gumma

DESCRIPTION Subcutaneous tuberculous nodule that becomes fluctuant and drains with underlying ulceration and sinus formation. Usual course - acute.

SYNONYMS
• scrofulous gumma
• cutis colliquativa tuberculosis

CAUSES
• mycobacterium tuberculosis

TREATMENT
• surgery
• incision
• drainage
• isoniazid
• rifampin

ICD-9-CM
017.0 tuberculous gumma

Tuberculous meningitis

DESCRIPTION Severe meningitis caused by mycobacterium tuberculosis following rupture of a metastatic subependymal focus of tuberculosis into the subarachnoid space. Incidence highest in children aged 1 to 5 years. Usual course: acute.

CAUSES
• mycobacterium tuberculosis

TREATMENT
• isoniazid
• ethambutol
• rifampin

ICD-9-CM
013.0 tuberculous meningitis

Tuberculous pericarditis

DESCRIPTION Results from direct extension of tuberculous mediastinal nodes or to hematogenous dissemination. Characteristics — pericardial friction rib, pericardial effusion, fever, tachycardia, chest pain, tachypnea.

CAUSES
• caseous lymph node rupture
• lymphohematogenous dissemination
• hematogenous spread
• mycobacterium tuberculosis

TREATMENT
• isoniazid
• ethambutol
• rifampin
• streptomycin
• kanamycin
• capreomycin
• pyrazinamide
• pyridoxine
• ethionamide
• cycloserine

ICD-9-CM
017.9 420.0 tuberculosis of pericardium

Tuberculous peritonitis

DESCRIPTION Tuberculosis spread from adjacent lymph nodes, a gastrointestinal focus, or tuberculous salpingo-oophoritis. Characteristics — indolent illness, doughy-feeling abdomen, local tenderness. Peritoneoscopy will differentiate from peritoneal carcinomatosis. Usual course: progressive.

CAUSES
• mycobacterium tuberculosis
• hematogenous seeding
• local extension from abdominal lymph node
• local extension from urinary tract
• debilitation
• alcoholism
• corticosteroids
• diabetes mellitus

TREATMENT
• antituberculous chemotherapy

ICD-9-CM
014.0 tuberculous peritonitis

Tuberculous pleurisy

DESCRIPTION Pleural tuberculosis. Characteristics — occurs soon after initial infection. Hypersensitive necrotizing effect causes a subpleural focus to rupture suddenly into a pleural space and produces an allergic effusion of mononuclear cells, protein, and pleural fluid enzyme. Usual course: -acute.

SYNONYMS
• tuberculosis of the pleura

CAUSES
• subpleural tuberculous foci rupture into pleural space
• miliary tuberculosis

TREATMENT
• antituberculous chemotherapy

ICD-9-CM
012.0 tuberculous pleurisy

Tubular necrosis, acute

DESCRIPTION Acute renal tubular necrosis is a syndrome with multiple causes accounting for 70% of renal failure patients. Types include - stage 1: onset azotemia; stage 2: oliguria; stage 3: diuresis; stage 4: resolving diuresis
Usual course - acute; reversible;

SYNONYMS
• lower nephron nephrosis
• vasomotor nephropathy

CAUSES
• ischemia
• disseminated intravascular coagulation
• nephrotoxins
• trauma
• dehydration
• circulatory insufficiency

TREATMENT
• hemodialysis
• maintain renal perfusion
• maintain euvolemia
• diuretics
• vasopressors
• alkalinization

ICD-9-CM
584.5 acute renal failure with lesion of tubular necrosis

Uterine bleeding postmenopausal

DESCRIPTION Bleeding from female genital tract beginning one or more years following menopause. Characteristics - may occur from any part of the reproductive tract including uterus, cervix, vagina, vulva; bleeding may be heavy or light.

CAUSES
• Iatrogenic as a result of estrogen replacement therapy
• Infection, atrophy, tumors (benign or malignant), polyps, adnexal pathology. Endometrial carcinoma is the cause of 1/3 of all cases of postmenopausal bleeding.

ICD-9-CM 627.1

Ventricular fibrillation

DESCRIPTION Ventricular rhythm rapid and chaotic. QRS complexes wide and irregular.

CAUSES Myocardial infarction or ischemia, untreated ventricular tachycardia, electrolyte imbalances, digitalis or quinidine toxicity, electric shock, hypothermia

Treatment If pulse is absent, follow protocol using defibrillation, epinephrine, lidocaine, bretylium. Pronestyl, and sodium bicarbonate as indicated.

 Ventricular standstill

DESCRIPTION No QRS complexes. Symptoms include loss of consciousness. No peripheral pulses, blood pressure or respirations. Death.

SYNONYMS
• Asystole

CAUSES Myocardial infarction or ischemia, untreated ventricular tachycardia, electrolyte imbalances, digitalis or quinidine toxicity, electric shock, hypothermia

 Ventricular tachycardia (VT)

DESCRIPTION Symptoms include chest pain, anxiety, palpitations, dyspnea, shock, coma, death. Ventricular rate usually regular at 140-220 beats per minute. QRS complexes are wide and bizarre.

CAUSES Myocardial ischemia, infarction, or aneurysm, ventricular catheters, drug toxicity (digitalis or quinidine), hypokalemia, hypercalcemia, anxiety

---

 Vernal keratoconjunctivitis

DESCRIPTION Bilateral conjunctivitis associated with corneal epithelial changes. Most likely to occur in spring and fall in males aged 5-20.
• Characteristics - signs and symptoms include tearing; intense itching; redness of the conjunctiva; and a tenacious, mucoid discharge containing numerous eosinophils. Symptoms usually disappear during cold months.

CAUSES Allergies (probably)

 Von Gierke's disease

DESCRIPTION An autosomal recessive glycogen storage disease, (Type Ia) Glucose-6-phosphatase deficiency affecting liver and kidneys. Characteristics — hepatomegaly, hypoglycemia, hyperuricaemia, xanthomas, bleeding, adiposity. Patients live into adulthood. May lead to symptomatic hypoglycemia. Patients needed added precautions when taking many drugs. Usual course - chronic; progressive.

SYNONYMS
• glucose-6-phosphatase deficiency type Ia
• hepatorenal glycogen storage disease

CAUSES
• genetic enzyme deficiency

TREATMENT
• frequent feeding
• allopurinol

ICD-9-CM
271.0 von gierke's disease

 Von Hippel-Lindau disease

DESCRIPTION 20% autosomal dominant chronic disease with variable expression. Characteristics — headache, loss of vision, unilateral ataxia, dizziness, retinal detachment, papilledema, macular star. Usual course - chronic.

SYNONYMS
• angioblastomatosis
• cerebelloretinal hemangioblastomatosis
• angiophakomatosis retinae et cerebelli

TREATMENT
• surgery
• radiotherapy

ICD-9-CM
759.6 von hippel-lindau disease

 Von Willebrand's disease

DESCRIPTION Group of hemorrhagic disorders in which the von Willebrand factor is either quantitatively or qualitatively abnormal. Usually inherited as an autosomal dominant trait though rare kindreds are autosomal recessive. Symptoms vary depending on severity and disease type but may include prolonged bleeding time, deficiency of factor VIII, and impaired platelet adhesion. Usual course - chronic.

SYNONYMS
• pseudohemophilia
• vascular hemophilia
• angiohemophilia

CAUSES
• No factor VIII associated proteins
• DECR factor VIII associated proteins activity

TREATMENT
• factor VIII replacement
• epsilon-aminocaproic acid
• DDAVP
• oral contraceptives to suppress menses

ICD-9-CM
286.4 von willebrand's disease

 Waldenstrom's macroglobulinemia

DESCRIPTION Malignant neoplasm of cells with lymphocytic, plasmacytic or intermediate morphology which secrete an IgM M component. Usual course - slowly progressive; death 3-10 years. Genetics - slight increased familial incidence.

CAUSES
• IgM M-component secretion

TREATMENT
• chlorambucil
• plasmapheresis for hyperviscosity
• prednisone

ICD-9-CM
273.3 waldenstrom's macroglobulinemia

 Werner's syndrome

DESCRIPTION Premature senility in an adult. Characteristics — early graying and some hair loss, cataracts, hyperkeratinization, and scleroderma-like changes in the skin of the lower extremities. Usual course - chronic.

SYNONYMS
• adult progeria
• progeria adultorum

CAUSES
• altered glycosaminoglycan turnover
• chromosomal instability

TREATMENT

ICD-9-CM
259.8 werner's disease or syndrome

Wernicke's encephalopathy

DESCRIPTION Acute, subacute, or chronic neurological disorder. Characteristics — confusion, apathy, drowsiness, ataxic, nystagmus, ophthalmoplegia. Most commonly results from chronic alcohol abuse and accompanied by organic amnesia and other nutritional polyneuropathies. Usual course - acute; subacute; chronic.

SYNONYMS
• Wernicke syndrome
• Wernicke's disease
• Gayet-Wernicke syndrome

CAUSES
• thiamine deficiency

TREATMENT
• intravenous thiamine supplementation
• supportive measures

ICD-9-CM
265.1 wernicke's encephalopathy

 Whipple's disease

DESCRIPTION A malabsorption disorder. Characteristics — diarrhea, steatorrhea, skin pigmentation, arthralgia, arthritis, lymphadenopathy, and central nervous system lesions. Usual course - progressive; curative with treatment.

SYNONYMS
• lipophagic intestinal granulomatosis
• intestinal lipodystrophy
• secondary nontropical sprue

CAUSES
• probable bacterial infection

TREATMENT
• penicillin G
• ampicillin
• tetracycline
• corticosteroids

ICD-9-CM
040.2 whipple's disease

 Wilson's disease

DESCRIPTION An inherited metabolic disorder characterized by excessive amounts of copper in the liver, brain, kidneys, and corneas. It can lead to tissue necrosis and fibrosis, which in turn can cause hepatic disease and neurologic changes. Without treatment, it leads to fatal hepatic failure. Usual course - chronic.

SYNONYMS
• progressive lenticular degeneration
• Westphal-Struempell pseudosclerosis

TREATMENT
• avoid copper-rich foods, penicillamine, potassium sulfide, pyridoxine, zinc acetate as alternative to penicillamine

ICD-9-CM
275.1 Wilson's disease

 Wolff-Parkinson-White syndrome

DESCRIPTION A form of pre-excitation characterized by a short PR interval and long QRS interval with a delta wave associated with paroxysmal tachycardia (or atrial fibrillation). Usual course - intermittent.

SYNONYMS
• preexcitation syndrome
• anomalous atrioventricular excitation

CAUSES
• accessory atrioventricular pathway
• circus movement conduction due to AV reentrant tachycardia

TREATMENT
• vagal maneuvers
• antiarrhythmic agents
• cardioversion
• electrical pacing
• surgical ablation

ICD-9-CM
426.7 wolff-parkinson-white syndrome

 Yaws

DESCRIPTION Non-venereal, infectious, tropical disease usually affecting persons under the age of 15. Spread by direct contact. Characteristics — painless papule that grows into a papilloma. The papule heals, leaving a scar. Late manifestations: deforming lesions of bones, joints, and skin. Usual course - chronic; progressive. Endemic areas - tropical regions.

SYNONYMS
• frambesia
• buba
• pian

CAUSES
• skin contact
• treponema pertenue

TREATMENT
• penicillin

ICD-9-CM
102.9 yaws

 Yellow fever

DESCRIPTION An acute infectious disease primarily of the tropics, caused by a virus and transmitted to man by mosquitoes of the genus Aedes and Haemagogus. Usual course - acute. Endemic areas - Africa; South America.

CAUSES
• flavivirus
• mosquito bite
• aedes aegypti

TREATMENT
• fluid replacement

ICD-9-CM
060.9 yellow fever

 Yersinia enterocolitica infection

DESCRIPTION Gram negative, facultatively anaerobic bacteria causing acute gastroenteritis and mesenteric lymphadenitis in children, and arthritis, septicemia, and erythema nodosum in adults. Transmitted through food, water, and person-to-person contact. Usual course - acute.

SYNONYMS
• yersinosis
• pasteurella pseudotuberculosis infection

CAUSES
• contaminated food ingestion

TREATMENT
• streptomycin
• gentamycin
• tetracycline
• chloramphenicol
• sulfamethoxazole-trimethoprim
• fluid replacement

ICD-9-CM
027.2 pasteurellosis

Index

Index

Index

Index

Index

Index

Index

Index

Index

Index

Index

Index

Index

Index

Index

-E-

Index

Index

Index

Index

-G-

Index

Index

Index

Index

Index

Index

Index

Index

Index

Index

Index

Index

Index

Index

Index

Index

Index

Index

Index

Index

Index

Index

Index

Index

Index

Index

Index

Index

of tendon sheath, Giant cell 970
pituitary epidermoid 1127
Pregnancy 422
primary malignant, Bone 114
rathke pouch 1127
syndrome, Pancreatic ulcerogenic 1110
Ulcerogenic islet cell 1110
Wilms' 1104
Tumoral hypercalcemia 478
tumors
Bladder 1122
Esophageal 362
Salivary gland 900
tunnel syndrome, Carpal 160
Turner's syndrome 1044
TWAR 196
type
1, Mobitz 1156
dissociative 306
I diabetes mellitus 288
I, Diabetes mellitus insulin-dependent IDDM or 288
I, glucuronyl transferase deficiency 1127
I, Primary hyperlipoproteinemia 1152
Ia, glucose-6-phosphatase deficiency 1164
II diabetes mellitus 292
II, Primary hyperlipoproteinemia 1152
III, Primary hyperlipoproteinemia 1152
IV, Primary hyperlipoproteinemia 1152
Senile dementia, Alzheimer's 24
V, Primary hyperlipoproteinemia 1152
Typhoid 1046
fever 1046
Typhus
abdominalis 1046
african tick 1122
fever, recrudescent 1123
fevers 1048
Louse-borne 1048
Murine 1048
recrudescent 1123
Tick 890
typus degenerativus amstelodamensis 1127

-U-

ulcer
Anal 1119
Decubitus 804
disease, Peptic 738
Duodenal 738
Gastric 738
Pressure 804
Rodent 102
siberian 1119
Trophic 804
with hemorrhage, Peptic 1149
with penetration, Peptic 1149
ulceration, Corneal 244
Ulcerative colitis 1050
Ulcerogenic
islet cell tumor 1110
tumor syndrome, Pancreatic 1110
Ulcus molle 190

Ullrich-Turner syndrome 1044
unconjugated hyperbilirubinemia, familial 1127
Undescended testes 252
undifferentiated lymphoma, Monomorphic 598
Undulant fever 140
unguium, Tinea 684
Unilocular hydatid disease 976
Unipolar affective disorder 270
univentricular heart 1127
unknown origin FUO, Fever of 372
upper
airway occlusion, Nocturnal 934
respiratory infection, Acute 226
urinary tract infection, Acute 842
urate, Nephropathy 668
Uremia 864
Ureterectasis 476
urethritica, Arthritis 856
Urethritis 1052
Trichomonal 1032
Urethro-oculo-articular syndrome 856
Urge incontinence 1054
URI 226
Urinary
incontinence 1054
tract infection in men 1056
tract infection in women 1058
tract infection, Acute upper 842
tract obstruction 476
urine disease, Maple syrup 1143
urogenital schistosomiasis 1156
urohepatic syndrome 1136
Urolithiasis 1060
Urologic stone 858
uropathy, Obstructive 476
Urticaria 1062
uterine
bleeding DUB, Dysfunctional 316
bleeding postmenopausal 1163
cancer 1064
cervix, Cancer 176
descensus 1068
malignancy 1064
myomas 1066
prolapse 1068
uterus, Dropped 1068
UTI 1056
Uveitis 1070
Anterior 1070
hilar adenopathy plus 904
posterior 1070

-V-

V, Primary hyperlipoproteinemia Type 1152
Vaccinations 526
Vaginal
adenosis 1072
bleeding during pregnancy 1074
intraepithelial neoplasia 1076
malignancy 1076
vaginalis
Corynebacterium 1090

Index